Holland–Frei Cancer Medicine

Tenth Edition

Dedication

The 10th edition of *Cancer Medicine* has grown from the vision and dedication of James F. Holland and his fellow pioneer Emil "Tom" Frei. Jim and Tom were among the founding fathers of medical oncology and life-saving combination chemotherapy for which they shared the Albert Lasker Award for Clinical Medical Research. Jim had originally planned a career in cardiology after graduating from Princeton and Columbia University College of Physicians and Surgeons. When he returned from the United States Army Medical Corps in 1951, he took what was to be a temporary position at Frances Delafield Hospital where he cared for children with leukemia, drawing him to the mission of making pre-curable cancers curable for more than six decades. After conducting research at the National Cancer Institute, he became the chief of medicine at Roswell Park Memorial Institute at the age of 28. With Tom Frei, then at NCI, Jim created the first cancer chemotherapy cooperative trials group, the Acute Leukemia Group B, that became the Cancer and Leukemia Group B (CALGB) and now Alliance for Clinical Trials in Oncology. In 1972, he had represented the United States in a Mission to Russia studying Soviet oncology and training of Soviet oncologists. The next year he established a department of neoplastic diseases at the Tisch Cancer Institute at Mt. Sinai in New York where he was later named a distinguished professor. Having served as the president of the American Association for Cancer Research and the American Society of Clinical Oncology, he inspired the creation of the T.J. Martell Foundation for Cancer Research. With his wife Jimmie Holland, founder of the field of onco-psychiatry, Jim helped to found and nurture AORTIC, the African Organization for Research and Training in Cancer, promoting cancer control and palliation in Africa for more than 25 years. Jim's contributions to oncologic research extended beyond treatment of leukemia to therapy of breast cancer and to the possible role of viruses in the development of that disease. A master clinician and extraordinary human being, Jim Holland inspired generations of oncologists and the editors of this text with his wisdom and insatiable drive to continue to help people with cancer. He was indeed a giant who we miss, but who will be remembered by everyone who had the privilege of knowing him.

Waun Ki Hong was born in 1942, the sixth of seven children, in a small suburb of Seoul, North Korea. After attending medical school at Yon Sei University, Ki served as a flight surgeon in the Vietnam War prior to training in internal medicine residency at the Boston VA medical center. After completing a medical oncology fellowship at Memorial Sloan Kettering Cancer Center, Ki headed back to Boston in 1976 as chief of oncology and hematology at the Boston VAMC where he led the first clinical chemoprevention studies in solid tumors while launching the VA Larynx preservation study with Greg Wolf. In 1984, he moved to the University of Texas MD Anderson Cancer Center as chief of the head and neck cancer division, soon combined with the lung cancer section to become the first department of lung and head and neck (aerodigestive cancers) in the country. Over a 30-year career at MD Anderson, Ki led as senior author dozens of seminal papers in premiere journals such as the *New England Journal of Medicine*, establishing himself with Bernard Fischer as fathers of clinical cancer chemoprevention. Ki led major collaborative program projects and SPORE grants, establishing a series of biomarker-based clinical trials that helped unlock our understanding of the impact of molecular agents on premalignancies, while providing substantial contributions to targeted therapy. Over the course of his career, Ki Hong mentored a veritable who's who of lung and aerodigestive track clinical and translational investigators and received numerous major honors. He served as the president of AACR and was one of very few individuals to deliver AACR's Joseph Burchenal Award and ASCO's David Karnofsky Lecture in the same academic year. Ki joined the editorial leadership of *Cancer Medicine* for the seventh edition and was remarkably persistent and effective at recruiting many of the world-class authors who have led its chapters. Perhaps even more notable than his stellar scientific contributions was his unstinting devotion to his proteges, trainees and friends, and especially his wife Mihwa, children Burt and Ed, and their families.

We editors who treasure these oncology giants miss them sorely and dedicate this 10th Edition of *Cancer Medicine* to these preeminent leaders in cancer practice, research, education, and training and diversity, equity, and inclusion.

Robert C. Bast Jr.
John C. Byrd
Carlo M. Croce
Ernest Hawk
Fadlo R. Khuri
Raphael E. Pollock
Apostolia M. Tsimberidou
Christopher G. Willett
Cheryl L. Willman

Holland–Frei Cancer Medicine

Tenth Edition

EDITORS

Robert C. Bast Jr., MD
Vice President for Translational Research
Professor of Medicine
Harry Carothers Wiess Distinguished University Chair for Cancer Research
Division of Cancer Medicine
Department of Experimental Therapeutics
The University of Texas MD Anderson Cancer Center
Houston, Texas

John C. Byrd, MD
The Gordon and Helen Hughes Taylor Professor and Chair
Department of Internal Medicine
University of Cincinnati College of Medicine
Cincinnati, Ohio

Carlo M. Croce, MD
Distinguished University Professor
John W. Wolfe Chair in Human Cancer
Department of Cancer Biology and Genetics
The Ohio State University
Comprehensive Cancer Center
Columbus, Ohio

Ernest Hawk, MD, MPH
Vice President and Head
Division of Cancer Prevention & Population Sciences
The University of Texas MD Anderson Cancer Center
Houston, Texas

Fadlo R. Khuri, MD
President
Professor of Internal Medicine
American University of Beirut
Beirut, Lebanon

Raphael E. Pollock, MD, PhD
Klotz Family Chair in Cancer Research
Professor and Director
Ohio State University Comprehensive Cancer Center
The Ohio State University Medical Center
Columbus, Ohio

Apostolia M. Tsimberidou, MD, PhD
Professor
Department of Investigational Cancer Therapeutics
The University of Texas MD Anderson Cancer Center
Houston, Texas

Christopher G. Willett, MD
Professor and The Mark W. Dewhirst Distinguished Professor of Radiation Oncology
Department of Radiation Oncology
Duke University School of Medicine
Durham, North Carolina

Cheryl L. Willman, MD
Executive Director
Mayo Clinic Cancer Programs: Rochester, Minnesota/Midwest, Arizona, Florida, London, Abu Dhabi
Director
Mayo Clinic Comprehensive Cancer Center
Professor of Laboratory Medicine and Pathology
College of Medicine
Mayo Clinic Cancer Center
Rochester, Minnesota

ASSOCIATE EDITORS

Jene' Reinartz
Administrator
Department of Translational Research
The University of Texas MD Anderson Cancer Center
Houston, Texas

Michael S. Ewer, MD, JD, PhD
Professor of Medicine
Department of Cardiology
The University of Texas MD Anderson Cancer Center
Houston, Texas

Anthea Hammond, PhD
Science Writer/Editor
Department of Hematology and Medical Oncology
Emory University
Atlanta, Georgia

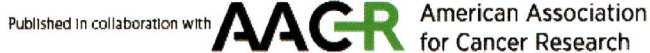
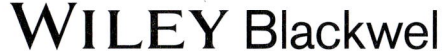

This edition first published 2023
© 2023 John Wiley & Sons, Inc.

© 2016 John Wiley & Sons, Inc (9e); © 2010 John Wiley & Sons, Inc (8e)

Published by John Wiley & Sons, Inc., Hoboken, New Jersey.
Published simultaneously in Canada.

No part of this publication may be reproduced, stored in a retrieval system, or transmitted in any form or by any means, electronic, mechanical, photocopying, recording, scanning, or otherwise, except as permitted under Section 107 or 108 of the 1976 United States Copyright Act, without either the prior written permission of the Publisher, or authorization through payment of the appropriate per-copy fee to the Copyright Clearance Center, Inc., 222 Rosewood Drive, Danvers, MA 01923, (978) 750-8400, fax (978) 750-4470, or on the web at www.copyright.com. Requests to the Publisher for permission should be addressed to the Permissions Department, John Wiley & Sons, Inc., 111 River Street, Hoboken, NJ 07030, (201) 748-6011, fax (201) 748-6008, or online at http://www.wiley.com/go/permission

Limit of Liability/Disclaimer of Warranty
While the publisher and author have used their best efforts in preparing this book, they make no representations or warranties with respect to the accuracy or completeness of the contents of this book and specifically disclaim any implied warranties of merchantability or fitness for a particular purpose. No warranty may be created or extended by sales representatives or written sales materials. The advice and strategies contained herein may not be suitable for your situation. You should consult with a professional where appropriate. Further, readers should be aware that websites listed in this work may have changed or disappeared between when this work was written and when it is read. Neither the publisher nor authors shall be liable for any loss of profit or any other commercial damages, including but not limited to special, incidental, consequential, or other damages.

For general information on our other products and services or for technical support, please contact our Customer Care Department within the United States at (800) 762-2974, outside the United States at (317) 572-3993 or fax (317) 572-4002.

Wiley also publishes its books in a variety of electronic formats. Some content that appears in print may not be available in electronic formats. For more information about Wiley products, visit our web site at www.wiley.com

Library of Congress Cataloging-in-Publication Data has been applied for:

Print ISBN: 9781119750680

Cover Design: Wiley
Cover Image(s): Hiep T. Vo and Apostolia Maria Tsimberidou

Set in 9/11pt MinionPro by Straive, Chennai, India

Printed in Singapore
M112757_300123

Contents

List of contributors   xi

Preface   xxvii

Acknowledgments   xxix

Part 1: INTRODUCTION

1. Cardinal manifestations of cancer   3
   James F. Holland, Robert C. Bast, Jr., John C. Byrd, Carlo M. Croce, Ernest Hawk, Fadlo R. Khuri, Raphael E. Pollock, Apostolia M. Tsimberadou, Christopher G. Willett, and Cheryl L. Willman

2. Biological hallmarks of cancer   7
   Douglas Hanahan and Robert A. Weinberg

Part 2: TUMOR BIOLOGY

3. Molecular biology, genetics, and translational models of human cancer   19
   Benno Traub, Florian Scheufele, Srinivas R. Viswanathan, Matthew Meyerson, and David A. Tuveson

4. Oncogenes   49
   Marco A. Pierotti, Milo Frattini, Samantha Epistolio, Gabriella Sozzi, and Carlo M. Croce

5. Tumor suppressor genes   73
   Fred Bunz and Bert Vogelstein

6. Epigenetic contributions to human cancer   89
   Stephen B. Baylin

7. Cancer genomics and evolution   101
   William P. D. Hendricks, Aleksandar Sekulic, Alan H. Bryce, Muhammed Murtaza, Pilar Ramos, Jessica D. Lang, Timothy G. Whitsett, Timothy K. McDaniel, Russell C. Rockne, Nicholas Banovich, and Jeffrey M. Trent

8. Chromosomal aberrations in cancer   125
   Megan E. McNerney, Ari J. Rosenberg, and Michelle M. Le Beau

9. MicroRNA expression in cancer   143
   Serge P. Nana-Sinkam, Mario Acunzo, and Carlo M. Croce

10. Aberrant signaling pathways in cancer   151
    Luca Grumolato and Stuart A. Aaronson

11. Differentiation therapy   161
    Sai-Juan Chen, Xiao-Jing Yan, Guang-Biao Zhou, and Zhu Chen

12. Cancer stem cells   177
    Grace G. Bushnell, Michael D. Brooks, and Max S. Wicha

13. Cancer and cell death   187
    John C. Reed

14. Cancer cell immortality: targeting telomerase and telomeres   201
    Ilgen Mender, Zeliha G. Dikmen, and Jerry W. Shay

15. Cancer metabolism   211
    Natalya N. Pavlova, Aparna D. Rao, Ralph J. DeBerardinis, and Craig B. Thompson

16. Tumor angiogenesis   223
    John V. Heymach, Amado Zurita-Saavedra, Scott Kopetz, Tina Cascone, Monique Nilsson, and Irene Guijarro

Part 3: QUANTITATIVE ONCOLOGY

17. Cancer bioinformatics   247
    John N. Weinstein

18. Systems biology and genomics   261
    Saima Hassan, Joe W. Gray, and Laura M. Heiser

19. Statistical innovations in cancer research   269
    J. Jack Lee and Donald A. Berry

20. Biomarker based clinical trial design in the era of genomic medicine   285
    R. Donald Harvey, Yuan Liu, Taofeek K. Owonikoko, and Suresh S. Ramalingam

21. Clinical and research informatics data strategy for precision oncology   293
    Douglas Hartman, Uma Chandran, Michael Davis, Rajiv Dhir, William E. Shirey, Jonathan C. Silverstein, and Michael J. Becich

Part 4: CARCINOGENESIS

22. Chemical carcinogenesis   305
    Lorne J. Hofseth, Ainsley Weston, and Curtis C. Harris

23. Ionizing radiation   325
    David J. Grdina

24. Ultraviolet radiation carcinogenesis   333
    James E. Cleaver, Susana Ortiz-Urda, and Sarah Arron

25. Inflammation and cancer   339
    Jelena Todoric, Atsushi Umemura, Koji Taniguchi, and Michael Karin

26. RNA tumor viruses   347
    Robert C. Gallo and Marvin S. Reitz

27. Herpesviruses   359
    Jeffrey I. Cohen

28 Papillomaviruses and cervical neoplasia 367
  Michael F. Herfs, Christopher P. Crum, and Karl Munger

29 Hepatitis viruses and hepatoma 373
  Hongyang Wang

30 Parasites 379
  Mervat El Azzouni, Charbel F. Matar, Radwa Galal, Elio Jabra, and Ali Shamseddine

Part 5: EPIDEMIOLOGY, PREVENTION, AND DETECTION

31 Cancer epidemiology 391
  Veronika Fedirko, Kevin T. Nead, Carrie Daniel, and Paul Scheet

32 Hereditary cancer syndromes: risk assessment and genetic counseling 403
  Rachel Bluebond, Sarah A. Bannon, Samuel M. Hyde, Ashley H. Woodson, Nancy Y.-Q. You, Karen H. Lu, and Banu Arun

33 Behavioral approaches to cancer prevention 425
  Roberto Gonzalez and Maher Karam-Hage

34 Diet and nutrition in the etiology and prevention of cancer 433
  Steven K. Clinton, Edward L. Giovannucci, Fred K. Tabung, and Elizabeth M. Grainger

35 Chemoprevention of cancer 453
  Ernest Hawk, Karen C. Maresso, Powel Brown, Michelle I. Savage, and Scott M. Lippman

36 Cancer screening and early detection 473
  Otis W. Brawley

Part 6: CLINICAL DISCIPLINES

37 Clinical cancer genomic diagnostics and modern diagnostic pathology 493
  Katherine Roth, Stephen B. Gruber, and Kevin McDonnell

38 Molecular diagnostics in cancer 505
  Zachary L. Coyne, Roshni D. Kalachand, Robert C. Bast Jr., Gordon B. Mills, and Bryan T. Hennessy

39 Principles of imaging 519
  Lawrence H. Schwartz

40 Interventional radiology for the cancer patient 521
  Zeyad A. Metwalli, Judy U. Ahrar, and Michael J. Wallace

41 Principles of surgical oncology 531
  Todd W. Bauer, Kenneth K. Tanabe, and Raphael E. Pollock

42 Principles of radiation oncology 543
  Scott R. Floyd, Justus Adamson, Philip P. Connell, Ralph R. Weichselbaum, and Christopher G. Willett

43 Principles of medical oncology 553
  Apostolia M. Tsimberidou, Robert C. Bast, Jr., Fadlo R. Khuri, and John C. Byrd

44 Pain and palliative care 567
  Laura Van Metre Baum and Cardinale B. Smith

45 Psycho-oncology 577
  Diya Banerjee and Andrew J. Roth

46 Principles of cancer rehabilitation medicine 585
  Michael D. Stubblefield, Miguel Escalon, Sofia A. Barchuk, Krina Vyas, and David C. Thomas

47 Integrative oncology in cancer care 593
  Gabriel Lopez, Wenli Liu, Santhosshi Narayanan, and Lorenzo Cohen

48 Health services research 599
  Michaela A. Dinan and Devon K. Check

Part 7: INDIVIDUALIZED TREATMENT

49 Precision medicine in oncology drug development 613
  Apostolia M. Tsimberidou, Elena Fountzilas, and Razelle Kurzrock

Part 8: CHEMOTHERAPY

50 Drug development of small molecule cancer therapeutics in an Academic Cancer Center 631
  Christopher C. Coss, Jeffrey T. Patrick, Damien Gerald, Gerard Hilinski, Reena Shakya, and John C. Byrd

51 Principles of dose, schedule, and combination therapy 641
  Joseph P. Eder and Navid Hafez

52 Pharmacology of small-molecule anticancer agents 655
  Zahra Talebi, Sharyn D. Baker, and Alex Sparreboom

53 Folate antagonists 667
  Lisa Gennarini, Peter D. Cole, and Joseph R. Bertino

54 Pyrimidine and purine antimetabolites 679
  Robert B. Diasio and Steven M. Offer

55 Alkylating agents and platinum antitumor compounds 693
  Zahid H. Siddik

56 DNA topoisomerase targeting drugs 701
  Anish Thomas, Susan Bates, William D. Figg, Sr., and Yves Pommier

57 Microtubule inhibitors 717
  Giuseppe Galletti and Paraskevi Giannakakou

58 Drug resistance and its clinical circumvention 731
  Jeffrey A. Moscow, Shannon K. Hughes, Kenneth H. Cowan, and Branimir I. Sikic

Part 9: BIOLOGICAL AND GENE THERAPY

59 Cytokines, interferons, and hematopoietic growth factors 739
  Narendranath Epperla, Walter Hanel, and Moshe Talpaz

60 Monoclonal antibody and targeted toxin therapy 755
  Robert C. Bast, Jr. and Michael R. Zalutsky

61 Vaccines and immunomodulators 781
  Jeffrey Schlom, Sofia R. Gameiro, Claudia Palena, and James L. Gulley

62 T cell immunotherapy of cancer   789
M. Lia Palomba, Jae H. Park, and Renier Brentjens

63 Cancer immunotherapy   799
Padmanee Sharma, Swetha Anandhan, Bilal A. Siddiqui, Sangeeta Goswami, Sumit K. Subudhi, Jianjun Gao, Karl Peggs, Sergio Quezada, and James P. Allison

64 Cancer gene therapy   817
Haruko Tashiro, Lauren Scherer, and Malcolm Brenner

65 Cancer nanotechnology   825
Xingya Jiang, Yanlan Liu, Danny Liu, Jinjun Shi, and Robert Langer

66 Hematopoietic cell transplantation   833
Qaiser Bashir, Elizabeth J. Shpall, and Richard E. Champlin

Part 10: SPECIAL POPULATIONS

67 Principles of pediatric oncology   847
Theodore P. Nicolaides, Elizabeth Raetz, and William L. Carroll

68 Cancer and pregnancy   867
Jennifer K. Litton

69 Cancer and aging   877
Ashley E. Rosko, Carolyn J. Presley, Grant R. Williams, and Rebecca L. Olin

70 Disparities in cancer care   885
Otis W. Brawley

71 Neoplasms in people living with human immunodeficiency virus   895
Chia-Ching J. Wang and Elizabeth Y. Chiao

72 Cancer survivorship   911
Lewis Foxhall

Part 11: DISEASE SITES

73 Primary neoplasms of the brain in adults   921
Matthew A. Smith-Cohn and Mark R. Gilbert

74 Neoplasms of the eye and orbit   933
Erica R. Alvarez, Claudia M. Prospero Ponce, Patricia Chevez-Barrios, and Dan S. Gombos

75 Neoplasms of the endocrine glands and pituitary neoplasms   943
Rui Feng, Chirag D. Gandhi, Margaret Pain, and Kalmon D. Post

76 Neoplasms of the thyroid   949
Matthew D. Ringel

77 Malignant tumors of the adrenal gland   961
Jeffrey E. Lee, Mouhammed A. Habra, and Matthew T. Campbell

78 Tumors of the diffuse neuroendocrine and gastroenteropancreatic system   971
Evan Vosburgh

79 Neoplasms of the head and neck   981
Robert L. Ferris, Adam S. Garden, and Nabil F. Saba

80 Cancer of the lung   1005
Daniel Morgensztern, Daniel Boffa, Alexander Chen, Andrew Dhanasopon, Sarah B. Goldberg, Roy H. Decker, Siddhartha Devarakonda, Jane P. Ko, Luisa M. Solis Soto, Saiama N. Waqar, Ignacio I. Wistuba, and Roy S. Herbst

81 Malignant pleural mesothelioma   1029
Michele Carbone, Daniel R. Gomez, Anne S. Tsao, Haining Yang, and Harvey I. Pass

82 Thymomas and thymic tumors   1043
Mayur D. Mody, Gabriel L. Sica, Suresh S. Ramalingam, and Dong M. Shin

83 Tumors of the heart and great vessels   1055
Moritz C. Wyler von Ballmoos and Michael J. Reardon

84 Primary germ cell tumors of the thorax   1061
John D. Hainsworth and Frank A. Greco

85 Neoplasms of the esophagus   1065
Max W. Sung and Virginia R. Litle

86 Carcinoma of the stomach   1083
Carl Schmidt, Nour Daboul, Carly Likar, and Joshua Weir

87 Primary neoplasms of the liver   1095
Hop S. Tran Cao, Junichi Shindoh, and Jean-Nicolas Vauthey

88 Gallbladder and bile duct cancer   1109
Mariam F. Eskander, Christopher T. Aquina, and Timothy M. Pawlik

89 Neoplasms of the exocrine pancreas   1123
Robert A. Wolff, Donghui Li, Anirban Maitra, Susan Tsai, Eugene Koay, and Douglas B. Evans

90 Neoplasms of the appendix and peritoneum   1139
Annie Liu, Diana Cardona, and Dan Blazer

91 Carcinoma of the colon and rectum   1147
Yota Suzuki, Douglas S. Tyler, and Uma R. Phatak

92 Neoplasms of the anus   1169
Alexandre A. A. Jácome and Cathy Eng

93 Renal cell carcinoma   1181
Claude M. Grigg, Earle F. Burgess, Stephen B. Riggs, Jason Zhu, and Derek Raghavan

94 Urothelial cancer   1191
Derek Raghavan, Richard Cote, Earle F. Burgess, Derek McHaffie, and Peter E. Clark

95 Neoplasms of the prostate   1201
Ana Aparicio, Patrick Pilie, Devaki S. Surasi, Seungtaek Choi, Brian F. Chapin, Christopher J. Logothetis, and Paul G. Corn

96 Tumors of the penis and the urethra   1239
Jad Chahoud, Andrea Necchi, and Philippe E. Spiess

97 Testis cancer   1245
Michael Hawking, Gladell Paner, Scott Eggener, and Walter M. Stadler

98 Neoplasms of the vulva and vagina   1261
Michael Frumovitz and Summer B. Dewdney

99 Neoplasms of the cervix 1275
   Anuja Jhingran

100 Endometrial cancer 1299
   Shannon N. Westin, Karen Lu, and Jamal Rahaman

101 Epithelial ovarian, fallopian tube, and peritoneal cancer 1311
   Jonathan S. Berek, Malte Renz, Michael L. Friedlander, and Robert C. Bast, Jr.

102 Nonepithelial ovarian malignancies 1329
   Jonathan S. Berek, Malte Renz, Michael L. Friedlander, and Robert C. Bast, Jr.

103 Molar pregnancy and gestational trophoblastic neoplasia 1343
   Neil S. Horowitz, Donald P. Goldstein, and Ross S. Berkowitz

104 Gynecologic sarcomas 1351
   Jamal Rahaman and Carmel J. Cohen

105 Neoplasms of the breast 1361
   Debu Tripathy, Sukh Makhnoon, Banu Arun, Aysegul Sahin, Nicole M. Kettner, Senthil Damodaran, Khandan Keyomarsi, Wei Yang, Kelly K. Hunt, Mark Clemens, Wendy A. Woodward, Melissa P. Mitchell, Rachel Layman, Evthokia A. Hobbs, Bora Lim, Megan Dupuis, Rashmi Murthy, Omar Alhalabi, Nuhad Ibrahim, Ishwaria M. Subbiah, and Carlos Barcenas

106 Malignant melanoma 1413
   Michael J. Carr, Justin M. Ko, Susan M. Swetter, Scott E. Woodman, Vernon K. Sondak, Kim A. Margolin, and Jonathan S. Zager

107 Other skin cancers 1437
   Stacy L. McMurray, William G. Stebbins, Eric A. Millican, and Victor A. Neel

108 Bone tumors 1451
   Timothy A. Damron

109 Soft tissue sarcomas 1477
   Katherine A. Thornton, Elizabeth H. Baldini, Robert G. Maki, Brian O'Sullivan, Yan Leyfman, and Chandrajit P. Raut

110 Myelodysplastic syndromes 1501
   Uma M. Borate

111 Acute myeloid leukemia in adults: mast cell leukemia and other mast cell neoplasms 1517
   Richard M. Stone, Charles A. Schiffer, and Daniel J. DeAngelo

112 Chronic myeloid leukemia 1537
   Jorge Cortes, Richard T. Silver, and Hagop Kantarjian

113 Acute lymphoblastic leukemia 1547
   Elias Jabbour, Nitin Jain, Hagop Kantarjian, and Susan O'Brien

114 Chronic lymphocytic leukemia 1559
   Jacqueline C. Barrientos, Kanti R. Rai, and Joanna M. Rhodes

115 Hodgkin lymphoma 1569
   David J. Straus and Anita Kumar

116 Clonal hematopoiesis in cancer 1579
   Philipp J. Rauch and David P. Steensma

117 Non-Hodgkin's lymphoma 1587
   Arnold S. Freedman and Ann S. LaCasce

118 Mycosis fungoides and Sézary syndrome 1603
   Walter Hanel, Catherine Chung, and John C. Reneau

119 Plasma cell disorders 1611
   Andrew J. Yee, Teru Hideshima, Noopur Raje, and Kenneth C. Anderson

120 Myeloproliferative disorders 1633
   Jeanne Palmer and Ruben Mesa

Part 12: MANAGEMENT OF CANCER COMPLICATIONS

121 Neoplasms of unknown primary site 1647
   John D. Hainsworth and Frank A. Greco

122 Cancer cachexia 1659
   Assaad A. Eid, Rachel Njeim, Fadlo R. Khuri, and David K. Thomas

123 Antiemetic therapy 1673
   Michael J. Berger and David S. Ettinger

124 Neurologic complications of cancer 1683
   Luis Nicolas Gonzalez Castro, Tracy T. Batchelor, and Lisa M. DeAngelis

125 Dermatologic complications of cancer chemotherapy 1701
   Anisha B. Patel, Padmavathi V. Karri, and Madeleine Duvic

126 Skeletal complications 1715
   Michael A. Via, Ilya Iofin, Jerry Liu, and Jeffrey I. Mechanick

127 Hematologic complications and blood bank support 1729
   Roger Belizaire and Kenneth C. Anderson

128 Coagulation complications of cancer patients 1739
   Tzu-Fei Wang and Kristin Sanfilippo

129 Urologic complications related to cancer and its treatment 1747
   Omar Alhalabi, Ala Abudayyeh, and Nizar M. Tannir

130 Cardiac complications 1757
   Michael S. Ewer, Steven M. Ewer, and Thomas M. Suter

131 Respiratory complications 1779
   Vickie R. Shannon, George A. Eapen, Carlos A. Jimenez, Horiana B. Grosu, Rodolfo C. Morice, Lara Bashoura, Ajay Sheshadre, Scott E. Evans, Roberto Adachi, Michael Kroll, Saadia A. Faiz, Diwakar D. Balachandran, Selvaraj E. Pravinkumar, and Burton F. Dickey

132 Gastrointestinal and hepatic complications in cancer patients 1811
   Robert S. Bresalier, Emmanuel S. Coronel, and Hao Chi Zhang

133 Oral complications of cancer and their treatment 1827
   Stephen T. Sonis, Anna Yuan, and Alessandro Villa

134 Gonadal complications 1839
   Robert W. Lentz and Catherine E. Klein

135 Sexual dysfunction   1849
Leslie R. Schover

136 Endocrine complications and paraneoplastic syndromes   1855
Sai-Ching J. Yeung and Robert F. Gagel

137 Infections in patients with cancer   1869
Harrys A. Torres, Dimitrios P. Kontoyiannis, and Kenneth V.I. Rolston

138 Oncologic emergencies   1883
Sai-Ching J. Yeung and Carmen P. Escalante

Part 13: THE FUTURE OF ONCOLOGY

139 A vision for twenty-first century healthcare   1907
Leroy Hood, Nathan D. Price, and James T. Yurkovich

Index   1915

List of contributors

Stuart A. Aaronson, MD
Jane B. and Jack R. Aron Professor and Founding Chair Emeritus
Department of Oncological Sciences
Icahn School of Medicine at Mount Sinai
New York, New York

Ala Abudayyeh, MD
Associate Professor
Department of Nephrology
The University of Texas MD Anderson Cancer Center
Houston, Texas

Mario Acunzo, PhD
Assistant Professor
Division of Pulmonary Diseases and Critical Care Medicine
Virginia Commonwealth University
Richmond, Virginia

Roberto Adachi, MD
Professor of Medicine
Department of Pulmonary Medicine
The University of Texas MD Anderson Cancer Center
Houston, Texas

Justus Adamson, PhD
Associate Professor
Department of Radiation Oncology
Duke University School of Medicine
Durham, North Carolina

Judy U. Ahrar, MD
Associate Professor
Department of Interventional Radiology
The University of Texas MD Anderson Cancer Center
Houston, Texas

Omar Alhalabi, MD
Assistant Professor
Department of Genitourinary Medical Oncology
The University of Texas MD Anderson Cancer Center
Houston, Texas

James P. Allison, PhD
Professor and Chair
Department of Immunology
The University of Texas MD Anderson Cancer Center
Houston, Texas

Erica R. Alvarez, MD
Assistant Professor
Medical Retina and Ocular Oncology Department of Surgery
Texas Tech University Health Sciences Center El Paso
Paul L. Foster School of Medicine
El Paso, Texas

Swetha Anandhan, MSc
Graduate Research Assistant
Department of Genitourinary Medical Oncology
The University of Texas MD Anderson Cancer Center
Houston, Texas

Kenneth C. Anderson, MD
Kraft Family Professor of Medicine
Harvard Medical School
Jerome Lipper Multiple Myeloma Center and LeBow Institute for Myeloma Therapeutics
Dana-Farber Cancer Institute
Boston, Massachusetts

Ana Aparicio, MD
Professor
Genitourinary Medical Oncology
The University of Texas MD Anderson Cancer Center
Houston, Texas

Christopher T. Aquina, MD, MPH
Assistant Professor of Surgery
Rutgers Cancer Institute of New Jersey
New Brunswick, New Jersey

Sarah Arron, MD, PhD
Associate Professor Dermatology
Department of Dermatology UCSF Cancer Center
University of California San Francisco
San Francisco, California

Banu Arun, MD
Professor
Breast Medical Oncology and Clinical Cancer Genetics
The University of Texas MD Anderson Cancer Center
Houston, Texas

Sharyn D. Baker, PharmD, PhD
Professor
Division of Pharmaceutics and Pharmacology
College of Pharmacy
The Ohio State University
Columbus, Ohio

Diwakar D. Balachandran, MD
Professor of Medicine
Department of Pulmonary Medicine
The University of Texas MD Anderson Cancer Center
Houston, Texas

Elizabeth H. Baldini, MD, MPH, FASTRO
Professor of Radiation Oncology
Harvard Medical School
Center for Sarcoma and Bone Oncology
Dana-Farber Cancer Institute and Brigham and Women's Hospital
Boston, Massachusetts

Diya Banerjee, MD
Clinical Instructor
Department of Psychiatry and Behavioral Sciences
Memorial Sloan Kettering Cancer Center
New York, New York

Sarah A. Bannon, MS
Genetic Counselor
Clinical Cancer Genetics
The University of Texas MD Anderson Cancer Center
Houston, Texas

Nicholas Banovich, PhD
Associate Professor
Integrated Cancer Genomics Division
Translational Genomics Research Institute
Phoenix, Arizona

Carlos Barcenas, MD
Associate Professor
Department of Breast Medical Oncology
The University of Texas MD Anderson Cancer Center
Houston, Texas

Sofia A. Barchuk, DO
Physical Medicine and Rehabilitation Resident
Department of Rehabilitation and Human Performance
Icahn School of Medicine at Mount Sinai
New York, New York

Jacqueline C. Barrientos, MD, MS
Professor of Medicine
Donald and Barbara Zucker School of Medicine at Hofstra/Northwell Health
New Hyde Park, New York

Qaiser Bashir, MD
Associate Professor
Department of Stem Cell Transplantation and Cellular Therapy
The University of Texas MD Anderson Cancer Center
Houston, Texas

Lara Bashoura, MD
Professor of Medicine
Department of Pulmonary Medicine
The University of Texas MD Anderson Cancer Center
Houston, Texas

Robert C. Bast Jr., MD
Vice President for Translational Research
Professor of Medicine
Harry Carothers Wiess Distinguished University Chair for Cancer Research
Division of Cancer Medicine
Department of Experimental Therapeutics
The University of Texas MD Anderson Cancer Center
Houston, Texas

Tracy T. Batchelor, MD
Professor of Neurology
Harvard Medical School
Neurologist-in-Chief
Department of Neurology
Brigham and Women's Hospital
Boston, Massachusetts

Susan Bates, MD
Professor of Medicine
Division of Hematology/Oncology
Columbia University Medical Center
New York, New York

Todd W. Bauer, MD, FACS
Professor of Surgery and Chief
Division of Surgical Oncology
University of Virginia
Charlottesville, Virginia

Laura Van Metre Baum, MD, MPH
Assistant Professor of Medicine
Division of Medical Oncology
Yale School of Medicine
New Haven, Connecticut

Stephen B. Baylin, MD
Professor of Oncology and Medicine
Virginia and D.K. Ludwig Professor for Cancer
The Johns Hopkins Medical Institutions
Baltimore, Maryland

Michael J. Becich, MD, PhD
Professor
Department of Biomedical Informatics
University of Pittsburgh
Pittsburgh, Pennsylvania

Roger Belizaire, MD, PhD
Assistant Professor of Pathology
Harvard Medical School
Department of Pathology
Dana-Farber Cancer Institute
Boston, Massachusetts

Jonathan S. Berek, MD, MMS
Laurie Kraus Lacob Professor and Director
Stanford Women's Cancer Center
Stanford University School of Medicine
Stanford, California

Michael J. Berger, PharmD, BCOP
Specialty Practice Pharmacist—Breast Medical Oncology
The James Cancer Hospital at The Ohio State University Medical Center
Columbus, Ohio

Ross S. Berkowitz, MD
Director of Gynecology
William H. Baker Professor of Gynecology
Harvard Medical School
Boston, Massachusetts

Donald A. Berry, PhD
Professor
Department of Biostatistics
The University of Texas MD Anderson Cancer Center
Houston, Texas

Joseph R. Bertino, MD (deceased)
American Cancer Society Professor
University Professor of Medicine & Pharmacology
Rutgers Robert Wood Johnson Medical School
Rutgers
The State University of New Jersey
New Brunswick, New Jersey

Dan Blazer, MD
Associate Professor
Department of Surgery
Duke University
Durham, North Carolina

Rachel Bluebond, MS
Genetic Counselor
Clinical Cancer Genetics
The University of Texas MD Anderson Cancer Center
Houston, Texas

Daniel Boffa, MD
Professor and Chief
Thoracic Surgery
Department of Surgery
Yale University
New Haven, Connecticut

Uma M. Borate, MD, MS
Associate Professor
Division of Hematology/Oncology
The Ohio State University
Columbus, Ohio

Otis W. Brawley, MD, MACP
Bloomberg Distinguished Professor of Oncology and Epidemiology
Johns Hopkins University
Baltimore, Maryland

Malcolm Brenner, MA, MB, BChir, PhD
Professor
Center for Cell and Gene Therapy, and Departments of Medicine, Human and Molecular Genetics and Pediatrics
Baylor College of Medicine
Houston, Texas

Renier Brentjens, MD, PhD
Professor and Chair
Department of Medicine
Roswell Park Cancer Institute Corporation
Buffalo, New York

Robert S. Bresalier, MD
Professor and Vice Chair for Research
Department of Gastroenterology, Hepatology and Nutrition
Birdie J and Lydia J Resoft Distinguished Professor in Gastrointestinal Oncology
The University of Texas MD Anderson Cancer Center
Houston, Texas

Michael D. Brooks, PhD
Postdoctoral Researcher
Department of Internal Medicine
University of Michigan
Ann Arbor, Michigan

Powel Brown, MD, PhD
Professor and Chair
Department of Clinical Cancer Prevention
The University of Texas MD Anderson Cancer Center
Houston, Texas

Alan H. Bryce, MD
Associate Professor and Chair
Division of Hematology/Oncology
Department of Internal Medicine
Mayo Clinic Arizona
Scottsdale, Arizona

Fred Bunz, MD, PhD
Associate Professor
Department of Radiation Oncology and Molecular Radiation Sciences
The Sidney Kimmel Comprehensive Cancer Center
Johns Hopkins University School of Medicine
Baltimore, Maryland

Earle F. Burgess, MD
Associate Professor & Chief
Genitourinary Medical Oncology
Department of Solid Tumor Oncology and Investigational Therapeutics
Levine Cancer Institute
Atrium Health
Charlotte, North Carolina

Grace G. Bushnell, PhD
Postdoctoral Research Fellow
Department of Internal Medicine
University of Michigan
Ann Arbor, Michigan

John C. Byrd, MD
The Gordon and Helen Hughes Taylor Professor and Chair
Department of Internal Medicine
University of Cincinnati College of Medicine
Cincinnati, Ohio

Matthew T. Campbell, MD
Assistant Professor
Department of Genitourinary Medical Oncology
The University of Texas MD Anderson Cancer Center
Houston, Texas

Michele Carbone, MD, PhD
Professor and William & Ellen Melohn Chair in Cancer Biology
Department of Pathology
University of Hawaii Cancer Center
Honolulu, Hawaii

Diana Cardona, MD
Associate Professor and Associate Director
Duke Health Clinical Laboratories
Duke University Medical Center
Durham, North Carolina

Michael J. Carr, MD, MS
Surgical Oncology Research Fellow
Moffitt Cancer Center
Tampa, Florida

William L. Carroll, MD
Julie and Edward J. Minskoff Professor of Pediatrics and Pathology
NYU Grossman School of Medicine
New York, New York

Tina Cascone, MD, PhD
Assistant Professor
Department of Thoracic/Head and Neck Medical Oncology
The University of Texas MD Anderson Cancer Center
Houston, Texas

Luis Nicolas Gonzalez Castro, MD, PhD
Instructor of Neurology
Harvard Medical School
Boston, Massachusetts

Jad Chahoud, MD, MPH
Assistant Member
Department of GU Oncology
Moffitt Cancer Center
Tampa, Florida

Richard E. Champlin, MD
Professor
Department of Stem Cell Transplantation and Cellular Therapy
The University of Texas MD Anderson Cancer Center
Houston, Texas

Uma Chandran, PhD
Research Associate Professor
Department of Biomedical Informatics
University of Pittsburgh
Pittsburgh, Pennsylvania

Brian F. Chapin, MD
Associate Professor
Urology
The University of Texas MD Anderson Cancer Center
Houston, Texas

Devon K. Check, PhD
Assistant Professor
Department of Population Health Sciences
Duke University School of Medicine
Durham, North Carolina

Alexander Chen, MD
Associate Professor
Division of Cardiothoracic Surgery
Department of Surgery
Division of Pulmonary and Critical Care
Department of Medicine
Washington University School of Medicine
St. Louis, Missouri

Sai-Juan Chen, MD, PhD
Professor and Director
State Key Laboratory of Medical Genomics
Shanghai Institute of Hematology
National Research Center for Translational Medicine
Ruijin Hospital Affiliated with Shanghai Jiao Tong University School of Medicine
Shanghai, China

Zhu Chen, PhD
Professor and Honorary Director
State Key Laboratory of Medical Genomics
Shanghai Institute of Hematology
National Research Center for Translational Medicine
Ruijin Hospital Affiliated with Shanghai Jiao Tong University School of Medicine
Shanghai, China

Patricia Chevez-Barrios, MD, FCAP
Professor
Department of Pathology and Genomic Medicine
Houston Methodist Hospital
Houston, Texas
Weill Cornell Medical College of Cornell University
New York, New York

Elizabeth Y. Chiao, MD, MPH
Professor
Departments of Epidemiology and General Oncology
The University of Texas MD Anderson Cancer Center
Houston, Texas

Seungtaek Choi, MD
Professor
Radiation Oncology
The University of Texas MD Anderson Cancer Center
Houston, Texas

Catherine Chung, MD
Associate Professor
Departments of Medicine and Pathology
The Ohio State University Wexner Medical Center
Columbus, Ohio

Peter E. Clark, MD
Professor and Chair
Department of Urology
Atrium Health
Levine Cancer Institute
Charlotte, North Carolina

James E. Cleaver, PhD
Emeritus Professor Dermatology
Department of Dermatology UCSF Cancer Center
University of California
San Francisco, California

Mark Clemens, MD
Professor
Department of Plastic Surgery
The University of Texas MD Anderson Cancer Center
Houston, Texas

Steven K. Clinton, MD, PhD
Professor
Departments of Internal Medicine, Human Sciences and Human Nutrition
Division of Medical Oncology
The Ohio State University College of Medicine and Comprehensive Cancer Center
Columbus, Ohio

Carmel J. Cohen, MD
Professor Emeritus
Division of Gynecologic Oncology
Icahn School of Medicine at Mount Sinai
New York, New York

Jeffrey I. Cohen, MD
Chief
Laboratory of Infectious Diseases
National Institute of Allergy and Infectious Diseases
Bethesda, Maryland

Lorenzo Cohen, PhD
Professor
Department of Palliative
Rehabilitation, and Integrative Medicine
Director
Integrative Medicine Program
The University of Texas MD Anderson Cancer Center
Houston, Texas

Peter D. Cole, MD
Professor of Pediatrics
Embrace Kids Foundation Endowed Chair in Pediatrics and Hematology/Oncology
Rutgers Robert Wood Johnson Medical School
Rutgers Cancer Institute of New Jersey
New Brunswick, New Jersey

Philip P. Connell, MD
Professor
Department of Radiation and Cellular Oncology
University of Chicago
Chicago, Illinois

Paul G. Corn, MD, PhD
Professor and Chair
Genitourinary Medical Oncology
The University of Texas MD Anderson Cancer Center
Houston, Texas

Emmanuel S. Coronel, MD
Assistant Professor
Department of Gastroenterology, Hepatology and Nutrition
The University of Texas MD Anderson Cancer Center
Houston, Texas

Jorge Cortes, MD
Director
Georgia Cancer Center at Augusta University
Professor of Medicine
Department of Medicine
Augusta University
Augusta, Georgia

Christopher C. Coss, PhD
Associate Professor
College of Pharmacy
The Ohio State University
Columbus, Ohio

Richard Cote, MD, FRCPath, FCAP
Professor & Chair
Department of Pathology and Immunology
Washington University in St. Louis School of Medicine
St. Louis, Missouri

Kenneth H. Cowan, MD, PhD
Professor and Director
Eppley Institute and Fred and Pamela Buffett Cancer Center
University of Nebraska
Omaha, Nebraska

Zachary L. Coyne, BMBS, BSc
Specialist Registrar
Department of Medical Oncology
Beaumont Hospital
Dublin, Ireland

Carlo M. Croce, MD
Distinguished University Professor
John W. Wolfe Chair in Human Cancer
Department of Cancer Biology and Genetics
The Ohio State University
Comprehensive Cancer Center
Columbus, Ohio

Christopher P. Crum, MD
Professor
Department of Pathology
Brigham and Women's Hospital
Harvard Medical School
Boston, Massachusetts

Nour Daboul, MD
Assistant Professor of Medicine
Department of Medicine
West Virginia University
Morgantown, West Virginia

Senthil Damodaran, MD, PhD
Associate Professor
Department of Breast Medical Oncology
The University of Texas MD Anderson Cancer Center
Houston, Texas

Timothy A. Damron, MD, FACS
Professor and Vice-Chairman
The David G. Murray Endowed Professor of Orthopedic Surgery
Department of Orthopedic Surgery
State University of New York
Syracuse, New York

Carrie Daniel, PhD, MPH
Associate Professor
Department of Epidemiology
The University of Texas MD Anderson Cancer Center
Houston, Texas

Michael Davis, MS
Software Integration Architect
Department of Biomedical Informatics
University of Pittsburgh
Pittsburgh, Pennsylvania

Lisa M. DeAngelis, MD
Professor of Neurology
Weill Cornell Medical College
New York, New York

Physician-in-Chief and Chief Medical Officer
Memorial Sloan Kettering Cancer Center
New York, New York

Daniel J. DeAngelo, MD/PhD
Professor of Medicine
Harvard Medical School
Chief of the Division of Leukemia
Department of Medical Oncology
Dana-Farber Cancer Institute
Boston, Massachusetts

Ralph J. DeBerardinis, MD, PhD
Professor
Children's Medical Center Research Institute
University of Texas Southwestern Medical Center
Dallas, Texas

Roy H. Decker, MD, PhD
Professor & Vice Chair of Therapeutic Radiology
Associate Cancer Center Director for Clinical Science
Department of Therapeutic Radiology
Yale University Medical School
New Haven, Connecticut

Siddhartha Devarakonda, MD
Assistant Professor
Division of Medical Oncology
Department of Medicine
Washington University School of Medicine
St. Louis, Missouri

Summer B. Dewdney, MD
Assistant Professor
Gynecologic Oncology
Rush University Medical Center
Chicago, Illinois

Andrew Dhanasopon, MD
Assistant Professor
Thoracic Surgery
Department of Surgery
Yale University
New Haven, Connecticut

Rajiv Dhir, MD
Professor
University of Pittsburgh
Pittsburgh, Pennsylvania

Robert B. Diasio, MD
William J and Charles H Mayo Professor and Director Emeritus Mayo Clinic Cancer Center
Department of Molecular Pharmacology and Experimental Therapeutics and Oncology
Mayo Clinic College of Medicine
Rochester, Minnesota

Burton F. Dickey, MD
Professor of Medicine
Department of Pulmonary Medicine
The University of Texas MD Anderson Cancer Center
Houston, Texas

Zeliha G. Dikmen, MD, PhD
Professor
Department of Biochemistry
Faculty of Medicine
Hacettepe University
Ankara, Turkey

Michaela A. Dinan, PhD
Associate Professor
Department of Chronic Disease Epidemiology
Yale University School of Public Health
New Haven, Connecticut

Megan Dupuis, MD
Assistant Professor
Department of Medicine
Vanderbilt University
Nashville, Tennessee

Madeleine Duvic, MD
Professor
Department of Dermatology
The University of Texas MD Anderson Cancer Center
Houston, Texas

George A. Eapen, MD
Professor of Medicine
Department of Pulmonary Medicine
The University of Texas MD Anderson Cancer Center
Houston, Texas

Joseph P. Eder, MD
Professor
Department of Medicine
Yale Cancer Center
Yale University
New Haven, Connecticut

Scott Eggener, MD
Bruce and Beth White Family Professor
Department of Surgery
University of Chicago Medicine and Biological Sciences
Chicago, Illinois

Assaad A. Eid, DSc., MBA
Professor and Founding Director AUB Diabetes Anatomy
Cell Biology and Physiological Sciences
American University of Beirut
Beirut, Lebanon

Mervat El Azzouni, MD, PhD
Professor of Medical Parasitology
Faculty of Medicine
Alexandria University
Alexandria Governorate, Egypt

Cathy Eng, MD, FACP, FASCO
Professor
Hematology and Oncology
Department of Medicine
Vanderbilt-Ingram Cancer Center
Nashville, Tennessee

Samantha Epistolio, PhD
Researcher
Institute of Pathology
Cantonal Hospital EOC
Locarno, Switzerland

Narendranath Epperla, MD, MS
Assistant Professor
Department of Internal Medicine
Division of Hematology at Ohio State University Comprehensive Cancer Center
Columbus, Ohio

Carmen P. Escalante, MD
Professor and Chair
Department of General Internal Medicine
The University of Texas MD Anderson Cancer Center
Houston, Texas

Miguel Escalon, MD, MHPE
Associate Professor
Department of Rehabilitation and Human Performance and Department of Medical Education
Icahn School of Medicine at Mount Sinai
New York, New York

Mariam F. Eskander, MD, MPH
Assistant Professor
Department of Surgery
Rutgers Cancer Institute of New Jersey
New Brunswick, New Jersey

David S. Ettinger, MD, FACP, FCCP
Alex Grass Professor of Oncology
Professor of Medicine, Radiation Oncology and Molecular Radiation Sciences
The Sidney Kimmel Comprehensive Cancer Center at Johns Hopkins
Johns Hopkins University School of Medicine
Baltimore, Maryland

Douglas B. Evans, MD
Ausman Family Foundation Professor of Surgery and Chair
Department of Surgery
Medical College of Wisconsin
Milwaukee, Wisconsin

Scott E. Evans, MD
Professor of Medicine
Department of Pulmonary Medicine
The University of Texas MD Anderson Cancer Center
Houston, Texas

Michael S. Ewer, MD, JD, PhD
Professor of Medicine
Department of Cardiology
The University of Texas MD Anderson Cancer Center
Houston, Texas

Steven M. Ewer, MD
Associate Professor
Division of Cardiovascular Medicine
Department of Internal Medicine
University of Wisconsin School of Medicine and Public Health
University of Wisconsin-Madison
Madison, Wisconsin

Saadia A. Faiz, MD
Professor of Medicine
Department of Pulmonary Medicine
The University of Texas MD Anderson Cancer Center
Houston, Texas

Veronika Fedirko, PhD, MPH
Associate Professor
Department of Epidemiology
The University of Texas MD Anderson Cancer Center
Houston, Texas

Rui Feng, MD
Resident
Department Neurosurgery
Icahn School of Medicine
Mount Sinai Health System
New York, New York

Robert L. Ferris, MD, PhD
Professor and Director
UPMC Hillman Cancer Center
Eye & Ear Institute
University of Pittsburgh
Pittsburgh, Pennsylvania

William D. Figg, Sr., PharmD
Senior Investigator
Genitourinary Malignancies Branch
Center for Cancer Research
National Cancer Institute
National Institutes of Health
Bethesda, Maryland

Scott R. Floyd, MD, PhD
Gary Hock and Lyn Proctor Associate Professor
Department of Radiation Oncology
Duke University School of Medicine
Durham, North Carolina

Elena Fountzilas, MD, PhD
Clinical Assistant Professor
European University Cyprus
Cyprus, Greece

Lewis Foxhall, MD
Professor and Vice President
Health Policy
Department of Clinical Cancer Prevention
The University of Texas MD Anderson Cancer Center
Houston, Texas

Milo Frattini, PhD
Head
Molecular Pathology Service
Laboratory of Molecular Pathology
Institute of Pathology
EOC
Locarno, Switzerland

Arnold S. Freedman, MD
Professor of Medicine
Department of Medical Oncology
Dana Farber Cancer Institute
Harvard Medical School
Boston, Massachusetts

Michael L. Friedlander, MD, PhD
Conjoint Professor of Medicine
Department of Medical Oncology
The Prince of Wales Hospital
University of New South Wales
Randwick
New South Wales, Australia

Michael Frumovitz, MD, MPH
Professor
Gynecologic Oncology and Reproductive Medicine
The University of Texas MD Anderson Cancer Center
Houston, Texas

Robert F. Gagel, MD
Professor
Department of Endocrine Neoplasia & Hormonal Disorders
The University of Texas MD Anderson Cancer Center
Houston, Texas

Radwa Galal, MD, MBBCH, PhD
Assistant Professor of Medical Parasitology
Alexandria University
Alexandria Governorate
Egypt

Giuseppe Galletti, MD, PhD
Instructor
Department of Medicine
Weill Cornell Medicine
New York, New York

Robert C. Gallo, MD
Professor and Director
The Homer and Martha Gudelsky Distinguished Professor in Medicine
Institute of Human Virology
University of Maryland School of Medicine
Baltimore, Maryland

Sofia R. Gameiro, PhD
Staff Scientist
Laboratory of Tumor Immunology and Biology
Center for Cancer Research
National Cancer Institute
National Institutes of Health
Bethesda, Maryland

Chirag D. Gandhi, MD, FACS, FAANS
Professor and Chairman
Department Neurosurgery
Westchester Medical Center
New York Medical College
Valhalla, New York

Jianjun Gao, MD, PhD
Associate Professor
Department of Genitourinary Medical Oncology
The University of Texas MD Anderson Cancer Center
Houston, Texas

Adam S. Garden, MD
Professor
Department of Radiation Oncology
The University of Texas MD Anderson Cancer Center
Houston, Texas

Lisa Gennarini, MD
Assistant Professor of Pediatrics
Albert Einstein College of Medicine
The Children's Hospital at Montefiore
New York, New York

Damien Gerald, PhD
Sr. Director
Cancer Biology
Drug Development Institute
Comprehensive Cancer Center
The Ohio State University
Columbus, Ohio

Paraskevi Giannakakou, PhD
Professor of Pharmacology
Department of Medicine
Weill Cornell Medicine
New York, New York

Mark R. Gilbert, MD
Chief
Neuro-Oncology Branch
National Cancer Institute
National Institutes of Health
Bethesda, Maryland

Edward L. Giovannucci, MD, ScD
Associate Professor
Department of Medicine
Channing Division of Network Medicine
Brigham and Women's Hospital and Harvard Medical School
Boston, Massachusetts

Sarah B. Goldberg, MD
Associate Professor
Department of Medicine
Section of Medical Oncology
Yale University
New Haven, Connecticut

Donald P. Goldstein, MD
Director Emeritus of New England Trophoblastic Disease Center
Brigham and Women's Hospital and Dana-Farber Cancer Institute
Boston, Massachusetts

Professor Emeritus of Obstetrics
Gynecology and Reproductive Biology
Harvard Medical School
Boston, Massachusetts

Dan S. Gombos, MD, FACS
Professor and Chief
Section of Ophthalmology
Department of Head and Neck Surgery
The University of Texas MD Anderson Cancer Center
Houston, Texas

Daniel R. Gomez, MD, MBA
Director
Thoracic Radiation Oncology
Memorial Sloan Kettering Cancer Center
New York, New York

Roberto Gonzalez, MD
Assistant Professor
Department of Behavioral Science
The University of Texas MD Anderson Cancer Center
Houston, Texas

Sangeeta Goswami, MD, PhD
Assistant Professor
Departments of Immunology and Genitourinary Medical Oncology
The University of Texas MD Anderson Cancer Center
Houston, Texas

Elizabeth M. Grainger RD, PhD
Research Specialist
Department of Internal Medicine
Division of Medical Oncology
The Ohio State University College of Medicine and Comprehensive Cancer Center
Columbus, Ohio

Joe W. Gray, PhD
Professor Emeritus
Department of Biomedical Engineering and Knight Cancer Institute
Oregon Health & Science University
Portland, Oregon

David J. Grdina, PhD
Professor Emeritus
Radiation and Cellular Oncology
The University of Chicago
Chicago, Illinois

Frank A. Greco, MD
Partner
Tennessee Oncology PLLC
Nashville, Tennessee

Co-Founder
Sarah Cannon Research Institute
Nashville, Tennessee

Claude M. Grigg, MD
Attending Physician
Department of Solid Tumor Oncology and Investigational Therapeutics
Levine Cancer Institute
Atrium Health
Charlotte, North Carolina

Horiana B. Grosu, MD
Associate Professor
Department of Pulmonary Medicine
The University of Texas MD Anderson Cancer Center
Houston, Texas

Stephen B. Gruber, MD, PhD, MPH
Director
Center for Precision Medicine and Department of Medical Oncology and Therapeutics Research
City of Hope National Medical Center
Duarte, California

Luca Grumolato, PhD
Associate Professor
INSERM U1239-University of Rouen Normandie
Mont Saint Aignan, France

Irene Guijarro, PhD
Research Project Manager
Department of Thoracic/Head and Neck Medical Oncology
The University of Texas MD Anderson Cancer Center
Houston, Texas

James L. Gulley, MD, PhD, FACP
Chief
Genitourinary Malignancies Branch; Director
Medical Oncology Service; Deputy Director
Center for Cancer Research
National Cancer Institute
National Institutes of Health
Bethesda, Maryland

Mouhammed A. Habra, MD
Professor
Department of Endocrine Neoplasia and Hormonal Disorders
The University of Texas MD Anderson Cancer Center
Houston, Texas

Navid Hafez, MD, MPH
Assistant Professor
Department of Medicine
Yale Cancer Center
Yale University
New Haven, Connecticut

John D. Hainsworth, MD
Co-Founder and Senior Medical Advisor
Sarah Cannon Research Institute
Nashville, Tennessee

Douglas Hanahan, PhD
Professor of Molecular Oncology and Former Director
Swiss Institute for Experimental Cancer Research (ISREC)
School of Life Sciences
Swiss Federal Institute of Technology Lausanne (EPFL)
Swiss Cancer Center Leman (SCCL)
Lausanne, Switzerland

Walter Hanel, MD, PhD
Assistant Professor
Department of Internal Medicine
Division of Hematology at Ohio State University Comprehensive Cancer Center
Columbus, Ohio

Curtis C. Harris, MD
Senior Investigator and Chief
Laboratory of Human Carcinogenesis
National Cancer Institute
National Institutes of Health
Bethesda, Maryland

Douglas Hartman, MD
Associate Professor
Department of Pathology
University of Pittsburgh
Pittsburgh, Pennsylvania

R. Donald Harvey, PharmD, BCOP, FCCP, FHOPA
Professor
Departments of Hematology/Medical Oncology and Pharmacology
Emory University School of Medicine
Atlanta, Georgia

Saima Hassan, MD, PhD, FRCSC
Scotia Bank Chairperson in Breast Cancer
Centre Hospitalier de l'Université de Montréal
Montréal, Canada

Ernest Hawk, MD, MPH
Vice President and Head
Division of Cancer Prevention & Population Sciences
The University of Texas MD Anderson Cancer Center
Houston, Texas

Michael Hawking, MD
Fellow
Hematology-Oncology
Department of Medicine
University of Chicago Medicine & Biological Sciences
Chicago, Illinois

Laura M. Heiser, PhD
Associate Professor
Department of Biomedical Engineering and Knight Cancer Institute
Oregon Health & Science University
Portland, Oregon

William P. D. Hendricks, PhD
Assistant Professor
Integrated Cancer Genomics Division
Translational Genomics Research Institute
Phoenix, Arizona

Bryan T. Hennessy, MD
Consultant Medical Oncologist
Department of Medical Oncology
Beaumont Hospital and Our Lady of Lourdes Hospital
Drogheda, Ireland

Roy S. Herbst, MD, PhD
Ensign Professor of Medicine and Chief
Medical Oncology
Department of Medicine
Section of Medical Oncology
Yale University
New Haven, Connecticut

Michael F. Herfs, PhD
Associate Professor
Laboratory of Experimental Pathology
GIGA-Cancer
University of Liege
Liege, Belgium

John V. Heymach, MD, PhD
Professor and Chair
Department of Thoracic/Head and Neck Medical Oncology
The University of Texas MD Anderson Cancer Center
Houston, Texas

Teru Hideshima, MD, PhD
Principal Associate of Medicine
Harvard Medical School
Institute Scientist
Dana-Farber Cancer Institute
Boston, Massachusetts

Gerard Hilinski, PhD
Sr. Director
Biochemistry
Drug Development Institute
Comprehensive Cancer Center
The Ohio State University
Columbus, Ohio

Evthokia A. Hobbs, MD
Assistant Professor
Department of Medicine
Oregon Health & Science University
Portland, Oregon

Lorne J. Hofseth, PhD
Professor
College of Pharmacy
University of South Carolina
Columbia, South Carolina

James F. Holland, MD, ScD (hc) (deceased)
Distinguished Professor of Neoplastic Diseases
Director, Emeritus of the Derald H. Ruttenberg Cancer Center
Icahn School of Medicine at Mt Sinai
New York, New York

Leroy Hood, MD, PhD
Chief Strategy Officer
Co-founder and Professor
Institute for Systems Biology
Seattle, Washington

Neil S. Horowitz, MD
Associate Professor and Director of Clinical Research
Division of Gynecologic Oncology
Department of Obstetrics and Gynecology
Brigham and Women's Hospital and Dana-Farber Cancer Institute
Harvard Medical School
Boston, Massachusetts

Shannon K. Hughes, PhD
Deputy Director
Division of Cancer Biology
National Cancer Institute
Bethesda, Maryland

Kelly K. Hunt, MD
Professor and Chair
Department of Breast Surgical Oncology
The University of Texas MD Anderson Cancer Center
Houston, Texas

Samuel M. Hyde, MS
Genetic Counselor
Clinical Cancer Genetics
The University of Texas MD Anderson Cancer Center
Houston, Texas

Nuhad Ibrahim, MD
Professor
Department of Breast Medical Oncology
The University of Texas MD Anderson Cancer Center
Houston, Texas

Ilya Iofin, MD
Assistant Professor and Chief
Orthopaedic Oncology Service
Department of Orthopaedic Surgery
Icahn School of Medicine at Mount Sinai
New York, New York

Elias Jabbour, MD
Professor
Department of Leukemia
The University of Texas MD Anderson Cancer Center
Houston, Texas

Elio Jabra, MD
Medical Resident
Hematology and Oncology Division
Department of Internal Medicine
American University of Beirut
Beirut, Lebanon

Alexandre A. A. Jácome, MD, PhD
Postdoctoral Fellow
Department of Gastrointestinal Medical Oncology
The University of Texas MD Anderson Cancer Center
Houston, Texas

Nitin Jain, MD
Associate Professor
Department of Leukemia
The University of Texas MD Anderson Cancer Center
Houston, Texas

Anuja Jhingran, MD
Professor
Department of Radiation Oncology
The University of Texas MD Anderson Cancer Center
Houston, Texas

Xingya Jiang, PhD
Postdoctoral Fellow
Center for Nanomedicine and Department of Anesthesiology
Harvard Medical School
Brigham and Women's Hospital
Boston, Massachusetts

Carlos A. Jimenez, MD
Professor of Medicine
Department of Pulmonary Medicine
The University of Texas MD Anderson Cancer Center
Houston, Texas

Roshni D. Kalachand, MBBCh
Specialist Registrar/Research Fellow
Department of Medical Oncology
Beaumont Hospital
Dublin, Ireland

Hagop Kantarjian, MD
Professor and Chair
Department of Leukemia
The University of Texas MD Anderson Cancer Center
Houston, Texas

Maher Karam-Hage, MD
Professor
Department of Behavioral Science
The University of MD Anderson Cancer Center
Houston, Texas

Michael Karin, PhD
Distinguished Professor
Department of Pathology
University of California San Diego
San Diego, California

Padmavathi V. Karri, MD
Intern
Department of Internal Medicine
Baylor College of Medicine
Houston, Texas

Nicole M. Kettner, PhD
Post-Doctoral Fellow
Department of Experimental Radiation Oncology
The University of Texas MD Anderson Cancer Center
Houston, Texas

Khandan Keyomarsi, PhD
Professor
Department of Experimental Radiation Oncology
The University of Texas MD Anderson Cancer Center
Houston, Texas

Fadlo R. Khuri, MD
President
Professor of Internal Medicine
American University of Beirut
Beirut, Lebanon

Catherine E. Klein, MD
Professor and Chief
Section of Hematology/Medical Oncology
Rocky Mountain Regional VA Medical Center
University of Colorado School of Medicine
Aurora, Colorado

Jane P. Ko, MD
Professor
Department of Radiology
Thoracic Imaging
Grossman School of Medicine
New York University
New York, New York

Justin M. Ko, MD, MBA
Director and Chief of Medical Dermatology
Stanford University Medical Center
Redwood City, California

Eugene Koay, MD, PhD
Associate Professor
Department of GI Radiation Oncology
The University of Texas MD Anderson Cancer Center
Houston, Texas

Dimitrios P. Kontoyiannis, MD, ScD, FACP, FIDSA
Professor
Department of Infectious Diseases
The University of Texas MD Anderson Cancer Center
Houston, Texas

Scott Kopetz, MD, PhD
Professor
Department of Gastrointestinal Medical Oncology
The University of Texas MD Anderson Cancer Center
Houston, Texas

Michael Kroll, MD
Professor
Department of Pulmonary Medicine
The University of Texas MD Anderson Cancer Center
Houston, Texas

Anita Kumar, MD
Assistant Attending Physician
Lymphoma Service
Memorial Sloan Kettering Cancer Center
New York, New York

Razelle Kurzrock, MD
Associate Director
Clinical Research
Medical College of Wisconsin Cancer Center
Genomic Science and Precision Medicine Center
Milwaukee, Wisconsin

Ann S. LaCasce, MD
Associate Professor
Department of Medical Oncology
Dana Farber Cancer Institute
Harvard Medical School
Boston, Massachusetts

Jessica D. Lang, PhD
Assistant Professor
Department of Pathology and Laboratory Medicine and Center for Human Genomics and Precision Medicine
University of Wisconsin-Madison
Madison, Wisconsin

Robert Langer ScD
David H. Koch Professor
Harvard-MIT Division of Health Sciences and Technology
Institute for Integrative Cancer Research
Massachusetts Institute of Technology
Cambridge, Massachusetts

Rachel Layman, MD
Associate Professor
Department of Breast Medical Oncology
The University of Texas MD Anderson Cancer Center
Houston, Texas

Michelle M. Le Beau, PhD
Arthur and Marian Edelstein Professor Emerita
Section of Hematology/Oncology
Department of Medicine
University of Chicago
Chicago, Illinois

J. Jack Lee, PhD, MS, DDS
Professor
Department of Biostatistics
The University of Texas MD Anderson Cancer Center
Houston, Texas

Jeffrey E. Lee, MD
Professor
Department of Surgical Oncology
Irving and Nadine Mansfield and Robert David Levitt Cancer Research Chair
Vice President
Medical and Academic Affairs
Cancer Network
The University of Texas MD Anderson Cancer Center
Houston, Texas

Robert W. Lentz, MD
Hematology/Oncology Fellow
University of Colorado School of Medicine
Aurora, Colorado

Yan Leyfman, MD
Clinical Research Fellow
Department of Hematology Oncology
Icahn School of Medicine at Mount Sinai
New York, New York

Donghui Li, PhD
Professor of Medicine
Department of GI Medical Oncology
The University of Texas MD Anderson Cancer Center
Houston, Texas

Carly Likar PA-C
Physician Assistant
Department of Surgery
West Virginia University
Morgantown, West Virginia

Bora Lim, MD
Associate Professor
Baylor Medical College
Houston, Texas

Scott M. Lippman, MD
Professor and Director
Moores Cancer Center
University of California San Diego
San Diego, California

Virginia R. Litle, MD
Chief of Thoracic Surgery
Medical Director of Thoracic Surgery
Intermountain Healthcare
Murray, Utah

Jennifer K. Litton, MD
Vice President for Clinical Research
Professor
Department of Breast Medical Oncology
The University of Texas MD Anderson Cancer Center
Houston, Texas

Annie Liu, MD, PhD
Resident
Department of Surgery
Duke University
Durham, North Carolina

List of contributors   xix

Danny Liu, BS
Postdoctoral Fellow
Center for Nanomedicine and Department of Anesthesiology
Harvard Medical School
Brigham and Women's Hospital
Boston, Massachusetts

Jerry Liu, MD
Assistant Professor
Department of Radiation Oncology
Icahn School of Medicine at Mount Sinai
New York, New York

Wenli Liu, MD
Associate Professor
Department of Palliative
Rehabilitation, and Integrative Medicine
The University of Texas MD Anderson Cancer Center
Houston, Texas

Yanlan Liu, PhD
Postdoctoral Fellow
Center for Nanomedicine and Department of Anesthesiology
Harvard Medical School
Brigham and Women's Hospital
Boston, Massachusetts

Yuan Liu, PhD, MS
Research Associate Professor
Department of Biostatistics and Bioinformatics
Rollins School of Public Health of Emory University
Atlanta, Georgia

Christopher J. Logothetis, MD
Professor
Department of Genitourinary Medical Oncology
The University of Texas MD Anderson Cancer Center
Houston, Texas

Gabriel Lopez, MD
Associate Professor
Department of Palliative Care
Rehabilitation, and Integrative Medicine
The University of Texas MD Anderson Cancer Center
Houston, Texas

Karen H. Lu, MD
Professor and Chair
Department of Gynecologic Oncology and Reproductive Medicine
The University of Texas MD Anderson Cancer Center
Houston, Texas

Anirban Maitra, MBBS
Professor
Department of Pathology
The University of Texas MD Anderson Cancer Center
Houston, Texas

Sukh Makhnoon, PhD, MS
Post-Doctoral Fellow
Department of Behavioral Science
The University of Texas MD Anderson Cancer Center
Houston, Texas

Robert G. Maki, MD, PhD, FACP, FASCO
Professor and Director
Developmental Therapeutics and Sarcoma Medical Oncology
Abramson Cancer Center
Perelman School of Medicine
University of Pennsylvania
Philadelphia, Pennsylvania

Karen C. Maresso, MPH
Scientific Project Director
Department of Clinical Cancer Prevention
The University of Texas MD Anderson Cancer Center
Houston, Texas

Kim A. Margolin, MD
Professor Emeritus
City of Hope National Cancer Center
Duarte, California

Professor and Co-director
Melanoma Program
St John's Cancer Institute
Santa Monica, California

Charbel F. Matar, MD
Clinical Fellow
Hematology and Oncology Division
Department of Internal Medicine
American University of Beirut
Beirut, Lebanon

Timothy K. McDaniel, PhD
Adjunct Professor
Vice President
Emerging Technologies
Translational Genomics Research Institute
Phoenix, Arizona

Kevin McDonnell, MD, PhD
Assistant Professor
Center for Precision Medicine and Department of Medical Oncology and Therapeutics Research
City of Hope National Medical Center
Duarte, California

Derek McHaffie, MD
Head
Section of Genitourinary Radiation Oncology
Levine Cancer Institute
Atrium Health
Charlotte, North Carolina

Stacy L. McMurray, MD
Assistant Professor
Department of Dermatology
Perelman School of Medicine
University of Pennsylvania
Philadelphia, Pennsylvania

Megan E. McNerney, MD, PhD
Associate Professor
Departments of Pediatrics and Pathology
Comprehensive Cancer Center
University of Chicago
Chicago, Illinois

Jeffrey I. Mechanick, MD
Professor and Director
Metabolic Support
Division of Endocrinology
Diabetes and Bone Disease
Icahn School of Medicine at Mount Sinai
New York, New York

Ilgen Mender, PhD
Postdoctoral Researcher
Department of Cell Biology
University of Texas Southwestern Medical Center
Dallas, Texas

Ruben Mesa, MD
Executive Director of the Cancer Center
Division of Hematology/Oncology
Mays Cancer Center
UT Health San Antonio
The University of Texas MD Anderson Cancer Center
San Antonio, Texas

Zeyad A. Metwalli, MD
Assistant Professor
Department of Interventional Radiology
The University of Texas MD Anderson Cancer Center
Houston, Texas

Matthew Meyerson, MD, PhD
Professor and Director of the Center for Cancer Genomics
Meyerson Laboratory
Department of Medical Oncology
Dana-Farber Cancer Institute
Harvard Medical School
Boston, Massachusetts

Eric A. Millican, MD
Assistant Professor
Department of Dermatology
University of Utah School of Medicine
Salt Lake City, Utah

Gordon B. Mills, MD, PhD
Professor and Wayne and Julie Drinkward Endowed Chair in Precision Oncology
Director of Precision Oncology and SMMART Trials Development and Cancer Biology in the Knight Cancer Institute
Oregon Health Sciences University
Portland, Oregon

Melissa P. Mitchell, MD
Associate Professor
Department of Radiation Oncology
The University of Texas MD Anderson Cancer Center
Houston, Texas

Mayur D. Mody, MD
Fellow
Department of Hematology and Medical Oncology
Emory University School of Medicine
Atlanta, Georgia

Daniel Morgensztern, MD
Professor and Clinical Director of Thoracic Oncology
Division of Medical Oncology
Department of Medicine
Washington University School of Medicine
St. Louis, Missouri

Rodolfo C. Morice, MD
Professor
Department of Pulmonary Medicine
The University of Texas MD Anderson Cancer Center
Houston, Texas

Jeffrey A. Moscow, MD
Chief
Investigational Drug Branch
Cancer Therapy Evaluation Program
Division of Cancer Treatment and Diagnosis
National Cancer Institute
Bethesda, Maryland

Karl Munger, PhD
Professor and Chair
Department of Developmental
Molecular and Chemical Biology
Tufts University School of Medicine
Boston, Massachusetts

Muhammed Murtaza, MBBS, PhD
Associate Professor
Department of Surgery
Assistant Director of the Center for Human Genomics and Precision Medicine
University of Wisconsin-Madison
Madison, Wisconsin

Rashmi Murthy, MD
Associate Professor
Department of Breast Medical Oncology
The University of Texas MD Anderson Cancer Center
Houston, Texas

Serge P. Nana-Sinkam, MD
Professor and Chair
Division of Pulmonary Diseases and Critical Care Medicine
Virginia Commonwealth University
Richmond, Virginia

Santhosshi Narayanan, MD
Assistant Professor
Department of Palliative, Rehabilitation, and Integrative Medicine
The University of Texas MD Anderson Cancer Center
Houston, Texas

Kevin T. Nead, MD, MPhil
Assistant Professor
Department of Epidemiology
The University of Texas MD Anderson Cancer Center
Houston, Texas

Andrea Necchi, MD
Associate Professor
Department of Genitourinary Oncology
Vita-Salute San Raffaele University
IRCCS San Raffaele Hospital and Scientific Institute
Milan, Italy

Victor A. Neel, MD, PhD
Assistant Professor
Department of Dermatology
Harvard Medical School
Boston, Massachusetts

Theodore P. Nicolaides, MD
Otto and Marguerite Manley and Making Headway Foundation Associate Professor of Pediatrics
Stephen D. Hassenfeld Children's Center for Cancer and Blood Disorders
NYU Grossman School of Medicine
New York, New York

Monique Nilsson, PhD
Senior Research Scientist
Department of Thoracic/Head and Neck Medical Oncology
The University of Texas MD Anderson Cancer Center
Houston, Texas

Rachel Njeim, MSC, PharmD
PhD Candidate Anatomy
Cell Biology and Physiological Sciences
American University of Beirut
Beirut, Lebanon

Susan O'Brien, MD
Professor
Division of Hematology/Oncology, Medicine
Chao Family Comprehensive Cancer Center
University of California – Irvine
Orange, California

Brian O'Sullivan, MD
Professor
Department of Radiation Oncology and Otolaryngology/Head and Neck Surgery
University of Toronto
Toronto, Ontario, Canada

Steven M. Offer, PhD
Assistant Professor
Department of Molecular Pharmacology and Experimental Therapeutics
Mayo Clinic College of Medicine
Rochester, Minnesota

Rebecca L. Olin, MD, MSCE
Associate Professor
Department of Medicine
Division of Hematology/Oncology
University of California San Francisco
San Francisco, California

Susana Ortiz-Urda, MD, PhD
Associate Professor
Department of Dermatology UCSF Cancer Center
University of California San Francisco
San Francisco, California

Taofeek K. Owonikoko, MD, PhD, MSCR
Professor and Vice-Chair for Faculty Development
Department of Hematology and Medical Oncology
Emory University School of Medicine
Atlanta, Georgia

Margaret Pain, MD
Assistant Professor
Department of Neurosurgery
Robert Wood Johnson Medical School
New Brunswick, New Jersey

Claudia Palena, PhD
Senior Investigator
Laboratory of Tumor Immunology and Biology
Center for Cancer Research
National Cancer Institute
National Institutes of Health
Bethesda, Maryland

Jeanne Palmer, MD
Section Head of Hematology
Division of Hematology/Oncology
Mayo Clinic
Phoenix, Arizona

M. Lia Palomba, MD
Hematologic Oncologist
Department of Medicine
Memorial Sloan-Kettering Cancer Center
New York, New York

Gladell Paner, MD
Professor
Department of Pathology
University of Chicago Medicine & Biological Sciences
Chicago, Illinois

Jae H. Park, MD
Hematologic-Oncologist
Department of Medicine
Memorial Sloan-Kettering Cancer Center
New York, New York

Harvey I. Pass, MD
Stephen E. Banner Professor of Thoracic Oncology and Chief
Thoracic Oncology
NYU Langone Medical Center
New York, New York

Anisha B. Patel, MD
Associate Professor
Department of Dermatology
The University of Texas MD Anderson Cancer Center
Houston, Texas

Jeffrey T. Patrick, PharmD
Senior Director
Drug Development Institute
Comprehensive Cancer Center
The Ohio State University
Columbus, Ohio

Natalya N. Pavlova, PhD
Postdoctoral Research Fellow
Cancer Biology and Genetics Program
Memorial Sloan Kettering Cancer Center
New York, New York

Timothy M. Pawlik, MD, MPH, PhD
Colon & Rectal Surgery Fellow
AdventHealth Central Florida
Orlando, Florida

Karl Peggs, MB, BCh
Professor
University College London Cancer Institute
London, UK

Uma R. Phatak, MD
Assistant Professor
Department of Surgery
University of Texas Medical Branch
Galveston, Texas

Marco A. Pierotti, PhD
Senior Consultant
Cogentech/IFOM
Milan, Italy

Patrick Pilie, MD
Assistant Professor
Genitourinary Medical Oncology
The University of Texas MD Anderson Cancer Center
Houston, Texas

Raphael E. Pollock, MD, PhD
Klotz Family Chair in Cancer Research
Professor and Director
Ohio State University Comprehensive Cancer Center
The Ohio State University Medical Center
Columbus, Ohio

Yves Pommier, MD, PhD
Senior Investigator
Developmental Therapeutics Branch
Center for Cancer Research
National Cancer Institute
National Institutes of Health
Bethesda, Maryland

Kalmon D. Post, MD, FACS, FAANS
Chairman Emeritus
Department of Neurosurgery
Mount Sinai Health System
New York, New York

Selvaraj E. Pravinkumar, MD, FRCP
Professor of Medicine
Department of Pulmonary Medicine
The University of Texas MD Anderson Cancer Center
Houston, Texas

Carolyn J. Presley, MD, MHS
Assistant Professor
Department of Internal Medicine
The Ohio State University
Columbus, Ohio

Nathan D. Price, PhD
Professor
Institute for Systems Biology
Seattle, Washington

Claudia M. Prospero Ponce, MD
Assistant Professor
Neuro-Ophthalmology and Ocular Pathology
Department of Neurology
Texas Tech University Health Sciences Center El Paso
Paul L. Foster School of Medicine
El Paso, Texas

Sergio Quezada, PhD
Professor
University College London Cancer Institute
London, UK

Elizabeth Raetz, MD
KiDS of NYU Foundation Professor of Pediatrics
Stephen D. Hassenfeld Children's Center for Cancer and Blood Disorders
NYU Grossman School of Medicine
New York, New York

Derek Raghavan, MD, PhD, FACP, FRACP, FASCO, FAAAS
Professor and President
Levine Cancer Institute
Atrium Health
Charlotte, North Carolina

Jamal Rahaman, MD
Clinical Professor
Division of Gynecologic Oncology
Icahn School of Medicine at Mount Sinai
New York, New York

Kanti R. Rai, MD
Joel Finkelstein Cancer Foundation Professor of Medicine
Zucker School of Medicine at Hofstra/Northwell Health
New Hyde Park, New York

Noopur Raje, MD
Professor of Medicine
Harvard Medical School
Center for Multiple Myeloma
Massachusetts General Hospital Cancer Center
Boston, Massachusetts

Suresh S. Ramalingam, MD, FACP, FASCO
Professor and Roberto C. Goizueta Distinguished Chair for Cancer Research
Department of Hematology and Medical Oncology
Emory University School of Medicine
Executive Director
Winship Cancer Institute of Emory University
Atlanta, Georgia

Pilar Ramos, PhD
Postdoctoral Fellow
Integrated Cancer Genomics Division
Translational Genomics Research Institute
Phoenix, Arizona

Aparna D. Rao, MBBS, PhD
Honorary Fellow
Sir Peter MacCallum Department of Oncology
The University of Melbourne
Melbourne, Australia

Philipp J. Rauch, MD
Hematology-Oncology Senior Fellow
Department of Medical Oncology
Harvard Medical School
Dana-Farber Cancer Institute
Boston, Massachusetts

Chandrajit P. Raut, MD, MSc, FACS
Professor of Surgery
Harvard Medical School
Boston, Massachusetts
Chief
Division of Surgical Oncology
Department of Surgery
Brigham and Women's Hospital
Boston, Massachusetts

Michael J. Reardon, MD
Professor and Allison Family Distinguished Chair of Cardiovascular Research
Department of Cardiac Surgery
Houston Methodist DeBakey Heart & Vascular Center
Houston, Texas

John C. Reed, MD, PhD
Executive Vice President and Global Head Research and Development
Sanofi
Paris, France

Marvin S. Reitz, PhD
Adjunct Professor
School of Medicine
University of Maryland
Baltimore, Maryland

John C. Reneau, MD, PhD
Assistant Professor
Clinical Division of Hematology
Department of Medicine
The Ohio State University Wexner Medical Center
Columbus, Ohio

Malte Renz, MD, PhD
Instructor
Department of Obstetrics and Gynecology
Stanford University School of Medicine
Stanford, California

Joanna M. Rhodes, MD, MSCE
Assistant Professor
Department of Medicine
Donald and Barbara Zucker School of Medicine at Hofstra/Northwell Health
New Hyde Park, New York

Stephen B. Riggs, MD, MBA, FACS
Attending Urologist
Department of Uro-oncology
Levine Cancer Institute, and Department of Urology
Atrium Health
Charlotte, North Carolina

Matthew D. Ringel, MD
Professor and Ralph W. Kurtz Chair
Director Division of Endocrinology, Diabetes and Metabolism
The Ohio State University Wexner Medical Center and Arthur G. James Comprehensive Cancer Center
Columbus, Ohio

Russell C. Rockne, PhD
Associate Professor
Department of Computational and Quantitative Medicine
City of Hope National Medical Center
Duarte, California

Kenneth V.I. Rolston, MD, FACP
Professor
Department of Infectious Diseases
The University of Texas MD Anderson Cancer Center
Houston, Texas

Ari J. Rosenberg, MD
Assistant Professor
Section of Hematology/Oncology
Department of Medicine
University of Chicago
Chicago, Illinois

Ashley E. Rosko, MD
Associate Professor
Department of Internal Medicine
The Ohio State University
Columbus, Ohio

Andrew J. Roth, MD
Clinical Instructor
Department of Psychiatry and Behavioral Sciences
Memorial Sloan Kettering Cancer Center
New York, New York

Katherine Roth, MD
Department of Medical Oncology and Therapeutics Research
City of Hope National Medical Center
Duarte, California

Nabil F. Saba, MD, FACP
Professor
Department of Hematology and Medical Oncology
Winship Cancer Institute
Emory University
Atlanta, Georgia

Aysegul Sahin, MD
Professor
Department of Anatomic Pathology
The University of Texas MD Anderson Cancer Center
Houston, Texas

Kristin Sanfilippo, MD, MPHS
Assistant Professor
Department of Internal Medicine
Washington University School of Medicine
Saint Louis, Missouri

Michelle I. Savage, BA
Program Director
Department of Clinical Cancer Prevention
The University of Texas MD Anderson Cancer Center
Houston, Texas

Paul Scheet, PhD
Professor
Department of Epidemiology
The University of Texas MD Anderson Cancer Center
Houston, Texas

Lauren Scherer, MD
Instructor
Department of Pediatrics
Baylor College of Medicine
Houston Methodist Hospital and Texas Children's Hospital
Houston, Texas

Florian Scheufele, MD
Post-Doctoral Fellow
Tuveson Laboratory
Cold Spring Harbor Laboratory
Cold Spring Harbor, New York

Charles A. Schiffer, MD
Professor
Department of Hematology-Oncology
Barbara Ann Karmanos Cancer Institute
Detroit, Michigan

Jeffrey Schlom, PhD
Chief
Laboratory of Tumor Immunology and Biology
Center for Cancer Research
National Cancer Institute
National Institutes of Health
Bethesda, Maryland

Carl Schmidt, MD, FACS
Professor
Department of Surgery
West Virginia University
Morgantown, West Virginia

Leslie R. Schover, PhD
Professor (retired)
Department of Behavioral Sciences
The University of Texas MD Anderson Cancer Center
Houston, Texas

Lawrence H. Schwartz, MD
James Picker Professor
Department of Radiology
Columbia University Vagelos
The New York Presbyterian Hospital
Columbia, South Carolina

Aleksandar Sekulic, MD, PhD
Associate Professor and Vice Chair
Department of Dermatology
Mayo Clinic Arizona
Scottsdale, Arizona

Reena Shakya, PhD
Director
Target Validation Shared Resource
Comprehensive Cancer Center
The Ohio State University
Columbus, Ohio

Ali Shamseddine, MD, FRCP, ESCO
Professor
Department of Internal Medicine
American University of Beirut
Beirut, Lebanon

Vickie R. Shannon, MD
Professor
Department of Pulmonary Medicine
The University of Texas MD Anderson Cancer Center
Houston, Texas

Padmanee Sharma, MD, PhD
Professor
Departments of Immunology and Genitourinary Medical Oncology
The University of Texas MD Anderson Cancer Center
Houston, Texas

Jerry W. Shay, PhD
Professor
Department of Cell Biology
University of Texas Southwestern Medical Center
Dallas, Texas

Ajay Sheshadre, MD
Assistant Professor
Department of Pulmonary Medicine
The University of Texas MD Anderson Cancer Center
Houston, Texas

Jinjun Shi, PhD
Associate Professor
Center for Nanomedicine and Department of Anesthesiology
Harvard Medical School
Brigham and Women's Hospital
Boston, Massachusetts

Dong M. Shin, MD, FACP, FAAAS
Professor
Department of Hematology and Medical Oncology
Emory University School of Medicine
Atlanta, Georgia

Junichi Shindoh, MD, PhD
Surgeon-in-Chief
Hepatobiliary-Pancreatic Surgery Division
Department of Digestive Surgery
Toranomon Hospital
Tokyo, Japan

William E. Shirey, MS
Chief Architect in Department of Biomedical Informatics
University of Pittsburgh
Pittsburgh, Pennsylvania

Elizabeth J. Shpall, MD
Professor and Chair ad interim
Department of Stem Cell Transplantation and Cellular Therapy
The University of Texas MD Anderson Cancer Center
Houston, Texas

Gabriel L. Sica, MD, PhD
Professor
Department of Pathology
University of Pittsburgh School of Medicine
Pittsburgh, Pennsylvania

List of contributors xxiii

Zahid H. Siddik, PhD
Professor
Department of Experimental Therapeutics
The University of Texas MD Anderson Cancer Center
Houston, Texas

Bilal A. Siddiqui, MD
Assistant Professor
Department of Genitourinary Medical Oncology
The University of Texas MD Anderson Cancer Center
Houston, Texas

Branimir I. Sikic, MD
Professor
Department of Medicine-Oncology
Stanford University School of Medicine
Stanford, California

Richard T. Silver, MD
Professor
Department of Medicine
Weill Cornell Medical College
Cornell University
New York, New York

Jonathan C. Silverstein, MD, MS
Professor
Department of Biomedical Informatics
University of Pittsburgh
Pittsburgh, Pennsylvania

Cardinale B. Smith, MD, PhD
Associate Professor
Department of Geriatrics and Palliative Medicine
Icahn School of Medicine at Mount Sinai
New York, New York

Matthew A. Smith-Cohn, DO
Staff Neuro-Oncologist
The Ben & Catherine Ivy Center for Advanced Brain Tumor Treatment
Swedish Neuroscience Institute
Swedish Health Services
Seattle, Washington

Luisa M. Solis Soto, MD
Assistant Professor
Department of Translational Molecular Pathology
The University of Texas MD Anderson Cancer Center
Houston, Texas

Vernon K. Sondak, MD
Professor and Richard M. Schulze Family Foundation Distinguished Endowed Chair in Cutaneous Oncology
Moffitt Cancer Center
University of South Florida Morsani College of Medicine
Tampa, Florida

Stephen T. Sonis, DMD, DMSc
Professor
Division of Oral Medicine and Dentistry
Brigham and Women's Hospital
Boston, Massachusetts

Gabriella Sozzi, PhD
Head of Tumor Genomics Unit
Department of Research
Fondazione IRCCS Istituto Nazionale Tumori
Milan, Italy

Alex Sparreboom, PhD
Professor
Division of Pharmaceutics and Pharmacology
College of Pharmacy
The Ohio State University
Columbus, Ohio

Philippe E. Spiess, MD, MS
Assistant Chief Surgical Services
Department of Genitourinary Oncology
Moffitt Cancer Center
Tampa, Florida

Walter M. Stadler, MD
Fred C. Buffett Professor
Department of Medicine
University of Chicago Medicine & Biological Sciences
Chicago, Illinois

William G. Stebbins, MD
Associate Professor
Department of Dermatology
Vanderbilt University School of Medicine
Nashville, Tennessee

David P. Steensma, MD
Edward P. Evans Chair in MDS Research
Department of Medical Oncology
Harvard Medical School
Dana-Farber Cancer Institute
Boston, Massachusetts

Richard M. Stone, MD
Professor
Department of Medicine
Harvard Medical School
Boston, Massachusetts

David J. Straus, MD
Attending Physician
Lymphoma Service
Memorial Sloan Kettering Cancer Center
New York, New York

Michael D. Stubblefield, MD
Clinical Professor
Department of Physical Medicine and Rehabilitation
Rutgers New Jersey Medical School
Newark, New Jersey

Ishwaria M. Subbiah, MD, MS
Assistant Professor
Department of Palliative, Rehabilitation and Integrated Medicine
The University of Texas MD Anderson Cancer Center
Houston, Texas

Sumit K. Subudhi, MD, PhD
Associate Professor
Department of Genitourinary Medical Oncology
The University of Texas MD Anderson Cancer Center
Houston, Texas

Max W. Sung, MD
Associate Professor
Division of Hematology and Medical Oncology
Icahn School of Medicine at Mount Sinai
New York, New York

Devaki S. Surasi, MBBS
Assistant Professor
Department of Nuclear Medicine
The University of Texas MD Anderson Cancer Center
Houston, Texas

Thomas M. Suter, MD
Professor
Department of Cardiology
Inselspital/University Hospital of Bern
Bern, Switzerland

Yota Suzuki, MD
General Surgery Resident
Department of Surgery
University of Texas Medical Branch
Galveston, Texas

Susan M. Swetter, MD
Professor
Department of Dermatology
Stanford University Medical Center and Cancer Institute
Stanford, California

Fred K. Tabung, MSPH, PhD
Assistant Professor
Department of Internal Medicine
The Ohio State University College of Medicine and Comprehensive Cancer Center
Columbus, Ohio

Zahra Talebi, PharmD
Postdoctoral Researcher
College of Pharmacy
The Ohio State University
Columbus, Ohio

Moshe Talpaz, MD
Professor
Internal Medicine and Medical Oncology
University of Michigan Medical School
Ann Arbor, Michigan

Kenneth K. Tanabe, MD, FACS
Professor
Department of Surgery
Harvard Medical School
Boston, Massachusetts

Koji Taniguchi, MD, PhD
Professor
Department of Pathology
University of California San Diego
San Diego, California

Nizar M. Tannir, MD, FACP
Professor
Department of Genitourinary Medical Oncology
The University of Texas MD Anderson Cancer Center
Houston, Texas

Haruko Tashiro, MD, PhD
Associate Professor
Department of Hematology/Oncology
Teikyo University School of Medicine
Tokyo, Japan

Anish Thomas, MD
Investigator
Developmental Therapeutics Branch
Center for Cancer Research
National Cancer Institute
National Institutes of Health
Bethesda, Maryland

David C. Thomas, MD, MHPE
Professor
Department of Medicine
Medical Education and Rehabilitation and Human Performance
Mt Sinai Hospital
New York, New York

David K. Thomas, MD
Director
Cachexia Discovery and Therapeutic Development
Broad Institute of MIT & Harvard
Cambridge, Massachusetts

Craig B. Thompson, MD
President and CEO
Memorial Sloan Kettering Cancer Center
New York, New York

Katherine A. Thornton, MD
Medical Oncologist
Department of Medicine
Memorial Sloan Kettering Cancer Center
New York, New York

Jelena Todoric, MD, PhD
Senior Scientist
Department of Pathology
University of California San Diego
San Diego, California

Harrys A. Torres, MD, FACP, FIDSA
Professor
Department of Infectious Diseases, Infection Control, and Employee Health
The University of Texas MD Anderson Cancer Center
Houston, Texas

Hop S. Tran Cao, MD, FACS
Associate Professor
Department of Surgical Oncology
The University of Texas MD Anderson Cancer Center
Houston, Texas

Benno Traub, MD
Post-Doctoral Fellow
Tuveson Laboratory
Cold Spring Harbor Laboratory
Cold Spring Harbor, New York

Jeffrey M. Trent, PhD
President and Research Director
Head
Melanoma Therapeutics Laboratory
Integrated Cancer Genomics Division
Translational Genomics Research Institute
Phoenix, Arizona

Debu Tripathy, MD
Professor and Chair
Department of Breast Medical Oncology
The University of Texas MD Anderson Cancer Center
Houston, Texas

Susan Tsai, MD
Associate Professor
Department of Surgery
Medical College of Wisconsin
Milwaukee, Wisconsin

Anne S. Tsao, MD
Professor
Department of Thoracic/Head & Neck Medical Oncology
The University of Texas MD Anderson Cancer Center
Houston, Texas

Apostolia M. Tsimberidou, MD, PhD
Professor
Department of Investigational Cancer Therapeutics
The University of Texas MD Anderson Cancer Center
Houston, Texas

David A. Tuveson, MD, PhD
Cancer Center Director
Roy J. Zuckerberg Professor of Cancer Research
Tuveson Laboratory
Cold Spring Harbor Laboratory
Cold Spring Harbor, New York

Douglas S. Tyler, MD
Professor and John Woods Harris Distinguished Chair
Department of Surgery
University of Texas Medical Branch
Galveston, Texas

Atsushi Umemura, MD, PhD
Professor
Departments of Pathology and Pharmacology
University of California San Diego
San Diego, California

Jean-Nicolas Vauthey, MD
Professor
Department of Surgical Oncology
The University of Texas MD Anderson Cancer Center
Houston, Texas

Michael A. Via, MD
Associate Professor of Medicine
Division of Endocrinology, Diabetes, and Bone Disease
Icahn School of Medicine at Mount Sinai/Beth Israel
New York, New York

Alessandro Villa, DDS, PhD, MPH
Associate Professor
Department of Orofacial Sciences
University of California San Francisco
San Francisco, California

Srinivas R. Viswanathan, MD, PhD
Assistant Professor
Department of Medical Oncology
Dana-Farber Cancer Institute
Harvard Medical School
Boston, Massachusetts

Bert Vogelstein, MD
HHMI Investigator
Clayton Professor of Oncology and Pathology
Department of Oncology
The Sidney Kimmel Comprehensive Cancer Center of Johns Hopkins University School of Medicine
Baltimore, Maryland

Evan Vosburgh, MD
Clinical Associate Professor of Medicine
Department of Medicine
Yale University School of Medicine
New Haven, Connecticut

Krina Vyas, MD
Physical Medicine and Rehabilitation Resident
Rutgers-New Jersey Medical School/Kessler Institute for Rehabilitation
Newark, New Jersey

Michael J. Wallace, MD (deceased)
Chair
Department of Interventional Radiology
The University of Texas MD Anderson Cancer Center
Houston, Texas

Chia-Ching J. Wang, MD
Associate Clinical Professor
Department of Hematology/Oncology
University of California San Francisco
San Francisco, California

Hongyang Wang
Vice President
Chinese Anti-Cancer Association
Beijing, China

Tzu-Fei Wang, MD, MPH
Associate Professor
Department of Medicine
University of Ottawa
The Ottawa Hospital and Research Institute
Ottawa, Ontario, Canada

Saiama N. Waqar, MBBS, MSCI
Associate Professor
Department of Medicine
Washington University School of Medicine
St. Louis, Missouri

Ralph R. Weichselbaum, MD
Daniel K. Ludwig Distinguished Service Professor
Department of Radiation and Cellular Oncology and the Ludwig Center for Metastasis Research
University of Chicago
Chicago, Illinois

Robert A. Weinberg, PhD
Professor and Director
MIT Ludwig Center for Molecular Oncology
Cambridge, Massachusetts

John N. Weinstein, MD, PhD
Professor and Hubert L. Stringer Chair in Cancer Research and Chair
Department of Bioinformatics and Computational Biology
The University of Texas MD Anderson Cancer Center
Houston, Texas

Joshua Weir, DO, MBA, MS
Assistant Professor
Department of Radiation Oncology
West Virginia University
Morgantown, West Virginia

Shannon N. Westin, MD, MPH
Professor
Department of Gynecologic Oncology and Reproductive Medicine
The University of Texas MD Anderson Cancer Center
Houston, Texas

Ainsley Weston, PhD
National Institute for Occupational Safety and Health
Centers for Disease Control and Prevention
Morgantown, West Virginia

Timothy G. Whitsett, PhD
Senior Scientific Writer
Neurogenomics Division
Integrated Cancer Genomics Division
Translational Genomics Research Institute
Phoenix, Arizona

Max S. Wicha, MD
Madeline and Sidney Forbes Professor of Oncology
Director, Forbes Institute for Cancer Discovery
Founding Director Emeritus, Rogel Cancer Center
Department of Internal Medicine
University of Michigan
Ann Arbor, Michigan

Christopher G. Willett, MD
Professor and The Mark W. Dewhirst Distinguished Professor of Radiation Oncology
Department of Radiation Oncology
Duke University School of Medicine
Durham, North Carolina

Grant R. Williams, MD, MSPH
Assistant Professor
Division of Hematology/Oncology
Geriatrics, and Palliative Care
Institute of Cancer Outcomes and Survivorship
O'Neal Comprehensive Cancer Center at UAB
University of Alabama at Birmingham
Birmingham, Alabama

Cheryl L. Willman, MD
Executive Director
Mayo Clinic Cancer Programs: Rochester, Minnesota/Midwest, Arizona, Florida, London, Abu Dhabi
Director
Mayo Clinic Comprehensive Cancer Center
Professor of Laboratory Medicine and Pathology
College of Medicine
Mayo Clinic Cancer Center
Rochester, Minnesota

Ignacio I. Wistuba, MD
Head ad interim
Division of Pathology and Laboratory Medicine
Professor and Chair
Department of Translational Molecular Pathology
The University of Texas MD Anderson Cancer Center
Houston, Texas

Robert A. Wolff, MD
Professor of Medicine
Department of GI Medical Oncology
The University of Texas MD Anderson Cancer Center
Houston, Texas

Scott E. Woodman, MD, PhD
Assistant Professor
Department of Melanoma Medical Oncology
The University of Texas MD Anderson Cancer Center
Houston, Texas

Ashley H. Woodson, MS
Genetic Counselor
Genome Medical, Inc.
Austin, Texas

Wendy A. Woodward, MD
Professor
Department of Radiation Oncology
The University of Texas MD Anderson Cancer Center
Houston, Texas

Moritz C. Wyler von Ballmoos, MD, PhD
Associate Professor
Department of Cardiac Surgery
Houston Methodist DeBakey Heart & Vascular Center
Houston, Texas

Xiao-Jing Yan, MD, PhD
Professor and Director
Department of Hematology
The First Affiliated Hospital of China Medical University
Shenyang, Liaoning, China

Haining Yang, PhD
Professor
Department of Thoracic Oncology
University of Hawaii Cancer Center
Honolulu, Hawaii

Wei Yang, MBBS, FRCR, MD
Professor and Chair
Department of Breast Imaging
The University of Texas MD Anderson Cancer Center
Houston, Texas

Andrew J. Yee, MD
Assistant Professor
Department of Medicine
Harvard Medical School
Massachusetts General Hospital Cancer Center
Boston, Massachusetts

Sai-Ching J. Yeung, MD, PhD, FACP
Professor
Department of Emergency Medicine
The University of Texas MD Anderson Cancer Center
Houston, Texas

Nancy Y.-Q. You, MD
Professor
Surgical Oncology and Clinical Cancer Genetics
The University of Texas MD Anderson Cancer Center
Houston, Texas

Anna Yuan, DMD, PhD
Assistance Professor
Division of Oral Medicine
Tufts University
Boston, Massachusetts

James T. Yurkovich
Translational Research Fellow
Institute for Systems Biology
Seattle, Washington

Jonathan S. Zager, MD
Professor and Chair
Department of Oncological Sciences
University of South Florida Morsani School of Medicine
Tampa, Florida

Michael R. Zalutsky, PhD, MA
Jonathan Spicehandler M.D. Professor of Neuro-Oncology Research
Departments of Radiology, Radiation Oncology, Pathology and Biomedical Engineering
Duke University School of Medicine
Durham, North Carolina

Hao Chi Zhang, MD
Assistant Professor
Department of Gastroenterology, Hepatology and Nutrition
The University of Texas MD Anderson Cancer Center
Houston, Texas

Guang-Biao Zhou, MD, PhD
Professor and Deputy Director
State Key Laboratory of Molecular Oncology
National Cancer Center/National Clinical Research Center for Cancer/Cancer Hospital
Chinese Academy of Medical Sciences and Peking Union Medical College
Beijing, China

Jason Zhu, MD
Medical Oncologist
Department of Solid Tumor Oncology and Investigational Therapeutics
Levine Cancer Institute
Atrium Health
Charlotte, North Carolina

Amado Zurita-Saavedra, MD
Associate Professor
Department of Genitourinary Medical Oncology
The University of Texas MD Anderson Cancer Center
Houston, Texas

Preface

Our understanding of cancer at the molecular, cellular, and clinical levels continues to expand. Translation of molecular diagnostics and therapeutics to the clinic has begun to realize the promise of precision medicine with the development and approval of dozens of new targeted drugs, antibodies, and predictive biomarkers. Assimilating this knowledge poses an acute challenge for students, residents, fellows, established practitioners of oncology, and other health care providers. Laboratory-based investigators seeking to translate their discoveries to human application require an accurate overview of clinical oncology, informed by cancer biology. As new diagnostics, therapies, and preventive strategies may now be applicable across multiple disease sites, it is essential that pharmaceutical and biotechnology companies understand the new advances and the unmet needs across the entire field of oncology.

This 10th Edition of *Cancer Medicine* provides a comprehensive synthesis of clinical oncology and the principles underlying approaches to prevention, early detection, diagnosis, and therapeutic management of cancer. Biological hallmarks of cancer and the clinical manifestations of neoplastic diseases are described. Pathways and processes that explain the origin and pathogenesis of neoplasms are presented. Transformational technologies are discussed in depth to improve the understanding of technical procedures such as deep sequencing, methods for measuring epigenetic modification of DNA and histones, transcriptional profiling, ncRNAs, specific functions of RNAs, proteomics, and metabolomics. The heterogeneity within and between cancers and their metastases is described, and the implications for clinical management are discussed. Quantitative oncology is explained in simple terms, providing an introduction to systems biology, biostatistics, bioinformatics, and novel trial design.

This work includes concise guidelines for the use of both drugs that are approved by the Food and Drug Administrations and novel agents. As in the past editions, there is an emphasis on multidisciplinary patient care including surgical and radiation oncology, psycho-oncology, survivorship, and population science. This volume should be of value to oncologists of every discipline.

The editors have chosen experts who have written authoritatively about the disciplines and diseases covered in their respective chapters. As the world of science and medicine chip away the unknowns of the cancer process and its prevention and therapy, we believe this work will provide a platform for the current status of oncology and will prepare the reader for a critical evaluation of discoveries still to come.

The Editors
2022

Acknowledgments

The editors gratefully acknowledge the exceptional contributions of Jene' Reinartz, associate editor, whose tireless efforts have been critical to the organization and completion of CM10. Her high level of competence, her patience, and equanimity have been an inspiration.

We thank Dr. Michael Ewer, associate editor, for his effort and expertise in reviewing multiple chapters. His dedication has been exemplary.

The editors thank Dr. Anthea Hammond, associate editor, for her exceptional efforts in editing many chapters for this edition.

We greatly appreciate our assistants Ruby Robinson, Sue Scott, Nathan Wentling, Marika Arledge, Cheri McClellan, Mary Jaber, Paula Chalhoub, Robby Stephens, Mary Nowak, Henry Vo, Donna Wimberley, Beatrice Montoya, Alexandria Chang, and Samira Habibovich who have helped to make this volume possible.

We also thank our loved ones who both supported us and enabled time for us to perform our editorial duties of calls and writing on weekend mornings and nights.

Working with John Wiley, Inc., has been a particular pleasure. Mandy Collison has been outstanding in bringing the book to completion. The Wiley staff has been most helpful.

Our authors have utilized their extraordinary knowledge, experience, and judgment to capture the critical points regarding each topic and disease site. The editors are grateful for their efforts and are proud of each chapter.

Finally, we must acknowledge the contribution of our patients and their supportive families from whom we have learned. It is their courage, equanimity, and strength in coping with illness that inspire us every day. For patients still to come, we hope that Cancer Medicine, 10th Edition, will benefit them by helping their doctors.

PART 1

Introduction

1 Cardinal manifestations of cancer

James F. Holland, MD, ScD (hc) (deceased) ■ Robert C. Bast, Jr., MD ■ John C. Byrd, MD ■ Carlo M. Croce, MD ■ Ernest Hawk, MD, MPH ■ Fadlo R. Khuri, MD ■ Raphael E. Pollock, MD, PhD ■ Apostolia M. Tsimberadou, MD, PhD ■ Christopher G. Willett, MD ■ Cheryl L. Willman, MD

> **Overview**
>
> Cancer is a singular word that embraces a vast diversity of diseases that can occur in any organ system throughout the animal kingdom. The unique characteristic of cancer is the proliferation of cells of a type different from, if ever so slightly, the normal complement of the organism. The proliferation may be rapid or slow, the accumulation of cells may be massive or miniscule. The essence of the matter, however, is that aberrant cells, distinct from the ordinary evolution of cell types, appear, and accumulate. Thus, a cancer differs from hypertrophy and hyperplasia, which involve normal cells.

A cancer cell does not obey the complex rules of architecture and function that govern the usual placement and behavior of cells within a tissue. The wondrous coexistence of cells and tissues of multiple types that make up the eye, the finger, or the kidney, for example, each with appropriate anatomic location with all connections intact to fulfill their appointed tasks, is part of the miracle we call life. The explanation for this marvelous organization is the field of continuing exploration seeking the messages and exquisite controls that exist in multicellular organisms.

Cancer is distinguished from other abnormal cellular growths that lead to benign tumors in its characteristic independence from the restrictions present in normal tissues. Benign tumors expand and compress but do not attack or invade adjacent tissues. Accumulated cancer cells make a tissue that ignores the anatomic barriers of adjacent cell membranes and basement membranes. Through chemical and mechanical means, the cancer cell insinuates itself between and into the space of the normal cells, killing them by chemical and physical means, the grand usurper. Even though the placenta in mammals shows this behavior, there is self-limitation in location and in survival of the placental invasion. Although leukocytes normally extravasate and permeate tissues, they do not share the other characteristics of cancer. The cancer cell is partially or absolutely insensitive to such normal constraints and may continue its invasiveness indefinitely.

Upon reaching a circulatory conduit, either a lymphatic or capillary vessel, a process that may not be entirely haphazard, cancer cells often penetrate the wall as part of their invasive behavior. They then may be carried by the lymphatic or venous circulation to remote sites where the possibility of adherence, extravasation, and colonization can occur, establishing metastases. In the absence of an intervening event, and given enough time, with few exceptions, the cancer process, as described, can lead to such anatomic or functional distortions that death ensues.

The cancer process does not start with a fully invasive cancer cell. A disorder in molecular instructions for protein synthesis is the common precursor lesion, nearly always because of qualitatively or quantitatively aberrant ribonucleic acid (RNA) messages transcribed from nuclear deoxyribonucleic acid (DNA). This occurs because of a mutation of the DNA, or because of overexpression of particular genes that encode proteins important as catalysts in pathways for stimulating growth, or because of under-expression of genes whose coded proteins control and inhibit growth. Portions of genes may be lost, translocated, or amplified. Indeed, entire chromosomes may be deleted, replicated, or fused in abnormal ways. All such distortions of DNA can give rise to abnormal or unbalanced RNA messages, leading to qualitative or quantitative differences in proteins that result in disordered cellular function. Sometimes the functional abnormality is so extreme as to be lethal to the cell, initiating the suicidal mechanism of apoptosis. In other instances, the functional abnormality results in disease. Some of these diseases display the characteristics of cancer. Mutation, overexpression, and under-expression of genes can result from a wide spectrum of intrinsic and extrinsic causes, with various pathways that lead not to one final common pathway but by several converging routes to cells with the phenotypic characteristics of cancer. When these cells are limited to an epithelial layer above the basement membrane, they are called *carcinoma-in-situ* or *intraepithelial neoplasia*. Similar changes probably occur, but are more difficult to recognize, in the mesenchymal tissues. Even cancer cells that do not penetrate the basement membrane, and thus lack one of the cardinal features of true cancer, represent a long series of antecedent molecular abnormalities that eventually lead to this optically recognizable cellular change. Furthermore, these evolving cancer cells are the common, if not the exclusive, precursor of invasive cancer.

In their earliest stages, as proliferating cells accumulate, cancers are almost always asymptomatic. Cancers cause symptoms as they advance as a consequence of their mass, because they ulcerate on an epithelial surface, or because of change in function of the affected structure or organ. Nearly all the symptoms that can be caused by cancer can also be caused more commonly by noncancerous diseases. The astute clinician must include cancer in the differential diagnosis of virtually every symptom, albeit a benign disease may usually explain it. Doctors never diagnose diseases they do not think of. Cancers occur at any age. A longer life span provides greater opportunity for intrinsic organic events or an encounter with environmental carcinogens, however, and greater opportunity for initial DNA mutations to be fully realized as invasive cancers. Thus, age is the principal risk factor for most, but not all, cancers.

Holland-Frei Cancer Medicine, Tenth Edition. Edited by Robert C. Bast, John C. Byrd, Carlo M. Croce, Ernest Hawk, Fadlo R. Khuri, Raphael E. Pollock, Apostolia M. Tsimberidou, Christopher G. Willett, and Cheryl L. Willman.
© 2023 John Wiley & Sons, Inc. Published 2023 by John Wiley & Sons, Inc.

Such common symptoms as sore throat, runny nose, or a chest cold can sometimes be a result of cancers of pharynx, sinuses, or bronchi, respectively. Indeed, patients with these cancer diagnoses usually have been treated, often repeatedly and for extended periods, for the benign disease because cancer was not considered in the differential diagnosis, and appropriate observations were not made. Cancer symptoms such as diarrhea, constipation, or mild pain often seem commonplace. Cancer symptoms may be intermittent, with spontaneous temporary improvement, a phenomenon that is usually misinterpreted by patients and often by physicians as evidence against the diagnosis of cancer. In fact, recurrent appearance or chronicity of a symptom which in short duration is characteristic of a common benign disease markedly heightens the possibility of an underlying dysfunction caused by cancer.

Cancers cause their symptoms by a few readily understandable mechanisms.

Occlusion of an essential conduit, partial or complete, can be caused by tumor. A tumor mass grows to such a size that it partially or completely occludes an essential conduit. Classic presentations are cancer of the bronchus where partial bronchial occlusion causes cough, diminishes ciliary clearance of secretion, and sometimes leads to bronchopneumonia. Complete bronchial occlusion leads to atelectasis and chronic pneumonia. Compromise of the esophageal lumen by tumor mass or muscular dysfunction resulting from infiltration causes dysphagia, which, in its early presentation, is far too often attributed to benign cause. Gastric tumors rarely cause complete obstruction, but often impair normal gastric motility. This defect may lead to easy satiety, anorexia, indigestion, and nausea. Decrease in caliber of the transverse and descending colon, sigmoid, or rectum by tumor mass can lead to change in bowel habit, including diminished caliber of stools, constipation, and bouts of cramps and/or diarrhea from peristaltic efforts of the proximal gut. Compromise of the lumen of the common bile duct by carcinoma of the head of the pancreas or of the bile duct itself produces obstructive jaundice, not infrequently after minor antecedent digestive complaints or unexplained pruritus ascribed to accumulated bile salts.

Ureteral obstruction by compression from retroperitoneal masses or bladder tumor leads to hydroureter and hydronephrosis, often asymptomatic or revealed by vague discomfort in flank or loin, or by urinary tract infection. Bilateral obstruction leads to uremia with its protean symptomatology. Compromise of the urethra as it courses through the prostate causes diminished urinary stream, inadequate bladder emptying, frequency, urgency, nocturia, and when severe, obstructive uropathy and uremia.

Tumors in the cecum and ascending colon and in the urinary bladder, because their content is not solid and because of greater luminal diameter, uncommonly cause obstruction, but may distort normal function enough to alter bowel or urinary habits.

A mass discovered by palpation or X-ray may be a presenting finding, as in breast carcinoma. Dysfunction from replacement of the substance of a parenchymatous organ by tumor is a subset of mass presentation. The classic example is a primary or, more commonly, metastatic brain tumor, which becomes identified by abnormal brain function. Seizure or paralysis, sensory or coordination abnormality, memory defect, and personality change may all be consequences of space occupation. These changes may occur not only because a specific area of the brain is affected, but since the calvarium is not distensible, because of increased intracranial pressure. In other patients, headache may be the only symptom of increased intracranial pressure. Similar dysfunction of the spinal cord with distal motor and sensory phenomena can reflect space occupation by a mass within or impinging on the cord or cauda equina. Hepatic dysfunction from space occupation by primary or metastatic tumor, often with related intrahepatic bile duct compression, can present as jaundice. Sometimes the liver enlarges to enormous size, causing digestive disorders, pain, and a visible and palpable mass in the upper abdomen. Thyroid cancer usually presents as a mass, and uncommonly this results in hypothyroid laboratory values, but rarely in clinical hypothyroidism.

A sarcoma of the soft tissues usually presents as a palpable mass. Testicular cancer ordinarily presents as a mass: the testicle may only be slightly larger than its fellow, but harder and heavier in the examiner's hand. Ovarian cancer may be detected as an adnexal mass.

A new lump or mass, or a changing one, requires exclusion of cancer based on clinical examination, imaging studies, or a biopsy. Most lipomas, and self-discovery of the xiphoid, are two types of lumps that can usually be dismissed on clinical grounds. A dominant breast mass or even a questionable one, requires assessment by appropriate imaging, and often by cytologic or histologic means. A thyroid nodule, an enlarged lymph node that is hard, a node that remains enlarged without infectious explanation for 2 weeks, a skin mass with the characteristics of melanoma or carcinoma, especially if ulcerated, a new subcutaneous or abdominal or scrotal mass all require consideration of cancer and appropriate diagnostic study.

Ulceration, on the skin or on an epithelial surface, can lead to blood loss and occasionally can serve as a portal of infection. Skin ulcerations are commonly ignored for weeks or months and are often interpreted as a common injury of unremembered origin that did not heal. Bronchial ulceration results in hemoptysis, usually blood-tinged sputum, and only rarely massive bleeding. Any of the upper alimentary canal cancers can ulcerate and bleed. Usually, the bleeding is slow, intermittent, and silent, leading to iron deficiency anemia. Hematemesis or massive melena is uncommon. Carcinomas of the cecum and ascending colon often present with the symptoms of anemia because of ulceration and bleeding.

Carcinoma of the bladder and carcinoma of the kidney commonly manifest as hematuria. Sometimes this is fortuitously discovered as a microscopic or chemical abnormality on routine urinalysis. Clots from renal bleeding can lead to ureteral colic. Hematuria less often heralds prostate cancer, but hematospermia implies prostate disease, benign, or malignant, because carcinoma of the seminal vesicle is exceedingly rare.

Endometrial carcinoma most often presents as postmenopausal vaginal bleeding, although any vaginal bleeding outside the normal menstrual cycle is worthy of suspicion. Contact bleeding during intercourse is suggestive of cervical ulceration, most commonly a result of cancer.

Pain is commonly thought of as a surrogate for early cancer, although this is mistaken. Most cancers are initially painless. Pain occurs when a tumor invades, presses on, or stretches a nerve, or when proximal smooth muscle contracts in an attempt to bypass an obstructed or dysfunctional distal segment of a conduit. Most pains of short duration that disappear are not caused by cancer. Cancer must enter the differential diagnosis, however, when pain is recurrent or persistent without ready explanation, or atypical, or present when there is no other recognizable cause. New pain, not necessarily severe, must be carefully interpreted. Abdominal pain and skeletal pain distinct from joint symptomatology deserve particular attention, and early rather than late studies to establish a cause. Pain in a breast mass does not exclude its being cancer.

Weight loss may first indicate an unsuspected cancer, and when combined with grumbling low-grade discomforts, malaise, and fatigue, is a cause for particular scrutiny. A wide variety of other diseases can also cause these common symptoms, but cancer should not be at the bottom of the list. If a diagnosis is not established after initial studies a second complete history and physical examination after a short interval is imperative.

Effusion caused by cancer in the pleural, pericardial, or peritoneal cavities can lead to dyspnea and discomfort. Increasing abdominal girth, often with malaise, oliguria, constipation, and weight gain, is a cardinal symptom of ascites. In the thorax, bronchogenic carcinoma, mesothelioma, metastatic breast or ovarian cancer, and primary carcinoma of serous membranes are the frequent causes of malignant effusion. Ascites as a presenting symptom is characteristic of ovarian cancer and cancer of the serous membranes. Pancreatic cancer, mesothelioma, metastatic carcinoma on the peritoneum and in the liver, and several nonneoplastic diseases also enter the differential diagnosis.

Perforation caused by invasion of the wall of a hollow viscus causes pain, usually sudden. Cancer is not suspected in most cases when this rare event occurs. Pneumothorax from perforation of the pleura by a primary or metastatic pulmonary tumor is an uncommon emergency. Fistulization of gastric cancer into the transverse colon leads to vague abdominal discomfort, which is misinterpreted or neglected, and then sudden onset of diarrhea with prominent gastrocolic reflex. Appendiceal cancer, albeit a rare tumor, frequently presents as acute appendicitis with peritonitis because of rupture. Perforation of the colon is more frequently caused by diverticulitis than by colon cancer. Ruptured ectopic pregnancy due to choriocarcinoma has been reported. Tracheoesophageal fistula formation in the course of esophageal or bronchogenic cancers is almost always late in the course.

Fever of unknown origin that persists for more than 1 week must include cancer among its possible causes. Hodgkin disease, other lymphomas, acute leukemia, cancer of the kidney, and cancers of the liver are high on the list of neoplasms that can cause fever. Certain cancers predispose to infections because of ulceration, obstruction, or disordered leukopoiesis.

Endocrine hyperactivity syndromes may occasionally turn out to be caused by cancer. Hyper-adrenalism, sometimes first manifest as hirsutism, can indicate adrenal cancer. Cushing syndrome can also result from small cell carcinoma of the lung. Hyperparathyroidism rarely comes from parathyroid cancer but can be mimicked by ovarian cancer and squamous carcinomas. Tumors that secrete thyroid hormone, estrogens, insulin, glucagon, aldosterone, epinephrine, or norepinephrine are often benign tumors of the parent endocrine organ, but cancer must always be considered. Functional neuroendocrine tumors may secrete serotonin and other vasoactive principles that cause the carcinoid syndrome.

Paraneoplastic syndromes may be early symptoms of cancer. Myasthenia gravis, Raynaud syndrome, hypertrophic osteoarthropathy and clubbing, and refractory anemia may herald thymoma, myeloma, lung cancer, and hematologic dyscrasia (and thymoma), respectively. A diligent search must be made for these and other causes.

Absence of cardinal manifestations is usual for cancers detected by screening by Papanicolaou smears, mammography, prostate-specific antigen determinations, colonoscopy, computed tomography, lung scanning, and total skin examination. Asymptomatic cancers discovered by these methods are generally far less advanced than those that cause symptoms. Occasionally, routine chemical or hematologic laboratory data in asymptomatic patients suggest cancer or leukemia. Such incidental discovery reinforces the proposition that early in their pathogenesis most cancers are asymptomatic.

Predisposition to cancer characterizes a broad spectrum of diseases, exposures, and lifestyle behaviors. Patients who have had inflammatory bowel disease, human papillomavirus infection of the cervix, hepatitis B or C infection, those with prior radiation exposure, earlier treatment with alkylating agents, anthracyclines, or podophyllotoxin derivatives, or specific environmental exposures such as asbestos, those who have smoked, heavily imbibed alcohol, or sun worshipped, and those with a strong family history of cancer, particularly those neoplasms known in part to be heredo-familial all are in groups that deserve special consideration for the particular cancers that occur in them at a higher frequency than normal.

Cancerophobia does not predispose to cancer. Depression occurs more frequently with carcinoma of the pancreas than with gastric carcinoma, however, and may be an early symptom of pancreatic neoplasia.

The present

By the time cancer is diagnosed, it is often past the stage of easy curability. Frequently the earliest symptoms were ignored or rationalized. Technical improvements in imaging, early surgery, and hormonal, chemotherapeutic, and immunologic treatment have decreased mortality from breast cancer; viral discovery, cytology, and early treatment have diminished cervical cancer mortality, and colonoscopy and polypectomy have decreased colon cancer mortality. Other screening programs portend similar promise by diagnosing cancers before they become symptomatic. Cancer has replaced syphilis as the great imitator. Many symptomatic patients with cancer are still curable with today's therapies. Delay cannot possibly help, however, once an early symptom occurs that eventually proves to be caused by cancer. Inclusion of cancer as a possibility in every differential diagnosis can save lives.

The future

The expansion of diagnostic techniques based on genomics and proteomics augurs well for earlier identification of cancers. Not only is it reasonable to believe that clinical diagnosis will be accelerated by laboratory methods, but genomic and proteomic discoveries are likely to alter our understanding of the cancer process as it occurs in humans. It is hoped that the consequent impact of this knowledge on cancer prevention and on cancer therapy will be revolutionary. The cardinal manifestations of cancer may then become principally of historical interest while laboratory abnormalities are instrumentally detectable well before clinical presentation. Indeed, departure from a population norm may be less significant than departure from an individual's prior proteomic profile taken as a baseline during health. If such a blue-sky future ever unfolds, public understanding and compliance will still be critical determinants of cancer prevention and early diagnosis.

Acknowledgments

The authors gratefully acknowledge the previous contributors to this article including Emil Frei III, MD, Waun Ki Hong, MD, William N. Hait, MD, Donald W. Kufe, MD, Donald L. Morton, MD, and Ralph R. Weichselbaum, MD.

2 Biological hallmarks of cancer

Douglas Hanahan, PhD ■ Robert A. Weinberg, PhD

Overview

A perplexing enigma for cancer medicine lies in its complexity and variability, at all levels of consideration. The hallmarks of cancer constitute an organizing principle that provides a conceptual basis for distilling the complexity of this disease in order to better understand it in its diverse presentations. This conceptualization involves eight biological capabilities—the hallmarks of cancer—acquired by cancer cells during the long process of tumor initiation and development and malignant progression. Two characteristic traits of cancer cells facilitate the acquisition of these functional capabilities. The eight distinctive hallmarks consist of sustaining proliferative signaling, evading growth suppressors, resisting cell death, enabling replicative immortality, inducing angiogenesis, activating invasion and metastasis, deregulating cellular energetics and metabolism, and avoiding immune destruction. The principal facilitators of their acquisition are genome instability with consequent gene mutation and tumor-promoting inflammation. The integration of these hallmark capabilities involves heterotypic interactions amongst multiple cell types populating the "tumor microenvironment," which is composed of cancer cells and a tumor-associated stroma, including three prominent classes of recruited support cells—angiogenic vascular cells, various subtypes of fibroblasts, and infiltrating immune cells. In addition, the neoplastic cells populating individual tumors are themselves typically heterogeneous, in that cancer cells can assume a variety of distinctive phenotypic states and undergo genetic diversification during tumor progression. Accordingly, the hallmarks of cancer—this set of necessarily acquired capabilities and their facilitators—constitute a useful heuristic tool for elucidating mechanistic bases and commonalities underlying the pathogenesis of diverse forms of human cancer, with potential and rational applications to cancer therapy.

Distilling the dauntingly complex manifestations of cancer

As outlined in the preceding article, and comprehensively described elsewhere in this encyclopedic textbook, the manifestations of cancer are disconcertingly complex and diverse. Cancers affecting different organs vary dramatically, in regard to genetics, histopathology, effects on systemic physiology, prognosis, and response to therapeutic intervention, explaining why the discipline of oncology is largely balkanized into organ-specific specialties, and why the articles of this textbook are largely aligned as individualistic descriptions of organ-specific cancers.

In the face of this disconcerting diversity and complexity of disease manifestations, one might ask whether there are underlying principles—mechanistic commonalities—masked by the genetic and phenotypic complexities that span the multitude of cancer types and forms. In 2000, and again in 2011, we put forward a hypothesis that the vast complexity of human cancers reflects different solutions to the same set of challenges, namely that the lesions we observe in the forms of symptomatic neoplastic disease have all necessarily acquired, by varying strategies, a common set of distinctive functional capabilities that enable inappropriate, chronic cell proliferation, and the focal or disseminated growth of populations of "cancer cells." We proposed to call this set of acquired capabilities "hallmarks of cancer".[1,2] We further suggested that two characteristic traits of neoplastic growths—elevated mutability of cancer cell genomes, and inflammation by complex arrays of immune cells—are key facilitators used by incipient neoplasias to acquire essential hallmark capabilities. Our current conceptualization of the biological hallmarks of cancer incorporates the eight distinct functional capabilities, and the two enabling facilitators, these being schematized in Figure 1.

The following sections describe these ten key aspects of cancer pathophysiology. Then we introduce the realization that cancer cells recruit a variety of normal cell types that contribute in various ways to the acquisition of hallmark functionalities. We conclude with a brief discussion on potential clinical implications of the hallmarks concept. For further detail and background, the reader is referred to our initial publications laying out the concept of the hallmarks of cancer,[1,2] as well as to another perspective that expands on the roles of stromal cells in enabling the hallmarks of cancer.[3] Notably, only a few recent publications not cited in these three perspective articles are referenced herein. A textbook on the biology of cancer[4] may provide additional detail on many of the mechanisms of cancer pathogenesis described in outline in this article.

Acquired functional capabilities embody biological hallmarks of cancer

In our current conceptualization, there are eight hallmark capabilities that are common to many if not most forms of human cancer (Figure 1). Each capability serves a distinct functional role in supporting the development, progression, and persistence of tumors and their constituent cells, as summarized briefly below.

Hallmark 1: sustaining proliferative signaling

The defining criterion of cancer as a disease is chronic, inappropriate cell proliferation, which results from corruption of cellular regulatory networks that normally orchestrate (transitory) proliferation of cells during embryonic development, physiological growth, and homeostatic maintenance of tissues throughout the body. Both positive (inductive) and negative (repressive) signals govern cell division and proliferation. Thus this first hallmark capability embodies a complex set of inductive signals that instruct entry into and progression through the cell growth-and-division cycle to produce daughter cells. In the context

---

Holland-Frei Cancer Medicine, Tenth Edition. Edited by Robert C. Bast, John C. Byrd, Carlo M. Croce, Ernest Hawk, Fadlo R. Khuri, Raphael E. Pollock, Apostolia M. Tsimberidou, Christopher G. Willett, and Cheryl L. Willman.
© 2023 John Wiley & Sons, Inc. Published 2023 by John Wiley & Sons, Inc.

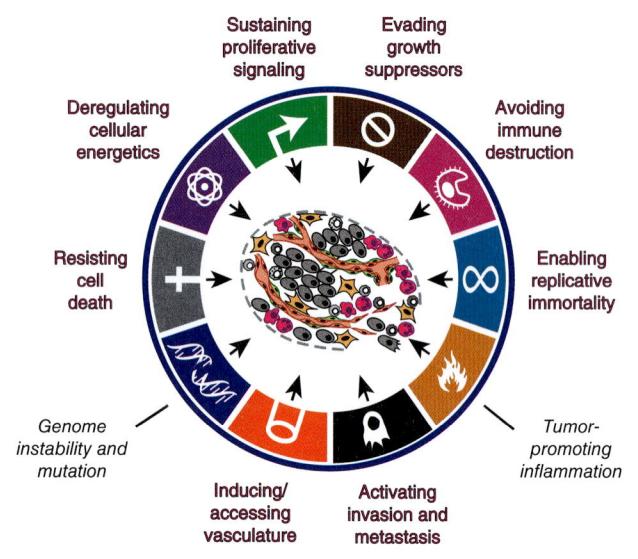

Figure 1 The biological hallmarks of cancer. The schematic illustrates what are arguably necessary conditions to manifest malignant disease—the hallmarks of cancer—comprising eight distinctive and complementary functional capabilities, and two facilitators (in black italics) of their acquisition [1,2]. These hallmark traits may be acquired at different stages in the multistep development of cancer, via markedly distinctive mechanisms in different forms of human cancer. Two aberrant characteristics of cancerous lesions are demonstrably involved in facilitating the acquisition during tumorigenesis of these functional capabilities: genome instability and the resultant mutation of regulatory genes, and the infiltration of immune-inflammatory cells endowed by their biology with one or another hallmark capability, for example, to support their roles in wound healing. Different forms of cancer may be more or less dependent on a particular hallmark. Thus adenomatous tumors typically lack the capability for invasion and metastasis. Leukemias may not require angiogenesis or invasive ability, although progression to lymphoma almost certainly requires both. The necessity of evading tumor immunity may be less important for certain cancers, but is increasingly appreciated to be widespread.

of cancer, such stimulatory signals are activated and, in contrast to normal situations in which proliferative signaling is transitory, the signals are sustained chronically.

The most well-established and widespread mechanism of sustaining proliferative signaling involves mutational alteration of genes within cancer cells that convert such genes into active "drivers" of cell proliferation. These activated genes—defined as oncogenes—render otherwise transitory proliferation-promoting signals chronic. Such oncogenes typically encode proteins altered in structure and function or abundance compared to their normal cellular counterparts, which are responsible for receiving proliferative signals from extracellular sources and transmitting the signals through complex regulatory circuits operating within the cell.

Prominent examples of mutated driver oncogenes that sustain proliferative signaling in human cancers include the epidermal growth factor (EGF) receptor as well as signal transducers in the downstream KRAS-RAF-MEK-MAPK pathway that process and transmit growth-stimulatory signals via a succession of protein phosphorylations to the cell division machinery operating in the nucleus. Mutations that render one or another of these proteins chronically active are found in many forms of human cancer, including the aforementioned *EGFR* and related receptor tyrosine kinases such as *HER2* and *ALK*; similarly acting mutations result in chronic activation of the downstream signal transducers *KRAS*, *BRAF*, and *MEK*. We note, however, that activation in cancer cells of this central mitogenic pathway does not invariably depend on genetic changes acquired during the course of tumor progression. In certain instances, epigenetic deregulation of autocrine (autostimulatory) and paracrine (cell-to-cell) signaling circuits can also provide cancer cells with chronic growth-promoting signals, doing so in the apparent absence of underlying somatic mutations.

Hallmark 2: evading growth suppressors

The essential counterbalance to proliferative signals in normal cells is braking mechanisms that either overrule the initiation of, or subsequently block the cell division process instigated by such signals. The genes encoding these proteins are often termed tumor suppressor genes (TSGs). The most prominent brakes are the direct regulators of progression through the cell growth-and-division cycle, embodied in the retinoblastoma protein (pRb) and several "cyclin-dependent" kinase-inhibitor proteins. The activity of this molecular braking system is itself normally regulated by the integration of extracellular pro- and antigrowth signals transduced by receptors on the cell surface, along with monitors of the intracellular physiologic state of the cell, in order to modulate tissue homeostasis and orchestrate transitory physiological proliferation.

The intracellular monitoring system, which is centered upon the p53 protein, serves to ensure that cells only advance through their growth-and-division cycles when the physiologic state of the cell is appropriate. Thus p53 detects unrepaired damage to a cell's genome as well as "stressful" physiologic imbalances that could impair accurate genome duplication, chromosomal segregation, and cell division, and responds by activating repressors of the cell cycle machinery. In cases of severe genomic damage or stressful physiological abnormalities, p53 and its associates can instead induce programmed cell death (see below), an extreme form of putting on the brakes to cell proliferation.

A number of component genes in both of these generic braking mechanisms—the Rb and p53 pathways—are classified as TSGs by virtue of their frequent loss-of-function via deletion or inactivating intragenic mutations, or via alternative mechanisms that achieve the same end by shutting down expression of these genes through epigenetic mechanisms, notably those involving DNA and histone methylation or by overexpressing microRNAs that target these genes. For example, the p53 gene is mutated in ~40% of all human cancers, and many of the remaining tumors with wild-type p53 instead carry genetic lesions or epigenetic alterations that compromise p53 signaling in other ways.

Genetic profiling of genomes and transcriptomes indicates that a majority of human tumors contain defects—genetic or epigenetic—in the functions of the Rb and p53 tumor suppressor pathways. Moreover, a large body of functional studies involving manipulation of these pathways in cultured cancer cells and mouse models of tumor initiation, growth, and malignant progression have clearly established the critical importance of TSGs in these pathways as significant barriers to the development of cancer. As such, evasion of growth suppressors is clearly a hallmark capability, necessary to ensure that continuing cancer cell proliferation and consequent tumor growth is not halted by braking mechanisms that, under normal circumstances, limit the extent of cell proliferation in order to maintain tissue homeostasis.

Hallmark 3: resisting cell death

There exists a second, fundamentally distinct barrier to aberrant cell proliferation, which involves intrinsic cellular mechanisms that can orchestrate the programmed death of cells deemed to be either aberrant or, in the case of development and homeostasis, superfluous. The most prominent form of programmed cell death is apoptosis, the genetically regulated fragmentation of a cell destined to die. Included among the situations where normal cells activate their apoptotic program to die are ones where the cell is damaged in various ways, or mislocalized, or inappropriately migrating or proliferating. The apoptotic program can be triggered by cell intrinsic as well as non-cell-autonomous signals that detect different forms of cellular abnormality.

The apoptotic cell death program involves the directed degradation of the chromosomes as well as other critical cellular organelles by specialized enzymes (e.g., caspases), the shriveling and fragmentation of the cell, and its engulfment, either by its neighboring cells or by tissue-surveying phagocytes, notably macrophages. The apoptotic cascade is completed in less than an hour in mammalian tissues, explaining why apoptotic cells are often surprisingly rare when visualized in tissue sections, even in a population of cells experiencing apoptosis-inducing environmental conditions, such as cancer cells in tumors subjected to cytotoxic chemotherapy, or to acute hypoxia consequent to vascular insufficiency.

The rapid engulfment of apoptotic cell bodies ensures that their death does not release subcellular components that would otherwise provoke an immune response; this "immune silence" contrasts with a second form of programmed cell death: necroptosis. Long known as necrosis and envisioned as the passive dissolution of a dying cell, necrosis can also be an active, programmed process that is governed by cellular regulators and effectors distinct from those regulating apoptosis. Necroptosis can be activated by various conditions, including oxygen and energy deprivation, viral infection, and inflammation.[5] Cells dying by necroptosis (or passive necrosis) rupture, releasing their contents and leaving their carcasses as immunogenic debris, attracting (or exacerbating) an immune-inflammatory response that, as discussed below, can have both tumor-promoting and tumor-antagonizing effects.

A third program capable of inducing cell death, termed autophagy, serves as a recycling system for cellular organelles that can help cells respond to conditions of nutrient deprivation, by degrading nonessential cellular organelles and recycling their component parts. Thus autophagy generates metabolites and nutrients necessary for survival and growth that cells may be unable to acquire from their surroundings. Additionally, while generally a survival system, extreme nutrient deprivation or other acute cellular stresses can lead to a hyperactivation of autophagic recycling that drives a cell to a point-of-no return, in which its complement of organelles falls below the minimum level required for viability; as a consequence, the cell dies via "autophagy-associated" cell death, distinct in its characteristics from both apoptosis and necroptosis. Stated differently, depending on the physiologic state of a neoplastic cell, autophagy may either sustain its survival and facilitate further proliferation, or eliminate it via autophagy-associated cell death.[6]

These three distinct protective mechanisms for triggering cell death must be variably circumvented or attenuated by cancer cells if they and their descendants are to continue their proliferative expansion in number and phenotypic evolution to states of heightened malignancy.

Hallmark 4: enabling replicative immortality

A third intrinsic barrier to chronic proliferation is integral to the linear structure of mammalian chromosomes: the telomeres at the ends of chromosomes record—by progressive reduction of their length during each cell division cycle—the number of successive cell generations through which a cell lineage has passed. The telomeres are composed of thousands of tandem copies of a specific hexanucleotide DNA sequence located at the ends of every chromosome, associated with a specialized set of DNA-binding proteins. Operating together, these nucleoprotein complexes protect the ends of chromosomes both from degradation by the DNA repair machinery which would otherwise sense DNA damage, and from end-to-end fusions with other chromosomes catalyzed by naked DNA ends.

Notably, when the number of telomere repeats erodes below a certain threshold, a tripwire is triggered, causing cell cycle arrest or apoptosis mediated by the p53 tumor suppressor protein, operating in its role to sense DNA damage and other cellular abnormalities. Circumventing these p53-induced antiproliferative responses (e.g., by mutational inactivation of the p53 gene) allows cancer cells with eroding telomeres to ignore the short telomere checkpoint and continue proliferating but only transiently: Sooner or later, the continuing erosion of telomeric DNA leads to loss of the protective nucleoprotein caps protecting the chromosomal DNA ends, which allows end-to-end fusions of chromosomes, breakage-fusion-bridge cycles during mitosis, and resultant karyotypic chaos that leads to cell death instead of cell division.

The cancer cells in many fully developed tumors circumvent the proliferative barrier presented by telomere erosion and the imminent mitotic catastrophe of telomere dysfunction by activating a system for telomere maintenance and extension that is normally used to preserve the replicative capacity of normal embryonic and tissue stem cells. This system involves expression of the telomere-extending enzyme telomerase. Less frequently, they engage an alternative interchromosomal recombination-based mechanism for preserving telomere length. Thus, through one strategy or another, cancer cells acquire the capability to maintain their telomeres, avoiding the barrier of intolerably shortened telomeres, thereby enabling the unlimited replicative potential—termed cellular immortality—that is required for continuing expansion of populations of cancer cells.

Hallmark 5: inducing or accessing vasculature

Like normal organs, tumors require a steady supply of oxygen, glucose, and other nutrients, as well as a means to evacuate metabolic wastes, in order to sustain cell viability and proliferation. The tumor-associated vasculature serves these purposes. The deleterious effect that ischemia has in normal tissue is well established clinically and experimentally: cells die, via one form of programmed cell death or another, causing tissue and organ degradation and dysfunction. Similarly, the growth of developing nests of cancer cells halts when their ability to acquire blood-borne nutrients becomes inadequate, typically when the nearest capillary is more than 200 μm away. Angiogenesis—the formation of new blood vessels—is commonly activated, and demonstrably beneficial for many tumor types.

Cells at the diffusion limit from the nearest capillary activate various stress response systems, of which the most prominent involves the hypoxia-inducible transcription factors (HIF), which regulate hundreds of genes, including ones that directly or indirectly induce angiogenesis and other stress-adaptive capabilities. Much like cells in ischemic tissues, cancer cells starving for lack of oxygen and glucose will typically die, by necrosis/necroptosis, apoptosis, or rampant autophagy. This explains why most vigorously growing tumors are well vascularized with evidence of ongoing angiogenesis.

Of note, the tumor-associated neovasculature is usually aberrant, both morphologically and functionally. Tumor blood vessels are tortuous, dilated, and leaky, with erratic flow patterns and "dead zones" in which no blood flow is detectable, in marked contrast to the seamless blood flow operating in the normal vasculature. Moreover, the degree of vascularity varies widely from one tumor type to another, ranging from intensely vascularized renal carcinomas to poorly vascularized pancreatic ductal adenocarcinomas.

Finally, we note that while chronic angiogenesis is a hallmark of most solid tumors, some may devise an alternative means to acquire access to the vasculature: in certain cases, cancers co-opt normal tissue vasculature, by employing the hallmark capability for invasion and metastasis. Thus, particular types of cancer cells can proliferate and grow along normal tissue capillaries, creating sleeves whose outer diameters are dictated by the 200-μm diffusion limit. While vascular cooption is evident in certain cases (e.g., glioblastoma) and in some tumors treated with potent angiogenesis inhibitors, most tumors rely to a considerable extent on chronic angiogenesis to support their expansive growth. Still, others may adapt to living in quasi-hypoxic environments where most cancer cells would perish. In light of these increasingly well-recognized alternative mechanisms, we have renamed this hallmark capability – originally designated as 'inducing angiogenesis' – to more accurately describe 'inducing or accessing vasculature'.

Hallmark 6: activating invasion and metastasis

The five hallmarks detailed above stand as logical necessities for the chronic proliferative programs of cancer cells. The sixth is less intuitive: high-grade cancer cells become invasive and migratory. These interrelated programs enable cancer cells to invade into adjacent tissue as well as into blood and lymphatic vessels (intravasation); these vessels serve thereafter as pipelines for dissemination to nearby and distant anatomical sites. The tissue-draining lymphatic vasculature can transport cancer cells to lymph nodes, where metastatic growths—lymph note metastases—can form; such cell colonies may serve, in turn, as staging areas for further dissemination by entering the bloodstream. Cells entering the bloodstream by direct intravasation within a tumor or indirectly via lymph nodes may soon become lodged in the microvessels of distant organs and extravasate across the vessel walls into the nearby tissue parenchyma. The resulting seeded micrometastases may die or lay dormant in such ectopic tissue locations or, with extremely low efficiency, generate macroscopic metastases—the process of "colonization."

The regulation of the intertwined capabilities for invasion and metastasis is extraordinarily complex, involving both cell-intrinsic programs and assistance from accessory cells in the tissue microenvironment. Prominent among the cancer cell-intrinsic regulatory mechanisms is the activation in epithelial cancer cells (carcinomas) of a developmental program termed the epithelial–mesenchymal transition (EMT),[2,4] which is associated with cell migrations and tissue invasions during normal organogenesis. A second overlapping regulatory program engaged by some invasive and metastatic cancer cells is the aforementioned hypoxia response system, which triggers the activation of the hypoxia-inducible transcription factors HIF1α and HIF2α, consequently altering expression of hundreds of genes.[7,8] Both transcriptional programs control genes that can facilitate invasive migration as well as survival in the blood and lymphatic systems, and in ectopic tissue locations.

Notably, the acquisition of this hallmark capability can occur at various points along the pathways of multistep tumor development and progression that lead incrementally from normal cells of origin to those found in aggressive high-grade malignancies. In some cases, the capability for invasion and metastasis arises late, reflecting mutational or epigenetic evolution of the cancer cell, whereby rare subsets of cells populating such primary tumors are enabled to become invasive/metastatic. In other cases, this capability is acquired early, such that many cancer cells within a tumor may already be capable of invasion and metastasis. Moreover, there are indications that the EMT program may in some cases be transiently active and functionally important for dissemination and seeding, and then switched off in macro-metastatic colonies.[9,10] It remains unclear whether the acquired traits of invasion and metastasis are beneficial and hence actively selected during the evolution of primary tumors; alternatively, these malignancy-defining capabilities may represent incidental by-products of activating global regulatory networks (e.g., proliferative signaling, EMT, HIF) that are selected because they facilitate primary tumor formation by contributing to the acquisition of other hallmark functions.

Hallmark 7: deregulating cellular energetics and metabolism

The concept that cancer cells alter their utilization of energy sources—notably glucose—to support their proliferation was introduced almost 90 years ago by Otto Warburg, who observed that certain cultured cancer cells have enhanced uptake of glucose, which is metabolized via glycolysis, even in the presence of oxygen levels that normally should favor oxidative phosphorylation. The result was counterintuitive, since glycolysis is far less efficient at producing ATP, the primary currency of intracellular energy. However, we now appreciate that the "aerobic" glycolysis described by Warburg produces, in addition to ATP, many of the building blocks for the cellular macromolecules that are required for cell growth and division. Hence, the metabolism of cancer cells resembles that of actively dividing normal cells rather than being a novel invention of neoplasia. Moreover, it is important to appreciate that there is not a binary switch from oxidative phosphorylation to aerobic glycolysis in cancer cells; rather, cancer cells continue to utilize oxidative phosphorylation in addition to incorporating differing rates of glycolysis, the proportions of which may well prove to be dynamic in time and variable amongst the cancer cells in different subregions within a tumor, as well as in different tissue microenvironments.

Aerobic glycolysis can be indirectly monitored by positron-emission tomography (PET) using radiolabeled analogs as tracers. PET involving [^{18}F]-fluorodeoxyglucose is commonly used to visualize glycolytic tumors via their elevated expression of glucose transporters and a resulting increase in the uptake of glucose. Although glucose is the primary fuel source used by most cancer cells, glutamine is also emerging as another key blood-borne source of energy and a precursor of lipids and amino acids. In most cases, glutamine likely supplements and enhances glucose in supplying energy and biomaterials for growth and proliferation of cancer cells, although in some cases of glucose insufficiency, glutamine uptake and metabolism may be able to compensate.[11]

A third player in metabolic fueling is lactate. While long considered to be toxic waste that is secreted by cells undergoing aerobic and anaerobic glycolysis, lactate is now appreciated to have diverse tumor-promoting capabilities.[12] In certain cancer cells, particularly those suffering glucose deprivation, extracellular lactate can be imported via specific transporters and used as fuel for generation of ATP and biomaterials. Similarly, some cancer-associated fibroblasts (CAFs) can utilize lactate. Hence, metabolic symbioses may be operative in some tumors, involving partnerships between glucose-importing/lactate-exporting cells and lactate-importing cells.[12]

Finally, we note a still unresolved question, about whether this hallmark is significantly independent of the six cited above in terms of its regulatory mechanisms, or conversely is concordantly regulated under the auspices of these other hallmark traits. Thus, oncogenes such as *KRAS* and *cMYC* and the loss of function of tumor suppressor genes such as *p53* can function to reprogram the energy metabolism of cancer cells. For these reasons, the reprogramming of cellular energetics and metabolism was initially defined as an "emerging hallmark".[2] Irrespective of this qualification, it is clearly a crucial property of the neoplastic cell phenotype.[13]

Hallmark 8. Avoiding immune destruction

The eighth hallmark has been on the horizon for decades, originally conceived as the proposition that incipient neoplasias must find ways to circumvent active surveillance by the immune system that would otherwise eliminate aberrantly proliferating premalignant cells. While clearly demonstrable in highly antigenic tumors in mouse models, and implicated in virus-induced human cancers, the generality of immune surveillance of incipient cancer as a barrier to neoplastic progression is unresolved. One factor is immune self-tolerance: the vast majority of antigens expressed by spontaneously arising cancer cells are likely shared with those expressed by their cells-of-origin in normal tissues and thus are ignored, reflecting the tolerance of the immune system for self-antigens. Nonetheless, some cancer cells demonstrably express antigens for which the immune system has failed to develop tolerance, including embryonic antigens, and novel-antigens produced by rampant mutation of the genome; such antigens can indeed elicit antitumor immune responses and are an increasing focus for strategies aimed to elicit efficacious tumor immunity.

By contrast, the immune response to the ~20% of virus-induced human tumors is clear: oncogenic viruses express foreign antigens (including oncoproteins responsible for driving cell transformation) to which the immune system is not tolerant, resulting in humoral and cellular immune responses that can kill virus-infected precancer cells and thereby eradicate incipient neoplasias. The fact that virus-transformed cells can nevertheless succeed in evading immune elimination to produce overt cancer testifies to immune-evasive capabilities evolved by such tumor viruses or selected for in virus-transformed cancer cells. Nevertheless, the immune system likely serves as a significant barrier to virus-induced tumors, as indicated by the increased rates of cancer in individuals who are immune-compromised for various reasons, including organ-graft recipients and AIDS patients.

Although the incidence of nonvirus induced human cancers is not markedly increased in the context of immunodeficiency, suggesting a lack of immune surveillance of incipient neoplasias in the other 80% of human cancers, various lines of evidence suggest that some tumor types must indeed deal with immune recognition and attack during later stages of tumor progression and, in response, acquire immune-evasive strategies. Here, histopathological and epidemiological analyses have shed light on the potential role of immune attack and immune evasion. For example, among patients with surgically resected colorectal carcinomas, those whose tumors contained dense infiltrates of cytotoxic T-lymphocytes (CTLs) have a better prognosis than patients with tumors of similar grade and size that have comparatively few infiltrating CTLs.[14] Such data implicate the actions of the immune system as a significant obstacle to the progressive growth and dissemination of cancer cells, one that is necessarily blunted or circumvented in some aggressive tumor types.[14] Indeed, immune phenotyping of tumors, including their associated stroma, is being evaluated as new metric in the evaluation of tumors that may enable, when combined with traditional criteria, more accurate assessments of prognosis and more effective treatment decisions.[15,16] Accordingly, it is reasonable to view antitumor immune responses as a significant barrier to be circumvented during the lengthy multistage development of many forms of human cancer.

Nevertheless, the rules of immune engagement remain ambiguous when viewing the spectrum of human cancers. Thus it is generally unclear when during different organ-specific tumor development pathways the attention of the immune system is attracted, or what the precise characteristics and efficacy of resultant immune responses are, or how the genetic constitutions of patients and the tumors that they harbor affect the development of antitumor immunity. Nevertheless, evading immune destruction seems increasingly to be an important mandate for developing tumors and thus an evident hallmark of cancer.

Taken together, we envision these capabilities acquired by most forms of human cancer to constitute a set of eight distinct hallmarks that define a necessary condition for malignancy (Figure 1), along with the two associated facilitators of their acquisition described below. Importantly, however, one cannot ignore the complex mechanisms underlying this conceptual simplicity: different tumors acquire these hallmarks by diverse mechanisms, doing so by co-opting and subverting a diverse array of mechanisms normally responsible for cell, tissue, and organismic homeostasis.

Aberrations that enable acquisition of the necessary functional capabilities

The lengthy process of tumor development and malignant progression, long appreciated to involve a succession of rate-limiting steps, reflects the need of evolving cancer cells to acquire the eight hallmark capabilities discussed above. How then are these functional capabilities acquired? Currently, there are two clearly established means by which the hallmarks are acquired: (1) genome instability and the resulting mutation of hallmark-enabling genes in the overt cancer cells and (2) inflammation by cells of the immune system that help provide these capabilities cooperatively.

Genome instability and the consequent mutation of hallmark-enabling genes is the primary modality of acquiring hallmark capabilities. The cell genome is subject to routine DNA damage, from a variety of chemically reactive products of normal metabolism, from environmental insults, and from its replication during every cell division. The resulting defects, if left unrepaired, become cell-heritable mutations, explaining the need of an elaborate consortium of proteins that continuously monitor DNA integrity and, in response to damage, undertake repair. Irreparable damage provokes the elimination of cells, a task orchestrated by the p53 tumor suppressor gene, which has for this reason been dubbed the "guardian of the genome."

This highly efficient genome integrity machine normally keeps the rates of gene mutation and genome rearrangement at low levels, which is likely incompatible with the efficient acquisition of hallmark functions by genetic evolution and phenotypic selection for these necessary capabilities. This dichotomy provides a compelling explanation for the frequent observation of genome instability in cancer cells. Indeed, many tumor types contain neoplastic cells that carry readily identifiable defects in the complex machinery designed to monitor and repair genomic damage. Most apparent are the frequently documented mutant alleles of p53 that have been found in perhaps 40% of all cancers; without p53 on duty, damaged DNA can persist unrepaired and mutant cells can survive and pass their damaged genomes on to their progeny. Numerous other specialized DNA repair and genome maintenance enzymes are also found to be defective in many tumors, and inherited familial defects in DNA repair often lead to elevated risk of cancer development, again by enabling the acquisition of tumor-promoting mutations.

The elevated rates and persistence of proliferation in neoplastic lesions create cell lineages that have undergone far more successive growth-and-division cycles than is typical of cells in normal tissues, accentuating the potential for mutagenic errors occurring during DNA replication. Among these consequences is one that we described earlier: critically shortened and thus dysfunctional telomeres can trigger chromosomal rearrangements and fusions that can affect gene function in various ways. Mutant cancer cells that survive this karyotypic chaos may have acquired advantageous phenotypes and thus the capability to undergo clonal expansion.

The foundation of cancer in genetic mutation is being further substantiated by the development of high-throughput DNA sequencing technologies and the consequent ability to systematically analyze large numbers of independently arising cancer cell genomes. Complemented by other methods for genome scanning, such as comparative genomic hybridization to identify copy number variations, and "chromosome painting" to detect translocations, the derangements of the cancer cell genome are being revealed in unprecedented detail (https://tcga-data.nci.nih.gov/tcga/tcgaHome2.jsp; https://www.sanger.ac.uk/group/cancer-genome-project/; http://icgc.org). The results substantiate the fact that almost every form of human cancer involves cancer cells whose genomes have been mutated either through chromosomal rearrangements or more localized intragenic mutations or both. The density of genetic alterations varies over many orders of magnitude, from very low numbers detected in certain pediatric cancers to the blizzards of mutations present in the genomes of UV-induced melanomas and tobacco-induced lung cancers. Thus, the aberrations can range from dozens of point mutations to hundreds of thousands, and from quasi-diploid chromosomal karyotypes to widespread aneuploidy, translocations, and multiple large-scale amplifications and deletions.

The data generated by these increasingly high-throughput genomic technologies is presenting a major challenge to clarify which of the plethora of mutational alterations in the cancer cell genome actually contribute causally to the acquisition of hallmark capabilities. The numbers of mutations that are being cataloged in many cancer cells greatly exceed those that are likely to be important in reshaping cell phenotype. The recurrence of specific mutations in cohorts of patients with the same cancer type or subtype provides one clue into functional involvement. Many other mutations, however, may reflect alternative solutions utilized in one individual's tumor but not another's, and thus are less frequently recurrent. And yet other mutations—often the great majority in a cancer cell's genome—may simply be ancillary consequences of genomic instability, having been carried along for the ride with other function-enabling mutations that do indeed afford selective advantage and thus clonal expansion during tumor growth and progression. Thus, the concept is emerging that cancer cells contain two classes of mutations: drivers, and passengers. One future imperative will be to leverage such genome profiling data to identify the driver mutations and their mechanistic contributions to the acquisition of hallmark capabilities, not only mutations that are frequent in a particular cancer type but also others—perhaps rare—that are nevertheless functionally important for an individual patient's tumor growth and progression. A second imperative will be to clarify the potential of both recurrent and rare driver mutations as therapeutic targets in different tumor types. An added complexity is that advantageous hallmark traits conferred by driver mutations in some tumors may be acquired in other tumors by changes in the epigenome—the spectrum of heritable changes in chromatin that are not reflected by changes in nucleotide sequence.[17,18] Indeed, it has been argued that all eight of the hallmark capabilities can be conveyed by epigenetic changes in gene regulation, occurring both in the overt cancer cells as well as in the supporting cells of the tumor-associated stroma.[19] While the prevalence of epigenetic mechanisms as primary orchestrators of tumorigenesis is currently unresolved, genomic instability may prove to play less prominent roles in some tumors, where mutational alterations in DNA may be consequential of hallmark functions rather than causal of them.

The field of cancer genetics is poised for an extraordinary decade during which tens of thousands of cancer cell genomes will be comprehensively analyzed for multiple parameters (alterations in DNA sequence and copy number, changes in gene transcription, splicing, and translation as well as re-patterning of histone and DNA methylation (and other modifications) that mediate regional alterations in chromosome condensation to govern gene accessibility for transcription). The challenge and the opportunity will be to distill the identity and contributions of specific alterations—genetic and epigenetic—to hallmark-enabling functions from increasingly massive datasets and to exploit such knowledge for improved detection, evaluation, and informed treatment of human cancers.

Tumor-promoting immune cell infiltration (Inflammation) is the second important modality through which developing cancers acquire hallmark capabilities. Remarkably, most tumors are infiltrated by a variety of cell types of the immune system (so-called infiltrating immune cells, or infiltrative immune (inflammatory) cells (IIC)[3]). While the inflammation caused by IIC might reasonably be considered a failed attempt to eradicate a tumor, recent evidence now clearly makes a far more insidious point: IIC help convey multiple hallmark capabilities, encompassing seven of the eight hallmarks.[3] Thus IICs can variously supply proliferative and survival signals, pro-angiogenic factors, and facilitate local invasion and blood-borne metastasis. In addition, some of these IIC (T-regulatory cells and myeloid-derived suppressor cells) can actively suppress the cytotoxic T lymphocytes that have been dispatched by the immune system to eradicate cancer cells.

Tumor-promoting IICs are recruited by a variety of means in different tumor types and at various stages of multistep tumorigenesis. The roster of the recruiting signals—including an ensemble of chemokine and cytokine signaling factors—is still incompletely understood. In some cases, the nature of the neoplastic lesion may trigger tissue abnormality or damage signals that attract IIC, in particular, innate immune cells but also in some cases B and T lymphocytes. In other cases, oncogenic signaling, by activating transcriptional networks, induces expression of cytokines and chemokines that recruit IIC. In early-stage lesions, the recruited IIC can help incipient cancer cells to proliferate, survive, evade antigrowth controls, or activate angiogenesis. At later stages of progression, IIC at the margins of tumors can facilitate invasiveness. Some experiments reveal that IICs can pair with cancer cells as they migrate through the circulation and become established in distant locations.[20] Additionally, certain IIC, such as macrophages, can subject cancer cells to DNA-damaging reactive oxygen species, thereby contributing to the mutational alteration and selective evolution of the cancer cell genome.

Most types of solid tumors are associated with tumor-promoting immune infiltrations that range from histologically subtle to the obvious inflammatory responses recognized by pathologists. In addition, the long-appreciated epidemiologic association between chronic inflammation and carcinogenesis supports the proposition that preexisting inflammatory conditions can be fertile breeding grounds for the inception and progression of certain forms of cancer. Chronically inflamed tissues share features with wound healing; both involve induction of angiogenesis and stimulation of cell survival, proliferation, and migration/invasion, involving the inflammatory IIC and other cell types (e.g., fibroblasts) that they activate in the affected tissue. These functions are of course hallmark capabilities, indicating that IIC can also inadvertently foster neoplastic initiation and/or progression of incipient cancer cells present in inflammatory tissue microenvironments.

The histopathological complexity of cancer, manifested in tumor microenvironments (TMEs)

Pathologists have long recognized that solid tumors are complex histological structures, incorporating not only cancer cells but also a variety of morphologically distinct cells and cellular structures recognizable because they are similar to constituents of noncancerous tissues, both normal and affected by conditions such as infections or wound healing. In analogy to the stroma that supports epithelia in many normal tissues, the apparently noncancerous component of tumors has been labeled as the tumor stroma. As in normal tissue stroma, the tumor-associated stroma can be seen to contain blood vessels, assemblages of fibroblastic cells, and in many cases IIC. Historically, a simplistic view of the tumor stroma posited that endothelial cells, through the process of angiogenesis that produced a tumor neovasculature, provided oxygen and nutrients, while CAFs were either passengers or provided structural support, and the IIC, discussed above, represented ineffectual antitumoral immune responses. As described in part above, we now appreciate the fact that the diverse stromal cells inside tumors can contribute functionally to the acquisition of seven of the eight hallmarks.[3]

In analogy to normal tissues, tumors are often conceptually compartmentalized into the parenchyma (formed by the cancer cells) and the stroma (formed by the ostensibly normal supporting cells); the assemblage of these two compartments, incorporating as well extracellular material (including extracellular matrix, ECM, and basement membrane, BM) is increasingly referred to as the "tumor microenvironment" (TME), as illustrated in Figure 2; some also refer to the TME exclusively as the noncancerous stromal compartment, although conceptually the microenvironment incorporates the entirety of the tumor, that is, both its neoplastic and stromal compartments.

The three classes of stromal cell—angiogenic vascular cells (AVCs), consisting of endothelial cells and supporting pericytes; CAFs, and IIC—constitute the bulk of the stromal component of the TME.[3] These simple classifications, however, mask important diversity in cellular phenotypes. Thus there are a number of CAF subtypes, of which the two most prevalent are derived either from myofibroblasts, mesenchymal stem cells, and tissue stellate cells that all characteristically express alpha-smooth muscle actin, or from connective tissue-derived fibroblasts that do not. Both subtypes of CAF are evidently induced by epigenetic reprogramming of their respective normal cells of origin by paracrine signals emanating from the TME; these inductive signals reflect similar signaling circuits used to engage fibroblasts in wound healing or inflammatory responses. A growing number of IIC subtypes are being recognized, each with distinctive functions and characteristics; some may be lineage derived (e.g., expressed by definition

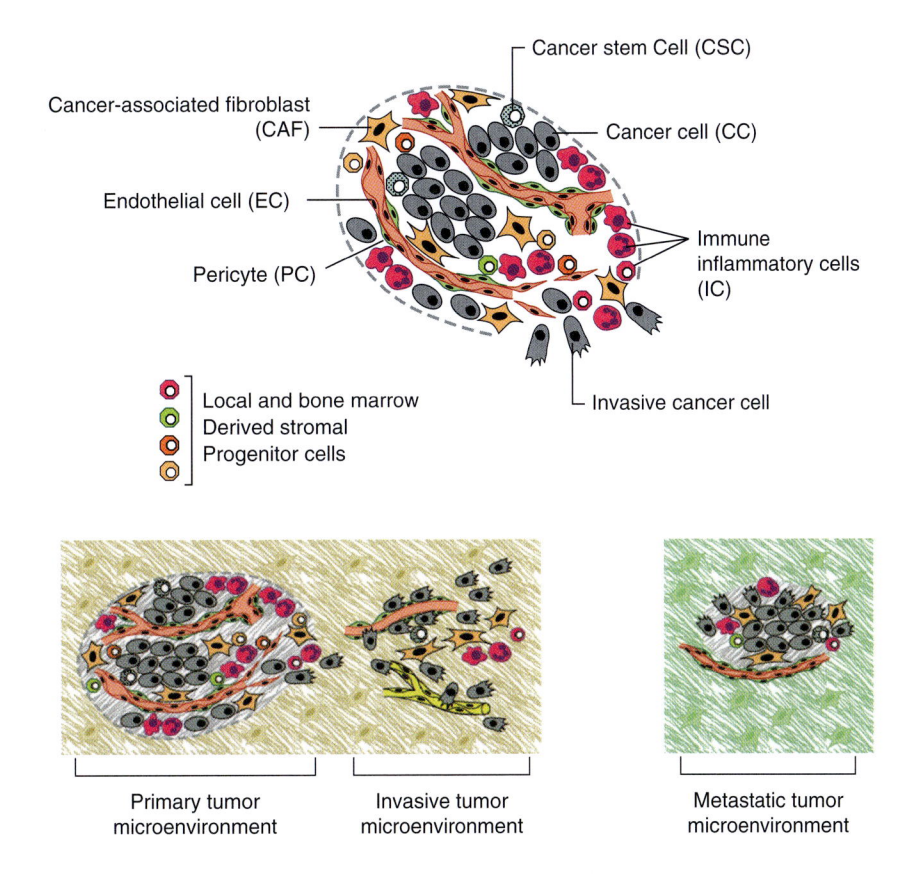

Figure 2 The constitution of the hallmark-enabling tumor microenvironment. An assemblage of distinct cell types constitutes the TME of most solid tumors, involving two distinct compartments—the parenchyma of cancer cells, and the stroma of supporting cells. Both compartments contain distinct cell and sub-cell types that collectively enable tumor growth and progression.[2,3] Notably, the immune-inflammatory cells present in tumors can include both tumor-promoting and/or immuno-suppressive as well as tumor-killing subclasses.

in immune cell progenitors recruited from the bone marrow), and others the result of "local education" by particular inductive signals in the TME. The list of tumor-promoting IIC includes distinctive forms (sub-types) of macrophages, neutrophils, partially differentiated myeloid progenitors, and in some cases specialized subtypes of B and T lymphocytes. The endothelial cells and pericytes of the tumor vasculature are comparatively less diverse, although both epitope and gene expression profiling have revealed tissue and tumor type-specific features of both endothelial cells and pericytes, likely with subtle functional implications in regard to tumor biology. A second distinct class of endothelial cells forms the lymphatic vascular network, which becomes enlarged via lymphangiogenesis proximal to many tumors, and is implicated in lymphatic metastasis.

This recent and more nuanced view of stromal cells elevates their importance in understanding the disease, by virtue of their hallmark-enabling functional contributions.[2,3] CAFs, as an example not discussed above, can in different neoplastic contexts secrete proteases, proliferative signaling ligands, and/or other bioactive molecules that contribute to different tumor phenotypes. CAFs have been variously documented to liberate epithelial cells from the growth-suppressive effects imposed by normal tissue architecture, to induce tumor-promoting inflammation, to facilitate both local invasion and metastatic seeding, and to provide cancer cells with metabolic fuel. CAFs can also induce angiogenesis and, remarkably, act in an immune-suppressive fashion to blunt the attacks of tumoricidal CTLs.

Looking to the future, an important goal will be to continue mapping the multidimensional landscape of stromal cell types and sub-types operative within different forms of cancer and at different stages of progression.

Another dimension to the TME involves genetic and functional heterogeneity within populations of cancer cells. Indeed, the cancer cells within individual neoplastic lesions have long been recognized to be morphologically and genetically heterogeneous. Genome profiling technologies (karyotyping, comparative genomic hybridization, allelic loss analysis, exome (gene) sequencing, and more recently whole genome sequencing, now at the single-cell level), have documented the mutational evolution of the genome as nascent cancer cells in incipient neoplasias progress to more fully developed cancer cells populating solid tumors and clonally distinct subdomains therein.

A second dimension of intratumoral heterogeneity is evident at the epigenetic level. Thus, in many carcinomas, cancer cells at the margins of invasive tumors are phenotypically distinct, having undergone an EMT that renders them more fibroblastic, with attendant capability for invasion. Others retain various degrees of differentiation characteristic of the cell type from which they originated, for example, squamous epithelia. Additionally, the regional variation in histological characteristics seen in various tumor types is now realized to reflect (at least in some cases) genetically distinct clones of cancer cells, the result of mutational alteration of unstable genomes and clonal outgrowth, presumably reflecting different genetic solutions within the same neoplasia to the challenge of acquiring hallmark-enabling capabilities that enable malignant progression.

Additionally, most cancers are now appreciated to contain distinct subpopulations—often comparatively rare—of cancer cells exhibiting phenotypic similarity, at least superficially, to normal tissue stem cells. These cancer stem-like cells (CSCs) typically proliferate comparatively slowly, express cell-surface markers diagnostic of tissue stem cells, and have enhanced capability to form new cancers upon ectopic transplantation of small numbers of cells into appropriate animal hosts, as compared to their more abundant counterparts, who proliferate more rapidly but are inefficient at or incapable of seeding transplant tumors.[9,21] (This latter assay operationally defines such cells as tumor-initiating cells, TICs.) The initial concept was that the cell of origin of a cancer was a normal tissue stem or progenitor cell, which became transformed into a CSC that in turn spawned cancer cells much like normal tissue stem cells spawn differentiated cell types, and indeed there are such cases. For example, the CSCs in squamous cell carcinomas of the skin produce partially differentiated cancer cells with features of squamous cells much as normal skin stem cells produce the squamous epithelium. A number of hematopoietic malignancies evidently also arise from transformation of normal stem/progenitor cells into CSCs. In certain other cases, however, there appears to be a dynamic bidirectional relationship between CSCs and cancer cells, in that cancer cells can be converted into CSCs, and vice versa; in some such cases, the EMT appears to switch on the CSC phenotype in cancer cells, while its converse (the mesenchymal-to-epithelial transition, MET) reduces the abundance of CSCs in tumors.[9,21] There are indications that the comparatively less proliferative CSC may be more resistant to some genotoxic anticancer drugs, providing an avenue for drug resistance and clinical relapse. As such, therapeutic targeting of CSCs may be crucial to achieving enduring cancer therapies.

Therapeutic targeting (and co-targeting) of cancer hallmarks

An important question for cancer medicine is whether there are the clinical applications of the hallmarks conceptualization? The most apparent benefit of this concept is in helping cancer researchers to appreciate the common principles and thereby rationalize the diverse molecular and cellular mechanisms by which particular forms of human cancer develop and progress to malignancy. A wealth of data is being generated by multi-platform analysis of cancer cells and neoplastic lesions in different tumor types (see, e.g., ref 22, and chapters throughout this textbook). Moreover, there will be other extrapolations of increasingly powerful analytic technologies, including the systems-wide comparison of lesional stages in tumorigenesis and tumor progression, in particular metastases, as well as comparisons of tumors and metastases during the response and relapse phases to mechanism-targeted therapies. The challenge will be to integrate all of this information in order to understand the key determinants of particular carcinogenesis pathways, to identify new therapeutic targets, to identify modes of adaptive resistance to therapy, and then to use the data for diagnosis, prognosis, and treatment decisions. It is possible, although as yet unproven, that the hallmarks of cancer will prove useful in this integration and distillation: perhaps, by filtering such cancer "omics" data through the growing knowledge base of effector mechanisms and regulatory pathways that functionally contribute to the eight hallmark capabilities and the facilitators of their acquisition, it will be possible to recognize and appreciate molecular genetic, cellular, and microenvironmental signatures as reflective of "hallmark-enabling" changes in individual human cancers, potentially informing more precise management of the disease.

A second application of the hallmarks concept to cancer medicine is envisioned to be in the form of new therapeutic designs. Indeed, there are either approved drugs or drugs in late-stage clinical trials that target each of the eight hallmark

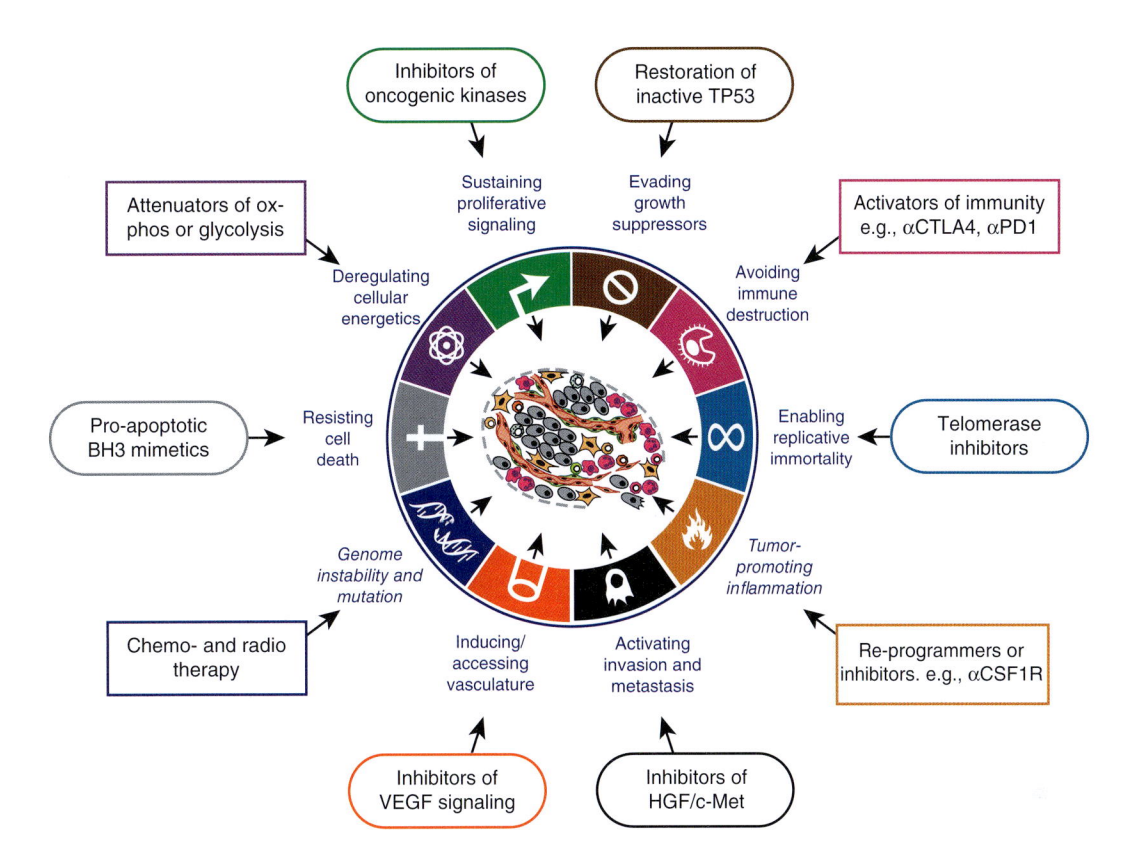

Figure 3 Therapeutic targeting of the hallmarks of cancer. Drugs have been developed that disrupt or interfere with all eight of the hallmark capabilities, and with the two enabling facilitators (genome instability and tumor-promoting inflammation). Some of these hallmark-targeting drugs are approved for clinical use, while others are being tested in late-stage clinical trials; moreover, there is a pipeline full of new hallmark-targeting drugs in development and preclinical evaluation. Recognizing that eventual adaptive resistance during therapeutic treatment is apparent for virtually all of these hallmark-targeting drugs, a hypothesis has emerged: perhaps, by co-targeting multiple independent hallmarks, it will be possible to limit or even prevent the emergence of simultaneous adaptive resistance to independent hallmark-targeting drugs[23]; clinical and preclinical trials are beginning to assess the possibilities.

capabilities and both of the enabling facilitators of those hallmarks (Figure 3); moreover, for most of the 10, there are multiple distinctive drugs targeting the same mechanistic effectors of these hallmarks. Although this is a provocative development in cancer therapeutics, these mechanism-based therapies targeting individual hallmarks have not in general been transformative for the treatment of late stage, aggressive forms of human cancer. An exception to this rule may be in the exciting ascendance of therapeutic immunomodulation to activate and sustain antitumoral immunity, involving most notably inhibitors of immune checkpoint receptors expressed on T lymphocytes (CTLA4 and PD1). Signaling from these checkpoint receptors can disable cytotoxic T cells, evidently rendering antitumoral immune responses ineffectual, thereby contributing to the hallmark capability for evading immune destruction. Notably, exciting clinical responses are being observed in melanoma and select other tumors[24,25] treated with therapeutic antibodies that inhibit checkpoint activation, particularly when both checkpoints are co-targeted with therapeutic antibody cocktails.[26] Nevertheless, not all patients respond to such immunotherapies, and the duration of response remains to be ascertained, as does the prevalence of adaptive resistance to such immunotherapies.

For other hallmark-targeting therapies, it is typical, after a period of response, to see adaptive resistance mechanisms kick in, enabling the surviving cancer cells (and cancer stem cells) to circumvent the mechanistic blockade imposed by the treatment and resume progressive growth. While different solutions can be proffered to the insufficiency of therapeutic targeting of cancer hallmarks, one future strategy might involve applying the concept of the hallmarks as independent and necessary components of a malignant cancer: by co-targeting multiple hallmarks concomitantly, it may be harder for resistance toward each to develop concurrently, and thus both efficacy and its duration might be improved.[23] Certainly, an important issue will be effectively managing the toxicities of such combinations. Thus, in addition to simple cocktails, it may be necessary to use hallmark-targeting drugs sequentially, episodically, or in layers, fine-tuned to maximize efficacy while managing toxicity and limiting adaptive resistance (Figure 3b). It is further envisioned that refined preclinical mouse models—both genetically engineered *de novo* and patient-derived xenograft (PDX) transplants—will have utility in testing alternative therapeutic trials designs aimed to reduce the matrix of possibilities to clinically feasible numbers, taking the best performing trial arms from preclinical trials into clinical trials and personalized treatments.[27–29]

In conclusion, the hallmarks of cancer may provide the student of modern oncology with a foundation and a framework for absorbing the subsequent topical articles of this encyclopedic textbook, and more generally for investigating and interpreting pathogenic mechanisms, and applying such knowledge toward the development of more effective diagnosis and treatment of human cancers.

References

1. Hanahan D, Weinberg RA. The hallmarks of cancer. *Cell*. 2000;**100**:57–70.
2. Hanahan D, Weinberg RA. Hallmarks of cancer: the next generation. *Cell*. 2011;**144**:346–674.
3. Hanahan D, Coussens LM. Accessories to the crime: functions of cells recruited to the tumor microenvironment. *Cancer Cell*. 2012;**21**:309–322.
4. Weinberg RA. *The Biology of Cancer*. New York: **Garland Press**; 2013.
5. Vanden Berghe T, Linkermann A, Jouan-Lanhouet S, et al. Regulated necrosis: the expanding network of non-apoptotic cell death pathways. *Nat Rev Mol Cell Biol*. 2014;**15**:135–147.
6. Rebecca VW, Amaravadi RK. Emerging strategies to effectively target autophagy in cancer. *Oncogene*. 2015. doi: **10.1038/onc.2015.99 [Epub ahead of print]**.
7. Keith B, Johnson RS, Simon MC. HIF1α and HIF2α: sibling rivalry in hypoxic tumour growth and progression. *Nat Rev Cancer*. 2011;**12**:9–22.
8. Semenza GL. Hypoxia-inducible factors: mediators of cancer progression and targets for cancer therapy. *Trends Pharmacol Sci*. 2012;**33**:207–214.
9. Reddy KB. Stem cells: current status and therapeutic implications. *Genes*. 2020;**11**(11):1372.
10. Dongre A, Weinberg RA. New insights into the mechanisms of epithelial-mesenchymal transition and implications for cancer. *Nat Rev Mol Cell Biol*. 2019 Feb;**20**(2):69–84.
11. Faubert B, Solmonson A, DeBerardinis RJ. Metabolic reprogramming and cancer progression. *Science*. 2020;**368**:6487.
12. Dhup S, Dadhich RK, Porporato PE, Sonveaux P. Multiple biological activities of lactic acid in cancer: influences on tumor growth, angiogenesis and metastasis. *Curr Pharm Des*. 2012;**18**:1319–1330.
13. Ward PS, Thompson CB. Metabolic reprogramming: a cancer hallmark even Warburg did not anticipate. *Cancer Cell*. 2012;**21**:297–308.
14. Fridman WH, Pagès F, Sautès-Fridman C, Galon J. The immune contexture in human tumours: impact on clinical outcome. *Nat Rev Cancer*. 2012;**12**:298–306.
15. Galon J, Mlecnik B, Bindea G, et al. Towards the introduction of the 'Immunoscore' in the classification of malignant tumours. *J Pathol*. 2014;**232**:199–209.
16. Galon J, Angell HK, Bedognetti D, Marincola FM. The continuum of cancer immunosurveillance: prognostic, predictive, and mechanistic signatures. *Immunity*. 2013;**39**:11–26.
17. You JS, Jones PA. Cancer genetics and epigenetics: two sides of the same coin? *Cancer Cell*. 2012;**22**:9–20.
18. Easwaran H, Tsai HC, Baylin SB. Cancer epigenetics: tumor heterogeneity, plasticity of stem-like states, and drug resistance. *Mol Cell*. 2014;**54**:716–727.
19. Sahai E et al. A framework for advancing our understanding of cancer-associated fibroblasts. *Nat Rev Cancer*. 2020 Mar;**20**(3):174–186.
20. Labelle M, Hynes RO. The Initial hours of metastasis: the importance of cooperative host-tumor cell interactions during hematogenous dissemination. *Cancer Discov*. 2012;**2**:1091–1099.
21. Batlle E, Clevers H. Cancer stem cells revisited. *Nat Med*. 2017;**23**(10):1124–1134.
22. The Cancer Genome Atlas Network. Comprehensive molecular portraits of human breast tumours. *Nature*. 2012;**490**:61–70.
23. Hanahan D. Rethinking the war on cancer. *Lancet*. 2013;**383**:558–563.
24. Sharma P, Allison JP. The future of immune checkpoint therapy. *Science*. 2015;**348**:56–61.
25. Topalian SL, Drake CG, Pardoll DM. Immune checkpoint blockade: a common denominator approach to cancer therapy. *Cancer Cell*. 2015;**27**:450–461.
26. Sharma P, Allison JP. Immune checkpoint targeting in cancer therapy: toward combination strategies with curative potential. *Cell*. 2015;**161**:205–214.
27. De Palma M, Hanahan D. The biology of personalized cancer medicine: facing individual complexities underlying hallmark capabilities. *Mol Oncol*. 2012;**6**:111–127.
28. Das Thakur M, Pryer NK, Singh M. Mouse tumour models to guide drug development and identify resistance mechanisms. *J Pathol*. 2014;**232**:103–111.
29. Siolas D, Hannon GJ. Patient-derived tumor xenografts: transforming clinical samples into mouse models. *Cancer Res*. 2013;**73**:5315–5319.

PART 2

Tumor Biology

3 Molecular biology, genetics, and translational models of human cancer

Benno Traub, MD* ■ Florian Scheufele, MD* ■ Srinivas R. Viswanathan, MD, PhD ■
Matthew Meyerson, MD, PhD ■ David A. Tuveson, MD, PhD

Overview

Cancer is a disease of abnormal cellular behavior and characterized by molecular aberrations that promote cellular proliferation and survival. Neoplastic progression ultimately produces tumor masses that compromise local organ function, and the invasion and metastasis of malignant cells away from their tissue of origin and spread throughout the body cause a diverse array of pathophysiologic sequelae that compromise the quality and length of life of patients. A background knowledge of cancer pathogenesis and cancer models should help oncologists understand the developing approaches for optimal patient care, including the new concept of personalized medicine.

This article is a basic, "methods-oriented" survey of molecular biology directed toward the clinician or trainee who wants a fundamental understanding of this discipline. It describes the principles that underlie the procedures used most commonly by molecular biologists and provides examples of clinically relevant situations that draw on particular techniques. Molecular biology already plays an important role in clinical cancer medicine, both in terms of diagnosis (e.g., in the analysis of tumors for prognostic or pathogenetic information) and in treatment (e.g., in the production of pharmacologic and biologic agents, such as recombinant growth factors and monoclonal antibodies).

We will begin with an overview of genes, gene expression, and gene cloning. Our discussion of techniques will follow the flow of genetic information as we explain the procedures used to analyze gene expression at the levels of DNA, ribonucleic acid (RNA), and protein. We conclude with a discussion of current cancer modeling systems *in vitro* and *in vivo*. Good general overviews of these topics can be found in several books.[1-3]

Overview: gene structure

Genes and gene expression

The gene is the fundamental unit of inheritance and the ultimate determinant of all phenotypes. The DNA of a normal human cell contains an estimated 20,000–25,000 protein-coding genes, but only a fraction of these are used (or expressed) in any particular cell at any given time. For example, genes specific for erythroid cells, such as the hemoglobin genes, are not expressed in brain cells. The identity of each gene expressed in a particular cell at a given time and its level of expression are defined as the "transcriptome."

According to the central dogma of molecular biology, the flow of genetic information usually runs from DNA to RNA to protein. A gene exerts its effects by having its DNA transcribed into a messenger ribonucleic acid (mRNA) copy (a "transcript") using the DNA of the gene as a template. The mRNA transcript is then translated into a protein, the final effector of the gene's action, by the ribosome, which decodes the sequence information contained within the transcript to build a corresponding protein composed of amino acids. Thus, molecular biologists often investigate gene expression or activation, which is the process of transcribing DNA into RNA or translating RNA into protein.

Functional components of the gene

Every gene consists of several functional components, each involved in a different facet of gene expression (Figure 1). Broadly speaking, there are two main functional units: the promoter region and the coding region.

The promoter region controls when and in what tissue a gene is expressed. For example, the hemoglobin gene promoter is responsible for its expression in erythroid cells and not in brain cells. In the DNA of the gene's promoter region, there are specific structural and sequence elements (see section titled "Structural considerations") that permit the gene to be expressed only in an appropriate cell. These structures are referred to as "*cis*-acting elements" because they reside on the same molecule of DNA as the gene. In some cases, other tissue type-specific *cis*-acting elements, called enhancers, reside on the same DNA molecule but at a great distance from the coding region of the gene.[4,5] In the appropriate cell, the *cis*-acting elements bind protein factors that are physically responsible for transcribing the gene. These proteins are called *trans*-acting factors because they reside in the cell's nucleus separate from the DNA molecule bearing the gene. For example, brain cells do not have the *trans*-acting factors that bind to the hemoglobin promoter and activate gene expression; therefore, brain cells do not express hemoglobin. They do, however, have *trans*-acting factors that bind to neuron-specific gene promoters.

The structure of a gene's protein is specified by the gene's coding region. The coding region contains the information that directs an erythroid cell to assemble amino acids in the proper order to make the hemoglobin protein. As described in detail later, DNA is a linear polymer consisting of four distinguishable subunits called nucleotides. In the coding region of a gene, the linear sequence of nucleotides encodes the amino acid sequence of the protein. This genetic code is in triplet form so that every group of three nucleotides encodes a single amino acid. The 64 triplets that can be formed by four nucleotides exceed the 20 distinct amino acids used to make proteins. This makes the code degenerate and allows some amino acids to be encoded by several different triplets.[6] The nucleotide sequence of any gene can be determined using a variety of methods (see section titled "Nucleotide sequencing" of this article). By translating the code, one can therefore derive

*Shared First-Author.

Holland-Frei Cancer Medicine, Tenth Edition. Edited by Robert C. Bast, John C. Byrd, Carlo M. Croce, Ernest Hawk, Fadlo R. Khuri, Raphael E. Pollock, Apostolia M. Tsimberidou, Christopher G. Willett, and Cheryl L. Willman.
© 2023 John Wiley & Sons, Inc. Published 2023 by John Wiley & Sons, Inc.

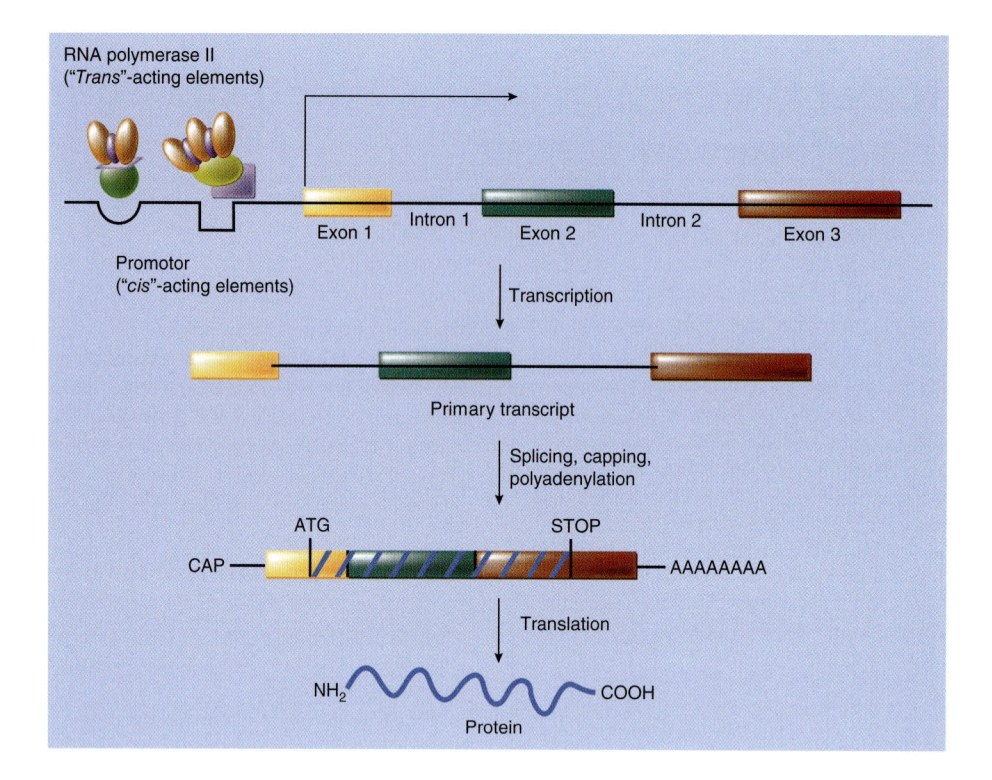

Figure 1 Gene expression. A gene's DNA is transcribed into messenger ribonucleic acid (mRNA), which, in turn, is translated into protein. The functional components of a gene are schematically diagrammed here. Areas of the gene destined to be represented in mature mRNA are called exons, and intervening areas of DNA between exons are called introns. The portion of the gene that controls transcription, and therefore expression, is the promoter. This control is exerted by specific nucleotide sequences in the promoter region ("cis"-acting factors) and by proteins ("trans"-acting factors) that must interact with promoter DNA and/or ribonucleic acid (RNA) polymerase II for transcription to occur. The primary transcript is the RNA molecule made by RNA polymerase II that is complementary to the entire stretch of DNA containing the gene. Before leaving the nucleus, the primary transcript is modified by splicing together exons (thus removing intronic sequences), adding a cap to the 5′ end and a poly-A tail to the 3′ end. Once in the cytoplasm, mature mRNA undergoes translation to yield a protein.

a predicted amino acid sequence for the protein encoded by a gene.

Structural considerations

Fine structure
Four nucleotides assembled in a distinct sequence make out the whole DNA (Figure 2). They consist of an invariant portion, a five-carbon deoxyribose sugar with a phosphate group, and a variable portion, the base. Two of the nucleotides are purines, adenine (A) and guanine (G), and two are pyrimidines, cytosine (C) and thymine (T). Nucleotides are connected to each other in the DNA polymer through their phosphate groups, leaving the bases free to interact with each other through hydrogen bonding. This base-pairing is specific, so that A interacts with T and C with G. DNA is ordinarily double-stranded; that is, two linear polymers of DNA are aligned so that the bases of the two strands face each other. Base pairing makes this alignment specific, so that one DNA strand is perfectly complementary to the other. This complementarity means that each DNA strand carries the information needed to make an exact replica of itself.

In every strand of DNA polymer, the phosphate substitutions alternate between the 5′ and 3′ carbons of the deoxyribose molecules. Thus, there is directionality to DNA: the genetic code reads in the 5′–3′ direction. In double-stranded DNA, the strand that carries the translatable code in the 5′–3′ direction is called the sense strand, whereas its complementary partner is termed the antisense strand.[7]

Gross structure
In eukaryotes, the coding regions of most genes are not continuous. Rather, they consist of areas that are transcribed into mature mRNA ("exons") interrupted by stretches of DNA that do not appear in mature mRNA ("introns") (see Figure 1). The exact functions of introns are not known with certainty. Some may contain regulatory sequences, and their conservation across evolution implies an important purpose. The overall physical structure of introns might be more important than their specific nucleotide sequences, because the sequences of introns diverge more rapidly in evolution than do those of exons. Recent findings in yeast cell showed regulatory functions of excised introns on cell growth under stressful conditions.[8,9] Overall, the DNA that encodes for protein comprises only a tiny minority of total DNA. Between genes, there are vast stretches of untranscribed DNA that are assumed to play an important structural role. There are also many regions that give rise to transcribed "noncoding" regulatory RNA species, which are functionally active without being translated into proteins.[10–12]

In the nucleus, DNA is not present as naked nucleic acid. Rather, it is found in close association with a number of accessory proteins that allow for the correct packaging of DNA, such as histones, and in this form is called chromatin.[13] DNA's double helix is ordinarily twisted on itself to form a supercoiled structure[14] that must partially unwind during DNA replication and transcription.[15] Accessory proteins such as topoisomerases, histone acetylases, and histone deacetylases, are involved in regulating this process.

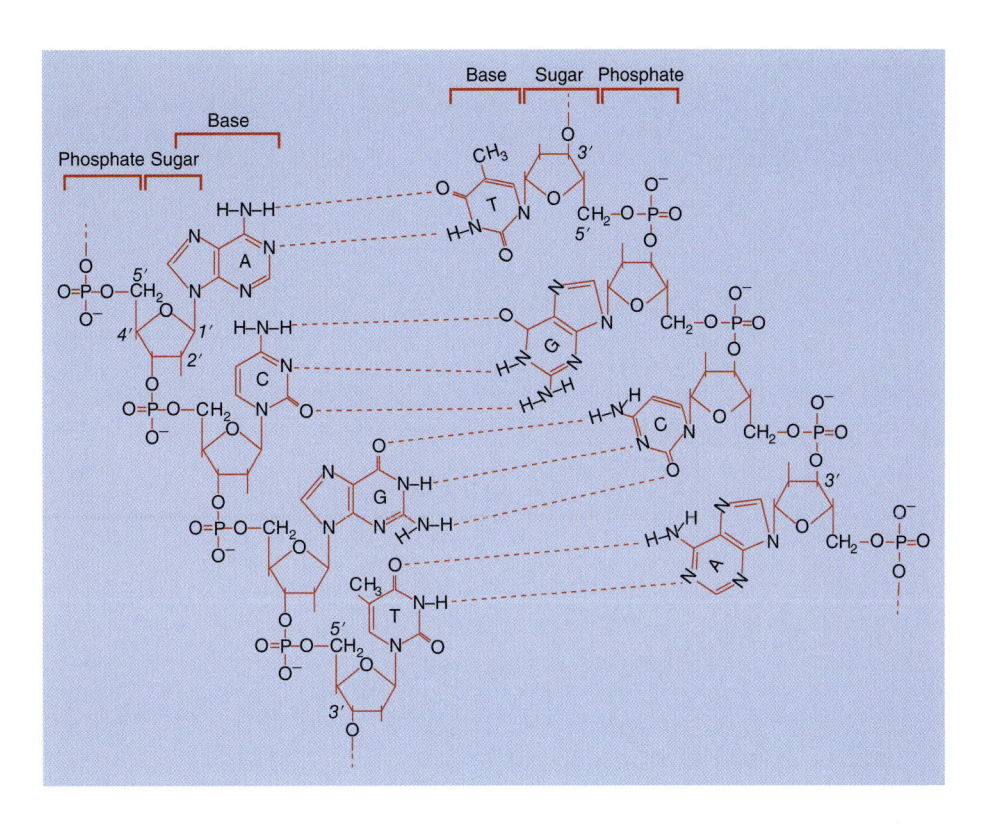

Figure 2 Structure of base-paired double-stranded DNA. Each strand of DNA consists of a backbone of five-carbon deoxyribose sugars connected to each other through phosphate bonds. Note that as one follows the sequence down the left-hand strand (A–C to G–T), one is also following the carbons of the deoxyribose ring, going from the 5′ carbon to the 3′ carbon. This is the basis for the 5′ to 3′ directionality of DNA. The one carbon of each deoxyribose is substituted with a purine or pyrimidine base. In double-stranded DNA, bases face each other in the center of the molecule and base pair via hydrogen bonds (dotted lines). Base-pairing is specific so that adenine pairs with thymine and guanine pairs with cytosine.

General techniques

Restriction endonucleases and recombinant DNA

In eukaryotic chromosomes, individual molecules of DNA are several million base pairs long. Because these molecules are far too large to analyze directly, scientists typically cut the DNA into fragments of more manageable size. Fortunately, bacteria have evolved a highly diverse set of enzymes, the restriction endonucleases, which cleave DNA internally within the polymer.[16] In nature, these enzymes have evolved to protect bacteria from invasion by foreign species, such as bacteriophages. To discriminate between "domestic" and "foreign" DNA, individual restriction endonucleases recognize specific sequences, usually 4–6 bases in length and often palindromic (i.e., the 5′–3′ sequences in the upper and lower strand are identical) (Figure 3).[17] DNA without such specific sequences is left undisturbed by the enzymes. However, when a restriction endonuclease spots a recognition site, it binds to the site and cleaves both strands of the DNA to which it has bound.

There is a lower limit to the size of useful DNA fragments, below which the informational content of each piece is negligible. Statistically, the longer a restriction endonuclease's recognition sequence, the less frequently this sequence will occur in a stretch of DNA. Therefore, the enzymes most commonly used to cut DNA into fragments of useful size are those that recognize a 6-nt recognition site ("six-base cutters"). For example, an endonuclease isolated from *Escherichia coli*, called EcoRI, recognizes the sequence GAATTC, and wherever this occurs in double-stranded DNA, it will cleave between the G and A (see Figure 3). (Note that the antisense strand, which reads CTTAAG in the 3′–5′ direction, will read GAATTC in the 5′–3′ direction, as this is a palindromic sequence.)

Gene cloning

Mechanics
The most powerful technique available for gene analysis, and the cornerstone for all others, is gene cloning (see Figure 3). In this process, a discrete piece of DNA is faithfully replicated in the laboratory. Cloning provides quantities of specific DNA sufficient for biochemical analysis or for any other manipulation, including joining to a foreign piece of DNA. In the early 1970s, Cohen et al.[18] drew on two fundamental properties of bacteria and their viruses (phages) that made this innovation possible: plasmids and DNA ligases.

Plasmids are circular molecules of DNA that replicate in the cytoplasm of bacterial cells, separate from the bacteria's own DNA. In nature, plasmids often carry genetic information useful to the host bacterium, such as genes that confer resistance to antibiotics. For the purposes of gene cloning, plasmids are important because they contain all of the information necessary for directing bacterial enzymes to replicate the plasmid DNA, in some cases, to many thousands of copies per bacterium.

DNA ligases are enzymes produced by bacteria (and some phages when they infect bacteria) that can link or ligate together separate pieces of DNA. A DNA ligase can join any two pieces of DNA together, even ones that are not ordinarily connected to each other in nature. Indeed, the power of cloning comes in the ability

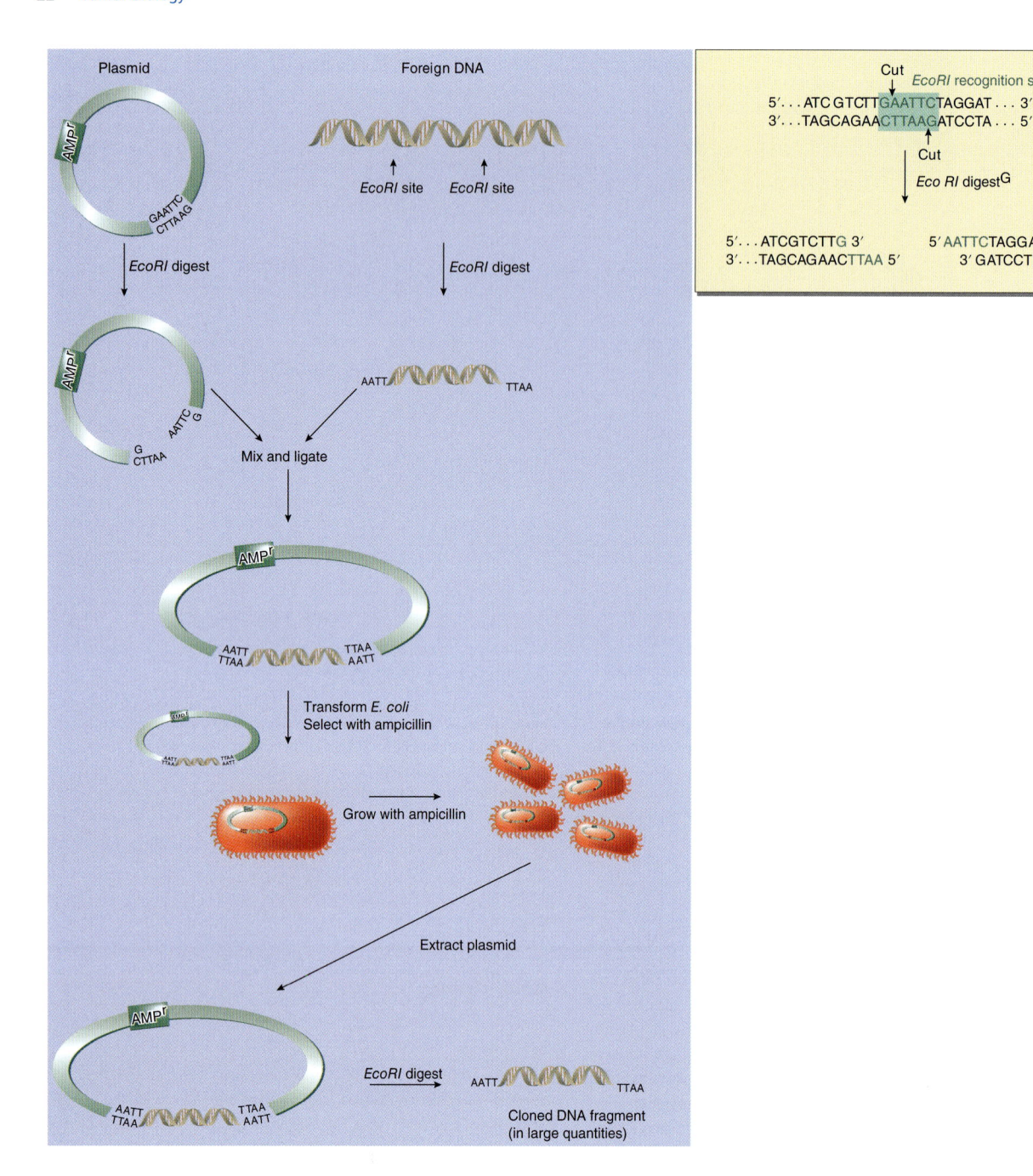

Figure 3 Digestion of DNA with the restriction endonuclease EcoRI and gene cloning. In this example, a small amount of foreign DNA (a few nanograms) is digested with EcoRI. The nucleotide sequence of this stretch of DNA contains the recognition sequence for EcoRI, GAATTC (boxed). EcoRI cuts the DNA in both strands between the indicated nucleotides, resulting in fragments with 5′ single-stranded tails. This foreign DNA can come from any source, the only requirement being that it contains the same restriction endonuclease recognition sites as the vector. Plasmid vector is also digested with EcoRI to create a linear DNA molecule. The "sticky" single-stranded ends of the foreign DNA can align and base-pair with the complementary "sticky ends" of the plasmid, after which DNA ligase covalently bonds foreign DNA to plasmid DNA. This recombinant DNA is introduced into E. coli by a process called transformation. Because the bacteria themselves are not resistant to ampicillin, growth in ampicillin will select only those bacteria that have taken up the plasmid DNA (which carries an ampicillin resistance gene). The plasmid contains a bacterial origin of replication so that as the bacterial culture grows, plasmids replicate, resulting in several copies in each bacterium. When the culture has grown to sufficient size, plasmid DNA can be isolated biochemically, foreign DNA can be cut from the plasmid using EcoRI, and the resulting yield will often be milligrams of DNA, that is, greater than a 10^6-fold amplification.

to "mix and match" segments of DNA in a fashion tailored to the desired use.

Cloning with restriction endonucleases

In the traditional form of gene cloning, a restriction endonuclease is used to cut open the circular plasmid DNA in a region not necessary for replication (see Figure 3). For example, the enzyme EcoRI recognizes the sequence GAATTC and cuts both DNA strands of the plasmid between the G and the A nucleotides in such a nonessential area. Protruding from the cut ends will be single-stranded DNA "tails" with the sequence AATT. (Note that the tail's sequence in the sense strand is the same as that in the antisense strand when read in the 5′–3′ direction.) Any other piece of DNA that has been cut with EcoRI will also have single-stranded AATT tails, which can be base-pair with the complementary TTAA tails (reading 3′–5′) on the cut plasmid. When this happens, the foreign DNA piece physically closes the gap in the plasmid, forming a closed circular plasmid again (which is necessary for plasmid propagation).

Although the nucleotides at the ends of the plasmid and foreign DNA know about each other, they are not covalently connected. This is an unstable situation that the DNA ligase rectifies. The DNA ligase covalently joins the plasmid and foreign DNA to create a recombinant plasmid, which still has all of the information needed to be replicated in a bacterium but also contains a foreign DNA insert.

When a recombinant plasmid is reintroduced into a host bacterium (by a process called transformation), the foreign DNA insert is replicated along with the plasmid into which it was inserted. When growing the bacteria culture, each cell division increases the amount of plasmid and as soon as the bacterial culture contains the desired quantity (this may be milligrams of plasmid DNA in a 1 L culture), it can be re-isolated as pure DNA. The cloned foreign piece of DNA can then be cut out (with EcoRI, in our example) for further analysis or manipulation. Similarly, host bacteria can be infected with recombinant bacteriophage bearing foreign DNA sequences. The plasmid or phage is called a vector because it is the vehicle that directs the foreign DNA into the host bacterium.

These extraordinarily powerful tools, which are now part of the standard armamentarium of all molecular biology laboratories, have been responsible for the development of nearly all of the analytic techniques described later. Several excellent manuals have been published that describe these techniques in detail.[19,20]

Gateway cloning
Gateway cloning is a proprietary commercial system that has gained widespread popularity for the ease with which it allows researchers to transfer DNA fragments between plasmids. A DNA fragment of interest is appended with specific Gateway sequences on the 5′ and 3′ ends ("attB1" and "attB2," respectively). A proprietary recombinase that recognizes these Gateway sequences is then used to transfer the fragment into a Gateway Donor vector, which contains sequences "attL1" and "attL2" flanking the fragment of interest. Once in the Gateway Donor vector, the fragment can be transferred to any of thousands of available Gateway Destination vectors using a proprietary recombinase mix.[21] This recombinase-based technology therefore allows gene fragments to be easily shuttled between plasmids without the need for restriction digestion and purification steps.

Gibson cloning
A recent development in cloning called the Gibson Assembly method allows for the assembly of multiple overlapping DNA fragments. Two or more fragments to be assembled are mixed together with a combination of three DNA enzymes—an exonuclease, polymerase, and ligase. The exonuclease removes the 5′ ends of the fragments, thereby exposing a 3′ single-stranded DNA overhang. Overlapping fragments then anneal via their 3′ overhangs, and the gaps and nicks are filled in by the DNA polymerase and DNA ligase, respectively. These fragments can be joined together in a one-step isothermal reaction. This powerful synthetic biology method can be routinely used to enzymatically assemble multiple DNA fragments of up to several hundred kilobases.[22]

Recently, it was even applied to synthesize the entire mouse mitochondrial genome, a size of 16.3 kilobases, using 600 overlapping fragments.[23]

Gene probes and hybridization

The ability to identify a specific gene (or mRNA) in a complex mixture of all of the DNA (or RNA) in a cell or tissue lies at the heart of gene analysis. This can only be achieved using a cloned fragment of DNA, called a probe, from the gene of interest. Such fragments are usually obtained from gene libraries constructed from genomic DNA or complementary DNA (cDNA) or generated using polymerase chain reaction (PCR, described below). These DNA fragments can be almost any size, from a few hundred or even fewer nucleotides to the size of an entire gene (several thousand nucleotides).

To be useful, a gene probe must contain a sufficient number of nucleotides so that it will recognize the sequences of its corresponding gene. Recognition occurs by a process called nucleic acid hybridization, in which two pieces of DNA can align themselves (or "anneal") by base-pairing of A to T and G to C bases (see Figure 2). Perfectly matched sequences pair more tightly than sequences containing mismatches, and long-matched sequences pair more tightly than shorter-matched sequences. Hybridization is the concept that underlies many molecular biology methods, such as Southern blotting, Northern blotting, microarray analysis, PCR, and others (see below).

Gene analysis: DNA

Southern blotting

One of the most useful techniques for analyzing a gene at the level of genomic DNA is Southern blotting, named for its inventor, E. M. Southern.[24] It allows one to determine whether specific nucleotide sequences in a cloned probe are present in a sample of genomic DNA, which usually means that the gene itself is present in the genomic DNA (Figure 4). Purified genomic DNA is digested with a specific restriction endonuclease to produce an array of differently sized DNA fragments. Electrophoresis through an agarose gel then separates these fragments according to size. (Because the phosphate groups in DNA make the molecules negatively charged, they migrate toward the anode in an electric field. The semiporous agarose allows DNA molecules to pass at a rate inversely proportional to their size. Thus, smaller molecules will be closer to the anode than larger molecules.) Because the agarose gel used in electrophoresis is thick and the DNA fragments can move within it, DNA in the gel is not in a suitable form for further analysis. The DNA fragments must therefore be irreversibly bound to a solid support to carry out nucleic acid hybridization studies. Thus, after electrophoresis, a paper-thin membrane microfilter (made of nitrocellulose or nylon) is placed over the flat gel. Liquid is forced through the agarose gel in a direction perpendicular to the direction in which the DNA moved during electrophoresis. As the liquid perfuses the gel, it carries DNA fragments with it, depositing them on the membrane filter, to which the DNA sticks. After transfer, the DNA fragments are arrayed by size on the solid support.

Next, a fragment of cloned DNA (the probe) is radiolabeled using any of a variety of techniques. The membrane containing the transferred DNA is soaked in a solution containing the radiolabeled probe. The probe hybridizes to any complementary sequences in the genomic DNA on the filter. The unbound probe

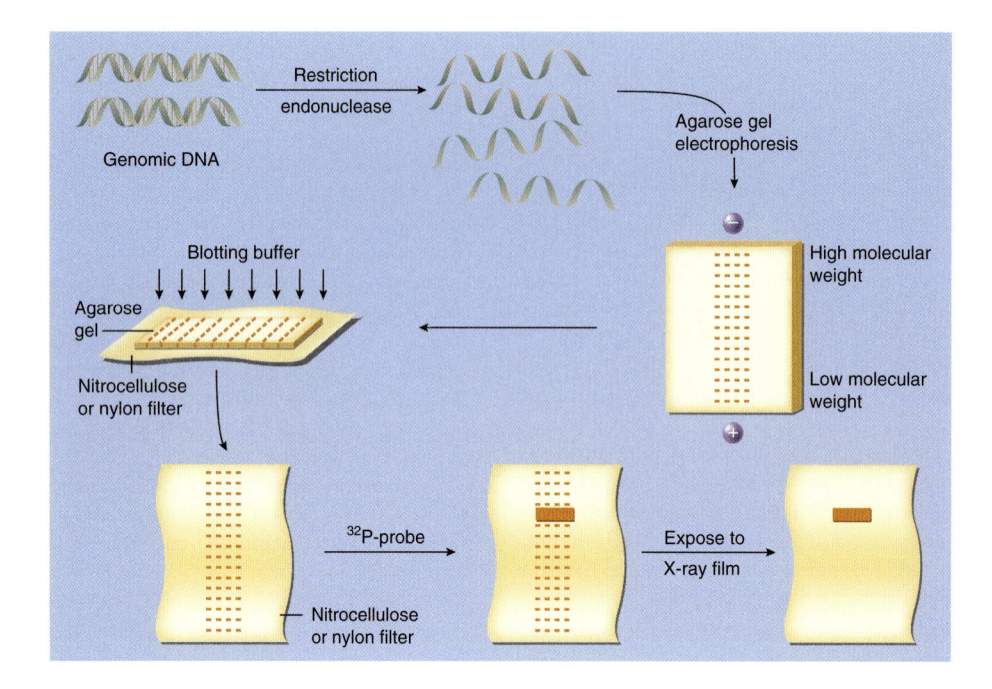

Figure 4 Genomic Southern blotting. Genomic DNA is digested with a single restriction endonuclease, resulting in a complex mixture of DNA fragments of different sizes, that is, molecular weights. Digested DNA is arrayed by size using electrophoresis through a semisolid agarose gel. Because DNA is negatively charged, fragments will migrate toward the anode, but their progress is variably impeded by interactions with the agarose gel. Small fragments interact less and migrate farther; large fragments interact more and migrate less. The arrayed fragments are then transferred to a sheet of nitrocellulose or nylon-based filter paper by forcing buffer through the gel as shown. The DNA fragments are carried by capillary action and can be made to bind irreversibly to the filter. Now the DNA fragments, still arrayed by size on the filter, can be probed for specific nucleotide sequences using a ^{32}P-radiolabeled nucleic acid probe. The probe will hybridize to complementary sequences in the DNA, and the position of the fragment that contains these sequences can be revealed by exposing the filter to X-ray film.

is washed away, and the remaining specifically hybridized probe can be visualized by exposing the filter to X-ray film. A pattern of one or more bands is visible, each corresponding to a restriction endonuclease-generated DNA fragment containing nucleotide sequences complementary to those in the radioactive probe. For any particular gene probe, the size (i.e., length) of the band it identifies will be the same from individual to individual (see below for restriction fragment length polymorphisms (RFLPs), an important exception). Therefore, if a gene has undergone a structural rearrangement, the pattern may change.

Because the amount of the radiolabeled probe that hybridizes to a Southern blot is proportional to the number of copies of the specific gene present in the target DNA, this technique can also be used quantitatively. For example, Southern blotting was used to determine that 30% of primary breast cancer tissue samples contained multiple copies of HER-2/neu oncogene DNA—that is, the gene was amplified.[25]

Polymerase chain reaction (PCR)

The detection of gene sequences by Southern blotting requires at least 1–2 mg of genomic DNA. This translates into several milligrams of tissue that must be used fresh or freshly frozen. PCR is a powerful technique that can amplify specific fragments of DNA (Figure 5), thus lowering the theoretic limit of detectable DNA sequences in a sample to a single molecule of DNA. With some advanced knowledge of the nucleotide sequences in the DNA to be detected, microscopically small amounts of tissue, even a single cell, contain enough DNA to be amplified, and the amplified DNA can be easily used for downstream analysis. Even fixed tissue in paraffin blocks or on slides can yield sufficient DNA for analysis using PCR.[26] Two short single-stranded DNA fragments, called primers, are designed with sequences complementary to those that flank the stretch of DNA to be amplified. Primers and target DNA are mixed, the mixture is heated to dissociate the paired double strands of target DNA, and the temperature is then lowered to permit hybridization, or annealing, of the primers to their complementary sequences on the target DNA. A DNA polymerase enzyme (Figure 6) is added to the mixture, which adds nucleotides to the 3′ end of the primers using the target DNA as a sequence template. This step generates one copy of each of the strands of one target DNA molecule. The mixture is heated again to dissociate the strands and then cooled to allow more primers to anneal to the target sequences on both the original and new pieces of DNA. DNA polymerase is added again and now generates four copies of the target sequences. These steps are repeated, resulting in a geometrically increasing amount of target DNA, that is, a chain reaction. With the discovery and cloning of the "Taq" DNA polymerase from the thermophilic bacterium *Thermus aquatic*, which retains activity after being heated to 95 °C, heating, and cooling steps could be carried out on the same mixture without adding a new enzyme for each cycle.[27,28] This allowed the PCR procedure to be automated.

Nucleotide sequencing

Sanger sequencing

The nucleotide sequence of a gene can be used to predict the structure and function of its protein product. Historically, the major method used for sequencing DNA has been the "enzymatic chain termination" method devised by Sanger et al.[29] This method relies on enzymes called *DNA polymerases* (Figure 6) that create new DNA polymers from individual nucleotides. DNA polymerase

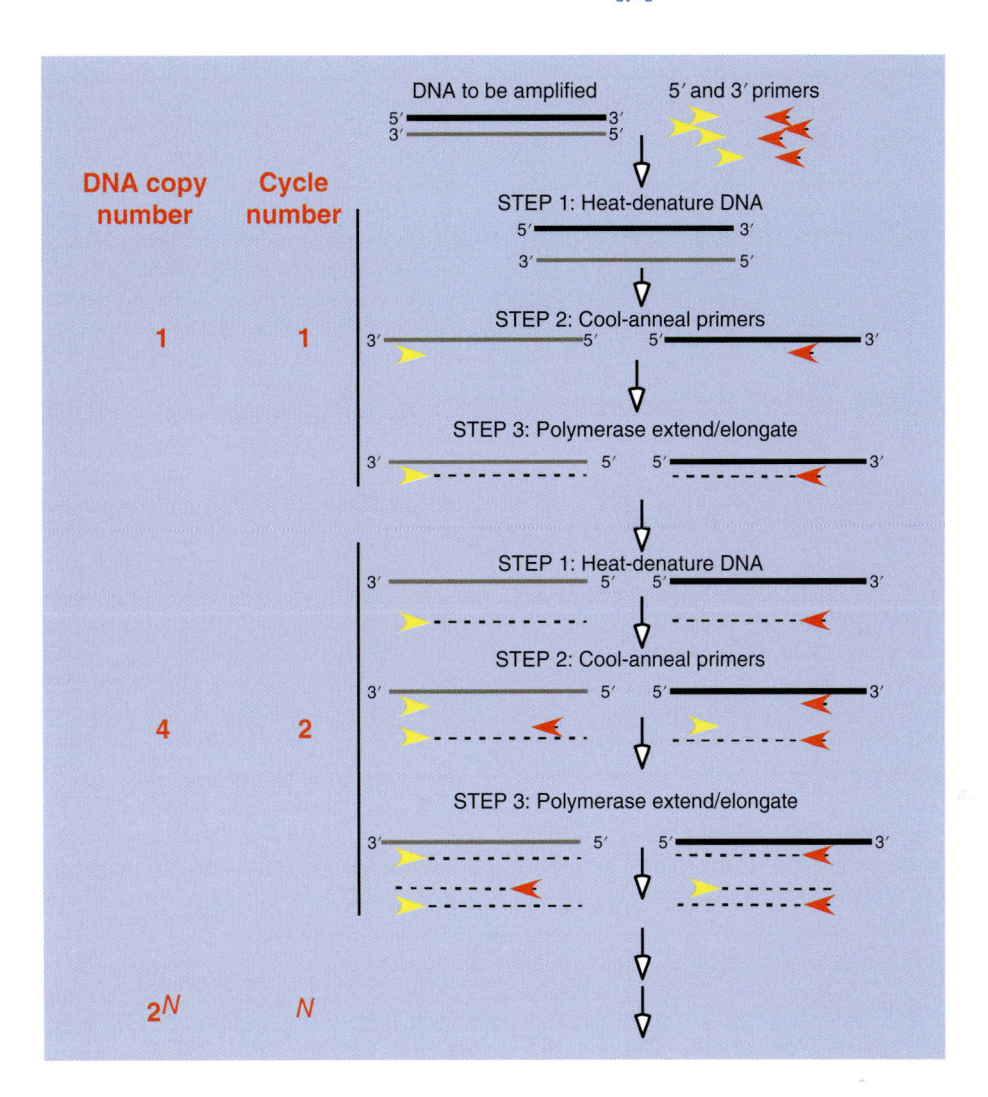

Figure 5 Polymerase chain reaction (PCR). DNA is mixed with short (10–20 base) single-stranded oligonucleotide primers that are complementary to the 5′ and 3′ ends of the sequence to be amplified. The mixture is heated to denature or "melt" all double-stranded DNA and then cooled to permit the primers to anneal to their complementary sequences on the DNA to be amplified. Note that the 5′ primer will anneal to the lower strand and the 3′ primer will anneal to the upper strand. A heat-resistant (thermostable) DNA polymerase (Taq polymerase; see text) was present in the original mixture, and it now synthesizes DNA by starting at the primers and using the strands to which the primers are annealed as a template. This results in the formation of two double-stranded DNA copies for every molecule of double-stranded DNA in the original mixture. The reaction is then heated to melt double-stranded DNA and cooled to allow reannealing, and the polymerase makes new double-stranded DNA again. There are now four double-stranded DNA copies for each original DNA molecule. This process can be repeated n times (usually 20–50) to result in $2n$ copies of double-stranded DNA.

activity requires a template of single-stranded DNA on which to create the new polymer. DNA polymerase sequentially adds new nucleotides to the 3′ end of a growing DNA chain. The base of each new nucleotide must be able to base-pair (i.e., be complementary) to the base on the template over which the polymerase is positioned. When the process is completed, the DNA polymerase will have made a new DNA chain whose nucleotide sequence is completely complementary to the template DNA (Figure 7).

Nucleotide sequencing is based on the observation that when DNA polymerase adds a synthetic abnormal nucleotide to a growing chain, the polymerization stops. The synthetic "terminating" nucleotides used most commonly are dideoxynucleotides that have no alcohol substitutions on the 3′ carbon of their deoxyribose groups and thus cannot be joined by a phosphate bridge to the next nucleotide (see Figure 2). For example, in the presence of dideoxyadenosine triphosphate (ddATP), chain termination will occur wherever an A appears in the new DNA sequence (a T in the template) (Figure 8). These reactions are performed *in vitro* in a test tube, where millions of new DNA molecules are being made at once. If normal deoxy-ATP is mixed with dideoxy-ATP in the proper proportion, only a few of these molecules will terminate at each T in the template. This will generate a series of new DNA polymers, each one stretching from the beginning of the chain to the position of an A (i.e., a T in the template). If the newly formed DNA is fluorescently labeled, the products can be separated electrophoretically in a polyacrylamide gel or capillary gel (see below). Each step of the ladder is a fragment of DNA that stretches from the start of the new polymer to the position of an A. Four separate reactions are performed using each of the four dideoxynucleotides, each coded with a distinct fluorescent color. The four reactions are run together in a capillary gel, and the order of nucleotides is read by the order of the different colors.

Sanger sequencing has served as the backbone for a generation of biological discovery and was instrumental to the Human Genome Project, which launched in 1990 and was completed in 2003. Following the successful assembly of the human genome sequence,

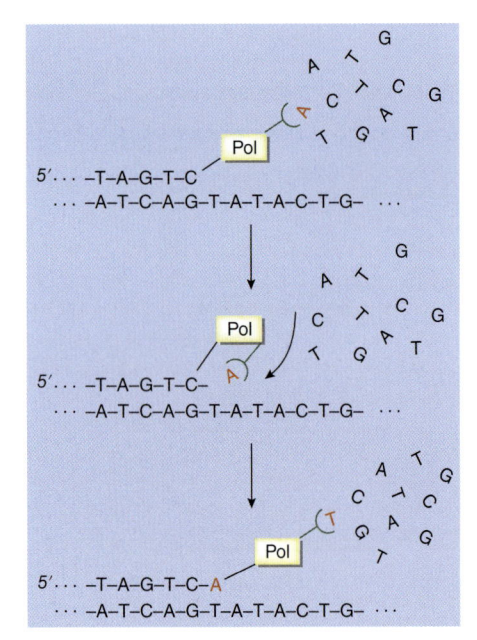

Figure 6 DNA polymerase. In this schematic, the enzyme DNA polymerase creates a new DNA chain (upper strand) using a template (lower strand). Specific nucleotides are added from the 5′ to the 3′ direction as determined by the next nucleotide in the template.

genome researchers shifted their efforts from *de novo* to comparative sequencing. These studies have aimed to sequence the genome in both its normal and diseased states, with the aim of understanding the genomic changes associated with disease.

Perhaps the most active area of comparative sequencing has been in cancer genomics. Early sequencing studies targeted to particular genes or gene families identified key differences between cancer and normal genomes; in many cases, these discoveries provided the rationale for targeted therapeutics. For example, the discovery of mutations in the c-kit protein tyrosine kinase gene by DNA sequencing of gastrointestinal stromal tumors (GISTs)[30] led to the successful treatment of GIST with the c-kit inhibitor imatinib.[31] In lung adenocarcinoma, activating mutations in the epidermal growth factor receptor (*EGFR*) tyrosine kinase gene are common, especially in East Asian populations,[32–34] and predict response to the kinase inhibitors gefitinib and erlotinib.[32–34] Activating mutations in the B homolog rapidly accelerated fibrosarcoma (*BRAF*) serine–threonine kinase gene have been found in over half of all melanomas[35] and subsequently in other cancer types, including colorectal, lung, and thyroid carcinomas. The *BRAF* inhibitor vemurafenib leads to improved overall survival in patients with metastatic melanoma harboring an activating BRAF *V600E* mutation.[36] Mutations in the phosphatidylinositol 3-kinase catalytic subunit gene *PIK3CA* mutations have been discovered in colorectal carcinoma, glioblastoma,[37] and breast carcinomas. In myeloproliferative diseases such as polycythemia vera, the *JAK2* V617F activating mutation is a pathognomonic finding.[38–40]

Next-generation sequencing

More recent cancer genomics studies have employed "next-generation" sequencing (NGS) technologies, which far surpass traditional Sanger sequencing in throughput, scale, and resolution. NGS methods allow for millions of short-fragment sequencing reactions to proceed in parallel.[41–44] Thus, all coding regions of

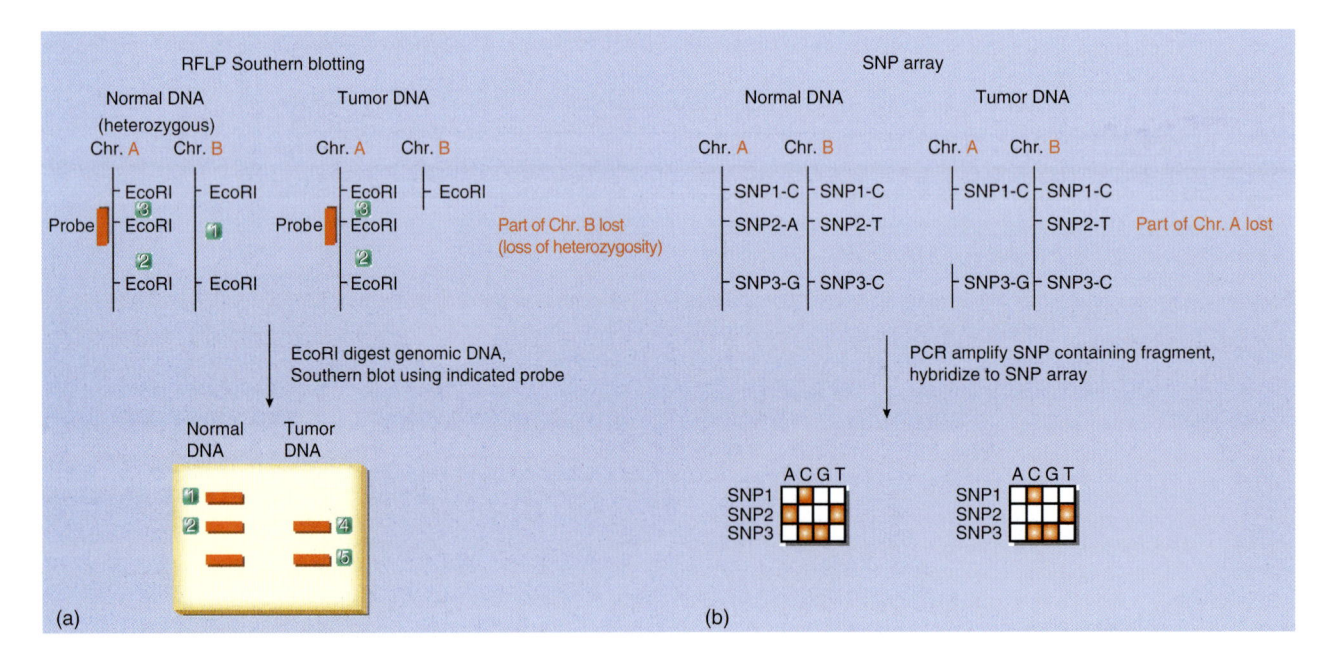

Figure 7 Methods to detect loss of heterozygosity in tumor tissue. (a) Restriction fragment length polymorphism (RFLP) and Southern blotting. In this example, an individual is heterozygous for an EcoRI recognition site: the second EcoRI site on chromosome A is absent on its diploid partner, chromosome B. The individual's tumor is assumed to be clonal and to have arisen from a cell that lost the region of chromosome B displayed in the figure. Southern blotting can then be performed using genomic DNA from the individual's normal DNA and tumor DNA in separate lanes of the agarose gel. Probing the DNA with the probe (indicated on the figure) reveals a heterozygous banding pattern in normal DNA (reflecting the presence of both polymorphisms, one on each chromosome pair) and a loss of that pattern in the tumor DNA. This is one of the hallmarks of a tumor suppressor gene. (b) Single nucleotide polymorphism (SNP) array. In this example, an individual is heterozygous for SNPs 2 and 3 and homozygous for SNP 1. Following the polymerase chain reaction (PCR) amplification of genomic fragments containing each SNP individually, these fragments are hybridized to an array composed of oligonucleotides complementary to the ones amplified. The loss of a heterozygous SNP signal on the array indicates loss of the chromosomal region containing this SNP.

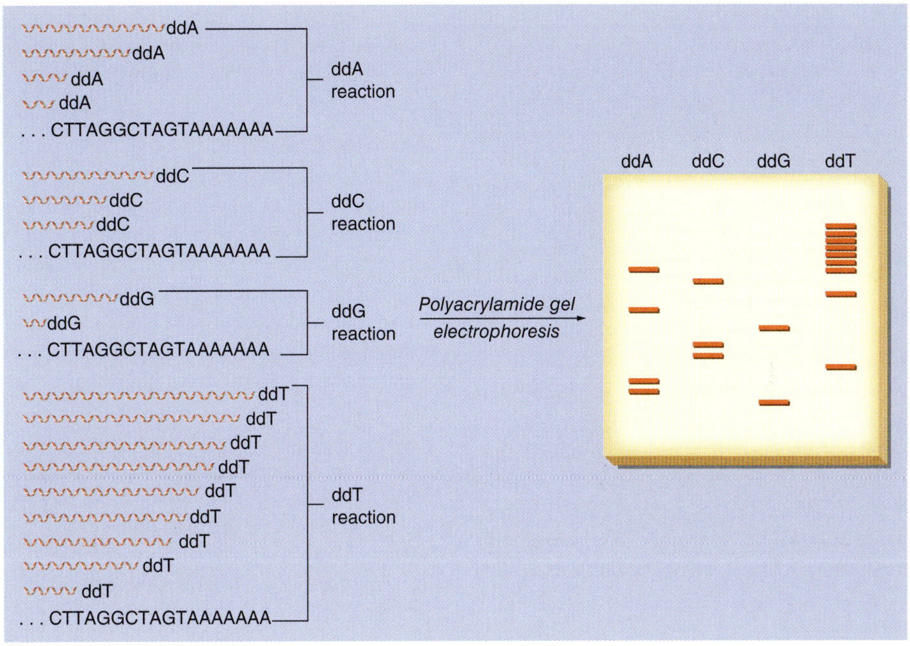

Figure 8 DNA sequencing using the chain termination method. In this example, DNA ending with the sequence CTTAGGCTAGTAAAAAAA is analyzed. Four reactions are performed, each using this DNA as a template for a DNA polymerase reaction and each containing one of the four dideoxynucleotides (dideoxyadenosine triphosphate [ddA], dideoxycytidine triphosphate [ddC], dideoxyguanosine triphosphate [ddG], and dideoxythymidine triphosphate [ddT]). In each reaction, chain elongation will terminate when the dideoxynucleotide is incorporated at the position of its complementary nucleotide in the template. This will result in a family of chains of differing lengths that correspond to the position at which polymerization terminated. In this example, these chains can be resolved by electrophoresis through a urea-containing polyacrylamide gel, in which longer chains run near the top of the gel and shorter chains near the bottom. Each new chain is radioactively labeled, and after autoradiography, the pattern of bands can be read from X-ray film. By noting the order in which bands appear, starting at the bottom of the gel, one can read the sequence of the template by substituting the complement of each dideoxynucleotide at every position. Reading from the bottom yields GAATCCGATCATTTTTTT, and substituting the complementary base at each position yields CTTAGGCTAGTAAAAAAA, the sequence of the template. The use of fluorescent labels in capillary gel electrophoresis is conceptually similar.

a sample can be completely and deeply sequenced in a single analysis. One of the biggest advantages of NGS is the ability to effectively detect the numerous mutations present in a heterogeneous cancer sample[45] without the need for purification of a clonal DNA template. Indeed, NGS assays have become the technology of choice for cancer mutation detection in the research arena, and are beginning to be incorporated in clinical diagnostic testing.

NGS was employed to sequence the first cancer genome, acute myeloid leukemia, in 2008.[46] Since then, the coding regions ("exomes") or whole genomes of a number of other tumor types have been sequenced. Many of these efforts have been coordinated through The Cancer Genome Atlas (TCGA) and the International Cancer Genome Consortium (ICGC) initiatives.

Most commercially available sequencing platforms employ "cyclic array sequencing," in which iterative cycles of enzymatic-based sequencing and imaging-based sequence detection are performed in parallel on a large array of DNA molecules.[43] These include the Illumina (Solexa), Pacific Bio, 454/Roche, SOLiD, and Ion Torrent platforms. In all of these approaches, the DNA sample is initially sheared into a library of small DNA fragments. Common adapter sequences are ligated to each of the fragments and serve as the initiating points for PCR-based amplification. This results in spatially clustered clonal amplicons of each fragment. The amplicons are then sequenced by synthesis, with imaging done at the end of each cycle across the entire array. In this manner, a large number of DNA fragments can be sequenced in parallel in a high-throughput fashion.

Each of the cyclic array sequencing approaches differs in the method used to generate PCR amplicons of DNA fragments and in the biochemistry underlying the sequencing process. There are also variations in read length, throughput, cost, and accuracy between the different methods. Currently, the Illumina sequencing platform is the most widely used for a majority of applications. Illumina sequencing generates clonal amplicons through a method known as "bridge PCR." In this method, forward and reverse primers complementary to adapter sequences are immobilized to a glass slide. PCR-based amplification results in a spatial cluster of approximately 1000 copies of each DNA fragment. Cyclic sequencing then occurs. In each cycle of sequencing, a DNA polymerase incorporates fluorescently labeled deoxyribonucleoside triphosphates (dNTPs) with a reversible 3′ termination moiety. Similar to the Sanger sequencing concept, the 3′ termination moiety allows only a single base to be added to each fragment. All fragments (or "features") are then imaged in four colors, with each color corresponding to one of the deoxyribonucleoside triphosphate species. The reversible 3′ termination moiety is then cleaved, and then next cycle of sequencing begins anew. At the end of this process, one is able to obtain the DNA sequence for each of the many fragments, all sequenced in parallel.

Target enrichment and clinical panel testing
While the methodology above can be used to sequence an entire genome, this is not always technically or computationally feasible, cost-effective, or necessary. "Target-enrichment" refers to the enrichment of the library for selected genomic regions prior to sequencing. Target enrichment can be performed through several methods, including PCR, molecular inversion, and hybrid capture;

hybrid capture is the most popular method in most situations. An excellent review is available on this topic.[47]

In hybrid capture target enrichment, oligonucleotide probes for genomic regions of interest are hybridized to a fragmented DNA library, and nonbinding fragments are washed away. The hybridization reaction may occur either on a surface (i.e., a slide) or in solution. In cancer genomics, hybrid capture is commonly used to reduce a full genome library to only those fragments that correspond to exomes. So-called "whole-exome" sequencing reduces the total amount of DNA to be sequenced from 3 Gb to 30 Mb. This reduces computational demands, cost, and sequencing time while still elucidating the majority of somatic mutations likely to occur in human cancers.

As NGS has decreased in cost and increased in reliability, it is being increasingly incorporated into clinical testing. The broad applicability is of special interest in the field of precision medicine. DNA sequencing in a broad field of stage IV solid tumors revealed possible combination therapies in 49% of patients, which significantly prolonged patient survival.[48] DNA sequencing can also be applied on circulating tumor DNA in order to identify druggable mutations without invasive procedures.[49]

DNA alterations and their ways of detection

In order to link diseases to genetic drivers, detecting DNA alterations is crucial. All of the techniques above have brought cancer research forward. Therefore, knowing strengths and weaknesses of the chosen assay is crucial. Exemplary DNA alterations and their way of detection are discussed in Table 1.

Gene expression: mRNA transcript analysis

Structural considerations

The first step in gene expression is transcription of the genetic information from DNA into RNA. The individual building blocks of RNA, ribonucleotides, have the same structure as the deoxyribonucleotides in DNA, except that: (1) the 2′ carbon of the ribose sugar is substituted with an –OH group instead of H and (2) there are no thymine bases in RNA, only uracil (demethylated thymine), which also pairs with adenine by hydrogen bonding. Just like DNA polymerases, the enzyme RNA polymerase II uses the nucleotide sequence of the gene's DNA as a template to form a polymer of ribonucleotides with a sequence complementary to the DNA template.

For accurate transcription, RNA polymerase II must: (1) use the antisense strand of DNA as a template, (2) begin transcription at the start of the gene, and (3) end transcription at the end of the gene. The signals that ensure faithful transcription are provided to RNA polymerase II by DNA in the form of specific nucleotide sequences in the promoter of the gene. After reading and interpreting these signals, the RNA polymerase generates a primary RNA transcript that extends from the initiation site to the termination site in a perfect complementary match to the DNA sequence used as a template. However, not all transcribed RNA is destined to arrive in the cytoplasm as mRNA. Rather, sequences complementary to introns are excised from the primary transcript, and the ends of exon sequences are joined together in a process termed splicing.[67] In addition to splicing, the primary transcript is further modified by the addition of a methylated guanosine triphosphate "cap" at the 5′ end[68] and by the addition of a stretch of anywhere from 20 to 40 adenosine bases at the 3′ end ("poly(A) tail").[69] These modifications appear to promote the translatability[70,71] and relative stability of mRNAs and help direct the subcellular localization of mRNAs destined for translation.

Northern blotting

The fundamental question in the analysis of gene expression at the RNA level is whether RNA sequences derived from a gene of interest are present in a cell type of interest under conditions of interest. Detecting specific RNA sequences can be accomplished by Northern blotting, the whimsically named RNA analog of Southern blotting. Intact RNA can be isolated from cells, free from significant amounts of DNA.[72] Messenger RNA is much smaller than genomic DNA, so it can be analyzed by agarose gel electrophoresis without the enzymatic digestion steps that are necessary for the analysis of high-molecular-weight DNA.

RNA is single-stranded and has a tendency to fold back on itself, allowing complementary bases to base-pair with each other and form what is termed secondary structure. Because secondary structure can lead to aberrant electrophoretic behavior, RNA is electrophoretically separated by size in the presence of a denaturing agent, such as formaldehyde or glyoxal/dimethyl sulfoxide. The RNA is then transferred to a nitrocellulose or nylon-based membrane in the same manner as DNA for Southern blotting (see Figure 4). Hybridization schemes and blot washing for Northern blotting are essentially the same as for Southern blotting. In this manner, specific RNA sequences corresponding to those in cloned DNA probes can easily be identified.

There is a lower limit to the sensitivity of Northern blotting so that only moderately abundant mRNAs can be detected. The sensitivity can be increased by nearly two orders of magnitude by enriching the RNA preparation for mRNA. Ordinarily, mRNA makes up <10% of the total RNA content of a cell or tissue; the remainder is made up primarily of ribosomal RNA and transfer RNA. An RNA preparation can be enriched for mRNA species by removing all RNA molecules that lack the 3′ poly(A) tail,[73] by exposing the preparation to a tract of poly(U) or poly(T) bound to an immobilized support, such as a plastic bead. The poly(A) portion of mRNA will bind to the poly(U) or poly(T) material, and non-poly(A)-containing RNA can be washed away. After washing, the poly(A)-containing mRNA can be recovered from the solid support and used in Northern blot analysis.

A dramatic use of Northern blotting in cancer research has been the demonstration of oncogene expression in RNA isolated from some human tumors. The earliest observations included expression of c-abl and c-myc in human tumor cell lines and leukemic blasts.[74,75] Since these early discoveries, a large number of proto-oncogenes have been shown to be transcribed in primary human tumor tissue.

Complementary DNA

There are exceptions to the central dogma of molecular biology (DNA–RNA–protein), the most prominent of which involves the life cycle of retroviruses. These viruses encode their genetic information in RNA rather than DNA. When they invade a susceptible host cell, they direct the synthesis of a DNA intermediate that is a complimentary copy of their genomic RNA. The enzyme that accomplishes this task, reverse transcriptase (RT), is a DNA polymerase (see above) that uses RNA, rather than DNA, as a template to form a cDNA copy of the RNA.[76,77] This enzyme can be used *in vitro* to make cDNA copies of any available RNA.

One important application of cDNA synthesis has been the construction of cDNA libraries, which are basically gene libraries

Table 1 Exemplary DNA alterations and their way of detection.

	DNA polymorphism (Two or more normal alleles for a single locus with lowest frequency of at least 1% of the population and usually associated with normal phenotype (unlike mutations).)		Copy-number variations	Structural rearrangements

Genotype	Single-nucleotide variants (SNVs) and small insertion–deletions[50]
	Change in DNA sequence
	• Noncoding region
	• Coding region
	  • With changes to AA sequence (nonsynonymous)
	  • Without AA changes (synonymous)
	Detectable both as single nucleotide polymorphism as well as sporadic mutation
		Microsatellites (short tandem repeats, STRs):
		Tandem dC-dA repeats (10–60 times) dispersed in about 50,000 copies throughout the human genome (31), varying in a polymorphic way among individuals
			Restriction fragment length polymorphisms (RFLPs):
			Restriction enzyme recognition sites characteristic for individuals, stably inherited:
			• Creation or loss of restriction site by SNV
			• Sequences of 1–5 kbp with 15–100 nucleotide tandem repeats, varying between individuals (variable number of tandem repeats (VNTRs, minisatellite DNA))[51]
				Change in gene copy numbers (allele loss, duplicates, triplicates, or even quadruplicates) changes gene dosage and may be associated with disease	Gross structural changes (deletions, insertions, duplications, inversions, and translocations (TRAs)) with a size range of 1 kb–3 Mb

Exemplary phenotype	Association of AA change from glycine to arginine at codon 388 in the coding domain of FGFR4 with cancers of breast, skin, prostate, lung, and others[52]	Microsatellite instability in colorectal cancer: differences in number of STR between normal and tumor tissue from the same patient suggest overall genetic instability,[53,54] caused by a mutation in mismatch repair genes. In humans, MSH2 is responsible for hereditary nonpolyposis colorectal cancer[55,56]	Loss of heterozygosity: detection of RFLP loss on one chromosome in tumor tissue implies loss of genetic material in the tumor, typically in tumor suppressor genes, such as retinoblastoma (Rb) or TP53,[57,58] (Figure 7a)	Mutant KRAS dosage promotes initiation, metastasis, and subtype differentiation of pancreatic cancer[59]	Bcr-Abl translocation (Philadelphia chromosome) in CML), parts of the c-abl gene are moved from Chr 22 to Chr 9[60]
Detection in Southern blotting	Not detectable (resolution of 100 nucleotides)	Only longer repeat expansions detectable (resolution of 100 nucleotides)	Alteration of Southern blot pattern between individuals (e.g., SNV change of AGGATTCGA to AGGAATTCGA creates EcoRI recognition site) (see Figure 3)	Deletion or duplication changes band intensity compared to normal control[6]	After translocation of restriction enzyme, Southern blot analysis may now detect • A larger fragment than normal if the recipient chromosome has another EcoRI site farther away or • A smaller fragment if there is a closer EcoRI site
Detection in (real-time) PCR	1. Allele-specific PCR (ASPCR): 3′-terminal base of primer matching wild-type or mutant allele, limited to known mutations or SNPs 2. High-resolution melting (HRM) curve analysis: heat dissociation of dsDNA to ssDNA based on DNA sequence 3. Preferential amplification for one allele by blocking WT amplification or varying denaturing temperature, favoring dissociation of mutant-wildtype alleles over WT-WT alleles (COLD-PCR)[64]	PCR-primer flanking repeat region reveals variable length, standard-of-care method in STR genotyping	Differences in size of PCR-amplification products after restriction enzyme digestion (similar to Southern blotting)	qPCR reveals difference in necessary cycles signal detection (c_q-value) region of interest and control Digital PCR (limiting dilution PCR, diluting DNA content so about only every second well of a microplate contains template), can lower CNV detection limit.[62] Suitable for targeted CNV scans	Translocation with fusion of exons results in chimeric transcript and protein, mRNA based PCR detection with primer spanning exon junction Translocation between genes can result in overexpression of oncogene without chimeric product, only detectable at DNA level, challenging due to multiple possible break-points and large size amplicons.[63] Overall inferior to NGS
Detection in nucleotide sequencing	Statistical differences of nucleotide sequence to reference genome increased specificity by increasing read depth in NGS	Pros: whole-genome sequencing can target multiple loci on one run, identification of insertions/deletions Cons/challenges: repetitive sequence is prone to sequencing errors ("stutter noise"), makes correct alignment difficult, and requires costly long-read sequencing[66]	Underlying genotype change can be detected in NGS, broad applicability of NGS has mostly abolished use of RFLPs in gene mapping	Comparison of read number compared to normal locus.[65] Suitable for whole-genome scans	Paired-end sequencing (from 5′ to 3′ end) result in split reads

consisting only of the genes that are expressed in a cell or tissue of interest,[78,79] and excluding the large proportion of the cell's DNA composed of intronic sequences, promoters, and "noncoding" DNA that lies between genes. One way to construct a library of tissue-specific expressed genes is to clone all of the mRNA in a specific cell or tissue of interest. To make a cDNA library, all of the mRNA is isolated from a cell or tissue. Using this as a template, RT is used to make cDNA copies of each mRNA molecule in the mixture. The cDNA is ligated into a plasmid or phage vector as described earlier (see Figure 3), and the recombinant vectors are introduced into bacteria. After growth on agar plates, each bacterial colony or phage plaque of a cDNA library houses a unique recombinant vector containing the cDNA copy of a single mRNA transcript. Desired clones can be detected by nucleic acid hybridization to the plaques or colonies using a radiolabeled gene probe.[80,81] Alternatively, if the vector containing the cDNA molecules can direct transcription of mRNA by host bacterial cells, mRNA will be synthesized and translated. In this case, each bacterial colony or plaque will produce a different protein, each encoded by an mRNA from the original cell or tissue being investigated. If an antibody directed against a protein of interest is available, the cDNA clone corresponding to the mRNA that encodes that protein can be identified by binding the antibody to the colonies or plaques of the cDNA library. This technique, called expression cloning, often employs the bacteriophage λgt11 as the cloning vector.[82]

cDNA libraries can be used to clone cDNA for a known gene to discover the sequence of the mRNA it encodes. One application of this is the generation of expressed sequence tag databases by sequencing clones of various cDNA libraries. Alternatively, cDNA libraries can be used to identify previously unknown genes. In a process called differential screening, cDNAs can be discovered that owe their existence to a particular differentiation or activation state in the cell of origin. For example, this technique has been used to identify genes whose expression is turned on by hormones or by growth factors.[83]

Sequence-based gene expression profiling

The most comprehensive way to display a unique pattern of gene expression that determines the identity of a cell or tissue would be to construct a cDNA library from it and sequence every clone. This was originally thought to be an impossible task and a technique called serial analysis of gene expression (SAGE) was developed to approximate this goal. In SAGE, a small and unique fragment (10–17 nucleotides in length) of each expressed gene (called a SAGE tag) is sequenced and the number of times it appears quantified (called the SAGE tag number). The SAGE tag numbers, therefore, directly reflect the abundance of the corresponding transcript.

The sensitivity and the quantitative accuracy of SAGE are theoretically unlimited. The generation of a SAGE library does not require any prior knowledge of what genes are expressed in the cell of interest. Therefore, SAGE is able to detect and quantify the expression of previously uncharacterized genes.

The generation of a SAGE library (Figure 9) used to be a technically challenging multistep procedure that has been described in detail elsewhere.[84] However, it has become much more feasible with (and in many cases, has been replaced by) the emergence of single-molecule sequencing platforms.[41]

SAGE has been used for the comparison of gene expression profiles of different cell types from normal and tumor tissue[85] and is one of the techniques used by the National Cancer Institute-funded Cancer Gene Anatomy Project (CGAP),[86] an international database aimed at cataloging the genes expressed in various normal and cancerous tissue types. SAGE libraries generated as part of the CGAP project are deposited on the National Center for Biotechnology Education/CGAP SAGE map web site (http://cgap.nci.nih.gov/SAGE).[86,87]

DNA microarray analysis

Another approach to comparative gene expression profiling employs the use of DNA microarrays (Figure 10), often referred to as DNA chips. Two basic types of DNA microarrays are currently available: oligonucleotide arrays[88,89] and cDNA arrays.[90,91] Both involve the immobilization of DNA sequences in a gridded array on the surface of a solid support, such as a glass microscope slide or silicon wafer. In the case of oligonucleotide arrays, 25-nt long fragments of known DNA sequence are synthesized *in situ* on the surface of the chip using a series of light-directed coupling reactions similar to photolithography. As many as 400,000 distinct sequences representing over 18,000 genes can be synthesized on a single 1.3×1.3 cm microarray. In the case of cDNA microarrays, cDNA fragments are deposited onto the surface of a glass slide using a robotic spotting device. For both approaches, the next step involves the purification of RNA from the source of interest (e.g., from a tumor), enzymatic fluorescent labeling of the RNA, and hybridization of the fluorescently labeled material to the microarray. Hybridization events are captured by scanning the surface of the microarray with a laser-scanning device and measuring the fluorescence intensity at each position in the microarray. The fluorescence intensity of each spot on the array is proportional to the level of expression of the gene represented by that spot.

Microarray analysis has proven to be a powerful method for the analysis of gene expression patterns in human cancer and for cancer classification. Gene expression profiles have been used for class prediction, for determining which samples belong to which tumor class, and for class discovery of new tumor types. The first proof of principle for gene expression analysis in cancer was the demonstration that acute myeloid leukemias and acute lymphoid leukemias could be accurately distinguished on the basis of their gene expression profile.[92] Since then, new cancer classes have been discovered in leukemias,[93] lymphomas,[94,95] brain cancer,[96] breast cancer,[97,98] prostate cancer,[99,100] lung cancer,[101,102] and others.

The challenge in interpreting microarray data is in recognizing meaningful gene expression patterns and in distinguishing those patterns from noise. Such noise (random gene expression levels) can be generated by (1) variability among microarrays, (2) variability in RNA labeling and hybridization methods, and, perhaps most importantly, (3) biologic variability among samples. It is likely that all of the above sources of variability are significant. Many of the problems associated with array-based technologies are eliminated with the use of sequence-based methods described in the section titled "Transcriptomic sequencing". Thus, as sequencing technologies have improved and become more affordable and widely available, microarray technology has become less used.

Reverse-transcriptase polymerase chain reaction (RT-PCR)

Another important use of cDNA technology has allowed PCR to be applied to RNA. DNA polymerases cannot use RNA as a template. However, if an RNA of interest is made into cDNA, then PCR can proceed as usual. The first step is generating a cDNA copy of the mRNA of interest using RT. This can be done using a primer consisting of Ts (complementary to the poly(A) tail) or of another sequence complementary to some portion of the 3′ region

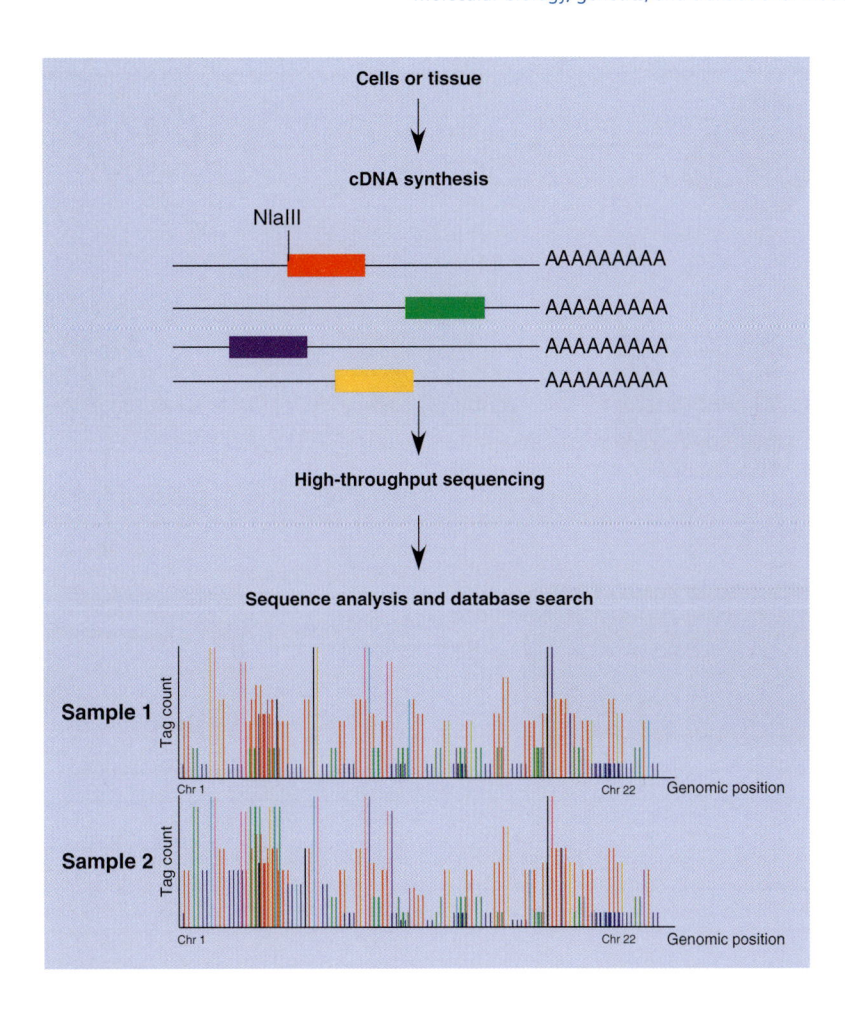

Figure 9 Construction and analysis of serial analysis of gene expression (SAGE) libraries. In step 1, a complementary deoxyribonucleic acid (cDNA) library is constructed from the cells or tissue of interest, and the cDNAs are immobilized on magnetic beads at their 3′ ends. In step 2, the cDNAs are subjected to restriction enzyme digestion with a so-called anchoring enzyme. This anchoring enzyme is a frequent cutter restriction endonuclease (usually NlaIII) that ensures that all of the cDNAs are cut at least once. Subsequently, another linker is ligated to the cDNA ends that contains a recognition site for a tagging enzyme. This tagging enzyme is a type two restriction endonuclease (usually MmeI) that cuts at some distance to the 3′ side of the actual recognition site. These tags are then directly processed for single-molecule DNA sequencing platform. Data are analyzed using software that reads the sequence obtained, derives the tags, matches them to their cognate cDNA, and gives the gene expression profile in a numeric format.

of the mRNA. Once the single-stranded cDNA is produced, it can be amplified in a standard PCR reaction using Taq polymerase as described earlier (see Figure 5). In one of the first applications of this technique, Philadelphia chromosome–positive leukemias were diagnosed by identifying chimeric bcr-abl mRNA species in clinical material using PCR. Since then, Reverse-transcriptase polymerase chain reaction (RT-PCR) has come into widespread clinical and laboratory use.[103]

One inherent problem in using standard PCR to monitor mRNA expression is quantitation of the amplified PCR products. In Northern blotting analysis, the intensity of the hybridization signal is directly proportional to the amount of target RNA in the sample. Thus, one can compare the number of RNA molecules in one sample with another. With PCR, however, a slight change in the efficiency of polymerization in an early cycle will lead to a geometrically increasing discrepancy between the amount of amplified product in that sample compared with another sample, and the amounts of PCR product when the reaction reaches saturation can also differ significantly. Fortunately, a number of techniques have been described for normalizing the products of PCRs to allow quantitative comparisons.

Most notably, quantitative RT-PCR[104] is a method for continuous monitoring of amplification. This method makes quantitative comparisons of amplifications during the unbiased linear range in which each cycle gives a constant increase in amplification. In one common method of quantitative RT-PCR, a fluorogenic probe that contains a fluorescent tag on one end and a quencher on the other end is designed within the amplified region. Amplification leads to digestion of the probe, thus liberating a free fluorescent molecule; the increase in fluorescence with each cycle is measured and is proportional to the amplification.

Transcriptomic sequencing

Within the last decade, RNA-sequencing ("RNA-Seq") has become the standard tool for transcriptome analysis, as it allows for precise characterization of the transcripts in a cell at single-nucleotide resolution. While microarray analysis, SAGE, quantitative RT-PCR, and Northern blotting can be used to quantify known transcript abundance, RNA-Seq allows for novel transcript discovery. This affords the ability to discover mutant genes in cancer cells, identify new RNA species, analyze alternative-splicing patterns, and interrogate RNA-editing and other RNA-processing events.

General technique and workflow

After RNA isolation from a sample of interest, the desired RNA species should be enriched. For example, mRNA, most commonly

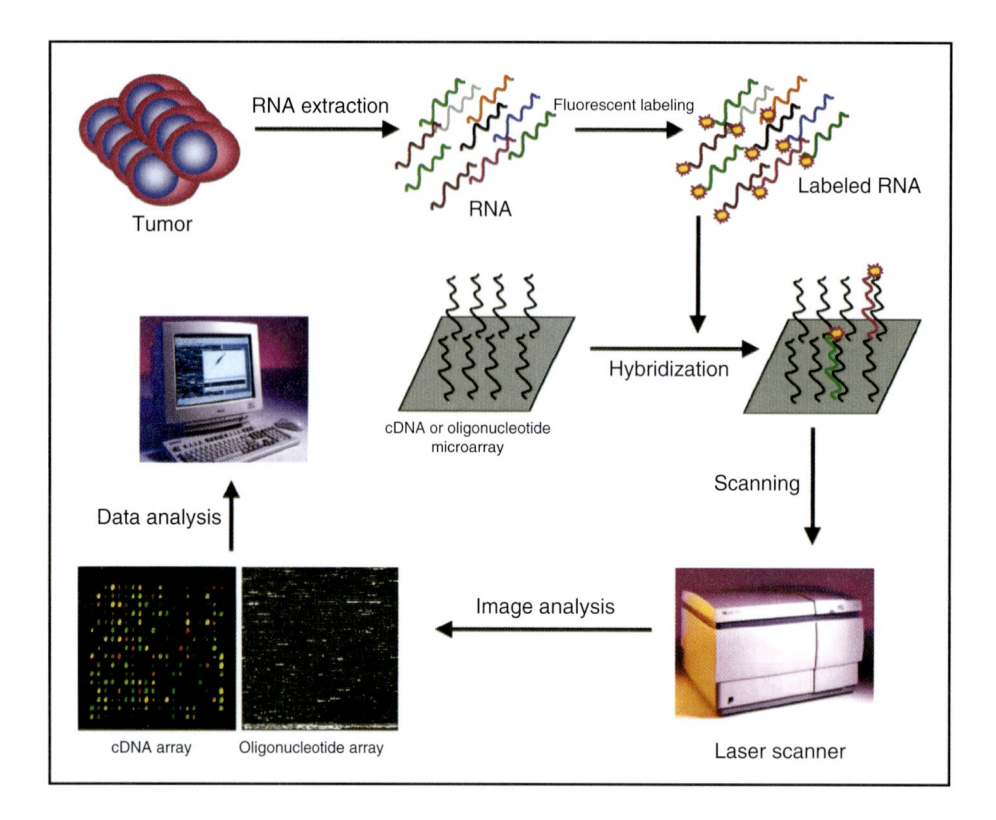

Figure 10 DNA microarray analysis. In this example, RNA extracted from a tumor is end-labeled with a fluorescent marker and then allowed to hybridize to a chip derivatized with complementary DNA (cDNAs) or oligonucleotides, as described in the text. The precise location of RNA hybridization to the chip can be determined using a laser scanner. Because the position of each unique cDNA or oligonucleotide is known, the presence of a cognate RNA for any given unique sequence can be determined.

the species of interest, is enriched by using probes that hybridize to the poly(A) 3′ tail and thereby depletes ribosomal and transfer RNAs. Generally, the isolated RNA is first reverse-transcribed into cDNA, and platform-specific sequencing adaptors are ligated to both 3′ and 5′ end. These are needed in order to amplify and sequence previously unknown transcripts sequences as the use of only poly(A) primers would lead to a 3′ bias and the use of only random primers may cause a substantial loss of information. Next, PCR amplification reduces the initial RNA amount required and enables the sequencing of transcripts with low abundance. This whole process is termed RNA-seq library preparation, and this library can now be sequenced using NGS (Figure 11).

RNA sequences must be "assembled" to reconstruct the transcripts that comprise the transcriptome. This is usually done by aligning the reads to a reference genome. Read alignments are assembled into transcript models using computational methods and expression levels of individual transcripts are quantified.[105–107]

RNA-Seq offers excellent dynamic range and the opportunity to identify unannotated transcripts, splice variants, gene-fusions, nonhuman transcripts, and somatic mutations, among other events. This is a significant advantage over microarray analysis, which is limited by a defined set of predesigned probes.[65]

Short-read sequencing
Short-read sequencing refers to the length of the cDNA sequence prepared during the library preparation and is necessary due to length limitations of certain sequencing platforms, for example <600 bp on the Illumina.[108] Therefore, before cDNA synthesis, RNA will be intentionally fragmented. This can be done by alkaline solutions, solutions containing divalent cations, such as Mg++, Zn++, or enzymatical cleavage including RNases,[109] and ideally results in random fragments. cDNA copies following RT are mostly within the 50–250 bp range. The library is then sequenced to an average of 20–30 million reads per sample. This form of RNA sequencing represents the most widely used form and has been used for the vast majority of all published RNA sequencing data. The sequencing data are bioinformatically processed using differential gene expression analysis (DGEA), in order to compare transcriptional differences between different experimental conditions. Additionally, short-range cDNA sequencing is also used in most other RNA-seq applications, including single-cell RNA-seq, and sequencing of additional non-mRNA species including small RNAs.

Long-read sequencing (cDNA and direct RNA sequencing)
Unlike the commonly used Illumina platform for short-read sequencing, the Pacific Biosciences and Oxford Nanopore platforms offer long-read sequencing. These novel approaches do not first fragment the RNA, and instead, sequence full-length transcripts. The Pacific Biosciences platform requires a full-length cDNA transcript, which is subjected to single-molecule real-time sequencing (SMRT). The name refers to a single molecule of DNA polymerase inside a so-called zero-mode waveguide (ZMV). The polymerase uses fluorescently labeled dNTPs, and the emitted signal during DNA synthesis can be detected in the ZMVs.[110] The Oxford Nanopore platform uses a different approach from other sequencing platforms. A protein nanopore in an electrically resistant membrane forms the basis of the nanopore device and a voltage is set across the membrane. Once the nucleotide sequence passes through the pore, the change in electric current can be detected.

In regular RT, premature termination of reverse transcription is a known problem, so the 5′ end tends to be underrepresented

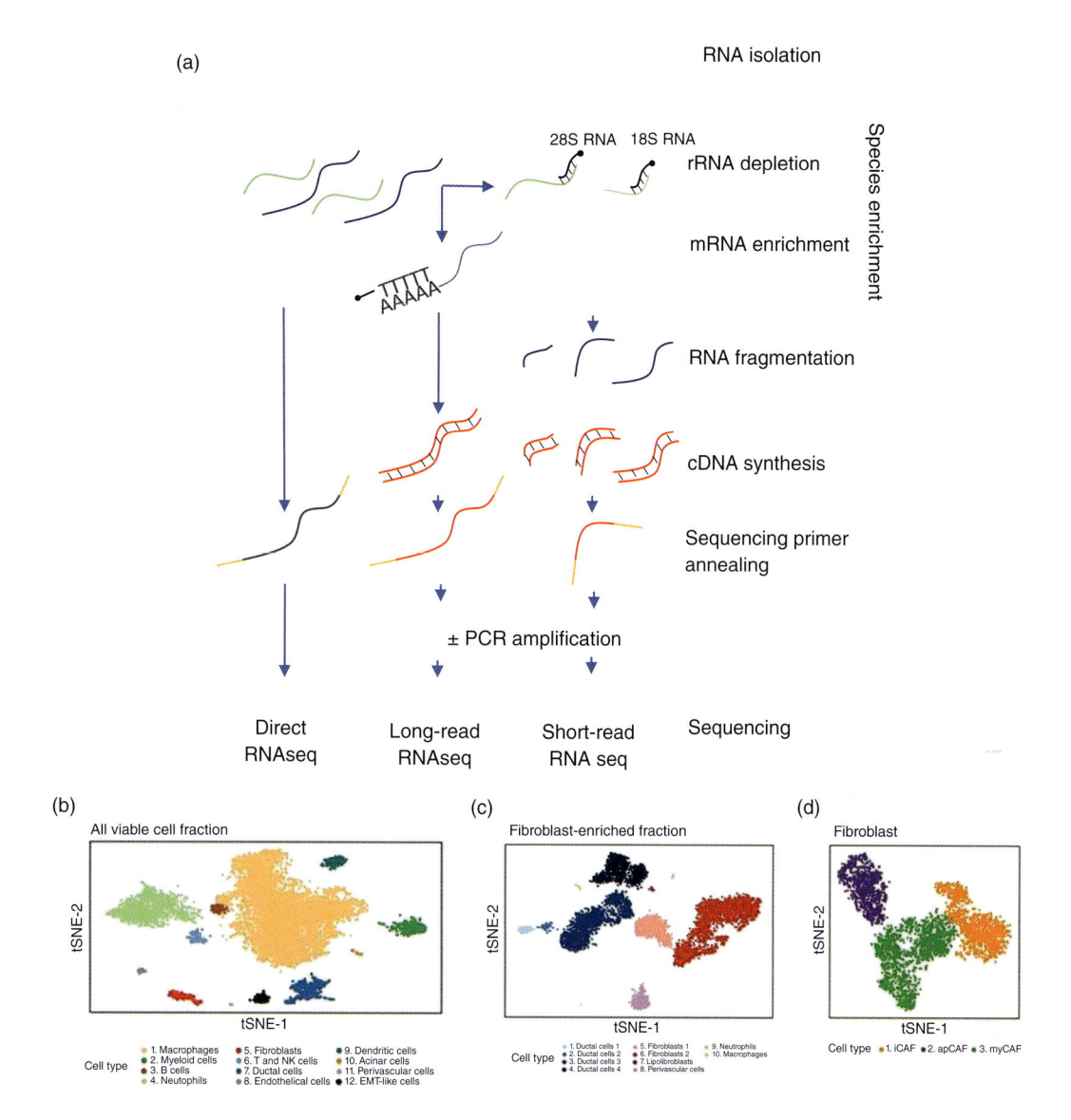

Figure 11 General workflow of RNAseq library preparation: After RNA isolation, the species of interest is enriched for (green, ribosomal RNA; blue, mRNA; red, cDNA). For short-read sequencing, RNA is fragmented. Except ONT, sequencing platforms need DNA templates (therefore cDNA synthesis). Sequencing primers (yellow) are annealed to all forms of RNA preparation. PCR amplification can reduce the initial amount of RNA needed. (a) Exemplary single-cell analysis of pancreatic cancer derived from a KPC mouse with unsupervised clustering of all viable cells displayed in different colored clusters. (b) Unsupervised clustering of the fibroblast-enriched fraction from (b), containing Fibroblasts but also EpCAM negative ductal cells and others (c) Identification of a new CAF-subtype (apCAF, purple) through unsupervised clustering of fibroblast fraction (clusters 5 and 6) from (c). (b–d) is obtained from Elyada et al[123] with kind permission from the American Association for Cancer Research.

(3′ bias) and no full-length cDNA copies are synthesized. Therefore, conversion to cDNA is achieved by template-switching RT. The reverse transcription and template switching properties of the Moloney murine leukemia virus (MMLV) RT is exploited for that cause: Once MMLV-RT reaches the 5′ end of the RNA template, it adds additional nucleotides to the 3′ end of the newly synthesized cDNA strand, mainly dCTPs (terminal transferase activity). This sequence pairs with an additionally added Oligonucleotide containing a GGG sequence, and MMLV-RT now switches templates from the original RNA strand to the Oligonucleotides. Replication is continued until RT reaches the end of the oligonucleotide.[111] The resulting cDNA strand now has one known primer site for PCR amplification on both ends. If RT pauses before reaching the 5′ end, the addition of nucleotides is less efficient and without pairing to the Oligonucleotide, the second priming site is absent and thus the truncated cDNA will not be exponentially amplified.

The Oxford Nanopore platform even offers direct RNA-seq. By removing the RT step, information on the RNA strand itself can be retained. This includes epigenetic modification and poly(A) tail length analysis. Although posttranscriptional RNA-modification has been known since the 1950s, its physiologic functions and associated diseases have only been studied more extensively through the development of epi-transcriptomic sequencing in recent years.[112,113] The most abundant mRNA modification is N6-methyl adenosine (m^{6}A) and has been associated with pro- and anti-tumorigenic functions, for example accumulation of m^{6}A on MYC transcripts decreased RNA stability and thus reduced MYC signaling in leukemic diseases.[114]

Overall, long-read sequencing offers the opportunity of sequencing complete individual RNA stands with up to 50 kb and is therefore especially useful in detecting different splice forms and alternative start sites of genes.

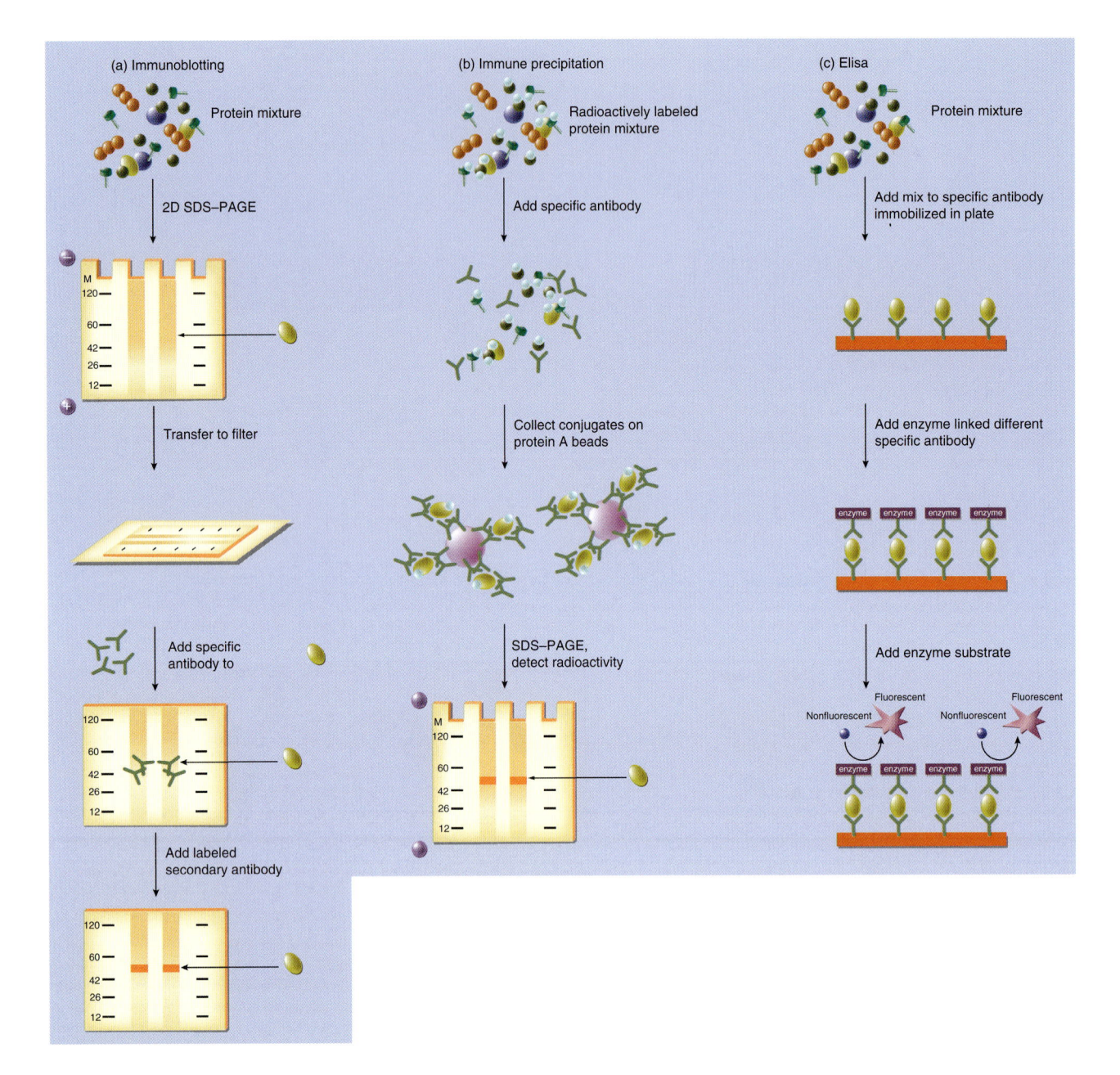

Figure 12 Methods of protein identification and detection. (a) Immune (Western) blotting. A complex mixture of proteins can be separated by size using electrophoresis (SDS–PAGE). The separated proteins are then transferred to a nitrocellulose or nylon filter in an electric field, maintaining their size-specific spatial orientation on the filter. Antibodies directed against one specific protein (in this case, the gray ellipsoid) in the original mixture are added to the filter and bind to the specific protein. Bound antibodies can be radiolabeled or enzymatically labeled themselves, or they can be visualized by incubating the filter with labeled anti-immunoglobulin antibodies. (b) Immunoprecipitation. A complex mixture of radiolabeled proteins (indicated by different geometric shapes) is incubated with antibodies specific for one of those proteins (in this case, the gray ellipsoid). After the antibodies have bound to their protein, small polystyrene or agarose beads containing staphylococcal protein A are added to the mixture. Protein A binds to the antibodies, and when centrifuged, the beads to which the protein A is bound will sediment to the bottom of the centrifuge tube, taking along the antibodies and the specific protein to which they have bound. The unbound proteins remain in the supernatant and can be removed. After boiling to dissociate the protein A/antibody/protein complex, specifically precipitated radiolabeled protein can be visualized by electrophoresis (SDS–PAGE) and autoradiography. (c) Enzyme-linked immunosorbent assay (ELISA). To perform ELISA, one needs to develop two independent antibodies that bind to the protein to be detected (gray ellipsoid in this example) with high specificity and affinity. One of these antibodies is then coupled to a plate, which is then incubated with the protein mix to be analyzed (this can be tissue, blood, or another body fluid). The specifically bound protein is retained on the plate and is detected with the second antibody generated against it that is coupled to an enzyme or isotope, allowing quantitation of the bound protein. ELISAs are usually very sensitive and can detect picomolar amounts of proteins.

Advantages and disadvantages of sequencing techniques
Short-read sequencing excels in robust, reliable, and affordable sequencing and very high sequencing depth with up to 20 billion reads per sample. Thereby, it enables the discovery of transcripts at the lowest transcription levels and large-scale DGEA.

Long-read sequencing, on the other hand, by sequencing ideally the whole transcript strand is especially useful in discovering different isoforms. However, long-read sequencing cannot reach the depth and high throughput of short reads.

In the end, besides availability, the technique to use depends on the question the experiment seeks to answer: High throughput screens and the search for genes at low transcript levels remain in the arms of short-read platforms; while in isoform discovery, the lower read depth is not an issue and long-read sequencing can be performed.

Single-cell sequencing (scRNA seq)
The high throughput opportunities in novel sequencing platforms enabled the development of the rapidly evolving field of single-cell RNA sequencing. In regular RNA-seq, bulk RNA extraction is performed. Within tissues, this fails to preserve information on cellular localization, and obviously does not give any information on the transcriptome of an individual cell. In scRNA sequencing, the tissue is dissociated into single cells, for example by mechanical disaggregation or enzymatic digestion.[115] For separation, labeling and RNA extraction of the single cells, various techniques have been developed.[116] The following library preparation steps are comparable to bulk RNA sequencing.

The major strength of scRNA seq lies within the analysis of tissue heterogeneity. It enables the identification of previously unknown cell subtypes and cell substates. During the computational analysis, cells can be grouped into unsupervised clusters or lined up along trajectories of cellular fate. The clusters can be dissected into subpopulations of cells, and rare, unknown cell populations can be identified. Similarly, different states of the same cell lineage can be studied on the cellular trajectories. This includes evolutionary processes but also states of oncogenic progression.[117] The applications of scRNA seq in cancer research have become extremely diverse.

First, in the sense of oncogenic trajectories: scRNA seq can be applied at all stages of the disease. In comparison of biopsies from premalignant lesions of gastric cancer at the scRNA level,[118] Zhang et al.[118] were able to identify cells at risk of oncogenic transformation including goblet cells, a hallmark of cells in intestinal metaplasia; and, furthermore, discovered a signature of six genes that are specific for early gastric cancer. By seeking these genetic alterations, detection of early gastric cancer might be facilitated. Similarly, in lung adenocarcinoma, single-cell comparisons of normal tissue with primary and metastatic cancers identified different tumor cell trajectories and gene sets of late-stage signatures were predictive for poor patient outcomes.[119]

Second, multiple studies have revealed intratumoral heterogeneity by applying scRNA seq,[120] including the discovery of previously unknown tumor cell subtypes. In the stroma-rich pancreatic cancer, cancer-associated fibroblasts (CAFs) increasingly drew attention through the discovery of two different subtypes with distinct phenotypes and gene expression profiles.[121,122] By using scRNA seq, not only could the presence of these subtypes be confirmed in various patient tissues, but also an additional subtype was identified[123] (Figure 11). The clinical importance comes through the discovery of their distinct functions. Up to now, most clinical studies targeting stromal components in pancreatic cancer have failed, and a clinical trial targeting the Hedgehog pathway in fibroblasts surprisingly showed adverse effects.[124] Indeed, one possibility that is currently being evaluated using scRNA seq is whether Hedgehog inhibitors differentially diminish tumor-suppressing CAFs while expanding tumor-promoting CAF subtypes.

Third, scRNA seq has also been used in multiple studies to address the question of therapy resistance. The comparison of a primary melanoma cell line with BRAF-inhibitor-resistant daughter clones revealed a small subpopulation that was initially present in the parental line, developing this approach as a predictive method for BRAF resistance.[125] Similarly, scRNA seq analysis of a patient-derived xenograft (PDX) derived from a metastatic, muscle-invasive urothelial bladder cancer before and after treatment with Tipifarnib (Farnesyltransferase inhibitor) showed PDL-1 upregulation in surviving cancer cells. The subsequent treatment of the donor patient with the PDL-1 inhibitor atezolizumab showed a favorable response.[126]

Clinical application of gene expression profiling
A number of gene expression profiling-based diagnostic tests have been approved by the Federal Drug Administration (FDA), and these are increasingly being incorporated into the clinical management of patients diagnosed with early-stage breast cancer.[127,128] Examples include the Oncotype DX,[129] Mammaprint,[130] PAM50,[131] and the H : I ratio Breast Cancer Index.[132] Each of these tests uses the expression level of a set of genes (from 2 to 70 genes) to provide prognostic information about a patient's breast cancer recurrence risk. These and other expression-based tests vary in their clinical utility, indications, and diagnostic validity. The Oncotype DX, or 21-gene recurrence score, is the most widely used and has been incorporated into management guidelines from the American Society of Clinical Oncology (ASCO).

The Oncotype DX score was developed based on testing of the expression of a candidate gene set (250 cancer-related genes) by quantitative RT-PCR in fixed tissue from a large number of patients collected from three different datasets. The score was validated in an independent dataset derived from samples banked on a large prospective randomized trial (NSABP B-14) designed to test the benefit of adjuvant tamoxifen in hormone-receptor-positive, node-negative breast cancer.[129] A gene signature composed of 21 genes was found to predict 10-year breast cancer recurrence. The expression levels of these 21 genes measured by quantitative RT-PCR combined with a quantitative algorithm are used to produce a number between 0 and 100, termed the recurrence score. The recurrence score is categorized into low (score <18), intermediate (score >18 but <30), and high (score ≥30). Several follow-up studies in various cohorts have confirmed that the Oncotype DX recurrence score is among the best-validated prognostic assays available. It is currently used to guide prognosis in women with node-negative, estrogen receptor (ER)-positive breast cancer, and to inform the decision about whether these women are likely to glean benefit from adjuvant chemotherapy. In practice, women with a low recurrence score have a favorable prognosis and are unlikely to derive significant absolute benefit from adjuvant chemotherapy.

As more and more genomic and transcriptomic data are generated and curated, increasing effort has been placed on developing molecular prognostic tests for a variety of tumor types. It is important to carefully consider the clinical utility, exact indications, and precisely defined patient population for application of these tests. At present, molecular prognostic profiles available can supplement, but not replace, clinical prognostic factors.

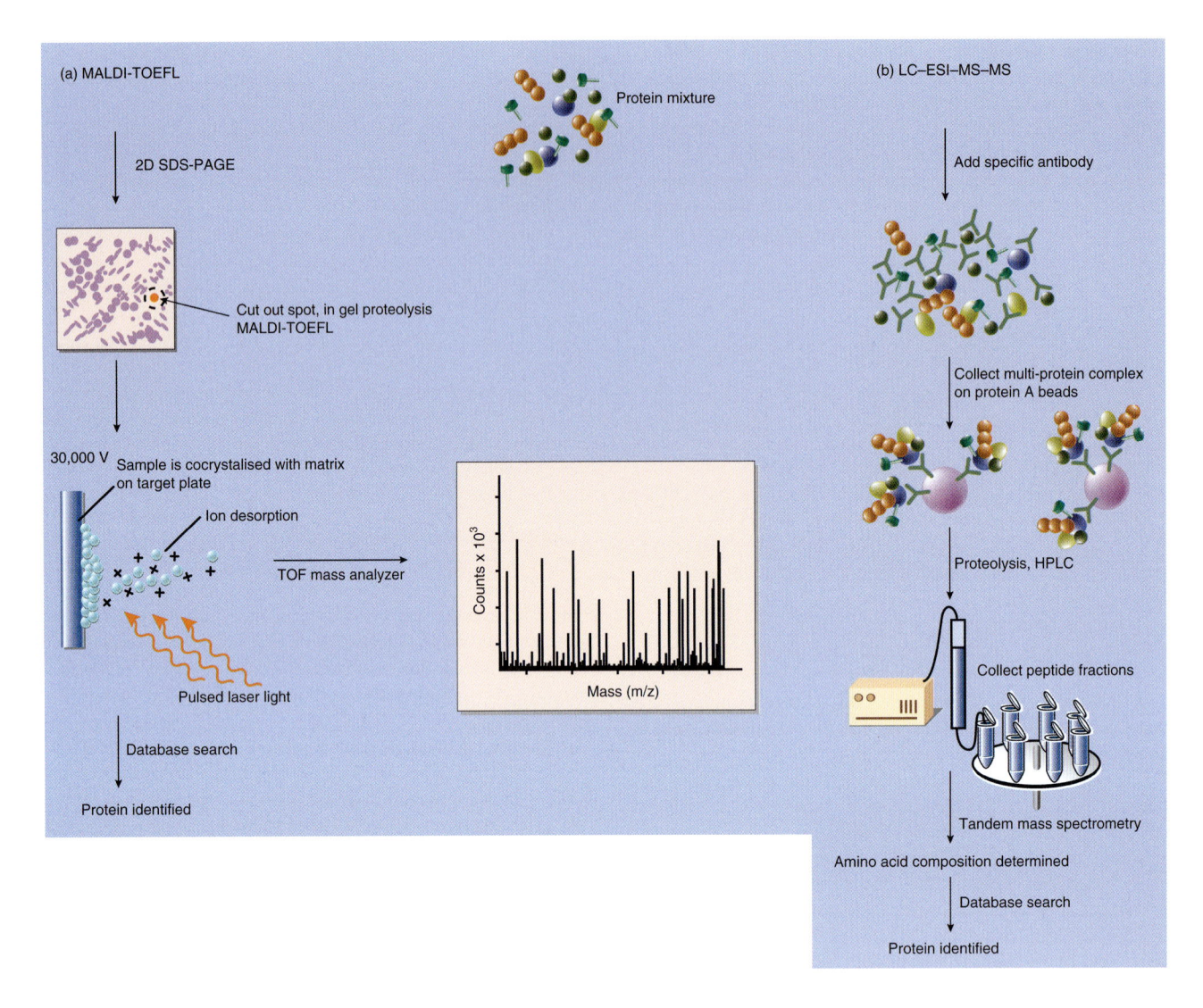

Figure 13 Mass spectrometry. (a) Matrix-assisted laser desorption ionization time-of-flight mass spectrometry (MALDI-TOF). For organisms whose genome sequence is known, the identification of "interesting" protein spots from a two-dimensional gel is routinely performed using MALDI-TOF. A complex mixture of proteins is separated by size and charge using two-dimensional electrophoresis. Protein spots are excised from the gel, digested with a protease, mixed with a matrix solution, and allowed to cocrystallize on a target plate. When a laser is fired at the target plate, the matrix absorbs the laser light's energy and vaporizes, carrying some of the sample with it into a vacuum space. At the time the laser is fired, a high voltage is applied to the target plate to accelerate the ionized sample's movement toward the time-of-flight (TOF) mass analyzer. The resulting peptide fingerprint can then be used to search databases to determine the identity of the protein. (b) The liquid chromatography-electrospray ionization tandem mass spectrometry (LC–ESIMS–MS) can be used to obtain amino acid sequence information, allowing highly refined database searches. The approach employs capillary high-performance liquid chromatography (HPLC), which allows very slow (submicroliter/min) flow rates that are essential for obtaining high-sensitivity ESI–MS–MS of peptides. Following the liquid chromatography and electrospray ionization, the ions are analyzed by linearly linked tandem mass spectrometers that yield amino acid composition information.

Epigenetic regulation

In recent decades, the search for genes implicated in tumorigenesis has focused on genes that are genetically altered in tumors. However, recent studies suggest that epigenetic modifications are also likely to play a role in tumorigenesis. Epigenetic modifications affect the expression of genes without causing any alterations in DNA sequence. Epigenetic regulatory programs depend on DNA methylation, chromatin (histone) modification, and noncoding RNAs, each of which plays a role in regulating cellular differentiation and tumorigenesis. For example, DNA methylation plays an important role in silencing gene expression, imprinting, and X-chromosome inactivation.[133–135] Inherited defects in DNA methylation and imprinting result in developmental defects and increase the risk of tumorigenesis. Recent data also implicate DNA methylation and chromatin changes as initiating events in neoplasia preceding the occurrence of genetic alterations.[136–138] Introducing a hypomorphic allele of the DNA methyltransferase gene *DNMT1* into the mouse germline led to 90% decrease in DNA methylation and subsequently to cancer development.[139]

Several novel technologies allow the comprehensive analysis of epigenetic modifications at a genome-wide scale. Methylation-sensitive arbitrarily primed polymerase chain reaction (MS-AP-PCR),[140] methylated CpG island amplification followed by restriction difference analysis (MCARDA),[141] CpG island arrays coupled with differential methylation hybridization (DMH),[142] restriction length genome scanning (RLGS) using methylation-sensitive enzymes,[143] methyl-CpG binding domain affinity chromatography,[144] and gene expression profiling following demethylation/deacetylation treatment,[145] all have been successfully used for the identification of novel methylated loci in different cancer types.[146] Methylation-specific digital karyotyping (MSDK) is a sequence-based technology that enables comprehensive and unbiased genome-wide DNA methylation analysis.[147] Using a combination of a methylation-sensitive mapping enzyme (e.g., EagI) and a fragmenting enzyme (e.g., NlaIII), short sequence tags can be obtained and uniquely mapped to genome location. The number of MSDK tags obtained from a sample reflects the methylation status of the mapping enzyme sites.

Methylations sensitive sequencing

DNA methylation and chromatin modification are interrelated processes that may be linked by noncoding RNAs.[146,148] Recently, the number and type of known histone modifications have increased dramatically, and a large set of enzymes has been identified that play a role in mediating these processes. The four core histones (H2A, H2B, H3, and H4) have been found to be subject to various posttranslational modifications, including acetylation, methylation, phosphorylation, ubiquitination, sumoylation, adenosine diphosphate (ADP) ribosylation, deimination, and proline isomerization. Most of these modifications regulate transcription by influencing the recruitment of other proteins, and a few are also involved in DNA repair and chromatin condensation. Using antibodies specifically recognizing methylated histone H3-lys9 and the recently developed ChIP-on-chip,[149] GMAT (genome-wide mapping technique),[150] and ChIP-Seq[151] technologies, it is now possible to analyze heterochromatin changes at a genome-wide scale.

Several recent studies suggest that cancers display a profound genome-wide epigenetic dysregulation.[152] Interestingly, several large-scale cancer genome sequencing projects have also revealed somatic mutations in epigenetic modifier proteins. Examples include mutation of the DNA methyltransferase DNMT3A in acute myeloid leukemia,[153,154] mutation of enzymes involved in DNA demethylation (e.g., TET2, IDH1, IDH2) in myeloid leukemias and gliomas,[155–157] mutation of the histone methyltransferase SETD2 in renal cell carcinoma,[158] mutation of the histone demethylase KDM6A in bladder cancer,[159] and many others. This highlights the fact that tumorigenesis is likely promoted through cooperation between aberrant epigenetic modifications and genetic mutations, with mutations at times occurring in the epigenetic modifiers themselves.

Gene expression: protein analysis

Regardless of genetic and transcriptomic changes, the protein is the final effector of the cellular phenotype, so adequate ways of analyzing protein expression and modification are essential.

Sodium dodecyl sulfate–polyacrylamide gel electrophoresis (SDS–PAGE)

The most common analytic technique applied to proteins is separation by size using electrophoresis. Proteins do not show a uniform charge-to-mass ratio like nucleic acids. Therefore, before running the gel, the anionic detergent sodium dodecyl sulfate (SDS) is added, which binds uniformly to proteins. Thus, all proteins become polyanions and the number of negative charges (supplied by the sulfate group in SDS) is directly proportional to the size, or molecular weight, of the protein. In the presence of an electric field, proteins in SDS will migrate toward the anode at a rate inversely proportional to the log of their molecular weights.[160] SDS–PAGE forms an integral component of most protein analysis techniques summarized in Table 2.

Engineered protein expression

The final goal of many molecular biology experiments is engineered protein expression, or the use of biologic systems to synthesize the protein encoded by the gene being studied. When the expressed protein synthesized by recombinant DNA methods is shown to have all of the properties of the natural protein, this is considered proof that the proper gene was cloned. Alternatively, expression can be an end in itself when one wants to produce large amounts of a particular protein that might be difficult to obtain from natural sources.

In vitro translation

One simple expression method is *in vitro* translation, which occurs entirely in a test tube. All of the components necessary for translating mRNA can be obtained from cells that are highly efficient in protein synthesis, such as reticulocytes (usually from rabbits) or wheat germ. Under the appropriate conditions, and in the presence of all 20 amino acids, a synthetic or purified RNA added to such a system will be efficiently translated into protein. If a radioactive amino acid, such as [^{35}S]methionine, is included in the mix, the reaction products can be analyzed by SDS–PAGE and autoradiography. Demonstrating an appropriately sized protein or one that is recognized by a specific antibody constitutes good evidence that the mRNA is the one desired.

Large-scale production of recombinant proteins

In vitro translation can be applied only at a small-scale analytic level. Producing large amounts of protein requires *in vivo* expression systems. One of the simplest involves cloning the cDNA for the desired protein into a bacterial plasmid or phage that contains a transcriptional promoter active in bacteria. When introduced into the appropriate bacterial host, large amounts of mRNA will be transcribed and translated into protein. The recombinant protein can be purified away from all of the bacterial proteins. Some clinically available interferons[170–172] have been produced by this method.

Bacteria do not have the machinery required to accomplish complex posttranslational modifications required by many eukaryotic proteins, such as the addition of specific carbohydrate groups. Moreover, the interior milieu of a bacterial cell is a reducing environment so that disulfide bonds essential to the structure and function of many eukaryotic proteins cannot form. When these modifications are required, mammalian cells can be used for expression. The basic concept is the same as in bacterial systems: a cDNA is cloned into a vector with a eukaryotic transcriptional promoter, and the resulting recombinant DNA is introduced into mammalian cells.[173] However, there are still significant disadvantages in the use of mammalian cells for large-scale recombinant protein production. Mammalian cells are expensive to grow *in vitro* because they require a medium rich in nutrients and growth factors. Yeast, insect, and even plant cells are being exploited as an attractive compromise between mammalian and bacterial cell culture for protein expression. These eukaryotic cells can execute most of the posttranslational modifications required by mammalian proteins, including disulfide bonding, while being easier and more economical to grow *in vitro*. A number of expression vectors analogous to those described for bacteria and animal cells have been developed for these alternative hosts. Interested readers are referred to in-depth articles.[174,175]

Table 2 Protein analysis techniques.

	Separation technique	Readout	Exemplary application
Immunoblotting (western blotting) (Figure 12)	SDS electrophoresis, followed by electrophoretic transfer to immobilized membrane	Antibody binding to proteins on membrane, followed by detection due to enzymatic assay or radioisotope emission	"Gold standard" for detecting protein overexpression; detection of HER2 OE in breast cancer[25]
Immune-precipitation	Antibody-based pulldown of proteins of interest in protein mixture followed by SDS electrophoresis separation	Antibody labeling or autoradiography for radiolabeled proteins	Discovery of virus-based oncologic transformation[161,162]
Enzyme-linked immunosorbent assay (ELISA)	Immobilized antibodies on test plates bind protein of interest	Secondary, enzyme-linked antibody binds proportional to captured amount of protein; fluorescent, chemiluminescent, or colorimetric substrate gives proportional readout	Measurement of serum protein levels (PSA)[163]
Mass spectrometry[164] (Figure 13)	Sample purification for example, by SDS–PAGE, followed by protein ionization and magnetic separation	Mass-to-charge ratio, alignment with reference database can identify protein of interest	Stable isotope labeling by amino acids in cell culture (SILAC): culturing cells with or without heavy AA can quantify protein abundance between samples[165]
Protein sequencing	Purification for example, by SDS–PAGE	• Edman degradation: sequential cleavage of N-terminal AA[166] • Mass spectrometry (see above) • Future directions: single-molecule detection for example by nanopore sequencing[169] (insights into protein sequencing with an α-hemolysin nanopore by atomistic simulations, Giovanni Di Muccio)	Simian sarcoma virus' transforming gene shows nearly identical AA sequence as B chain of human PDGF[167,168]

Methods for analyzing protein–protein interactions

An important and challenging task in postgenomic biology is to understand the function of proteins encoded by the genome and to determine their involvement in signaling pathways and cellular networks. One approach is to investigate the interaction of a protein with other proteins of known function. By performing such analysis at a genome-wide level, one can create protein–protein physical interaction networks.[176] These networks can be combined with gene expression or other genomic data to generate regulatory and signaling networks at the cellular level. Several methods allow the characterization of protein–protein interactions at a genome-wide scale. These include comprehensive protein pull-down assays, protein chips, and two-hybrid screens. Comprehensive protein pull-down assays use the combination of immunoprecipitation and mass spectrometric methods, whereas protein chips apply microarray technology originally used for DNA or RNA profiling for protein interaction analysis.

The classic two-hybrid screen is performed in yeast and is based on the Gal4 system. Gal4 is a yeast transcriptional factor with well-defined and functionally distinct DNA binding (DB) and trans-activator (TA) domains and a DNA target sequence. In the two-hybrid screen, the two proteins to be analyzed are fused to the DB and TA domains of Gal4, respectively. The resulting fusion proteins are referred to as "bait" and "prey." If the two proteins interact, then the DB and TA domains are brought into close proximity and create a functional transcriptional activator, the activity of which can be monitored using various reporter genes. The two-hybrid screen can be performed at three different levels: (1) testing the interaction of two known proteins, (2) testing the interaction of a known protein with all proteins, and (3) testing the interaction among all proteins. Unlike other approaches used for analyzing protein–protein interactions, the yeast two-hybrid screen does not require the expression and purification of any recombinant proteins. Thus, it is fairly straightforward to perform at a genome-wide scale and is applicable for nearly all protein interaction studies. A few such genome-wide studies were recently performed, and the resulting "interactome" maps greatly facilitate the functional annotation of the genome.[177–179]

Functional screens for the identification of therapeutic targets in cancer

One consequence of the sequencing of the human genome is that we now have a comprehensive catalog of all of the genes that can be expressed. Cancer genome sequencing efforts have also given us a catalog of the genes most commonly mutated in cancer. The challenge going forward is to integrate this data with functional studies and to systematically compile a list of genes whose mutation or aberrant expression drives cancer initiation or maintenance. Recent technical advances provide the means to search systematically for genes involved in cancer development. Broadly, these efforts can be divided into loss-of-function approaches (i.e., assessment of cellular phenotype after inhibition of gene expression) or gain-of-function approaches (i.e., assessment of cellular phenotype after enforcement of gene expression).

Loss-of-function approaches

RNA interference

RNA-interference (RNAi) refers to an ancient biological pathway by which small (18–21 nt), double-stranded RNA (dsRNA) molecules, of two types, can catalytically induce degradation of complementary mRNA molecules in a sequence-specific manner. First, in plants and some other lower eukaryotes, "short interfering RNAs" (siRNAs) may be endogenously processed from longer dsRNA substrates. These longer dsRNA molecules are often derived from viruses, and so RNAi represents a form of viral immunity in these organisms.[180,181] Second, microRNAs (miRNAs) are components of the eukaryotic genome, and many are deeply conserved across evolution (including in humans).[182,183] miRNAs are transcribed from the genome, much like mRNAs, and are processed into a mature form that is about 22 nt in length. In their final processed forms, siRNAs and miRNAs function similarly, as sequence-specific negative regulators of gene expression.

Soon after the discovery of miRNAs and the report of sequence-specific endogenous silencing by dsRNAs, it became clear that siRNAs could be designed to inhibit the expression of any gene of interest.[184] Indeed, over the last 15 years, RNAi technology has become a staple of loss-of-function analysis in research laboratories. RNAi has been widely adopted for applications ranging from inhibiting the function of single genes in cell culture to developing gene therapy techniques *in vivo* to specifically target disease-associated alleles.

In mammalian cells, RNAi-mediated gene suppression can be induced by the transfection of chemically synthesized siRNAs, or by the use of plasmids expressing short hairpin RNAs (shRNAs), which get processed to siRNAs endogenously by the Drosha and Dicer ribonucleases.[185,186] shRNAs can be expressed from a plasmid containing an RNA polymerase III promoter, or from an miRNA-like context as part of a longer transcript, under the control of an RNA polymerase II promoter.[187] In either case, the siRNA becomes incorporated into the RNA-induced silencing complex (RISC) and directs sequence-specific degradation or translational suppression of the target mRNA, resulting in decreased protein expression.[188] Although siRNAs are easily synthesized and highly effective, they are relatively expensive and can only be used for transient loss-of-function experiments. Vector-based systems offer the possibility of adding selectable markers, such as drug resistance, stable expression of the RNAi construct, as well as being a renewable resource through propagation in bacteria. More recently, inducible RNAi vectors have been developed, allowing fine temporal and spatial regulation of RNAi-induced gene knockdown.[189]

Both siRNA and shRNA libraries have been used successfully in transfection-based arrayed screens looking at phenotypes that develop shortly after gene suppression, such as apoptosis, cell signaling events, or cell cycle distribution.[190–192] For many other cancer-related phenotypic assays, such as anchorage-independent colony formation, bypass of senescence, or tumor xenografts, long-term gene suppression is essential, requiring stable integration, and expression of the RNAi vector. An additional significant advantage of retroviral-based libraries is the ability to work with cells that are refractory to transfection. This is particularly true for lentiviral-based systems, which can even be used to infect postmitotic and other difficult to transduce cells, including primary or differentiated cells.[193,194]

Gene editing with CRISPR/Cas9 for research and diagnostics of cancer

An additional approach which evolved over the last decades is the CRISPR/Cas9 (clustered regularly interspaced short palindromic repeats and CRISPR-associated protein 9) technology. It constitutes a powerful tool for gene-editing and also bears potential for application in precision medicine.

CRISPR was initially discovered by Ishino and coworkers[195,196] in 1987 and further investigation revealed that CRISPR confers resistance of bacteria toward phage infection dependent on the abundance of spacer-phage sequences. By forming a CRISPR RNA (crRNA) and trans-activating crRNA (tracrRNA) hybrid (also called a single guide RNA sequence or sgRNA), the CRISPR Cas system can direct the Cas9 enzyme to hybridize with specific DNA sequences and introduce double-stranded breaks in the region of interest.[197] Besides bacteria, the CRISPR/Cas9 technology was also shown to be successful in editing genes in human and mouse eukaryotic cells.[198,199]

CRISPR gene editing in cancer
After targeting specific DNA sequence, the cell repairs the double-stranded break using ether nonhomologous end joining or homology-directed repair (HDR). The first mechanism is failure-prone and gives rise to deletion or insertion of bases. The latter uses the homologous DNA sequence leading to correct damage repair, resulting in sequence substitution when a repair template is present. Thus, the CRISPR/Cas9 technology can be used for knockouts (KOs) or knockins through the depletion, addition, or replacement of DNA sequences. By the means of specific gene KOs using the CRISPR/Cas system, the biological function and relevance of a specific protein can be deciphered in a very efficient way leading to better understanding of molecular drivers of cancer in migration, proliferation, chemotherapy resistance, and invasion as well as cellular signaling processes. Furthermore, CRISPR/Cas is also capable of generating novel animal models (Figure 14).

Pooled library screening
The pooled library screen using CRISPR is a powerful tool to discover new dependencies of cancer based on a loss-of-function model. Thousands of specific genes are targeted by plasmids in these CRISPR libraries and the effect on a specific phenotype can subsequently be studied in different conditions. The first step in this approach consists of lenti- or retroviral delivery of the sgRNA into the cells followed by a selection step by certain growth conditions for selection of the phenotype of interest. After this selection step, the DNA is isolated from the cells and subjected to DNA sequencing. These data are then mapped to a library with the gene-specific gRNAs and further analyzed *in silico* by computational approaches. The phenotypes of the cells and the respective target genes are then compared to the phenotype of known controls within the library, to identify changes introduced by targeting the respective gene of interest. These CRISPR pooled screening approaches are capable of identifying new dependencies in tumorigenesis by checking a broad number of potential genes and pathways leading to the development of novel treatment options. Although for generating reliable results a sufficient number of cells have to be transduced and kept in maintenance based on the size of the library used in the screen. Furthermore, appropriate selection methods, sequencing technology, and the computational analysis tools have to be taken into account, when interpreting these data.

CRISPR/Cas9 gene therapy of cancer
Immunotherapy of various cancers is a field which can be directed by CRISPR/Cas9 through the generation of chimeric antigen receptor T (CAR-T) cells. Here, the chimeric antigen receptor has two domains executing its main functions, namely recognition of the cancer antigen and activation of the respective T cell.[200] For the production of autologous CAR-T cells, the patient's T-cells are isolated, genetically edited *ex vivo* to recognize and attack cancer antigens, and transferred back into the patient. Alternatively, allogenic CAR-T cells can be used. Therefore, T-cells from healthy donors are used and modified *ex vivo*. The chimeric antigen receptor is introduced preferably into the T-cell receptor α constant (TRAC) locus using the CRISPR/Cas9 method.[201] Further, the endogenous T cell receptor of the donor cell is knocked out using CRISPR to eliminate graft versus host reactions, and the MHC I complex of the donor cells is targeted to increase the life span of the CAR-T cell in the recipient's body. To further increase the efficiency of the CAR-T cells, PD-1 can be deleted in the T cells by CRISPR/Cas9, as tumors tend the upregulate PD-L1 thereby mitigating the effect of CAR-T treatment.[202] The CAR-T therapy using CRISPR is an evolving field and there are multiple phase I and II studies ongoing to date to explore the safety and efficiency of CAR-T treatment in cancer.[203] These would pave the way to exploitation of the patients' immune system for cancer treatment alongside with therapy improvement by reduction of cancer immune escape mechanisms.

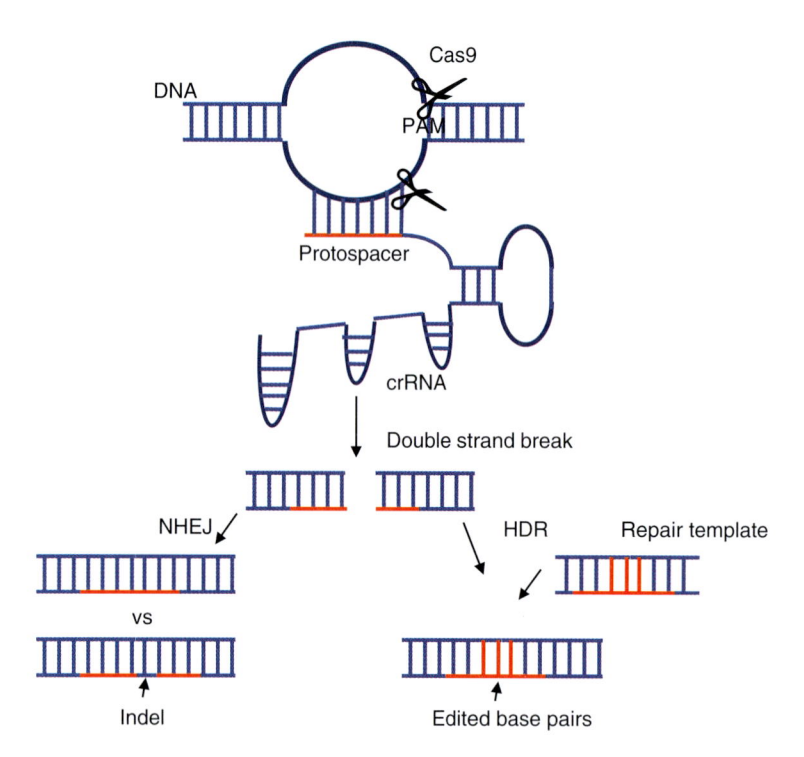

Figure 14 Schematic mechanism of *CRISPR/Cas9* gene editing: the crRNA recognizes the target sequence on the DNA and facilitates cleavage of the DNA in the presence of a PAM motif resulting in double-stranded breaks (DSB). DSB are repaired by nonhomologous end joining (NHEJ) resulting in insertions or deletions (INDELs) or by homology-directed repair (HDR) in the presence of a template for base editing.

Limitations of CRISPR/Cas9
Before using the CRISPR/Cas9 technology in clinical applications and in order to carefully interpret research results, potential off-target effects should be considered. There are some promising efforts to reduce these off-target effects, but further work has to be done to improve safety of this technology.[204,205]

SHERLOCK as a diagnostic method for cancer
Besides the usage of CRISPR Cas system to generate KOs and knock-ins, the system may also function as a diagnostic tool for cancer. Indeed, the ability of CRISPR Cas system to detect nucleic acids can be exploited for CRISPR-based diagnostics (CRISPR-Dx). To achieve this, an alternative nuclease, known as Cas13a, can be used together with crRNA to sense specific RNA sequences, resulting in a cleavage of proximate nontargeted RNAs.[206–209] This causes cell death *in vivo* or degradation of labeled RNA *in vitro*, indicating the presence of a specific target RNA.[207] For example, Gootenberg et al.[210] demonstrated the detection of specific strains of Zika and Dengue virus *in vitro* by degradation of a reporter RNA using the Cas13a based molecular detection method SHERLOCK (specific high sensitivity enzymatic reporter unlocking).[210] They used an ortholog of Cas13a derived from *Leptotrichia wadei* (LwCas13a) with increased activity and attomolar sensitivity. Hereby they were able to reach single-molecule sensitivity for RNA as well as DNA, which was even maintained when all steps were performed in a single reaction.[210] Further, the SHERLOCK system showed lower variation when compared to other detection methods for nucleic acids like qPCR or ddPCR.[210] This was validated by the detection of viral fragments at a concentration of 2 aM, still granting the differentiation between the used Zika and Dengue viruses.[210] Further, they demonstrated that SHERLOCK can also be used to detect virus from serum, urine, or saliva.[210] By introduction of synthetic mismatches into the crRNA target duplex, Cas13a was able to discriminate single-base differences, which was specific enough to be used in human genotyping of single-nucleotide polymorphisms (SNPs).[210] Given this specificity, SHERLOCK was also capable of testing cell-free DNA (cfDNA) fragments in patient blood. Here, SHERLOCK was able to identify cancer mutations EGFR L858R and BRAF V600E in cfDNA at allelic fractions of 0.1%, lying in the clinical range of application.[210] The work of Myhrvold et al.[211] in 2018 also demonstrated the sensitivity and specificity of SHERLOCK in detecting extracted nucleic acids. To also use SHERLOCK for detection of viral nucleic acids in body fluids (including urine or saliva) they developed HUDSON (heating unextracted diagnostic samples to obliterate nucleases), to lyse viral particles, and protect nucleic acids from degradation by RNase through chemical and heat reduction.[211] This enabled detection of ZIKA Virus in urine, blood, serum, saliva, or plasma without purification or dilution (only blood samples were diluted 1 : 3) using a colorimetric readout.[211] Furthermore, they were able to identify at known point mutation in the ZIKA virus pandemic, S139N, as wells as six known drug resistance mutation in HIV RT using SHERLOCK with a visual readout.[211] Thus, the combination of SHERLOCK with HUDSON proved as a robust field-deployable diagnostic tool, combining the sensitivity and specificity of amplification-based nucleic acid diagnostics and the speed and simplicity of rapid antigen testing.[211] A similar assay based on CRISPR–Cas12 with simultaneously performed reverse transcription and isothermal amplification (loop-mediated amplification; RT-LAMP) has recently been developed and validated for diagnostic of severe acute respiratory syndrome coronavirus type 2 (SARS-CoV-2) for RNA isolated from nasopharyngeal or oropharyngeal swabs of patients.[212]

Thus, the CRISPR–Cas based SHERLOCK tool could also be a powerful tool for detection of mutations associated with tumorigenesis such as oncogenic kirsten rat sarcoma (KRAS) alleles in pancreatic, lung, and colorectal cancer, comprising the three most lethal cancers in the United States.[213] Identification of those Ras-addicted tumors from patient samples may also further be simplified when combined with HUDSON to create a colorimetric rapid testing procedure.[211,213] As the KRAS mutation depicts a critical and initial step in tumorigenesis of various cancers, this may constitute a first screening diagnostic test followed by further diagnostics like cross-sectional imaging.

CRISPR–Cas9 to prioritize cancer drug targets using cancer driver events and MSI

Individual molecular aberrations in a patient's tumor hold the potential for identifying personalized therapeutic targets, although many dependencies in a tumor are not mutated and are instead synthetic lethal targets that are oftentimes empirically determined.[214,215] The application of the CRISPR–Cas9 system using libraries of sgRNAs to study gene function constitutes a method to robustly generate null alleles to identify and prioritize novel cancer drug candidates in an unbiased manner.[216] Behan et al.[216] performed a CRIPSR–Cas9 screen in 339 cancer cell lines with 18,009 targets to evaluate cellular fitness and were able to accurately identify crucial genetic dependencies. In their analysis, they distinguished between context-specific fitness genes and core fitness genes, the latter also showing higher expression in healthy tissue and thus being at risk for higher toxicity.[216] They prioritized their candidates into three groups according to their tractability for the development of small molecules and antibodies.[217] Here, the first group showed targets of approved drugs or drugs in development, the second group showed drugs without clinical development and the third group did not have supporting information for tractability of targets.[216] Within group 1 the class of protein kinases was enriched, while the targets of groups 2 and 3 were more diverse.[216] Thus, CRISPR–Cas9 screening combined with assessment of genomic mutational data (cancer driver events and microsatellite instability (MSI)) and tractability data can be a promising tool to identify and develop novel powerful drug targets in various cancer types. MSI resulting from defects in the DNA mismatch repair system is a common feature of cancer cells and is—in conjunction with altered immune checkpoint as well as factors mutational burden—positively linked to efficacy of immunotherapy.[218] This susceptibility of MSI cancer toward immune checkpoint inhibitors in concert with wide-spanning CRISPR screens can pave the way toward the discovery and development of novel highly specific anti-cancer drugs and treatment options.[219,220]

Drug discovery by CRISPR–Cas9 protein domain screening

When deleting potential targets by using CRISPR–Cas9 most strategies use sgRNAs designed to bind to the 5′ exons of the gene.[221-224] Here, Shi et al.[225] observed considerable variance in performance of individual sgRNAs for the same gene lying between >20-fold depletion and 2-fold depletion of cells. When targeting Brd4 those sgRNAs which bind to the BD1 domain caused the biggest effect while sgRNA targeting outside of the domain had a weaker phenotype.[225] Thus, they further evaluated whether targeting protein domains would have a stronger effect on negative selection.[225] After targeting all exons in Brd4, the sgRNAs with a depletion of >10-fold were found to be directed toward exons encoding for domains BD1, BD2, or the C-terminal motif, as wells as extra-terminal domains at a later timepoint.[225] A weak phenotype was observed in sgRNAs binding outside of domains.[225] Furthermore, SURVEYOR assay and deep-sequencing revealed that the phenotype severity was not through robustness of mutagenesis between domain-targeting and 5′ exon targeting sgRNAs as well as off-target effects.[225] But genes edited by CRISPR within domains get depleted faster from the cells than genes edited outside of domains, raising the hypothesis of higher chance of null mutations if critical domains are targeted.[225] Here deep sequencing showed, that frame shift mutations in Brd4 caused negative selection. On the other hand, in-frame mutations only caused negative selection when targeting a functional domain (BD1), suggesting that in-frame mutations within a domain may hinder proper protein function, while in-frame mutations outside of a domain may leave protein function unaffected.[225] When retaining functionality in a diploid cell population, in-frame mutations will leave about 56% of the cells with at least one functional allele, while in-frame mutations causing loss of function would affect nearly every cell.[225] This work highlighted domain-targeted CRISPR–Cas9 screening as a robust tool to discover novel cancer dependencies.[225]

CRISPR for generation of genetically modified animal models

There are various applications of the CRISPR technology to generate genetically modified animal models. Therefore, the fertilized 1-cell-stage embryo model, using electroporation, microinjection, or genome oviductal nucleic acid delivery (GONAD), is a very common method. While electroporation facilitates genome editing via electoral stimulation of fertilized 1-cell-stage embryos with the CRISPR Cas9/sgRNA complex, the microinjection method relies on direct injection of the Cas9/sgRNA complex into the pronucleus or the cytoplasm of the fertilized 1-cell stage embryos.[226,227] Besides this, the GONAD technology utilizes direct injection of the Cas9/gRNA complex into the oviduct of pregnant mice in combination with electroporation.[228] An advantage of the Cas9 systems is further, that it is capable of using multiple sgRNAs and thus can target multiple genes.[197-199] Using CRISPR Cas9 for genome editing *in vivo* remains a challenge, as the Cas9 and associated sgRNAs exceed the capacity of adeno-associated or lentiviral vectors.[229,230] To overcome these limitations Platt et al.[231] created a Cre-dependent Rosa26 Cas9 knockin mouse. Therefore, a *Streptococcus pyogenes* Cas9 cassette was inserted into the Roas26 locus driven by the CAG promotor.[231] Further, the expression of Cas9 was restricted by a loxp-stop-loxP transcriptional silencer upstream of the Cas9 sequence to facilitate Cre-dependency.[231] This Cre-dependency was validated in a ubiquitous (β-actin Cre) as well as tissue-specific manner (tyrosine hydroxylase-Cre, parvalbumin-Cre).[231] Further, an adeno-associated virus (AAV) 1/2 vector containing sgRNA targeting NeuN and Cre was delivered by stereotactic injection into the prefrontal cortex of mice. This resulted in indel formation at the injecting site evidenced by deep sequencing as well as reduction in protein expression of NeuN.[231] To this end, they designed a single AAV vector with a Kras^{G12D} HDR donor sequence, and a U6-sgRNA for Kras, p53, and Lkb1.[231] Delivery of the contract was facilitated by intratracheal applications of AAV9 into Cre-dependent Cas9 animals.[231] Analysis after four weeks revealed 0.1% indels in p53 and 0.4% indels in Lkb1 as well as 0.1% HDR for KrasG12D.[231] Further, observation showed tumor formation in the animals harboring loss of function on p53 and Lkb1 as well as mutant Kras^{G12D}, and pathological examination revealed invasive lung adenocarcinoma within less than 60 days.[231] These data underscore the ability of the CRISPR Cas9 gene editing system in conjunction with Cre-dependent expression of Cas9 as well as AAV-mediated sgRNA delivery in generating complex model organisms of human cancer. This may facilitate the way for generation of genetically modified animal models and a better understanding of tumorigenesis.

Gain-of-function approaches

Most gain-of-function screens involve transient or stable introduction of a cDNA library into cells, ideally resulting in the hyperactivation of pathways positively regulated by the gene corresponding to the introduced cDNA. Several large collections of cloned cDNAs have been used successfully to this end.[232,233] Several of these are compatible with recombination-mediated transfer systems, allowing shuttling of the open reading frames (ORFs) of interest into different vectors, facilitating adaptation of the system to individual needs.

Gain-of-function approaches have been used for a variety of purposes, including to identify modulators of signal transduction pathways as assessed by transcriptional reporters,[234] to identify genes whose expression can bypass senescence,[233] and to identify genetic programs conferring drug resistance phenotypes.[235] Depending on the goal of the screen, the cDNA can be transiently expressed by transfection (an approach that works well with transcriptional reporter-driven systems focused on short-term events) or stably integrated by using a viral cDNA expression vector (an approach that is often needed for many screens relevant to oncogenic transformation that require long-term expression and selection).

Another type of gain-of-function approach utilizes miRNA expression libraries to screen using phenotypic assays. miRNAs implicated in cancer include let-7, a negative regulator of RAS, c-Myc, and other oncogenes[236]; the miR-17-92 cluster, which is upregulated in lymphomas and can promote lymphomagenesis[237]; and miR-15 and miR-16, negative regulators of BCL2, that are downregulated in chronic lymphocytic leukemia.[238] The full extent of the contribution of miRNAs to tumorigenesis is not yet known; thus, further functional studies are necessary. For example, work using a retroviral expression library of miRNAs identified miR-372 and miR-373 in a Ras-induced senescence bypass screen, suggesting possible oncogenic function for these miRNAs.[239] Future applications of this approach will likely yield many more cancer-relevant miRNAs and the identification of their respective targets are also likely to provide further insight into the oncogenic process.

Organoids as an evolving tool for research and clinical application

Background

Culturing malignant cells for cancer research has been used for multiple decades. Starting from one cervical cancer cell line, Hela cells, the American Type Culture Collection now maintains nearly 4000 human cell lines. These cells are grown as a monolayer on a tissue culture plate and can usually be passaged indefinitely. Studying these cell lines has revealed numerous insights into oncologic transformation. However, these cell lines have certain limitations. The two-dimensional growth in tissue culture dishes leads to clonal selection and genetic instability.[240] Culturing established cell lines in a three-dimensional matrix has resolved some of these limitations, like the lack of three-dimensional cell-to-cell interactions, cell polarization, as well as nutrient and oxygen deprivation within three-dimensional structures. Nevertheless, by originating from monolayer lines, these three-dimensional cultures, so-called spheroids, share many of the same limitations as their originating cell lines.[241] Therefore, alternative, 3D culture systems are needed, which ideally recapitulate the cellular and genetic heterogeneity as it is found *in vivo* in human humors. One tractable culture system that aims to address these challenges is the so-called organoids.

The term organoids (organ-like) is meant to reflect the close resemblance of the culture system to the originating tissue in terms of morphology and cellular heterogeneity.[242] Benign organoids can be generated from pluripotent stem cells (PSCs) by embedding PSCs in a three-dimensional matrix and adding a nutrient-rich media composed of tissue-specific growth factors to enable the differentiation into organoids. Theoretically, organoids can be generated from all epithelial tissues, where progenitors can be derived from PSCs.[242,243] The cocktail of growth hormones differs from organoid line to organoid line as it is thought to mimic the organ's stem cell niche. Alternatively, tissue-specific organoids can be generated from adult stem cells (ASCs) obtained directly from an adult organ.[244] Additionally, patient-derived organoids (PDOs) are cultured from patient tumors that contain neoplastic cells. The tissue can be retrieved surgically and also using small fine needle biopsies (Figure 15).

The 3D matrix in which the organoids are grown prevents cellular attachment and cell differentiation. Although there is a large variety of possible matrices, ranging from collagen-based matrices to completely synthetic matrices, the vast majority of researchers use Matrigel®, a scaffold derived from the murine Engelbreth-Holm-Swarm (EHS) sarcoma, rich in components of the basement membrane.

Cancer research applications

The ability to culture normal, nonmalignant cells in cell culture without immortalization offers the ability to compare all stages of neoplastic progression to wild-type cells. Additionally, normal cells from normal human and animal tissues can be genetically modified to allow the *in vitro* evaluation of stages of progressive oncologic transformation. In colorectal cancer as well as in pancreatic cancer, the sequential introduction of driver mutations leads to increased oncogenic potential and is paralleled by histopathologic resemblance with the respective preneoplastic and neoplastic lesions. Toshiro Sato and his group used human epithelial intestinal organoids and introduced mutations of APC, KRAS, SMAD4, p53, and PIK3CA using CRISPR/Cas9 which led to increased oncogenic potential, paralleled by reduced niche dependency so that organoids are able to sustain their growth with reduced media supplements, such as the loss of EGF dependence in KRAS mutant cells. Similarly, mouse pancreatic organoids with a defined genetic background have been used to develop organoids recapitulating pancreatic tumorigenesis, ranging from normal ductal structures to preinvasive and invasive neoplasms as sequential genetic mutations are incorporated.[246,247] Similar studies have developed engineered tumor organoid models for breast,[248] liver,[249] gastric,[250] and esophageal cancer. These models enable studying oncologic transformation with an isogenic background, something that cannot be achieved when comparing patient-derived lines. By studying various stages of cancer, up- and downregulation of genes during oncologic transformation can be discovered. In pancreatic cancer, this led to the discovery of tumor dependencies in redox and lipid metabolism, which can potentially be targeted therapeutically.[251,252]

Alternatively, neoplastic organoids can also be generated from malignant cells obtained from cancer patients. An increasing number of research institutions have established tumor

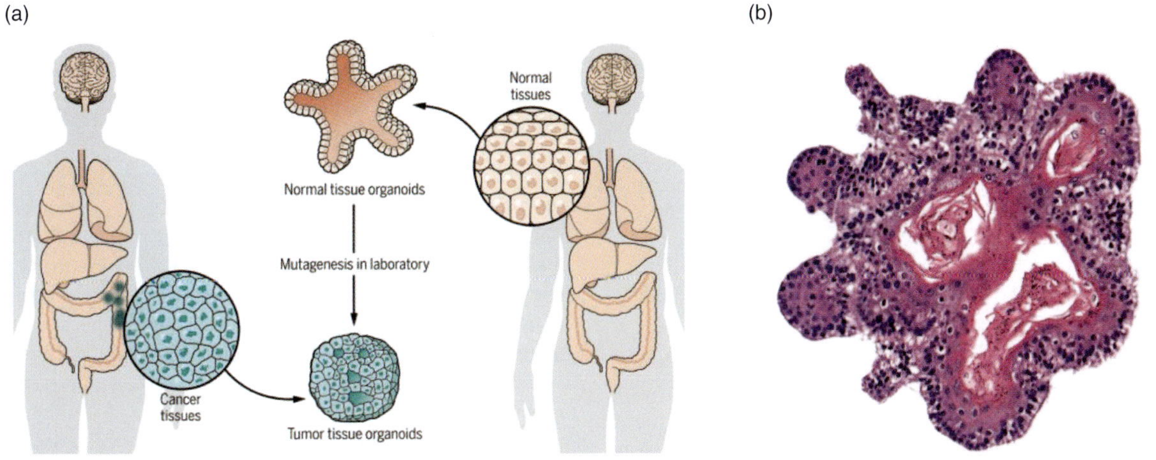

Figure 15 (a) Tumor organoid generation through genetic engineering of normal organoids (right) or derived from tumor patients (left). (b) Exemplary H&E staining of squamous cell carcinoma derived from oral mucosa. Figure adapted from Tuveson and Clevers[245] with kind permission from the American Association for the Advancement of Science.

organoid biobanks. Previously, the low efficiency of generating patient-derived cell lines or PDXs only made surgically resected specimens with copious amounts of starting tissue eligible. Now, the possibility of generating PDOs from the limited amount of tissue from a fine needle biopsy enables researchers and clinicians to study cancer at all stages, especially in metastatic patients who would not typically undergo surgery. Organoid biobanks have been generated from esophageal,[253] gastric,[254] and colon[253,255] cancer as well as hepatocellular,[256] cholangiocarcinoma,[257] and pancreatic cancer,[258,259] as well as breast,[260] endometrial,[261] prostate,[262] and childhood kidney cancer.[263]

These biobanks have been shown to resemble the primary tumors, however, it is not yet clear to which extent intratumoral heterogeneity is captured.[245] Organoids appear to capture some features of the subtypes of certain cancers, including pancreatic cancer where transcriptional profiling has revealed several different subtypes differing in gene expression patterns of pathways like TGF-β, MYC, and KRAS. Although the nomenclature differs between studies, these patterns overlap and the squamous or basal-like subtype confer the worst prognosis while the classical or progenitor subtype progresses more slowly. These subtypes are highly clinically relevant as they differ significantly regarding therapy response and survival. However, in established cell lines, the subtypes are not represented evenly with a tremendous bias toward the basal-like phenotype.[264,265] In contrast, pancreatic organoids have been shown to better reflect both subtypes of human pancreatic cancer.[258]

Organoids in their natural habitat—the tumor microenvironment

Although organoids have excelled in recapitulating the malignant lesions, cancer is more than just neoplastic cells. The interaction with the so-called tumor microenvironment (TME) is crucial and its composition has been shown to have a significant impact on a patient's prognosis.[266–268] The TME consists of both extracellular matrix (ECM) components as well as nonneoplastic cells (immune cells, stroma cells, endothelial cells). The immune component consists of a mixture of cells, with some cells showing a tumor-suppressing phenotype like CD8+ T-cells, and some showing rather a tumor promoting, immune suppressant phenotype including CD4+ T-regulatory cells and M2 macrophages.

In the stroma compartment, endothelial cells educated by the tumor tissue can lack adhesion markers and thereby prevent immune cell invasion. Likewise, stroma fibroblasts, in this context also called CAFs, can secrete immunomodulatory cytokines and chemokines including TGF-β and CXCL12, also promoting a tumor-suppressive phenotype.[269]

In order to mechanistically study these interactions, two distinct approaches of either maintaining the original TME or reconstituting a TME have been developed.

Kuo and colleagues[270] have developed air-fluid organoid cultures where tumor fragments can be maintained in a viable state for weeks to several months. In a recent publication, they reported that multiple human air-fluid organoid cultures could also maintain lymphocytes and fibroblast contents over the span of several weeks, if the cultures were supplemented with IL-2 and other factors.[271]

An alternative approach is to first generate a tumor organoid culture, and then to add TME components in effort to recapitulate the original tumor architecture and cellular dynamics. The Tuveson group was able to dissect the heterogeneity of CAFs in pancreatic cancer and group them into at least three groups with distinct gene expression and secretome patterns. Fibroblasts in close proximity to neoplastic cells showed high αSMA expression and are thereby called myofibroblastic CAFs (myCAFs). Inflammatory Fibroblasts (iCAF) on the other hand lost αSMA expression and were located more distant from the tumor cells. While myCAFs contribute to ECM deposition, iCAFs secreted paracrine effectors like IL-6, IL-11, CXCL12, and LIF and thereby created an immunosuppressive, tumor-promoting phenotype.[121–123] Importantly, these findings could also be validated in other cancer types like colorectal cancer and breast cancer.[261,272] Similarly, co-culturing of immune cells has been performed with intestinal organoids and breast cancer organoids.[273,274]

An alternative way of exposing tumor organoids to an intact TME is the mouse xenograft. Organoid transplants have been successful for colon, pancreatic, breast, bladder, and prostate cancer among others.[260,275–277]

When planning *in vivo* studies, choosing the right recipient mouse is crucial. Studies involving an intact immune system require syngeneic transplantations (tumor and recipient from same species), so commonly cell lines derived from genetically engineered mouse models (GEMMs) are used. Alternatively, humanized mice can be used for transplantation of human tumors. Here, immunocompromised mice are injected with human hematopoietic stem cells which results in reconstitution of the hematopoietic lines.[278] In studies not focused on the immune system, immunocompromised mice can be used. Their immunodeficiency ranges from athymic nude mice with reduced T-cells to severe combined immunodeficient (SCID) mice with compromised B- and T-cell lineage and IL2rg mutant SCID mice (NSG) that are deficient in mature lymphocytes and NK cells.[279,280]

The most accessible model is the heterotopic subcutaneous implantation. This is commonly used for simple, usually, cell-line-based xenografts to address questions like engraftment rate and tumor growth, but also for s.c. implantation of larger tumor pieces (PDX).[279] However, differences regarding tumor growth as well as drug response have been observed when s.c. tumors are compared to tumors implanted into their originating organ (orthotopic implantation).[281] Here, the interaction of tumor cells with the correct stromal compartment can be studied and pharmacologically targeted.[282]

However, even the orthotopic engraftment has a major drawback: Cells are directly injected into the stromal compartment, whereas epithelial neoplasms originate from neoplastic cells above the basement membrane, and it has been previously unclear to which extent this may bias findings in xenograft models. To address this problem, Miyabayashi et al.[283] developed an alternative in situ orthotopic model: By injecting human pancreatic tumor organoids directly into the pancreatic ducts of NSG mice, the tumor cells were able to populate within the ductal epithelial compartment. Thereby, intraductal transplants were primarily influenced by murine ductal cells while orthotopic transplantations interacted with all stromal components (fibroblasts, vasculature, and nerves). Classic orthotopic transplantation of organoids (OGOs) and intraductal transplanted organoids (IGOs) showed various phenotypic differences: OGOs relatively uniformly developed high-grade-lesions and quickly progressed to invasive pancreatic ductal adenocarcinoma (PDAC). IGOs on the other hand differed from organoid line to organoid line with about half of the lines showing fast tumor progression and invasion while the other half showed a noninvasive, glandular morphology. This is also reflected in the survival curves where OGOs were more homogenous while IGOs showed a bimodal distribution of so-called fast-progressors and slow-progressors. While proliferation in fast-progressing IGOs resembled proliferation in the corresponding OGOs, slow-progressing IGOs only proliferated when in contact with murine ductal cells. Furthermore, in some organoid lines, a heterogenous pattern was observed. Even from single-cell clones, transplants showed both invasive areas as well as glandular areas. While the invading cells showed expression of squamous markers, the glandular areas showed expression of basal markers. Mechanistically, the invasive areas were associated with hyperactivation of the KRAS pathway and increased KRAS signaling leading to activation of epithelial–mesenchymal transition (EMT), ECM remodeling, and axon guidance pathways. Thereby, the importance of these pathway genes like AMIGO2 and KLK-6 was discovered as they might represent druggable targets. When transcriptional profiles are compared, squamous/basal-like gene signatures and pathways like EMT are enriched in the OGOs while classical signatures and pathways were enriched in IGOs. Although both subtypes are present in each model, when compared to the transcription phenotypes reported in the COMPASS trial (analyzing gene expression in advanced pancreatic cancer patients in order to capture all stages of the disease), the IGO profile matched the reported human population best. Overall, these results underline the high plasticity of tumor organoids and highlight both the TME influence as well as the need for an adequate modeling system in order to recapitulate tumor subtypes.

New therapeutic strategies

Organoids for precision medicine

Using the collected data of an organoid biobank in order to bring new therapeutic strategies from bench to bedside is a major translational goal in cancer research. One approach is the development of individualized treatment strategies. In retrospective studies, organoids have been shown to recapitulate the patient's response toward common therapeutics. This includes a similar sensitivity or resistance pattern toward standard-of-care chemotherapeutic agents as well as especially high sensitivity toward targeted therapies which have been matched with oncologic driver mutations (Figure 16).[255,284–286] Furthermore, drug screening responses in pancreatic organoids suggested potential therapies even in patients that showed resistance toward all standard-of-care drugs in pancreatic cancer.[258] To this date, PDOs can suggest alternative treatment options in second- or third-line therapies, if only because PDO generation takes up to 4–6 weeks. In order to be able to offer PDO-derived therapies as first-line therapies, the development time for organoid preparation needs to be shortened and evidence that organoids are truly predictive of patient's responses needs to be established. Therefore, prospective clinical trials need to be carried out that can measure and evaluate a group of patients' responses toward identical chemotherapeutic agents and match these results with the PDO treatment results.[245]

The cumulative results from drug screens in organoid libraries can also be used to identify groups of patients with common response molecular signatures. This approach has been applied to 66 PDOs of pancreatic cancer. Their gene expression pattern was matched to the organoid drug responses and thereby, gene signatures potentially predicting drug response were identified.[258]

Disease monitoring

With pancreatic cancer being a prime example, a major challenge in clinical oncology is to detect cancerous lesions at early, curable stages. In pancreatic cancer, only 15–20% of patients are eligible for potentially curative surgical resection.[287] For this type of cancer, no feasible way of early detection is currently available. Organoids and organoid biobanks can help to identify new biomarkers for early disease detection. Using a proteomic screen of PanIN organoids, Kim et al.[288] identified 107 proteins produced and secreted by these organoids. Within these proteins, they identified thrombospondin-2 (THBS2) to be able to differentiate between normal controls, and resectable and progressed disease. The combination of THBS2 with CA19-9 led to a specificity of 98% and a sensitivity of 87% for discriminating PDAC patients from healthy controls.

Longitudinal generation of organoids can also be used for disease monitoring. Tiriac et al.[258] showed a single patient's series in pancreatic cancer where organoids were generated at the time of diagnosis, the first clinical relapse, and from a rapid autopsy. The first organoid line showed broad sensitivity to chemotherapeutic agents which was paralleled by a positive patient response. Interestingly, the organoids generated after disease progression showed KRAS amplification and increased drug resistance. Alternatively, Gao et al.[262] showed the feasibility of generating organoids from circulating tumor cells (CTCs) in prostate cancer. Longitudinal studies of CTCs could enable noninvasive early detection of

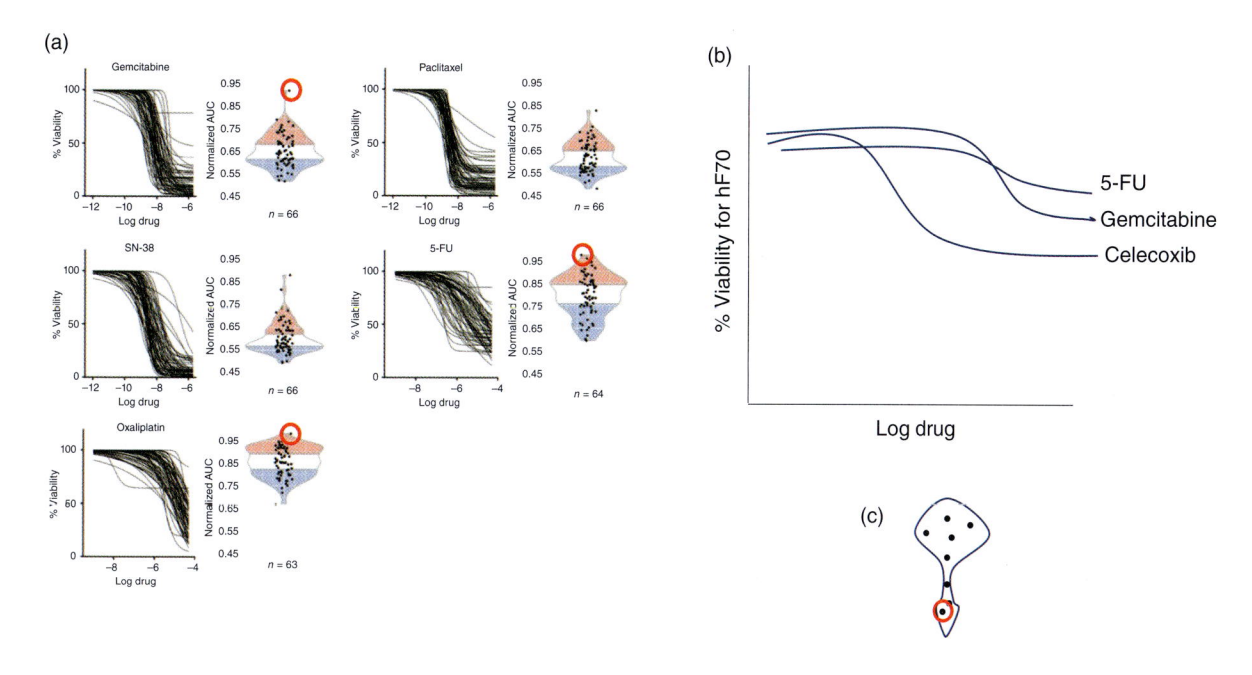

Figure 16 (a) Differential response of pancreatic tumor organoids to standard-of-care drugs in pancreatic cancer. (b) Exemplary Drug–response curve of pan-resistant human tumor organoid hF70 including response to targeted therapy Celecoxib. (c) Exemplary Normalized AUC for human tumor organoid response to Celecoxib. Red circles mark hF70 in AUC distribution of human tumor organoids. Note the differential response to standard of care drugs (highly resistant) and targeted therapy Celecoxib (top 10% most sensitive). Figure adapted from Tiriac et al.[258] with kind permission from the American Association for Cancer Research.

increasing therapy resistance. As CTCs are very rare (as few as 1 cell in 10^9 nucleated cells) in peripheral blood draws and can hardly be studied directly,[289] expanding them as organoids will enable the study of molecular alterations as well as therapy monitoring.

Mouse models of human cancer

Despite advances in our understanding of the biology of cancer at the molecular level, the application of this knowledge to the clinical management of cancer patients has been lagging. One factor limiting the translation of discoveries made in the laboratory to the clinic has been the availability of *in vivo* animal models of cancer that faithfully reproduce the human disease. Animals, particularly rodents, have been used in cancer research for decades to explore fundamental biological properties of tumors and to evaluate anti-neoplastic therapies.[290] Initially, such rodent models were largely limited to spontaneous or carcinogen-induced neoplasms, or more commonly the ectopic or orthotopic transplantation of murine or human tumor cells into syngeneic or immunodeficient mice. Although none of these approaches accurately represents the complexity of human cancer, preclinical studies with these models are nonetheless traditionally required during the regulatory approval of investigational antineoplastic agents.

Improved animal cancer models became available with the advent of GEMMs of cancer in the early 1980s. GEMMs enabled the direct investigation of potential tumorigenic genes *in vivo*, and today, models that accurately represent nearly every major human cancer exist.[291] The first generation of GEMMs was transgenic tumor-prone mice produced through the ectopic introduction of activated oncogenes. Indeed, such "oncomice" confirmed the tumorigenic properties of c-Myc, Ras, and several viral oncoproteins; mice transgenic for these oncogenes developed lymphoma, breast cancer, and pancreatic cancer.[292] However, most human cancers could not be accurately modeled using this approach, likely due to the nonphysiological properties inherent in ectopic expression cassettes and tissue mosaicism. An early alternative approach was through the disruption or "KO" of endogenous putative tumor suppressor alleles that were identified in cancer-prone kindreds. Indeed, KO mice confirmed Knudsen's hypothesis of tumor suppressor gene function, although the tumor spectrum in such KO mice oftentimes was quite distinct from the cognate human condition. A detailed description of the basic methodologies required for the generation of transgenic and KO mice can be found in an excellent manual.[293] A major drawback of these early mouse models is that genetically engineered mutations are present in every cell of the mouse. This is problematic for multiple reasons. First, it can lead to embryonic lethality or abnormalities if the affected oncogene or tumor suppressor gene is required for normal development. Second, with the exception of hereditary cancer predisposition syndromes, the modus operandi of these mutational events does not reproduce the human disease because the majority of human tumors evolve owing to acquired somatic genetic changes. Third, it does not allow interrogation of the role of cancer-relevant genes in a particular organ type or stage of tumorigenesis. Recognizing these deficiencies, investigators are developing ever more sophisticated mouse models that more faithfully reflect the human disease.

Current state-of-the-art mouse models employ new genetic tools to address the shortcomings of classic oncomice and KO mice.[294] The advent of inducible and conditional mutant alleles enables the sophisticated spatial and temporal control of cancer gene expression. A common type of inducible cancer allele is transcriptionally regulated by variants of the *E. coli* tetracycline (TET) operon, usually with the chemical analog doxycycline. It has two different variations, TET-OFF and TET-ON, depending on whether the expression of the targeted gene (regulated by a TET-responsive transactivator) is expressed in the presence (TET-ON) or absence

(TET-OFF) of doxycycline.[295] Doxycycline-sensitive alleles can include putative oncogenes, and such alleles were used to demonstrate a causal role for oncogenes in the development and maintenance of many tumor types in mouse models.[291,296] Additionally, doxycycline-dependent alleles can reversibly suppress gene expression through the expression of dominant-negative tumor suppressor genes and shRNAi constructs.[297] To control the cell lineage in which the doxycycline-dependent genetic element is expressed, cell-type-specific promoters are used to encode the TET transactivator.[295] Another inducible gene expression system utilizes chimeric proteins containing the gene of interest fused to the ligand-binding portion of the ER. Such fusion proteins are held in a latent state in the cytoplasm in complex with heat shock proteins and are released following the addition of estrogenic analogs such as tamoxifen. ER fusions with Myc and P53 have been used to generate a variety of clever mouse models of various cancer types.[298,299] Conditional mutant alleles are employed to directly modulate gene expression through either deleting putative tumor suppressor genes or expressing a single allele of an activated oncogene from its endogenous promoter. Conditional mutant alleles are controlled by the bacteriophage P1 Cre/loxP system, whereby the Cre recombinase directs the looping and excision of DNA elements that are flanked by 34 bp LoxP sites. Conditional tumor suppressor alleles thus consist of genes that contain exons surrounded by intronic LoxP sites, and these alleles are expressed at diploid levels until Cre recombinase is introduced and mediates deletion of the gene with loss of mRNA and protein. Conditional oncogenes are latent alleles that are not expressed until Cre recombinase causes the removal of transcriptional silencing or "Stop" elements, and in this scenario, the gene dosage changes from haploid to diploid with half of the gene dosage consisting of the oncogenic alleles. Additional recombinases are available for mouse modeling, and there are a variety of related strategies to control conditional gene expression. Inducible cancer alleles can be used alone or in tandem with conditional mutant alleles such that added ligands can control the expression of Cre recombinase, enabling exquisite spatial and temporal control of cancer gene expression.[300,301] Using these state-of-the-art strategies, GEMMs have been developed that faithfully model the development of preinvasive and invasive carcinomas of the lung, pancreas, prostate, ovary, and breast.[291] Such models oftentimes demonstrate additional pathophysiological sequelae, including cachexia and metastasis, and somatic biochemical and genomic alterations that are common in the cognate human malignancy. A major advance using these GEMMs is the identification of new pathways in human cancers by cross-species comparisons.[302] Studies are investigating the role of cancer GEMMs in diagnostic and therapeutic development. Unanswered questions about GEMMs include the absence of evidence demonstrating their superior predictive therapeutic utility compared to xenografted tumor models, and whether species-specific differences in drug metabolism, TME, and cell-intrinsic pathways will preclude the translation of information from GEMMs to the clinical setting. Nonetheless, several publications suggest that these models will be informative in the preclinical assessment of anti-neoplastic agents.

CRISPR in mouse models of cancer

With the advances of the CRISPR/Cas9 technology, the expensive and complex process of generation GEMMs be simplified. Therefore, the prokaryotic adaptive immune machinery is used to introduce double-stranded breaks at the genetic location of interest using sgRNA. Those double-stranded breaks are subsequently repaired by the cell's nonhomologous enjoining (NHEJ) and HDR. While NHEJ results in deletions and insertions causing knock out of the gene, HDR is capable of introducing an edited sequence in the presence of a proper repair template.

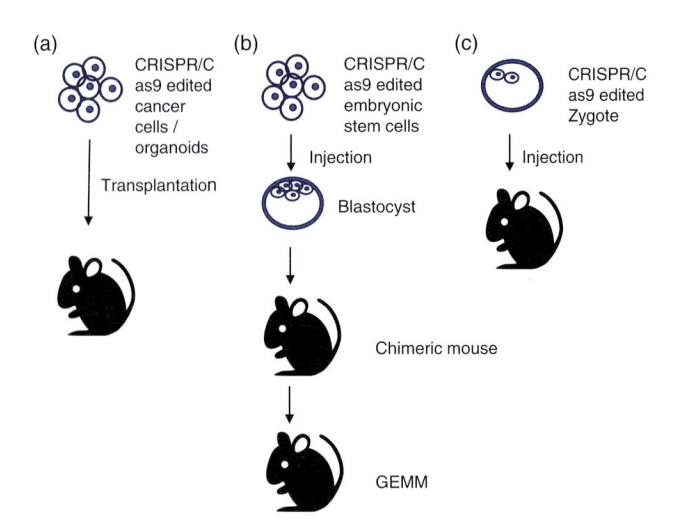

Figure 17 Generation of genetically modified mouse models using CRISPR/Cas9: (a) cancer cell lines or organoids are modified *ex vivo* and transplanted into mice. (B) Embryonic stem cells can be isolated from wild-type or GEMM mice, edited by CRISPR/Cas9, and injected into blastocysts for the generation of GEMM via a chimeric mouse stage. (c) Manipulation of the Zygote via CRISPR/Cas9 for generation of GEMM[310].

Transplantation of CRISPR engineered cells

An efficient way to generate GEMM is its transplantation of *ex vivo* CRISPR-engineered cells into mice. This approach has been successfully used to generate hematopoietic neoplasms like Myc-associated B-cell lymphoma or acute myeloid leukemia.[303–305] For solid tumors, orthotopic tumor cell transplantation after manipulation *ex vivo* represents a powerful approach to study tumorigenesis at the appropriate anatomic site. Here, models for several solid tumors have been established including pancreas, colorectal, liver, intestine, and tumors of the nervous system.[306–309] When mouse cells lines are used for tumor cell generation, transplantation into immunocompetent mice is possible, while transplantation of human cancer cell lines requires transplantation into immunodeficient mice, the latter hampering investigation of tumor-immune cell interaction (Figure 17a).

Editing of germline cells using CRISPR

While traditional targeting of embryonic stem (ES) cells with subsequent *in vitro* fertilization to generate GEMMs is very time consuming, targeting ES cells using CRISPR is capable of producing reliable KO and knockin models.[311] Further, CRISPR-based approaches also harbor the possibility to generate GEMMs with multiple edited genes. Additionally, when using EC from GEMMs carrying conditional oncogenic alleles (e.g., Cre-dependent) this process can further be accelerated.[312] Mice zygotes demonstrate another possible approach for gene editing in GEMMs using CRISPR. Here, targeting a gene with subsequent NHEJ results in ubiquitous KO of the gene, while HDR in the presence of a repair template results in knockin of an altered sequence.[226,313] This method can further be used for the knockin of a loxP flanked sequence for possible conditional gene manipulation[313] (Figure 17b,c).

Generation of somatic GEMM using CRISPR

CRISPR technology also offers the possibility to edit genes *in vivo* in somatic cells. This generation of somatic GEMMs is superior to germline edited cancer models as it models the development of cancer in a more natural and precise way. Crucial for the generation of somatic GEMMs by CRISPR is the specific targeting of relevant cells or organs. For the delivery transfection of DNA encoding, the CRISPR elements can be achieved by hydrodynamic tail vein injection for transfection to the liver or electroporation of the pancreas.[314,315] Besides this direct transfection of DNA, viral delivery using adeno viruses, AAVs, and also integrating viruses like lentiviruses are suitable for selective organ delivery of the respective CRISPR components. To tackle limited packing size of viral vectors, compact *Staph. aureus* Cas9 can be used.[316] Alternatively, Cas9 expressing mouse lines can be used to overcome limited packing space of the viral vectors. Also, when using conditional Cas9 expressing mice, gene editing can be controlled in a spatial and temporal manner.[231,317] Further, delivery of CRISPR components can be achieved using nanoparticles with high transport capacity and varying systems (gold, PEGylated, lipid).[318–320] CRISPR is also capable to generate large structural rearrangement and mega-base scale deletions as wells as chromosomal translocations, making the modeling of complex alterations *in vivo* possible.[315,321,322]

Key references

The complete reference list can be found on Vital Source version of this title, see inside front cover.

7. Watson JD, Crick FHC. Molecular structure of nucleic acids: a structure for deoxyribose nucleic acid. *Nature*. 1953;**171**(4356):737–738.
21. Hartley JL, Temple GF, Brasch MA. DNA cloning using *in vitro* site-specific recombination. *Genome Res*. 2000;**10**(11):1788–1795.
24. Southern EM. Detection of specific sequences among DNA fragments separated by gel electrophoresis. *J Mol Biol*. 1975;**98**(3):503–517.
25. Slamon DJ, Godolphin W, Jones LA, et al. Studies of the HER-2/neu proto-oncogene in human breast and ovarian cancer. *Science (New York, NY)*. 1989;**244**(4905):707–712.
29. Sanger F, Nicklen S, Coulson AR. DNA sequencing with chain-terminating inhibitors. *Proc Natl Acad Sci U S A*. 1977;**74**(12):5463–5467.
35. Davies H, Bignell GR, Cox C, et al. Mutations of the *BRAF* gene in human cancer. *Nature*. 2002;**417**(6892):949–954.
39. Kralovics R, Passamonti F, Buser AS, et al. A gain-of-function mutation of JAK2 in myeloproliferative disorders. *N Engl J Med*. 2005;**352**(17):1779–1790.
46. Ley TJ, Mardis ER, Ding L, et al. DNA sequencing of a cytogenetically normal acute myeloid leukaemia genome. *Nature*. 2008;**456**(7218):66–72.
48. Sicklick JK, Kato S, Okamura R, et al. Molecular profiling of cancer patients enables personalized combination therapy: the I-PREDICT study. *Nat Med*. 2019;**25**(5):744–750.
54. Thibodeau SN, Bren G, Schaid D. Microsatellite instability in cancer of the proximal colon. *Science (New York, NY)*. 1993;**260**(5109):816–819.
60. Nowell P, Hungerford D. Chromosome studies on normal and leukemic human leukocytes. *JNCI: J Natl Cancer Inst*. 1960;**25**:85–109.
65. Meyerson M, Gabriel S, Getz G. Advances in understanding cancer genomes through second-generation sequencing. *Nat Rev Genet*. 2010;**11**(10):685–696.
67. Sharp PA. Split genes and RNA splicing. *Cell*. 1994;**77**(6):805–815.
74. Westin EH, Wong-Staal F, Gelmann EP, et al. Expression of cellular homologues of retroviral onc genes in human hematopoietic cells. *Proc Natl Acad Sci U S A*. 1982;**79**(8):2490–2494.
79. Rougeon F, Mach B. Stepwise biosynthesis *in vitro* of globin genes from globin mRNA by DNA polymerase of avian myeloblastosis virus. *Proc Natl Acad Sci U S A*. 1976;**73**(10):3418–3422.
109. Hrdlickova R, Toloue M, Tian B. RNA-Seq methods for transcriptome analysis. *Wiley Interdiscip Rev RNA*. 2017;**8**(1). doi: 10.1002/wrna.1364.
116. Ziegenhain C, Vieth B, Parekh S, et al. Comparative analysis of single-cell RNA sequencing methods. *Mol Cell*. 2017;**65**(4):631–643 e4.
120. Lawson DA, Kessenbrock K, Davis RT, et al. Tumour heterogeneity and metastasis at single-cell resolution. *Nat Cell Biol*. 2018;**20**(12):1349–1360.
121. Ohlund D, Handly-Santana A, Biffi G, et al. Distinct populations of inflammatory fibroblasts and myofibroblasts in pancreatic cancer. *J Exp Med*. 2017;**214**(3):579–596.
124. Ozdemir BC, Pentcheva-Hoang T, Carstens JL, et al. Depletion of carcinoma-associated fibroblasts and fibrosis induces immunosuppression and accelerates pancreas cancer with reduced survival. *Cancer Cell*. 2014;**25**(6):719–734.
129. Paik S, Shak S, Tang G, et al. A multigene assay to predict recurrence of tamoxifen-treated, node-negative breast cancer. *N Engl J Med*. 2004;**351**(27):2817–2826.
134. Feinberg AP, Tycko B. The history of cancer epigenetics. *Nat Rev Cancer*. 2004;**4**(2):143–153.
144. Shiraishi M, Sekiguchi A, Terry MJ, et al. A comprehensive catalog of CpG islands methylated in human lung adenocarcinomas for the identification of tumor suppressor genes. *Oncogene*. 2002;**21**(23):3804–3813.
161. Whyte P, Buchkovich KJ, Horowitz JM, et al. Association between an oncogene and an anti-oncogene: the adenovirus E1A proteins bind to the retinoblastoma gene product. *Nature*. 1988;**334**(6178):124–129.
163. Engvall E, Perlmann P. Enzyme-linked immunosorbent assay (ELISA) quantitative assay of immunoglobulin G. *Immunochemistry*. 1971;**8**(9):871–874.
164. Mann M, Hendrickson RC, Pandey A. Analysis of proteins and proteomes by mass spectrometry. *Annu Rev Biochem*. 2001;**70**:437–473.
165. Ong SE, Blagoev B, Kratchmarova I, et al. Stable isotope labeling by amino acids in cell culture, SILAC, as a simple and accurate approach to expression proteomics. *Mol Cell Proteomics*. 2002;**1**(5):376–386.
184. Elbashir S. Analysis of gene function in somatic mammalian cells using small interfering RNAs. *Methods*. 2002;**26**(2):199–213.
195. Ishino Y, Shinagawa H, Makino K, et al. Nucleotide sequence of the iap gene, responsible for alkaline phosphatase isozyme conversion in *Escherichia coli*, and identification of the gene product. *J Bacteriol*. 1987;**169**(12):5429–5433.
196. Barrangou R, Fremaux C, Deveau H, et al. CRISPR provides acquired resistance against viruses in prokaryotes. *Science*. 2007;**315**(5819):1709–1712.
197. Jinek M, Chylinski K, Fonfara I, et al. A programmable dual-RNA-guided DNA endonuclease in adaptive bacterial immunity. *Science*. 2012;**337**(6096):816–821.
198. Cong L, Ran FA, Cox D, et al. Multiplex genome engineering using CRISPR/Cas systems. *Science*. 2013;**339**(6121):819–823.
199. Mali P, Yang L, Esvelt KM, et al. RNA-guided human genome engineering via Cas9. *Science*. 2013;**339**(6121):823–826.
201. Eyquem J, Mansilla-Soto J, Giavridis T, et al. Targeting a CAR to the TRAC locus with CRISPR/Cas9 enhances tumour rejection. *Nature*. 2017;**543**(7643):113–117.
202. Choi BD, Yu X, Castano AP, et al. CRISPR-Cas9 disruption of PD-1 enhances activity of universal EGFRvIII CAR T cells in a preclinical model of human glioblastoma. *J Immunother Cancer*. 2019;**7**(1):304.
204. Ran FA, Hsu PD, Lin CY, et al. Double nicking by RNA-guided CRISPR Cas9 for enhanced genome editing specificity. *Cell*. 2013;**154**(6):1380–1389.
205. Shen B, Zhang W, Zhang J, et al. Efficient genome modification by CRISPR-Cas9 nickase with minimal off-target effects. *Nat Methods*. 2014;**11**(4):399–402.
210. Gootenberg JS, Abudayyeh OO, Lee JW, et al. Nucleic acid detection with CRISPR-Cas13a/C2c2. *Science*. 2017;**356**(6336):438–442.
211. Myhrvold C, Freije CA, Gootenberg JS, et al. Field-deployable viral diagnostics using CRISPR-Cas13. *Science*. 2018;**360**(6387):444–448.
216. Behan FM, Iorio F, Picco G, et al. Prioritization of cancer therapeutic targets using CRISPR-Cas9 screens. *Nature*. 2019;**568**(7753):511–516.
220. Le DT, Durham JN, Smith KN, et al. Mismatch repair deficiency predicts response of solid tumors to PD-1 blockade. *Science*. 2017;**357**(6349):409–413.
225. Shi J, Wang E, Milazzo JP, et al. Discovery of cancer drug targets by CRISPR-Cas9 screening of protein domains. *Nat Biotechnol*. 2015;**33**(6):661–667.
226. Wang H, Yang H, Shivalila CS, et al. One-step generation of mice carrying mutations in multiple genes by CRISPR/Cas-mediated genome engineering. *Cell*. 2013;**153**(4):910–918.
227. Qin W, Dion SL, Kutny PM, et al. Efficient CRISPR/Cas9-mediated genome editing in mice by zygote electroporation of nuclease. *Genetics*. 2015;**200**(2):423–430.
228. Gurumurthy CB, Takahashi G, Wada K, et al. GONAD: a novel CRISPR/Cas9 genome editing method that does not require *ex vivo* handling of embryos. *Curr Protoc Hum Genet*. 2016;**88**:15.8.1–15.8.12.
229. Kumar M, Keller B, Makalou N, et al. Systematic determination of the packaging limit of lentiviral vectors. *Hum Gene Ther*. 2001;**12**(15):1893–1905.
230. Wu Z, Yang H, Colosi P. Effect of genome size on AAV vector packaging. *Mol Ther*. 2010;**18**(1):80–86.
231. Platt RJ, Chen S, Zhou Y, et al. CRISPR-Cas9 knockin mice for genome editing and cancer modeling. *Cell*. 2014;**159**(2):440–455.
244. Sato T, Vries RG, Snippert HJ, et al. Single Lgr5 stem cells build crypt-villus structures *in vitro* without a mesenchymal niche. *Nature*. 2009;**459**(7244):262–265.
247. Boj SF, Hwang C-I, Baker LA, et al. Organoid models of human and mouse ductal pancreatic cancer. *Cell*. 2015;**160**(1–2):324–338.

255 van de Wetering M, Francies HE, Francis JM, et al. Prospective derivation of a living organoid biobank of colorectal cancer patients. *Cell*. 2015;**161**(4):933–945.

264 Bailey P, Chang DK, Nones K, et al. Genomic analyses identify molecular subtypes of pancreatic cancer. *Nature*. 2016;**531**(7592):47–52.

269 Giraldo NA, Sanchez-Salas R, Peske JD, et al. The clinical role of the TME in solid cancer. *Br J Cancer*. 2019;**120**(1):45–53.

271 Neal JT, Li X, Zhu J, et al. Organoid modeling of the tumor immune microenvironment. *Cell*. 2018;**175**(7):1972–1988.e16.

283 Miyabayashi K, Baker LA, Deschenes A, et al. Intraductal transplantation models of human pancreatic ductal adenocarcinoma reveal progressive transition of molecular subtypes. *Cancer Discov*. 2020;**10**(10):1566–1589.

292 Hanahan D, Wagner EF, Palmiter RD. The origins of oncomice: a history of the first transgenic mice genetically engineered to develop cancer. *Genes Dev*. 2007;**21**(18):2258–2270.

293 Behringer R, Gertsenstein M, Nagy KV, et al. *Manipulating the Mouse Embryo: A Laboratory Manual*. New York: Cold Spring Harbor Laboratory Press; 2014.

310 Weber J, Rad R. Engineering CRISPR mouse models of cancer. *Curr Opin Genet Dev*. 2019;**54**:88–96. doi: 10.1016/j.gde.2019.04.001.

4 Oncogenes

Marco A. Pierotti, PhD ■ Milo Frattini, PhD ■ Samantha Epistolio, PhD ■ Gabriella Sozzi, PhD ■ Carlo M. Croce, MD

> **Overview**
>
> The initiation and the progression of human neoplastic disease is a multistep process involving the accumulation of genetic changes, characterized by the activation of oncogenes and the inactivation of tumor suppressor genes, in somatic cells. Oncogenes are altered versions of the proto-oncogenes involved in the regulation of cell growth that are activated by mutation, chromosomal rearrangement, or gene amplification. In this article, at first we describe the methods that have been applied for the discovery and the identification of oncogenes. Then, we present the genetic mechanisms of proto-oncogenes activation with several examples and the role played by oncogenes in the initiation and progression of various cancers.
>
> The identification of oncogene abnormalities has provided tools for the molecular diagnosis and monitoring of cancer. Most important, oncogenes represent potential targets for new types of cancer therapies that permit to kill cancer cells selectively while sparing normal cells. These therapies display an evident benefit for the treatment of several tumors; however, mainly due to the occurrence of secondary resistance mechanisms, they are not able to kill 100% of neoplastic cells. In the last part of the article, we review all the genes for which a targeted therapy has been developed.

Introduction

The origin of cancer has been a long-debated issue opposing two models, one based on the evidence of tight relationships between exposure to chemical compounds and occurrence of some forms of cancers. Historically, the first of such evidence was provided by Sir Percival Pott, who in 1775 recognized the association between the scrotum carcinoma and chimney sweeps. The second model started to take place in 1911 when a pathologist, Francis Peyton Rous, made a seminal observation that a sarcoma growing on a domestic chicken could be transferred to another fowl simply by injecting the healthy animal with a cell-free filtrate derived from the original sarcoma. It took some decades to recognize that the agent causing the tumor was an RNA virus named Rous sarcoma virus, RSV. That it could be present as integrated into the cell genome thanks to the enzyme reverse transcriptase, and for this reason, it has been named retrovirus and that its transforming capability relayed on the presence of a gene additional to those normally present in nontransforming RNA virus, that is pol-gag-env, the additional gene causing cancer was named v-src. The surprising discovery was that a cellular homolog of v-src, named c-src, is present in all the cells of different species including human beings. Both models thus implied that cancer was due to external causes, environmental exposure to dangerous chemicals or tumor viruses. However, a third possibility was risen by a German biologist, Theodor Boveri, who in 1902 noticed that in tumor cells the chromosomes became scrambled. He thus proposed that cancer is the result of aberrant mitoses and uncontrolled growth caused by physical or chemical insults or by microscopic pathogens. Somehow, Boveri anticipated the existence of the cancer genes. Since his visionary proposal, multiple experimental proofs have confirmed that, at the molecular level, cancer is due to lesions in the cellular DNA. First, it has been observed that a cancer cell transmits to its daughter cells the phenotypic features characterizing the "cancerous" state. Second, most of the recognized mutagenic compounds are also carcinogenic. Finally, as Boveri anticipated, the karyotyping of several types of human tumors, particularly those belonging to the hematopoietic system, led to the identification of recurrent chromosomal aberrations, reflecting pathologic rearrangements of the cellular genome. Taken together, these observations suggest that the molecular pathogenesis of human cancer is due to structural and/or functional alterations of specific genes whose normal function is to control cellular growth and differentiation or, in different terms, cell birth and cell death.[1,2] The identification and characterization of the genetic elements playing a role in the scenario of human cancer pathogenesis have been made possible by the development of a cell-based technique, the DNA transfection, originally developed by two Dutch researchers, Frank Graham and Alex van der Erb. They found that they could obtain a precipitated of micro-crystal salt including the DNA after treatment of the purified cellular DNA with calcium phosphate. By deposing the latter on a monolayer of acceptor cells, usually NIH 3T3, they found that the DNA could be absorbed like it was carried by a viral vector. By employing this technique, the first human oncogene was isolated in 1982 and resulted to be the human homolog of a cancer gene isolated in 1964 by Jennifer J. Harvey from a rat sarcoma and designated as v-Ha-ras. As the prototype src, a series of human oncogenes were then shown to be the cellular homolog of the transforming genes picked up from the genome of the infected cancer cells by retroviruses in rodents and birds. The discovery of the nature and origin of the human oncogenes has, therefore, reconciled the two models, environmental factors and viruses, by showing that both have the same target, the proto-oncogenes, so-called to mean that after alteration normal cellular genes could switch into oncogene, thus contributing to cause cancer.[3] Subsequently, it was discovered that most cellular transforming genes do not have a viral counterpart.[4] Therefore, a second relevant experimental approach to identify human oncogenes has regarded the identification and characterization of clonal and recurrent cytogenetic abnormalities (including translocations, inversions, etc.) in cancer cells, especially those derived from the hematopoietic system. Here, a molecular analysis has discovered alterations of the gene function associated to the chromosomal aberrations. The first described cancer-associated cytogenetic aberration was the translocation t(9,22) found in 1960 by Peter Nowell in all the chronic myelogenous leukemia (CML) cells and subsequently

---

Holland-Frei Cancer Medicine, Tenth Edition. Edited by Robert C. Bast, John C. Byrd, Carlo M. Croce, Ernest Hawk, Fadlo R. Khuri, Raphael E. Pollock, Apostolia M. Tsimberidou, Christopher G. Willett, and Cheryl L. Willman.
© 2023 John Wiley & Sons, Inc. Published 2023 by John Wiley & Sons, Inc.

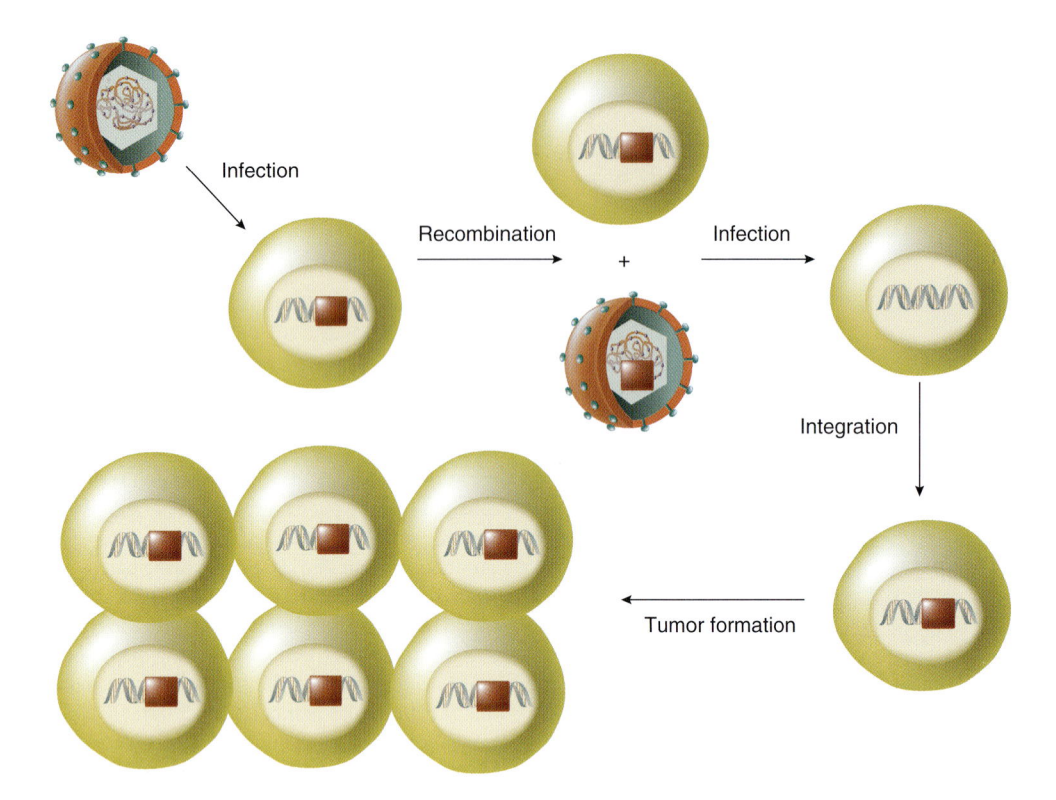

Figure 1 Retroviral transduction. An RNA tumor virus infects a human cell carrying an activated *src* gene (red box). After the process of recombination between retroviral genome and host DNA, the oncogene *c-src** is incorporated into the retroviral genome and is re-named *v-src*. When the retrovirus carrying *v-src* infects a human cell, the viral oncogenesis rapidly transcribes and is responsible for the rapid tumor formation.

shown to fuse together bcr-abl genes being the latter an oncogene of an avian tumor retrovirus. Additional oncogenes have been identified through the analysis of anomalously stained chromosomal regions (homogeneously staining regions [HSR]), representing gene amplification.[5] Furthermore, the detection of chromosome deletions has been instrumental in the process of identification and cloning of a second class of cancer-associated genes, the tumor suppressors (which act in the normal cell as negative controllers of cell growth and are inactive in tumor cells).[4,5] Lastly, using automated sequencing instruments, it has been demonstrated that point mutations are a frequent mechanism of oncogene activation as well.[6] In the last subgroup, we can also include those obtained by the analysis of the protein kinases (kinome)[7] or phosphatases (phosphatome)[8] of the human genome or of several isoforms of a relevant protein involved in cancer development (such as PI3K).[9] In this article, the methods by which oncogenes were discovered, which have been only briefly anticipated, will be described. The various functions of cellular proto-oncogenes will then be presented, and the genetic mechanisms of proto-oncogene activation will be summarized. The role of specific oncogenes in the initiation and progression of human tumors will be then illustrated. Lastly, the discovery that oncogenes may represent relevant target for new drugs will be discussed.

Discovery and identification of oncogenes

The first oncogenes were discovered through the study of *retroviruses,* RNA tumor viruses whose genomes are reverse-transcribed into DNA in infected animal cells.[10] During the course of infection, retroviral DNA is inserted into the chromosomes of host cells. The integrated retroviral DNA, called the provirus, replicates along with the cellular DNA of the host, leading to the production of viral progeny that bud through the host cell membrane to infect other cells.[10] Acutely transforming retroviruses can rapidly cause tumors within days after injection. Chronic or weakly oncogenic retroviruses can cause tissue-specific tumors in susceptible strains of experimental animals after a latency period of many months.

Retroviral oncogenes are altered versions of host cellular proto-oncogenes that have been incorporated into the retroviral genome by recombination with host DNA, a process known as retroviral *transduction*.[4] This surprising discovery was made through study of the RSV (Figure 1), revealing that the transforming gene of RSV was not required for viral replication.[11] Molecular hybridization studies then showed that the RSV transforming gene (designated *v-src*) was homologous to a host cellular gene (*c-src*) that was widely conserved in eukaryotic species.[12] Studies of many other acutely transforming retroviruses from fowl, rodent, feline, and nonhuman primate species have led to the discovery of dozens of different retroviral oncogenes (Table 1). In every case, these retroviral oncogenes are responsible for the rapid tumor formation and efficient *in vitro* transformation activity, characteristic of acutely transforming retroviruses.

In contrast, weakly oncogenic retroviruses do not carry viral oncogenes. These retroviruses, which include mouse mammary tumor virus (MMTV) and various animal leukemia viruses, induce tumors by a process called *insertional mutagenesis* (Figure 2).[13] This process results from the integration of the provirus DNA into the host genome in infected cells and acquires relevance when (rarely) the provirus is inserted near a proto-oncogene, whose expression is then abnormally driven by the transcriptional regulatory elements contained within the long terminal repeats of the provirus.[13] Therefore, proviral integration represents a mutagenic

Table 1 Oncogenes.

Oncogene	Chromosome	Identification	Method neoplasm	mechanism of activation	Protein function
Growth factors					
v-sis	22q12.3-13.1	Sequence homology	Glioma/fibrosarcoma	Constitutive production	B-chain PDGF
int2	11q13	Proviral insertion	Mammary carcinoma	Constitutive production	Member of FGF family
KS3	11q13.3	DNA transfection	Kaposi sarcoma	Constitutive Production	Member of FGF family
HST	11q13.3	DNA transfection	Stomach carcinoma	Constitutive production	Member of FGF family
Growth factor receptors					
Tyrosine kinases: integral membrane proteins					
EGFR	7p1.1-1.3	DNA amplification/DNA sequencing	Squamous cell carcinoma	Gene amplification/protein/point	EGF receptor
v-fms	5q33-34 (FMS)	Viral homologue	Sarcoma	Constitutive activation	CSF1 receptor
v-kit	4q11-21 (KIT)	Viral homologue/DNA sequencing	Sarcoma/GIST	Constitutive activation/point mutation	Stem cell factor receptor
v-ros	6q22(ROS)	Viral homologue	Sarcoma	Constitutive activation	?
MET	7p31	DNA transfection	MNNG-treated human osteocarcinoma cell line	DNA rearrangement/ligand-independent constitutive activation (fusion proteins)	HGF/SF receptor
TRK	1q32-41	DNA transfection	Colon/thyroid carcinomas	DNA rearrangement/ligand-independent constitutive activation (fusion proteins)	NGF receptor
NEU	17q11.2-12	Point mutation/DNA amplification	Neuroblastoma/breast carcinoma/NSCLC	Gene amplification/point mutation	?
RET	10q11.2	DNA transfection	Carcinomas of thyroid Men 2A/Men 2B	DNA rearrangement/point mutation (ligand-independent constitutive activation/fusion proteins)	GDNF/NTT/ART/PSP receptor
Receptors lacking protein kinase activity					
mas	6q24-27	DNA transfection	Epidermoid carcinoma	Rearrangement of 5' noncoding region	Angiotensin receptor
Signal transducers					
Cytoplasmic tyrosine kinases					
SRC	20p12-13	Viral homologue	Colon carcinoma	Constitutive activation	Protein tyrosine kinase
v-yes	18q21-3 (YES)	Viral homologue	Sarcoma	Constitutive activation	Protein tyrosine kinase
v-fgr	1p36.1-36.2 (FGR)	Viral homologue	Sarcoma	Constitutive activation	Protein tyrosine kinase
v-fes	15q25-26 (FES)	Viral homologue	Sarcoma	Constitutive activation	Protein tyrosine kinase
ABL	9q34.1	Chromosome translocation	CML	DNA rearrangement (constitutive activation/fusion proteins)	Protein tyrosine kinase

(*continued overleaf*)

Table 1 (Continued)

Oncogene	Chromosome	Identification	Method neoplasm mechanism of activation	Protein function	
Membrane-associated G proteins					
H-RAS	11p15.5	Viral homologue/DNA transfection	Colon, lung, pancreas carcinomas	Point mutation	GTPase
K-RAS	12p11.1-12.1	Viral homologue/DNA transfection	AML, thyroid carcinoma, melanoma/colon/lung	Point mutation	GTPase
N-RAS	1p11-13	DNA transfection	Carcinoma, melanoma	Point mutation	GTPase
BRAF	6	DNA sequencing	Melanoma, thyroid, colon, ovary	Point mutation	Ser/Thr kinase
gsp	20	DNA sequencing	Adenomas of thyroid	Point mutation	Gs alpha
gip	3	DNA sequencing	Ovary, adrenal carcinoma	Point mutation	Gi alpha
GTPase exchange factor (GEF)					
Dbl	Xq27	DNA transfection	Diffuse B-cell lymphoma	DNA rearrangement	GEF for Rho and Cdc42Hs
Vav	19p13.2	DNA transfection	Hematopoietic cells	DNA rearrangement	GEF for Ras?
Serine/threonine kinases: cytoplasmic					
v-mos	8q11 (MOS)	Viral homologue	Sarcoma	Constitutive activation	Protein kinase (ser/thr)
v-raf	3p25 (RAF-1)	Viral homologue	Sarcoma	Constitutive activation	Protein kinase (ser/thr)
pim-1	6p21 (PIM-)	Insertional mutagenesis	T-cell lymphoma	Constitutive activation	Protein kinase (ser/thr)
Cytoplasmic regulators					
v-crk	17p13 (CRK)	Viral homologue		Constitutive tyrosine phosphorylation of cellular substrates (e.g., paxillin)	SH-2/SH-3 adaptor
Transcription factors					
v-myc	8q24.1 (MYC)	Viral homologue	Carcinoma myelocytomatosis	Deregulated activity	Transcription factor
N-MYC	2p24	DNA amplification	Neuroblastoma: lung	Deregulated activity	Transcription factor
L-MYC	1p32	DNA amplification	Carcinoma of lung	Deregulated activity	Transcription factor
v-myb	6q22-24	Viral homologue	Myeloblastosis	Deregulated activity	Transcription factor
v-fos	14q21-22	Viral homologue	Osteosarcoma	Deregulated activity	Transcription factor API
v-jun	p31-32	Viral homologue	Sarcoma	Deregulated activity	Transcription factor API
v-ski	1q22-24	Viral homologue	Carcinoma	Deregulated activity	Transcription factor
v-rel	2p12-14	Viral homologue	Lymphatic leukemia	Deregulated activity	Mutant NF-kappa B
v-ets-1	11p23-q24	Viral homologue	Erythroblastosis	Deregulated activity	Transcription factor
v-ets-2	21q24.3	Viral homologue	Erythroblastosis	Deregulated activity	Transcription factor
v-erbA1	17p11-21	Viral homologue	Erythroblastosis	Deregulated activity	T3 Transcription factor
v-erbA2	3p22-24.1	Viral homologue	Erythroblastosis	Deregulated activity	T3 Transcription factor
Others					
BCL2	18q21.3	Chromosomal translocation	B-cell lymphomas	Constitutive activity	Antiapoptotic protein
MDM2	12q14	DNA amplification	Sarcomas	Gene amplification/increased protein	Complexes with p53

Abbreviations: AML, acute myeloid leukemia; CML, chronic myelogenous leukemia; GTPase, guanosine triphosphatase; PDGF, platelet-derived growth factor.

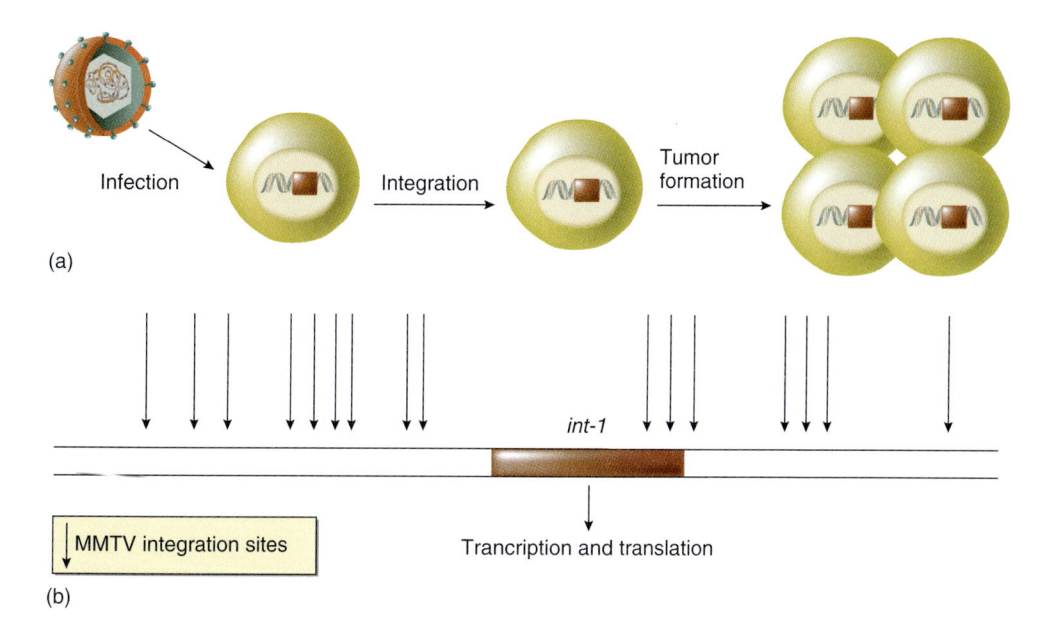

Figure 2 Insertional mutagenesis. (a) The process is independent from genes carried by the retrovirus. Retrovirus, e.g., MMTV, infects a human cell. The proviral DNA is integrated into the host genome in infected cells. Rarely, the provirus inserts near a proto-oncogene (e.g., int-1) and activates the proto-oncogene. Activated proto-oncogene results in cell transformation and in tumor formation. (b) Sites of integration of MMTV retrovirus near the proto-oncogene int-1. All sites determine int-1 activation.

event that activates a proto-oncogene. The long latent period of tumor formation of weakly oncogenic retroviruses is, therefore, due to the rarity of the provirus insertional event that leads to tumor development from a single transformed cell. Insertional mutagenesis by weakly oncogenic retroviruses, first demonstrated in bursal lymphomas of chickens, frequently involves the same oncogenes (such as myc, myb, and erb B) that are carried by acutely transforming retroviruses.[13,14] In many cases, however, insertional mutagenesis has been used as a tool to identify new oncogenes, including int-1, int-2, pim-1, and lck.[13]

The demonstration of activated proto-oncogenes in human tumors was first shown by the DNA-mediated transformation technique.[15,16] This method, also called gene-transfer or transfection assay, assesses the ability of donor DNA from a tumor to transform a recipient strain of rodent cells called NIH 3T3, an immortalized mouse cell line (Figure 3).[17] This sensitive assay, which can detect the presence of single-copy oncogenes in a tumor sample, also enables the isolation of the transforming oncogene by molecular cloning techniques.[18] Overall, approximately 20% of individual human tumors have been shown to induce transformation of NIH 3T3 cells in gene-transfer assays. The value of transfection assay was reinforced by Weinberg's laboratory, which showed that the ectopic expression of the telomerase catalytic subunit (hTERT), in combination with the simian virus 40 large T product and a mutated oncogenic H-ras protein, resulted in the direct tumorigenic conversion of normal human epithelial and fibroblast cells.[19] Many of the oncogenes identified by gene-transfer studies are identical or closely related to oncogenes transduced by retroviruses.[20] A number of new oncogenes (such as neu, met, ret, and trk) have also been identified by the gene-transfer technique.[21] In some cases, however, oncogenes identified by gene transfer were shown to be activated by rearrangement during the experimental procedure and were not found activated in the original human tumors that served as the source of the donor DNA. This was the case of ret (= REarranged during Transfection),

isolated from a human lymphoma but subsequently found genuinely rearranged and activated in papillary thyroid carcinomas.[22] Chromosomal translocations have served as guideposts for the discovery of new oncogenes, mainly in hematological but also in some solid tumors.[23,24] These abnormalities include chromosomal rearrangements (such as translocations, inversions, etc.) as well as the gain or loss of whole chromosomes or chromosome segments. The first consistent karyotypic abnormality identified in a human neoplasm was a characteristic small chromosome in the cells of patients with CML.[23] Later identified as a derivative of chromosome 22, this abnormality was designated the Philadelphia chromosome, after its city of discovery. The application of chromosome banding techniques in the early 1970s enabled the precise cytogenetic characterization of many chromosomal translocations in human leukemia, lymphoma, and solid tumors.[25] The subsequent development of molecular cloning techniques then enabled the identification of proto-oncogenes at or near chromosomal breakpoints in various neoplasms. Some of these proto-oncogenes, such as myc and abl, had been previously identified as retroviral oncogenes. In general, however, the cloning of chromosomal breakpoints has served as a rich source of discovery of new oncogenes involved in human cancer. More recently, the use of high-throughput sequencing technologies and bioinformatics from the Human Genome Project led to the discovery of new genes involved in cancer development, such as BRAF and PIK3CA.[6,9]

Oncogenes, proto-oncogenes, and their functions

Proto-oncogenes encode proteins that are involved in the control of cell growth. Alteration of the structure and/or expression of proto-oncogenes can activate them to become oncogenes capable of inducing in susceptible cells the neoplastic phenotype. Oncogenes can be classified into five groups based on the functional and biochemical properties of protein products of their normal counterparts (proto-oncogenes). These groups are (1) growth factors, (2) growth factor receptors, (3) signal transducers, (4) transcription

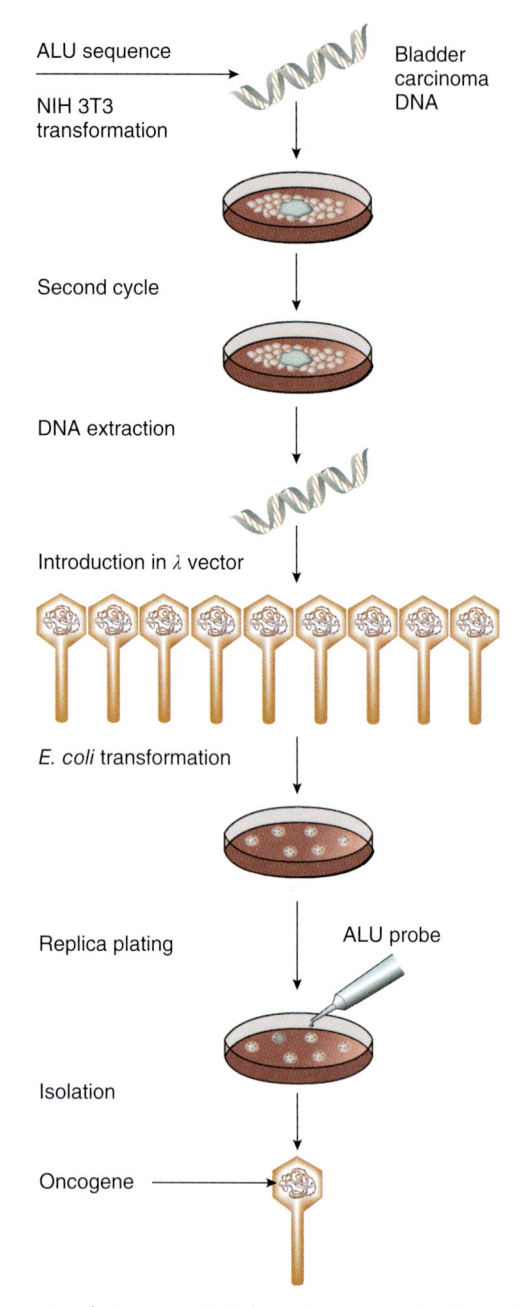

Figure 3 Transfection assay. DNA from a tumor (e.g., bladder carcinoma) is used to transform a rodent immortalized cell line (NIH 3T3). After serial cycles, DNA from transformed cells was extracted and then inserted into p vector, which was subsequently used to transform an appropriate *Escherichia coli* strain. Using a specific probe (Alu in the figure) it was possible to isolate and then characterize the involved human oncogene.

factors, and (5) others, including programmed cell death regulators. Table 1 lists examples of oncogenes according to their functional categories.

Growth factors

Growth factors are secreted polypeptides that function as extracellular signals to stimulate the proliferation of target cells which possess a specific receptor in order to respond to a specific type of growth factor.[2] A well-characterized example is platelet-derived growth factor (PDGF), an approximately 30-kd protein consisting of two polypeptide chains.[26] PDGF, released from platelets during the process of blood coagulation, stimulates the proliferation of fibroblasts, a cell growth process that plays an important role in wound healing. Other well-characterized examples of growth factors include nerve growth factor (NGF), epidermal growth factor, and fibroblast growth factor.

The link between growth factors and retroviral oncogenes was revealed by study of the *sis* oncogene of simian sarcoma virus, a retrovirus first isolated from a monkey fibrosarcoma. Sequence analysis showed that *sis* encodes the β-chain of PDGF.[26] This discovery established the principle that inappropriately expressed growth factors may constitutively activate their receptor, resulting in self-sustained aberrant cell proliferation and therefore functioning as oncogenes. The mechanism behind this is called *autocrine stimulation* (Figure 4).[26] This model, derived from experimental animal systems, has been demonstrated in a human tumor, dermatofibrosarcoma protuberans (DP), an infiltrative skin tumor that was demonstrated to present specific cytogenetic features: reciprocal translocation and supernumerary ring chromosomes, involving chromosomes 17 and 22.[26] Molecular cloning of the breakpoints revealed a fusion between the *collagen type Ia1 (COL1A1)* gene and *PDGF-b* gene. The fusion gene resulted in a deletion of *PDGF-b* exon 1 and a constitutive release of this growth factor. Subsequent experiments of gene transfer of DP's genomic DNA into NIH 3T3 cells directly demonstrated the occurrence of an autocrine mechanism by the human rearranged *PDGF-b* gene involving the activation of the endogenous PDGF receptor.[26] Another example of a growth factor that can function as an oncogene is *int-2*, a member of the fibroblast growth factor family. *Int-2* is sometimes activated in mouse mammary carcinomas by MMTV insertional mutagenesis.[27]

Growth factor receptors

Some viral oncogenes are altered versions of normal growth factor receptors that possess intrinsic tyrosine kinase (TK) activity.[28] Receptor tyrosine kinases (RTK), as these growth factor receptors are collectively known, have a characteristic protein structure consisting of three principal domains: (1) the extracellular ligand-binding domain, (2) the transmembrane domain, and (3) the intracellular TK catalytic domain (Figure 5). RTK are molecular machines that transmit information in a unidirectional fashion across the cell membrane. The binding of a growth factor to the extracellular ligand-binding domain of the receptor results in the activation of the intracellular TK catalytic domain, usually after dimerization, leading to the activation of downstream proteins which physically interact with RTK, mainly represented by the mitogen-activated protein kinases (MAPK) pathway, by the PI3K/AKT axis and by STAT proteins. These pathways are activated differently, depending on the specific RTK, overall resulting in abnormal cell duplication and in escaping from programmed cell death (apoptosis).[28]

The list of RTK includes *erb B1, erb B2, fms, kit, met, ret, ros, alk,* and *trk*, which can be *conver*ted into oncogenes through different mechanisms, often depending on tumor type.[28] *erb B1* (the epidermal growth factor receptor [EGFR]) can be oncogenically activated by deletion of the ligand-binding domain, by point mutations in the TK domain in a subgroup of patients affected by non-small-cell lung cancer (NSCLC) (more commonly in Japan than in other Western countries, suggesting that ethnic differences may have a significant impact on *erb B1* activation),[29] or at germ-line level in patients showing multiple lung adenocarcinomas,[30] by overexpression of ligands or by gene amplification in colorectal cancer (CRC) patients.[31]

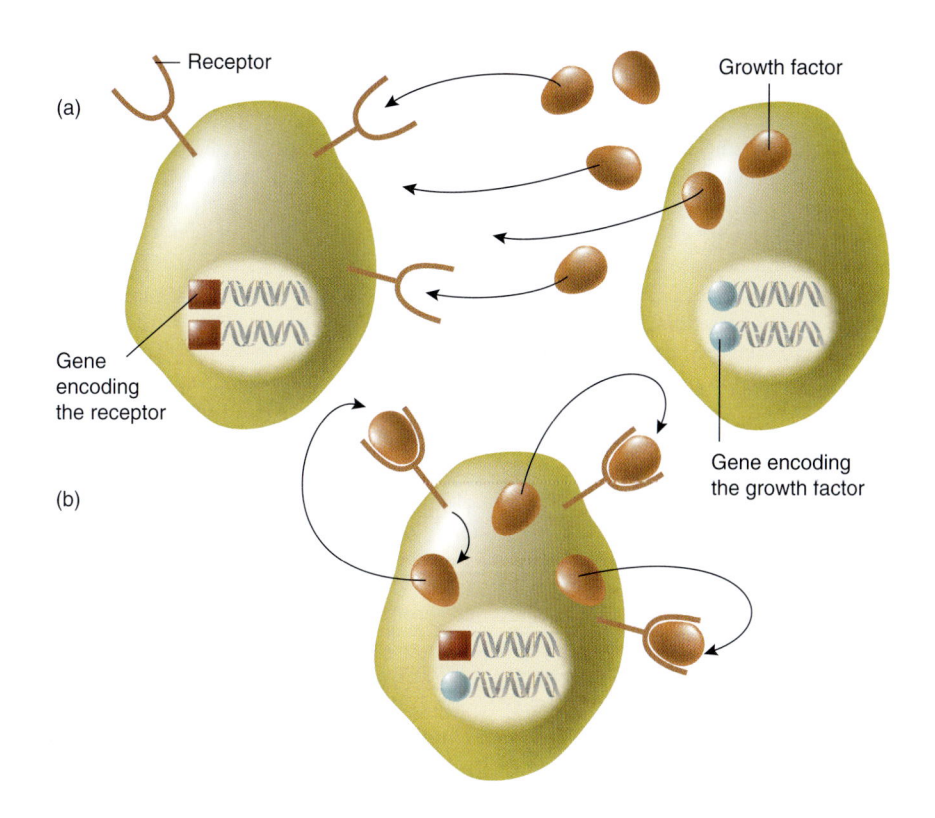

Figure 4 Paracrine and autocrine stimulation. (a) A growth factor produced by the cell on the right stimulates another cell carrying the appropriate receptor (left) on cell membrane. This process is named paracrine stimulation. (b) A growth factor is produced by the same cell expressing the cognate receptor. This process is designated autocrine stimulation.

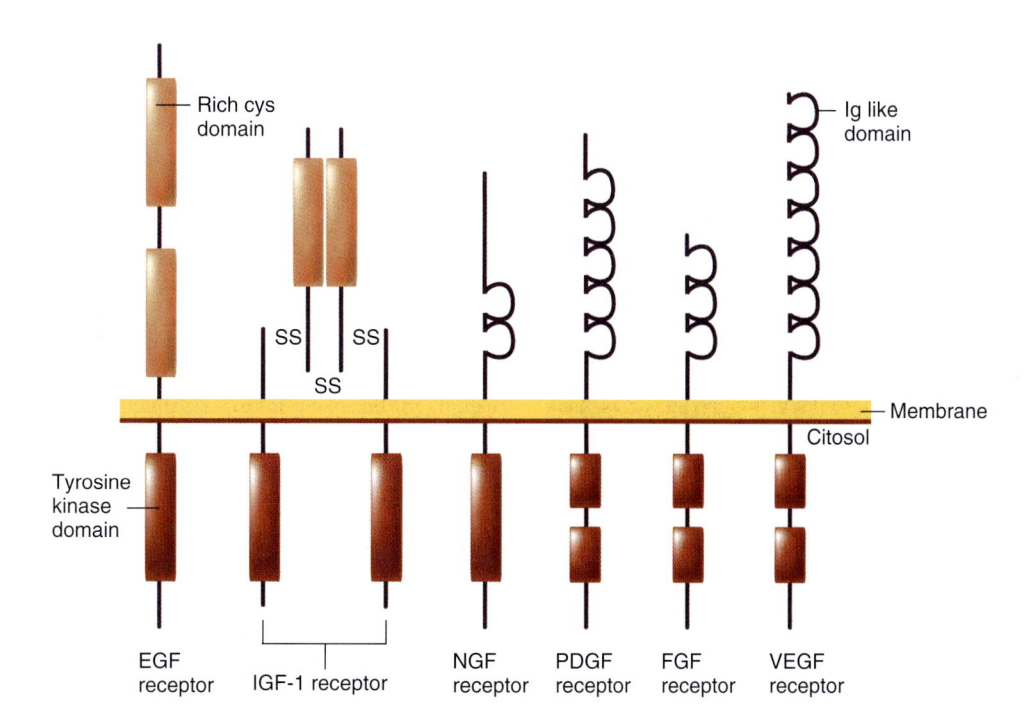

Figure 5 Representative examples of tyrosine kinase receptor families.

Another example is represented by *erb B2*, whose growth factor is still unknown, which is altered by gene amplification in breast and gastric cancer, and by point mutations in gastric, colorectal, and breast cancers. Interestingly, immunohistochemical staining for *erb B2* revealed no differences between tumors with or without *erb B2* mutations, indicating that overexpression probably does not accompany the mutation.[32]

Last example is *kit*, whose activation in tumor cells can be due to three different mechanisms: (1) autocrine and/or paracrine stimulation of the receptor by its ligand, SCF; (2) cross-activation by other kinases and/or loss of regulatory phosphatase activity; and (3) acquisition of activating mutations of several different exons of the *kit* gene.[33] *kit* mutations (typically in exon 17) are most commonly found in mastocytosis/mast cell leukemia, acute myelogenous leukemia (AML), seminoma/dysgerminoma, and sinonasal natural killer/T-cell lymphoma. In gastrointestinal stromal tumors (GIST), more heterogeneous mutations are described: mutations most commonly occur in exon 11 (encoding the juxtamembrane region) (in about 65% of all GISTs) whereas about 10% of GISTs have kit exon 9 mutations and 2% exon 13 or exon 17 mutations. In GIST showing any alterations in the *kit* gene, point mutations may occur in *pdgfra*, a gene belonging to the same family as *kit*. Approximately 5% of GIST have a constitutively activating mutations in *pdgfra*, mostly (80%) found in exon 18 and the rest either in exon 12 (10–15%) or 14 (1–5%).[33] *kit* and *pdgfra* mutations are mutually exclusive. Gastric GISTs with exon 11 deletions are more aggressive than those with substitutions. The less common *kit* exon 9 codons 502–503 duplication occurs predominantly in small intestinal GISTs. pdgfra mutations are associated with gastric GISTs, epithelioid morphology, and a less malignant course of disease.[33] Germ-line mutations in kit gene have been found in patients manifesting multiple GIST arising at earlier age, urticaria pigmentosa, melanocytic nevi, melanomas, achalasia, or neuronal hyperplasia of the mesenteric plexus.

Signal transducers

Mitogenic signals are transmitted from RTK on the cell surface to the cell nucleus through a series of complex interlocking pathways collectively referred to as the signal transduction cascade.[28] This relay of information is accomplished in part by the stepwise phosphorylation of interacting proteins in the cytosol. Signal transduction also involves guanine nucleotide-binding proteins and second messengers such as the adenylate cyclase system. The first retroviral oncogene discovered, *src*, was subsequently shown to be involved in signal transduction.[12,28]

Many proto-oncogenes are members of signal transduction pathways.[34] These consist of two main groups: nonreceptor protein kinases and guanosine triphosphate (GTP)-binding proteins. The nonreceptor protein kinases are subclassified into TKs (e.g., *abl*, *lck*, and *src*) and serine/threonine kinases (e.g., *raf-1*, *mos*, and *pim-1*). GTP-binding proteins with intrinsic guanosine triphosphatase (GTPase) activity are subdivided into monomeric and heterotrimeric groups. Monomeric GTP-binding proteins are members of the important *ras* family of proto-oncogenes that includes H-*ras*, K-*ras*, and N-*ras*.[35] Heterotrimeric GTP-binding proteins (G proteins) implicated as proto-oncogenes currently include *gsp* and *gip*. Signal transducers are often converted to oncogenes by mutations that lead to their unregulated activity, which in turn leads to uncontrolled cellular proliferation.[35]

Transcription factors

Transcription factors are nuclear proteins that regulate the expression of target genes or gene families.[36] Transcriptional regulation is mediated by protein-binding to specific DNA sequences or DNA structural motifs (such as zinc fingers), usually located upstream of the target gene. The mechanism of action of transcription factors also involves binding to other proteins, sometimes in heterodimeric complexes with specific partners. Transcription factors are the final link in the signal transduction pathway that converts extracellular signals into modulated changes in gene expression.

Many proto-oncogenes are transcription factors that were discovered through their retroviral homologues.[36] Examples include *erb* A, *ets*, *fos*, *jun*, *myb*, and *c-myc*. Together, fos and jun form the AP-1 transcription factor, which positively regulates a number of target genes whose expression leads to cell division.[37] *Erb A* is the receptor for the T3 thyroid hormone, triiodothyronine.[38] Proto-oncogenes that function as transcription factors are often activated by chromosomal translocations in hematologic and solid neoplasms. In certain types of sarcomas, chromosomal translocations cause the formation of fusion proteins involving the association of *EWS* gene with various partners and resulting in an aberrant tumor-associated transcriptional activity. Interestingly, a role of the adenovirus *E1A* gene in promoting the formation of fusion transcript fli1/ews in normal human fibroblasts was recently reported.[39] An important example of a proto-oncogene with a transcriptional activity in human hematologic tumors is the *c-myc* gene, which helps to control the expression of genes leading to cell proliferation.[40] As will be discussed later in this article, the *c-myc* gene (which is encoded for a nuclear DNA-binding protein belonging to the helix-loop-helix/ leucine zipper superfamily, involved in transcriptional regulation) is frequently activated by chromosomal translocations in human leukemia and lymphoma.

Programed cell death regulation

Normal tissues exhibit a regulated balance between cell proliferation and cell death. Programmed cell death is an important component in the processes of normal embryogenesis and organ development. A distinctive type of programmed cell death, called apoptosis, has been described for mature tissues.[41] Studies of cancer cells have shown that both uncontrolled cell proliferation and failure to undergo programmed cell death can contribute to neoplasia and insensitivity to anticancer treatments.

The first proto-oncogene shown to regulate programmed cell death is *bcl-2, discovered in* human lymphomas. Experimental studies show that *bcl-2* activation inhibits (in a dominant mode) programmed cell death in lymphoid cell populations. The *bcl-2* gene encodes a protein localized to the inner mitochondrial membrane, endoplasmic reticulum (ER), and nuclear membrane. The mechanism of action of the bcl-2 protein has not been fully elucidated but studies indicate that it functions in part as an antioxidant that inhibits lipid peroxidation of cell membranes,[42] and in part through protein–protein interaction with homologue proteins. Site-directed mutagenesis of BH1 and BH2 domains showed that these two regions are important for binding of bcl-2 to bax, a member of the bcl-2-family that promotes cell death and whose interaction with bcl-2 is necessary to regulate the apoptotic pathway (Figure 6). Although translocation is the main mechanism of *bcl-2* gene activation, *bcl-2* point mutations (in high-grade B-cell lymphomas) and amplification (in about 30% of high-grade diffuse large cell lymphomas (DLCL) lacking bcl-2 translocation) have been reported.[42] Clinical relevance of bcl-2 expression has been shown in solid tumors, such as breast, prostate, thyroid, and lung.[42]

The second oncogene involved in apoptosis is caspase-9, which is activated by the following intrinsic pathway. Release of cytochrome c into the cytosol results in activation of the caspase adaptor Apaf-1 and procaspase-9, which form a holoenzyme complex named apoptosome.[43] Caspase-9, in turn, activates downstream caspases, especially caspase-3 and also caspase-6, 7, and 8, leading to DNA fragmentation and apoptosis. It has been demonstrated that Akt may regulate apoptosome function by phosphorylation of caspase-9 at the Ser-196 level.[44,45] This phosphorylation event has relevant functional consequences, leading to the suppression of apoptosis caspase-9-mediated. The Akt suppression is specific for caspase-9 and probably is due to the inactivation of the intrinsic

Oncogenes

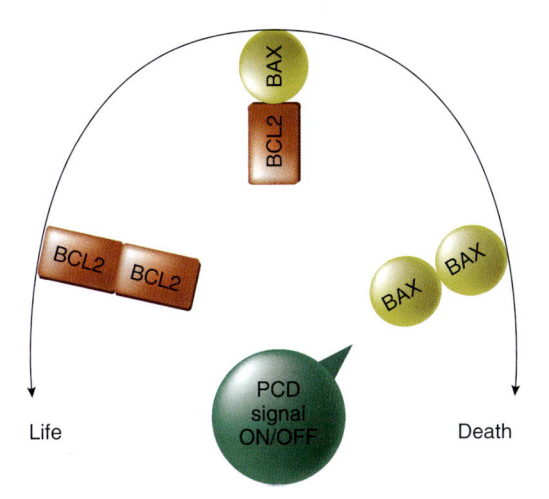

Figure 6 Effect of bcl-2 activity on the control of the cell life. In the presence of BAX only, the cell goes to apoptosis. bcl-2 regulates the cycle of the cell by the interaction with BAX. When bcl-2 is overexpressed, the cell cycle is deregulated and the apoptosis is prevented, eventually leading to tumor formation. This is an important cause for tumor formation. *Abbreviation:* PCD, program cell death or apoptosis.

catalytic activity. Furthermore, it has been demonstrated that bax is also involved, leading to caspase-9 stimulation (through Apaf-1) in response to mitochondrial membrane damage.[44,45]

Mechanisms of oncogene activation

The activation of oncogenes involves genetic changes to cellular proto-oncogenes. The consequence of these genetic alterations is to confer a growth advantage to the cell. Four genetic mechanisms activate oncogenes in human neoplasms: (1) mutation, (2) gene amplification, (3) chromosome rearrangements, and (4) overexpression. The first three mechanisms result in either an alteration of proto-oncogene structure or an increase in proto-oncogene expression (Figure 7). Because neoplasia is a multistep process, more than one of these mechanisms may occur, leading to a combination of proto-oncogene activation and tumor suppressor gene loss or inactivation.

Mutation

Mutations activate proto-oncogenes through structural alterations in their encoded proteins. These alterations, which usually involve critical protein regulatory regions or directly the catalytic domain, often lead to the uncontrolled, continuous activity of the mutated protein. Various types of mutations, such as base substitutions, deletions, and insertions, are capable of activating proto-oncogenes.[46] Retroviral oncogenes, for example, often have deletions that contribute to their activation. Examples include deletions in the amino-terminal ligand-binding domains of the *erb B*, *kit*, *ros*, *met*, and *trk* oncogenes. In human tumors, however, most characterized oncogene mutations are base substitutions (point mutations) that change a single amino acid within the protein.

Point mutations are frequently detected in the ras family of protooncogenes (*K-ras*, *H-ras*, and *N-ras*). The human *ras* genes encode for membrane-bound 21 kd proteins (189 amino acids) involved in signal transduction, with a guanine nucleotide-binding activity as well as an intrinsic GTPase activity. When activated, ras proteins transduce the signal by linking TKs to downstream serine/threonine kinases, such as raf, and MAP kinases (Figure 8).[47]

Stabilization of ras proteins in their active state causes a continuous flow of signal transduction, which results in malignant transformation. This status can be achieved after point mutation, mainly at codon 12 (in *K-ras* gene), 13, and 61 (mainly in *N-ras* gene) level. Rare mutations can be detected in codons 59, 117, and 146.[47] Mutations of *ras* in human tumors have been linked to carcinogen exposure: for example, the occurrence of *K-ras* mutations in NSCLC seems to be due to smoking exposure, in particular to benzopyrene.[47] It has been estimated that as many as 15–20% of unselected human tumors may contain a *ras* mutation. Mutations in *K-ras* predominate in tumors derived from endodermal tumors, including carcinomas of pancreas (90%), colorectal (40%), and lung.[47] This finding is due to the fact that *K-ras*, but not *H-ras* or *N-ras*, promotes the expansion of an endodermal stem/progenitor cell and blocks its differentiation.[47] N-*ras* mutations are preferentially found in hematologic malignancies, with up to a 25% incidence in AMLs and myelodysplastic syndromes, or in melanoma and in a subgroup of CRC.[47] The majority of thyroid carcinomas have been found to have *ras* mutations distributed among K-*ras*, H-*ras*, and N-*ras*, without preference for a single *ras* family member, but showing an association with the follicular type of differentiated thyroid carcinomas.

In addition to cancer, *ras* mutations are involved in other diseases. Specifically, N-*ras* mutations cause a human autoimmune lymphoproliferative syndrome,[48] while *H-ras* and *K-ras* germ-line mutations underlie disorders of the Noonan syndrome spectrum.[47] The last data, coupled with the evidence that cancers rarely occur in these individuals, are leading to a re-evaluation of the effective role played by *ras* genes in carcinogenesis.

Another example of activating point mutations is represented by those occurring in *BRAF* gene, the first result of the human genome project in the screening of cancer genes using high-throughput genomic technologies.[7] The *BRAF* gene product is recruited to the plasma membrane upon binding to ras-GTP and represents a key point in the signal transduction through the MAP kinase pathway (see Figure 8). The most common oncogenic mutation of *BRAF*, occurring in more than 90% of cases, is the valine to glutamic acid change at codon 600, which mimics the phosphorylation of threonine 599 and serine 602, required for BRAF activation. In tissue specimens, *BRAF* mutations occur in melanomas (75%), thyroid (45%), colorectal (12%), ovarian cancer (14%), and in acute lymphoblastic leukemia (ALL).[43] Furthermore, it has been shown that *BRAF* mutations occur in CRC only when tumors do not carry mutations in the *K-ras* gene, and in papillary thyroid carcinoma when *RET* or *TRK* rearrangements are absent. These mutual exclusions have led to the assumption that *BRAF* and K-*ras* alterations, or *BRAF*, *RET*, and *TRK* alterations, could have the same functional effect in colorectal or in thyroid carcinogenesis, respectively.[43] As regards CRC, *BRAF* mutations are frequently present in sporadic cases with methylated hMLH1 promoter, but not in HNPCC-related cancers, thus representing a possible strategy for exclusion criteria for HNPCC.[43] Moreover, *BRAF* mutations are frequently found in hyperplastic polyps and in serrated adenomas,[43] suggesting that they represent an early and critical event in these types of lesions. *BRAF* mutations may have an influence on patients' prognosis depending on the tumor type where they occur: in ovarian cancer *BRAF* mutations are associated with type I tumors, that are slow growing and generally confined to the ovary at diagnosis,[43] and with the aggressive papillary thyroid and colorectal carcinomas.[43] *Beside BRAF mutations, there is a number of additional molecular marker alterations that have been proposed to be included in a diagnostic algorithm for thyroid cancers.*[49,50] Thyroid cancers are indeed often characterized by

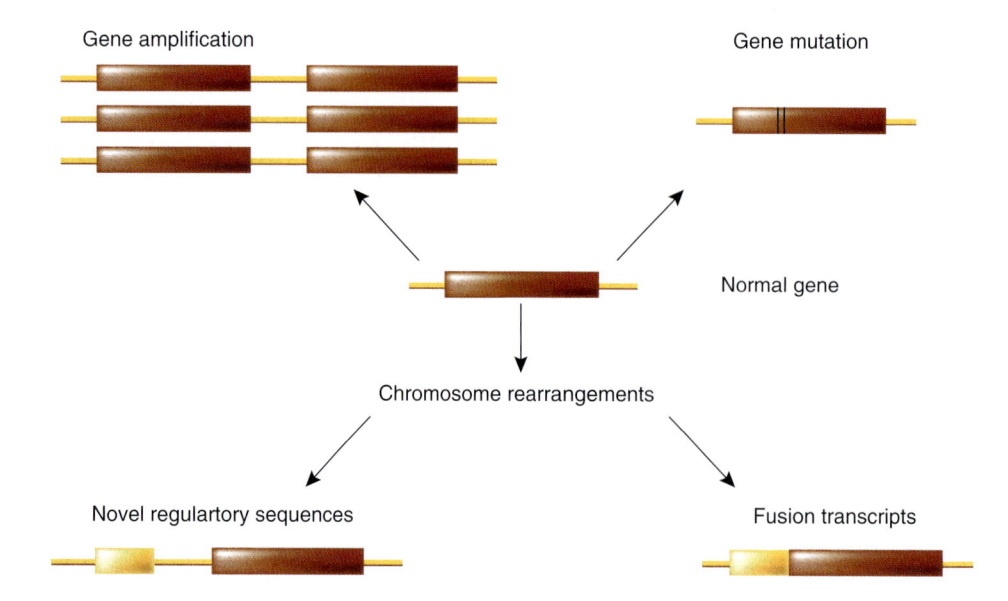

Figure 7 Schematic representation of the main mechanisms of oncogene activation (from proto-oncogenes to oncogenes). The normal gene (proto-oncogene) is depicted with its transcribed portion *(rectangle)*. In the case of gene amplification, the latter can be duplicated 100-fold, resulting in an excess of normal protein. A similar situation can occur when following chromosome rearrangements such as translocation, the transcription of the gene is now regulated by novel regulatory sequences belonging to another gene. In the case of point mutation, single amino acid substitutions can alter the biochemical properties of the gene product, causing, in the example, its constitutive enzymatic activation. Chromosome rearrangements, such as translocation and inversion, can then generate fusion transcripts resulting in chimericoncogenic proteins.

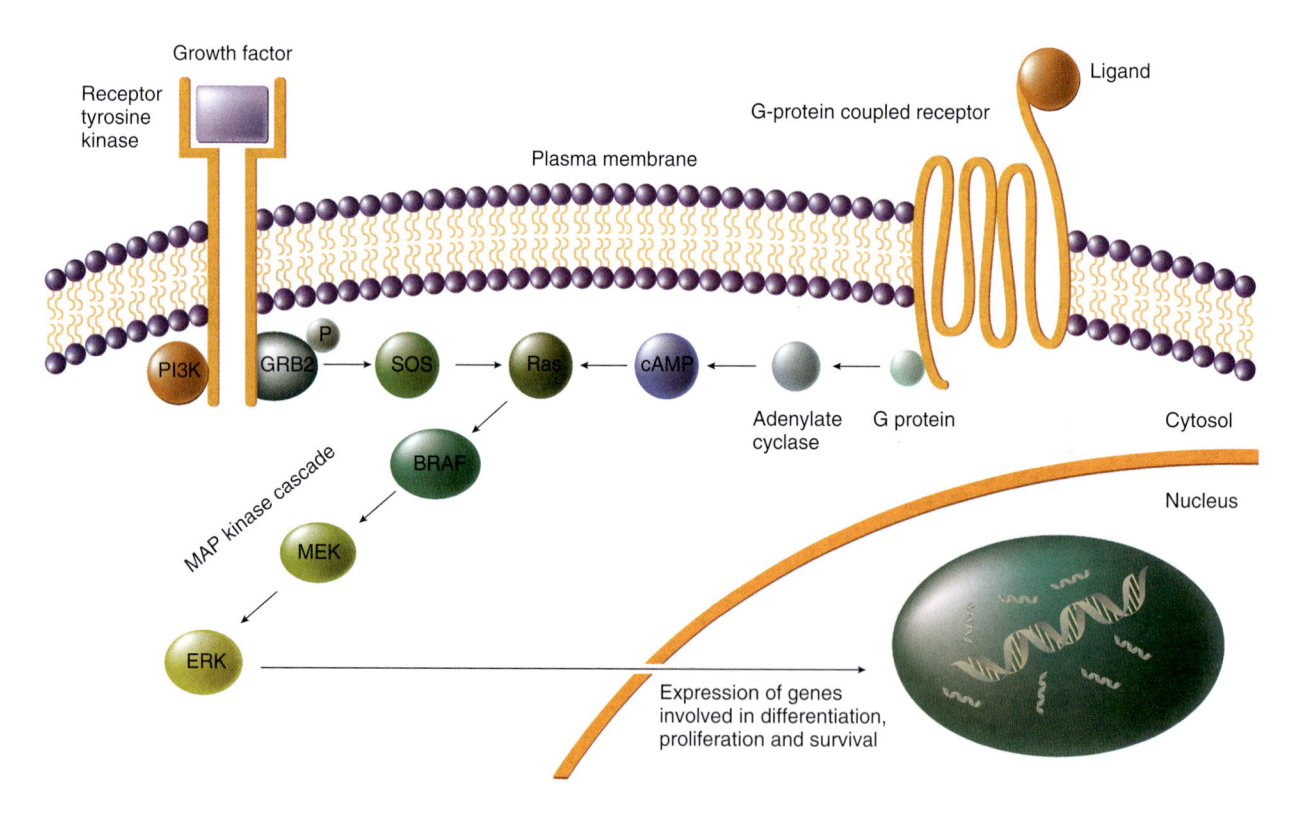

Figure 8 The ras-raf-MAPK signaling pathway.

RET/PTC or PAX8/PPARG chromosomal rearrangements, or point mutation in RAS and BRAF proto-oncogenes. Mutations of the BRAF, RAS, or RET genes occur generally in papillary thyroid carcinomas, accounting for 70% of these tumors.[49,50] To date, there are at least 13 different forms of RET/PTC rearrangements that have been detected, and they vary according to the different genetic fusion partners. Among the rearrangements, RET/PTC1 and RET/PTC3 are apparently the most common ones, accounting for more than 90% of all RET/PTC rearrangements (Table 4).[49,50] Concerning RAS gene family, three members (H-ras, K-ras, and N-ras) have been shown to be mutated in thyroid cancer. The most common RAS mutations were detected in the N-ras gene, followed by H-ras, and least frequently, K-ras. However, it became clear that the RAS mutations are predominantly related to poorly differentiated thyroid carcinomas and anaplastic thyroid cancers than papillary thyroid cancer, which suggests that RAS should be mainly involved in cancer progression rather than in early phases of thyroid cancerogenesis.[49,50]

Another significant example of activating point mutations is represented by those affecting the *ret* proto-oncogene in multiple endocrine neoplasia (MEN) type 2 (2A and 2B) syndrome and familial medullary thyroid carcinomas (FMTC). MEN 2A is associated most frequently with mutations of codon 634 (85%), particularly C634R. This germ-line point mutation affecting one of the cysteine residues located in the juxtamembrane domain of the ret receptor has been found to confer an oncogenic potential through the abnormal formation of intermolecular disulfide bonding, resulting in a ligand-independent activation of the TK activity of the receptor. Most MEN2B patients carry the M918T mutation in the kinase domain, which confers an aggressive phenotype to MEN2B subtype. Sporadic mutations of V804, M918, and E768 occur in about 50% of sporadic medullary thyroid carcinomas, whereas FMTC mutations are evenly distributed among the various cysteines in the extracellularly cysteine-rich domain, and occasionally in the TK domain. M918T mutation leads to a ligand-independent activation of the kinase without causing a constitutive dimerization of the receptor and alters also the substrate specificity of the kinase. More recently, two mutations (V804 and E805) in tandem were found in a MEN2B subtype, affecting the hinging motion of the kinase lobes.[51]

Gene amplification

Gene amplification refers to the expansion in copy number of a gene within the genome of a cell. Gene amplification was first discovered as a mechanism by which some tumor cell lines can acquire resistance to growth-inhibiting drugs. The process of gene amplification occurs through redundant replication of genomic DNA, often giving rise to karyotypic abnormalities called double-minute chromosomes (DMs) and HSRs.[52] DMs are characteristic minichromosome structures without centromeres. HSRs are segments of chromosomes that lack the normal alternating pattern of light and dark staining bands. Both DMs and HSRs represent large regions of amplified genomic DNA, containing up to several hundred copies of a gene. Amplification leads to the increased expression of genes, conferring a selective advantage for cell growth.

The frequent observation of DMs and HSRs in human tumors suggested that the amplification of specific protooncogenes may be a common occurrence in cancer.[53] Studies then demonstrated that three proto-oncogene families—*myc*, *erb B*, and *ras*—are amplified in a significant number of human tumors (Table 2). About 20–30% of breast and ovarian cancers show *c-myc* amplification.[53] N-*myc* was discovered as a new member of the *myc* proto-oncogene family through its amplification in neuroblastomas.[53] Amplification of *N-myc* correlates strongly with advanced tumor stage in neuroblastoma (Table 3), suggesting a role for this gene in tumor progression.[53] *L-myc* was discovered through its amplification in small-cell lung carcinoma and in bladder neoplasia.[53] Furthermore, *c-myc* activation may be mediated by APC and/or b-catenin alterations in several tumors, leading to an increase of *c*-myc transcription through an accumulation of b-catenin into the cytoplasm and the nucleus.[53] A nuclear accumulation of c-myc may identify high-risk subsets of patients with synovial sarcoma of the extremities.[53] Amplification and overexpression of *c-myc*, in combination with *erb B2* alterations, have been reported to be

Table 2 Oncogene amplification in human cancers.

Tumor type	Gene amplified	%
Neuroblastoma	MYCN	20–25
Small-cell lung cancer	MYC	15–20
Glioblastoma	ERB B1 (EGFR)	33–50
Breast cancer	MYC	20
	ERB B2 (EGFR2)	~20
	FGFR1	12
	FGFR2	12
	CCND1 (cyclin d1)	15–20
Esophageal cancer	MYC	38
	CCND1 (cyclin d1)	25
Gastric cancer	K-RAS	10
	CCNE (cyclin e)	15
Hepatocellular cancer	CCND1 (cyclin d1	13
Sarcoma	MDM2	10–30
	CDK4	11
Cervical cancer	MYC	25–50
Ovarian cancer	MYC	20–30
	ERB B2 (EGFR2)	15–30
	AKT2	12
Head and neck cancer	MYC	7–10
	ERB B1(EGFR)	10
	CCND1(cyclin d1)	~50
Colorectal cancer	MYB	15–20
	H-RAS	29
	K-RAS	22

Table 3 Correlation of N-myc copy number with stage and survival in neuroblastoma.

Tumor type	No. of cases	%
Benign ganglioneuromas	0/64	0
Low stages	31/772	4
Stage 4-S	15/190	8
Advanced stages	612/1.974	31
Total	658/3000	22

associated with tumor progression from noninvasive to invasive and with poor prognosis[53] in patients with breast carcinoma. In melanoma[53] and in medulloblastoma,[53] c-myc expression seems to be a useful prognostic marker able to identify high-risk patients. Amplification of *erb B* is found in up to 50% of glioblastomas (often accompanied by the loss of the exons 2-7, leading to the so-called *erb B1* variant III, which is constitutively activated),[54] in 10–20% of head and neck squamous carcinomas, and in about 50% of CRC.[55] Gene amplification and overexpression of *erb B2* have been reported in approximately 25% of breast, ovarian, endometrial, gastric, and salivary gland carcinomas.[32] It was detected also in 16% of non-small-cell lung carcinoma and in a subset of malignant pancreatic endocrine tumor (gastrinoma).

In breast cancer, *erb B2* amplification correlates with advanced stage and poor prognosis. Members of the *ras* gene family, including K-*ras* and N-*ras*, are sporadically amplified in various carcinomas.[32]

Chromosomal rearrangements

Recurring chromosomal rearrangements are often detected in hematological malignancies as well as in some solid tumors.[56] These rearrangements consist mainly of chromosomal translocations and, less frequently, chromosomal inversions. Chromosomal rearrangements can lead to hematological malignancy by two different mechanisms: (1) the transcriptional activation of proto-oncogenes or (2) the creation of fusion genes. Transcriptional activation results from chromosomal rearrangements that move a proto-oncogene close to an immunoglobulin or T-cell receptor gene (see Figure 7). Therefore, the proto-oncogene is constitutively activated in blood cells, leading to cancer development.

Fusion genes can be created by chromosomal rearrangements when the chromosomal breakpoints fall within the loci of two different genes, leading to a composite structure consisting of the head of one gene and the tail of another gene. Fusion genes encode chimeric proteins with transforming activity. In general, both genes involved in the fusion contribute to the transforming potential of the chimeric oncoprotein. Mistakes in the physiologic rearrangement of immunoglobulin or T-cell receptor genes are thought to give rise to many of the recurring chromosomal rearrangements found in hematologic malignancy.[57] Examples of molecularly characterized chromosomal rearrangements in hematologic and solid malignancies are given in Table 4. In some cases, the same proto-oncogene is involved in several different translocations (i.e., c-myc, ews, and *ret*).

Gene activation
The t(8;14)(q24;q32) translocation, found in about 85% of cases of Burkitt's lymphoma, is a well-characterized example of the transcriptional activation of a proto-oncogene. This chromosomal rearrangement places the c-myc gene, located at chromosome band 8q24, under the control of regulatory elements from the immunoglobulin heavy-chain locus located at 14q32. The c-myc gene is also activated in some cases of Burkitt's lymphoma by translocations involving immunoglobulin light-chain genes. These are t(2;8)(p12;q24), involving the κ locus located at 2p12, and t(8;22)(q24;q11), involving the λ locus at 22q11 (Figure 9). The position of the chromosomal breakpoints relative to the c-myc gene may vary considerably in individual cases of Burkitt's lymphoma, but with the same effect. An alternative mechanism of c-myc alteration is represented by gene mutations, which can occur in the gene transactivation domain and in the coding region after translocation into the *Ig* gene[58] or in the noncoding gene exon 1 and at the exon 1/intron 1 boundary with or without c-myc gene translocation.[59] In T-cell ALL (T-ALL), the c-myc gene is activated by the t(8;14)(q24;q11) translocation, when it is placed under the control of regulatory elements within the T-cell receptor.[60] In this tumor, several other proto-oncogenes encoding nuclear proteins are activated by various chromosomal translocations involving α or β loci of the T-cell receptor. These include *HOX11, TAL1, TAL2,* and RBTN1/Tgt1.[60] The proteins encoded by these genes are thought to function as transcription factors through DNA-binding and protein–protein interactions, whose inappropriate expression leads to uncontrolled cellular proliferation.

A number of other proto-oncogenes are also activated by chromosomal translocations in leukemia and lymphoma.

Gene fusion
The first example of gene fusion was discovered through the cloning of the breakpoint of the Philadelphia chromosome in CML.[61] The t(9;22)(q34;q11) translocation in CML fuses the c-abl gene, normally located at 9q34, with the *bcr* gene at 22q11 (Figure 10). The *bcr/abl* fusion, created on the der(22) chromosome, encodes a chimeric protein of 210 kD with increased TK activity and abnormal cellular localization.[61] The precise mechanism by which the *bcr/abl* fusion protein contributes to the expansion of the neoplastic myeloid clone is not yet known. The t(9;22) translocation is also found in up to 20% of cases of ALL. In these cases, the breakpoint in the *bcr* gene differs somewhat from that found in CML, resulting in a 185-kD bcr/abl fusion protein.[61] It is unclear at this time why the slightly smaller bcr/abl fusion protein leads to such a large difference in neoplastic phenotype. Inhibition of bcr/abl TK activity has been introduced as a chemotherapeutic approach in patients with CML. Administration of imatinib resulted in an antileukemic effect in CML patients in whom treatment with standard chemotherapy had failed.[62] However, cases of imatinib resistance have also been recently documented.[63] Cause of such a failure is due to either bcr/abl gene amplification or single amino acid substitutions affecting residues that are in direct contact with ATP or are within the ATP pocket of the kinase domain of abl, resulting in structural changes that could influence inhibition sensitivity. Strategies for overcoming resistance have been suggested, exploiting dependence of bcr/abl protein on the molecular chaperone heat shock protein 90.[63]

Additional genes encoding TKs involved in gene fusion events in hematologic malignancy are represented by the t(2;5)(p23;q35) translocation in anaplastic large cell lymphomas fusing the *NPM* gene (5q35) with the *ALK* gene (2p23),[64] and the t(5;12)(q33;p13) translocation fusing the tel gene (12p13) with the TK domain of the platelet-derived growth factor receptor *b* gene (PDGFR-b at 5q33) in chronic myelomonocytic leukemia (CMML) (Table 4).[65]

Gene fusions sometimes lead to the formation of chimeric transcription factors.[66] The t(1;19)(q23;p13) translocation, found in childhood pre-B-cell ALL, fuses the *E2A* transcription factor gene (19p13) with the *PBX1* homeodomain gene (1q23).[67] The E2A/PBX1 fusion protein consists of the amino-terminal transactivation domain of the E2A protein and the DNA-binding homeodomain of the PBX1 protein. Another gene fusion leading to a chimeric transcription factor is represented by the t(15;17)(q22;q21) translocation in acute promyelocytic leukemia, fusing the *PML* gene (15q22) with the *RARA* gene at 17q21.[68] Leukemia patients with the *PML/RARA* gene fusion respond well to retinoid treatment. In these cases, treatment with all-trans retinoic acid induces differentiation of promyelocytic leukemia cells.

The *ALL1* gene, located at chromosome band 11q23, is involved in approximately 5–10% of acute leukemia cases overall in children and adults.[69] *ALL1* is unique because it participates in fusions with a large number of different partner genes on the various chromosomes. Over 20 different reciprocal translocations involving the *ALL1* gene at 11q23 have been reported, the most common of which are those involving chromosomes 4, 6, 9, and 19. In approximately 5% of cases of acute leukemia in adults, the *ALL1* gene is fused with a portion of itself. This special type of gene fusion is called self-fusion.[70] Self-fusion of the *ALL1* gene, which is thought to occur through a somatic recombination mechanism, is found in high incidence in acute leukemias with trisomy 11 as a sole cytogenetic abnormality. The *ALL1* gene encodes a large protein with DNA-binding motifs, a transactivation domain, and a region with homology to the *Drosophila trithorax* protein (a regulator of homeotic gene expression). The various partners in *ALL1* fusions encode a diverse group of proteins, some of which appear to be nuclear proteins with DNA-binding motifs.[70] The ALL1 fusion protein consists of the amino terminus of ALL1 and the carboxyl terminus of one of a variety of fusion partners. It appears that the critical feature in all ALL1 fusions, including self-fusion, is the uncoupling of the ALL1 amino-terminal domains from the remainder of the ALL1 protein.

Solid tumors, especially sarcomas, sometimes have consistent chromosomal translocations that correlate with specific histological types of tumors.[52] In general, translocations in solid tumors result in gene fusions that encode chimeric oncoproteins. Studies

Table 4 Molecularly characterized chromosome rearrangements in tumors.

Affected gene	Rearrangements	Disease	Protein type
Hematopoietic tumor			
Gene fusion			
c-ABL (9q34) bcr (22q11)	t(9:22) (q34:q11)	Chronic myelogenous leukemia and acute Leukemia	Tyrosine kinase activated by BCR
ALK (2p23) NPM (5q35)	t(2;5)(p23;q35)	Anaplastic large cell lymphomas	Tyrosine kinase activated by NPM
PDGFR-b (5q33) tel (12p13)	t(5;12)(q33;p13)	Chronic myelomonocytic leukemia	Tyrosine kinase activated by tel
PBX1(1q23) E2A(19p13.3)	t(1:19)(q23:p13.3)	Acute pre-B-cell leukemia	Homeodomain (HLH)
PML(15q21) RAR(17q21)	t(15:17) (q21:q11-22)	Acute myeloid leukemia	Zn finger
CAN(6p23) DEK(9q34)	t(6:9) (p23:q34)	Acute myeloid leukemia	No homology
REL	ins(2:12) (p13:p11.2-14)	Non-Hodgkin's lymphoma	NF-κB family
NRG		No homology	
Oncogenes juxtaposed with IG loci			
c-MYC	t(8:14) (q24:q32) t(2:8) (p12:q24) t(8:22) (q24:q11)	Burkitt's lymphoma. BL-ALL	HLH domain
BCL-1 (PRADI?)	t(11:14) (q13:q3	B-cell chronic lymphocyte leukemia	PRADI-GI cyclin
BCL-2	t(14:18) (q32:21)	Follicular lymphoma	Inner mitochondrial membrane
BCL-3	t(14:19) (q32:q13.1)	Chronic B-cell leukemia	CDC10 motif
IL-3	t(5:14) (q31:q32)	Acute pre-B-cell leukemia	Growth factor
Oncogenes juxtaposed with TCR loci			
c-MYC	t(8:14) (q24:q11)	Acute T-cell leukemia	HLH domain
LYLA	t(7:19) (q35:p13)	Acute T-cell leukemia	HLH domain
TALA/SCL/TCL-5	t(1:14) (q32:q11)	Acute T-cell leukemia	HLH domain
TAL-2	t(7:9) (q35:q34)	Acute T-cell leukemia	HLH domain
Rhombotin 1/Ttg-1	t(11:14) (p15:q11)	Acute T-cell leukemia	LIM domain
Rhombotin 2/Ttg-2	t(11:14) (p13:q11) t(7:11) (q35:p13)	Acute T-cell leukemia	LIM domain
HOX 11	t(10:14) (q24:q11) t(7:10) (q35:q24)	Acute T-cell leukemia	Homeodomain
TAN-1	t(7:9) (q34:q34.3)	Acute T-cell leukemia	Notch homologue
TCL-1	t(7q35-14q32.1) or inv t(14q11-14q32.1) or inv	B-cell chronic lymphocyte leukemia	
Solid tumors			
Gene fusions in sarcomas			
FLI1,EWS	t(11:22) (q24:q12)	Ewing's sarcoma	Ets transcription factor family
ERG,EWS	t(21:22) (q22:q12)	Ewing's sarcoma	Ets transcription factor family
ATV1,EWS	t(7:21) (q22:q12)	Ewing's sarcoma	Ets transcription factor family
ATF1,EWS	t(12:22) (q13:q12)	Soft-tissue clear cell sarcoma	Transcription factor
CHN,EWS	t(9:22) (q22 31:q12)	Myxoid chondrosarcoma	Steroid receptor family
WT1,EWS	t(11:22) (p13:q12)	Desmoplastic small round cell tumor	Wilms' tumor gene
SSX1,SSX2,SYT	t(X:18) (p11.2:q11.2)	Synovial sarcoma	HLH domain
PAX3,FKHR	t(2:13) (q37:q14)	Alveolar	Homeobox homologue
PAX7,FKHR	t(1:13) (q36:q14)	Rhabdomyosarcoma	Homeobox homologue
CHOP,TLS	t(12:16) (q13:p11)	Myxoid liposarcoma	Transcription factor
var,HMG1-C	t(var:12) (var:q13-15)	Lipomas	HMG DNA-binding protein
HMG1-C?	t(12:14) (q13-15)	Leiomyomas	HMG DNA-binding protein
Gene fusions in thyroid carcinomas			
RET/ptc1	inv(10) (q11.2:q2.1)	Papillary thyroid carcinomas	Tyrosine kinase activated by H4
RET/ptc2	t(10:17) (q11.2:q23)	Papillary thyroid carcinomas	Tyrosine kinase activated by RIa(PKA)
RET/ptc3	inv(10) (q11.2)	Papillary thyroid carcinomas	Tyrosine kinase activated by ELE1
TRK	inv(1) (q31:q22-23)	Papillary thyroid carcinomas	Tyrosine kinase activated by TPM3
TRK–T1(T2)	inv(1) (q31:q25)	Papillary thyroid carcinomas	Tyrosine kinase activated by TPR
TRK–T3	t(1q31:3)	Papillary thyroid carcinomas	Tyrosine kinase activated by TFG
Hematopoietic and solid tumors			
Oncogenes juxtaposed with other loci			
PTH deregulates PRAD1	inv(11)(p15:q13)	Parathyroid adenoma	PRADI-GI cyclin
BTG1 deregulates MYC	t(8:12)(q24:q22)	B-cell chronic lymphocytic	MYC-HLH domain

Abbreviations: IG, immunoglobulin; TCR, T-cell receptor; HLH, helix-loop-helix structural domain; Zn, zinc; HMG, high mobility group; H4; ELE1; TPR and 1TFG, partially uncharacterized genes with a dimerizing coiled-coil domain; RIa, regulatory subunit of PKA enzyme; TPM3, isoform of nonmuscle tropomyosin.

thus far indicate that in sarcomas, the majority of genes fused by translocations encode transcription factors.[71] Table 4 summarizes translocations in solid tumors, with the most relevant represented by the t(12;16)(q13;p11) translocation fusing the *FUS (TLS)* gene at 16p11 with the *CHOP* gene at 12q13 in myxoid liposarcomas,[72] and the t(11;22)(q24;q12) translocation, fusing the *EWS* gene at 22q12 with the *FLI1* gene at 11q24 in Ewing's sarcoma.[73]

In DP, both a reciprocal translocation t(17;22)(q22;q13) and supernumerary ring chromosomes derived from the t(17;22) have been described.[74]

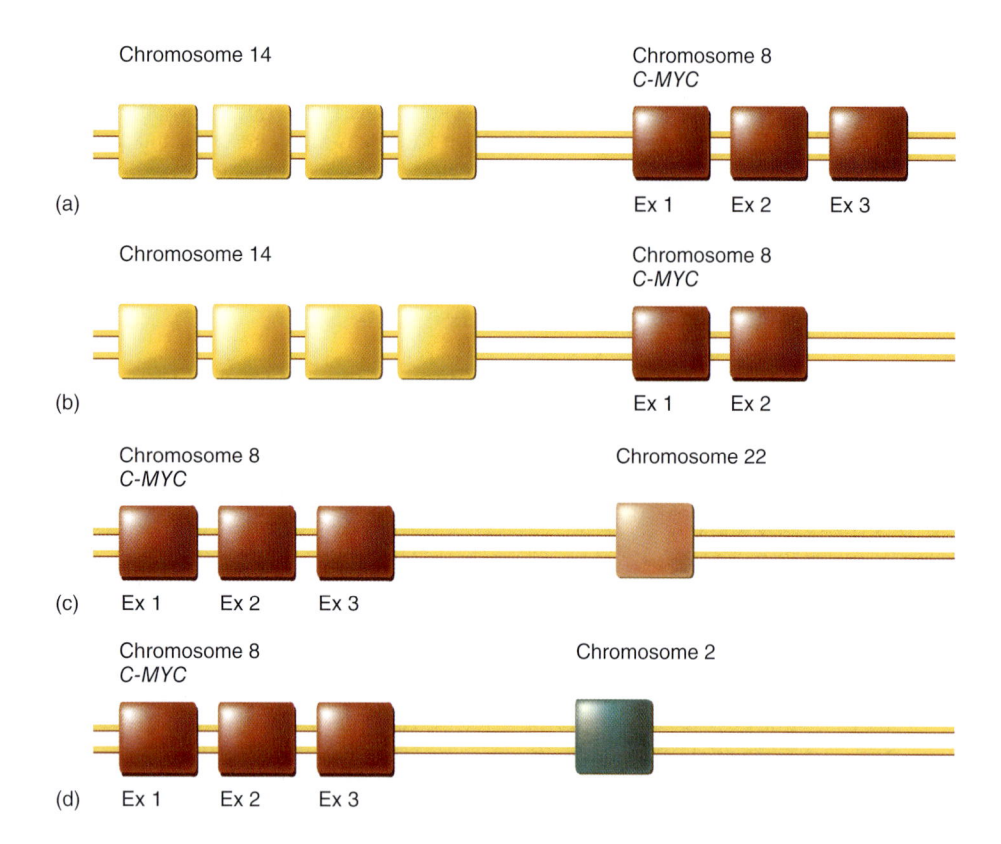

Figure 9 c-myc translocations found in Burkitt lymphoma. (a) t(8;14)(q24;q32) Translocation involving the locus of immunoglobulin heavy chain gene located at 14q32. (b) t(8;14)(q24;q32) translocation where only 2 exons of c-myc are translocated under regulatory elements from the immunoglobulin heavy chain locus located at 14q32. (c) t(8;22) (q24;q11) translocation involving the *l* locus of immunoglobulin light chain gene at 22q11. (d) t(2;8)(p12;q24) translocation involving the *k* locus of immunoglobulin light chain gene located at 2p12.

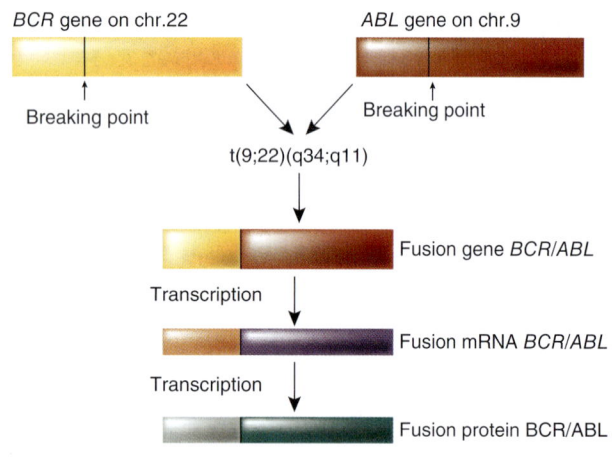

Figure 10 Gene fusion. The t(9;22) (q34;q11) translocation in CML determines the fusion of the c-abl gene with the bcr gene. Such a gene fusion encodes an oncogenic chimeric protein of 210 kD.

Although early successful studies in this field have been performed with lymphomas and leukemia, as we have discussed before, the first chromosomal abnormality in solid tumors to be characterized at the molecular level as a fusion protein was an inversion of chromosome 10 found in papillary thyroid carcinomas.[75] In this tumor, two main recurrent structural changes have been described, including inv(10) (q112.2; q21.2), as the more frequent alteration, and a t(10;17) (q11.2; q23). These two abnormalities represent the cytogenetic mechanisms which activate the proto-oncogene *ret* on chromosome 10, forming the oncogenes ret/ptc1 and RET/ptc2, respectively. Moreover, other chromosomal rearrangements leading to ret activation were recently described, especially in children of the Chernobyl-contaminated areas.[76,77] Virtually all breakpoints in the *RET* gene occur within intron 11, leading intact the TK domain of the receptor and enabling the *RET/PTC* oncoprotein to bind to SHC via Y1062 and activate the downstream cascade.[78] Somatic chromosomal rearrangements involving the *RET* gene represent the most frequent genetic alteration in PTC, although wide variations in frequency ranging from 5% to 70% have been observed in different geographic areas.[79] Recent results suggest that a broad variability in the reported prevalence of RET/PTC rearrangements is at least in part a result of the use of different detection methods and tumor genetic heterogeneity.[80] Alterations of chromosome 1 in the same tumor type have then been associated to the activation of NTRK1 (chromosome 1), an NGF receptor, which, like *RET*, forms chimeric fusion oncogenic proteins in PTC.[81] A comparative analysis of the oncogenes originated from the activation of these two TK receptors has allowed the identification and characterization of common cytogenetic and molecular mechanisms of their activation. In all cases, chromosomal rearrangements fuse the TK portion of the two receptors to the 5′-end of different genes that, because of their general effect, have been designated as "activating genes." In the majority of cases, the latter belong to the same chromosome where the related receptor is located, 10 for RET and 1 for NTRK1.

Furthermore, although functionally different, the various activating genes share the following three properties:

1. They are ubiquitously expressed.
2. They display domains demonstrated or predicted to be able to form dimers or multimers.
3. They translocate the signal from the membrane to the cytoplasm.

These characteristics can explain the mechanism(s) of oncogenic activation of *ret* and *NTRK1* proto-oncogenes. In fact, following the fusion of their TK domain to the activating gene (1) *ret* and *NTRK1*, whose tissue-specific expression is restricted to subsets of neural cells, become expressed in the epithelial thyroid cells; (2) their dimerization triggers a constitutive, ligand-independent trans-autophosphorylation of the cytoplasmic domains and, as a consequence, the latter can recruit SH2- and SH3-containing cytoplasmic effector proteins, such as Shc and Grb2 or phospholipase C gamma (PLC), thus inducing a constitutive mitogenic pathway; and (3) the relocalization in the cytoplasm of *ret* and *NTRK1* enzymatic activity could allow their interaction with unusual substrates, perhaps modifying their functional properties. RET rearrangements are mutually exclusive with NTRK1 rearrangements and BRAF mutations and show similar but distinct gene expression patterns in PTC.[78] Overall, papillary carcinomas with RET/PTC rearrangements typically present at younger age and have a high rate of lymph-node metastases, clinical papillary histology, and possibly more favorable prognosis.[78]

Protein overexpression and constitutive phosphorylation

Protein overexpression refers to a general deregulation driven by a mechanism not understood or not investigated. An example is Akt, three serine-threonine kinases that represent major effectors mediating survival signal. Generally, Akt proteins possess six sites of phosphorylation: Ser124 and Thr450 are basally phosphorylated, Tyr315 and Tyr316 depend on Src, Thr308 represents the major site of regulation and is phosphorylated by 3-phosphoinositides-dependent protein kinase 1, Ser473 is only required for maximal Akt activity but the mechanism by which it is phosphorylated remains controversial. Akt is phosphorylated and therefore activated after cell stimulation from different growth factors and from a series of interleukins, while its action is inhibited by PTEN. Once activated, Akt dissociates from the plasma membrane and translocates to both the cytoplasm and the nucleus. Akt inhibits directly, through phosphorylation of Bad and caspase-9, and indirectly, by inducing *de novo* gene expression of IKK protein kinase and transcription factors. Akt determines cell survival also by virtue of its involvement in cell-cycle progression.[82] Analyses of tissue specimens pointed out that the protein encoded by Akt3 is overexpressed in poorly differentiated breast and prostate cancers and may contribute to the progression of sporadic melanoma.[83] Akt1 is especially involved in the pathogenesis of sporadic thyroid cancer, whereas Akt2 seems to be the isoform which plays a pivotal role in ovarian, pancreatic, thyroid, and CRC. Mutations in Akt genes are rare.[84]

New markers from large-scale genomic analysis

Kinases

A recent analysis organized the protein kinase complement of the human genome (the so-called "kinome") into a dendrogram containing nine broad groups of genes.[85] Using high-throughput sequencing technologies and bioinformatics from the human genome project, one major branch of the histogram, containing three of the nine major groups, was selected for mutational analysis. The selected groups included the 90 TK genes (TK group), the 43 TK-like genes (TKL group), and the 5 receptor guanylate cyclase genes (RGC group). The analysis took into consideration all exons encoding their predicted kinase domains in 35 CRC cell lines and in 147 colorectal specimens.[7] Thirty-five different types of somatic mutations were identified in seven genes (*NTRK3, FES, KDR, EPHA3, NTRK2* belonging to the TK group, *MLK4* to *TKL*, and *GUCY2F* to *RGC*) representing an attractive target for chemotherapeutic intervention.[7]

Phosphatases

The protein tyrosine phosphatases (PTPs), gene superfamily (the so-called "phosphatome") is composed of three main families: (1) the classic PTPs, including the receptor protein tyrosine phosphatase (RPTPs) and the nonreceptor protein tyrosine phosphatase (NRPTPs); (2) the dual-specificity phosphatases (DSPs), which can dephosphorylate serine and threonine in addition to tyrosine residues; and (3) the low molecular weight phosphatases (LMPs).[86] Using high-throughput technologies, a mutational analysis of all the coding exons of 53 classic PTPs (21 RPTPs and 32 NRPTPs), 32 DSPs, and 1 LMP was performed in 175 CRCs.[8] Six genes containing somatic mutations were identified, including three members of the RPTP subfamily (*PTPRF, PTPRG,* and *PTPRT*), and three members of the NRPTP subfamily (*PTPN3, PTPN13,* and *PTPN14*). Overall, 77 mutations were identified, in aggregate, affecting 26% of colorectal tumors analyzed. The great majority of the mutations would result in proteins devoid of phosphatase catalytic activity.[8] The identification of protein phosphatases mutated could lead to reactivation of their activity through new targeted pharmacologic treatments or, better, inactivate the corresponding kinases that phosphorylate substrates normally regulated by the mutant phosphatases.

PI3K isoforms

Phosphatidylinositol 3-kinases (PI3K) belong to the lipid kinase family that regulate signal transduction.[87] Hidden Markov models identified eight *PI3K* and *PI3K*-like genes, including two uncharacterized genes, in the human genome. By the analysis of the predicted kinase domains, it has been found that *PIK3CA* was the only gene with somatic mutations.[9] Hyperactivating *PIK3CA* mutations were also identified in several cancers from colon, lung, ovaries, liver, brain, stomach, and breast.[88–90] The analysis of *PIK3CA* mutations in patients affected by hereditary CRCs revealed alteration in 21% of FAP invasive carcinomas, in 21% of HNPCC invasive carcinomas and in 15% of sporadic invasive carcinomas, thus demonstrating that *PIK3CA* mutations are involved in both type of familial colorectal carcinogenesis [familial adenomatous polyposis (FAP) and hereditary non-polyposis colorectal cancer (HNPCC)] without an evident segregation (at odds with *BRAF*), and with a similar extent that seen in sporadic patients.[91] In addition to point mutations, *PIK3CA* may be altered through gene amplification, especially in ovarian cancer.[92]

miRNA

MicroRNAs (miRNAs) are small noncoding RNAs with 19–25 bases of length that control gene expression by destroying messenger RNA or inhibiting its translation.[93] They target the expression of many cellular regulators, including those controlling programmed cell death via the intrinsic (Bcl-2 and Mcl-1), extrinsic (TRAIL and

Fas), p53-and ER stress-induced apoptotic pathways, as well as the necroptosis cell death pathway.[94] Most miRNAs are located in regions between genes, but they can be also located within intron regions and even within protein-coding exon regions.[93]

miRNAs were discovered in 1993, when it was found that small RNAs encoded by the lin-4 locus control the development of *Caenorhabditis elegans* by modulating the expression of lin-14 proteins. The importance of these small RNA molecules was recognized in 2000, upon the discovery of a small RNA molecule named let-7, highly conserved between species, from worms to humans. By forming a regulatory complex (RNA-induced silencing complex, RISC) with Argonaute proteins, miRNAs are involved in a variety of biological processes, including cell proliferation, cell death, cell lineage determination, stem cell maintenance, and temporal regulation of developmental stages, by triggering the degradation and translational repression of target messenger RNAs (mRNAs) with complementary sequences.[93]

miRNAs are frequently present in unstable regions of chromosomes that are prone to deletion and amplification in cancer cells, and it has been suggested that abnormalities in miRNAs are not limited to some cancers but are directly related to the oncogenic mechanism itself. The first finding showing a relationship between cancer and miRNA was in chronic lymphocytic leukemia (CLL). In CLL, deletions are often found in the chromosomal region 13q14, but no protein-coding gene has been found at this deletion site and the pathologic significance of the deletion has long been unclear. Calin et al. showed that two miRNAs were localized in this region, miR-15a and miR-16-1, and their expression was reduced in CLL with 13q14 deletion.[95,96] Cimmino et al. also showed that this reduced miRNA expression was involved in the development of CLL because miR-15a and miR-16-1 targeted the apoptosis inhibitor BCL-2.[97] In addition, in multiple myeloma, many studies have demonstrated that miRNAs might be involved in drug resistance.[93] Interestingly the development of miRNA microarrays, beads-based flow cytometry, and high-throughput deep sequencing, in the near future could permit to investigate how genome-wide miRNA profiles (miRNome) can aid in tumor classification, diagnosis, and prognosis prediction.[93]

Oncogenes in the initiation and progression of neoplasia

Human neoplasia is a complex multistep process involving sequential alterations in proto-oncogenes (activation) and in tumor suppressor genes (inactivation). Statistical analysis of the age incidence of human solid tumors indicates that five or six independent mutational events may contribute to tumor formation. In human leukemias, only three or four mutational events may be necessary, presumably involving different genes.

The study of chemical carcinogenesis in animals provides a foundation for our understanding of the multistep nature of cancer.[98] In the mouse model of skin carcinogenesis, tumor formation involves three phases, termed *initiation, promotion,* and *progression*. Initiation of skin tumors can be induced by chemical mutagens such as 7,12-dimethyl-benzanthracene (DMBA) (Figure 11). After application of DMBA, the mouse skin appears normal. If the skin is then continuously treated with a promoter, such as the phorbol ester TPA, precancerous papillomas will form. Chemical promoters such as TPA stimulate growth but are not mutagenic substances. Over a period of months of continuous application of the promoting agent, some of the papillomas will progress to skin carcinomas. Treatment

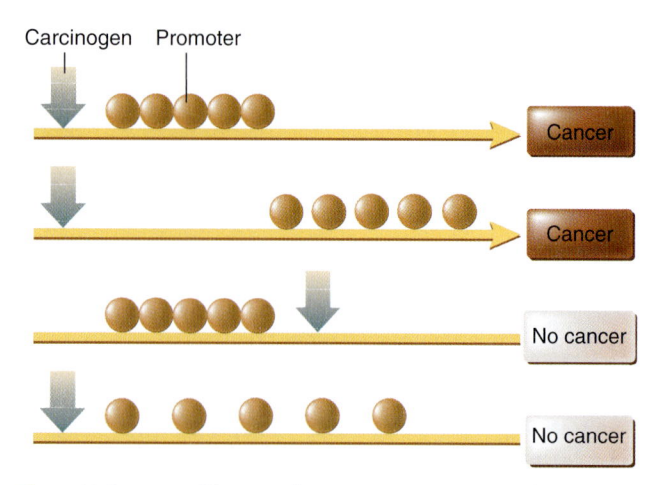

Figure 11 Some possible ways of exposure to a mutagen and to a tumor promoter and their effects. Cancer develops exclusively when the exposure to promoter follows the exposure to carcinogen (mutagen, e.g., 7,12-dimethyl-benzanthracene) and only when the intensity of the exposure to promoter is higher than a threshold.

with DMBA or TPA alone does not cause skin cancer. Mouse papillomas initiated with DMBA usually have H-*ras* oncogenes with a specific mutation in codon 61 of the H-*ras* gene. The mouse skin tumor model indicates that initiation of papillomas is the result of mutation of the H-*ras* gene in individual skin cells by the chemical mutagen DMBA. For papillomas to appear on the skin, however, growth of mutated cells must be continuously stimulated by a promoting agent. Additional unidentified genetic changes must then occur for papillomas to progress to carcinoma.

Although a single oncogene is sufficient to cause tumor formation, transformation by a single oncogene is not usually seen in experimental models of cancer. On the contrary, different oncogenes frequently cooperate in producing the neoplastic phenotype.[99] Cooperation between oncogenes can also be demonstrated by *in vitro* transformation studies using nonimmortalized cell lines. For example, studies have shown cooperation between the nuclear myc protein and the cytoplasmic-membrane-associated ras protein in the transformation of rat embryo fibroblasts.[100]

Collaboration between two different categories of oncogenes (e.g., nuclear and cytoplasmic) can often be demonstrated but is not strictly required for transformation.[101] These transgenic mice strains, in fact, generally show an increased incidence of neoplasia and the tumors that result frequently are clonal, implying that other events are necessary.[102]

Cytogenetic studies of the clonal evolution of human hematologic malignancies have provided much insight into the multiple steps involved in the initiation and progression of human tumors.[103] The evolution of CML from chronic phase to acute leukemia is characterized by an accumulation of genetic changes seen in the karyotypes of the evolving malignant clones. The early chronic phase of CML is defined by the presence of a single Philadelphia chromosome. The formation of the *bcr/abl* gene fusion as a consequence of the t(9;22) translocation is thought to be the initiating event in CML.[25] The biologic progression of CML to a more malignant phenotype corresponds with the appearance of additional cytogenetic abnormalities such as a second Philadelphia chromosome, isochromosome 17, or trisomy 8.[104] Although the karyotypic changes in evolving CML are somewhat variable from patient to patient, the accumulation of genetic changes always correlates with progression from differentiated cells of low malignancy to undifferentiated cells of high malignancy.

The initiation and progression of human neoplasia involve the activation of oncogenes and the inactivation or loss of tumor suppressor genes. The mechanisms of oncogene activation and the time course of events, however, vary among different types of tumors. In hematologic malignancies, soft-tissue sarcomas, and the papillary type of thyroid carcinomas, initiation of the malignant process predominantly involves chromosomal rearrangements that activate various oncogenes. Many of the chromosomal rearrangements in leukemia and lymphoma are thought to result from errors in the physiologic process of immunoglobulin or T-cell receptor gene rearrangement during normal B-cell and T-cell development. Late events in the progression of hematologic malignancies involve oncogene mutation, mainly of the *ras* family, inactivation of tumor suppressor genes such as *TP53,* and sometimes additional chromosomal translocations.[105]

In lung cancers, the initiation of neoplasia has been shown to involve oncogene and tumor suppressor gene mutations. These mutations are generally thought to result from chemical carcinogenesis, especially in the case of tobacco-related lung cancers, where a novel tumor suppressor gene (designated *FHIT*) has been found to be inactivated in the majority of cancers, particularly in those from smokers.[106] Later, K-ras (especially in the adenocarcinoma subtype) and *TP53* alterations drive the malignant transformation of lung cancer.[107]

As far as CRC is concerned, intensive screening for genetic alteration led to the identification of two major types of CRC that are distinct by their carcinogenic process. One is characterized by normal karyotype, normal DNA index, and genetic instability at microsatellite loci (MSI) and was called RER-positive tumor for replicative error-positive phenotype and now is called MSI-positive cancer.[108] The second one is represented by alterations of *APC, K-ras,* and *TP53* genes and genetic losses at MSI.[109] The second type led to the association between the stepwise progression from normal to dysplastic epithelium to carcinoma and the accumulation of multiple clonally selected genetic alterations. This model, first proposed by Vogelstein in 1990,[110] suggests that APC (or, better, the APC-b-catenin pathway) represents the initial mutational event that determines hyperplastic proliferation and then early adenoma formation. The stage of late adenoma is achieved with K-ras protein stabilization. Loss of tumor suppressor genes at chromosome 18q (such as *DCC*) and mutations in the *TP53* gene lead to carcinoma *in situ* formation (Figure 12).[108,109]

In melanoma, *BRAF* mutations occur in the vast majority of cases and represent a very early event, since they were also detected in preneoplastic lesions such as Spitz and Blue nevi.[6]

Although there is variability in the pathways of human tumor initiation and progression, studies of various types of malignancy have clearly confirmed the multistep nature of human cancer.

Oncogenes as target of new drugs

Several oncogenes act in key points of cell life. Most of them, in fact, codify for growth factor receptors or are involved in the signal transduction. Therefore, they represent a natural target for the development of new drugs, that are able to block selectively the cells carrying a deregulation in the drug target. Here are summarized the new insights in targeted therapies.

ERB B2

ERB B2 gene amplification occurs in a consistent fraction of breast cancers. A monoclonal antibody (MoAb) against erb B2 receptor, trastuzumab, was the first anti-erb B2 drug that entered clinical practice, with evident benefit for patients harboring erb B2 gene amplification/overexpression. Trastuzumab is indicated for patients affected by a metastatic breast cancer and, more recently, also for the adjuvant and neo-adjuvant setting. Currently, additional targeted therapies, both MoAbs (pertuzumab and a second-generation trastuzumab named T-DM1, with trastuzumab conjugated with emtansine) and small-molecule tyrosine kinase inhibitors (TKIs) (lapatinib) have been developed and are routinely used for the treatment of metastatic patients and in the neo-adjuvant setting. Unfortunately, not all patients showing *erb B2* gene amplification may benefit from trastuzumab administration. This is probably due to the deregulation of *erb B2* downstream members. Indeed, at preclinical level, it has been demonstrated that activating point mutations in the *PIK3CA* gene as well as the loss of expression of PTEN protein lead to trastuzumab resistance.[32]

More recently, it has been demonstrated that *erb B2* can be deregulated in other solid tumors, with a putative relevant clinical role. Erb B2 gene amplification or protein overexpression occurs in up to 34% of patients affected by an advanced gastric or gastroesophageal junction cancers, and trastuzumab is approved for erb B2 positive patients (as evaluated by fluorescent *in situ* hybridization or by immunohistochemistry).[32] In CRC, *erb B2* gene amplification is a rare phenomenon (observed in less than 5% of cases), linked to resistance to EGFR-targeted therapies.[111]

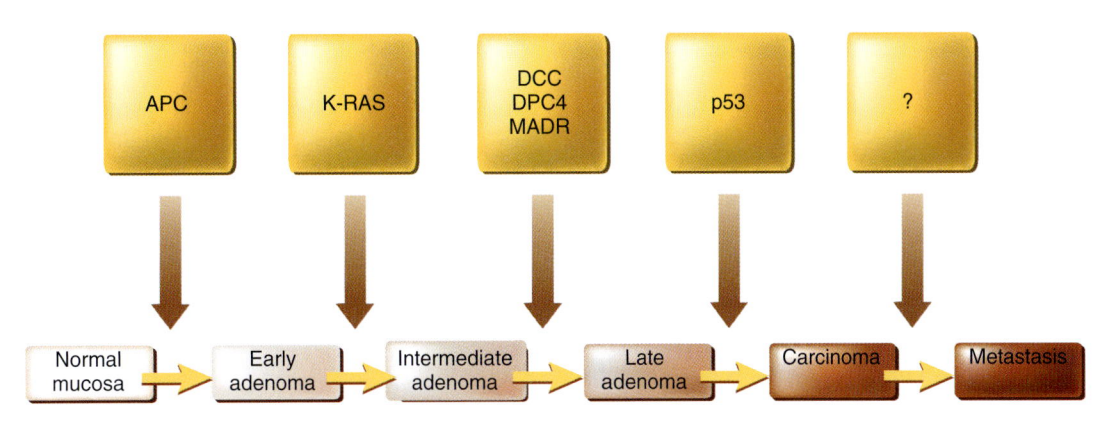

Figure 12 Colorectal cancer development. Colorectal cancer results from a series of pathological changes that transform normal colonic epithelium into invasive carcinoma. Specific genetic events, shown by vertical arrows, accompany this multistep process.

However, the efficacy of trastuzumab in CRC, proposed in *in vivo* models (xenografts), deserves additional confirmatory studies. In lung adenocarcinoma, a recent retrospective study showed that patients with *erb B2* gene mutations (occurring in about 1% of cases) may benefit from the administration of trastuzumab. Furthermore, the occurrence of *erb B2* gene mutations or amplification seems to be represented by a mechanism of secondary resistance to anti-EGFR therapies.[112]

ERB B1

ERB B1 codifies for a RTK playing an important role in cancer cell proliferation, angiogenesis, and metastasis. Therefore, targeting erb B1 is a valuable molecular approach in cancer therapy. Two classes of erb B1 antagonists have been successfully tested in phase III trials and are now in clinical use: MoAbs and TKIs. MoAbs, represented by cetuximab and panitumumab, are able to bind to the extracellular domain of the receptor when it is in the inactive configuration, compete for receptor binding by occluding the ligand-binding region, and thereby block ligand-induced TK of the receptor. On the contrary, TKIs compete reversibly (first generation) or irreversibly (second generation) with ATP to bind to the intracellular catalytic domain of the receptor and, therefore, inhibit receptor autophosphorylation and downstream signaling.[54]

In NSCLC, only 10–20% of patients have a partial response to first-generation TKI gefitinib/erlotinib. Several retrospective and prospective studies confirmed that patients carrying an *EGFR* mutation were particularly sensitive to gefitinib/erlotinib, with a response rate up to 80% of mutated patients. Many types of mutations in the *erb B1* have been reported, but so far only four drug-sensitive mutations have been ascertained, including exon 19 deletions, and exon 18 (G719A/C), exon 21 L858R, and exon 21 L861Q substitutions. The role of the S768I mutation is still undefined. *Erb b1* mutations typically occur in patients with a never-smoking history, Asian ethnicity, female gender, and adenocarcinoma histology. In the majority of cases, the primary (before first-generation TKIs administration) and the secondary (in patients initially responsive to gefitinib/erlotinib) drug resistance has been linked to a specific somatic mutation (*T790M*) occurring in exon 20. In addition, other mutations in *erb B1* (i.e., exon 20 insertions), as well as *MET* and *erb B2* gene amplification represent alternative mechanisms of TKIs resistance.[113] Based on the evidence that the T790M change occurs in a consistent number of TKIs-treated patients, it has been developed a third-generation TKI specifically addressed against such a mutation, osimertinib.[114] However, it has also been demonstrated that the T790M change cannot occur in all the metastases nor in a homogeneous manner and, therefore, small biopsies cannot be representative of the overall molecular situation of the patients. Starting from a very comprehensive study that showed that cancers are able to release DNA mutant alleles in the blood (this type of DNA has been named "circulating-tumor DNA" or ctDNA),[115] it has been proposed, and then demonstrated, that the identification of the T790M mutation in plasma may be extremely useful in the identification of patients who can be positively addressed to the treatment with osimertinib: indeed, the analysis of blood derivates (serum or, better, plasma) may be done serially with less invasive techniques as compared to the standard biopsy collection.[116] More recently, however, it has been discovered that the efficacy of third-generation TKIs in T790M-mutant patients can be compromised by newly acquired mutations, such as those occurring in the codons 796–797. In particular, the most important mutation that has been correlated with third-generation TKIs resistance is C797S: when this mutation occurs (in about 15–20% of osimertinib-treated, T790M mutant patients), the third-generation TKI is not able to enter into the catalytic domain and to block the EGFR kinase activity. However, the C797S mutant protein may be sensitive to first- and second-generation TKIs against EGFR: therefore, if the C797S mutation occurs *in trans* with respect to the T790M, a combination of first/second and third-generation TKIs may lead to cancer cell death. On the contrary, if the two alterations occur *in cis*, the resultant protein has a catalytic domain that is completely refractory to all the so-far developed TKI drugs.[117]

In CRC, the class of erb B1 inhibitors showing clinical efficacy is represented by MoAbs. Cetuximab or panitumumab monotherapy is associated with response rates of 9–12%, that increase to 20–30% when the drugs are used in combination with irinotecan in patients who did not benefit from a previous therapy with irinotecan. Recent data indicate that erb B1 protein expression as evaluated by immunohistochemistry, as well as *erb B1* gene status by fluorescent *in situ* hybridization, cannot be used to predict the efficacy of EGFR-targeted therapies (in contrast with earlier studies), essentially due to the fact that these two methodologies are not reproducible. On the contrary, *K-ras* and *N-ras* gene mutations are negative predictors of EGFR-targeted therapies efficacy and are mandatory to be tested before MoAbs administration.[118] In addition, the detection of gene or protein alterations of *other erb B1* downstream members, such as *BRAF* and *PIK3CA* point mutations, and the loss of expression of PTEN protein, has been proposed to be additional mechanisms of the resistance to cetuximab/panitumumab, but the data reported so far are controversial and therefore their test is not required before drug administration.[119]

Cetuximab and panitumumab are effective also in 10–13% of patients affected by head and neck squamous cell carcinoma, and EGFR-targeted therapy is the first and only molecularly targeted therapy to demonstrate a survival benefit for patients with recurrent or metastatic disease.[120]

KIT and PDGFRA

It has been clearly demonstrated that imatinib, an inhibitor of TK activity in bcr-abl-positive leukemia was effective in treating GIST (Figure 13). In this pathology, *kit* and *pdgfra* mutational status predicts for the likelihood of achieving response to such a targeted drug. Patients with a *kit* exon 11 mutation have a partial response rate up to 85–90%, while those with a *kit* exon 9 mutation have a partial response rate of around 50%. Recent data points out that for patients with *kit* exon 9 mutation the better treatment is represented by a double dose of imatinib. Patients who have GIST with *kit* exon 11 mutation also have longer median time to treatment failure as compared to those with GIST harboring other types of mutations. Patients who have no detectable mutation of *kit* or *pdgfra* respond less frequently to imatinib than those with exon 11 mutants, but still up to 39% do respond. The rare patients who have GIST with *kit* exon 13 or 17 mutation of *pdgfra* mutation may also respond to imatinib. The rare patients who have GIST with a mutation known to be resistant to imatinib, such as D842V *pdgfra* exon 18 mutation, may be the only exception to this rule. Interestingly, the D842V *pdgfra* exon 18 mutation is functionally equivalent to the D816V *kit* exon 17 mutation, never found in GIST, but which confers resistance to imatinib treatment in leukemia.[33] A majority of patients with a GIST metastatic disease ultimately cease to respond to imatinib. The reasons for failure usually include secondary mutations at the ATP/imatinib binding pocket (exon 13 or exon 14) or in the activation loop (exon 17) of the kit protein kinase that prohibit imatinib binding. Patients who progress despite imatinib dose escalation are candidates for a trial with other TKIs. Sunitinib (SU11248) is an inhibitor of kit, pdgfra,

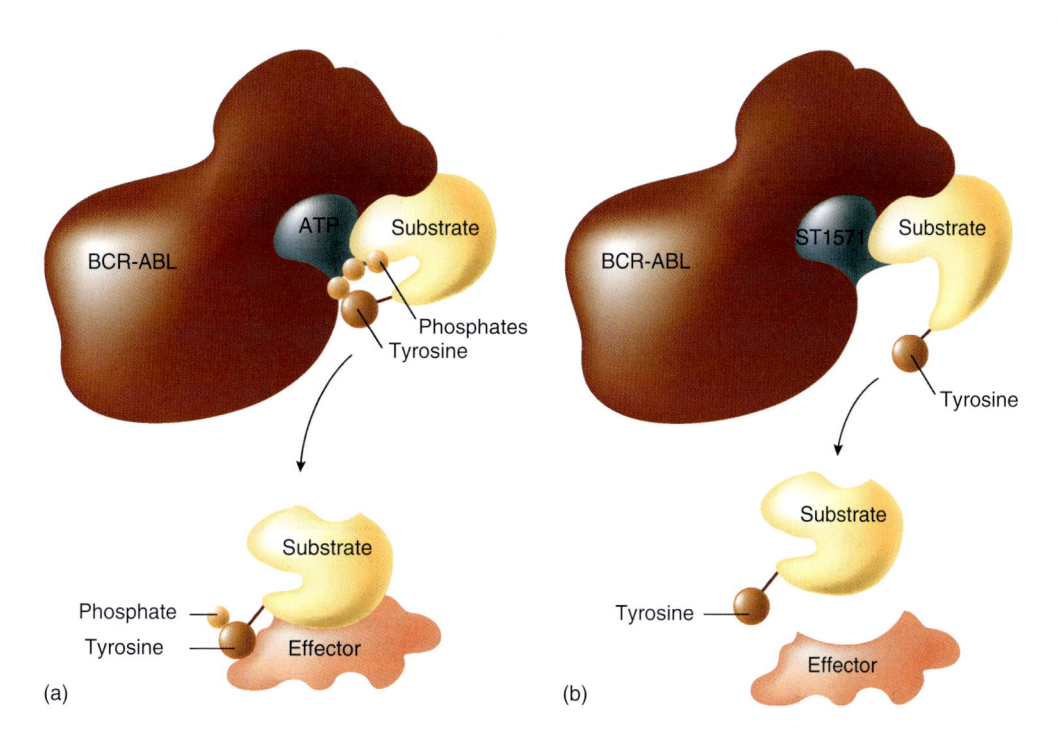

Figure 13 Mode of action of imatinib. (a) The effect of ATP binding on the oncoprotein BCR-ABL is depicted. The fusion protein binds the molecule of ATP in the kinase pocket. Afterward, it can phosphorylate a substrate, that can interact with the downstream effector molecules. When imatinib is present (b), the oncoprotein binds imatinib in the kinase pocket (competing with ATP), and then the substrate cannot be phosphorylated.

fms-like TK-3, and vascular EGFR-2, and has been approved by the Food and Drug Administration for the treatment of GIST patients whose disease has progressed on imatinib or are unable to tolerate treatment with imatinib.

More recently, the clinical role of *kit* mutations has expanded to melanoma. It has been shown that *kit* mutations occur in specific subtypes of melanoma patients, in the majority of uveal, in up to in 39% of mucosal, 36% of acral, and 28% of melanomas arising from chronically sun-damaged skin, but not in any (0%) cutaneous melanomas without chronic sun damage.[121] The typical alteration is represented by the L576P point mutation. Results from case reports and from human uveal melanoma cell lines demonstrated that imatinib inhibits cell proliferation and invasion rates.[122] These results justify the need for clinical trials (which are now under evaluation) to investigate *in vivo* the response of uveal melanoma to imatinib.

RET

Recently, various kinds of therapeutic approaches, including TKIs, gene therapy with dominant-negative *RET* mutants, MoAbs, and nuclease-resistant aptamers that recognize and inhibit RET, have been developed. The use of these strategies in preclinical models has provided evidence that RET is indeed a potential target for selective cancer therapy. In clinical cases, in addition to papillary thyroid cancers where they play a relevant role, *RET* rearrangements have been found in a small subgroup of lung cancers (1–2%). Two specific gene fusions (*CCDC6-RET* and *KIF5B-RET*) have been described. *RET* rearrangements appear limited to adenocarcinoma histology and are not seen concurrently with *erb B1* or *K-ras* mutations, or *ALK* rearrangements. In last years, retrospective studies demonstrated that five multikinase inhibitors (Cabozantinib, vandetanib, sunitinib, lenvatinib, and nintedanib) achieved tumor responses in about 30% of RET-rearranged NSCLC patients.[123] Most of these therapies have received FDA approval. Selective RET inhibitor drugs LOXO-292 (selpercatinib) and BLU-667 (pralsetinib) are also undergoing phase I/II clinical trials.[124]

RAS

A number of different approaches aimed at abrogating K-*ras* activity have been explored in clinical trials. Usually, the inhibitors directly addressed to K-ras are too toxic for human cells. Currently, the most promising agents are represented by aminobiphosphonates, which have entered clinical practice in the treatment of bone metastases from several neoplasms, including breast and prostate adenocarcinomas.

K-*ras* mutations play also a role in the prediction of efficacy of treatment targeted to upstream activated RTK, such as EGFR. Indeed, K-*ras* mutations represent an independent predictive factor in cetuximab or panitumumab-treated advanced CRC patients.[125] Until 2013, only the characterization of *K-ras* codons 12 and 13, located in exon 2, was mandatory before the administration of EGFR-targeted therapies. But, starting from the evidence that also different *K-ras* mutations (at codons 59, 61, 117, and 146, located in exons 3 and 4, which can be cumulatively found in up to 5% of cases) can be detected in CRC and that also these regions are important for K-ras activity, the analysis of large cohorts demonstrated that also *K-ras* exons 3–4 mutations are negative predictors of efficacy of MoAbs against EGFR.[125] Furthermore, *N-ras* mutations may occur in CRC patients (in up to 5% of cases, in the same codons altered in *K-ras* gene), and recently it has been demonstrated that also patients carrying mutations in this gene are resistant to anti-EGFR therapies.[125] Overall, therefore, the combined analysis of *K-ras* and *N-ras* gene mutations is now mandatory before the administration of EGFR-targeted therapies in CRC patients with a metastatic disease. Unfortunately, it has been demonstrated that after approximately 6 months of therapy, the majority of RAS wild-type cases develops resistance to anti-EGFR therapies, mainly following the emergence of RAS mutant clones, as a consequence of either *de novo* mutations or clonal selection of a mutant clone present at the beginning, but undetectable with the standard methodologies used for the analysis of tissue specimens. Therefore, these patients must exit from the administration of EGFR targeted therapies and are usually addressed to a second-line therapy including a different chemotherapy backbone combined with an antiangiogenic MoAb (e.g., bevacizumab).[126] However, a recent prospective clinical trial demonstrated that a rechallenge strategy with cetuximab and irinotecan may be active in patients with RAS wild-type metastatic CRC with acquired resistance to first-line irinotecan- and cetuximab-based therapy, especially in patients showing a RAS wild-type status at liquid biopsy level at the end of the second-line therapy.[127] In addition, a preliminary study, conducted on a small cohort of metastatic CRC patients, reported that about half of the RAS mutant patients treated with bevacizumab-based chemotherapies are able to revert their RAS status to RAS wild-type, at least in plasma, leading to their availability for a cetuximab-based chemotherapic scheme.[128] Indeed, these patients achieved a PFS from 6 to 12 months in the patients treated in second-line setting and a PFS of 4 months in the patients treated in fourth-line, thus opening to the possibility of cetuximab administration in the course of disease also in RAS mutant patients.[129]

For the treatment of patients affected by a *K-ras* mutant NSCLC, a new therapeutic option is now available: the mutation-specific inhibitors. In particular, the most promising drug seems to be SII-P inhibitors, targeting K-ras G12C mutations: this is of particular relevance because G12C mutation represents the most prevalent type of alteration occurring in *K-ras* gene in NSCLC, accounting for more than one-third of *K-ras* mutant NSCLC patients.[130]

BRAF

BRAF now provides a critical new target for drugs treating malignant melanoma, including antisense oligonucleotides and small molecules. These inhibitors block the expression of BRAF protein, block the BRAF/ras interaction, block its kinase activity or the kinase activity of the *BRAF* target protein MAP kinase.[110] Besides these approaches, vemurafenib is a selective BRAF TKI inhibitor approved for the treatment of melanoma patients. The Food and Drug Administration approved this drug for the administration to patients carrying the V600E specific mutation, whereas the European Medicine Agency approved it for all the patients carrying any mutation at codon 600 (therefore including V600K, V600D, and V600G, overall accounting for more than 10% of melanoma cases). The effect of vemurafenib on *BRAF* mutant patients is extremely fast in terms of tumor regression, but after 10–12 months secondary alterations (represented by abnormally spliced BRAF proteins or other *BRAF* somatic mutations) lead to a rapid re-appearance of metastatic lesions.[131]

A recent role has been proposed also in NSCLC. *BRAF* mutations occur only in a small proportion of cases (up to 2%), mainly at codon 600, but also in other hot-spot codons (466, 469, 594): therefore, lung cancer represents the tumor with the widest spectrum of *BRAF* mutations. A number of BRAF inhibitors, including sorafenib, vemurafenib, and dabrafenib are under clinical development in V600E *BRAF* mutant lung cancer patients, with vemurafenib showing the most promising results, at least on the basis of few case reports. Finally, and not only in NSCLC but it also seems that vemurafenib is more active when combined with inhibitors targeting BRAF downstream effectors, the MEK inhibitors, in BRAF mutant patients.[132,133]

AKT

Deregulation of Akt expression seems to be involved into Akt drug response and radioresistance in several tumors,[134] especially in metaplastic cancer, where it confers resistance to hormone therapy,[135] and in ovarian cancer, where it confers resistance to cisplatin by modulating the direct action of p53 on the caspase-dependent mitochondrial death pathway.[136] Moreover, recent efforts have been made in the development of small-molecule inhibitors that directly bind to Akt, such as triciribine and pyridine derivatives. However several drawbacks have been found because of issues toxicity due to the involvement of Akt in insulin signaling.[83]

PIK3CA

Due to the relevance in carcinogenesis, PIK3CA represents a natural target for specific therapies and has been extensively investigated in many solid tumors. *PIK3CA* mutations are linked, at least at preclinical level, to resistance against trastuzumab in metastatic breast cancers,[137] whereas it *has been proposed that only specific mutations* (ie, those occurring in exon 20) represent a mechanism of primary resistance to cetuximab or panitumumab in metastatic CRC patients, without large confirmation.[119] The investigation of *PIK3CA* mutations can be useful in clinical diagnosis in CRC patients before the administration of aspirin in an adjuvant setting. Aspirin, in fact, is a drug efficiently preventing colorectal adenomas and carcinomas, and the effect is thought to be driven by the inhibition of cyclooxygenase enzymes. This anticancer effect has been reported to be restricted to patients with cyclooxygenase overexpression. Two large prospective studies demonstrated that a stronger effect is observed in patients additionally carrying a *PIK3CA* mutation, probably because it seems that *PIK3CA* gene product further induces cyclooxygenase expression. A more recent study based on retrospective analysis has confirmed the predictive value of *PIK3CA* mutations for patients treated with aspirin in adjuvant treatment. Interestingly, this effect could not be observed in patients taken the specific cyclooxygenase inhibitor rofecoxib.[138] But the major clinical application of *PIK3CA* mutations in clinical diagnosis is in ovarian cancer patients. In particular, the orally available PI3K inhibitor alpelisib has shown antitumor activity in combination with fulvestrant as treatment for hormone receptor (HR)-positive, *erbB2*-negative breast cancer in patients with a PIK3CA mutation and received FDA approval.[139–142] Furthermore, the efficacy of alpelisib on other PIK3CA-altered advanced solid tumors is under investigation and preliminary studies demonstrate encouraging signs of the antitumor activity of these drugs.[143]

BCL-2

Many groups have been working to develop anticancer drugs that block the function of antiapoptotic bcl-2 members, thus favoring cell death. Methods include the downregulation of bcl-2 expression through antisense oligonucleotides, or the use of peptides or small organic molecules to the bcl-2 binding pocket, preventing its sequestration of proapoptotic proteins. One of the most promising aspects of these small-molecule inhibitors in treating cancer is that their targets and mechanisms of action are different from those of cytotoxic drugs and radiation. This makes it feasible to combine small-molecule inhibitors with other treatments, creating a synergistic therapy, without likely development of cross-resistance or increased toxicity.[144]

MET

MET is a RTK activated by the hepatocyte growth factor. MET protein overexpression has been observed in a number of neoplastic diseases, usually associated with poor prognosis. *MET* gene amplification is responsible of protein overexpression in only a subgroup of MET-positive cancers. In NSCLC, *MET* gene amplification occurs in 2–4% of both squamous and non-squamous cancers. Interestingly MET amplification represents one of the main mechanism of secondary resistance to TKIs against EGFR. Besides MET can be characterized by extremely different alterations in exon 14. In particular base substitutions, insertions, deletions involve several gene positions important for splicing out introns flanking exon 14, including the branch point, polypyrimidine tract, 3′ splice site of intron 13, and the 5′ splice site of intron 14, generally leading to MET exon 14 skipping.[145] This alteration has a much higher incidence in older patients with a lower percentage of never-smokers compared to patients with tumors harboring other oncogenes and occurs predominantly in pulmonary sarcomatoid carcinomas, indeed about 20–30% of sarcomatoid carcinomas harbor MET exon 14 skipping. *MET* exon 14 skipping is mutually exclusive with other lung cancer drivers (*EGFR, K-ras, ALK, ROS1,* or *RET*).[145]

Several MET inhibitors have been developed, both TKI (such as crizotinib and tivantinib) and MoAbs (such as onartuzumab), but the efficacy of these compounds has to be still proven in lung as well as in other cancers.[146] Very recent data seem to outline that *MET* exon 14 skipping and MET amplification are associated with clinical response to MET inhibitor therapy in a substantial proportion of patients.[145]

FGFR

FGFR family includes four members, with FGFR1 showing the most promising clinical role in cancers. In particular, in NSCLC, FGFR1 gene amplification occurs in approximately 20% of cases with a squamous histology but in less than 2% of adenocarcinoma. These amplifications appear to confer an FGFR1-addiction to tumoral cells. FGFR1 inhibitors (such as AZD4547, JNJ-42756493, BGJ398, and ponatinib) are under evaluation.[147,148] FGFR is a relevant marker also in genitourinary neoplasms with FGFR3 mutations playing the pivotal role in these tumors. Urothelial cancer cluster I subtypes are enriched with FGFR3 mutations and are generally associated with immunologically cold tumors that do not respond to checkpoint inhibitors.[149] Small-molecule TKIs of FGFR3 are currently in development and seem to show promising results. The FGFR3 TKI erdafitinib was recently reported in a phase II trial to have an overall response rate of 40%.[149] Given that this is a population that has poorer responses to immunotherapy and minimal therapeutic options, erdafitinib may represent a potential breakthrough for patients with urothelial cancer.[149]

ALK

Rearrangements of ALK primarily occur as fusion to *EML4* gene. These fusion proteins can be found in approximately 3–7% of lung adenocarcinoma. Among EML4-ALK fusion proteins, several *EML4* breakpoints have been described. In rare cases, other fusion partners have been observed, including *TFG* and *KIF5B* genes.[150] The first ALK selective inhibitor was represented by the multitargeted inhibitor crizotinib. The first clinical trial including ALK-positive patients showed very attractive results: 61% of overall survival, 71% of disease control rate, and increased progression-free survival, leading a rapid approval of crizotinib by the FDA for the treatment of lung adenocarcinomas characterized by *ALK* translocation, as evaluated by fluorescent *in situ* hybridization.[151] Unfortunately, the duration of clinical benefit of crizotinib is limited, due to the occurrence of variable systemic resistance mechanisms: occurrence of secondary point mutations in ALK active site, ALK fusion gene amplifications, erb B family pathway activation, *ALK* copy number gain, *kit* gene amplification, *K-ras* mutations. In 30% of ALK-rearranged cases, the resistance to crizotinib is associated with a secondary mutation in the kinase domain of ALK that interferes with the drug binding or ATP affinity. Several ALK mutations have been identified, but the most common ones are L1196M and G1269A. Other, rarer ALK mutations leading to crizotinib resistance are L1152R, C1156Y, I1171T, F1174L, V1180L, D1203N, S1206Y.[152] Recently, second-generation ALK TKIs have been developed to overcome resistance to crizotinib, such as ceritinib and alectinib. Ceritinib and alectinib have been approved for metastatic ALK-positive NSCLC patients and are more prone to prevent the development of brain metastasis, at odds with crizotinib: this is the main reason for their introduction in first-line treatment. Furthermore, also a novel highly selective and potent inhibitor of ALK and ROS1, brigatinib, showed efficacy in crizotinib-resistant ALK-positive patients in two preliminary studies, which led to its approval in this setting, and it is currently being investigated as the first-line therapy versus crizotinib in TKI-naïve patients.[153] ALK rearrangements are also considered one (but not the most frequent) of the mechanisms of acquired resistance to TKI against EGFR in *erb B1*-mutant lung adenocarcinoma.[150]

ROS1

Rearrangements of *ROS1* oncogene appear to occur in approximately 1–2% of lung adenocarcinoma. *ROS1* has a high degree of homology with *ALK* (49% within the TK domain and 77% with the ATP-binding site) and patients with *ROS1* rearrangements display superimposable clinicopathological features with whom carrying *ALK* translocations.[149] The multitargeted inhibitor crizotinib has demonstrated efficacy in *ROS1* rearranged patients, with preliminary response rate of 57% and disease control rate of 79%. As a consequence, *ROS1* rearrangements have entered clinical diagnosis for lung adenocarcinoma patients. Despite excellent initial responses to crizotinib, the majority of NSCLC patients develop disease progression. Identification of resistance mechanisms to crizotinib, and newer generation TKIs with increased activity against ROS1 and ROS1-resistance mutations are under evaluation in several clinical trials.[153]

NTRK

The NTRK family is made up of 3 genes crucial to nervous system development and physiology. These genes—*NTRK1*, *NTRK2*, and *NTRK3*—encode the receptors TRKA, TRKB, and TRKC, respectively. Each receptor is activated by a different binding factor, which triggers phosphorylation of the proteins' intracellular kinase domain, setting off various signaling pathways that maintain normal nervous system function.[154]

In cancer, NTRK family alterations are characterized by gene fusions. NTRK fusions are highly promiscuous: so far, over 80 different 5′ fusion partners have been discovered. *NTRK1* partners are mostly found on chromosome 1, indicating that intrachromosomal rearrangements are the main drivers of *NTRK1* fusions. *NTRK2* and *NTRK3* fusions, on the other hand, usually occur via interchromosomal rearrangements.[155]

Recent studies have shown that NTRK fusions contribute to tumorigenesis in over 90% of infantile fibrosarcoma, congenital mesoblastic nephroma, breast secretory carcinoma, and salivary gland carcinoma. They also occur with lower frequency in the majority of the most diffused cancers, including the big killer CRC and NSCLC.[156]

Many new molecules, specifically addressed against NTRK alterations, are under evaluation in clinical trials: of these, larotrectinib, an oral NTRK inhibitor, was approved in 2018 in the United States for the management of patients with locally advanced or metastatic solid tumors carrying NTRK gene rearrangements.[157] The efficacy of larotrectinib has been proved in adults and children characterized by fusions of these genes.[158]

In addition to larotrectinib, another drug that is under regulatory review in Europe and the United States is entrectinib, an oral selective inhibitor of NTRK, ROS1, and ALK. In 2019, this drug received its first global approval in Japan, for the treatment of adult and pediatric patients with NTRK fusion-positive, advanced or recurrent solid tumors. Entrectinib has shown potent antineoplastic activity and tolerability in various neoplastic conditions, particularly in NSCLC positive for NTRK fusions.[159]

IDH

Isocitrate dehydrogenases, IDH1 and 2, are enzymes that catalyze the reversible oxidative decarboxylation of isocitrate to yield α-ketoglutarate as part of the TCA cycle in glucose metabolism. In cancer, IDH1 and 2 can be altered following the occurrence of point mutations, which leads to the hyperaccumulation of 2-hydroxyglutarate that, in turn, causes widespread changes in histone and DNA methylation.

IDH genes are especially relevant in gliomas. In brain tumors, the main alteration in IDH1 is the point mutations R132H (rare mutations are R132C/G/S/L) and in IDH2 the point mutation R172K (rarer mutations are R172M/S/W). IDH1 and IDH2 molecular status has diagnostic relevance because it differentiates glioma from gliosis.[160] These genes are mutated in nearly 50% of astrocytomas, or grade II/III oligodendroglioma, and even in 10% of glioblastoma, especially following a recurrence after primary astrocytoma.[160] Alterations in IDH1 and IDH2 genes are associated with better prognosis, but their role in the prediction of response to therapies is still debated.[161] The identification of IDH mutations is now a prerequisite for the classification of brain tumors, that, therefore, are the first type of cancer with a molecular-based, instead of only a cyto/pathological-based, classification.

ESR1

ESR1 gene encodes for the estrogen receptor 1; in HR-positive breast cancer, mutations, and rearrangements in this gene have emerged as a key mechanism of resistance to endocrine therapy, and in the future, they will probably become a prognostic and predictive biomarker, used in clinical practice for breast cancer, especially in the metastatic setting.[162,163]

Summary and conclusions

The initiation and progression of human neoplasia are a multistep process involving the accumulation of genetic changes in somatic cells. These genetic changes then consist of the activation of cooperating oncogenes and the inactivation of tumor suppressor genes, which both appear necessary for a complete neoplastic phenotype. Oncogenes are altered versions of normal cellular genes called proto-oncogenes. Proto-oncogenes are a diverse group of genes involved in the regulation of cell growth. The functions of proto-oncogenes include growth factors, growth factor receptors, signal transducers, transcription factors, and regulators of programmed cell death. Proto-oncogenes may be activated by mutation, chromosomal rearrangement, or gene amplification. Chromosomal rearrangements that include translocations and inversions can activate proto-oncogenes by deregulation of their transcription (e.g., transcriptional activation) or by gene fusion. Tumor suppressor genes, which also participate in the regulation of normal cell growth, are usually inactivated by point mutations or truncation of their protein sequence coupled with the loss of the normal allele.

The discovery of oncogenes represented a breakthrough for our understanding of the molecular and genetic basis of cancer. Oncogenes have also provided important knowledge concerning the regulation of normal cell proliferation, differentiation, and programmed cell death. The identification of oncogene abnormalities has provided tools for the molecular diagnosis and monitoring of cancer. Most important, oncogenes represent potential targets for actually approved and for new types of cancer therapies. The goal of these drugs is to kill cancer cells selectively while sparing normal cells. One promising approach entails using specific oncogene targets to trigger programmed cell death. The first example of the accomplishment of such a goal is represented by the inhibition of the tumor-specific TK bcr/abl in CML, by imatinib. The same compound has been proven active also in a different tumor type, GIST where it inhibits the TK receptor *c-kit* and in chordomas, where it switches off the PDGFR.[24] Another example is represented by gefitinib and cetuximab, which inhibit the intracellular TK and the extracellular domain, respectively, of erb B1. Thereafter, a plethora of new targeted drugs has entered clinical trials, with evident benefit for the treatment of several neoplastic diseases that were, before targeted therapies development, very hard to be treated and cured. Nowadays, the analysis of oncogenes alterations has been simplified by the introduction of next-generation sequencing, characterized by the capability to detect a large number of alterations with a multigene approach in only one experiment starting from a small amount of genomic DNA, thus rendering this methodology highly attractive especially when only small biopsies are available. Another advantage of next-generation sequencing is the fact that this technology is able also to characterize gene alterations in liquid biopsies, which are less invasive samples that can be repeated serially overtime. The use of high-throughput technologies for the identification of new oncogenes (in tissue samples and plasma) and the rapidly expanding knowledge of the molecular mechanisms of cancer hold great promise for the development of better-combined methods of cancer therapy in the near future.

Key references

The complete reference list can be found on Vital Source version of this title, see inside front cover.

3. Vogt PK. Retroviral oncogenes: a historical primer. *Nat Rev Cancer*. 2020;**12**(9):639–648.
22. Santoro M, Moccia M, Federico G, et al. RET gene fusions in malignancies of the thyroid and other tissues. *Genes (Basel)*. 2020;**11**(4):424.
26. Kazlauskas A. PDGFs and their receptors. *Gene*. 2017;**614**:1–7.
27. Callahan R, Smith GH. MMTV-induced mammary tumorigenesis: gene discovery, progression to malignancy and cellular pathways. *Oncogene*. 2000;**19**(8):992–1001.
29. Zhang YL, Yuan JQ, Wang KF, et al. The prevalence of EGFR mutation in patients with non-small cell lung cancer: a systematic review and meta-analysis. *Oncotarget*. 2016;**7**(48):78985–78993.
30. Ohtsuka K, Ohnishi H, Kurai D, et al. Familial lung adenocarcinoma caused by the EGFR V843I germ-line mutation. *J Clin Oncol*. 2011;**29**(8):e191–e192.
31. Lee HS, Kim WH, Kwak Y, et al. Molecular testing for gastrointestinal cancer. *J Pathol Transl Med*. 2017;**51**(2):103–121.
33. von Mehren M, Joensuu H. Gastrointestinal stromal tumors. *J Clin Oncol*. 2018;**36**(2):136–143.

36 Laham-Karam N, Pinto GP, Poso A, et al. Transcription and translation inhibitors in cancer treatment. *Front Chem*. 2020;**8**:276.

40 Nguyen L, Papenhausen P, Shao H. The role of c-MYC in B-cell lymphomas: diagnostic and molecular aspects. *Genes (Basel)*. 2017;**8**(4):116.

42 Knight T, Luedtke D, Edwards H, et al. A delicate balance - The BCL-2 family and its role in apoptosis, oncogenesis, and cancer therapeutics. *Biochem Pharmacol*. 2019;**162**:250–261.

43 Dankner M, Rose AAN, Rajkumar S, et al. Classifying BRAF alterations in cancer: new rational therapeutic strategies for actionable mutations. *Oncogene*. 2018;**37**(24):3183–3199.

44 Dorstyn L, Akey CW, Kumar S. New insights into apoptosome structure and function. *Cell Death Differ*. 2018;**25**(7):1194–1208.

47 Chen S, Li F, Xu D, et al. The function of RAS mutation in cancer and advances in its drug research. *Curr Pharm Des*. 2019;**25**(10):1105–1114.

49 D'Cruz AK, Vaish R, Vaidya A, et al. Molecular markers in well-differentiated thyroid cancer. *Eur Arch Otorhinolaryngol*. 2018;**275**(6):1375–1384.

50 Abdullah MI, Junit SM, Ng KL, et al. Papillary Thyroid Cancer: Genetic Alterations and Molecular Biomarker Investigations. *Int J Med Sci*. 2019;**16**(3):450-460.

59 Lancho O, Herranz D. The MYC enhancer-ome: (2018). Long-range transcriptional regulation of MYC in cancer. *Trends Cancer*;**4**(12):810–822.

62 Shin H, Choi SY, Kee KM, et al. Comprehensive analyses of safety and efficacy toward individualizing imatinib dosage in patients with chronic myeloid leukemia. *Int J Hematol*. 2020;**111**(3):417–426.

67 Hu Y, He H, Lu J, et al. E2A-PBX1 exhibited a promising prognosis in pediatric acute lymphoblastic leukemia treated with the CCLG-ALL2008 protocol. *Onco Targets Ther*. 2016;**9**:7219–7225.

68 Suguna E, Farhana R, Kanimozhi E, et al. Acute myeloid leukemia: diagnosis and management based on current molecular genetics approach. *Cardiovasc Hematol Disord Drug Targets*. 2018;**18**(3):199–207.

70 Arber DA, Orazi A, Hasserjian R, et al. The 2016 revision to the World Health Organization classification of myeloid neoplasms and acute leukemia. *Blood*. 2016;**127**(20):2391–2405.

74 Saab J, Rosenthal IM, Wang L, et al. Dermatofibrosarcoma protuberans-like tumor With COL1A1 copy number gain in the absence of t(17;22). *Am J Dermatopathol*. 2017;**39**(4):304–309.

93 Handa H, Murakami Y, Ishihara R, et al. The role and function of microRNA in the pathogenesis of multiple myeloma. *Cancers (Basel)*. 2019;**11**(11):1738.

94 Shirjang S, Mansoori B, Asghari S, et al. MicroRNAs in cancer cell death pathways: apoptosis and necroptosis. *Free Radic Biol Med*. 2019;**139**:1–15.

95 Aqeilan RI, Calin GA, Croce CM. miR-15a and miR-16-1 in cancer: discovery, function, and future perspectives. *Cell Death Differ*. 2010;**17**:215–220.

96 Calin GA, Dumitru CD, Shimizu M, et al. Frequent deletions and down-regulation of micro-RNA genes miR15 and miR16 at 13q14 in chronic lymphocytic leukemia. *Proc Natl Acad Sci USA*. 2002;**99**:15524–15529.

97 Cimmino A, Calin GA, Fabbri M, et al. miR-15 and miR-16 induce apoptosis by targeting BCL2. *Proc Natl Acad Sci*. 2005;**102**:13944–13949.

108 Evrard C, Tachon G, Randrian V, et al. Microsatellite instability: diagnosis, heterogeneity, discordance, and clinical impact in colorectal cancer. *Cancers (Basel)*. 2019;**11**(10):1567.

109 Recio-Boiles A, Waheed A, Cagir B. Cancer, Colon. In: *StatPearls*. Treasure Island (FL): StatPearls Publishing; 2020.

110 Fearon ER, Vogelstein B. A genetic model for colorectal tumorigenesis. *Cell*. 1990;**61**:759–767.

111 Lee MKC, Loree JM. Current and emerging biomarkers in metastatic colorectal cancer. *Curr Oncol*. 2019;**26**(Suppl 1):S7–S15.

112 Díaz-Serrano A, Gella P, Jiménez E, et al. Targeting EGFR in lung cancer: current standards and developments. *Drugs*. 2018;**78**(9):893–911.

113 Takezawa K, Pirazzoli V, Arcila ME, et al. HER2 amplification: a potential mechanism of acquired resistance to EGFR inhibition in EGFR-mutant lung cancers that lack the second-site EGFRT790M mutation. *Cancer Discov*. 2012;**2**(10):922–933.

114 Saad N, Poudel A, Basnet A, et al. Epidermal growth factor receptor T790M mutation-positive metastatic non-small-cell lung cancer: focus on osimertinib (AZD9291). *Onco Targets Ther*. 2017;**10**:1757–1766.

115 Bettegowda C, Sausen M, Leary RJ, et al. Detection of circulating tumor DNA in early- and late-stage human malignancies. *Sci Transl Med*. 2014;**6**(224):224ra24.

116 Oellerich M, Christenson RH, Beck J, Walson PD. Plasma EGFR mutation testing in non-small cell lung cancer: A value proposition. *Clin Chim Acta*. 2019;**495**:481–486.

117 Del Re M, Crucitta S, Gianfilippo G, et al. Understanding the mechanisms of resistance in EGFR-positive NSCLC: from tissue to liquid biopsy to guide treatment strategy. *Int J Mol Sci*. 2019;**20**(16):3951.

121 Meng D, Carvajal RD. KIT as an oncogenic driver in melanoma: an update on clinical development. *Am J Clin Dermatol*. 2019;**20**(3):315–323.

123 Bronte G, Ulivi P, Verlicchi A, et al. Targeting RET-rearranged non-small-cell lung cancer: future prospects. *Lung Cancer (Auckl)*. 2019;**10**:27–36.

124 Li AY, McCusker MG, Russo A, et al. RET fusions in solid tumors. *Cancer Treat Rev*. 2019;**81**:101911.

125 Zhao B, Wang L, Qiu H, et al. Mechanisms of resistance to anti-EGFR therapy in colorectal cancer. *Oncotarget*. 2017;**8**(3):3980–4000.

126 Goldberg RM, Montagut C, Wainberg ZA, et al. Optimising the use of cetuximab in the continuum of care for patients with metastatic colorectal cancer. *ESMO Open*. 2018;**3**:e000353.

127 Cremolini C, Rossini D, Dell'Aquila E, et al. Rechallenge for patients with RAS and BRAF wild-type metastatic colorectal cancer with acquired resistance to first-line cetuximab and irinotecan: a phase 2 single-arm clinical trial. *JAMA Oncol*. 2019;**5**(3):343–350.

128 Gazzaniga P, Raimondi C, Nicolazzo C, et al. ctDNA might expand therapeutic options for second line treatment of KRAS mutant mCRC. *Ann Oncol*. 2017;**28**(5):568.

129 Raimondi C, Nicolazzo C, Belardinilli F, et al. Transient disappearance of RAS mutant clones in plasma: a counterintuitive clinical use of EGFR inhibitors in RAS mutant metastatic colorectal cancer. *Cancers*. 2019;**11**(42):1–10.

130 O'Bryan JP. Pharmacological targeting of RAS: recent success with direct inhibitors. *Pharmacol Res*. 2019;**139**:503–511.

132 Garbe C, Eigentler TK. Vemurafenib. *Recent Results Cancer Res*. 2018;**211**:77–89.

133 O'Leary CG, Andelkovic V, Ladwa R, et al. Targeting BRAF mutations in non-small cell lung cancer. *Transl Lung Cancer Res*. 2019;**8**(6):1119–1124.

138 Paleari L, Puntoni M, Clavarezza M, et al. PIK3CA Mutation, aspirin use after diagnosis and survival of colorectal cancer. A systematic review and meta-analysis of epidemiological studies. *Clin Oncol (R Coll Radiol)*. 2016;**28**(5):317–326.

139 André F, Ciruelos E, Rubovszky G, et al. Alpelisib for PIK3CA-mutated, hormone receptor-positive advanced breast cancer. *N Engl J Med*. 2019;**380**(20):1929–1940.

140 Markham A. Alpelisib: first global approval. *Drugs*. 2019;**79**(11):1249–1253.

141 Juric D, Janku F, Rodón J, et al. Alpelisib plus fulvestrant in PIK3CA-altered and PIK3CA-wild-type estrogen receptor-positive advanced breast cancer: a phase 1b clinical trial. *JAMA Oncol*. 2019;**5**(2):e184475.

142 Stirrups R. Alpelisib plus fulvestrant for PIK3CA-mutated breast cancer. *Lancet Oncol*. 2019;**20**(7):e347.

143 Juric D, Rodon J, Tabernero J, et al. Phosphatidylinositol 3-kinase α-selective inhibition with Alpelisib (BYL719) in PIK3CA-altered solid tumors: results from the first-in-human study. *J Clin Oncol*. 2018;**36**(13):1291–1299.

145 Drilon A, Cappuzzo F, Ou SI, et al. Targeting MET in lung cancer: will expectations finally be MET? *J Thorac Oncol*. 2017;**12**(1):15–26.

149 Devitt ME, Dreicer R. Evolving role of genomics in genitourinary neoplasms. *Acta Med Acad*. 2019;**48**(1):68–77.

150 Rosas G, Ruiz R, Araujo JM, et al. ALK rearrangements: biology, detection and opportunities of therapy in non-small cell lung cancer. *Crit Rev Oncol Hematol*. 2019;**136**:48–55.

152 Toyokawa G, Seto T. Updated evidence on the mechanisms of resistance to ALK inhibitors and strategies to overcome such resistance: clinical and preclinical data. *Oncol Res Treat*. 2015;**38**(6):291–298.

153 Mezquita L, Planchard D. The role of brigatinib in crizotinib-resistant non-small cell lung cancer. *Cancer Manag Res*. 2018;**10**:123–130.

154 Amatu A, Sartore-Bianchi A, Siena S. NTRK gene fusions as novel targets of cancer therapy across multiple tumour types. *ESMO Open*. 2016;**1**(2):e000023.

155 Hsiao SJ, Zehir A, Sireci AN, et al. Detection of tumor NTRK gene fusions to identify patients who may benefit from tyrosine kinase (TRK) inhibitor therapy. *J Mol Diagn*. 2019;**21**(4):553–571.

156 Cocco E, Scaltriti M, Drilon A. NTRK fusion-positive cancers and TRK inhibitor therapy. *Nat Rev Clin Oncol*. 2018;**15**(12):731–747.

157 Scott LJ. Larotrectinib: first global approval. *Drugs*. 2019;**79**(2):201–206.

158 Drilon A, Laetsch TW, Kummar S, et al. Efficacy of larotrectinib in TRK fusion-positive cancers in adults and children. *N Engl J Med*. 2018;**378**(8):731–739.

159 Al-Salama ZT, Keam SJ. Entrectinib: first global approval. *Drugs*. 2019;**79**(13):1477–1483.

160 Gupta A, Dwivedi T. A simplified overview of World Health Organization classification update of central nervous system tumors 2016. *J Neurosci Rural Pract*. 2017;**8**:629–641.

161 van den Bent MJ, Dubbink HJ, Marie Y, et al. IDH1 and IDH2 mutations are prognostic but not predictive for outcome in anaplastic oligodendroglial tumors: a report of the European Organization for Research and Treatment of Cancer Brain Tumor Group. *Clin Cancer Res*. 2010;**16**(5):1597–1604.

162 Carausu M, Bidard FC, Callens C, et al. ESR1 mutations: a new biomarker in breast cancer. *Expert Rev Mol Diagn*. 2019;**19**(7):599–611.

163 De Santo I, McCartney A, Migliaccio I, et al. The emerging role of ESR1 mutations in luminal breast cancer as a prognostic and predictive biomarker of response to endocrine therapy. *Cancers (Basel)*. 2019;**11**(12):1894.

5 Tumor suppressor genes

Fred Bunz, MD, PhD ■ Bert Vogelstein, MD

> **Overview**
>
> Cancer is a genetic disease caused by alterations in proto-oncogenes and tumor suppressor genes. Oncogenes, the first type of gene to be associated with cancer, are activated by somatic mutations and promote unregulated cell growth. In contrast, tumor suppressor genes encode proteins that maintain tissue homeostasis and are inactivated in tumors. Inactivated tumor suppressor genes can be acquired by somatic mutation, during the life of an individual, or transmitted via the germline from one generation to the next, causing familial cancer predisposition syndromes. Tumor suppressor genes thus provide a conceptual link between inherited cancer risk and sporadic cancers.

A genetic basis for the development of cancer has been hypothesized for over a century. This hypothesis is supported by familial, epidemiologic, and cytogenetic studies. It is now known that at ~200 genes in the human genome can, when mutated, promote the growth of cancers.[1] Malignant tumors arise through a multistage process in which an individual cell initially acquires a mutation that confers a relative growth advantage; the clonal expansion of that cell, followed by the acquisition of a second mutation constitutes the next stage of tumor growth. Successive waves of clonal selection and expansion eventually lead to the formation of an invasive, disseminated cancer.

Two classes of genes, oncogenes and tumor suppressor genes, are required for maintaining the balance between cell proliferation and cell death in adult tissues, a status known as tissue homeostasis. Mutations in oncogenes and tumor suppressor genes upset this balance in a variety of ways and thereby perturb tissue homeostasis. (A distinct subtype of tumor suppressor gene does not affect tissue homeostasis directly, but rather controls the rate at which subsequent mutations are acquired.) The activation of oncogenes and the inactivation of tumor suppressor genes cause the relative growth advantages that underlie the stages of tumor development.

The majority of the mutations that contribute to tumor development are acquired somatically (i.e., in the body during the life of the individual). A relatively small fraction of cancers is caused by tumor suppressor gene mutations that are present in the germline and therefore harbored in all somatic cells of the individual. Such alleles are heritable and can be passed on to progeny, increasing cancer risk in subsequent generations.

The identification and function of proto-oncogenes and oncogenes are reviewed in other articles of this encyclopedia. Here, we provide a brief summary of their general properties in order to highlight how they differ from tumor suppressor genes. The oncogenes present in cancers have sustained gain-of-function alterations. Oncogenes harbor mutations that increase or deregulate the activity of the wild type allele (sometimes referred to as the proto-oncogene). These mutations most commonly involve single base substitutions that cause constitutive activation of the protein product. Alternative mechanisms of activation are gene fusion and gene amplification, which can each cause the encoded protein to be overexpressed.

In contrast to oncogenes, tumor suppressor genes are defined by their functional inactivation during tumorigenesis. Inactivating mutations in tumor suppressor genes can include missense or nonsense mutations, small insertions or deletions (indels) that may disrupt a functional domain or cause frameshifts, or larger deletions that eliminate part or all of the coding exons. Tumor suppressor gene mutations are most often acquired somatically but can also be inherited via the germline. Because they involve gains in function that would presumably interfere with normal embryogenesis, mutations in oncogenes almost always arise somatically in the cells of a developing tumor. Germline oncogene mutations have been described, notably affecting rearranged during transfection (RET) and metastasis (MET), and leading to familial medullary thyroid cancer and hereditary papillary renal cell carcinoma, respectively. These are rare exceptions. Genetic risk factors for cancer nearly always involve germline tumor suppressor gene mutations.

The aims of this article are to review the landmark studies that established the existence of tumor suppressor genes, to describe the identification and cloning of representative tumor suppressor genes, to highlight selected functions of tumor suppressor genes and their relationship to cancer cell phenotypes, and to highlight the important role of genome maintenance in tumor suppression.

Genetic basis for tumor development

The inherited basis of human cancer has been appreciated for more than 150 years.[2] In 1866, Broca described a family with a high prevalence of breast and liver cancer. He proposed that an inherited abnormality within the affected tissue allowed for tumor development. Following the rediscovery of Mendel's work, Haaland, who studied the rates of spontaneous mammary tumor formation in various inbred strains of mice, argued that tumorigenesis could be considered a Mendelian genetic trait. Between 1895 and 1913, Warthin identified four multigenerational families with susceptibilities to specific cancer types that appeared to be transmitted in an autosomal dominant fashion (Figure 1).[3] These and other studies suggested the existence of an inherited genetic basis for some cancers. However, it remained difficult to firmly rule out other explanations for familial clustering, such as shared exposure to a carcinogenic agent in the environment or diet. It was

---

Holland-Frei Cancer Medicine, Tenth Edition. Edited by Robert C. Bast, John C. Byrd, Carlo M. Croce, Ernest Hawk, Fadlo R. Khuri, Raphael E. Pollock, Apostolia M. Tsimberidou, Christopher G. Willett, and Cheryl L. Willman.
© 2023 John Wiley & Sons, Inc. Published 2023 by John Wiley & Sons, Inc.

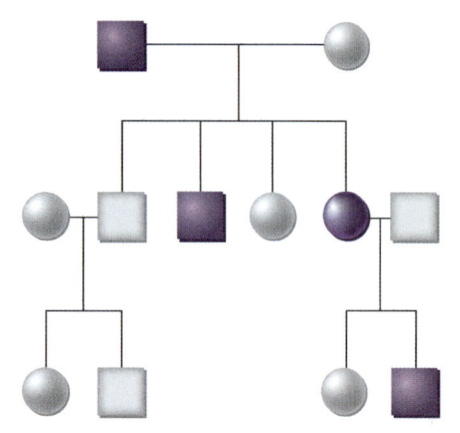

Figure 1 The inheritance of cancer in a family. The affected members with cancer are indicated by shaded squares (males) or circles (females). This family demonstrates a dominant pattern of inheritance, meaning that each offspring has a 50% chance of inheriting a germline mutation that confers a high probability of developing cancer.

also apparent that most cancers in humans appeared to arise as sporadic, isolated cases.

A role for somatic mutations in the development of cancer was first proposed by Boveri.[3] He observed that sea urchin eggs fertilized by two sperm cells would exhibit abnormal mitotic divisions, leading to the loss of chromosomes in daughter cells. Atypical tissue masses would then appear in the resulting gastrula. Boveri believed that these abnormal tissues were physically similar to the poorly differentiated tissue masses seen in tumors and hypothesized that cancer arose from a cellular aberration producing abnormal mitotic figures. Boveri's hypothesis found experimental support decades later, when the majority of cancers were shown to have karyotypic abnormalities. For decades thereafter, uncertainty remained as to whether the changes in chromosome number and structure found in tumors were a cause or an effect of the neoplastic process.

A landmark observation in the search to identify a genetic basis for cancer was made by Rous in 1911 when he reported that sarcomas could be reproducibly induced in hens by the application of cell-free filtrates of tumor tissues. This seminal observation provided evidence that tumors could be virally induced, and in later years would provide support for the emerging view that cancer could be attributed to discrete genetic elements.[4]

The potent oncogene harbored by the Rous sarcoma virus was identified six decades later, by Bishop and Varmus. Molecular characterization and cloning of the transforming sequences of the virus demonstrated that its oncogenicity depended on an element designated *V-SRC*. Bishop and Varmus discovered that *V-SRC* was in fact a transduced and mutated copy of a cellular proto-oncogene, *C-SRC* (now simply designated *SRC*). Subsequently, it was found that all oncogenes associated with acutely transforming ribonucleic acid (RNA) tumor viruses originated as cellular genes that were appropriated in mutant form during the virus life cycle.

In human cancers, activated oncogenes are not transmitted by retroviruses but instead result from somatic mutations of endogenous proto-oncogenes. Oncogenes play a role in most forms of human cancer but are particularly prominent in so-called "liquid" tumors, such as leukemias and lymphomas, as well as in sarcomas. Such cancers often have characteristic chromosomal translocations that alter oncogenes at the breakpoints, fusing them with unrelated genes and endowing the fusion product with new properties that increase cell birth or decrease cell death.

Somatic cell genetic studies of tumorigenesis

Studies of mouse tumor models that began in the 1960s provided experimental evidence that the ability of cells to form a tumor behaves as a recessive phenotypic trait.[5] Hill and Ephrussi independently observed that the growth of murine tumor cells in syngeneic animals, a trait known as tumorigenicity, could be suppressed when the malignant cells were fused to nonmalignant cells, thereby creating what are known as intraspecies hybrid cells. Significantly, reversion to tumorigenicity often occurred when the hybrid cells were propagated for extended periods in culture. The reappearance of the tumorigenic phenotype was shown to be associated with specific chromosome losses in the revertant hybrid cells. These seminal observations implied the existence of dominant genetic elements that could suppress the ability of cells to form tumors. Thus, tumorigenicity was a recessive phenotype that was expressed in the absence of these dominant genes. Similar conclusions were drawn from subsequent experiments with mouse, rat, and hamster intraspecies somatic cell hybrids, as well as by interspecies hybrids between rodent tumor cells and normal human cells.

The cell hybridization approach was next used to identify human chromosomal elements that could suppress tumorigenesis. However, the karyotypic instability of rodent-human hybrids complicated the analysis of the human chromosomes involved in tumor suppression. Stanbridge and his colleagues overcame this technical problem by studying hybrids made by fusing human tumor cell lines to normal, diploid human fibroblasts. Their cytogenetic analysis confirmed that interspecies hybrids retaining both sets of parental chromosomes were nontumorigenic. Tumorigenic revertants arose only rarely after chromosome losses.

Importantly, the loss of specific chromosomes, and not simply chromosome loss in general, correlated with the reversion to tumorigenicity. Tumorigenicity was suppressed even if activated oncogenes were expressed in the hybrids, which appeared to affirm the dominance of these genetic elements. The observation that the loss of specific chromosomes was associated with the reversion suggested that a single chromosome, and perhaps even a single gene, might be sufficient to suppress tumorigenicity. Accordingly, many subsequent studies demonstrated that transfer of even very small chromosome fragments could specifically suppress the tumorigenic properties of some human cancer cell lines.

It is important to understand that the experiments in syngeneic mice could capture only a subset of the complex cellular phenotypes that are responsible for tumor evolution. Although tumorigenic growth in immunocompromised animals can be experimentally suppressed in hybrids resulting from fusion between malignant and normal cells or by transfer of unique chromosome fragments, many other traits that are characteristic of naturally occuring cancer cells were likely retained. Suppression of tumorigenicity following cell fusion or microcell chromosome transfer thus represented correction of only some of many alterations that give rise to cancers in humans. Nonetheless, these landmark studies provided an elegant demonstration that supported the existence of suppressive genetic elements and their dominant effects on tumorigenesis.

Retinoblastoma: a paradigm for tumor suppressor gene function

The contemporary studies by Knudson forged a crucial theoretical link between the experimental analysis of rodent tumor hybrids and human cancer patients. A physician by training, Knudson, exhaustively analyzed the age-specific incidence of the ocular cancer retinoblastoma in sporadic and inherited forms of the disease.[6] His observation of the early onset of bilateral or multifocal disease in patients with familial retinoblastoma led him to propose that two "hits" or mutagenic events were necessary for retinoblastoma development.

Retinoblastoma occurs sporadically in most cases, but in some families, it displays an autosomal dominant mode of inheritance. In individuals with the inherited form of the disease, Knudson proposed that the first hit is present in the germline, and thus in all cells of the body. However, Knudson argued, the presence of a single mutation was insufficient for tumor formation; a second, somatically acquired mutation was necessary for the development of a tumor. Thus, the elevated risk of cancer in mutation carriers could be explained by the high likelihood of a somatic mutation occurring in at least one retinal cell during development. In contrast, the sporadic form of retinoblastoma was caused by two somatic mutations within the same founder cell, an event that would be statistically improbable and therefore extremely rare. Although each of the two hits could theoretically have been in different genes, the molecular cloning of the *RB1* gene ultimately demonstrated that both hits involved the same genetic locus. Knudson's insights into the genetic basis of inherited and sporadic cases of retinoblastoma illustrated the mechanisms through which germline and somatic genetic changes could contribute to tumorigenesis. The "two-hit" hypothesis also provided a unifying link to between the epidemiology of retinoblastoma, and other cancer predisposition syndromes, and the illuminating phenotypes of somatic cell hybrids.

The first clue to the location of a putative gene responsible for inherited retinoblastoma was revealed by karyotypic analyses of patients with retinoblastoma.[7] Deletions within chromosome 13 were observed in the normal blood cells obtained from a subset of patients. The common region of deletion included chromosome band 13q14. When compared with karyotypically normal family members, patients with deletions of 13q14 were found to have reduced levels of esterase D, an enzyme of unknown physiologic function that is expressed in multiple forms. This enzyme was irrelevant to the disease, but analysis of esterase D proteins provided a straightforward means of tracking the deletion. An analysis of the segregation patterns of esterase D isozymes and retinoblastoma development in families with inherited retinoblastoma established that the esterase D and *RB1* loci were genetically linked.

One child with inherited retinoblastoma was found to have esterase D levels that were approximately one-half of normal. However, no microscopically evident deletion of chromosome 13 was seen upon karyotypic analysis of his blood cells and skin fibroblasts. Interestingly, tumor cells from this patient exhibited a complete absence of esterase D activity, despite harboring one grossly intact copy of chromosome 13. Based on these findings, it was proposed that the copy of chromosome 13 retained in the tumor cells had a submicroscopic deletion that inactivated both the esterase D and *RB1* loci. Moreover, it was concluded that the initial *RB1* mutation in the child was recessive at the cellular level (i.e., cells with inactivation of one *RB1* allele had a normal phenotype). The effect of the predisposing mutation could be unmasked in the tumor cells by a second event, the somatic loss of the chromosome 13 region that harbored the wild-type *RB1* allele. This explanation was entirely consistent with Knudson's two-hit hypothesis.

To establish the generality of these observations, Cavenee and colleagues undertook studies of inherited and sporadic retinoblastomas, by using deoxyribonucleic acid (DNA) probes from chromosome 13.[8] Probes detecting DNA polymorphisms were used, so that the two parental copies of chromosome 13 in the cells of the patient's normal and tumor tissues could be distinguished. By using such markers to compare paired normal and tumor samples from each patient, the Cavenee group was able to demonstrate that loss of heterozygosity (LOH, the loss of one parental set of markers) for chromosome 13 alleles had occurred during tumorigenesis in more than 60% of the cases studied. LOH on chromosome 13, and specifically for the region of chromosome 13 containing the *RB1* gene, occurred via a number of different mechanisms (Figure 2). In addition, through study of inherited cases, it was shown that the copy of chromosome 13 retained in the tumor cells was derived from the affected parent and that the chromosome carrying the wild-type *RB1* allele had been lost. These data established that the unmasking of a predisposing mutation at the *RB1* gene, whether the initial mutation had been inherited or had arisen somatically in a single developing retinoblast, occurred by the same underlying mechanisms.

Patients with the inherited form of retinoblastoma were known to be at an increased risk for the development of other cancer types, particularly osteosarcoma. LOH for the chromosome 13q region containing the *RB1* locus was detected in osteosarcomas arising in patients with the inherited form of retinoblastoma. This finding proved that inactivation of both *RB1* alleles was also critical to the development of osteosarcomas in those with inherited retinoblastoma. Chromosome 13q LOH was also frequently observed in sporadic osteosarcomas. These molecular studies of retinoblastomas and osteosarcomas were entirely consistent with Knudson's two-hit hypothesis and suggested that the inactivation of a single tumor suppressor gene could contribute to many forms of cancer. The genetic basis of retinoblastoma stands as a paradigm for understanding the role of tumor suppressor genes in sporadic and inherited forms of the same type of cancer.

Analysis of the *RB1* gene

The molecular cloning of the *RB1* gene was facilitated by the identification in the chromosome 13q14 region of a DNA marker that segregated with the disease. Analysis of the DNA sequences flanking this DNA marker revealed a gene with 27 exons spanning more than 200 kb of DNA, which expressed an RNA transcript of about 4.7 kb. The *RB1* gene appears to be expressed ubiquitously, and notably is not restricted to retinoblasts and osteoblasts.

The positional cloning of *RB1* facilitated the subsequent study of mutations that inactivate the gene and the functions of the encoded protein. Although gross deletions of *RB1* sequences are observed in a small subset of retinoblastoma and osteosarcoma cases, most tumors appear to express full-length *RB1* transcripts and lack detectable gene rearrangements. Hence, the detection of inherited and somatic mutations in the *RB1* gene in most cases requires detailed characterization of its sequence. As predicted, patients with inherited retinoblastoma have one mutated and one normal allele in their normal cells (blood cells were usually used for this type of analysis). In tumor tissues, the remaining *RB1* allele is inactivated by somatic mutation, usually by loss of the normal allele through a gross chromosomal event (Figure 2), but in some cases by a point mutation that impairs the function of the expressed protein. In cases where multiple tumors arose in an individual patient with inherited retinoblastoma, each of the tumors was found to contain the same germline mutation. However, different somatic mutations affected the remaining *RB1* allele. The vast majority of patients with a single retinoblastoma

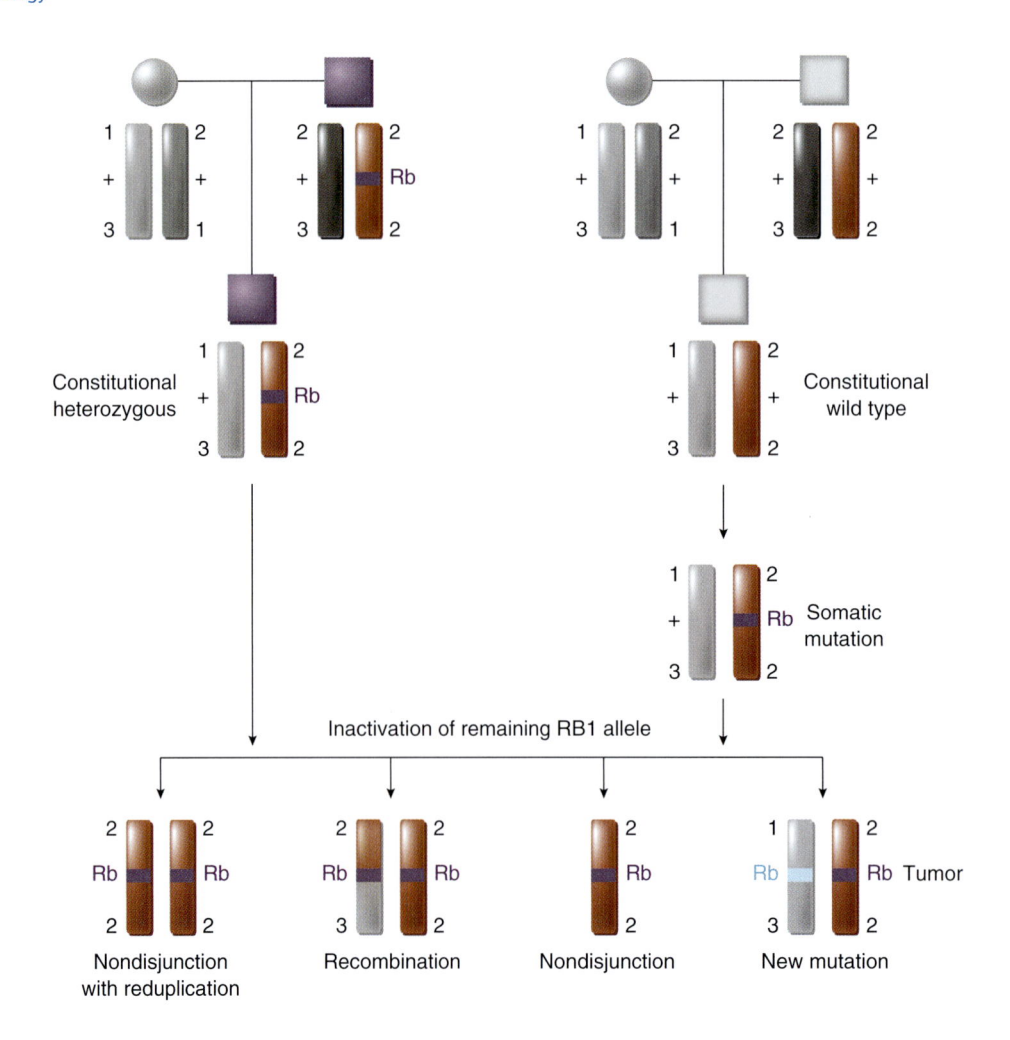

Figure 2 Chromosomal mechanisms that result in loss of heterozygosity (LOH) at the retinoblastoma predisposition (*RB1*) locus at chromosomal band 13q14. In the inherited form of the disease (top left), the affected son inherits a mutant *RB1* allele (rb) from his affected father and a normal *RB1* allele (+) from his mother. Thus, all of his cells contain one wild-type and one mutant *RB1* allele. His constitutional genotype at the *RB1* locus is rb/+). The maternal and paternal copies of chromosome 13 in his normal cells can be distinguished with the use of polymorphic DNA markers flanking the *RB1* locus (the polymorphic alleles are designated by number). A retinoblastoma can arise after inactivation of the remaining wild-type *RB1* allele. Among the genetic mechanisms found to inactivate the remaining wild-type *RB1* allele during tumor development are chromosome nondisjunction and reduplication of the remaining copy of chromosome 13, mitotic recombination, nondisjunction, and new RB mutations that inactivate the remaining *RB1* allele. Shown at the top right is the situation in the noninherited (sporadic) form of the disease. A somatic mutation arises in a developing retinal cell and inactivates one of the *RB1* alleles. A retinoblastoma will develop if the remaining wild type *RB1* allele is inactivated by one of the mechanisms shown in the figure.

and no family history of the disease harbour two mutant alleles in their tumors and two normal alleles in their normal cells.

Patients with germline mutations of *RB1* are at elevated risk for the development of a limited number of tumor types, including retinoblastoma in childhood, osteosarcoma, soft-tissue sarcoma, and melanoma later in life. Despite the near ubiquity of *RB1* expression in human tissues, *RB1* germline mutations fail to predispose to most common cancers. Interestingly, *RB1* mutations have been observed in a wide variety of sporadic cancers, including breast, small-cell lung, bladder, pancreas, and prostate cancers. It thus appears that the retinoblastoma protein functions as a critical factor in the maintenance of homeostasis in the cells of the developing retina, but plays a less critical role in most other developing tissues.

Function of retinoblastoma protein P105-RB

The protein product of the *RB1* gene is a 105 kDa nuclear phosphoprotein known as p105-Rb or, more commonly, pRB. Studies by Whyte and colleagues provided critical insights into pRB function.[9] They demonstrated that pRB formed a complex with the E1A oncoprotein encoded by the DNA tumor virus adenovirus type 5. (Unlike retroviral oncogenes, the oncogenes present in DNA tumor viruses have no cellular homologs.) E1A has many effects on cell growth, including cell immortalization and cooperation with other oncogenes (e.g., mutated RAS oncogene alleles) in neoplastic transformation of rodent cells in vitro. It was therefore hypothesized that functional inactivation of pRB, through its interaction with E1A might account for the observed ability of adenoviruses to transform cells in culture. Accordingly, engineered mutations that inactivated the ability of E1A to bind to pRB also eliminated the ability of E1A to transform cells. The significance of the physical interaction between pRB and adenovirus E1A was further supported by the subsequent demonstration that other DNA tumor virus oncoproteins also formed complexes with pRB,[10] including SV40 T antigen and the E7 proteins of human papillomavirus (HPV) types 16 and 18, which are the etiological agents of several types of human cancer, including cervical carcinoma

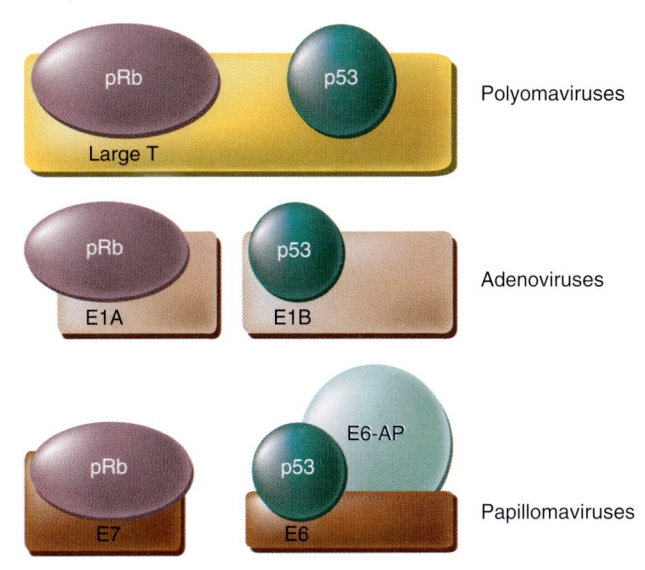

Figure 3 Schematic representation of interactions between tumor suppressor gene products and proteins encoded by DNA tumor viruses. Large T antigen from polyomaviruses such as simian virus 40 (SV40) bind both the retinoblastoma (pRB) and p53 proteins. For the adenoviruses and the high-risk HPVs (types 16 and 18), various viral protein products complex with pRB and p53. A cellular protein known as E6-associated protein (E6-AP) cooperates with the HPV E6 protein to complex and degrade p53.

(Figure 3). Engineered mutations that inactivated the transforming activities of these oncoproteins also inactivated their ability to interact with pRB. E7 proteins from "high-risk" HPVs (i.e., those linked to cancer development), such as HPV 16 and 18, formed complexes more tightly with pRB than did E7 proteins of "low-risk" viruses (e.g., HPV types 6 and 11). These interactions provided compelling evidence that DNA tumor viruses might transform cells by inactivating tumor suppressor gene products. In addition, given the critical dependence of DNA tumor viruses on the host cell DNA synthesis machinery for replication of the viral genome, the studies supported the hypothesis that pRB might impact normal cell growth by interacting with cellular proteins that control entry into the DNA synthesis (S) phase of the cell cycle.

The functional activity of pRB is regulated by phosphorylation during normal progression through the cell cycle. pRB appears to be predominantly unphosphorylated or hypophosphorylated during G1 phase and maximally phosphorylated in G2 (Figure 4). The critical phosphorylation events that regulate pRB occur during the transition from G1 phase to S phase of the cell cycle, and are mediated by cyclin-dependent kinase (Cdk) protein complexes. When unphosphorylated, pRB binds to proteins in the E2F family and inhibits transcription. When phosphorylated by Cdk complexes, pRB dissociates from E2Fs, thereby allowing these transcription factors to activate the expression of genes that are required during S-phase for DNA replication, such as DNA polymerase α, thymidylate synthase, ribonucleotide reductase, cyclin E, and dihydrofolate reductase.

TP53 gene

In the late 1970s a cellular phosphoprotein with a relative molecular mass of 53 kDa was identified in a complex with a protein expressed by a DNA virus known as SV40. SV40 is a member of a class of viruses that was notable for their ability to induce cancer-like phenotypes in experimental models. Soon thereafter, it was established that this cellular protein, simply designated p53 in reference to its apparent molecular weight, similarly bound to oncoproteins expressed from other DNA tumor viruses, including the adenovirus E1B55K protein.[11] Antibodies that could uniquely identify p53 in cell lysates facilitated the analysis of this protein in a variety of cell types and growth conditions. p53 was detected at low levels in normal cells and high levels in many tumors and tumor-derived cell lines. These initial observations suggested that increased levels of p53 might contribute to cancer. Consistent with that notion, *TP53* (the gene found to encode the p53 protein) appeared to function as an oncogene in *in vitro* assays. However, subsequent studies, including detailed analysis of recurrent regions of loss in colorectal cancers, definitively showed that *TP53* was in fact a tumor suppressor gene.[12] We now know that p53 is the most frequently altered gene in human cancers in general and is inactivated in a large number of diverse cancer types.

In 1988, LOH at chromosome 17p had previously been observed in colorectal, bladder, breast, and lung cancers. Detailed physical mapping showed that the *TP53* gene was present in the common region of loss. Analysis of the sequence of the *TP53* alleles retained in those cancers with 17p LOH demonstrated that the remaining *TP53* allele was invariably mutated. These observations were soon extended to other cancer types. The high frequency of *TP53* mutations across many common types of cancer explained the confusion surrounding the earlier designation of p53 as an oncogene product. Some of the *TP53* clones that had previously been studied were derived from mouse and human cancer cells. These alleles were in fact mutants that had lost their wild type function.

It was subsequently discovered that germline mutations in the *TP53* gene are the cause of Li–Fraumeni syndrome (LFS).[13] Affected individuals are at risk for developing soft-tissue sarcoma, osteosarcoma, brain tumors, breast cancer, and leukemia. Between one-half and two-thirds of patients with LFS have germline mutations in the central core domain of the *TP53* coding sequences that resemble the somatic mutations seen in sporadic cancers.

In addition to somatic and inherited mutations in the gene, the function of *TP53* can be inactivated by other mechanisms. As noted earlier, most cervical cancers contain high-risk or cancer-associated HPV genomes (i.e., HPV type 16 or 18). The *E6* gene product of high-risk, but not low-risk, HPV types binds to a cellular protein known as E6-AP (for E6-associated protein) and stimulates p53 degradation. A cellular p53-binding protein known as mouse double minute 2 (MDM2) is overexpressed in a subset of soft-tissue sarcomas as a result of gene amplification involving chromosome 12q sequences.[14] MDM2 encodes an enzyme known as an E3 ubiquitin ligase that catalyzes the posttranslational modification of p53, thus targeting it for degradation by the proteasome. Sarcomas with MDM2 amplification and overexpression rarely harbor somatic mutations in *TP53*, presumably because such mutations do not confer an additional growth advantage during tumor evolution. Experimental disruption of MDM2 in the germline of mice is lethal because it allows the unregulated expression of p53; conversely, disruption of *TP53* rescues MDM2-deficient mice from embryonic lethality. The interaction between p53 and its negative regulator MDM2 is a classic example of how a tumor suppressor protein and an oncogene product can function in the same pathway.

p53 function

p53 is a transcriptional regulatory protein that binds specific promoter elements within a large and functionally diverse set

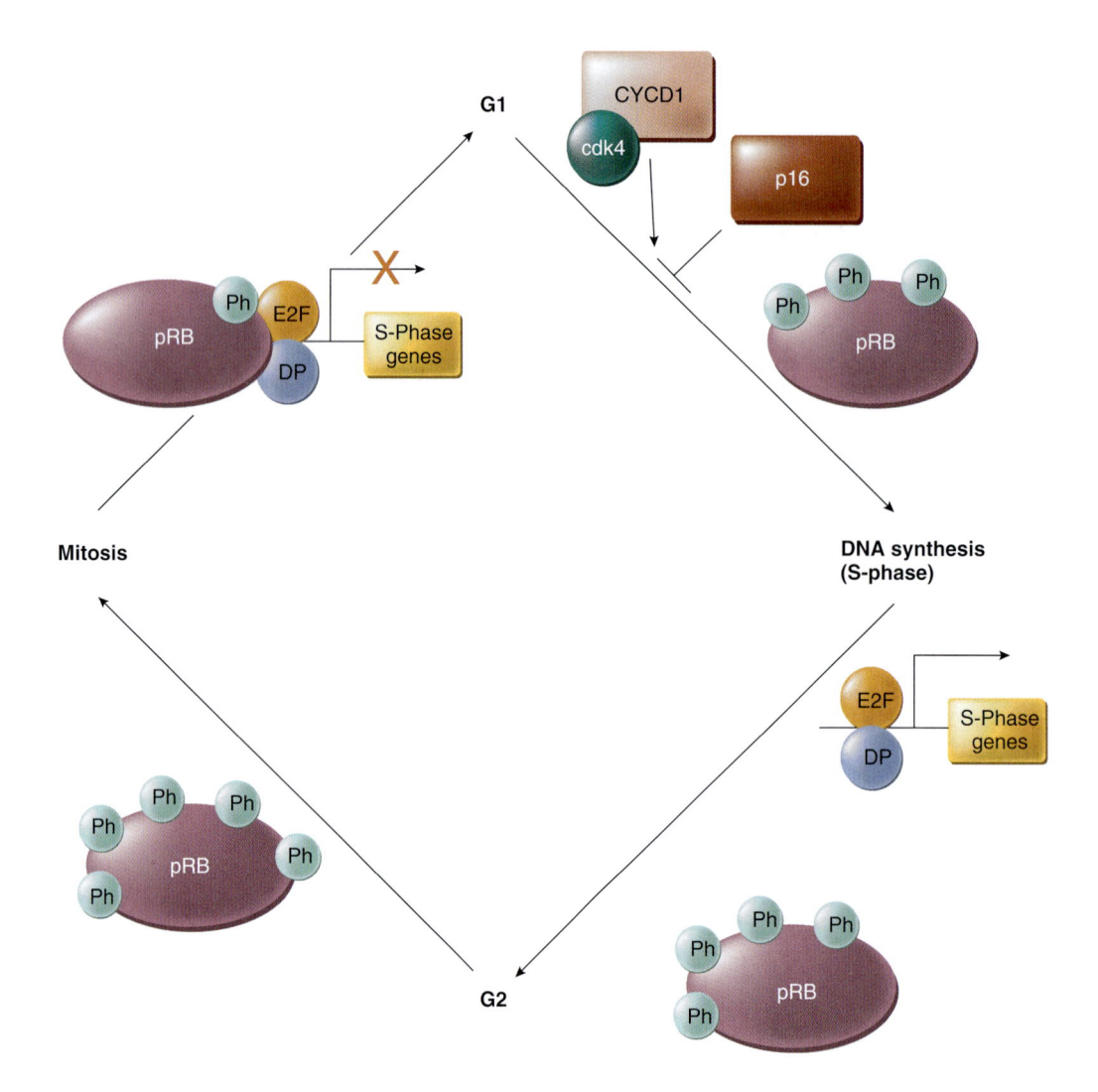

Figure 4 The function of the retinoblastoma protein (pRB) is regulated during the cell cycle by phosphorylation. The pRB protein is hypophosphorylated in the G1 phase of the cell cycle, and phosphorylation (Ph) of specific sites appears to increase during progression through the cell cycle. A protein complex that appears to phosphorylate pRB before DNA synthesis (S-phase) includes a cyclin (Cyc) and a cyclin-dependent kinase (Cdk)—for example, cyclin D1 and Cdk4. The CycD1/Cdk4 complex is regulated by the p16 inhibitor protein, which is itself the product of a tumor suppressor gene on chromosome 9p, known as CDKN2 (see text). In its hypophosphorylated state, pRB binds to E2F transcriptional regulatory proteins. When pRB is brought to the promoter regions of genes via its interaction with E2F proteins, pRB represses the expression of the E2F/DP target genes. Phosphorylation of pRB releases it from the E2F/DP protein complex and results in gene activation, including those genes involved in DNA synthesis. The figure also indicates that pRB phosphorylation increases in G2 with pRB dephosphorylated at or near anaphase.

of downstream target genes. In its wild-type conformation, p53 is capable of binding to specific DNA sequences via a central core domain (Figure 5). The amino terminal sequences of p53 constitute a transcriptional activation domain, and the carboxyl terminal sequences are required for the formation of a transcriptionally active tetramer. p53 activates the transcription of a large number of genes that collectively mediate cell growth, cell death and cellular metabolism. Among the first p53 target genes to be described was *CDKN1A*, which encodes the Cdk inhibitor p21.[15] By increasing the levels of p21, p53 can negatively regulate Cdk activity and thereby trigger the arrest of the cell cycle. MDM2, which encodes a negative regulator of p53 stability, is also a p53 target gene. By increasing the abundance of MDM2, p53 can limit its own activity. p53 also controls a number of downstream genes that promote apoptosis, including *PUMA*, *FDXR*, and *NOXA*. Many other transcriptional targets of p53 have been identified in recent years, some of which appear to be cell-type specific. These genes have surprisingly diverse functions, a finding that underscores the remarkable breadth of p53 function.[16]

The majority of the somatic and germline mutations in *TP53* are missense mutations leading to amino acid substitutions in the central portion of the protein (encoded by exons 5–9). These mutations have marked effects on the ability of p53 to bind to its cognate DNA recognition sequence and stimulate transcription. Some mutations (e.g., mutations at codons 248 or 273) alter *TP53* sequences that are directly responsible for sequence-specific DNA binding. Other mutations (e.g., codon 175) appear to affect the folding of p53 and thus indirectly affect its ability to bind to DNA. Interestingly, a disproportionate number of *TP53* mutations occur at just six codons, which together account for approximately 30% of the total *TP53* mutations identified. Previous experimental evidence suggests that mutations at these positions, known as hotspots, can confer oncogenic gains of function, but this does not appear to be the case in human cancers.[17,18]

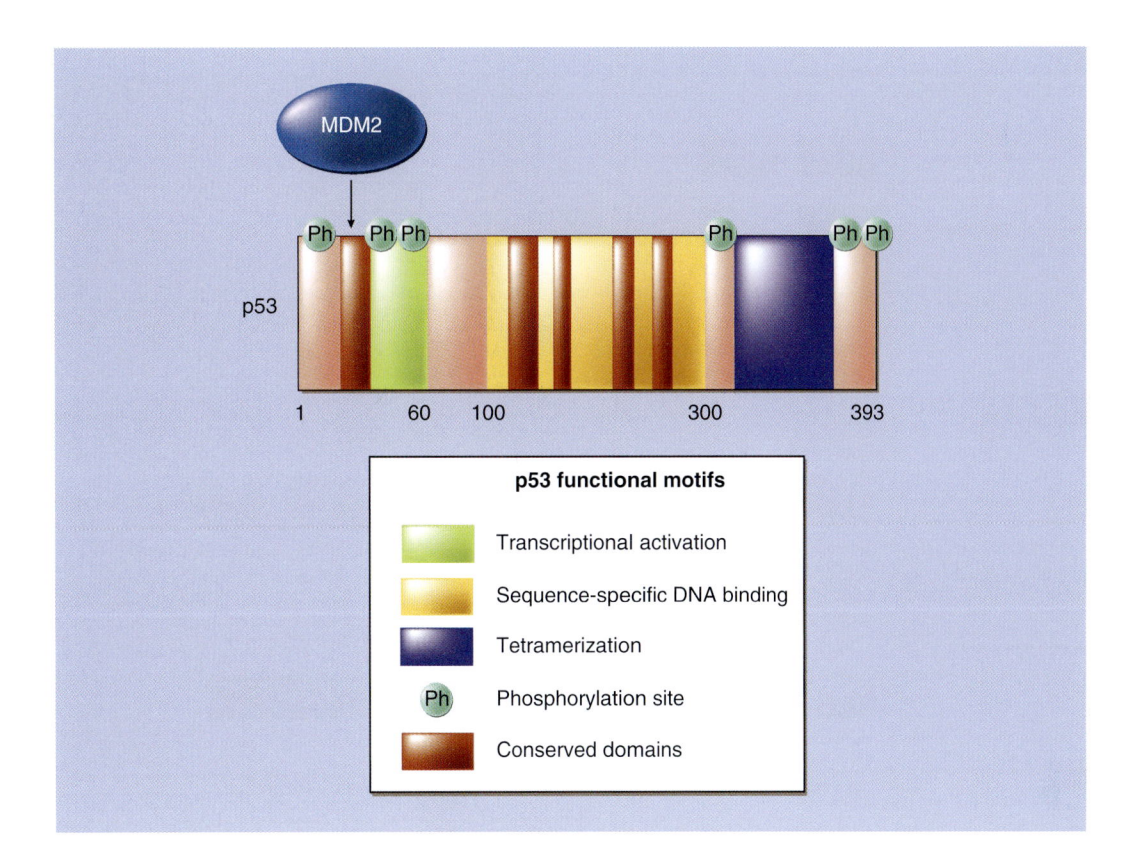

Figure 5 p53 functional motifs. Regions of p53 involved in transcriptional activation, sequence-specific DNA binding, tetramerization, and binding by the MDM2 protein are indicated. The five distinct regions of p53 that are highly conserved among diverse species are indicated. In addition, the locations of several sites in the protein that are phosphorylated (Ph) and that regulate p53-mediated transcription are indicated.

Complexity at the cyclin-dependent kinase inhibitor 2A locus

Studies of the cyclin-dependent kinase inhibitor 2A (*CDKN2A*) locus on chromosome 9p illustrate how observations from initially disparate lines of investigation often converged on a particular locus as a critical factor in cancer development.[19] LOH at chromosome 9p was frequently observed in many different tumor types, including melanoma, glioma, non-small-cell lung, bladder, head and neck cancers, and leukemia. Of particular interest were observations establishing that a subset of such tumors had homozygous (biallelic) deletions affecting the 9p21 region. The earlier studies of retinoblastoma had firmly established the functional significance of homozygous deletions, and the recurrent, overlapping deletions localized to chromosome 9p, therefore, suggested the existence of a tumor suppressor gene in the region. In addition to the frequent somatic alterations of chromosome 9p in cancers, linkage studies of families with inherited melanoma had identified a melanoma predisposition locus that mapped to essentially the same region. One of the genes identified in the region as a result of positional cloning efforts was initially termed multiple tumor suppressor 1 (MTS1). Sequence analysis of MTS1 showed that it was identical to a previously described gene that encoded a small Cdk inhibitor protein known as p16. Because the p16 protein functioned by inhibiting Cdk4 and Cdk6, it was termed inhibitor of cyclin-dependent kinase 4 (INK4) protein. Interestingly, a related Cdk inhibitor locus mapped immediately next to the *p16/MTS1* gene on chromosome 9p encoded a second protein, known as p15 (Figure 6). The gene encoding the p16 protein was formerly termed *INK4A*, and the gene for p15 was termed *INK4B*. The approved symbols are *CDKN2A* and *CDKN2B*, respectively.

CDKN2A is a classic tumor suppressor gene that is involved in both sporadic and inherited forms of cancer. Somatic mutations in *CDKN2A* are present in many different cancer types, including but not limited to melanoma, glioma, pancreatic and bladder cancers, and leukemia. In many tumors, deletions affecting the *CDKN2A* gene also involve the *CDKN2B* gene. The prevalence and specific nature of *CDKN2A* mutations vary markedly from one tumor type to another. In contrast to other tumor suppressor genes, such as *RB1* and *TP53*, homozygous deletion is a fairly common mechanism of *CDKN2A* inactivation in cancer. Heterozygous mutations in *CDKN2A* are present in families with inherited predispositions to melanoma or pancreatic cancer.

Detailed studies of the *CDKN2A* locus led to the identification of a novel alternative transcript containing nucleotide sequences identical to those in transcripts for the p16^{INK4A} protein, but with evidence of a unique upstream exon (Figure 6).[20] The alternative *CDKN2A* locus transcript encodes a protein known as p14 Alternative Reading Frame (p14^{ARF}). The orthologous protein in the mouse is somewhat larger, and accordingly known as p19^{ARF}.

As illustrated in Figure 6, the p14^{ARF} protein contains sequences from a distinct first exon (exon 1β) located upstream of exon 1α, the first exon present in transcripts for p16. Exon 1β is spliced to exon 2, which, along with exon 3, is present in the transcripts for both the p14^{ARF} and p16^{INK4A} proteins. However, the splice between exon 1β and exon 2 creates a different open reading frame in the resulting transcript. As a result, p14^{ARF} shares no amino acid sequence similarity with p16^{INK4A}.

Somatic and inherited mutations at the *CDKN2A* locus that result in the inactivation or deletion of the p16^{INK4A} protein are common in human cancer, but localized mutations that solely

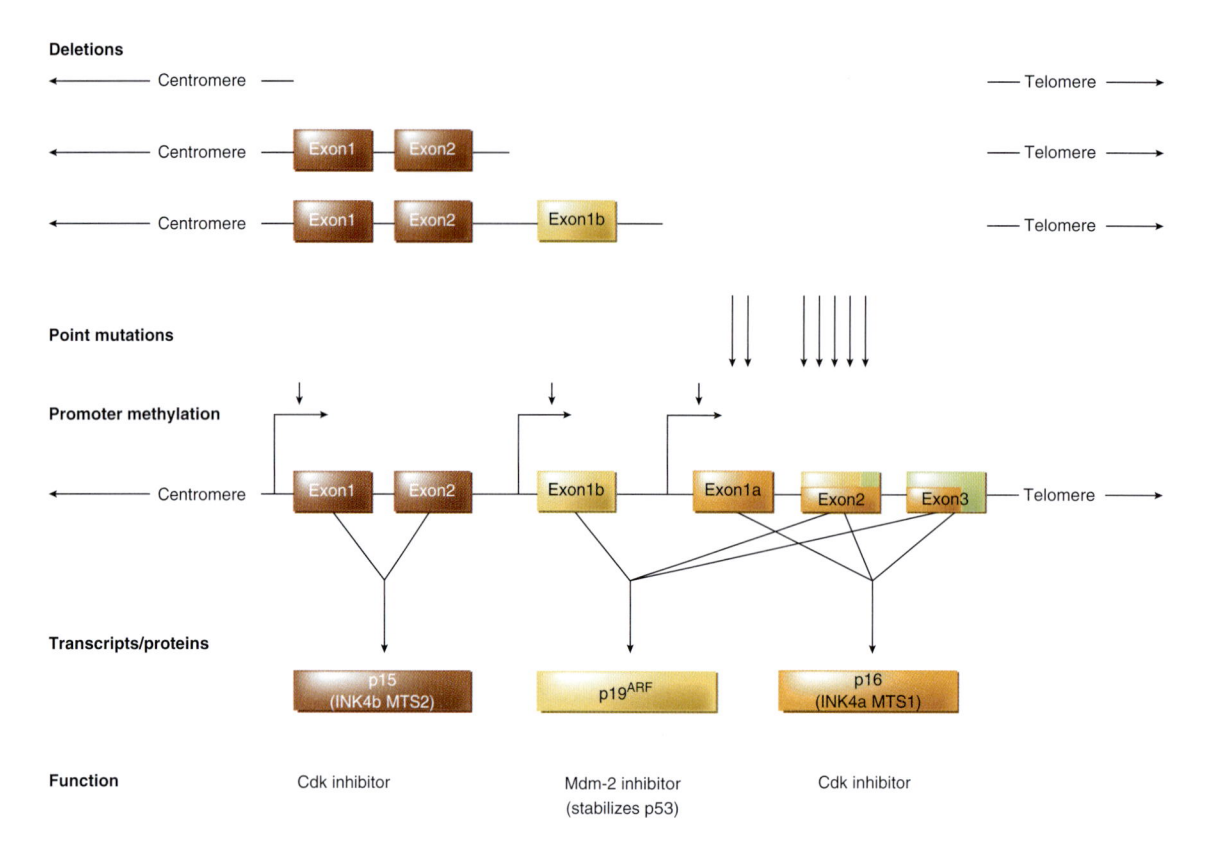

Figure 6 Genomic structure, mutations, and transcripts of the *CDKN2B* (p15) and *CDKN2A* (p16/p19^{ARF}) locus. The origins of the p15, p16, and p19^{ARF} transcripts are shown schematically, along with a representative depiction of genomic deletions, point mutations (arrows), and promoter methylation (arrowheads) noted in human cancers. The exons of the *CDKN2B* and *CDKN2A* loci are shown as rectangles. The transcripts/proteins and presumed functions of the transcripts/proteins are indicated. The red rectangles indicate the open reading frame in transcripts encoding p15; the yellow rectangles indicate the open reading frame present in transcripts encoding p19ARF; and the lavender rectangles indicate the open reading frame present in transcripts encoding p16. The size of the locus, exons, and transcripts are not shown to scale.

inactivate p14^{ARF} are uncommon. The frequent occurrence of homozygous deletions at the *CDKN2A* locus implies that mutational loss of both proteins—and of neighboring p15^{INK4B}—may provide a strong selective advantage during tumor development. Studies of mice with engineered disruption of the genes that encode p19^{ARF} and p16^{INK4A} suggest that these proteins can independently function as tumor suppressor genes *in vivo*.

The p16^{INK4A} protein suppresses tumorigenesis through its inhibition of Cdk4 activity. Phosphorylation of pRB by activated Cdk4 impedes its ability to regulate E2F-target genes (Figure 4). The p16^{INK4A} protein, by virtue of its negative regulation of Cdk4 activity, is a critical factor in regulating pRB phosphorylation. Loss of p16^{INK4A} results in the hyperphosphorylation of pRB and its subsequent inability to bind E2Fs. Unbound by pRB, the E2F proteins promoter the expression of proteins that favor the transition from G1 to S phase.

The cell cycle phase transition from G1 to S phase is also controlled indirectly by p14^{ARF}. The p14^{ARF} protein binds to MDM2 and inhibits the MDM2-mediated degradation of p53.[21] The stabilization of p53 results in the induction of its downstream target *CDKN1A*, which encodes the Cdk inhibitor p21. Thus increased, p21 binds to several Cdk complexes that control cell cycle transitions, including the transition from G1 to S. The convergence of multiple tumor suppressor pathways on the G1-S transition suggests that the deregulation of this event is a critical requirement for tumor growth in general.

Genetic alterations that affect p16^{INK4A} and p53 frequently coexist in cancer cells, suggesting that these losses of function are not equivalent. In contrast, mutations that inactivate *RB1* and *CDKN2A* tend to be mutually exclusive, suggesting that they function in a singular pathway (Figure 7).

The genetic basis of adenomatous polyposis coli

Familial adenomatous polyposis (FAP), alternatively known as adenomatous polyposis coli (APC), is an autosomal dominant disorder affecting about 1 in 10,000 individuals in the United States. The syndrome is characterized by the development of hundreds to thousands of adenomatous polyps in the colon and rectum of affected individuals by early adulthood. Many FAP patients also develop extracolonic tumors known as jaw osteomas and desmoid tumors. The lifetime risk of colorectal cancer in those with the classic form of FAP is extremely high, approaching 100% by age 60 years.

An interstitial deletion at chromosome 5q in a patient with features of FAP, but without any family history of the syndrome, guided efforts to localize the *APC* gene.[22] Subsequent DNA linkage studies confirmed that, in multiple kindreds with FAP, or the subtype known as Gardner syndrome, the polyposis phenotype segregated with DNA markers near 5q21. In 1991, the *APC* gene was successfully cloned by positional approaches and was confirmed as the specific gene responsible for FAP. The *APC* gene is large, with more than 15 exons. The predominant *APC* transcript encodes a 2843-amino acid protein expressed in many adult tissues.

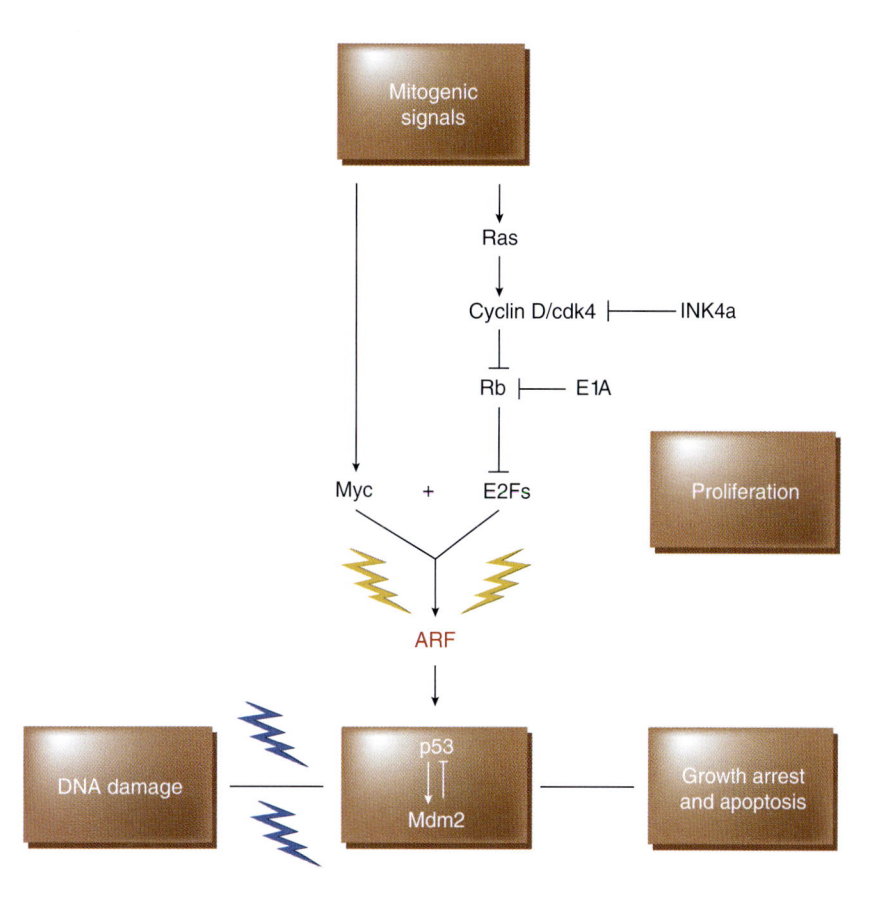

Figure 7 Role of the p14*RF protein in checkpoint control. The p14^ARF protein (ARF) responds to proliferative signals normally required for cell proliferation. When these signals exceed a critical threshold, the ARF-dependent checkpoint (yellow lightning bolts) is activated, and ARF triggers a p53-dependent response that induces growth arrest or apoptosis, or both. Oncoproteins, such as products of mutated RAS alleles, constitutively activated receptors, or cytoplasmic signal transducing oncoproteins, can trigger ARF activity via the cyclin D-Cdk4-RBE2F or Myc-dependent pathways, both of which are normally necessary for S-phase entry. In inhibiting cyclin D-dependent kinases, p16^{INK4A} can dampen the activity of mitogenic signals. In the figure, the adenovirus oncoprotein E1A is shown to work, at least in part, by opposing pRB function. For simplicity, Myc and E2F-1 are shown to activate p53 via the effects on ARF, though highly overexpressed levels of these proteins can activate TP53 in ARF-negative cells, albeit with an attenuated efficiency. ARF activation of p53 depends on inactivation of MdM2. DNA damage signals (e.g., ionizing and ultraviolet radiation, hypoxic stress) activate (blue lightning bolts) p53 through multiple signaling pathways.

In most individuals with FAP, heterozygous germline mutations of the *APC* gene can be identified. The germline *APC* mutations in affected individuals lead to truncations of the open reading frame that inactivate the function of the encoded protein (Figure 8). Consistent with Knudson's two-hit hypothesis, inactivation of the remaining wild-type *APC* allele by somatic mutation in those carrying a germline *APC* mutation is observed in the polyps that arise. Mutations in the 5' region of the *APC* gene appear to correlate with an attenuated phenotype, attributable to re-entry of the ribosome downstream of the premature stop codon, resulting in an APC protein that retains some of its normal activity. Mutations in the 3' third of the *APC* gene are also associated with a milder polyposis phenotype than mutations in the central third of the gene, presumably because the large truncated APC proteins similarly retain some tumor suppressor activity.

A germline missense mutation in the middle of the *APC* gene has been found to predispose to colorectal cancers in Ashkenazi Jewish families. This mutation does not directly alter the function of the gene product, but instead appears to be highly mutable, resulting in somatic deletions or insertions of surrounding nucleotides that produce truncations.

APC is mutationally inactivated in a majority of sporadic colorectal adenomas and carcinomas. These somatically acquired mutations are similar in nature and location to the germline *APC* mutations found in individuals with FAP.

Germline mutations in the *MUTYH* gene cause an autosomal recessive syndrome that phenotypically resembles an attenuated form of FAP (alternatively called MYH-associated polyposis or MAP).[23] The *MUTYH* protein functions in DNA repair. Biallelic inactivation of *MUTYH* prevents cells from repairing errors that arise during genomic DNA replication.

Function of APC

The *APC* gene encodes a large protein of roughly 300 kDa that regulates cell adhesion, cell migration, and apoptosis in the colonic crypt. APC binds to a number of regulatory proteins including β-catenin, a protein that coordinates cell–cell interactions with gene regulation by the TCF/LEF family of growth-promoting transcription factors.[24]

In cooperation with β-catenin, APC functions in developmental signaling via a mechanism known as the WNT/APC pathway (Figure 9). In the absence of WNT signals, APC binds to β-catenin along with the proteins Axin and the protein kinase GSKβ, which form a complex that mediates destruction of β-catenin. During normal development, the WNT/APC pathway is activated by extracellular ligands. Ligand binding stimulates the dissociation

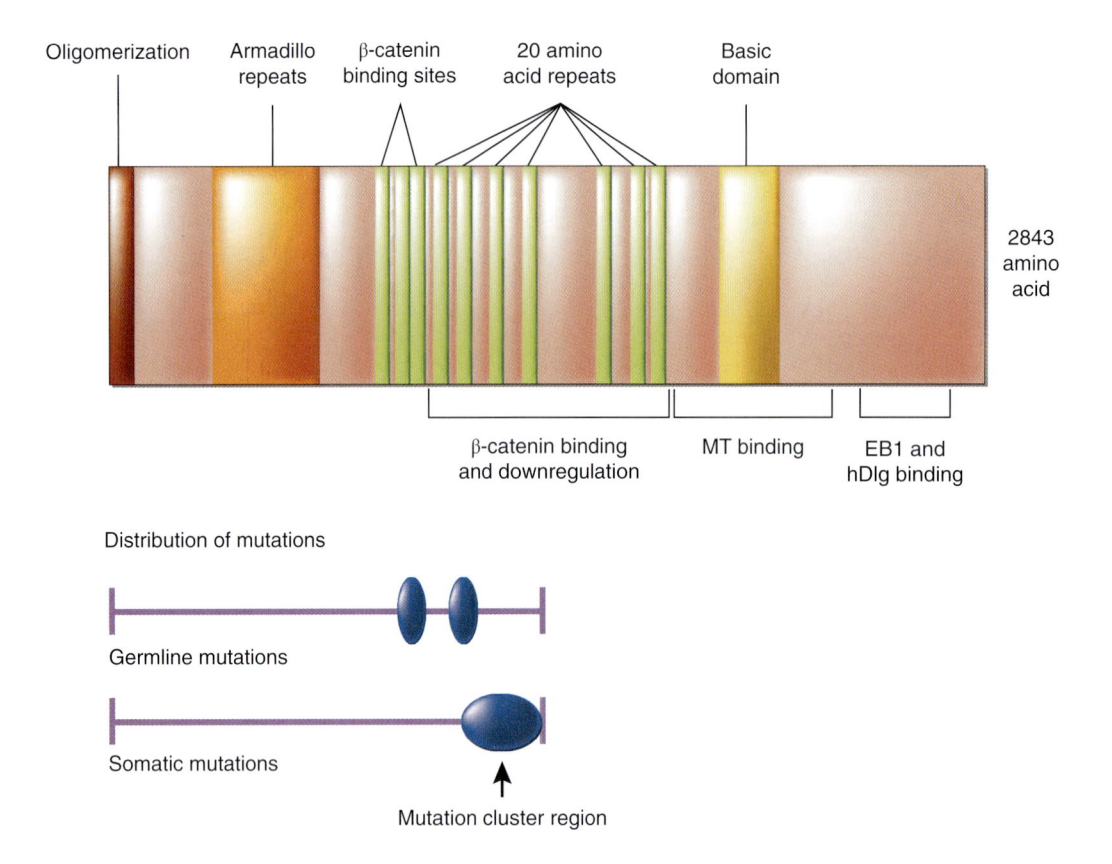

Figure 8 Schematic representation of APC protein domains with respect to the distribution of mutations. A putative domain involved in homo-oligomerization of APC is located at the amino-terminus. A series of repeats of unknown function with similarity to the *Drosophila* armadillo protein, sequences known to mediate binding to β-catenin and its downregulation, a basic domain in the carboxy-terminal third of the protein that appears to facilitate complexing with microtubules (MT), and sequences near the carboxy terminus of APC that are known to interact with the EB1 and human homolog of the *Drosophila* discs large protein. Chain terminating mutations in the *APC* gene are dispersed throughout the 5′ half of the sequence, with two apparent "hot spots" at codons 1061 and 1309. Somatic mutations in the *APC* gene in colorectal cancer appear to cluster in a region termed the "mutation cluster region," and mutations at codons 1309 and 1450 are most common.

of the destruction complex, leading to the increased abundance of β-catenin and an increase in TCF/LEF activity. The truncated APC proteins expressed in many colorectal cancers lack some or all of the peptide motifs crucial for binding to β-catenin. Thus, β-catenin is constitutively stabilized in a ligand-independent manner by the loss of APC.

Consistent with the role of the APC/β-catenin complex in tumor suppression, somatic mutations in *CTNNB1*, the gene that encodes β-catenin, are found in most of the small fraction of colorectal cancers that lack *APC* mutations. These mutations consistently alter GSK3β phosphorylation consensus sites near the amino terminus of the β-catenin protein, and render the mutant β-catenin protein resistant to degradation by APC and GSK3β. Thus, *CTNNB1* is a proto-oncogene that functions in concert with the tumor suppressor *APC*.

Wilms tumor gene

Wilms tumor, also known as nephroblastoma, is the most common renal malignancy in children and constitutes 7% of all childhood cancers. These pediatric tumors are similar to retinoblastomas in several respects. Both types of tumor can occur bilaterally or unilaterally, with single or multiple foci, and in a sporadic or inherited fashion. The two-hit model originally proposed for retinoblastoma was also proposed to apply to Wilms tumor.[25] However, hereditary cases are not as common among Wilms tumor patients as they are in retinoblastoma patients. Almost all patients inheriting a mutation at the *RB1* locus develop a retinoblastoma, but only approximately 50% of individuals carrying a germline mutation predisposing to Wilms tumor develop the disease. Therefore, the germline mutations that underlie Wilms tumor have a lower penetrance compared to the mutations that cause retinoblastoma.

Insight into the inherited genetic basis for Wilms tumor was provided by a report describing six patients with Wilms tumor and sporadic aniridia (i.e., congenital absence of the iris). It was proposed that the simultaneous occurrence of these two very rare conditions might result from chromosomal aberrations affecting two or more adjacent loci, a situation now often called a contiguous gene syndrome—mutation of one locus presumably leading to aniridia and mutation of another leading to Wilms tumor. Similar linkage had previously been found between *RB1* and the functionally irrelevant but adjacent locus that encoded esterase D. The physical linkage between Wilms tumor and aniridia was subsequently supported by the discovery of interstitial deletions of chromosome 11p13 in peripheral blood samples from children with the WAGR syndrome (Wilms tumor with aniridia, genitourinary abnormalities, and mental retardation). Subsequent studies of paired samples of Wilms tumor and normal cells from patients, using probes that detect restriction fragment length polymorphisms (RFLPs) on chromosome 11p, revealed that LOH of 11p occurred frequently in Wilms tumors of both the inherited and sporadic types.

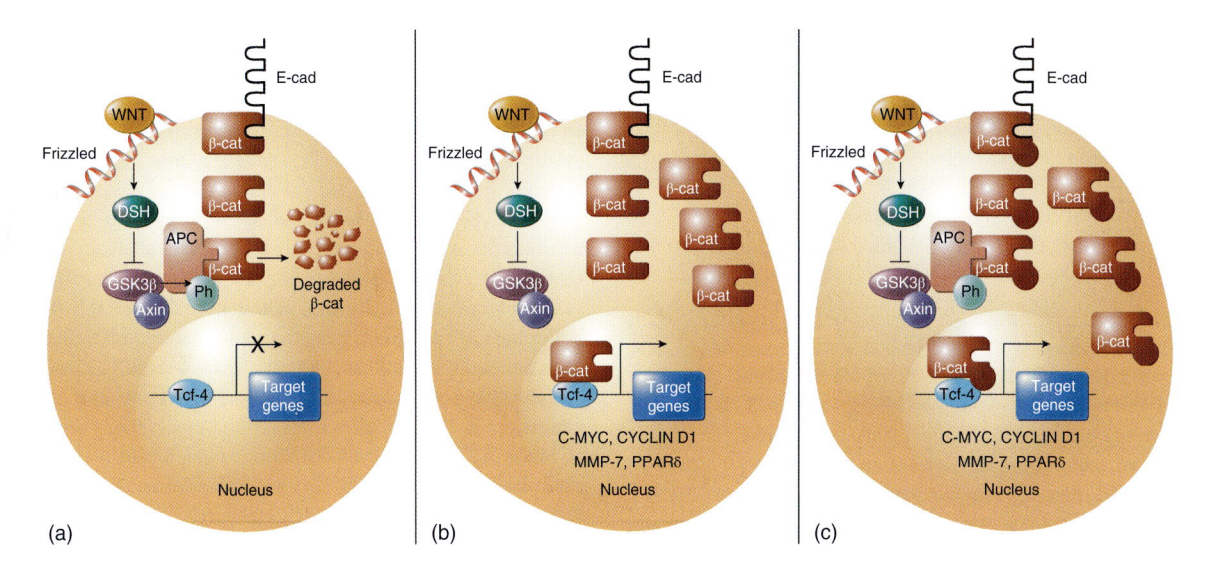

Figure 9 A model indicating the function of the APC, axin, and Gsk3β proteins in the regulation of β-catenin (β-cat) in normal cells, and the consequence of Apc or β-cat defects in cancer cells. β-Cat is an abundant cellular protein, and much of it is often bound to the cytoplasmic domain of the E-cadherin (E-cad) cell–cell adhesion protein. (a) In normal cells, the proteins glycogen synthase kinase 3β(Gsk3β), APC, and Axin function to promote degradation of free cytosolic β-cat, probably as a result of phosphorylation of the N-terminal sequences of β-cat by Gsk3β. Gsk3β activity and β-cat degradation are inhibited by activation of the wingless (Wnt) pathway, as a result of the action of the Frizzled receptor and disheveled (Dsh) signaling protein. (b) Mutation of *APC* in colorectal and other cancer cells results in accumulation of β-cat, binding to Tcf-4, and transcriptional activation of Tcf-4 target genes, such as *MYC*, cyclin D1, *MMP-7*, and PPARS (see text). (c) Point mutations and small deletions in β-cat in cancer cells inhibit phosphorylation and degradation of β-cat by Gsk3β and APC, with resultant activation of *MYC* and other Tcf-4 target genes.

The Wilms tumor 1 (*WT1*) gene was identified in 1990 by virtue of mutations that inactivated the gene in patients with the WAGR syndrome and by analysis of somatic mutations in the gene in tumors from patients with unilateral Wilms tumor and no associated congenital malformation.[25] In contrast to the rather ubiquitous expression of the *RB1*, *TP53*, and *APC* genes, expression of the *WT1* gene is found only in embryonic kidneys and a few other tissues. Because of alternative splicing, multiple related proteins are expressed from the *WT1* locus.

Wilms tumor has a complex genetic landscape.[26] In stark contrast to retinoblastoma, in which a single locus is implicated in all cases of the disease, Wilms tumor is caused by many different germline and somatic alterations involving many different genes. Mutations in *WT1* therefore account for only a small proportion of all cases.

The protein encoded by *WT1* is a transcription factor that plays a central role in the developing kidney. The other genes involved in sporadic and inherited forms of Wilms tumor functionally converge on the signaling pathways that mediate fetal nephrogenesis.

Neurofibromatosis 1 and 2 genes

Neurofibromatosis 1 gene
Neurofibromatosis 1 (NF1), also known as Von Recklinghausen's disease, is a rare, dominantly inherited syndrome characterized by the development of multiple benign tumors of the nerves and skin, which are commonly derived from the embryonic neural crest. In addition to the nearly uniform development of neurofibromas, NF1 patients are at elevated risk for developing pheochromocytomas, schwannomas, neurofibrosarcomas, and primary brain tumors. The *NF1* gene was initially localized to the pericentromeric region of chromosome 17q by linkage analyses.[27] Intensive positional cloning efforts in this chromosome region led to the identification of the *NF1* gene in 1991. The *NF1* gene is large, spanning roughly 350 kb, and encodes a protein product with a molecular mass of about 300 kDa called neurofibromin. Neurofibromin negatively regulates RAS activity, thereby providing another cogent example of complementary roles of oncogenes and tumor suppressor genes that participate in the same pathway.

Approximately one-half of NF1 cases are inherited. Somatic mutations in *NF1* that occur during embryonic development account for the remaining half of cases. In such cases, the disease tends to be more localized, as only a portion of the cells in the child or adult harbour the underlying mutation.

Neurofibromatosis 2 gene
Neurofibromatosis 2 (NF2—also known as central neurofibromatosis) is an autosomal dominant disorder that is distinct from NF1 in both genetic and clinical features.[28] A hallmark of NF2 is the occurrence of bilateral schwannomas that affect the vestibular branch of the eighth cranial nerve (acoustic neuromas). NF2 patients are also at elevated risk for meningiomas, spinal schwannomas, and ependymomas. The *NF2* gene was mapped to chromosome 22q by a combination of linkage analyses and LOH studies and was cloned in 1993. Germline mutations inactivating the *NF2* gene are the cause of NF2. Somatic *NF2* mutations are observed in a subset of sporadic schwannomas and meningiomas.

von Hippel–Lindau gene
von Hippel–Lindau (VHL) syndrome is a rare dominant disorder predisposing affected individuals to the development of hemangioblastomas of the central nervous system and retina, renal carcinomas of the clear cell type, and pheochromocytomas. The *VHL* gene was mapped to chromosome 3p by linkage analysis.[29] LOH studies established that the *VHL* gene behaves as a typical tumor suppressor gene, with both alleles inactivated during tumorigenesis. Positional cloning efforts led to the identification of the *VHL*

gene in 1993. Germline mutations inactivating one *VHL* allele are seen in the majority of affected individuals in tumor-prone families.

The *VHL* gene encodes a 213-amino acid protein that functions in the oxygen-sensing pathway. The protein encoded by VHL is part of a ubiquitin ligase complex that degrades hypoxia-inducing factor 1a (HIF-1a) in the presence of oxygen. In the absence of oxygen in normal cells, or when *VHL* is mutated in tumor cells, the HIF-1a transcription factor is stabilized, leading to the expression of cytokines such as vascular endothelial growth factor and the stimulation of angiogenesis, a critical facet of tumorigenesis.

Tumor suppressor genes required for the maintenance of genetic stability

DNA mismatch repair gene defects and hereditary nonpolyposis colorectal cancer (HNPCC)
Hereditary nonpolyposis colorectal cancer (HNPCC), also known as Lynch syndrome, is an autosomal dominant disorder associated with an elevated risk of colon cancer.[30] Affected individuals often develop cancer at early ages. HNPCC patients are also at higher risk of endometrial cancer and cancers of the ovary, stomach, small intestine, hepatobiliary tract, urinary tract, and other sites. The underlying defect in HNPCC patients is inherited mutations in genes that are required for DNA mismatch repair (MMR).

Four different genes (*MSH2, MLH1, MSH6,* and *PMS2*) are associated with HNPCC, with mutations in *MSH2* and *MLH1* the most common. The proteins encoded by these genes each contribute to the complex enzymatic machinery that recognizes and repairs base-pair mismatches that result from base misincorporation during DNA replication.

The protein products of the *MSH2* and *MLH1* genes have critical roles in the recognition and repair of DNA mismatches (Figure 10). In cells with one normal and one mutant allele of a DNA MMR gene, DNA repair is impaired minimally, if at all. A "second hit" eliminates MMR function, leading to significant elevation of the error rate of DNA replication. The resulting genetic instability is highly manifest in mononucleotide, dinucleotide, and trinucleotide repeat tracts, which are known as microsatellites. Therefore, microsatellite instability (MSI) is a phenotypic hallmark of MMR deficiency. This hypermutable phenotype of MMR-deficient cancers represents a distinctive pathway to tumorigenesis.

HNPCC is a relatively common cancer predisposition syndrome that accounts for about 3% of all colorectal cancers. Among individuals with early onset colorectal cancer (occurring in individuals <50 years), about 20% harbour germline mutations in MMR genes. Overall, about 15% of colorectal tumors exhibit a hypermutable phenotype as a result of the inactivation of MMR genes. The majority of these are sporadic. Recent clinical trials show that this hypermutable phenotype can be exploited for therapeutic purposes with immune checkpoint inhibitors (ICIs). MMR-deficient cancers often harbor more than 1000 somatic mutations that are present in every cancer cell (i.e., clonal). Cancers with this many mutations are more likely to harbor neoantigens that can be recognized by the immune system, and ICIs can stimulate the immune system to kill these cancer cells.

Familial breast cancer
Breast cancer is among the most common cancers in women, second only to skin cancer. While most breast cancers arise sporadically in individuals with little or no prior family history of the disease, approximately 5–10% occur in familial clusters and are hereditary in nature. In affected families, the trait of cancer predisposition is passed down in an autosomal dominant manner. Those who have a history of breast cancer in multiple first-degree relatives are at highest risk. These patterns were evident for decades, but only in the late 1980s was genetic evidence obtained that predisposition to breast cancer in some families could be attributed to a penetrant autosomal dominant allele.

The first chromosomal region to be conclusively linked to familial breast cancer was chromosome 17q21 in 1990 by King and colleagues.[31] The *BRCA1* gene was subsequently identified within this region by positional cloning. Germline *BRCA1* mutations substantially increase the risk of breast cancer and also of ovarian cancer.

Mutations in *BRCA1* account for a large proportion of all familial breast cancer kindreds. By focusing on cancer-prone kindreds that did not carry mutant *BRCA1* alleles, a consortium of investigators was able to map a separate susceptibility locus on chromosome 13q12. The *BRCA2* gene was subsequently cloned in 1995. Mutations in *BRCA1* or *BRCA2* together account for more than one-half of all familial breast cancers.

The germline mutations in *BRCA1* and *BRCA2* are incompletely penetrant; not all carriers will develop disease. Depending on the precise mutation and other factors, approximately 50–85% of women who inherit a mutant allele will develop breast cancer by age 70.[32] The risk of ovarian cancer is similarly elevated. Notably, men with germline mutations in *BRCA2* are at increased risk of male breast cancer and prostate cancer. In both men and women, *BRCA2* mutations also confer an increased risk of pancreatic cancer and melanoma.

The frequency of mutated BRCA alleles varies among various human subpopulations. For example, approximately 2% of Ashkenazi Jews carry one of three high risk mutations (*BRCA1 185delAG, BRCA1 5382insC,* or *BRCA2 6174delT*). The high frequency of these alleles is the result of a founder effect. All living Ashkenazim are descended from a relatively small group of individuals that must have harbored these alleles.

As with most tumor suppressor genes and their associated familial cancer syndromes, germline mutations of *BRCA1* lead to the presence of a mutant allele in every cell of the body. Cancers then arise through inactivation of the second wild-type allele by the mechanisms outlined in Figure 2. LOH of the remaining wild-type allele is usually responsible for the second "hit" leading to biallelic inactivation.

One distinctive feature of *BRCA1* and *BRCA2* mutations is that they are generally found in the germline of predisposed individuals. Unlike tumor suppressor genes like *TP53* and *APC*, which are inactivated in the germline of cancer-prone individuals as well as in a large proportion of sporadic cancers, *BRCA1* and *BRCA2* are much less often mutated somatically during tumorigenesis.

The *BRCA1* and *BRCA2* genes encode large nuclear proteins that are required for the efficient repair of DNA double-strand breaks. Interestingly, germline mutations in the genes that encode the DNA damage response signalling proteins *ATM* and *CHEK2* are also associated with an elevated risk of breast cancer. The common functions of these breast cancer genes suggest that the ability to sense and repair DNA damage is an important factor in the maintenance of tissue homeostasis in the epithelia of breast and other tissues. Moreover, this defect in sensing and repairing DNA damage has been exploited through drugs that further compromise DNA repair, thereby establishing synthetic lethality and affording new treatment modalities for patients with BRCA mutations.

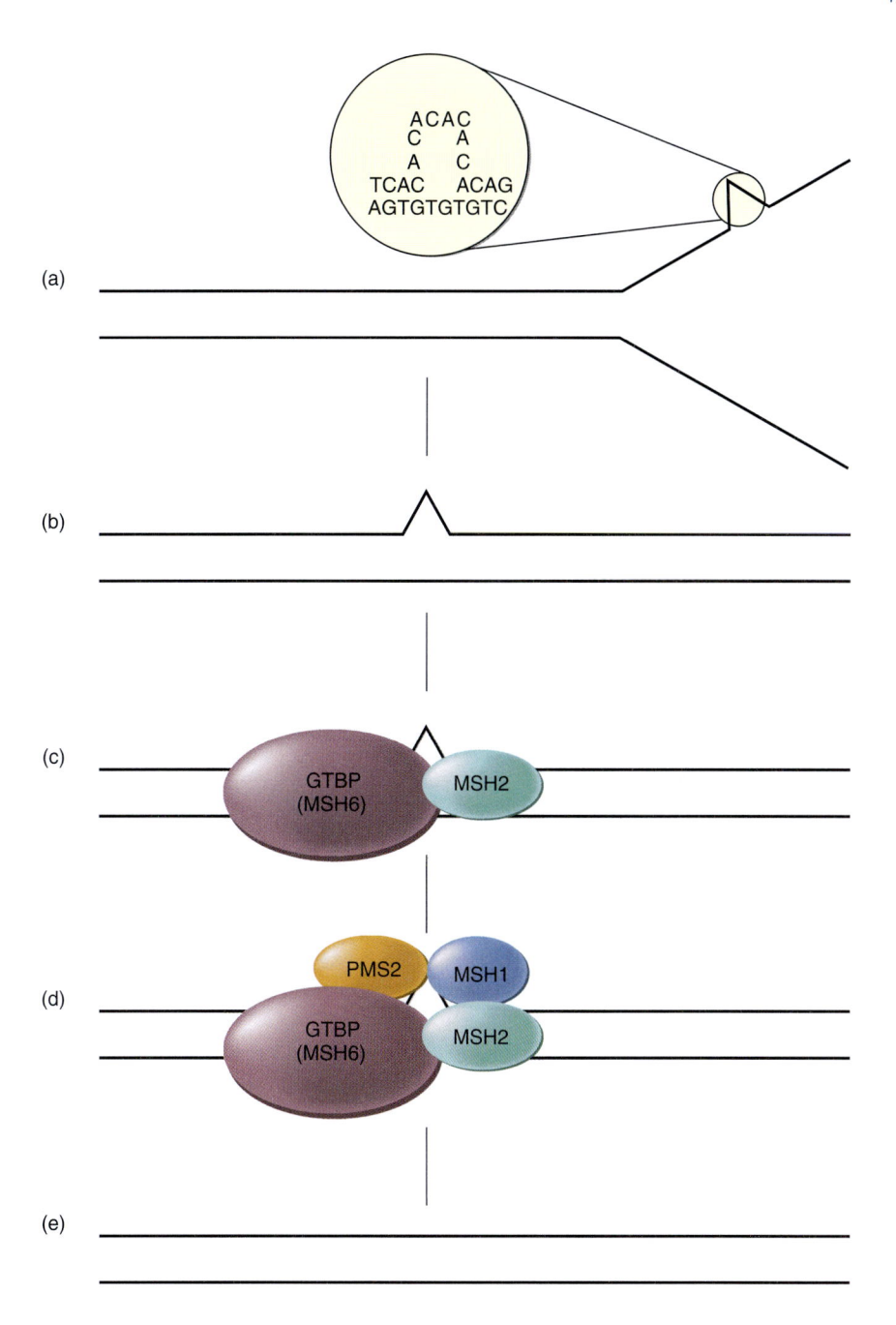

Figure 10 Mismatch repair pathway in human cells. (a,b) During DNA replication, DNA mismatches may arise from strand slippage (shown) or misincorporation of bases (not shown). (c) The mismatch is recognized by a complex that includes MSH2. (d,e) MLH1 is recruited to the complex, and the mismatch is repaired through the action of a number of proteins, including an exonuclease, helicase, DNA polymerase, and ligase.

Recessive cancer predisposition syndromes

A limited number of cancer predisposition syndromes are inherited in an autosomal recessive pattern and are therefore found primarily in populations with high rates of consanguinity.[33] Among these syndromes are ataxia telangiectasia, Bloom syndrome, xeroderma pigmentosum, and Fanconi anemia. These disorders are rare and, interestingly, commonly caused by defects in various mechanisms of DNA damage sensing and repair. The highly elevated risk of cancer in homozygous individuals, in some cases approaching 100%, underscores the importance of genome maintenance in tissue homeostasis.

Tumor suppressor genes and hereditary cancers

The validation of Knudson's two-hit hypothesis by the positional cloning of *RB1* and the identification of *TP53* as the target of LOH together created an enduring paradigm for understanding the genetic basis of inherited and sporadic cancers. Tumor suppressor genes, their associated heritable cancer syndromes, and the predominant tumor types are listed in Table 1. In many but not all cases, somatic mutations of these tumor suppressors lead to sporadic tumors of the same type as those that arise in heterozygous mutation carriers.

Table 1 Select tumor suppressor genes associated with inherited cancer predisposition syndromes.

Gene[a]	Syndrome	Hereditary pattern	Pathway[b]	Major hereditary tumor types[c]
APC	Familial adenomatous polyposis	Dominant	APC	Colon, thyroid, stomach, intestine
AXIN2	Attenuated polyposis	Dominant	APC	Colon
CDH1	Familial gastric carcinoma	Dominant	APC	Stomach
CYLD	Familial cylindromatosis	Dominant	CC/AP	Pilotrichomas
EXT1, EXT2	Hereditary multiple exostoses	Dominant	HH	Bone
PTCH1	Gorlin	Dominant	HH	Skin, medulloblastoma
SUFU	Medulloblastoma predisposition	Dominant	HH	Skin, medulloblastoma
FH	Hereditary leiomyomatosis	Dominant	RAS	Leiomyomas
SDHB, SDHC, SDHD	Familial paraganglioma	Dominant	RAS	Paragangliomas, pheochromocytomas
VHL	von Hippel–Lindau	Dominant	PI3K	Kidney
TP53 (p53)	Li–Fraumeni	Dominant	DDR/CC/AP	Breast, sarcoma, adrenal, brain, medulloblastoma, others
WT1	Familial Wilms tumor	Dominant	CM	Wilms
STK11 (LKB1)	Peutz–Jeghers	Dominant	PI3K	Intestinal, ovarian, pancreatic
PTEN	Cowden	Dominant	PI3K	Hamartoma, glioma, uterus
TSC1, TSC2	Tuberous sclerosis	Dominant	PI3K	Hamartoma, kidney
CDKN2A (p16INK4A, p14ARF)	Familial malignant melanoma	Dominant	CC/AP	Melanoma, pancreas
CDK4	Familial malignant melanoma	Dominant	CC/AP	Melanoma
RB1	Hereditary retinoblastoma	Dominant	CC/AP	Eye
NF1	Neurofibromatosis	Dominant	RAS	Neurofibroma
BMPR1A	Juvenile polyposis	Dominant	TGFB	Gastrointestinal
MEN1	Multiple endocrine neoplasia type I	Dominant	TGFB	Parathyroid, pituitary, islet cell, carcinoid
SMAD4	Juvenile polyposis	Dominant	TGFB	Gastrointestinal
NF2	Neurofibromatosis	Dominant	APC	Meningioma, acoustic neuromas
MUTYH	Attenuated polyposis	Recessive	DDR	Colon
ATM	Ataxia telangiectasia	Recessive	DDR	Leukemias, lymphomas, brain
BLM	Bloom	Recessive	DDR	Leukemias, many solid tumors
BRCA1, BRCA2	Hereditary breast cancer	Dominant	DDR	Breast, ovary
FANCA, FANCC, FANCD2, FANCE, FANCF, FANCG	Fanconi anemia A, C, D2, E, F, and G	Recessive	DDR	Leukemias
NBS1	Nijmegen breakage	Recessive	DDR	Lymphomas, brain
RECQL4	Rothmund-Thomson	Recessive	DDR	Bone and skin
WRN	Werner	Recessive	DDR	Bone and brain
MSH2, MLH1, MSH6, PMS2	HNPCC	Dominant	MMR	Colon, uterus
XPA, XPC; ERCC2, ERCC3, ERCC4, ERCC5; DDB2	Xeroderma pigmentosum	Recessive	DDR	Skin

Abbreviations: APC, WNT/adenomatous polyposis coli pathway; CC/AP, pathways involved in cell cycle regulation and/or apoptosis; DDR, DNA damage sensing and repair; HH, Hedgehog signalling; MMR, mismatch repair; PI3K, phosphatidylinositol 3-kinase pathway; RAS, receptor tyrosine kinase pathway-RAS signalling pathway; TGFB, TGF-β signalling pathway.
[a]Representative genes of all major pathways and hereditary cancer predisposition types are listed. Approved gene symbols are provided for each entry; alternative names are in parentheses.
[b]In many cases, the gene has been implicated in several pathways. The single pathway that is listed for each gene represents a "best guess" (when one can be made) and should not be regarded as conclusive.
[c]In most cases, the nonfamilial tumor spectrum caused by somatic mutations of the gene includes those occurring in familial cases but also additional tumor types. For example, mutations of TP53 and CDKN2A are found in many more tumor types than those to which Li–Fraumeni and familial malignant melanoma patients, respectively, are predisposed.

Summary

The inactivation of tumor suppressor genes is a pivotal event in the evolution of cancers. With the exception of several of the leukemias, virtually all cancers arise as a result of genetic losses of function. The identification of tumor suppressor genes, by seminal clinical observations and a variety of experimental approaches, has provided important insights into the phenotypes that make cancer cells dangerous and revealed new approaches to anticancer therapy. From a theoretical standpoint, tumor suppressor genes represent a link between the hereditary and sporadic forms of cancer. With few exceptions, tumor suppressor gene mutations can be found in cancer-prone individuals and in sporadic tumors of the same type.

Acknowledgment

The authors gratefully acknowledge the past contributions of David Cosgrove and Ben Ho Park to earlier versions of this article.

References

1 Vogelstein B, Papadopoulos N, Velculescu VE, et al. Cancer genome landscapes. *Science*. 2013;**339**(6127):1546–1558.
2 Lynch HT, Shaw TG, Lynch JF. Inherited predisposition to cancer: a historical overview. *Am J Med Genet C Semin Med Genet*. 2004;**129C**(1):5–22.
3 Balmain A. Cancer genetics: from boveri and mendel to microarrays. *Nat Rev Cancer*. 2001;**1**(1):77–82.
4 Vogt PK. Retroviral oncogenes: a historical primer. *Nat Rev Cancer*. 2012;**12**(9):639–648.
5 Anderson MJ, Stanbridge EJ. Tumor suppressor genes studied by cell hybridization and chromosome transfer. *FASEB J*. 1993;**7**(10):826–833.
6 Knudson AG. Hereditary cancer: two hits revisited. *J Cancer Res Clin Oncol*. 1996;**122**(3):135–140.
7 Weinberg RA. The molecular basis of retinoblastomas. *Ciba Found Symp*. 1989;**142**:99–11.
8 Cavenee WK, Dryja TP, Phillips RA, et al. Expression of recessive alleles by chromosomal mechanisms in retinoblastoma. *Nature*. 2002;**305**(5937):779–784.
9 Cooper JA, Whyte P. RB and the cell cycle: entrance or exit? *Cell*. 1989;**58**(6):1009–1011.
10 DeCaprio JA. How the rb tumor suppressor structure and function was revealed by the study of adenovirus and SV40. *Virology*. 2009;**384**(2):274–284.
11 Levine AJ. The common mechanisms of transformation by the small DNA tumor viruses: the inactivation of tumor suppressor gene products: p53. *Virology*. 2009;**384**(2):285–293.

12. Baker SJ, Vogelstein B. P53: a tumor suppressor hiding in plain sight. *J Mol Cell Biol*. 2019;**11**(7):536-538.
13. Guha T, Malkin D. Inherited *TP53* mutations and the li-fraumeni syndrome. *Cold Spring Harb Perspect Med*. 2017;7(4). doi: 10.1101/cshperspect.a026187.
14. Iwakuma T, Lozano G. MDM2, an introduction. *Mol Cancer Res*. 2003;**1**(14): 993-1000.
15. el-Deiry WS, Tokino T, Velculescu VE, et al. WAF1, a potential mediator of p53 tumor suppression. *Cell*. 1993;**75**(4):817-825.
16. Kastenhuber ER, Lowe SW. Putting p53 in context. *Cell*. 2017;**170**(6):1062-1078.
17. Lane DP. How to lose tumor suppression. *Science*. 2019;**365**(6453):539-540.
18. Boettcher S, Miller PG, Sharma R et al. A dominant-negative effect drives selection of TP53 missense mutations in myeloid malignancies. *Science*. 2019;**365**:599-604.
19. Serrano M. The tumor suppressor protein p16INK4a. *Exp Cell Res*. 1997;**237**(1): 7-13.
20. Haber DA. Splicing into senescence: the curious case of p16 and p19ARF. *Cell*. 1997;**91**(5):555-558.
21. Sherr CJ. Tumor surveillance via the ARF-p53 pathway. *Genes Dev*. 1998;**12**(19): 2984-2991.
22. Kinzler KW, Vogelstein B. Lessons from hereditary colorectal cancer. *Cell*. 1996;**87**(2):159-170.
23. Ma H, Brosens LAA, Offerhaus GJA, et al. Pathology and genetics of hereditary colorectal cancer. *Pathology*. 2018;**50**(1):49-59.
24. Barker N, Morin PJ, Clevers H. The yin-yang of TCF/beta-catenin signaling. *Adv Cancer Res*. 2000;**77**:1-24.
25. Lee SB, Haber DA. Wilms tumor and the WT1 gene. *Exp Cell Res*. 2001;**264**(1): 74-99.
26. Treger TD, Chowdhury T, Pritchard-Jones K, Behjati S. The genetic changes of wilms tumour. *Nat Rev Nephrol*. 2019;**15**(4):240-251.
27. Goldberg NS, Collins FS. The hunt for the neurofibromatosis gene. *Arch Dermatol*. 1991;**127**(11):1705-1707.
28. Halliday D, Parry A, Evans DG. Neurofibromatosis type 2 and related disorders. *Curr Opin Oncol*. 2019;**31**(6):562-567.
29. Semenza GL. The genomics and genetics of oxygen homeostasis. *Annu Rev Genom Hum Genet*. 2020;**21**:183-204.
30. Lynch HT, Lynch PM, Lanspa SJ, et al. Review of the lynch syndrome: History, molecular genetics, screening, differential diagnosis, and medicolegal ramifications. *Clin Genet*. 2009;**76**(1):1-18.
31. King MC. "The race" to clone BRCA1. *Science*. 2014;**343**(6178):1462-1465.
32. Domchek SM, Armstrong K, Weber BL. Clinical management of BRCA1 and BRCA2 mutation carriers. *Nat Clin Pract Oncol*. 2006;**3**(1):2-3.
33. Vermeij WP, Hoeijmakers JH, Pothof J. Genome integrity in aging: human syndromes, mouse models, and therapeutic options. *Annu Rev Pharmacol Toxicol*. 2016;**56**:427-445.

6 Epigenetic contributions to human cancer

Stephen B. Baylin, MD

> **Overview**
>
> The ever-expanding body of work aimed at understanding the components and roles of the epigenome in normal and neoplastic cells is increasingly being translated for possibilities of enriching cancer management. It is ever more clear that the evolution of cancer from its earliest origins in benign risk states through initiation and progression represents an interplay between epigenetic and genetic alterations. Although the number of FDA-approved epigenetic therapy agents is still small, and largely for hematopoietic malignancies, a large increase in clinical trials for older and newer drugs that target epigenome abnormalities, often given in combinations, shows promise for the emergence of new therapy paradigms in the near future. New platforms for sensitive detection of epigenetic abnormalities in DNA from blood and other sites are refining our abilities to monitor cancer risk states and predict and monitor therapy responses. All of this above progress accompanies profound advances in other cancer management paradigms, such as immune checkpoint therapy for which epigenetic drugs may enhance the efficacy of these approaches and help reverse resistance which often emerges. The study of the epigenome and the potential for use of the knowledge for translation to improve cancer care is thus an ever more vibrant area of basic and clinical research.

Over the past 25 years, our understanding of the mechanisms underlying cancer initiation and progression continue to expand including the appreciation that multiple epigenetic processes and not just genetic alterations drive the process.[1-3] In turn, there is rapid progress in defining, for both tumor development and control of normal development and maintenance of normal tissue homeostasis, what constitutes epigenetics and what is termed the "epigenome" and its constituents. Strictly speaking, the term epigenetic refers to heritable changes in gene expression, during embryonic development and for adult tissue maintenance that do not involve changes in the primary base sequence of DNA.[4,5] This definition encompasses two critical, translationally relevant characteristics, expanded upon later, concerning epigenetic alterations in cancer and their clinical importance. First, the coding and noncoding genes and DNA sequences affected by epigenetic changes in cancer remain wild type for DNA sequence rather than harboring irreversible mutations. Second, and closely related, the changes are, then, potentially reversible if normal expression of the involved DNA regions can be restored such that key functions associated with them can emerge.[1-6] This recognition of epigenetic changes, which are fundamental to cancer initiation and progression, is occurring in the midst of a dynamic explosion of knowledge as to how the human epigenome is normally controlled, via DNA methylation and chromatin packaging of DNA, to regulate gene expression in different tissues and during development.[4,5]

For example, epigenetic processes play a fundamental role during normal embryonic development and adult cell renewal. In the involved dynamics, these processes control the emergence of different cellular phenotypes, all with same underlying DNA sequences. This knowledge of gene regulation continues to grow rapidly, including building our understanding of the spectrum of epigenetic changes that are key to cancer development. Still, for understanding many basic aspects of the constitution of the normal and cancer epigenomes and especially for translating the information to improving the management of cancer, we may still be in early stages. However, there is ever progressing ability to marry our understanding of epigenetics in basic cancer biology with development of cancer biomarkers and epigenetic-based therapies. Emerging paradigms are increasingly entering clinical use, and many more are being tested for efficacy in a growing number of clinical trials.

Mechanisms involved in epigenetic regulation of gene expression

For considering translation implications of epigenetics for cancer management, it is essential to have some understanding of basic mechanisms that establish control of the normal and cancer epigenomes. These involve a series of intertwined molecular events, virtually any of which can become altered during the initiation and/or progression of virtually all cancer types. It is important to note that the role of the above control must be considered in the context that the epigenome has a dynamic structure that entails not only a linear distribution along DNA but also a three-dimensional one[7] (Figure 1). The latter is essential for regulating transcription activity through facilitating DNA interactions and looping connections across the entire genome[7] (Figure 1). This structural arrangement ensures that regulation of canonical gene expression occurs not only at their start sites but also from their connecting to more distal control elements, or enhancers fundamental to coordinated gene control (Figure 1). Also, there are spatial aspects of the epigenome in which boundary regions protect long segments of DNA between them to protect encompassed genes to ensure maintenance of their normal expression (Figure 1). Finally, the majority of genome contains DNA, which does not function in canonical gene expression. Formerly thought to be space filling "junk" DNA for which the epigenome ensures repression of unwanted expression, and indeed this is a major role for epigenetic control, there are many regions which are indeed transcribed which are now recognized to produce key regulatory RNA species vital to cellular function (Figure 1). All of these points will be visited throughout this article with respect to the abnormal epigenome of cancers and how critical proteins and

---

Holland-Frei Cancer Medicine, Tenth Edition. Edited by Robert C. Bast, John C. Byrd, Carlo M. Croce, Ernest Hawk, Fadlo R. Khuri, Raphael E. Pollock, Apostolia M. Tsimberidou, Christopher G. Willett, and Cheryl L. Willman.
© 2023 John Wiley & Sons, Inc. Published 2023 by John Wiley & Sons, Inc.

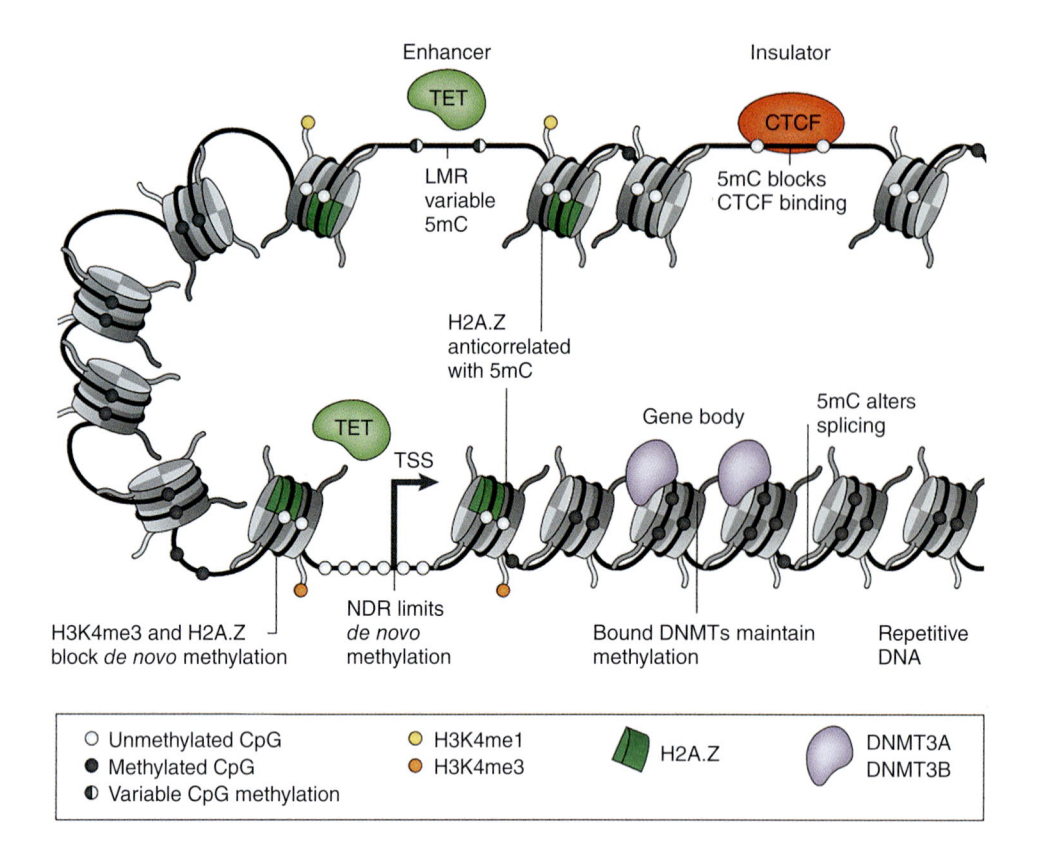

Figure 1 Molecular anatomy of CpG sites in chromatin and their roles in gene expression. About 60% of human genes have CpG islands (CGIs) at their promoters and frequently have nucleosome-depleted regions (NDRs) at the transcriptional start site (TSS). The nucleosomes flanking the TSS are marked by trimethylation of histone H3 at lysine 4 (H3K4me3), which is associated with active transcription, and the histone variant H2A.Z, which is antagonistic to DNA methyltransferases (DNMTs). Downstream of the TSS, the DNA is mostly CpG-depleted and is predominantly methylated in repetitive elements and in gene bodies. CGIs, which are sometimes located in gene bodies, mostly remain unmethylated but occasionally acquire 5-methylcytosine (5mC) in a tissue-specific manner (not shown). Transcription elongation, unlike initiation, is not blocked by gene body methylation, and variable methylation may be involved in controlling splicing. Gene bodies are preferential sites of methylation in the context CHG (where H is A, C, or T) in embryonic stem cells, but the function is not understood (not shown). DNA methylation is maintained by DNMT1 and also by DNMT3A and/or DNMT3B, which are bound to nucleosomes containing methylated DNA99. Enhancers tend to be CpG-poor and show incomplete methylation, suggesting a dynamic process of methylation or demethylation occurs, perhaps owing to the presence of ten-eleven translocation (TET) proteins in these regions, although this remains to be shown. They also have NDRs, and the flanking nucleosomes have the signature H3K4me1 mark and also the histone variant H2A.Z32,100. The binding of proteins such as CTCF to insulators can be blocked by methylation of their non-CGI recognition sequences, thus leading to altered regulation of gene expression, but the generality of this needs further exploration. The sites flanking the CTCF sites are strongly nucleosome-depleted, and the flanking nucleosomes show a remarkable degree of phasing. The figure does not show the structure of CpG-depleted promoters or silenced CGIs, although in both cases the silent state is associated with nucleosomes at the TSS. LMR, low-methylated region. Source: Reproduced by permission from Jones.[7]

complexes encompassing them regulate this complex control of DNA function. A brief review of these processes is provided in this section, and more detailed information is contained in multiple cited reviews and book chapters.

Formation of chromatin

While the primary base sequence of DNA can be viewed as a "hard drive" for storing all the information required for cell function, the patterns of gene expression are determined by how this DNA is modified following synthesis and replication and how it is packaged by the epigenome into the nucleus by interacting proteins, or chromatin.[3–5,7,8] The packaging might be viewed as "software," which provides the readout of the hard drive information contained in the DNA sequence. The primary role of the DNA modification and chromatin packaging is to balance the genome such that the majority of DNA is encompassed in a silent or low transcription state to guard against unwanted expression of repeat sequences, potential transposable elements, and viral insertions accrued over evolution.[5,9–11] The fundamental scaffolding proteins for chromatin are histone proteins and their assembly with DNA into structures termed nucleosomes[7,8,12] (Figure 2). The latter are essential for establishing the three-dimensional arrangement and functional readout of DNA in the nucleus.[7,8,12] Nucleosomes consist of ~146 bp of DNA wrapped twice around an octamer of the core histone proteins, H2A, H2B, H3, and H4.[7,8,12] For functional mediation of gene expression profiles from DNA, nucleosomes must not only be properly distributed linearly along DNA but must also be arranged into higher order, multinucleosomal structures[7,8,12] (Figure 2). These dynamics are mediated by chromatin remodeling proteins, and the more widely and irregularly spaced, the nucleosomes are in their linear placement along DNA, and the less compacted, the more "open" the chromatin is and allows the DNA to be available for active transcription (Figure 2). This is often the case in areas in and around active gene promoters. Conversely, the more regular and evenly the nucleosomes are spaced, the more compacted their higher order structures (Figure 1); the more "closed" is the chromatin, the more repressive for transcription (Figure 2). This latter configuration

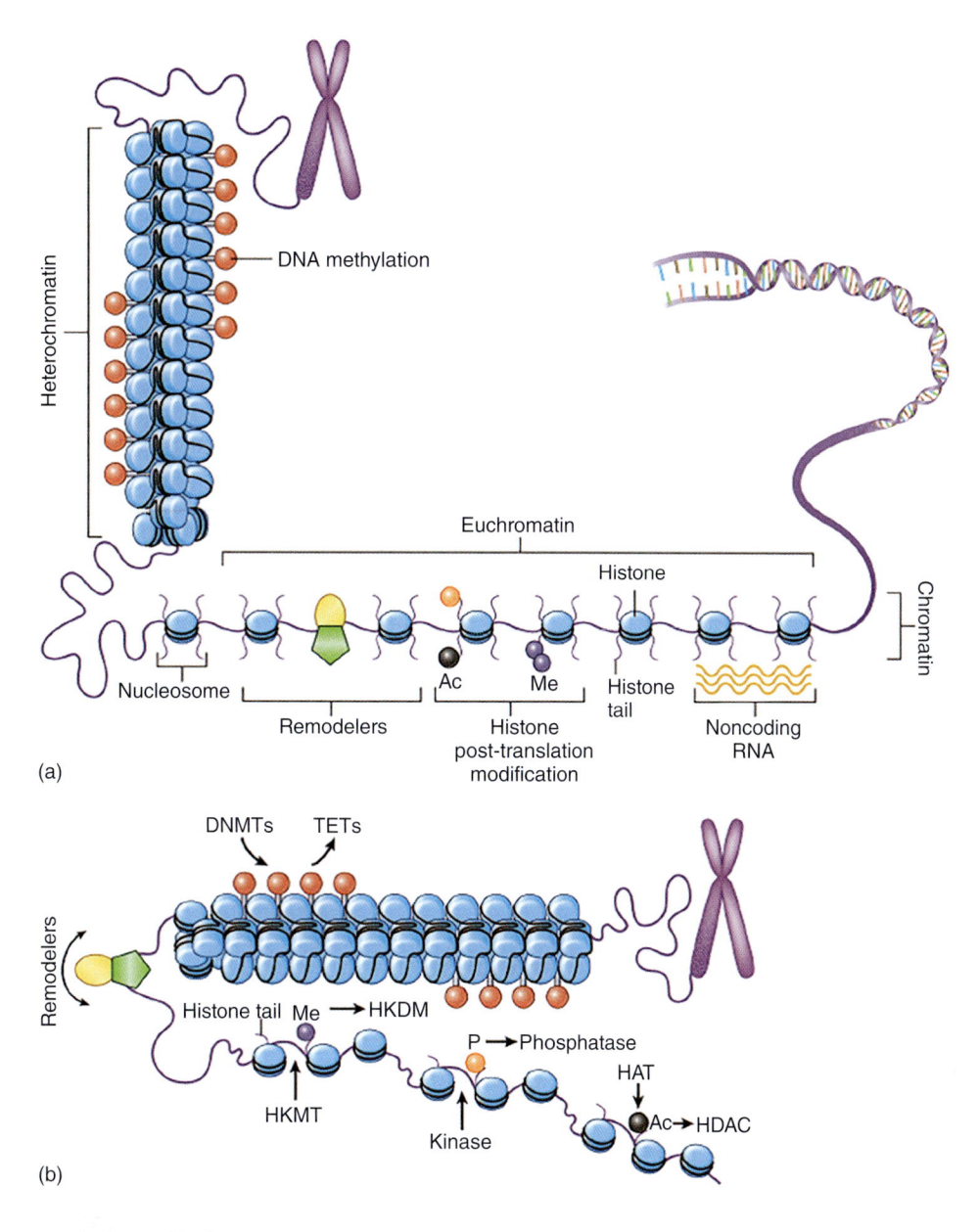

Figure 2 The epigenome landscape. (a) Chromatin states support either transcriptional activation or silencing of genes, allowing gene regulatory regions to switch these states through positioning of nucleosomes (blue ovals). More open conformations leave the transcription start site nucleosome free. Modifications of nucleosome histone tails (purple lines extending from ovals) regulate the process, including DNA methylation (red lollipops), serine phosphorylation (orange circle), lysine acetylation (black circle) and lysine methylation (purple circle), and nucleosome remodeler complexes (green pentagon with yellow oval). Additionally, noncoding RNAs (yellow waves) can participate in these regulatory steps through recruitment of chromatin proteins and DNA methylation. (b) Control of histone modifications and of DNA methylation by proteins: writers (DNMTs, HKMTs, HATs, kinases for phosphorylation), readers (shown in subsequent figures for binding to and interpreting each mark for function), erasers (TETs for DNA methylation, HKDMs for lysine methylation, HDACs, phosphatases for removing phosphorylation), and nucleosome remodelers. Red lollipops indicate DNA methylation; green pentagon with yellow oval indicates nucleosome remodeler complexes; purple circle indicates histone lysine methylation; orange circle indicates serine phosphorylation; black circle indicates lysine acetylation. *Abbreviations*: DNMT, DNA methyltransferase; HAT, histone acetylates; HDAC, histone deacetylases; HKDM, histone lysine demethylase; HKMT, histone lysine methyltransferase; TET, ten-eleven translocation protein. Source: Reproduced by permission from Ahuja et al.[8]

dominates most of the human genome, as noted earlier, to prevent unwanted gene expression and to facilitate chromosome structure.

Integrally involved with this dynamic chromatin structure is a dependency of nucleosome function on "states" of chromatin, which are determined by differing ratios of active and repressive histone "modifications"[4,5,7,8,10] (Figure 2). These consist of additions or modifications to key amino acids, primarily located in the tails of the histones that stick out from the nucleosome assembly, in the form of lysine acetylation, lysine and arginine methylation, serine and threonine phosphorylation, glutamic acid ADP-ribosylation, and lysine ubiquitination and sumoylation.[4,5,7,10] The balance of these marks forms what was initially termed a "histone code," now realized to be more complex than originally envisioned. Thus, nucleosome positioning and histone modifications mediate packaging of the genome such that both constitutive and cell-type-dependent chromatin patterns of open and/or closed configurations are maintained from cell division to cell division, ensuring that these patterns remain stable and heritable in nondividing cells unless cell signaling dictates otherwise.[4,5,7,10] This way cells maintain a "memory" for patterns of gene expression and chromosome structure that facilitate normal patterns of development and the maintenance of mature cell renewal and differentiation states.[4,5,7,10]

The histone modifications introduced above are established and maintained by a series of enzymes, the most characterized of which include lysine methylation and acetylation.[3,8] These enzymes first can act as "writers" that establish key modifications for repression or activation of genes and include histone acetylases (HATs) for histone acetylation of, for example, histone three (H3) lysines 4, 9, and 7 (H3K4, 9, 27 acetyl), and these marks generally facilitate transcription, whereas their deacetylated states accompany transcriptional repression. For histone methylation, writers include histone methyltransferases (HMTs) for establishing methylation states, which can be transcriptionally activating, including for lysine 4 of histone 3 (H3K4me3), or repressive states such as states of methylation for H3K9 (H3K9me1, 2, 3) and 27 (H3K27me1, 2, 3).[3,8] The H3K27 methylation events for transcriptional repression involve key writer proteins, the EZH2 enzymes, which are present in the polycomb group (PcG) protein complex.[3,8] The establishing of these modifications is balanced by a series of enzymes that function as "erasers" to remove the marks, and they include histone deacetylases (HDACs) and histone demethylases that reverse histone acetylation and methylation, respectively.[3,8] Finally, there are a series of proteins or "readers" that can recognize and interact with all of the above histone modification markers to recruit protein complexes that facilitate establishing active and repressive transcription states.[3,8] In addition to PcG, another key example is the NuRD complex that contains the HDAC enzymes and that facilitates histone deacetylation events, which generally serve to repress transcription.[13]

DNA methylation

While not present in all multicellular organisms, humans, other mammals, and other higher organisms add an additional layer of epigenetic regulation, DNA methylation, to the above chromatin events. Working in close concert with chromatin states to package the human genome, DNA methylation is added to postreplicated DNA primarily at the C5 position of the base, cytosine in the context of the CpG dinucleotide in the mammalian genome.[6,14,15] Similar to establishment of chromatin histone modifications, a series of writer proteins, the family of DNA methyltransferase (DNMT) enzymes[14–16] catalyze donation of the methyl group to DNA by transferring it from S-adenosyl methionine. As for chromatin, there are reader proteins and DNA methyl binding proteins such as MBD2 and MBD3, that recognize DNA methylation and recruit protein complexes that allow the DNA modification, especially when located in gene promoter sequences or in the repeat sequences, which were noted previously to be silenced in the genome, to help mediate transcriptional repression. Importantly, the above protein complexes are those that contain some of the histone-modifying writers and readers outlined in previous sections that control chromatin function such as the NURD complex.[13,17,18]

It is important for understanding the role of DNA methylation changes in cancer to understand that its distribution in the genome is closely tied to a nonrandom, but uneven distribution of the CpG dinucleotide.[14,15] This is related to the fact that there has been global and progressive depletion of CpGs over evolution because the deamination of methylated CpGs converts the cytosines (Cs) into thymidines.[15,16] Failure to repair these thymidine changes then results in transition of the Cs to Ts. However, there remains interspersed conservation of nondepleted, CpG-rich stretches (~0.4 to several thousand kb) or the so-called "CpG islands," which are particularly important, as will be discussed later, to the DNA methylation patterns in cancer.[15,16] These islands, especially when found in the 5′ end of about 50–60% of human genes,[15,16] remain non-DNA methylated and transcriptionally available, while the majority of the CpG' sites in the remainder of DNA are methylated and associated with transcriptionally repressed regions[2,8,15,16] (Figures 1 and 2).

The above patterns of DNA methylation, depicted in Figure 1, work in tight concert with the nucleosome positioning and histone modifications previously discussed to determine the epigenetic regulation of the epigenome. Thus, methylated DNA helps maintain a tight heritable state to ensure the transcriptionally inert status of the majority of the genome. This function is most apparent in the closed chromatin or "heterochromatic regions" concentrated in pericentromeric parts of chromosomes. In contrast, the non-DNA methylated CpG islands associated with gene start sites appear to reflect and facilitate a transcriptional ready and/or active transcription state.[8,19] This tight interaction between histone modifications and DNA methylation helps maintain the repression of many closed chromatin states. Thus, deacetylated histone lysines, such as for H3K9, and repressive methylation marks, such as H3K9me2 and 3, associate with methylated DNA.[8,19–21] In turn, such marks, and particularly H3K9me, appear important for targeting of DNA methylation in cancer therapy.[8,20,21] It is important to note that there is at least one important exception to the above role of DNA methylation in repression of gene transcription in that 5mC is present in the body, rather than at start sites or promoter regions, and is found in active and expressed genes. This methylation appears to work with another histone mark, H3K36me3, to allow transcriptional elongation and enhanced gene expression.[22]

There have been recent and most important advances in our understanding of how DNA methylation patterns are established and maintained for DNA methylation in the epigenome. It has long been recognized, as mentioned earlier, that there are three biologically active DNMTs for establishing and maintaining sites of DNA methylation.[14] In this regard, DNMT 1 is predominantly a maintenance DNMT, which is responsible for preserving patterns of established DNA methylation during DNA replication. DNMT3A and DNMT3B are predominantly de novo DNMTs, which can establish new sites of DNA methylation. However, much data suggest a more complex scenario in which there can be cooperativity between the three DNMTs and interacting proteins such that they can, in some instances, replace each other in function when stress situations require this.[23,24] For example, DNMT3A and DNMT3B may function to repair errors made by DNMT1 during DNA synthesis.[24]

Like for the control of chromatin modifications, in addition to the above-discussed writers and readers for the process, an eraser function has been recently recognized for DNA methylation that can foster the removal of this mark. For decades, it was believed that erasure of this modification is a passive event accomplished only by failure to replace methylation sites during DNA replication. Now, it is firmly established that a family of enzymes, termed TET (Ten-Eleven Translocations) family proteins, can, through oxidative steps, convert 5-methyl cytosine (5MT) into 5-hydroxylmethyl cytosine (5hMT), which through subsequent DNA repair steps convert 5MT back into cytosine.[4,14,25,26] These conversions are important during normal development and adult cell functions,[4,14,25,26] and we outline their importance in cancer later.

Histone acetylation

This key feature of chromatin control is, as for the other aspects reviewed above and for DNA methylation, dynamically controlled by a series of writers readers and erasers. Generally, acetylated histone lysines associate with more open chromatin regions, which are more accessible for transcription, while deacetylation at such sites facilitates more closed and transcriptionally repressive domains. For ongoing clinical translation, focus has been on targeting the HDACs, which help establish the repressive state, which is increased in many cancers. For this activity, the proteins work as members of key protein complexes, such as NURD and those harboring MBDs[17,27] and those target key histone lysines and DNA methylation sites to facilitate gene repression. HDACs comprise a complex family of proteins that can reside in the cell nucleus or cytoplasm depending on their function.[20,28–30] The nuclear proteins, HDACs 1 through 3, are mostly involved in transcriptional repression and are being extensively targeted for cancer therapies, which will be reviewed later in this article.

Another key determinant of histone acetylation status is the bromodomain (BRD 2, 3, and 4) and extraterminal domain (BET) protein family. These epigenetic readers are important in cancer development and help maintain acetylation of lysines on histone 4.[31,32] This acetylation occurs at gene promoter and enhancer regions where these proteins can be recruited by their interaction with proteins with HAT activity, which modify the lysine residues.[31,32] For cancer, much attention has been paid to studies demonstrating that BET proteins can maintain the active expression of the cMYC oncogene, but they can also foster expression of other genes.[31,32] A series of BET inhibitors have been developed over the past 15 years, which in preclinical studies reduced BET levels at enhancers and promoters, promoted genome-wide transcription changes, and induced accompanying antitumor activities.[31–34] A series of BET inhibitors have thus entered clinical trials, predominantly in liquid tumors, with targeting of cMYC most suggested as the leading, potential mechanism underlying antitumor activity.[31–34] Although, BET inhibitors are still promising cancer drugs, when used alone they have induced unacceptable toxicities in patients, and how they will contribute to cancer management in the future remains to be determined.

Altered DNA methylation and chromatin in the "Cancer Epigenome"

Loss of DNA methylation

Virtually all cancer types harbor what appears to be a marked shift away from the normal epigenetic patterns for normal cells, described in the previous sections.[2,35] This has been best studied to date for DNA methylation, where there are at least two major changes that are now well appreciated. First, there are global losses of this modification from the widespread regions of the genome, which harbor DNA methylation in normal cells.[6,35–37] Indeed, this was the first chromatin abnormality well cataloged for cancer[38] although much still remains to be learned about the ramifications of this change. Since these are generally areas of closed chromatin where the DNA methylation helps to maintain transcriptionally repressed DNA, such losses could associate with abnormal transcription.[1,2,36,37] Indeed, a number of genes with oncogenic potential, and which normally have low expression in normal cells, have now been reported to be upregulated in association with cancer-specific decreases in promoter DNA methylation.[1,35] Also, regions of DNA methylation loss have also been recently associated with upregulation of antitumor genes.[39] Also, pericentromeric regions are a target for DNA methylation losses in multiple cancer types, and this may play a role in the genesis of chromosomal instability and/or abnormal transcription of genes and repeat sequences in neoplasia.[1,2,36,37,40] Most recently, losses of DNA methylation from gene body regions have also been observed in tumors. This can have an opposite effect on gene expression to those above as methylation in these regions, as discussed earlier above, actually facilitates gene expression through enhancing transcriptional elongation.[22,41] Finally, losses of DNA methylation can occur in cancer cells in regions that act as "insulator" regions to protect genes within their boundaries from being inappropriately repressed or expressed.[42,43] Losses of DNA methylation from such sites have now been associated with aberrant upregulated, constitutive expression of oncogenes, and this can behave as a driver event for promoting tumor initiation and/or progression.[42,43]

Cancer DNA hypermethylation

One of the most investigated epigenetic abnormalities in cancer entails localized increases in DNA methylation in gene promoter CpG islands, which are protected from this change, as discussed earlier, in virtually all normal, postembryonic development cells (Figure 1).[1,2,35–37] This change is associated with tight transcriptional repression, or repression of inducibility of genes and thus, can provide an alternative to gene mutations for loss of function of a number of well-characterized tumor-suppressor genes.[1,2,35–37] In addition to these classic-suppressor genes, data derived from random screens of cancer cell DNA for DNA hypermethylated genes, such as in the Cancer Genome Atlas Project (TCGA), indicate that hundreds of such genes appear to exist, for multiple cancer types analyzed, in a given patient's tumor.[1,2,35–37,44,45] While all of these gene changes may not be pivotal for driving the initiation or progression of the particular cancers that harbor them, many, including the classic-suppressor genes, do encode for genes for which loss of function would be important for tumor development.[1,2,35] Many such genes, which are seldom mutated in cancers, may still have important roles in tumorigenesis, since they undergo promoter DNA hypermethylation and silencing during tumor progression.[2,35] In this regard, virtually every critical pathway known to play a role in tumorigenesis is involved with genes bearing cancer-specific DNA hypermethylation in one or more tumor types.[1,2,35] Finally, many of the genes involved exhibit the DNA methylation change in preinvasive lesions, which have the potential for malignant progression, as demonstrated for "benign" colon polyps.[2,35–37,46] In these preinvasive colon lesions, repression of the involved genes leads to deregulation of key pathways and their inherent cellular signaling, which are well known to drive the initiation and progression of all colon cancers.[2,35–37,46] Experimental data are accruing for several hypotheses concerning the functional significance for promoter DNA hypermethylation in preinvasive lesions. First, these methylation changes appear tightly linked to states associated with cancer risk including chronic inflammation including scenarios for enhanced DNA damage[2,46–48] and aging[49] and loss of function for the involved genes appear to help drive tumor initiation.[50]

Importantly, cancer-specific promoter region CpG island hypermethylation involves genes which are biased toward those which play key roles, in the absence of promoter DNA methylation in normal embryonic development. Thus, maintaining their availability for proper induction of expression is critical to allow blocking of stem cell renewal and accompanying cell lineage commitment and differentiation.[50,51] The loss of this induction capacity via cancer-specific promoter methylation may then foster, during tumor initiation and/or progression, the appearance of abnormally expanding stem-like cells with poor differentiation capacity, thus enhancing stages of tumor initiation and/or progression.[50,51] These control events, operative during normal embryonic development, and renewal processes in normal adult tissues are tightly linked to the key chromatin, repressive PcG protein complex introduced earlier. PcG occupancy of many CpG island containing gene promoters, in the absence of DNA methylation in these regions, helps maintain the genes in a low but inducible expression state until gene activation is needed for cells to leave the stem cell state and contribute to the appearance of differentiating cells.[50,51] During tumor initiation, many such genes evolve a quantitative switch wherein abnormal DNA methylation comes to occupy the promoter regions and the position of the PcG complex is altered in position.[50,51] The result is a tightening of a transcriptionally repressive state that hinders proper induction of the genes, and this can render, for a tumor suppressor gene, loss of function.[50,51] It is estimated that, depending on the tumor type, well over half of the abnormally DNA hypermethylated genes with promoter CpG islands represent these normally PcG controlled genes.[50,51] The resultant loss of gene expression or capacity of induction potential is then permissive for changes in cell signaling pathways that maintain stem cell-like properties and can predispose the cells to sensitization to transformation by mutations in oncogenes or tumor suppressor genes.[50,51] Thus, gene silencing may be permissive but not sufficient for cancer evolution by cooperating with genetic changes.[50,51]

Specific patterns of abnormal, gene promoter hypermethylation are recognized that are important to the numbers and function of genes involved. The best known of these is the CpG island methylator phenotype or CIMP.[52–56] Originally described for CRC, this state is now recognized as a quantitative accrual of the promoter methylation that can be recognized in subsets of virtually all major cancer types.[52–56] Importantly, these subsets are often linked to key tumor characteristics with examples including a high association with proximal colon CRC and those with BRAF mutations and mismatch repair deficiency. Endometrial cancers can also harbor CIMP,[52] as can glioblastomas with *IDH1* mutations.[57] Although the full translational significance of CIMP in cancer is still to be determined, tumors with the highest quantitative degree of CIMP appear to have a worse prognostic outcome as best established for CRC.[52–56]

Finally, there is a building body of data for cancer-specific increases of DNA methylation in gene enhancer regions, which can alter binding of key proteins and histone modifications in these regulatory sequences that serve as master regulators of gene expression.[7] These sequences can lie at variable, and often large, distances away from gene proximal promoters.[58–60] De novo DNA methylation changes at enhancers may then also contribute to key gene expression abnormalities in cancer and, again especially for increasing cancer risk states.[61,62] While the theme of differential enhancer DNA methylation in cancer is under intense investigation, the role of these changes, and their balance with gene promoter CpG island hypermethylation, must continue to be clarified.

Long-range changes in DNA methylation and chromatin in cancer

A recent exciting advance in studying both normal and cancer epigenomes, stemming from in-depth analyses of CpG methylation and chromatin changes throughout the cancer genome, is that there are nonrandom regional configurations that can be altered between neoplastic and normal cells (Figure 1). They occupy megabase regions in many chromosomes (100 kb–10 Mb).[1,2,35,63–65] They are largely CpG poor regions, and the constituent CpGs are heavily methylated but to degrees that vary significantly throughout different normal tissues, leading to the term partially methylated domains.[1,2,35,63–65] Cancers characteristically have losses of normal DNA methylation throughout these areas, creating so-called megabase islands or canyons of hypomethylated domains as particularly defined to date in colon and other cancers.[1,2,35,63–65] Within these blocks of sequences, cancers can establish long-range appearance of repressive histone modifications, such as for H3K9methylation as well.[1,2,35,63–65] In some regions, there may be long-range areas of nonrepressive or more open chromatin.[64,66–69] Intriguingly, much smaller regions containing embedded genes within these large domains that harbor promoter CpG islands can have the de novo gains in DNA methylation discussed in detail earlier.[1,2,35,64] Thus, in essence, hypomethylated canyons in cancer often exhibit many of the cancer-associated losses and more focal CpG island gains of DNA methylation in cancer.[1,2,64] Moreover, these large domains may harbor a much higher than expected percentage of genes with a history of embryonic and adult stem cell chromatin regulation that are particularly vulnerable in cancer to abnormal, promoter CpG island DNA hypermethylation.[1,2,35,47,64,70,71]

Another key facet of chromatin dynamics, which can be greatly altered in cancer, is the advancing knowledge about regulation of the noncoding regions of the genome that do not encompass canonical coding genes (Figure 1) and comprise of over about 80% of the human genome. There are a myriad of rapidly emerging advances for understanding this regulation, which are not yet approved targets for cancer therapies but are already in clinical trials which may establish their promise. Thus, there are a large series of noncoding long RNAs (lnRNAs) that can act locally at gene sites, or at a distance, to enhance or repress gene expression.[72] Another small-size class of noncoding RNAs, microRNAs (miRNA), which are only 20 or so nucleotides long, are the most studied for these type of noncoding regions in cancer.[73,74] These nucleotides, processed through a complex series of steps to become mature miRNAs, can then recognize specific sites in transcripts of canonical coding genes and induce gene silencing.[73,74] This silencing involves blunting of protein translation and/or promoting degradation of the target gene mRNA.[73,74] Importantly, the target sites for a given miRNA can engage with hundreds of transcripts, allowing modulation of multiple key signaling pathways simultaneously.[73,74] The effect for cancer, when miRNA expression is abnormally controlled, is to play a potential role at many points in initiation and progression of tumorigenesis.[73,74]

Connections between epigenetic and genetic alterations in cancer

One of the most intriguing themes to emerge over the past several years is the recognition that, in virtually all tumor types, one of the most frequent types of mutations is in genes encoding for proteins that establish and maintain the epigenome.[1,2,75,76] While the exact implications of most of these remain to be defined, there are now several key links between these genetic alterations and tumorigenesis, DNA methylation abnormalities, or chromatin changes. Important examples are mutations in IDH 1 and 2 genes and the TET genes. They are now recognized in low-grade gliomas in younger patients[77,78] and in hematologic cancers[79–81] and are associated with altered DNA and histone demethylation pathways. IDH2 mutations particularly associate with the previously introduced CIMP phenotype.[57,82–84] These IDH mutations lead to massive accumulation of a metabolite, 2-hydroxy-glutarate formed at the expense of depleting ketoglutarate,[85–87] a cofactor for multiple enzymes that help regulate and maintain key chromatin marks including for TET proteins to protect against abnormal DNA methylation.[88,89] This combination of events then incites repressive histone marks and CIMP.[85–87] Mouse studies indicate that IDH mutations are drivers for early tumor progression events[90] by blocking normal differentiation of normal stem/progenitor cells and thus facilitate abnormal self-renewal and diminished lineage commitment and differentiation.[57,85,91] Use of IDH mutation inhibitors has reached clinical use as outlined later in this article.

Another fascinating type of epigenetic mutations, first recognized in a subset of pediatric glioblastomas, occurs in genes encoding for histones themselves and function in a novel manner. Although these mutations occur in only one multiple copies of histone H3, they robustly disrupt the activity of an individual enzyme, EZH2 responsible for establishing the repressive histone modification, H3K27me3.[92] The resultant cancers thus, profoundly lose this transcriptional repression and have marked activation of genes, which can then drive steps in tumor initiation and/or progression.[1,93,94] A recurrent feature of these altered tumorigenesis events is that the mutations induce expansion of a primitive, stem-like group of cells, suggesting the tumors arise because of the arrest of a key developmental step important for normal brain development.[92] Subsequent to this H3K27 mutation, other histone mutations have been defined such as for H3K36, and, in the last 3 to 4 years, over 100 similar mutations were defined.[92] They all appear to function by disrupting proteins that act as writers or erasers of affected histone modifications.[92] Similarly, even more related such mutations will be recognized, which drive important steps in the development of a full spectrum of cancers.

Connections between DNA methylation and chromatin for immune regulation in cancer

During the past several years, a remarkably expanded emphasis has been placed on studies of how epigenetic processes regulate both immune-related signaling from cancer cells and how key immune cell types function and mediate antitumor immunity. From a translational standpoint, these interactions, as will be elaborated upon in a later section, are fundamental to driving an expanding number of clinical trials for combining epigenetic therapy and immunotherapy to increase the efficacy of the latter.

In terms of immune-related signaling from cancer cells, it has been noted for many years that drugs which can reverse DNA methylation and/or block histone deacetylation can upregulate antigens that could signal to the immune system.[20,95] In the past several years, investigators have found that this immune attraction is upregulated by epigenetic therapy drugs by a systematic signaling process termed as "viral mimicry".[96,97] This term arises because the drug response initiates induction of type I and III interferon signaling induced by increased levels of cytoplasmic viral RNAs due to activating transcription from normally silenced endogenous retroviruses or ERVs, which are DNA sequences that have been incorporated into the human genome over millennia. These DNA sequences actually constitute ~8% of the genome, and their silencing for expression in somatic cells is a normal process facilitated by maintaining DNA methylation and/or repressive histone modifications at their transcription start sites.[9] Thus, epigenetic therapy drugs such as DNMTis and HDACis, especially when used in combination, induce DNA demethylation of these ERV sites, allowing transcription of these viral gene products which enter the cytoplasm and form double-stranded RNA structures to viral defense responses triggered by type I and III interferon signaling (Table 1). An aggregate consequence of the above drug responses, seen in mouse models of important cancers, including non-small-cell lung (NSCLC) and ovarian cancer, is that combination of DNMTis and HDACis results in attraction of key immune cells to the tumors and diminish other such cells, which actually promote tumor growth.[28,98] Simultaneously, the treatment stokes release of key cytokines from the tumor cells that have the potential for recruiting immune cells for cytotoxic effects against cancer cells and also converting the status of such cells from an ineffective or "exhausted" state to an immune functional effector state. This latter aspect of exhaustion is expanded upon below.

Another major link to epigenetic control of immune responses with high translational significance is direct drug effects on DNA methylation and chromatin organization, which regulate the function of key immune cell subsets. Such epigenetic regulation has been a rapidly growing research enterprise, for both normal and cancer-related immunology over the past decade. Pertinent current details are the subject of multiple recent reviews[99–101] but brief, important summary information is as follows. The most studied and a critical immune cell type for mounting an immune attack against cancer cells is the T cell and particularly CD8+ T cells. These cells are attracted to tissues, including cancer cells, in scenarios wherein the cells are targeted to the tissue of interest by ongoing inflammation and antigen presentation to the cells by antigen-presenting immune cells. Epigenetic steps through a dynamic series of normal changes involving genome-wide DNA methylation alterations and histone modifications[102–104] modulate each of the steps by which T cell differentiation and ultimate fates occur (Figure 2). These epigenetic states, in turn, mediate this control by guiding how key transcription factors induce or repress regulatory regions of genes that guide T-cell development, maturation, and lineage commitment.[105] The differentiation and cell fate outcomes then occur through responses of cell signaling pathways, which determine the conversion of immune naive CD8+ T cells to become CD8+ memory cells, which can rapidly respond to antigens to which the cells have previously been exposed, or become effector T cells that can quickly mount an immune attack.[105] From the standpoint of DNA methylation, the above changes involve losses of this modification to reverse repression of naive T-cell-associated genes followed by maintenance of demethylation to allow their expression in CD8+ effector T cells.[102–104]

In the context of immunotherapy, another important set of epigenetic control dynamic key to the above-discussed T cell states involves regulation of the "immune checkpoint" setting. This relates to the fact that immune-exhausted T cells upregulate molecules on their cell surfaces and on other key subsets of immune cells, which inhibit this setting including PD-1 and CTLA-4, and other collaborating proteins such as LAG3 and TIM3.[99–101] These proteins interact with receptors on interactor cells and on tumors particularly PD-L1 for achieving immune checkpoint inhibition.[99–101] For transient infections that are adequately cleared, this is a normal process that can block activation of damaging autoimmune responses.[99–101] However, the interaction between PD-1 on immune cells and PD-L1 on tumor cells invokes a state of immune tolerance in the former.[99–101] Discovery of these interactions earned the Nobel Prize for Drs. Allison and Honjo with a predominant reason being that they greatly helped explain why, over many years, tumor immune therapies had not been greatly efficacious.[99–101] This recognition spawned a new era for "immune checkpoint therapy," which has been revolutionary for cancer treatment. The above immune checkpoint interactions were initially discovered using viral infection models. For

Table 1 Epigenome-targeting drugs that are approved or in clinical trials.

Inhibitor	Mechanism	Rationale	Drug	Target	Cancer type	Approval or trial status	Pharmaceutical company
DNMTi	Inhibition of DNA methylation	Removes hypermethylation of tumor suppressor genes	Azacitidine (Vidaza)	Pan-DNMT	MDS	EMA and FDA	Celgene Corporation (and generic)
			Decitabine (Dacogen)	Pan-DNMT	AML MDS	EMA (for AML) and FDA (for MDS)	Otsuka Pharmaceutical (and generic)
			Guadecitabine	Pan-DNMT	AML	FDA	Astex Pharmaceuticals
			Onureg	Pan-DNMT	AML	FDA	Bristol-Myers Squibb/Celgene
			Inqovi	Pan-DNMT	MDS	FDA	Astex Pharmaceuticals
HDACi	Inhibition of histone deacetylation	Reduces oncogene transcription and signaling, and promotes cell-cycle arrest and apoptosis	Belinostat (Beleodaq)	HDAC class I and class II	Peripheral T cell lymphoma	FDA	Spectrum Pharmaceuticals
			Panobinostat (Farydak)	HDAC class I, class II, and class IV	Multiple myeloma	FDA	Novartis
			Romidepsin (Istodax)	HDAC class I	Cutaneous T cell lymphoma	FDA	Bristol-Myers Squibb/Celgene
			Vorinostat (Zolinza)	HDAC class I, class II, and class IV	Cutaneous T cell lymphoma	FDA	Merck & Co.
IDH Inhibitors	Inhibition of IDH mutations		TIBSOVO	IDH 1 and IDH 2 Mutations	AML	FDA	Agios Pharmaceuticals
Abbott Real-time IDH Assay	Assay for IDH mutations	Screens for IDH mutations for patients with AML			AML	FDA	Abbott
Tazverik	Inhibitor of EZH2	Blocks EZH2 in patients with soft tissue sarcoma with mutations in the SWI/SNF			Soft tissue sarcoma including epithelial sarcomas	FDA	Epizyme

a transient infection, in the interactions between CTLA4 on key immune cells and PD-1 on immune cells and PD-L1 on infected cells, these proteins are upregulated in a normal response to the virus to allow immune tolerance to follow a successful infection resolution.[99–101] In the host, this also guards against induction of autoimmune responses.[99–101] However, if infection persists, the chronic interaction between CTLA4 and its receptors or PD1 and PD-L1 renders sustained immune tolerance, or ineffective immune attack capacity in T cells and other immune cell subsets.[99–101] These chronic effects were subsequently discovered for chronic interactions of the above proteins in the setting of immune attack against tumor cells with an emerging understanding that this was the key explanation for diminished efficacy of immunotherapy.[99–101] This understanding opened the way for the tremendous impact that immune checkpoint therapy has had on cancer treatment.[99–101]

In epigenetics, there is now growing understanding that there are both the transient and chronic interactions between virally infected and immune cells, and these interactions between tumor and immune cells are epigenetically modulated in a reversible manner.[102–104] Losses of DNA methylation and accompanying activating chromatin states occur at start sites of the immune checkpoint mediating genes to create active immune cells and are then reversed to restore basal-state normal tolerance.[102–104] However, during chronic infection and chronic immune tolerance of T cells diminishing tumor immune attack, exhausted CD8+ T cells retain DNA methylation-mediated silencing of immune checkpoint genes. A more detailed outline of the concept is beyond the scope of this article but is reviewed elsewhere.[99] These include epigenetic control of exhaustion or activation states of other immune cells for key tumor immune control including NK, macrophages, and other antigen-presenting cells, and myeloid tumor suppressor cells or MDSCs. Reversing chronic epigenetic regulation of these cell types may be essential for effective immune checkpoint therapy. Thus, epigenetic therapy drugs can experimentally achieve treatment paradigms to facilitate efficacy of immune checkpoint cancer therapy. The current position of clinical trials to explore this is addressed later in this article.

Clinical implications of altered DNA methylation in cancer

As indicated in the preceding sections, more and more information is accumulated regarding the basic biology of epigenetic control of normal and neoplastic cells as are endeavors to translate this information to the clinical arena. For cancer, two areas have received the most attention: first is use of data for developing biomarkers to facilitate means for detection of cancer risk, achieving early cancer detection, predicting disease course, and monitoring responses to therapies. The second major area is exploiting our knowledge of epigenetic biology to develop cancer therapies targeting key aspects of the cancer epigenome. Approaches are generally based on "reprogramming" the cancer epigenome to allow major changes in gene expression that can induce antitumor effects and/or enhance immune recognition and attack upon tumor cells. Both of these above translational categories are briefly reviewed in the following sections.

Cancer DNA methylation biomarkers

General comments
To date, assays for changes in DNA methylation have dominated the field of using epigenetic assays for biomarker approaches

to cancer. DNA and methylated sequences within, as opposed to proteins and RNA, represent stable molecules, thus providing for optimal use in tumors and tumor products that enter the bloodstream or into sputum, urine, stool, and other available peripheral sites. Moreover, alterations in DNA methylated sequences have much higher frequencies in the cancer genome than do genetic changes including specific mutations.[1,44,75,106] Over a decade ago, sensitive PCR-based approaches for individual sites of cancer-specific DNA methylation changes were derived and increasingly used for detecting and utilizing markers analyzed as a sensitive means of cancer biomarker strategies.[106–108] Over the past several years, refinement of these platforms, including ever increasingly more quantitative assays, and development of new ones have been introduced for novel biomarker approaches for virtually all major cancer types.[108,109] Subsequently, multiple approaches have been derived to explore the entire epigenome for DNA methylation, and this has much expanded derivation of marker strategies employing many more DNA regions that can be queried in the assays above and beyond probing just promoters of cancer-specific, DNA hyper- or hypo-methylated genes. These efforts have been greatly enhanced by expanding numbers of publicly available databases for genome-wide DNA methylation analyses, and some with associated gene expression correlations, which can be utilized to explore virtually every cancer type for derivation of biomarker possibilities.[110] The most utilized database has been the Cancer Genome Atlas project or TCGA, which contains genome-wide DNA methylation and gene expression data for tumor and normal samples for virtually all major cancer types.[110] Also, the assays for DNA methylation in TCGA employ the most commonly used platform for genome-wide queries, arrays developed by Illumina.[110] Finally, while detection of DNA methylation dominates current approaches, various means for assessing changes in chromatin parameters are coming into play.[111]

DNA methylation biomarkers in current clinical use

DNA methylation clock for aging and its link to cancer risk
One emerging use of DNA methylation markers, although not standard as yet in the cancer biomarker space, involves the very tight link of DNA methylation changes and the risk over decades for many cancer types and especially colorectal cancer (CRC). For the chronological age link, multiple studies have utilized panels composed of the most variable methylation levels at sequences of the epigenome, gains, and losses, to tightly predict chronological age.[112] In fact, the relationship is so tight, within ±3 years, that many states in the United States use this to analyze DNA samples available at crime scenes to predict the age of suspects.[112] For cancer risk, similar panels from analyses of normal colon matched to the age of individuals track for CRC in a curve that virtually overlaps a marked increase of this malignancy from 60 years of age and on.[49,113] This relationship is very tight for promoter methylation levels of genes with the hypermethylation patterns discussed earlier for appearance in CRC.[82] The overall hope for such research data is that such methylation assays have potential use in screening populations to identify individuals at highest risk for developing CRC. In such approaches, individuals with a methylation score reflective of a higher age than their actual chronological age may encourage more frequent screening with stool and blood tests and a more aggressive schedule for scheduling colonoscopies.

Clinical use of DNA methylation markers
The fact that cancer-specific abnormalities of DNA methylation occur early in preinvasive stages and early stages of cancer allows for uses of such markers in early diagnosis. Those with versions of approval are now predominantly employed for CRC and prostate cancer diagnoses. They all use variations of the PCR procedures introduced earlier that quantitate methylation levels in specific gene promoter sequences. Detection of CRC has been particularly enhanced by detection of altered DNA methylation in stool and blood DNA. The FDA initially approved in 2014 the widely used Cologuard stool test from Exact Sciences[9] with an update in 2019 for age ranges.[114,115] This platform is then currently recommended for individuals 45 years or older who are at typical average risk, and such individuals must lack a history of inflammatory bowel diseases (IBDs) such as chronic ulcerative colitis or Crohn's disease with their high propensity for CRC development or who lack a family history of germline mutations which produce a high frequency for CRC emergence in syndromes such as familial adenomatous polyposis (FAP) or inherited, proximal colon, serrated polyps in Lynch syndrome. The test employs detection of both epigenetic and genetic abnormalities consisting of gene promoter methylation markers for *BMP3* and *NDRG4,* and a genetic change, *KRAS* mutations plus an immunochemical assay for detection of blood in the stool.[114,115] In most recent data, sensitivity of Cologuard for CRC detection, including advanced, premalignant adenomas, was 92.3% with a specificity of 84.5%.[114–116] In addition to detection of CRC in stool DNA, use of a specific promoter methylation mark for *SEPT9* is FDA approved.[117] This *SEPT9* test represents the most widely studied individual gene methylation biomarker in CRC and reported sensitivity for CRC detection ranges from 48.2% to 95.6% and specificity from 79.1% to 99.1%.[117]

Another clinically available, CLIA-approved use of DNA methylation markers is for prostate cancer. ConfirmMDx is developed by MDxHealth and can be performed on formalin-fixed, paraffin-embedded (FFPE) biopsy tissues.[118,119] The test is employed after an initial negative biopsy to help determine whether a repeat biopsy should be performed. Fourteen different prostate areas are utilized for the repeat biopsy and the promoter methylation status of three genes frequently hypermethylated in prostate cancer, *GSTP1, APC,* and *RASSF1* with *ACTB* as a normal control gene, assessed by real-time quantitative methylation-specific PCR (MSP).[118,119] An EpiScore is determined and predicts, from multiple published studies, the presence of low- to high-grade prostate cancer with sensitivities and specificities ranging, respectively, from 62% and 64% or greater over multiple studies.[118,119]

Another biomarker use for DNA methylation biomarkers in cancer is for predicting cancer cell sensitivity to different therapies. Again, the DNA methylation status for the promoter region of individual genes has been utilized for this purpose and a clinically available test is for the DNA damage repair gene *O6MGMT* in patients with glioblastoma.[120–122] Hypermethylation of this gene associates with abnormal silencing and GSTP is otherwise needed to facilitate removal of alkyl adducts from the O6 position of guanine. This loss of function sensitizes to the cell-killing effects of alkylating agents.[120,121] Detection of the *O6MGMT* hypermethylation then predicts a higher likelihood of response and longer length of time to posttreatment disease recurrence after use of such treatments with and without radiation therapy.[122] The *O6MGMT* methylation test is available for clinical use in glioblastoma patients as PredictMDx™ from MDxHealth.

"Epigenetic" cancer therapy
Epigenetic therapy is based on the concept of altering cancer-specific changes to reprogram the epigenome as it is defined in

the previous sections. This section focuses on several classes of drugs in clinical trials to achieve this purpose and several that have been approved by the FDA over the past 20 years. The two most employed are those that inhibit the DNMTs which establish and maintain DNA methylation (DNMTi's) and that inhibit HDACs which block acetylation of chromatin (HDACis). Most approaches are potential ones, especially for solid tumors, and are still the subject of clinical trials. We briefly outline some of the most promising ones.

Approved uses of DNA hypomethylating agents in hematologic neoplasms

Approved DNMTis are all for hematologic-related diseases and include 5-aza-cytidine (Vidaza from BMS-Celgene) and 5-aza-2′-deoxycytidine (DAC) (Dacogen from Otsuka), approved for use in the pre-leukemic disease, myelodysplasia (MDS).[3,123,124] Most recently, a newer demethylating agent, Guadecitabine (SG110 from Astex Pharmaceuticals and Otsuka Pharmaceutical Co., Ltd.) has received FDA approval for MDS. This agent, a dinucleotide that links DAC to deoxyguanosine, acts effectively as a prodrug, which releases DAC upon in vivo exposure.[3,123-125] The resultant effective half-life for DAC increases fourfold compared to intravenous DAC. Although the drug does not increase overall survival, the FDA has granted an orphan drug designation to Guadecitabine for patients with MDS based on its acceptable pharmacokinetics. Most recently, two new FDA approvals of DNMTis bring in a needed patient more benefits than those discussed above, both of which are oral agents and eliminate the need for intravenous or subcutaneous administration as opposed to each of those discussed above. The first drug Onureg (BMS/Celgene)[126-128] is essentially an oral form of Vidaza for treatment of patients with AML, which is approved for patients who, first, have achieved remission including with incomplete blood count recovery (CRi), following intensive induction chemotherapy, and who cannot tolerate intensive curative therapy approaches such as bone marrow transplant.[126-128] The second approved drug C-DEC (Astex Pharmaceuticals and Otsuka Pharmaceutical Co., Ltd) is a single tablet containing cedazuridine and DAC.[123,124] This is approved for use in patients with previously treated and untreated, *de novo*, and secondary MDS induced by previous chemotherapies and for chronic myelomonocytic leukemia (CMML). The cedazuridine component of the combination is an inhibitor of cytidine deaminase, an enzyme that otherwise degrades DAC and thus shortens its half-life.[123,124,128] Despite early response rates of 10% to 20% for MDS, as for most epigenetic therapy approaches, the effects of DNMTis rely on reprogramming of the epigenome rather than initial cytotoxic effects. Thus, responses usually emerge only after several month treatment cycles.[3,124,129,130] In addition, while the effects of these drugs are occasionally curative and/or achieve very long-term stable disease and survival, none are yet optimal. Treatment failures are common, and resistance usually emerges in patients who do well initially.[3,124,129,130] For the trials leading to FDA approval of the initial DNMTis in MDS, Vidaza provides a doubling of survival advantage in higher-risk patients with MDS, but Dacogen failed to achieve benefit in this regard.[3,124,129,130] The reasons for the survival differences are not clear but could reflect differences in the precise patient populations involved. Neither drug has been approved for treating AML in multiple trials and is not specifically FDA approved for this disease. Both DAC and Vidaza and all currently employed DNMTis have significant bone marrow toxicities, and patients must be observed closely for neutropenia and thrombocytopenia and need for hematologic support and/or dose reductions when these toxicities warrant.[3,129,130]

Importantly, a major shift has recently occurred leading to what will be assuredly become the standard approach for using Dacogen and Vidaza in patients with acute AML, exhibiting some promise but not yet established for MDS. The FDA has provided breakthrough approval for combining either DAC or Vidaza with the BCL2 inhibitor, Venetoclax from AbbVie in the AML clinical setting.[127,128,131,132] Venetoclax blunts the role of BCL2 as an inhibitor of apoptosis, but the precise mechanisms for treatment efficacy when combined with DNMTis remain to be determined. Nevertheless, the combination in patients with AML who have never received a DNMTi and who are not eligible for standard high-dose chemotherapy induction treatment produces response rates from around 60% to over 70% in trials to date with promising results for a benefit in overall survival.[131,132] The combined regimens are well tolerated without increasing the bone marrow toxicity standard for the DNMTis, and it also occurs with Venetoclax alone.[131,132] Response rate for the combinations is lower in patients who previously received either Dacogen or Vidaza but still reaches around 40% in the ongoing trials to date.[131,132]

The demonstration that DNMTis can constitute effective agents for treatment of solid tumors has proven it difficult to achieve especially when these drugs are used alone. While many clinical trials, some with promising results, have been implemented to test DNMTis for achieving such efficacy, no FDA approvals for this purpose have yet been established. The greatest potential of these drugs is displayed when they are combined with other therapeutic approaches, which are discussed in a later section.

Approved uses of histone deacetylase inhibitors (HDACis)

The second and largest class of FDA-approved epigenetic drugs for cancer therapy, again primarily for hematologic neoplasms, are HDACis that inhibit multiple histone deacetylases. Several of these agents, discussed earlier as targeting multiple classes of HDACs in this family of enzymes, are approved for treatment of diseases, predominantly peripheral T cell lymphomas.[3,20,133] Responses for this disease can be dramatic[3,20,133,134] with response rates for vorinostat approaching ORR 30% and a median time to tumor progression 202 days[3,20,133] with the HDACi, vorinostat. For romidepsin, approved for PTCL patients who have failed at least one prior systemic therapy, patients have shown an ORR of 25% including 15% CR/ unconfirmed CR (CRu), with a durable median duration of response (DOR) of 28 months in responders. Belinostat is also approved to treat peripheral T cell lymphoma in patients whose disease has recurred or is refractory.[135] However, the above responses to all the above HDACis are generally not durable and resistance usually emerges. Many other HDACis are in various stages in clinical trials, especially when combined with other agents and likely more FDA approvals will be pending. The mechanisms underlying the clinical efficacies leading to their approval are complex and under investigation. Certainly, restoration of chromatin acetylation to enhance expression of tumor suppressor genes may be involved, but these processes can enhance antigen expression and other immune processes as well.[3,20,133] These multifold activities underlie the fact that HDACis, such as DNMTis, are in clinical trials for multiple combinatorial therapy approaches. There is extensive experimental evidence for synergy of DNA demethylating, and histone deacetylase inhibition, for re-expression of DNA-hypermethylated cancer genes.[28,99,136] However, there are no current FDA approvals for these approaches. Multiple clinical trials have been exploring combination therapies with these agents. Probably, over the next few years, all of these clinical studies will determine the true position of these drugs, and their mechanism of clinical efficacy, in the clinical arena.

Approved uses of IDH mutant inhibitors

Importantly, drugs directly targeting the IDH mutations have been developed, and two years ago, the FDA approved the drug ivosidenib or TIBSOVO, from Agios Pharmaceuticals, for treatment of newly diagnosed AML in patients 75 years or older whose cancers harbor a functional IDH1 mutation as determined by an FDA-approved assay from Abbot Laboratories and who are not able to undergo intensive induction chemotherapy.[80,81]

The use of epigenetic therapy in solid tumors, while less well explored, has been introduced in the past[137,138] and continues to be a major focus of clinical trials with some promising and important results.[19,139] As discussed in many sections of this article, preclinical data suggest the potential of such approaches is as compelling in these cancers as in the hematologic malignancies. For example, recent preclinical studies have investigated how low doses of DNMT inhibitors can affect solid tumor cells and suggest that nanomolar doses of both Vidaza and Dacogen can yield antitumor responses, which may reflect the ability of these drugs to "reprogram" cancer cells with little off-target effects.[140] Such low-dose approaches, plus the availability of new DNA-demethylating agents discussed earlier, and combining these drugs with other epigenetic therapy agents such as histone deacetylase inhibitors (HDACis) and other agents targeting the epigenome are the likely directions to prove high efficacy. For example, combined DNMTis and HDACis in recent trials in 65 patients with advanced, pretreated, non-small-cell lung cancer resulted in robust, durable responses in a small subset.[141] In addition, results in these same trials suggest that the epigenetic therapy could prime a larger group of patients for better responses to subsequent therapies[141] including standard chemotherapies, and immune checkpoint approaches.[142,143] Combining these epigenetic drugs is now being explored in many trials for patients with most common solid tumor types and also hematologic malignancies to improve the efficacy of immune checkpoint inhibitors and to meet major unmet needs to reverse resistance to the latter agents.[99–101] It is certain that, over the next few years, the results of these trials, including those introduce new drugs targeting the epigenome, will determine the efficacy of the strategies and their potential for introducing them into the clinical management of cancer. Examples of the latter, including proteins discussed in the previous sections, include those explore the use of inhibitors of BET proteins and EZH2. In fact, the latter has become the first FDA-approved epigenetic therapy for solid tumors, an uncommon form of soft tissue sarcoma.[144]

Key references

The complete reference list can be found on Vital Source version of this title, see inside front cover.

1. Shen H, Laird PW. Interplay between the cancer genome and epigenome. *Cell*. 2013;**153**(1):38–55.
2. Baylin SB, Jones PA. A decade of exploring the cancer epigenome biological and translational implications. *Nat Rev Cancer*. 2011;**11**(10):726–734.
3. Jones PA, Issa JP, Baylin S. Targeting the cancer epigenome for therapy. *Nat Rev Genet*. 2016;**17**(10):630–641.
5. Allis C, Jenuwein T, Reinberg D, Caparros M. Overview and concepts. In: Caparros M, ed. *Epigenetics*, 2nd ed. New York: Cold Spring Harbor Laboratory Press; 2015.
7. Jones PA. Functions of DNA methylation: islands, start sites, gene bodies and beyond. *Nat Rev Genet*. 2012;**13**(7):484–492.
9. Ohtani H, Liu M, Zhou W, et al. Switching roles for DNA and histone methylation depend on evolutionary ages of human endogenous retroviruses. *Genome Res*. 2018;**28**(8):1147–1157.
12. Kornberg RD, Lorch Y. Twenty-five years of the nucleosome, fundamental particle of the eukaryote chromosome. *Cell*. 1999;**98**(3):285–294.
14. Li E, Zhang Y. DNA methylation in mammals. *Cold Spring Harb Perspect Biol*. 2014;**6**(5):a019133.
15. Bird A. DNA methylation patterns and epigenetic memory. *Genes Dev*. 2002;**16**(1):6–21.
18. de Dieuleveult M, Yen K, Hmitou I, et al. Genome-wide nucleosome specificity and function of chromatin remodellers in ES cells. *Nature*. 2016;**530**(7588):113–116.
20. Zahnow CA, Topper M, Stone M, et al. Inhibitors of DNA methylation, histone deacetylation, and histone demethylation: a perfect combination for cancer therapy. *Adv Cancer Res*. 2016;**130**:55–111.
28. Topper MJ, Vaz M, Chiappinelli KB, et al. Epigenetic therapy ties MYC depletion to reversing immune evasion and treating lung cancer. *Cell*. 2017;**171**(6):1284–1300 e21.
29. Cappellacci L, Perinelli DR, Maggi F, et al. Recent progress in histone deacetylase inhibitors as anticancer agents. *Curr Med Chem*. 2020;**27**(15):2449–2493.
31. Stathis A, Bertoni F. BET proteins as targets for anticancer treatment. *Cancer Discov*. 2018;**8**(1):24–36.
32. Genta S, Pirosa MC, Stathis A. BET and EZH2 inhibitors: novel approaches for targeting cancer. *Curr Oncol Rep*. 2019;**21**(2):13.
33. Dawson MA, Kouzarides T. Cancer epigenetics: from mechanism to therapy. *Cell*. 2012;**150**(1):12–27.
35. Jones PA, Baylin SB. The epigenomics of cancer. *Cell*. 2007;**128**(4):683–692.
40. Feinberg AP, Tycko B. The history of cancer epigenetics. *Nat Rev Cancer*. 2004;**4**(2):143–153.
46. Baylin SB, Ohm JE. Epigenetic gene silencing in cancer – a mechanism for early oncogenic pathway addiction? *Nat Rev Cancer*. 2006;**6**(2):107–116.
47. Ohm JE, McGarvey KM, Yu X, et al. A stem cell-like chromatin pattern may predispose tumor suppressor genes to DNA hypermethylation and heritable silencing. *Nat Genet*. 2007;**39**(2):237–242.
55. Advani SM, Advani P, DeSantis SM, et al. Clinical, pathological, and molecular characteristics of CpG island methylator phenotype in colorectal cancer: a systematic review and meta-analysis. *Transl Oncol*. 2018;**11**(5):1188–1201.
56. Issa JP. CpG island methylator phenotype in cancer. *Nat Rev Cancer*. 2004;**4**(12):988–993.
57. Turcan S, Rohle D, Goenka A, et al. IDH1 mutation is sufficient to establish the glioma hypermethylator phenotype. *Nature*. 2012;**483**(7390):479–483.
60. Cowie P, Hay EA, MacKenzie A. The noncoding human genome and the future of personalised medicine. *Expert Rev Mol Med*. 2015;**17**:e4.
64. Berman BP, Weisenberger DJ, Aman JF, et al. Regions of focal DNA hypermethylation and long-range hypomethylation in colorectal cancer coincide with nuclear lamina-associated domains. *Nat Genet*. 2012;**44**(1):40–46.
70. Schlesinger Y, Straussman R, Keshet I, et al. Polycomb-mediated methylation on Lys27 of histone H3 pre-marks genes for de novo methylation in cancer. *Nat Genet*. 2007;**39**(2):232–236.
71. Widschwendter M, Fiegl H, Egle D, et al. Epigenetic stem cell signature in cancer. *Nat Genet*. 2007;**39**(2):157–158.
74. Di Leva G, Garofalo M, Croce CM. MicroRNAs in cancer. *Annu Rev Pathol*. 2014;**9**:287–314.
77. Yan H, Parsons DW, Jin G, et al. IDH1 and IDH2 mutations in gliomas. *N Engl J Med*. 2009;**360**(8):765–773.
80. DiNardo CD, Stein EM, de Botton S, et al. Durable remissions with ivosidenib in IDH1-mutated relapsed or refractory AML. *N Engl J Med*. 2018;**378**(25):2386–2398.
82. Issa JP. Aging and epigenetic drift: a vicious cycle. *J Clin Invest*. 2014;**124**(1):24–29.
92. Nacev BA, Feng L, Bagert JD, et al. The expanding landscape of 'oncohistone' mutations in human cancers. *Nature*. 2019;**567**(7749):473–478.
94. Lewis PW, Muller MM, Koletsky MS, et al. Inhibition of PRC2 activity by a gain-of-function H3 mutation found in pediatric glioblastoma. *Science (New York, NY)*. 2013;**340**(6134):857–861.
96. Chiappinelli KB, Strissel PL, Desrichard A, et al. Inhibiting DNA methylation causes an interferon response in cancer via dsRNA including endogenous retroviruses. *Cell*. 2015;**162**(5):974–986.
97. Roulois D, Loo Yau H, Singhania R, et al. DNA-demethylating agents target colorectal cancer cells by inducing viral mimicry by endogenous transcripts. *Cell*. 2015;**162**(5):961–973.
98. Stone ML, Chiappinelli KB, Li H, et al. Epigenetic therapy activates type I interferon signaling in murine ovarian cancer to reduce immunosuppression and tumor burden. *Proc Natl Acad Sci USA*. 2017;**114**(51):E10981–E10990.
99. Topper MJ, Vaz M, Marrone KA, et al. The emerging role of epigenetic therapeutics in immuno-oncology. *Nat Rev Clin Oncol*. 2020;**17**(2):75–90.
100. Topalian SL, Taube JM, Anders RA, Pardoll DM. Mechanism-driven biomarkers to guide immune checkpoint blockade in cancer therapy. *Nat Rev Cancer*. 2016;**16**(5):275–287.

101 Demaria O, Cornen S, Daëron M, et al. Harnessing innate immunity in cancer therapy. *Nature*. 2019;**574**(7776):45–56.
102 Youngblood B, Hale JS, Ahmed R. T-cell memory differentiation: insights from transcriptional signatures and epigenetics. *Immunology*. 2013;**139**(3):277–284.
104 Blank CU, Haining WN, Held W, et al. Defining 'T cell exhaustion'. *Nat Rev Immunol*. 2019;**19**(11):665–674.
106 Laird PW. The power and the promise of DNA methylation markers. *Nat Rev Cancer*. 2003;**3**(4):253–266.
112 Horvath S, Raj K. DNA methylation-based biomarkers and the epigenetic clock theory of ageing. *Nat Rev Genet*. 2018;**19**(6):371–384.
116 Tepus M, Yau TO. Non-invasive colorectal cancer screening: an overview. *Gastrointest. Tumors*. 2020;**7**(3):62–73.
119 Uhr A, Glick L, Gomella LG. An overview of biomarkers in the diagnosis and management of prostate cancer. *Can J Urol*. 2020;**27**(S3):24–27.
120 Hegi ME, Diserens AC, Gorlia T, et al. MGMT gene silencing and benefit from temozolomide in glioblastoma. *N Engl J Med*. 2005;**352**(10):997–1003.
124 Stomper J, Rotondo JC, Greve G, Lübbert M. Hypomethylating agents (HMA) for the treatment of acute myeloid leukemia and myelodysplastic syndromes: mechanisms of resistance and novel HMA-based therapies. *Leukemia*. 2021;**6**:1–7.
125 Daher-Reyes GS, Merchan BM, Yee KWL. Guadecitabine (SGI-110): an investigational drug for the treatment of myelodysplastic syndrome and acute myeloid leukemia. *Expert Opin Investig Drugs*. 2019;**28**(10):835–849.
127 Wei AH, Döhner H, Pocock C, et al. Oral azacitidine maintenance therapy for acute myeloid leukemia in first remission. *N Engl J Med*. 2020;**383**(26):2526–2537.
128 Short NJ, Konopleva M, Kadia TM, et al. Advances in the treatment of acute myeloid leukemia: new drugs and new challenges. *Cancer Discov*. 2020;**10**(4):506–525.
130 Issa JP. Optimizing therapy with methylation inhibitors in myelodysplastic syndromes: dose, duration, and patient selection. *Nat Clin Pract Oncol*. 2005;**2**(Suppl 1):S24–S29.
131 Guo Y, Liu B, Deng L, et al. The efficacy and adverse events of venetoclax in combination with hypomethylating agents treatment for patients with acute myeloid leukemia and myelodysplastic syndrome: a systematic review and meta-analysis. *Hematology (Amsterdam, Netherlands)*. 2020;**25**(1):414–423.
132 Winters AC, Gutman JA, Purev E, et al. Real-world experience of venetoclax with azacitidine for untreated patients with acute myeloid leukemia. *Blood Adv*. 2019;**3**(20):2911–2919.
133 Ho TCS, Chan AHY, Ganesan A. Thirty years of HDAC inhibitors: 2020 insight and hindsight. *J Med Chem*. 2020;**63**(21):12460–12484.
136 Cameron EE, Bachman KE, Myohanen S, et al. Synergy of demethylation and histone deacetylase inhibition in the re-expression of genes silenced in cancer. *Nat Genet*. 1999;**21**(1):103–107.
140 Tsai HC, Li H, Van Neste L, et al. Transient low doses of DNA-demethylating agents exert durable antitumor effects on hematological and epithelial tumor cells. *Cancer Cell*. 2012;**21**(3):430–446.
141 Juergens RA, Wrangle J, Vendetti FP, et al. Combination epigenetic therapy has efficacy in patients with refractory advanced non-small cell lung cancer. *Cancer Discov*. 2011;**1**(7):598–607.
142 Brahmer JR, Tykodi SS, Chow LQ, et al. Safety and activity of anti-PD-L1 antibody in patients with advanced cancer. *N Engl J Med*. 2012;**366**(26):2455–2465.
143 Topalian SL, Hodi FS, Brahmer JR, et al. Safety, activity, and immune correlates of anti-PD-1 antibody in cancer. *N Engl J Med*. 2012;**366**(26):2443–2454.
144 Rothbart SB, Baylin SB. Epigenetic therapy for epithelioid sarcoma. *Cell*. 2020;**181**(2):211.

7 Cancer genomics and evolution*

William P. D. Hendricks, PhD ■ Aleksandar Sekulic, MD, PhD ■ Alan H. Bryce, MD ■ Muhammed Murtaza, MBBS, PhD ■ Pilar Ramos, PhD ■ Jessica D. Lang, PhD ■ Timothy G. Whitsett, PhD ■ Timothy K. McDaniel, PhD ■ Russell C. Rockne, PhD ■ Nicholas Banovich, PhD ■ Jeffrey M. Trent, PhD

Overview

Over 100 years ago, the Nobel Prize for Physiology and Medicine was given to Paul Ehrlich for postulating that "magic bullets" could specifically target and kill cells such as cancer cells based on their unique molecular features. The completed Human Genome Project and the cancer genomics revolution have now mapped many of the genetic changes underlying the unique features of common malignancies. Although cancer has long been recognized to be heterogeneous in its clinical presentation, course, pathology, and response to therapy, we now recognize that it is far more molecularly heterogeneous than anticipated and that such variability will require an individualized approach to patient care. Rather than a single magic bullet, we need an arsenal requiring precise delivery. While inter- and intratumoral genomic heterogeneity present significant challenges to cancer management and drug development, a number of developments foster hope for accelerated progress in the war on cancer. First, our catalogue of genomic targets underlying diverse cancers is rapidly growing. Second, we are beginning to understand how diverse mutations converge on a small number of druggable pathways. Third, we continue to develop drugs and biologic agents (e.g., immune checkpoint inhibitors) that target an increasingly diverse array of genomic subtypes of cancer. Finally, advances in "next-generation" sequencing technologies now enable far earlier detection of disease and disease recurrence. This article focuses on these developments and how their integration is aiding in the precise delivery of "magic bullets."

Precis

Cancer is a genetic disease in which the stepwise accumulation of oncogene and tumor suppressor gene mutations in clonally expanding cell populations drives malignant transformation and progression. Throughout the twentieth century, overwhelming evidence accumulated in support of this model, while a growing understanding of the mutations underlying cancer subtypes helped to guide innovation in clinical cancer management. The genomics revolution begun in the twenty-first century has now transformed our understanding of cancer by generating exhaustive catalogues of cancer-driving mutations and identifying the vast genomic diversity existing between and within individual tumors. These data are enabling targeted drug development, genomics-guided clinical management, and new approaches to early disease detection. Yet, gaps nonetheless remain in our knowledge of the causative mutations underlying some cancers, in our understanding of the biology of the mutations we have identified, in developing drugs

*William P. D. Hendricks and Aleksandar Sekulic are contributed equally to this work.

capable of targeting many of these diverse mutations, in shifting mutational profiles across progression and metastasis, and in fending off the inevitable emergence of drug resistance. In this article, we review the history and methods of cancer genetics and genomics, summarize the current knowledge of the spectrum of mutations in cancers, discuss the emerging concepts in cancer evolution and genomic heterogeneity, discuss the emergence of immunotherapy and its role combating genomic diversity, and present a case study on the clinical impact of melanoma genomics.

Introduction

As detailed in previous articles, cancer is a genetic disease resulting from the stepwise accumulation of mutations that confer upon cells a selective growth advantage.[1] Such mutations alter the birth and death rates of cells as well as the genomic stability of cells as they undergo waves of clonal expansion. With the accumulation of mutations in cancer genes, cell populations acquire increasingly malignant phenotypes in successive generations. These hallmark cancer phenotypes include sustained proliferation, evasion of growth suppression, evasion of the immune system, promotion of inflammation, activation of invasion and metastasis, induction of genomic instability, immortal replication, induction of angiogenesis, deregulation of cellular energetics, and resistance to cell death.[2] Cancer genes in which mutation confers a growth advantage are classified as oncogenes or tumor suppressor genes. Oncogenes, when activated through mutation, often in recurrent hotspots, drive constitutive activation of cell-signaling pathways, accelerating the cell birth rate. Tumor suppressor genes, when mutationally silenced or inactivated, are no longer able to promote cell death and thereby decrease the cell death rate. This model has been well characterized in colorectal cancer in which mutations in the *APC* tumor suppressor have been shown in most cases to drive adenoma formation. Additional mutations in cancer genes (e.g., oncogenic *RAS*) comprising proliferative, cell cycle, and apoptosis pathways then result in the formation of malignant tumors capable of invasion and metastasis.[3,4] Additional cancers have also been shown to follow this model, although we now know that there are many disparate evolutionary paths to malignancy even within the same cancer type (Figure 1).

While some mutations in cancer genes occur in the germline and are heritable, the majority (90%) arise sporadically in somatic tissues over an individual's lifetime (i.e., they are tumor specific) due to replication error, genotoxic stress, and/or environmental damage.[5] These mutations may result from subtle sequence alterations (single-base substitutions and insertions or deletions of one or a few bases), changes in chromosome copy number

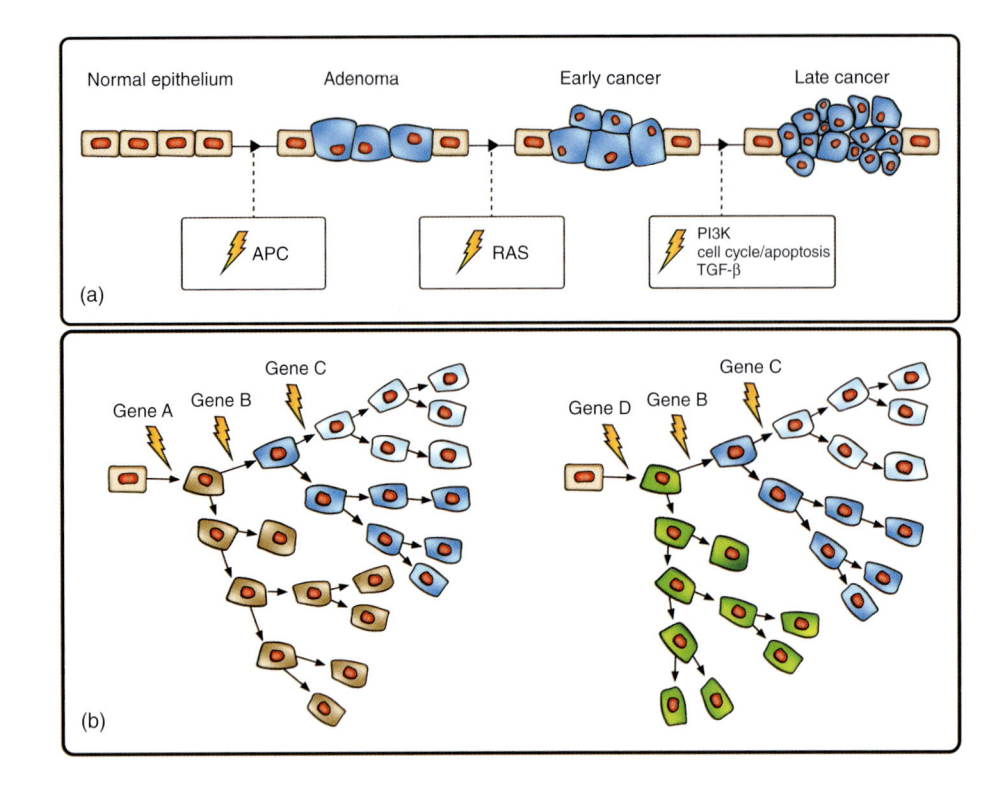

Figure 1 Cancer results from the stepwise accumulation of diverse, branching mutations. (a) "Vogelgram" model of progressive development of colorectal cancer.[3] Inactivation of the tumor suppressor *APC* is commonly observed in colorectal cancer precursor lesions. Subsequent mutational activation of the *RAS* oncogene is associated with transition from early adenoma to early cancer. Progressive accumulation of molecular alterations eventually leads to a malignant tumor that can invade the basement membrane and metastasize to lymph nodes and distant organs. (b) Expanded model depicting disparate cancer-initiating mutations as well as stepwise branching evolution in which cells accumulate secondary mutations followed by clonal expansion leading to both inter- and intratumoral heterogeneity.

(amplification, deletion, chromosome loss, or duplication), or changes in chromosome structure (inter- and intrachromosomal translocation, inversion, or other types of rearrangement). For the remainder of this article, we refer to these alterations as somatic single-nucleotide variants (SNVs), copy number variants (CNVs), or structural variants (SVs). Classic examples of SNVs, CNVs, and SVs are shown in Figure 2 and include an activating missense SNV in *NRAS* (one of the most commonly mutated oncogenes), an inactivating homozygous deletion CNV in one of the most commonly inactivated tumor suppressors *TP53*, and an activating translocation SV involving *BCR* and *ABL*. Epigenomic modifications of cancer genes can also significantly alter gene function. These modifications of DNA, while not altering the DNA sequence itself, can include DNA methylation changes, chromatin modifications, and noncoding RNA-dependent gene regulation that may be heritable and play a role in tumorigenesis. These increasingly important areas, intensely aided by "next-generation" sequencing technologies, will be discussed in other articles. We focus here on DNA sequence-altering mutations.[6–9] In this article, we use specific examples to highlight the state of cancer genomics knowledge by describing the current methods in genomic analysis, compiling results from landmark cancer genomic studies, assessing the role of cancer evolution in determining its clinical management, and introducing the interaction of immunotherapy interacts with cancer genomics and evolution. We then conclude with a detailed case study of melanoma genomics, evolution, and genomics-guided medicine.

The history and methods of cancer genomics

The early history of cancer genetics

The elucidation of cancer's genetic etiology and mapping the breadth of its diversity has paralleled seminal advances in genetics and genetic technology (Figure 3a). Many landmark studies in the late nineteenth to early twentieth century laid the groundwork for cancer genomics—development of the theory of evolution by natural selection,[10] discovery of heritable biological units,[11] identification of chromosomes,[12] chromosomal heredity[13,14] and chromosomal genes,[15] and modern evolutionary synthesis linking biology, genetics, and evolutionary theory.[16] The subsequent discovery of DNA's structure then provided a framework for understanding the genetic code and the mechanism for molecular transmission of genetic information.[17] Meanwhile, reports of heritable breast and colorectal cancers had arisen,[18] and the causal nature of the chemical, physical, and biological agents such as coal tar,[19] cigarette smoke,[20] radiation,[21] and viruses[22] was increasingly identified in specific cancer types. Discovery that these carcinogenic agents were also mutagenic drove speculation that cancer was a disease of mutation. Ultimately, although cancer had been suggested by some to be a chromosomal disease or a disease of mutation, the concept of cancer as a genetic disease did not gain traction until later in the twentieth century when cytogenetic and sequencing technology alongside experimental transformation of normal cell lines with oncogenes enabled assessment of cancer gene mutations at the molecular level and establishment of their

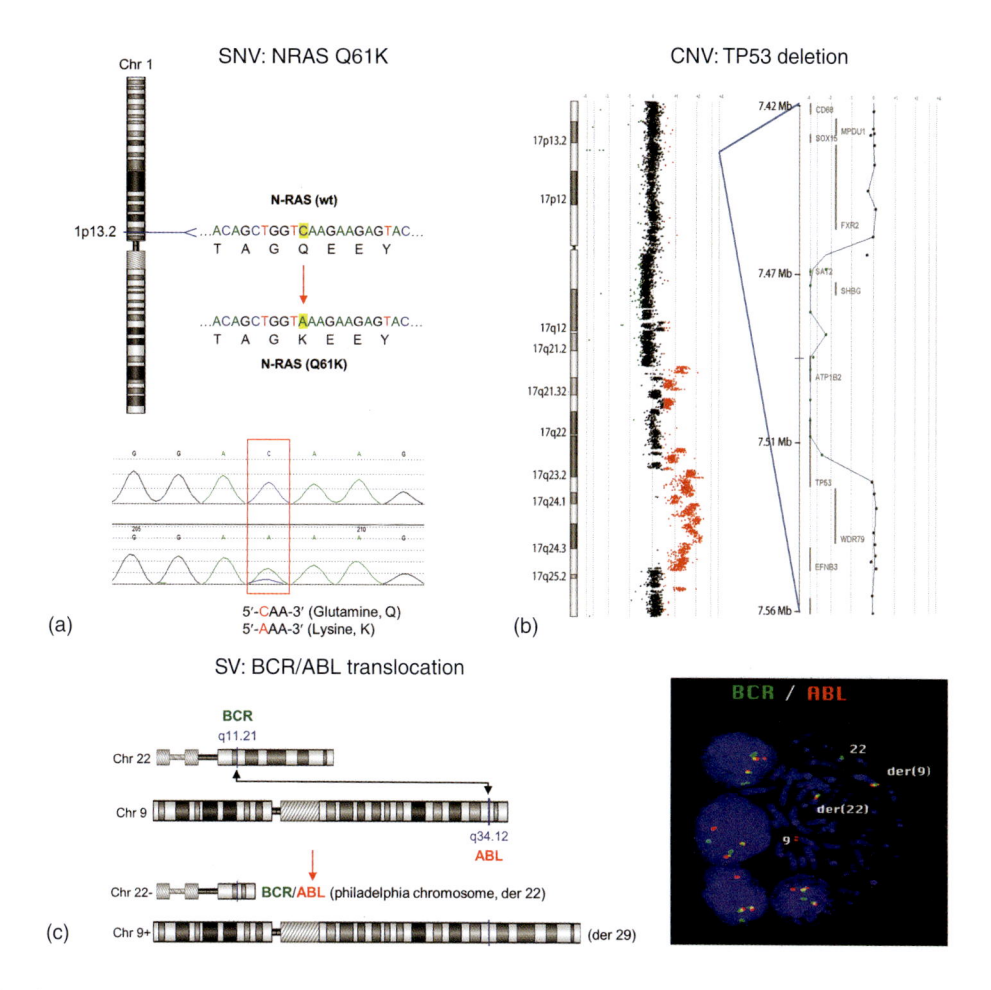

Figure 2 Examples of cancer mutation types. (a) The *NRAS* oncogene, located on chromosome 1, is commonly mutationally activated in diverse cancers. An SNV results in a codon alteration and substitution of glutamine (Q) for lysine (K) at amino acid 61—Q61K (top figure). Shown below is the chromatogram from Sanger sequencing analysis of a tumor sample harboring the *NRAS* Q61K mutation. (b) CGH log2 ratio data are plotted for chromosome 17 (left) as well as a focal region of homozygous deletion with a breakpoint within the TP53 tumor suppressor (right). Regions of DNA copy loss are plotted to the left of the axis, and regions of gain are plotted to the right. Individual log2 ratio data (dots) and log2 ratio moving average (line) are shown. (c) Schematic of the DNA translocation that occurs between the genes *BCR* and *ABL*, leading to the formation of the *BCR–ABL* gene fusion known as the Philadelphia chromosome (left). Shown on the right is inter- and metaphase FISH detection of the *t* (9;22) BCR–ABL gene fusion using fluorescently labeled genomic probes for *BCR* (green) and *ABL* (red). Note that the fusion of *BCR* and *ABL* probes results in a yellow signal indicating colocalization of the red and green probes as a result of the *t* (9;22). The BCR–ABL micrograph is the courtesy of Dr. Susana Raimondi of St. Jude Children's Research Hospital.

causal role in tumorigenesis. Some of these landmark studies are shown in Figure 3a.

Molecular cytogenetics: identification of recurrent chromosomal alterations in cancer

Mid-twentieth century developments in the field of cytogenetics such as chromosome staining in fixed leukocytes from peripheral blood finally enabled empirical observation of the chromosomal complement of a cell.[23,24] Using this approach, Nowell was the first to discover a specific recurrent genetic change associated with a cancer type—the "Philadelphia chromosome" fragment in nearly all evaluated cases of chronic myelogenous leukemia (CML).[25] Over a decade later, Rowley then used chromosome banding to map the components of this fragment, determining the Philadelphia chromosome to be a balanced reciprocal translocation between chromosomes 9 and 22.[26,27] These discoveries drove a search for recurrent structural aberrations both within and across cancer types. This led to the identification of characteristic translocations in sarcomas, leukemias, and lymphomas. However, most carcinomas were found to possess few recurrent alterations, instead displaying great variety in the number and type of chromosome aberrations.[28]

After Nowell and Rowley's discoveries, rapid innovation in chromosomal banding and tools using spectral karyotyping (SKY) allowed progressively detailed views of chromosome aberrations in cancer cells using techniques based on fluorescence *in situ* hybridization (FISH) using fluorescent DNA probes that hybridize to specific chromosomal regions.[29–38] Approaches for genome-wide cytogenetic analysis have also been developed including SKY,[29] multiplex FISH (M-FISH),[39] chromosome microdissection,[38] and comparative genomic hybridization (CGH).[40] CGH is a particularly powerful fluorescent molecular cytogenetic technique for screening genome-wide chromosomal copy number changes in tumor genomes (Table 1).

Novel approaches for printing nucleic acids on slides (microarrays) soon revolutionized molecular cytogenetics by reducing cost and increasing throughput. Array CGH (aCGH) originally involved spotting large probes (large-insert clones or artificial chromosomes)[41,42] onto slides in intervals (1–3 Mb resolution) across chromosomal regions. This was replaced by high-resolution, genome-wide platforms consisting of small,

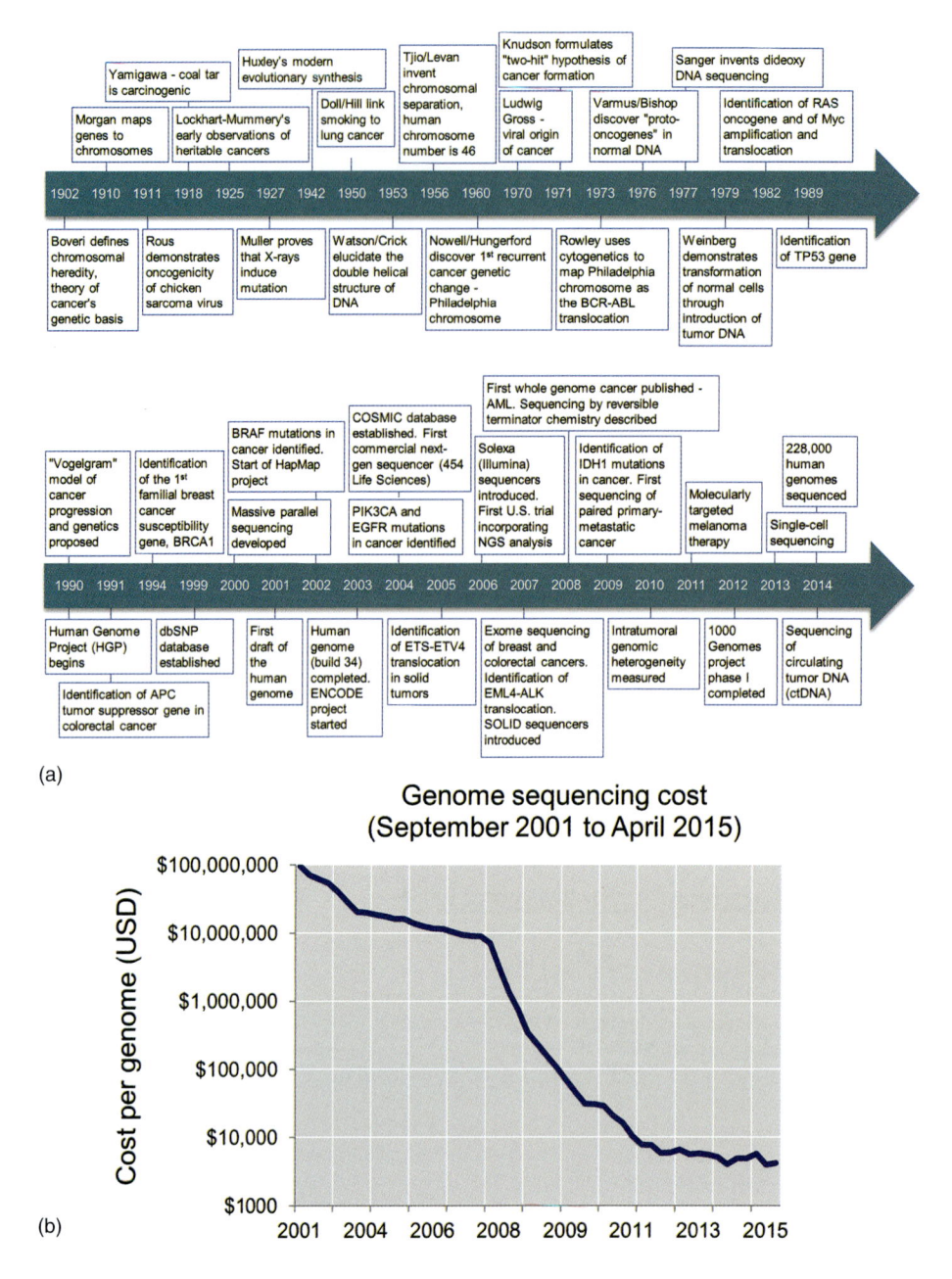

Figure 3 The history of cancer genomics. (a) Timeline of landmark studies in cancer genetics and genomics from Boveri's formulation of the chromosomally aberrant nature of cancer in 1902 to the advent of 228,000 human genomes sequenced in 2014. (b) Cost of sequencing a 3000-Mb genome (i.e., the size of the human genome) over time. Source: Data from the NHGRI Genome Sequencing Program (Wetterstrand KA; see http://www.genome.gov/sequencingcosts/).

customizable oligonucleotide probes[43,44] that demonstrated increased throughput and sensitivity in characterizing cancers such as breast,[45–47] melanoma,[48–50] and B-cell lymphoma.[51,52] Similarly, oligonucleotide arrays designed to genotype thousands of single-nucleotide polymorphisms (SNPs) are useful for characterizing tumor genome complexity with rapid genotyping of over millions of SNPs now possible (Affymetrix, Illumina). Similar to CGH arrays, SNP arrays quantitate locus-specific hybridization signals and can be used to estimate copy number or loss of heterozygosity (LOH).[53–55] Notable cancer studies incorporating SNP arrays include genotyping of the NCI-60 cell line panel[56] as well as lung cancer,[57] acute myeloid leukemia (AML),[55,58] neuroblastoma,[59] melanoma,[56,60,61] basal cell carcinoma,[54] breast cancer,[62] colorectal cancer,[62–64] glioblastoma,[65,66] and pancreatic cancer.[67]

Both SVs and CNVs can be characterized using the tools of molecular cytogenetics and cytogenomics. Translocations are some of the most common SVs observed in cancer and, as in the case of the Philadelphia chromosome in CML, are signature aberrations for many liquid cancers and sarcomas. They involve the movement of a chromosomal segment from one position to another, either within the same chromosome (intra-chromosomal) or a different chromosome (interchromosomal). Other types of SVs include chromosomal deletions, duplications, inversions, insertions, rings, and isochromosomes. These SVs may result from errors in double-stranded break (DSB) repair or other means of intra- or interchromosomal recombination.[68] Translocations and other SVs can either activate oncogenes (such as when the *ABL* tyrosine kinase is constitutively activated by fusion with the *BCR* gene) or inactivate tumor suppressor genes (such as when

Table 1 Glossary.

Term	Definition
Array comparative genomic hybridization (CGH)	Microarray platform optimized to identify genome-wide DNA copy number changes
Chromothripsis	Phenomenon by which extensive chromosomal rearrangements occur in a single event in one or a few chromosomes
Copy number variant (CNV)	Change in DNA copy number such as amplification or deletion relative to a reference sequence
Driver mutation	A mutation that confers a selective growth advantage on the cell in which it occurs
Epigenomics	Global study of epigenetic changes throughout the genome
Exome sequencing	Application of NGS for the parallel sequencing of many exons (coding areas of the genome)
Fluorescence in situ hybridization (FISH)	Cytogenetic technique for detecting specific DNA sequences on chromosomes using fluorescent probes
Gene expression array	Oligonucleotide microarray platform designed to probe for the transcriptome-wide abundance of RNA messages
Genomics	Study of the structure, function, evolution, and sequence of genomes
Germline mutation	Mutation in the germ cell lineage present in all cells of the body and transmitted to offspring
Loss of heterozygosity	Loss of the normal, functional allele at a heterozygous locus via deletion or other mutational event
Massively parallel sequencing (also known as next-generation sequencing or NGS)	High-throughput sequencing methodologies based on simultaneous sequencing of large numbers of genes or entire genomes
Mutational hills	Mutations that occur at low frequency
Mutational mountains	Mutations such as BRAF V600E that are frequent in a single cancer type or across multiple cancer types
Single-nucleotide polymorphism (SNP) array	Microarray platform that probes for genome-wide SNPs used to characterize allelic variation, LOH, or CNVs in cancers
Oncogene	Gene which, when activated by mutations, promotes cancerous phenotype
Passenger mutation	A mutation that does not confer a selective growth advantage to the cell in which it occurs
Sanger sequencing	An approach for targeted DNA sequencing of individual genes or sets of genes using dideoxy chain termination and agarose gel electrophoresis
Single-nucleotide polymorphism (SNP)	Single-nucleotide sequence difference occurring in germlines of individuals across populations
Single-nucleotide variant (SNV)	Change in the DNA sequence relative to a reference sequence including point mutations and small insertions and deletions
Somatic mutation	Mutation acquired after conception in a subset of cells (e.g., in a cancer)
Structural variant (SV)	Structural DNA change rearrangement translocations, inversions, and so on
Transcriptomics	Study of all RNA transcripts in a cell or population of cells
Tumor suppressor	A gene safeguarding cellular processes that, when inactivated, facilitates oncogenesis

translocations involving the *TP53* tumor suppressor interrupt the gene and lead to loss of function). CNVs involving a gain or loss of an entire chromosome are some of the simplest and most common chromosomal aberrations and result from defective chromosomal segregation. The functional consequence of CNVs can be difficult to establish because the aberrations may extend over tens of thousands of megabases and may affect hundreds to thousands of genes. It has been easier to establish the cancer relevance of more limited regions of chromosomal gain and loss, created by amplification or deletion, as these smaller aberrations have been shown to alter the dosage of known oncogenes or tumor suppressor genes. Classic examples of oncogene amplification in solid tumors discovered through molecular cytogenetics include *ERBB2* in breast cancers and *MYC* in a variety of tumor types, while loss of specific regions of the genome is often associated with loss of tumor suppressor genes such as *TP53*, *RB1*, *PTEN*, and *CDKN2A*. Inactivation of the remaining normal allele of carriers with inherited mutations of *RB1*, *BRCA1*, *BRCA2*, *TP53*, and *PTPRJ*, or in somatic cancer cells that have acquired mutations in one allele of these genes, is critical for the promotion of tumorigenesis.

Molecular genetics: identification of recurrent sequence alterations in cancer

While some molecular cytogenetic techniques are capable of detecting chromosomal breakpoints at base pair resolution, advances in molecular genetics were required to allow detection of subtle sequence changes in DNA itself. These advances were enabled by developments in molecular cloning and the invention of the polymerase chain reaction (PCR) capable of generating the millions of DNA copies necessary for detection of these mutations.[69] Coupled with the Sanger sequencing method based on dideoxynucleotide chain termination and agarose gel electrophoresis,[70] progressive advances in this methodology, including fluorescently labeled nucleotides, capillary electrophoresis, paired-end sequencing, shotgun sequencing, and improved laboratory automation, have allowed scaling required to sequence entire genomes. This technology enabled the Human Genome Project (HGP), launched in 1990 as a $3 billion, publicly funded, international collaboration. The rough draft of the human genome, covering 94% of the genome, was published in 2001[71,72] with the complete draft finished ahead of schedule in 2003.[73] In addition to establishing genome-wide ground truth for the locations, organization, and sequences of all human genes, the technical and informatic lessons learned in the course of this project enabled the initial ambitious cancer mutation screens on the level of entire gene families[74–77] and the majority of the protein-coding genome.[62,66,67] Nonetheless, genome sequencing projects using Sanger-based sequencing techniques continued to be expensive and logistically challenging and thereby limited the application of this approach toward large-scale characterization of cancer genomes until the advent of massively parallel sequencing.

Gene expression microarrays: cancer signatures and pathways

Microarrays such as those employed in aCGH studies were originally developed for high-throughput gene expression studies. Complementary DNA (cDNA formed from reverse transcription of RNA) and later oligonucleotide microarrays were implemented in high-throughput quantitation of mRNA transcripts. Advances in this technology paralleled improvements in automated Sanger sequencing in the 1990s and through the turn of the millennium.

They provided some of the initial insights into gene signatures and pathways correlating to specific cancer subtypes. A parallel method, serial analysis of gene expression (SAGE), was developed to enable high-throughput digital quantitation of transcripts.[78] While originally designed to assay the expression of individual genes, gene expression profiling methods were later adapted to profile and map global transcription at the exon and genome levels[79] as well as to profile the expression of mature human microRNAs (miRNAs).[80] Gene expression patterns have been widely used to subclassify cancers into homogeneous entities not easily discernable using traditional histopathologic or cytogenetic techniques, for instance, in diffuse large B-cell lymphoma (DLBCL),[81,82] lung cancer,[83] melanoma,[84] and breast cancer.[85,86] Certain subgroups have been shown to represent distinct disease states with differing outcomes and responding differently to standard therapies. Gene expression profiles have also been widely mined to specifically identify sets of genes predictive of disease progression, response to therapy, or metastasis,[87–89] as well as the presence of specific recurrent cytogenetic abnormalities,[90–92] or gene mutations.[93–96] Although advances in massively parallel sequencing have largely supplanted microarrays in sensitivity and robustness, if not cost and clinical readiness, gene expression profiling continues to play a significant role in cancer biology and medicine. In fact, commercially available clinical tests based on microarray signatures (OncoType DX and MammaPrint) are available for breast cancer profiling.

Massively parallel sequencing: charting cancer genome landscapes

Explosive growth in our understanding of cancer genomics has been built on the backbone of the advances that emerged from the completion of the human genome at the turn of the twenty-first century. Although these advances had driven the cost of one genome down from an estimated $1 billion to the $1 million mark at the time of the HGP's completion, this extraordinary cost nonetheless held back large-scale genomic studies[97] and the application of genomic sequencing to individual patients. Thus, beginning in the 2000s, the National Human Genome Research Institute (NHGRI) initiated a $70 million sequencing technology program intended to drive the price down toward the $1000 mark. The cost of a human genome sequence now lies slightly below $1000 (Figure 3b).

The quest for the $1000 genome required a fundamental rethinking of the approach to DNA sequencing. Sanger sequencing, even in its most expert execution, faced insurmountable bottlenecks including (1) the need for molecular cloning steps and/or individual PCRs to generate sequencing templates and (2) the fact that every sequencing reaction can only accommodate a relatively small genomic region. Therefore, cloning/amplifying and sequencing many regions, even when run in parallel with the most efficient automation, requires large amounts of labor, materials, equipment, and analysis time. The paradigm shift in sequencing cost and throughput was brought about by the invention of approaches that allowed the generation of sequencing templates without cloning or individual PCRs, immobilization of entire sequencing libraries in a single reaction chamber, and massively parallel sequencing of millions (and with today's advances billions) of templates in that chamber. The ability of this approach to sequence clones derived from single DNA molecules additionally provides great power for detection of rare variants from heterogeneous tumor samples. These rapid, accurate, and inexpensive approaches are also referred to as next-generation sequencing (NGS).

The key inventions in the 1990s and early 2000s such as sequencing-by-synthesis, pyrosequencing, colony sequencing, and emulsion PCR enabled the development of the first NGS platforms.[98–101] The first such platform was described by Lynx Therapeutics (later acquired by Solexa) in 2000, although it did not achieve widespread adoption.[102] 454 Life Sciences offered the first commercially available system—the 454 FLX Pyrosequencer—in 2004,[103] followed by Solexa's (now Illumina) Genome Analyzer in 2006[104] and Applied Biosystems' Supported Oligonucleotide Ligation and Detection (SOLiD) System in 2007 that also incorporated colony sequencing.[105,106] The Solexa system was used in 2008 to sequence James Watson's genome within a single laboratory in only 2 months.[107] These platforms at last made the possibility of sequencing and assembling multiple cancer genomes a reality as evidenced by the characterization of genome-wide SVs in two lung cancer genomes.[108] This study utilized a paired-end approach, demonstrating strikingly complex genomic rearrangements including those resulting in previously unreported fusion transcripts. Importantly, this study also demonstrated that DNA copy number can be estimated by the relative local abundance of genomic fragments sequenced, providing sensitivity comparable to aCGH platforms while at the same time providing DNA sequence information. Massively parallel sequencing methods have now dramatically decreased the cost of sequencing while greatly increasing the throughput. Presently, sequencing of 6 trillion bases (e.g., sequencing equivalent to 1872 human genomes or 1872X average genome coverage) within a single 2-day commercial instrument run is standard, with throughput still steadily increasing.

Many massively parallel sequencing platforms exist today and are reviewed in more detail elsewhere.[109] Table 2 provides an overview of some of the most common platforms in use today. They have been adapted to a variety of purposes ranging from diverse DNA sequence, copy number, and structural analyses to transcriptomics and epigenomics. While sequencing the entire genome is routinely performed, it is not always necessary or informative to do so, and thus, a number of targeted strategies have been conceived that enable more cost-effective and focused analyses. New enrichment methods using nucleic acid hybridization or PCR to select the desired regions of the genome prior to sequencing are common.[110–113] A relatively small fraction of the human genome has been functionally characterized, and therefore, it is often most expedient to assess the <2% of the genome containing coding regions (all exons—aka the exome). Thus, a number of commercially available human exome and other targeted capture kits (such as panels of common cancer genes) are available. This ability to target specific genes to enable rapid, accurate, and affordable sequencing is aiding not only in biological discovery but also in clinical laboratory testing.

Cancer genome landscapes

Landmark cancer genomic studies

Enabled by such high-throughput technologies, the genomic studies of the past decade have provided a surprisingly complex view of human cancer. The first large-scale cancer mutation screens implemented high-throughput Sanger sequencing of individual genes such as *BRAF* in large cohorts[114,115] or focused on gene families such as protein kinases in diverse cancer types.[74–77,116,117] Notably, such early screens led to the identification of activating *BRAF* mutations in a large percentage of human melanomas[114] and

Table 2 Selected massively parallel sequencing platforms.

Company	System platform[a]	Release	Template prep.	Seq. chemistry	Max. read length	Bases per run (Gb)	Accuracy	Run time	Application
Illumina	Illumina NovaSeq 6000	2017	Emulsion PCR	Reversible terminator	250	6000	>99%	13–44 h	WGS, E-S, RNA-S, T-S, C-S, MG
	Illumina NextSeq 2000	2020	Solid-phase	Reversible terminator	300	300	>99%	2 days	E-S, RNA-S, T-S, C-S, MG, Microbial WGS
	Illumina NextSeq 550	2015	Solid-phase	Reversible terminator	150	120	>99%	30 h	E-S, RNA-S, T-S, C-S, MG, Microbial WGS
	Illumina MiSeq	2014	Solid-phase	Reversible terminator	600	15	>99%	4–55 h	T-S, C-S, DN-S
	Illumina MiniSeq	2016	Solid-phase	Reversible terminator	200	7.5	>99%	4–24 h	DN-S, T-S
	Illumina iSeq 100	2018	Solid-phase	Reversible terminator	300	1.2	>99%	9.5–19 h	DN-S, T-S
Thermo fisher scientific	Ion torrent GeneXus	2019	Emulsion PCR	Proton detection	400	6	>99%	24 h	DN-S, T-S
	Ion GeneStudio S5	2018	Emulsion PCR	Proton detection	600	15–50	>99%	6.5–19 h	DN-S, T-S
PacBio	Sequel	2015	Single molecule	Real-time sequencing	30,000	20	>99%	20 h	DN-S, T-S, RNA-S
	Sequel II	2019	Single molecule	Real-time sequencing	20,000	160	>99.9%	30 h	DN-S, T-S, RNA-S
Oxford nanopore technologies	PromethION	2018	PCR or no-PCR liquid phase	Nanopore ion	Variable (up to 2,000,000)	8600	>99.99%	<72 h	WGS, E-S, RNA-S, T-S, C-S, MG
	GridION	2017	PCR or no-PCR liquid phase	Nanopore ion	Variable (up to 2,000,000)	150	>99.99%	<48 h	WGS, E-S, RNA-S, T-S, C-S, MG
	MinION	2015	PCR or no-PCR liquid phase	Nanopore ion	Variable (up to 2,000,000)	30	>99.99%	<48 h	E-S, RNA-S, T-S, C-S, MG

WGS, whole-genome sequencing; E-S, exome sequencing; RNA-S, RNA-sequencing; T-S, targeted sequencing; C-S, ChIP-sequencing; MG, metagenomics; DN-S, *de novo* sequencing.
There are many companies developing novel platforms that are or will become available in the near future.
[a]Additional versions are available for some models.

nevi[118] as well as *ERBB2* mutations in human breast cancer.[117] The first cancer exomes were completed in 140 AML samples in 2003.[119] This study identified six previously described and, strikingly, seven previously unknown coding mutations in AML genomes. Soon after, the results of Sanger-based exome sequencing of 13,023 genes in 11 breast and 11 colorectal cancers were published in 2006.[120] This study revealed a total of 189 frequently mutated genes with an average of 90 mutant genes per tumor, although only a subset were thought to be causally related to tumorigenesis or progression (an average of 11 per tumor). In a follow-up analysis of an additional 7000 genes in the same tumors, it was confirmed that a handful of commonly mutated genes (the "mountains" in the genomic landscape) existed among a large number of less-frequently mutated "hills." In 2008, four Sanger-based exome projects additionally characterized over 20,000 genes in glioblastoma multiforme (GBM)[62,66,67] and pancreatic cancer.[67] Amidst an average of 63 and 47 mutations per pancreatic tumor or glioblastoma, these studies identified novel genes bearing low-frequency but recurrent mutations in such genes as *IDH1* and *PIK3R1* in glioblastoma. Strikingly, these studies uncovered few unknown genes recurrently mutated at high rates. In these and future studies, it was found that the frequently mutated mountains of cancer had already largely been identified using the low-throughput genetic technologies of the past decades. The growing challenge has since been interpretation and characterization of the many hills. Lending some order to this confusion, these studies all show that multiple genes within core signaling pathways, rather than single genes, tend to be mutated in these cancers, suggesting an avenue for treating tumors based on aberrant pathways instead of individual aberrant genes.

Following these landmark studies, the number, breadth, and size of cancer genome projects rapidly accelerated, in keeping with the advent of massively parallel sequencing. The first whole-genome sequences in cancer generated by massively parallel sequencing were those of two lung cancers published in 2008[108] followed shortly by those of individual AML cases published in 2008 and 2009.[121,122] These studies focused on assessment of genome-wide SVs and missense mutations, respectively. The first analysis of paired primary and metastatic tumors enabling genome-wide assessment of evolution was conducted in breast cancer in 2009, identifying both shared and exclusive mutations in each sample.[123] The first studies to systematically assess genome-wide mutations of all classes, published in 2010, were conducted in cell lines from melanoma[124] and small-cell lung cancer.[125] These studies uncovered an extraordinary mutation burden (over 33,000 mutations in melanoma and 23,000 in lung) and mutational signatures supporting ultraviolet (UV) radiation etiology in melanoma and tobacco smoke etiology in lung. Discovery continued at a rapid pace, and as discussed later, large genomic analyses having been completed in all common cancers, many rare cancers, primary/recurrent/metastatic matched cohorts, and even cancers undergoing treatment.

Large-scale cancer genomic studies have also been powered by national and international consortia. Notably, the US National Cancer Institute (NCI) and NHGRI launched a large collaborative project in 2005, The Cancer Genome Atlas (TCGA; see http://cancergenome.nih.gov/). The TCGA effort began with large pilot studies in GBM,[66] ovarian cancer,[126] and squamous cell lung cancer.[127] TCGA studies have since included colorectal,[128] breast,[129] endometrial,[130] AML,[131] clear cell renal cell,[132] expanded glioblastoma,[133] urothelial bladder,[134] lung adenocarcinoma,[135] gastric,[136] chromophobe renal cell,[137] papillary thyroid,[138] head and neck squamous cell,[139] low-grade glioma,[140] cutaneous melanoma,[141] and a suite of 18 pan-cancer (PANCAN) studies.[142] Across 34 cancer types, data have been collected from more than 11,000 cases. These PANCAN studies have afforded the opportunity to characterize genomic drivers across tumor types,[143] enhancer expression,[144] alternative splicing,[145] and oncogenic pathways[146-148] and pathogenic germline variants across tumor types.[149] Similarly, ambitious studies have been undertaken by members of the International Cancer Genome Consortium (ICGC; see http://icgc.org)[150] launched in 2010 to comprehensively catalog all genomic aberrations associated with at least 50 different cancers. This consortium currently encompasses 55 projects covering 33 cancer types with over 13,000 donors and has produced publications on epigenomic sequencing techniques,[151,152] DLBCL,[153] Burkitt lymphoma,[154] X-chromosome hypermutation,[155] signatures of mutational processes,[156] and primary central nervous system (CNS) lymphoma.[157] The MSK-IMPACT study employed a targeted sequencing strategy to characterize more than 10,000 patients with advanced cancers, with 11% of patients matched to genomically guided clinical trials.[158] These comprehensive, large-scale projects will continue to rapidly advance our understanding of cancer genetics and genomics and will potentially revolutionize our approach to the diagnosis and treatment of cancer.

Cancer genomic data repositories and analysis tools

Data generated by the TCGA, ICGC, and other curated genomic repositories are publicly available. Systematic analysis of these data remains challenging, but improved web-based tools both for general academic and clinical users and specialized data scientists are greatly democratizing cancer genomics research (Table 3). One of the oldest and most comprehensive resources for mining such data is the Catalogue of Somatic Mutations in Cancer (COSMIC; see http://www.sanger.ac.uk/genetics/CGP/cosmic) maintained by the Wellcome Trust Sanger Institute Cancer Genome Project.[159] COSMIC is manually curated from publications and therefore entails a broad reach across targeted studies and genome projects (currently more than 20,000 such studies). The current build (27 August 2020) describes over 70 million mutations in more than 1.4 million samples encompassing 38,000 cancer genomes. In addition to SNVs, it details over 22 million noncoding mutations, 19,000 fusions, 61,000 SVs, 1.2 million CNVs, and 9.2 million expression variants. These data are easily queried using key words or by gene or cancer type. COSMIC also includes more advanced tools that are in some cases linked to other databases. These include a detailed census of all human genes that have been causally linked to tumorigenesis (Cancer Gene Census; see www.sanger.ac.uk/genetics/CGP/Census)[5,160] as well as tools to assess mutation signatures and drug sensitivity. Another highly versatile data portal is the cBioPortal for Cancer Genomics maintained by Memorial Sloan-Kettering Cancer Institute.[161] This portal primarily contains highly processed Cancer Cell Line Encyclopedia (CCLE)[162] and TCGA datasets but provides a powerful, intuitive web interface enabling queries by gene or cancer type as well as more advanced interfaces for data specialists. A similar portal is available for ICGC data (see http://dcc.icgc.org).

While the above portals offer access to the generalist, additional repositories exist for advanced users to access various levels of raw data. The Cancer Genomics Hub (CGHub), hosted by the University of California Santa Cruz (UCSC), is a secure central repository for data generated through the NCI including TCGA, CCLE, and Therapeutically Applicable Research to Generate Effective Treatments (TARGET).[163] The European Genome–Phenome Archive (see http://ega.crg.eu) similarly collects and distributes sequencing and genotyping data, primarily cancer data emerging

Table 3 Cancer genomics databases.

Name	Detail	Link
canEvolve	Analysis of mRNA, miRNA, protein expression, and CNA data in 10,000 patient samples from TCGA, GEO, and array express	www.canevolve.org/
canSAR	Integrated analysis of biological, chemical, and pharmacological data from COSMIC, chEMBl, UniProt, BindingDB, array express, and STRING	https://cansar.icr.ac.uk/
cBioPortal	TCGA data portal; graphical visualization and analysis	http://www.cbioportal.org/public-portal/
CGAP	Graphical summary and bioinformatics analysis of gene expression; Integration of cytogenetic data	https://mitelmandatabase.isb-cgc.org/
CGHub	Secure, comprehensive data repository; TCGA, CCLE, and TARGET projects	https://xena.ucsc.edu/
CPRG	Integrative analysis tools for cancer research	http://www.broadinstitute.org/software/cprg
COSMIC	Largest genomics data repository; manually curated publications and output from large sequencing studies	http://www.sanger.ac.uk/genetics/CGP/cosmic
EBI array express	Annotated functional genomics data; data generated via microarray and high-throughput sequencing projects	http://www.ebi.ac.uk/microarray-as/ae/
EGA	Comprehensive data repository; restricted access; ICGC output; SNP and can data	https://www.ebi.ac.uk/ega/
GDAC	Pipelines for genomic analysis; user-friendly interface	http://gdac.broadinstitute.org/
GEO	Gene expression microarray and functional genomics data repository	http://www.ncbi.nlm.nih.gov/geo/
ICGC	Visualization tool; genomic, transcriptomic, and epigenomic characterization of 50 tumor types	http://dcc.icgc.org
MethylCancer	Methylation database; interprets the correlation of methylation, gene expression, and cancer biology	http://methycancer.psych.ac.cn
SomamiR	Archive of experimentally validated somatic mutations in noncoding RNA	http://compbio.uthsc.edu/SomamiR/
UCSC cancer genome browser	Multipurpose data viewer incorporating multiple data types including clinical information	https://xena.ucsc.edu/

from the ICGC. Data repositories and analysis tools are also available for other data types. Cytogenetic aberrations and fusions observed in over 65,000 human tumors have been compiled and are maintained online (The Mitelman Database of Chromosome Aberrations in Cancer at the US NCI Cancer Genome Anatomy Project [CGAP] Web site: https://mitelmandatabase.isb-cgc.org/).[28] Data from numerous gene expression microarray studies are warehoused by multiple entities, including the US National Center for Biotechnology Information (NCBI Gene Expression Omnibus; see http://www.ncbi.nlm.nih.gov/geo/) and the European Bioinformatics Institute (EBI Array Express; see http://www.ebi.ac.uk/microarray-as/ae/). Additional data repositories and web resources are outlined in Table 3.

The vast and varied landscapes of human cancers

Although few new mutational "mountains" have been discovered in the past decade, the systematic study of cancer genomes has revealed many new "hills" as well as mutational processes, signatures, and dysregulated pathways. The total mutation burden itself can reflect cancer etiology and has bearing on clinical course and is much more variable than originally anticipated. In some pediatric cancers such as rhabdoid tumors[164] and small-cell carcinoma of the ovary,[165] cases with only a single coding SNV have been discovered, while leukemias such as AML bear a median of nine coding SNVs (Figure 4). Conversely, cancers with mutagenic etiology, such as bladder, lung, and melanoma, bear high mutation rates with medians of 148, 217, and 254 coding SNVS, while tumors with mismatch repair defects can contain thousands of coding SNVs. Distinct mutational signatures can also reflect these external and internal mutagenic factors. For instance, enrichment for C>T transition in dipyrimidines, a hallmark of UV light damage, is seen in cancers from UV-damaged sites.[156] Overall, coding SNVs are generally more common in cancers than coding CNVs and SVs, although broad variability in CNV and SV profiles also exists across cancer types. Thirty seven percent of cancers experience tetraploidy, with a quarter of most solid tumor genomes containing large-scale chromosomal variations and 10% containing focal CNVs. Over 140 genomic regions have been found to contain recurrent CNVs, only 38 of which contain known tumor suppressors or oncogenes.[166–168] Whole-genome sequencing has also uncovered chromothripsis events, occurring in 2–3% of cancers, when errors in chromosome segregation during mitosis lead to shattering of a single or a few chromosomes and massive rearrangement in a single-cell generation.[169–171]

In addition to mutagenic etiology, variability in mutation burden is the likely result of mutation timing, patient age, and the number of divisions that had occurred in precursor cells, with mutations accumulating in dividing cells over time,[164,165] although a "punctuated evolution" model has also been proposed.[172–174] Ultimately, only a few such mutations can "drive" cancer (driver mutations) insofar as they confer a selective fitness advantage on the cells that carry them. Other mutations are "passengers" with no known relevance to cancer development or the cancerous state.[175] Several methods have been developed to classify mutations as drivers or passengers based on the pattern and frequency with which they arise across cancers,[4,176,177] but experimental validation is required to confirm the role of these mutations in cancer.

It has been estimated that more than 138 cancer driver genes exist,[4] with 571 genes causally implicated in cancer catalogued in the Cancer Gene Census (see https://cancer.sanger.ac.uk/census).[5] The 10 most commonly mutated cancer oncogenes and tumor suppressor genes are shown in Table 4, and cancer genes associated with the most lethal cancers in the United States are shown in Table 5. While this vast array of mutations may seem overwhelmingly complex, particularly from the therapeutic perspective, there is nonetheless reason for optimism. For example, dramatic clinical responses are seen even in highly complex cancers using agents targeting mutant proteins, such as mutant *BRAF* in melanoma and ALK receptor tyrosine kinase (*ALK*) in lung cancer.[202,203] Further, multiple cancer genes often converge on an individual signaling pathway and may be functionally equivalent. Thus, a specific pathway may be subject to genomic aberrations at a frequency far higher than any of its individual gene components. More recently,

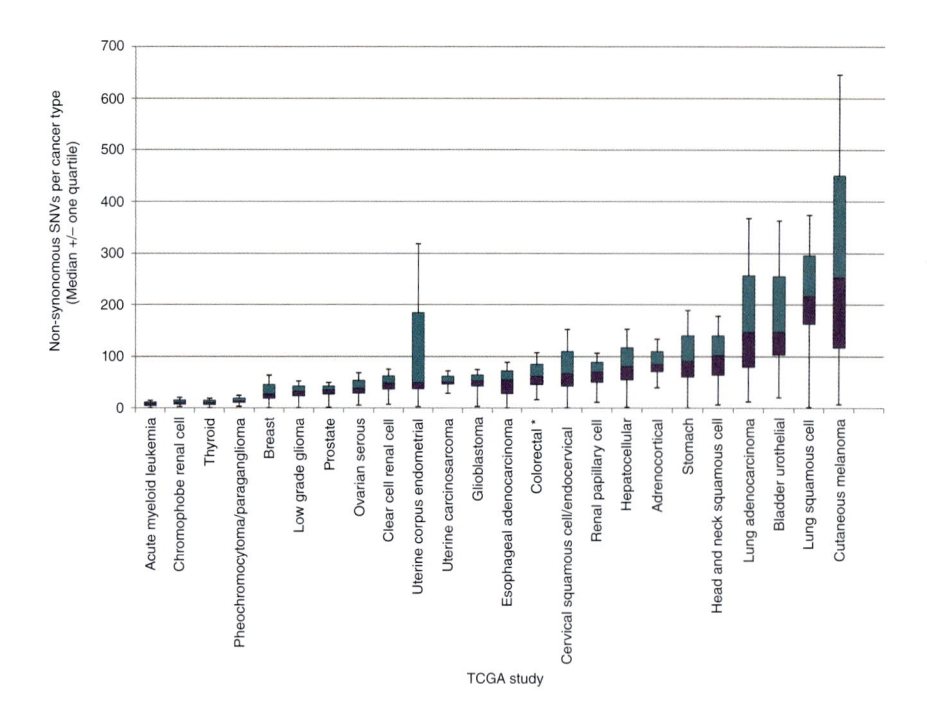

Figure 4 Number of coding single-nucleotide variants (SNVs) per tumor type across a selection of human cancers. DNA sequencing data obtained from published TCGA studies were used to calculate the distribution and median number of coding SNVs mutations in each cancer type. Colored bars indicate the 25% and 75% quartiles. Outlier values (values below Q1−1.5 × IQR or above Q3 + 1.5 × IQR) are not shown, and asterisks represent studies with more than 10% outliers.

Table 4 Ten most commonly mutated oncogenes and tumor suppressor genes (TSG) in the COSMIC database.

Gene	Classification[a]	SNVs in COSMIC	Homozygous deletions (TSGs) or amplifications (oncogenes) in COSMIC[b]	Fusions in COSMIC
TP53	TSG	50,046	1445	1
LRP1B	TSG	35,149	1245	0
PTPRT	TSG	14,142	249	0
APC	TSG	13,996	726	0
KMT2C	TSG	12,061	723	0
FHIT	TSG	11,947	3092	1
ZFHX3	TSG	11,187	984	0
PTEN	TSG	7646	1072	0
NOTCH1	TSG	7592	668	3
CAMTA1	TSG	6833	1075	0
BRAF	Oncogene	57,926	765	643
JAK2	Oncogene	53,142	353	28
KRAS	Oncogene	46,865	1006	1
EGFR	Oncogene	33,398	1299	0
FLT3	Oncogene	19,141	577	0
ERBB4	Oncogene	16,049	723	1
PIK3CA	Oncogene	15,064	1168	0
IDH1	Oncogene	11,246	485	0
KIT	Oncogene	10,855	472	0
CTNNB1	Oncogene	8761	352	17

[a] Oncogene and TSG status were determined by the 20/20 rule (4) using sample data in the COSMIC database (see http://cancer.sanger.ac.uk/cosmic/; COSMIC v91, accessed 21 August 2020). Only those classified as Tier 1 oncogene or TSGs were included in analysis.
[b] Amplifications shown for samples in which the average genome ploidy ≤ 2.7 and the total gene copy number ≥ 5 or the average genome ploidy > 2.7 and the total gene copy number ≥ 9. Homozygous deletions shown for samples in which the average genome ploidy ≤ 2.7 and the total gene copy number = 0 or the average genome ploidy > 2.7 and the total copy number < (average genome ploidy - 2.7).

the introduction of immunotherapeutic agents provides hope to cancers with increased tumor mutation burden (TMB).

The complexity is reduced still further by the fact that most driver genes converge on the hallmark pathways and can ultimately be reduced to those impacting cell differentiation, cell proliferation, cell death, and genomic maintenance.[2] These pathways can be perturbed directly by mutation of their constituents and indirectly by mutation of regulatory genes or elements, epigenomic dysregulation, microenvironmental factors such as T-cell exhaustion, or even changes to the patient's microbiome. Thus, the integration of multiple types of genomic data will clearly be necessary to reduce the initial complexity of somatic

Table 5 Commonly mutated cancer genes in the deadliest cancers.

Cancer[a]	Familial cancer genes	Common somatically mutated genes	References
Breast	BRCA1, BRCA2, PTEN, TP53	PIK3CA, TP53, MAP3K1, GATA3, MLL3, CDH1, PTEN, ERBB2, MAP2K4, CDKN2A, PTEN, RB1	62,120,129,178–180
Colorectal	APC, MSH2, MLH1, MSH6, PMS2, MUTYH, LKB1, SMAD4, BMPR1A, PTEN, KLLN	APC, TP53, KRAS, PIK3CA, FBXW7, SMAD4, TCF7L2, NRAS, ARID1A, SOX9, FAM123B, ERBB2, IGF2, NAV2, TCF7L1	62,120,128,181,182
Liver	HFE, SLC25A13, ABCB11, FAH, HMBS, UROD	TP53, CTNNB1, AXIN1, RPS6KA3, RB1, FAM123A, CDKN2A, MYC, RSPO2, CCND1, FGF19, ARID1A, ARID1B, ARID2, MLL, MLL3	183–186
Lung	EGFR, BRAF, KRAS, TP53	TP53, KRAS, STK11, EGFR, ALK, BRAF, AKT1, DDR2, HER2, MEK1, NRAS, PI3CA, PTEN, RET, ROS1, EML4, NTRK1, FHIT, FRA3B, FGFR1, HER2	57,75,115,117,125,127,135,187
Pancreatic	BRCA2, PALB2	KRAS, TP53, CDKN2A, SMAD4, MLL3, TGFRB2, ARID1A, SF3B1, ROBO2, KDM6A, PREX2	67,188–191
Prostate	BRCA2, BRCA1, HOXB13	EPHB2, ERG, TMPRSS2, PTEN, TP53, SPOP, FOXA1, MED12, NKX3-1	174,192–196
Ovarian	STK11, BRCA1, BRCA2	FBXW7, AKT2, ERBB2, TGFBR1, TGFBR2, BRAF, KRAS, PIK3CA, PTEN, ARID1A, BRCA1, MMP-1, BRCA1, BRCA2, MLPA, MAPH	126,197–200

[a] The seven cancers estimated to cause the greatest number of deaths in the United States in 2015.[201]

cancer genetics into a tractable understanding of the affected hallmark pathways.

While it seems possible that the majority of cancer genes have now been discovered, new genes are occasionally implicated in cancer, although at low frequency across many cancer types or at high frequency in a rare and previously uncharacterized cancer. However, most cancers require five to eight driver mutations based on epidemiological studies,[204] and only three to six drivers have been found in most cancers with notable exceptions (such as pediatric cases) in which three or fewer drivers have been discovered.[4] These gaps are likely due to both technical limitations of sequencing technology and study design and limitations in our growing understanding of mutations occurring in noncoding regions of DNA or through epigenomic mechanisms, or even stable biological events occurring outside of the cancer cell in the tumor microenvironment, or, more distantly still, in the patient's microbiome. Clearly, the catalogue of cancer-driving mutations and other biological factors is still incomplete, and although the maps of cancer genome landscapes have been broadly charted, much work remains to characterize these vast and still largely unexplored landscapes in detail in order to guide clinical cancer management.

Clinical implications of cancer genome landscapes

The information currently available from cancer genomics projects has greatly improved our comprehension of the development, progression, and clinical behavior of human neoplasms. These data and the technology used to generate them are also impacting cancer screening, diagnostics, and treatment. As sequencing costs continue to decline, routine personal exome- and genome-wide screening becomes increasingly affordable, and it is likely that each patient's personal genome sequence will comprise a key component of their medical record. Such screening of germline DNA may reveal inherited mutations that would otherwise go undiagnosed until disease presentation and the power of this approach will grow exponentially as we continue to connect genetic variants to disease phenotypes. It is the combination of both germline and somatic cancer analysis that is at the vanguard of genomic cancer care. The NIH has acknowledged the importance of this new healthcare approach through the establishment of the Precision Medicine Initiative within the NCI cancer Moonshot program.[205] Germline targeted Sanger sequencing using small gene panels is already commonly used in familial cancer screening. In cases such as germline BRCA1/2 or MLH1/MSH2 mutations, which dramatically increase lifetime risk for breast/ovarian or colorectal cancer, genomic testing can guide clinical decisions about surveillance and prophylactic surgery. Now, NGS-based sequencing of hundreds of genes can be completed at a similar cost, and the turn-around time thereby enables the detection of lower penetrance rare variants not detectable with smaller panels. For example, in a study of 141 BRCA1/2-negative patients with a family or personal history of breast cancer, a panel of 40 additional genes identified 16 patients with pathogenic variants in 9 genes other than BRCA1/2 such as TP53 and PTEN.[206] These findings have shaped new guidelines from the National Comprehensive Cancer Network recommending targeted panels for patient's breast or ovarian cancer family history who are negative for common hereditary mutations.[207] Targeted NGS panels have also shown greater sensitivity and specificity than traditional diagnostic tools in genetic testing of familial cancer genes such as BRCA1/2, TP53, and APC in additional studies.[178,208–210] NGS panels may also facilitate differential diagnosis and patient stratification, given that the diagnostic yields of NGS panels, exomes, or even whole genomes have been shown in multiple studies to more sensitively identify inherited cancer predispositions than do small Sanger-based panels.[211,212]

Detection of genetic cancer susceptibility through germline testing significantly impacts clinical management, including the approaches to prognosis, screening, prophylactic interventions, and therapeutic selection. In 2005 and 2006, several groups demonstrated antitumor activity of PARP inhibition (PARPi) in the setting of BRCA1/2-mutated cancers, with associated homologous recombination deficiencies (HRDs).[213–215] Ten years later, the FDA would approve three different PARP inhibitors in the treatment of BRCA1/2-mutated ovarian cancers.[216] The study of olaparib that led to approval looked at ~300 patients with BRCA1/2 mutations across cancer types.[217] Overall, there was a 26% response rate (RECIST 1.1), with a 31% response rate in ovarian cancers. Rucaparib and niraparib were approved shortly after in ovarian cancer. Rucaparib further demonstrated that HRD correlates with progression-free survival (PFS).[218] While niraparib showed PFS improvements to both BRCA1/2 wild-type and mutant ovarian cancer patients, BRCA1/2 mutant tumors or those with increased HRD demonstrated the largest PFS.[219] Since, PARPi in combination with DNA damaging agents, molecular targeted agents, or immunotherapeutics continue being explored in clinical trials across a wide spectrum of tumor types, many with HRD.[220]

The next *BRCA1/2*-mutant-driven approvals for PARPi include that for olaparib in metastatic prostate cancer with *BRCA1/2* or *ATM* mutations[221,222] and rucaparib for metastatic prostate cancer with *BRCA* mutations after failing androgen receptor therapy.[223] Foundation Medicine's FoundationOne CDx panel, which can identify HRD, was approved as a companion diagnostic to olaparib.[224] A host of other germline and somatic panels (e.g., the Myriad genomic instability score) have been developed to determine HRD and germline alterations or signatures associated with therapeutic response to PARPi.[220,225] This has led to testing of an HRD score, the sum of the LOH, telomeric–allelic imbalance, and large-scale state transitions scores, though with mixed clinical results in response to PARPi.[225] Finally, the demonstration that PARPi could reach the brain in clinical trials has prompted exploration in GBM settings and CNS metastasis,[226,227] settings with known subsets harboring DNA damage response dysregulation.[228] Interestingly, metastatic breast tumors showed increased HRD compared to patient-matched primary tumors,[229] suggesting PARPi usage in the metastatic setting. As whole-genome sequencing of tumor/normal pairs becomes standard practice in clinical settings, novel associations of germline alterations with therapeutic response would be expected across a wide range of tumor types.

Cancer genetics discoveries have driven targeted drug development since the first report of a recurrent chromosomal abnormality—the *BCR–ABL* translocation in CML. The selective tyrosine kinase inhibitor (TKI) imatinib, designed to target the constitutively active chimeric tyrosine kinase protein product of the *BCR–ABL* fusion gene in CML, was the first successful targeted therapy.[230–232] The paradigm of targeting cancer-specific mutations to improve the therapeutic index of chemotherapy has now been repeated with dramatic success. Examples include expansion of the indication of imatinib to treat *PDGFR*- and *KIT*-mutated gastrointestinal stromal tumors (GISTs) and hypereosinophilic syndromes;[233–235] two additional BCR–ABL inhibitors, dasatinib and nilotinib, in primary and imatinib-resistant CML;[236–238] trastuzumab, an inhibitor of the Her2/ERBB2 tyrosine kinase receptor whose encoding gene *ERBB2* is amplified and overexpressed in 25–30% of breast carcinomas;[239,240] the multitargeted TKI sunitinib in renal cell carcinoma, GIST, and pancreatic neuroendocrine tumors;[241–243] gefitinib and erlotinib with striking efficacy in the 5–10% of lung adenocarcinoma patients with European ancestry and 25–30% of Japanese patients who harbor activating mutations in epidermal growth factor receptor (*EGFR*);[244,245] crizotinib in *ALK*-rearranged lung cancer;[246,247] vismodegib in basal-cell carcinoma bearing hedgehog pathway mutations;[248] and vemurafenib in *BRAF*-mutant melanoma.[249] Cancer gene mutations have also been associated with innate or acquired resistance to these targeted therapies. For example, amplification of the *BCR–ABL* gene is common in CML patients resistant to imatinib.[230,250] Preclinical studies and clinical trials are ongoing for numerous novel therapeutic agents directed against genomic targets in cancer in addition to agents capable of circumventing or treating drug-resistant disease.

The success in targeted drug development has largely grown around mutations occurring with appreciable frequency in individual cancers, such as frequent *BRAF* mutations in melanoma. However, not all cancers of a given type harbor "typical" mutations and may, in fact, carry uncommon but targetable genomic alterations. As the fundamental goal of personalized oncology is to recommend the most appropriate treatment for an individual, patient's genomic data may enable such personalized tailoring of care. However, despite the completion of the HGP in 2003, genomic medicine's entrance into the cancer care stream has been painstakingly slow. In 2010, Von Hoff et al.[251] published results from one of the first pilot studies using personalized molecular profiling to guide treatment selection in refractory metastatic cancer. Despite considerable challenges including the absence of a precedent for the novel trial design, overall patient attrition, and a diverse pharmacopeia, it was found that in 27% of 68 patients, treatment selection guided by molecular profiling (gene expression microarray analysis) resulted in a longer PFS than that during the most recent regimen on which the patient had progressed. The next major step in bringing genomic tools to the patient was a novel study combining whole-genome sequencing and comprehensive RNA sequencing to individualize the treatment of metastatic triple-negative breast cancer (TNBC) patients.[252] TNBC is characterized by the absence of expression of estrogen receptor (ER), progesterone receptor (PR), and HER-2. This study identified somatic mutations in the RAS/RAF/MEK and PI3K/AKT/mTOR signaling pathways which have led to clinical trials combining agents targeting MEK and/or mTOR genes with encouraging results.

Implementation of personalized genomics in cancer care required new trial designs such as described earlier. Over the recent years, multiple innovative large academic observational and interventional trials have been published[253–258] or are ongoing (see http://clinicaltrials.gov). These include adaptive trials such as I-SPY 2 (Investigation of Serial Studies to Predict Your therapeutic response with imaging and molecular analysis) in which treatment arms are modified in the course of the study based on patient response.[259] Basket trials such as the NCI MATCH trial have assigned >1000 patients with various advanced cancers to treatment baskets based on mutational profiles and then treat with agents matched to their tumor's mutations.[256] Umbrella trials are also ongoing in which multiple drugs are studied in a single disease. For example, the recently completed Stand-Up-To-Cancer and the Melanoma Research Alliance Dream Team Clinical trial assessed molecularly guided therapy in a single-histology patient population: metastatic melanoma patients whose tumors lack the disease's most common targetable mutation, *BRAF* V600. In a randomized treatment study, a combination of whole-genome and whole-transcriptome sequencing was used to identify molecular aberrations matched to an appropriate clinical treatment from a pharmacopeia composed of standard of care and FDA-approved and investigational agents.[255] The challenges of returning accurate and actionable information during a clinically relevant time period in such studies are considerable. This includes patient consent, tumor biopsy, quality DNA/RNA extraction, DNA and RNA sequencing, data integration, report generation, and tumor board review to formulate a treatment plan (Figure 5). Scaling such processes and assuring coverage in national reimbursement programs such as Medicare has, over the past 2 years, made such approaches available to large numbers of patients outside of the major national medical centers.

Large-scale genomic characterization of tumors in the context of clinical trials has allowed identification of predictive biomarkers—recurrent genomic alterations that identify patients most likely to benefit from a particular drug. These provide tremendous clinical value by allowing patient stratification to the most relevant treatment option and have been rapidly commercialized. A broadening array of sequencing tests that may aid in the diagnosis and treatment decisions is available to oncologists and their patients. Over 100 academic centers and 50 commercial laboratories have made such tests available. Examples of such

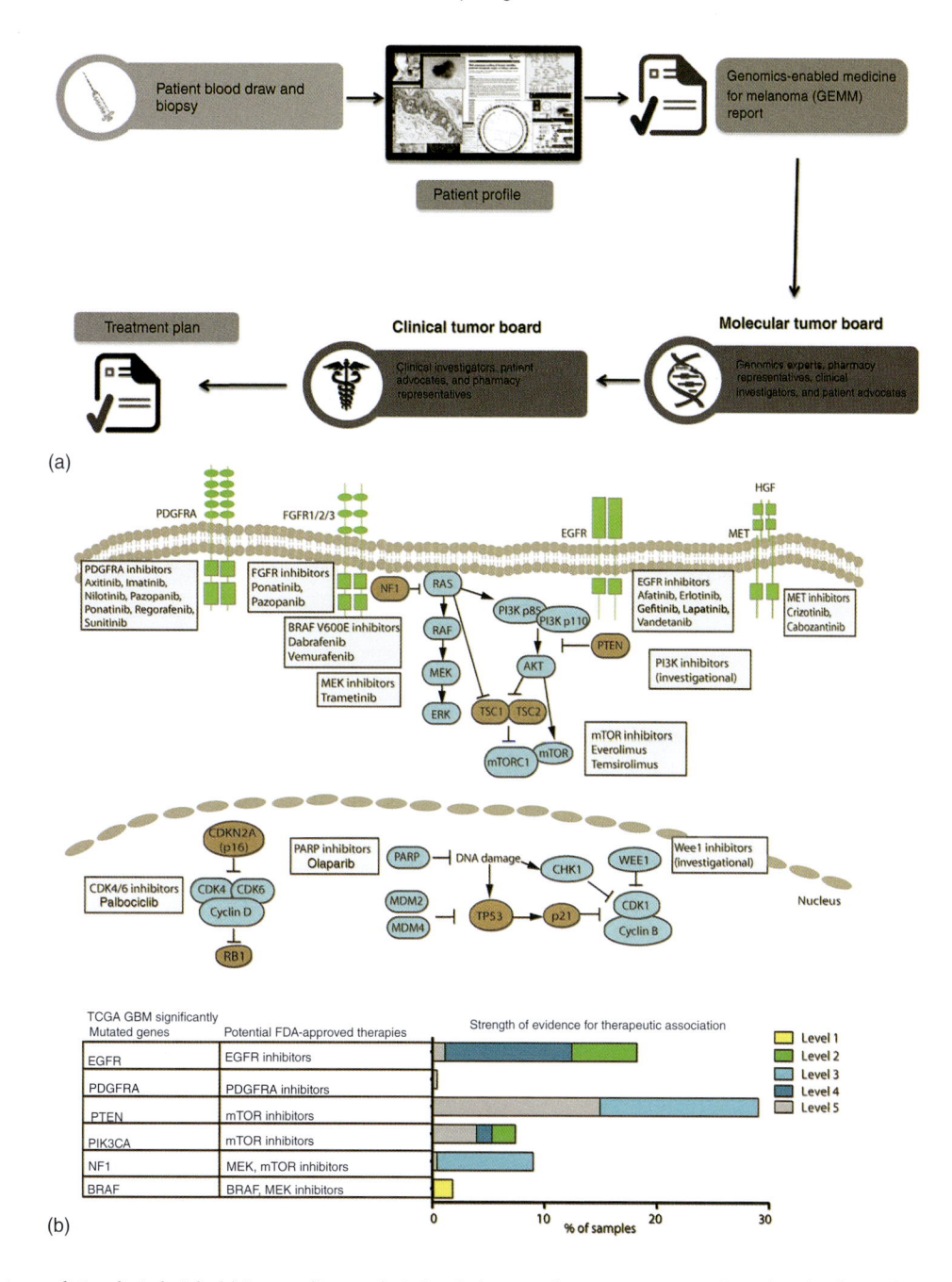

Figure 5 Precision medicine clinical trials. (a) Process diagram depicting the key steps from patient consent through molecular profiling and treatment plan generation. The entire process from biopsy to treatment plan is designed to be performed in less than 5 weeks. Source: From LoRusso et al.[255] Reprinted with permission. (b) Potential therapeutic implications of significantly mutated genes identified in the primary glioblastoma TCGA dataset. (Top) Pathway representation of frequently altered pathways and selected potential therapeutic agents. (Bottom) Table of frequently mutated genes from TCGA mapped to potential FDA-approved therapeutic agents. (Right) Bar chart of the level of evidence for the association between an alteration and therapeutic implication. Source: Adapted from Prados et al.[253] Reprinted with permission.

commercial tests are provided in Table 6. Now that there is nationwide Medicare coverage for such testing, expanded panel-, exome-, or whole-genome-based sequencing will continue to transform screening and diagnostics in the coming years. However, routine clinical use will require an expanded incorporation of genomic testing into guidelines, physician education, and better evidence to illustrate the benefit of such testing for off-label drug use. Finally, in the absence of germline genomic analysis (whether part of hereditary cancer testing or conducted in tumor-matched normal tissue) there is a high likelihood that germline variants may be misinterpreted as targetable somatic alterations. Widespread controversy exists over the balance between patient autonomy and the perception that a patient's knowledge of this information would result in physical or mental harm.[260]

Cell-free tumor-specific DNA (ctDNA)

Unlike relative differences in mRNA or protein expression between tumor and normal tissue, somatic mutations in cancer genes are exclusive and specific markers of cancer cells. This has been recently leveraged to use cell-free, tumor-specific DNA (ctDNA) in plasma as an accurate circulating biomarker that could be leverage in early detection, monitoring tumor burden/therapeutic response, and therapeutic selection. The value of ctDNA for monitoring tumor burden, treatment response, and recurrence was first recognized in colorectal cancer.[261] This study identified somatic mutations in patient tumors in recurrently mutated colorectal cancer genes (TP53, PIK3CA, APC, and KRAS) and retrospectively analyzed plasma samples using highly sensitive assays specifically design for each patient. The results showed that ctDNA levels reflect changes in tumor burden during treatment when compared with imaging and carcinoembryonic antigen. Another study used NGS of tumors and digital PCR and found that ctDNA levels during treatment reflected disease progression in metastatic breast cancer.[262] In these results, ctDNA was found to be more responsive and applicable to the largest fraction of patients when compared with the enumeration of circulating tumor cells or CA-125, a glycoprotein biomarker of breast cancer. Similar results supporting the role of the serial analysis of ctDNA for monitoring tumor burden have been published for lung cancer,[263,264] melanoma,[265] osteosarcoma,[266] and a number of other disease types.[267,268]

As mutations in known cancer-driver genes have been detected in circulation, the FDA has recently approved a number of single-gene (EGFR and PIK3CA) or multigene panels (e.g., Archer Reveal ctDNA 28, FoundationOne Liquid CDx, Guardant360 CDx, Inivata InVision, and MSK-ACCESS) as companion diagnostics for targeted therapeutic selection.[268] Further, as ctDNA assays allow for longitudinal follow-up, the ability of liquid biopsy to monitor or discover therapeutic resistance mechanisms is also under investigation.[268] An example was demonstrated by Murtaza et al.,[269] who demonstrated that a PIK3CA mutation arose in the ctDNA of a breast cancer patient who progressed on paclitaxel.

To achieve the maximal clinical utility of liquid biopsies in early-stage disease, where tumor burden is low, continued advancements in ctDNA detection sensitivity are necessary. Advances in molecular methods including the use of high-depth, noise-corrected, and targeted NGS assays are enabling the study of patients with localized, potentially resectable cancers.[270,271] Recent work in localized breast cancer shows that ctDNA can predict postoperative recurrence of cancer, a median of 8 months before tumors become detectable on imaging.[272] This study and others describing ctDNA in localized cancers demonstrate novel opportunities for optimizing treatment of cancer with curative intent by individualizing therapeutic strategies.[273] The prognostic value of liquid biopsy has been studied in more than 800 early-stage breast cancer patients.[268] While early successes were demonstrated, prospective, multicenter trials are needed. Approaches that employ multiplexed PCR and NGS (such as the Signatera assay[274]) or targeted digital sequencing (TARDIS)[275] allow personalized tracking for mutations in clinically relevant sample volumes. The diagnostic and prognostic roles of ctDNA are currently under clinical evaluation across a spectrum of tumor types.

Prospective trials are needed to establish the benefit of guiding clinical cancer management using ctDNA as a biomarker. Nevertheless, observational studies reported have shown superior performance of ctDNA to monitor tumor burden compared to the numbers of circulating tumor cells or glycoprotein biomarkers.[276] With some variations between cancer types, ctDNA has a promise of wide applicability across patients as shown in a recent comprehensive survey of 640 patients.[276] This study found that ctDNA was detectable in 55% of patients with potentially curable disease. These results suggest that improved molecular assays may enable detection of ctDNA in presymptomatic individuals with cancer, potentially leading to a screening test with higher specificity than traditional methods.[277–280]

Cancer evolution

The ability to sequence cancer genomes has shed light on the process of molecular evolution and its importance for understanding cancer biology and treatment. Although not new, historical consideration of this concept has largely been confined to a process of linear clonal evolution driving the development of an increasingly malignant cancer phenotype.[1] However, it is increasingly clear that cancer evolution generates tremendous heterogeneity by continuously generating clonal diversity. As a result, multiple related but distinct clonal lineages may coexist within a single patient.[281] These lineages differ in their ability to progress and metastasize[282] as well as to respond to or resist therapy.[283] The implications of this complex, branched evolution model will be critically important for understanding cancer biology and developing better treatment approaches.

The cornerstone of cancer evolution lies in the accumulation of genomic mutations, ultimately impacting cellular phenotype. Although the majority of acquired cancer mutations are likely to be passengers, a small proportion will impact critical cellular pathways and processes, thereby acting as disease drivers. However, the exact molecular mechanisms leading to increased mutagenesis in cancer are incompletely understood. Recent analysis, carried out on thousands of cancer genomes, identified at least 20 distinct mutational signatures pointing to diverse processes driving mutagenesis in various cancers, with most cancers showing evidence of more than one such process at play.[156] Although the factors leading to several identified mutational signatures such as UV, smoking, and exposure to chemotherapy agents are well known, many are not associated with known causative processes. Elucidating such novel mechanisms of mutagenesis will be important for facilitating development of better prevention and treatment strategies.

The accumulation of mutations clearly provides the raw material (population diversity) for cancer evolution. However, this accumulation often contributes to the process of clonal evolution within temporal and spatial constrains. The order in which mutations are acquired can dramatically impact the cell fate. For example, a loss of BRCA1 or BRCA2 leads to cell cycle arrest in the context of normal TP53 but not in the setting of TP53 loss.[284] Consistent with this observation, a loss of the second copy of BRCA1 in breast cancer typically occurs after the loss of TP53. The order of mutational events may also depend on the cell type and the state of differentiation. This is seen with KRAS or NRAS mutations, which occur early in colon cancer development, while similar NRAS mutations are seen mainly at a late stage in myelodysplastic syndrome.[285,286] Spatial constraints of clonal diversification, on the other hand, have been noted in clear cell renal cell carcinoma and non-small cell lung cancer (NSCLC),[287,288] where divergent clones develop in specific geographic locations of the tumor. In fact, such spatial separation could lead to "parallel evolution" characterized by distinct mutations arising independently in individual clones, but targeting the same gene or the same pathway, as observed in a variety of cancers.[289] An important practical implication of such parallel evolution is that a full spectrum of mutational driver

Table 6 Commercial cancer genome tests.

Provider	Product	Description[a]
Ambry genetics	Exome next	Full exome + mitochondrial genome, SNVs, CNVs
Ambry genetics	BRCA1 and BRCA2 gene sequencing	SNVs, CNVs, BRCA1/2 SVs
Arup laboratories	Gastrointestinal hereditary cancer panel	15 genes + intron/exon junctions, SNVs, CNVs
Ashion analytics	GEM cancer panel	562 genes, tumor/germline, SNVs, CNVs
	GEM GW	Whole exome, tumor/germline, SNVs, CNVs, SVs
	RNA sequencing	RNA, tumor/germline. Gene expression, fusions, alternative splicing, SNVs
Cancer genetics incorporated (CGI)	FOCUS:CLL	7 actionable CLL targets
	FOCUS:Myeloid	54 genes, prognostic and therapeutic assessment
Caris	MI Profile	47 genes, SNVs
Foundation medicine	Foundation one	236 genes, 47 introns from 19 genes associated with SV. SNVs, CNVs, SVs
	Foundation one heme	405 genes, 31 introns associated with SV, and RNA-seq of 265 genes. SNVs, CNVs, SVs, fusions and gene expression in hematologic tumors
GeneDx	XomeDx	Full exome, SNVs
	XomeDx Plus	Full exome + mitochondrial genome, SNVs
	XomeDx Slice	Targeted exome, SNVs
	Comprehensive cancer panel	29 genes, SNVs, CNVs
GPS@WUSTL	Comprehensive cancer gene set analysis	Sequencing of 42 genes. Mutation analysis
Agendia	Mammaprint	Microarray gene expression analysis of 70 genes. Predicts chemotherapy benefit and risk of recurrence of breast cancer
Myriad genetics	BRACAnalysis	Sanger, BRCA1/2, breast and ovarian cancer risk
	COLARIS	Sanger, 6 genes, hereditary colorectal cancer
	COLARIS AP	Sanger, APC and MYH genes, adenomatous polyposis colon cancer risk
	MELARIS	Sanger, CDKN2A, hereditary melanoma
	PANEXIA	Sanger, PALB2 +BRCA2 genes, pancreatic cancer risk
	Myriad myRisk hereditary cancer	Sanger, 25 genes, breast, ovarian, gastric, colorectal, pancreatic, melanoma, prostate, and endometrial cancer risk
NeoGenomics laboratories	NeoTYPE cancer exome profile	4813 genes, identify SNVs
	NeoTYPE profiles	Custom gene panels, SNVs
OncotypeDX	OncotypeDX breast cancer assay	RT-PCR, 21 genes, gene expression, chemotherapy benefit, and likelihood of recurrence for invasive breast cancer
	OncotypeDX colon cancer assay	RT-PCR, 18 genes, gene expression, recurrence risk in stage II and stage III colon cancer
	OncotypeDX prostate cancer assay	RT-PCR< 17 genes, gene expression, treatment selection for prostate cancer
Paradigm	PCDx	# of genes not specified, DNA and RNA analysis, SNVs, CNVs, SVs, gene expression, fusions, alternative splicing
Personal genome diagnostics (PGDX)	Whole genome analysis	Whole genome, tumor or ctDNA and germline, SNVs, CNVs, SVs
	CancerXome	Full exome, SNVs, CNVs, SVs
	Cancer select (R88, R203)	88 or 203 genes, SNVs, CNVs, SVs
	ImmunoSelect-R	Exome, ineoantigen prediction to asses utility of immunotherapy
	PlasmaSelect-R	58 genes in ctDNA, SNVs
Quest Diagnostics	OncoVantage	34 genes, SNVs

[a]These descriptions are derived from company websites and may not be complete. They also do not constitute endorsement of any particular product.

events may need to be identified, and effective targeted therapeutic strategy capable of simultaneously inhibiting independent and molecularly distinct clones within a single patient may be required.

Characterizing the clonal and subclonal diversity of tumors remains nontrivial. Using standard bulk sequencing technologies, all the cells from within a sample are processed together. Thus, DNA and/or RNA from all the cells processed is combined. To identify distinct populations of cells with unique mutation profiles or gene expression changes, researchers rely on computational approaches to identify somatic mutations that cosegregate together at similar frequencies.[290–292] While these inference-based approaches can be quite useful, they can be difficult to interpret, and some information is invariably lost. Recent advances in technology allow researchers to profile DNA and RNA within single cells.[293–295] These approaches work by physically separating individual cells during processing and adding barcodes to the RNA or DNA that can be used to identify which molecule came from which cell after sequencing. The rapid advance and adoption of this technology has enabled cancer researchers to profile the RNA and DNA of tumors at single-cell resolution across thousands or even hundreds of thousands of cells in parallel.[293–295]

These methods are enabling researchers to assess tumor evolution at unprecedented granularity. Indeed, a number of studies have used this technology to profile overall tumor heterogeneity, profile differences in cell populations between primary and metastatic lesions, and explore changes driving treatment resistance.[296-303] A powerful approach to uncovering mechanisms of treatment resistance is to pair single-cell genomics with patient-derived cell lines, ex vivo tumor models, or patient-derived xenograft (PDX) models and subject these models to relevant treatment conditions. Indeed, one such study treatment resistance in NSCLC was able to demonstrate the complexity of resistance mechanisms, with an increase in intratumor heterogeneity driving treatment resistance.[302] Another study examining vemurafenib resistance in BRAF melanoma cells lines was able to identify rare populations of cells that existed in before treatment that were driving resistance.[296] Continuing advances in single-cell genomics technologies and accompanying computational methods are likely to further advance these findings over the next 5 years.

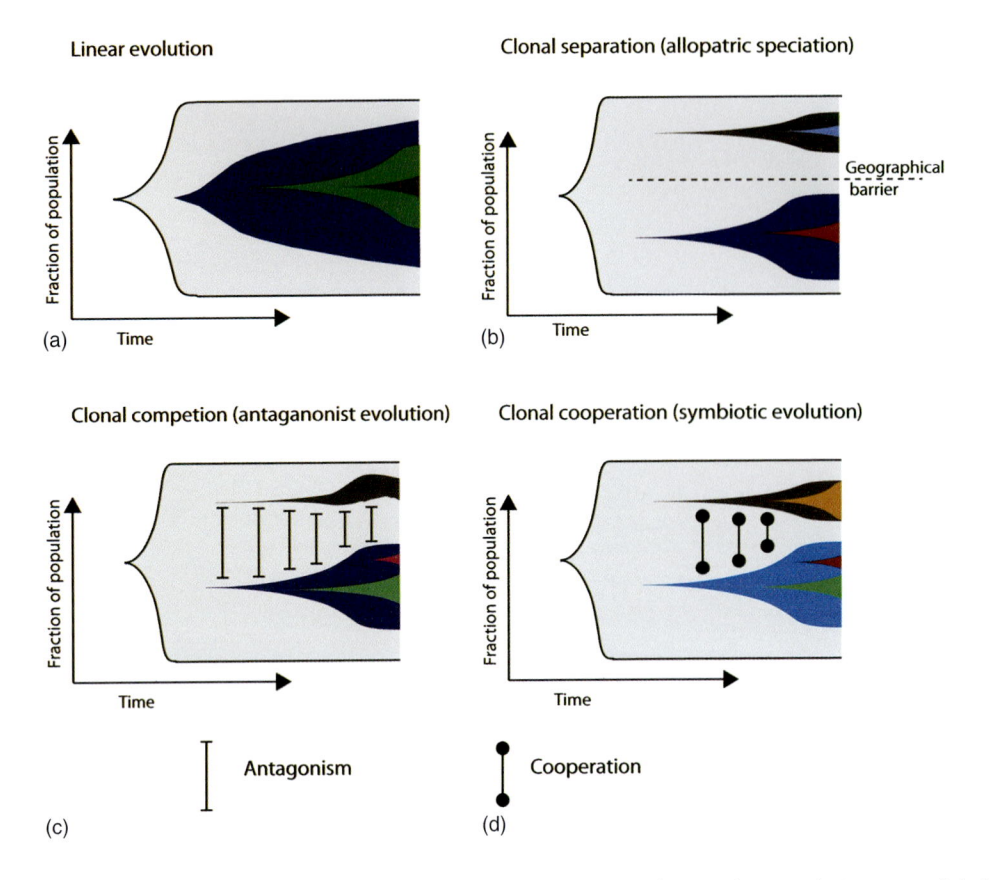

Figure 6 (a) Linear evolution involves sequential accumulation of mutations over time. As can be seen, linear evolution can result in heterogeneity if a subclone has failed to outcompete its predecessors. (b) Tumor subclones may evolve through a process equivalent to allopatric speciation when subclonal populations are geographically distinct within a tumor. (c) Clonal competition can occur between subclonal populations, where distinct subclones compete for growth advantages (equivalent to an antagonistic relationship). (d) Subclonal populations may cooperate, resulting in a symbiotic relationship. Source: From McGranahan and Swanton,[289] Reprinted with permission.

Although clonal diversification is crucial, recent data indicates that simple outgrowth of the most aggressive clones does not fully account for the extent of clonal evolution in cancer. Indeed, similar to the principles of evolutionary biology in general, where no species evolves in isolation, cancers seem to evolve within an ecosystem of interactions not only with the host but also with other coexisting tumor clones. For example, in an experimental model of glioblastoma a minor clone harboring an *EGFR* mutation appears to support the major *EGFR*-wt clone through paracrine mechanisms.[304] Similarly, within heterogeneous tumors in zebrafish melanoma xenograft models a phenomenon of "cooperative invasion" is seen. Here, the presence of an invasive clone enables invasion by another, otherwise poorly invasive clone.[305] Such clonal cooperation does not only apply to tumor survival and progression but also extends into the realm of therapeutic resistance. In a model of colon cancer, for instance, the presence of an EGFR inhibitor-resistant, *KRAS*-mutated minor clone appears to support the survival of a drug-sensitive, *KRAS*-wt clone through paracrine mechanisms involving transforming growth factor α and amphiregulin.[283]

Based on the above temporal and spatial constraints as well as clonal interactions, several models of clonal evolution have been proposed.[289] These range from (1) a simple model of linear evolution, where successive accumulation of mutations leads to increasingly aggressive clones that outcompete their predecessors, to (2) models of allopatric speciation, where subpopulations evolve in geographically distinct areas of the tumor, to the models incorporating clonal interactions including (3) a model of clonal competition with distinct clones competing for growth advantages in the form of antagonistic evolution and (4) a model of clonal cooperation with a symbiotic relationship between individual clones (Figure 6). The complexity of clonal dynamics and evolution have necessitated the application of mathematical models born from the foundations of population genetics.

Mathematical models have been used to quantify and predict clonal evolution in cancer.[306,307] Beginning with an initiating event, such as a DNA mutation, the principles of population genetics such as mutation rates, evolutionary selection, and trait fixation can be used to compute the probabilities of clonal emergence and heterogeneity within the tumor.[308] Classical population genetics models such as the Wright–Fisher model translate these concepts into a mathematical framework.[309,310] These methods have been extended to include spatial structures in tissues and evolution through heterogeneous populations[311,312] and as a theoretical and mathematical structure to discover functional evolutionary dependencies in human cancers.[313]

The variant allelic fraction of mutations identified genome-wide or within exomes is often used to identify subclonal populations within bulk tumor samples. Mathematical models can be used to hypothesize the temporal evolution of clones within the cancer and are able to produce linear, branched, neutral, or punctuated evolutionary dynamics, depending on the strength of the selection pressures and fitness advantages conferred or removed by different classes of mutations.[314] These models also provide predictions of cancer evolution and immune evasion such as the evolution of neoantigens produced by a tumor.[315]

Recently, evolutionary game theory (EGT) has been used to adapt the concept of fitness into cancer clonal dynamics.[316] The EGT framework has been used to improve treatment through two mechanisms: (1) mitigation of the emergence of resistant clones in the tumor and (2) taking advantage of collateral sensitivity.

An evolutionary strategy to treat cancer is to control, rather than eradicate, all cancer cells. Gatenby and colleagues have shown how resistant clones may be prevented from dominating the tumor through treatment-induced selection pressure using an adaptive treatment strategy based on EGT.[317,318] Instead of applying the principle of maximum tolerated dose, leaving behind a subset of resistant clones resulting in treatment failure and tumor recurrence, Gatenby suggests intermittent low-dose treatments aimed at maintaining a low tumor burden consisting of both sensitive and resistant tumor clones. Zhang et al.[319] have implemented this treatment design in a clinical trial in the setting of castrate-resistant metastatic prostate cancer with promising results. Bridging the modeling with experiments, Kaznatcheev et al. proposed a method to estimate the parameters of a given EGT model in the cocultures of NSCLC cells that are sensitive and resistant to the kinase inhibitor alectinib that may be used to design treatment strategies that incorporate the dynamics of sensitive and resistant clones during treatment.[320]

Another approach to cancer treatment optimization through evolutionary principles and mathematical modeling is the principle of collateral sensitivity, wherein evolution under a first drug induces susceptibility to a second. Dhawan et al. demonstrated this concept by evolving the ALK rearranged NSCLC line H3122 to a panel of 4 ALK TKIs and showed that all ALK inhibitor resistant cell lines displayed significant cross-resistance to all other ALK inhibitors.[321] Zhao et al.[322] then showed how the temporal dynamics of collateral sensitivity may be exploited by resulting in hypersensitivity to diverse small molecules. Nichol et al.[323] then used *Escherichia coli* bacteria to show that collateral sensitivity depends on the repeatability of evolution, suggesting that evolutionary dynamics should first be predictable before collateral sensitivity can be effectively used as a tool to control tumor evolution through combination treatment approaches. This work led to a novel application of counterdiabatic driving, first used in quantum mechanics with applications to quantum computing, to hypothetically control the speed and trajectory of cancer evolution through, for example, modulation of drug concentrations.[324] Taken all together, theoretical and computational models of tumor clonal evolution can be used to (1) better understand the clonal architecture of tumors arising from selection pressures and spatial constraints in order to (2) mitigate the emergence of resistance to single or combination treatments[325,326] and (3) identify vulnerabilities that either preexist or result from treatment-induced selection pressures with the ultimate goal of improving therapeutic response and eliminating tumor recurrence.

Understanding of the molecular spectrum and mechanisms of cancer evolution impacts our ability to treat cancer. Molecular heterogeneity and clonal evolution limit the benefits derived from targeted treatments. The repertoire of clones with distinct molecular signatures within each patient's tumor(s) allows for treatment-driven selection, manifesting as acquired therapeutic resistance even in patients who initially respond to treatment. Preexisting somatic mutations (even passenger events) or new mutations acquired during therapy can drive therapeutic resistance. While improvements in experimental models have enhanced our ability to understand and perturb complex patterns of clonal evolution in the laboratory, development of methods such as ctDNA analysis in plasma can allow monitoring of clonal evolution in the clinic.[327] In patients who progress on targeted therapies, multiple studies have shown that somatic mutations driving resistance are detectable in plasma. For instance, lung cancer patients treated with erlotinib or gefitinib (an EGFR inhibitor) most often develop acquired treatment resistance due to a second mutation in *EGFR* T790M that affects drug binding. This resistance-driving mutation is detectable in ctDNA up to 16 weeks before disease progression is evident on routine imaging.[264] Similar data has been reported for patients with colorectal cancer who progress on cetuximab (an anti-EGFR antibody) where *KRAS* mutations are evident weeks before disease progression.[328] A recent study of colorectal cancer patients confirmed that if targeted therapy is discontinued upon disease progression (a drug holiday) and replaced with chemotherapy, circulating levels of the *KRAS* mutation in ctDNA recede (suggesting recession of *KRAS*-mutation bearing tumor subclone).[329] While these studies used deep targeted sequencing strategies to investigate hypothetical genes driving treatment resistance, hypothesis-free genome-wide analysis to discover novel drivers of treatment resistance has also been described.[269] These proof-of-principle results describing ctDNA analysis to track clonal evolution warrant investigation of ctDNA-based personalized adaptive, sequential, or combination treatment strategies.

Cancer genomics and evolution in clinical practice: a case study in melanoma

Background

Malignant melanoma is the fifth most common cancer in males and sixth most common in females in the United States and is one of few that is increasing in incidence.[330] Although detection and surgical resection of early-stage disease can be curative, a primary tumor with thickness of merely 1 mm can result in metastatic disease and an abysmal prognosis. Dramatic recent progress in melanoma precision medicine powerfully illustrates the potential for genomics to impact clinical cancer management. In this section we focus on this progress and its impact on melanoma treatment, while clinical features will be discussed in detail elsewhere. Melanoma is a disease of transformed melanocytes and is clinically subdivided by anatomic location, histopathology, sun exposure, and progression (using tumor-node-metastasis staging).[331] By site, cutaneous melanoma most commonly originates on the sun-exposed skin and is further categorized based on the type of sun exposure of the primary site in areas with chronic sun exposure (e.g., face and forearms) and those with intermittent sun exposure (e.g., back). Less-common subtypes include acral melanoma, occurring on non-hair-bearing areas of the skin on the hands and feet; ocular melanoma, which is predominantly uveal with a smaller proportion of conjunctival melanomas; mucosal (nasopharyngeal, bowel, anorectal, or vulvovaginal); and primary CNS melanoma. Although historically all metastatic melanomas were treated with largely ineffective cytotoxic chemotherapies, recent insights into molecular differences among melanoma subtypes have ushered a new era in the management of this disease.[332]

The genetic basis of melanoma

Where variation in clinical course by melanoma histopathologic subtype is confounding, genomic characterization is now helping to clarify the etiology, biology, and optimal treatment. Just

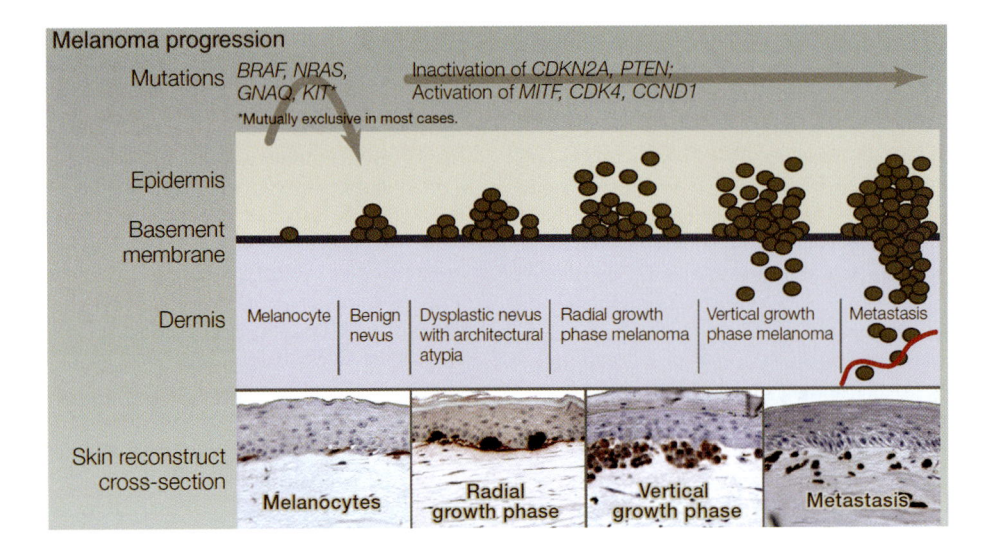

Figure 7 The genetic basis of cutaneous melanoma. Melanoma, the deadliest of skin cancers, is caused by the transformation of melanocytes (pigment-producing cells) that accumulate genetic alterations, leading to abnormal proliferation and dissemination. Clinically, melanoma lesions can be classified based on the location and progression, which range from benign nevi to metastatic melanoma. Important driver genes in melanomas are shown in the figure. MAPK signaling is often constitutively activated through alterations in membrane receptors or through mutations of RAS or BRAF. Source: Adapted from Vultur and Herlyn.[333] Reprinted with permission.

as breast cancer can best be characterized according to the ER, PR, and Her2 status, the genotype should now take a prominent role in the clinical approach to melanoma due to its implications for treatment. Although the genesis of melanoma is still poorly understood, melanoma is known to occur through the stepwise accumulation of mutations in cancer genes within melanocytes (Figure 7).[333] Most melanomas are sporadic with 5–10% of cases due to familial predisposition predominantly driven by germline variants in the first familial melanoma gene identified—the tumor suppressor *CDKN2A* (40% of the familial cases).[334-336] Additional rare variants in other cancer genes have since been found in familial cases (*CDK4, BRCA2, BAP1, TERT* promoter, *MITF*, and *POT1*[337-342]). Beyond heredity, UV radiation is recognized as the greatest risk factor for cutaneous melanomas, although not for sun-shielded mucosal, acral, or ocular disease.[343] In keeping with UV etiology, additional melanoma risk factors include fair skin, increased freckling and benign nevi, *MC1R* germline variants, and tanning.[344-347]

Early genetic and functional characterization of melanoma determined that it is driven both by mutations that inactivate cell cycle gatekeepers and also by those that activate cell proliferation pathways. Building on the discovery of familial mutations in *CDKN2A*, a locus that regulates the p53 and RB proteins, these tumor suppressors were found to be frequently disrupted by disparate mutations that enable unconstrained cell growth such as *CDKN2A, CDK4, RB1, TP53,* and *MDM2* mutations.[348-352] Meanwhile frequent mutations in the proliferation pathway genes *BRAF, KIT, NRAS,* and *PTEN* were identified and found to cooperate with the inactivation of cell cycle tumor suppressors to promote malignancy.[114,118,353-366] Cytogenetic and molecular studies further pointed to as-yet unidentified genes in recurrently altered regions of chromosomes 1p, 6q, 7p, and 11q.[352,367-375] As with many early genetic analyses of human cancers, these studies were typically performed in disparate small cohorts or model systems, focused on only one or several genes in a single clinical subtype, and often produced inconclusive results.

Melanoma genomic landscapes

The striking genetic complexity between the subtypes and within individual tumor genomes revealed by the above analyses was soon confirmed at high resolution through a succession of genomic studies. Genome-wide aCGH profiling and targeted sequencing of *BRAF* and *NRAS* in 126 tumors first revealed the distinct patterns of somatic mutation based on the subtype. *BRAF* and *NRAS* mutations were found to be enriched in sun-shielded cutaneous melanoma but rare in sun-exposed, mucosal, and acral melanomas. The patterns of mutation also varied by the subtype with CNVs enriched in mucosal melanoma. Subsequent analyses identified patterns of CNV correlating with poor prognosis[49,353] as well as subtype-specific *KIT* mutations occurring in 10–20% of mucosal and acral as well as at low frequency in cutaneous melanoma in sun-damaged sites.[48,376] The existence of molecular subsets of disease was also borne out by gene expression microarray studies,[84,377,378] and such molecular subsetting of clinical melanoma categories seeded hope that these types could be tied to clinical outcome or exploited for therapeutic targeting.[379]

A spate of massively parallel sequencing studies beginning in 2011 spurred explosive growth in the genomic understanding of cutaneous melanoma, recently culminating in two large multiplatform studies that jointly span over 500 cases.[141,339,379-389] These studies corroborate prior identification of important melanoma drivers (*BRAF, NRAS, NF1, TP53, CDKN2A,* and *RB1*) and also point to new genes not previously linked to the disease including *RAC1, PREX2, PPP6C, ARID2, TACC1, GRM3, MAP3K4, MAP3K9, IDH1, MRPS31, RPS27,* and the *TERT* promoter. Melanoma is now predominantly categorized according to *BRAF, RAS,* and *NF1* status, all of which, when mutated, constitutively activate the mitogen-activated protein kinase (MAPK) pathway, a central regulator of cell proliferation (Figure 8, 141). These mutations tend to be mutually exclusive and account for all but 10% of cases, suggesting four genomic subtypes: BRAF, NRAS, NF1, and "triple wild type" (TWT). Genome-wide sequencing has also enabled the characterization of mutation signatures in melanoma, shedding further light on the role of UV radiation in various subtypes. Melanomas on sun-exposed skin are characterized by UV

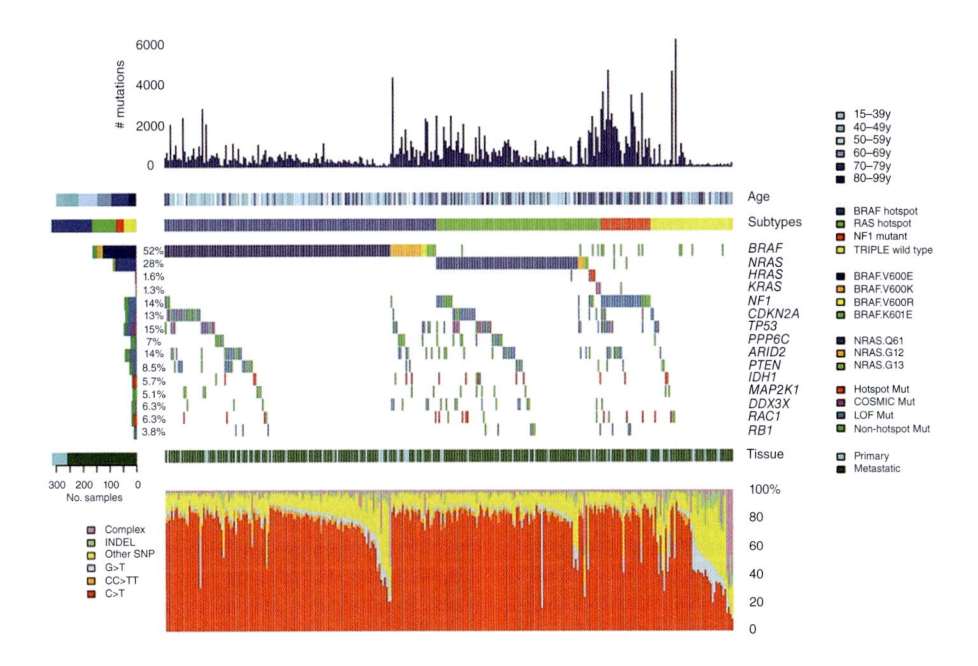

Figure 8 The genomic landscape of cutaneous melanoma. The total number of mutations, age at melanoma accession, and mutation subtype (BRAF, RAS [N/H/K], NF1, and Triple-WT) are indicated for each sample (top). (Not shown are one hypermutated and one cooccurring NRAS BRAF hot-spot mutant). The color-coded matrix of individual mutations (specific BRAF and NRAS mutations indicated) (middle), the type of melanoma specimen (primary or metastasis), and mutation spectra for all samples (bottom) are indicated. For the two samples with both a matched primary and metastatic sample, only the mutation information from the metastasis was included. Source: From The Cancer Genome Atlas Network.[141] Reprinted with permission.

signature mutations—cytosine to thymine (C>T) substitutions occurring in dipyrimidines as more than 60% of the total mutation burden.[141,382,390] Curiously, most common mutations in BRAF and NRAS are not C>T substitutions despite their driver roles in the majority of sun-exposed melanomas.[381] While it is often noted that melanoma has one of the highest average mutational burden of any cancer type, the mutation frequency can range from 0.1 to 100 mutations per megabase.[177] This marked heterogeneity tracks with the clinical heterogeneity of the disease, with the highest mutational rate in melanoma on sun-exposed skin at >100/Mb, intermediate rates in mucosal melanoma at 2–5/Mb, and the lowest rates in uveal and CNS melanoma at <0.1/Mb.[380,391,392]

Cutaneous BRAF melanomas account for over 50% of tumors and predominantly bear the hotspot missense mutation V600E, although other activating BRAF mutations, amplifications, and even fusions do occur. BRAF-mutated melanomas are characterized by higher incidence in younger patients; UV signature in 91%; relatively fewer CNVs compared to TWT; amplifications of BRAF, MITF, PD-1, and PD-L1; enrichment for TP53 mutations; and more frequent PTEN deletions. RAS melanomas are the second most common (30%), typically NRAS Q61R/K/L and with occasional mutations in KRAS or HRAS. These mutations are nearly always mutually exclusive with BRAF mutations although molecular features of this category otherwise resemble the BRAF subtype. NF1 melanomas comprise 15% of cases, the majority of which contain inactivating NF1 mutation. Among the above three subtypes, NF1-mutated melanomas bear the highest SNV burden, occur in older patients, and contain a UV signature. It can cooccur with BRAF and NRAS mutations and tends to show a pattern of cooccurrence with other mutated "RASopathy" genes such as RASA2.[383] Similar to BRAF and RAS mutations, in most NF1 mutation can drive MAPK pathway activation. Finally, TWT melanoma is a heterogeneous subtype that lacks recurrent driver mutations although KIT, CTNNB1, GNAQ, GNA11, and EZH2 mutations have been found at low frequency. Notable characteristics of this subtype include higher numbers of SVs, fusions, and CNVs; amplifications containing KIT, PDGFRA, KDR, CDK4, CCND1, MDM2, and TERT; and only few (7%) with TERT promoter mutations and only 30% containing UV signature mutations.[141] It is important to highlight that despite diversity across genomic subtypes, the vast majority of melanoma driver mutations converge on the MAPK and PI3K pathways, such that approximately 91% of cutaneous melanomas depend on aberrant activation of this single pathway.[141]

Despite exhaustive characterization of cutaneous melanoma, genomic landscapes of less-common clinical subtypes remain poorly characterized. Several small studies of uveal, acral, desmoplastic, and mucosal melanoma have identified recurrent mutations, but much still remains unknown. Uveal melanoma, the most common ocular tumor, has been shown in studies encompassing nearly 80 cases to have one of the lowest melanoma mutation burdens and to be characterized by mutations in GNAQ (50%) as well as frequent BAP1, EIF1AX, and SF3B1 mutations in tumors with high metastatic propensity.[388,389,393–395] Acral melanoma occurs on the non-hair-bearing skin of the palms, soles, and nail beds; is the most common melanoma subtype in non-Caucasians; and has a poorer prognosis than cutaneous melanoma on the hair-bearing skin due to later diagnosis.[396] Although known to be largely BRAF wild type for nearly a decade, acral melanoma is rarely included in larger cutaneous genomics studies, and limited focused data sets are available. Now, hundreds of acral melanomas have been characterized across a number of studies both in the United States and China. These studies have identified the following characteristics: about 30% KIT mutant, 20% BRAF mutant, 10% NRAS mutant, low SNV burden, high CNV and SV burden, and the absence of UV signature.[49,380–382,395,397,398] Data on mucosal melanoma, another rare and aggressive subtype that is predominantly BRAF wild type, is sparse with few cases comprehensively assessed.[391] This study largely confirmed prior targeted and cytogenomic analyses,

Table 7 Therapeutic options in melanoma by genomic subtype.

Genotype	Approved treatments	Selected phase I or II data
BRAF mutant	• Vemurafenib (BRAFi) + cobimetinib (MEKi) for BRAF V600E/K mutated melanoma • Dabrafenib (BRAFi) + trametinib (MEKi) for BRAF V600E/K mutated melanoma • Encorafenib (BRAFi) + binimetinib (MEKi) for BRAF V600E/K mutated melanoma In combination with immunotherapy[a] • Atezolizumab (anti-PD-L1) + vemurafenib (BRAFi) + cobimetinib (MEKi) for BRAF V600E/K mutated melanoma	
NRAS mutant	Targeted therapy—none	Trametinib, MEK162
Triple wild type[b]	Targeted therapy—none	None
KIT mutant or overexpressed	Targeted therapy—none	Imatinib, Nilotinib, Dasatinib
GNAQ/GNA11 mutant	Targeted therapy—none	Selumetinib, Trametinib, MEK 162
Other targets	Larotrectinib (NRTK fusions)	
Immunotherapy/high tumor mutational burden (TMB)	Monotherapy: • Ipilimumab: CTLA4 inhibitor • Nivolumab: PD-1 Inhibitor • Pembrolizumab: PD-1 Inhibitor • Atezolizumab: PD-L1 inhibitor Combination: • Nivolumab + ipilimumab • Atezolizumab (anti-PD-L1) + vemurafenib (BRAFi) + cobimetinib (MEKi) for BRAF V600E/K mutated melanoma High mutational burden • Pembrolizumab—tumors with high TMB (≥10 mut/MB)	

[a]Phase III studies for immunotherapy have not included genotyping beyond BRAF. FDA approval for these does not specify genotype and thus is inclusive of all genotypes.
[b]No trials to date have specifically identified TWT patients, although KIT and GNAQ/GNA11 cases do occur in this category.

showing a low SNV frequency; high CNV and SV burden; absence of UV signature; and recurrent mutations in KIT, PTEN, and other putative cancer genes in two or fewer samples. Desmoplastic melanoma, a rare and invasive fibrous form of dermal melanoma, has also recently been characterized (62 cases), and preliminary results reveal a notably high SNV burden (one of the highest to date at 62 mutations/Mb), UV signatures, absence of BRAF or NRAS mutations, and a diverse array of mutations that activate the MAPK and PI3K pathways.[399] Notable similarities and differences between these rare tumor types support their potentially distinct etiology and may help guide therapeutic management.

Clinical implications of melanoma genomics

Although no definitive correlation with outcome has been identified based on the above genomic subtyping or other molecular classifications in melanoma, these genomic subtypes have direct bearing on the treatment of advanced metastatic melanoma (Table 7). The BRAF subtype carries the greatest array of clinical options. Mutant BRAF has now proven to be an effective therapeutic target, with BRAF V600E/K and K601 targetable by the inhibitors of BRAF or MEK. As of 2015, three such small molecule inhibitors have demonstrated an overall survival (OS) benefit in randomized clinical trials. Vemurafenib and dabrafenib are BRAF inhibitors (BRAFis) with demonstrated response rates greater than 90% in mutant BRAF melanoma.[249,400] Trametinib is a MEK inhibitor (MEKi) which, while less dramatically effective than BRAFi, nevertheless triples PFS versus chemotherapy.[401] The best results to date from trials of targeted agents in mutant BRAF melanoma have come from combined BRAFi and MEKi use, illustrated by dabrafenib and trametinib, a combination with marked improvement in PFS and OS with an overall reduction in toxicity.[402,403] Today, BRAFi and MEKi are used principally in combinations, rather than monotherapies.

In addition, emerging combinations of immunotherapy with targeted therapy have led to the approval of triple combination treatment including anti-PD1 antibodies with BRAFi and MEKi (e.g., atezolizumab + vemurafenib + cobimetinib).[404,405]

Development of targeted agents to treat melanomas driven by NRAS, NF1, TWT, and rare histological melanoma subtypes has lagged behind that for mutant BRAF melanoma, with no completed phase III studies. Nevertheless, early-phase clinical studies have shown sufficient efficacy to encourage the ongoing efforts at developing agents for these patients. NRAS melanoma has been treated with a variety of MEKis in clinical trials including trametinib,[406] MEK162,[407] and selumetinib.[408] Of these, only MEK162 has shown a significant response rate (around 20%), with the others showing a best response of stable disease. No trials have been conducted specifically in NF1 melanoma, in part due to the emerging understanding of this subtype and overlap with RAF and RAS subtypes. Conflicting preclinical reports have suggested that NF1 mutation and/or loss confers sensitivity or resistance to MEKi, and that this relationship is also dependent on the RAF/RAS status.[383,409–411] KIT-mutant melanoma (which is common in TWT cutaneous as well as acral and mucosal subtypes) has been shown in two randomized Phase II studies to have an overall response rate to imatinib of 19–29%, with the best responses in cases with canonical KIT SNVs rather than amplifications.[350,412] The most robust data in GNAQ/GNA11-mutant disease comes from a randomized phase II study with the MEKi selumetinib.[413] Selumetinib induced tumor regression in 49% of patients and led to a nonstatistically significant improvement in OS to 11.8 months versus 9.1 months. Additional agents in the development that are relevant to many subtypes and/or may motivate additional subtyping include CDK, MDM2, and PI3K/Akt/mTOR inhibitors in clinical trials in addition to ERK, IDH1, EZH2, and aurora kinase inhibitors in various stages of preclinical or clinical development.[141]

In addition to targeted agents against commonly mutated proteins in melanoma, additional targeted agents may have relevance for treatment of melanomas based on individual molecular aberations. For example, larotrectinib, which was approved by the FDA in October of 2020 for patients with solid tumors that have a *NTRK* gene fusion, may have role in the treatment of individual melanoma patients harboring these fusions.[414] Although such fusions are rare in typical cutaneous melanomas, they may be significantly more common in certain melanoma subtypes, such as Spitzoid melanoma.[415]

Immunotherapies, especially immune checkpoint inhibitors (ICIs) in the case of melanoma, have revolutionized standard-of-care treatment regimens. The initial clinical data around the CTLA-4 inhibitor, ipilimumab,[416,417] followed by the PD1 inhibitors, pembrolizumab[418,419] and nivolumab,[420–422] have demonstrated improved, durable responses not only in melanomas but in a host of solid tumor types as well.[423,424] Despite these improvements in outcomes, many patients do not respond to single agent or combination therapies that include ICIs, while significant adverse events have been observed in other patients.[425] Thus, there is a growing need for predictive and prognostic markers associated with ICI treatment. The role of genomics in guiding response/resistance to immunotherapeutic regimens is just beginning to be elucidated.[426–428]

As ICIs are approved for a number of indications, including melanoma, there are established biomarkers, such as the protein levels of PD-L1, the cognate ligand to PD-1.[429] The KEYNOTE 024 trial demonstrated improved outcomes in NSCLC patients whose tumor harbored a PD-L1 protein expression above 50%.[430] However, disparities among assays, biopsy specimens, varied levels across multiple tumors from a single person, and mixed results across tumor types have complicated a sole reliance on PD-L1 expression level.[429,431] Two more established biomarkers associated with ICI response are TMB and mismatch repair deficiency (dMMR)/microsatellite instability (MSI). Checkmate 227 demonstrated that TMB (defined as 10 mutations per megabase in that trial) predicted benefit, irrespective of PDL1 expression.[432] Likewise, colorectal cancer studies revealed that dMMR/MSI high tumors had improved overall response rates.[433] Despite these results, patients with low TMB and/or low dMMR/MSI respond to ICI treatment, necessitating refinement of these strategies. Access to more comprehensive sequencing (such as those described earlier in this article) will incorporate accurate algorithms for TMB calculation and dMMR/MSI assessment.

Though in its infancy, studies are now comparing ICI response in the context of specific genomic alterations. In melanoma, *BRAF* mutation has no significant effect on the response to approved ICI regimens.[434] Ongoing and future trials that employ combinations of ICIs with targeted therapeutics (e.g., BRAFis and MEKis) may show differences in response based on mutational profiles. Outside of melanoma, there are a few examples of molecular alterations impacting ICI response rates. In a study of ~250 patients with solid tumors, Miao et al. showed that inactivating mutations in the tumor suppressor *PTEN* clustered in patients with primary ICI resistance.[435] In smaller clinical studies, mutations in *POLE* confer a favorable response to ICIs.[436,437] Given that *POLE* mutations can lead to an "ultramutated" phenotype, there is compelling rationale for exploring this rare mutation in response to ICIs. One compelling biological vignette is the response of NSCLC harboring *KRAS* mutations with and without loss of the tumor suppressor *STK11*. Both in preclinical models and patients, the overall response rate in patients with concomitant KRAS and STK11 mutations is significantly worse than patients whose tumors harbor KRAS mutations alone or KRAS with loss of TP53.[438,439] Thus, even in settings with clear genomic driver events, secondary mutations may impact ICI response rates. Finally, exome sequencing affords the opportunity to elucidate molecular signatures correlated with ICI response. A 105-gene, immune signature differentiated responders from nonresponders in response to CTLA-4 inhibition in melanoma.[440]

As the number of immunotherapeutic options (ICIs, CAR-T, etc.) increase, and the approval of ICIs in combination with cytotoxic therapies and/or targeted agents continues, there will be an unmet need to identify and clinically deploy molecular predictors of response/resistance to these new therapies. The continued increase in trials incorporating WGS, single-cell sequencing, and cell-free DNA sequencing will certainly provide opportunities to elucidate such biomarkers.

Table 8 Hypothetical treatment approaches to acquired BRAFi/MEKi resistance.

Mechanism of resistance	Therapeutic strategy
EGFR activation	EGFR inhibitor—erlotinib, gefitinib, afatinib, dasatinib PIK3 inhibitor—in trials
IGF-1R activation	PIK3Ca inhibitor—in trials
PTEN loss	
PTEN mutation	
PIK3CA activation	
cMET activation	cMET inhibitor—crizotinib
PDGFR-β activation	RTK inhibitor—dasatinib, sunitinib
FGFR activation	FGFR inhibitors—ponatinib, dasatinib
COT activation	ERK inhibitor—in trials

Drug resistance and evolution in melanoma

Despite the activity of targeted agents in *BRAF* melanoma, drug resistance (both innate and acquired) remains a key challenge. Only about 50% of patients respond to BRAFi, and in those who do respond, acquired resistance to BRAFi invariably develops.[249] BRAFi resistance is driven by a diverse range of mechanisms, most of which reactivate MAPK activity or redirect proliferative signaling through the PI3K pathway. Resistance can occur through further mutation in *NRAS*,[441] *MEK1*,[442,443] *MEK2*,[443] *NF1*,[409] or *BRAF* (via amplification).[444] *BRAF* splice variants,[445] *EGFR* activation,[446,447] and *COT* activation[448] have also been implicated. Activation of other receptor tyrosine kinases such as *PDGFR-β* and *IGF-1R* or loss of *PTEN* has also been demonstrated in laboratory models.[443,449–453] Clinical trials are ongoing to test whether identification of these resistance mechanisms in the clinical setting will allow for targeted therapeutic approaches that may circumvent resistance to BRAFi. The hypothetical approaches to circumvent specific resistance mechanism after progression on dual inhibition with BRAFi and MEKi are shown in Table 8.

With the recent approval of new targeted and immunologic therapies for metastatic disease, it is now critically important to clearly identify the genetic signature of the patient's disease in order to optimize outcomes. Likewise, genomic testing can accelerate new drug development and target identification for the less-common subtypes of melanoma and potentially lead to identification of resistance pathways to guide drug selection in individual patients. Thus, the genomic landscape of melanomas conforms to the clinical heterogeneity of the disease, with melanomas of different locations having markedly different genotypic signatures that speak to distinct etiologies. The challenge, then, is to use available genomic technologies in a real-time clinical setting. In theory, one could identify and follow the disease mechanisms active in the individual patient to guide treatment selection over time.

In addition to molecular diversity across melanoma subtypes and even between individual patients within the same disease subtype, a higher order of complexity is becoming apparent. As outlined in the previous section on cancer evolution, recent data indicates that development of melanoma cannot be fully explained by a linear model of accumulating mutations leading to an increasingly aggressive phenotype. Instead, an emerging picture points to cancer as a complex ecosystem driven by the process of branched clonal evolution. As a result, multiple related but distinct clonal lineages may exist within a single patient,[281] with some lineages being more likely to progress and metastasize.[282] Furthermore, this diversity may provide an escape mechanism leading to therapeutic resistance. This is well illustrated by almost universal development of resistance to BRAF inhibition in melanoma, where rapidly relapsing disease can harbor multiple resistance mechanisms differing between individual subclones even within a single patient.[454] This challenge is potentiated by the fact that, while some mechanisms of resistance are driven by mutations, others appear to be mediated through epigenetic or posttranslational processes.[455] The obvious and critical question raised by these observations is whether a single tumor biopsy in a metastatic setting can capture the full spectrum of disease heterogeneity, its drivers, and potential therapeutic targets. The solution to this conundrum may lie in approaches with the potential to monitor the clonal complexity on a larger scale, such as "liquid biopsies," which attempt to molecularly characterize circulating tumor DNA in patient's bloodstream. Emerging data evaluating the detection of ctDNA and the concordance of *BRAF* mutation status between the tumor and plasma samples is encouraging.[276,456,457] In addition, anecdotal evidence suggests that serial ctDNA analysis may be a useful marker of treatment response to immunotherapy.[265]

Summary

The detailed characterization of the genomic lesions underlying cancer has led to the identification of biological pathways driving tumorigenesis, improved cancer diagnosis through molecular classification, enhanced selection of therapeutic targets for drug development, promoted the development of faster and more efficient clinical trials using targeted agents and sophisticated biomarkers, and created markers for early detection and recurrence surveillance. Yet, gaps nonetheless remain in our knowledge of the causative mutations underlying some cancers, in our understanding of the biology of the mutations we have identified, in developing drugs capable of targeting many of these diverse mutations, and in fending off the inevitable emergence of drug resistance. As summarized in this article, genomics has already made extraordinary contributions to our understanding of cancer biology and cancer medicine. Nevertheless, the enormous potential of cancer genomics has only just begun to be realized.

Acknowledgments

The authors thank the patients who have supported these studies and also Matthew Taila, Victoria Zismann, Jessica Lang, and Jim Schupp for assistance in the preparation and proofreading of this article as well as Jeffrey Watkins for assistance in creation of figures. WPDH, AS, AHB, and JMT received research support from a Stand Up To Cancer—Melanoma Research Alliance/Melanoma Dream Team Translational Cancer Research Grant (SU2C-AACR-DT0612). Stand Up To Cancer is a program of the Entertainment Industry Foundation administered by the American Association for Cancer Research (AACR). WPDH, AS, PR, and JMT are supported by NIH R01CA195670. AS is additionally supported by the Pardee Foundation, NIH R01CA179157, and NIHR01CA185072. MM is additionally supported by a grant from the Science Foundation Arizona. JMT is additionally supported by the Komen Breast Cancer Foundation KG111063 and the Melanoma Research Alliance VUMC42693-R with additional generous support from The Entertainment Industry Foundation, Dell, Inc. through the Dell Powering the Possible Program, and Yale Cancer Center's UM1 CA186689.

Key references

The complete reference list can be found on Vital Source version of this title, see inside front cover.

1. Nowell PC. The clonal evolution of tumor cell populations. *Science*. 1976;**194**(4260):23–28.
2. Hanahan D, Weinberg RA. Hallmarks of cancer: the next generation. *Cell*. 2011;**144**(5):646–674.
3. Fearon ER, Vogelstein B. A genetic model for colorectal tumorigenesis. *Cell*. 1990;**61**(5):759–767.
4. Vogelstein B, Papadopoulos N, Velculescu VE, et al. Cancer genome landscapes. *Science*. 2013;**339**(6127):1546–1558.
33. Gracia E, Ray ME, Polymeropoulos MH, et al. Isolation of chromosome-specific ESTs by microdissection-mediated cDNA capture. *Genome Res*. 1997;**7**(2):100–107.
34. Guan XY, Trent JM, Meltzer PS. Generation of band-specific painting probes from a single microdissected chromosome. *Hum Mol Genet*. 1993;**2**(8):1117–1121.
35. Guan XY, Zhang HE, Zhou H, et al. Characterization of a complex chromosome rearrangement involving 6q in a melanoma cell line by chromosome microdissection. *Cancer Genet Cytogenet*. 2002;**134**(1):65–70.
37. Meltzer PS, Guan XY, Trent JM. Telomere capture stabilizes chromosome breakage. *Nat Genet*. 1993;**4**(3):252–255.
38. Meltzer PS, Guan X-Y, Burgess A, Trent JM. Rapid generation of region specific probes by chromosome microdissection and their application. *Nat Genet*. 1992;**1**(1):24–28.
71. Lander ES, Linton LM, Birren B, et al. Initial sequencing and analysis of the human genome. *Nature*. 2001;**409**(6822):860–921.
72. Venter JC, Adams MD, Myers EW, et al. The sequence of the human genome. *Science*. 2001;**291**(5507):1304–1351.
78. Velculescu VE, Zhang L, Vogelstein B, Kinzler KW. Serial analysis of gene expression. *Science*. 1995;**270**(5235):484–487.
84. Bittner M, Meltzer P, Chen Y, et al. Molecular classification of cutaneous malignant melanoma by gene expression profiling. *Nature*. 2000;**406**(6795):536–540.
85. Sorlie T, Perou CM, Tibshirani R, et al. Gene expression patterns of breast carcinomas distinguish tumor subclasses with clinical implications. *Proc Natl Acad Sci U S A*. 2001;**98**(19):10869–10874.
95. Pavey S, Johansson P, Packer L, et al. Microarray expression profiling in melanoma reveals a BRAF mutation signature. *Oncogene*. 2004;**23**(23):4060–4067.
96. Hedenfalk I, Duggan D, Chen Y, et al. Gene-expression profiles in hereditary breast cancer. *N Engl J Med*. 2001;**344**(8):539–548.
101. Dressman D, Yan H, Traverso G, et al. Transforming single DNA molecules into fluorescent magnetic particles for detection and enumeration of genetic variations. *Proc Natl Acad Sci U S A*. 2003;**100**(15):8817–8822.
107. Wheeler DA, Srinivasan M, Egholm M, et al. The complete genome of an individual by massively parallel DNA sequencing. *Nature*. 2008;**452**(7189):872–876.
118. Pollock PM, Harper UL, Hansen KS, et al. High frequency of BRAF mutations in nevi. *Nat Genet*. 2003;**33**(1):19–20.
144. Chen H, Li C, Peng X, et al. A pan-cancer analysis of enhancer expression in nearly 9000 patient samples. *Cell*. 2018;**173**(2):386–99 e12.
158. Zehir A, Benayed R, Shah RH, et al. Mutational landscape of metastatic cancer revealed from prospective clinical sequencing of 10,000 patients. *Nat Med*. 2017;**23**(6):703–713.
165. Ramos P, Karnezis AN, Hendricks WP, et al. Loss of the tumor suppressor SMARCA4 in small cell carcinoma of the ovary, hypercalcemic type (SCCOHT). *Rare Diseases*. 2014;**2**(1):e967148.

172. Tomasetti C, Vogelstein B, Parmigiani G. Half or more of the somatic mutations in cancers of self-renewing tissues originate prior to tumor initiation. *Proc Natl Acad Sci U S A*. 2013;**110**(6):1999–2004.
175. Bozic I, Antal T, Ohtsuki H, et al. Accumulation of driver and passenger mutations during tumor progression. *Proc Natl Acad Sci U S A*. 2010;**107**(43):18545–18550.
202. Bollag G, Tsai J, Zhang J, et al. Vemurafenib: the first drug approved for BRAF-mutant cancer. *Nat Rev Drug Discov*. 2012;**11**(11):873–886.
205. Collins FS, Varmus H. A new initiative on precision medicine. *N Engl J Med*. 2015;**372**(9):793–795.
224. Zhu J, Tucker M, Marin D, et al. Clinical utility of FoundationOne tissue molecular profiling in men with metastatic prostate cancer. *Urol Oncol*. 2019;**37**(11):813e1–e9.
231. Druker BJ, Talpaz M, Resta DJ, et al. Efficacy and safety of a specific inhibitor of the BCR-ABL tyrosine kinase in chronic myeloid leukemia. *N Engl J Med*. 2001;**344**(14):1031–1037.
244. Paez JG, Janne PA, Lee JC, et al. EGFR mutations in lung cancer: correlation with clinical response to gefitinib therapy. *Science*. 2004;**304**(5676):1497–1500.
251. Von Hoff DD, Stephenson JJ, Rosen P, et al. Pilot study using molecular profiling of patients' tumors to find potential targets and select treatments for their refractory cancers. *J Clin Oncol*. 2010;**28**(33):4877–4883.
252. Craig DW, O'Shaughnessy JA, Kiefer JA, et al. Genome and transcriptome sequencing in prospective metastatic triple-negative breast cancer uncovers therapeutic vulnerabilities. *Mol Cancer Ther*. 2013;**12**(1):104–116.
253. Prados MD, Byron SA, Tran NL, et al. Toward precision medicine in glioblastoma: the promise and the challenges. *Neuro-Oncology*. 2015;**17**:1051–1063.
254. Borad MJ, Champion MD, Egan JB, et al. Integrated genomic characterization reveals novel, therapeutically relevant drug targets in FGFR and EGFR pathways in sporadic intrahepatic cholangiocarcinoma. *PLoS Genet*. 2014;**10**(2):e1004135.
255. LoRusso PM, Boerner SA, Pilat MJ, et al. Pilot trial of selecting molecularly guided therapy for patients with non-V600 BRAF-mutant metastatic melanoma: experience of the SU2C/MRA melanoma dream team. *Mol Cancer Ther*. 2015;**14**(8):1962–1971.
261. Diehl F, Schmidt K, Choti MA, et al. Circulating mutant DNA to assess tumor dynamics. *Nat Med*. 2008;**14**(9):985–990.
262. Dawson SJ, Tsui DW, Murtaza M, et al. Analysis of circulating tumor DNA to monitor metastatic breast cancer. *N Engl J Med*. 2013;**368**(13):1199–1209.
269. Murtaza M, Dawson SJ, Tsui DW, et al. Non-invasive analysis of acquired resistance to cancer therapy by sequencing of plasma DNA. *Nature*. 2013;**497**(7447):108–112.
270. Forshew T, Murtaza M, Parkinson C, et al. Noninvasive identification and monitoring of cancer mutations by targeted deep sequencing of plasma DNA. *Sci Transl Med*. 2012;**4**(136):136ra68.
275. McDonald BR, Contente-Cuomo T, Sammut SJ, et al. Personalized circulating tumor DNA analysis to detect residual disease after neoadjuvant therapy in breast cancer. *Sci Transl Med*. 2019;**11**(504):eaax7392.
282. Gerlinger M, Rowan AJ, Horswell S, et al. Intratumor heterogeneity and branched evolution revealed by multiregion sequencing. *N Engl J Med*. 2012;**366**(10):883–892.
311. Allen B, Lippner G, Chen YT, et al. Evolutionary dynamics on any population structure. *Nature*. 2017;**544**(7649):227–230.
317. Rockne RC, Hawkins-Daarud A, Swanson KR, et al. The 2019 mathematical oncology roadmap. *Phys Biol*. 2019;**16**(4):041005.
327. Aparicio S, Caldas C. The implications of clonal genome evolution for cancer medicine. *N Engl J Med*. 2013;**368**(9):842–851.
331. Balch CM, Gershenwald JE, Soong S-j, et al. Final version of 2009 AJCC melanoma staging and classification. *J Clin Oncol*. 2009;**27**(36):6199–6206.
333. Vultur A, Herlyn M. SnapShot: melanoma. *Cancer Cell*. 2013;**23**(5):706–706.e1.
350. Hodi FS, Corless CL, Giobbie-Hurder A, et al. Imatinib for melanomas harboring mutationally activated or amplified KIT arising on mucosal, acral, and chronically sun-damaged skin. *J Clin Oncol*. 2013;**31**(26):3182–3190.
352. Pollock PM, Trent JM. The genetics of cutaneous melanoma. *Clin Lab Med*. 2000;**20**(4):667–690.
365. Pollock P, Walker G, Glendening J, et al. PTEN inactivation is rare in melanoma tumours but occurs frequently in melanoma cell lines. *Melanoma Res*. 2002;**12**(6):565–575.
367. Lee J-H, Miele ME, Hicks DJ, et al. KiSS-1, a novel human malignant melanoma metastasis-suppressor gene. *J Natl Cancer Inst*. 1996;**88**(23):1731–1737.
368. Millikin D, Meese E, Vogelstein B, et al. Loss of heterozygosity for loci on the long arm of chromosome 6 in human malignant melanoma. *Cancer Res*. 1991;**51**(20):5449–5453.
370. Trent JM, Meyskens FL, Salmon SE, et al. Relation of cytogenetic abnormalities and clinical outcome in metastatic melanoma. *N Engl J Med*. 1990;**322**(21):1508–1511.
371. Trent JM, Rosenfeld SB, Meyskens FL. Chromosome 6q involvement in human malignant melanoma. *Cancer Genet Cytogenet*. 1983;**9**(2):177–180.
372. Trent JM, Stanbridge EJ, McBride HL, et al. Tumorigenicity in human melanoma cell lines controlled by introduction of human chromosome 6. *Science*. 1990;**247**(4942):568–571.
373. Trent JM, Thompson FH, Meyskens FL. Identification of a recurring translocation site involving chromosome 6 in human malignant melanoma. *Cancer Res*. 1989;**49**(2):420–423.
374. Wiltshire RN, Duray P, Bittner ML, et al. Direct visualization of the clonal progression of primary cutaneous melanoma: application of tissue microdissection and comparative genomic hybridization. *Cancer Res*. 1995;**55**(18):3954–3957.
400. Hauschild A, Grob JJ, Demidov LV, et al. Dabrafenib in BRAF-mutated metastatic melanoma: a multicentre, open-label, phase 3 randomised controlled trial. *Lancet*. 2012;**380**(9839):358–365.
401. Flaherty KT, Robert C, Hersey P, et al. Improved survival with MEK inhibition in BRAF-mutated melanoma. *N Engl J Med*. 2012;**367**(2):107–114.
402. Flaherty KT, Infante JR, Daud A, et al. Combined BRAF and MEK inhibition in melanoma with BRAF V600 mutations. *N Engl J Med*. 2012;**367**(18):1694–1703.
418. Hamid O, Robert C, Daud A, et al. Safety and tumor responses with lambrolizumab (anti-PD-1) in melanoma. *N Engl J Med*. 2013;**369**(2):134–144.
454. Shi H, Hugo W, Kong X, et al. Acquired resistance and clonal evolution in melanoma during BRAF inhibitor therapy. *Cancer Discov*. 2014;**4**(1):80–93.

8 Chromosomal aberrations in cancer

Megan E. McNerney, MD, PhD ■ *Ari J. Rosenberg, MD* ■ *Michelle M. Le Beau, PhD*

> **Overview**
>
> The malignant cells of most patients who have leukemia, lymphoma, or a solid tumor have acquired clonal chromosomal abnormalities, the identification of which can aid in establishing the correct diagnosis and prognosis, and in the selection of therapy. Today, our arsenal of approaches to characterize an individual's malignant disease combines pathologic evaluation, cytogenetic analysis, and molecular studies. The advent of high-throughput methods, such as next-generation sequencing, capable of surveying the entire genome or large panels of cancer-related genes presents new options for a revolutionary change in the way we diagnose, characterize, and treat cancer. The vision for the future entails an integrated molecular profile, i.e., chromosomal pattern, gene/miRNA expression, DNA methylation/epigenomic pattern, gene mutation status, pharmacogenomic profile, and chemosensitivity of each patient's tumor, as well as predisposition to disease, facilitating the development of an individualized treatment plan with decreased toxicities and prolonged survival.

Introduction

Cancer is a heterogeneous group of diseases caused by the stepwise accumulation of numerous genetic and epigenetic aberrations altering the function of genes that regulate genome stability, cell proliferation and differentiation, cell death, adhesion, angiogenesis, invasion, and metastasis in complex cell and tissue microenvironments. The analysis of metaphase chromosomes provided our first broad glimpse into the genetic anatomy of a malignant cell and identified many of the basic abnormalities that characterize cancer, such as deletions, translocations, and gene amplifications. Specific cytogenetic abnormalities have been identified that are very closely, and sometimes uniquely, associated with morphologically distinct subsets of leukemia, lymphoma, or solid tumors.[1,2] The detection of one of these recurring abnormalities is helpful in establishing the diagnosis and adds information of prognostic importance. In the hematologic malignancies, patients with favorable prognostic features benefit from standard therapies with a well-known spectra of toxicities, whereas those with less favorable clinical and cytogenetic characteristics may be better treated with more intensive or investigational therapies. The disappearance of an abnormal clone is an important indicator of complete remission following treatment; whereas, the appearance of new abnormalities signals clonal evolution and, often, more aggressive behavior. Similarly, in solid tumors, the detection of a recurring cytogenetic abnormality or genetic change may inform the selection of targeted therapy, or an investigational clinical trial. Given the rapid progress in genomic analysis, one can envision a new approach to patients with cancer based on molecular profiling of the malignant cells as well as host factors that influence the development and treatment of the disease.[3] This article focuses on the key role of cytogenetic analysis in the context of diagnosis, prognosis, and molecular pathobiology of human tumors.

Genetic consequences of genomic rearrangements

Recurring chromosomal translocations result in alterations of the genes located at the breakpoints and play an integral role in the process of malignant transformation.[2] The altered genes fall into several functional classes, including tyrosine or serine protein kinases, cell surface receptors, growth factors and, the largest class, transcription regulators, which regulate growth and differentiation via the induction or repression of gene transcription. There are two general mechanisms by which chromosomal translocations result in altered gene function in a dominant fashion. The first is deregulation of gene expression, characteristic of the translocations in lymphoid neoplasms that involve the immunoglobulin genes in B lineage tumors and the T cell receptor genes in T lineage tumors, that result in the inappropriate or constitutive expression of an oncogene. The second mechanism is the expression of a novel, fusion protein, resulting from the juxtaposition of coding sequences from two genes, typically located on different chromosomes. Thus, these tumor-specific fusion proteins are therapeutic targets. Examples are the chimeric BCR-ABL1 protein resulting from the t(9;22) in chronic myeloid leukemia (CML), or the anaplastic lymphoma kinase (ALK) fusion proteins in lung cancer.

A number of human tumors, particularly solid tumors, result from homozygous, recessive mutations. The hallmark of these genes, known as "tumor suppressor genes" (TSGs), whose normal role(s) is to limit cellular proliferation, promote differentiation, or repair DNA, is the loss of genetic material, resulting from chromosomal loss or deletion, as well as by other genetic mechanisms.[2] A growing number of TSGs act by haploinsufficiency, whereby loss of one allele results in a reduction in the level of the protein product by half, perturbing normal cellular processes.[4] This mechanism is common in the recurring deletions in myeloid neoplasms. Conversely, alterations in copy number resulting from gain of a whole, or part of a, chromosome, or from gene amplification, e.g., *ERBB2/HER2* in breast cancer, result in increased expression of one or more critical genes.

More than one mutation is typically required for the pathogenesis of human tumors; thus, an important aspect of cancer biology is the elucidation of the spectrum of chromosomal and molecular mutations that cooperate in the pathways leading to disease and drug resistance. Where known, we describe the cooperating mutations associated with specific cytogenetic subsets of leukemia, lymphoma, or solid tumors.

Holland-Frei Cancer Medicine, Tenth Edition. Edited by Robert C. Bast, John C. Byrd, Carlo M. Croce, Ernest Hawk, Fadlo R. Khuri, Raphael E. Pollock, Apostolia M. Tsimberidou, Christopher G. Willett, and Cheryl L. Willman.
© 2023 John Wiley & Sons, Inc. Published 2023 by John Wiley & Sons, Inc.

Table 1 Glossary of cytogenetic and genetic terminology.[a]

Amplification	An increase in the number of copies of a DNA segment
Aneuploidy	An abnormal chromosome number, due to either gain or loss
Banded chromosomes	Each chromosome pair has a unique pattern of alternating dark and light segments due to special stains or pretreatment with enzymes before staining
Breakpoint	A specific site on a chromosome that is involved in a structural rearrangement, such as a translocation or deletion
Centromere	The chromosome constriction that is the site of the spindle fiber attachment, enabling chromatid separation by shortening of the spindle fibers attached to opposite poles during mitosis
Clone	Defined as two cells with the same additional or structurally rearranged chromosome, or three cells with loss of the same chromosome
Deletion	A segment of a chromosome is missing, typically as the result of two breaks and loss of the intervening piece (interstitial deletion)
Diploid	Normal chromosome number and composition of chromosomes
Epigenetics	The study of the heritable changes in gene function that result from modifications to the genome, such as DNA or histone methylation, rather than changes in the primary DNA sequence
Fluorescence in situ hybridization	A molecular-cytogenetic technique based on the visualization of fluorescently labeled DNA probes hybridized to complementary DNA sequences from metaphase or interphase cells, used to detect numerical and structural abnormalities
Haploid	Only one-half the normal complement, i.e., 23 chromosomes
Hyperdiploid	Additional chromosomes; therefore, the modal number is 47 or greater
Hypodiploid	Loss of chromosomes with a modal number of 45 or less
Inversion	Two breaks occur in the same chromosome with rotation of the intervening segment
Isochromosome	A chromosome that consists of identical copies of one chromosome arm (separated by the centromere) with loss of the other arm
Karyotype	Arrangement of chromosomes from a cell according to an internationally established system, such that the largest chromosomes are first and the smallest ones are last. A normal female or male karyotype is described as 46,XX or 46,XY, respectively
Loss of heterozygosity (LOH)	Typically results from a gross chromosomal abnormality, such as a deletion, that results in loss of one parental copy of a locus or segment (also called hemizygosity). Copy-neutral LOH is the presence of two copies of a chromosome (or segment) originating from one parent, with loss of the copy contributed by the other (also called uniparental disomy)
Single nucleotide polymorphisms (SNPs)	These are common, heritable DNA sequence variations that occur when a single nucleotide (A, T, C, or G) is changed, occurring every 100–300 base pairs
Pseudodiploid	A diploid number of chromosomes accompanied by structural abnormalities
Recurring abnormality	A numerical or structural abnormality noted in multiple patients who have a similar neoplasm
Translocation	A break in at least two chromosomes with exchange of material
Nomenclature symbols	
p	Short arm
q	Long arm
+	Indicates a gain of a whole chromosome (e.g., +8)
−	Indicates a loss of a whole chromosome (e.g., −7)
t	Translocation
del	Deletion
inv	Inversion
i	Isochromosome
mar	Marker chromosome
r	Ring chromosome

[a]Source: Modified from Ouyang and Le Beau.[2]

Chromosome nomenclature

Chromosomal abnormalities are described according to the International System for Human Cytogenetic Nomenclature (Table 1).[5] The total chromosome number is listed first, followed by the sex chromosomes, and numerical and structural abnormalities in ascending order. The observation of at least two cells with the same structural rearrangement, e.g., translocations, deletions, or inversions, or gain of the same chromosome, or three cells each showing loss of the same chromosome, is considered evidence for the presence of an abnormal clone. An exception to this is a single cell characterized by a recurring structural abnormality, which likely represents the karyotype of the malignant cells. One cell with a normal karyotype is considered evidence for a normal cell line.

Methods that complement karyotype analysis

Fluorescence *in situ* hybridization (FISH)

Fluorescence *in situ* hybridization (FISH) is widely used in cancer diagnostics and is based on the ability of a labeled DNA probe to anneal to complementary DNA from interphase cells, or metaphase chromosomes that are affixed to a glass microscope slide.[6] FISH can be performed on marrow or blood smears, or fixed and sectioned tissue, e.g., formalin-fixed paraffin-embedded (FFPE) tissue, since it does not require dividing cells. Probes are now commercially available for most clinically relevant abnormalities, such as centromere-specific probes to detect numerical abnormalities as well as the sex chromosome complement in the stem cell transplant setting, and locus-specific probes to detect translocations, deletions, and amplifications (Figure 1a–e). Most laboratories have developed FISH panels for each disease, e.g., acute myeloid leukemia (AML), acute lymphoblastic leukemia (ALL), Ph-like ALL, and myeloma, enabling the rapid evaluation of concurrent abnormalities. Advantages of FISH include (1) the rapid nature of the method; (2) its high sensitivity and specificity—cytogenetic abnormalities have been identified by FISH in samples that appeared to be normal by conventional cytogenetic analyses; and (3) the ability to obtain cytogenetic data from samples with a low mitotic index or terminally differentiated cells. The major disadvantage is the inability to interrogate more than a few abnormalities. FISH is often used to assess therapeutic efficacy by evaluating abnormalities identified by karyotyping at diagnosis, e.g., detection of the *BCR-ABL1* fusion in CML patients following therapy with an oral tyrosine kinase inhibitor (TKI). Applications in solid tumors include the detection of gene amplification, e.g., *ERBB2* in breast cancer and epidermal growth factor receptor (*EGFR*) or *ALK* in lung cancer, or the UroVysion™ test in bladder cancer.

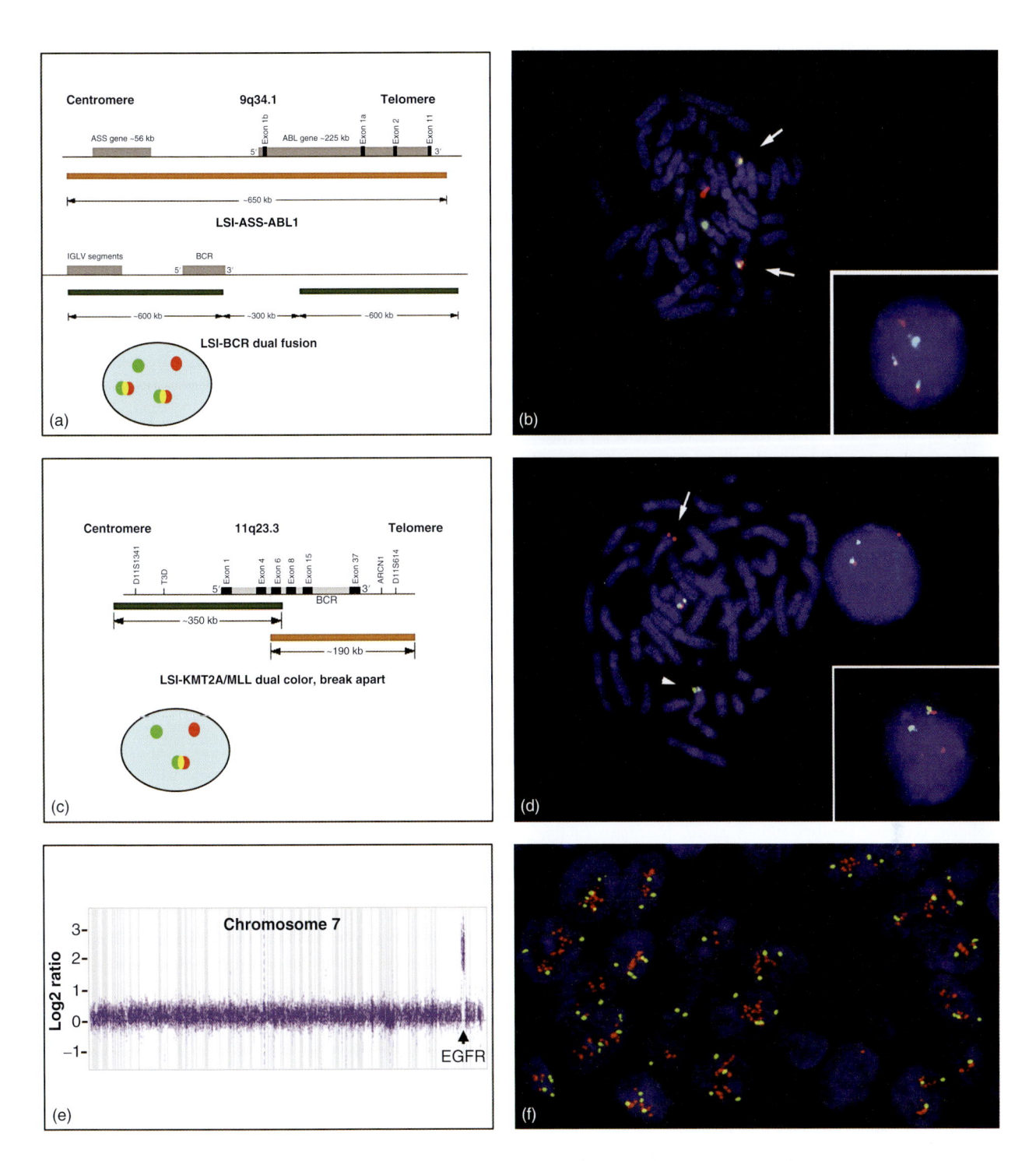

Figure 1 Fluorescence *in situ* hybridization and SNP array analysis. Panels (b), (d), and (e) illustrate images of metaphase or interphase cells following FISH; the cells are counterstained with 4,6-diamidino-2-phenylindole-dihydrochloride (DAPI). (a) Schematic diagram of the genomic origin of the *BCR* and *ABL1* dual fusion probe (Abbott Molecular), and configuration of signals in interphase cells. (b) In cells with the t(9;22), one green and one red signal is observed on the normal 9 and 22 homologs, and two yellow fusion signals (arrows) are observed on the der(9) and the der(22) (Ph) chromosomes as a result of the juxtaposition of the *ABL1* and *BCR* sequences. (c) Schematic diagram of the *KMT2A/MLL* break-apart probe (Abbott Molecular), and configuration of signals in interphase cells. (d) In cells with a translocation of 11q23.3, a yellow fusion signal is observed for the germline configuration on the normal chromosome 11 homolog, a green signal is observed in the der(11) chromosome, and a red signal is observed on the partner chromosome. (e, f) Detection of gene amplification. (e) SNP array analysis for DNA copy number aberrations in a glioblastoma reveals amplification of the *EGFR* locus. (f) FISH analysis for *ERBB2/HER2* amplification in breast carcinoma. The probe labeled with Spectrum Green (green signal) is a centromere-specific probe for chromosome 17 (CEP17). Most cells have two copies of the centromere of chromosome 17; however, polyploid cells have more copies. The probe labeled with Spectrum Orange (red signal) is a locus-specific probe for the *ERBB2/HER2* gene, with an estimated average of 10–20 copies per cell (Abbott Molecular). The *ERBB2/HER2*:CEP17 ratio was reported as ≥ 2.0. Images for panels (e, f) were kindly provided by Dr. Carrie Fitzpatrick, Department of Pathology, University of Chicago.

Other low-throughput methods

In addition to FISH, other low-throughput tests, such as ISH, reverse-transcription polymerase chain reaction (RT-PCR), and immunohistochemistry (IHC) comprise the bulk of clinical molecular tests to detect translocations or copy number aberrations (CNAs). For example, they provide rapid diagnosis of acute promyelocytic leukemia (APL) or diagnosis of ER/PR and *ERBB2* status in breast cancer. The main disadvantage of these assays is that the number of clinically relevant gene alterations per tumor has grown to the extent that high-throughput assays are becoming more efficient and cost-effective.

Single nucleotide polymorphism (SNP) arrays

Single nucleotide polymorphism (SNP) arrays probe for the presence of common SNPs genome wide. They provide sensitive detection of CNAs, on the order of kilobases, providing higher resolution than karyotyping (3–5 Mb resolution) (Figure 1e). Unlike karyotyping, they do not require dividing cells, an advantage for solid tumors. SNP arrays also detect copy-number neutral loss-of-heterozygosity (CN-LOH) but not balanced translocations. SNP arrays are currently clinically available as an adjunct test to karyotyping and FISH analysis of leukemias and lymphomas, and they facilitate detection of genomic abnormalities in a substantial proportion of cases with a normal karyotype.[7]

Next-generation sequencing (NGS)

Next-generation sequencing (NGS) is sequencing in a massively parallel manner, analyzing over one billion DNA fragments simultaneously, and has revolutionized clinical cancer diagnosis. NGS enables the most comprehensive testing, providing data on a spectrum of genetic alterations and often within a single assay. The capabilities of NGS assays include assessing CNAs, LOH, translocations, single nucleotide mutations, small insertions and deletions (indels), tumor mutation burden, microsatellite instability, germline predisposition variants, pharmacogenomic information, and oncogenic virus identification. NGS assays enable "liquid biopsies"—the molecular assessment of circulating tumor DNA—which promise to improve early detection of cancer, monitoring of treatment response, tumor evolution, and relapse. Assays are rapidly evolving, driven by advances in instrumentation, assay design, software, and dropping costs. In-house NGS is routine at some centers, and academic and commercial providers have enabled NGS to become more broadly used in oncology.

Tumor DNA or RNA can be obtained from fresh tissue, FFPE tissue, slide scrapings, biopsies, or even peripheral blood for circulating tumor DNA. Generally, small amounts of material are required, and some tests are available even for fine-needle aspirates. High tumor cellularity is preferred, although lower cellularity can be compensated for by greater sequencing depth.[8] Extracted nucleic acids are converted into sequencing libraries and 75–250 base pair paired-end reads are generated, which are then aligned to the reference genome.

CNAs are detected by counting the number of reads that align to a region, and comparing that number to data collected from a panel of normal diploid samples (Figure 2a). Regions of LOH are determined by examining SNP allele frequencies within the region. Homozygous deletions and amplifications greater than seven have been detected with 99% sensitivity and 100% specificity by NGS, comparing favorably to IHC and FISH.[8] Being higher-resolution than other methods, NGS has the advantage of detecting smaller CNAs. Of note, however, NGS provides average DNA content, similar to arrays. In contrast, ISH is performed on a cell-by-cell basis; thus, ISH may have higher sensitivity for samples with low tumor cellularity or intratumoral heterogeneity.

Translocations can be characterized by (1) read pairs that map to discordant portions of the genome; or (2) reads that map directly to a breakpoint (Figure 2b). NGS can achieve comparable sensitivity and specificity as FISH and provides finer-scale information.[9] Although FISH is the gold standard for translocation identification, NGS is more practical and sensitive for cases with a large number of potential fusion partners, for instance, in the detection of TRK fusion-positive cancers.[10]

Targeted gene panels

Targeted gene panels cover ~0.05% of the genome and are comprised of tens to hundreds of clinically significant genes. Some panels are comprehensive, whereas others are tailored for the tumor type. Compared to whole-genome sequencing (WGS), they are cost-effective, provide greater sequencing depth, high sensitivity, the shortest turn-around-time, and decreased bioinformatics burden, as well as circumventing issues of incidental findings.[11]

For identification of CNAs, target genes are typically enriched from DNA by probe-hybridization. Targeting translocations is less straightforward, because most translocations have breakpoints in introns, which can be significantly longer than NGS reads. Thus, capture probes for DNA must target introns, which increases the territory of DNA surveyed (Figure 2a). RNA-based sequencing avoids the problem of intervening introns, but is limited to detecting expressed chimeric fusion transcripts, and will fail to detect common translocations in B or T cell neoplasms, such as *IGH-MYC*. Additionally, RNA suffers degradation in FFPE specimens.

Exome sequencing

Exome capture is enrichment by hybridization-capture of all protein-coding DNA, ~1% of the genome. Some clinical labs offer this as an unbiased assay of mutations and CNAs in all potentially pathogenic genes. The cost is lower than WGS, but there is limited utility in detecting translocations.

Whole-genome sequencing (WGS)

WGS is sequencing of the entire tumor genome without a prior enrichment step and identifies all structural changes in coding and noncoding regions. Although used for research purposes and some clinical trials,[12] WGS is encumbered by cost, data size, and computational requirements. As sequencing costs decrease and laboratories gain more experience with NGS data, WGS may eventually become more widely used.

Specific clonal disorders

Chronic myeloid leukemia (CML)

The first consistent chromosomal abnormality in any malignant disease was identified in CML.[13] The Philadelphia (Ph) chromosome results from a reciprocal t(9;22)(q34.1;q11.2) (Figures 1a,b, and 4a), and arises in a pluripotent stem cell that gives rise to both lymphoid and myeloid lineage cells. The standard t(9;22) is identified in about 95% of CML patients, whereas 5% have variant translocations that also involve a third chromosome. The genetic consequences are to move the 3′ portion of the *ABL1* oncogene on chromosome 9 next to the 5′ portion of the *BCR* gene on 22. Rare patients with CML who lack the t(9;22) have a rearrangement

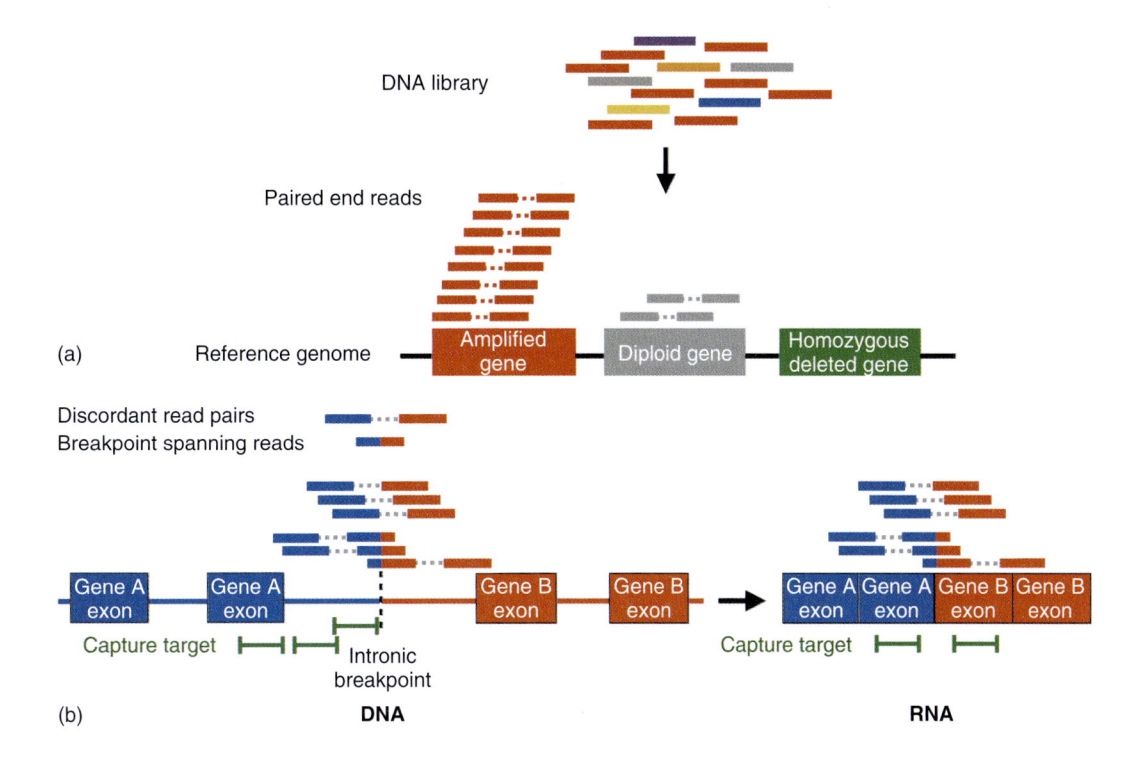

Figure 2 Detection of chromosomal aberrations by next-generation sequencing (NGS). (a) Copy number alterations are determined from a DNA library, that can be derived from whole-genome DNA, or enriched by exome-capture or a smaller, targeted gene panel. Paired-end or single-end (not shown) NGS is performed on the tumor sample, and reads are aligned to a reference human genome. The number of reads that align to a region is compared to either normal tissue from the same patient, or a database of normal, diploid patient samples. Regions of amplification will have a higher number of reads as compared to normal. Regions with heterozygous or homozygous deletions will have relatively fewer reads than expected. (b) Translocations can be identified by discordant read pairs that map to two different regions of the genome, or from reads that span breakpoints. Structural changes can be detected from DNA (left panel) or RNA (right panel). In the case of DNA, translocations can be identified by whole-genome sequencing or by an initial capture step. As translocations involving two genes often have heterogeneous breakpoints occurring in large regions of intronic sequence, capture probes have to be designed to span this intervening sequence. The advantage of using RNA is that the introns are spliced out; thus, capture probes are only required for exons, which are shorter than introns.

involving *ABL1* and *BCR* that is detectable only at the molecular level (~0.5% of cases).[14]

The t(9;22) and resultant *BCR-ABL1* fusion is the *sine qua non* of CML.[14] The BCR-ABL1 fusion protein acquires a novel function in transmitting growth-regulatory signals to the nucleus via the RAS/MAPK, PI3K/AKT, and JAK/STAT pathways. The tyrosine kinase activity of BCR-ABL1 can be specifically inhibited by several commercially available oral TKIs: imatinib mesylate (Gleevec/STI571, Novartis Pharmaceuticals), dasatinib (Sprycel, BMS-354825, Bristol-Myers Squibb), and nilotinib (Tasigna, AMN107, Novartis Pharmaceuticals).[15,16] Additional oral agents are also being tested in clinical trials.[17] Imatinib has shown remarkable activity in all phases of CML and is the preferred therapy for most patients with newly diagnosed CML, who can be monitored by FISH analysis or quantitative reverse-transcription polymerase chain reaction (qRT-PCR).[18] Several types of genetic changes are associated with imatinib resistance, including point mutations leading to amino acid substitutions in the ABL1 kinase domain that interfere with imatinib binding, as well as the acquisition of additional copies of the Ph chromosome or *BCR-ABL1* gene amplification, both of which can be detected by FISH.[18]

Historically, most CML patients in the accelerated or acute phases (80%) showed karyotypic evolution, commonly a gain of chromosomes 8 or 19, or a second Ph (by gain of the first), or an i(17q), as well as mutations in the *TP53, RB1, MYC, CDKN2A (p16), KRAS/NRAS*, or *RUNX1/AML1* genes.[14] With the advent of TKI therapy, the natural history of CML has been altered, and the karyotype in blast phase differs, but is not yet well described due to the scarcity of patients.

Interestingly, because each of the oral TKIs blocks kinase activities in addition to ABL1, they have proven to be effective in other hematologic malignancies, including myeloproliferative neoplasms with rearrangements of *PDGFRB*, a myeloproliferative variant of hypereosinophilic syndrome that expresses the FIP1L1-PDGFRA fusion protein, and in patients with mast cell malignancies that demonstrate *KIT* activation, as well as in some solid tumors, e.g., *KIT*-mutated melanoma and GIST.[19]

Other myeloproliferative neoplasms (MPNs)

A cytogenetically abnormal clone is present in 15% of untreated, and 40% of treated polycythemia vera (PV) patients, compared with 100% when the disease progresses to AML (Table 2).[20] Common changes are +8 or +9, del(13q), or del(20q), noted in 30% of patients.[20] A del(5q) (40%) or −7 (20%) are often observed in the leukemic phase. Cytogenetic analysis has revealed clonal abnormalities in 60% of primary myelofibrosis (MF), commonly +8, −7, or a del(7q), del(11q), del(13q), and del(20q).[21] A change in the karyotype may signal evolution to AML. $JAK2^{V617F}$ mutations leading to activation of the STAT, PI3K, and MAPK signaling pathways occur in PV (90–95%), essential thrombocythemia (ET, 50–70%), and MF (40–50%).[21–23] More recently, the majority of ET and MF cases with nonmutated *JAK2* have been shown to carry somatic mutations in the calreticulin gene (*CALR*).[24,25]

Table 2 Recurring chromosomal abnormalities in malignant myeloid diseases.

Disease[a]	Chromosome abnormality	Frequency	Involved genes[b]		Consequence
CML	t(9;22)(q34.1;q11.2)	~99%[c]	ABL1	BCR	Fusion protein—altered cytokine signaling pathways, genomic instability[c]
PV	+8	20% (combined)			
	+9				
	del(20q)				
	del(13q)				
	Partial trisomy 1q				
MF	+8	30% (combined)			
	+9				
	−7/del(7q)				
	del(5q)/t(5q)				
	del(20q)				
	del(13q)				
	Partial trisomy 1q				
AML	t(8;21)(q22;q22.1)	10%	RUNX1T1/ETO	RUNX1/AML1	Fusion protein—altered transcriptional regulation
	t(15;17)(q24.1;q21.2)	9%	PML	RARA	Fusion protein—altered transcriptional regulation
	inv(16)(p13.1q22) or t(16;16)(p13.1;q22)	5%	MYH11	CBFB	Fusion protein—altered transcriptional regulation
	t(9;11)(p21.3;q23.3)	5–8% for all t(11q23.3)	MLLT3/AF9	KMT2A/MLL	Fusion proteins—altered chromatin structure and transcriptional regulation
	t(10;11)(p12;q23.3)		MLLT10/AF10	KMT2A	
	t(11;19)(q23.3;p13.3)		KMT2A	MLLT1/ENL	
	t(11;19)(q23.3;p13.1)		KMT2A	ELL	
	t(6;11)(q27;q23.3)		MLLT4/AF6	KMT2A	
	Other t(11q23.3)		KMT2A		
	del(11)(q23)				
	+8	8%			
	−7 or del(7q)	14%			
	del(5q)/t(5q)	12%			
	t(6;9)(p23;q34.1)	1%	DEK	NUP214/CAN	Fusion nuclear pore protein
	inv(3)(q21.3q26.2) or t(3;3)	2%	MECOM/EVI1		Overexpression of MECOM
	del(20q)	5%			
Therapy-related MN	−7 or del(7q)	45%			
	del(5q)/t(5q)	40%			
	der(1;7)(q10;p10)	2%			
	dic(5;17)(q11.1–13;p11.1–13)	5%		TP53	Loss of function—DNA damage response
	t(9;11)(p21.3;q23.3)/t(11q23)	3%	MLLT3	KMT2A	Fusion proteins—altered transcriptional regulation
	t(11;16)(q23.3;p13.3)	2% (t-MDS)	KMT2A	CREBBP	
	t(21q22.1)	2%	RUNX1/AML		
	t(3;21)(q26.2;q22.1)	3%	MECOM	RUNX1	Overexpression of MECOM
MDS (unbalanced)	+8	10%			
	−7/del(7q)[d]	12%			
	del(5q)/t(5q)[d]	15%			
	del(20q)	5–8%			
	−Y	5%			
	i(17q)/t(17p)[d]	3–5%	TP53		Loss of function, DNA damage response
	−13/del(13q)[d]	3%			
	del(11q)[d]	3%			
	del(12p)/t(12p)[d]	3%			
(Balanced)	t(1;3)(p36.3;q21.2)[d]	1%	MMEL1	RPN1	Deregulation of MMEL1—Transcriptional activation?
	t(2;11)(p21;q23.3)/t(11q23.3)[d]	1%		KMT2A	KMT2A fusion—altered transcriptional regulation
	inv(3)(q21.3q26.2)/t(3;3)[d]	1%	RPN1	MECOM/EVI1	Altered transcriptional regulation by MECOM
CMML	t(5;12)(q32;p13.2)	~2%	PDGFRB	ETV6/TEL	Fusion protein—altered signaling pathways

[a]AML, acute myeloid leukemia; CML, chronic myeloid leukemia; CMML, chronic myelomonocytic leukemia; MDS, myelodysplastic syndrome.
[b]Genes are listed in order of citation in the karyotype, e.g., for CML, ABL1 is at 9q34.1 and BCR at 22q11.2.
[c]Rare patients with CML have an insertion of ABL1 adjacent to BCR in a normal-appearing chromosome 22.
[d]Considered in the WHO 2016 Classification as presumptive evidence of MDS in patients with persistent cytopenias(s), but with no dysplasia or increased blasts.

Primary myelodysplastic syndromes (MDS)

The myelodysplastic syndromes (MDS) are a heterogeneous group of diseases.[26,27] Clonal chromosome abnormalities can be detected in marrow cells of 40–60% of patients with primary MDS at diagnosis, including MDS with single lineage dysplasia (MDS-SLD, 20–50%), MDS with multilineage dysplasia (MDS-MLD, 50%), MDS with ring sideroblasts (MDS-RS, 20–50%), MDS with excess blasts (MDS-EB-1,2, 30–50%), MDS with isolated del(5q) (100%), MDS-unclassifiable (MDS-U), and childhood myelodysplastic syndrome, including refractory cytopenia of childhood (Table 2).[28–30] The common changes, +8, del(5q), −7/del(7q), and del(20q), are similar to those seen in AML de novo (Figure 3a).

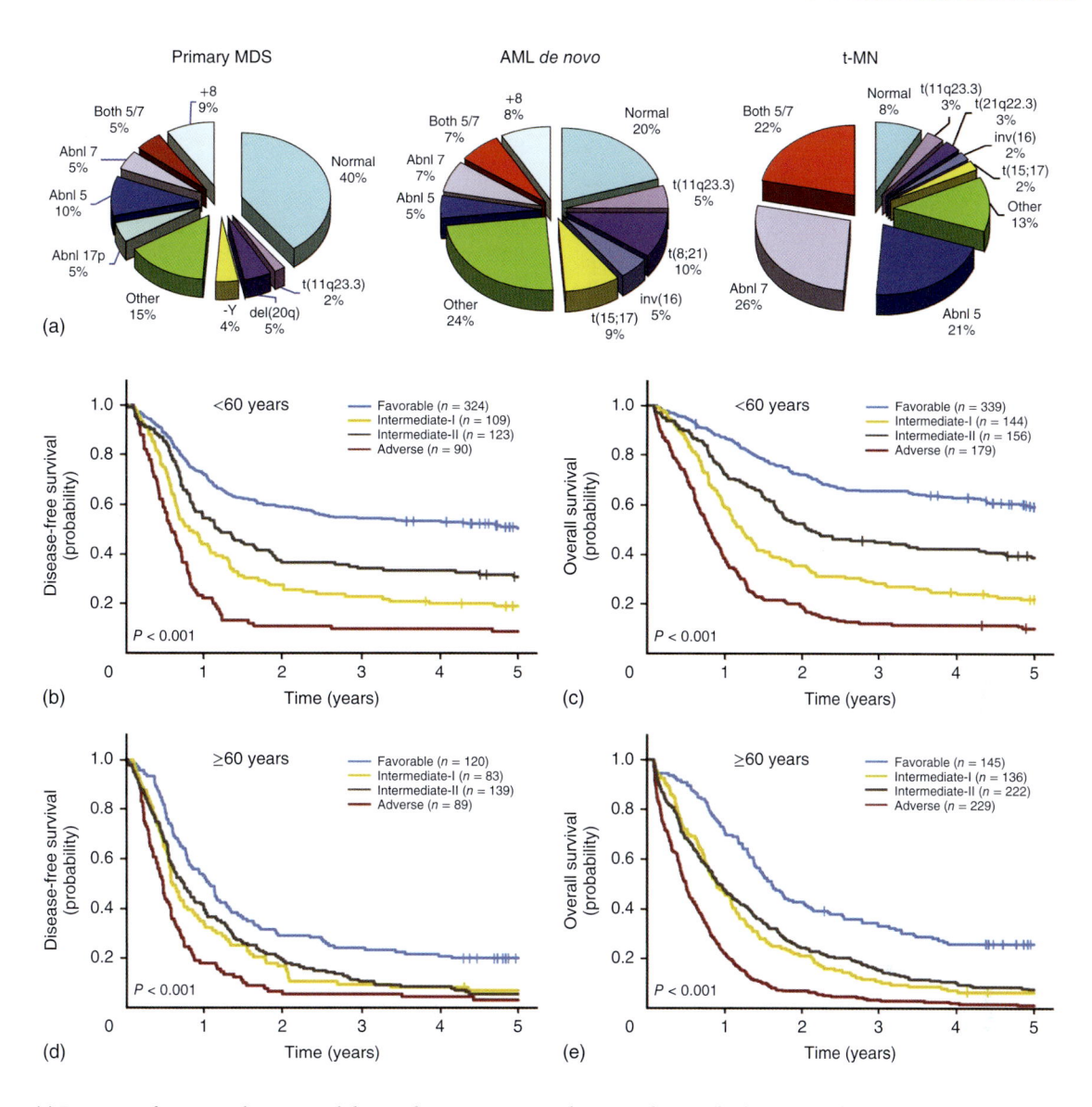

Figure 3 (a) Frequency of recurring chromosomal abnormalities in MDS, AML *de novo*, and t-MN. (b–e) Outcome of patients with AML classified according to the four European LeukemiaNet groups. (b) Disease-free survival and (c) overall survival of AML patients younger than 60 years of age. (d) Disease-free survival and (e) Overall survival of patients aged 60 years or older. Source: Adapted from Mrozek et al.[31]

The recurring translocations that are closely associated with the distinct morphologic subsets of AML *de novo* are almost never seen in MDS.

MDS with isolated del(5q) occurs in a subset of older patients, frequently women, with RA, generally low blast counts, and normal or elevated platelet counts.[30,32] These patients have an interstitial deletion of 5q, as the sole abnormality, or with one or two additional abnormalities, and typically have a relatively benign course that extends over several years.[32]

SNP microarrays can detect abnormalities in 10–15% of cases with a normal karyotype. Of these, LOH of 7q, 11q, and 17p are associated with a poor outcome.[33,34] As defined by the International Prognostic Scoring System Revised, patients with a "very good outcome" have -Y or del(11q) as the sole abnormality; those with a "good outcome" have normal karyotypes, del(5q) alone or with one or two additional abnormalities, del(12p) alone, or del(20q) alone; those with an "intermediate outcome" have del(7q), +8, +19, i(17q), or any other single or double abnormality; those with a "poor outcome" have −7, inv(3q)/t(3;3), double abnormalities, including −7/del(7q), and complex karyotypes with 3 abnormalities; and those with a "very poor outcome" have complex karyotypes with >3 abnormalities, typically with abnormalities of chromosome 5.[28,35]

Acute myeloid leukemia (AML) *de novo*

Clonal chromosomal abnormalities are detected in ~75% of patients with AML and have prognostic and therapeutic implications.[36–39] The most frequent abnormalities are +8 and −7 (Figure 3a).[2] The recurring translocations occur in younger patients with a median age in the 30s, whereas other abnormalities, such as del(5q), or −7/del(7q), occur in patients with a median age over 50. The WHO classification now recognizes specific recurring abnormalities together with their molecular counterparts as separate disease entities within AML (Table 2).[2] These entities include the core-binding factor (CBF) leukemias characterized by the t(8;21)(q22;q22.1) (Figure 4b) occurring in 5% of AML, and the inv(16)(p13.1q22) (Figure 4c) in 5% of AML (25% of AMMoL), the t(15;17)(q24.1;q21.2) (Figure 4d) in APL, the t(9;11)(p21.3;q23.3) (Figure 4e), the t(6;9)(p23;q34.1), the

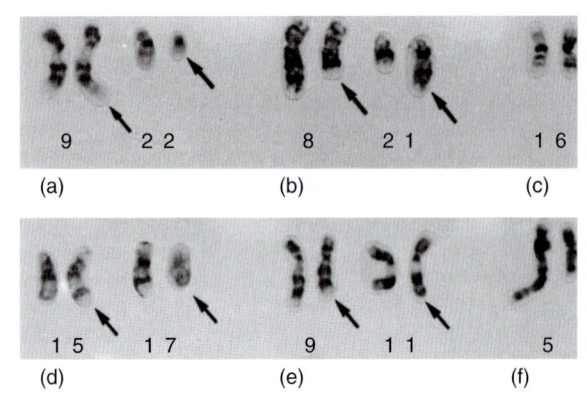

Figure 4 Partial karyotypes from trypsin-Giemsa-banded metaphase cells depicting select recurring chromosomal rearrangements observed in myeloid leukemias. The rearranged chromosomes are identified with arrows. (a) t(9;22)(q34.1;q11.2), CML. (b) t(8;21)(q22;q22.1), AML-M2. (c) inv(16)(p13.1q22), AMMoL-M4Eo. (d) t(15;17)(q24.1;q21.2), APL. (e) t(9;11)(p21.3;q23.3), AMoL-M5. (f) del(5)(q15q35), t-MN.

inv(3)(q21.3q26.2) or t(3;3)(q21.3;q26.2), the t(1;22)(p13.3;q13.1), and the t(9;22)(q34.1;q11.2) with the BCR-ABL1 fusion.[30] At the molecular level, CBF rearrangements disrupt the two genes encoding the subunits of the CBF transcription factor (*RUNX1* at 21q22.1, and *CBFB* at 16q22) essential for hematopoiesis.[40] CBF-AML has a favorable prognosis in adults (overall 5-year survival of 70% for t(8;21); 60% for inv(16)), but the outcome in children with a t(8;21) is poor.[40] Secondary mutations of *KIT*, *KRAS*, and *NRAS* are common in CBF-AML, although only *KIT* mutations confer a poor prognosis.[40]

The t(15;17) results in a fusion retinoic acid receptor-alpha protein (PML-RARA), the oncogenic potential of which results from the aberrant repression of RARA-mediated gene transcription through histone deacetylase (HDAC)-dependent chromatin remodeling.[41] *FLT3* internal tandem duplications (ITDs), are observed in 35% of patients. Establishing the diagnosis of APL with the typical t(15;17) is important, because this disease is sensitive to therapy with all-trans retinoic acid (ATRA) and arsenic trioxide. Translocations of 11q23.3 are associated with acute monoblastic leukemia and are 4-times more common in children less than 1 year of age than in adults.[42] They result in fusion proteins of *KMT2A/MLL*, which encodes a histone methyltransferase that regulates transcription of target genes, e.g., *HOX* genes, via chromatin remodeling.[43]

In an international effort, the European LeukemiaNet (ELN) has proposed a standardized system integrating cytogenetic and molecular abnormalities.[36] The favorable group includes patients with the t(8;21), inv(16), mutated *NPM1* without *FLT3-ITD* (normal karyotype), and biallelic mutated *CEBPA* (normal karyotype); intermediate includes patients with a normal karyotype with mutated *NPM1* and *FLT3-ITD*, wild type *NPM1* with or without *FLT3-ITD*, patients with the t(9;11) or abnormalities not classified as favorable or adverse; and the adverse group includes patients with the inv(3q)/t(3;3), t(6;9), t(11q23.3), t(9;22), del(5q), −7, loss of 17p, or complex karyotype (≥3 abnormalities), wild type NPM1 and FLT3-ITD[high], and mutated *RUNX1*, *ASXL1*, or *TP53*. Several large studies have validated this classification in predicting outcome, and support the view that these genetic groups should be applied to younger (<60 years old) and older (≥60 years old) patients separately (Figure 3b–e).[31] Other studies have provided evidence that the mutation analysis of additional genes, i.e., *DNMT3A* and *TET2*, may refine the ELN risk stratification.[44]

Therapy-related myeloid neoplasms (t-MN)

Therapy-related myeloid neoplasms (t-MN), comprised of t-MDS/t-AML, is a late complication of cytotoxic therapy used in the treatment of both malignant and nonmalignant diseases.[45] Loss of part of chromosome 5, del(5q) (Figure 4f), and/or part or all of chromosome 7 [−7/del(7q)] are characteristic in patients who received alkylating agents (Figure 3a). Clinically, these patients have a long latency period (5 years), present with MDS, which often progresses rapidly to AML with multilineage dysplasia and a poor prognosis (median survival 8 mos.). In our experience, 92% of t-MN patients had an abnormal karyotype, and 70% had an abnormality of one or both chromosomes 5 and 7,[46] and these observations have been confirmed in other series.[47] In contrast, only about 20% of patients with AML *de novo* have a similar abnormality of chromosomes 5 or 7 or both.[2] There are two minimally deleted regions (MDRs) on 5q: 5q31.2 (containing *EGR1*) is deleted in patients with t-MN, AML, *de novo*, and high-risk MDS,[48] whereas loss of 5q32 (containing *RPS14*, *MIR145*, *MIR146A*, and *CSNK1A1*) is associated with MDS with an isolated del(5q).[32,48] However, the deletion in virtually all patients is large (~70 Mb) spanning 5q14–q33, and encompassing both MDRs. Moreover, it is becoming clear that genes outside the MDR, such as *APC*, also contribute to disease. Molecular analysis of the genes within the deleted segment of chromosome 5 is compatible with a haploinsufficiency model in which the coordinate loss of more than one gene on 5q in HSCs cooperate in disease pathogenesis, i.e., a contiguous gene syndrome, and drive distinct disease characteristics, namely anemia (*RPS14* and *APC*), megakaryocytic dysplasia (*MIR145* and *MIR146A*), HSC expansion (*EGR1*, *APC*, and *CSNK1A1*), and clonal dominance (*CSNK1A1*).[48,49]

A second subtype of t-MN is seen in patients receiving drugs known to inhibit topoisomerase II, e.g., etoposide, teniposide, and doxorubicin. Clinically, these patients have a shorter latency period (1–2 years), present with overt leukemia, often with monocytic features, without an antecedent MDS, and have a more favorable response to intensive induction therapy. Translocations involving *KMT2A* at 11q23.3, or *RUNX1* at 21q22.1 are common in this subgroup.[45]

Acute lymphoblastic leukemia (ALL)

The identification of prognostic subgroups based on recurring cytogenetic abnormalities (Table 3, Figure 5) and molecular markers has resulted in the application of risk-adapted therapies in ALL.[50,51] The Children's Oncology Group has defined four risk groups: lower risk (5-year event-free survival [EFS], at least 85%), with either the *ETV6-RUNX1* fusion or simultaneous trisomies of chromosomes 4 and 10; standard and high risk (those remaining in the respective National Cancer Institute risk groups); and very high risk (5-year EFS, 45% or below) with extreme hypodiploidy (<44 chromosomes), or the *BCR-ABL1* fusion, and induction failure.[52,53] Genome-wide profiling studies using CMA have revealed a high frequency of submicroscopic CNAs in pediatric ALL, including deletions of *PAX5* (32%), *IKZF1* (IKAROS, 29%), *CDKN2A/B* (50%), *BTG1*, and *EBF1* (8%) that disrupt genes and pathways controlling B cell development and differentiation.[51] Genetic alterations of *IKZF1* are associated with a very poor outcome in B cell progenitor ALL.[51]

Translocation 9;22
The incidence of the t(9;22) in ALL is 30% in adults overall, ~50% in adults over 60 years of age, and 5% in children, and is associated with a very poor prognosis. About 70% of the patients show additional abnormalities, commonly with +der(22)t(9;22),+21, or −7

Table 3 Cytogenetic-immunophenotypic correlations in malignant lymphoid diseases.

Disease[a]	Chromosome abnormality	Frequency[b]	Involved genes[c]		Consequence
Acute lymphoblastic leukemia					
Precursor B	t(12;21)(p13.2;q22.1)	25%	ETV6/TEL	RUNX1/AML1	Fusion protein—TF
	t(9;22)(q34.1;q11.2)	10%[d]	ABL1	BCR	Fusion protein—Altered cytokine signaling pathways
	t(4;11)(q21.3;q23.3)	5%	AFF4	KMT2A	Fusion protein—TF
Pre-B	t(1;19)(q23;p13.3)	6% (30%)	PBX1	TCF3 (E2A)	Fusion protein—TF
Ph-like ALL	t(X;14)(p22.3;q32.3)	CRLF2- 30% of Ph-Like ALL	CRLF2	IGH	Deregulated expression (CRLF2)-cytokine receptor
	del(X)(p22.3p22.3)		P2RY8	CRLF2	Deregulated expression (CRLF2))—cytokine receptor
B (SIg+)	t(8;14)(q24.2;q32.3) or variant	7% (100%)	MYC	IGH	Deregulated expression—TF
Other	Hyperdiploidy (50–60)	10%			
	del(12p),t(12p)	10%			
T	t(11;14)(p15.4;q11.2)	1%	LMO1		Deregulated expression—TF
	t(11;14)(p13;q11.2)	3%	LMO2	TRA	Deregulated expression—TF
	t(10;14)(q24.3;q11.2)	3%	TLX1	TRA	Deregulated expression—TF
	del(9p),t(9p)	<1% (10%)	CDKN2A, CDKN2B	TRA	Tumor suppressor gene—cell cycle regulation
Non-Hodgkin lymphoma					
B cell NHL					
Burkitt	t(8;14)(q24.2;q32.3)	95%	MYC	IGH	Deregulated expression—TF
	t(2;8)(p12;q24.2)	1%	IGK	MYC	Deregulated expression—TF
	t(8;22)(q24.2;q11.2)	4%	MYC	IGL	Deregulated expression—TF
Follicular SNCL	t(14;18)(q32.3;q21.3)	80%	IGH	BCL2	Deregulated expression—Anti-apoptosis protein
DLBCL		20%			
DLBCL	t(3;22)(q27;q11.2)	45% for all t(3q27)	BCL6	IGL	Deregulated expression—TF
	t(3;14)(q27;q32.3)		BCL6	IGH	Deregulated expression—TF
MCL	t(11;14)(q13.3;q32.3)	~100%	CCND1	IGH	Deregulated expression—TF
LPL	t(9;14)(p13.2;q32.3)		PAX5	IGH	Deregulated expression—TF
MALT	t(11;18)(q22.2;q21.3)	40–50%	BIRC3/API2	MALT1	Fusion protein—NFkB activation
	t(1;14)(p22.3;q32.3)	10%	BCL10	IGH	Deregulated expression—Increased NFkB activation
	t(14;18)(q32.3;q21.3)	10–20%	IGH	MALT1	Deregulated expression—Increased NFkB activation
	t(3;14)(p13;q32.3)	10%	FOXP1	IGH	Deregulated expression—TF
PCFCL	t(14;18)(q32.3;q21.3)	40%	IGH	BCL2	Deregulated expression—anti-apoptosis protein
T cell NHL					
ALK+ ALCL	t(2;5)(p23.2;q35.1)	75%	ALK	NPM1	Deregulated expression Tyrosine kinase
ALK− ALCL	t(6;7)(p25.3;q32.3)	10–15%	IRF4, DUSP22		Deregulated expression of TF (IRF4) and phosphatase (DUSP22)
Nasal/NK cell	i(1q), i(7q), i(17q)				
Hepatosplenic	i(7q)	>95%			
Peripheral	t(5;9)(q33.3;q22.2)	15%	ITK	SYK	Constitutively active tyrosine kinase (SYK)
Chronic lymphocytic leukemia					
B	t(11;14)(q13.3;q32.3)	10%	CCND1	IGH	Deregulated expression—Cell cycle regulation
	t(14;19)(q32.3;q13.2)	5%	IGH	BCL3	Deregulated expression—Increased NFkB activation
	t(2;14)(p13;q32.3)	5%		IGH	
	t(14q32.3)	15%	IGH		
	del(13q)	30%			
	+12	25%			
T	t(8;14)(q24.2;q11.2)	5%	MYC	TRA	Deregulated expression—TF
	inv(14)(q11.2q32.3)	5%	TRA/TRD	IGH	Deregulated expression
	inv(14)(q11.2q32.1)	5%	TRA/TRD	TCL1A	Deregulated expression—TF
Multiple myeloma					
B	−13/del(13q)	40%			
	t(4;14)(p16.3;q32.3)	15%	FGFR3 NSD2	IGH IGH	Deregulated expression—Growth factor receptor and histone methyltransferase
	t(14;16)(q32.3;q23)	5%	IGH	MAF	Deregulated expression—TF
	t(6;14)(p21;q32.3)	4%	CCND3	IGH	Deregulated expression—Cell cycle regulation
	t(11;14)(q13.3;q32.3)	15%	CCND1	IGH	Deregulated expression—Cell cycle regulation
	t(14q32.3)	50%	IGH		
	del(17p)/t(17p)	30%	TP53		Loss of DNA damage response
	gain of 1q	20%			
	hyperdiploidy: +3,+5,+7,+9,+11				

(continued overleaf)

Table 3 (Continued)

Disease[a]	Chromosome abnormality	Frequency[b]	Involved genes[c]		Consequence
Adult T-cell leukemia/lymphoma					
	t(14;14)(q11.2;q32.3)		TRA	IGH	Deregulated expression
	inv(14)(q11.2q32.3)		TRA/TRD	IGH	Deregulated expression
	+3				

[a]DLBCL, diffuse large B cell lymphoma; MCL, mantle cell lymphoma; LPL, lymphoplasmacytoid lymphoma; SLL, small lymphocytic lymphoma; MALT, mucosa-associated lymphoid tumor; PCMZL, primary cutaneous marginal zone lymphoma; PCFCL, primary cutaneous follicular center lymphoma; ALCL, anaplastic large cell lymphoma; CTCL, cutaneous T-cell lymphoma.
[b]The percentage refers to the frequency within the disease overall. The number in the parentheses refers to the frequency within the morphological or immunological subtype of the disease.
[c]Genes are listed in order of citation in the karyotype, e.g., for precursor B ALL, *ETV6* is at 12p13.2 and *RUNX1* is at 21q22.1.
[d]By cytogenetic analysis, the frequency in children is about 5%, and in adults is about 25%; using molecular probes, this frequency is 30% in adults overall, and 50% in adults over 60 years of age.

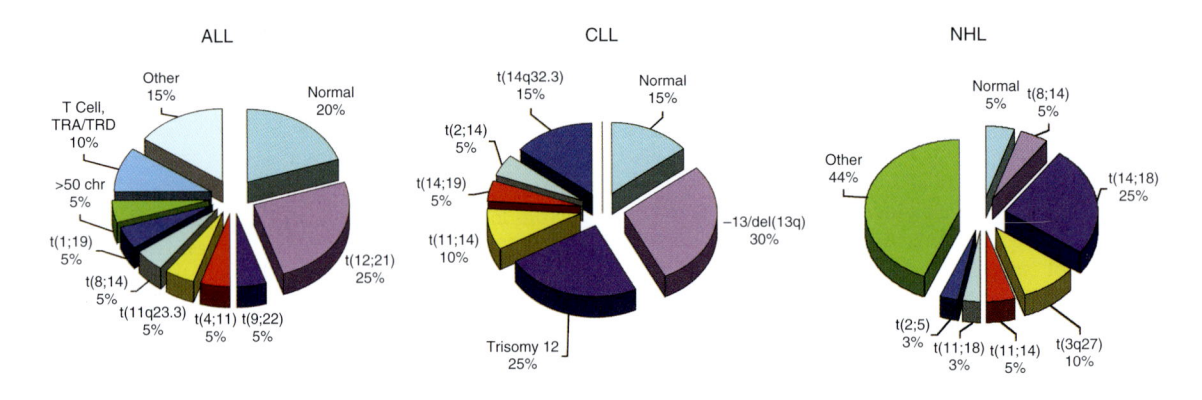

Figure 5 Frequency of recurring chromosomal abnormalities in ALL, CLL, and NHL.

(associated with a poorer outcome).[54] Most cases have a B lineage phenotype (CD10+, CD19+, and TdT+), but there is frequent expression of myeloid-associated antigens (CD13 and CD33). In over half of the patients, the break in *BCR* is more proximal, resulting in a smaller BCR-ABL1 fusion protein with even greater tyrosine kinase activity (BCR-ABL1^{p190}). Genetic alterations of the *IKZF1* gene are detectable in up to 80% of Ph+ ALL cases and are associated with an unfavorable outcome even with the use of TKIs.[14,55]

Translocations involving 11q

Translocations involving the *KMT2A* gene at 11q23.3 are observed in 5% of ALL patients, but in 80% of ALL in infants.[43,56] Of these, the most common is the t(4;11)(q21.3;q23.3) (Figure 6a), followed by the t(11;19)(q23.3;p13.3). Patients with the t(4;11) have a pro B phenotype (CD10−, CD19+), with co-expression of monocytic (CD15+) or, less commonly, T cell markers, and a poor response to conventional chemotherapy (adults: remission rate of 75% with EFS of only 7 months).[43,56]

Translocation 12;21

The t(12;21)(p13.2;q22.1) has been identified in a high proportion (∼25%) of childhood precursor B leukemia but is uncommon in adults (∼4% of ALL cases).[57] This cryptic translocation is not detectable by cytogenetic analysis but can be detected reliably using RT-PCR or FISH analysis. The t(12;21) defines a distinct subgroup of patients aged 1–10 years, with a B lineage immunophenotype (CD10+, CD19+, HLA-DR+), and a favorable outcome (5-year EFS of 91% vs 65% for other ALL). The t(12;21) results in a fusion protein containing the N-terminus of ETV6/TEL, a transcriptional repressor of the ETS family, and most of the RUNX1 transcription factor.

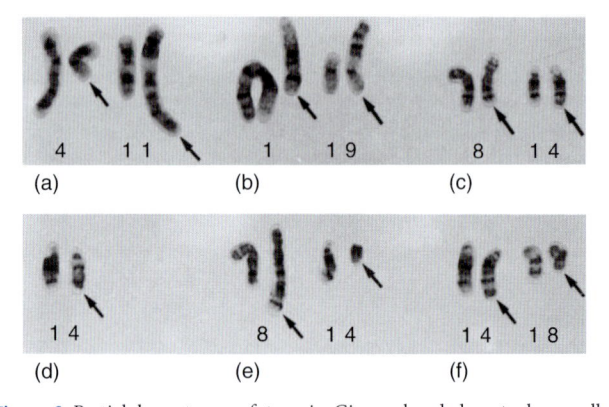

Figure 6 Partial karyotypes of trypsin-Giemsa-banded metaphase cells depicting select recurring chromosomal rearrangements observed in lymphoid neoplasms. The rearranged chromosomes are identified with arrows. (a) t(4;11)(q21.3;q23.3) in ALL. (b) t(1;19)(q23;p13.3) in pre-B cell ALL. (c) t(8;14)(q24.2;q32.3) in B cell ALL and Burkitt lymphoma. (d) inv(14)(q11.2q32.3) in T cell leukemia/lymphoma. (e) t(8;14)(q24.2;q11.2) in T cell leukemia/lymphoma. (f) t(14;18)(q32.3;q21.3) in B cell lymphoma.

Hyperdiploidy

The leukemia cells of some patients with ALL are characterized by a gain of many chromosomes. Two distinct subgroups are recognized: a group with 1–4 extra chromosomes (47–50 chromosomes), and the more common group with >50 chromosomes (typically 51–60 chromosomes). The latter subgroup is common in children (~30%) but is rarely observed in adults (<5%). Certain additional chromosomes are common (X chromosome, and chromosomes 4, 6, 10, 14, 17, 18, and 21). Patients with >50 chromosomes with +4, +10, and +17 have favorable clinical features, including age between 1 and 9 years, low white blood cell count (median 6700/μL), and favorable immunophenotype (early pre-B or pre-B).[58,59]

Translocation 1;19 and translocation 8;14
The t(1;19)(q23;p13.3) is associated with a good prognosis and has been identified in about 6% of children with a B lineage leukemia (Figure 6b). The leukemia cells have cytoplasmic immunoglobulin and are CD10+, CD19+, CD34−, and CD9+. The t(8;14)(q24.2;q32.3) is observed in mature B cell ALL (Figure 6c). These patients have a high incidence of central nervous system involvement and/or abdominal nodal involvement at diagnosis. Historically, the outcome has been poor, but the use of high-intensity chemotherapy has markedly improved the outcome (EFS of 80% in children).

Ph-like ALL
Ph-like ALL is a novel subgroup of high-risk ALL (15% of pediatric, and 30% of adult ALL), characterized by increased expression of HSC genes, a similar gene expression profile to Ph-positive ALL, and by a high frequency of *IKZF1* deletions and mutations, which confer a poor prognosis. Genetic alterations responsible for the activated kinase and cytokine receptor signaling signature in Ph-like ALL include point mutations and gene fusions affecting *CRLF2, JAK2, ABL1, ABL2, PDGFRB, CSF1R, NTRK3, EPOR, EBF1, FLT3, IL7R, SH2B3*, and other genes.[60,61] FISH probes that detect the most common abnormalities are commercially available and can be used to form a diagnostic panel.

T-cell acute lymphoblastic leukemia

T lymphoblastic leukemia/lymphoma has a distinct pattern of recurring abnormalities, involving the T cell receptor loci at 14q11.2 (Figure 6d,e) and two regions of chromosome 7 (7q34.3) and 7p14) (Table 3).[62,63] The most common are the t(10;11)(q24.3;q11.2) (7% of childhood and 30% of adult patients, *TLX1* gene), and the cryptic t(5;14)(q35.1;q32.1) (*TLX3*, 20% of childhood, and 10–15% of adult cases). About 30% of patients have activating mutations of the *NOTCH1* gene. Patients with T-cell ALL are most often young males and often have a mediastinal tumor mass, high white blood cell count, and leukemia cells in the cerebrospinal fluid.

Chronic lymphocytic leukemia (CLL)

Only 50% of CLL patients have detectable abnormalities by cytogenetic analysis, which increases to 80% when FISH analysis is used (Table 3, Figure 5).[64] The most frequent changes seen by FISH are: −13/del(13q) (55%), deletion of *ATM* on 11q (18%), +12 (16%), deletion of *TP53* on 17p, and deletion of 6q (6%).[65] The median survival is shorter in patients with 17p (32 months) or 11q (79 months) loss, than in those with no detectable abnormality (111 months), +12 (114 months), or −13/del(13q) (133 months). ZAP-70, an enzyme critical for T cell activation, is upregulated in CLL cells that contain unmutated *IGH* genes, conferring a poor prognosis.[66] Patients whose CLL cells have mutated *IGH* and lack expression of ZAP-70 and CD38 have the longest treatment-free period after diagnosis.[67]

T-cell CLL and large granular lymphocytic leukemia are uncommon disorders. Rearrangements involving 14q11.2, with or without an accompanying break in 14q32.1, have been reported in T-CLL as well as in T-cell lymphomas (Table 3).[62] The most common is inv(14)(q11.2q32.1) (Figure 6d).

Non-Hodgkin lymphoma (NHL)

More than 90% of non-Hodgkin lymphoma (NHL) cases are characterized by clonal chromosomal abnormalities, which correlate with histology and immunophenotype (Table 3, Figure 5).[68] For example, the t(14;18) is observed in a high proportion of follicular small cleaved cell lymphomas (70–90%), most patients with a t(3;22)(q27;q11.2) or t(3;14)(q27;q32.3) have diffuse large B cell lymphomas (DLBCL), and patients with a t(8;14)(q24.2;q32.3) have either small noncleaved cell or DLBCL. *IGH* at 14q32.3 is frequently involved in translocations in B-cell neoplasms (~70%). Similarly, a large proportion of T cell neoplasms are characterized by rearrangements of the TCR genes at 14q11.2, 7q34.3, or 7p14. Gene expression profiling has proven useful in distinguishing unique genetic subtypes of lymphoma. For example, gene expression profiling has shown that DLBCL comprises at least three different sub-types (germinal center B-cell-like, activated B-cell-like, and primary mediastinal B-cell lymphoma), each with a distinct oncogenic mechanism, prognosis, and response to therapies.[69]

The t(8;14), or variant t(2;8) or t(8;22), is characteristic of both endemic and nonendemic Burkitt tumors, as well as Epstein–Barr virus-negative and -positive tumors (Figure 6c). Moreover, the t(8;14) has also been observed in other lymphomas, particularly small noncleaved cell (non-Burkitt) and large cell immunoblastic lymphomas, HIV-associated BL (100%), and HIV-related DLBCL (30%).[70] The t(8;14) results in constitutive expression of *MYC* (8q24.2) via juxtaposition of the coding exons with *IGH* sequences (14q32.3). MYC is a transcription factor that plays a critical role in a number of cellular processes including DNA replication, proliferation, and apoptosis.

Between 70% and 90% of follicular lymphomas and 20% of DLBCL have the t(14;18) (Figure 6f), in which the *BCL2* gene at 18q21.3 is juxtaposed to the *IGH* J segment, leading to the deregulated expression of BCL2, an anti-apoptotic mitochondrial membrane protein.[71] Common secondary abnormalities include −7, +18, and del(6q). Double-hit lymphomas arising from the progression of a follicular lymphoma to a DLBCL have both a *BCL2* and *MYC* translocation.[72]

The t(11;14) (q13.3;q32.3) is observed in virtually all cases of mantle cell lymphoma, a poor prognostic group with a median survival of 3 years, in 3% of myeloma, and in up to 20% of prolymphocytic leukemias.[73] This translocation results in the activation of the cyclin D1 (*CCND1*) gene, located 100–130 Kb away from the breakpoint, by the *IGH* gene. The D-type cyclins act as growth factor sensors, regulating cell division via phosphorylation and inactivation of RB1.

Rearrangements leading to overexpression of *BCL6* at 3q27 occur in 40% of DLBCL, and in up to 10% of follicular lymphomas, and result most commonly from a t(3;22)(q27;q11.2) or t(3;14)(q27;q32.3).[68,69] BCL6 is a 96 kD POZ/Zn finger transcriptional repressor and may suppress genes involved in lymphocyte activation, differentiation, cell cycle arrest, and apoptosis. Somatic mutations have been identified in the 5′ regulatory regions of *BCL6* in ~20% of DLBDL without translocations, suggesting that overexpression of *BCL6* is more broadly involved than initially recognized.[74]

Extranodal marginal zone B-cell lymphomas of mucosa-associated lymphoid tissue (MALT lymphoma) are comprised of several genetic subgroups, one characterized by +3 plus other abnormalities (60%), and another by the t(11;18)(q21.2;q21.3) (25–50%) and its variants.[75] The t(11;18) results in the fusion of the apoptosis-inhibitor gene *BIRC3 (API2)*, to a novel gene at 18q21.3, *MALT1*, whose product activates the NFkB pathway.

Anaplastic large cell lymphoma (ALCL) is characterized by a young age at presentation, and skin and/or lymph node infiltration by large, often bizarre lymphoma cells, which preferentially involve the paracortical areas and lymph node sinuses. The majority of such tumors express one or more T-cell antigens, a minority express B-cell antigens, and some express both T- and B-cell antigens (the null phenotype). The t(2;5)(p23.2;q35.1), t(1;2)(q25;p23), or variant rearrangement involving the *ALK* tyrosine kinase gene at 2p23 occurs at a high frequency in ALCL of either T-cell or null phenotype.[76] The tumor cells are positive for CD30 on the cell membrane and in the Golgi region, and ALK expression is detectable in 60–85% of cases, where it confers a more favorable outcome (5-year survival, 80% in ALK+ vs 40% in ALK- tumors).

Multiple myeloma

The application of FISH in combination with plasma cell enrichment techniques has led to the discovery of abnormalities in a high proportion of myeloma, a monoclonal malignancy of postfollicular B cells, preceded by a premalignant monoclonal gammopathy of undetermined significance (MGUS) (Table 3).[77–80] MGUS is characterized by chromosomal aneuploidy, *IGH* translocations (45%), hyperdiploidy, and deletions of 13q (15–50%), leading to dysregulation of the cyclin D/RB1 pathway, also seen as the earliest changes in plasma cell myeloma.[77,79–82]

A molecular cytogenetic classification for myeloma recognizes three major groups: (1) Nonhyperdiploid with *IGH* translocations (40% of myeloma patients and 10% of MGUS patients); (2) hyperdiploid; and (3) other abnormalities.[77,81] The t(11;14)(q13.3;q32.2) is found in 15% of cases and results in *CCND1* overexpression. The t(4;14)(p16.3;q32.3) is noted in about 15% of patients and deregulates the expression of the fibroblast growth factor receptor 3 gene *(FGFR3)* translocated to the der(14), and the *NSD1* domain remaining on the der(4) chromosome. The t(14;16)(q32.3;q23), noted in 5% of cases, results in the overexpression of the *MAF* transcription factor gene. The t(4;14) and t(14;16) are both associated with a poor clinical outcome, whereas the t(11;14) confers a favorable prognosis. Nearly half of myeloma cases are hyperdiploid (45%), most commonly with 49–56 chromosomes, including trisomy for three or more odd-numbered chromosomes (chromosomes 3, 5, 7, 9, 11, 15, 19, or 21), a genetic subgroup that is associated with older patients and a more favorable outcome.

Deletions of *TP53* on 17p are noted in 10% of myeloma by FISH and are associated with a poor prognosis (37% of these patients also have mutations of *TP53*). Chromosome 1 abnormalities frequently resulting in both gain of 1q and loss of 1p *(CDKN2C)* are associated with a shorter survival.[79] Thus, a comprehensive FISH testing panel for myeloma should include probes for 1p and, particularly, 1q.

Additional events occur with disease progression in myeloma, including mutations of *NRAS* and *KRAS* (30–40%), *MYC* deregulation, and epigenetic alterations. Several genes are silenced through aberrant promoter hypermethylation in both MGUS and multiple myeloma, including *DAPK1* (67%), *SOCS1*, *CDKN2B (p15)*, and *CDKN2A (p16)*.[79,81]

Solid tumors

In contrast to the hematologic malignancies, our understanding of the contribution of chromosomal alterations to solid tumors has lagged behind, largely due to technical constraints. With recent advances in genetic analysis, however, it has become clear that chromosomal changes also play a significant role in solid tumors (Table 4). Although simple karyotypes with disease-specific gene fusions are the norm in hematologic malignancies and sarcomas, chromosomal aberrations in other solid tumors often involve a larger fraction of the genome. Indeed, the median number of somatic CNAs in solid tumors is 39, a much higher number than in hematologic malignancies.[83] Extreme cases of CNAs have been described as "chromothripsis" and "chromoplexy," involving highly complex rearrangements,[84,85] that are frequently associated with *TP53* mutations and a poor prognosis. As with hematologic malignancies, many recurring alterations in solid tumors involve genes encoding transcriptional regulators or tyrosine kinases, the latter creating potentially druggable proteins. In addition to providing potential therapeutic targets, chromosomal alterations can give insight into the biology of solid tumors, improve disease classification, assist in diagnosis of cancer of unknown primary, predict response to therapy, and inform our understanding of prognosis. Representative diseases and associated recurring chromosomal aberrations are discussed below.

Sarcomas

Sarcomas are a heterogeneous group of diseases that over time have come to be recognized as comprising an increasing number of distinct entities. Histologic similarity does not always translate to similar clinical behavior, and knowledge of the genetic basis of these diseases has assisted in improving disease classifications and contributed to our understanding of how these separate diseases are related.

In 1983, the t(11;22)(q24.3;q12.2) was identified in Ewing sarcomas.[86,87] This translocation results in an in-frame fusion of Ewing Sarcoma Breakpoint Region 1 (*EWSR1*), a member of the FET family, and Friend Leukemia Virus Integration Site 1 (*FLI1*), a member of the ETS transcription factor family. The resultant EWS-FLI1 fusion protein consists of the N-terminal transactivation domain of EWS fused with the DNA-binding domain of FLI1, forming an oncogenic transcription factor that upregulates or downregulates thousands of genes, and is required for tumorigenesis.[88,89] The fusion breakpoint is variable, and the functional significance of the different fusion products is not entirely characterized.[90]

A decade later, the *EWSR1* and ETS-Related Gene (*ERG*) fusion was identified in ~10% of Ewing sarcomas. *ERG* encodes another ETS family member that has 98% identity with *FLI1* in the DNA-binding ETS domain.[91] Together with EWS-FLI1, these account for 95% of Ewing sarcomas. The remaining 5% contain other fusions of FET family members, particularly *EWSR1* or *FUS*, with ETS family members, including *FLI1, ERG, ETV1, ETV4,* or *FEV*.[89] These fusions are mutually exclusive, suggesting that the resulting proteins function in a similar manner.

Ewing-like sarcomas are histologically similar to Ewing sarcomas but do not contain a detectable FET/ETS chromosomal rearrangement. They are characterized by other rearrangements, involving *EWSR1* and non-ETS family members.[89] It is likely that diagnostic definitions of these diseases will change as we improve our understanding of the fusion genes and the associated disease. Complicating the diagnostic challenge is the association of *EWSR1* rearrangements with other sarcomas, including *EWSR1-ATF1* and clear cell sarcoma, *EWSR1-WT1* and desmoplastic round cell tumor, *EWSR1-NR4A3* and extraskeletal myxoid chondrosarcoma, *EWSR1-DDIT3* and myxoid liposarcoma, and *EWSR1-ZNF278* and small round cell sarcoma. As with Ewing Sarcoma, a single

Table 4 Recurring chromosomal abnormalities in solid tumors.

Tumor type	Chromosome abnormality	Frequency	Fusion product or candidate gene affected[a]		Consequence
Bladder	t(4;4)(p16.3;p16.3)	3%	FGFR3	TACC3	Kinase activation
	t(12;17)(q13.1;q12)	3%	DIP2B	ERBB2	Kinase activation
	add(6p22.3)	20%	E2F3/SOX4		
	add(7p12)	10–15%	EGFR		Kinase activation
	add(3q26.3)	20%	PIK3CA		
	add(12q13.2)	10–15%	ERBB3		Kinase activation
	del(9p21.3)	50%	CDKN2A		
	del(17p11.2)	25%	NCOR1		
	del(10q23.3)	10–15%	PTEN		Kinase activation
	del(13q14.2)	15%	RB1		
	del(9q34.1)	5–10%	TSC1		Kinase activation
Breast	t(1;1)(p12;q44)	2%	MAGI3	AKT3	Kinase activation
	add(11q13.3)	15%	CCND1		Luminal subtype
	add(8p11.23)	15%	ZNF703		Luminal subtype
	add(8q24.2)	20%	MYC		Basal-like subtype
	add(17q12)	15%	ERBB2		Kinase activation
	add(7p12)	3%	EGFR		Kinase activation
	del(8q23.2)	10%	CSMD1		
	del(13q14.2)	5%	RB1		
	del(10q23.3)	5%	PTEN		Kinase activation
Cervical	add(8q24.2)	8%	MYC		
	add(11q13.3)	3%	CCND1		
	add(7p12)	3%	EGFR		Kinase activation
	add(17q12)	3%	ERBB2		Kinase activation
Colon	t(2;11)(p11.2;p15.1)	3%	TCF7L1	NAV2	
	t(10;10)(q25.2;q25.3)	3%	VTI1A	TCF7L2	
	add(17q12)	5%	ERBB2		Kinase activation
	add(8q24.2)	6%	MYC		
	add(11p15.5)	4%	IGF2, miR-483		
	add(1q)	17%			
	del(3p14.2)	10%	FHIT		
	del(16p13.3)	25%	RBFOX1		
	del(6q26)	10%	PRKN2		
	del(5q22.2)	2%	APC		
	del(14q)	30%			
	del(15q)	30%			
Endometrial	i(1)(q10)				
	add(15q26.3)	2%	IGF1R		Poor prognosis
	add(8q24.2)	5%	MYC		Serous-like
	add(17q12)	4%	ERBB2		Serous-like
	add(19q12)	4%	CCNE1		Serous-like
Esophagus	add(11q13.3)		CCND1		
Head and neck	t(4;4)(p16.3;p16.3)	<5%	FGFR3	TACC3	
	add(3q26.3)	20%	SOX2		
	add(7p12)	15%	EGFR		Kinase activation
	add(11q13.3)	35%	CCND1		
	del(9p21.3)	25%	CDKN2A		
Lung cancer, small cell	inv(1)(p32p34.3)	10%	RLF	MYCL1	
	add(3q26.2)	25–30%	SOX2		
	add(1p34.3)		MYCL		
	add(8q24.2)		MYC		
	add(6p22.3)		SOX4		
	add(19q12)		URI1		
	del(13q14.2)		RB1		
	del(8p21.1)		ESCO2		
	del(5q31.3)		ANKHD1		
	del(5q12.1)		KIF2A		
Lung cancer, non-small cell	inv(2)(p21p23.2)	5%	EML4	ALK	Kinase activation
	t(4;6)(p15.2;q22.1)	all ROS1 2%	SLC34A2	ROS1	Kinase activation
	t(6;20)(q22.1;q12)		ROS1	SDC4	Kinase activation
	t(5;6)(q32;q22.1)		CD74	ROS1	Kinase activation
	inv(10)(p11.2q11.2)	all RET 1%	KIF5B	RET	Kinase activation
	inv(6)(q22.1q25)		ROS1	EZR	Kinase activation
	inv(10)(q11.2q21.2)		RET	CCDC6	Kinase activation
	add(12q15)	5–10%	MDM2		
	add(7p12)	8%	EGFR		Kinase activation
	del(9p21.3)	25%	CDKN2A		

(continued overleaf)

Table 4 (Continued)

Tumor type	Chromosome abnormality	Frequency	Fusion product or candidate gene affected[a]		Consequence
Prostate	t(1;7)(q32.1;p21)	1%	SLC45A3	ETV1	
	t(7;7)(q32;q34)	1%	NRF1	BRAF	Kinase activation
	t(1;17)(q32.1;q21.3)	1%	SLC45A3	ETV4	
	t(21;21)(q22.3;q22.3)	all TMPRSS2-ERG 45%	TMPRSS2	ERG	ETS family member fusions—Altered transcription
	del(21)(q22.3q22.3)		TMPRSS2	ERG	
	t(1;21)(q32.1;q22.3)	1%	SLC45A3	ERG	
	t(3;21)(q27.2;q22.3)	1%	ETV5	TMPRSS2	
	t(7;21)(p21;q22.3)	1%	ETV1	TMPRSS2	
	t(17;21)(q21;q22)	1%	ETV4	TMPRSS2	
	t(1;7)(q32.1;q34)	1%	SLC45A3	TMPRSS2	
	trisomy 7			BRAF	Kinase activation
	monosomy 8				
Renal cell	t(X;17)(p11.2;q23.1)	all TFE translocations ~2%	TFE3	CLTC	Translocation type
	t(X;1)(p11.2;p34.3)		TFE3	SFPQ	Translocation type
	inv(X)(p11.2q13.1)		TFE3	NONO	Translocation type
	t(X;17)(p11.2;q25)		TFE3	ASPSCR1	Translocation type
	add(5q)	69%			
	add(7q)	20%			
	del(3p25.3)	95%	VHL		
	del(14q)	42%			
	del(8p)	32%			
	del(9p)	29%			
Thyroid carcinoma	inv(10)(q11.2q21)	25%	RET	CCDC6	Kinase activation
	inv(10)(q11.2q11.2)	10%	RET	NCOA4	Kinase activation
	t(10;17)(q11.2;q24.2)	2%	RET	PRKAR1A	Kinase activation
	inv(1)(q21.3q23.1)		TPM3	NTRK1	
	t(1;3)		NTRK1	TPR/TFG	
	inv(7)(q21.2q34)		AKAP9	BRAF	Kinase activation
Salivary gland mucoid carcinoma	t(11;19)(q21;p13.2)	35–70%	MAML2	CRTC1	Good prognosis
Lipoma	add(12q)	80–90%	HMGA2, MDM2		
Synovial sarcoma	t(X;18)(p11.2;q11.2)		SSX1	SYT1	Altered chromatin remodeling
Rhabdomyosarcoma, alveolar type	t(2;13)(q36.1;q14.1)		PAX3	FOXO1	
	t(1;13)(p36.1;q14.1)		PAX7	FOXO1	
Extraskeletal myxoid chondrosarcoma	t(9;22)(q22;q12.2)	50–60%	NR4A3	EWSR1	
	t(9;17)(q22;q12)	15–20%	NR4A3	TAF15	
Myxoinflammatory fibroblastic scarcoma	t(1;10)(p22.1;q24.3)	~95%	TGFBR3	OGA	
	add(3p12.1)		VGLL3		
Congenital fibrosarcoma	t(12;15)(p13.2;q25.3)	~95%	ETV6	NTRK3	Altered transcription
Fibromyxoid sarcoma	t(7;16)(q34;p11.2)	~95%	CREB3L2	FUS	
Anaplastic astrocytoma	trisomy 7	30%			
	del(9p)	30%			
	del(10q)	30–40%			
Glioblastoma	trisomy 7	50–60%			
	del(9p)	30–40%			
	monosomy 10	50–60%			
	monosomy 13	30–40%			
Schwannoma	del(22q12.2)	45%	NF2		
	add(9q34)	10%			
	add(17q)	5%			
Ewing tumor	t(11;22)(q24.3;q12.2)	85%	FLI1	EWSR1	Altered transcription
	t(21;22)(q22.3;q12.2)	10%	ERG	EWSR1	Altered transcription
Medulloblastoma	monosomy 6				Good prognosis
	add(8q24)				Poor prognosis
	i(17q)				
Neuroblastoma	add(2p24.3)	60%	MYCN		
	add(2p23.2)	10%	ALK		
Wilms tumor	add(1q)	25–30%			Poor prognosis
	del(11p13)	10–30%	WT1		
	del(Xq11.1)	13%	AMER1		
	del(16q)	10–15%			
Mesoblastic nephroma (cellular subtype), Infantile fibrosarcoma, Secretory breast carcinoma, Mammary analog secretory carcinoma of the salivary gland	t(12;15)(p13.2;q25.3)	80–90%	ETV6	NTRK3	Kinase activation
Retinoblastoma	del(13q14.2)	~3%	RB1		
Clear cell sarcoma of soft parts	t(12;22)(q13.1;q12.2)		ATF1	EWSR1	Altered transcription
	t(2;22)(q33.3;q12.2)		CREB1	EWSR1	Altered transcription

Table 4 (Continued)

Tumor type	Chromosome abnormality	Frequency	Fusion product or candidate gene affected[a]		Consequence
Testicular tumors	i(12p) add(12p)	Together nearly 100%			
Dermatofibrosarcoma protuberans	t(17;22)(q21.3;q13.1) Ring chromosome		COL1A1	PDGFB	Kinase activation

[a]Genes are listed in order of citation in the karyotype, e.g., for bladder cancer, DIP2B is at 12q13.1 and ERBB2 at 17q12.

rearrangement is most common for each diagnosis, but fusion partners can be variable.

A translocation involving SS18 at 18q11.2 and SSX1 at Xp11.23 was identified in synovial sarcoma in 1986.[92] A large family of genes and pseudogenes are homologous with SSX1, such as SSX2, or SSX4, and many of them can form fusion oncogenes with SS18. The resulting fusion proteins regulate transcription through interactions with the SWI-SNF chromatin remodeling complex and the polycomb group protein complex.[93–95] The various fusion gene products appear to have subtle functional differences and result in morphologically distinct tumor variants. Clinically, this identification is critical as synovial sarcoma is particularly sensitive to alkylating agents, such as ifosfamide.

Our understanding of other chromosomal aberrations in sarcoma histologic subtypes is evolving but is critical in the era of novel therapeutics.[96] Alveolar soft-part sarcoma is characterized by a translocation involving the ASPSCR1 gene on chromosome 17 and the TFE3 gene on the X chromosome resulting in a nonreciprocal translocation t(X;17)(p11.2;q25.3). Alveolar rhabdomyosarcoma is characterized by recurring translocations involving FOXO1 on chromosome 13—t(2;13) or t(1;13)—leading to a PAX3 or PAX7 fusion protein with FOXO1. Dermatofibrosarcoma protuberans is characterized by a nonreciprocal translocation between chromosome 17 and 22 leading to the COL1A1-PDGFB fusion protein, which may in part explain the responsiveness of this disease to TKIs, such as imatinib.[97] Solitary fibrous tumor is characterized by recurrent inversion of chromosome 12 resulting in fusion of NAB2 and STAT6 and is a distinct molecular feature of this disease. Epithelioid hemangioendothelioma is a rare vascular neoplasm characterized by a translocation between WWTR1 and CAMTA1 leading to a disease-defining fusion gene.[98] With multiple systemic options for soft tissue sarcoma, such as trabectedin[99] and eribulin,[100] with differential activity across subtypes of soft tissue sarcoma, identification of disease-defining fusion proteins are critical to diagnosis and treatment.

Renal cell carcinoma

Conventional renal cell carcinoma (RCC) refers to clear cell carcinoma, which comprises ~85% of cases. Almost all clear cell RCCs are associated with disruption of VHL, through deletion, mutation, and/or epigenetic silencing. VHL is typically altered in every cell within the tumor, indicating that these genetic changes occur in the parental clone, and are likely to be essential for tumor initiation.[101] In addition to loss of VHL, 90% or more of clear cell RCCs harbor a deletion of other genes located on 3p, including PBRM1, SETD2, and BAP1.[102]

Oncocytomas and chromophobe RCCs are thought to originate from the intercalated cells of the collecting ducts, and they can be difficult to distinguish histologically. Oncocytomas, however, rarely metastasize, suggesting that prior reports of metastatic oncocytomas may have been incorrectly diagnosed. Both can harbor a variety of chromosomal abnormalities; oncocytomas, but not chromophobe RCC, frequently have rearrangements leading to overexpression of CCND1 (11q13.3). Identifying these alterations can have a major impact on predicting risk of metastatic potential and, therefore, clinical management.[103]

Gliomas

Oligodendrogliomas are well-differentiated tumors that are associated with an unbalanced translocation involving 1q and 19p, with subsequent loss of 1p and 19q. Anaplastic oligodendrogliomas and oligoastrocytomas are somewhat less differentiated, and their prognosis appears to be related to the presence of the codeletion. Among oligodendrogliomas, those that harbor this codeletion are sensitive to chemotherapy, and patients have a median survival that exceeds 10 years. In contrast, tumors without these changes are more likely to have astrocytic features, and shorter survival (2–3 years).[104] Thus, assessment for the codeletion is recommended for all oligodendrogliomas at the time of diagnosis.

Testicular cancer

Testicular and other extragonadal germ cell tumors are characterized by an isochromosome of the short arm of chromosome 12—i(12)(p10). This finding is of particular importance given the high responsiveness of this malignancy to cisplatin-based chemotherapy and the high cure rate associated with multiagent chemotherapy. Even in the absence of a clear clinical and histologic presentation consistent with testicular cancer, a finding of i(12p) in cancer of unknown primary, in particular, associated with mediastinal adenopathy in a young man should be considered a germ cell tumor until proven otherwise.[105]

Non-small-cell lung cancer (NSCLC)

In addition to predicting response to cytotoxic therapy, the protein products resulting from a number of chromosomal alterations have emerged as drug targets. A decade ago, small molecule inhibitors of EGFR were found to be effective for ~10% of patients with non-small-cell lung cancer (NSCLC), a subset that appeared to be comprised of never-smokers with adenocarcinoma, especially in Asian patients.[106] It was subsequently found that most responders have EGFR mutations with frequent amplification of the mutated allele.[107] Prior to this discovery, KRAS mutations were the sole driver mutation identified in NSCLCs, presenting a challenging drug target. In 2007, the EML4-ALK fusion oncogene was identified in ~5% of patients, typically in young, never, or light smokers.[108] Just 4 years later, crizotinib was approved by the FDA for patients with EML4-ALK translocations. Since that time, second-generation ALK inhibitors such as brigatinib and alectinib have been approved and received FDA approval for treatment of ALK-rearranged NSCLC.[109] In patients with genetic alterations predicting response, targeted inhibitors of EGFR and ALK are preferred over cytotoxic therapy.

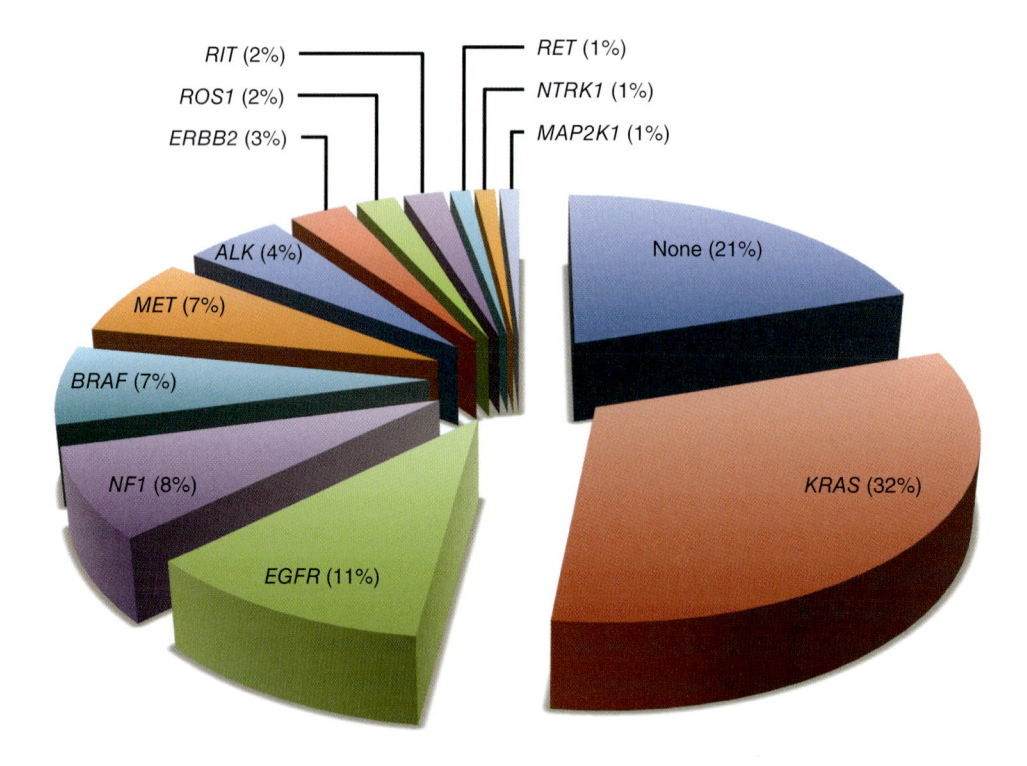

Figure 7 Frequency of driver gene alterations in lung adenocarcinoma. Genes that are involved in chromosomal abnormalities are identified with bold text.

Although the percent of patients with each driver oncogene is low, there is a growing number of driver oncogenes in adenocarcinomas (Figure 7). These include fusions of *ALK* with other fusion partners; *CD74-ROS1, SLC34A2-ROS1,* and other fusions involving *ROS1*; *KIF5B-RET* and other *RET* fusions; fusions involving *NTRK1*; and others. Recent sequencing efforts have also identified amplifications of *MET* and *ERBB2*.[110] *FGFR3-TACC3* mutations were first identified in glioblastoma but have also been found in squamous cell carcinoma of the lung, as well as urothelial cancers.[111] Patients with fusions involving *ALK* and *ROS1* respond to crizotinib, brigatinib, and alectinib. Testing for alterations of driver genes is recommended for patients with newly diagnosed NSCLC, especially those with adenocarcinoma or young age at diagnosis. As the number of identified driver mutations has grown, multiplex evaluation or more comprehensive sequencing techniques have replaced PCR-based assays of individual genes.

Prostate cancer

Given the high prevalence of prostate cancer, the *TMPRSS2-ERG* fusion found in ~40–50% of patients with prostate cancer is the most common gene fusion in human neoplasms.[112,113] It leads to high expression of *ERG*, driven by the androgen receptor-regulated *TMPRSS2* promoter, which is otherwise expressed at very low levels. Like the *EWSR1* fusion genes in sarcoma, multiple other *ETS* family members also form fusion genes in prostate cancer, including *ETV1, ETV4, ETV5,* and *ELK4*, and these fusions are mutually exclusive. Each of these *ETS* family members can form fusions with 5′ fusion partners, including *TMPRSS2* or *SCL45A3*, or other fusion partners. In total, 60% of prostate cancers harbor *ETS*-family fusions (Figure 8).

ETS-family rearrangements appear to be an early event in tumor initiation and have been demonstrated in preneoplastic prostatic intraepithelial neoplasm (PIN) lesions.[114] Initially, ETS-family rearrangements were associated with a poor prognosis; subsequent reports refuted this finding, and it remains a topic of debate. Recent preclinical data have demonstrated sensitivity of *ETS*-rearranged cell lines and xenograft models to PARP1 inhibitors, now under evaluation in clinical trials.[115]

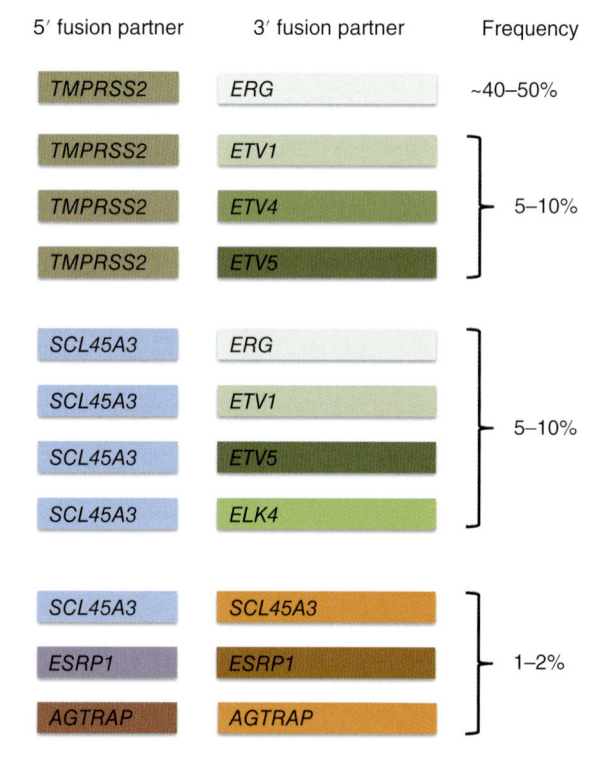

Figure 8 Fusion genes identified in prostate cancer.

Approximately 1% of prostate cancers harbor fusions involving each of *CRAF* and *BRAF* and are sensitive to sorafenib.[116] It is estimated that virtually 100% of advanced prostate cancers harbor alterations in the PTEN-PI3K-Akt pathway, and *PTEN* deletion in localized prostate cancer portends a worse prognosis.[117] *PTEN* deletion together with *MYC* amplification predicts a 50-fold increase in prostate cancer mortality compared to the absence of both abnormalities.[118] To date, however, PI3K and AKT inhibitors have not demonstrated clinical benefit.

Approximately 5% of localized prostate cancers have amplifications of *AURKA* or *MYCN*. In the aggressive neuroendocrine variant, however, the amplification rate is ~40%.[119] Preclinical models have demonstrated sensitivity of neuroendocrine tumors to AURKA inhibitors, and ongoing clinical trials are testing these agents for this aggressive subtype. Although evaluation for chromosomal aberrations in prostate cancer seldom occurs outside of a clinical trial, more widespread analysis will likely occur with the implementation of NGS and fusion-specific panels.

NTRK-fusion-positive cancers

Chromosomal translocations involving the genes (*NTRK1*, *NTRK3*, and *NTRK3*) encoding the neurotrophin tyrosine kinase receptors occur at a low frequency in several common tumors, e.g., lung and thyroid cancer and gliomas, but molecularly define other rare tumors, including cellular congenital mesoblastic nephroma, infantile fibrosarcoma, secretory breast cancer, and mammary analog secretory carcinoma of the salivary gland.[120] The most common of these, the t(12;15)(p13.2;q25.3), occurs in ~85% of these rare tumors, and results in the ETV6-NTRK3 fusion, and constitutive expression of the TRK3 kinase. The treatment of patients with first-generation TRK inhibitors, such as larotrectinib or entrectinib, is associated with a high rate of response (>75%) regardless of tumor histology, representing a compelling example of the histology-independent activity of targeted therapy in a molecularly defined subset of cancers.

Key references

The complete reference list can be found on Vital Source version of this title, see inside front cover.

1. Heim S, Mitelman F. *Cancer Cytogenetics: Chromosomal and Molecular Genetic Aberrations of Tumor Cells.* New York: Wiley; 2015.
2. Ouyang KJ, Le Beau MM. Role of cytogenetic analysis in the diagnosis and classification of hematopoietic neoplasms. In: Orazi A, Weiss LM, Foucar K, Knowles DM, eds. *Knowles' Neoplastic Hematopathology.* Philadelphia, PA: Lippincott Williams & Wilkins; 2014:232–264.
5. McGowan-Jordan J, Simons A, Schmid W. *An International System for Human Cytogenetic Nomenclature.* Basel: Karger AG; 2016.
6. Gozzetti A, Le Beau MM. Fluorescence in situ hybridization: uses and limitations. *Semin Hematol.* 2000;**37**(4):320–333.
7. Mikhail FM, Biegel JA, Cooley LD, et al. Technical laboratory standards for interpretation and reporting of acquired copy-number abnormalities and copy-neutral loss of heterozygosity in neoplastic disorders: a joint consensus recommendation from the American College of Medical Genetics and Genomics (ACMG) and the Cancer Genomics Consortium (CGC). *Genet Med.* 2019;**21**(9):1903–1916.
8. Frampton GM, Fichtenholtz A, Otto GA, et al. Development and validation of a clinical cancer genomic profiling test based on massively parallel DNA sequencing. *Nat Biotechnol.* 2013;**31**(11):1023–1031.
10. Penault-Llorca P-L, F., Rudzinski ER, Sepulveda AR. Testing algorithm for identification of patients with TRK fusion cancer. *J Clin Pathol.* 2019;**72**(7):460–467.
14. Chereda B, Melo JV. Natural course and biology of CML. *Ann Hematol.* 2015;**94**(Suppl 2):S107–S121.
17. Rossari F, Minutolo F, Orciuolo E. Past, present, and future of Bcr-Abl inhibitors: from chemical development to clinical efficacy. *J Hematol Oncol.* 2018;**11**(1):84.
21. Tefferi A, Pardanani A. Myeloproliferative neoplasms: a contemporary review. *JAMA Oncol.* 2015;**1**(1):97–105.
24. Nangalia J, Massie CE, Baxter EJ, et al. Somatic CALR mutations in myeloproliferative neoplasms with nonmutated JAK2. *N Engl J Med.* 2013;**369**(25):2391–2405.
25. Klampfl T, Gisslinger H, Harutyunyan AS, et al. Somatic mutations of calreticulin in myeloproliferative neoplasms. *N Engl J Med.* 2013;**369**(25):2379–2390.
26. Bejar R, Stevenson K, Abdel-Wahab O, et al. Clinical effect of point mutations in myelodysplastic syndromes. *N Engl J Med.* 2011;**364**(26):2496–2506.
27. Weinberg OK, Hasserjian RP. The current approach to the diagnosis of myelodysplastic syndromes. *Semin Hematol.* 2019;**56**(1):15–21.
30. Arber DA, Orazi A, Hasserjian R, et al. The 2016 revision to the World Health Organization classification of myeloid neoplasms and acute leukemia. *Blood.* 2016;**127**(20):2391–2405.
36. Dohner H, Estey E, Grimwade D, et al. Diagnosis and management of AML in adults: 2017 ELN recommendations from an international expert panel. *Blood.* 2017;**129**(4):424–447.
39. Eisfeld AK, Mrozek K, Kohlschmidt J, et al. The mutational oncoprint of recurrent cytogenetic abnormalities in adult patients with de novo acute myeloid leukemia. *Leukemia.* 2017;**31**(10):2211–2218.
41. de The H, Pandolfi PP, Chen Z. Acute promyelocytic leukemia: a paradigm for oncoprotein-targeted cure. *Cancer Cell.* 2017;**32**(5):552–560.
45. Godley LA, Larson RA. Therapy-related myeloid leukemia. *Semin Oncol.* 2008;**35**(4):418–429.
48. McNerney ME, Godley LA, Le Beau MM. Therapy-related myeloid neoplasms: when genetics and environment collide. *Nat Rev Cancer.* 2017;**17**(9):513–527.
51. Roberts KG. Genetics and prognosis of ALL in children vs adults. *Hematology Am Soc Hematol Educ Program.* 2018;**2018**(1):137–145.
53. Reshmi SC, Harvey RC, Roberts KG, et al. Targetable kinase gene fusions in high-risk B-ALL: a study from the Children's Oncology Group. *Blood.* 2017;**129**(25):3352–3361.
59. Paulsson K, Lilljebjorn H, Biloglav A, et al. The genomic landscape of high hyperdiploid childhood acute lymphoblastic leukemia. *Nat Genet.* 2015;**47**(6):672–676.
60. Roberts KG, Gu Z, Payne-Turner D, et al. High frequency and poor outcome of philadelphia chromosome-like acute lymphoblastic leukemia in adults. *J Clin Oncol.* 2017;**35**(4):394–401.
63. Liu Y, Easton J, Shao Y, et al. The genomic landscape of pediatric and young adult T-lineage acute lymphoblastic leukemia. *Nat Genet.* 2017;**49**(8):1211–1218.
64. Caporaso N, Goldin L, Plass C, et al. Chronic lymphocytic leukaemia genetics overview. *Br J Haematol.* 2007;**139**(5):630–634.
68. Dave BJ, Nelson M, Sanger WG. Lymphoma cytogenetics. *Clin Lab Med.* 2011;**31**(4):725–761.
69. Pasqualucci L, Dalla-Favera R. Genetics of diffuse large B-cell lymphoma. *Blood.* 2018;**131**(21):2307–2319.
77. Fonseca R, Bergsagel PL, Drach J, et al. International Myeloma Working Group molecular classification of multiple myeloma: spotlight review. *Leukemia.* 2009;**23**(12):2210–2221.
80. Kumar SK, Rajkumar SV. The multiple myelomas - current concepts in cytogenetic classification and therapy. *Nat Rev Clin Oncol.* 2018;**15**(7):409–421.
85. Marcozzi A, Pellestor F, Kloosterman WP. The genomic characteristics and origin of chromothripsis. *Methods Mol Biol.* 1769;**2018**:3–19.
89. Pappo AS, Dirksen U. Rhabdomyosarcoma, Ewing sarcoma, and other round cell sarcomas. *J Clin Oncol.* 2018;**36**(2):168–179.
98. Rosenberg A, Agulnik M. Epithelioid hemangioendothelioma: update on diagnosis and treatment. *Curr Treat Opt Oncol.* 2018;**19**(4):19.
99. Patel S, von Mehren M, Reed DR, et al. Overall survival and histology-specific subgroup analyses from a phase 3, randomized controlled study of trabectedin or dacarbazine in patients with advanced liposarcoma or leiomyosarcoma. *Cancer.* 2019;**125**(15):2610–2620.
100. Schoffski P, Chawla S, Maki RG, et al. Eribulin versus dacarbazine in previously treated patients with advanced liposarcoma or leiomyosarcoma: a randomised, open-label, multicentre, phase 3 trial. *Lancet.* 2016;**387**(10028):1629–1637.
106. Herbst RS, Morgenszstern D, Boshoff C. The biology and management of non-small cell lung cancer. *Nature.* 2018;**553**(7689):446–454.
109. Peters S, Camidge DR, Shaw AT, et al. Alectinib versus crizotinib in untreated ALK-positive non-small-cell lung cancer. *N Engl J Med.* 2017;**377**(9):829–838.
113. Wang G, Zhao D, Spring DJ, DePinho RA. Genetics and biology of prostate cancer. *Genes Dev.* 2018;**32**(17-18):1105–1140.
117. Cancer Genome Atlas Research N. The molecular taxonomy of primary prostate cancer. *Cell.* 2015;**163**(4):1011–1025.
120. Albert CM, Davis JL, Federman N, et al. TRK fusion cancers in children: a clinical review and recommendations for screening. *J Clin Oncol.* 2019;**37**(6):513–524.

9 MicroRNA expression in cancer

Serge P. Nana-Sinkam, MD ∎ Mario Acunzo, PhD ∎ Carlo M. Croce, MD

> **Overview**
>
> In the last two decades, researchers have identified a new group of non-coding RNAs (ncRNAs) classified according to their function and size. The best studied of these ncRNAs termed microRNAs (miRNAs) are short non-coding RNAs that are approximately 22 nucleotides in length and play key roles in the regulation of a large number of biological processes and diseases, including cancer. Since the initial description of an association between miRNA and cancer in 2002, miRNAs have emerged as central regulators of processes fundamental to the initiation and progression of cancer. More recently, miRNAs have been detected in bodily fluids including blood, sputum, and urine, thus making them potential noninvasive diagnostic and prognostic biomarkers of disease. The application of miRNAs in human cancer therapy represents one of the newest frontiers for cancer treatment and thus, the intense focus on investigation. However, our knowledge of these small molecules and their application to human cancers is still growing. In this article, we provide an overview of the connection between miRNAs and cancer with a focus on translation to human application.

Background

As investigators increasingly recognize the inherent complexities of cancer initiation and progression, they continue to search for novel molecular pathways in cancer that may be leveraged for the development of clinically informative biomarkers and therapeutics, with the ultimate goal of saving lives. For decades, investigators have held the belief that a large percentage of the human genome was composed of "junk-DNA" or "dark matter" due to its inability to code for proteins. In the last two decades, researchers have now identified functions for regions of the human genome previously considered to be nonfunctional. Some genes located within these regions indeed encode for noncoding RNAs (ncRNAs), with microRNAs (miRNAs) representing the most researched member of this group. Since their initial discovery two decades ago in *Caenorhabditis elegans*, miRNAs have emerged as key regulators of biological processes fundamental to the initiation and progression of cancers.[1,2] Approximately, 22 nucleotides (nt) in length, miRNAs tend to be highly conserved across species and often demonstrate global deregulation in solid and hematological malignancies.[3,4] By directly binding to either the 3′ or 5′ untranslated region (UTR) of target mRNAs, miRNAs can either degrade target mRNA or inhibit translation. In addition, based on their relatively short size, miRNAs have the capacity for the simultaneous regulation of tens to hundreds of genes, thus interdicting in numerous biological pathways. In fact, the estimate that miRNAs may regulate up to 60% of the human genome is likely inaccurate, and miRNA may regulate over 90% of protein-coding genes.[4,5] miRNAs are often located in fragile regions of the chromosome and thus susceptible to regulation through chromosomal amplifications, deletions, or rearrangements.[6] The mechanisms for the regulation of miRNAs in the setting of cancer are complex and remain only partially understood. However, increasing lines of investigation indicate that miRNA regulation may occur by several mechanisms, including alterations in key components of processing, epigenetic silencing, and polymorphisms in either miRNAs or target mRNAs interfering with binding and regulation.[7] The mechanisms for miRNA regulation and function are further complicated by their tumor and cell specificity. We are now approaching the identification of nearly 3000 miRNAs. This number, however, could be an overestimation due to the challenges associated with defining "true miRNAs." In a recent investigation conducted by Alle et al.,[8] the investigators validated approximately 2300 true human mature miRNA sequences. Consequently, these challenges in defining miRNAs have driven popular databases, such as miRBase, to become more stringent in order to minimize the inclusion of potential false positives. Collectively, miRNAs may function either as tumor suppressors or oncogenes depending on tumor and cell type and regulate processes fundamental to tumorigenesis (hallmarks of cancer) including differentiation, proliferation, and angiogenesis.[7] While the use of high-throughput profiling strategies for the identification of clinically relevant miRNA-based biomarkers has been useful, this approach to miRNA investigation remains limited by issues of reproducibility and the need for improved algorithms for miRNA-target prediction and validation. Thus, there is still considerable work required to translate miRNAs into markers for clinical decision-making. One must also consider the inherent difficulties in achieving tumor-specific miRNA delivery. As miRNA biology transitions to the clinic, there is encouraging evidence suggesting that human applications for miRNAs, particularly as therapeutics, are in the not-too-distant future. For instance, nanotechnology-based carriers for miRNA delivery represent a new promising tool for the effective shuttling of miRNAs in the human body. Santaris/miRNA Therapeutics Inc. and Regulus Therapeutics have tested human delivery of an antagomir against miR-122 for the treatment of hepatitis C. More recently, investigators have initiated phase II trials testing human delivery of an antagomir against miR-155 for treating subcutaneous T-cell lymphoma as well as a phase I trial testing miR-16 replacement in recurrent malignant mesothelioma. Such studies represent the first of hopefully a series of future applications for the treatment of human cancer.

Biogenesis and production of microRNAs

miRNAs are short ncRNAs with a length of approximately 22 nucleotides encoded by evolutionarily conserved genes. miRNAs are more frequently located within the introns or exons of protein-coding genes (about 70%) or in intergenic regions (30%). The expression of intragenic miRNAs is related to their

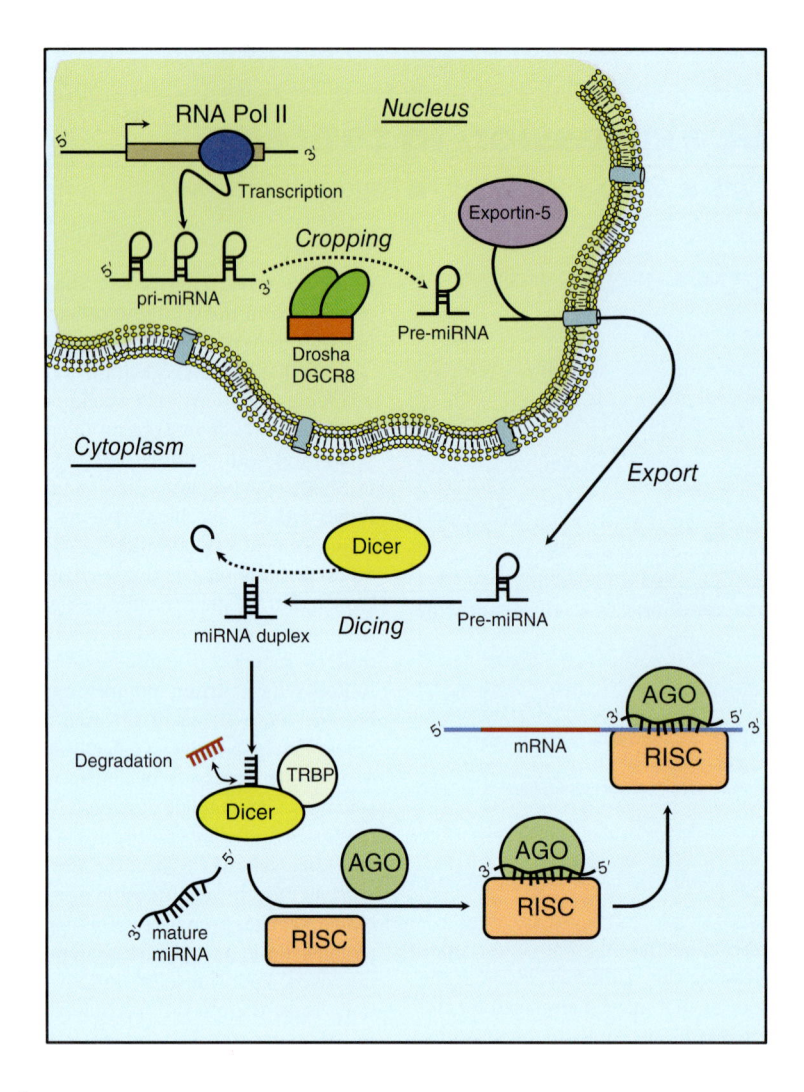

Figure 1 MicroRNA biogenesis.

host gene expression, all intergenic miRNAs having independent transcription units.[9] miRNAs are processed and generated through a well-orchestrated series of interrelated steps, each of which is currently being investigated (Figure 1). In the first step, a long primary transcript termed the pri-miRNA undergoes transcription by RNA polymerase II. The pri-miRNAs are then bound to the double-stranded RNA-binding domain (dsRBD) protein known as DiGeorge syndrome critical region gene 8 (DGCR8) for vertebrates.[10] An RNase III endonuclease termed The Drosha/DGCR8 complex cleaves the pri-miRNA into a smaller stem-loop ~70-nucleotide (nt) precursor miRNA (pre-miRNA). Pre-miRNAs are then exported from the nucleus to the cytoplasm using the double-stranded RNA-binding protein, Exportin 5 (XPO5).[11] Once in the cytoplasm, the pre-miRNA is cleaved into a mature 18–25 nucleotide miRNA by a complex that includes RNAase Dicer, Argonaute 2 (Ago 2), and transactivation-responsive RNA-binding protein (TRBP). The Ago2 protein belongs to the Argonaute family of proteins that bind fragments to guide RNA (including miRNAs). The resultant miRNA sequence, which consists of two strands, is then loaded into the RNA-induced silencing complex (RISC), with the mature strand being maintained while the complementary strand is degraded. The remaining strand possesses complementarity either to the 3′ or 5′ UTR of a target gene leading to degradation through endonuclease activity or to translational inhibition. Recently, investigators have shown that a miRNA can also bind to the coding sequence of a transcript, leading to translational repression.[12] The degree of complementarity between the "seed" sequence of the mature miRNA and the target is the primary determinant of the biological effect. It is important to recognize that investigators have now identified additional mechanisms for miRNA biogenesis. For example, in a recent study by Kim et al.,[13] the investigators observed canonical miRNA biogenesis, even following the ablation of DICER. Moreover, they found that pre-miRNA sequences were able to directly load into AGO, which led to the preferential selection of 5p miRNA over 3p miRNA. This direct loading of pre-miRNA into AGO may represent an overlooked pathway in miRNA biogenesis, which further illustrates that we are just beginning to understand the complexities of this process.

MicroRNA deregulation in cancer

Calin et al.[14] made the first observations linking miRNA deregulation to cancer in a study. While investigating the mechanisms for chronic lymphocytic leukemia (CLL), this team of investigators made the startling observation that a pair of miRNAs, miR-15a/16-1 which, along with the deleted in leukemia (DLEU) gene, are located at the chromosomal region 13q14.3, was either deleted or down-regulated in 68% of patients with CLL.[14]

In addition, both of these miRNAs were highly expressed in normal CD5+ B cells. Both findings suggested that these miRNAs were in fact important to the pathogenesis of the disease. This initial observation was corroborated by independent investigators who identified a functional link between miR-15a/16-1 and the prosurvival molecule B-cell lymphoma 2 (Bcl2). They validated *in vitro* that miR-15a/16-1 targeted Bcl2 to induce apoptosis. Since this initial discovery of miRNAs in CLL, investigators have observed patterns of global dysregulation of miRNAs across both solid and hematological malignancies. In the last few years, researchers have determined that the causes of such dysregulation are multifactorial. For instance, the altered expression and/or function of the proteins involved in the biogenesis of miRNAs, such as Drosha and Dicer, can lead to aberrant expression of miRNAs and, thus to cancer.[15] A decreased expression level of Drosha and Dicer has been found in a high percentage of ovarian cancer patients.[16] Moreover, epigenetic changes within miRNA promoters, such as changes in their methylation, can also induce changes in miRNA expression levels.[17] Like other deregulated genes that cover an important role as oncogenes or tumor suppressors, the epigenetic deregulated expression of a single miRNA can be the triggering event for carcinogenesis. One such example involves the intensely studied miR-155, whose dysregulation can induce leukemia in miR-155 transgenic mice.[18] The tumor-suppressor miR-127 in primary prostate cancer and bladder tumors causes the upregulation of the proto-oncogene BCL6, which is a direct target of miR-127.[19] On the other hand, miRNAs can also act as protagonists in the control of the global cellular methylation status by acting on the enzymes responsible for epigenetic control. For example, the miR-29 family is able to modulate methylation levels by affecting the *ex novo* expression of DNA methyltransferases DNMT3a and DNMT3B in lung cancer.[17] Another important and complex regulative mechanism of miRNAs is related to the transcriptional control of gene expression.[20] The activation of the miR-17/92 cluster induced by the MYC oncogene modulates the antiapoptotic action of E2F Transcription Factor 1 (E2F1), thus mediating the MYC proliferative effect.[21] Recently, the effect of the membrane tyrosine-kinase receptors on miRNA expression has been studied. For instance, the hepatocyte growth factor receptor mesenchymal-epithelial transition factor (c-MET) is able, through the transcriptional factor activator protein 1 (AP1), to induce the expression of the onco-miRNA miR-221/222 cluster, suggesting that the important effect of deregulated c-MET in cancer is at least in part linked to a deregulated miRNA expression pathway.[22] Finally, considering that the loss of p53 is one of the most represented genetic abnormalities in cancer, the link between the miR-34a family and p53 is another important example of miRNA transcriptional regulation.[23] p53 stimulates the transcription of the miR-34 family, inducing apoptosis and senescence. The loss of p53 function induces the downregulation of the miR-34 family in a very high percentage of ovarian cancer patients with a p53 mutation.[24] Hence, the primary theme is that patterns of miRNA expression are globally deregulated in cancer, this event being potentially a cause as well as a consequence of cancer itself. The global deregulation of miRNA in cancer has a dramatic effect on the downstream targets of several cellular pathways.

Recently, investigators have also determined that miRNA function may be altered through mutations in target gene-seed sequences. Such mutations can render a miRNA incapable of regulating a given mRNA and have been identified as biomarkers of clinical outcome. Mutations in the 3′ UTR have been identified in several solid malignancies, including ovarian, lung, breast, and colon cancers. Conversely, single nucleotide polymorphisms (SNPs) in miRNA gene sequences can change miRNA functions. We know that mRNA functional regulation by miRNAs is highly sensitive to base-pair mismatches within nucleotides two to eight of the miRNA, which has been defined as the seed region.[25] Therefore a single point mutation on a miRNA gene or a posttranscriptional modification such as RNA editing can change the function or modify the targetome of a miRNA.[25,26] For example, it was determined that a SNP in a let-7 (lethal-7) miRNA complementary site in the Kirsten rat sarcoma virus (KRAS) 3′ UTR increases non-small-cell lung cancer risk.[27] A mutation of let-7 binding site in the Kras 3′ UTR has also been detected in juvenile myelomonocytic leukemia (JMML).[28]

MicroRNA as biomarkers in cancer

Over the last several years, miRNAs have been implicated in virtually every type of cancer. Early studies have focused on applying high-throughput platforms as a means for linking patterns of miRNA deregulation to clinical parameters. One of the first such approaches was made in 2005 by Volinia and colleagues who profiled the miRNA signatures of six solid human tumors, detecting miR-21, miR-17-5p, and miR-191 overexpressed in some tumors.[29] Since that initial study, investigators have conducted multiple similar studies with the primary goal of identifying a prognostic miRNA signature. Yanaihara and colleagues conducted high-throughput profiling of cases of stage 1 adenocarcinoma of the lung. They identified over 40 miRNAs that distinguished lung tumors from the adjacent uninvolved lung.[30] A broader study conducted on 22 different tumor types showed how a miRNA expression profile is able to classify tumors according to the tissue of origin with high accuracy.[31] Studies have also focused on preselected miRNAs as potential prognostic markers. For example, Nadal et al.[32] examined the tumor-suppressive miR-34 as a prognostic biomarker in early-stage adenocarcinoma of the lung. They identified methylation and reduced expression of miR-34b/c in nearly half (46%) of early-stage lung adenocarcinomas and determined that reduced expression and methylation of miR-34b/c correlated with shorter disease-free survival and overall survival. For example, in a separate study, investigators showed that miRNA expression levels may correlate with BCR-ABL kinase activity in chronic myeloid leukemia (CML),[33] suggesting, therefore, a potential application in the adjustment of the therapy during treatment to improve the outcome. Another very intriguing application of miRNAs as biomarkers consists of the integration of both protein-coding and noncoding gene expressions in order to develop a prognostic signature in the early stages of cancer. Akagi et al.[34] examined 148 cases of stage 1 lung adenocarcinoma for 42 preselected genes as predictive biomarkers. Through testing and subsequent validation in independent cohorts, the authors developed a four-gene classifier (DLC1, XPO1, HIF1A, and BRCA1) that correlates to survival in stage 1 lung adenocarcinoma. In addition, they determined that miR-21 expression was independently associated with survival in the same cohorts. Lastly, the combination of the four-gene classifier and miR-21 expression was superior to either biomarker alone. Despite the multitude of very encouraging miRNA profiling studies, investigators have yet to reach a consensus on which miRNAs confer the most accurate prognostic information. A primary reason for the lack of reproducibility is that similarly to other high-throughput analyses, miRNA profiling studies are susceptible to certain biases, including small cohort sizes, varying platforms [array, sequencing,

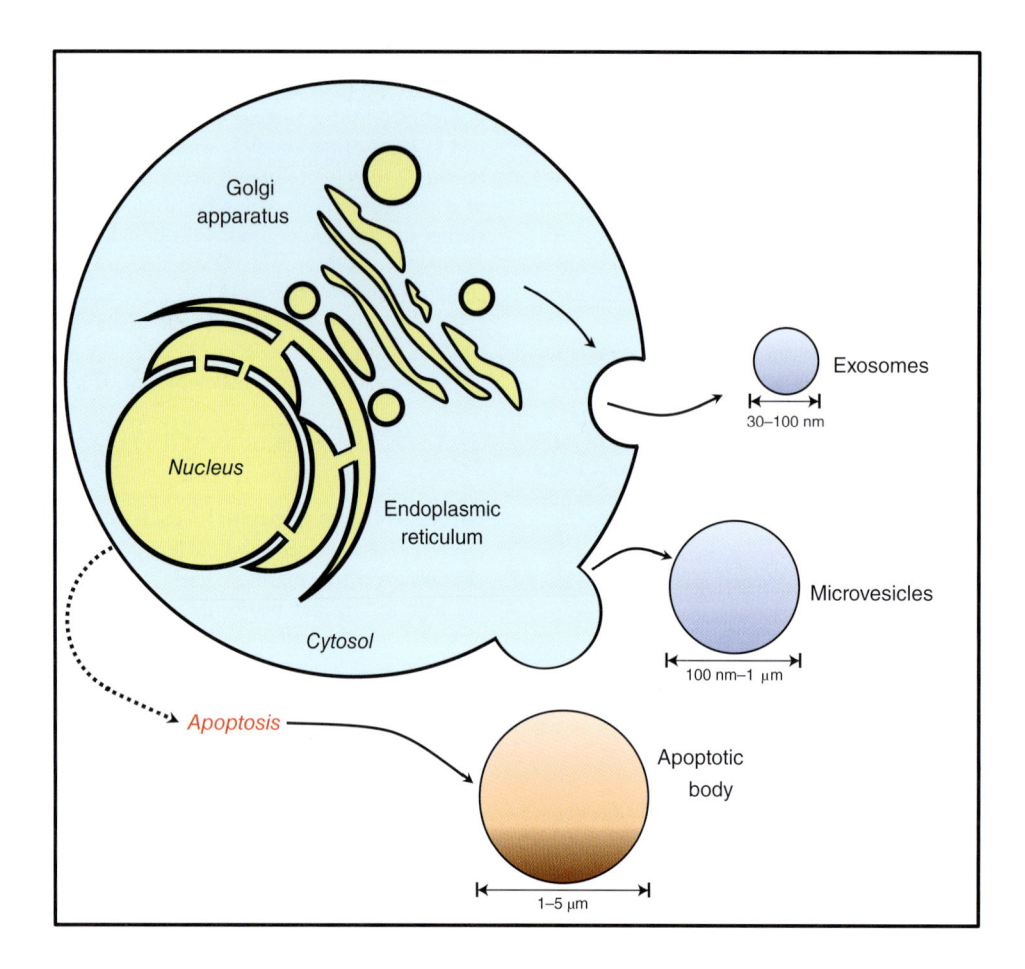

Figure 2 Process of extracellular vesicles release from cells. Apoptotic cells release apoptotic bodies.

reverse transcription polymerase chain reaction (RT-PCR)], and variability in data interpretation.

MicroRNAs as noninvasive biomarkers in cancer

The development of noninvasive biomarkers in cancer that may inform clinical decision-making remains elusive and the subject of continued study. Several studies have demonstrated that miRNAs exist in body fluids (serum, plasma, urine, sputum, cerebrospinal fluid, and bronchoalveolar lavage) in a relatively stable form at different conditions of pH and temperature.[35–37] miRNAs are also present in the blood, where they were detected in plasma, platelets, erythrocytes, and nucleated blood cells. One of the earliest studies revealed that miRNAs were detectable in circulation in prostate cancer.[38] Shen et al.[39] demonstrated that plasma-based miRNAs could be used as biomarkers to distinguish solitary lung nodules. A subsequent larger study further validated the concept that circulating miRNAs could be used in the setting of lung cancer early detection.[40] Remarkably, in a similarly large study conducted by Asakura et al.,[41] the investigators identified and validated the ability of a combined classifier of serum miRNAs for predicting resectable lung cancer cases with high sensitivity and specificity, regardless of histology and TNM status. Collectively, these miRNA-based classifier systems represent potentially valuable clinical tools for informing the detection and treatment of cancer patients.

The compartment-specific location of miRNAs in circulation remains the subject of debate. However, circulating miRNAs have been found packaged in extracellular vesicles (EVs) as well as associated with RNA-binding proteins like Argonaute 2 or lipoprotein complexes, which prevent their degradation (Figure 2).[42–45] EVs are small membrane-encapsulated fluid particles comprised of a family shedding vesicles and exosomes that are released from a wide variety of cell types mechanisms that are cell dependent.[46] Investigators to date have focused primarily on exosomes, which are 30–100 nm vesicles. These particles consist of a lipid bilayer, generated from secretory multivesicular bodies (MVB) that fuse with the plasma membrane for release into the extracellular environment. Exosomes contain various molecular constituents of their cell of origin, including lipids, proteins, messenger RNA (mRNA), and miRNA, which may be transferred from donor to target cells to facilitate direct cell-to-cell communication and subsequent reprogramming of the tumor microenvironment.[43] In pathological states, such as cancer, exosomes cross-talk, and/or influence major tumor-related pathways such as epithelial-mesenchymal transition (EMT), cancer stemness, angiogenesis, and metastasis involving many cell types within the tumor microenvironment.[47–50] Exosomes have also been detected in a number of human body fluids, including plasma, urine, breast milk, amniotic fluid, malignant ascites, and bronchoalveolar lavage fluid, suggesting their potential importance as biomarkers of disease.[51]

Selected miRNAs implicated in cancer

Following a multitude of miRNA in cancer studies, several miRNAs, miR-15 and miR-16, miR-155, let-7, miR-21, and miR-34, for example, have emerged as fundamental contributors to tumor development. These miRNAs are now being integrated into clinical trials as biomarkers for clinical diagnosis and therapy.

MiR-15/16
The miR-15 and miR-16 family is a gene cluster located on chromosome 13 (13q14.3). In 2002, investigators first identified this cluster as the target of a deletion in chromosome 13q in CLL, thereby discovering the first association between microRNAs and cancer.[14] The deletion of chromosome 13q is present in 55% of human CLL[52] and is associated with the indolent phenotype of disease.[53] Often downregulated in CLL, miR-15 and miR-16 were later determined to have tumor suppressor properties by targeting BCL2[54] and Cyclin D1.[55] Bcl2 is a mitochondrial membrane protein that blocks apoptosis and promotes the oncogenesis of several cells, including lymphocytes.[56] High levels of BCL2, have been found in CLL[57] as an additional consequence of miR-15 and miR-16 deletion.[54] Recently, a specific BCL2 inhibitor, ABT-199 (Venetoclax), was developed and approved by the U.S. Food and Drug Administration (FDA) for CLL treatment.[58,59]

Let-7
The let-7 gene was first discovered in *C. elegans* as a key regulator of development.[60] The mature form of let-7 family members is highly conserved across species. let-7 miRs family plays an essential role in regulating cell proliferation and differentiation during development in different species. In addition, let-7 is a marker of fully differentiated cells while undetectable in stem cells.[61] The human let-7 family contains 12 members located on nine different chromosomes; they map to fragile sites associated with different types of solid cancers.[62] Indeed, the deregulation of these miRs has been shown as a feature of many types of cancer.[63–65] There is a well-known double negative feedback between let-7 and the c-Myc oncogene, which is one of the most studied target and regulator of let-7.

MiR-21
MiR-21 is one of the most studied oncomiRs, as most of its validated targets are tumor suppressors (i.e., PTEN, Bcl2, and Sprouty1 and 2). This miR is probably one of the most dynamic miRNAs, being responsive to various stimuli, given its involvement in positive and negative feedback loops. miR-21 is one of the most altered miRNAs in solid tumors, including breast, ovaries, cervix, colon, lung, liver, brain, esophagus, prostate, pancreas, and thyroid.[29,66–68] miR-21 is also upregulated in leukemic cancers,[69] indicating an important key role for this miRNA in cancer development and progression. Moreover, a recent study established circulating miR-21 as a biomarker of various carcinomas, unveiling its potential as a tool for cancer diagnosis.[70]

MiR-34
The miR-34 family consists of three highly related miRNAs: miR-34a, miR-34b, and miR-34c. miR-34a is expressed at higher levels than miR-34b/c in all tissues, particularly the brain, with the exception being the lung.[62] These miRNAs are directly induced by p53 in response to DNA damage or oncogenic stress[71] and contribute to the p53 downstream effect by targeting c-Myc, Bcl2, C-Met, and Src.[72] MiR-34a plays a fundamental role not only in tumor suppression but also in modulation of drug response in a number of cellular models, including hepatocellular carcinoma (HCC), breast cancer, bladder carcinoma, head and neck squamous For example, overexpression of miR-34a in NSCLC restores TRAIL-induced apoptosis by mechanism of downregulating platelet-derived growth factor receptor (PDGFR)[73]

MiR-200 family
The miR-200 family consists of five members: miR-200a, miR-200b, miR-200c, miR-141, and miR-429. These miRs are highly expressed in epithelial tissues and are involved in tumor suppression by inhibiting EMT, migration, invasion, tumor cell adhesion, and metastasis.[74] Among miR-200 family targets, ZEB1 and ZEB2, two central mediators of EMT, are two of the most studied. Moreover, there is a double-negative ZEB/miR-200 feedback loop, given the ability of ZEB1 to suppress the expression of miR-200 family members.[75] Furthermore, there is evidence that breast cancer metastases may be under the control of the Akt-miR200-E-cadherin axis. Specifically, the balance of the three Akt isoforms can control the expression of miR-200 and that of the E-cadherin mRNA in primary and metastatic human breast cancers.[76]

Therapeutic targeting and miRNA
Given that deregulation of a single or group of miRNAs can drive malignancy, it is hypothesized that through directed targeting of their deregulation, at least *in vitro*, one can attenuate carcinogenesis. Alternatively, patterns of miRNA deregulation may drive chemoresistance to traditional agents. For example, strategies aimed at using global miRNA expression profiling of selectively created drug-resistant cell lines have been utilized to identify which specific miRNAs are responsible for the acquired resistance. These findings have translated to miRNAs serving both as directed targets and predictors of response to chemotherapeutic agents. Importantly, the contribution of specific miRNAs to chemoresistance can be highly cell tumor-specific. As mentioned, miRNAs have the capacity to simultaneously target and regulate multiple biological pathways. In the case of CLL, selected patterns of miRNA expression could clinically predict which patients would respond to the selected agent fludarabine.[77] In solid tumors such as lung cancer, miRNAs including miR-21, miR-30, miR-221, and miR-222 have been associated with response to chemotherapeutic agents. Recently, Vecchione et al.[78] profiled a miRNA signature that is able to define chemoresistance in ovarian cancer. It has been reported that miRNA profiling is useful to identify a subtype of temozolomide-resistant glioblastoma.[79] Furthermore, in addition to informing treatment response, investigators have also examined the potential of co-administering miRNAs with traditional chemotherapies to increase cancer cell sensitivity to the chemotherapy treatment.[80]

In the last few years, the majority of applications of miRNAs as directed therapies in human disease have taken place in *in vitro* and murine models of disease settings. The primary goal of directed therapeutics is to manipulate miRNAs that are known to be deregulated in tumors and thus alter their downstream targets and biological pathways. This approach may occur through the selected targeting of a miRNA or as a strategy for augmenting the effects of an established therapeutic agent. The manipulation of miRNAs via either selective gain of function (e.g., mimics) for the purposes of repletion or silencing (e.g., antagonists) has been applied with variable results. miRNAs may be delivered by several modalities, including viral vectors and nanoparticles (NPs). Viral-based carriers have been effectively used to deliver miRNAs in solid tumors, including let-7 in lung cancer.[81] However, viral carriers for small molecule delivery are not without limitations, including the potential immunogenic and toxic effects of the carrier to the host. More recently, investigators have employed lipid-based NPs as carriers for small molecules, including miRNA. NPs represent smaller engineered particles that are particularly suitable for drug delivery based on their modifiable composition allowing for optimal binding and absorption. Several recent studies have demonstrated the efficacy of NPs as vehicles for miRNA delivery in vivo. For example, Wu et al. recently showed that lipid-based NPs could be utilized to effectively deliver miR-29 in lung cancer both in vitro and in vivo.[82] In an independent study, Trang et al. showed that delivery of let-7 could reduce tumor growth and many oncogenes.[83] Issues of off-target effects, stability of carriers, and toxicity all remain germane to miRNA-based therapeutics. The use of miRNA sponges represents an alternative strategy to antagomirs. RNA sponges are able to simultaneously repress a large number of miRNA molecules. The existence of circular RNA (circRNA) has been already established in nature and can represent an example of a miRNA sponge. circRNA is a type of RNA, which forms a covalently closed continuous loop, forming a circRNA whereby the 3′ and 5′ ends are attached together, forming a round RNA molecule. This structural characteristic confers stability to circRNAs in the cytosol while also ensuring the ability to bind a variable number of miRNA molecules simultaneously thus inhibiting their action. circRNAs are derived from protein-coding genes but do not encode for any protein and thus are identified as ncRNA.[84] Recently, investigators determined that a circRNA called R1as/CiRS-7 could serve as a sponge for miR-7. This circRNA was able to downregulate miR-7 by acting as a specific sponge for it through 63 miR-7 binding sites.[85] The design of synthetic sponges able to mimic natural circRNA action represents a novel approach for the modulation of aberrant miRNA expression in cancer. This technology is very useful in satisfying the need to simultaneously downregulate several miRNAs or miRNA families.[86]

Recently, investigators have developed novel computational tools for the design of synthetic miRNAs capable of effectively and simultaneously targeting multiple specific mRNAs of choice (multitarget, multisite targeting). Lagana et al.[86] in 2014 developed and validated a bioinformatic tool termed "miR-Synth," which represents a single synthetic miRNA able to target MET and epidermal growth factor receptor (EGFR) simultaneously. Interestingly, this tool can be applied to create synthetic miRNAs for a wide variety of different target combination choices. The concept of modulating miRNA in cancer through the reintroduction or the repression of deregulated miRNAs combined with the use of synthetic technology for the modulation of miRNA expression (miRNA sponges) and, finally, the employment of synthetic miRNA that can modulate simultaneously the expression of different genes of choice does not represent a strategy void of issues. The off-target problem and difficulties in delivery make miRNA-centered cancer therapy a promising technology not yet applicable.

Human applications for miRNAs

While the majority of miRNA-focused lines of investigation have been laboratory-based, an increasing number of human clinical trials have begun to incorporate miRNAs as predictive/therapeutic biomarkers or as directed therapeutics. Currently, there are almost 400 clinical trials incorporating miRNAs that are either actively recruiting or completed recruiting. The majority of such studies are utilizing miRNAs as potential clinical biomarkers. However, in the last few years, we have witnessed the emergence of clinical studies directed at utilizing miRNAs as therapeutics in humans. The most recognized such study involves the application of an antagomir for miR-122 to treat hepatitis C.[87] Both phase I and phase II trials have been completed using the agent SPC3649 (Miravirsen) in both healthy volunteers and those with chronic Hepatitis C.[88] Currently, studies are ongoing to examine the utility of Miravirsen in chronic Hepatitis C nonresponders. In terms of using miRNAs as therapeutics for cancer treatment, the first such study is an ongoing phase I trial, which is a multicenter phase I trial using a liposomal formulation of miR-34 (MRX34) for primary unresectable liver cancer or advanced metastatic solid malignancies with or without metastases. Ultimately, the clinical trials were suspended due to the adverse immunological reactions in patients.[89,90] The disappointing results of the MRX34 trials reflect the challenges associated with preparing for and interpreting the observed toxicity effects in humans. In addition to MRX34, there are two exciting studies on the horizon that have the potential for clinical application. The first study identified as MesomiR-1 is a phase I trial involving the use of an EGFR-targeting delivery vehicle harboring miR-16 in individuals with malignant pleural mesothelioma or advanced non-small-cell lung cancer who have failed previous therapies.[91] The second study involves Cobomarsen, an oligonucleotide inhibitor of miR-155, which is currently being used for treating mycosis fungoides (MF), a type of cutaneous T-cell lymphoma. Thus far, the patients exhibit tolerance and promising clinical activity in response to the drug molecule.[92] Moving forward with phase II clinical trials, this study is expanding to include patients presenting with other hematological malignancies.

Key references

The complete reference list can be found on Vital Source version of this title, see inside front cover.

1 Lee RC, Feinbaum RL, Ambros V. The C. elegans heterochronic gene lin-4 encodes small RNAs with antisense complementarity to lin-14. *Cell*. 1993;**75**:843–854.

3 Croce CM. Causes and consequences of microRNA dysregulation in cancer. *Nat Rev Genet*. 2009;**10**:704–714.

4 Lagos-Quintana M, Rauhut R, Lendeckel W, Tuschl T. Identification of novel genes coding for small expressed RNAs. *Science*. 2001;**294**:853–858.

6 Calin GA, Croce CM. MicroRNA signatures in human cancers. *Nat Rev Cancer*. 2006;**6**:857–866.

7 Nana-Sinkam SP, Croce CM. Non-coding RNAs in cancer initiation and progression and as novel biomarkers. *Mol Oncol*. 2011;**5**:483–491.

9 Rodriguez A, Griffiths-Jones S, Ashurst JL, Bradley A. Identification of mammalian microRNA host genes and transcription units. *Genome Res*. 2004;**14**:1902–1910.

10 Gregory RI, Yan KP, Amuthan G, et al. The microprocessor complex mediates the genesis of microRNAs. *Nature*. 2004;**432**:235–240.

11 Bohnsack MT, Czaplinski K, Gorlich D. Exportin 5 is a RanGTP-dependent dsRNA-binding protein that mediates nuclear export of pre-miRNAs. *RNA*. 2004;**10**:185–191.

14 Calin GA, Dumitru CD, Shimizu M, et al. Frequent deletions and down-regulation of micro- RNA genes miR15 and miR16 at 13q14 in chronic lymphocytic leukemia. *Proc Natl Acad Sci U S A*. 2002;**99**:15524–15529.

17 Fabbri M, Garzon R, Cimmino A, et al. MicroRNA-29 family reverts aberrant methylation in lung cancer by targeting DNA methyltransferases 3A and 3B. *Proc Natl Acad Sci U S A*. 2007;**104**:15805–15810.

22 Garofalo M, Romano G, Di Leva G, et al. EGFR and MET receptor tyrosine kinase-altered microRNA expression induces tumorigenesis and gefitinib resistance in lung cancers. *Nat Med*. 2011;**18**:74–82.

23 He L, He X, Lowe SW, Hannon GJ. microRNAs join the p53 network--another piece in the tumour-suppression puzzle. *Nat Rev Cancer*. 2007;**7**:819–822.

25 Brennecke J, Stark A, Russell RB, Cohen SM. Principles of microRNA-target recognition. *PLoS Biol*. 2005;**3**:e85.

29 Volinia S, Calin GA, Liu CG, et al. A microRNA expression signature of human solid tumors defines cancer gene targets. *Proc Natl Acad Sci U S A*. 2006;**103**:2257–2261.

31 Rosenfeld N, Aharonov R, Meiri E, et al. MicroRNAs accurately identify cancer tissue origin. *Nat Biotechnol*. 2008;**26**:462–469.

38 Mitchell PS, Parkin RK, Kroh EM, et al. Circulating microRNAs as stable blood-based markers for cancer detection. *Proc Natl Acad Sci U S A*. 2008;**105**:10513–10518.

40 Boeri M, Verri C, Conte D, et al. MicroRNA signatures in tissues and plasma predict development and prognosis of computed tomography detected lung cancer. *Proc Natl Acad Sci U S A*. 2011;**108**:3713–3718.

43 Valadi H, Ekstrom K, Bossios A, et al. Exosome-mediated transfer of mRNAs and microRNAs is a novel mechanism of genetic exchange between cells. *Nat Cell Biol*. 2007;**9**:654–659.

46 Turchinovich A, Weiz L, Langheinz A, Burwinkel B. Characterization of extracellular circulating microRNA. *Nucleic Acids Res*. 2011;**39**:7223–7233.

51 Cazzoli R, Buttitta F, Di Nicola M, et al. microRNAs derived from circulating exosomes as noninvasive biomarkers for screening and diagnosing lung cancer. *J Thorac Oncol*. 2013;**8**:1156–1162.

52 Pekarsky Y, Croce CM. Role of miR-15/16 in CLL. *Cell Death Differ*. 2015;**22**:6–11.

54 Cimmino A, Calin GA, Fabbri M, et al. miR-15 and miR-16 induce apoptosis by targeting BCL2. *Proc Natl Acad Sci U S A*. 2005;**102**:13944–13949.

55 Jiang QQ, Liu B, Yuan T. MicroRNA-16 inhibits bladder cancer proliferation by targeting cyclin D1. *Asian Pac J Cancer Prev*. 2013;**14**:4127–4130.

59 Uchida A, Isobe Y, Asano J, et al. Targeting BCL2 with venetoclax is a promising therapeutic strategy for "double-protein expression" lymphoma with MYC and BCL2 rearrangements. *Haematologica*. 2019;**104**:1417–1421.

60 Reinhart BJ, Slack FJ, Basson M, et al. The 21-nucleotide let-7 RNA regulates developmental timing in *Caenorhabditis elegans*. *Nature*. 2000;**403**:901–906.

62 Calin GA, Sevignani C, Dumitru CD, et al. Human microRNA genes are frequently located at fragile sites and genomic regions involved in cancers. *Proc Natl Acad Sci U S A*. 2004;**101**:2999–3004.

69 Fulci V, Chiaretti S, Goldoni M, et al. Quantitative technologies establish a novel microRNA profile of chronic lymphocytic leukemia. *Blood*. 2007;**109**:4944–4951.

70 Wu K, Li L, Li S. Circulating microRNA-21 as a biomarker for the detection of various carcinomas: an updated meta-analysis based on 36 studies. *Tumour Biol*. 2015;**36**:1973–1981.

71 Di Leva G, Garofalo M, Croce CM. MicroRNAs in cancer. *Annu Rev Pathol*. 2014;**9**:287–314.

73 Garofalo M, Jeon YJ, Nuovo GJ, et al. MiR-34a/c-dependent PDGFR-alpha/beta downregulation inhibits tumorigenesis and enhances TRAIL-induced apoptosis in lung cancer. *PLoS One*. 2013;**8**:e67581.

74 Mongroo PS, Rustgi AK. The role of the miR-200 family in epithelial-mesenchymal transition. *Cancer Biol Ther*. 2010;**10**:219–222.

77 Ferracin M, Zagatti B, Rizzotto L, et al. MicroRNAs involvement in fludarabine refractory chronic lymphocytic leukemia. *Mol Cancer*. 2010;**9**:123.

78 Vecchione A, Belletti B, Lovat F, et al. A microRNA signature defines chemoresistance in ovarian cancer through modulation of angiogenesis. *Proc Natl Acad Sci U S A*. 2013;**110**:9845–9850.

84 Li J, Yang J, Zhou P, et al. Circular RNAs in cancer: novel insights into origins, properties, functions and implications. *Am J Cancer Res*. 2015;**5**:472–480.

86 Lagana A, Acunzo M, Romano G, et al. miR-Synth: a computational resource for the design of multi-site multi-target synthetic miRNAs. *Nucleic Acids Res*. 2014;**42**:5416–5425.

87 Janssen HL, Reesink HW, Lawitz EJ, et al. Treatment of HCV infection by targeting microRNA. *N Engl J Med*. 2013;**368**:1685–1694.

88 Janssen HL, Kauppinen S, Hodges MR. HCV infection and miravirsen. *N Engl J Med*. 2013;**369**:878.

90 Beg MS, Brenner AJ, Sachdev J, et al. Phase I study of MRX34, a liposomal miR-34a mimic, administered twice weekly in patients with advanced solid tumors. *Investig New Drugs*. 2017;**35**:180–188.

91 van Zandwijk N, Pavlakis N, Kao SC, et al. Safety and activity of microRNA-loaded minicells in patients with recurrent malignant pleural mesothelioma: a first-in-man, phase 1, open-label, dose-escalation study. *Lancet Oncol*. 2017;**18**:1386–1396.

92 Seto AG, Beatty X, Lynch JM, et al. Cobomarsen, an oligonucleotide inhibitor of miR-155, co-ordinately regulates multiple survival pathways to reduce cellular proliferation and survival in cutaneous T-cell lymphoma. *Br J Haematol*. 2018;**183**:428–444.

10 Aberrant signaling pathways in cancer

Luca Grumolato, PhD ■ *Stuart A. Aaronson, MD*

> **Overview**
>
> Most, if not all, human cancers harbor aberrant activation of one or several signaling pathways, contributing to tumor initiation and/or progression. In this article, we describe how growth factors signal to receptors with intrinsic tyrosine kinase activity to promote cell proliferation and survival, largely through activation of the phosphatidylinositol-3′-kinase(PI-3-K)/Akt and Ras/MAPK pathways. Using different paradigmatic examples of oncogenic alterations in growth factor signaling, we discuss functional implications and relevance of these pathways for human cancer. General cell signaling principles in both normal and tumor cells will be addressed, and we briefly discuss how the initiation and progression of specific cancer types can be affected by the deregulation of certain other pathways.
>
> Finally, we discuss the concepts of oncogene addiction and targeted therapy and provide a few representative examples to illustrate how increased understanding of the mechanisms underlying signaling pathway aberrations in cancer has been translated to the clinic.

Intercellular communication in multicellular organisms is required for processes such as embryonic development, tissue differentiation, and systemic responses to wounds and infections. These complex signaling networks are in large part mediated by growth factors, cytokines, and hormones. Such factors can influence cell proliferation in positive or negative ways, as well as induce a series of differentiated responses in appropriate target cells. Cytoplasmic molecules that mediate these responses have been termed second messengers. The eventual transmission of biochemical signals to the nucleus leads to effects on the expression of genes involved in mitogenic and differentiation responses.

The pathogenic expression of critical genes in growth factor signaling pathways can also contribute to altered cell growth associated with malignancy. The v-*sis* oncogene of simian sarcoma virus, which encodes a growth factor homologous to the B chain of human platelet-derived growth factor (PDGF-B), is the paradigm for such genes.[1] The normal counterparts of other retroviral oncogenes were subsequently shown to encode membrane-spanning growth factor receptors.[2,3] Other genes that act early in intracellular pathways of growth factor signal transduction have been implicated as oncogenes as well. Present knowledge indicates that the constitutive activation of growth factor signaling pathways through genetic alterations affecting these genes contributes to the development and progression of most human cancers.

Because of space limitations, this article primarily focuses on growth factor signaling mediated by receptors with intrinsic tyrosine (Tyr) kinase activity, while other pathways relevant to cancer biology are more briefly summarized.

Growth factor receptors with Tyr kinase activity

Hormones that act at great distances from the cells producing them have been known for many years. Hormones as signaling molecules were isolated from tissue fluids and readily characterized by their *in vivo* effects. The initial discoveries of growth factors indicated more subtle activities capable of stimulating the growth of chicken embryonic nerve cells in the case of nerve growth factor (NGF),[4] or promotion of eyelid opening and incisor eruption in the case of epidermal growth factor (EGF).[5] An important discovery concerning growth factors came from the demonstration of a unique enzymological activity associated with binding of EGF to its receptor.[5] Studies of the product of the viral oncogene, v-*src*, had led to the demonstration of its ability to act as a protein kinase.[6,7] It was well established that phosphorylations and dephosphorylations affected the activities of a variety of proteins, and many protein kinases capable of phosphorylating serine (Ser) and/or threonine (Thr) residues had been previously identified. However, the *src* product was shown to instead phosphorylate Tyr residues, thus representing the prototype of a new class of kinases.[8] Cohen then showed that addition of EGF led to phosphorylation of its purified receptor on Tyr residues,[5] and subsequent studies demonstrated that Tyr kinase activity is central to the functions of a large number of mitogenic signaling molecules.

More than 50 receptor Tyr kinases (RTKs) belonging to at least 18 different receptor families have been identified[9,10] (Figure 1). All RTKs contain a large, glycosylated, extracellular ligand-binding domain, a single transmembrane region, and a cytoplasmic portion with a conserved protein Tyr kinase domain. In addition to the catalytic domain, a juxtamembrane region and a carboxyl-terminal tail can be identified in the cytoplasmic portion. Because of their structure, RTKs can be visualized as membrane-associated allosteric enzymes with the ligand binding and protein Tyr kinase domains separated by the plasma membrane. Their role is to catalyze the transfer of the γ-phosphate of adenosine triphosphate (ATP) to Tyr residues of other proteins, as well as within their own polypeptide chain. Tyr phosphorylation represents the language that these receptors use to transduce the information carried by the growth factor.

RTKs are activated by their ligands through receptor oligomerization, which stabilizes interactions between adjacent cytoplasmic domains and controls the activation of kinase activity.[10] Dimerization can take place between two identical receptors

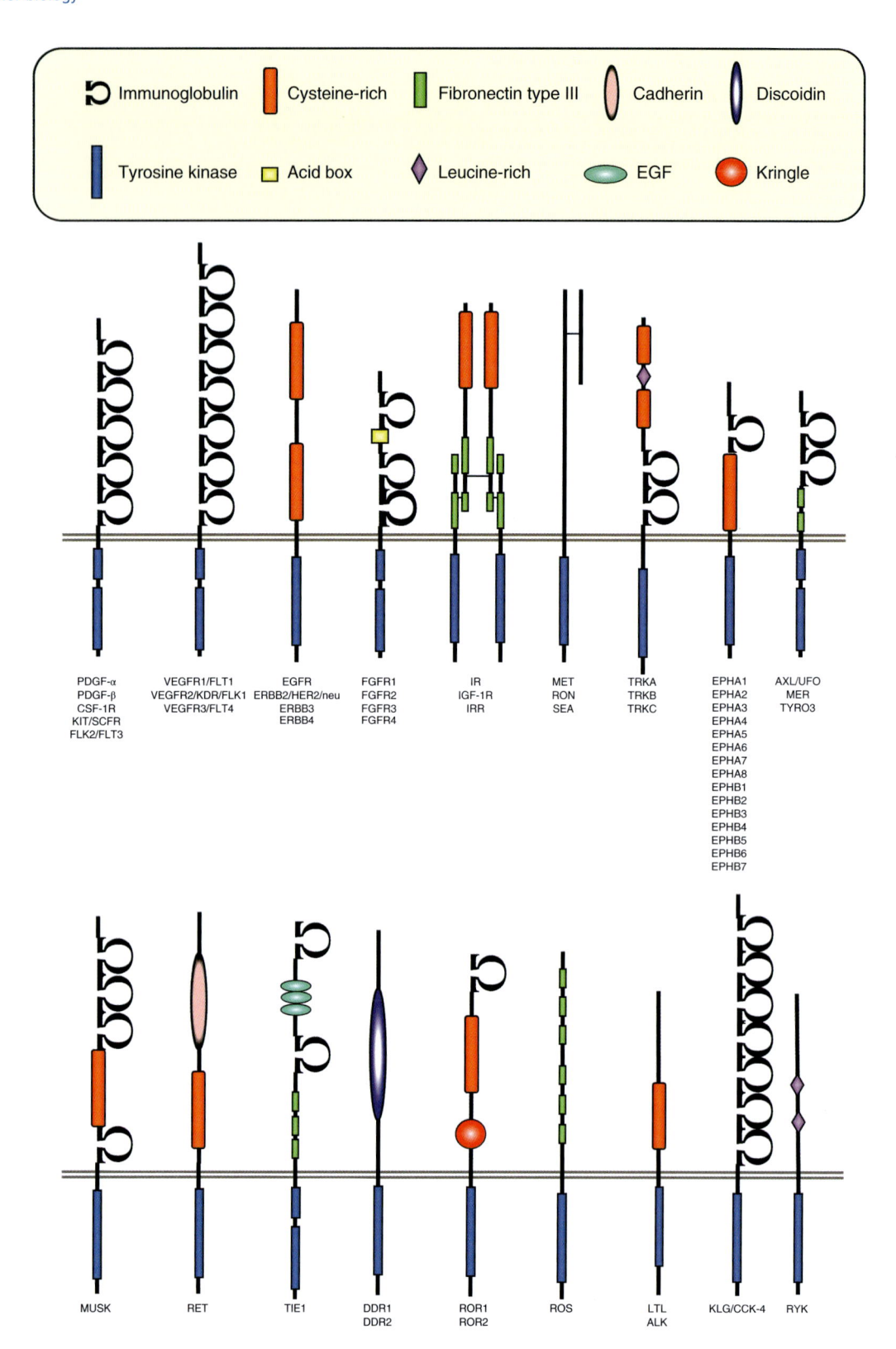

Figure 1 Families of receptor tyrosine kinases.

(homodimerization), between different members of the same receptor family, or, in some cases, between a receptor and an accessory protein (heterodimerization),[10] thus expanding both the repertoire of ligands recognized by each receptor and the diversity of signaling pathways recruited by a given receptor.

How ligands bind to induce receptor oligomerization varies for each class of RTKs.[10,11] PDGF, for example, induces receptor dimerization by virtue of its dimeric nature.[12] EGF induces instead a conformational change in the extracellular domain of the epidermal growth factor receptor (EGFR), resulting in the exposure of a dimerization domain that is masked in the absence of the ligand.[10] Fibroblast growth factor (FGF), which is a monomeric ligand like EGF, needs an accessory molecule, heparan sulfate proteoglycan, to induce receptor dimerization.[13,14] In contrast, the insulin receptor (IR) family exists as disulfide-bonded homo- or heterodimers of receptor subunits, and ligand binding causes a conformational change in the preformed dimeric receptor, which leads to receptor activation.[15,16]

In the unphosphorylated state, the receptor possesses a low catalytic activity due to the particular conformation of a specific domain in the kinase region, which interferes with the phosphotransfer event. Upon receptor dimerization induced by the ligand, trans-autophosphorylation of the kinase domain removes this inhibition, and the catalytic activity is enhanced and persists for some time independently of the presence of the ligand. In addition to this mechanism, different RTKs contain *cis*-inhibitory elements outside the kinase domain, such as in the juxtamembrane domain (for example in KIT and MuSK) or the C-terminal tail (for example in Tie2), that can be disrupted by trans-phosphorylation following receptor dimerization. The full activation of the catalytic domain induces the phosphorylation of a series of other Tyr residues to create specific docking sites for downstream molecules that participate in the transduction of the signal (see below).

Aberrations affecting growth factor receptors in tumor cells

Although growth factor receptors can be constitutively activated by autocrine/paracrine loops, a number of other mechanisms have been identified by which growth factor receptors can become transforming. The paradigm for such alterations is the avian erythroblastosis viral oncogene *v-erbB*, corresponding to a truncated form of EGFR, in which the deletion of the ligand-binding domain results in the constitutive activation of the receptor.[2] Alterations affecting a large number of RTKs have been implicated in different human malignancies. One mechanism involves the amplification or overexpression of a normal receptor, such as in the case of EGFR, ErbB2, and MET.[17–20] ErbB2 was initially identified as an amplified gene in a primary human breast carcinoma and a salivary gland tumor.[21,22] Clinical studies have indicated that the normal ErbB2 gene is frequently amplified and/or overexpressed in human breast carcinomas and in ovarian carcinomas,[23] and detection in breast carcinomas of high ErbB2 levels was initially a prognostic indicator of poor survival.[17,18] Whereas ErbB2 overexpression has been observed primarily in adenocarcinomas, overexpression of a normal EGFR has been reported frequently in squamous cell carcinomas and glioblastomas.[17,24] In many cases, the EGFR appears to be activated by autocrine stimulation by one of its ligands, most commonly transforming growth factor-α (TGF-α).

Genomic alterations, such as mutation or rearrangement, have also been shown to activate the transforming capacity of RTKs in different human malignancies.[25] For example, mutations in the EGFR kinase domain[26,27] are associated with the constitutive activation of this receptor in non-small cell lung cancer (NSCLC).[24] While such mutations are not common in other types of tumors, glioblastomas often contain partial deletions of the EGFR extracellular domain, including the constitutively active EGFRvIII variant.[28] The *ret* gene is activated by rearrangement, as a somatic event, in about one-third of papillary thyroid carcinomas, while germline mutations of cysteine residues in the extracellular region, which affect receptor dimerization, are responsible for multiple endocrine neoplasia (MEN) 2A and for the familial medullary thyroid (FMTC) carcinoma syndrome.[29]

Of note, point mutations in the RET kinase domain are associated with MEN 2B,[30] indicating that the catalytic function of a RTK can be upregulated by oncogenic alterations affecting distinct domains of the receptor. Another example of an RTK activated by genetic alterations in the germline is the receptor for the hepatocyte growth factor (HGF), MET, which is responsible for hereditary papillary renal carcinomas.[31] Aberrant activation of MET through amplification/overexpression or mutations is also found in a variety of sporadic tumors including renal, liver, and gastric cancer.[20] Moreover, alterations affecting splice donor or acceptor sites are responsible for skipping of exon 14, which encodes MET juxtamembrane domain, resulting in the expression of an activated receptor in different types of cancer, including 3–4% of NSCLC.[32,33] Finally, several other receptors, including the anaplastic lymphoma kinase (ALK), ROS1, and the neurotrophic receptor tyrosine kinases (NTRKs), have been shown to be oncogenically activated in human malignancies by chromosomal rearrangements that lead to fusion products containing the activated TK domain.[25,34,35]

> **KEY POINTS:**
> - RTKs are activated by growth factors through receptor dimerization and subsequent trans-phosphorylation.
> - Tyr phosphorylation represents the language used by these receptors to transduce their signals, allowing specific recruitment of different effector or adaptor proteins.
> - Different mechanisms are responsible for constitutive RTK activation in tumor cells. These include receptor/ligand overexpression, RTK amplification/mutation, and chromosomal translocation, which results in the formation of a constitutively active fusion protein.

Signaling pathways of RTKs

Molecules, known as adaptor and scaffolding proteins,[36] play an integral role in intracellular signaling by both recruiting various proteins to specific locations, and by assembling networks of proteins particular to RTK cascades. These adaptor proteins often contain a variety of motifs that mediate protein–protein interactions, including Src homology 2 (SH2) and phosphoTyr-binding (PTB) domains, which bind to specific phosphorylated Tyr-containing sequences, or SH3 domains, which recognize and bind to proline-rich sequences in target proteins.[36,37] One such adaptor, Grb2, is important in the activation of the small G-protein Ras (Figure 2).

The PDGF system has served as the prototype for identification of the components of signaling cascades. Certain molecules become physically associated and/or phosphorylated by the activated platelet-derived growth factor receptor (PDGFR) kinase. These include phospholipase C (PLC)-γ,[38] phosphatidylinositol-3′-kinase (PI-3-K) regulatory subunit (p85),[39] NCK,[40] the phosphatase SHP-2,[41] Grb2,[42] CRK,[43] *RAS* p21 GTPase-activating protein (GAP),[44] SRC, and SRC-like Tyr kinases.[45] Many of these molecules contain SH2 or SH-3 domains.

PI-3-K and survival signaling

The regulation of cell survival and cell death is essential for both normal development and tissue homeostasis in adult organisms, where damaged cells must be removed and terminally differentiated cells must be sustained. PI-3-K is a lipid kinase that catalyzes the transfer of the γ-phosphate from ATP to the D3 position of

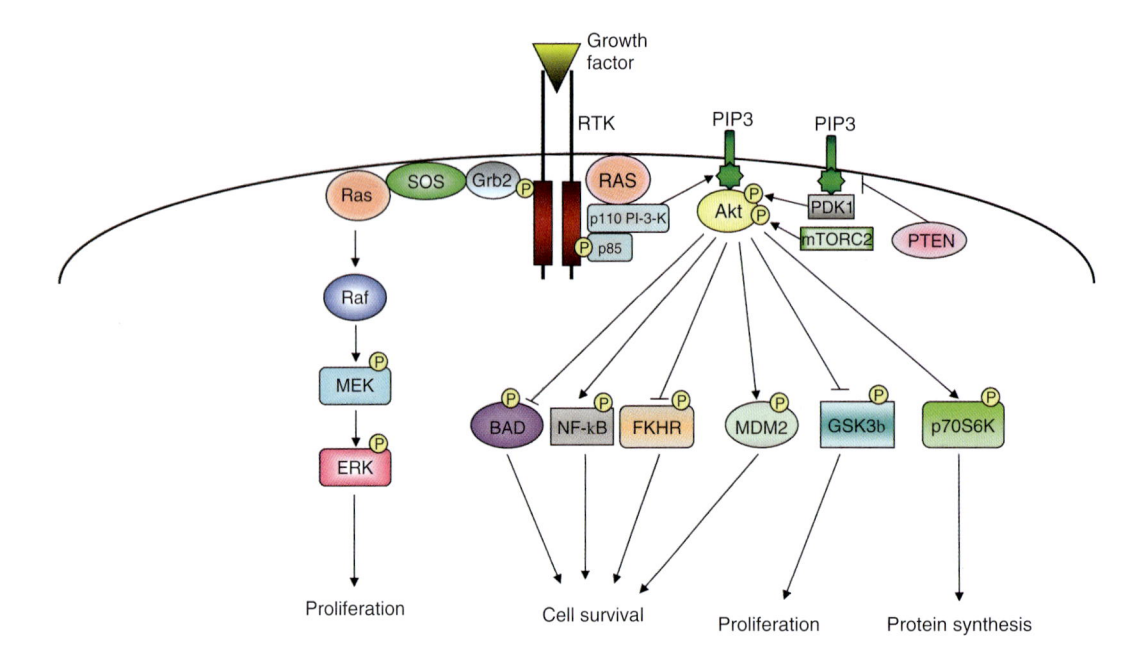

Figure 2 Intracellular effectors of receptor tyrosine kinases.

the phosphoinositide (PtdIns), generating PtdIns(3,4,5)P$_3$. These lipids can act in a variety of cascades, promoting the activation of several proteins (Figure 2). PI-3-K activation has been demonstrated to play an important role in survival signaling in a number of cell types.[46,47] The prototypical class 1 PI-3-K consists of two tightly associated subunits encoded by two distinct loci: a regulatory and a catalytic subunit. The classic mode of PI-3-K activation involves binding of the regulatory subunit to the phosphorylated Tyr residues of RTKs through SH2 domains, resulting in a conformational change that facilitates activation of the catalytic subunit. There are several known downstream effectors of PI-3-K. These include Rac, certain isoforms of protein kinase C, and, most relevant to cell survival, Akt, the cellular homolog of the viral oncogene *v-Akt*.[46,47] Three human homologues encode 57 kDa Ser/Thr kinases that contain an N-terminal pleckstrin homology (PH) domain, which binds to the activated PtdIns products of PI-3-K. Upon recruitment to the plasma membrane, AKT is phosphorylated by phosphoinositide-dependent protein kinase 1 (PDK1) at Thr 308, which is essential for kinase activation, and by the target of rapamycin complex 2 (mTORC2) at Ser 473, further enhancing its activity[46–48] (Figure 2).

Akt promotes survival and prevents apoptosis in various cell types through the regulation of different downstream pathways and effectors.[49] It phosphorylates the pro-apoptotic protein BAD (B-cell lymphoma 2-associated agonist of cell death), thus creating a docking site for the cytosolic protein 14-3-3, which sequesters BAD and inhibits its activity. Akt also phosphorylates forkhead box O (FOXO) transcription factors, creating a binding site for 14-3-3, which retains them in the cytoplasm, thus inhibiting their transcriptional targets, including pro-apoptotic proteins such as BIM and FAS ligand. Moreover, Akt can increase p53 degradation through phosphorylation of MDM2, and there is evidence that Akt can increase the pro-survival functions of the nuclear factor-κB (NF-κB) transcription-factor complex and inhibit the pro-apoptotic c-Jun N-terminal kinase (JNK) and p38 pathways.[49] Besides promoting cell survival, Akt can also exert positive effects on cell growth and metabolism through inhibitory phosphorylations of the tuberous sclerosis complex 2 (TSC2), resulting in the activation of the mTOR pathway, or GSK3, which normally targets cyclin D1 for degradation[48,50] (Figure 2).

PI-3-K signaling in cancer

PIK3CA, which encodes the p110α catalytic subunit, was originally found to be amplified in a high percentage of ovarian tumors and ovarian tumor cell lines.[51] Later studies revealed that PIK3CA is one of the most frequently mutated oncogenes across several different human cancer types, including colon, breast, endometrial, brain, and gastric tumors.[52–54] While far less frequently mutated in cancer, Akt can also play a role in human malignancies. Akt1 was found to be amplified 20-fold in a primary gastric adenocarcinoma.[55] Additional studies have shown genomic amplification and overexpression of Akt2 in pancreatic and ovarian carcinoma cell lines, as well as in some ovarian and breast carcinomas.[56] Overexpression of Akt2 occurs more frequently in undifferentiated more aggressive tumors. Missense mutations in the Akt1 PH domain were identified in breast, colon, and ovarian cancers, resulting in prolonged Akt activation due to its pathological localization to the plasma membrane.[57]

Further evidence of the involvement of the PI-3-K/Akt pathway in cancer stems from the discovery of the PTEN (phosphatase and tensin homolog) tumor suppressor, a gene inactivated by mutation in a high fraction of glial and endometrial tumors, as well as in melanoma, prostate, renal, and small-cell lung carcinomas.[50,53,58] By dephosphorylating the 3 position of phosphatidylinositol, PTEN directly opposes PI-3-K activity, thus inhibiting Akt activation (Figure 2). Inactivating mutations resulting in pathway upregulation can also affect the p85 regulatory subunit, encoded by the *PIK3R1* gene, as observed fairly frequently in glioblastoma, adrenocortical, and endometrial carcinoma.[54]

Ras

Ras proteins are a major point of convergence in RTK signaling, as well as important components of the machinery necessary to transduce extracellular signals (Figure 2). These small GTP-binding proteins are membrane-bound intracellular signaling molecules that mediate a wide variety of cellular functions, including proliferation, differentiation, and survival. Ras acts as a molecular switch alternating from an inactive guanosine diphosphate (GDP)-bound state to an active GTP-bound state. The paradigm for Ras activation involves the recruitment of a guanine nucleotide exchange factor (GEF) to the membrane in response to growth factor binding and subsequent activation of a RTK.[59] GEFs promote the release of GDP from the catalytic pocket of Ras, and the relative abundance of intracellular GTP as compared to GDP ensures preferential binding of GTP. The best example of a Ras GEF is SOS (son of sevenless, Figure 2), which is brought to the membrane by its stable association with the adaptor protein Grb2.[60] Although Ras is a GTPase, its intrinsic GTPase activity is actually quite low and requires additional proteins known as GTPase-activating proteins (GAPs) to promote GTP hydrolysis. GAPs can accelerate GTP hydrolysis by several orders of magnitude and are, thus, negative regulators of Ras functions.[59,61]

Ras mediates its multitude of biologic effects *via* a number of downstream effectors. Several proteins have been shown to directly bind to Ras in a GTP-dependent manner, including Raf and PI-3-K.[61] In fact, Ras can activate PI-3-K independently of RTKs, providing a direct connection between Ras and PI-3-K prosurvival signaling.[59]

Ras and cancer

Ras has been shown to be oncogenically activated by mutations in over 15% of all human tumors, and in some cancers such as pancreatic carcinoma the frequency is as high as 90%.[61,62] The initial evidence for Ras involvement in cancer came from the discovery of transforming retroviruses, Harvey and Kirsten sarcoma viruses, which contained H- and K-ras cellular-derived oncogenes. The first human oncogenes were identified by transfecting genomic DNA from human tumor cell lines into NIH3T3 mouse fibroblasts and isolating the DNA fragments from the transformed foci. These were shown to be the human homologues of the viral ras genes.[63]

The major hotspots for activating Ras mutations decrease the intrinsic rate of GTP hydrolysis by Ras and make the molecule significantly less sensitive to GAP-stimulated GTP hydrolysis. Thus, the outcome is a predominantly GTP-bound form that is constitutively active and essentially independent of growth factor stimulation.[61,62]

While *Ras* amplification is less frequent,[64] another mechanism of activation of this GTPase involves loss-of-function mutations of the *NF1* gene encoding the Ras GAP neurofibromin, observed in glioblastoma and lung cancer, as well as in the familial tumor syndrome, neurofibromatosis type I.[59,65]

Signaling downstream of Ras: Ras > Raf > MAPK cascade

The most well-studied effector of Ras is the Ser/Thr kinase Raf. Raf has been shown to bind to Ras and, in many cases, has been demonstrated to be indispensable for Ras functions, such as cellular transformation.[66–68] There are three known mammalian Raf isoforms, designated A-, B-, and C-Raf (also known as Raf-1), displaying distinct expression patterns.[66] Ras-GTP binds to the amino terminus of Raf and promotes its activation, resulting in Raf homo- or heterodimerization and the phosphorylation of different Ser/Thr and Tyr residues participating in the regulation of Raf activity.[68,69] Once activated, Raf can phosphorylate MEK (mitogen/extracellular-signal-regulated kinase kinase), also known as mitogen activated protein kinase kinase (MAPKK), a dual-specificity kinase, leading to its activation[66,69] (Figure 2). MEK can, in turn, activate MAPK, also named extracellular signal-regulated kinase (ERK) through tandem phosphorylations on both Thr 183 and Tyr 185. ERK then translocates to the nucleus, where it can activate a variety of proteins through phosphorylation on Ser or Thr, including the ETS family of transcription factors and the kinase p90 RSK, involved in protein translation.[69,70] Activation of the Ras-Raf-mitogen activated protein kinase (MAPK) pathway results in an increase of DNA synthesis and cell proliferation, exemplified by the induction of cyclin D1,[71] a major regulator of early cell cycle progression. In fact, cyclin D1 is also one of the most frequently amplified genes in cancer.[72]

Raf and cancer

The direct implication of Raf in human cancer came with the identification of B-Raf mutations in more than half of melanoma cell lines and primary tumors.[73] B-Raf mutations, which generally affect few specific residues, such as valine 600, were subsequently found in other malignancies, including thyroid (60%), colorectal (10%), and lung (6%) cancer.[66] While B-Raf is one of the most commonly activated oncogenes, mutated in about 8% of all cancers, the frequency of A-Raf and C-Raf mutations is far lower, probably because of their weaker basal kinase activity compared to B-Raf.[66] Of note, oncogenic activation of B-Raf can also occur following chromosome translocations, which result in the expression of fusion proteins containing the catalytic carboxy terminus of B-Raf. Such translocations have been found in pediatric astrocytoma, glioma, and thyroid cancers.[66]

Other MAPKs

In addition to the ERKs, there are other MAPKs belonging to distinct MAPK cascades with both different upstream activators and downstream effectors. JNK and p38 are stress-activated kinases involved in the cellular responses to a wide variety of extracellular stimuli, including mitogens, inflammatory cytokines, and UV irradiation.[74,75] In contrast to its ability to activate the MAPK/ERK cascade, Ras only minimally perturbs JNK and p38, whose activity is mainly induced by the Rho family of small G-proteins, including Rac1, Cdc42, and RhoA. The pathways leading to JNK or p38 activation mirror those seen for ERK, with a variety of MAPKKs that can phosphorylate the various JNK isoforms.[74,75]

As with the ERKs, the end result of JNK and p38 activation is the phosphorylation of different transcription factors, resulting in increased expression of their target genes. Examples of transcription factors directly phosphorylated by either JNK or p38, or both, include activating transcription factor 2 (ATF2), ELK1, JUN, MYC, and MEF2.[74,76] Of note, some of these factors were initially discovered as retroviral oncogenes.

KEY POINTS:

- Activated RTKs promote PI-3-K mediated synthesis of PtdIns3P, resulting in the recruitment and activation of the kinase Akt. Through the regulation of different downstream effectors, Akt promotes survival in various cell types.

- RTKs stimulate cell proliferation largely through activation of the Ras/Raf/MAPK pathway.

- In human cancer, these downstream pathways can be frequently activated independently of RTKs, generally through mutations in the genes encoding various key effectors, including PI-3-K, Ras, and Raf.

Other signaling pathways aberrantly deregulated in cancer

While activation of the RTK pathway is common in most types of cancer, other signaling pathways can also play instrumental roles in tumor initiation and progression. During embryonic development and in adulthood, these pathways exert diverse physiological functions, but, as with RTK signaling, they can be aberrantly activated (or inactivated) in cancer, as a result of mutations, chromosomal rearrangements, or other mechanisms.

Although RTKs represent the largest family of surface receptors possessing an enzymatic activity, other ligands can also signal through receptors with such activities. For example, transforming growth factor-β (TGFβ) ligands induce the formation of a tetrameric complex containing two type I and two type II TGFβ receptors, both Ser/Thr kinases. Type II receptors can then phosphorylate type I receptors, which propagate the signal through binding and the subsequent phosphorylation of the suppressor of mothers against decapentaplegic (SMAD) transcription factors, resulting in SMAD activation.[77] Depending on the cellular context, the TGFβ pathway can play a role in either tumor suppression or progression. In premalignant cells, TGFβ signaling can promote apoptosis, thus explaining the frequent inactivating mutations of TGFβ receptors or SMADs found in certain tumors, including colorectal and pancreatic carcinomas. Other tumors, including glioma, melanoma, and breast carcinoma, can use other mechanisms to circumvent this tumor-suppressive activity of TGFβ, while maintaining a functional pathway, which, in more advanced tumors, can favor progression and metastasis through crosstalk between tumor cells and their microenvironment.[77]

Other surface receptors lack an intrinsic catalytic activity, but instead directly interact with enzymatic adaptor proteins that mediate propagation of the signal. This is the case, for example, with cytokine receptors, which bind to the Janus kinase (JAK) family of Tyr kinases.[78] Upon cytokine-induced dimerization of their receptors, JAKs transphosphorylate each other, as well as the C-terminus of the receptors, thus creating docking sites for a family of transcription factors, the signal transducers and activators of transcription (STATs). Following JAK-mediated phosphorylation, STATs form homo- or heterodimers through their SH2 domains and translocate to the nucleus to transcriptionally activate their target genes.[78,79] Activating mutations of JAK2 are common in patients with different types of myeloproliferative neoplasms, including polycythemia vera and essential thrombocythaemia, resulting in cytokine hypersensitivity and cytokine-independent proliferation.[80] While STAT mutations are far less common, different mechanisms have been shown to promote STAT3 and STAT5 activation in various types of cancer, affecting not only the growth and invasion of the tumor cells but also the relationship between the tumor and the immune system.[79] Another example of receptors directly interacting with proteins possessing enzymatic activity is represented by the G-protein coupled receptors (GPCRs), a large family of seven membrane-spanning domain proteins, which signal through very different types of ligands, including hormones, neurotransmitters, and chemokines.[81] While certain tumors contain mutations in GPCRs or their G proteins, the most common mechanism of aberrant activation of this signaling pathway in cancer is through receptor overexpression and autocrine stimulation.[81] The GPCR pathway is particularly relevant in tumors of the endocrine system, and ligands signaling through these receptors, such as certain chemokines, are among the major modulators of the tumor microenvironment.[82]

Activation of other signaling pathways with well-established roles in cancer occurs through more complex mechanisms, which may involve different co-receptors, adaptor proteins, and cytoplasmic complexes, with or without enzymatic activity. This is the case with Wnt, Hedgehog, Hippo, Notch, and tumor necrosis factor (TNF)/NF-κB signaling. A common feature of these diverse signaling pathways is that ligand activation of the receptor results in stabilization or activation at or near the cell membrane of a transcription or co-transcription factor, such as NF-κB (TNF)[83] and GLI (Hedgehog),[84] or yes-associated protein (YAP)/transcriptional co-activator with PDZ binding motif (TAZ) (Hippo)[85] and β-catenin (Wnt).[86] A variation on this theme is represented by the Notch pathway, where binding by Delta/Jagged ligands induces the cleavage of the Notch receptor and the release of its cytoplasmic region, which translocates to the nucleus and activates the CBF1, Suppressor of Hairless, Lag-1 transcription factors.[87] These highly conserved signaling pathways regulate fundamental physiological processes required for normal embryonic development and maintain different types of stem/progenitor cells in the adult. Their capacity to regulate cell proliferation, survival, and differentiation helps to explain why these pathways are frequently targeted in tumorigenesis. For example, mutations of genes resulting in aberrant activation of Wnt/β-catenin signaling can be found in almost all colorectal carcinomas.[86,88,89] Of note, aberrant activation of Wnt signaling through different mechanisms has also been identified in significant fractions of diverse tumor types, including breast, adrenocortical, and hepatocellular carcinoma.[86,90–92]

A different class of ligands bind, in the cytoplasm or in the nucleus, to a large family of transcription factors, which serve as the receptors. Once bound to their ligands, these nuclear receptors can activate, as homo- or heterodimers, the expression of specific target genes through interaction with different co-activators.[93] The nuclear receptor family includes around 50 members and regulates diverse physiological processes, which can play a crucial role in some types of cancer. For example, the proliferation and growth of a large fraction of breast and prostate tumors depend on estrogen/progesterone and androgen receptors, respectively. These findings have important implications for the treatment of these tumors, which respond to sex hormone antagonists or inhibitors of sex hormone synthesis.[94–96] Another example of the involvement of nuclear receptors in cancer is the chromosomal translocation of the *promyelocytic leukemia* (PML) and the *retinoid acid receptor* α (RARα) genes resulting in a PML-RAR fusion protein. This fusion protein deregulates transcription of RARα target genes and leads to the disruption of PML nuclear bodies, stress-sensitive nuclear domains involved in senescence and p53 activation. This results in accumulation of immature granulocyte precursors and to a deadly form of blood malignancy, acute promyelocytic leukemia (APL).[97] The discovery of this tumorigenic mechanism translated into the design of a new therapy based on the treatment with all-trans RA and/or arsenic trioxide, which provoke degradation of the PML-RAR fusion protein, thus resulting in cure of 70–80% of APL patients.[97,98] The example of APL illustrates how signaling pathways aberrantly activated in cancer can be specifically targeted in the clinic to block or restrain the growth and/or the spread of tumors, a concept discussed further below.

> **KEY POINTS:**
> - Other ligand families signal through their receptors to activate diverse effector pathways.
> - In most cases, such receptors directly or indirectly activate specific transcription factors at or near the cell surface, and these factors regulate the expression of specific target genes.
> - Certain ligands penetrate the cell to bind their cognate receptors, which function as *bona fide* transcription factors.
> - These pathways control a wide range of physiological processes, and their aberrant deregulation through different mechanisms plays an instrumental role in the initiation and/or progression of various tumors.

Growth factor signaling and cancer therapy

Since many of the signaling pathways involved in cellular transformation by oncogenes have been elucidated, efforts are underway to develop treatment strategies that target these specific signaling molecules or their downstream effectors. The major advantage of rationally based targets is that these agents have less inherent toxicities than standard chemotherapeutic regimens. Another advantage is that approaches are generally available to monitor *in vivo* the specific effects of the drug, enabling correlation of clinical response with pharmacodynamic analyses of target inhibition, thus speeding the process of clinical testing.

Targeted strategies rely on the concept of "oncogene addiction," which implies that tumor cells, despite their complex pattern of mutational events, can become particularly dependent on one or a few signaling pathways for their growth and/or survival.[99] These pathways are thought to counterbalance other pro-apoptotic signals also triggered by the oncogenic alterations in the tumor: once the pro-survival signal is blocked, the tumor cell undergoes what has been defined as "oncogenic shock" and dies.[100] This idea is supported by studies with tumor cell lines[101] as well as in genetically modified mice, in which complete regression of tumors induced by oncogenes, such as K-Ras, was achieved by switching off expression of the oncogene.[102] Treatments targeting aberrantly activated signaling pathways, either alone or in combination with traditional chemo- or radiation therapy, have yielded extraordinary clinical benefit for certain types of malignancies. However, in most of the cases, additional genetic lesions, often activating the same signaling pathway, have been shown, to eventually bypass the targeted oncogene, resulting in disease progression (see below).

Monoclonal antibodies

One possible target for therapeutic intervention is the initial triggering of growth factor signaling at the surface of tumor cells. Monoclonal antibodies can be generated to specifically neutralize the activities of growth factors or interfere with ligand–receptor interactions. Monoclonal antibodies have also been applied to interfere with receptors overexpressed in certain types of cancer[103] (Table 1). Trastuzumab (herceptin, Genentech), a humanized monoclonal antibody against ErbB2, became the first clinically approved drug targeting an oncogene product. Experimental evidence further indicated that trastuzumab enhances the responsiveness of ErbB2 overexpressing breast cancer cells to taxanes, anthracyclines, and platinum compounds.[104] Thanks to this monoclonal antibody, invasive breast cancers with ErbB2 amplification (~20% of the cases), once corresponding to the type with the worst prognosis, now display a 10-year survival rate of 85%.[105]

Cetuximab (erbitux, ImClone Systems), a chimeric monoclonal antibody against EGFR has been approved for the treatment of colorectal and head and neck cancers in combination with chemotherapy and radiotherapy, respectively.[104,106,107] Of note, it was shown that cetuximab significantly increased the survival of colorectal cancer patients with wild-type K-Ras. However, it had no benefit in the presence of K-Ras mutations, accounting for 40% of the tumors,[108] thus emphasizing the need to identify the particular genetic context of a given tumor for a successful therapeutic intervention. Mutation of the *K-Ras* gene is also the most common mechanism responsible for acquired resistance to cetuximab treatment, while in other patients the tumors develop mutations in the extracellular domain of the EGFR that interfere with antibody recognition.[109,110]

Another example is bevacizumab (avastin, Genentech), a monoclonal antibody targeting vascular endothelial growth factor (VEGF), a ligand that promotes angiogenesis. Bevacizumab has been approved by the FDA for the treatment of different tumor types, including glioblastoma, colorectal, renal, and lung cancer (Table 1). Contrary to trastuzumab and cetuximab, bevacizumab acts on vascular endothelial cells in the tumor microenvironment, with the double advantage that drug resistance is less likely to develop in such normal cells than in the genetically unstable tumor cells, and that the therapy may be applicable to a wider range of tumors.[111] Of note, recent findings suggest that targeting VEGF may also directly affect tumor cells, which can express VEGF receptors.[112]

Tyr kinase inhibitors

Increased understanding of the important role of growth factor signal transduction in cancer has also led to intensive efforts focused on the development of small-molecule inhibitors of constitutively activated Tyr kinases (Table 1). The most striking example is imatinib (gleevec, Novartis), a small molecule inhibitor of the non-receptor Tyr kinase Abl. *Abl* is translocated in chronic myelogenous leukemia (CML) as part of the Philadelphia (Ph) chromosome to create the *Bcr-Abl* oncogene.[113] Imatinib interacts with the ATP-binding pocket of the Abl kinase domain and stabilizes a catalytically inactive conformation of this oncogene product.[114] Clinical trials rapidly confirmed the efficacy of this compound in CML and, therefore, Bcr-Abl as a target in this disease. Remarkable responses were observed in the chronic phase of the disease with complete clearing of Ph+ cells from the circulation in 95% of patients, who had failed standard therapy. Only 9% of patients relapsed over a median follow-up of 18 months,[115] leading to regulatory approval. Imatinib was subsequently shown to inhibit other related Tyr kinases, in particular Kit and PDGFR, for which activating mutations have been identified in gastrointestinal stromal tumor (GIST), leading to FDA approval for use in therapy of this tumor type as well. In leukemia patients, imatinib is most effective in the chronic phase, with fewer responses and more relapses with patients in myeloid blast crisis. During the progression of the disease, tumor cells can develop resistance, either through mutations that interfere with the binding of imatinib to Abl or by Bcr-Abl gene amplification.[114] To overcome resistance, second (dasatinib, nilotinib, bosutinib) and third (ponatinib) generation Abl inhibitors have been developed that can now be used either as a first-line therapy, or to treat patients that relapsed to imatinib.[116]

Table 1 Cancer therapeutics targeting the RTK signaling pathway.[a]

Cancer drug	Target	Disease
Monoclonal antibodies		
Bevacizumab (Avastin)	VEGF	Colorectal cancer, NSCLC, RCC, glioblastoma, cervical cancer, ovarian epithelial cancer, peritoneal cancer, fallopian tube cancer
Cetuximab (Erbitux)	EGFR	Colorectal cancer, head and neck cancer
Necitumumab (Portrazza)	EGFR	NSCLC
Panitumumab (Vectibix)	EGFR	Colorectal cancer
Pertuzumab (Perjeta)	ERBB2	Breast cancer
Ramucirumab (Cyramza)	VEGFR2	Stomach adenocarcinoma, NSCLC, hepatocellular carcinoma, colorectal cancer
Trastuzumab (Herceptin)	ErbB2	Breast cancer, gastric cancer
Secreted proteins		
Aflibercept (Zaltrap)	Part of VEGFR1 and VEGFR2 fused to Fc of human IgG1	Colorectal cancer
Palifermin (Kepivance)	Recombinant form of KGF	Oral mucositis
Small molecule inhibitors		
Acalabrutinib (Calquence)	BTK	Chronic lymphocytic leukemia, mantle cell lymphoma
Afatinib (Gilotrif)	EGFR, ErbB2, ErbB4	NSCLC
Alectinib (Alecensa)	ALK	NSCLC
Alpelisib (Piqray)	PI3K	Breast cancer
Avapritinib (Ayvakit)	PDGFR, c-KIT	GIST
Axitinib (Inlyta)	VEGFR, PDGFR, c-KIT	RCC
Binimetinib (Mektovi)	MEK1/2	Melanoma
Brigatinib (Alunbrig)	ALK, EGFR	NSCLC
Bosutinib (Bosulif)	Abl, Src	CML
Cabozantinib (Cometriq)	MET, RET, VEGFR, c-KIT, FLT-3, TIE-2, TRKB, AXL	Thyroid cancer
Ceritinib (Zykadia)	ALK	NSCLC
Cobimetinib (Cotellic)	MEK1	Melanoma
Copanlisib (Aliqopa)	PI3K	Follicular lymphoma
Crizotinib (Xalkori)	ALK, MET	NSCLC
Dabrafenib (Tafinlar)	B-Raf	Melanoma, NSCLC, anaplastic thyroid cancer
Dacomitinib (Vizimpro)	pan-EGFR	NSCLC
Dasatinib (Sprycel)	Abl, Src	CML, ALL
Duvelisib (Copiktra)	PI3K delta/gamma	Chronic lymphocytic leukemia or small lymphocytic lymphoma, follicular lymphoma
Encorafenib (Braftovi)	RAF	Melanoma
Entrectinib (Rozlytrek)	TrkA, TrkB, TrkC, ROS1 and ALK	NSCLC (ROS1 positive) and solid tumors with NTRK fusions
Erdafitinib (Balversa)	FGFR	Urothelial carcinoma
Erlotinib (Tarceva)	EGFR	NSCLC, pancreatic carcinoma
Everolimus (Afinitor)	mTOR	RCC, astrocytoma, PNET, breast cancer
Fedratinib (Inrebic)	FLT3, JAK2	Myelofibrosis
Gefitinib (Iressa)	EGFR	NSCLC
Gilteritinib (Xospata)	FLT3, AXL, ALK, and LTK	Acute myeloid leukemia
Ibrutinib (Imbruvica)	BTK	CLL, mantle cell lymphoma
Idelalisib (Zydelig)	PI3K	CLL, non-Hodgkin lymphoma
Imatinib (Gleevec)	Abl, PDGFR, c-Kit	CML, GIST, ALL, dermofibrosarcoma protuberans, chronic eosinophilic leukemia, myeloproliferative neoplasm
Lapatinib (Tykerb)	EGFR, ErbB2	Breast cancer
Larotrectinib (Vitrakvi)	Trk	Solid tumors with NTRK fusions
Lenvatinib (Lenvima)	RET, VEGFR, KIT, PDGFR, FGFR	Endometrial carcinoma, hepatocellular carcinoma, RCC, thyroid cancer
Lorlatinib (Lorbrena)	ALK and ROS1	NSCLC
Neratinib (Nerlynx)	EGFR, ErbB2	Breast cancer
Nilotinib (Tasigna)	Abl, PDGFR, c-Kit	CML
Osimertinib (Tagrisso)	EGFR	NSCLC
Pazopanib (Votrient)	VEGFR, PDGFR, c-KIT	RCC, soft tissue sarcoma
Ponatinib (Iclusig)	ABL, VEGFR, FGFR, TIE2 and Flt3	ALL, CML
Regorafenib (Stivarga)	VEGFR, RET, c-KIT, PDGFR, RAF	Colorectal cancer, GIST
Sorafenib (Nexavar)	VEGFR, PDGFR, FLT3, c-KIT, RAF, RET	RCC, hepatocellular carcinoma, thyroid cancer
Sunitinib (Sutent)	VEGFR, PDGFR, FLT3, c-KIT, RET	GIST, RCC, PNET
Temsirolimus (Torisel)	mTOR	RCC
Trametinib (Mekinist)	MEK	Melanoma
Vandetanib (Caprelsa)	VEGFR, EGFR, RET	Thyroid cancer
Vemurafenib (Zelboraf)	B-Raf	Melanoma
Zanubrutinib (Brukinsa)	BTK	Mantle cell lymphoma

Abbreviations: ALK, anaplastic lymphoma kinase; ALL, acute lymphoblastic leukemia; APL, acute promyelocytic leukemia; BCC, basal cell carcinoma; BTK, Bruton's tyrosine kinase; CLL, chronic lymphocytic leukemia; CML, chronic myeloid leukemia; EGFR, epidermal growth factor receptor; FGFR, fibroblast growth factor receptor; GIST, gastrointestinal stromal tumor; KGF, keratinocyte growth factor; MEK, mitogen-activated protein kinase kinase; mTOR, mechanistic target of rapamycin; NTRK, neurotrophic tyrosine receptor kinase; NSCLC, non-small cell lung cancer; PDGFR, platelet-derived growth factor receptor; PI3K, phosphoinositide-3 kinase; PNET, pancreatic neuroendocrine tumor; RCC, renal cell carcinoma; Trk, tropomyosin receptor kinase; VEGFR, vascular endothelial growth factor receptor.
Drugs included in this table have been approved by the Food and Drug Administration (FDA).
[a] Source: https://www.cancer.gov/about-cancer/treatment/drugs

Examples of other small molecules targeting RTKs include gefitinib (iressa, AstraZeneca), erlotinib (tarceva, OSI/Genentech), afatinib (gilotrif, Boehringer-Ingelheim), and osimertinib (tagrisso, AstraZeneca), which were approved for the treatment of lung cancers displaying EGFR mutations.[117] Crizotinib (xalkori, Pfizer) inhibits ALK, a receptor activated by chromosome translocations or mutations in different tumors, including lung cancer and neuroblastoma.[118] Other more promiscuous small molecule inhibitors that target different Tyr kinases involved in both tumorigenesis and angiogenesis, such as sorafenib (nexavar, Bayer) and sunitinib (sutent, Pfizer), have been approved for the treatment of certain cancers, including advanced renal cell carcinoma, hepatocellular carcinoma, and imatinib-refractory GIST. In 2018, the FDA approved the first "tumor-agnostic" inhibitor: larotrectinib (vitrakvi, Bayer) can be used for the treatment of any pediatric and adult solid tumor containing a *NTRK* gene fusion.[119]

Inhibition of growth factor downstream signaling

Downstream components of growth factor signaling pathways activated in cancer cells are also potential therapeutic targets. While extensive efforts to generate efficient and specific Ras inhibitors for the clinic have not yet been successful, this approach has paid off with the approval of small molecules targeting downstream effectors of RTK signaling (Table 1). One striking example is vemurafenib (zelboraf, Plexxikon/Roche), approved in 2011 for the treatment of melanomas harboring B-Raf V600E mutation. Vemurafenib is paradigmatic in that it was specifically developed to selectively block the mutant, but not the wild-type, B-Raf, with the aim of reducing the debilitating secondary effects that usually accompany cancer treatments. Similarly to other targeted therapeutic agents, after an initial response, the tumors often become unresponsive to the inhibitor and relapse. Several mechanisms have been described for the acquired resistance to vemurafenib, including mutation of Ras, expression of particular B-Raf splice-variants, or the overexpression of RTKs, such as the PDGFR,[66,68] all resulting in the reactivation of the MAPK pathway. Besides acquired mutations, it has been shown that MAPK reactivation in the presence of B-Raf inhibition can also occur through the release of negative feedback loops.[120] These compensatory mechanisms, which regulate the strength and duration of the signaling in physiological conditions, can provoke a rebound in ERK activity in a subset of cancer cells.[121] Such persister or tolerant cells constitute a sort of reservoir, from which fully resistant cells can emerge through acquisition of *de novo* mutations.[122] To enhance MAPK inhibition and prevent feedback reactivation, melanoma patients are now treated with combinations of B-Raf and MEK inhibitors, which proved better and more durable responses.[123,124] Feedback reactivation in response to B-Raf inhibition can have even stronger consequences in other types of cancer: consistent with its poor response in B-Raf-V600E mutant colon cancer patients, vemurafenib induces a rapid activation of EGFR signaling in these tumors.[125] Indeed, clinical trials have shown that the effects of B-Raf inhibitors in colon cancer patients can be significantly improved when combined with MEK[126] or EGFR and MEK[127] inhibitors. Combinations of EGFR and MEK inhibitors have also been proposed to treat EGFR mutant NSCLC,[128] indicating that preventing pathway reactivation could be a general strategy to delay acquired resistance in most types of tumors.

It has been shown that prolonged vemurafenib treatment can sensitize melanoma cells to drug withdrawal, due to a compensatory mechanism that provokes excessive activation of the MAPK pathway.[129] This study suggests that an intermittent dosing may forestall the clonal expansion of resistant/tolerant cells. This type of adaptive therapy,[130] in which modulation of the treatment is optimized to preserve a balance between subpopulations of cancer cells displaying different sensitivities to the drug, may help preventing or delaying tumor relapse through acquisition of a resistant phenotype.[131]

Since the isolation of the first growth factor more than 60 years ago, the knowledge gained on RTK signaling has translated into the development of over 50 clinically approved cancer drugs targeting this pathway (Table 1). Thanks to the astonishing advances in DNA sequencing of the last two decades, treatment can now be individually tailored based on the evolving genetic profile of the tumor, significantly extending patient response and survival, even for extremely aggressive types of cancer.

> **KEY POINTS:**
> - Tumor cells can become dependent, or addicted to a particular signaling pathway for their growth and survival.
> - The pathways aberrantly deregulated in tumor cells can be specifically targeted in the clinic through different therapeutic strategies, including monoclonal antibodies, Tyr kinase inhibitors, and inhibitors of downstream effectors.

> **Summary**
>
> In multicellular organisms, physiological processes are regulated through a complex and interconnected network of signaling pathways, generally mediated by hormones, cytokines, and growth factors. These molecules normally act in a timely and precise manner to specifically control the phenotype of a well-defined population of cells, including their proliferation, differentiation, survival, and motility. When a signaling pathway goes awry, this tight regulation is lost, resulting in an aberrant cell behavior that can lead to cell transformation. Most human cancers contain aberrant activation (or, less commonly, inhibition) of more than one such pathway, contributing to increased proliferation, survival, invasiveness, and metastatic spread. Such aberrations occur through different mechanisms, including autocrine/paracrine deregulation or genetic alterations affecting a particular component of the pathway. In this article, we will discuss growth factor signaling through receptors exhibiting intrinsic tyrosine kinase activity and focus on two major downstream pathways activated by these receptors to promote cell proliferation and survival, that is, the PI-3-K/Akt and Ras/MAPK pathways. General principles in cell signaling in both normal and tumor cells will be addressed, and we will briefly discuss how the initiation and progression of particular types of cancer can be affected by the deregulation of other signaling pathways.
>
> Finally, we will discuss the concepts of oncogene addiction and targeted therapy, providing paradigmatic examples to illustrate how increased understanding of the mechanisms responsible for aberrant deregulation of particular signaling pathways in cancer has been translated to the clinic.

Acknowledgments

Luca Grumolato was supported by grants from "Institut National du Cancer," "Agence Nationale de la Recherche" and "Ligue contre le cancer." Stuart A. Aaronson was supported by grants from the NCI, NICHD, and Breast Cancer Research Foundation.

Key references

The complete reference list can be found on Vital Source version of this title, see inside front cover.

9. Aaronson SA. Growth factors and cancer. *Science*. 1991;**254**(5035):1146–1153.
10. Lemmon MA, Schlessinger J. Cell signaling by receptor tyrosine kinases. *Cell*. 2010;**141**(7):1117–1134.
16. Pollak M. The insulin and insulin-like growth factor receptor family in neoplasia: an update. *Nat Rev Cancer*. 2012;**12**(3):159–169.
17. Citri A, Yarden Y. EGF-ERBB signalling: towards the systems level. *Nat Rev Mol Cell Biol*. 2006;**7**(7):505–516.
18. Arteaga CL, Engelman JA. ERBB receptors: from oncogene discovery to basic science to mechanism-based cancer therapeutics. *Cancer Cell*. 2014;**25**(3):282–303.
19. Trusolino L, Bertotti A, Comoglio PM. MET signalling: principles and functions in development, organ regeneration and cancer. *Nat Rev Mol Cell Biol*. 2010;**11**(12):834–848.
20. Gherardi E, Birchmeier W, Birchmeier C, Vande WG. Targeting MET in cancer: rationale and progress. *Nat Rev Cancer*. 2012;**12**(2):89–103.
24. Tebbutt N, Pedersen MW, Johns TG. Targeting the ERBB family in cancer: couples therapy. *Nat Rev Cancer*. 2013;**13**(9):663–673.
25. Shaw AT, Hsu PP, Awad MM, Engelman JA. Tyrosine kinase gene rearrangements in epithelial malignancies. *Nat Rev Cancer*. 2013;**13**(11):772–787.
26. Lynch TJ, Bell DW, Sordella R, et al. Activating mutations in the epidermal growth factor receptor underlying responsiveness of non-small-cell lung cancer to gefitinib. *N Engl J Med*. 2004;**350**(21):2129–2139.
29. Drilon A, Hu ZI, Lai GGY, Tan DSW. Targeting RET-driven cancers: lessons from evolving preclinical and clinical landscapes. *Nat Rev Clin Oncol*. 2018;**15**(3):151–167.
46. Engelman JA, Luo J, Cantley LC. The evolution of phosphatidylinositol 3-kinases as regulators of growth and metabolism. *Nat Rev Genet*. 2006;**7**(8):606–619.
48. Hoxhaj G, Manning BD. The PI3K-AKT network at the interface of oncogenic signalling and cancer metabolism. *Nat Rev Cancer*. 2020;**20**(2):74–88.
52. Samuels Y, Wang Z, Bardelli A, et al. High frequency of mutations of the PIK3CA gene in human cancers. *Science*. 2004;**304**(5670):554.
53. Kandoth C, McLellan MD, Vandin F, et al. Mutational landscape and significance across 12 major cancer types. *Nature*. 2013;**502**(7471):333–339.
54. Zhang Y, Kwok-Shing Ng P, Kucherlapati M, et al. A pan-cancer proteogenomic atlas of PI3K/AKT/mTOR pathway alterations. *Cancer Cell*. 2017;**31**(6):820–832.e3.
61. Pylayeva-Gupta Y, Grabocka E, Bar-Sagi D. RAS oncogenes: weaving a tumorigenic web. *Nat Rev Cancer*. 2011;**11**(11):761–774.
68. Karoulia Z, Gavathiotis E, Poulikakos PI. New perspectives for targeting RAF kinase in human cancer. *Nat Rev Cancer*. 2017;**17**(11):676–691.
73. Davies H, Bignell GR, Cox C, et al. Mutations of the BRAF gene in human cancer. *Nature*. 2002;**417**(6892):949–954.
74. Wagner EF, Nebreda AR. Signal integration by JNK and p38 MAPK pathways in cancer development. *Nat Rev Cancer*. 2009;**9**(8):537–549.
77. Massague J. TGFbeta signalling in context. *Nat Rev Mol Cell Biol*. 2012;**13**(10):616–630.
78. Stark GR, Darnell JE Jr. The JAK-STAT pathway at twenty. *Immunity*. 2012;**36**(4):503–514.
82. Lappano R, Maggiolini M. G protein-coupled receptors: novel targets for drug discovery in cancer. *Nat Rev Drug Discov*. 2011;**10**(1):47–60.
83. Perkins ND. The diverse and complex roles of NF-κB subunits in cancer. *Nat Rev Cancer*. 2012;**12**(2):121–132.
84. Briscoe J, Therond PP. The mechanisms of Hedgehog signalling and its roles in development and disease. *Nat Rev Mol Cell Biol*. 2013;**14**(7):416–429.
85. Harvey KF, Zhang X, Thomas DM. The Hippo pathway and human cancer. *Nat Rev Cancer*. 2013;**13**(4):246–257.
86. Clevers H, Nusse R. Wnt/beta-catenin signaling and disease. *Cell*. 2012;**149**(6):1192–1205.
87. Guruharsha KG, Kankel MW, Artavanis-Tsakonas S. The Notch signalling system: recent insights into the complexity of a conserved pathway. *Nat Rev Genet*. 2012;**13**(9):654–666.
93. Evans RM, Mangelsdorf DJ. Nuclear receptors, RXR, and the Big Bang. *Cell*. 2014;**157**(1):255–266.
96. Mills IG. Maintaining and reprogramming genomic androgen receptor activity in prostate cancer. *Nat Rev Cancer*. 2014;**14**(3):187–198.
97. de The H, Pandolfi PP, Chen Z. Acute promyelocytic leukemia: a paradigm for oncoprotein-targeted cure. *Cancer Cell*. 2017;**32**(5):552–560.
99. Weinstein IB. Cancer. Addiction to oncogenes—the Achilles heal of cancer. *Science*. 2002;**297**(5578):63–64.
100. Sharma SV, Settleman J. Oncogene addiction: setting the stage for molecularly targeted cancer therapy. *Genes Dev*. 2007;**21**(24):3214–3231.
105. Sawyers CL. Herceptin: a first assault on oncogenes that launched a revolution. *Cell*. 2019;**179**(1):8–12.
109. Misale S, Di Nicolantonio F, Sartore-Bianchi A, et al. Resistance to anti-EGFR therapy in colorectal cancer: from heterogeneity to convergent evolution. *Cancer Discov*. 2014;**4**(11):1269–1280.
112. Goel HL, Mercurio AM. VEGF targets the tumour cell. *Nat Rev Cancer*. 2013;**13**(12):871–882.
114. Druker BJ. Translation of the Philadelphia chromosome into therapy for CML. *Blood*. 2008;**112**(13):4808–4817.
118. Hallberg B, Palmer RH. Mechanistic insight into ALK receptor tyrosine kinase in human cancer biology. *Nat Rev Cancer*. 2013;**13**(10):685–700.
130. Gatenby RA, Silva AS, Gillies RJ, Frieden BR. Adaptive therapy. *Cancer Res*. 2009;**69**(11):4894–4903.
131. Amirouchene-Angelozzi N, Swanton C, Bardelli A. Tumor evolution as a therapeutic target. *Cancer Discov*. 2017. doi: 10.1158/2159-8290.CD-17-0343.

11 Differentiation therapy

Sai-Juan Chen, MD, PhD ■ *Xiao-Jing Yan, MD, PhD* ■ *Guang-Biao Zhou, MD, PhD* ■ *Zhu Chen, PhD*

> **Overview**
>
> Abnormal differentiation is one of the main features of human cancers, especially in hematological malignancies. Many aberrant genetic and epigenetic factors have been shown to disrupt the regulation of cell differentiation in a variety of cancers and play an important role in oncogenesis. Differentiation therapy refers to the application of therapeutic agents selectively targeting the key molecules involved in the process of cell differentiation, leading to the restoration of normal cellular homeostasis and the eventual clearance of cancer cells. Over the past four decades, investigations of the molecular mechanisms underlying cancer cell differentiation arrest or blockage have allowed the identification of an array of drug targets. On the other hand, many physiological or pharmacological agents have been tested using *in vitro* and *in vivo* systems as the inducers of differentiation and maturation of cancer cells. The translational research in this field has gradually turned the differentiation therapy from a concept to clinical practices. The most successful model of cancer differentiation therapy is the development of synergistic targeted therapy for acute promyelocytic leukemia (APL) with all-trans-retinoic acid (ATRA) and arsenic trioxide (ATO). This article discusses the basic theories of differentiation therapy and the clinical achievements of this therapeutic approach.

Molecular mechanisms underlying differentiation blockage in cancer

It has long been recognized that in human cancers, there exists some relationship between the clinical aggressiveness and their differentiation status, with poorly differentiated tumors being usually more aggressive. To understand the biology of differentiation arrest or blockage in cancer, it is necessary to elucidate how the related functions are regulated in normal cells and how they become disrupted in cancer cells.

These studies are of importance for identifying meaningful therapeutic targets.

It is well established that pluripotent embryonic stem cells are capable of self-renewal and differentiating into various cells with specific functions in an organism. These cells can then develop into distinct cell types, tissues, and organs, which are under accurate regulation in a finely organized manner. A large body of evidence has been obtained that the underlying mechanisms entail the sequential action of cell-/tissue-specific or time-specific transcription factors (TFs) that activate or repress the differentiation-associated genes under appropriate conditions.[1-3] The transcriptional expression of genes is also orchestrated by complex mechanisms designated as epigenetic regulation. Notably, many pathways and networks that regulate cell differentiation during normal development are affected by genetic and epigenetic abnormalities during tumorigenesis. As a result, cancer cell population generally bears an aberrant expression of regulators for embryonic morphogenesis and maintains a subset with properties of stem cells. Meanwhile, cancer cells often show defects in programs that keep cells in differentiated state (Figure 1).

Transcriptional factors (TFs)

Cellular differentiation can be defined by a sequential process of acquisition of different functions, and cell fate is largely determined by control of gene expression through the combination of TFs and epigenetic modifiers.[3,4] TFs are nuclear proteins capable of DNA binding and trans-activating or trans-repressing the transcription of target genes. They are often assembled into multiprotein complex with cofactors (activators or repressors) and play decisive roles in regulating the gene expression profiles of stem/progenitor cells and determining their ability to differentiate into mature cell lineages.[4] TFs are also essential for the control of cell proliferation and programmed cell death (apoptosis, etc.). Recently, cellular reprogramming and induction of pluripotency across differentiated lineages have been achieved using combinations of TFs, which provide strong evidence for the key role that TFs play in the decisions of cell fate.[5-10] In addition, that cell differentiation can be directed by lineage-specific TFs has also been supported by a large amount of experimental data.[3,5,12] In contrast, abnormalities of differentiation-associated TFs due to dysregulated expression or aberrant functions imposed by gene point mutations or fusions may disturb the differentiation program of normal stem/progenitor cells.[4] As a result, immature descendants with growth and survival advantages may be produced, eventually leading to the development of cancer.

The cancer-associated TFs can be divided into distinct classes according to structural and/or functional features,[11] such as leucine zipper factors (bZIP, e.g., c-JUN), helix-loop-helix factors (bHLH, e.g., MYC), Cys4 zinc fingers [e.g., nuclear receptors (NRs), GATA factors], helix-turn-helix factors (HTH, e.g., HOX family, OCT-1/2), and Rel homology region (e.g., NF-κB). These TFs are considered as key regulators of cell proliferation, differentiation, and apoptosis, and their mutations and/or aberrant expression have been shown to play an essential role in malignant transformation. A special class of ligand-activated zinc finger proteins known as superfamily of NRs is worth particular attention, as they are major regulators in the initiation and/or maintenance of differentiated status of many cell/tissue types.[12] This family contains the receptors for different ligands including steroid/thyroid hormones, retinoids, vitamin D3, and certain fatty acids. Notably, many of these receptors are subject to dysregulated expression or structural abnormalities in various cancers. These abnormalities subsequently lead to aberrant repression of target gene expression in the presence of physiological concentrations of ligand, undesired activation of the normally hormone-regulated genes in a hormone-independent way, or even activation of some genes unrelated to hormone regulation, which will be discussed in detail in the section entitled "Agents targeting aberrant TFs."

Holland-Frei Cancer Medicine, Tenth Edition. Edited by Robert C. Bast, John C. Byrd, Carlo M. Croce, Ernest Hawk, Fadlo R. Khuri, Raphael E. Pollock, Apostolia M. Tsimberidou, Christopher G. Willett, and Cheryl L. Willman.
© 2023 John Wiley & Sons, Inc. Published 2023 by John Wiley & Sons, Inc.

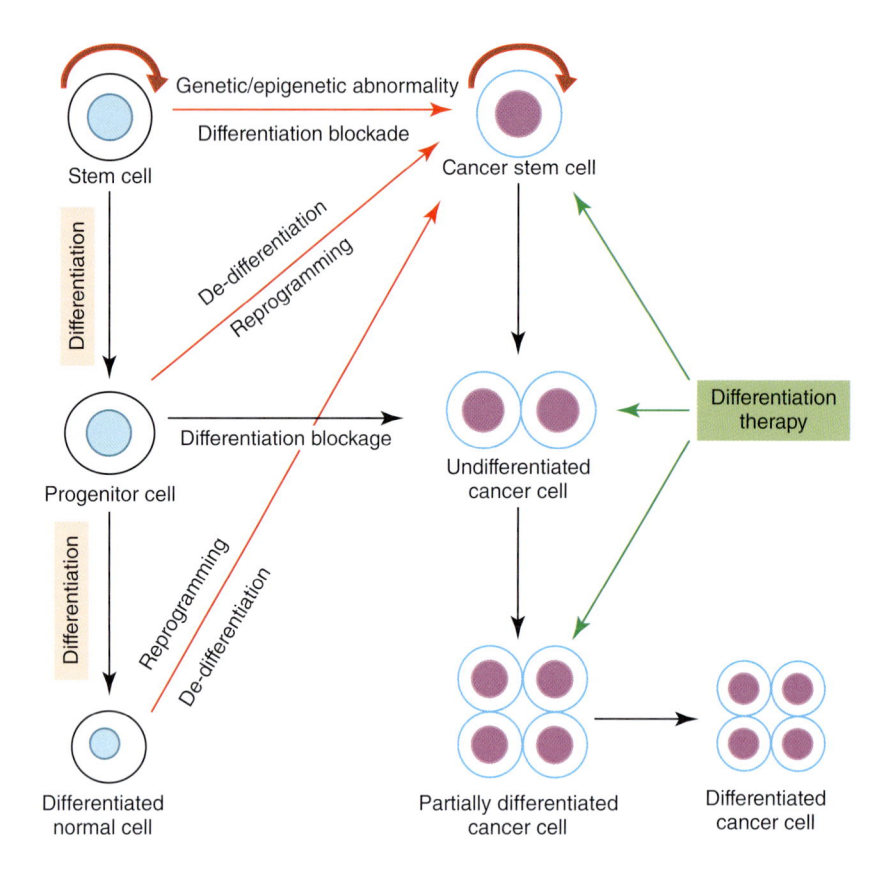

Figure 1 Differentiation blockade and differentiation therapy in cancer. In addition to self-renewal, normal stem cells are capable of differentiating into specific mature cells, while differentiation blockade may lead to the development of cancer. Cancer stem cells may originate from normal stem cells acquiring genetic and/or epigenetic abnormalities, or from normal progenitor or differentiated cells undergoing de-differentiation and reprogramming also due to genetic and/or epigenetic abnormalities. Differentiation therapy exerts therapeutic efficacy by inducing differentiation of cancer stem cells and undifferentiated cancer cells.

For a long time, hematopoiesis has been at the frontline of research in the biology of normal and abnormal cell differentiation,[4,13,14] owing to the discoveries of hematopoietic hormones and related signaling pathways and the specific TFs that regulate the fate of hematopoietic stem/progenitor cells (HSPCs) (Figure 2). Each stage of myeloid and lymphoid differentiation shows particular TFs signatures that function in networks. For example, RUNX1, GATA1, C/EBPα, C/EBPβ, MYB, E2A, PAX5, TAL1/SCL, or PU.1 is turned on or turned off in an orchestrated manner to ensure blood cell lineage specification.[3,14] Some of these TFs were originally identified following the molecular characterization of gene point mutations or fusion in leukemia, such as C/EBPα in *CEBPA* mutation of acute myeloid leukemia (AML), *RUNX1* in the *RUNX1(AML1)–ETO* fusion gene of t(8;21) AML, and *SCL(TAL1)* in t(1;14) T-cell acute lymphoblastic leukemia (ALL).[15–17] Disruption of these hematopoietic TFs in leukemia blocks hematopoietic cells in their early stages of differentiation.

The fact that abnormal TFs disturbing cell differentiation are "drivers" in oncogenesis has aroused interest for these proteins to be potential targets for therapeutic intervention. However, most current anticancer research activities are concentrated on cell-surface receptors because they offer a relatively straightforward way for drugs to affect cellular behavior, whereas agents acting at the level of transcription need to penetrate the cell membrane and enter into the nucleus. Efforts should be supported to design drugs affecting cancer-associated transcriptional patterns for re-establishing differentiation. Small-molecule drugs directed against well-defined interacting sites between TFs and DNA or between TFs and other proteins in transcription machinery can be developed, so as to modulate the key TF target genes. On the other hand, the re-introduction of differentiation-related wild-type TFs with gene therapy might also serve as a strategy for cancer differentiation therapy.

Epigenetic modifiers

Epigenetic regulation constitutes crucial mechanisms governing the variability in gene expression, which is heritable through mitosis and potentially also meiosis, without changes of genomic sequence.[18,19] All cells of an organism share the same genome information but exhibit different phenotypes with diverse functions. This phenotypic diversity is due to distinct gene expression patterns among different cell types. It is well established that chromatin states are primary determinants for the turn-on or turn-off of genes. The assembly and compaction of chromatin require multiple regulatory mechanisms, including DNA methylation (cytosine methylation and hydroxymethylation) or demethylation, posttranslational modifications of histones (phosphorylation, acetylation, methylation, and ubiquitylation), and noncoding RNA-mediated pathways.[19–21] A large number of enzymes have been identified to be regulatory factors in the mechanisms, such as DNA methyltransferases (DNMTs), DNA demethylases (DNDMs), histone deacetylases (HDACs), histone acetyltransferases (HATs), histone methyltransferases (HMTs), and histone demethylases (HDMs) (Figure 3a, b). Now, it is recognized that the HMT category comprises lysine methyltransferases (KMTs) and arginine methyltransferases (PRMTs). The different modifications

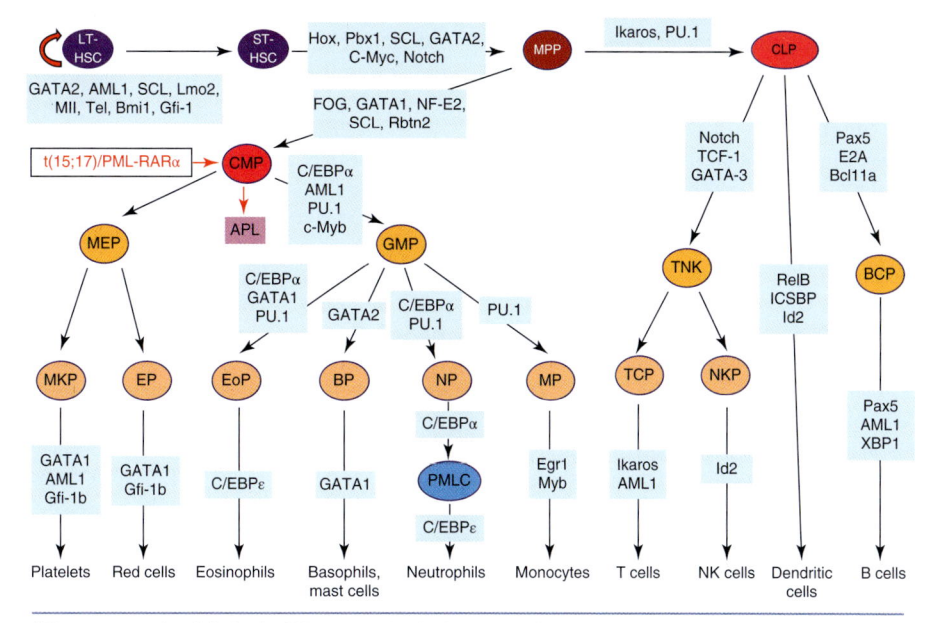

Figure 2 Signaling pathways and transcriptional factors (TFs) regulating the differentiation of HSPCs. Differentiation block may result in leukemia, exemplified by development of acute promyelocytic leukemia (APL), a subtype of acute myeloid leukemia (AML) characterized by accumulation of abnormal promyelocytes in bone marrow/peripheral blood, the presence of t(15;17)/PML-RARα fusion gene, and severe bleeding syndrome. In fact, almost all the listed signaling molecules and TFs are subject to mutations (gene fusions, point mutations, gene amplifications/deletions) and/or dysregulation of expression in hematological malignancies.

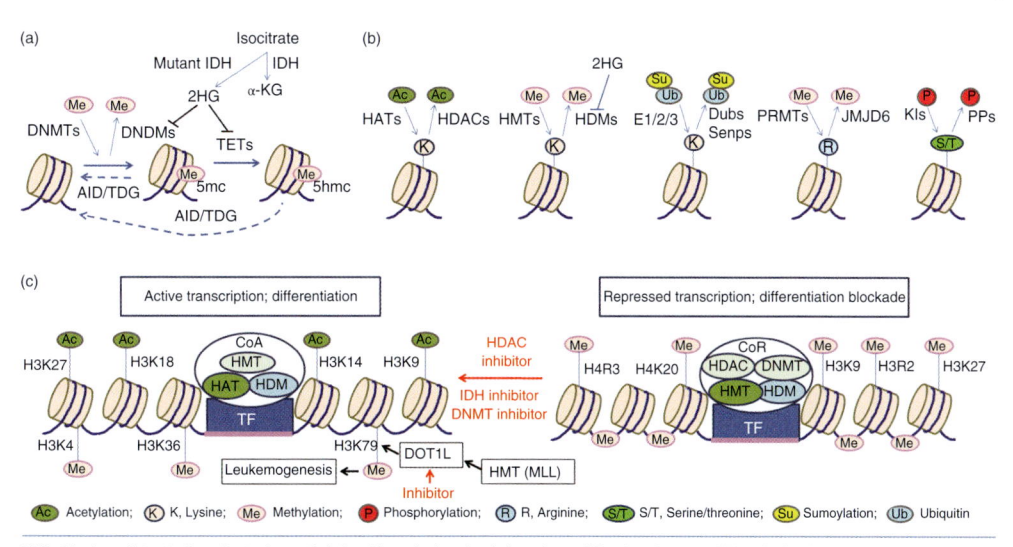

Figure 3 Epigenetic regulation involved in the cell differentiation and tumorigenesis. (a) DNA methylation (cytosine methylation and hydroxymethylation) are regulated by different enzymes DNMTs, TETs, and IDH. (b) Posttranslational modifications of histones include phosphorylation, acetylation, methylation, and ubiquitylation or sumoylation, which are regulated by a variety of factors HATs, HDACs, HMTs, HDMs, and so on. Notably, most of these epigenetic modifier genes have been found to be mutated in human cancers including solid tumors and hematological malignancies. (c) Gene expression is controlled in the promoter regions by a combination of chromatin modification and transcriptional factor (TF). In tumor cells, gene expression is silenced by condensing chromatin, methylating DNA, and deacetylating histones, which results in the differentiation blockade. Inhibition of HDACs, DNMTs, and IDH may result in active transcription and differentiation of cancer cells. Some HMTs (e.g., MLL and related fusion proteins) may enhance H3K79methylation by promoting DOT1L to activate transcription of some leukemogenic genes, and inhibitors of DOT1L may suppress the leukemogenic genes to treat leukemia.

of DNA or histones are closely interrelated and can both reinforce each other and inhibit each other. Many histone-modifying enzymes are components of cofactor complexes and function cooperatively with TFs to modulate gene expression (Figure 3c).

New technological platforms have allowed a comprehensive epigenomic map to be made in pluripotent and differentiated cells, which provide further support to the concept that cell differentiation is accompanied by dynamic features of chromatin states.[21-24] Genetic studies in different model organisms have shown the importance of chromatin regulators in key developmental transitions and cell fate decision. Cancer cells are characterized by typical genome-wide aberrations at the epigenetic level, such as the hypomethylation, the hypermethylation of specific promoter regions, the histone deacetylation, the downregulation of microRNAs (miRNAs), and the dysregulation of certain components of epigenetic machinery.[19,20,25] Recently, accumulating evidences showed that global alterations in DNA methylation patterns and enhancer deregulation were linked to AML clonal expansion, further supporting the notion that epigenetic heterogeneity better explains leukemia identity compared to the genetic background.[26,27] With the advent of next-generation sequencing technologies, somatic alterations of many epigenetic modifiers have been identified as common genetic events in cancers including solid tumors and hematopoietic malignancies.[28-31] In acute leukemia and myelodysplastic syndrome (MDS), besides the already known aberrations of mixed lineage leukemia (MLL1) located on 11q23, mutations in a subset of epigenetic modifiers, including other SET domain-containing proteins (MLL2, SETD2),[32] tet methylcytosine dioxygenase 2 (TET2),[33-35] isocitrate dehydrogenase (IDH1/IDH2),[36] additional sex combs-like1 (ASXL1),[37,38] enhancer of zeste homolog 2 (EZH2),[39,40] and DNA methyltransferase 3A (DNMT3A),[41,42] have been discovered. These mutations have been shown not only to contribute to the leukemogenesis but also serve as the biomarker of clinical prognosis since they often predict a poor overall survival (OS) of patients.[29-31] Based on the clinical observation and basic research, it could be concluded that the coordinated action of epigenetic modification factors with those of genetic regulators are important for tight regulation of gene expression through downstream molecular effectors, thus confer the cancer cells a selective advantage to differentiation block, apoptotic deficiency, and uncontrolled cell growth. Because the epigenetic modifications are usually dynamic and reversible, therapies targeting epigenetic modifiers hold the promise of being clinically effective.

Cancer stem cells (CSCs)

Most cancers are heterogeneous in terms of cell proliferation and differentiation status. In recent years, evidence has been accumulated to suggest that the existence of less-differentiated, stem cell-like cells within the cancer cell population in solid tumors (lung, colon, prostate, ovarian, and brain cancers and melanoma) and leukemia.[43-46] These cells are now referred to as cancer stem cells (CSCs) or tumor-initiating cells capable of self-renewal and contributing to tumor onset, expansion, resistance, recurrence, and metastasis after therapy.[47] Indeed, a single leukemia-initiating cell (LIC) from human being can cause a full-blown AML in animal model.[48] As a result, malignant cells in a given cancer are highly hierarchical, with the unique self-renewing CSCs at the top of the hierarchy, while all other cells are derived from differentiated CSCs (Figure 1).

Investigation of the properties of CSCs and their roles in disease mechanisms occupies a central position in cancer research nowadays. Generally speaking, CSCs represent the driving force behind cancer initiation, progression, metastasis, recurrence, and drug resistance.[44,49] It is nevertheless not easy to define the phenotypes of CSCs in that they are variable from one cancer to another and are affected by the initial transformation as well as different stages of neoplastic development. Currently, fluorescence-activated cell sorting using cell surface markers or intracellular molecules represents the common method to identify CSCs.[43,44] There are still problems to be tackled: CSC biomarkers are lacking in some cancers; not all CSCs express the markers or marker sets; some differentiated cancer cells also express the same marker sets as CSCs do; some currently used marker sets are not specific to CSC since they are also expressed by stem/progenitor cells in normal tissues. On the other hand, gene expression patterns may be of value because dysregulation of certain pathways or networks can be seen in CSCs but not in differentiated cancer cell compartments, which can eventually be used as new CSC markers. So far, PI3K/Akt, PTEN, JAK/STAT, TGF-β, Wnt/β-catenin, hedgehog, Notch, NF-κB, and Bcl-2 have been included in the pathways that are involved in the control of self-renewal and differentiation of CSCs.[43,44]

Traditional cytotoxic chemotherapy (CT) or radiation therapy is designed to target cancer cells with rapid proliferative or dividing abilities. These therapies are usually unable to eliminate CSCs, which are in a relatively quiescent state and divide slowly, and can consequently regenerate cancers and drive disease recurrence.[49-51] It is believed that only when CSCs are eradicated can cancer patients actually be cured. In recent years, great attention has been given to the characteristics of CSCs by both scientific and medical communities because these cells provide a unique target for cancer treatment. The CSCs-targeted strategy focuses on the elimination of CSCs by acting on specific surface molecules, signaling pathways, or microenvironments, which are indispensable for the maintenance of stem cells, or by inducing CSCs into the more differentiated state.[46,49,50,52] A number of existing agents have been investigated in this regard and high-throughput screening of chemical libraries has also been used to find novel CSC-targeted chemicals.[53,54]

Potential cancer cell differentiation-inducing agents

The concept of differentiation therapy was pioneered by the work of Pierce and Verney in 1961 when they observed differentiation of teratocarcinoma cells.[55] In the 1970s, important reports were made to demonstrate the differentiating capability of DMSO on erythropoiesis, the differentiation of neuroblastoma cells with some inducers, and the morphologic and functional maturation of leukemia cells induced by certain agents.[56-59] Many substances have thus been shown to possess the potential of cancer differentiation inducer with *in vitro* cell line experiments. Cancer differentiation therapy aims at using appropriate therapeutic agents to induce cell cycle arrest and a commitment to the cell differentiation program toward terminal cell division, specific function gaining, and ultimately apoptosis.[54] This concept applies relatively clearly to hematologic malignancies, whereas "authentic" differentiation therapy for solid tumors is sometimes difficult to define and often refers to the processes that convert malignant cells to a more benign phenotype, accompanied by diminished proliferative and metastatic abilities and the expression of mature cell markers.[52] Interestingly, some initially defined differentiation inducers have turned out to be compounds targeting oncoproteins, while some newly developed targeting therapeutics have been found to trigger significant differentiation of cancer cells. Thus far, more than 80 agents of differentiation induction have been identified and biosynthesized, and most of them are under investigations *in vitro* or on animal models, among which only a fraction have been used in clinical practice.

Agents targeting aberrant TFs

As discussed previously, TFs play a powerful role in physiological cellular differentiation and can be abnormally regulated or functionally disturbed in cancers. The modulation and/or restoration of the functions of differentiation-associated TFs constitute one of the main strategies for cancer differentiation therapy. Here, we introduce some differentiation-induction agents, which specifically target hormone-regulated TFs.

Retinoids

Retinoids are a group of vitamin A derivatives. Retinoic acids (RAs) are the physiologically existing active metabolite of retinol, which regulate a wide range of biological processes including development, differentiation, proliferation, and apoptosis in normal or cancer cells.[12,60–62] The most important isomers of RAs are all-trans-retinoic acid (ATRA), 13-*cis*-retinoic acid (13-cRA), and 9-*cis*-retinoic acid (9-cRA), which have different spectrums of biological activity and ligand affinity.[63,64] Synthetic retinoids include bexarotene and fenretinide. The effects of RAs on cell differentiation are exerted mostly via their NRs. Two types of receptors, the retinoic acid receptors (RARs, with three major isoforms RAR-α/-β/-γ) and the retinoid X receptors (RXRs, with three main isoforms RXR-α/-β/-γ), mediate RA signaling as heterodimer RAR/RXR.[12,62] These receptor heterodimers are able to bind, at the genomic level, to the specific motifs defined as retinoic acid response elements (RAREs) on the promoters of target genes. RAR/RXR differentially activates or represses gene transcription while recruiting co-activators (CoA) or corepressors (CoR) complexes. These different modes of action depend on the presence or absence of the ligands, RAs. Physiological concentrations of RA (1 pmol/L) are able to release CoR (such as N-CoR/SMRT complex and the chromatin remodeling complexes, e.g., HDACs, DNMTs) from the RAR/RXR and recruit CoA (such as p300/CBP complex with HAT activity), leading to the transcriptional activation of genes involved in cell differentiation (e.g., C/EBPα and PU.1), growth, and apoptosis.[56,62,65–70]

Retinoid signaling is often disrupted during carcinogenesis, suggesting that restoration of this pathway may be a viable option for cancer treatment.[60,61,64,71] The effects of RA-induced differentiation are particularly observed on promyelocytic leukemia cell-like cell lines such as HL60 and APL cell lines such as NB4, or fresh primary APL (acute promyelocytic leukemia) cells.[57,72] These cells can undergo terminal differentiation to morphologically and functionally mature granulocytes after incubation with pharmacological concentrations (0.1–1 μmol/L) of RAs, especially ATRA.[57] Myeloblasts from other AML subtypes are generally not affected by RAs, whereas only limited differentiating effects of retinoids are seen on cell lines such as THP-1 (monoblastic leukemia), K562 (blastic phase of CML), HEL (erythroleukemia), and U937 (monocytic leukemia).[56,72] Until now, the most successful clinical practice of differentiation therapy is the use of ATRA in APL, which will be discussed in detail in the following section.

Retinoids have been reported to induce the differentiation of many solid tumor cell lines *in vitro* and suppress carcinogenesis in tumorigenic animal models, including human teratoma, melanoma, neuroblastoma, osteosarcoma, and rhabdomyosarcoma.[63,73,74] In thyroid carcinoma cell lines, retinoids were shown to induce the expression of type I iodothyronine-5′-deiodinase and sodium/iodide symporter, which are the thyroid differentiation markers.[75–77] In early clinical studies, patients with poorly differentiated, inoperable thyroid carcinoma with lacking or insufficient iodine uptake were treated with 13-cRA at oral doses of 0.3–1.5 mg/kg/day over 5 weeks and up to 9 months. The results showed an increased radioiodide uptake in 20–40% of patients.[77–79] In some of these trials, a fluorine-18 fluorodeoxyglucose positron emission tomography (18 F-FDG PET) was used for the evaluation of therapy with 13-cRA in thyroid cancer. These data indicate retinoids as promising differentiation therapy agents for the treatment of thyroid cancer.

In addition to induction of differentiation, retinoids exert antitumor effects through other modes of action: repressing cell proliferation, promoting cell apoptosis, and inhibiting angiogenesis and metastasis.[62,63] Notably, retinoids are used effectively in the treatment of certain cutaneous premalignancies and malignancies with good results.[80] Bexarotene, the first synthetic highly selective RXR agonist, has been shown to induce apoptosis of cutaneous T-cell lymphoma (CTCL) cells with downregulation of its receptors and of survivin, an inhibitor of apoptosis.[81]

In clinical practice, systemic retinoids are approved by the US Food and Drug Administration (FDA) for the treatment of APL and CTCL.

Vitamin D compounds

Vitamin D is known to have a variety of actions at cell proliferation and differentiation.[82] These actions are mainly mediated by vitamin D receptor (VDR), a member of NR superfamily. While performing physiological functions, VDR forms a heterodimer with RXR. The VDR/RXR heterodimer binds to vitamin D response elements (VDREs) in the promoter regions of target genes.[77] In the absence of physiologically active form of vitamin D, 1,25 dihydroxy vitamin D3 [$1,25(OH)_2D_3$](1,25D), the VDR/RXR heterodimer recruits CoR including HDACs and results in transcriptional repression.[71] However, once the ligand binds to VDR/RXR, the resultant conformational change of the receptor heterodimer triggers the transcriptional activation of the target genes. It has been demonstrated that the recruitment of several coactivators to VDR/RXR is indispensable for this trans-activation. The VDR also directly interacts with a number of other proteins (e.g., β-catenin) and regulates their activities.[83] Besides, 1,25D can trigger "rapid responses" via activating membrane-initiated signaling pathways, such as MAPK pathways, the lipid signaling pathways, or PI3K/AKT pathway.[84–86]

Similar to the differentiation-inducing effects of retinoids, 1,25D has been shown to dispose differentiating actions on various types of human AML cells,[82] including HL-60, U937, NB4, THP-1, and KG-1. Animal model studies have shown that 1,25D strongly promotes cell differentiation and thereby significantly prolongs the survival of mice transplanted with leukemic cells. However, the results of clinical trials are unsatisfactory. Neither 1,25D nor vitamin D analogs (VDAs) showed clear beneficial effects on patients with AML or MDS.[87,88] An important issue for these failures could be the heterogeneous nature of the diseases. The clinical utility of 1,25D has also been limited by the severe toxicity of its therapeutic doses, primarily due to fatal drug-induced hypercalcemia.[89] Some types of solid tumors, such as colon, breast, and prostate cancers and osteosarcoma, were also reported to respond to *in vitro* applied VDAs.[90,91] Nevertheless, little is known about how VDAs mediate their antiproliferation or pro-differentiation activity.[90] Moreover, the results of clinical trials of VDAs across a variety of cancers have been disappointing with regard to efficacy.[92] Thus, the routine recommendation of vitamin D for cancer treatment is premature.

PPARγ agonists
Peroxisome proliferator-activated receptor gamma (PPARγ) is also a member of the NR superfamily.[93] PPARγ forms heterodimer with RXR, which then binds to PPARγ response elements in the promoter regions of target genes. It is well established that PPARγ is important in the regulation of proliferation, differentiation, and apoptosis in many cell types.[93] Synthetic PPARγ agonists have been developed, including drugs used in the treatment of type 2 diabetes [e.g., troglitazone, rosiglitazone (TGZ)] and nonsteroidal anti-inflammatory agents (e.g., indomethacin).[56,73]

Activation of PPARγ with agonists was shown to be able to suppress the growth and induce the differentiation of several types of tumors in vitro and in animal models for colon, breast, prostate, thyroid cancers, liposarcoma (LPS), pituitary adenomas, and acute leukemia.[94-96] Antitumor effects of PPARγ agonists could be associated with regulation of cell cycle, apoptosis, and expression of tumor suppressor genes (TSGs) (e.g., *PTEN* and *BRCA1*).[54,97,98] Besides, there has been evidence for "off-target" effects of PPARγ agonists, which is independent of the PPARγ receptor activity.[56]

Clinical trials of PPARγ agonists have been carried out in several human malignancies. A few studies reported that TGZ could induce the differentiation of cancer cells in patients with LPS.[99] It was initially found that terminal adipocytic differentiation was induced in a few patients with intermediate to high-grade LPS. However, such responses and clinical benefit could not be confirmed in a subsequent trial.[100] Clinical investigations in breast, prostate, colon, lung, and thyroid cancers and LPS did not reveal a meaningful benefit of TGZ therapy.[56,77,100-102] Although the clinical effects of PPARγ agonists have not been convincing, their low toxicity profile and potential additive or synergistic effects combined with other anticancer agents such as retinoids make them reasonable candidates in combination therapy trials.

Agents targeting epigenetic modifiers
It has been shown that the aberration of epigenetic regulation and TFs governing differentiation occurs in many cancers. Recurrent somatic alterations in epigenetic modifiers are also observed in solid tumors and hematological malignancies. Hence, there has been substantial interest in preclinical and clinical studies for epigenetic regulating agents to be considered as differentiation inducers.[103] A large amount of epigenetic agents are currently under investigation and a few have received FDA approval. Promising results have already been yielded in certain cancer types.

Compounds targeting DNA methylation

DNMTs inhibitors
DNA methylation is the most characterized epigenetic modification and is described as a stable epigenetic marker.[104] As mentioned previously, DNA methylation levels are under the control of enzymes able to modulate the addition (by DNA methyl transferases; DNMTs) or the removal (by the indirect action of TET and IDH1/2 proteins) of methyl groups to cytosine or adenine residues. DNMT3A, a de novo methyltransferase, is mutated in the patients with AML (20–25%) and other hematological malignancies.[105] It has been reported by several studies that DNMT3A mutations are associated with inferior OS.[106,107] As hypermethylation of TSGs and overexpression of DNMTs have been established as the key factors in carcinogenesis, demethylating agents seem especially promising as anticancer drugs.[108,109] To date, 5-azacytidine (5-Aza) and 5-aza-2′-deoxycytidine (decitabine) are the most explored DNMTs inhibitors (DNMTi), already approved by the FDA for the treatment of patients with MDS or AML, and 5-Aza has also been approved by the FDA and the European Medicines Agency (EMA) for the treatment of chronic myelomonocytic leukemia (CMML).[108] Of note, azacytidine is predominantly incorporated into RNA with a more evident effect on gene translation. Chemical DNMT inhibition significantly alters DNA methylation patterns with consequent induction of cell cycle arrest, DNA damage accumulation, apoptosis, differentiation, and immune cell activation.[110] The mode of action on AML cells seems dose-dependent and a "dual mechanism" has been identified: the cytotoxicity and/or the inhibition of cell proliferation at high doses, and the DNA hypomethylation effect on the induction of gene expression at low doses.[108,109] Numerous studies have described terminal differentiation of AML cells treated with 5-Aza or decitabine.[109,111,112] Moreover, it has been demonstrated that decitabine-induced killing of myeloid leukemia cells is independent of DNA damage and apoptosis.[109] In some solid tumor cells, 5-Aza or decitabine induces cancer cell apoptosis and senescence through multiple mechanisms.[113]

Recent clinical studies indicated that repeated exposure to these agents at low doses (decitabine: 20 mg/m^2 for 5 days every 28 days; 5-Aza: 75 mg/m^2 for 7 days every 28 days) could induce DNA demethylation with a better antineoplastic effect than when used at higher doses (decitabine: 45 mg/m^2 for 3 days every 42 days).[109,114-117] In MDS patients, 5-Aza induced an overall response rate of 20–30% and significantly improved survival compared with standard care, while decitabine induced cytogenetic remission (Cyto-CR) rates of 35–50% at optimal doses and prolongs survival when compared with historical controls.[109,114-119] Clinical trials of DNMTi in combination with other agents also obtained promising results in solid tumors such as non-small-cell lung cancer and refractory ovarian cancer.[112,120,121] More recently, guadecitabine (SGI-110), a novel DNMTi with improved stability, has been developed and tested in clinical trials with promising results.[122,123] This agent showed antileukemia effects by promoting apoptosis and altering the immune microenvironment in AML, instead of inducing cell differentiation. To date, the efficacy of DNMTi as single agents for AML treatment is limited, possibly due to the fact that targeting a single layer of epigenetic deregulation cannot be sufficient to reach a complete rescue of the epigenetic landscape of malignant cells. Therefore, efforts to develop new DNMTi with more selective effects and fewer toxicities or combinatorial treatments of DNMTi and other agents should be continued. Furthermore, investigation of the potential differentiation effects and underlying mechanism of novel DNMTi is needed.

IDH1/2 inhibitors
Somatic mutations of the metabolic enzyme IDH1/2 have recently been reported in myeloid neoplasms (such as AML and MDS) and other solid tumors (such as glioma, melanoma, thyroid cancer, and chondrosarcoma).[36,124-126] Almost all mutations are located at arginine residues in the catalytic pockets of IDH1 (R132) or IDH2 (R140 and R172) and thus confer on the enzymes a new activity: catalysis of α-ketoglutarate (α-KG) to 2-hydroxyglutarate (2-HG).[126,127] High concentrations of 2-HG, known as an "oncometabolite," have been shown to inhibit α-KG-dependent dioxygenases, including histone and DNDMs, which are main modifiers of the epigenetic state of cells (Figure 3a).[126-129] It has been suggested that IDH1/2 mutations can impair hematopoietic

differentiation and promote leukemia development.[128,130] The differentiation block and increased proliferation were reversible upon silencing of mutated IDH2 in AML.[131] In solid tumors, likewise, cancer-associated IDH mutations could induce a block of cellular differentiation to promote tumorigenesis and therefore might be potential targets of differentiation therapy.[120,132] Indeed, it was shown that a selective IDH1/R132H inhibitor (AGI-5198) could induce the expression of genes associated with gliogenic differentiation and trigger astroglial differentiation of IDH1/R132H mutant (mIDH1) cells.[132] Blockade of mIDH1 suppressed the growth of glioma cells with IDH1/R132H or in IDH1/R132H glioma xenograft mice but not those with wild-type IDH1 *in vitro*. It is worth noting that AGI-6780, a small molecule that potently and selectively inhibits the tumor-associated mutant IDH2/R140Q, was capable of inducing differentiation of TF-1 erythroleukemia and primary human AML cells *in vitro*.[133] These findings provide proof of concept that inhibitors targeting mutant IDH1 or IDH2 may have potential applications as cancer differentiation inducers.

Recently, it was found that inhibitors specific for mutant IDH2 could trigger differentiation of leukemic blasts into granulocytes and impair self-renewal of IDH2-mutant leukemia cells *ex vivo* or *in vivo*,[134,135] while inhibition of IDH1 was able to promote differentiation and regression of AML xenografts *in vivo*.[136] Promising results of clinical studies on ivosidenib (AG-120, the first inhibitor of mutated IDH1) and enasidenib (AG-221, the inhibitor of the mutated IDH2 protein) were reported.[135,137–140] Based on the reasonable results, from 2017-2019, the FDA approved ivosidenib for adult patients with relapsed or refractory (R/R) or newly diagnosed AML with IDH1 mutation, and enasidenib for the treatment of adult patients with R/R AML with an IDH2 mutation. Consistent with the preclinical data, around 20% of patients with AML treated with ivosidenib experienced differentiation syndrome (DS).[137] Similarly, enasidenib induced leukemic cell differentiation with the emergence of functional mutant IDH2-containing neutrophils in R/R AML patients and differentiation syndrome occurred in about 12% of patients.[141]

Although IDH inhibitors have shown good clinical response in AML with relevant gene mutations, patients still face resistance and relapse. The mechanisms of acquired resistance remain unclear. It was shown that many granulocytes still harbored the driving mutation upon treatment, suggesting that similar to low-dose RA therapy of APL, terminal blast differentiation could have a debulking effect but might not be sufficient for full leukemia clearance.[142] Furthermore, the second site mutations of the allele and the mutual conversion of IDH mutant subtypes are the two possible mechanisms. Hence, a combined treatment with other effective drugs or development of more powerful IDH inhibitors might, to some degree, resolve the problems.

Compounds targeting histone acetylation

HDAC inhibitors

As enzymes catalyzing the deacetylation of histones, HDACs are involved in the control and regulation of cell growth and differentiation. Abnormal expression or mutations of HDACs, together with aberrant histone acetylation patterns, have been found in a broad range of cancer types.[143] HDACs have thus become a novel class of targets in cancer therapy (Figure 3c). Histone deacetylase inhibitors (HDACis) comprise diverse compounds such as suberoylanilide hydroxamic acid (SAHA, vorinostat), valproic acid (VPA), or panobinostat. It has been reported that HDACis promote growth arrest, differentiation, and apoptosis of many solid tumor cells (e.g., lung, prostate, thyroid, and breast cancers, chondrosarcoma, and glioblastoma) and cell lines of hematopoietic malignancy, and exhibit only minimal effects on normal tissues.[73,144–150] For instance, SAHA and VPA were able to induce *in vitro* myeloid differentiation and early apoptosis of Kasumi-1 AML cells, which express AML1-ETO. Similar effects were also reported in a murine xenograft tumor model. Treatment of mice bearing AML1-ETO9a (A/E9a) AML with panobinostat caused an antileukemic response and panobinostat triggered terminal myeloid differentiation via proteasomal degradation of A/E9a.[151] Inspired by preclinical data, many researchers have investigated the effects of HDACis in clinical trials. An early study of SAHA showed efficacy in a panel of hematologic diseases.[152] The compound was applied to the treatment for refractory CTCL and became the first HDACi approved by FDA for this disease. A pilot study combining VPA and ATRA in eight refractory or high-risk AML patients demonstrated clinical benefits in seven cases, with myelomonocytic differentiation of circulating blasts. Although initial promising results were obtained in phase I trials, HDACi as monotherapy or in combination with other drugs failed to improve responses or survival.[153,154] In the future, the effects of the combination of HDACi with conventional cancer treatment should be further explored.

BRD4 inhibitors

BRD4 belongs to the bromodomain and extra-terminal (BET) domain protein family. In addition to serving as a scaffold protein that links acetylated histones and TFs,[155,156] it may also possess HAT activity.[157] BRD4 has been found to be involved not only in numerous physiological processes including development and cellular differentiation but also in driving aberrant transcriptional programs in cancer cells.[155] In 2011, several independent studies showed that BET inhibitors exhibit anti-AML activity in animal models.[158,159] A modest knockdown of BRD4 was sufficient to trigger terminal differentiation and apoptosis in AML cells, and depletion of BRD4 elicited an antiproliferation effect on AML cells.[159] Based on these findings, a number of inhibitors targeting BET proteins have been developed and tested against several tumor types, including leukemia.[160] Among these, small molecules JQ1 showed robust antileukemic effects *in vitro* and *in vivo*, accompanied by terminal myeloid differentiation and elimination of leukemia stem cells.[159] Recently, the first Phase I study of a BET bromodomain inhibitor (OTX-015) in R/R acute leukemia patients was published.[160–162] Clinical responses were identified in a small subset (about 10%) of patients treated at doses near or below the maximum tolerated dose.[160,161] However, all of these patients who obtained a complete remission eventually relapsed while receiving therapy. Hence, although BET inhibition remains a therapeutic strategy for human AML, challenges should be dealt with in exploring more effective BET inhibitors, in determining optimal combination drug regimens to make responses more durable, as well as in identifying predictive correlates of BET inhibitor sensitivity.

Compounds targeting histone methylation

DOT1L inhibitors

MLL gene is one of the epigenetic modifier genes identified through molecular cloning of chromosomal translocations involving 11q23. This gene encodes a SET domain HMT, which catalyzes the methylation of lysine 4 of histoneH3 (H3K4) at specific gene loci.[163] MLL is essential for fetal and adult hematopoiesis in that it regulates the expression of HOX genes and some cofactors key to the expansion and differentiation of HSPCs.[164–166] Abnormalities of MLL gene account for over 70% of infant leukemia and approximately 10% of adult AML, and are correlated to a particularly worse clinical outcome.[167] In addition to MLL translations, MLL partial tandem duplication (PTD) is also reported as a recurrent genetic defect. In the chimerical genes, the catalytic SET domain of MLL is lost and the fusion partners are capable of interacting with a histone H3K79 methyltransferase DOT1L.[168,169] As a result, fusion products not only retain gene-specific recognition elements within the MLL moiety but also gain the ability to recruit DOT1L to these locations. The ectopic H3K79 methylation due to recruitment of DOT1L leads to enhanced expression of leukemogenic genes, such as HOXA9 and MEIS1.[170] Of particular interest is that DOT1L contributes to the transforming activity of MLL fusion and thus functions as a catalytic driver of leukemogenesis.

It has been proposed that inhibition of DOT1L may provide a pharmacologic basis for therapeutic intervention in MLL-related leukemia (Figure 3c). *In vitro* and *in vivo* experiments have demonstrated that EPZ-5676, a specific inhibitor of DOT1L, can selectively kill cells carrying on the MLL gene translocation by causing cell cycle arrest and promoting cell differentiation.[171] Data of phase 1 clinical trial of EPZ-5676 for the treatment of R/R MLL rearranged acute leukemia patient reported that the compound was generally safe and well tolerated (NCT01684150). Eight of the 34 MLL-related patients showed biological or clinical responses,[172] including two complete responses (CRs) and one partial response (PR). Other DOT1L inhibitors such as EPZ4777 and SYC-522 also have been documented to promote differentiation and apoptosis.[173–175] Interestingly, bioinformatics analysis suggested that DOT1L may play a role in the pathogenesis of breast cancer. *In vitro* study has shown that DOT1L inhibition selectively inhibited proliferation, self-renewal, and metastatic potential of breast cancer cells and induced cell differentiation.[176]

LSD1 inhibitors
Histone lysine demethylase LSD1 (also known as KDM1A) demethylates di- and mono-methylated K4 on histone H3, leading to reduced levels of H3K4me3. It has been shown that LSD1 exerts a wide range of impact on transcriptional programs, acting either as a transcriptional repressor or as an activator depending on the cellular context.[105] Pharmacological inhibition or genetic depletion of LSD1 induced differentiation of MLL-driven AML stem cells and that of other genetically defined AML subtypes.[177] Tranylcypromine (TCP), a LSD1 inhibitor, could induce the expression of myeloid differentiation genes in AML cells and reactivate the ATRA-driven therapeutic response in non-APL AML.[178] Recently, two novel LSD1 inhibitors, NCD25 and NCD38, were identified for their ability to inhibit leukemia growth and induce myeloid differentiation.[179] The LSD1 inhibitors GSK2879552 and IMG-7289, alone or in combination with ATRA, showed promising activity against AML *in vitro*,[180] leading to two ongoing phase I trials for patients with R/R AML (NCT0217782, NCT02842827) and to a phase I/II trial for MDS patients (NCT02929498).

PRMT5 inhibitors
Arginine residues within H3 or H4 histone can be methylated by protein arginine methyltransferases (PRMTs). Moreover, PRMTs could also modify nonhistone substrates, such as AML1 and ASH2L proteins, and may thus play pivotal roles in a wide range of cellular processes.[105] Overexpression of PRMTs is often present in various cancers including leukemia, rendering these enzymes particularly intriguing as therapeutic targets.[181] Within the PRMT family members, PRMT5 catalyzes symmetric dimethylarginine of histone proteins to induce gene silencing by generating repressive histone markers, including H2AR3me2s, H3R8me2s, and H4R3me2s. PRMT5 can also methylate nonhistone proteins such as the TFs p53, E2F1, and p65, indicating the multiple roles of this enzyme in physiological and pathological situations.[182] Of note, PRMT5 specific inhibitor EPZ015666 was recently reported to rescue the differentiation block of human leukemic cells *in vitro* and in a mouse model of MLL-rearranged leukemia,[183] shedding light on its potential clinic application.

Agents targeting other pathways for potential differentiation therapy

DHODH inhibitors
The application of inhibitors of the de novo nucleotide biosynthetic pathways, crucial for the proliferation of living entities, offers therapeutic opportunities for the treatment of autoimmune diseases and cancer.[184] Dihydroorotate dehydrogenase (DHODH), a rate-limiting enzyme in *de novo* pyrimidine biosynthesis, converts L-dihydroorotate (DHO) to orotate (ORO). Recently, high-throughput drug screening was performed to identify new differentiation inducers for AML cells, and inhibitors targeting DHODH attracted attention.[185] Brequinar, a potent and selective DHODH inhibitor, was found to induce the differentiation of AML cells accompanied by a decrease albeit not a complete depletion of LICs, an effect similar to the one observed with RA treatment of APL mouse models. Then, BAY 2402234, also a selective and orally bioavailable DHODH inhibitor, showed monotherapeutic efficacy and differentiation-inducing effect across multiple AML subtypes.[186] Meanwhile, a compound with highly potent DHODH inhibitory effect, ASLAN003, was announced to induce differentiation and to reduce the proliferation/viability of AML cells *ex vivo* and in mice models.[187] These discoveries highlighted the potential of DHODH as an *in vivo* therapeutic target for AML differentiation therapy, raising the possibility of advancing them to future clinical trials. Until now, three Phase 1b/2a multi-center clinical trials are ongoing respectively to assess the safety, tolerability and efficacy of brequinar (NCT03760666), BAY 2402234 (NCT03404726), and ASLAN003 (NCT03451084) in adult AML patients.

FLT3 inhibitors
FLT3 ligand (FL) has a significant role in the proliferation and differentiation of hematopoietic cells. Mutations in the FLT3 receptor gene have been reported in 30% of patients with AML, including FLT3-ITD (internal tandem duplication) and FLT3-TKD (tyrosine kinase domain) point mutations.[188] It has been well established that FLT3-ITD confers a poor prognosis in AML patients with standard CT regimens. Given the pathological and prognostic role that FLT3-ITD mutations play in AML, mutant FLT3 represents an attractive therapeutic target. In fact, several FLT3 inhibitors have been developed and are currently in clinical trials. These agents work largely through competitive inhibition of ATP-binding sites in the FLT3 receptor, leading to cell cycle arrest and differentiation. Notably, in 13 of 14 FLT3-ITD AML patients with normal karyotype treated with quizartinib, a potent and selective FLT3 inhibitor, terminal myeloid differentiation of BM blasts was observed in association with a clinical DS.[189] This clinical DS was nevertheless different from that observed in APL. The increase of WBC count during the ATRA treatment of APL is presumably because of a much larger fraction of the leukemic burden undergoing differentiation, whereas in FLT3-ITD AML,

the majority of the malignant cells undergo apoptosis relatively rapidly, followed by gradual differentiation of the residual BM blasts. The "surge" of the absolute neutrophil count after this differentiation is, therefore, much more modest than that seen in APL. Sorafenib is one of the first-generation FLT3 inhibitors, which is less specific for FLT3 and has a broad kinase inhibitory effect with more off-target toxicities. Sorafenib had limited single-agent activity in AML, with marrow remissions observed in <10% of patients.[190] The clinical results with sorafenib were more promising when used in combination.[191] Recently, *in vitro* treatment combing low doses of sorafenib and selinex, an XPO1 (Exportin 1, a NR exporter) inhibitor, promoted myeloid differentiation of AML cells without noticeable cell killing.[192] The combinatorial therapy demonstrated profound *in vivo* antileukemia efficacy in a human FLT3-mutated xenograft model. In an ongoing Phase IB clinical trial the selinex/sorafenib combination induced complete/partial remissions in 6 of 14 refractory AML patients (ClinicalTrials.gov: NCT02530476).

MAPK inhibitors
As mentioned previously, assessing differentiation is more difficult in solid tumors than in leukemia, because the genetic basis of most solid tumors involves the cooperation of multiple oncogenic pathways and is thus considerably more complex than that of leukemia. In addition, tissue sampling cannot be easily repeated and *ex vivo* cultures are rarely possible for solid tumors. Thus, differentiation therapy for some solid tumors refers to the processes that induce CSCs into terminally differentiated cancer cells, or convert malignant cells to a more benign phenotype, and then re-sensitize the patients to current therapy. Metastatic thyroid cancers that are refractory to radioiodine (iodine-131) are associated with a poor prognosis. Several trials have evaluated strategies to "re-differentiate" metastatic thyroid cancers and render them responsive to radioiodine, including trials evaluating retinoids and lithium, which only yielded a modest clinical benefit. Recently, the MAPK pathway inhibitors showed promising effects on thyroid cancer. Approximately 70% of papillary thyroid cancers had mutually exclusive gene mutations encoding the growth factor receptors RET or NTRK1, the three RAS family genes (N, H, K), and BRAF. Constitutive activation of these proteins stimulated mitogen-activated protein kinase (MAPK) signaling, which inhibited the expression of thyroid hormone biosynthesis genes.[193] In mouse models of thyroid cancer, selective MAPK pathway inhibitors increased the expression of the sodium–iodide symporter and uptake of iodine.[194] A clinical study showed that the MAPK kinase (MEK) 1 and MEK2 inhibitor selumetinib (AZD6244, ARRY-142886) could reverse refractoriness to radioiodine in patients with metastatic thyroid cancer.[193] Combination of selumetinib with EZH2 inhibitor tazemetostat enhanced differentiation of papillary thyroid cancer cells harboring BRAF V600E mutation through synergistically decreasing global trimethylation of H3K27.[195] These studies demonstrated modest clinical and biologic activity of MEK inhibitors in thyroid tumors. However, to eradicate cancer and prevent recurrence, differentiation strategies require additional research and development.

In the past decades, the studies on cancer differentiation inducers gradually take momentum. Of particular interest is the model disease APL, where differentiation-inducing agents have been demonstrated to exert a curative effect in the great majority of patients. Besides, some other differentiation-induction agents have shown promising effects in preclinical experiments and clinical trials. Differentiation therapy for cancers, although still in its relative infancy, has given hope to a large number of cancer patients.

APL as a successful model of cancer differentiation therapy

APL is the M3 subtype of AML, characterized not only by distinct clinical manifestations but also by unique molecular pathogenesis and effective target-based differentiation therapy.

Clinical treatment strategies in APL

APL was first described in 1957 as the most malignant form of acute leukemia.[196] Patients with APL show specific features: a very rapid fatal natural course of only a few weeks' duration, an accumulation of abnormal promyelocytes in bone marrow, and a severe bleeding syndrome due to disseminated intravascular coagulation (DIC) or hyperfibrinolysis. In the era before ATRA-based therapy, only 23–35% of the APL patients could have a 5-year survival by CT.[197] Inspired by the Chinese philosophy of educational approach in health maintenance and the Western medical science of induction of cancer cell differentiation, scientists from Shanghai Institute of Hematology (SIH) carried out the research on leukemia differentiation therapy since the late 1970s.[197]

In 1980, a group from the United States published the results of *in vitro* terminal differentiation of HL-60 cells upon the effect of 13-cRA.[57] Clinical improvement or CR after treatment with 13-cRA in a few isolated cases of APL were then reported, accompanied by maturation of promyelocytes with disappearance of signs of coagulopathy.[198–200] The SIH group, on the other hand, was focused on the potential therapeutic effects of ATRA. The first clinical trial of ATRA was reported in 24 APL cases (16 newly diagnosed and 8 anthracycline refractory cases) who were treated with ATRA alone.[201] CR was achieved in all patients and the evidence of *in vivo* blast differentiation with Auer's rods in polynucleated granulocytes was documented. The results have been quickly confirmed by a large amount of clinical practices around the world.[56,197] ATRA therapy became the standard for induction of newly diagnosed APL patients, which was then further improved stepwise through the effective combination regimen of ATRA with CT. Moreover, the roles of ATRA and CT in consolidation or maintenance therapy have been verified to reduce the incidence of relapse. By using this protocol, 5-year OS was up to about 70%.[73,197,202–204] The routine prescription of ATRA is 45 mg/m^2/day, while the recommended dosage of ATRA in the SIH is 25 mg/m^2/day. The reason to reduce the initial dose of ATRA is to avoid ATRA toxicity but to achieve the same therapeutic effects as the conventional dosage.[205]

Even though the ATRA/CT combination was considered a very efficient anti-APL therapy, up to about 30% of APL patients still ended with relapse.[206–208] The introduction of arsenic trioxide (ATO) since the early 1990s has further changed the clinical landscape of APL. *In vitro* studies showed that ATO exerts dose-dependent effects on APL cells including differentiation and apoptosis, although the differentiation is only a partial one compared with that induced by ATRA.[209] Clinically, refractory or relapsed APL after ATRA/CT therapy as well as newly diagnosed APL could achieve CR, suggesting an absence of cross-resistance between ATRA and ATO.[210] Therefore, new therapeutic strategies have focused on minimizing CT and administering ATRA plus ATO as primary therapy. Indeed, the ATRA-/ATO-based protocol yielded a much longer survival in newly diagnosed APL compared with therapy with ATRA or ATO alone.[197,211,212] These outcomes

Table 1 Sanz score for APL risk stratification.[a]

Characteristic	Low risk	Intermediate risk	High risk
WBC (×10^9/L)	≤10	≤10	>10
Platelets (×10^9/L)	>40	≤40	≤40

[a]Source: Data from Krivtsov and Armstrong.[165]

were even not influenced by FLT3 mutation status, which was a poor prognostic factor in APL patients treated with ATRA and CT.[213] Combination of ATRA and ATO have obtained about 95% of CR rate and 5-year OS were more than 90%.[211] Of note, the combination therapy with ATRA and ATO improved outcomes compared with ATRA and CT with very high EFS and OS rates (97% and 99%, respectively) in low-to-intermediate risk APL by Sanz Score (Table 1).[214–216] Furthermore, the latest clinical study showed that combination of ATRA and ATO could replace or reduce chemotherapy in consolidation therapy for the APL patients in different risk subgroups (Ref. 259). The classical stratification system (Sanz model) is widely used in estimating the APL risk in many clinical trials and daily practice, however, the concept of risk stratification should be renewed with the evolving of the treatment paradigm. Recently, a systematic analysis of APL genomics and transcriptomics in the APL2012 trial allowed to establish a comprehensive risk stratification system for precision treatment of APL by combining the three parameters, namely NRAS mutation, levels of APL22 score and WBC count (Ref. 260). Based on the results of these studies, both the US Food and Drug Administration (FDA) and the European Medicines Agency (EMA) have recently approved ATO for the treatment of newly diagnosed patients with low-to-intermediate risk APL (defined as WBC count ≤10 × 10^9/L). The conventional administration of ATO is the intravenous route. An oral formulation of ATO was also found to be active in relapsed APL and has subsequently been evaluated in upfront management. Another formulation of arsenic in advanced clinical investigation is tetra-arsenic tetra-sulfide ($A_{S4}S_4$) and an oral $A_{S4}S_4$-containing formula named the Realgar–Indigo naturalis formula (RIF) in traditional Chinese Medicine was used in APL patients.[217,218] No significant differences were noted between the RIF and intravenously administered ATO groups with regard to the CR rate, OS or DFS.[219–222] These trials have established the feasibility and safety of prolonged oral arsenic administration, but long-term safety data are still required. Oral arsenic formulations are not currently available in the United States or Europe. Based on these results, now the combination of ATRA and arsenic has been the first-line strategy for APL patients. The recommendation of APL treatment is listed in Tables 2 and 3.

As the prognosis of APL patients is getting much better, the issues of early mortality (related to bleeding, DS, or infection) and relapse [including central nerve system (CNS) relapse] becomes increasingly important. In patients with clinical and pathologic features of APL, ATRA should be started upon first suspicion of APL without waiting for genetic confirmation of the diagnosis.[223] Early initiation of ATRA may prevent the lethal complication of bleeding. DS is a common complication in the ATRA or ATO treatment, with a frequency being around 25% both in the United States and in Europe,[224,225] but relatively rare in East Asian populations (5–10%).[203,211] Signs and symptoms of this syndrome include hyperleukocytosis, dyspnea with interstitial pulmonary infiltrates, peripheral edema, unexplained fever, weight gain, hypotension, and acute renal failure. The mortality could be down to 3% or lower if DS is recognized early and treated promptly with CT and high dose of dexamethasone (10 mg twice daily).[225,226] In addition, patients with a high white blood cell count (WBC > 30 × 10^9/L) at diagnosis may benefit from prophylactic steroids. A common practice to avoid CNS prophylaxis (methotrexate 5–10 mg, cytarabine 40–50 mg, and dexamethasone 5 mg) for APL patients are recommended, four to six times for non-high-risk APL and six to eight times for the patients with high WBC counts.[223] Another issue is side effects of ATO because the compound has long been considered as a very strong poison. In fact, the protocol incorporating ATO proves to be quite safe. The common adverse effects such as minor bone marrow myelosuppression, hepatotoxicity, gastrointestinal reactions, and neurotoxicity can be controlled and are generally reversible without need of the discontinuation of the drug.[211,223] In very rare situations, clinically significant

Table 2 The recommendation of APL treatment (Chinese guideline in 2018).

	Non-high-risk APL	High-risk APL
Induction therapy	ATRA 25 mg/m^2/d + ATO 0.16 mg/kg/d or RIF 60 mg/kg/d until complete remission (about 1 month) HU 20–40 mg/kg/d (when WBC > 10 × 10^9/L)	ATRA 25 mg/m^2/d + ATO 0.16mg/kg/d or RIF 60 mg/kg/d until complete remission (about 1 month) + IDA 8 mg/m^2/d or DNR 45 m/m^2/d × 1–3
Consolidation therapy	Strategy 1 ATRA 25 mg/m^2/d for 2 weeks every 4 weeks × 7 cycles + ATO 0.16 mg/kg/d or RIF 60 mg/kg/d for 4 weeks every 8 weeks × 4 cycles Strategy 2 Chemotherapy for 2–3 cycles until MRD (−) DA: DNR 45 mg/m^2/d × 3 + Ara-C 100 mg/m^2/d × 5 Or MA: MTZ 6–8 mg/m^2/d × 3 + Ara-C 100 mg/m^2/d × 5 Or HA: HHT 2 mg/m^2/d × 7 + Ara-C 100 mg/m^2/d × 5 Or IA: IDA 8 mg/m^2/d × 3 + Ara-C 100 mg/m^2/d × 5	Strategy 1 Chemotherapy for 2–3 cycles until MRD (−) DA: DNR 45 mg/m^2/d × 3 + Ara-C 100 mg/m^2/d × 5 Or MA: MTZ 6–8 mg/m^2/d × 3 + Ara-C 100 mg/m^2/d × 5 Or HA: HHT 2 mg/m^2/d×7 + Ara-C 100mg/m^2/d×5 Or IA: IDA 8 mg/m^2/d × 3 + Ara-C 100 mg/m^2/d × 5 Strategy 2 ATRA 25 mg/m^2/d + ATO 0.16 mg/kg/d days 1–28 × 2 cycles
Maintenance therapy	Strategy 1 (Optional) ATRA 25 mg/m^2 for 2 weeks of weeks 1–4, then ATO 0.16 mg/kg/d or RIF 60 mg/kg/d for 2 weeks every 4 weeks of weeks 5–12 × 3 cycles Strategy 2 ATRA 25 mg/m^2 for 2 weeks of weeks 1–4, then ATO 0.16 mg/kg/d or RIF 60 mg/kg/d for 2 weeks every 4 weeks of weeks 5–12 × 8 cycles	Strategy 1 ATRA 25 mg/m^2 for 2 weeks of weeks 1–4, then ATO 0.16 mg/kg/d or RIF 60 mg/kg/d for 2 weeks every 4 weeks of weeks 5–12 × 8 cycles Strategy 2 ATRA 25 mg/m^2/d for 2 weeks, then 6-MP 50–90 mg/m^2/d for 3 months + MTX 5–15 mg/m^2 once weekly × 11 weeks × 8 cycles

Abbreviations: BM, bone marrow; HU, hydroxyurea; IDA, idarubicin; DNR, daunorubicin; Ara-C, cytarabine; MTZ, mitozantrone; HHT, homoharringtonine; IDA, idarubicin; 6-MP, 6-mercaptopurine; MTX, methotrexate; MRD (−), minimal residual disease negative, qPCR result negative for PML-RARα.

Table 3 The recommendation of APL treatment (NCCN guideline 2020).

	Induction therapy	Consolidation therapy
High-risk APL[a]	ATRA 45 mg/m²/d (days 1–36) + Idarubicin 6–12 mg/m²/d on days 2, 4, 6, 8 + ATO 0.15 mg/kg/d (days 9–36) until BM remission (bone marrow aspirate and biopsy day 28)	ATRA 45 mg/m²/d × 28 + ATO 0.15 mg/kg/d × 28 days × 1 cycle, then ATRA 45 mg/m²/d × 7 days/2 weeks × 3 + ATO 0.15 mg/kg/d × 5 days for 5 weeks × 1 cycle)
	ATRA 45 mg/m²/d + ATO 0.15 mg/kg/d until BM remission (bone marrow aspirate and biopsy day 28) + a single dose of gemtuzumab ozogamicin 9 mg/m² one day 1 or day 2 or day 3 or day 4	ATO 0.15 mg/kg/d × 5 days/week for 4 weeks every 8 weeks × 4 cycles + ATRA 45 mg/m²/d for 2 weeks every 4 weeks × 7 cycles. If ATRA or ATO discontinued due to toxicity, a single dose of gemtuzumab ozogamicin 9 mg/m² once every 4–5 weeks until 28 weeks from CR
	ATRA 45 mg/m²/d + ATO 0.3 mg/kg/d IV on days 1–5 of week one and 0.25 mg/kg twice weekly in weeks 2–8 until BM remission (bone marrow aspirate and biopsy day 28) + a single dose of gemtuzumab ozogamicin 9 mg/m² one day 1 or day 2 or day 3 or day 4	ATRA 45 mg/m²/d for 2 weeks every 4 weeks × 4 cycles ATO 0.3 mg/kg/d IV on days 1–5 of week 1 and 0.25 mg/kg twice weekly in weeks 2–4 × 4 cycles. If ATRA or ATO discontinued due to toxicity, a single dose of gemtuzumab ozogamicin 9 mg/m² once every 4–5 weeks until 28 weeks from CR
	ATRA 45 mg/m²/d until BM remission (bone marrow aspirate and biopsy day 28) + DNR 50 m/m²/d × 4 days (days 3–6) + Ara-C 200 mg/m²/d × 7 days (days 3-9)	ATO 0.15 mg/kg/d × 5 days/week × 5 weeks × 2 cycles, then ATRA 45 mg/m²/d × 7 days + DNR 50 mg/m²/d × 3 days for 2 cycles
	ATRA 45 mg/m²/d until BM remission (bone marrow aspirate and biopsy day 28) + DNR 60 m/m²/d × 3 days + Ara-C 200 mg/m²/d × 7 days	DNR 60 mg/m²/d × 3 days + Ara-C 200 mg/m²/d × 7 days, then DNR 45 mg/m²/d × days + Ara-C 1.5–2 g/m² Q12h × 3 days)
	ATRA 45 mg/m²/d until BM remission (bone marrow aspirate and biopsy day 28) + idarubicin 12 mg/m²/d on days 2, 4, 6, 8	ATRA 45 mg/m²/d × 15 days + IDA 5 mg/m²/d × 3 days + Ara-C 1 g/m²/d × 4 days, then ATRA × 15 days + MTZ 10 mg/m²/d × 5 days, then ATRA × days + IDA 12 mg/m²/d × 1 day + Ara-C 150 mg/m² Q8h × 4 days
Low-risk APL	ATRA 45 mg/m²/d + ATO 0.15 mg/kg/d until BM remission (bone marrow aspirate and biopsy day 28–35 if cytopenia)	ATO 0.15 mg/kg/d × 5 days/week for 4 weeks every 8 weeks × 4 cycles + ATRA 45 mg/m²/d for 2 weeks every 4 weeks × 7 cycles
	ATRA 45 mg/m²/d + ATO 0.3 mg/kg/d IV on days 1–5 of week one and 0.25 mg/kg twice weekly in weeks 2–8 until BM remission (bone marrow aspirate and biopsy day 28–35 if cytopenia)	ATRA 45 mg/m²/d × 2 weeks/4 weeks × 4 cycles ATO 0.3 mg/kg/d IV on days 1–5 of week one and 0.25 mg/kg twice weekly in weeks 2–4/4 weeks × 4 cycles
	ATRA 45 mg/m²/d until clinical remission + Idarubicin 12 mg/m²/d on days 2, 4, 6, 8	ATRA 45 mg/m²/d × 15 days + IDA 5 mg/m²/d × 4 days, then ATRA 45 mg/m²/d × 15 days + MTX 10 mg/m²/d × 3 days, then (ATRA 45 mg/m²/d × 15 days + IDA 12 mg/m²/d × 1 day

Abbreviations: NCCN, US National Comprehensive Cancer Network; DNR, daunorubicin; Ara-C, cytarabine; BM, bone marrow; IDA, idarubicin; MTZ, mitozantrone; HHT, homoharringtonine; 6-MP, 6-mercaptopurine; MTX, methotrexate.
[a]For the high-risk APL, if the patient has low ejection fraction, chemotherapy should be avoided; if the patient has prolonged QTc, ATO and chemotherapy should be avoided.

arrhythmias due to prolongation of the QT interval on the ECG are observed, which can be avoided with appropriate precautions and withdrawal of the medicine.[227] At the same time, arsenic concentrations in the urine of patients who had ceased maintenance treatment for 2 years were below the safety limits recommended by government agencies in several countries or regions, whereas arsenic levels in plasma, nails, and hair were only slightly higher than those found in healthy controls.[211]

Leukemogenesis and therapeutic mechanisms of APL

It has been well known that PML-RARα resulting from t(15;17)(q22;q21) translocation is the key driver of APL leukemogenesis, which exerts dominant-negative effects on RARα-and PML-related pathways.[228] The functional regulation of retinoids and their receptors (including RARα) has been described in the previous part (agents targeting aberrant TFs). While, PML belongs to the TRIM family of protein, defined by the presence of a RING domain, one or two other zinc fingers (B boxes), and a long coiled-coil domain. In normal cells, PML proteins multimerize to form multiprotein subnuclear structures called PML-nuclear bodies (PML-NBs).[229] PML-NBs have been shown to play an important role in DNA damage repair, apoptosis, growth, senescence, and angiogenesis, and more recently, in the maintenance of HSPCs.[230] Recently, it was reported that RING domain tetramerization is required for PML-NBs biogenesis and PML sumoylation.[231] The fusion protein interferes with the normal functions of both RARα and PML, which represses the transcriptional expression of target genes essential for hematopoietic differentiation and yields an increasing proliferation and self-renewal of LICs.[228,232,233] PML-RARα binding to RXR co-receptor functions as a constitutive transcriptional repressor at RAREs of target genes through recruitment of CoR, which leads to the characteristic differentiation block.[197,232,234] In APL cells, PML-NBs are disrupted owing to the formation of PML/PML-RARα heterocomplex, interfering with the normal biological functions of PML.[234] This mechanism probably cooperates with the disruption of the RAR/RXR pathway to enforce the APL-specific differentiation block and acquisition of self-renewal, thus transforming the committed HSPCs into immortal, fully transformed LICs (Figure 4).

Combining the discovery of PML-RARα in APL pathogenesis with special effective treatment of ATRA and ATO has pointed to a possible molecular mechanism underlying PML-RARα-specific therapy. Indeed, a large number of studies have revealed that ATRA and ATO act through distinct but complementary mechanisms, providing a biologic rationale for the two agents to be used in combination to achieve synergistic efficacy with low toxicity. At pharmacological level (10^{-7}–10^{-6} mol/L), ATRA binds to the ligand-binding domain (LBD) of RARα portion in the fusion protein and induces a conformational change of the chimerical receptor.[235,236] This leads to displacement of CoR complexes and recruitment of CoA complexes and clearance of PML-RARα from promoters of target genes, thereby restoring wild-type RARα function and subverting the differentiation block.[68,197,234,237] ATRA also leads to the degradation of PML-RARα oncoprotein,[238–240] which may contribute to the response, and generate a restoration

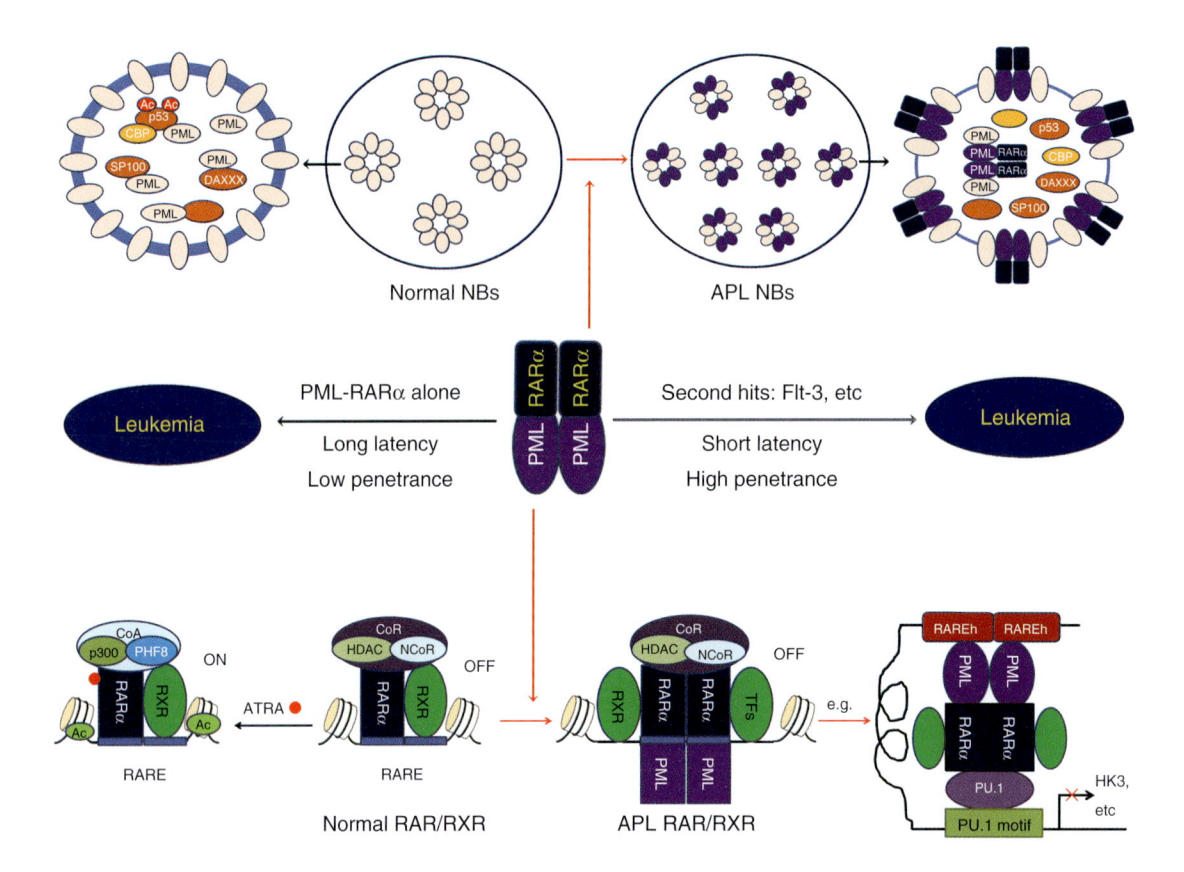

Figure 4 Molecular pathogenesis of APL. PML-RARα plays a key role in leukemogenesis of APL, which exerts dominant-negative effects on RARα- and PML-related pathways. Under physiological condition, RAR/RXR heterodimers bind to the specific motifs defined as RAREs on the promoters of target genes and differentially activates or represses gene transcription while recruiting CoA or CoR complex depend on the presence or absence of the ligands, such as ATRA. The fusion protein binding to RXR co-receptor functions as a constitutive transcriptional repressor at RAREs of target genes through recruitment of CoR. On the other hand, PML proteins multimerize to form multiprotein subnuclear structures called PML-nuclear bodies (PML-NBs) in normal cells. In APL cells, PML-NBs are disrupted owing to the formation of PML/PML-RARα heterocomplex.

of nuclear architecture with the reformation of PML-NBs. Re-establishment of RARα signaling allows differentiation of APL blasts and yields short-term disease management. Even though ATRA and anthracyclines are very efficient anti-APL therapies, APL patients can relapse, perhaps due to ATRA failing to affect LICs. ATO exerts dose-dependent effects on APL cells in initial cellular and molecular mechanistic studies.[209,241] At low concentrations, ATO induces partial morphologic differentiation in APL cells, whereas at high concentrations, apoptosis induction occurs predominantly. Both effects are associated with a degradation of PML-RARα. Arsenic efficiently triggers the degradation of PML-RARα and PML through direct binding to the RBCC domain of PML moiety, which induces the conformational changes of PML proteins, leading to protein–protein aggregation and sumoylation of these proteins.[241–243] In addition, ATO-induced oxidative stress promotes PML homodimerization by cross-linking PML via disulfide bonds.[244] Sumoylated PML and PML-RARα recruit the ubiquitin ligase RNF4 and are subject to proteasome-mediated proteolysis.[245,246] Besides, arsenic can act through other mechanisms independent of PML-RARα status, such as pro-apoptotic effects mediated by the mitochondria-mediated pathway, DNA damage, telomerase activity, autophagy, and so on.[197,247] Notably, ATO could induce LIC eradication in APL through several pathways, which may be a key factor in the success of ATO for APL patients.[197,233,237,247,248] Sufficient and rapid degradation of PML and PML-RARα is required for LIC clearance and long-term disease eradication,[248,249] which can be obtained by ATO treatment.

Arsenic can also facilitate the elimination of LICs through inhibiting Notch pathway, antagonizing the Hedgehog–Gli pathway, and repressing NF-κB and β-catenin. The pleiotropic behaviors may be the reason why arsenic is very active in APL, as a single agent as well as in combination.

Because ATRA and ATO target respectively the C- and N-terminals of PML-RARα, enhanced degradation of PML-RARα oncoprotein might provide a plausible explanation for the superior efficacy of combination therapy in patients. Intriguingly, consistent with the mechanistic researches, genetic mutations in the LBD of the RARα moiety that interfere with ATRA binding or nuclear coregulators binding are observed in about 40% of relapsed APL patients treated with ATRA/CT,[250–252] while genetic mutations in the PML moiety of the PML-RARα oncogene that probably impair the direct binding of ATO to PML-RARα in patients with clinical ATO resistance have been described after treatment with ATRA/ATO/CT.[253,254] A small number of APL patients harbor PLZF-RARα fusion gene resulting from t(11;17)(q23;q21), which are resistant to ATRA and ATO therapy.[255,256] These data further support that PML-RARα is the direct target of both ATRA and ATO. Several groups have shown that ATRA and ATO display a synergy in many pathways including TFs and cofactors, activation of calcium signaling, stimulation of the IFN pathway, activation of the proteasome system, cell cycle arrest, gain of apoptotic potential, downregulation of telomerase, and telomere length, upregulation of cAMP/PKA activity, and enhanced arsenic uptake by APL cells through induced expression of cell membrane arsenic

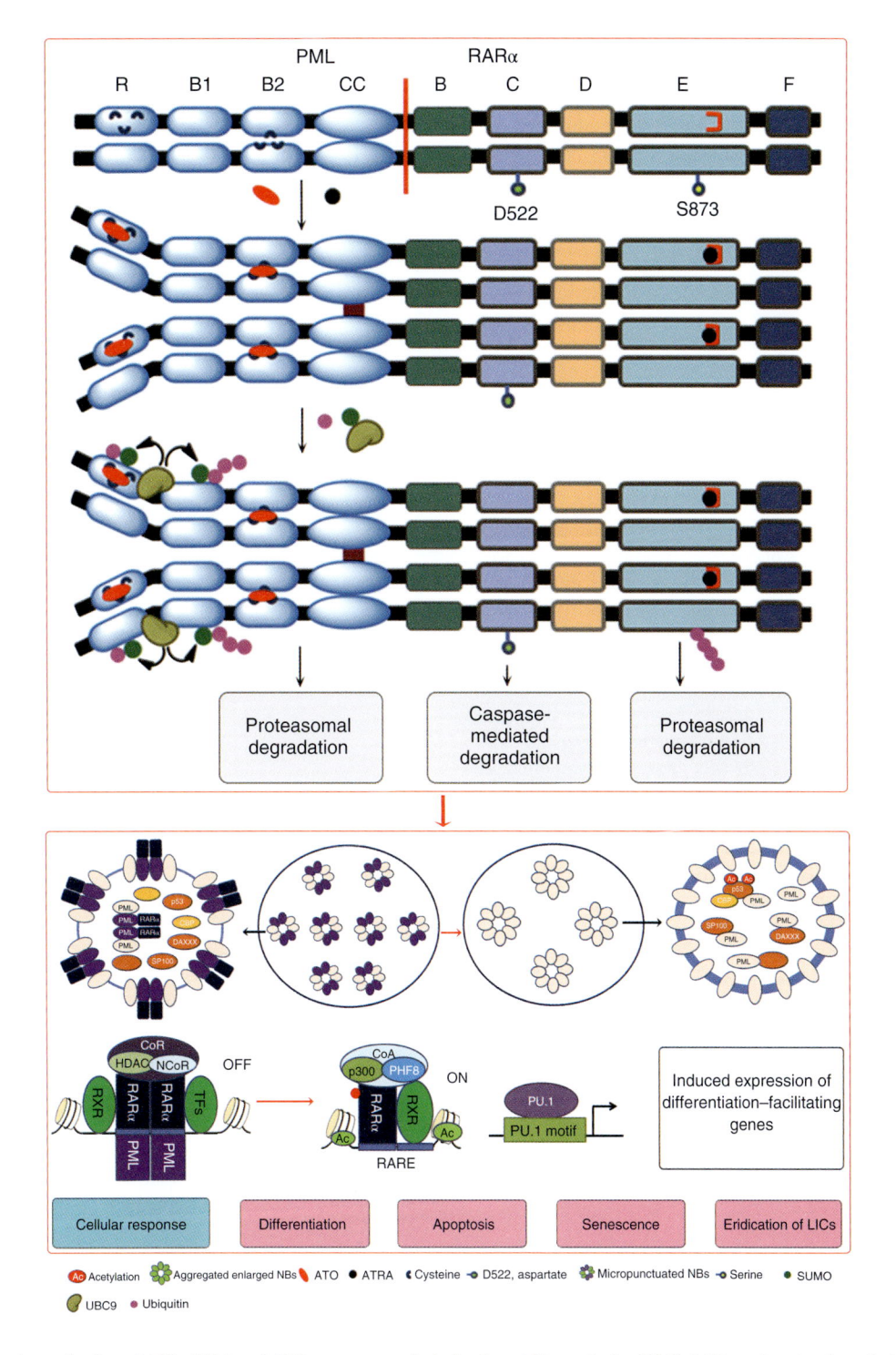

Figure 5 Therapeutic mechanism of APL. ATRA and ATO target respectively the C- and N-terminals of PML-RARα, enhancing degradation of PML-RARα oncoprotein. ATRA binds to the LBD of RARα portion in the fusion protein and ATO binds to the RBCC domain of PML moiety, which induces the conformational change and the consequential degradation of the fusion protein. The degradation of PML-RARα generates a restoration of nuclear architecture with the reformation of PML-NBs. ATRA binding also leads to displacement of CoR complexes and recruitment of CoA complexes and clear PML-RARα from promoters of target genes, thereby restoring wild-type RARα function. The synergistic effects of ATRA and ATO result in a variety of cellular response including differentiation, apoptosis, and senescence of leukemic cells, and importantly, the eradication of leukemia-initiating cells LICs.

transporter (AQP9).[197,232,257,258] Recent studies have shown that the ATRA/ATO combination rapidly clears PML-RARα+ LICs, resulting in APL eradication and obviously prolonged survival in murine models.[233,249] All these findings may contribute to the dramatically improved response from APL patients under the treatment of ATRA and ATO combination.

In conclusion, ATRA and ATO exert different but cross-linked actions on APL cells. ATRA mainly works through transcriptional modulation, and the main effects of ATO occur at the protein level, while both agents target PML-RARα. These data may further explain the lack of cross-resistance between the two agents (Figure 5). Therapy of APL with ATRA and ATO is to date the most successful example of cancer differentiation therapy, and key factor can be the synergistic targeting of the oncoprotein by the two agents. This scientific history may hence serve as a template for subsequent development of similar treatments in other leukemias and solid tumors. More importantly, the story of APL provides a new way for thinking that differentiation therapy is essentially target therapy on the molecules affecting differentiation pathway and combination or synergistic targeting strategy is highly effective to eliminate CSCs.

Perspectives

Taken together, differentiation therapy against cancer has the potential to make tumor cells convert from a malignant path to a benign course, which has given hope to scientists and clinicians on a much better cancer treatment outcome. However, interest and application of differentiation-based therapy for solid tumors and hematological malignancies other than APL are just at the beginning. One major challenge is the complexity of histopathological subtypes and clinical stages of cancers, resulting in the absence of developmental models of cancer progression. The re-establishment of the genotype that characterizes the original tissue types and the morphological transformation of tumor cells to the normal cells may help determine more successful differentiation induction. In addition, there have not yet been definite markers for evaluating the effects of differentiation inducers. Assessment of the precise therapeutic role of agents is often hampered by the difficulties in distinguishing *in vivo* cytotoxicity from differentiation. The classic evaluation of therapeutic responses mainly focuses on the shrinkage of the tumor mass, but this is not suitable for the response evaluation of differentiation therapy that just restores the differentiation program of tumor cells. Consequently, identifying accurate novel biomarker sets of response to differentiation therapy becomes urgent for clinical application. Recent evidence suggests that targeting leukemia driver proteins other than PML-RARα can induce cell differentiation in some other types of AML and can eventually yield high-quality CR, paving the way for enlarging this approach in hematological malignancies. Nevertheless, solid tumors are still viewed as much more heterogeneous aberrant tissues than most leukemia, and much more complex molecular mechanisms are involved in their pathogenesis. Hence, the development of differentiation therapy in solid tumors may need a more comprehensive approach to combine CT, immunotherapy, and differentiation agents in order to produce multiplied synergistic targeting effects.

Summary

Most human cancers show characteristics of abnormal cell differentiation, often coupled with dysregulation of proliferation, apoptosis, and/or senescence. Cancer cells may be blocked at a particular stage of differentiation along with the involved cellular lineage, or they may differentiate into an inappropriate cell type. Hence, cancer differentiation therapy represents the approach aimed at the re-activation of endogenous differentiation programs or subverting differentiation/maturation blockage within cancer cells, often accompanied by the loss of malignant phenotype and the restoration, at least in part, of the normal phenotype.

Many agents have been identified to show differentiation-inducing effect on cancer cells *in vitro* and *ex vivo*. Therapy-induced differentiation can be easily monitored in AML because normal hematopoietic cells differentiate rapidly and a broad range of surface markers and well-defined morphological features for differentiated cells exist. To trigger malignant cells to overcome their differentiation block and to enter the apoptotic pathways has become an elegant alternative to the therapies simply killing malignant cells. However, initial differentiation therapy attempts in patients failed to induce reasonable clinical remission because it had historically been hampered by many factors, especially due to the insufficient understanding of the pathways of normal cell differentiation and the much higher complexity of the process of cancer cell reversion to "normal" cells/tissues induced by differentiation therapy than the cytotoxic approaches. Of note, terminal maturation rapidly clears tumor bulk, while modifying the self-renewal of cancer-initiating cells has a delayed impact. Thus, only full, and not partial, differentiation-driven loss of self-renewal of clonogenic cells would be predicted to have a long-term impact on cancer eradication. The advancement of differentiation therapy to a real successful clinical practice was not realized until the use of ATRA and ATO in the treatment of APL. This breakthrough has transformed APL from once a fatal disease to one of the most curable human cancers, with 5-year OS rates of more than 90%. In addition, over the past several years, progress has been made in understanding the differentiation pathways that are also cross-talking with those of the regulation of cell proliferation and survival, and the development of some targeted therapies on other types of leukemia has already yielded promising differentiation-inducing effects, which need to be further explored clinically.

This article focuses on the basic theories of differentiation therapy, and the clinical achievements of this novel therapeutic approach.

Key references

The complete reference list can be found on Vital Source version of this title, see inside front cover.

1. Boyer LA, Lee TI, Cole MF, et al. Core transcriptional regulatory circuitry in human embryonic stem cells. *Cell.* 2005;**122**:947–956.
5. Takahashi K, Yamanaka S. Induction of pluripotent stem cells from mouse embryonic and adult fibroblast cultures by defined factors. *Cell.* 2006;**126**:663–676.
10. Riddell J, Gazit R, Garrison BS, et al. Reprogramming committed murine blood cells to induced hematopoietic stem cells with defined factors. *Cell.* 2014;**157**:549–564.
21. Chen T, Dent SY. Chromatin modifiers and remodellers: regulators of cellular differentiation. *Nat Rev Genet.* 2014;**15**:93–106.
27. Corces M, Buenrostro J, Wu B, et al. Lineage-specific and single-cell chromatin accessibility charts human hematopoiesis and leukemia evolution. *Nat Genet.* 2016;**48**:1193–1203.
31. Patel JP, Gönen M, Figueroa ME, et al. Prognostic relevance of integrated genetic profiling in acute myeloid leukemia. *N Engl J Med.* 2012;**366**:1079–1089.
36. Mardis ER, Ding L, Dooling DJ, et al. Recurring mutations found by sequencing an acute myeloid leukemia genome. *N Engl J Med.* 2009;**361**:1058–1066.
42. Yan XJ, Xu J, Gu ZH, et al. Exome sequencing identifies somatic mutations of DNA methyltransferase gene DNMT3A in acute monocyticleukemia. *Nat Genet.* 2011;**43**:309–315.
48. Barabe F, Kennedy JA, Hope KJ, et al. Modeling the initiation and progression of human acute leukemia in mice. *Science.* 2007;**316**:600–604.
53. Gupta PB, Onder TT, Jiang G, et al. Identification of selective inhibitors of cancer stem cells by high-throughput screening. *Cell.* 2009;**138**:645–659.
56. Nowak D, Stewart D, Koeffler HP. Differentiation therapy of leukemia: 3 decades of development. *Blood.* 2009;**113**:3655–3665.
59. Sachs L. Control of normal cell differentiation and the phenotypic reversion of malignancy in myeloid leukaemia. *Nature.* 1978;**274**:535–539.
72. Breitman TR, Collins SJ, Keene BR. Terminal differentiation of human promyelocytic leukemic cells in primary culture in response to retinoic acid. *Blood.* 1981;**57**:1000–1004.
111. Flotho C, Claus R, Batz C, et al. The DNA methyltransferase inhibitors azacitidine, decitabine and zebularine exert differential effects on cancer gene expression in acute myeloid leukemia cells. *Leukemia.* 2009;**23**:1019–1028.
130. Lu C, Ward PS, Kapoor GS, et al. IDH mutation impairs histone demethylation and results in a block to cell differentiation. *Nature.* 2012;**483**:474–478.
133. Wang F, Travins J, DeLaBarre B, et al. Targeted inhibition of mutant IDH2 in leukemia cells induces cellular differentiation. *Science.* 2013;**340**:622–626.

178 Schenk T, Chen WC, Göllner S, et al. Inhibition of the LSD1 (KDM1A) demethylase reactivates the all-trans-retinoic acid differentiation pathway in acute myeloid leukemia. *Nat Med.* 2012;**18**:605–611.

185 Sykes DB, Kfoury YS, Mercier FE, et al. Inhibition of dihydroorotate dehydrogenase overcomes differentiation blockade in acute myeloid leukemia. *Cell.* 2016;**167**:171–186.e15.

189 Sexauer A, Perl A, Yang X, et al. Terminal myeloid differentiation in vivo is induced by FLT3 inhibition in FLT3/ITD AML. *Blood.* 2012;**120**:4205–4214.

196 Hillestad LK. Acute promyelocytic leukemia. *Acta Med Scand.* 1957;**159**:189-194.

197 Wang ZY, Chen Z. Acute promyelocytic leukemia: from highly fatal to highly curable. *Blood.* 2008;**111**:2505–2515.

198 Daenen S, Vellenga E, van Dobbenburgh OA, et al. Retinoic acid as antileukemic therapy in a patient with acute promyelocytic leukemia and Aspergillus pneumonia. *Blood.* 1986;**67**:559–561.

201 Huang ME, Ye YC, Chen SR, et al. Use of all-trans retinoic acid in the treatment of acute promyelocyticleukemia. *Blood.* 1988;**72**:567–572.

205 Chen GQ, Shen ZX, Wu F, et al. Pharmacokinetics and efficacy of low-dose all-trans retinoic acid in the treatment of acute promyelocytic leukemia. *Leukemia.* 1996;**10**:825–828.

209 Chen GQ, Shi XG, Tang W, et al. Use of arsenic trioxide (As2O3) in the treatment of acute promyelocytic leukemia (APL): I. As2O3 exerts dose-dependent dual effects on APL cells. *Blood.* 1997;**89**:3345–3353.

210 Shen ZX, Chen GQ, Ni JH, et al. Use of arsenic trioxide (As2O3) in the treatment of acute promyelocytic leukemia (APL): II. Clinical efficacy and pharmacokinetics in relapsed patients. *Blood.* 1997;**89**:3354–3360.

211 Hu J, Liu YF, Wu CF, et al. Long-term efficacy and safety of all-trans retinoic acid/arsenic trioxide-based therapy in newly diagnosed acute promyelocyticleukemia. *Proc Natl Acad Sci U S A.* 2009;**106**:3342–3347.

217 The Cooperation Group of Phase IIII. Clinical trial of compound Huangdai tablet: phase II clinical trial of compound Huangdai tablet in newly diagnosed acute promyelocytic leukemia. *Chin J Hematol.* 2006;**27**:801–804.

218 Wang L, Zhou GB, Liu P, et al. Dissection of mechanisms of Chinese medicinal formula Realgar-Indigo naturalis as an effective treatment for promyelocyticleukemia. *Proc Natl Acad Sci U S A.* 2008;**105**:4826–4831.

219 Zhu HH, Wu DP, Jin J, et al. Oral tetra-arsenic tetra-sulfide formula versus intravenous arsenic trioxide as first-line treatment of acute promyelocytic leukemia: a multicenter randomized controlled trial. *J Clin Oncol.* 2013;**31**:4215–4221.

225 Montesinos P, Bergua JM, Vellenga E, et al. Differentiation syndrome in patients with acute promyelocytic leukemia treated with all-trans retinoic acid and anthracycline chemotherapy: characteristics, outcome, and prognostic factors. *Blood.* 2009;**113**:775–783.

230 de Thé H, Pandolfi PP, Chen Z. Acute promyelocytic leukemia: a paradigm for oncoprotein-targeted cure. *Cancer Cell.* 2017;**32**:552–560.

239 Zhu J, Gianni M, Kopf E, et al. Retinoic acid induces proteasome-dependent degradation of retinoic acid receptor alpha (RARalpha) and oncogenic RARalpha fusion proteins. *Proc Natl Acad Sci U S A.* 1999;**96**:14807–14812.

241 Chen GQ, Zhu J, Shi XG, et al. In vitro studies on cellular and molecular mechanisms of arsenic trioxide (As2O3) in the treatment of acute promyelocytic leukemia: As2O3 induces NB4 cell apoptosis with downregulation of Bcl-2 expression and modulation of PML-RAR alpha/PML proteins. *Blood.* 1996;**88**:1052–1061.

242 Zhang XW, Yan XJ, Zhou ZR, et al. Arsenic trioxide controls the fate of the PML-RARalphaoncoprotein by directly binding PML. *Science.* 2010;**328**:240–243.

247 Chen SJ, Zhou GB, Zhang XW, et al. From an old remedy to a magic bullet: molecular mechanisms underlying the therapeutic effects of arsenic in fighting leukemia. *Blood.* 2011;**117**:6425–6437.

254 Zhu HH, Qin YZ, Huang XJ. Resistance to arsenic therapy in acute promyelocytic leukemia. *N Engl J Med.* 2014;**370**:1864–1866.

255 Chen SJ, Zelent A, Tong JH, et al. Rearrangements of the retinoic acid receptor alpha and promyelocytic leukemia zinc finger genes resulting from t(11;17)(q23;q21) in a patient with acute promyelocytic leukemia. *J Clin Invest.* 1993;**91**:2260–2267.

259 Chen L, Zhu HM, Li Y, et al. Arsenic trioxide replacing or reducing chemotherapy in consolidation therapy for acute promyelocytic leukemia (APL2012 trial). *Proc Natl Acad Sci U S A.* 2021;**118**(6):e2020382118.

260 Lin X, Qiao N, Shen Y, et al. Integration of Genomic and Transcriptomic Markers Improves the Prognosis Prediction of Acute Promyelocytic Leukemia. *Clin Cancer Res.* 2021;**27**(13):36836–3694.

12 Cancer stem cells

Grace G. Bushnell, PhD ■ Michael D. Brooks, PhD ■ Max S. Wicha, MD

> **Overview**
>
> There is substantial evidence that many, if not most, tumors contain a subpopulation of cells that display stem cell properties. These "cancer stem cells" (CSC) play an important role in tumor initiation and propagation. Furthermore, these cells may mediate metastasis and resistance to cancer therapeutic agents and therefore play a fundamental role in cancer relapse. This highlights the importance of developing therapeutic approaches to target this cell population. In this article, we will review current thoughts on the role of tissue stem cells in carcinogenesis and the pathways that regulate the plasticity and heterogeneity of these cells. We will then review clinical implications of CSC in dormancy and metastasis and current efforts to therapeutically target these cells.

Cancer stem cell hypothesis

The idea that cancer originated from "primitive embryonic-like cells" dates back over a hundred years.[1] However, it is only within the past several decades that cellular and molecular technologies have permitted the direct testing of these concepts. The "cancer stem cell (CSC) hypothesis" consists of two separate but inter-related concepts. The first concerns the cellular origins of cancer and the second the cellular organization of established cancers.

Models of carcinogenesis and cellular origin of cancer

Currently, two main models of carcinogenesis have been proposed, which are summarized in Figure 1. The classical "stochastic/clonal" model proposes that cancer may arise from any cell and that carcinogenesis evolves through random stochastic processes of mutation followed by clonal selection. As illustrated in the sequential accumulation of mutations during carcinogenesis, disease development is driven by the Darwinian selection of the fittest clones of cancer cells. In contrast to stochastic models, the CSC model posits that this process originates in those cells that possess or acquire the stem cell property of self-renewal. It is important to emphasize that the CSC model does not hold that tissue stem cells are the sole cellular source of cancer initiation. Although cancers may arise in normal tissue stem cells,[2,3] there is evidence that some cancers arise in tissue progenitor cells through mutations that endow these cells with self-renewal capabilities.[4] This process generates tumors that display a degree of hierarchical organization. At the apex of this hierarchy are CSCs, which are operationally defined as cancer cells that maintain the ability to self-renew. These CSCs are capable of generating tumors that recapitulate the phenotypic heterogeneity of the original tumor when transplanted into mouse models.

Although the "stochastic" and "CSC model" were initially described as mutually exclusive, elements drawn from both models might better describe tumor development. Reports by the Vogelstein group suggest that the incidence of cancers in many organs is directly proportional to their number of tissue stem cell divisions.[5] The latter is reflective of their stem cell frequency and division rate. As tissue stem cell mutations are themselves stochastic, this work unifies the two models where stem cells may be a functional unit of mutation and subsequent clonal selection. CSCs may then also undergo mutation during tumor evolution, generating tumors that contain multiple CSCs and their clonal progeny. Finally, CSCs may also be generated by de-differentiation of bulk tumor cells into cells with the ability to self-renew. The combination of these concepts, derived from both models of carcinogenesis and with the emerging idea of CSC plasticity, may provide a molecular explanation for the generation of intratumor heterogeneity; a phenomenon with considerable therapeutic implications.

Cancer stem cells as a unifying concept in multiple cancers

CSCs were first identified in human leukemia in 1997.[6] In seminal studies, John Dick et al. demonstrated that only a small fraction of primary human leukemia cells were capable of regenerating the leukemia when transplanted into immune-suppressed NOD/SCID (nonobese diabetic/severely compromised immunodeficient) mice.[6] Further, these tumor-initiating leukemia cells were prospectively identified by virtue of their phenotypic characterization as CD34+/CD38−, a phenotype resembling that found on normal hematopoietic stem cells. Although the frequency of these leukemia-initiating cells was found to be approximately 1 in 250,000, the leukemias generated in transplanted mice recapitulated the phenotypic heterogeneity of the initial tumor. Utilizing similar tumor transplantation technologies, investigators have subsequently identified CSC in a wide variety of solid tumors. These include cancers of the breast,[7] brain,[8] prostate,[9,10] colon,[11,12] pancreas,[13] liver,[14,15] lung,[16] melanoma,[17] and head and neck.[18] In fact, evidence suggests that the majority of tumors are hierarchically organized and contain cell populations that display stem cell properties.

Isolation, identification, and characterization of CSCs

In order to study the basic attributes of CSCs, it is necessary to first identify, purify, and characterize these cells by employing techniques that enable one to distinguish them from the bulk tumor cell population. The functional characteristics of CSCs, including self-renewal capability and differentiation potential, can be exploited by various *in vitro* and *in vivo* assays to identify and characterize this important cell population. Several methods or techniques exist to identify and isolate stem cell-like cancer cells;

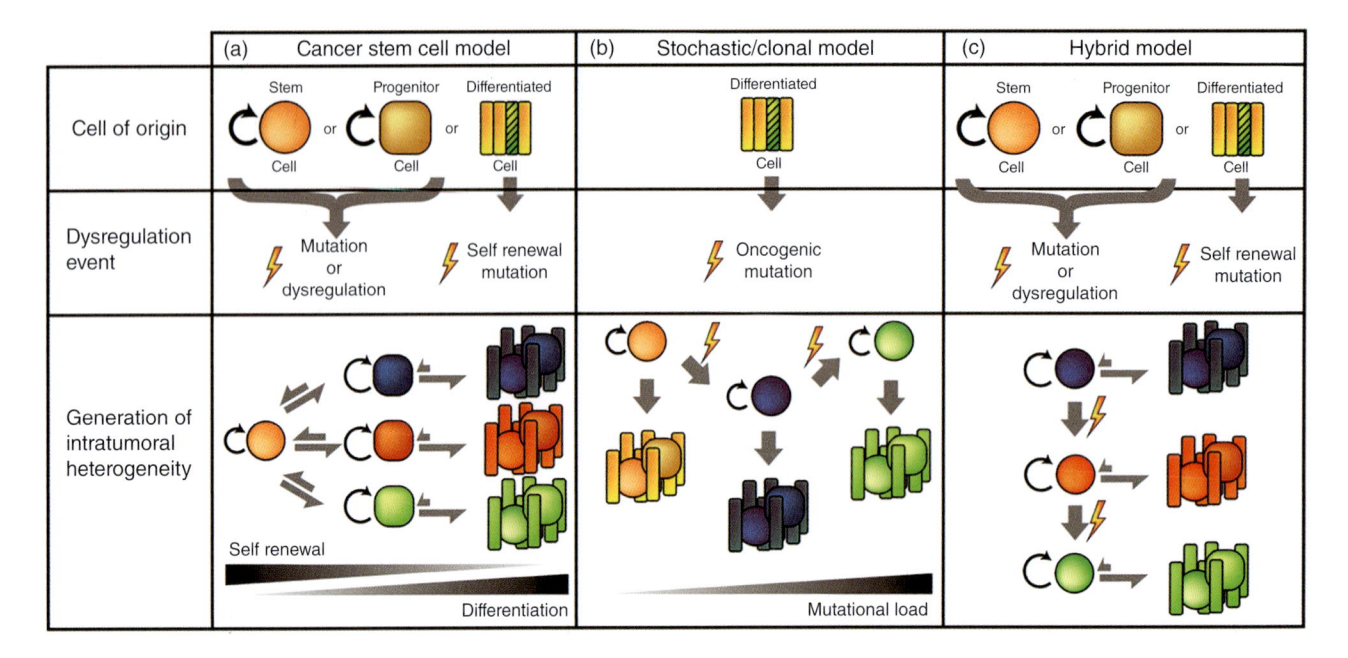

Figure 1 Schematic representation of two models of tumorigenesis. (a) Depicts "cancer stem cell model" where tumors arise in cells with stem cell properties or a differentiated cell acquires mutations that confer the ability to self-renew. These CSCs are then at the top of the differentiation hierarchy and produce differentiated progeny that form the tumor bulk. (b) Depicts the "stochastic/clonal model" of tumorigenesis where random mutations in any cell generate cancerous clonal populations, which evolve through further mutation. (c) Depicts the "hybrid model" where generation of heterogeneity is both by differentiation of cancer stem cells and evolution through mutation.

flow cytometry detecting expression of CSC-related markers, dye exclusion, ALDH (aldehyde dehydrogenase) assay, label retention (PKH staining), and autofluorescence in the presence of riboflavin. CSCs, enriched by these techniques, may be functionally validated by sphere formation assays or serial transplantation assays *in vivo* for evaluation of tumorigenic and self-renewal potential. The details of the methods are listed in the following sections.

CSC marker expression
The first CSCs in solid tumors were described in human breast cancer based on cellular expression of CD44 and lack of expression of CD24 (i.e., CD44+/CD24−).[7] Interestingly, these markers have proven useful for the isolation of CSC from a variety of other solid tumors. In parallel, CD133 has been shown to be useful in enriching for CSC in brain and lung cancers.[8,16] Another stem cell marker, ALDH, is also used along with CD44/CD24 or CD133 to identify the CSC population in several tumors. ALDHs are a family of enzymes that are involved in the oxidation of retinol to retinoic acid.[19] ALDH activity can be readily determined using the commercially available Aldefluor assay and was shown to be a useful CSC marker in cancers of the breast,[20] ovary,[21] colon,[22] head and neck,[23] and melanoma.[24]

Dye exclusion assays
Dye exclusion is based on the ability of stem cells to efflux lipophilic dyes, such as Rhodamine or Hoechst, owing to the high expression of the ATP-binding cassette transporter proteins such as ABCG2/BCRP1.[25] Utilizing flow cytometry analysis, cells that do not retain dye are observed as a side population.[26] Several studies have demonstrated that such side populations are enriched in cells with tumor-initiating capacity and are capable of regenerating heterogeneous cell populations.[27] This stem cell-like side population has been observed in several cancer types, as well as bone marrow and normal solid tissues.[28,29] The cellular toxicity of Hoechst dye limits their ability to be combined with functional studies.

Label retention
Another dye-based method used to characterize CSCs *in vitro* is the cell membrane, label-retaining assay using fluorescent PKH dye. This dye consists of a fluorophore that binds to the cell membrane lipid bilayer.[30] Upon cell division, the dye becomes distributed equally among daughter cells. Subsequent continuous cell divisions lead to decreased intensity.[31] Stem cells, including CSCs, normally undergo an asymmetric self-renewal process generating a stem cell and a daughter cell. The generated stem cells are quiescent and thus retain PKH due for a longer time period, whereas the daughter cells proliferate and differentiate leading to decreased intensity of PKH due. These daughter cells are then identified and sorted by flow cytometry. This method has been used successfully to isolate murine hematopoietic and mammary stem cells.[32]

Additionally, CSCs demonstrate autofluorescence in the presence of riboflavin.[33] The authors isolated this population using flow cytometry, distinguished these cells from the side population, and demonstrated that these putative CSCs had greater tumor sphere-forming ability, increased chemo-resistance, were highly metastatic, and possessed long-term *in vivo* tumorigenicity. Further, in support of the CSC model, this autofluorescent CSC-like population was detected in several cancers.[33]

Sphere formation assays
The sphere formation assay is another *in vitro* assay that has proven useful for the identification of CSC populations. This is based on a property shared by both normal and malignant stem cells: survival when cultured in suspension and generation of spheroids at clonal density.[34] These spheres can be serially passaged and display stem cell properties with each passage. It has also been

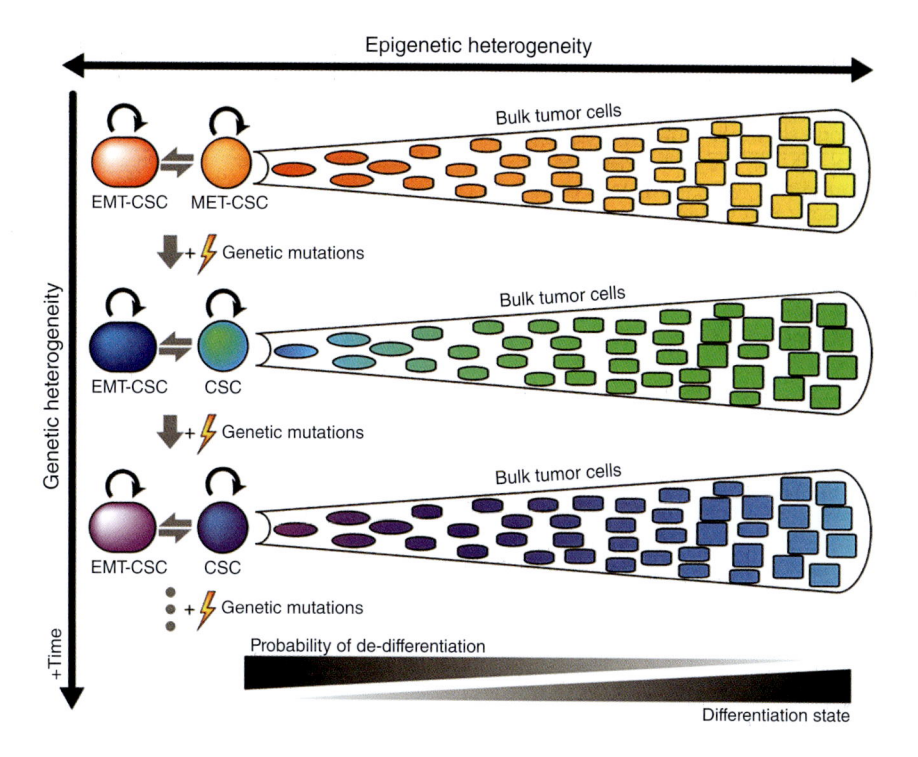

Figure 2 Cancer stem cell plasticity. Cancer stem cells exhibit both genetic and epigenetic heterogeneity.

possible to combine a number of *in vitro* CSC assays. For instance, the addition of PKH dye during sphere formation results in the formation of spheres that often contain a single label-retaining sphere-initiating cell.[35]

In vivo serial dilution CSC assays
Although the use of CSC markers and *in vitro* assays has proven useful in the isolation and characterization of CSCs, all of these techniques have limitations. The expression of CSC markers Is variable and may be influenced by culture conditions or the tumor microenvironment (TME).[36] Further, sphere formation assays may not correlate with tumor initiation capacity.[37] In light of these limitations, the "gold standard" for CSC identification is demonstration of tumor initiation upon implantation into immunosuppressed mice.[37] The tumor-initiating frequency in any cell population may be assessed by the ability of cells to initiate development in mice using limiting dilution of cell suspensions. Thus, the definition of CSCs is ultimately an operational one.

It is important to note that immunosuppressed mouse models also have limitations. In human melanoma, the frequency of tumor-initiating cells was strongly influenced by the degree of immune competence of the mouse model utilized.[38] Studies have indicated that the immune system plays an important role in CSC regulation.[39,40] Studies elucidating these roles have been carried out in mouse tumors transplanted into syngeneic immune-competent mice. Such studies have confirmed the existence of CSC as determined by serial transplantation.[41]

Lineage tracing studies
One criticism of all transplantation studies is that they perturb the normal microenvironment where tumors develop. To circumvent this limitation, a series of studies using cell markers and lineage tracing have been performed. Such studies have confirmed the existence of CSC in tumors of the skin,[42] brain,[43] and colon.[44]

Cancer stem cell plasticity and heterogeneity

In addition to genetic heterogeneity driven by mutation and clonal selection, there is emerging evidence that CSCs are heterogeneous and display cellular plasticity or the ability to interconvert between cell states (Figure 2). In particular, the concept of bulk tumor cells, without CSC properties, dedifferentiating into CSCs is an important area of study in CSC biology. The following sections will discuss the concepts of plasticity and heterogeneity as they relate to the epigenetic state, stemness signaling pathways, the epithelial to mesenchymal transition, signal transduction, and the microenvironment in CSCs.

Epigenetic state of cancer stem cells

The last two decades of research have generated evidence that cancer is not only a disease driven by genetics but also by epigenetics. The focus of epigenetics in cancer and developmental biology has revealed further links between the behavior and state of cancer cells and that of normal stem cells and in particular embryonic stem cells (ESCs). In ESCs, chromatin is generally less compact and in a more open, "permissive" state compared to differentiated cells.[45] Additionally, promoters of nonexpressed developmental genes in ESCs are poised in what has been termed a "bivalent" state where there exist histone modifications associated with both gene transcription and repression. The histone modification associated with gene repression is trimethylation of histone H3 lysine 27, which is created by the polycomb repressive complex 2 (PRC2). This, in turn, provides a binding site for the polycomb repressive complex 1 (PRC1). ESCs that have mutant components of PRC1/2 show de-repression of tissue-specific genes and an inability to maintain the de-differentiated state.[46] Cancer cells have been found to share some of these features with ESCs. In particular, polycomb group targets are 12 times more likely to demonstrate DNA hypermethylation in cancer cells, compared to nonpolycomb group targets indicating a repression of tissue-specific genes and induction of an epigenetic state similar to that of ESCs.[47] These features have also been found to be specific to CSCs. For example, key genes involved in transcriptional repression in ESCs including PRC2, EZH2, and SUZ12 are all overexpressed in ovarian, breast, prostate, and colon cancers and are crucial for the maintenance of the CSC population in each.[48–51] Additionally, in breast cancer ectopic expression of SUZ12 in differentiated breast cancer cells results in CSC formation[49] and DNA methyltransferase 1 (DMNT1) was found to be crucial for the maintenance of breast CSCs.[52] In glioblastoma, BMI1 and EZH2 are highly expressed in CD133+ CSCs and their knockdown disrupts CSC function.[53] Finally, in melanoma, histone demethylase JARID1B was found to be crucial in the dynamics of the CSC population.[54] Taken together this evidence suggests, CSCs and ESCs maintain the dedifferentiated state through epigenetic modifications, and these modifications, in turn, provide a foundation for both plasticity and heterogeneity.

Core stemness signaling in cancer stem cells

Not only do CSCs and ESCs share key epigenetic features, but they also share key pluripotency transcription factors including OCT4, NANOG, and SOX2, among others.[55,56] There is evidence that overexpression of these genes is linked to tumor initiation, progression, resistance to therapy, and prognosis.[57,58] These transcription factor networks can be used to define stemness from a gene expression standpoint. In addition to their role in maintaining CSC phenotype, these signaling pathways may be another source of heterogeneity and plasticity, and specifically may be partially responsible for the dedifferentiation of bulk tumor cells into CSC. Reprogramming of mature terminally differentiated cells occurs in normal tissues and thus may also occur in tumors.[59] Injury can drive dedifferentiation of normal tissue cells in order to repair the stem cell pool in the brain, colon, and lung.[60–62] Though these reprogramming events are less extreme than the dedifferentiation that occurs in CSC, it may indicate that bulk tumor cells could dedifferentiate to the CSC state in tumors. A more extreme example of reprogramming is the conversion of somatic cells to induced pluripotent stem cells by ectopic expression of OCT3/4, SOX2, KLF4, and cMyc.[63] While highly inefficient *in vitro*, this process does illustrate the extreme ability of cellular reprogramming and plasticity to alter stemness. Activation of iPSC reprogramming factors has been identified in many types of CSCs of the breast, prostate, liver, brain, and lung.[64–67] Finally, it has also been shown that transcription factors associated with stemness and pluripotency can reprogram bulk cancer cells into CSCs. In bulk glioma cells ectopic expression of core developmental transcription factors including POU3F2, SOX2, SALL2, and OLIG2 induced stem cell properties.[66] In colorectal cancer cells OCT3/4, SOX2, and KLF4 overexpression enhanced CSC properties including sphere formation, CSC marker expression, chemoresistance, and tumorigenicity.[68] Differentiated breast cancer cells can also be converted back to stem-like cells through combined expression of SLUG and SOX9.[69]

EMT/MET and cancer stem cells

Epithelial–mesenchymal transition (EMT) is a physiological process of particular importance during embryonic development whereby epithelial cells acquire mesenchymal properties, characterized by a loss of cell adhesion and the acquisition of invasive properties. The EMT process was initially described during development, where it induced the migration of mesodermal cells during gastrulation or the delamination of the neural crest cells from the dorsal neural tube.[70] Similarly in cancer, EMT has been associated with the process of metastasis where epithelial cells from the primary tumor acquire mesenchymal phenotype and invade to other tissues.[71]

EMT is regulated by signals from the microenvironment that mediate epigenetic alterations driven by core transcription factors. Microenvironmental factors include tissue hypoxia, TGF-β (transforming growth factor-β), and other inflammatory molecules with subsequent induction of EMT-related transcription factor expression such as TWIST1, TWIST2, SNAI1, SNAI2, ZEB1, and ZEB2, among others.[72,73] Overexpression of these transcription factors induces a mesenchymal and invasive phenotype through repression of cell adhesion molecules, such as E-cadherin.[74] Twist1, which is involved in mesenchymal development during embryogenesis, has been shown to induce metastasis in breast cancer.[75] Several studies suggest that the EMT process generates CSC-like cells.[76,77] In this regard, overexpression of SNAI1 or TWIST1 alone was shown to induce EMT in MCF10 and immortalized human mammary epithelial cells.[78] In addition, there was increased expression of the stem cell marker CD44 and a decrease in CD24 expression, which suggests induction of CSC-like phenotype. Moreover, TWIST1 has been associated with an increased ability of breast cancer cells to form mammospheres and secondary tumors in oncogenic HRAS-g12V model.[79] Based on the molecular classification of breast cancer, a basal subtype, particularly claudin-low are known to possess an EMT-like gene expression signature. Such cancers have a high proportion of CD44+/24− cells that are locked within the mesenchymal state. These tumors display a highly aggressive behavior accompanied by a greater propensity to develop metastasis. Further, TWIST1 upregulated BMI expression, when suppressed by the miR-200 microRNA cluster, decreased CSC self-renewal, and cellular differentiation. Similarly, BMP signaling induced MET via induction of mir-205 and the miR-200 family of microRNAs that are key regulators of MET.[80]

The aforementioned studies strongly suggest the role of EMT in the acquisition of a stem cell phenotype. It is plausible that the CSC possesses alternative phenotypes; one involved in tumor invasion and metastasis while another state maintains the bulk of the tumors. This is evident from the studies that used gene expression analysis to compare ALDH+ and CD44+/24− BCSCs isolated from different subtypes of breast cancer. This comparative gene expression analysis suggested that, although each population was independently capable of tumor initiation in NOD/SCID mice, yet they were quite distinct both functionally and anatomically in the original primary tumors. ALDH+ CSCs usually populated the interior of the tumors where they self-renewed and proliferated at a higher rate, whereas CD44+/24− CSCs were more mesenchymal, displayed an EMT phenotype located on the tumor margins or invasive front, and were more quiescent.[81] Further characterization of these two populations showed that CD44+/24− cells were highly vimentin-positive and E-cadherin negative, whereas an ALDH+ population was highly positive for E-cadherin and negative for vimentin. Therefore, these CD44+/24− cells were more EMT-like and may be poised to invade the blood vessels when triggered by stromal factors such as hypoxia, TGF-β, and other inflammatory agents.

These studies also demonstrated that BCSCs maintain the plasticity to transition between EMT and MET states in a process regulated by the TME. The interconversion of BCSCs from the EMT-like to MET-like state has also been shown to be regulated by microRNA networks. Such networks included EMT-inducing mir-9, mir-100, mir-221, and mir-155 as well as MET-inducing mir-200, mir-205, and mir-93.[82] The plasticity of BCSCs from a quiescent mesenchymal state to a proliferative epithelial-like state is critical for formation of tumor metastases at distant sites. The knockdown of TWIST1 in a spontaneous squamous-cell carcinoma model reversed EMT and allowed cells to proliferate and form metastasis.[83] Similarly, the loss of the EMT inducer Prrx1 was required for cancer cells to form lung macrometastasis.[84] In addition, MET-promoting factors, such as miR-200 family members, were found to promote metastatic colonization of breast cancer cells and induce epithelial differentiation.[85] Furthermore, expression of Id1 gene in breast cancer cells reconverted EMT cells into MET by downregulating TWIST1, which is required for establishing macrometastasis.[86] EMT may also regulate the conversion between CSC and non-CSC or bulk states. For example, Chaffer et al. found that basal breast cancer non-CSCs are plastic and can generate CSC de novo in a ZEB1 dependent manner.[87] The above studies provide evidence that two alternative states of CSCs display plasticity and are regulated by microenvironmental factors that modulate the genetic regulators and several transcription factors. They also provide preliminary evidence that some breast cancer non-CSC may convert to the CSC state through EMT. The existence of multiple CSC states and plasticity between the CSC and non-CSC state has important therapeutic implications as elimination of CSC may require successful targeting of multiple CSC populations and conversion to the CSC state.

Signal transduction pathways in cancer stem cells

Like their normal counterparts, a number of evolutionarily conserved developmental pathways play a significant role in the regulation of CSCs in several cancer types. The conservation of these pathways in CSCs of different tumor types further strengthens the cancer stem model. Moreover, these pathways could provide common potential therapeutic targets irrespective of the tumor type.

Hedgehog signaling

The Hedgehog (Hh) family of proteins controls cell growth, survival, pattern of the vertebrate body, and stem/progenitor cell maintenance. Dysregulation of Hh signaling, including that arising from somatic mutation, has been linked to several cancer types. The binding of Hh proteins to the receptor Patched (Ptc) activates a signaling cascade that leads to the upregulation of a zinc-finger transcription factor GLI1–3 and its downstream gene targets.[88-90] Of the three mammalian Hh ligands, sonic hedgehog (SHH), Indian hedgehog (IHH), and desert hedgehog (DHH), SHH is the most highly expressed Hh signaling molecule and is involved in the regulation of many epithelial tissues. Aberrant activation of Hh signaling has been linked to basal cell carcinoma,[91,92] medulloblastoma,[93,94] rhabdomyosarcoma,[95] and other cancers, such as glioma, breast, esophageal, gastric, pancreatic, prostate, and small-cell lung carcinoma.[96] GLI1 amplifications are also known to occur in gliomas.[97]

The Hh signaling pathway plays a major role in mammary gland development both in humans and in mice. In mice, constitutive activation of Gli1 or inactivation of Gli3 resulted in mammary bud formation defects.[98] Ectopic expression of Gli1 has been shown to induce the nuclear Snail expression resulting in loss of E-cadherin expression in mouse mammary glands tissue during pregnancy.[99] In addition, the transcription factor FOXC2 also promoted mesenchymal differentiation via the Hh pathway and Snail upregulation.[100] Similarly, SHH overexpression in mouse mammary glands leads to mammary bud defects.[101] Perturbation of other Hh pathway molecules, such as activation of SMO or loss of PTCH1, has resulted in terminal end bud abnormalities.[102] Normal human mammary stem cells expressed PTCH1, Gli1, and Gli2 during mammosphere formation, a pathway that is downregulated during the process of differentiation. Hh signaling played an important role in stem cell regulation as activation of Hh signaling through Hh ligand, or Gli1/Gli2 overexpression, increased mammosphere formation and size through activation of BMI-1, a member of the polycomb gene family.[103] The similar activation of SMO, driven by an MMTV (mouse mammary tumor virus) promoter, increased mammosphere formation of primary mammary epithelial cells in transgenic mice.[102] Hh ligands are also known to exert mitogenic effects on mammary stem cells through paracrine interactions. This process may be involved in the regulation of mammary differentiation during pregnancy, in a process regulated by TP63.[104] Apart from TP63, the transcription factor Runx2 has been shown to regulate the expression of Hh ligands.[105]

Hh signaling pathway members SHH, PTCH1, and GLI1 were highly expressed in invasive breast carcinomas suggesting a role for this pathway in human breast cancers.[106] Further, Hh ligand expression was associated with basal-like breast cancer; an aggressive phenotype with relatively poor outcome. These findings were corroborated in mouse models where ectopic expression of Hh ligand in BLBC mice induced high-grade invasive tumors.[107] Similarly, SHH upregulation due to hypomethylation of the SHH promotor has been observed in breast carcinomas that were associated with expression of NF-κB in breast cancer clinical samples.[108] Hh signaling has also been linked to bone metastasis in this disease. In bone metastases, secretion of Hh ligand by tumor cells activates the transcription of osteopontin (OPN) by bone osteoclasts. This further promotes osteoclast maturation and resorptive activity, facilitating metastasis.[109]

The most commonly used antagonist of the Hh pathway is the plant alkaloid cyclopamine that binds to SMO and downregulates Gli1.[110] Other antagonists that bind to SMO include SANTs 1–4;[111] KAAD-cyclopamine,[110] compound-5 and compound-Z,[112] and Cur-61414.[113] Further, 5E1 monoclonal antibody targeting SHH treated tumors in small-cell lung carcinoma.[114] GDC-0449 (Vismodegib, trade name: Erivedge®), the first Hh pathway inhibitor approved by FDA, was used in clinical trials in combination with the Notch signaling inhibitor RO4929097 (a γ-secretase inhibitor, GSI).[115]

Notch signaling

Notch is another evolutionarily conserved signaling pathway that is involved in the regulation of cell fate determination, proliferation, and differentiation in many tissues. The core components of the Notch signaling cascade include the ligands-Delta-like-1, -3, and -4 (DLL1, DLL3, and DLL4), Jagged-1 and -2 (JAG1 and JAG2), and four transmembrane receptors (Notch 1 to Notch 4). After ligand binding, the receptor undergoes two proteolytic events. First, cleavage occurs in close proximity to the extracellular side of the plasma membrane. This is followed by a second cleavage within the transmembrane domain, mediated by a γ-secretase complex, which leads to the release of the intracellular domain of the receptor from the membrane. Upon cleavage, the intracellular Notch domain translocates to the nucleus where it forms a complex with the ubiquitously expressed transcription factor CSL and recruits co-activators such as mastermind-like (MAML-1, -2, and -3).[116] The transcriptional targets of Notch signaling include not only differentiation-related factors, such as Hairy/enhancer of split (Hes) and Hes-related (HRT/HRP/Hey) families but also cell cycle regulators (p21 and cyclin D1) and regulators of apoptosis.[116,117]

The oncogenic role of Notch 1 was first discovered in T-ALL where the translocation of t(7;9)(q34;q34.3) led to juxtaposition of Notch 1 with TCR-β (T cell receptor-beta). This translocation led to the ligand-independent activity and deregulated expression of intracellular Notch 1 regulated by TCR-β that impacted T-cell differentiation.[118] Overexpression of Notch 4 in mouse mammary glands utilizing an MMTV promotor blocked cellular differentiation with aberrant lactation and poorly differentiated mammary and salivary adenocarcinomas occurred between two and seven months of age.[119] This evidence again underscores the role that Notch signaling plays in the differentiation and tumorigenesis of several tissues. A correlation between Ras overexpression and elevated Notch 1 levels has been reported.[120] Furthermore, expression of Numb, a negative regulator of Notch signaling, was lost in approximately 50% of primary human mammary carcinomas and these tumors showed increased Notch 1 activity.[121] Overexpression of several Notch signaling molecules was reported in several tumors such as pancreatic cancer, renal cell carcinoma, prostate cancer, multiple myeloma, and Hodgkin's and anaplastic lymphoma.[122-126] In lung cancer, Notch signaling had a differential effect based on the cell type: in small lung cancer, Notch signaling is inactive but Hes1 and Hash1 are active[127] and introduction of constitutively active intracellular Notch induces Notch signaling resulting in growth arrest.[128] In contrast, Notch signaling is active in nonsmall lung cancer with high expression of Hes1 and Hey1.[127]

CD24+/24− breast CSCs have been reported to display Notch pathway activation.[129] Notch 3 was found to be upregulated in CD44+ populations of normal and breast cancer cells via SAGE analysis.[130] Other studies have suggested that Notch 4 is the most important regulator of breast stem cells.[131] Moreover, aberrant activation of Notch signaling is an early event in breast cancer, as this has been observed in ductal carcinoma in situ (DCIS). Treatment of primary DCIS tissue with a γ-secretase inhibitor significantly reduced the mammosphere formation.[129] Similarly, in an in vitro mammosphere culture system, activation of Notch signaling via a DSL peptide promoted self-renewal and branching morphogenesis in three-dimensional Matrigel cultures,[132] a process that was inhibited by a Notch 4 blocking antibody or a γ-secretase inhibitor. Therefore, activated Notch signaling may maintain the epithelial cells in a proliferative state instead of differentiation leading to carcinoma.

Regulation of Notch pathways has also been attributed to epigenetic regulation through hypermethylation and hypomethylation. Notch ligand DLL1 gene is hypermethylated resulting in decreased NOTCH1 expression.[133] Similarly, reduced methylation of NOTCH4 gene promoter in tumors compared to surrounding tissue was observed.[134] Overexpression of JAG2 in multiple myeloma cells was correlated with hypomethylation in malignant cells from multiple myeloma patients and cell lines.[135] Knockdown of the canonical Notch effector Cbf-1 in mammary stem cells increased stem cell activity, whereas constitutive Notch signaling increased luminal progenitor cells, leading to hyperplasia and tumorigenesis.[136] In addition, co-expression of JAG1 and NOTCH1 was associated with poor overall survival.[137] In ESA+ CD24−CD44+ BCSCs, activity of Notch 4 and Notch 1 were eightfold and fourfold higher, respectively, compared to the differentiated bulk tumor cells and inhibition of this activity resulted in reducing tumor growth.[131]

The complexity of the Notch pathway increases through interaction with other oncogenic pathways such as ErbB2, Jak/Stat, TGF-β, NF-κB, Wnt, and Hh.[138] As ErbB2 induces Notch 1 activity through Cyclin D1,[139] combined treatment of DAPT and Lapatinib targeted stem/progenitor cells both in vitro and in vivo in DCIS.[140] The Wnt pathway also interacts with Notch through Jagged-1 (target of WNT/TCF pathway) and Mel-18, a negative regulator of Bmi-1. Knockdown of Mel-18 has been shown to enhance the self-renewal of BCSCs through upregulation of Jagged-1, consequently activating the Notch pathway.[141] The activation of Notch activity further activates the Hh pathway and increases expression of Ptch and Gli.[103] Taken together, these studies suggest that treatments aimed at targets affecting multiple stem cell pathways could present a novel strategy for targeted therapies. A variety of agents that inhibit Notch signaling are in early phase clinical trials. These include γ-secretase inhibitors that block Notch processing,[142] antibodies against specific Notch receptors,[143,144] and antibodies against the Notch ligand DLL4.[145,146]

Wnt signaling

The Wnt/β-catenin/TCF pathway is another complex evolutionarily conserved pathway involved not only in development and maintenance of adult tissue homeostasis but also cell proliferation, differentiation, migration, and apoptosis.[147] It also regulates the self-renewal and maintenance of embryonic and tissue-specific stem cells.[148-150] Dysregulation of Wnt signaling is a hallmark of several cancers where molecules involved in pathway could act as either tumor suppressors or enhancers depending on their activation status.[151-153] Wnt signaling involves both canonical and noncanonical pathways. The canonical Wnt pathway involves activation of β-catenin/TCF complex, resulting in its dissociation from APC (adenomatous polyposis coli) with subsequent translocation into the nucleus leading to activation of transcriptions including TCF/LEF.[154] This, in turn, leads to upregulation of oncogenic targets such as c-myc and cyclin D1. This canonical pathway has been extensively studied and found to be deregulated in many cancers. Noncanonical Wnt signaling involves a planer-cell polarity pathway that regulates the cytoskeleton and a Wnt-calcium-dependent pathway that regulates intracellular calcium levels.[155,156] Mutation of APC (Wnt pathway molecule regulating β-catenin stability) is associated with the majority of sporadic colorectal cancers.[157,158] Germline mutations in APC have been shown to be involved in familial polyposis syndromes, a condition associated with development of numerous intestinal polyps with a high propensity for further neoplastic transformation. In addition to colon cancer, oncogenic mutations in β-catenin have been described in cancers of the liver and colon, as well as in melanoma, thyroid, and ovarian cancers.[159] Epigenetic silencing through methylation of Wnt antagonist genes such as the secreted frizzled-related proteins (SFRPs) has been reported in colon, breast, prostate, lung, and other cancers.[147]

Wnt signaling has been shown to be involved in maintenance of CSCs in several cancers. In a transgenic mouse model, LRP5 (a key component of the Wnt co-receptor group) knockdown significantly reduced stem/progenitor cells.[160] In addition, transgenic mice overexpressing Wnt-1 developed mammary glands that were enriched for epithelial cells expressing keratin 6 and Sca1 markers of mammary stem cells. This suggests that mammary carcinogenesis may involve stem cell expansion secondary to Wnt activation. Wnt/β-catenin signaling is also involved in EMT regulation through downregulation of E-cadherin and upregulation of

Snail and Twist.[161] EMT has been shown to induce stem cell-like phenotype in breast cancer cells.[77] Wnt signaling has also been demonstrated to maintain pluripotency and neural differentiation of ESCs.[162] Wnt signaling may also contribute to stem cell expansion induced by tumor hypoxia, a process mediated by Hif 1-α.[163]

A number of drugs that inhibit Wnt signaling are in development. In preclinical models, two nonsteroidal anti-inflammatory drugs (NSAIDs), sulindac[164] and celecoxib,[165,166] have been found to inhibit Wnt signaling by targeting Dvl and cyclo-oxygenase, respectively. Sulindac is currently being investigated in phase II trials.[167] In addition, several non-NSAID inhibitors such as NSC668036 and PCN-N3, among others, have been shown to degrade β-catenin by inhibiting DVL and hence, stabilizing the destruction complex.[168,169] Further, antibodies targeting Wnt pathway members are also under development. A Wnt3A neutralizing antibody was shown to reduce proliferation and enhance apoptosis in prostate cancer mouse models.[170] Another monoclonal antibody-OMP-54F28 has been shown to inhibit patient-derived xenograft tumor growth by specifically targeting CSCs. A Wnt decoy receptor[171] and an antibody to the Wnt co-regulator R spondin[148] are also in development. These aforementioned Wnt inhibiting drugs are currently being tested in several early phase clinical trials.

Microenvironmental control of cancer stem cell plasticity

The microenvironment is emerging as a crucial determinant of CSC phenotype and plasticity.[172] The TME includes not only the tumor cells, but also stromal cells, immune cells, vasculature, and the extracellular matrix. Each of these has been shown to play a role in tumor cell phenotype and particularly the function of CSCs. Cancer-associated fibroblasts (CAFs) are part of the stroma of the TME.[173] They are normal fibroblasts that have been subverted to become "cancer associated" by the alterations in the microenvironmental signals caused by cancer cells and in turn they have various roles in supporting cancer cells, increasing tumorigenicity, and resistance to therapy. Specifically, CAFs have been shown to increase the gland forming ability of prostate CSC,[174] stimulate EMT and stemness in prostate cancer cells,[175] and regulate breast CSCs via CCL2.[176] Mesenchymal stem cells (MSCs) are multipotent progenitor cells that contribute to the maintenance and repair of many tissues including adipose, bone, cartilage, and muscle.[177] MSCs home to sites of injury and thus home to tumors. MSCs can induce stemness via chemokine loop with CXCL7 and IL6 as a reciprocal interaction between CSC and the most stem-like MSCs.[178] MSCs can also cause elevated miR-199a expressed which induces CSCs.[179] Immune cells are also emerging as crucial regulators of tumor cell phenotype. Both innate and adaptive immune cells may have both tumor-killing and tumor-promoting effects on the TME.[180] Tumor-associated macrophages have been shown to regulate CSCs via STAT3 in both liver[181] and breast cancer[182] and also promote stemness via promotion of EMT.[183] Myeloid-derived suppressor cells have also been shown to promote stemness via IL6/STAT3 signaling in breast CSC.[184] Finally vasculature can also promote CSC phenotype and plasticity via regulation of hypoxia, which promotes stemness.[163,185] While not an exhaustive review, these studies provide evidence that the microenvironment is a crucial regulator of CSC phenotype through reciprocal interactions with CSC and various TME host cells. Targeting interactions between CSC and the microenvironment is a promising avenue for CSC therapies.

Clinical significance of cancer stem cells

Cancer stem cells in treatment resistance

There is now substantial evidence that CSC plays an important role in treatment resistance; in addition to their role in tumor propagation and tumor metastasis, resistance of CSC to cytotoxic chemotherapy was first demonstrated in preclinical models[186,187] and later confirmed in clinical trials.[188] The relative resistance of CSC to radiation therapy has been demonstrated in a number of tumor types. In patients, it has been shown that the relative proportion of cells expressing CSC markers increases following chemotherapy or radiation therapy.[188] A number of mechanisms have been described that contribute to this resistance. These include alterations in cell cycle kinetics, increased expression of antiapoptotic proteins, increased in cellular transporters, and increased efficiency of DNA repair, as reviewed in Ref. 189. In addition to the relative therapeutic resistance of CSC, these cells may actually be stimulated by chemotherapy via stimulation of cytokine loops activated by these treatments. These inflammatory cytokines include IL-8 and IL-6. Inhibitors to these cytokines and their receptors have been developed, and several are entering clinical trials.

Cancer stem cells in metastasis

For most cancer, metastasis or spread of tumor cells to distant organs is ultimately the cause of death for patients. By the operational definition of CSCs as those cells that can initiate tumors, metastases must arise from CSCs initiating tumors in a foreign environment.[190] Metastasis occurs through a series of stages collectively defined as the metastatic cascade. An emerging preliminary step of the metastatic cascade is the premetastatic phase.[191,192] This is the phase at which the primary tumor conditions the immune system as well as distal metastatic sites to facilitate the arrival and survival of tumor cells in these locations. The metastatic cascade then continues with invasion of tumor cells into the surrounding tissue, a process that is facilitated by EMT and thus, is intimately associated with stemness. Following invasion, tumor cells may then intravasate into a blood or lymphatic vessel, which are often leaky at the site of tumors, and traverse throughout the vasculature as a circulating tumor cell (CTC). CTCs have been shown to have CSC marker expression and functional properties of CSC.[193-196] CTCs can then arrest in the vascular bed of a distant organ. Following arrest, tumor cells can then extravasate from inside of the vascular lumen into the tissue itself. At this point tumor cells are typically called disseminated tumor cells (DTCs). DTCs have also been shown to express CSC markers and to display functional properties of CSC.[197] In order to form a micro- or macro-metastasis the tumor cells must then proliferate and initiate a new tumor. The premetastatic niche functionally increases the ability of tumor cells to initiate new tumors in these hostile environments, and thus directly supports stemness.[198] Following formation of micro- or macro-metastasis CSCs has been found in metastasis which have similar heterogeneity to the primary tumor yet originated from subclones of the primary. There is also emerging evidence that tumor cells that have been selected for metastasis may have a greater proportion of CSC. This is in line with the idea that metastasis is really an extension of tumor initiating ability, just at distal metastatic sites instead of the organ of origin. It is clear that CSCs are crucial to metastasis and yet much of the research on CSCs has focused on primary tumor initiation rather than metastasis. A crucial avenue of future research is understanding the reciprocal interactions of metastatic CSCs with

Cancer stem cells in dormancy

Clinical dormancy is a crucial aspect of cancer care and monitoring of patients. Clinically dormancy refers to the time after treatment that a patient is asymptomatic but still carries tumor cells that do not grow into overt metastases. The majority of solid tumors and hematological malignancies undergo a period of dormancy that may be characterized by years to decades of minimal residual disease[199]. For breast cancer, patients with estrogen receptor-positive disease may recur with metastasis 20 or more years after initial diagnosis/treatment[200]. However, not all patients will recur. Understanding the biology of dormant DTCs is crucial to understanding how to prevent late recurrence. As with metastasis above, any tumor cell that is capable of initiating metastasis is, by the operational definition, a CSC. The ability of tumor cells to sit dormant may also imply that they have CSC characteristics as quiescence is a property of normal stem cells. There is evidence that CSCs are uniquely capable of dormancy via autophagy[201] and that CSC may be forced into dormancy by the microenvironment,[202] potentially by occupying the normal stem cell niche in host tissues.[172,203] There are still many unanswered questions regarding dormancy but the understanding of CSCs will play a role in furthering this field and therapeutics to address dormancy.

Therapeutic targeting of cancer stem cells

The CSC model has significant clinical implications. In addition to emphasizing the importance of successfully targeting these cells, acknowledgment of their existence implies a critical role in the TME, which merits thoughtful consideration for the future design of therapeutic trials and development of appropriate clinical endpoints. Currently, tumor shrinkage as accessed by RECIST (response evaluation criteria in solid tumors) is considered an important endpoint for accessing treatment efficacy. However, tumor shrinkage is only poorly correlated with ultimate patient survival across a wide spectrum of tumor types.[204] Tumor shrinkage is a measure of effects of treatments on bulk tumor populations. As CSC constitute only a minority of the tumor bulk, successful targeting of these cells will not necessarily lead to tumor shrinkage. For that reason, the current approach for CSC drug development involves accessing toxicity in Phase I trials followed by combining CSC-targeting drugs with more traditional agents that target bulk populations. As many of the pathways utilized by CSC are shared with normal tissue stem cells, caution is required when introducing such therapeutics in the clinic to access their safety profile. With this cautionary note, a number of CSC-targeting drugs summarized in Figure 3 are now in early phase clinical testing. Interestingly, preliminary data suggests that these agents are well tolerated at doses that reduce CSC number in serial biopsies.[205] This suggests that CSC may be more dependent on these pathways than their normal tissue stem cell counterparts, providing an advantageous therapeutic window. Novel methods are under development to achieve more direct measurement of CSC targeting agents' effects.

Another important prediction of the CSC model is that CSC-targeted therapies should have their greatest effect when they are deployed in the adjuvant setting. This is the case because the CSCs are unique in that they possess a sufficient self-renewal capacity to generate clinically significant disease from micrometastases. The efficacy of adjuvant therapies is directly related to their ability to eliminate micrometastasis. This concept is supported by studies demonstrating the remarkable ability of Her2-targeting

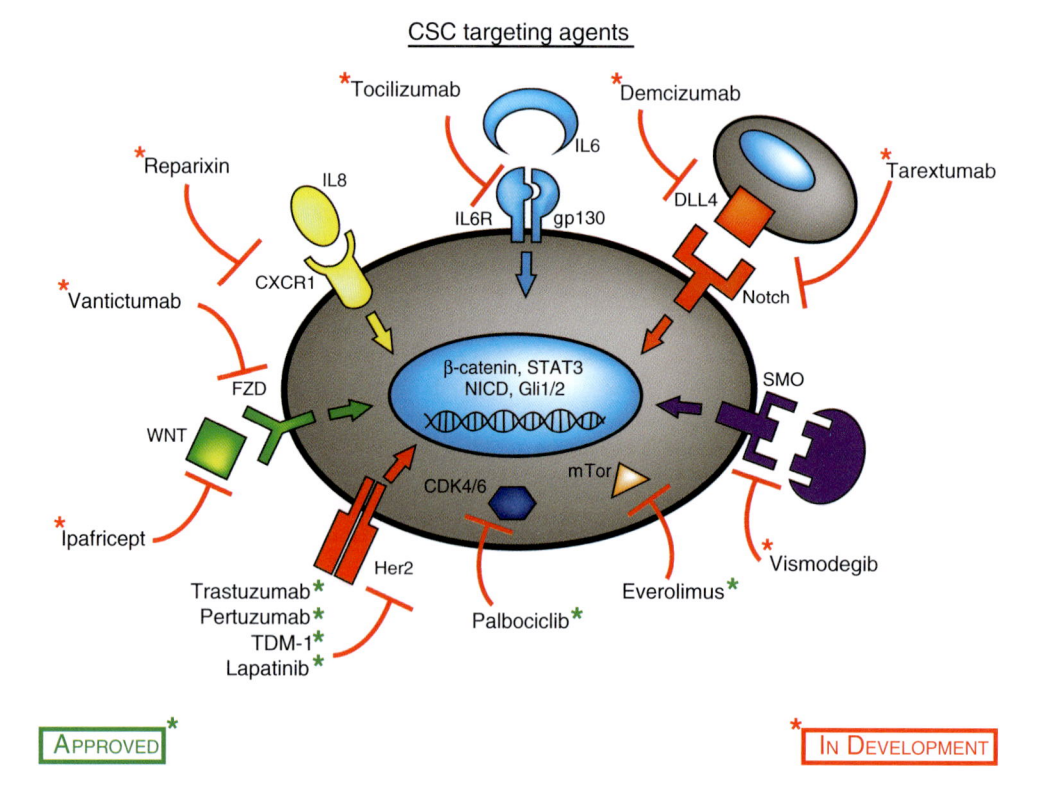

Figure 3 Cancer stem cell-targeted drugs and their cellular targets currently being evaluated in early phase clinical trials or FDA approved for other purposes.

drugs, such as trastuzumab, to prevent recurrence when utilized in the adjuvant setting in Her2+ breast cancer.[188] The clinical importance of Her2 in breast cancer may be due to its role as an important regulator of CSC in these tumors.[206]

One of the most exciting areas in cancer therapy is the development of cancer immunotherapies including immune checkpoint blockers. Interestingly, there is evidence that CSC may be particularly competent at evading immune surveillance. Several mechanisms have been proposed, including the high expression of PDL-1 or secretion of immunosuppressive TGF-β.[207] A number of approaches utilizing the immune system to target CSCs are being developed to circumvent these processes. These include CSC-based vaccines and peptides.[41,208] In the future, such approaches may be combined with immune checkpoint blockade to more effectively target CSCs.

Worldwide, there are currently over 70 clinical trials utilizing novel CSC targeting agents. Most of these studies are in their early stages but the next several years should yield exciting and potentially significant results. Ultimately, carefully controlled randomized clinical trials will be required to conclusively determine if the successful targeting of CSCs improves patient outcome.

Summary

Despite considerable progress in delineating the molecular underpinnings of cancer, this increased understanding has yet to translate into significant improvements in survival for patients with advanced disease. For most common cancers, the development of metastasis renders them incurable. There is now substantial evidence that many cancers are hierarchically organized and driven by a population of cells that display stem cell properties. These properties include the ability to self-renew and differentiate, forming the cells that constitute the tumor bulk. These cells, termed "tumor-initiating cells" or "CSCs," mediate tumor metastasis and contribute to treatment resistance. The existence of as well as understanding of molecular mechanisms regulating cancer stem cells is of clinical significance in that additional therapies targeting stem cell populations may be required to limit metastasis and significantly improve patient survival.

Key references

The complete reference list can be found on Vital Source version of this title, see inside front cover.

1. Huntly BJ, Gilliland DG. Cancer biology: summing up cancer stem cells. *Nature*. 2005;**435**:1169.
2. Sell S. On the stem cell origin of cancer. *Am J Pathol*. 2010;**176**:2584–2594.
3. Reya T, Morrison SJ, Clarke MF, Weissman IL. Stem cells, cancer, and cancer stem cells. *Nature*. 2001;**414**:105.
4. Pattabiraman DR, Weinberg RA. Tackling the cancer stem cells—what challenges do they pose? *Nat Rev Drug Discov*. 2014;**13**:497.
5. Tomasetti C, Vogelstein B. Variation in cancer risk among tissues can be explained by the number of stem cell divisions. *Science (New York, NY)*. 2015;**347**:78.
6. Bonnet D, Dick JE. Human acute myeloid leukemia is organized as a hierarchy that originates from a primitive hematopoietic cell. *Nat Med*. 1997;**3**:730.
7. Al-Hajj M, Wicha MS, Benito-Hernandez A, et al. Prospective identification of tumorigenic breast cancer cells. *Proc Natl Acad Sci U S A*. 2003;**100**:3983–3988.
8. Singh SK et al. Identification of human brain tumour initiating cells. *Nature*. 2004;**432**:396.
9. Collins AT, Berry PA, Hyde C, et al. Prospective identification of tumorigenic prostate cancer stem cells. *Cancer Res*. 2005;**65**:10946–10951.
10. Patrawala L et al. Highly purified CD44+ prostate cancer cells from xenograft human tumors are enriched in tumorigenic and metastatic progenitor cells. *Oncogene*. 2006;**25**:1696–1708.
11. O'Brien CA, Pollett A, Gallinger S, Dick JE. A human colon cancer cell capable of initiating tumour growth in immunodeficient mice. *Nature*. 2007;**445**:106.
12. Ricci-Vitiani L et al. Identification and expansion of human colon-cancer-initiating cells. *Nature*. 2007;**445**:111.
13. Li C et al. Identification of pancreatic cancer stem cells. *Cancer Res*. 2007;**67**:1030–1037.
20. Ginestier C et al. ALDH1 is a marker of normal and malignant human mammary stem cells and a predictor of poor clinical outcome. *Cell Stem Cell*. 2007;**1**:555–567.
31. Kusumbe AP, Bapat SA. Cancer stem cells and aneuploid populations within developing tumors are the major determinants of tumor dormancy. *Cancer Res*. 2009;**69**:9245–9253.
34. Dontu G et al. In vitro propagation and transcriptional profiling of human mammary stem/progenitor cells. *Genes Dev*. 2003;**17**:1253–1270.
36. Weiswald L-B, Bellet D, Dangles-Marie V. Spherical cancer models in tumor biology. *Neoplasia*. 2015;**17**:1–15.
37. Barrett LE et al. Self-renewal does not predict tumor growth potential in mouse models of high-grade glioma. *Cancer Cell*. 2012;**21**:11–24.
38. Quintana E et al. Efficient tumour formation by single human melanoma cells. *Nature*. 2008;**456**:593.
39. Boyle ST, Kochetkova M. Breast cancer stem cells and the immune system: promotion, evasion and therapy. *J Mammary Gland Biol Neoplasia*. 2014;**19**:203–211.
44. Schepers AG et al. Lineage tracing reveals Lgr5+ stem cell activity in mouse intestinal adenomas. *Science*. 2012;**337**:730–735.
47. Widschwendter M et al. Epigenetic stem cell signature in cancer. *Nat Genet*. 2007;**39**:157.
52. Pathania R et al. DNMT1 is essential for mammary and cancer stem cell maintenance and tumorigenesis. *Nat Commun*. 2015;**6**:6910.
54. Roesch A et al. A temporarily distinct subpopulation of slow-cycling melanoma cells is required for continuous tumor growth. *Cell*. 2010;**141**:583–594.
57. Malta TM et al. Machine learning identifies stemness features associated with oncogenic dedifferentiation. *Cell 173*. 2018;**e315**:338–354.
58. Miranda A et al. Cancer stemness, intratumoral heterogeneity, and immune response across cancers. *Proc Natl Acad Sci U S A*. 2019;**116**:9020–9029.
62. Tata PR et al. Dedifferentiation of committed epithelial cells into stem cells in vivo. *Nature*. 2013;**503**:218.
63. Takahashi K, Yamanaka S. Induction of pluripotent stem cells from mouse embryonic and adult fibroblast cultures by defined factors. *Cell*. 2006;**126**:663–676.
69. Guo W et al. Slug and Sox9 cooperatively determine the mammary stem cell state. *Cell*. 2012;**148**:1015–1028.
70. Acloque H, Adams MS, Fishwick K, et al. Epithelial-mesenchymal transitions: the importance of changing cell state in development and disease. *J Clin Invest*. 2009;**119**:1438–1449.
71. Kang Y, Massagué J. Epithelial-mesenchymal transitions: twist in development and metastasis. *Cell*. 2004;**118**:277–279.
74. Onder TT et al. Loss of E-cadherin promotes metastasis via multiple downstream transcriptional pathways. *Cancer Res*. 2008;**68**:3645–3654.
77. Mani SA et al. The epithelial-mesenchymal transition generates cells with properties of stem cells. *Cell*. 2008;**133**:704–715.
79. Morel A-P et al. EMT inducers catalyze malignant transformation of mammary epithelial cells and drive tumorigenesis towards claudin-low tumors in transgenic mice. *PLoS Genet*. 2012;**8**:e1002723.
81. Liu S et al. Breast cancer stem cells transition between epithelial and mesenchymal states reflective of their normal counterparts. *Stem Cell Rep*. 2014;**2**:78–91.
82. Liu S, Clouthier SG, Wicha MS. Role of microRNAs in the regulation of breast cancer stem cells. *J Mammary Gland Biol Neoplasia*. 2012;**17**:15–21.
87. Chaffer CL et al. Poised chromatin at the ZEB1 promoter enables breast cancer cell plasticity and enhances tumorigenicity. *Cell*. 2013;**154**:61–74.
100. Mani SA et al. Mesenchyme Forkhead 1 (FOXC2) plays a key role in metastasis and is associated with aggressive basal-like breast cancers. *Proc Natl Acad Sci*. 2007;**104**:10069–10074.
103. Liu S et al. Hedgehog signaling and Bmi-1 regulate self-renewal of normal and malignant human mammary stem cells. *Cancer Res*. 2006;**66**:6063–6071.
109. Kang Y et al. A multigenic program mediating breast cancer metastasis to bone. *Cancer Cell*. 2003;**3**:537–549.
131. Harrison H et al. Regulation of breast cancer stem cell activity by signaling through the Notch4 receptor. *Cancer Res*. 2010;**70**:709–718.
132. Dontu G et al. Role of Notch signaling in cell-fate determination of human mammary stem/progenitor cells. *Breast Cancer Res*. 2004;**6**:R605.
140. Farnie G, Willan PM, Clarke RB, Bundred NJ. Combined inhibition of ErbB1/2 and Notch receptors effectively targets breast ductal carcinoma in situ (DCIS) stem/progenitor cell activity regardless of ErbB2 status. *PLoS One*. 2013;**8**:e56840.

152 de La Coste A et al. Somatic mutations of the β-catenin gene are frequent in mouse and human hepatocellular carcinomas. *Proc Natl Acad Sci*. 1998;**95**:8847–8851.

154 Miller RK, et al. Beta-catenin versus the other armadillo catenins: assessing our current view of canonical Wnt signaling. *Progress in molecular biology and translational science*. 2013;**116**:1387–40.

161 Heuberger J, Birchmeier W. Interplay of cadherin-mediated cell adhesion and canonical Wnt signaling. *Cold Spring Harb Perspect Biol*. 2010;**2**:a002915.

176 Tsuyada A et al. CCL2 mediates cross-talk between cancer cells and stromal fibroblasts that regulates breast cancer stem cells. *Cancer Res*. 2012;**72**:2768–2779.

177 Spees JL, Lee RH, Gregory CA. Mechanisms of mesenchymal stem/stromal cell function. *Stem Cell Res Ther*. 2016;**7**:125.

178 Liu S et al. Breast cancer stem cells are regulated by mesenchymal stem cells through cytokine networks. *Cancer Res*. 2011;**71**:614–624.

180 Vesely MD, Kershaw MH, Schreiber RD, Smyth MJ. Natural innate and adaptive immunity to cancer. *Annu Rev Immunol*. 2011;**29**:235–271.

182 Yang J et al. Tumor-associated macrophages regulate murine breast cancer stem cells through a novel paracrine EGFR/Stat3/Sox-2 signaling pathway. *Stem Cells*. 2013;**31**:248–258.

184 Peng D et al. Myeloid-derived suppressor cells endow stem-like qualities to breast cancer cells through IL6/STAT3 and NO/NOTCH cross-talk signaling. *Cancer Res*. 2016;**76**:3156–3165.

190 Steinbichler TB et al. "The role of exosomes in cancer metastasis." *Seminars in cancer biology*. Vol. 44. Academic Press, 2017.

191 Sceneay J, Smyth MJ, Möller A. The pre-metastatic niche: finding common ground. *Cancer Metastasis Rev*. 2013;**32**:449–464.

192 Kaplan RN et al. VEGFR1-positive haematopoietic bone marrow progenitors initiate the pre-metastatic niche. *Nature*. 2005;**438**:820.

193 Aktas B et al. Stem cell and epithelial-mesenchymal transition markers are frequently overexpressed in circulating tumor cells of metastatic breast cancer patients. *Breast Cancer Res*. 2009;**11**:R46.

196 Theodoropoulos PA et al. Circulating tumor cells with a putative stem cell phenotype in peripheral blood of patients with breast cancer. *Cancer Lett*. 2010;**288**:99–106.

197 Balic M et al. Most early disseminated cancer cells detected in bone marrow of breast cancer patients have a putative breast cancer stem cell phenotype. *Clin Cancer Res*. 2006;**12**:5615–5621.

198 Williams K, Motiani K, Giridhar PV, Kasper S. CD44 integrates signaling in normal stem cell, cancer stem cell and (pre) metastatic niches. *Exp Biol Med*. 2013;**238**:324–338.

199 Sosa MS, Bragado P, Aguirre-Ghiso JA. Mechanisms of disseminated cancer cell dormancy: an awakening field. *Nat Rev Cancer*. 2014;**14**:611.

200 Pan H et al. 20-year risks of breast-cancer recurrence after stopping endocrine therapy at 5 years. *N Engl J Med*. 2017;**377**:1836–1846.

204 Reddy RM, Kakarala M, Wicha MS. Clinical trial design for testing the stem cell model for the prevention and treatment of cancer. *Cancer*. 2011;**3**:2696–2708.

13 Cancer and cell death

John C. Reed, MD, PhD

Overview

Cell death is a normal facet of human physiology, ensuring tissue homeostasis by offsetting cell production with cell demise. Neoplasms arise in part because of defects in physiological cell death mechanisms, contributing to pathological cell expansion when genetic or epigenetic alternations impart a selective survival advantage to premalignant or malignant cells. Defects in normal cell death pathways also contribute to cancer progression by permitting progressively aberrant cell behaviors, while also desensitizing tumor cells to immune-mediated attack, radiation, and chemotherapy. Multiple mechanisms have been identified that account for dysregulation of cell death mechanisms in human malignancies, providing insights into cancer pathogenesis and providing targets for therapeutic intervention based on the concept of restoring sensitivity to natural pathways for triggering cell suicide. Moreover, the extensive overlap of components of the cell death machinery with responses to pathogens has been implicated in tumor immunity mechanisms.

Introduction

Evasion of endogenous cell death processes represents one of the cardinal characteristics of cancer.[1] Enormous amounts of cell death occur on a daily basis within the human body, estimated at 50–70 billion cells per day for the average adult. In bulk terms, this amounts to a mass of cells equal to an entire body weight annually. This "programmed" cell death offsets daily cell production resulting from cell division, achieving tissue homeostasis. Cell death can proceed by several distinct mechanisms. Apoptosis and necrosis are the two broadest categories of cell death mechanisms, but specialized forms of cell death have also been described including necroptosis, pyroptosis, ferroptosis, autophagic cell death (autosis), lysosomal cell death, parthenatos, phagoptosis, and others.[2] Apoptosis is the most common nonpathological route of cell demise in the context of normal tissue homeostasis and mammalian development, where cell death is generally immunologically silent or even immune tolerizing.[3–5]

Numerous examples have been delineated whereby cancer cells place roadblocks in the way of endogenous cell death mechanisms, thus endowing neoplastic cells with a selective survival advantage. Several molecules that create barriers to cell death within tumors have been identified, providing insights into pathogenic mechanisms of human neoplasia and cancer—in addition to suggesting targets for drug discovery, with the aim to restore integrity of natural pathways for cell suicide and thereby stimulating auto-destruction of cancer cells.[5,6] Alternatively, malignant cells can escape demise by silencing or neutralizing endogenous activators of cell death, with several examples of such mechanisms already elucidated. Replacing or reawakening these endogenous stimulators of programmed cell death defines another emerging strategy for potentially eradicating tumors.[7,8]

Defects in natural mechanisms for cell death aid cancers in many ways.[5,6,9] First, activation of oncogenes such as *C-MYC* drives proliferation of transformed cells but also promotes apoptosis, unless counteracted by cell survival proteins—thus constituting a type of oncogene "complementation."[10] A second, closely related, benefit to tumors of defective cell death is that various cell cycle "checkpoints" trigger apoptosis of cells undergoing aberrant cell replication or division. Thus, defects in apoptosis and other cell death mechanisms can permit aberrant cell division. Third, genomic instability is also aided by defects in cell death mechanisms because mutations introduced by DNA replication errors and chromosome segregation errors would normally trigger cell suicide. Fourth, defects in cell death mechanism allow growth factor (or hormone)-independent cell survival, thus helping transformed cells to escape normal paracrine and endocrine growth control mechanisms. Fifth, cell death induced by hypoxia and metabolic stress, conditions that occur in the microenvironments of most rapidly growing solid tumors, are neutralized by defects in cell death machinery that occur in cancers. Sixth, invasion and metastasis of solid tumors may also be enabled by defects in cell death mechanisms, given that epithelial cells normally undergo apoptosis when they lose their attachment to extracellular matrix (ECM) through integrins.[11] Seventh, defects in cell death mechanisms contribute to avoidance of immune surveillance mechanisms by making it more difficult for cytolytic T cells (CTLs) and natural killer (NK) cells to kill tumor cells.

In this article, the major pathways for cell death are reviewed, and examples of their defects in cancers are described, including hypoexpression (hypoactivity) of pro-death genes and overexpression (hyperactivity) of cytoprotective genes. Also described are routes of cell demise that can be invoked in tumor cells by therapeutic agents, including apoptotic and nonapoptotic cell death. Insights into the mechanisms that lead to cell death dysregulation in cancers have also sparked a variety of oncology drug discovery and development efforts, which are also described briefly. With apology to the many contributors to the field of cell death biology, only representative references are cited for purposes of brevity.

Pathways for cell death

Several endogenous pathways for triggering cell suicide have been delineated and a variety of ways for cataloging these cell death mechanisms have been utilized by the research community.[9,12,13] A general construct for categorizing cell death mechanisms can be attributed to the essential involvement of a family of intracellular proteases called "caspases" (cysteine-dependent aspartate-specific proteases).[14] Broadly, cell death mechanisms can thus be divided

---

Holland-Frei Cancer Medicine, Tenth Edition. Edited by Robert C. Bast, John C. Byrd, Carlo M. Croce, Ernest Hawk, Fadlo R. Khuri, Raphael E. Pollock, Apostolia M. Tsimberidou, Christopher G. Willett, and Cheryl L. Willman.
© 2023 John Wiley & Sons, Inc. Published 2023 by John Wiley & Sons, Inc.

into caspase-dependent versus caspase-independent, though mixtures of these two basic mechanisms are commonly observed in various settings.

Caspase-dependent cell death

Caspase-dependent cell death culminates in the constellation of morphological changes meeting criteria for "apoptosis," where cells detach from the ECM, become rounded and shrunken in volume, with nuclear chromatin condensation and nuclear fragmentation, and the membrane "bubbling" with membrane protrusions (blebs) that can bud off to create apoptotic bodies. These morphological changes can be attributed directly or indirectly to the multitude of proteolytic cleavage events mediated by caspases, a full accounting of which is still under investigation using comprehensive proteomics methods.[15]

Caspases operate in hierarchical networks of upstream initiators and downstream effectors, where caspases cleave and activate each other to create amplifiable cascades of proteolysis.[16,17] These proteases are present as inactive zymogens within the cytosol of essentially all animal cells. Activation of the most proximal caspases typically occurs through protein interactions that encourage clustering of the inactive zymogens.[17] Once activated, these upstream initiators then cleave and activate downstream effector caspases. The upstream initiator caspases contain N-terminal prodomains that mediate protein interactions with other proteins involved in caspase regulation—namely CARDs (caspase-associated recruitment domains) and death effector domains (DEDs) (Table 1). Genomic mutations that inactive caspases have been described in a variety of cancers, though overall they are relatively rare—perhaps suggesting that loss of any one of these proteases is insufficient to endow cells with a selective growth advantage.

Multiple pathways that lead to caspase activation and that thereby cause apoptosis or variations of apoptosis have been delineated (Figure 1). For example, CTL and NK cells introduce apoptosis-inducing proteases, particularly granzyme B (a serine protease), into target cells via perforin-mediated pores.[18] Enzymologically, granzyme B is a serine rather than a cysteine protease. However, similar to the caspases, granzyme B cleaves its substrates at Asp residues.[19] Granzyme B is capable of cleaving and activating multiple caspases. Tumors overcome this pathway for cell death by expressing various immune ligands for checkpoint receptors expressed on T-cells (PD1, Tim3, LAG3, etc.) that suppress T-cell activation or by expressing ligands for inhibitory NK receptors (KIRs).

Another caspase-activation pathway is stimulated by tumor necrosis factor (TNF) family receptors. Eight of the ~30 known members of the TNF family in humans contain a so-called death domain (DD) in their cytosolic tails.[20,21] Several of these DD-containing TNF-family receptors use caspase-activation as a signaling mechanism, including TNFR1/CD120a, Fas/APO1/CD95, death receptor 3 (DR3)/Apo2/Weasle, DR4/TrailR1, DR5/TrailR2, and DR6. Ligation of these receptors at the cell surface results in receptor clustering and recruitment of several intracellular proteins, including certain pro-caspases, to the cytosolic domains of these receptors, forming a "death-inducing signaling complex" (DISC) that triggers caspase activation and leads to apoptosis.[22]

The specific caspases recruited to the DISC are caspase-8 and, in some cases, caspase-10. These caspases contain DEDs in their N-terminal prodomains that bind to a corresponding DED in FADD, a bipartite adapter protein containing a DD and a DED. FADD functions as a molecular bridge between the DD and DED domain families and is in fact the only protein in the human genome with this dual-domain structure. Consequently, cells from mice in which the *fadd* gene has been knocked out are resistant to apoptosis induction by TNF-family cytokines and their receptors. Cells derived from *caspase-8* knock-out mice also fail to undergo apoptosis in response to ligands or antibodies that activate TNF-family death receptors, demonstrating an essential role for this caspase in this pathway.[23,24] However, mice lack the highly homologous protease, caspase-10, which is found in humans, having arisen from an apparent gene duplication on chromosome 2.[16] Thus, caspases-8 and 10 may play redundant roles in human cells. Additionally, it would be an understatement to state that the complexity of roles characterizes these caspases, a topic that will be addressed later in this article when we touch on necroptosis.

Genomic mutations in genes encoding TNF-family ligands or receptors have been documented in some types of cancer. For example, somatic mutations in the *FAS (CD95)* gene have been found in lymphoid malignancies.[25,26] Missense mutations within the DD of Fas (CD95) are associated with retention of the wild-type allele, suggesting a dominant-negative mechanism, whereas missense mutations outside the DD are associated with allelic loss.

Mitochondria also play important roles in apoptosis, releasing cytochrome-c (Cyt-c) into the cytosol, which then causes the assembly of a multiprotein caspase-activating complex, referred to as the "**apoptosome**".[27–30] The central component of the apoptosome is Apaf1, a caspase-activating protein that oligomerizes upon binding Cyt-c and which specifically binds pro-caspase-9. Apaf1 and pro-caspase-9 interact with each other via their CARDs. Such CARD–CARD interactions play important roles in many steps in apoptosis pathways. The central importance of the Cyt-c-dependent pathway for apoptosis is underscored by the observation that cells derived from mice in which either the *apaf1* or *pro-caspase-9* genes have been ablated are incapable of undergoing apoptosis in response to agents that trigger Cyt-c release from mitochondria.[31,32] Nevertheless, such cells can die by non-apoptotic routes,[33] demonstrating that mitochondria control both caspase-dependent and caspase-independent cell death pathways (see below). Mitochondria can also participate in cell death pathways induced via TNF-family death receptors, through cross-talk mechanisms involving proteins such as Bid, which becomes activated upon proteolytic cleavage by caspase-8 and then stimulates Cyt-c release from mitochondria.[34] However, mitochondrial ("intrinsic") and death receptor ("extrinsic") pathways for caspase activation are fully capable of independent operation in most (but not all) types of cells.[35] Tumor cells can evolve a variety of mechanisms for averting mitochondria-dependent apoptosis, as outlined below.

Table 1 Domains associated with cell death proteins.

Domain	Proteins (examples)
Caspase catalytic domain	Caspase family cysteine proteases
Caspase-associated recruitment domain (CARD)	Caspases-1, -4, -5, -9; Apaf1; ASC; NLRP1, 4
Death domain (DD)	TNFR1, FAS, DR4, DR5, TRADD, RAIDD, RIP1
Death effector domain (DED)	Caspases-8, -10; FADD; c-FLIP
Baculovirus IAP repeat (BIR)	XIAP, c-IAP1, c-IAP2, Livin, Apollon, ML-IAP, NAIP
Bcl-2 homology (BH)	Bcl-2, Bcl-XL, Mcl-1, Bax, Bak, Bim, Bid
Pyrin domain (PYD)	ASC, NLRP1, NLRP3, etc., AIM2
Receptor homologous interaction motif (RHIM)	RipK1, RipK3

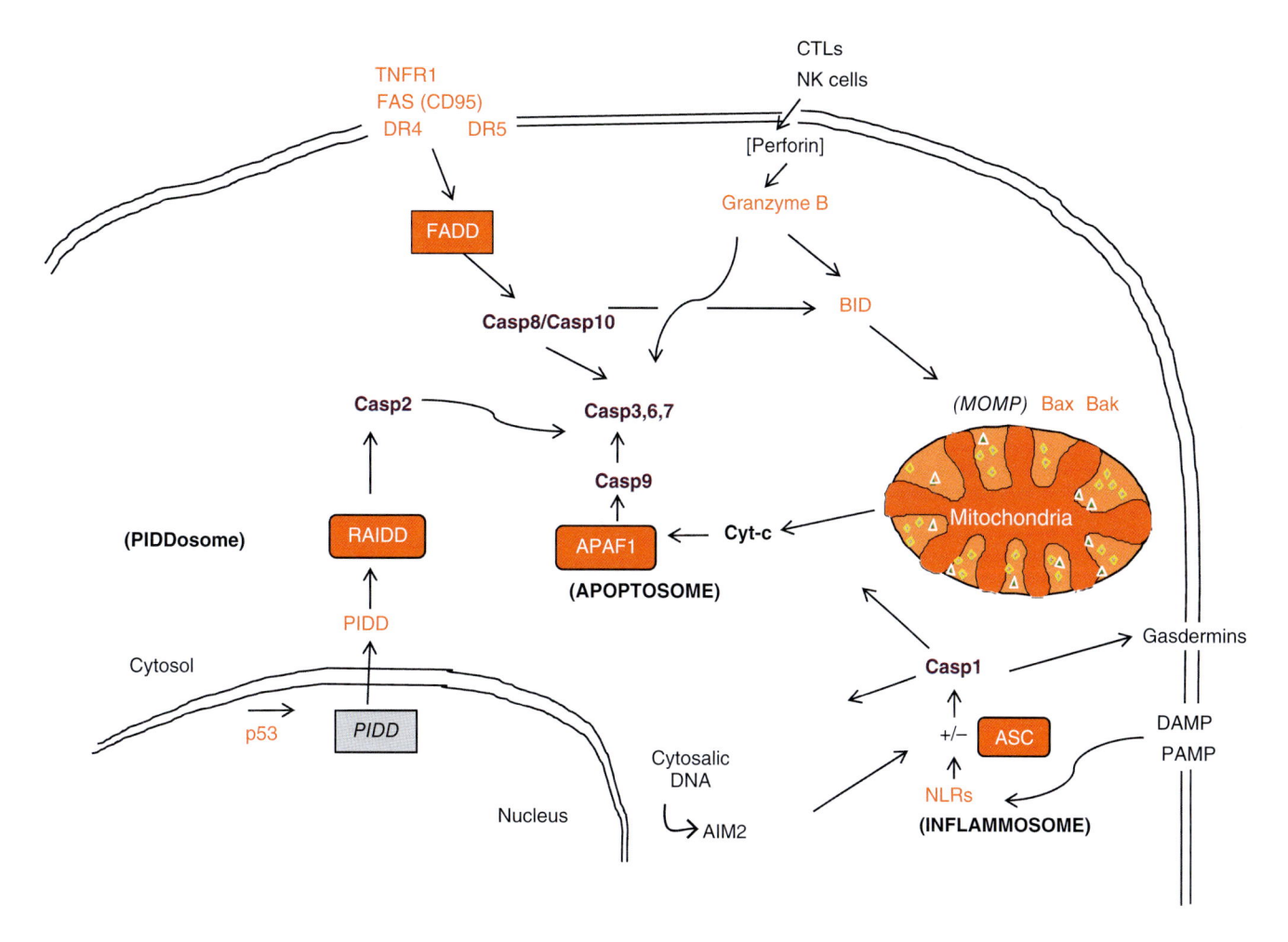

Figure 1 Caspase activation pathways. The major pathways for caspase activation in mammalian cells are presented. The schematic represents an oversimplification of the events that occur in vivo. The extrinsic (left, upper) is induced by members of the TNF-family of cytokine receptors such as TNFR1, Fas, and the TRAIL receptors, DR4, and DR5. These proteins recruit adapter proteins to their cytosolic DDs, including FADD, to assemble "death-inducing signaling complexes" (DISCs), which bind DED-containing pro-caspases, particularly pro-caspase-8, inducing their activation. Caspase-8 (and caspase-10 in humans) cleave downstream effector proteases, such as caspases-3, -6, and -7, as well as pro-apoptotic Bcl-2 family member Bid, which is an agonist of MOMP-inducing Bax and Bak. CTLs and NK cells introduce the protease granzyme B to target cells (right, upper). This protease cleaves and activates multiple members of the caspase family, as well as Bid. The intrinsic pathway (left, lower) is initiated by the release of Cyt-c from mitochondria, induced by various stimuli, including elevations in the levels of pore-forming pro-apoptotic Bcl-2 family proteins such as Bax and Bak. In the cytosol, Cyt-c binds and activates Apaf-1, allowing it to associate with and activate pro-caspase-9, forming "apoptosomes." Active caspase-9 directly cleaves and activates the effector proteases, caspase-3 and -7. Exogenous PAMPs and endogenous DAMPs active NLR family proteins to cause their oligomerization and assembly of "inflammasomes" that may contain PYD-containing adapter protein ASC in many cases, which binds pro-caspase-1. Activated caspase-1 cleaves a variety of cellular proteins, including cytokines as well as plasma membrane pore-forming proteins (particularly gasdermins) that promote osmotic stress and cell death. gasdermin-mediated pores contribute to NLR-based inflammasome activation through ionic flux changes. AIM2 senses cytosolic DNA and binds via its PYD to the PYD of adapter protein ASC, which in turn binds via its CARD to the CARD of pro-caspase-1, thereby inducing pyroptosis.

Activation of caspase-1 in the context of infection and inflammation has been shown to stimulate a caspase-dependent form of cell death called **pyroptosis**.[36] Caspase-1 has a CARD-containing prodomain that can bind directly to the CARDs of NLR (nucleotide-binding domain and leucine-rich repeat domain) proteins, such as NLRP1 (NALP1). Alternatively, the CARD of caspase-1 can bind the CARD of a bipartite adapter protein ASC (Pycard), which also contains a PRYIN domain (PYD) that binds PYDs of NLR family proteins such as NLRP3 (NALP3) or proteins such as AIM2. NLRs oligomerize in response to binding components of pathogens (pathogen-associated molecular patterns, PAMPs) or molecules elaborated during tissue injury (danger-associated molecular patterns, DAMPs), forming "**inflammasomes**" that recruit and activate caspase-1.[37–40] For purposes of completeness, the human genome encodes a very closely related, probably largely interchangeable protein, caspase-4, while mice have an alternative protein, caspase-11, that interestingly becomes activated via binding of bacterial lipopolysaccharide (LPS) together with other proteins. The ultimate route of cell death ascribed to pyroptosis entails cleavage of gasdermin B (and possibly other members of this family), which then forms pores in the plasma membrane.

The relevance of pyroptosis to cancer biology is still under investigation.[41] However, stressful conditions of the tumor microenvironment (TME), particularly after exposure to chemotherapy or radiation, can elaborate DAMPs that trigger inflammasome assembly and pyroptosis. Moreover, AIM2 and probably other intracellular sensors of DNA in aberrant cellular locations (e.g., cytosol) are purported to become relevant in aneuploid tumors where chromosomal nondisjunction events during

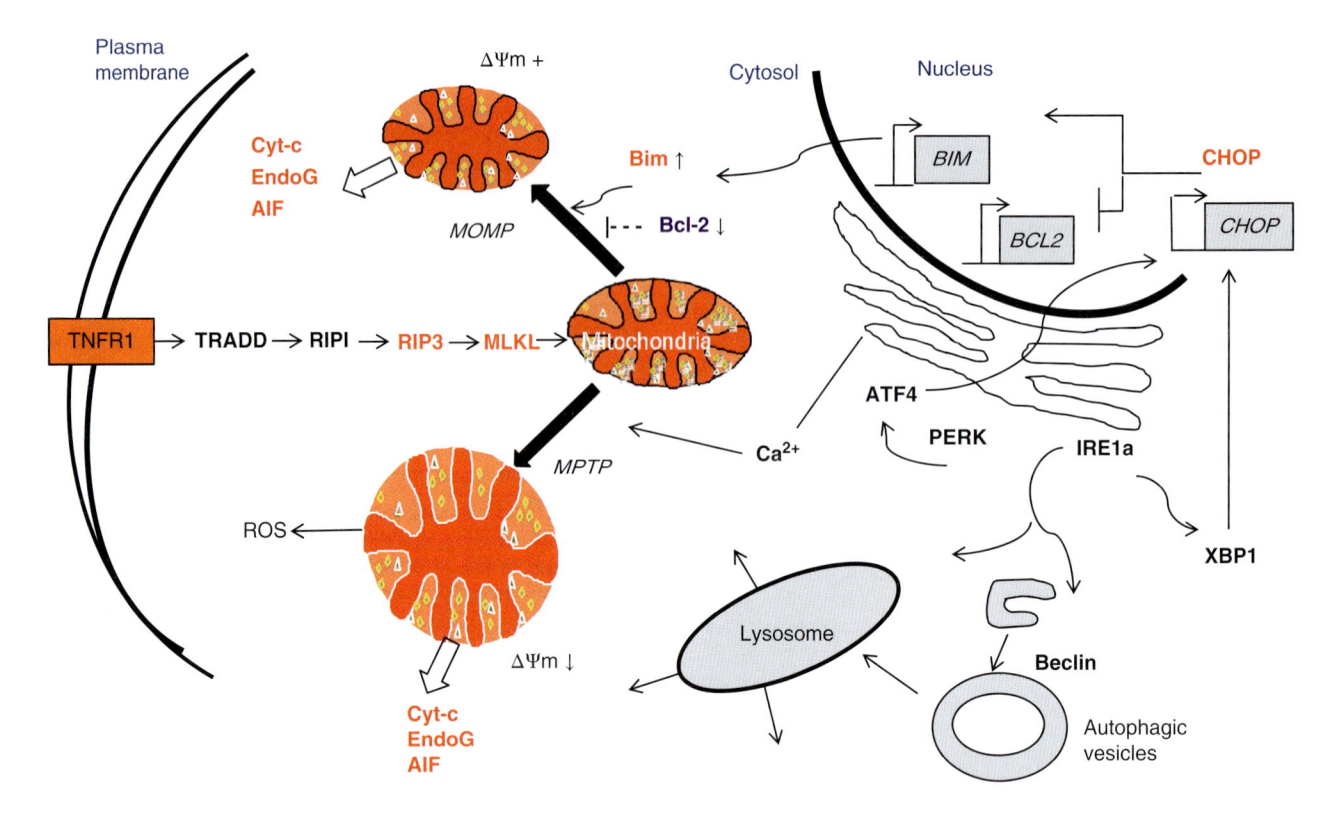

Figure 2 *Caspase-independent cell death pathways.* Some of the prominent caspase-independent cell death mechanisms are depicted. The TNFR1-mediated pathway for necrosis (necroptosis) involves a cascade of events that include recruitment of Rip1, which in turn activates Rip3, which activates MLKL and which causes mitochondrial and probably lysosomal changes that stimulate ROS generation and lead to necrosis. The cytosolic DD of TNFR1 binds the DD-containing adapter protein TRADD, which binds the DD of Rip1. The kinase cascade involves Rip1, followed by Rip3, followed by MLKL. Mitochondria release proteins stored in the inter-membrane space, including Cyt-c, endonuclease G, and AIF. The release can be induced by MOMP (*upper*), which is regulated by Bcl-2 family proteins and does not involve organelle swelling. Alternatively, the release of mitochondrial contents occurs as a result of MPTP complex opening, which leads to organelle swelling and loss of the electrochemical gradient ($\Delta\Psi_m$). MPTP opening is induced by Ca^{2+} influx and oxidative stress, among other stimuli. Accumulation of unfolded proteins in the ER results in UPR signaling, including activation of IRE1α, which splices XBP1 mRNA to generate XBP1 protein (transcription factor), and activation of the kinase PERK, which stimulates phosphorylation events that promote ATF4 mRNA translation and production of transcription factor ATF4. The UPR transcription factors (XBP1, ATF4, and (not shown) ATF6) converge on the promoter of the CHOP gene, which encodes a transcription factor that upregulates pro-apoptotic gene BIM and downregulates antiapoptotic gene BCL-2. Autophagic vesicles emerge from the ER and form double-membrane vesicles, which fuse with lysosomes (*bottom, right*).

cell division lead to mislocation of unpaired chromosomes and pieces of chromosomes.

Caspase-2 is another CARD-carrying member of the caspase family. Its CARD interacts specifically with the CARD of the bipartite adapter protein RIP-associated ICH/CED-3-homologous protein with a death domain (RAIDD), which additionally carries a DD.[42] Caspase-2 activation has been linked to genotoxic stress via a pathway whereby tumor suppressor p53 induces the expression of P53 induced protein with a death domain (PIDD), a DD-containing protein that binds the DD of RAIDD, oligomerizes, and assembles into a multiprotein complex termed the "PIDDosome."[43] However, in the grand scheme of cell death mechanisms that are triggered by genotoxic stress, this caspase-dependent mechanism is probably rather minor. Additional caspase activation mechanisms have been elaborated, though it is less clear how prominently they figure in the pathophysiology of cell death.[44–47]

Caspase-independent cell death

Multiple caspase-independent cell death mechanisms have been identified, with a few prominent examples mentioned here (Figure 2). **Necrosis** can be initiated by many stimuli. It occurs when cells are incapable of maintaining osmotic equilibrium such that plasma membrane integrity is compromised, resulting in cell swelling and rupture. Organelles within cells during necrosis also typically swell and rupture, including mitochondria and lysosomes, releasing molecules that promote cell death. Initiators of necrosis include circumstances that compromise bioenergetics such as hypoxia and hypoglycemia, resulting in inadequate ATP concentrations for powering plasma membrane ionic pumps and insults to the plasma membrane such as serum complement factors that create pores. Necrosis is relevant to cancer biology in the context of rapidly growing tumors that outstrip their vascular supply (insufficient angiogenesis), creating regions of hypoxia and nutrient insufficiency.

Mitochondria-initiated cell death pathways can also lead to caspase-independent cell death, in addition to the aforementioned caspase-dependent pathway downstream of Cyt-c.[48] In addition to Cyt-c, mitochondria also release several other proteins of relevance to apoptosis, including Endonuclease G, Apoptosis Inducing Factor (AIF) (an activator of nuclear endonucleases), and SMAC (Diablo) and Omi (HtrA2), antagonists of a family of caspase-inhibitory proteins known as the IAPs (*see below*).[49,50] Moreover, distinguishing mitochondria-driven apoptotic from nonapoptotic cell death can be challenging in many contexts due to the similar morphological features caused probably by some of the proteins released from these organelles such as EndoG and AIF, which promote chromatin condensation and DNA fragmentation. The mitochondrial mechanisms for apoptotic and nonapoptotic cell death are activated by myriad stimuli, including growth factor deprivation, oxidants, Ca^{2+} overload, DNA-damaging agents, microtubule-modifying drugs, and much more. In this sense, mitochondria are sometimes viewed as central integrators of cell stress signals that dictate ultimately cell life and death decisions.[51-53]

Uniformly, these mitochondrial cell death mechanisms involve compromises of mitochondrial membrane integrity, but the membrane permeability change can occur via different mechanisms.[54] In the context of insults such as ischemia-reperfusion injury (where oxidative stress occurs due to reactive oxygen species (ROS) and nitrosyl free radicals) and Ca^{2+} dysregulation where cytosolic free Ca^{2+} levels rise (due to loss of plasma membrane integrity or escape from the endoplasmic reticulum [ER]), osmotic homeostasis of mitochondria is perturbed due to opening of the **mitochondrial permeability transition pore** (MPTP) complex that spans inner and outer membranes at contact sites where they come into close apposition.[55-57] The change in permeability in the inner membrane of mitochondria allows water and electrolytes to enter the protein-rich matrix of mitochondria, resulting in swelling of the organelle and eventually popping of the outer membrane, whose surface area is smaller than the extensively folded inner membrane with it cristae. During the pathological opening of the MPTP complex, the electrochemical gradient (proton gradient) that is essential for ATP production is lost, and thus bioenergetics is severely compromised. An essential component of the MPTP complex is the adenine nucleotide translocator (ANT), which is thought to be chiefly responsible for the permeability transition that leads to mitochondrial swelling.

Alternatively, cell death mechanisms can involve the phenomenon of **mitochondrial outer membrane permeabilization** (MOMP), where the outer membrane becomes selectively permeabilized, allowing the release of Cyt-c and other proteins that reside in the inter-membrane space.[54,58,59] With MOMP, the electrochemical gradient is preserved, and mitochondrial osmotic homeostasis is maintained. MOMP is caused by pro-apoptotic members of the Bcl-2 family (see below), namely Bax and Bak (possibly also Bok).[60-63] Though others may exist, an established mechanism for triggering MOMP entails the interaction of pro-apoptotic proteins such as Bid, Bim, and Puma with Bax and/or Bak, causing oligomerization of Bax and Bak in the mitochondrial outer membrane and the formation of ill-defined pores that permit the escape of Cyt-c and other proteins. MOMP induced by Bax and/or Bak thus initiates the mitochondrial pathway for caspase-dependent cell death and apoptosis by releasing Cyt-c, but it also secondarily causes caspase-independent necrotic cell death by uncoupling of oxidative phosphorylation (when Cyt-c becomes limiting) and causing diversion of electrons from the respiratory chain into the production of toxic free radicals.[64]

Given the diversity of cell death mechanisms initiated by mitochondria, it is not surprising that tumors evolve a variety of alternations in these organelles and their regulation. The metabolic changes that convert the bioenergetic signature of tumor cells from dependence on aerobic respiration to nonaerobic glycolysis are well known (Warburg effect) and could be argued to make tumor cells less dependent on mitochondria. Indeed, some tumors seem to have a diminution in the numbers of mitochondria compared to normal cells of the same cell lineage.[65]

Cell death induced by CTL and NK cells can also occur via caspase-independent mechanism. In this regard, granzyme B directly cleaves some of the same substrates as caspases,[66,67] thereby potentially bypassing the need for caspases to cause proteolytic events associated with apoptosis. Also, the cytotoxic granules of CTLs and NK cells contain several other death-promoting molecules besides granzyme B.[18] Moreover, the perforin-mediated pores created in the plasma membrane of target cells by CTLs and NK cells can also lead to osmotic disequilibrium and thus caspase-independent cell death. The diversity of cytolytic mechanisms invoked by CTLs and NK cells bodes well for attempts to harness the immune system as a weapon for attacking cancers, since specific blocks to cell death in tumors (see below) might be overwhelmed by the multiple parallel cytotoxic mechanisms initiated by these immune cells.

Necroptosis is the term that has been applied to a caspase-independent cell death mechanism initiated by TNFR1 and selected other members of the TNF receptor family. When caspase-8 is incapacitated, TNFR1 can stimulate a nonapoptotic cell death signaling pathway that involves the serine/threonine protein kinases RipK1 and RipK3, and the pseudo-kinase mixed lineage kinase domain-like (MLKL).[68-70] The interactions of Rip1 and Rip3 interact via receptor homotypic interaction motif (RHIM) domains, which mediate the assembly of multiprotein amyloid structures called "necrosomes" (reviewed in).[71] Phosphorylation of MLKL by RipK3 promotes interaction of MLKL with lipids, where it oligomerizes to disrupt membrane integrity (reviewed in).[72] Rip3-dependent necroptosis occurs predominantly through a process involving ROS generated by mitochondria. Necroptosis was initially identified by studies of tumor cells where TNFα was shown to kill via a caspase-independent mechanism, suggesting that this cell death pathway could provide a conduit for attacking cancers via such cytokines.

Both caspase-dependent and caspase-independent cell death signaling mechanisms have been implicated in endoplasmic reticulum stress (**ER stress**). A wide variety of microenvironmental conditions (including those relevant to the TME) can cause the accumulation of unfolded proteins in the ER, triggering an adaptive signal transduction response called the **unfolded protein response** (UPR).[73-75] Among these UPR events is increased transcription of a gene encoding the pro-apoptotic transcription factor C/EBP homologous protein (CHOP), which in turn stimulates expression of the gene encoding DR5 (death receptor 5; TNF-related apoptosis-inducing ligand [TRAIL] receptor 2), causing caspase-8-dependent apoptosis. Additionally, CHOP has been reported to directly stimulate transcription of the gene encoding Bim, a pro-apoptotic member of the Bcl-2 family (see below) that stimulates Bax/Bak oligomerization in mitochondrial membranes to induce MOMP and release Cyt-c and other proteins from mitochondria. Finally, it has been suggested that ER stress leads to oligomerization in ER membranes of an integral membrane protein Bap31, which contains a DED-like domain and reportedly recruits caspase-8, constituting yet another potential apoptosis-inducing mechanism.[76] Thus, ER stress has multiple potential routes of stimulating both caspase-dependent and -independent cell death, with the predominant pathway probably varying among cell types and pathophysiological contexts.

Furthermore, the important role that the ER plays in regulating intracellular Ca^{2+} homeostasis provides another potential link to the cell death mechanism where changes in cytosolic free Ca^{2+} contribute (reviewed in[77,78]). When extreme, liberation of Ca^{2+} from the lumen of the ER can trigger a variety of downstream signaling events that promote cell death. Also, the ER collaborates with mitochondria in many ways that can either promote cell life or cause death. ER membranes from close contact with mitochondria to create structures where Ca^{2+} effluxes from ER into mitochondria, aiding bioenergetics. However, too much Ca^{2+} entry into mitochondria triggers the opening of the MPTP complex, such that mitochondria swell and eventually rupture.

Autophagy ("self-eating") is a catabolic mechanism where senescent proteins and organelles become entrapped in double-membrane vesicles that bud off from the ER and that are transported to lysosomes for degradation of their contents. The physiological roles of autophagy include protein homeostasis, supplementing the ubiquitin-proteasome system for removal of unfolded, defective, and aged proteins, as well as providing a source of substrates for maintaining metabolism during times of nutrient deprivation.[79,80] In the context of nutrient deprivation, autophagy can contribute to cell survival and is thought to aid tumors at some points in their evolution. However, when taken to an extreme, mechanisms that rely on components of the autophagy machinery have been reported to cause cell death via a process called autophagic cell death (also known as **autosis**), which is caspase-independent.[81] Under some conditions, exposure of tumor cells to cytotoxic chemotherapeutic drugs can trigger autophagic cell death.[82]

Tumor cells can be killed via phagocytic mechanisms, where macrophages engulf and destroy the eaten cell through lysosomal mechanisms. This process has been termed either **phagocytic cell death** or **entosis**.[2] A resistance mechanism used by tumors to avoid phagocytosis involves expression of CD47, a "don't eat me" signal (reviewed in[83]). Upon binding signal regulatory protein-alpha (SIRP-alpha) on macrophages, CD47 suppresses phagocytosis. Besides suppressing phagocytosis, the biology of CD47 is highly complex due to its interactions with a variety of proteins (e.g., integrins and thrombospondin) and its cell type- and cellular context-dependent roles in signal transduction, with reported implications for tumor migration and metastasis, angiogenesis, and evasion of antitumor immune responses.

Anoikis is a term used to describe apoptotic cell death induced by cell suspension, where epithelial cells lose their attachment to ECM.[84] In most experimental systems, anoikis does involve caspase activation, such that pharmacological inhibitors of these proteases delay cell death. However, caspase-independent mechanism probably attributable to MOMP also plays a role. For epithelial cells, integrin-mediated adhesion to ECM is critical for cell survival, thus forcing epithelial cells under normal circumstances to remain in their appropriate positions in the body. In normal physiology, anoikis has been reported for epithelial cells that become extruded from mucosal surfaces. Neoplastic cells must overcome anoikis to metastasize, thus constituting an important progression event in the bio-oncology of solid tumors.

Immunogenic cell death (ICD) is a term that has been used to describe processes by which tumor cell death can help to trigger anticancer immune responses (reviewed in).[85] ICD is caspase-independent. The basic concept stems in part from experiments where cultured tumor cells were treated with various chemotherapeutic agents in vitro at concentrations that all resulted in cell death regardless of the drug. These injured and dying cells were injected into immunocompetent mice as a sort of vaccine and thereafter challenged with viable tumor cells. Only some types of anticancer drugs resulted in immune protection, namely anthracyclines and oxaliplatin (as well as x-irradiation), leading to the concept that the cellular injury induced by certain chemotherapeutic agents endows the stressed and dying cancer cells with immunogenic properties. The concept is consistent with the observation from mouse experimental systems where eradication of tumors by chemotherapy was reported to be successful only in immunocompetent animals.

While molecular details remain a subject of experimental investigation, some of the features of ICD that likely contribute to the immunogenic mechanisms have emerged. Among these are the release of calreticulin from the ER where it gathers on the extracellular surface, release of HMGB1 (the most abundant of the nonhistone chromatin proteins), and excretion of ATP. HMGB1 and ATP are well-known DAMPs that trigger pyroptosis, along with elaboration with multiple cytokines that initiate an innate immune response. HMGB1 also interacts with innate immunity receptors of the toll-like receptor (TLR) and Receptor for advanced glycation end products (RAGE) classes, stimulating the production of multiple cytokines, lymphokines, and chemokines. ATP through purinergic receptors, particularly P2XR7, stimulates ionic changes (K^+ and Ca^{2+} efflux) that stimulate NLRP3 inflammasome assembly. Calreticulin on tumor cell surfaces binds CD91-positive immune cells in the TME, resulting in tumor cell phagocytosis (unless protected by high levels of CD47) and subsequent processing of tumor antigens for presentation by dendritic cells and macrophages.

Relevant to the topic of immune surveillance against tumors, and perhaps also to ICD in some circumstances, various DNA-sensing proteins stimulate an innate immunity mechanism in which STING-1 (TMEM173) plays a central role. STING is an integral membrane protein found in the ER that serves as an adaptor for the assembly of signal transduction complexes that include TBK-1, an activator of IRF-3, NF-kB, and STAT6, transcription factors that stimulate the expression of genes encoding interferons, cytokines, lymphokines. Multiple proteins that sense cytosolic DNA interact directly or indirectly with STING-1 to stimulate this pathway, including DAI, IFI16, and DDX41. An interesting additional pathway for STING-1 activation is initiated by the DNA sensor cGAS (cyclic GMP AMP synthase), which produces a second messenger (cyclic di-GMP) that binds to and activates STING-1.[81] As mentioned above, chromosomal instability in tumor cells is at least one source of ectopic DNA that stimulates the STING pathway, but some chemotherapeutic drugs may also enhance the mislocalization of DNA into the cytosol and thereby stimulate STING. Regardless, activation of the STING pathway is thought to be highly immunogenic. Moreover, STING reportedly can under some circumstances contribute to protein interaction cascades that result in Rip3 activation to stimulate necroptosis.

Additional caspase-independent cell death mechanisms have been described, including lysosome-dependent cell death,[86] iron-dependent cell death (ferroptosis),[87] netotic cell death, parthanatos, and others,[12] which are not reviewed here. All of them may be relevant to cancer biology at some level in some contexts.

Cell death resistance mechanisms used by cancers

Cancer cells have been shown to put the brakes on caspases and thereby suppress apoptosis by at least three fundamental mechanisms—(1) preventing activation of caspase zymogens (pro-enzymes), (2) neutralizing active caspases (active enzymes), and (3) suppressing the expression of genes encoding caspases or caspase-activating proteins (see below). Malignant cells also develop a variety of ways of counteracting caspase-independent cell death mechanisms. Some of the more prominent examples understood to date are outlined here.

IAPs

Endogenous suppressors of caspases include inhibitor of apoptosis proteins (IAPs) ($n = 8$ in humans),[16,88,89] an evolutionarily conserved family of proteins that directly bind active caspases and that either suppress their protease activity or that target active caspases for destruction.[88,90,91] Overexpression of IAPs occurs in cancers and leukemias, making it more difficult to propagate the caspase-dependent proteolytic events necessary for apoptotic cell death.

IAPs are characterized by the presence of protein interaction domains called BIRs (baculovirus internal repeats), numbering between 1 and 3 per protein[92] (Table 1). Most IAPs also carry RING domains that endow them with E3 ligase activity through interactions with ubiquitin-conjugating enzymes (UBCs). Some of the apoptogenic proteins released from mitochondria, notably SMAC and HtrA2,[93,94] bind certain BIRs and thereby compete for protein interactions on the surface of IAPs. In many cases, SMAC binding to IAPs induces their polyubiquitination and proteasomal degradation. Thus, factors that cause MOMP to take the breaks off the caspases by eliminating various IAP family proteins.

The most established caspase inhibitor among the IAP family members is XIAP (so-called because its encoding gene resides on the X-chromosome). The XIAP protein contains 3 BIR domains. BIR2 of XIAP (and an adjacent segment) binds downstream effector proteases, caspases-3 and -7, to potently suppress apoptosis at a distal point. BIR3 of XIAP binds upstream initiator protease, caspase-9, to suppress an apical step in the mitochondrial pathway for apoptosis. Overexpression of XIAP mRNA and protein has been reported in cancers and leukemias, apparently caused by epigenetic mechanisms rather than genomic lesions to the XIAP gene. XIAP protein stability may also be increased in tumors with Akt hyperactivity.[95]

The c-IAP-1 (BIRC2) and c-IAP2 (BIRC3) proteins are also capable of binding to caspases-3, 7, and 9, though they are far less potent as direct enzymatic inhibitors and may rely on their E3 ligase activity for controlling caspase degradation. However, these IAP family members also participate in other cell death-relevant mechanisms by impacting signal transduction by TNF family receptors.[68,69,96] Binding of cytokine TNFα to TNFR1 can trigger at least three different signaling pathways, each involving overlapping but distinct protein complexes that are assembled at the receptor.[97] In addition to the pathways for caspase-dependent and -independent cell death outlined above, TNFR1 also stimulates a cell survival pathway in which c-IAP1 and c-IAP2 participate. In this regard, the BIR3 domains of c-IAP1 and c-IAP2 directly bind the kinase Rip1. In the TNFR1-mediated survival pathway, Rip1 forms protein complexes that contain the E3 ligases c-IAP1, c-IAP2, and TRAF2, stimulating noncanonical (lysine 63, rather than lysine 48) ubiquitination of Rip1 to initiate a signal transduction pathway that causes activation of transcription factor NF-κB.[98,99] NF-κB influences the expression of many target genes involved in host defenses and immune regulation, among which are several genes that suppress apoptosis[100] (see below). As a result, this NF-κB pathway nullifies the caspase pathway, negating apoptosis, in addition to accounting for the untoward inflammatory actions of this cytokine. In addition, the Rip3-dependent pathway for necroptosis is suppressed by c-IAP1 and c-IAP2, probably via their roles as E3 ligases and possibly involving ubiquitin/proteasome-mediated reductions in Rip3 protein levels. In human cancers, chromosomal translocations that deregulate c-IAP2 by creating a chimeric protein (MALT-c-IAP2) have been described in lymphomas.[101,102] Additionally, the genomes of some cancers have amplification of the gene encoding TRAF2, the c-IAP1/c-IAP2-binding protein implicated in TNF-family receptor signaling. Overexpression of c-IAP1 and c-IAP2 mRNAs and proteins, presumably via epigenetic mechanisms, is also reported.

In this regard, c-IAP2 is among the direct transcriptional targets of NF-κB, and hyperactivity of the canonical (RelA) and alternative (RelB) pathways is well established in human malignancies of various types.

Additional members of the IAP family not described here (survivin, Apollon/BRUCE, ML-IAP, etc.) also have interesting mechanisms of interacting with components of cell death pathways and they also can have other roles beyond cell death regulation. For example, the survivin protein plays a fundamental role in chromosome segregation and cytokinesis.[103]

c-FLIP

The c-FLIP protein provides another example of an endogenous modulator of caspases whose overexpression is a common occurrence in tumors.[104,105] FLIP is structurally similar to certain caspases, containing a pair of DEDs analogous to caspases-8 and -10. It directly binds and suppresses activation of caspases-8 and -10 in the context of TNF-family death receptor signaling. However, the role of c-FLIP is more complex than merely suppressing caspase-8/10 activation, as it also collaborates with these caspases in poorly understood ways (probably involving caspase-8, MALT, and Bcl-10) to promote NF-κB activation.[106] Testimony to this complex interaction is also found in the observation that knockout of the genes encoding either c-FLIP or caspase-8 in mice results in similar embryonic lethal phenotypes. In addition to promoting NF-κB activation, the c-FLIP gene is itself also a direct transcriptional target of NF-κB, whose expression is strikingly upregulated (positive feedback).[107]

While c-FLIP interaction with caspase-8 prevents the proteolytic processing events that result in caspase-8-mediated apoptosis, it does not prevent caspase-8 from cleaving the deubiquitinase, CLYD in the context of TNFR1 signaling.[108–110] In this setting, caspase-8 serves as a switch between apoptosis and necroptosis. Specifically, when RipK1 is recruited to TNFR1 complexes, non-canonical ubiquitination of RipK1 promotes its association with the NF-kB activator NEMO, supporting cell survival. However, Cylindromatosis Deubiquitinase (CYLD)-mediated deubiquitination of RipK1 enables its association with RipK3, promoting the assembly of necrosomes that trigger caspase-independent necroptosis. In this context, caspase-8 protects against necroptosis by cleaving and inactivating CYLD. Thus, the c-FLIP/caspase-8 complex has a prosurvival role, by preventing caspase-8-mediated apoptosis and also cleaving CYLD to prevent necroptosis.

Though a requirement for c-FLIP is not demonstrated, caspase-8 also plays an essential survival promoting-role in the context of signal transduction downstream of T-cell and B-cell antigen receptors (TCRs, BCRs). In this regard, NF-kB downstream of these antigen receptors involves a large multimeric protein assembly called the "CBM Signalosome" (reviewed in.[71] Phosphorylation of CARD-carrying proteins such as CARMA-1 (CARD-11) promotes oligomerization of Bcl-10 via CARD-CARD interactions, creating large filamentous helical structures with a star-like pattern. Recruited to these assemblies is the para-caspase, MALT1, which in turn binds the E3 ligase TRAF6—a mediator of noncanonical ubiquitination (particularly K63 linked). Through unclear mechanisms, caspase-8 is recruited to these complexes along with FADD, with caspase-8 essential for NF-kB activation to thereby support cell survival. Thus, caspase-8 also plays a pro-survival role in this cellular context. Interestingly, chromosomal translocations and gene amplification involving MALT1 as well as genomic lesions in other components of the CBM signalosome play pathogenic mechanisms in some B-cell lymphomas.[111]

Bcl-2

Among the central regulators of MOMP are members of the Bcl-2 family, evolutionarily conserved proteins that either promote (e.g., Bax; Bak) or suppress (e.g., Bcl-2, Bcl-XL) MOMP.[112–114] The Bcl-2-family proteins (n = approximately 26 in humans)[15] physically interact with each other, forming complex networks of homo- and hetero-dimers that steer the cell toward either life or death.[115,116] Numerous examples of altered expression and function of Bcl-2-family proteins have been identified in cancers, accounting for intrinsic resistance to cell death induced by myriad stimuli, including most cytotoxic anticancer drugs and x-irradiation, growth factor deprivation, and therapeutic inhibitors of growth factor receptor signal transduction pathways.

Many members of the Bcl-2-family have a hydrophobic stretch of amino acids near their carboxyl-terminus that anchors them in the outer mitochondrial membrane. In contrast, other Bcl-2-family members such as Bid, Bim, and Bad lack these membrane-anchoring domains, but dynamically target to mitochondria in response to specific stimuli. Still, others have the membrane-anchoring domain but keep it latched against the body of the protein, until stimulated to expose it (e.g., Bax).

Based on their predicted (or experimentally determined) three-dimensional structures, Bcl-2 family proteins can be broadly divided into two groups. One subset of these proteins is probably similar in structure to the pore-forming domains of bacterial toxins, such as the colicins and diphtheria toxin.[117–119] These α-helical pore-like proteins include both antiapoptotic proteins (Bcl-2, Bcl-X_L, Mcl-1, Bfl-1, Bcl-W, and Bcl-B), as well as pro-apoptotic proteins (Bax, Bak, Bok, and Bid). Most of the proteins in this subcategory can be recognized by conserved stretches of amino acid sequence homology, including the presence of Bcl-2 homology (BH) domains, BH1, BH2, BH3, and sometimes BH4 (Table 1). However, this is not uniformly the case, as the Bid protein contains only a BH3 domain but has been determined to share the same overall protein-fold with Bcl-X_L, Bcl-2, and Bax. Where tested to date, these proteins have all been shown to form ion-conducting channels in synthetic membranes in vitro, including Bcl-2, Bcl-X_L, Bax, and Bid,[120] but the significance of this pore activity remains largely unclear. The other subset of Bcl-2 family proteins appears to have in common only the presence of the BH3 domain, including Bad, Bik, Bim, Hrk, Bcl-G_S, p193, APR (Noxa), and PUMA. These "BH3-only" proteins are uniformly pro-apoptotic. Their cell death-inducing activity depends, in most cases, on their ability to dimerize with antiapoptotic Bcl-2 family members, functioning as trans-dominant inhibitors of proteins such as Bcl-2 and Bcl-X_L.[114,115] However, a select group of them (Bim, Bid, and Puma) interact with pro-apoptotic proteins Bax and Bak, functioning as agonists that induce their oligomerization in mitochondrial membranes to stimulate MOMP.

The BH3 domains mediate dimerization among Bcl-2 family proteins (Figure 3). This domain consists of an amphipathic α-helix of ∼16 amino acids length that inserts into a hydrophobic crevice on the surface of antiapoptotic proteins such as Bcl-2 and Bcl-X_L.[117,118] The BH3-only proteins link a wide variety of environmental and iatrogenic stimuli to the mitochondrial pathway for apoptosis (see below).

While Bcl-2 family members clearly regulate MOMP, it has been proposed that they also regulate other aspects of mitochondrial biology. For example, components of the MPTP complex, including ANT and the voltage-dependent anion channel (VDAC), reportedly interact with Bcl-2 family members, with antiapoptotic proteins suppressing and proapoptotic facilitating MPTP complex opening.[121] Additionally, VDAC has been proposed as a facilitator of Cyt-c release from mitochondria, via a Bcl-2 suppressible mechanism[122] while Bcl-XL has been reported to enhance the delivery of ATP to the cytosol via effects on ANT and thereby support cell survival in the context of growth factor deprivation.[123] Antiapoptotic Bcl-XL also may regulate mitochondrial metabolism through poorly understood mechanisms to reduce the production of acetyl-CoA.[124] The significance of this reduction in acetyl-CoA has been attributed to reduce N-acetylation of apoptosis-relevant proteins, including certain caspases, which may make it more difficult to activate these proteases. Bcl-2 has also been proposed to regulate mitochondrial redox metabolism, though mechanistic details remain largely unclear.[125]

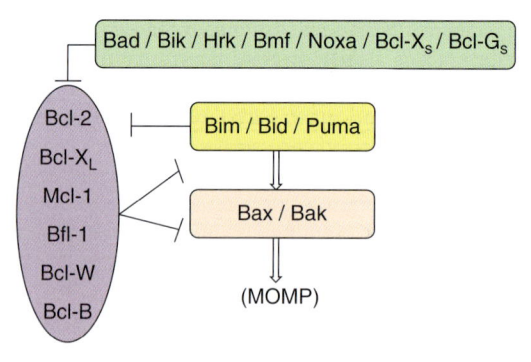

Figure 3 *Network of interactions among Bcl-2-family proteins.* The functional and physical interactions among pro-apoptotic and antiapoptotic Bcl-2-family proteins are depicted as pertains to their regulation of MOMP.

In addition to mitochondria, mechanistic links for Bcl-2 family proteins to ER stress have also been delineated.[126] For example, Bax and Bak can bind the ER stress signaling protein, IRE-1α, a central component of UPR signaling.[127] IRE-1α spans the ER membranes and possesses a protein kinase domain and a ribonuclease domain that reside on the cytosolic face of the ER membrane. Bax and Bak stimulate the intrinsic autokinase activity and the endoribonuclease activity of IRE1α, thus stimulating the production of CHOP-inducing transcription factor XBP-1 (by RNA splicing mechanisms) and also stimulating stress kinase activation (Ask1, p38MAPK, JNK1, etc.). Pro-apoptotic (Bak/Bax) and antiapoptotic (Bcl-2/Bcl-XL) family members also have opposing effects on basal ER Ca^{2+} levels, probably via effects on Ca^{2+} channel proteins in ER membranes (e.g., IP_3Rs, BI-1, and TmBim3).[78]

In addition to mitochondria- and ER-initiated cell death pathways, Bcl-2-family proteins have also been implicated in control of autophagic cell death. Antiapoptotic protein Bcl-2 binds the autophagy protein Beclin, preventing it from forming complexes with downstream autophagy proteins (e.g., ATG5) and apparently sequestering Beclin to preclude its participation in autophagy.[128] During nutrient deprivation, Bcl-2 can suppress cell death mechanisms that depend on components of the autophagy pathway.[129] Beclin has recently been recognized as a haploinsufficient tumor suppressor gene,[130] suggesting that suppression of autophagy contributes to tumorigenesis. These recent findings concerning links between autophagy, tumorigenesis, and antiapoptotic Bcl-2-family proteins indicate a master-switch role for Bcl-2-family proteins in controlling cell life and death decisions.

Genomic lesions involving members of the Bcl-2 family are well documented in human cancers.[6,131–133] These mechanisms include hyperactivation of antiapoptotic Bcl-2 family members by chromosomal translocations that cause overproduction of transcripts and proteins (Bcl-2), gene amplification (Bcl-2, Bcl-X, and Mcl-1), and deletion/mutational inactivation of microRNAs

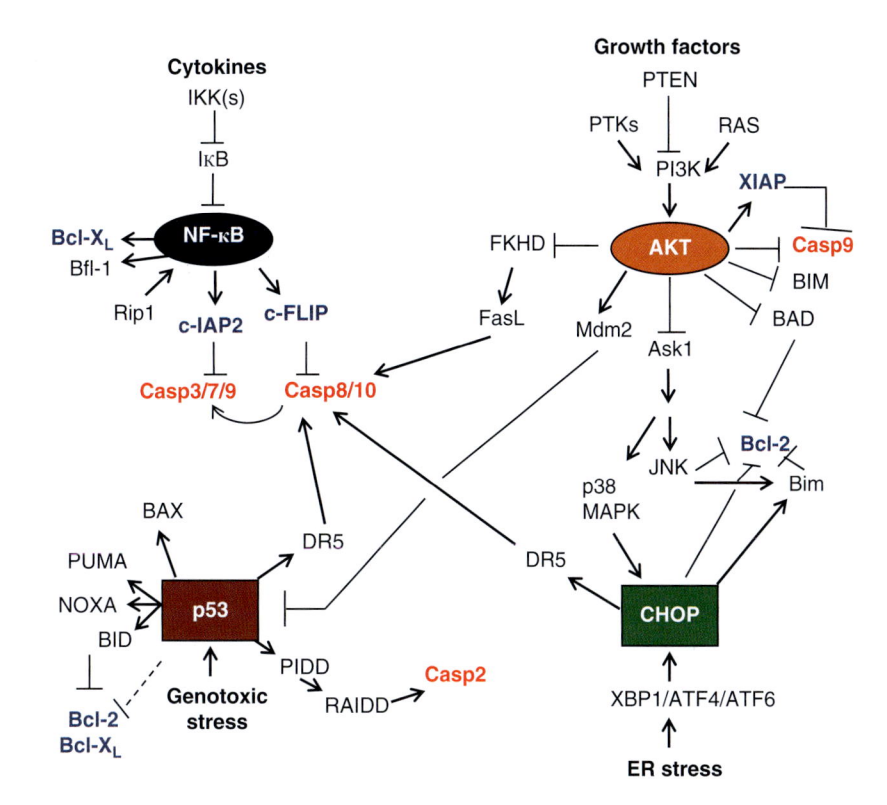

Figure 4 *Signal transduction and cell death regulation.* Some of the transcription factors and kinases that play prominent roles in apoptosis regulation are depicted, including kinases Akt (PKB) and the transcription factors p53, NF-κB, and CHOP. Illustrative examples of the connections to apoptosis-regulating proteins and genes are shown, without attempting to be comprehensive. The protein kinase Akt (PKB) is activated in response to second-messengers produced by PI3K, a lipid kinase that is activated by many growth factor receptors and oncoproteins. PTEN is a lipid phosphatase that prevents the accumulation of these second messengers, the expression of which is lost in many tumors through gene deletions, gene mutations, and other mechanisms[89]. Akt can phosphorylate and either activate (arrows) or inactivate (⊣) multiple proteins directly or indirectly relevant to apoptosis.[134] Expression of the transcription factor CHOP is stimulated by transcription factors that are elaborated during ER stress, including XBP1, ATF4, and ATF6. See text for additional details.

that suppress the expression of antiapoptotic Bcl-2 family genes (miR15-16 targeting Bcl-2 mRNA). Conversely, mutations inactivating pro-apoptotic members of the Bcl-2 family also occur in some human cancers (Bax). Additionally, a wide and diverse array of epigenetic mechanisms contributes to dysregulation of Bcl-2 family gene expression in cancers and leukemias, some of which are outlined below.

Signal transduction pathway alterations in cancers—impact on cell death machinery

Various receptor-mediated signal transduction pathways converge on the core components of the cell death machinery outlined above, including tyrosine kinase growth factor receptors and their downstream signaling pathways that become deregulated in many cancers. Some examples of the intimate links between growth factor receptor-mediated signal transduction and cell death pathways are described here (Figure 4).

Protein kinases

By catalyzing the phosphorylation of tyrosines on themselves and on various substrates, protein tyrosine kinases (PTKs) growth factor receptors uniformly transduce signals that lead to activation of the (1) phosphatidylinositol-3′kinase (PI3K) and Akt pathway and (2) Raf/MEK/Erk pathway (*reviewed elsewhere in this book*). One or both of these pathways is also activated by most nonreceptor PTKs (Src-family, Jak-family, c-Abl, etc.) and Ras-family GTPases.

The murine gene encoding Akt was first discovered by virtue of its similarity to the *v-akt* oncogene found in some murine leukemia viruses, where it becomes activated in thymomas caused by retrovirus insertions near the *c-akt* gene.[135] Humans contain three *AKT* genes. Akt can phosphorylate multiple proteins within the core apoptosis machinery.[136] For example, the pro-apoptotic Bcl-2 family member Bad is a target of Akt, where phosphorylation of Bad causes its sequestration by 14-3-3 family proteins, thus inhibiting Bad from heterodimerizing with Bcl-X$_L$.[137] Akt also phosphorylates Bax on serine 184, inhibiting its translocation from cytosol to mitochondrial membranes,[138] as well as Bim, suppressing its pro-apoptotic activity.[139] Akt also can phosphorylate human caspase-9, blocking apoptosis downstream of mitochondria.[140] Forkhead transcription factors (FKHDs) are another class of substrates of Akt relevant to apoptosis. Some FKHD family members such as Foxo-3 appear to control apoptosis, perhaps by affecting the transcription of genes encoding FasL and Bim.[141] Phosphorylation of FKHD by Akt prevents its entry into the nucleus. Akt also reportedly causes phosphorylation of XIAP, promoting the stability of the XIAP protein probably by reducing ubiquitin-dependent proteasomal degradation.[95]

Several growth factor receptors and lymphokine receptors signal via Jak/STAT pathways. STAT family transcription factors are known to stimulate transcription of the *BCL-X* gene as at least one of their mechanisms of suppressing apoptosis.[142] Additionally, Jak family nonreceptor PTKs are capable of stimulating PI3K activity, which in turn causes activation of Akt family kinases. These signaling mechanisms are also relevant to various oncogenes such as BCR-ABL, the oncogenic driver of certain types of leukemia.[143]

The Raf/MEK/Erk signaling pathway has important links to the cell death machinery. For example, phosphorylation by Erk of pro-apoptotic protein Bim on serine 69 promotes Bim protein degradation via proteasomal-dependent mechanisms.[144] Inhibitors of the Raf/MEK/Erk pathway, therefore, help to promote apoptosis by enabling the accumulation of Bim protein levels. MEK-dependent phosphorylation of antiapoptotic protein Bcl-2 has also been described, purportedly enhancing its survival-promoting function through unclear mechanisms.[145]

Protein acetylation

Acetylation of lysines in histones is a well-established mechanism for controlling chromatin structure and thus transcription of genes. However, acetylation of nonhistone proteins is increasingly recognized as a mechanism for impacting biological processes through diverse mechanisms. In terms of cell death regulation, examples of dysregulated protein acetylation impacting the core components of the cell death machinery are only just emerging. For example, acetylation of transcription factor FoxO1 was reported to be required for induction of Bim expression in the context of treatment of cancer cells with histone deacetylase (HDAC) inhibitors.[146] Acetylation also indirectly impacts the expression of multiple apoptosis and cell death-relevant genes through modification of lysines on a variety of other transcription factors, including STATs, NF-κB, and p53.[147] Additionally, acetylation of tumor suppressor p53 has also been reported to be required for a transcription-independent mechanism of Bax activation.[148] Acetylation of DNA damage repair protein Ku70 neutralizes its antiapoptotic functions by interfering with interactions with proteins constituting core components of the cell death machinery (see below). As mentioned above, via effects on mitochondrial acetyl-CoA production, Bcl-XL may also broadly impact N-alpha-acetylation of proteins, including certain caspases that require this posttranslational modification for interactions with upstream activators.[124]

Transcriptions factors

As expected, epigenetic dysregulation of expression of cell death genes is a common occurrence in human cancers, with mechanisms too abundant to catalog here. Among the cancer-relevant connections are steroid hormone receptors including estrogen, androgen, and vitamin D receptors, which regulate the expression of various cell death and cell survival genes. For example, estrogen receptor (ER) is a prominent transcriptional regulator of the *BCL-2* gene expression in mammary epithelial cells and in ER-positive breast adenocarcinomas.[149] Retinoid receptors and other nuclear receptors also regulate the expression of various cell death and cell survival genes through transcriptional mechanisms.[150] The roles of transcription factors such as FKHD family members (Foxo-3, FoxO1), CHOP, NF-κB family members, and p53 have been cited above.

Putting a brief spotlight on NF-kB, for example, this family of transcription factors becomes activated via multiple signaling pathways initiated by cytokine receptors, innate immunity receptors, and antigen receptors. NF-kB family transcription factors stimulate the expression of several pro-survival genes including *BCL-X, C-FLIP, C-IAP2*, and others.

Precedents also exist for nontranscriptional mechanisms of regulating cell death proteins, where transcription factors leave the nucleus and physically interact with Bcl-2 family members on the surface of mitochondria.[151] Chromatin-modifying enzymes responsible for histone acetylation and deacetylation have also been implicated in controlling core components of the cell death machinery. Therefore, cancer-associated aberrations in the regulation of transcription factors and chromatin-modifying enzymes are connected ultimately to perturbations in the core cell death machinery.

Cytotoxic chemotherapeutic oncology drugs

Chemotherapeutic cytotoxic drugs remain a foundational component of cancer therapy today, though giving way to more targeted agents and to cancer immunotherapeutics. These chemical agents were designed to interfere with the replication of rapidly dividing cells by inhibiting DNA synthesis, inducing DNA damage, or crippling microtubules. The cellular injuries induced by classical chemotherapeutic anticancer drugs, and x-irradiation, trigger molecular events with connections to the core cell death machinery. Some examples are described here. Cytoprotective proteins that blunt cell death pathways thus play important roles in chemoresistance.

Radiotherapy and DNA-damaging anticancer drugs potently stimulate the activation of the tumor suppressor p53, one of the principal mediators of apoptosis induced by genotoxic stress. The p53 protein is a tetrameric transcription factor, whose levels are controlled by the E3 ligase Mdm2. This transcription factor directly induces the expression of BH3-only proteins Bim, Bid, and PUMA, and the MOMP-inducing protein Bax, thus linking p53 to the death machinery.[152–155] Active p53 also stimulates transcription of DR5, a TNF-family death receptor, thus rendering tumor cells more sensitive to its ligand TRAIL.[156] Loss of p53 activity occurs in many human malignancies by a variety of mechanisms, including gene deletion, gene mutations that result in mutant p53 proteins lacking transcriptional activity, and *MDM2* gene amplification. Small-molecule drugs that block Mdm2 protein interaction with p53 have shown promising preclinical activity against hematological malignancies,[157] and are synergistic with Bcl-2 inhibitors.[158] As of this time, none of these chemical inhibitors of Mdm2, however, has successfully transited the clinical trial journey to approval.

Interestingly, in addition to its role as a nuclear transcription factor, evidence has emerged suggesting that p53 may promote apoptosis also via nontranscriptional mechanisms under some circumstances. Specifically, a cytoplasmic pool of p53 reportedly associates with mitochondria, directly inducing activation of the Bax and inhibiting Bcl-2 and Bcl-XL.[159,160] Importantly, even mutant p53 is capable of activating this cell death pathway, raising hopes of finding pharmacological interventions that agonize this mechanism for promoting cell death.

DNA damage is also linked to the regulation of the core cell death machinery via p53-independent mechanisms. For example, Ku70 plays an important role in repairing double strand DNA breaks. Ku70 binds Bax and suppresses its translocation to mitochondria, but after DNA damage, Ku70 becomes acetylated and dissociates from Bax.[161,162] Ku70 also interacts with c-FLIP and suppresses its ubiquitination and proteasomal degradation, where Ku70 acetylation releases c-FLIP and allows its degradation to promote apoptosis.[163] Another DNA repair protein RAD9 has been reported to translocate from the nucleus to mitochondria following DNA damage, where it reportedly binds and neutralizes antiapoptotic proteins Bcl-2 and Bcl-XL to promote cell death.[164]

Antimicrotubule drugs impact the cell death machinery via a variety of mechanisms. For example, the pro-apoptotic Bcl-2 family member Bmf-1 is sequestered on microtubules. When microtubules are disrupted by anticancer drugs, Bmf is released from microtubule-binding proteins (dynein light chains), allowing it to engage and neutralize antiapoptotic members of the Bcl-2 family.[165] A role for Bim in cell death induced by microtubule-targeting drugs has also been identified, facilitated perhaps by other BH3-only proteins Bmf and Puma.[166] Microtubule-targeting drugs also stimulate a stress kinase cascade that results in multisite phosphorylation of Bcl-2, which is proposed to impair its antiapoptotic function.[167,168]

Cancer drug discovery by targeting the cell death machinery

Multiple efforts have been made to devise therapeutics that neutralize antiapoptotic or activate pro-apoptotic components of the core cell death machinery. All drug targets can be approached by at least 3 means, involving an attack at the level of the gene, mRNA, or protein. The relative attractiveness of these alternative strategies depends on the nuances of the target and its biology. The discussion here is limited to therapeutic strategies that modulate protein targets, though nucleic acid-based therapeutics (RNA therapeutics, gene therapy) have been explored preclinically and some even taken into advanced clinical trials. Also, while a wide variety of signal-transducing proteins (e.g., protein kinases, transcription factors) provide inputs into cell death pathways described above and thus are attractive targets for indirectly promoting tumor cell death, the focus here is limited to direct modulators of components of the core cell death machinery.

Bcl-2-family inhibitors

In humans, six antiapoptotic members of the Bcl-2-family have been identified (Bcl-2, Bcl-XL, Mcl-1, Bcl-W, Bfl-1, and Bcl-B), with overexpression of various individuals occurring in a variety of cancers. Simultaneous overexpression of two or more antiapoptotic members of the Bcl-2 family in tumors has also been documented in some cases, raising the issue of redundancy. Overexpression of Bcl-2 or other antiapoptotic members of the Bcl-2 family has been associated with chemoresistant states, due to the ability of these proteins to block cell death induced by DNA-damaging agents, microtubule-modifying drugs, and antimetabolites. Thus, restoring chemosensitivity by nullifying Bcl-2 and related proteins has emerged as an attractive strategy for improving cancer therapy.

Chemicals that bind regulatory sites on antiapoptotic Bcl-2-family proteins and that directly neutralize the cytoprotective actions of these proteins have been identified and brought into clinical development. Some have progressed into advanced human clinical trials, and at least one molecule (venetoclax) has produced sufficiently compelling data to merit regulatory approval.[169] The compounds described to date target a crevice on the surface of antiapoptotic Bcl-2-family proteins that serves as a receptor for the BH3 peptidyl motif present in endogenous antagonists of the antiapoptotic Bcl-2 family proteins.[6,117,133] Compounds that mimic the BH3 peptidyl structure suppress antiapoptotic Bcl-2-family proteins, tapping into a natural pathway for defending against excessive Bcl-2. Several natural products and synthetic chemicals have been reported to occupy the BH3-binding site on Bcl-2 or Bcl-XL, and some of them have been shown to promote apoptosis of tumor cells in culture and to suppress tumor growth in mouse models.[170–176] The strategies for generating chemical antagonists of antiapoptotic Bcl-2 family proteins have ranged from highly selective inhibitors, which neutralize only 1 of the 6 human antiapoptotic Bcl-2 family proteins, to broad-spectrum that cross-react with multiple family members. The trade-offs with these opposing strategies are efficacy versus drug safety. For example, the development of a chemical inhibitor with activity against Bcl-2, Bcl-XL, and Bcl-W was terminated, because of thrombocytopenia—which has been attributed to the requirement for Bcl-XL for the longevity of platelets.[177–179] In contrast, a selective Bcl-2 inhibitor (venetoclax) is free of the thrombocytopenia side-effect, but with a narrower spectrum of activity.

Other approaches to tackling Bcl-2 family proteins for cancer therapy have been proposed, though most of those concepts are less validated. For example, direct agonists of Bax and Bak could be envisioned that mimic the actions of Bid, Bim, and Puma,[180] though this has not been reduced to practice to date. Indirect mechanisms for upregulating levels of pro-apoptotic Bcl-2 family members have also been explored. Small-molecule antagonists of the E3 ligase Mdm2 that prevent its interaction with p53 cause accumulation of this tumor suppressor, which in turn stimulates transcription of several pro-apoptotic Bcl-2 family genes including *BAX, BIM, BID*, and *PUMA*. Mdm2 antagonists have progressed to advanced clinical trials, but results have so far remained underwhelming. In addition, chemical inhibitors of MEK (Trametinib, Cobimetinib, etc.) can produce elevations in the levels of Bim protein by reducing its ubiquitination and proteasomal degradation. In another approach to restoring apoptosis sensitivity, small-molecule inhibitors of Akt that are currently in advanced clinical development also would be expected to help restore the activity of pro-apoptotic Bcl-2 family proteins that are phosphorylated by this protein kinase (e.g., Bad and Bax). Finally, compounds that stimulate an orphan member of the nuclear receptor family, Nur77 (NR4A1), have been described that cause this transcription factor to exit the nucleus and translocate to mitochondria, where it interacts with Bcl-2, Bfl-1, and Bcl-B to promote cell death.[151,181–183]

TRAIL

Cytokines of the TNF family have been extensively evaluated in preclinical studies for anticancer activity. Two general strategies for exploiting this endogenous mechanism for triggering apoptosis have been tested clinically, involving parenteral administration of either recombinant proteins constituting functional fragments of the cytokine ligands or agonistic monoclonal antibodies that bind the TNF-family death receptors and trigger their activation.

Attempts to apply TNFα, the founding member of the TNF family, as a cancer therapy provided highly toxic, due to the proinflammatory activity of this cytokine. At present, TNFα is employed only in rare circumstances for the treatment of melanomas and soft tissue sarcomas confined to specific limbs using tourniquet-based methods to prevent systemic exposure.[184]

TRAIL emerged as a possible alternative, owing to its ability to induce tumor cell apoptosis without inducing signals that cause inflammation. Preclinical studies, including data from primates, indicated that a soluble fragment of TRAIL (produced as a recombinant protein) was nontoxic, apparently sparing normal tissues, while showing potent preclinical activity against tumor xenografts in mice.[185] Moreover, TRAIL is sometimes synergistic when used in combination with cytotoxic anticancer drugs, at least in preclinical mouse models. Based on these promising data, a recombinant version of TRAIL was taken into clinical trials, but its lack of efficacy resulted in its eventual termination. Postulated reasons for the poor efficacy of TRAIL in the clinic are myriad, including intrinsic blocks in cancers to the downstream apoptotic signaling pathways, expression of "decoy" receptors that compete for TRAIL binding to function death receptors on tumor cells, insufficient expression levels of DR4 (TRAIL-R1) and DR5 (TRAIL-R2), and other explanations.[185]

Agonistic antibodies that bind DR4, DR5, or both have been reported, and several were taken into clinical development.[186,187] Clinical responses when tested as monotherapy were rare, and some of these antibodies showed hepatotoxicity,[188,189] which was theorized to be due to FcR-binding to Kupfer cells in the liver. In this regard, the agonist antibodies were uniformly dependent on FcR-binding to achieve cross-linking of receptors in tumor cells, and thus reliant on macrophages, NK cells, or other types of FcR-expressing immune cells to achieve the desired apoptotic signaling. More recently, highly engineered antibodies that utilize FcR-independent mechanisms to achieve death receptor cross-linking have been advanced into clinical studies, awaiting definitive results at the time of this writing.

TRAIL and TRAIL receptors can induce apoptosis via either mitochondria-dependent or -independent pathways, depending on the specifics of how apoptosis pathways are regulated in a given tumor.[190] The mitochondrial-dependent route of signaling entails cleavage by caspase-8 of Bid, which activates the protein such that it can interact with Bax and Bak to induce MOMP. The possible advantage of mitochondria-independent apoptosis is that roadblocks to apoptosis created by survival proteins such as Bcl-2 are bypassed, an attractive feature for chemorefractory cancers that often have defects in the mitochondrial pathway. Unfortunately, predicting whether TRAIL operates via a mitochondria-dependent versus -independent mechanism in a given tumor is still an empirical process, as no single predictive biomarker has emerged.

Among the roadblocks to TRAIL-induced apoptosis is c-FLIP, a protein that is produced as either longer or shorter isoforms (due to mRNA splicing) that associate with the caspases normally recruited into the TRAIL receptor complex. The longer c-FLIP protein is overexpressed in many cancers and is capable of squelching signaling by TNF-family death receptors by modulating caspase activation.[104] Chemical compounds that reduce c-FLIP protein levels have been identified, including HDAC inhibitors such as suberoylanilide hydroxamic acid (SAHA)[191] and synthetic triterpenoids such as bardoxolone (1[2-cyano-3,12-dioxooleana-1,9^{11}-dien-28-oyl]imidazole [CDDO]) and its analogs.[134,192–196] Preclinical studies have shown that bardoxolone analogs used in combination with recombinant TRAIL can synergistically suppress the growth of human tumor xenografts in mice, where the human tumor cells were resistant to treatment with TRAIL alone.[197] Thus, compounds such as CDDO can restore the sensitivity of cancer cells to TRAIL (and agonistic anti-TRAIL receptor antibodies), and therefore might serve as adjuncts to TRAIL therapy. At least in mice, the combination of TRAIL and CDDO analogs is a nontoxic therapy,[197] suggesting that combining these two targeted therapies provides a promising direction for future research. Bardoxolone (CDDO analog) was brought into the clinic for a nononcology indication but development was terminated.

Finally, onco-immunotherapies that stimulate either cytolytic (CD8+) T-cells (CTLs) or NK cells to attack tumors have emerged as a foundational element of cancer treatment, thanks in large part to the advent of checkpoint inhibitors. Tumor cell killing by CTLs and NK cells is thought to be largely dependent on perforin and granzyme-mediated mechanism, with contributions also by TNF-family death ligands such as FasL and TRAIL.

IAP inhibitors

The most common strategy employed for generating small-molecule inhibitors of IAPs is to mimic the effects of endogenous antagonists of IAPs, particularly the proteins SMAC and HtrA2. SMAC- and HtrA2-mimicking agents bind the BIRs of multiple IAP family members, thus disrupting their interactions with caspases (caspases-3, -7, -9) and kinases (Rip1, Rip2).[198] The active region of SMAC and HtrA2 has been reduced to a 4 amino acid peptide, that is necessary and sufficient to bind IAPs, displace caspases or kinases, and promote apoptosis or inhibit signal transduction.[199] Several peptidyl compounds have been described that occupy the same tetramer-binding site on IAPs,[200–202] as well as at least one natural product. Several of the synthetic compounds were taken into clinical development but abandoned due to lack of clinical activity. These SMAC-mimicking compounds show only occasional single-agent activity as apoptosis inducers when applied against cultured tumor cell lines, which has been the reason for the termination of several of these drug development programs. However, SMAC mimics often sensitize transformed cells very potently to apoptosis induced by cytotoxic anticancer drugs and TNF-family death receptors such as TRAIL and agonistic antibodies targeting TRAIL Receptors. In this sense, IAP antagonists take the brakes off the cell death pathways induced by TNF-family death receptors, providing a solid rationale for combination therapy.

Finally, an additional strategy for attacking IAPs has been suggested by interrogation of the actions of another apoptogenic protein released from mitochondria called ARTS.[203] The ARTS protein binds certain IAPs, including XIAP, c-IAP1, and c-IAP2. It has been shown to recruit an E3 ligase (Siah-1) to IAPs and promote their degradation.[204] Short peptides from ARTS purportedly can induce apoptosis,[205] though the translation of these observations into drug-like molecules remains an ambition to date. The structural nature of the ARTS-binding site on IAPs also remains to be determined, which would presumably provide important insights into the "druggability" of this protein–protein interface.

Some tumors overexpress simultaneously two or more members of the IAP family, suggesting that broad-spectrum inhibitors that address multiple IAPs may be preferable to selective agents. More extensive comparisons of the therapeutic indices of selective versus broad-spectrum inhibitors are needed to reveal the best path forward.[206,207]

Conclusions

Dysregulation of programmed cell death mechanisms plays critical roles in cancer pathogenesis and progression. Elaboration of the complex cell death pathways and the networks of proteins that modulate these pathways has provided insights into the underlying mechanisms of cell life-death decisions—though many mechanistic details remain still to be revealed. Tumor cell death can occur through either immunologically silent or immunogenic mechanisms, the latter having broad implications for efforts to expand the utility of cancer immunotherapy. The knowledge-base established and emerging has already sparked multiple efforts to translate mechanistic insights into therapeutic strategies, with success achieved so far for the Bcl-2 inhibitor venetoclax and with many other agents undergoing clinical evaluation.

List of abbreviations

BH	Bcl-2 homology domain
CARDs	caspase recruitment domains
caspases	cysteine aspartyl proteases
Cyt-c	cytochrome-c
CTL	cytolytic T cells
DD	death domain
DEDs	death effector domains
DISC	death-inducing signaling complex
DR	death receptor
ER	endoplasmic reticulum
FasL	Fas-ligand
FKHD	forkhead transcription factors
IAP	inhibitor of apoptosis
miRs	microRNAs
MOMP	mitochondrial outer membrane permeabilization
MPT	mitochondrial permeability transition
MLKL	mixed lineage kinase domain like
MALT	mucosa-associated lymphoid tissue
MMs	multiple myelomas
NK	natural killer
NHLs	non-Hodgkin lymphomas
PI3K	phosphatidylinositol-3′kinase
PCD	programmed cell death
ROS	reactive oxygen species
TNFR1	TNF receptor-1
TNF	tumor necrosis factor
UBCs	ubiquitin-conjugating enzymes

Key references

The complete reference list can be found on Vital Source version of this title, see inside front cover.

3 Danial NN, Korsmeyer SJ. Cell death: critical control points. *Cell*. 2004;**116**(2):205–219.
5 Reed JC. Apoptosis-targeted therapies for cancer. *Cancer Cell*. 2003;**3**:17–22.
12 Kroemer G, El-Deiry WS, Golstein P, et al. Classification of cell death: recommendations of the nomenclature committee on cell death. *Cell Death Differ*. 2005;**12**(Suppl 2):1463–1467.
14 Degterev A, Yuan J. Expansion and evolution of cell death programmes. *Nat Rev Mol Cell Biol*. 2008;**9**(5):378–390.
17 Boatright KM, Salvesen GS. Mechanisms of caspase activation. *Curr Opin Cell Biol*. 2003;**15**:725–731.
18 Lieberman J. The ABCs of granule-mediated cytotoxicity: new weapons in the arsenal. *Nat Rev Immunol*. 2003;**3**:361–370.
21 Kersse K, Verspurten J, Vanden BT, Vandenabeele P. The death-fold superfamily of homotypic interaction motifs. *Trends Biochem Sci*. 2011;**36**(10):541–552.
24 Wallach D, Varfolomeev EE, Malinin NL, et al. Tumor necrosis factor receptor and Fas signaling mechanisms. *Annu Rev Immunol*. 1999;**17**:331–367.
27 Zou H, Li Y, Liu X, Wang X. An APAF-1 cytochrome c multimeric complex is a functional apoptosome that activates procaspase-9. *J Biol Chem*. 1999;**274**:11549–11556.
29 Adams JM, Cory S. Apoptosomes: engines for caspase activation. *Curr Opin Cell Biol*. 2002;**14**:715–720.
34 Korsmeyer SJ, Wei MC, Saito M, et al. Pro-apoptotic cascade activates BID, which oligomerizes BAK or BAX into pores that result in the release of cytochrome c. *Cell Death Differ*. 2000;**7**:1166–1173.
35 O'Reilly LA, Strasser A. Apoptosis and autoimmune disease. *Inflamm Res*. 1999;**48**:5–21.
36 Bergsbaken T, Fink SL, Cookson BT. Pyroptosis: host cell death and inflammation. *Nat Rev Microbiol*. 2009;**7**(2):99–109.
37 Schroder K, Zhou R, Tschopp J. The NLRP3 inflammasome: a sensor for metabolic danger? *Science*. 2010;**327**(5963):296–300.
38 Franchi L, Eigenbrod T, Munoz-Planillo R, Nunez G. The inflammasome: a caspase-1-activation platform that regulates immune responses and disease pathogenesis. *Nat Immunol*. 2009;**10**(3):241–247.
41 Xia X, Wang X, Cheng Z, et al. The role of pyroptosis in cancer: pro-cancer or pro-"host"? *Cell Death Dis*. 2019;**10**:650–673.
49 Green DR, Galluzzi L, Kroemer G. Mitochondria and the autophagy-inflammation-cell death axis in organismal aging. *Science*. 2011;**333**(6046):1109–1112.
50 Penninger JM, Kroemer G. Mitochondria, AIF and caspases--rivaling for cell death execution. *Nat Cell Biol*. 2003;**5**:97–99.
51 Kroemer G, Reed JC. Mitochondrial control of cell death. *Nat Med*. 2000;**6**:513–519.
52 Ferri KF, Kroemer G. Organelle-specific initiation of cell death pathways. *Nat Cell Biol*. 2001;**3**:E255–E263.
58 Green DR, Kroemer G. The pathophysiology of mitochondrial cell death. *Science*. 2004;**305**:626–629.
59 Tait SW, Green DR. Mitochondria and cell death: outer membrane permeabilization and beyond. *Nat Rev Mol Cell Biol*;**11**(9):621–632.
60 Chao DT, Korsmeyer SJ. Bcl-2 family: regulators of cell death. *Annu Rev Immunol*. 1998;**16**:395–419.
61 Vaux D, Korsmeyer S. Cell death in development. *Cell*. 1999;**96**:245–254.
62 Wei MC, Zong WX, Cheng EH, et al. Proapoptotic BAX and BAK: a requisite gateway to mitochondrial dysfunction and death. *Science*. 2001;**292**(5517):727–730.
68 Zhang DW, Shao J, Lin J, et al. RIP3, an energy metabolism regulator that switches TNF-induced cell death from apoptosis to necrosis. *Science*. 2009;**325**(5938):332–336.
69 Declercq W, Vanden BT, Vandenabeele P. RIP kinases at the crossroads of cell death and survival. *Cell*. 2009;**138**(2):229–232.
74 Kaufman RJ. Orchestrating the unfolded protein response in health and disease. *J Clin Invest*. 2002;**110**:1389–1398.
75 Kim I, Xu W, Reed JC. Cell death and endoplasmic reticulum stress: disease relevance and therapeutic opportunities. *Nat Rev Drug Discov*. 2008;**7**(12):1013–1030.
77 Giorgi C, Romagnoli A, Pinton P, Rizzuto R. Ca2+ signaling, mitochondria and cell death. *Curr Mol Med*. 2008;**8**(2):119–130.
78 Sano R, Reed J. ER stress-induced cell death mechanisms. *Biochim Biophys Acta*. 2013;**1833**(12):3460–3470.
79 Mizushima N, Levine B, Cuervo AM, Klionsky DJ. Autophagy fights disease through cellular self-digestion. *Nature*. 2008;**451**(7182):1069–1075.
80 Levine B, Kroemer G. Autophagy in the pathogenesis of disease. *Cell*. 2008;**132**(1):27–42.
84 Frisch SM, Screaton RA. Anoikis mechanisms. *Curr Opin Cell Biol*. 2001;**13**(5):555–562.
85 Kroemer G, Galluzzi L, Kepp O, Zitvogel L. Immunogenic cell death in cancer therapy. *Annu Rev Immunol*. 2013;**31**:51–72.
88 Deveraux QL, Reed JC. IAP family proteins: suppressors of apoptosis. *Genes Dev*. 1999;**13**:239–252.
90 Salvesen GS, Duckett CS. IAP proteins: blocking the road to death's door. *Nat Rev Mol Cell Biol*. 2002;**3**:401–410.
93 Du C, Fang M, Li Y, et al. SMAC, a mitochondrial protein that promotes cytochrome c-dependent caspase activation by eliminating IAP inhibition. *Cell*. 2000;**102**:33–42.
94 Suzuki Y, Imai Y, Nakayama H, et al. A serine protease HtrA2/Omi, is released from the mitochondria and interacts with XIAP, induces cell death. *Mol Cell*. 2001;**8**:613–621.
97 Cho YS, Challa S, Moquin D, et al. Phosphorylation-driven assembly of the RIP1-RIP3 complex regulates programmed necrosis and virus-induced inflammation. *Cell*. 2009;**137**(6):1112–1123.
99 Karin M, Gallagher E. TNFR signaling: ubiquitin-conjugated TRAFfic signals control stop-and-go for MAPK signaling complexes. *Immunol Rev*. 2009;**228**(1):225–240.
100 Baud V, Karin M. Is NF-kappaB a good target for cancer therapy? Hopes and pitfalls. *Nat Rev Drug Discov*. 2009;**8**(1):33–40.
101 Wegener E, Krappmann D. CARD-Bcl10-Malt1 signalosomes: missing link to NF-kappaB. *Sci STKE*. 2007;**2007**(384):pe21.
102 Garrison JB, Samuel T, Reed JC. TRAF2-binding BIR1 domain of c-IAP2/MALT1 fusion protein is essential for activation of NF-kappaB. *Oncogene*. 2009;**28**(13):1584–1593.
104 Thome M, Tschopp J. Regulation of lymphocyte proliferation and death by FLIP. *Nat Rev Immunol*. 2001;**1**(1):50–58.
105 Yu JW, Shi Y. FLIP and the death effector domain family. *Oncogene*. 2008;**27**(48):6216–6227.
108 O'Donnell MA, Perez-Jimenez E, Oberst A, et al. Caspase 8 inhibits programmed necrosis by processing CYLD. *Nat Cell Biol*. 2011;**13**:1437–1443.
109 Dillon CP, Oberst A, Weinlich R, et al. Survival function of the FADD-Caspase-8-cFLIPL complex. *Cell Rep*. 2012;**1**(5):401–407.
113 Cory S, Huang DC, Adams JM. The Bcl-2 family: roles in cell survival and oncogenesis. *Oncogene*. 2003;**22**(53):8590–8607.

115 Strasser A. The role of BH3-only proteins in the immune system. *Nat Rev Immunol*. 2005;**5**:189–200.

117 Fesik SW. Insights into programmed cell death through structural biology. *Cell*. 2000;**103**:273–282.

128 Levine B, Pattingre S, Tassa A, et al. Bcl-2 antiapoptotic proteins inhibit Beclin 1-dependent autophagy. *Cell*. 2005;**122**(6):927–939.

129 Shimizu S, Kanaseki T, Mizushima N, et al. Role of Bcl-2 family proteins in a non-apoptotic programmed cell death dependent on autophagy genes. *Nat Cell Biol*. 2004;**6**(12):1221–1228.

144 Luciano F, Jacquel A, Colosetti P, et al. Phosphorylation of Bim-EL by Erk1/2 on serine 69 promotes its degradation via the proteasome pathway and regulates its proapoptotic function. *Oncogene*. 2003;**22**:6785–6793.

149 Teixeira C, Reed JC, Pratt MAC. Estrogen promotes chemotherapeutic drug resistance by a mechanism involving Bcl-2 proto-oncogene expression in human breast cancer cells. *Cancer Res*. 1995;**55**:3902–3907.

156 Wu GS, Burns TF, ERR MD, et al. KILLER/DR5 is a DNA damage-inducible p53-regulated death receptor gene. *Nat Genet*. 1997;**17**:141–143.

169 King AC, Peterson TJ, Horvat TZ, et al. Venetoclax: a first-in-class oral Bcl-2 inhibitor for the management of lymphoid malignancies. *Ann Pharmacother*. 2017;**51**(5):410–416.

198 Fesik SW, Shi Y. Structural biology. Controlling the caspases. *Science*. 2001;**294**:1477–1478.

202 Gonzalez-Lopez M, Welsh K, Finlay D, et al. Design, synthesis and evaluation of monovalent Smac mimetics that bind to the BIR2 domain of the anti-apoptotic protein XIAP. *Bioorg Med Chem Lett*. 2011;**21**(14):4332–4336.

203 Gottfried Y, Rotm A, Lotan R, et al. The mitochondrial ARTS protein promotes apoptosis through targeting XIAP. *EMBO J*. 2004;**23**(7):1627–1635.

204 Garrison JB, Correa RG, Gerlic M, et al. ARTS and Siah collaborate in a pathway for XIAP degradation. *Mol Cell*. 2011;**41**(1):107–116.

14 Cancer cell immortality: targeting telomerase and telomeres

Ilgen Mender, PhD ■ *Zeliha G. Dikmen, MD, PhD* ■ *Jerry W. Shay, PhD*

> **Overview**
>
> Finding specific targeted agents for cancer therapy remains a challenge. One of the hallmarks of cancer is the limitless proliferation (immortalization) of cancer cells, which correlates with the activation of the ribonucleoprotein enzyme complex called telomerase. Since 85–90% of primary human cancers express telomerase activity, while most normal cells do not, telomerase is a unique and almost universal therapeutic target for cancer. Although there have been several approaches developed for telomerase targeted therapies, there is still no successful therapeutic agent that has been approved. This article reviews the different approaches to target telomerase and summarizes preclinical and clinical results.

Telomere and telomerase

Telomeres $(TTAGGG)_n$ are repetitive hexameric nucleotide repeats that are found at the ends of linear chromosomes. Telomere length varies in different organisms such as humans (2–15 kb) and mice (up to 100 kb).[1] Telomeres are protected from being recognized as damaged or broken chromosomes by a special protein complex. This is termed the shelterin complex which stabilizes the chromosomal ends with six protein components (TRF1, TRF2, Rap1, TIN2, TPP1 (ACD), and POT1) to protect the telomeric ends from exonuclease activity and DNA damage recognition.[1-3] Shelterin proteins also have a role in the generation of a special lariat-like loop structure called telomere loops (T-loop). The single-stranded DNA overhangs at the ends of chromosomes bend backward and are believed to strand invade into the telomere duplex structure disrupting the double-stranded TTAGGG repeats and forming a triple-stranded structure called the displacement loop (D-loop). The D-loop is bound by a single stranded TTAGGG binding protein called POT1 and this entire T-loop and D-loop structure functions in part by hiding or masking the single stranded DNA from being recognized as broken DNA and thus is important in telomere maintenance.[4]

G-quadruplex formation is a secondary structure that is generated between guanine bases in telomeric DNA and is also proposed to protect the ends of chromosomes.[5] Since normal somatic cells have a limited capacity to divide in culture, they stop proliferating after a finite number of population doublings (the so-called Hayflick limit), which is related to DNA replication turnover.[6] Because DNA polymerase is unable to replicate the 3′ end of the DNA lagging strand (often referred to as the end replication problem), in the absence of a maintenance mechanism, telomeres shorten with each cell division until they become uncapped.[7] In addition to the end replication problem, oxidative stress and/or other unknown processes may accelerate telomeric shortening *in vitro* and *in vivo*. The telomeric sequence does not encode any gene, and its erosion will not cause loss of genomic information.[8] However, telomere position effect over long distances (TPE-OLD),[9] also termed telomere looping[10] as well as telomeric repeat-containing RNA (TERRA) can modulate gene expression.[8] It has been shown that transcription of certain genes that are far from telomeres can be regulated by telomere length. For instance, the presence of TRF2 (a shelterin protein that binds to duplex TTAGGG repeats) at telomere-distal gene promoters is relatively depleted when telomeres are long.[11] The nontelomeric binding effect of TRF2 near the *hTERT* promoter, results in transcriptional repression of *hTERT* when telomeres are long but is expressed in cells when telomeres are short. Thus, telomere shortening can initially be important to keep normal somatic cells from reactivating telomerase and triggering cancer cell immortality.[12] It has also been shown in some tumors that telomere-elongated cancer cells express higher levels of TERRA and influence gene expression.[8] In addition, telomere looping may involve interactions with blocks of interstitial telomeric sequences (ITS) through interaction with shelterin proteins or TERRA.[10]

It is believed that only a few short telomeres with uncapped ends is sufficient to trigger a p53-dependent G1/S cell cycle arrest, which is known as replicative senescence. A key biomarker of the onset of senescence is the length of the shortest telomere and it is correlated with age-associated pathologies. Therefore, methods that can measure the shortest telomere length instead of average telomere length become valuable to provide more information about telomere-associated aging disorders (Table 1). For instance, human laminopathies and telomeropathies often correlate with short telomeres.[19,20]

When cells enter senescence, the fate of normal cells is to remain in a quiescent phase. If other alterations occur in important cell cycle checkpoint genes such as TP53 or pRB, then senescence can be bypassed and cells continue to proliferate until many telomere ends become critically shortened leading to end fusions and chromosome bridge fusion breakage cycles (also referred to as crisis). Senescence and crisis are two fundamental mechanisms involving telomeres that help protect cells in large and long-lived organisms, such as humans, against the early development of cancer. Dysfunctional telomeres activate DNA damage response (DDR) signaling, leading to genomic instability and initially cellular senescence. Telomere-specific damage can be determined by using the **T**elomere dysfunction **I**nduced **F**oci (TIF) assay (Table 1).

Cells that escape from crisis almost universally express the enzyme telomerase; a ribonucleoprotein cellular reverse transcriptase, which has two essential components and other essential factors for the elongation of telomeres: the catalytic component **hTERT** (**TE**lomerase **R**everse **T**ranscriptase), the **TE**lomerase **R**NA **C**omponent (hTR or hTERC) (Figure 1a,b) and accessory proteins such as dyskerin (DKC1), TCAB1, NHP2, NOP10, and

---

Holland-Frei Cancer Medicine, Tenth Edition. Edited by Robert C. Bast, John C. Byrd, Carlo M. Croce, Ernest Hawk, Fadlo R. Khuri, Raphael E. Pollock, Apostolia M. Tsimberidou, Christopher G. Willett, and Cheryl L. Willman.
© 2023 John Wiley & Sons, Inc. Published 2023 by John Wiley & Sons, Inc.

Table 1 Some common techniques that are used in telomere biology.

Methods	Principle
TRF (terminal restriction fragment analysis)[13]	Telomeric sequences are detected by Southern blot analysis with a radioactive or nonradioactive telomeric probe. Intensity of telomeric signals is measured to determine an average telomere length
TIF (telomere-dysfunction-induced foci)[14]	This method is based on the co-localization of DNA damage marker by an antibody and telomeres using an antibody against one of the shelterin proteins or telomeric probe
TESLA (telomere shortest length assay)[15]	A ligation and PCR-based approach is used to detect the amplified TRFs from all chromosome ends from <1 to 18 kb. It is facilitated by user-friendly image-processing software
	TESLA provides information about the shortest telomeres without detecting ITSs
	TESLA can be used in T cells to use telomere length as a biomarker of high-performing centenarians[16]
ddTRAP (droplet digital telomere repeat amplification protocol)[17,18]	Two-step assay with whole-cell lysates that utilizes a telomerase-mediated primer extension followed by ddPCR detection of extended products
	Improved throughput, increased sensitivity, and better repeatability of the TRAP assay
	ddTRAP can be used in T cells to use telomerase activity as a biomarker of high-performing centenarians[16]

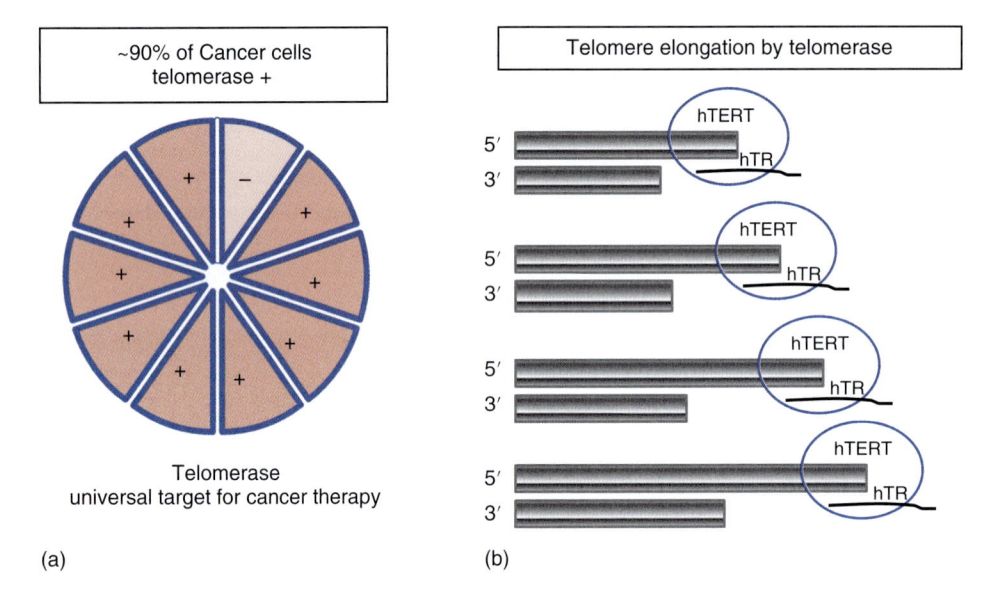

Figure 1 Normal cells that do not express telomerase activity cannot elongate their telomeres, hence their lifespan is limited whereas telomerase expressing cancer cells (~90% of cancer cells, (a)) can elongate their telomeres by telomerase (with hTERT and hTR subunits, (b)) resulting in unlimited proliferative lifespan (a hallmark of cancer). This important difference between normal and cancer cells makes telomerase almost a universal target.

GAR1.[19,21,22] Telomerase is active during early human fetal development, then becomes silent in most tissues (Figure 2a) except embryonic stem cells and some but not all proliferating progenitors (e.g., male germline spermatocytes, activated lymphocytes, and a few other transient amplifying cell types).[23] Telomerase is not required for cells to become malignant, however, 85–90% primary human tumors have telomerase activity while the vast majority of normal tissues do not have detectable enzyme activity (Figure 2a).[22] ddTRAP (droplet digital telomeric repeat amplification protocol) is a sensitive and quantitative method that can be used to determine telomerase activity even at the single-cell level (Table 1). A rarer (10–15%) mechanism to maintain telomere length in mostly rarer cancer cell types is called ALT, **A**lternative **L**engthening of **T**elomeres involve intra-telomeric recombination and perhaps T-loop resolution. ALT-positive cancer cells (commonly mesenchymal and neuroepithelial cell origins, such as osteosarcomas, soft tissue sarcomas, and astrocytomas) are characterized by telomere length heterogeneity and formation of the nuclear promyelocytic leukemia (PML) bodies.[24–27] While co-existence of telomerase-mediated telomere maintenance and ALT in ALT cells is possible, telomerase-positive cells have a factor that represses ALT.[28] At the genetic level, ATRX and DAXX are involved in chromatin remodeling at telomeres and loss-of-function mutations in ATRX and DAXX are associated with engaging the ALT-associated phenotype.[29]

There have been several studies on changes in telomerase expression/activation in normal and cancer cells. DNA rearrangement breakpoints within the telomerase reverse transcriptase (TERT) promoter region correlate with increased TERT expression in some cancers.[30] Also, mutations upstream of the TERT promoter lead to activated telomerase in nontumorigenic fibroblasts.[31] Mutations in the TERT promoter[32] and gene amplifications in TERT[33,34] correlate with increased TERT transcriptional activation and expression of telomerase activity. While it is difficult to regulate very low abundant transcripts such as TERT, it has been reported that another mechanism for telomerase regulation is by alternative splicing. Precursor mRNA (pre-mRNA) that is transcribed from DNA is processed to exclude introns (noncoding sequences) and join exons (coding sequences) to produce an mRNA for mature protein. However, during RNA splicing, exons may be included or excluded from the pre-mRNA to create diverse proteins with multifunctional roles. This process is known as alternative splicing.[35] Induction of hTERT cDNA in normal human cells causes reactivation of telomerase and unlimited proliferation,[36,37] indicating

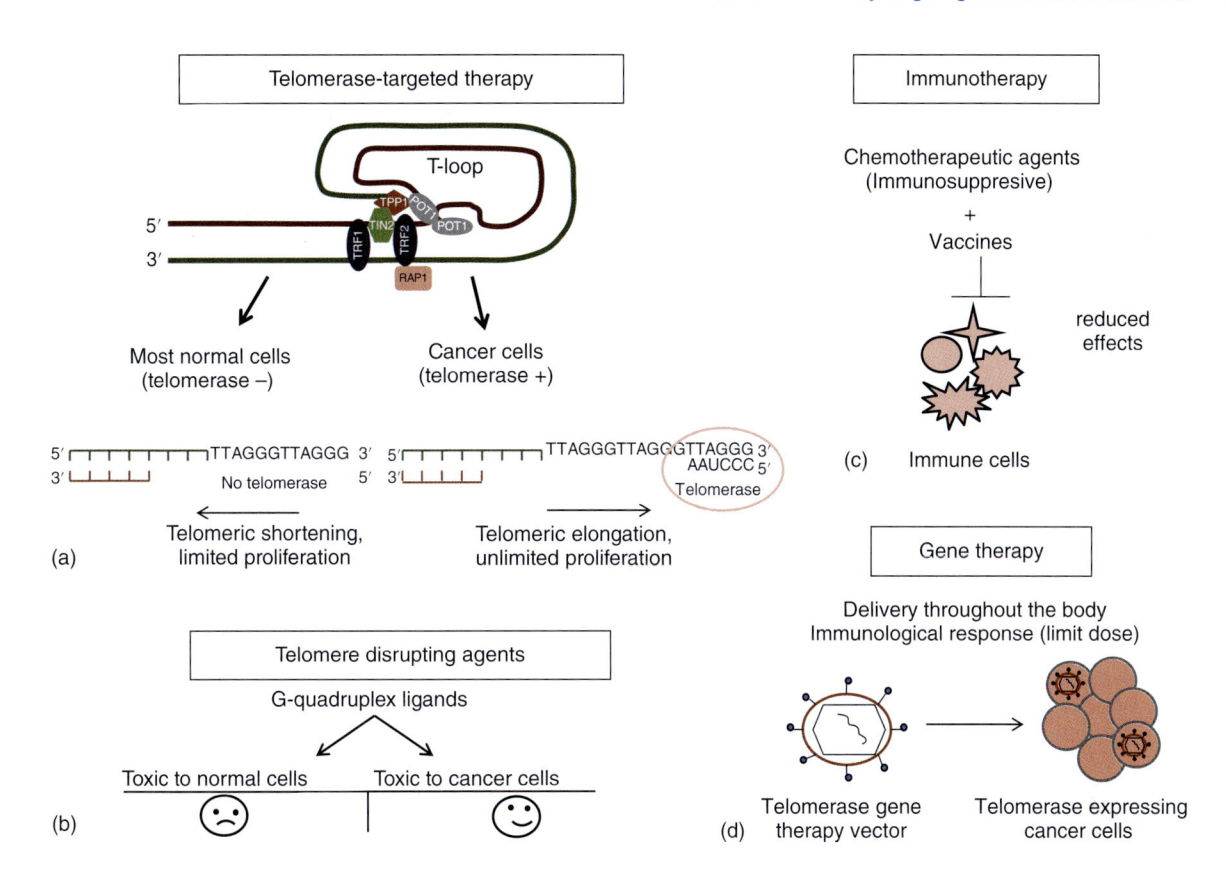

Figure 2 Diagram of hypothetical telomere demonstrating the T-loop structure. This structure is similar in normal and cancer cells but since normal cells generally do not express telomerase, telomeres shorten progressively while cancer cells expressing telomerase can maintain their telomeres (a). There are disadvantages of G-quadruplex stabilizers (b), immunotherapy (c), and gene therapy approaches (d). Since G-quadruplex stabilizers show their toxic effects by binding and stabilizing T-loop structures and they are also found at the other regions of chromosomes beside telomeres, these agents are toxic for both normal and cancer cells (b). One of the most important disadvantages for immunotherapy is that when combination chemotherapy is used with vaccines for cancer patients, some agents can block the effect of immunization since most chemotherapeutic agents are immunosuppressive (c). The challenge for gene therapy is the delivery of the gene therapy to the vast majority of cancer cells (d) throughout the body and immunologic responses to therapy can also be dose limiting. Gene therapies generally require more invasive approaches to delivery and are generally not orally available for systemic delivery.

that repression of telomerase activity is primarily regulated by transcriptional mechanisms, and generation of full-length hTERT is likely responsible for activation of telomerase.[38,39] However, it is also known that posttranscriptional and epigenetic alterations may play an important role in this dynamic process.[38] There is no known consensus mechanism to repress telomerase in developmental and reactivate telomerase in cancer progression, but alternative splicing is one of the potential mechanisms for repression or reactivation of telomerase.[40,41] Several groups have found that there are different hTERT splice forms such as minus alpha, minus beta or minus alpha beta,[35,40,42,43] which may have a role on regulating telomerase activity.[35,39] hTERTα is one of the known splice variants that inhibits telomerase activity by acting as a dominant-negative inhibitor. Thus, the balance between the hTERTα splice variant and full-length hTERT and other splice variants is important in the regulation of active telomerase.[38,44] For example, a 1.1-kb region of 38-bp variable number of tandem repeats (conserved among Old World primates) is essential for exclusion of hTERT exon 7 and 8 to produce the minus beta splicing form, and that RNA:RNA pairing between these repetitive sequences may be used to regulate decisions on hTERT splicing.[45,46] Importantly, misregulation of alternative splicing is a hallmark of nearly all cancers. Although hTR (hTERC), a functional RNA, is found in almost all cells, hTERT is only detected at extremely low levels even in cancer cells. How this is regulated to produce an optimal level for telomerase function in stem cells and cancer cells is still largely unknown. However, one could speculate that targeting hTERT at the splicing level could be a novel approach to reduce telomerase activity in cancer cells perhaps with minimal toxicity to normal cells.[35] It has been recently shown that neuro-oncological ventra antigen 1 (NOVA1) may regulate hTERT splicing. Reduction in NOVA1 levels shifts hTERT splicing toward inactive transcripts and reduces telomerase activity, leading to telomere shortening in vitro and in smaller tumors in vivo.[47,48] TERT expression can also be mediated by other transcription factors, such as MYC, SP-1, E2F, and AP1. Also, estrogen receptor α can induce TERT transcription by interacting with the TERT promoter.[8]

Compared to normal cells with long telomeres, most cancer cells have relatively short telomeres. Since normal stem cells generally have longer telomeres compared to cancer cells, this may facilitate cancer cells to undergo apoptosis with telomerase targeted drug administration without a significant effect on normal cells.[49] As an example, the transfection of an hTERT dominant-negative mutant into tumor cell lines resulted in apoptosis and reduced tumorigenic capacity.[50,51] The death by apoptosis in tumor cells correlates with initial telomere length, the tumor cells with short telomeres die before those with longer telomeres when treated with a telomerase inhibitor.[52] In addition, it has been proposed that tumors are less likely to develop resistance against telomerase-based therapies compared to other cancer targets.[53] All of these factors suggest that targeting telomerase is not only a unique and almost universal cancer target, but it is likely to be a relatively safe anticancer approach with fewer side effects compared to standard chemotherapy. Thus, more understanding of the relationships between telomeres, telomerase, and cancer will help to develop innovative therapeutic approaches in cancer. Cryo-EM structure studies of the human telomerase holoenzyme[54] will also help to advance our structural understanding of telomerase and for future drug design.

Telomerase as a potential target for cancer therapy

Although proof of concept of different approaches for telomerase-based therapies has repeatedly been achieved in the preclinical setting, there are no telomerase inhibitors that have been approved by the Food and Drug Administration (FDA). The most promising telomere/telomerase targeted strategies are summarized in Table 2 and Figure 2.

G-quadruplex stabilizers

G-quadruplexes are formed by the ability of guanosine self-assembly together with monovalent cations (e.g., potassium) in the presence of guanine tandem repeats. G-quadruplexes may form in telomeres, oncogene promoter sequences, and other biologically relevant regions of the genome.[55] It has been demonstrated that small molecules that target G-quadruplex structure in human telomeres cause telomerase inhibition (perhaps indirectly) and telomeric end disruption.[56] Thus, this secondary DNA structure is a popular target to design small-molecule ligands.

Telomestatin is isolated from *Streptomyces anulatus* 3533-SV4 and reported to be a telomerase inhibitor that interacts with G-quadruplex structures.[57,58] Nakajima and coworkers showed that telomestatin causes telomerase inhibition and induces apoptosis in primary leukemic blasts that were isolated from bone marrow of acute myeloid leukemia (AML-M2) patients.[59] Another reported G-quadruplex ligand is termed TMPyP4. Hurley and colleagues showed that telomestatin causes telomerase inhibition by stabilizing of intramolecular G-quadruplex structures and eventually telomere shortening, whereas TMPyP4 suppressed the proliferation of ALT-positive cells as well as telomerase positive cells by facilitating the formation of intermolecular G-quadruplexes leading to the induction of anaphase bridges. They also reported that telomestatin more tightly and specifically binds to the intramolecular G-quadruplexes compared to other G-quadruplex interactive compounds such as TMPyP4.[60] Another investigated telomeric G4 ligand is termed RHPS4 (pentacyclic acridine). RHPS4 reduces telomerase activity at sub-micromolar levels through stabilization of G-quadruplex structures formed by single stranded telomeric DNA.[61] Others report that RHSP4 causes telomere capping alterations in a telomere length-independent manner.[62] *In vivo* experiments demonstrate that RHSP4 is even more effective when compared with other antineoplastic drugs in terms of antitumoral and antimetastatic effects.[63] Although BRACO19 (trisubstituted acridine) is classified as a G-quadruplex stabilizer due to *in vitro* and *in vivo* anticancer effects,[52] the utility of this compound is limited because of its low permeability for biological barriers in the airways or intestinal epithelial cell cultures *in vitro*.[64] Several ligands induce growth inhibition of various cancer cells *in vitro* by causing cellular senescence and/or apoptosis. These ligands also exert short-term effects on telomere uncapping.[65] Over the past decade, many G-quadruplex ligands have been described including fluorenons, bisubstituted acridines, cationic porphyrins, a perylenetetracarboxylic diimide derivative, indolo-quinolines, and benzonaphtofurandione tetracyclic compounds. However, the evidence for specificity of these compounds for telomerase expressing cells is very limited and they poorly bind to the quadruplex structures compared to double DNA.[52] Thus, there is concern that many of these compounds may affect quadruplex structures in normal cells as well as cancer cells. Any compound that inhibits cell growth will decrease telomerase activity, so it is not sufficient to show telomerase inhibition to suggest specificity without also testing these compounds on normal cells without telomerase (Figure 2b).

Some of the proteins that interact with G-quadruplex stabilizers also have the ability to induce senescence and/or apoptosis. Although these structures appear to be good targets for anticancer therapy, one of the most common concerns is that G-quadruplex structures are observed during replication in chromosome regions besides telomeres. Because G-quadruplexes also have a large planar surface formed by terminal G-tetrad, most of the small molecules designed so far target this common structure instead of a specific target for a particular G-quadruplex. Thus, a general concern about these compounds is safety: while small-molecule ligands towards G-quadruplex structures affect cancer cells, they may also affect the telomere structure of normal cells[66,67] (Figure 2b).

Although there are two quadruplex-related small molecules that entered into clinical trials, there remains lack of direct evidence that these small molecules are specific for telomerase targeted therapy. The first agent CX-3543 (quarfloxin/quarfloxacin, Cylene Pharmaceuticals, San Diego, CA, USA) is a fluoroquinolone derivative, that selectively disrupts nucleolin/rDNA G-quadruplex complexes in the nucleolus by inhibiting Pol1 transcription,

Table 2 Telomere/telomerase targeted strategies.

Therapeutic approach	Inhibitors	Description
G-quadruplex stabilizers	BRACO19, RHPS4, Telomestatin, porphyrin, TMPyP4, CX-3543/quarfloxin, AS1411/Cytarabine/Ara-C	Recognize and stabilize G4s. Induce telomeric and nontelomeric DNA damage and transcriptional/translational perturbation of cancer-related genes
Immunotherapy	GV1001, VX-001, GRNVAC1/2	Vaccine approach aims to activate the immune system to recognize and kill cancer cells
Adenoviral gene therapies	Telomelysin/OBP-301, OBP-502, OBP-702	TERT promoter-driven oncolytic activities
Telomere and telomerase associated proteins	Geldanamycin (GA), Curcumin	Inhibits telomerase activity
PARP (poly (ADP-ribose) polymerase) inhibitors	XAV939, G007-LK, and RK-287107	Blocking tankyrase, a member of PARP family, downregulate Wnt/β-catenin signaling
Small-molecule inhibitors	BIBR1532	Noncompetitive telomerase inhibitor
Antisense oligonucleotides (ASO)	GRN163L	Competitive telomerase inhibitor
Telomerase based telomere uncapping approach	6-Thio-dG	Recognized by telomerase and rapidly incorporates toxic product in telomeres

resulting in decreased cancer cell proliferation and induction of apoptosis.[68,69] However, CX-3543 also interacts with MYC G-quadruplexes,[68] so the *in vitro* antiproliferative and *in vivo* antitumoral activity in xenograft models may not be related to G quadruplexes at telomeres. In addition, CX-3543 selectively targets Pol1, rather than telomere function, which further suggests that CX-3543 may have indirect or even no effect on telomere function.[69] The other quadruplex-forming agent in clinical trials is AS1411 (Cytarabine/Ara-C, Antisoma Research, London, UK), which specifically targets nucleolin.[70] Progress on these drugs have not been advanced and none are FDA approved.

Immunotherapy

Tumor-associated antigens (TAAs) specific immunotherapy has been investigated for several decades. However, since most TAAs immunotherapies have been restricted to only a few tumor types, telomerase-based immunotherapy would theoretically be a promising approach due to the ubiquitous expression of telomerase in most tumor cells.[71] Degradation of hTERT in proteasomes by E3 ubiquitin ligase results in protein fragments/peptides that are generated on the tumor cell surface as antigens by the major histocompatibility complex (MHC) class I pathway. Thus, targeting these antigens by a patient's own immune system (CD8+ T lymphocytes) is a direct way to kill the telomerase expressing tumor cells[72,73] (reviewed in Ref. 74). Several hTERT vaccines have already been developed, but GV1001 and GRNVAC1 were the most promising vaccines in clinical trials. GV1001 is a 16 mer TERT peptide (aa 611–626) that binds multiple human leukocyte antigen (HLA) class II molecules. Studies showed that vaccination with hTERT transfected dendritic cells helped to induce telomerase specific CD4+ and CD8+ T cell responses[75] and also vaccination with GV1001 induced hTERT specific T cell responses in nonresectable pancreatic cancer patients and non-small-lung cancer patients.[76,77] The combination treatment of GV1001 and cyclophosphamide in hepatocellular carcinoma failed to show partial or complete responses to treatment in a Phase 2 clinical trial.[78] In addition, GV1001 vaccination with chemotherapy together did not improve overall survival in advanced or metastatic pancreatic cancer in a Phase 3 clinical trial.[79] GRNVAC1 was also designed to induce CD4 and CD8 T cell responses. GRNVAC1 was prepared from autologous dendritic cells transduced with mRNAs encoding a near full-length hTERT protein *ex vivo*. The dendritic cells were reintroduced to the patient and predicted to recognize any hTERT peptide in a patient's tumor.[53] GRNVAC1 was also tested in Phase 2 clinical trials for acute myelogenous leukemia patients. Since monotherapy is likely to have limited efficacy, combination therapy might be a more effective approach to kill the heterogeneous nature of tumor cells. However, most chemotherapeutic agents are potentially immunosuppressive and they might reduce the immunization effect. For this reason, vaccines may be less effective when used in combination with chemotherapeutic agents[80] (Figure 2c). Hence, new strategies are required to improve clinical efficacy with enhanced immune response effects of telomerase vaccination during chemotherapy.

Gene therapy

Gene therapy is a technique that treats diseases by delivering therapeutic DNA into a patient's cells. Using DNA that encodes a therapeutic effect can be delivered to the target cells where the DNA becomes expressed by the cell machinery that ultimately makes a protein that in cancer results in apoptosis. Genes can be delivered via oncolytic viral vectors and can include prodrugs or suicide genes.[81] Although gene therapy can be highly tumor specific, there are challenges including manufacture/formulation which is often complex and often specialist clinical trial expertise is required[82] (Figure 2d). Some studies showed proof of concept in treating cancer, but there are some concerns about off-target effects and the need to target the vast majority of tumor cells to have tumor burden reduction and durable responses.[83,84] There are adenoviral vectors that have been engineered to kill the cancer cells by entering to the host cells that have telomerase activity. These adenoviral vectors have a TERT promoter that drives replication of the adenovirus. In these instances, the virus only replicates in telomerase positive cells thus sparing most normal cells.[85] After replication and amplification of the virus, the tumor cell will lyse and viral particles should spread to adjacent cells.[85–88] This approach is known as a tumor-specific replication-competent adenoviral (hTERTp-TRAD) gene therapy approach.[83,89] One of the examples for virus therapy is telomelysin (OBP-301), which is an hTERT promoter-driven modified oncolytic adenovirus. Preclinical studies demonstrated antitumor activity of telomelysin or similarly engineered adenoviruses on various cancer cells.[86,88,90,91] Phase 1 clinical trials did not show any significant toxic rate limiting events, but there were multiple adverse side effects such as fever, chills, fatigue, and injection site pain. Some patients with solid tumors developed asymptomatic transient decreased lymphocyte counts.[92] Thus, systemic treatment has the potential to have side effects on telomerase positive normal transient amplifying stem cells. Therefore, systemic hTERTp-TRAD is likely to cause some side effects on proliferating cells in the crypts of the intestine, hematological cells, and a subset of cells in the basal and suprabasal layer of the epidermis.[21,82] The other concern is the intratumoral injections may not be sufficient to spread and reduce the tumor burden systemically.[93] Suicide gene therapy (Ad-hTR-NTR), also called "gene-directed enzyme prodrug therapy," targets only tumor cells without affecting normal cells similar to oncolytic gene therapy.[53,94] Three general steps are required for this approach: first is targeting the vector, second is carrying an enzyme-encoding gene driven hTERT is transfected into the cells, third is a prodrug that was added and is activated by an enzyme, resulting in a release of toxins into the cytoplasm and causing telomerase positive cell death.[94] Although gene therapy (suicide gene or oncolytic vector) showed some promising results, they do not appear to be as effective as vaccines or oligonucleotides.[95] Future direction would be to make multi-functional viral vectors such as those only replicating in p53 mutant cells and with telomerase expression. This would potentially reduce the side effect on normal proliferating stem cells.

Small-molecule inhibitors and antisense oligonucleotides

Although millions of compounds have been screened to identify small-molecule inhibitors of telomerase, there are currently no potent/specific small-molecule inhibitors except one candidate compound, BIBR1532. While BIBR1532 showed promising results in some preclinical models,[96,97] it was not effective enough to enter clinical trials perhaps due to its short binding rate kinetics with telomerase.[98,99] After many years of screening new drugs, GRN163L (Imetelstat, Geron Corporation), was found as a parallel approach to small-molecule inhibitors. This telomerase targeted oligonucleotide approach uses a 13-mer lipid-modified N3′ → P5′ thio-phosphoramidate oligonucleotide and has shown highly potent telomerase inhibition as a competitive enzyme inhibitor by being designed to complement the hTR RNA template of telomerase that recognizes telomeres.[100] GRN163L was generated as a second improved generation of GRN163 to increase cellular uptake with a conjugating lipophilic palmitoyl (C16) group attached to the 5′ terminal.[49] The effects of GRN163L have been investigated in different cancer cell lines and xenograft models. GRN163L demonstrates both in vitro and in vivo effects by inhibiting telomerase activity resulting in progressive telomere shortening in a variety of cancer cell lines such as hepatocellular carcinoma,[101] lung cancer,[102] breast cancer,[103,104] bladder cancer,[93] multiple myeloma,[105] pancreatic cancer,[106] colorectal cancer,[107] glioblastoma,[108] and esophageal adenocarcinoma.[109] In vivo antimetastatic effects of GRN163L were tested in tumor xenograft models. When A549 human lung cancer cells were injected into immunosuppressed nude mice via the tail vein, lung tumor formation was not observed in the animals treated with 15 mg/kg GRN163L (intraperitoneal, three times per week for 3 weeks).[102] In mice having implanted hepatoma cancer cells, GRN163L inhibited tumor growth and also sensitized tumor cells to conventional chemotherapy.[101] In a xenograft model of breast cancer, administration of 30 mg/kg GRN163L for 12 treatments (three times per week, 4 weeks total) effectively reduced the proliferation of breast cancer cells and metastasis to the lungs.[104] Different studies showed that GRN163L reduced tumor size as well as improved survival in a human myeloma cell-derived xenograft model.[105] Although there are many studies showing promising effects of GRN163L in vitro and in vivo, GRN163L has not progressed in most clinical trials due to hematological side effects and liver function abnormalities as well as other adverse events. When patients have dose-limiting toxicities (DLT) such as thrombocytopenia, due to GRN163L, patients must go off trial until their platelet numbers return to the normal range. This results in telomeres re-elongating during the drug holiday period.

GRN163L (Imetelstat) is the first telomerase inhibitor in clinical trials and has involved multiple clinical trials (https://ClinicalTrials.gov shows 13 completed, 3 withdrawn, and 1 terminated trial due to intracranial hemorrhages). These are summarized in Table 3. The preliminary data in 50–74 years old patients with advanced solid tumors (6 colorectal, 3 lung, 2 mesothelioma, 2 pancreas, 7 others) showed aPTT prolongation (active prolonged thromboplastin), gastrointestinal side effects, fatigue, anemia, GGT elevation, and peripheral neuropathy. Although thrombocytopenia is a dose-limiting toxicity at 4.8 mg/kg, one death with unknown reasons was observed at 3.2 mg/kg dose.[110] Locally recurrent or metastatic breast cancer (MBC) patients were treated with GRN163L in combination with paclitaxel and bevacizumab (3 of 14 patients with de novo MBC and 6 of 14 patients with prior (neo) adjuvant taxane). Phase 1 clinical trials showed that the most common toxicities were cytopenia. The majority of patients had dose reduction or delays with GRN163L and/or paclitaxel due to neutropenia and/or thrombocytopenia or other adverse effects.[95] Main outcome from pediatric patients with solid tumors in Phase 1 clinical trials was that the reduction of telomerase activity in PBMCs (peripheral blood mononuclear cells) and telomerase positive tumors with the recommended Phase 2 dose, which is 285 mg/m^2 (MTD; maximum tolerated dose). In this study, intravenous injection was conducted for 2 h on days 1 and 8 of a 21-day cycle. As a result, DLT (360 mg/m^2) caused myelosuppression leading to a delay in the therapy more than 14 days. In addition, some patients also had anemia, lymphopenia, neutropenia, thrombocytopenia, leucopenia, or catheter-related infections depending on their grade level and cycle number of treatment.[111] The advanced breast cancer Phase 2 trial (NCT01256762) was stopped due to poorer overall survival in patients treated with GRN163L.[71] Since GRN163L (Imetelstat) is administered on days 1 and 8 of a 21-day cycle, it is possible that telomerase cannot be inhibited sufficiently and long-term so that a new telomere equilibrium length for cancer cells emerges. GRN163L has still efficacies against myelofibrosis and essential thrombocythemia and there are ongoing clinical studies in patients with myelodysplastic syndromes.[8]

Challenges for developing telomerase inhibitors

The other potential challenge for telomerase inhibitors, such as GRN163L, is that the response time which is needed to induce senescence or crisis is long since telomere attrition occurs following each cell replication cycle. Therefore, this delayed long-lag response may limit its utility as a first-line treatment for advanced cancer. It has been suggested that telomerase inhibitors following conventional therapy might be a good option to block the growth of residual cancer cells.[87] A Phase 2 study used GRN163L in a maintenance therapy setting after initial standard of care doublet chemotherapy for advanced non-small-cell lung cancer (NSCLC) was completed (https://clinicaltrials.gov: NCT01137968). This study was designed to evaluate whether GRN163L, given as maintenance therapy, prolonged progression-free survival (PFS) in

Table 3 GRN163L in clinical trials.

ClinicalTrials.gov Identifier/phase	Condition	Drug Intervention	Status
NCT01568632/Phase 1	Refractory or recurrent solid tumors/lymphoma	GRN163L	Withdrawn
NCT01273090/Phase 1	Refractory or recurrent solid tumors/lymphoma	GRN163L	Completed
NCT01243073/Phase 2	Essential thrombocythemia/polycythemia vera (ET/PV)	GRN163L	Completed
NCT00594126/Phase 1	Refractory or relapsed multiple myeloma	GRN163L	Completed
NCT01916187/Phase 1	Neuroblastoma	GRN163L, 13-cis retinoic acid	Withdrawn
NCT00732056/Phase 1	Recurrent or metastatic breast cancer	GRN163L, paclitaxel, bevacizumab	Completed
NCT00310895/Phase 1	Refractory or relapsed solid tumor malignancies	GRN163L	Completed
NCT00718601/Phase 1	Refractory or relapsed multiple myeloma	GRN163L and Velcade w/Decadron	Completed
NCT01242930/Phase 2	Multiple myeloma	GRN163L, standard of care	Completed
NCT00510445/Phase 1	Advanced or metastatic non-small-cell lung cancer	GRN163L, paclitaxel, carboplatin	Completed
NCT01265927/Phase 1	Her2+ breast cancer	GRN163L, trastuzumab	Completed
NCT00124189/Phase 1	Chronic lymphoproliferative disease (CLD)	GRN163L	Completed
NCT02011126/Phase 2	Relapsed or refractory solid tumors	GRN163L	Withdrawn
NCT01137968/Phase 2	Non-small-cell lung cancer	GRN163L, bevacizumab	Completed
NCT01731951/Phase 2	Primary or secondary myelofibrosis	GRN163L	Completed
NCT01256762/Phase 2	Recurrent or metastatic breast cancer	GRN163L, paclitaxel, w/wo bevacizumab	Completed
NCT01836549/Phase 2	Recurrent or refractory brain tumors	GRN163L	Terminated

NSCLC. Eligible stage IV or recurrent locally advanced NSCLC patients were randomized to GRN163L (9.4 mg/kg over a 2 h IV infusion on day 1 and day 8 of each 21-day cycle) with or without bevacizumab for day 1 of each 21-day cycle or observation) versus standard of care alone (patients who had received bevacizumab before randomization were continued with bevacizumab maintenance or had no follow-up maintenance treatment). This study while not achieving statistical significance showed a trend in PFS in the GRN163L arm and was most apparent in the cohort of patients with the shortest telomeres at the initiation of the trial.[112] Experience with these types of trials is important to more fully understand how to provide antitelomerase therapies going forward.

Overexpression of mutant hTERC and wild type hTERC-targeted siRNA by lentiviral vectors are different types of gene therapy strategies for telomerase-targeted therapies

The other strategy to disrupt telomere maintenance in cancer cells is to express mutant hTR (hTERC) in the template region (mutant-template human telomerase RNA; MT-hTERC). Wild-type telomere repeats contain DNA binding sites for direct telomeric-binding proteins such as POT1, TRF1, and TRF2 in humans.[113,114] It is predicted that mutated DNA that is directly synthesized by MT-hTERC disrupts the binding of telomeric proteins,[115–117] which might lead to rapid telomere uncapping. Studies showed that the uncapping of human telomeres by mutating TRF2 can induce growth arrest (p53-dependent) and apoptosis in cells.[118,119] Introduction of MT-hTERC via lentiviral vectors into telomerase-positive human cancer cells causes an alteration in the cancer cellular phenotype and reduced tumor growth in xenografts.[116,117] In another approach using siRNA (a hairpin short-interfering RNA) expressed from a lentiviral vector targeted wild-type human telomerase RNA (WT-hTERC) also caused cell growth inhibition and apoptosis (these effects are telomere length independent). Co-expression of MT-hTERC and anti-WT-hTERC-siRNA showed additive or perhaps synergistic effects on cancer cells. Therefore, mutant-hTERC and siRNA present promising anticancer therapy strategies due to the lack of dependency on p53, initial telomere length, or progressive telomere shortening.[120] However, these are still gene therapy approaches and require high efficiency in targeting to the cancer cells to be effective in the clinical setting.

Telomerase-based telomere uncapping approach

Ideal cancer targets are those that are expressed in cancer cells, but not in normal cells. Compared to other targets, telomerase is one of the most universal targets expressed in almost all tumor cells, but not in normal cells except proliferative progenitor stem cells. Therefore, telomerase is an important target to focus on new therapeutic strategies.

The strategy that directly targets telomerase inhibition is correlated with tumor telomere length, whereas telomere-targeted approaches are independent from initial telomere length (Figure 3). This makes an important difference between these two approaches. With direct telomerase inhibition, a long lag period is expected (the time between enzyme inhibition and biological effect). Thus treatment will generally be long and depend on significant reduction of telomere length before reduction of tumor growth, senescence, or apoptosis is observed.[50,51] Some approaches that target telomeres (not directly telomerase) leading to telomere uncapping (e.g., G-quadruplex), which is independent from p53 status and initial telomere length. However, normal tissue toxicity is still a big concern due to quadruplex formation in other regions of the genome and in normal cells.[121] Thus, approaches that do not target through telomerase may not have a therapeutic window of efficacy. In addition, using direct telomerase inhibitor or telomere-targeted therapies may need to be combined with other cytotoxic drugs to reduce the potential resistance capacity of heterogeneous tumor cells.[121] For example, the cells from mTR knock-out mice showed telomere dysfunction by sensitizing cells to some anticancer drugs (e.g., doxorubicin).[122] This result shows that telomerase-targeted therapy in combination with other chemotherapeutic agents may sensitize cells to other chemotherapies by reducing resistant capacity.

Other studies showed the effect of nucleotide analogs, including 5-fluoro-2′-deoxyuridine (5-FdU) triphosphate, in telomerase-positive cancer cells. 5-FdU is incorporated into a telomere DNA product by telomerase and this results in an increased number of TIFs, prevents binding of telomere shelterin proteins, activates the ATR-related DDR, and leads to cell death in a telomerase-dependent manner.[123] Another study showed the antitumor effects of 6-dithio-2′-deoxyguanosine analogs in colon cancer and melanoma cells by inhibiting thioredoxin1 (TRX1) and telomerase.[124]

In recent work, we focused on a novel approach to identify a small molecule that would uncap telomeres but only in telomerase-positive cells. This theoretical approach using a small molecule obviates some of the problems with gene therapy and could reduce the lag phase from initiation of treatment to tumor burden reduction. To test this concept, we decided to focus on nucleoside analogs that are good substrates for telomerase (not an inhibitor) and more specific to telomerase than other polymerases. 6-thio-2′deoxyguanosine (6-thio-dG) is a telomere-targeted nucleoside analogue prodrug, which is preferentially recognized by telomerase. Its incorporation into de novo synthesized telomeres by telomerase is known to induce damage on telomeric DNA.[125] This results in rapid tumor shrinkage or growth arrest in many tumor-derived xenograft models with minimal side effects.[125–127] The most important advantage of this telomere-targeting therapy over direct telomerase inhibitors is that 6-thio-dG does not have a long lag period for tumor-killing effects. In addition, it does not directly inhibit telomerase but is preferentially recognized by telomerase over other polymerases and incorporated into the telomeres resulting in immediate DNA chain termination. Importantly, its effect is independent of initial telomere length by using tumor telomerase to make unstable telomeres.[128] 6-Thio-dG, which induces telomere replication stress in telomerase-positive cancer cells, also triggers innate sensing and contributes to host antitumor immunity.[129] It has been shown that 6-thio-dG induces the cyclic guanosine monophosphate–adenosine monophosphate synthase (cGAS)-mediated cytosolic DNA sensing pathway in response to dysfunctional telomeres.[130] Additionally, 6-thio-dG overcomes chemotherapy and targeted therapy resistance including mutant EGFR resistance and PD-L1 blockade resistance in advanced tumors.[129,131] SLC43A3, an equilibrative nucleobase transporter, is downregulated in 6-thio-dG-resistant lung cancer cells, and is thus proposed as a biomarker for drug sensitivity.[132]

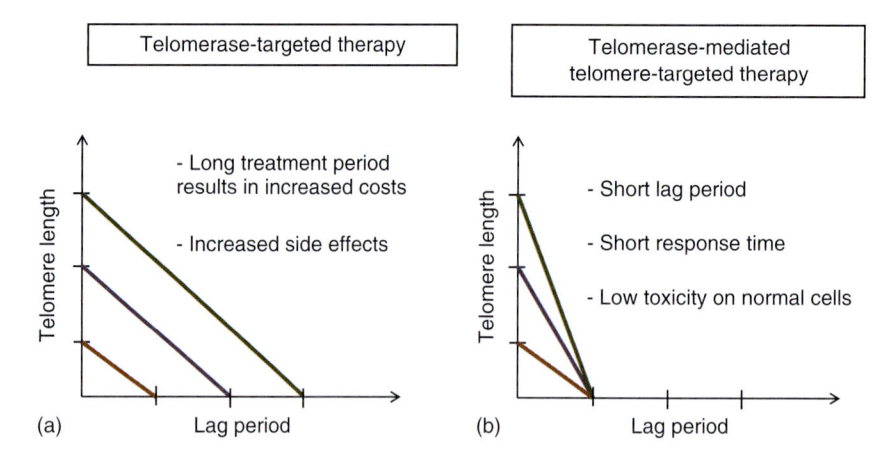

Figure 3 Telomerase targeted therapeutic responses (such as Imetelstat/GRN163L) are dependent on the initial tumor cell telomere length. Cancer cells have variable telomere lengths. Therefore, cells with long telomeres are predicted to take a longer treatment period to be sensitive to telomerase inhibitors compared to cells with shorter telomeres (a). As a result, any long-term treatment for telomerase may lead to unwanted side effects, high costs, and potentially re-establishing feedback upregulation of telomerase to a stable new telomere length. In contrast to telomerase targeted therapies, telomerase mediated telomere targeting therapies (such as 6-thio-dG or MT-hTERC gene therapy) do not need long treatment periods since they are independent of the initial telomere length, therefore short response time to tumor burden reduction is a key advantage of these approaches (b). The other most important advantage is that they may be less toxic to normal cells since quiescent stem cell and most somatic cells do not express telomerase. However, the MT-hTERC approach has the same obvious limitations of all gene therapy approaches of needing to reach almost all cells and delivery is a concern. However new approaches such as 6-thio-dG may be oral available and have the obvious advantage that all small molecules have in cancer therapies.

In summary, targeting telomeres and telomerase in cancer continues to be an area of increased interest. However, there are no drugs that have been approved so far. G-quadruplex stabilizers cause telomerase inhibition and telomeric end disruption. However, the specificity of these compounds is limited since they may also affect quadruplex structures in normal cells. The utility of vaccines (hTERT GV1001 (peptide vaccine) and GRNVAC1 (dendritic cell priming *ex vivo*) in combination with conventional therapy may be limited due to immunosuppressive effect of chemotherapeutic drugs. GRN163L (Imetelstat) is a direct telomerase inhibitor and causes progressive telomere shortening in cancer cells. Clinical trials in solid tumors have not progressed due to hematological toxicities. One of the potential challenges for GRN163L is the response time that is needed to kill cancer cells. Gene therapy targets cancer by delivering therapeutic DNA; mutant hTERT (dominant-negative approach) or siRNA directed at hTERT are some of the gene therapy approaches in preclinical studies. Gene therapy requires high efficiency to target almost every cancer cell. Telomerase-mediated telomere-targeted therapy is predicted to have a much shorter lag period compared to direct telomerase inhibitors. A nucleoside analogue 6-thio-dG is a promising anticancer treatment approach. It is preferentially recognized by telomerase and incorporated into telomeres resulting in damage on telomeres. This small-molecule results in rapid cell-killing effects but only in telomerase-expressing cells with minimal effects on telomerase silent normal cells (Figure 3). Importantly, 6-thio-dG overcomes drug resistance and enhances immune responses in advanced tumors.

Acknowledgments

Ilgen Mender was supported by T32 CA124334. These studies were also supported in part by NCI SPORE P50CA70907, the Simmons Cancer Center Support Grant 5P30 CA142543, and support from the Southland Financial Corporation Distinguished Chair in Geriatric Research (Jerry W. Shay). This work was performed in space constructed with support from National Institute of Health grant C06 RR30414. Jerry W. Shay is a founding scientists of Maia Biotech, Chicago, IL, that is advancing 6-thio-dG into clinical development.

Key references

The complete reference list can be found on Vital Source version of this title, see inside front cover.

2. Shay JW. Are short telomeres predictive of advanced cancer? *Cancer Discov.* 2013;**3**(10):1096–1098.
6. Shay JW, Wright WE. Hayflick, his limit, and cellular ageing. *Nat Rev Mol Cell Biol.* 2000;**1**(1):72–76.
9. Kim W, Ludlow AT, Min J, et al. Regulation of the human telomerase gene TERT by telomere position effect-over long distances (TPE-OLD): implications for aging and cancer. *PLoS Biol.* 2016;**14**(12):e2000016.
10. Kim W, Shay JW. Long-range telomere regulation of gene expression: telomere looping and telomere position effect over long distances (TPE-OLD). *Differentiation.* 2018;**99**:1–9.
13. Mender I, Shay JW. Telomere restriction fragment (TRF) analysis. *Bio Protoc.* 2015;**5**(22):e1656.
14. Mender I, Shay JW. Telomere dysfunction induced foci (TIF) analysis. *Bio Protoc.* 2015;**5**(22):e1658.
15. Lai TP, Zhang N, Noh J, et al. A method for measuring the distribution of the shortest telomeres in cells and tissues. *Nat Commun.* 2017;**8**(1):1356.
16. Tedone E, Huang E, O'Hara R, et al. Telomere length and telomerase activity in T cells are biomarkers of high-performing centenarians. *Aging Cell.* 2019;**18**(1):e12859.
17. Ludlow AT, Shelton D, Wright WE, Shay JW. ddTRAP: a method for sensitive and precise quantification of telomerase activity. *Methods Mol Biol.* 1768;**2018**:513–529.
18. Ludlow AT, Robin JD, Sayed M, et al. Quantitative telomerase enzyme activity determination using droplet digital PCR with single cell resolution. *Nucleic Acids Res.* 2014;**42**(13):e104.
19. Shay JW, Wright WE. Telomeres and telomerase: three decades of progress. *Nat Rev Genet.* 2019;**20**(5):299–309.
20. Shay JW. Telomeres and aging. *Curr Opin Cell Biol.* 2018;**52**:1–7.
21. Wright WE, Piatyszek MA, Rainey WE, et al. Telomerase activity in human germline and embryonic tissues and cells. *Dev Genet.* 1996;**18**(2):173–179.
22. Shay JW, Wright WE. Role of telomeres and telomerase in cancer. *Semin Cancer Biol.* 2011;**21**(6):349–353.

23 Shay JW, Wright WE. Implications of mapping the human telomerase gene (hTERT) as the most distal gene on chromosome 5p. *Neoplasia*. 2000;2(3):195–196.
24 Min J, Shay JW. TERT promoter mutations enhance telomerase activation by long-range chromatin interactions. *Cancer Discov*. 2016;6(11):1212–1214.
25 Min J, Wright WE, Shay JW. Clustered telomeres in phase-separated nuclear condensates engage mitotic DNA synthesis through BLM and RAD52. *Genes Dev*. 2019;33(13–14):814–827.
26 Min J, Wright WE, Shay JW. Alternative lengthening of telomeres can be maintained by preferential elongation of lagging strands. *Nucleic Acids Res*. 2017;45(5):2615–2628.
27 Min J, Shay JW. Telomere clustering drives ALT. *Aging (Albany, NY)*. 2019;11(19):8046–8047.
35 Wong MS, Wright WE, Shay JW. Alternative splicing regulation of telomerase: a new paradigm? *Trends Genet*. 2014;30:430–438.
38 Yi X, White DM, Aisner DL, et al. An alternate splicing variant of the human telomerase catalytic subunit inhibits telomerase activity. *Neoplasia*. 2000;2(5):433–440.
39 Aisner DL, Wright WE, Shay JW. Telomerase regulation: not just flipping the switch. *Curr Opin Genet Dev*. 2002;12(1):80–85.
45 Wong MS, Chen L, Foster C, et al. Regulation of telomerase alternative splicing: a target for chemotherapy. *Cell Rep*. 2013;3(4):1028–1035.
46 Wong MS, Shay JW, Wright WE. Regulation of human telomerase splicing by RNA:RNA pairing. *Nat Commun*. 2014;5:3306.
47 Ludlow AT, Wong MS, Robin JD, et al. NOVA1 regulates hTERT splicing and cell growth in non-small cell lung cancer. *Nat Commun*. 2018;9(1):3112.
48 Sayed ME, Yuan L, Robin JD, et al. NOVA1 directs PTBP1 to hTERT pre-mRNA and promotes telomerase activity in cancer cells. *Oncogene*. 2019;38(16):2937–2952.
82 Shay JW, Keith WN. Targeting telomerase for cancer therapeutics. *Br J Cancer*. 2008;98(4):677–683.
87 Ouellette MM, Wright WE, Shay JW. Targeting telomerase-expressing cancer cells. *J Cell Mol Med*. 2011;15(7):1433–1442.
89 Keith WN, Thomson CM, Howcroft J, et al. Seeding drug discovery: integrating telomerase cancer biology and cellular senescence to uncover new therapeutic opportunities in targeting cancer stem cells. *Drug Discov Today*. 2007;12(15-16):611–621.
93 Dikmen ZG, Wright WE, Shay JW, Gryaznov SM. Telomerase targeted oligonucleotide thio-phosphoramidates in T24-luc bladder cancer cells. *J Cell Biochem*. 2008;104(2):444–452.
100 Herbert BS, Pongracz K, Shay JW, Gryaznov SM. Oligonucleotide N3′–>P5′ phosphoramidates as efficient telomerase inhibitors. *Oncogene*. 2002;21(4):638–642.
102 Dikmen ZG, Gellert GC, Jackson S, et al. In vivo inhibition of lung cancer by GRN163L: a novel human telomerase inhibitor. *Cancer Res*. 2005;65(17):7866–7873.
103 Gellert GC, Dikmen ZG, Wright WE, et al. Effects of a novel telomerase inhibitor, GRN163L, in human breast cancer. *Breast Cancer Res Treat*. 2006;96(1):73–81.
125 Mender I, Gryaznov S, Dikmen ZG, et al. Induction of telomere dysfunction mediated by the telomerase substrate precursor 6-thio-2'-deoxyguanosine. *Cancer Discov*. 2015;5(1):82–95.
126 Sengupta S, Sobo M, Lee K, et al. Induced telomere damage to treat telomerase expressing therapy-resistant pediatric brain tumors. *Mol Cancer Ther*. 2018;17(7):1504–1514.
127 Zhang G, Wu LW, Mender I, et al. Induction of telomere dysfunction prolongs disease control of therapy-resistant melanoma. *Clin Cancer Res*. 2018;24(19):4771–4784.
128 Mender I, Gryaznov S, Shay JW. A novel telomerase substrate precursor rapidly induces telomere dysfunction in telomerase positive cancer cells but not telomerase silent normal cells. *Oncoscience*. 2015;2(8):693–695.
129 Mender I, Zhang A, Ren Z, et al. Telomere stress potentiates STING-dependent anti-tumor immunity. *Cancer Cell*. 2020;38(3):400–411.e6.
131 Mender I, LaRanger R, Luitel K, et al. Telomerase-mediated strategy for overcoming non-small cell lung cancer targeted therapy and chemotherapy resistance. *Neoplasia*. 2018;20(8):826–837.
132 Mender I, Batten K, Peyton M, et al. SLC43A3 Is a biomarker of sensitivity to the telomeric DNA damage mediator 6-thio-2'-deoxyguanosine. *Cancer Res*. 2020;80(5):929–936.

15 Cancer metabolism

Natalya N. Pavlova, PhD ■ Aparna D. Rao, MBBS, PhD ■ Ralph J. DeBerardinis, MD, PhD ■ Craig B. Thompson, MD

> **Overview**
>
> Successful cell proliferation is dependent on a profound remodeling of cellular metabolism, required to support the biosynthetic needs of a growing cell. Constitutive signaling through aberrantly activated oncogenes activates pro-growth metabolic circuits that can lock cancer cells into net macromolecular synthesis and resistance to cell death. Oncogenic signaling can induce cellular uptake of metabolic substrates, such as glucose and glutamine, as well as utilization of unconventional nutrient sources. In contrast to some nonproliferating tissues, which preferentially degrade metabolic substrates to carbon dioxide to maximize energy production, cancer cells prioritize the use of acquired metabolic substrates in anabolic processes, including fatty acid, cholesterol, nonessential amino acid, and nucleotide biosynthesis. The accumulation of these precursors supports the synthesis of the macromolecules necessary to sustain cell growth. Oncogene-directed increases in levels of select metabolites can also influence cellular processes beyond metabolic circuits, resulting in changes to the cellular epigenetic state as well as long-ranging effects on cells within the tumor microenvironment. As cancer progresses, the metabolic properties and liabilities of malignant cells evolve to support metastasis and therapy resistance. Recent studies suggest these alterations in tumor cell metabolism can be exploited to improve the diagnosis and treatment of a wide variety of cancers.

Malicious builders

A unifying characteristic of cancer is loss of extrinsic controls over cell proliferation. In normal tissues, the quantities of cells, as well as their relative positions, are maintained by extracellular signaling, which include tissue-specific soluble growth factors as well as signals from the extracellular matrix to which cells adhere. Together, these mechanisms control the timing and the extent of cell survival and proliferation. Basal level of signaling enables day-to-day tissue maintenance, while the upregulation of growth signaling in response to tissue perturbations leads to enhanced production of terminally differentiated cells—for instance, epidermal keratinocytes and dermal fibroblasts in a setting of a cutaneous injury, or T-cells in response to infection. In this manner, cell proliferation only takes place in response to a cell type-specific signal of a sufficient strength and duration, which ensures that the overall structural and biochemical integrity of a metazoan organism is maintained.

In a contrast to normal cells, genetic and epigenetic alterations acquired by cancer cells allow them to accumulate within tissues in a manner that is independent of extrinsic growth stimuli, at the same time becoming resistant to antigrowth signals.[1] Together, these adaptations enable survival and proliferation of cancer cells in settings where normal cell proliferation is strictly regimented. Mutations, copy number amplifications, and translocations targeting growth factor receptors are among the most frequently seen growth-promoting genetic alterations in tumors and are thus termed "driver alterations." For example, activating mutations in epidermal growth factor receptor (EGFR) are found in 10% of non-small-cell lung carcinoma in the US and up to 35% in Japan,[2] and amplifications of HER2 are found in 25–30% of breast carcinomas.[3] In addition to growth factor receptors, downstream integrators of growth factor and matrix attachment signals are often aberrantly activated in cancer as well: for instance, up to 70% of breast cancers have mutations in the PI-3 kinase pathway,[4] up to 90% of pancreatic tumors are driven by activating mutations in KRAS,[5] and amplification of c-Myc is seen in up to 50% of human cancers regardless of tissue of origin.[6]

A cell that had received a proper growth signal commits to creating two daughter cells. To accomplish this, it must synthesize a complete set of biomolecules sufficient to build a new, functional cell. This set of biomolecules is extremely diverse and includes not only a vast array of proteins but also lipids and their derivatives for building plasma and organelle membranes, hexose sugars for glycosylation of proteins, as well as pentose sugars, and nucleotide bases for genome replication. To ensure that a cell does not attempt to replicate itself without having ample supply of biomolecules, the same signals that control proliferation are in control of nutrient uptake and the biosynthesis of macromolecular precursors. Thus, a growth factor-stimulated cell undergoes remodeling of its metabolism in order to support the required biosynthesis. First, this remodeling involves acquiring a sufficient amount of building materials from the surrounding environment. Second, a proliferating cell must prioritize the use of these materials for biosynthesis, as opposed to catabolizing them for energy.

> **Box 1**
>
> Constitutive signaling via aberrantly activated oncogenes allows cancer cells to perpetually receive pro-growth stimuli, which for normal tissues are only transient in nature. As a consequence, cancer metabolism is constitutively geared towards supporting proliferation.

This article will describe the mechanisms of how oncogenic transformation reshapes cellular metabolism towards nutrient acquisition and biosynthesis. Furthermore, this article will demonstrate how the altered metabolic state of cancer cells, in turn, exerts profound effects on cellular epigenetic state and on tumor microenvironment, driving tumor expansion, and dissemination. To this end, we will explore how alterations in tumor metabolism can be exploited in cancer detection and therapy.

From yeast to mammals—same means to different ends

Metabolic pathways and enzymes that drive their progression are remarkably conserved throughout evolution, yet the way the metabolism of metazoan cells is regulated is fundamentally distinct from unicellular organisms. Unicellular organisms, such as bacteria or yeast, use external nutrient abundance as a signal to begin proliferating.[7] By attuning their proliferation to the environmental conditions, this strategy allows them to maximize their evolutionary success. For a metazoan organism, on the other hand, an evolutionary goal is not to multiply its cells to no end—which would lead to a loss of homeostatic control—but to maintain the functionality and structural integrity of its organs and tissues, repair injuries and fight infections. To serve this goal, metazoans had developed complex and tissue-specific control mechanisms which regulate cell survival and proliferation, yet allow for rapid induction of proliferation of specific cell populations when needed. Accordingly, the pro-proliferative metabolic state of cancer cells, driven by the loss of tissue-specific control mechanisms, can be best understood by first examining the differences in metabolic regulation in metazoans and in unicellular eukaryotes.

Metabolism of living cells is centered on the acquisition and stepwise biochemical transformation of molecules which consist of reduced carbon and nitrogen. Glucose is a major metabolic substrate that can be utilized by all living cells as a source of (1) bioenergetic equivalents in a form of high-energy phosphate bonds of adenosine triphosphate (ATP), and (2) carbon building blocks, which can be used to produce a variety of biomolecules. One key chemical constituent that a glucose molecule does not provide is nitrogen. Nitrogen is required for the biosynthesis of amino acids and nucleotide bases, thus, an access to a source of reduced nitrogen is critical for both unicellular eukaryotes and metazoans. While some bacteria can reduce atmospheric nitrogen to ammonia, most species must acquire a reduced form of nitrogen from the environment. Unicellular organisms can use free ammonia (NH_4^+) as a source of reduced nitrogen. For example, a wild-type, or prototrophic, yeast culture can proliferate in a so-called "synthetic complete" medium, which consists purely of glucose as a sole carbon source and ammonia as a sole nitrogen source. A yeast cell has all metabolic enzymes to synthesize a complete spectrum of biomolecules from the materials provided.

Metazoan organisms rely on glucose as a preferred carbon source and amino acids as the primary source of reduced nitrogen. In contrast to unicellular organisms, metazoans lost the ability to synthesize 9 out of 20 amino acids required for protein synthesis (these 9 amino acids are termed "essential," while the rest are termed "nonessential"). The amino acid glutamine, a carrier of two nitrogen atoms, is the predominant "nitrogen currency" for metazoan organisms. Because of its special importance as a reduced nitrogen source, glutamine is a "conditionally essential" amino acid for most proliferating metazoan cells.[8]

The significance of glucose and glutamine as key metabolic substrates for metazoan cells can be illustrated by the fact that in a mammalian organism, nearly constant levels of these two nutrients are maintained in plasma at all times: glucose levels are within the range of 4–6 mM and glutamine, the most abundant amino acid in plasma, ranges within 0.6–0.9 mM.[9] These steady levels of glucose and glutamine are maintained by a combination of hormone-mediated utilization of glycogen stores in muscle and liver, *de novo* synthesis of glutamine and glucose, as well as the stimulation of feeding behavior.

Unicellular organisms do not have steady levels of carbon and nitrogen sources around them at all times. Instead, they rely on nutrient-sensing mechanisms to assess the availability of nutrients in their environment. In yeast, for instance, glucose limitation leads to Snf1 kinase [a homolog of AMP-activated protein kinase (AMPK) in mammalian cells] activation, which promotes energy production and suppresses biosynthetic processes.[10] Addition of glucose to a yeast culture triggers a shift towards biosynthetic metabolism and proliferation.[11,12] When glucose is abundant, Ras1 and Ras2 GTPases, homologues of the mammalian RAS protein family, become active and promote cell cycle progression. Another signaling mediator downstream of glucose is Sch9 kinase, which is related to Akt and S6 kinases in mammals and plays a role in promoting the use of glucose for biosynthetic processes.[13] Concurrently, the amino acid status of a yeast cell is measured through Gcn2 serine/threonine kinase, which is homologous to mammalian GCN2. Gcn2 is activated by uncharged tRNA, which accumulates in cells when amino acid levels are insufficient. Activated Gcn2, in turn, inhibits protein translation rates and induces Gcn4 (ATF4 in mammals), a transcription factor which controls expression of a number of enzymes involved in *de novo* synthesis of amino acids.[14] In the absence of glucose, however, active Snf1 represses Gcn4 expression, thus coordinating the metabolism of nitrogen and carbon.[15] As intracellular amino acid levels rise, they, in turn, activate TOR1/2 (mTOR in mammalian cells), which acts as a coordinator of a number of anabolic processes, including protein translation and biosynthesis of fatty acids. If nutrient sources remain plentiful, cell growth is converted into cell division and the process is repeated until the extracellular nutrient supply falls below the necessary threshold.

Cells within a metazoan organism are surrounded by ample glucose and glutamine in plasma and interstitial fluid, yet in contrast to yeast, they do not proliferate unless a proper extrinsic growth signal is present. First of all, the very access of cells to the extracellular pools of glucose and glutamine is controlled by receptor tyrosine kinases, proteins which are absent in unicellular eukaryotes. We now appreciate that stimulation by a cytokine or a growth factor, for example, directs a cell to take up nutrients, providing it with a supply chain of metabolic substrates. To this end, signals from receptor tyrosine kinases converge on PI-3 kinase/Akt, activation of which triggers rapid translocation of glucose transporters (GLUTs) from the cytosol-localized endosomal vesicles to the plasma membrane,[16,17] as well as stimulates GLUT gene expression,[18] driving the entry of glucose into cells. In illustration of this paradigm, PI-3 kinase/Akt signaling facilitates glucose uptake by populations of cells that are induced to undergo proliferative expansion, for example activated T-cells mounting an immune response,[19] or those induced to synthesize massive amounts of macromolecules, such as milk-producing cells of the mammary gland during lactation.[20]

In addition to effects on glucose transport, growth factor-stimulated mammalian cells rapidly induce transcription of a set of immediate-early genes, one of which is the transcription factor c-Myc. C-Myc drives expression of a large set of metabolic genes and plays a role as a gatekeeper of cellular access to glutamine—the major metazoan source of nitrogen.[21] To this end, c-Myc facilitates the expression of glutamine transporters, ASCT2 and SN2,[22] as well as a glutaminase enzyme, GLS1, which catalyzes the breakdown of glutamine to glutamate and free ammonia.[23] Through facilitation of glutamine acquisition, c-Myc also indirectly influences the uptake of essential amino acids by the cell. Essential amino acid transport into cells is coupled to the efflux of glutamine into the extracellular space.[24] This mechanism allows cells to coordinate the import of essential amino acids to intracellular glutamine status.

Besides signals from receptor tyrosine kinases, cellular anchorage to the extracellular matrix is also needed to facilitate glucose uptake. Glucose consumption is suppressed in cells that are deprived of the matrix attachment even in the presence of soluble growth factors.[25] Shifting the mechanical properties of the extracellular matrix fine-tunes the rates of glucose utilization in epithelial cells.[26] These controls ensure that not only proliferation but also positions of cells within the tissue are controlled on a metabolic level.

Taken together, pro-growth signaling through receptor tyrosine kinases has emerged as a control point for nutrient acquisition. While conserved from yeast to mammals, mammalian RAS is no longer governed by glucose abundance, but by tissue-specific receptors. Similarly, mammalian TOR, while retaining its sensitivity to amino acid levels, had been harnessed by growth signaling control via Akt-dependent phosphorylation and inactivation of TSC2, a negative regulator of mTOR. Next, we will next examine how genetic alterations in growth signaling pathways influence the nutrient uptake in cancer cells.

> **Box 2**
>
> Nutrient abundance is sufficient to stimulate proliferation of unicellular organisms, but not of metazoan cells, which has relegated the control over the ability to access nutrients around them to extrinsic growth stimuli.

Bad table manners of cancer cells

Discovery of the fundamental differences in rates of nutrient uptake between tumors and nontransformed tissues was among the earliest in modern cancer research, predating the discovery of the oncogenes and the role of carcinogens in tumorigenesis. In the 1920s, biochemical characterization of cancer cells from peritoneal ascites and slices of normal, nonproliferating tissues by German physiologist Warburg[27] revealed that the rate of consumption of glucose by tumors far exceeds that of normal tissues. Some thirty years later, American pathologist Harry Eagle has shown that glutamine requirements of HeLa cells in culture exceed the needs for other amino acids by 10- to a 100-fold, far surpassing the quantity needed for protein synthesis.[28]

On a signaling level, cellular glucose uptake is controlled through PI-3 kinase/Akt, which targets GLUTs to plasma membrane, as well as promotes their expression on a transcriptional level.[17] Thus, cancer-specific alterations in PI-3 kinase/Akt signaling allow cancer cells to consume glucose constitutively. Activated RAS and c-Src can promote GLUT1 expression as well.[29] To match the supply of carbon with a supply of nitrogen, tumor cells concurrently increase their uptake of glutamine. As described above, the key driver of glutamine uptake and utilization in mammalian cells is c-Myc.[22,30] With c-Myc levels aberrantly elevated, cancer cells continuously import and utilize available glutamine for bioenergetic support, nucleotide biosynthesis, and to coordinate essential amino acid uptake and nonessential amino acid biosynthesis in support of protein production.

Tumors originate within the confines of a normal tissue, which is not suited to sustain uncontrolled cellular proliferation. Thus, tumors often lack adequate vasculature, as *de novo* angiogenesis within tissues is negatively regulated by tissue-specific factors.[31] Capillaries that do form in response to tumor-secreted pro-angiogenic molecules tend to be underdeveloped and inefficient in delivering oxygen and nutrients to a growing tumor.

As proliferation of cancer cells depletes the microenvironment around them of amino acids and glucose, growing tumors face increasingly unfavorable conditions for proliferation. One adaptation that cancer cells use to withstand nutrient limitations is *autophagy*—a regulated process of self-catabolism of proteins, lipids, and even whole organelles as a temporary means of sustaining viability during starvation.[32] A major cellular bioenergetic sensor, AMPK, initiates the process of autophagy in response to falling ATP/AMP levels, whereas mTOR, on the other hand, acts as an autophagy inhibitor.[33] The significance of autophagy for tumor growth *in vivo* has been demonstrated in mutant Kras^{G12D} and Braf^{V600E}-driven lung tumors, in which the genetic knockout of the autophagy machinery component Atg7 dramatically limits tumor cell accumulation and aggressiveness.[34,35]

While autophagy can serve as a temporary means to survive nutrient shortages and maintain cellular bioenergetics, it cannot be used as a source of new biomass. In addition to intracellular proteins, KRAS- and c-Src-transformed cells have been recently shown to recover amino acids from proteins dissolved in extracellular fluid, which are consumed via large (up to 1–2 µm in diameter) vesicles at sites of plasma membrane ruffling.[36] These vesicles are called macropinosomes (from latin *pino*—"to drink"). Under conditions of nutrient depletion, macropinosomes are targeted to lysosomes, where engulfed cargo is degraded. This alternative, "scavenging" form of nutrient uptake allows cells to survive amino acid limitations by unlocking otherwise inaccessible amino acid stores. RAS-driven macropinocytosis is an evolutionarily ancient mechanism of acquiring nutrients. In fact, it can be a primary pathway of nutrient acquisition in slime molds, such as *Dictyostelium*.[37] Thus, reactivation of macropinocytosis in oncogene-transformed cells can be viewed as yet another example of how cancer cells utilize evolutionarily ancient mechanisms of nutrient uptake.

Another problem that stems from the inadequacies of tumor vasculature is reduced supply of oxygen, or hypoxia. Lack of sufficient oxygen has a profound effect on cellular metabolism as it inhibits those biochemical reactions in which oxygen is consumed. One reaction that becomes inhibited in hypoxic conditions is stearoyl-CoA desaturase 1 (SCD1)-catalyzed desaturation of fatty acid carbon bonds to create unsaturated fatty acids, which are essential for proper fluidity of plasma and organelle membranes. To circumvent this problem, Ras-transformed cells were shown to be able to bypass the need for SCD1-catalyzed desaturation reaction by scavenging unsaturated lipids from the extracellular environment.[38]

> **Box 3**
>
> Oncogene signaling allows cancer cells to use conventional metabolic sources, glucose, and glutamine, in an unrestricted manner, as well as enables cells to access unconventional sources of biomolecules.

The traveling electrons

Most biochemical reactions within living cells are energetically unfavorable, and require catalysis by specific metabolic enzymes. Metabolic reactions can be divided into two types: (1) *catabolic*—in which complex biochemical substrates are degraded to simpler constituents, and (2) *anabolic*—in which complex biomolecules, such as amino acids, fatty acids, and nucleotides are produced from simpler constituents. Catabolic processes involve reactions in which substrates undergo oxidation. Electrons derived from these oxidative steps are captured in a form of hydride anions (:H⁻), which are carried by specialized enzyme cofactors NAD⁺ and FAD (NADH and FADH2 in their reduced forms), or NADP⁺ (NADPH in its reduced form). The chemical energy of electrons from NADH and FADH2 is then utilized by a series of enzyme complexes of *the electron transport chain*, which is located at the inner membrane of mitochondria. NADH/FADH2-derived electrons travel down the electron transport chain until they react with oxygen to produce water. The chemical energy of electrons that are being passed along the electron transport chain is used to create a proton gradient between the mitochondrial matrix and the mitochondrial intermembrane space. The resulting build-up of electrochemical potential across the inner mitochondrial membrane, in turn, fuels the activity of ATP synthase, a supramolecular complex which regenerates high-energy phosphate bonds of ATP from ADP. The coupling of electron transport to ADP conversion to ATP is termed *oxidative phosphorylation*.

In living cells, the ratio of ATP to ADP provides the thermodynamic driving force for a myriad of energetically unfavorable cellular processes, as well as for protein and lipid phosphorylation by kinases—a versatile mode of regulating functions of a variety of proteins and transmitting signals within a cell.

The maintenance of an electrochemical proton gradient through the electron transport chain is dependent on the availability of oxygen—the terminal acceptor of electrons, and ADP—a substrate for the ATP synthase. An excessive influx of electrons from NADH/FADH2 can deplete the supply of either of these, stopping oxidative phosphorylation. Consequently, electrons that become stalled in the electron transport chain can be lost over time from their intramembrane carriers, reacting with the aqueous environment of the cell to produce reactive oxygen species (ROS). ROS are avid oxidants, which readily react with a wide spectrum of biomolecules—including lipids, proteins, and nucleotides. To control their redox state, cells produce a variety of ROS-neutralizing molecules, or antioxidants. However, when ROS become elevated beyond the cellular antioxidant capacity, they can cause widespread damage to cellular organelles and DNA.

As noted above, most catabolic reactions couple the oxidation of their substrates to the reduction of NAD⁺ and FAD to NADH and FADH2. In contrast, a few metabolic reactions result in a transfer of electrons to a structurally related cofactor, NADP⁺, reducing it to NADPH. While NADH and FADH2 are mainly used for energy production, it is NADPH that replenishes the cellular antioxidant pool by sustaining the reduced state of glutathione and related sulfhydryl-containing molecules. In addition, the reducing power of NADPH is used in biosynthesis of complex biomolecules, such as fatty acids and nucleotides, which require sequences of reductive reactions. How does a cell choose to prioritize one class of such reactions over others? As it turns out, the allocation of substrates into processes that support bioenergetics versus those with biosynthetic outcomes is coordinated by many of the same pro-growth signals that promote the uptake of biochemical substrates by cells in the first place.

> **Box 4**
>
> A living cell maintains its viability by oxidizing biochemical substrates acquired from the environment. Catabolic reactions produce simple building blocks which can be consecutively utilized in biosynthetic reactions. In addition, catabolic reactions serve as sources of reducing power to fuel cellular energy production, enable biosynthetic reactions, and bolster the antioxidant defense.

Warburg effect: how to play safe while looking sloppy

Glucose catabolism takes place in two cellular compartments: its first stage, glycolysis, occurs in the cytosol, while the second stage is localized to mitochondria and involves a series of reactions of the tricarboxylic acid cycle (TCA cycle, which is also called citric acid or Krebs cycle). Phosphorylation of glucose by a hexokinase (HK) to produce glucose-6-phosphate is the first committed step of glycolysis (Figure 1a). The HK reaction prevents the exit of glucose back into the extracellular space. A second committed step of glycolysis is an irreversible phosphorylation catalyzed by phosphofructokinase enzyme (PFK1). Along with targeting the GLUT1 transporter to the plasma membrane, Akt potentiates the action of both HK[39] and PFK1,[40] thus acting as a coordinator of glucose progression through glycolysis. In fact, the ability of Akt to suppress apoptosis in response to growth factor withdrawal is dependent on glucose;[41] moreover, overexpression of GLUT1 and HK alone is sufficient to suppress growth factor withdrawal-induced cell death.[40] PFK1 activity in cancer cells is further enhanced by frequent overexpression of PFKFB3,[42] an enzyme which produces fructose-2,6-bisphosphate, an allosteric activator of PFK1.

Downstream of glucose capture and degradation, the various intermediates of glycolysis, and the TCA cycle provide the backbones of essentially all the amino acids, acyl groups, and nucleotides a cell can synthesize *de novo* to support macromolecular synthesis. When it was discovered that oncogenic mutations resulted in flooding the cell with glucose that can maintain a supply of these precursors, it became clear why the Warburg effect was selected for during tumorigenesis. A cell engaged in excessive glucose uptake becomes resistant to apoptosis, has virtually unlimited supply of macromolecular precursors, and simply secretes any carbon in excess of its needs by converting the end product of glycolysis, pyruvate, into lactate, which is expelled from the cell. This form of gluttony exhibited by tumors harboring mutations which increase glucose uptake became known as *aerobic glycolysis*—to distinguish it from the well-established increase in glucose uptake exhibited by normal cells when depleted of oxygen, or *anaerobic glycolysis*.

Recently, it has been shown that aerobic glycolysis is not restricted to tumor cells. When stimulated with growth factors, normal cells too, begin to display Warburg-like metabolism.[43] The discovery that the Warburg effect is a growth factor-driven phenomenon and not a peculiar "abnormality" of cancer cells warranted exploring whether it may be in fact, a part of a metabolic reprogramming aimed at increasing the cellular capacity for biosynthesis. Thus, it is now becoming appreciated that maximization of the bioenergetic yield from glucose catabolism to CO_2 would run contrary to the biosynthetic priorities of a growth factor-stimulated cell.[44]

How can glycolysis help biosynthesis? There are several ways through which glycolytic intermediates can act as substrates for producing both biosynthetic precursors and NADPH (Figure 1a). One such pathway is the *pentose phosphate pathway (PPP)*, which begins with glucose-6-phosphate. Glucose-6-phosphate is oxidized to produce two NADPH molecules and after a series of interconversions, produces ribose-5-phosphate—a structural component of nucleotides. Significantly, the PPP enzyme transketolase-like 1 (TKTL1) is required for growth of a number of cancer cell lines and is predictive of poor prognosis in patients.[45]

Another key branch point of glycolysis is at the level of 3-phosphoglycerate. In a series of three consecutive reactions, 3-phosphoglycerate is converted to the amino acid serine. As metabolic studies demonstrate, serine biosynthesis is massively

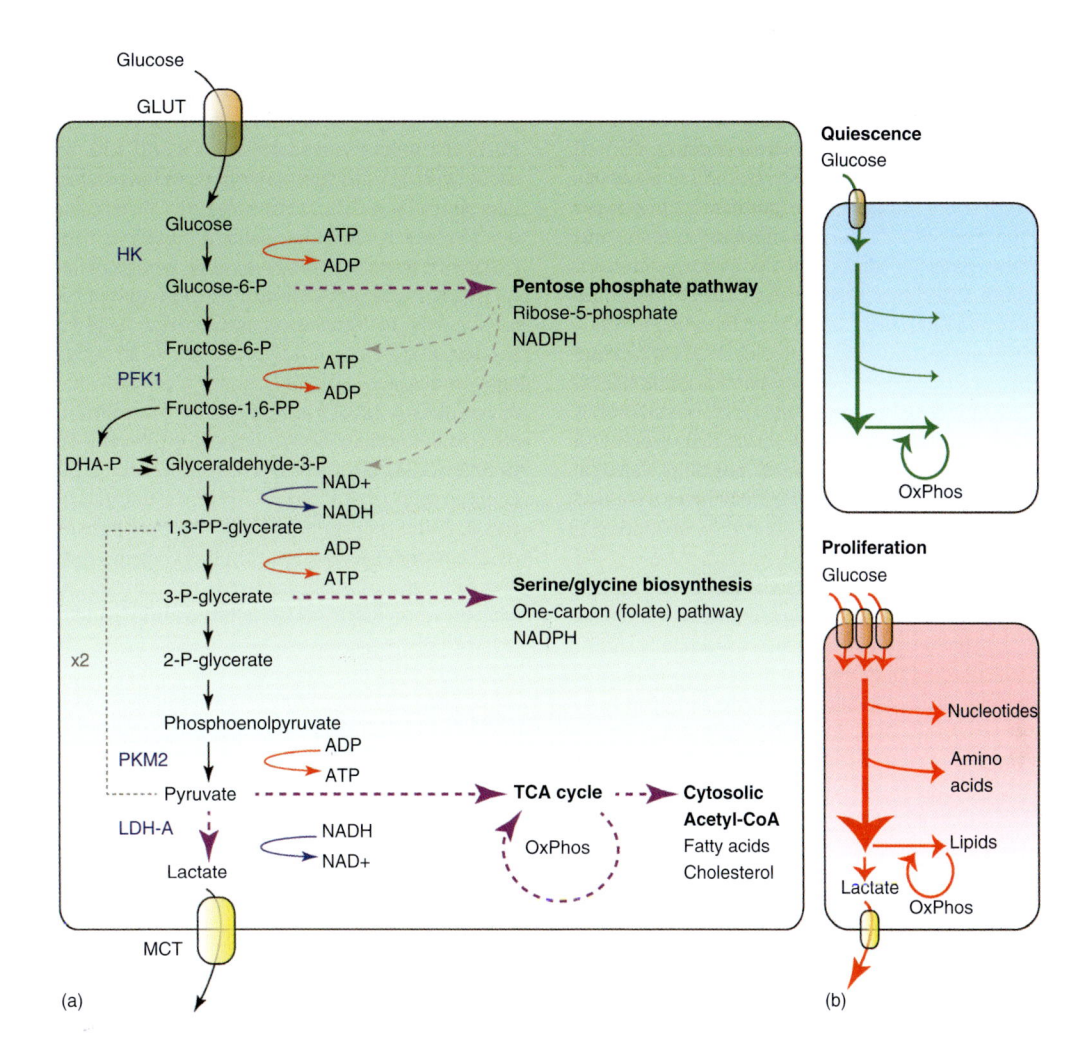

Figure 1 Glycolysis. (**a**) catabolism of one glucose molecule via glycolysis yields two molecules of pyruvate, which can then be transported to the mitochondria and used as a source of acetyl-CoA for the TCA cycle. Alternatively, pyruvate can be reduced to lactate and excreted out of the cell. Besides its bioenergetic uses, glycolysis also provides biosynthetic power to cells. Glucose-6-phosphate can be utilized in the pentose phosphate pathway to generate NADPH and ribose-5-phosphate for nucleotide biosynthesis; or, its intermediates can be shunted back into glycolysis (shown by grey dashed arrows). In addition, 3-phosphoglycerate can be converted to serine, a carbon donor for the folate (one-carbon) cycle. Folate cycle generates NADPH, as well as provides one-carbon units for the biosynthesis of nucleotide bases and for methylation reactions. *Abbreviations*: GLUT, glucose transporter; HK, hexokinase; PFK1, phosphofructokinase 1; PKM2, pyruvate kinase M2; LDH-A, lactate dehydrogenase A; MCT, monocarboxylate transporter; OxPhos, oxidative phosphorylation. (**b**) Quiescent cells consume moderate amount of glucose and preferentially catabolize it to pyruvate to fuel oxidative phosphorylation in mitochondria. In proliferating cells, growth factor signaling or constitutively active oncogenes facilitate the increase in glucose uptake. In contrast to a quiescent cell, the majority of glucose consumed by a growth-stimulated cell goes into biosynthetic pathways to produce nucleotides, amino acids, and lipids—or is expelled as lactate.

upregulated in tumors beyond the amount necessary for protein biosynthesis.[46] Moreover, the PHGDH gene, encoding the enzyme which catalyzes the limiting step in serine biosynthesis, is frequently amplified in breast cancer and in melanoma, predicts tumor aggressiveness, and is required for tumor growth *in vivo*.[47,48] Why do tumors produce so much serine? Serine is not only used as a building block in protein translation, but is also a key substrate in a so-called *one-carbon*, or *folate cycle*, where a serine-donated carbon is passed on to a tetrahydrofolate molecule. The folate cycle involves a complex series of oxidative-reductive transformations, which involve serine-donated methyl groups, and is indispensable for a number of processes that affect cellular growth and proliferation.[49] In particular, serine-derived carbon is used (1) as a carbon donor for purine synthesis; (2) a donor of methyl groups onto S-adenosylmethionine (SAM), a substrate for histone and DNA methyltransferase enzymes, and (3) as a donor of reducing power for the production of NADPH. As a recent study had demonstrated, up to 50% of all cellular NADPH may be generated via one-carbon pathway.[50] Taken together, diversion of glycolytic intermediates into pentose phosphate shunt and into serine biosynthesis pathway both provide building blocks for nucleotide generation as well as produce NADPH.

How does a cell regulate the rate at which glycolytic intermediates are diverted into biosynthetic pathways? Exploration of the interplay between growth factor signaling pathways and metabolism have led to a seminal discovery that has shed light on this question. Specifically, tumor cells express an M2 splice variant of pyruvate kinase M (called PKM2), while their normal counterparts preferentially express the M1 variant.[51] Pyruvate kinase is a rate-limiting enzyme that catalyzes the conversion of phosphoenolpyruvate (PEP) to pyruvate (Figure 1a). Intriguingly, the PKM2 isoform is a less active form of pyruvate kinase than PKM1. Moreover, PKM2, but not PKM1, is susceptible to further inhibition via binding to phosphorylated tyrosine residues through its unique C-terminal sequence.[52] Thus, the activity of PKM2 becomes dampened even further in response to increased tyrosine kinase signaling. Replacement of PKM2 with a PKM1 isoform reduces the tumorigenic potential of cancer cells, promotes oxygen consumption, and inhibits production of lactate.[51] The lower rate of catalysis by PKM2 creates a "traffic jam" at the level of PEP, facilitating the entry of accumulated glycolytic intermediates into the two pathways described above.[53] Reciprocally, products downstream of both PPP (succinylaminoimidazolecarboxamide ribose-5′-phosphate, or SAICAR)[54] and serine biosynthetic pathway (serine itself)[55] act as allosteric activators of PKM2, which allows a cell to balance the biosynthetic and bioenergetic uses of glycolysis. Besides its function as a gatekeeper of glycolysis, PKM2 also promotes glucose utilization at the level of gene expression. Thus, in EGF-treated cells, PKM2 becomes phosphorylated by Erk1/2 and is translocated to the nucleus, where it directly controls expression of GLUT1 and LDH-A genes, further contributing to the Warburg effect.[56]

It is important to recognize that the appearance of a Warburg effect does not require suppression of glucose oxidation from basal levels, but rather a disproportionate increase in lactate secretion relative to oxygen consumption.[57] Increased access to glucose in cells stimulated by growth factors allows glucose carbon to generate biosynthetic precursors both from glycolysis and from the TCA cycle. Nevertheless, several constraints exist to prevent excessive rates of glucose oxidation in this context, because overproduction of NADH/FADH2 in the TCA cycle would quickly deplete available ADP, overload the electron transport chain, and overproduce ROS.[58] To prevent this from happening, both NADH and ATP act as allosteric inhibitors of the mitochondrial gatekeeper enzyme PDH, attenuating the production of acetyl-CoA from pyruvate and ensuring that the electron transport chain does not produce more ATP than a cell can use at the moment.

Besides being allosterically controlled by ATP and NADH, PDH is also negatively regulated via phosphorylation by pyruvate dehydrogenase kinase 1 (PDK1). Expression of PDK1 is induced when cellular production of electron donors for the electron transport chain exceeds the amount that can be assimilated by the available oxygen. Specifically, PDK1 transcription is upregulated by HIF1α, a transcription factor induced under these conditions.[59,60] Concurrently, HIF1α activates transcription of LDH-A, re-routing the flux of carbon away from the TCA cycle and towards lactate production.[61] Even though HIF1α is classically activated by oxygen deficit, transformed cells exhibiting excess glycolysis induce HIF1α even in normoxic conditions.[62] Nor is HIF1α the only transcriptional activator of PDK1. Indeed, another commonly activated pathway in cancer, Wnt/β-catenin pathway, has been shown to promote the Warburg effect by upregulating the expression of PDK1, as well as the lactate transporter MCT1.[63]

A damaging effect of an unrestricted pyruvate catabolism has been recently proposed as a metabolic mechanism of oncogene-induced senescence (OIS). OIS is a phenomenon in which overexpression of mutant oncogenes, such as RAS or BRAF, triggers growth arrest, overproduction of ROS, and DNA damage response.[64] Interestingly, the onset of OIS is dependent on PDH activity. To this end, the modulation of the PDH activity by expressing PDK1 or inhibiting PDH phosphatase PDP2 was found to facilitate cellular escape from OIS.[65]

A decade ago, it was discovered that the role of mitochondria in the successful evolution of the eukaryotic cells depended more on their contributions to macromolecular biosynthesis than to ATP production. In an evolutionary sense, mitochondria became essential organelles because they supplied a variety of precursors for biosynthetic reactions. In what is referred to as *cataplerosis*, TCA cycle intermediates exit the mitochondria to be used as precursors for a variety of anabolic reactions—including biosynthesis of sugars, nonessential amino acids, and fatty acids. In addition, mitochondria support the synthesis of iron–sulfur (Fe–S) clusters, which are central for the function of a variety of mitochondrial as well as cytosolic enzymes.

Cytosol-localized biosynthesis of fatty acids and cholesterol is particularly essential for proliferating cells. A universal precursor for fatty acid and cholesterol biosynthesis is acetyl-CoA, but because the bulky Coenzyme A cannot cross the mitochondrial membrane, a cell cannot directly access the mitochondrial pool of acetyl-CoA for use in biosynthetic reactions. Instead, the TCA intermediate citrate is shuttled out of the mitochondria and into the cytosol, where it is cleaved by ATP citrate lyase (ACL), regenerating acetyl-CoA (Figure 2). ACL is essential for tumorigenesis, and its inhibition suppresses tumor growth in mice.[69,70] Notably, ACL enzyme becomes activated following Akt induction,[71] so that Akt not only enables glucose uptake and catabolism but also diverts carbon flux away from mitochondria and towards fatty acid biosynthesis.

> **Box 5**
>
> Pro-growth signals facilitate the uptake of glucose and remodel the glycolytic flux to satisfy the increased biosynthetic demands of a growing cell (Figure 1b).

The cavalry arrives!—glutamine and anabolic metabolism

As described earlier, besides glucose, many cancer cells (as well as normal cells that have received a signal to proliferate) avidly consume glutamine. Glutamine uptake and its hydrolysis to glutamate, termed *glutaminolysis*, are coordinated by the transcription factor c-Myc; in fact, amplification of c-Myc was shown to make cells critically dependent on glutamine supply. Why is glutamine so essential for dividing cells? First, the carbon skeleton of glutamine is used to restock the TCA cycle when its intermediates exit the mitochondria to participate in anabolic synthesis. Because proliferating cells continuously borrow TCA cycle intermediates, such as citrate, to support biosynthesis, cataplerotic processes must be balanced by the influx of carbons elsewhere in the cycle in a process termed *anaplerosis*. Two major anaplerotic inputs have been described: one is via glutamine-derived α-ketoglutarate and another is via pyruvate carboxylase (PC)-catalyzed carboxylation of pyruvate into oxaloacetate (Figure 2). Though glutamine is a preferential anaplerotic substrate in cancer cells, cells with high PC activity can use a PC-derived oxaloacetate to survive glutamine deprivation or glutaminase suppression.[72] In addition, besides replenishing the TCA cycle, glutamine-derived α-ketoglutarate can exit the TCA cycle halfway in the form of malate and become oxidized by malic enzyme (ME) in the cytosol to produce NADPH.[73] Together, malic enzyme, pentose phosphate pathway, and folate cycle produce virtually all of the cellular NADPH.

As discussed earlier, the entry of glycolysis-derived pyruvate into the TCA cycle may be restricted by negative regulatory inputs into PDH—for example, as a result of upregulated HIF1α or activation of Wnt signaling. This, however, creates a quandary—if pyruvate is diverted away from the TCA cycle by the coordinate inhibition of pyruvate dehydrogenase and activation of LDH-A and MCT, how

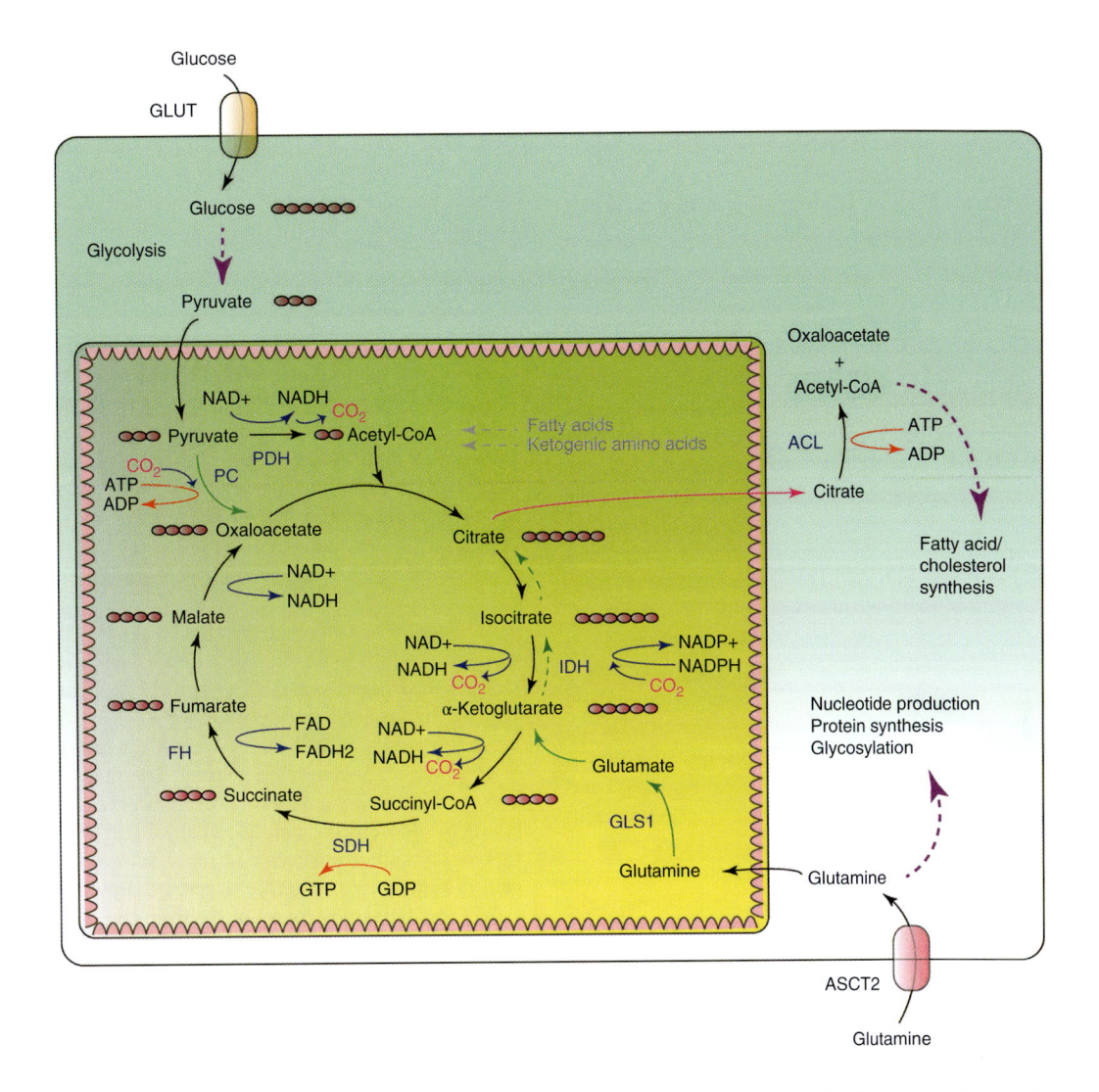

Figure 2 Carbon metabolism in mitochondria. Glycolysis-derived pyruvate serves as a donor of acetyl-CoA for the tricarboxylic acid (TCA) cycle. Cataplerotic efflux of citrate into the cytosol (shown by a maroon arrow) allows maintaining the extramitochondrial pool of acetyl-CoA for fatty acid and cholesterol biosynthesis. Glutamine and pyruvate function as anaplerotic substrates to restock the TCA cycle intermediates (shown by solid green arrows). In conditions when acetyl-CoA is limiting, citrate can be produced from the reductive carboxylation of glutamine-derived α-ketoglutarate (shown by dashed green arrows). Pink circles represent a number of carbon atoms in a molecule. *Abbreviations*: GLUT, glucose transporter; PDH, pyruvate dehydrogenase; PC, pyruvate carboxylase; IDH, isocitrate dehydrogenase; SDH, succinate dehydrogenase; FH, fumarate hydratase; ACL, ATP-citrate lyase; GLS1, glutaminase; ASCT2, glutamine transporter. Source: Based on Wise et al.;[66] Metallo et al.;[67] Mullen et al.[68]

can the TCA cycle produce enough citrate for biosynthesis? In fact, some cancer cells have found an unexpected solution to this problem by using glutamine-derived α-ketoglutarate to run a section of the TCA cycle in reverse, producing citrate for fatty acid biosynthesis in conditions where pyruvate-derived acetyl-CoA levels are limiting (Figure 2).[66–68]

Besides contributing its carbon skeleton to the TCA cycle, glutamine is a major donor of reduced nitrogen for cellular needs. While its amine nitrogen is used primarily in nonessential amino acid biosynthesis, amide nitrogen of glutamine contributes to the biosynthesis of purine and pyrimidine bases. Glutamine provides nitrogen for the synthesis of all four nucleotide bases: one molecule of glutamine is needed to build a thymine, adenine and cytosine use two, and guanine synthesis requires three glutamine molecules. Notably, together with promoting glutamine uptake for synthesis of nucleotide bases, c-Myc also controls the expression of a number of nucleotide biosynthetic enzymes—namely, thymidylate synthase (TS), inosine monophosphate dehydrogenase 2 (IMPDH2) and phosphoribosyl pyrophosphate synthetase 2 (PRPS2), a rate-limiting enzyme in the biosynthesis of nucleotides.[74,75]

In conclusion, the notion that pro-growth signaling is a central facilitator of the acquisition and use of extracellular nutrients by metazoan cells has overturned a long-held view that cellular metabolic networks are self-regulating and exist independently from signaling inputs. However, metabolic circuits themselves are not merely passive recipients of cellular signals. In fact, a cell continuously monitors rising and falling levels of select metabolites and integrates this information so as to coordinate global decisions including growth and differentiation.

Box 6

Glutamine fuels anabolic metabolism by serving as both a source of carbon to replenish the TCA cycle intermediates and maintain its biosynthetic capacity, as well as providing reduced nitrogen for the biosynthesis of nucleotides and nonessential amino acids.

The nucleus smells what's cooking

Metabolites are known to act as allosteric modulators of specific metabolic enzymes, providing regulatory feedback which allows a cell to adjust the output of its catabolic and anabolic reactions in response to fluctuations in metabolite levels. An example of such regulation is allosteric activation of glycolysis gatekeeper enzyme PKM2 by SAICAR and serine, products of two biosynthetic branches of glycolysis.

Notably, the signaling capacity of some metabolites extends far beyond the regulation of metabolic circuits. Thus, metabolites can act as cofactors or as substrates in a variety of nonmetabolic enzymatic reactions, and through changes in their abundance, convey a regulatory message to these processes.[76] Deposition and removal of epigenetic marks in particular are regulated by levels of select metabolites, allowing a cell to coordinately alter its gene expression programs in response to changes in its nutritional status.[77]

Eukaryotic cell chromatin is composed of genomic DNA wrapped around histone octamers. To serve as a template for transcription, select loci within genomic DNA must be temporarily unwound and become accessible to the assembly of transcriptional complexes. The accessibility of genomic loci for transcription is regulated through deposition and removal of epigenetic marks on (1) DNA itself, by covalently attaching methyl groups to carbon 5 of cytosine bases, and (2) select amino acid residues of histones, to which a variety of chemical groups can be added. Acetyl and methyl residues are among the most versatile epigenetic marks that can be deposited on histones. Acetylation marks are predominantly associated with enhanced gene transcription and have a rapid turnover rate (in the order of minutes). Methylation marks have slower turnover rate and can be either activating or repressive, depending on the residue on which the mark is deposited. Combinations of epigenetic marks influence the general accessibility of DNA loci for transcription as well as guide the recruitment and assembly of transcription complexes, thus exerting profound effects on gene expression. Both acetyl and methyl epigenetic marks originate directly from products of metabolic reactions, acetyl-CoA and SAM, respectively. Thus, histone acetyltransferase enzymes deposit acetyl groups of acetyl-CoA onto lysine and arginine residues of histones, while SAM, a product of one-carbon (folate) cycle, provides methyl groups for both histone and DNA methyltransferases.

Using metabolic intermediates as precursors for epigenetic marks allows a cell to respond to its "fed" status with targeted upregulation of metabolic genes. As an example, targeted depletion of extramitochondrial acetyl-CoA through genetic repression of ACL profoundly affects histone acetylation patterns, resulting in attenuated expression of GLUTs, HK, PFK1, and LDH-A.[78] In this manner, by affecting histone acetylation, high levels of acetyl-CoA can promote the utilization of glucose and reinforce the Warburg effect.

Not only the deposition but the removal of acetyl and methyl marks from histones is guided by the cellular metabolic status as well. Thus, sirtuin deacetylases, which catalyze the removal of acetyl groups from histones, as well as a variety of nonhistone proteins, use an oxidized form of NAD^+ as a cofactor;[79] similarly, oxidized FAD serves as a cofactor for a histone demethylase LSD1.[80] By sensing a shift in NAD^+/NADH ratio, sirtuins coordinate multiple genetic and posttranslational changes aimed at maximizing energy conservation and extraction from metabolic substrates.

A whole host of enzymes—some of which are epigenetic regulators, while others are involved in posttranslational modifications of nonhistone proteins—are regulated by the abundance of TCA cycle metabolites: α-ketoglutarate, succinate, and fumarate. Specifically, α-ketoglutarate acts as a cofactor for Jumonji C domain-containing family of histone demethylases, a TET family of methylcytosine hydroxylases, as well as prolyl hydroxylases (PHDs), a class of enzymes which regulate HIF1α levels, among other processes. In the course of reactions catalyzed by these enzymes, α-ketoglutarate itself is converted to succinate. Importantly, both succinate and its downstream product fumarate act as inhibitors of α-ketoglutarate-dependent enzymes.[81] In such a manner, changes in α-ketoglutarate abundance in relation to levels of succinate and fumarate may exert a broad influence on a variety of cellular processes. In fact, select tumor types take advantage of the signaling potential of TCA cycle metabolites by acquiring mutations in metabolic enzymes. These mutations, in turn, lead to unnatural elevations in levels of signaling-competent metabolites, which, in an analogy with oncogenes, are referred to as *oncometabolites*.[82]

To date, three groups of metabolic enzymes have been found to be recurrently mutated in cancer. TCA cycle enzymes succinate dehydrogenase (SDH) and fumarate hydratase (FH) are targeted by loss-of-function mutations, leading to the accumulation of succinate and fumarate, respectively. Biallelic loss of SDH underlies the development of hereditary paragangliomas and pheochromocytomas,[83] and loss of fumarate hydratase is responsible for the rare familial cancer syndrome HLRCC (hereditary leiomyomatosis and renal cell cancer).[84] Conversely, gain-of-function mutations in isocitrate dehydrogenase 1 and 2 (IDH1 and IDH2) are found in the majority of low-grade glioma cases, as well as in acute myelogenous leukemia (AML), chondrosarcoma, and cholangiosarcoma.[85–88] Oncogenic mutations in IDH1 and IDH2 convey an unusual neomorphic function to the enzyme. Whereas the wild-type isocitrate dehydrogenase catalyzes a conversion of isocitrate to α-ketoglutarate, the mutant form reduces α-ketoglutarate to a D-enantiomer of 2-hydroxyglutarate.[89,90] While D-2-hydroxyglutarate levels in cells are normally very low, IDH-mutant cells accumulate this metabolite to millimolar amounts, and owing to its structural similarity to α-ketoglutarate, D-2-hydroxyglutarate acts as a competitive inhibitor of α-ketoglutarate-dependent enzymes.[91]

As many α-ketoglutarate-driven enzymes are involved in epigenetic remodeling, oncometabolite-driven tumors have profoundly altered epigenomes. For instance, SDH loss is associated with the increase in DNA methylation (a so-called "hypermethylator" phenotype) in SDH-driven paragangliomas as well as in sporadic gastrointestinal stromal tumors, a fraction of which harbors SDH mutations as well.[92,93] Similarly, mutant alleles of IDH1 and 2 are strongly associated with the hypermethylator phenotype in glioma and AML.[94,95] In AML, in particular, IDH mutations are mutually exclusive with the loss-of-function mutations in methylcytosine hydroxylase TET2, further strengthening the mechanistic link between the two enzymes.[95] In various cellular settings, introduction of mutant IDH, or treatment with D-2-hydroxyglutarate, was sufficient to trigger alterations in DNA and histone methylation and suppress cell differentiation.[96,97] Conversely, targeted inhibition of mutant IDH enzymes promoted differentiation in glioma and AML cell models.[98,99] Taken together, through global remodeling of DNA and histone methylome, oncometabolites may contribute to tumorigenesis through locking cells in an undifferentiated state.

> **Box 7**
>
> Metabolic adaptations of cancer cells not only facilitate macromolecular biosynthesis but can also exert profound nonmetabolic effects on cellular fate.

From petty thieves to ringleaders—how cancer cells corrupt their neighbors

Even though composed of genetically stable cells, the tissue microenvironment in the vicinity of a tumor becomes profoundly altered during tumorigenesis. Most strikingly, its constituents—fibroblasts, endothelial cells, and components of innate and adaptive immunity—convert from being pro-homeostatic into active enablers of tumor growth.[100] Tumors use a variety of signals to corrupt normal cells, including secreted factors, cell–cell interactions, as well as changes in metabolite levels. Two prominent examples illustrating how altered tumor metabolism affects its microenvironment are discussed below.

Increased nutrient consumption by tumors is coupled to the secretion of large amounts of lactate into the extracellular fluid, which has wide-ranging effects on tumor microenvironment. Thus, lactate contributes to the induction of angiogenesis by stabilizing HIF1α in endothelial cells[101] and potentiating pro-angiogenic NF-κB and PI3-kinase signaling,[102–104] as well as by promoting vascular endothelial growth factor (VEGF) secretion from macrophages.[105] At the same time, lactate attenuates local antitumor immune responses by suppressing migration of monocytes[106] and activation of T-cells and dendritic cells,[107,108] as well as affecting the polarization state and localization patterns of tumor-associated macrophages.[109,110] Tumor-associated macrophages can assume two functional subtypes: M1, which is associated with secretion of pro-inflammatory cytokines, and M2, which is involved in immunosuppression and wound repair. Tumor-associated macrophages are predominantly M2-polarized, and M2 subtype has been shown to be directly induced by lactate.[109] Finally, accumulation of lactate contributes to a decreased pH of the tumor extracellular fluid, which, in turn, promotes the activity of numerous matrix-degrading enzymes and promotes invasion.[111,112]

Another strategy used by cancer cells to attenuate antitumor immune responses is through the selective depletion of the amino acid tryptophan from their microenvironment.[113] To this end, tumors upregulate the expression of tryptophan-degrading enzymes, indoleamine-2,3-dioxygenase (IDO) and tryptophan-2,3-dioxygenase (TDO), which both degrade tryptophan to its derivative kynurenine. Insufficient levels of tryptophan trigger apoptosis of effector T-cells;[114] in addition, accumulation of kynurenine promotes the emergence of immune-suppressive regulatory T cells (Tregs).[115] Finally, kynurenine-mediated signaling enhances invasiveness and extracellular matrix-degrading capacity of tumor cells themselves.[116]

> **Box 8**
>
> Cancer cells use the signaling capacity of select metabolites to influence the state of cells in their microenvironment and promote tumorigenesis.

Feeding habits in rogue travelers—from making your own to eating like a local

Recent advances have enabled the study of metabolic reprogramming during tumor progression and revealed a number of metabolic phenotypes and liabilities associated with metastasis, a critical process given how often it dictates clinical outcome. Alterations in metabolism have been observed at every stage of cancer metastasis, including the process of intravasation, in circulating tumor cells, and during eventual colonization and growth of metastases.[117]

The process of epithelial-mesenchymal transition (EMT), associated with enhanced migratory and invasive capacity, has been linked to altered metabolism in preclinical models of metastasis.[118,119] For example, EMT-associated proteins have a relatively high asparagine content and expression of asparagine synthetase, which converts aspartate to asparagine, can promote invasiveness and metastasis in breast cancer models. Conversely in the same models, systemic depletion of asparagine or silencing of asparagine synthetase in cancer cells led to decreased lung metastases.[119]

Understanding the factors that influence the ability of circulating tumor cells to form metastases highlights potential metabolic liabilities associated with this process. Although not relevant to every cancer type, oxidative stress in the bloodstream has emerged as an important factor dictating the ability of circulating cancer cells in eventually forming metastases. Studies using in vivo models of melanoma,[120] breast,[121] and lung cancer[122,123] have demonstrated that the suppression of oxidative stress promotes metastasis. In many cases, cancer cells metastasize to regional lymph nodes before hematogenous spread to distant organs. In mouse models of melanoma,[124] a comparison of lymphatic fluid and blood plasma revealed factors associated with decreased oxidative stress and ferroptosis in the lymphatic fluid, such as increased glutathione and oleic acid and decreased free iron. Oleic acid was shown to protect melanoma cells from ferroptosis and increase their capacity to form metastases. As such, metabolic features of the environment that a cancer cell is exposed to, in this example the lymphatic environment, can influence the ability of cells to survive in the bloodstream and enhance the process of subsequent distant metastasis.

Detailed studies of the utilization of specific fuels within a tumor can reveal important insights related to cancer progression and adaptation to the metabolic milieu of specific metastatic niches. For example, in addition to the previously described melanoma study, fatty acid metabolism has been studied in a variety of contexts. Ovarian cancers metastasize to the lipid-rich environment of the omentum and in mouse models of ovarian cancer, limiting transfer of fatty acids from adipocytes to ovarian cancer cells resulted in a reduced growth of metastases.[125] In a different tumor type, oral carcinoma, the expression of CD36 (a lipid transporter, that facilitates fatty acid import) occurs in a subset of human tumors and correlates with poor prognosis.[126] A high-fat diet increased the metastatic potential of CD36-positive cells and conversely, neutralizing antibodies to CD36 reduced metastatic burden in mouse models of oral carcinoma. Another example of metabolic reprogramming that enables cancer cells to adapt to a unique metabolic niche is metastasis of colorectal carcinoma cells to the liver.[127] Specifically, liver metastases arising from colorectal carcinomas markedly upregulate aldolase B. Aldolase B upregulation, in turn, enables cells to efficiently utilize fructose, a carbon source abundant in the liver, as a source of glycolytic intermediates. Notably, both aldolase B inhibition as well as dietary fructose restriction dramatically suppresses metastasis of colorectal carcinoma cells to the liver—but not to the lung, where fructose levels are low. Thus, metastatic clones are able to reprogram their metabolism in a way that helps them to take advantage of the nutritional composition of specific metastatic niches.

Finally, our understanding of tumor metabolism and metastasis has been enhanced by the application of novel approaches to study cancer metabolism in vivo, particularly using metabolic tracers such as the stable isotope ^{13}C. In non-small-cell lung cancer, the use of peri-operative isotope tracers (^{13}C-glucose and ^{13}C-lactate) at the time of primary tumor resection uncovered new aspects of metabolic heterogeneity and fuel utilization, including the finding that some lung tumors use both glucose and lactate as a carbon source for the TCA cycle.[128,129] Tumors with prominent lactate uptake were associated with rapid cancer progression. This observation was studied in mechanistic detail in mouse models of melanoma, where expression of monocarboxylate transporter 1 (MCT1) was associated with and required for efficient metastatic spread.[130] The inhibition of MCT1 resulted in a reduction in circulating melanoma cells and formation of metastases, as well as suppression of the oxidative pentose phosphate pathway and increased production of ROS. In this context, a metabolic feature is associated with metastatic potential that can be harnessed therapeutically.

Cancer metabolism comes into the clinic

For over three decades, increased uptake of glucose by cancer cells has been successfully exploited in tumor imaging, where the uptake of 2-deoxyglucose conjugated to ^{18}F, a radioactive isotope of fluorine, is detected by positron emission tomography (PET).[131] ^{18}F-fluorodeoxyglucose (^{18}F-FDG) is transported into cells and is phosphorylated by HK in the same manner as glucose, yet cannot be further catabolized, which leads to its intracellular accumulation. A noninvasive tumor detection approach, ^{18}F-FDG-PET is widely used in the clinic for tumor detection and staging as well as for monitoring tumor response to therapy. However, ^{18}F-FDG-PET has a number of limitations, which include false-positive signals from tissue infiltration by immune cells (for instance, in autoimmune thyroiditis), or inability to detect those tumors that are not markedly glycolytic (as is often the case in prostate cancer). In addition, some tissues, especially brain, exhibit high constitutive levels of glucose uptake, which precludes the detection of tumors localized to brain. Following the success of ^{18}F-FDG, other metabolite-based tracers, such as ^{18}F-fluoroglutamine,[132] ^{11}C-acetate,[133] α-^{11}C-methyl-L-tryptophan,[134,135] and 4-[^{18}F] fluorobenzyl triphenylphosphonium (^{18}FBnTP),[136] are currently being developed. Other metabolic imaging approaches, such as ^{1}H magnetic resonance spectroscopy (MRS) are being developed for the use in the clinic. MRS can detect endogenously abundant metabolites in select tissues. For instance, MRS has been adapted to the detection of gliomas with IDH1 mutation, by using accumulation of D-2-hydroxyglutarate as a marker.[137] A potential application of tumor imaging is its use as a predictive biomarker. For example, the novel tracer ^{18}FBnTP has been developed as a noninvasive tool to measure tumor oxidative phosphorylation and in preclinical models ^{18}FBnTP uptake can be used to predict response to inhibitors of Complex I of the electron transport chain.[136] Thus, in addition to providing valuable information about diagnosis and staging, metabolic imaging has important potential as a therapeutic decision-making and monitoring tool.

In addition to tumor imaging, at least two metabolic cancer therapies have been successfully used in the clinic for decades. L-asparaginase, a recombinant form of a bacterial enzyme which degrades the amino acid asparagine, was approved by the FDA in 1978 as an effective therapy for childhood acute lymphoblastic leukemia (ALL).[138] Leukemic cells lack the capacity to synthesize sufficient asparagine, so that the depletion of plasma asparagine (as well as, potentially, glutamine) sensitizes them to cell death. A class of drugs which inhibit nucleotide biosynthesis is another example of a successful metabolic therapy. These agents include 5-fluorouracil, an inhibitor of thymidine synthesis, gemcitabine and hydroxyurea, deoxyribonucleotide synthesis blockers, and an antifolate drug methotrexate, which interferes with dihydrofolate reductase (DHFR)-mediated synthesis of tetrahydrofolate (THF), disrupting the folate cycle-driven synthesis of nucleotides. The therapeutic efficacy of antifolate drugs was first demonstrated by Sidney Farber in Boston in the 1940s,[139] followed by the discovery of their mechanism of action in 1958.[140]

Dependence of cancer cells on glucose metabolism had prompted extensive testing of therapies that target the uptake of glucose or various steps in the glycolysis pathway. However, antiglycolytic interventions, such as, for example, inhibition of HK by a nonmetabolizable glucose analog 2-deoxyglucose or a drug lonidamine had shown mixed results in trials, and lonidamide had undesirable systemic effects.[141] Furthermore, 2-deoxyglucose was shown to trigger compensatory activation of IGF-I receptor-mediated signaling.[142] A snapshot of therapeutic agents targeting metabolic pathways that are currently being developed are shown in Table 1.

The most successful therapies targeting cancer metabolism to emerge recently are inhibitors of mutant IDH1 and IDH2. As described earlier, mutations in IDH represent an example of a genetic alteration which results in accumulation of an oncometabolite (D-2-hydroxyglutarate) that plays an important role in tumorigenesis. In the setting of acute myeloid leukemia, safety and efficacy of IDH inhibitors have been demonstrated in clinical trials,[143,144] leading to their approval for clinical use. Studies investigating the use of these agents in solid tumors are ongoing.

A significant practical challenge in the development of therapies targeting cancer metabolism is identifying those with an appropriate therapeutic window, given many metabolic processes also

Table 1 Recently-approved and investigational therapies capitalizing on reprogrammed cancer metabolism.

Enzyme target	Targeting compound	Metabolic pathway
GLUT family of glucose transporters	Phloretin, silybin	Glucose uptake
MCT (lactate transporter)	AZD3965	Glycolysis
PDK1	Dichloroacetate	Pyruvate catabolism
Mitochondrial complex I	Metformin, IACS-010759	Oxidative phosphorylation
PDH, aKGDH	Devimistat (CPI613)	TCA cycle
Glutaminase (GLS1)	CB-839	Glutaminolysis
Fatty acid synthase	TVB-2640	Fatty acid biosynthesis
HMGCR	Statins	Sterol biosynthesis
IDH1	Ivosidenib (AG-120)	Oncometabolite production
IDH2	Enasedenib (AG-221)	Oncometabolite production
IDH1/2	Vorasedinib (AG-881)	Oncometabolite production
IDO/TDO	INCB024360, Indoximod	Tryptophan degradation

play a critical role in normal tissues and organs. One proposed approach is to develop rational therapeutic combinations including metabolic interventions, including dietary interventions to novel inhibitors, and more conventional anticancer therapies. For example, by blocking glucose uptake systemically, PI3K inhibitors cause hyperglycemia and insulin release by the pancreas. The boost in circulating insulin may activate growth factor signaling pathways in cancer cells, hampering the therapeutic effect of PI3K inhibition. In mice, these systemic effects can be mitigated by implementing a low carbohydrate, ketogenic diet, and this improves the antitumor efficacy of the PI3K inhibitors.[145] Another example, which illustrates both an improvement in therapeutic window and potential benefits of combination with systemic therapy, is the novel inhibitor of glutamine metabolism JHU083, an analog of 6-diazo-5-oxo-L-norleucine (DON). JHU083 is a prodrug that is activated by esterases in the tumor microenvironment, thereby reducing the toxicity of systemic DON administration.[146] JHU083 not only impairs cancer cell growth by blocking glutamine metabolism but also enhances the antitumor immune response and was shown to increase the efficacy of immunotherapy in mouse tumor models. It remains to be seen whether dietary interventions or novel metabolic inhibitors will have clinical efficacy, but this represents an active area of ongoing research.

Box 9

The dependence of tumor cells on various aspects of their altered metabolism has formed a basis for a number of imaging and therapeutic strategies.

Conclusions

Discoveries of modern cancer metabolism have elucidated how tumor cells reprogram their metabolism to sustain growth, circumvent nutrient and oxygen limitations and alter their own fate as well as the fate of neighboring cells. There is, conceivably, a lot more left to learn about how a cell gauges the levels of its many metabolites and the complex ways in which it converts this information into decisions about nutrient acquisition, execution of cell death and differentiation programs, and a cross-talk with the microenvironment as well as the organism as a whole. In addition to macronutrients, the contribution of micronutrients, such as vitamins and metal ions, to metabolism and signaling of cancer cells is only beginning to be unraveled. Our growing understanding of cancer metabolism has already been translated into innovative imaging and therapeutic tools, and the arsenal of these applications will continue to grow in the foreseeable future.

Summary

Proliferation of cells within a metazoan organism is governed by external stimuli, including signals from soluble growth factors as well as from cellular attachments to the extracellular matrix. Pro-growth signals induce a profound shift in the metabolic state of a responding cell, increasing its capacity for de novo synthesis of macromolecules—namely, proteins, lipids, and nucleic acids, required for growth. Pro-growth signals directly facilitate the uptake of metabolic substrates from the surrounding environment, ensuring that a proliferating cell has an adequate supply of macromolecular precursors to grow. Pro-growth signals also dictate the downstream metabolic fate of acquired substrates, directing them towards the generation of precursors for a variety of biosynthetic reactions, which include fatty acid, cholesterol, nonessential amino acid, and nucleotide biosynthesis. In contrast to normal tissues, in which pro-growth signals are transient in nature, aberrantly activated oncogenes accumulated by cancer cells lock their metabolism in a constitutive state of nutrient acquisition and macromolecule biosynthesis.

Whereas pro-growth signals influence the uptake of metabolic substrates and their progression through cellular metabolic pathways, changes in levels of select metabolites, in turn, affect a diverse range of nonmetabolic processes in the cell. For example, intracellular metabolites act as either substrates or as cofactors for several classes of epigenetic enzymes. As a consequence, changes in levels of select metabolites exert changes upon the cellular epigenetic state. Some tumor types take advantage of this form of regulation by acquiring mutations in metabolic enzymes, leading to a newly discovered class of cancer-inducing intermediates, termed oncometabolites. In addition, metabolic alterations of cancer cells influence other cells within the tumor microenvironment, resulting in increased tumor expansion and dissemination.

A number of imaging and therapeutic agents which exploit cancer-specific metabolic alterations have been used in the clinic, and our developing understanding of the complexity of tumor-specific metabolic adaptations holds a promise for expanding the arsenal of such applications in the future.

Key references

The complete reference list can be found on Vital Source version of this title, see inside front cover.

1. Hanahan D, Weinberg RA. Hallmarks of cancer: the next generation. *Cell.* 2011;**144**(5):646–674.
7. Broach JR. Nutritional control of growth and development in yeast. *Genetics.* 2012;**192**(1):73–105.
9. Hensley CT, Wasti AT, DeBerardinis RJ. Glutamine and cancer: cell biology, physiology, and clinical opportunities. *J Clin Invest.* 2013;**123**(9):3678–3684.
12. Zaman S, Lippman SI, Schneper L, et al. Glucose regulates transcription in yeast through a network of signaling pathways. *Mol Syst Biol.* 2009;**5**:245.
17. Wieman HL, Wofford JA, Rathmell JC. Cytokine stimulation promotes glucose uptake via phosphatidylinositol-3 kinase/Akt regulation of Glut1 activity and trafficking. *Mol Biol Cell.* 2007;**18**(4):1437–1446.
19. Jacobs SR, Herman CE, Maciver NJ, et al. Glucose uptake is limiting in T cell activation and requires CD28-mediated Akt-dependent and independent pathways. *J Immunol.* 2008;**180**(7):4476–4486.
20. Boxer RB, Stairs DB, Dugan KD, et al. Isoform-specific requirement for Akt1 in the developmental regulation of cellular metabolism during lactation. *Cell Metab.* 2006;**4**(6):475–490.
22. Wise DR, DeBerardinis RJ, Mancuso A, et al. Myc regulates a transcriptional program that stimulates mitochondrial glutaminolysis and leads to glutamine addiction. *Proc Natl Acad Sci U S A.* 2008;**105**(48):18782–18787.
25. Schafer ZT, Grassian AR, Song L, et al. Antioxidant and oncogene rescue of metabolic defects caused by loss of matrix attachment. *Nature.* 2009;**461**(7260):109–113.
26. Park JS, Burckhardt CJ, Lazcano R, et al. Mechanical regulation of glycolysis via cytoskeleton architecture. *Nature.* 2020;**578**(7796):621–626.
27. Warburg O. On the origin of cancer cells. *Science.* 1956;**123**(3191):309–314.
30. Yuneva M, Zamboni N, Oefner P, et al. Deficiency in glutamine but not glucose induces MYC-dependent apoptosis in human cells. *J Cell Biol.* 2007;**178**(1):93–105.
33. Kim J, Kundu M, Viollet B, Guan KL. AMPK and mTOR regulate autophagy through direct phosphorylation of Ulk1. *Nat Cell Biol.* 2011;**13**(2):132–141.
36. Commisso C, Davidson SM, Soydaner-Azeloglu RG, et al. Macropinocytosis of protein is an amino acid supply route in Ras-transformed cells. *Nature.* 2013;**497**(7451):633–637.
40. Rathmell JC, Fox CJ, Plas DR, et al. Akt-directed glucose metabolism can prevent Bax conformation change and promote growth factor-independent survival. *Mol Cell Biol.* 2003;**23**(20):7315–7328.
41. Elstrom RL, Bauer DE, Buzzai M, et al. Akt stimulates aerobic glycolysis in cancer cells. *Cancer Res.* 2004;**64**(11):3892–3899.
44. Vander Heiden MG, Cantley LC, Thompson CB. Understanding the Warburg effect: the metabolic requirements of cell proliferation. *Science (New York, NY).* 2009;**324**(5930):1029–1033.

46 Locasale JW, Grassian AR, Melman T, et al. Phosphoglycerate dehydrogenase diverts glycolytic flux and contributes to oncogenesis. *Nat Genet.* 2011;**43**(9):869–874.

47 Possemato R, Marks KM, Shaul YD, et al. Functional genomics reveal that the serine synthesis pathway is essential in breast cancer. *Nature.* 2011;**476**(7360): 346–350.

51 Christofk HR, Vander Heiden MG, Harris MH, et al. The M2 splice isoform of pyruvate kinase is important for cancer metabolism and tumour growth. *Nature.* 2008;**452**(7184):230–233.

52 Christofk HR, Vander Heiden MG, Wu N, et al. Pyruvate kinase M2 is a phosphotyrosine-binding protein. *Nature.* 2008;**452**(7184):181–186.

59 Kim JW, Tchernyshyov I, Semenza GL, Dang CV. HIF-1-mediated expression of pyruvate dehydrogenase kinase: a metabolic switch required for cellular adaptation to hypoxia. *Cell Metab.* 2006;**3**(3):177–185.

62 Lum JJ, Bui T, Gruber M, et al. The transcription factor HIF-1alpha plays a critical role in the growth factor-dependent regulation of both aerobic and anaerobic glycolysis. *Genes Dev.* 2007;**21**(9):1037–1049.

65 Kaplon J, Zheng L, Meissl K, et al. A key role for mitochondrial gatekeeper pyruvate dehydrogenase in oncogene-induced senescence. *Nature.* 2013;**498**(7452):109–112.

76 Wellen KE, Thompson CB. A two-way street: reciprocal regulation of metabolism and signalling. *Nat Rev Mol Cell Biol.* 2012;**13**(4):270–276.

79 Imai S, Armstrong CM, Kaeberlein M, Guarente L. Transcriptional silencing and longevity protein Sir2 is an NAD-dependent histone deacetylase. *Nature.* 2000;**403**(6771):795–800.

89 Ward PS, Patel J, Wise DR, et al. The common feature of leukemia-associated IDH1 and IDH2 mutations is a neomorphic enzyme activity converting alpha-ketoglutarate to 2-hydroxyglutarate. *Cancer Cell.* 2010;**17**(3):225–234.

90 Dang L, White DW, Gross S, et al. Cancer-associated IDH1 mutations produce 2-hydroxyglutarate. *Nature.* 2010;**465**(7300):966.

95 Figueroa ME, Abdel-Wahab O, Lu C, et al. Leukemic IDH1 and IDH2 mutations result in a hypermethylation phenotype, disrupt TET2 function, and impair hematopoietic differentiation. *Cancer Cell.* 2010;**18**(6):553–567.

96 Lu C, Ward PS, Kapoor GS, et al. IDH mutation impairs histone demethylation and results in a block to cell differentiation. *Nature.* 2012;**483**(7390):474–478.

98 Rohle D, Popovici-Muller J, Palaskas N, et al. An inhibitor of mutant IDH1 delays growth and promotes differentiation of glioma cells. *Science.* 2013; **340**(6132):626–630.

109 Colegio OR, Chu NQ, Szabo AL, et al. Functional polarization of tumour-associated macrophages by tumour-derived lactic acid. *Nature.* 2014;**513**(7519): 559–563.

116 Opitz CA, Litzenburger UM, Sahm F, et al. An endogenous tumour-promoting ligand of the human aryl hydrocarbon receptor. *Nature.* 2011; **478**(7368):197–203.

117 Faubert B, Solmonson A, DeBerardinis RJ. Metabolic reprogramming and cancer progression. *Science (New York, NY).* 2020;**368**(6487):eaaw5473.

120 Piskounova E, Agathocleous M, Murphy MM, et al. Oxidative stress inhibits distant metastasis by human melanoma cells. *Nature.* 2015;**527**(7577):186–191.

137 Choi C, Ganji SK, DeBerardinis RJ, et al. 2-Hydroxyglutarate detection by magnetic resonance spectroscopy in IDH-mutated patients with gliomas. *Nat Med.* 2012;**18**(4):624–629.

143 DiNardo CD, Stein EM, de Botton S, et al. Durable remissions with ivosidenib in IDH1-mutated relapsed or refractory AML. *N Engl J Med.* 2018; **378**(25):2386–2398.

16 Tumor angiogenesis

John V. Heymach, MD, PhD ■ Amado Zurita-Saavedra, MD ■ Scott Kopetz, MD, PhD ■ Tina Cascone, MD, PhD ■ Monique Nilsson, PhD ■ Irene Guijarro, PhD

> **Overview**
>
> Angiogenesis, the growth of new capillary blood vessels, is central to cancer growth and metastasis and is recognized to be a potential therapeutic target for the treatment of cancer. Antiangiogenic agents have become part of the standard treatment armamentarium for many solid tumors, providing significant clinical benefits for some cancers (e.g., renal cell, colorectal) and modest or no benefit for others. This article is focused on principles of tumor angiogenesis that are intrinsic to the behavior of human cancer, and lessons that can be gleaned from the clinical testing and use of angiogenesis inhibitors alone and in combination with other agents to date.

Tumor angiogenesis

Angiogenesis, the growth of new capillary blood vessels, is central to the growth and metastatic spread of cancer. More than four decades ago, it was recognized to be a potential therapeutic target for the treatment of cancer.[1] Since that seminal observation, the field has undergone explosive growth that has taken it from theory to clinical validation of angiogenesis as a therapeutic target, and antiangiogenic therapy is now in routine clinical use. Bevacizumab, a monoclonal antibody targeting vascular endothelial growth factor (VEGF), has undergone the most extensive clinical evaluation to date and is now a standard agent for the treatment of colorectal, lung, renal cell, and other malignancies. Several other antiangiogenic agents are also in routine use for other cancers including ramucirumab, an antibody targeting VEGF receptor-2; the VEGF- and placental-growth factor (PlGF) targeting protein aflibercept; and a number of tyrosine kinase inhibitors targeting angiogenic pathways including sunitinib, pazopanib, sorafenib, vandetanib, and axitinib.

While the progress of the field is encouraging, the clinical benefits of antiangiogenic agents have been relatively modest thus far, and key questions remain unanswered: How should antiangiogenic therapy be combined with other therapeutic regimens and treatment modalities? In what tumor types, and at what stage(s), should these agents be used? Can markers be developed to identify patients most likely to benefit, or experience toxicities, from treatment? The ultimate impact of antiangiogenic therapy in the treatment of cancer will be determined at least in part by the ability of basic researchers and clinicians to address these questions.

An understanding of the cellular and molecular basis of tumor angiogenesis is, therefore, important for clinicians who diagnose and treat cancer by whatever modalities. This article is focused on certain general principles of tumor angiogenesis that are intrinsic to the behavior of human cancer, and lessons that can be gleaned from the clinical testing and use of angiogenesis inhibitors to date.

Rationale for targeting tumor vasculature

There has been enormous progress in understanding the molecular and cellular events that enable a preneoplastic cell to transform, grow into a macroscopic tumor, and metastasize. These events include, but are not limited to, the activation of certain oncogenes and/or the loss of specific suppressor genes; becoming self-sufficient in growth signals and unresponsive to apoptotic signals; the acquisition of limitless replicative potential; and the escape from immune surveillance.[2] Current evidence argues that these neoplastic properties may be necessary but not sufficient for a cancer cell to expand into a population that is symptomatic, clinically detectable, metastatic, and lethal. For a tumor to develop a metastatic and/or a lethal phenotype, it must first recruit and sustain its own private blood supply, a process called tumor angiogenesis.[2]

A tumor can recruit vessels through at least four mechanisms—(1) cooption of existing vessels; (2) sprouting from existing vessels (angiogenesis); (3) formation of new vessels de novo, typically from bone-marrow-derived cells in the adult (vasculogenesis); (4) intussusception, the insertion of interstitial tissue columns into the lumen of preexisting vessels (reviewed in Ref. 3).

Non-angiogenic tumors are harmless: prolonged survival with non-angiogenic, dormant tumors

There is an early stage of neoplastic development when tumors are not yet able to recruit new microvascular endothelial cells (ECs) and cannot induce angiogenesis. As a result, such tumors remain *in situ* and dormant at <1 mm size and are harmless to the host.[4] For over 100 years, pathologists performing autopsies on individuals who died of accidental causes have found that for a given age group, a large number of individuals harbor *in situ* carcinomas while a very small percentage in that age group are diagnosed with cancer during life.[5] For example, carcinoma *in situ* is found in the breasts of 39% of women age 40–50 years who died of trauma but only 1% are ever diagnosed with cancer in this age range. Carcinoma *in situ* of the prostate is diagnosed in 46% of men age 60–70 years who died of trauma but only 15% are diagnosed during life.

Disease of cancer requires expansion of tumor mass
Expansion of the tumor mass beyond the initial microscopic size is usually dependent on recruitment of a vascular supply. This angiogenic phenotype is likely dependent on the balance of endogenous

---

Holland-Frei Cancer Medicine, Tenth Edition. Edited by Robert C. Bast, John C. Byrd, Carlo M. Croce, Ernest Hawk, Fadlo R. Khuri, Raphael E. Pollock, Apostolia M. Tsimberidou, Christopher G. Willett, and Cheryl L. Willman.
© 2023 John Wiley & Sons, Inc. Published 2023 by John Wiley & Sons, Inc.

pro- and antiangiogenic factors,[6–9] including secreted factors such as VEGF and basic fibroblast growth factor (bFGF); recruitment of bone marrow-derived EC precursors; and decreased expression of endogenous angiogenesis inhibitors [i.e., thrombospondin (TSP)-1]. Other mechanisms will unquestionably be uncovered. Absence of tumor angiogenesis prevents expansion of the tumor mass beyond a microscopic size, thereby avoiding metastatic spread and tumor-related symptoms, and hence, "cancer without disease."[6] The therapeutic implications of this concept are profound. Therapeutic blockade of angiogenesis may not only slow the growth of clinically evident tumors but also may help prevent the emergence of microscopic lesions into clinically evident tumors.

Recruitment of microvascular ECs is also necessary for expansion of a normal tissue mass and for expansion of an organ mass, for example, after partial hepatectomy.[10] In fact, angiogenesis is fundamental to reproduction, development, and repair but such physiologic angiogenesis occurs mainly as short-lived capillary blood vessel growth that usually lasts only days (ovulation angiogenesis), weeks (wound healing angiogenesis), or months (fetal and placental angiogenesis) but then it is always downregulated spontaneously and on a predictable timetable.[11,12] These physiological roles for angiogenesis help explain some of the toxicities observed from the use of angiogenesis inhibitors in the clinic that are detailed below.

Historic background

More than 100 years ago, it was observed that tumors were often more vascular during surgery than normal tissues.[13] This was explained by simple dilation of existing host blood vessels.[14] Vasodilation was thought to be a side effect of metabolites or of necrotic tumor products escaping from the tumor. Three reports, although largely overlooked, suggested that tumor hyperemia could be related to neovascularization and not solely to vasodilation.[15,16] Nonetheless, debate continued in the literature for decades about whether a tumor could expand to a large size (centimeters) by simply living on preexisting vasculature (vessel cooption).[17] Even the few investigators who accepted the concept of tumor-induced neovascularization generally assumed that this was an inflammatory reaction, a side effect of tumor growth, not a requirement for tumor growth.[18] It is now recognized that the two processes are often linked and that the recruitment of inflammatory cells plays a key role in initiating and promoting tumor angiogenesis.

Beginning of angiogenesis research

Hypothesis: tumor growth depends on angiogenesis
In 1971, Judah Folkman proposed a new hypothesis that tumor growth is angiogenesis dependent.[1] This hypothesis suggested that tumor cells and vascular ECs within a neoplasm may constitute a highly integrated ecosystem and that ECs may be switched from a resting state to a rapid growth phase by a "diffusible" chemical signal from tumor cells. An additional speculation was that angiogenesis could be a relevant target for tumor therapy (i.e., antiangiogenic therapy). These ideas were based on experiments Folkman and Frederick Becker performed in the early 1960s, which revealed that tumor growth in isolated perfused organs was severely restricted in the absence of tumor vascularization (Figure 1).[19–23]

These concepts were not widely accepted at the time but eventual acceptance of Folkman's 1971 hypothesis, and the development of angiogenesis research as a field, was subsequently facilitated by a number of advances including the ability to reproducibly culture vascular ECs, the discovery of endogenous angiogenesis proteins, and the identification of drugs able to block angiogenesis.[24–28]

Experimental evidence
By the mid-1980s, considerable experimental evidence had been assembled to support the hypothesis that tumor growth is angiogenesis dependent. The idea could now be stated in its simplest terms: "Once tumor take has occurred, every further increase in tumor cell population must be preceded by an increase in new capillaries that converge upon the tumor."[29] The hypothesis predicted that if angiogenesis could be completely inhibited, tumors would become dormant at a small, possibly microscopic, size.[22] It forecasted that whereas the presence of neovascularization would be necessary, but not sufficient, for expansion of a tumor, the absence of neovascularization would prevent expansion of a primary tumor mass beyond 1–2 mm^3 and restrict a metastasis to a microscopic dormant lesion (Figure 1).

The hypothesis that tumors are angiogenesis dependent has been supported by a large body of preclinical evidence.[30] Some of the observations supporting the angiogenic hypothesis include:

1. Tumors implanted into subcutaneous transparent chambers grow slowly and linearly before vascularization. After vascularization, tumor growth is rapid and tumor volume may increase exponentially.[31,32]
2. Tumors grown in the vitreous of the rabbit eye remain viable but are restricted to diameters of less than 0.50 mm for as long as 100 days. Once the tumor reaches the retinal surface, it becomes neovascularized and within 2 weeks can undergo a 19,000-fold increase in volume over the avascular tumor.[33]
3. The limit of oxygen diffusion is approximately 100–200 μm. Tumor cells that exceed these distances from a capillary vessel become necrotic (Figure 2).[34]
4. A neutralizing antibody to VEGF inhibited tumor growth by more than 90%. The antibody had no effect on the tumor cells *in vitro*.[35] This observation has been replicated using different means to block VEGF, including a fusion protein engineered from VEGF receptors (VEGF trap).[36] Similar results were seen with an antibody directed against another angiogenic factor, bFGF.[37]

Biology of tumor angiogenesis

The role of angiogenesis in preneoplasia and early tumorigenesis

In the experiments with isolated perfused organs by Folkman and colleagues more than four decades ago, the growth of tumors was severely restricted in diameter in the absence of angiogenesis.[19,38] This and other studies led to the proposal that the growth of solid tumors is dependent on new capillary sprouts (angiogenesis) and that without angiogenesis solid tumors might become completely dormant.[1] This raised the possibility that angiogenesis might be a therapeutic target not only for the treatment of advanced cancers but potentially for chemoprevention as well.

Preneoplasia is associated with increased angiogenesis in human tumors

Studies from human specimens provide further support for the hypothesis that angiogenesis occurs early in tumor progression,

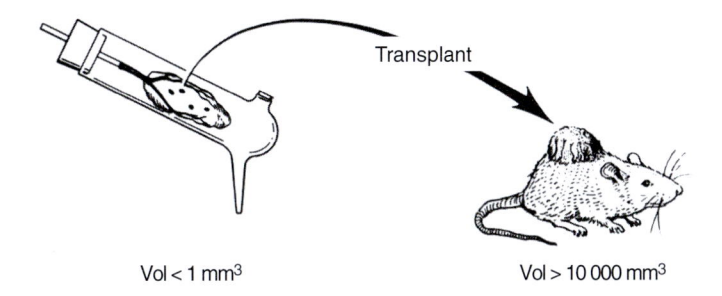

Figure 1 Tumors remain avascular in isolated perfused organs.[19] Whole organs, supported by perfusion, allow growth of tumors in isolation from a host. The tumor remains very small, less than 1 mm³ in an avascular environment compared to growth in mice which can exceed 10,000 mm³. Source: Based on Folkman et al.[19]

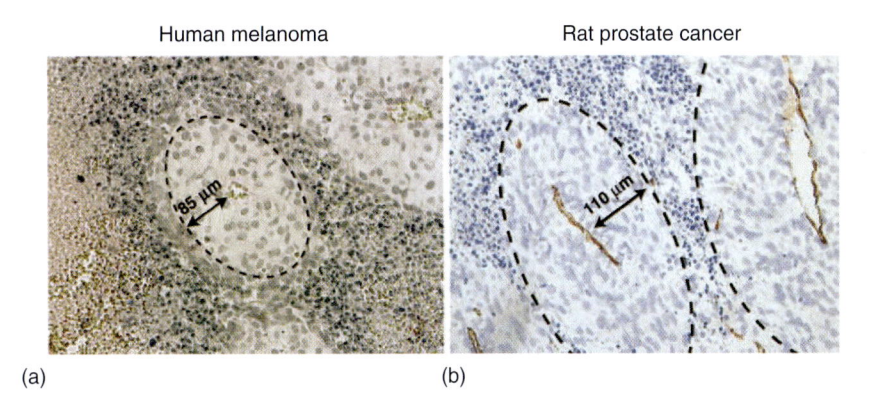

Figure 2 (a) A cuff of viable tumor cells surrounding a microvessel in a human melanoma growing in a SCID mouse has an average radius of 85 μm. The appearance of an ellipsoid is a result of the way the section is cut. (b) A cuff of rat prostate cancer cells surrounding a microvessel has an average radius of 110 μm.

typically during the preneoplastic stage. In cervix cancer, an initial mild increase in vessel density has been detected in the early dysplastic [cervical intraepithelial neoplasia (CIN) I] stage. Mid–late dysplasias (CIN II–III) exhibited a readily apparent angiogenic switch, wherein new vessels became densely apposed underlying the dysplastic epithelium.[39,40] Biopsies from lung cancer patients and high-risk individuals have shown that preneoplastic lesions ranging from hyperplasia and metaplasia to carcinoma are associated with increased microvessel density.[41–43] A distinctive pattern known as angiogenic squamous dysplasia[42] has also been identified. The specific angiogenic stimulators in bronchial preneoplastic lesions have not been established but elevated levels of VEGF,[41] epidermal growth factor receptor (EGFR),[44] and COX-2[45] have been observed.

Role of angiogenesis in the metastatic spread of cancer

In addition to its role in enabling the growth of premalignant or malignant lesions, angiogenesis contributes to the hematogenous metastatic spread of tumors. This spread may be facilitated by the presence of "mosaic" blood vessels in tumors, in which both endothelial and tumor cells form the luminal blood surface, facilitating the shedding of tumor cells into the circulation. In one study, approximately 15% of vessels in a colon cancer xenograft model were mosaic vessels in which tumor cells appeared to directly contact the luminal vessel surface without ECs acting as a barrier.[46] Similar numbers of mosaic tumor vessels were detected in human tumor biopsies. These observations suggest that the irregular architecture and function of tumor vessels may facilitate tumor cell shedding into the circulation and metastatic spread.

Micrometastases also appear to be dependent on angiogenesis in order to progress into clinically evident tumors. They may remain dormant in distant sites for an extended period of time but a small fraction of these acquire an adequate blood supply to permit the development of tumors; angiogenesis inhibitors can inhibit this process in a variety of murine models.[47–52] and they may offer benefit when used for chemoprevention as well as in treatment of early-stage or advanced disease.[53–55]

Taken together, these studies provide evidence that the induction of angiogenesis is an early and important step in tumor progression, likely occurring in precancerous lesions, and is involved in metastatic spread. For these reasons, angiogenesis is a rational target for chemoprevention. Additional studies will be needed to elucidate the key regulators of early angiogenesis, and to identify the optimal antiangiogenic agents for chemoprevention, advanced disease, and other applications.

Regulators of angiogenesis

The discovery of diffusible factors stimulating tumor angiogenesis

The observation in the 1970s that tumors implanted into the avascular cornea or onto the vascularized chick chorioallantoic membrane induced an ingrowth of new capillaries, indicated that tumors released diffusible angiogenic factors.[9] This result motivated the development of bioassays to guide the search for tumor-derived angiogenic factors.[56]

Fibroblast growth factors

Basic fibroblast growth factor (bFGF or FGF-2) was the first angiogenic protein to be isolated and purified from a tumor (1982), followed shortly by acidic FGF (aFGF or FGF-1).[28,57,58] In cancer mouse models, inhibition of the FGFR pathway results in inhibited angiogenesis and reduced tumor growth.[59]

Abnormally elevated levels of bFGF are found in the serum and urine of cancer patients and in the cerebrospinal fluid of patients with brain tumors.[60,61] High bFGF levels in renal carcinoma correlated with a poor outcome[62] and correlate with stage of disease and tumor grade of Wilms' tumor patients.[63]

In addition to contributing to tumor angiogenesis, multiple FGFR fusion proteins have been identified on diverse cancers and appear to be oncogenic drivers as its pharmacologic inhibition suppresses the growth of FGFR fusion-tumor models.[64] Additional reports have shown FGFR1 to be amplified in a subset of small-cell lung cancers among other malignancies, and tumor cells harboring FGFR amplification are sensitive to target inhibition.[65] The inhibition of FGFRs, will therefore have direct antitumor cell effects and indirect tumor cell effects through targeting of the tumor vasculature.

Vascular endothelial growth factor (VEGF) family

Harold Dvorak first proposed that tumor angiogenesis is associated with increased microvascular permeability.[66] This led to the identification of vascular permeability factor (VPF).[67–69] VPF was subsequently sequenced by Napoleone Ferrara and colleagues and in 1989 was reported to be a specific inducer of angiogenesis called VEGF.[68–70] At the same time, a novel angiogenic protein was first isolated and purified from a tumor (sarcoma 180) and was shown to be VEGF.[70] Since then, more than 40 angiogenic inducers have been identified, most as tumor products (Table 1).[3,71] VEGF is an EC mitogen and motogen that is angiogenic *in vivo*.[72–74] Its expression correlates with blood vessel growth during embryogenesis and is essential for development of the embryonic vascular system.[75,76] VEGF expression also correlates with angiogenesis in the female reproductive tract, and in tumors.[77–80] VEGF is a 40–45 kDa homodimeric protein secreted by a wide variety of cells and the majority of tumor cells. VEGF exists as five different isoforms of 121, 145, 165, 189, and 206 amino acids, of which $VEGF_{165}$ is the predominant molecular species produced by a variety of normal and neoplastic cells. Two receptors for VEGF are found mainly on vascular ECs, the 180 kDa fms-like tyrosine kinase (Flt-1, VEGFR-1)[81] and the 200 kDa human kinase insert domain-containing receptor (KDR) and its mouse homolog, Flk-1 (VEGFR-2).[82] VEGF binds to both receptors, but KDR/Flk-1 transduces the signals for endothelial proliferation and chemotaxis.[83–86] Other structural homologues of the VEGF family include VEGF-B, VEGF-C, VEGF-D, and VEGF-E.[87,88] VEGF-C and -D bind to VEGFR-3, which is preferentially expressed on lymphatic endothelium.[89,90]

Subsequent studies revealed that neuropilin-1, a neuronal guidance molecule, is also co-receptor for $VEGF_{165}$.[91,92] This finding provides a molecular mediator that coordinates growth in the vascular and the nervous system. Neuropilin is not a tyrosine kinase receptor and is expressed on tumor cells allowing tumor VEGF to bind to their surface. Surface-bound VEGF could make ECs chemotactic to tumor cells, or it could act in a juxtacrine manner to mediate cooption of microvessels. Neuropilin also binds placenta growth factor-2 (PlGF-2) and heparin is essential for the binding of $VEGF_{165}$ and PlGF-2 to neuropilin-1.[93,94]

VEGF signal transduction

While VEGF-A binds VEGFR-1 with a higher affinity than VEGFR-2, the majority of biological effects of VEGF-A on tumor endothelium are thought to be mediated through VEGFR-2. Upon ligand binding, VEGFR-2 dimerizes, resulting in activation of the tyrosine kinase and autophosphorylation of residues including Tyr^{951}, Tyr^{996}, Tyr^{1054}, Tyr^{1175}, and Tyr^{1214}.[95] Phosphorylation of these residues induces the activation of signal transduction molecules including PI3K, phospholipase C-γ (PLC-γ), Akt, Src, Ras, and mitogen-activated protein kinase (MAPK) (Figure 3). Phosphorylation of Tyr^{1175} results in the binding and phosphorylation of PLC-γ, which subsequently promotes the release of Ca^{2+} from internal stores and activation of protein kinase C (PKC). PKC activation and Ca^{2+} mobilization are considered to be critical for VEGF-A induced cell proliferation and nitric oxide (NO) production, respectively.[96]

The PI3K pathway is paramount in the regulation of cell proliferation, survival, and migration. VEGF-A has been shown to promote phosphorylation of the p85 subunit of PI3K and enhance PI3K enzymatic activity. The mechanism by which VEGF-A results in activation of PI3K remains unclear, although studies have implicated a role for Src kinases, β-catenin, and VE-cadherin.[97,98]

Table 1 Examples of regulators of angiogenesis.[a]

Proangiogenic molecules	Antiangiogenic molecules	Transcription factors, oncogenes, and other regulators
Vascular endothelial growth factor (VEGF)	Interferon-α,β,γ	Hypoxia-inducible factor (HIF)-1α, 2α
Basic fibroblast growth factor (bFGF)	Thrombospondin-1,2	Nuclear factor-κB (NFκB)
Transforming growth factor-α (TGF-α)	Angiopoietin 2	Epidermal growth factor receptor (EGFR)
Platelet-derived growth factor (PDGF)	Tissue inhibitors of MMPs (TIMPs)	Ras
Epidermal growth factor (EGF)	Endostatin	p53
Angiopoeitins	Angiostatin	Von Hippel–Lindau
Interleukin-6	Interleukin-12	Cadherin
Interleukin-8	Endostatin	Integrin
Matrix metalloproteinases (MMPs)	Thrombospondin-1	Semaphorin
Hepatocyte growth factor (HGF)		Id1, Id2
Stromal cell-derived factor-1α (SDF-1α)		Prolyl hydroxylases
Delta-like ligand 4 (DLL4)		myc
Ephrins		
Monocyte chemoattractant protein-1 and other chemokines		

[a]Source: Adapted from Carmeliet and Jain[3] and Bouck et al.[71]

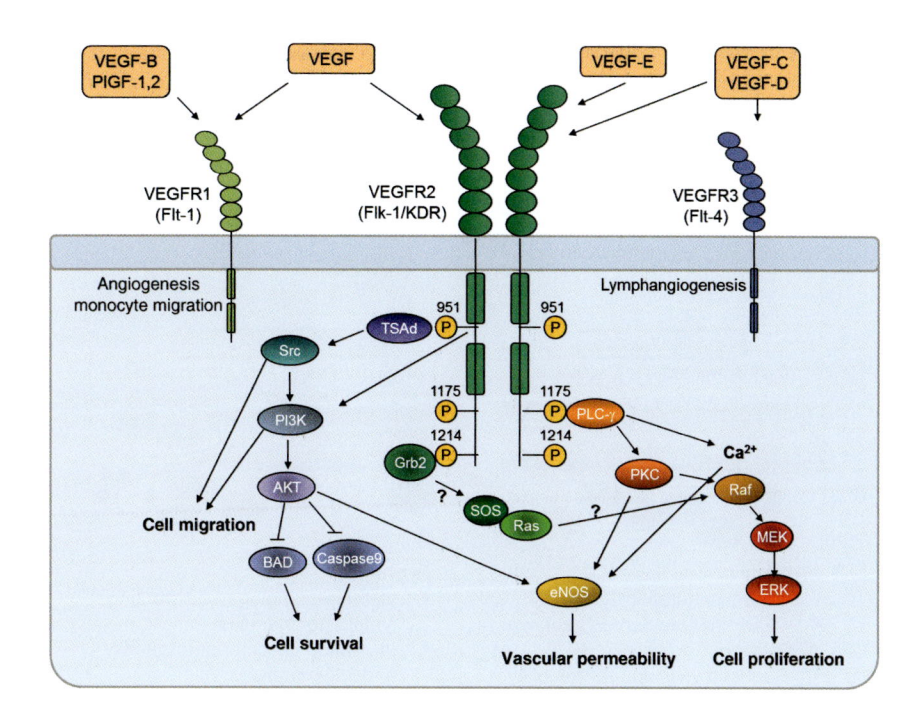

Figure 3 VEGFR signal transduction. VEGF family members, VEGF, VEGF-B, VEGF-C, VEGF-D, VEGF-E, and PlGF bind three VEGFR tyrosine kinases, resulting in dimerization, receptor autophosphorylation, and activation of downstream pathways. Signal transduction via VEGFR2 is shown. Ligand binding to VEGFR2 activates signal-transduction molecules phospholipase C-[gamma] (PLC-[gamma]), PI3K, Akt, Ras, Src, and MAPK and regulates cell proliferation, migration, survival, and vascular permeability.

VEGFR-2 induced activation of PI3K results in accumulation of phosphatidylinositol-3,4,5-triphosphate (PIP_3), which induces phosphorylation of Akt/PKB. Once activated, Akt/PKB phosphorylates and thus inhibits proapoptotic proteins BAD and caspase-9.

Members of the Src family kinases, Src, Fyn, and Yes, are expressed in ECs. Following VEGFR-2 autophosphorylation, T cell-specific adapter (TSAd) binds Tyr^{951} and then associates with Src. Src kinases control actin stress fiber organization and may mediate VEGF-A-induced PI3K activation. Ligand binding to VEGFR-2 also initiates activation of the Ras pathway, triggering signaling through the Raf-1-MEK-ERK signal cascade[95] known to be important in growth factor-induced cell proliferation. This activation may occur through multiple routes.[95,99]

Biological function of VEGF

In its initial discovery, VEGF was identified as a mediator of vessel permeability.[87,100] This capacity to render small veins and venules hyperpermeable is a critical function of VEGF. While the mechanisms by which VEGF increases microvascular permeability are incompletely understood, it may be at least in part due to VEGF-induced endothelial fenestrations,[76] opening of junctions between adjacent ECs,[101] and through NO production.[102–104]

Moreover, VEGF is a survival factor for ECs, inhibiting cell apoptosis through activation of the PI3K-Akt pathway[105] and increases in the antiapoptotic protein bcl-2.[106] In vivo, VEGF blockade has been demonstrated to cause apoptosis of immature, nonpericyte covered vessels.[107] VEGF is an EC mitogen though VEGFR-2-mediates signal transduction through Erk1/2, JNK/SAPK, and possibly PKC.[106,108] VEGF also induces expression of matrix metalloproteinases (MMPs) and serine proteinases involved in degradation of the basement membrane necessary for vascular sprouting[106] and facilitates EC migration through FAK and p38 MAPK-induced actin reorganization.[3,101,106,109]

Circulating VEGF may be one of the angiogenic signals by which tumors recruit bone marrow-derived cells, including endothelial progenitors and myeloid cells whose recruitment is thought to be mediated by VEGFR-2 and VEGFR-1, respectively.[110–114] A growing body of evidence suggests that VEGFR-bearing bone-marrow-derived cells contribute to initiating tumor formation, by creating a "metastatic niche," and/or help promote tumor angiogenesis[115–119] although there appear to be VEGFR-1 independent mechanisms as well.[120] Circulating endothelial and myeloid cells are being studied as potential biomarkers, as noted later in the article, and may contribute to resistance to VEGF inhibitors.[121,122] It is worth noting that not all VEGF in the circulation may be tumor derived. VEGF is stored in platelets and is transported by and released from them.[123] Furthermore, Pinedo and colleagues report that higher platelet counts correlate with a worse prognosis for cancer patients.[124,125] Therefore, it is possible that for those tumors that recruit bone marrow-derived ECs, communication from tumor to bone marrow may be mediated in part by the VEGF in circulating platelets.

Angiopoietins

Angiopoietin-1 (Ang1) is a 70 kDa ligand that binds to a specific tyrosine kinase expressed only on ECs, called Tie2 (also called Tek). Ang1 ligand binds Tie2 expressed on ECs, and Tie2 subsequently dimerizes and is phosphorylated. Activated Tie2 triggers activation of PI3K and Ras/Raf/MEK, promoting EC survival and proliferation/migration (Figure 4).[126] A ligand for Tie1 has not been discovered.[91,127–130] Ang1 is an EC-specific growth factor but it is not a direct endothelial mitogen in vitro, as it induces recruitment of pericytes and smooth muscle cells to become incorporated in the vessel wall. Pericyte and smooth muscle recruitment are

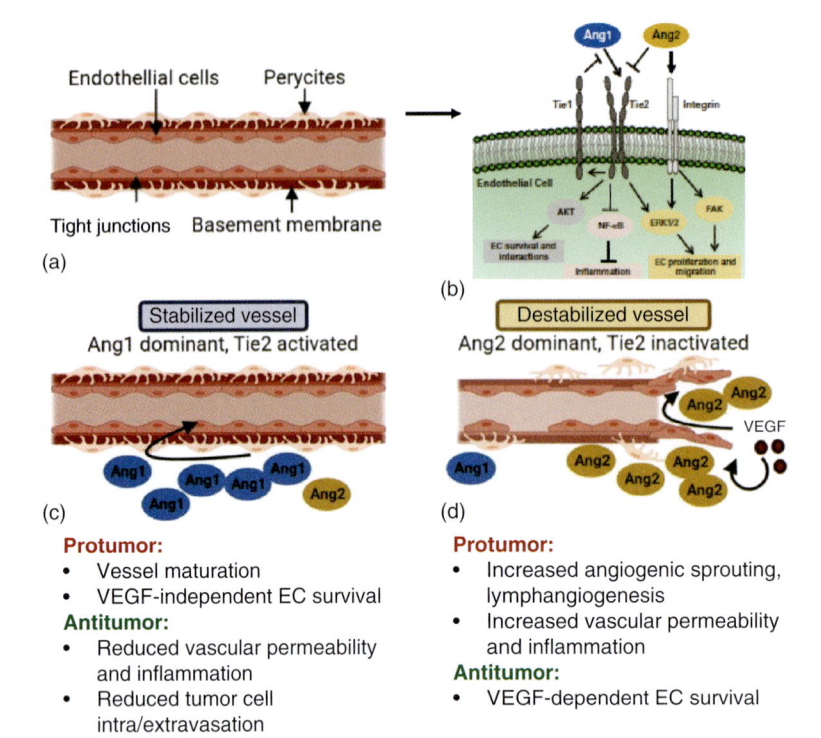

Figure 4 Ang/Tie2 signaling pathway. (a) Representation of nascent tumor blood vessel structure in quiescent state. Endothelial cells (ECs; green) are organized to form vessel lumen and tightly interact with perivascular cells (blue), separated by basement membrane. (b) Ang1 ligand binds Tie2 localized on ECs; Tie2 subsequently dimerizes and is phosphorylated. Activated Tie2 activates phosphatidylinositol 3-kinase and Ras/Raf/MEK, promoting EC survival and proliferation/migration. Generally, Ang2 functions as an Ang1 antagonist by inducing increased vascular permeability, sprouting vascularization. Autophosphorylated Tie2 activates Tie1, the extracellular domain of which in turn interferes with Ang1/Tie2 binding, therefore antagonizing Ang1 signaling. Ang1 has anti-inflammatory properties, whereas Ang2 plays a proinflammatory role. Ang1-activated Tie2 inhibits nuclear factor-κB–mediated inflammatory gene expression, whereas Ang2 promotes expression through blockade of Ang1 function. (c) Perivascular cells secrete Ang1, which binds Tie2 expressed on ECs. In this interaction, Ang1 contributes to vessel integrity, reduces vessel permeability, and maintains vasculature quiescence. (d) Ang2 plays a major role in angiogenesis by mediating dissociation of pericytes and destabilizing cellular junctions. In the presence of other proangiogenic factors (e.g., VEGF), ECs proliferate and/or migrate to form new sprouting, disorganized blood vessels. In the absence of proangiogenic factors, Ang2 signaling results in EC apoptosis and regression. Source: Cascone and Heymach[126].

mediated by endothelial production of PDGF-BB (and probably other factors) when Tie2 is activated by Ang1.[131] There is increased vascularization in mice that overexpress Ang1 in the skin[130] with larger vessels that are not leaky, in contrast to dermal vessels of mice overexpressing VEGF. In transgenic mice expressing both Ang1 and VEGF in the skin, dermal angiogenesis is increased in an additive manner, but the vessels do not leak.[132] This model mimics angiogenesis in healing wounds (i.e., relatively nonleaky vessels with pericytes and smooth muscle cells in the vascular wall). In contrast, tumor vessels are leaky and thin-walled with a paucity of pericytes. Angiopoietin-2 (Ang2), produced by tumor vascular endothelium, blocks the Tie-2 receptor and acts to repel pericytes and smooth muscle cells.[127] Nevertheless, tumor vessels remain thin "endothelium-lined tubes" even though some of these microvessels reach the diameter of venules. High levels of Ang2 are associated with metastases in melanoma patients, and in preclinical models, Ang2 promotes metastatis.[133,134] A key point is that angiopoietins and VEGF together play a role in angiogenesis, and the activity of both is context-dependent with different activities observed in angiogenic versus mature vessels. Because VEGF plays a key role in the proangiogenic activity of Ang2 targeting both the Ang/Tie2 and VEGF receptor pathways may provide clinical benefit. However, given that angiopoietins can apply either pro- or antitumorigenic effects, depending on the context, the best targeting approach remains unclear.[126]

Other factors regulating angiogenesis

Interleukin-8 (IL-8) is a proinflammatory chemotactic cytokine produced by monocytes, macrophages, and tumor cells.[135] IL-8 induces EC proliferation and chemotaxis as well as promotes cell survival.[135,136] The effects of IL-8 are mediated through interactions with two cell-surface G protein-coupled receptors, CXCR1 and CXCR2, and activation of subsequent downstream signaling molecules including PI3K and MAPK.[137] Hepatocyte growth factor/scatter factor (HGF/SF) is the ligand for c-Met,[138] and it has been shown to facilitate tumor angiogenesis. c-Met is expressed on ECs, and activation by tumor-secreted HGF/SF augments matrix degradation and EC invasion. NOTCH proteins and ligands are also elevated in several cancers, and NOTCH signaling has been shown to both promote and suppress tumor growth depending on the tumor type.[139] Interactions between NOTCH and its ligand DLL4 promote tumor angiogenesis through VEGF/VEGFR signal transduction pathways.[140,141]

Endogenous inhibitors of angiogenesis

Endogenous angiogenesis inhibitors block vascular ECs from proliferating, migrating, or increasing their survival in response to a spectrum of proangiogenic proteins. The first clue to the existence of endogenous angiogenesis inhibitors came from the discovery that interferon-α inhibited EC migration and that platelet factor 4 inhibited endothelial proliferation.[142–144] Both

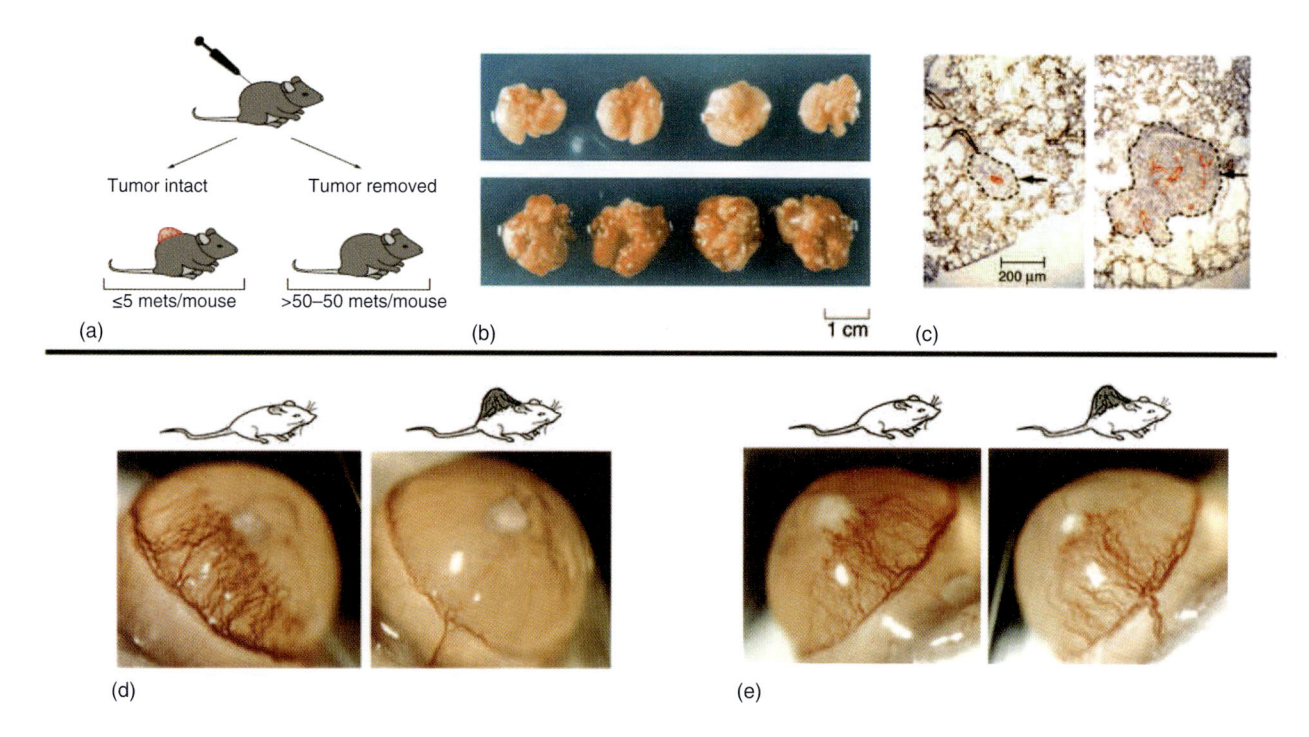

Figure 5 (a) Mice bearing Lewis Lung carcinoma.[164] Tumors were resected when tumor size reached 1.5–2 cm² and the animals were killed after 5 or 15 days. (b) Upper panel: lungs from animals still bearing the primary tumor. Lower panel: lungs removed at the same time from animals in which the tumor had been resected and the animals killed 15 days later. (c) Left panel: microscopic pulmonary metastasis in an animal in which a primary tumor is in place at the same time as the right panel. There is no evidence of angiogenesis as only a single central microvessel stained with antibody to von Willebrand factor. This dormant metastasis is 200 microns in its longest diameter. Right panel: lung metastasis from an animal euthanized 5 days after the primary tumor was removed, showing 8 or 9 new vessels in an enlarging metastasis. (d) A human prostate carcinoma (LNCaP) growing on the dorsum of a SCID mouse inhibits cornea neovascularization induced by an implanted sustained-release pellet of bFGF (80 ng) (right panel). Left panel depicts bFGF-induced corneal neovascularization at 5 days in the absence of a primary tumor. LNCaP prostate cancer generates angiostatin. (e) A human colon cancer that does not produce an angiogenesis inhibitor, growing in a SCID mouse as a control for (d). Source: Based on Holmgren et al.[164]

were subsequently shown to inhibit angiogenesis.[142–146] Since that time a number of other endogenous inhibitors have been described including interleukin-12, platelet factor 4, TSP-1, angiostatin, endostatin, arrestin, canstatin, tumstatin, MMP-2, pigment epithelium-derived factor, and antiangiogenic antithrombin III (an internal fragment of antithrombin III, named aaAT).[27,147–153]

Thrombospondin-1
Bouck and her colleagues initially proposed that a tumor could generate an angiogenesis inhibitor; they subsequently proposed that the angiogenic phenotype was the result of a net balance of endogenous inhibitors and stimulators of angiogenesis.[154] They studied a nontumorigenic line that secreted high levels of an angiogenesis inhibitor, a truncated form of TSP-1.[155] TSP-1 was shown to be regulated by the tumor suppressor *p53*.[156,157] Loss of p53 function in the transformed derivatives of these cells dramatically decreased the level of the angiogenesis inhibitor. Restoration of p53 upregulated TSP-1 and raised the antiangiogenic activity of the tumor cells. Deletion of TSP-1 led to accelerated growth of breast cancers that arise spontaneously in neu-transgenic mice.[158] The demonstration that the switch to an angiogenic phenotype involved a negative regulator of angiogenesis generated by the tumor per se suggested to Folkman a unifying angiogenic mechanism to explain a well-recognized but previously unsolved clinical and experimental phenomenon: the inhibition of tumor growth by the tumor mass. In this phenomenon, "the removal of certain tumors, for example, breast carcinomas, colon carcinomas, and osteogenic sarcomas can be followed by rapid growth of distant metastases."[159,160] In melanoma, partial spontaneous regression of the primary tumor may be followed by rapid growth of metastases, and when ionizing radiation is employed to regress a small-cell lung cancer, distant metastases may undergo rapid growth.[151,161] Once it was demonstrated that a tumor could generate a negative regulator of angiogenesis, then it became clear that a primary tumor, while stimulating angiogenesis in its own vascular bed, could possibly inhibit angiogenesis in the vascular bed of a distant metastasis.[155] In subsequent years, a number of other endogenous angiogenesis inhibitors were discovered including angiostatin, endostatin, and tumstatin.[149–151,162,163]

Angiostatin
Angiostatin is a 38 kDa internal fragment of plasminogen that was purified from the serum and urine of mice bearing a subcutaneous Lewis lung carcinoma that suppressed growth of its lung metastases by inhibiting their angiogenesis (Figure 5).[149] Angiostatin is not secreted by tumor cells but is generated through proteolytic cleavage of circulating plasminogen by a series of enzymes released from the tumor cells. Several potential mechanisms of its antiangiogenic activity have been reported including induction of endothelial apoptosis[165–167]; suppression of EC migration induced by plasmin binding to $\alpha_v\beta_3$-integrin[168,169]; inhibition of HGF-induced signaling via c-MET, Akt, and ERK-1/2 [170]; and downregulation of VEGF.[171]

Endostatin
A strategy similar to the one that uncovered angiostatin (e.g., suppression of tumor growth by tumor mass) was employed to identify

endostatin.[150,151,163] Like angiostatin, endostatin is generated from larger parent proteins by cleavage via enzymes released by tumor cells. Endostatin is a 20–22 kDa internal fragment of collagen XVIII.[150,163,172,173] It is the first of a group of endogenous angiogenesis inhibitors that are predominantly extracellular proteins, which generally require proteolytic processing to become active.[3,174] Endostatin appears to have both direct and indirect effects on tumor endothelium. It is a specific inhibitor of EC proliferation and migration.[175,176] Endostatin also inhibits integrin-dependent EC migration because it binds to α5β1-integrins on the EC surface.[177] It has been proposed that $\alpha_5\beta_1$-integrin may be a functional receptor for endostatin.[30] A wide variety of tumors have been inhibited by endostatin preclinically[178] including thyroid carcinoma, colon carcinoma, leukemia, non-small-cell lung cancer, pancreatic cancer, neuroblastoma, breast cancer, and spontaneous pancreatic islet carcinomas.[179–186]

Tumstatin

Tumstatin (28 kDa) is the NC1 domain fragment of the α_3 collagen molecule and exhibits antiangiogenic activity preclinically.[187–191] Tumstatin (α_3(IV)NC1) binds to ECs via $\alpha_v\beta_3$- and $\alpha_6\beta_1$-integrins[187,188,190,191] and induces apoptosis of ECs.[189] Experiments demonstrated that the antiangiogenic activity of tumstatin is dependent on $\alpha_v\beta_3$-integrin binding to ECs[187,191] and support the notion of its function as a negative regulator of angiogenesis.[187,192–194]

Other pathways regulating angiogenesis

Hypoxia-inducible factor-1

Expression of angiogenic factors including VEGF is positively regulated by hypoxia through the stabilization of the transcription factor hypoxia-inducible factor 1 (HIF-1).[195,196] HIF-1 is a transcription factor comprised of two subunits, HIF-1α and HIF-1β. While HIF-1β is expressed constitutively, expression of HIF-1α is tightly regulated. The stability of HIF-1α is primarily controlled by hypoxia. When oxygen is abundantly present, prolyl hydroxylases modify proline residues 402 and 564 on HIF-1α allowing it to bind the Von Hippel–Lindau (VHL) tumor suppressor gene which targets it for degradation.[196] Following binding of the HIF-1α and -β subunits, HIF-1 transverses to the nucleus and modulates the expression of genes involved in angiogenesis, cell survival, invasion, and glucose metabolism.[196] Indeed, HIF-1α is thought to be the key regulator of potent proangiogenic factors including VEGF.

Recent studies have revealed a number of non-hypoxic regulators including receptor tyrosine kinases such as EGFR,[197] the PI3K/Protein kinase B (AKT)/mechanistic target of rapamycin (mTOR) pathway, and metabolic pathways (reviewed in Refs [198,199]). Alterations in these pathways have been shown to contribute to inherited cancer syndromes, highlighting their role in carcinogenesis. For example, germline mutations in the VHL gene underlying VHL disease, lead to a markedly elevated risk of developing renal cell carcinoma (RCC), hemangioblastomas of the central nervous system (CNS), and other cancers. The VHL protein encoded by this gene is part of a protein complex that targets HIFs for degradation.[198] Sporadic mutations in the VHL gene also occur in clear-cell RCC. A second syndrome, hereditary leiomyomatosis and RCC, results from mutations in the fumarate hydratase (FH) gene.[200] FH is a mitochondrial protein involved in the tricarboxylic acid (TCA) cycle. Although the mechanism(s) are still under investigation, it appears that loss of FH function results in increased HIFs by causing a buildup of intracellular fumarate, which inhibits the enzymes (HIF hydroxylases, also known as EGLNs) that hydroxylate HIFs and target them for VHL-mediated degradation. A third hereditary syndrome, tuberous sclerosis complex, is caused by mutations in the tuberous sclerosis complex, resulting in elevated HIFs via the mTOR pathway.[201,202] Several other syndromes have also been identified that resulted in elevated HIF and downstream gene products, causing a "pseudohypoxic" state.[199,201] These observations support the hypothesis that dysregulation of the HIF pathways regulating angiogenesis are likely to play a role in driving early tumorigenesis. Several drugs targeting HIFs are currently in clinical development.

Oncogenes and tumor suppressors as regulators of angiogenesis

It is widely established that activation of proto-oncogenes can induce tumorigenesis. *In vitro*, expression of activated oncogenes increases cell proliferation and decreases apoptosis.[203] While these changes contribute to tumorigenesis by altering the equilibrium between cell proliferation and apoptosis, there is considerable evidence that this alone is not sufficient to produce expansive tumor growth.[204,205] Rather, tumors must also acquire an adequate vascular supply to grow, and published reports have demonstrated that transfection of tumor cells with oncogenes results in enhanced production of proangiogenic molecules,[206] and the *in vivo* growth of oncogene-driven tumors can be restricted with angiogenesis inhibitors.[207]

Ras

Ras is one of the most commonly activated oncogenes, occurring in 17–25% of all human tumors.[208] The transfection of transformed murine ECs with the Ras oncogene results in elevated production of VEGF, and treatment of these cells with the PI3K inhibitor, wortmannin, abrogates VEGF expression, indicating that mutated Ras regulates VEGF expression in a PI3K-dependent manner.[209] K-Ras gene mutations were positively associated with high VEGF expression in human non-small-cell lung cancer (NSCLC) specimens[210] and other disease types. In a doxycycline-inducible Ras melanoma model, downregulation of Ras led to massive apoptosis of microvascular endothelium in the tumor within 6 h and large tumors completely disappeared by 12 days.[211]

p53

p53 indirectly promotes tumor vascularization by altering the expression of both pro- and antiangiogenic factors. Evaluation of 73 NSCLC clinical specimens revealed a strong association between p53 nuclear localization and microvessel count.[212] Additionally, in an analysis of 107 NSCLC patients, p53 was significantly associated with VEGF expression and microvessel count.[213] It is likely that loss of wild-type p53 enhances tumor cell expression of additional proangiogenic factors in NSCLC. Wild-type p53 has been demonstrated to promote Mdm2-mediated ubiquitination and degradation of HIF-1α.[214] The loss of wild-type p53 is associated with elevated levels of HIF-1α in tissue culture and VEGF expression.[214] As previously noted, loss of p53 function also leads to a reduction in the expression of the angiogenesis inhibitor TSP-1.

EGFR family

EGFR is a member of the erbB family of receptor tyrosine kinases which also includes HER2/Neu, HER3 (ErbB3), and HER4 (ErbB4). Activation of EGFR can promote expression of proangiogenic molecules. Epidermal growth factor (EGF) has been shown to increase VEGF production in some tumor cell lines[215,216] and, conversely, treatment of tumor cells with EGFR inhibitors can decrease VEGF expression in various tumor types.[197,216–218] In NSCLC cell lines, EGF activates HIF-1α and induces expression of the chemokine receptor CXCR4 in tissue culture.[219] Moreover, in an immunohistochemical study of 172 NSCLC patients, expression of EGFR was associated with HIF-1α positivity,[220] and EGFR mutations causing constitutive receptor activation led to upregulated HIF-1α protein and increased VEGF levels.[221]

Like EGFR, HER2/Neu has also been shown to play a role in regulating angiogenesis. Blockade of HER2 using the monoclonal antibody trastuzumab (Herceptin) can block the production of multiple angiogenic factors and induce vessel normalization and regression in a murine model of human breast cancer, and enhance the effects of VEGF pathway blockade.[222,223]

Therapeutic approaches to targeting tumor vasculature

Angiogenesis inhibitors versus vascular targeting agents

Angiogenesis is the formation of new vessels from preexisting vasculature. Angiogenesis inhibitors are, therefore, typically targeted at the early stages in this process, including endothelial sprouting and survival mechanisms, which are often VEGF-dependent. Vascular targeting agents (VTAs), also known as vascular disrupting agents (VDAs), differ from angiogenesis inhibitors in that they target established abnormal tumor vasculature.[224] VTAs can induce rapid collapse of tumor vasculature, and their effects on normal vasculature can cause a host of side effects including acute coronary syndromes, thrombophlebitis, and tumor pain. None of these agents is currently in routine clinical use for cancer but several have undergone clinical testing. Vadimezan (ASA404) initially demonstrated positive results in combination with chemotherapy for patients with lung cancer in a Phase II trial[225] but was subsequently found to not prolong overall survival (OS) in Phase III testing.[226] Combretastatin A4 is another VTA undergoing evaluation for anaplastic thyroid cancer.

Antiangiogenic effects of chemotherapy and other therapeutic agents

Multiple preclinical studies have suggested that several "classical" chemotherapeutic agents may also have potent antiangiogenic effects, which may be enhanced by low dosing schedules.[227–229] It also appears that taxanes and vinca alkaloids may have relatively more potent antiangiogenic effects than other drugs,[229] which may help explain why there are differences in the degree of enhancement observed when antiangiogenic agents are added to chemotherapy. This prompted further examination of a wide variety of drugs which were found to also have antiangiogenic effects, prompting the term "accidental antiangiogenics."[230]

Targeting VEGF pathway

VEGF is the prototypic member of a family of structurally related, homodimeric growth factors that includes PlGF, VEGF-B, VEGF-C, VEGF-D, and VEGF-E. As described earlier, VEGF members bind to a family of transmembrane receptor tyrosine kinases that include VEGFR-1 (Flt-1), VEGFR-2 (KDR, Flk-1), and VEGFR-3 (Flt-4) (Figure 3). The effects of VEGF or VEGFR on vascular permeability and endothelial proliferation, migration, and survival are thought to be primarily mediated by VEGFR-2 while VEGFR-3 is primarily expressed on lymphatic endothelium (reviewed in Refs 95, 102). Agents targeting the VEGF pathway include monoclonal antibodies that bind the ligand (i.e., bevacizumab) or block the receptor (i.e., ramucirumab). In addition, many small-molecule receptor tyrosine kinase inhibitors (RTKIs) have been developed to target critical signaling pathways involved in angiogenesis. These RTKs, which include sorafenib, vandetanib (ZD6474), sunitinib (SU11248), axitinib (AG-013736) nintedanib (BIBF 1120), lenvatinib (E7080), regorafenib (BAY 73-4506), pazopanib (GW-786034), and cabozantinib (XL184) typically inhibit multiple receptors such as PDGFR, c-KIT, FGFR, and Axl in addition to VEGFR. These multi-targeting agents have demonstrated higher anticancer activity compared to single-target agents. Conversely, the off-target effects may have additive toxicities. The receptor specificity for each inhibitor, as well as their pharmacokinetics and potency, is likely to be the key determinants of their clinical activity. Representative agents targeting the VEGF pathway that are currently US Food and Drug Administration (FDA) approved are listed in Table 2.

Combinations of antiangiogenics with chemotherapy: mechanisms for enhanced antitumor activity

Preclinical and clinical studies have demonstrated that antiangiogenic therapy improves the outcome of cytotoxic therapies.[231,232] This finding is paradoxical. It was initially expected that targeting the tumor vasculature would drastically diminish the delivery of oxygen and therapeutics to the solid tumor, producing hypoxia that would cause many chemotherapeutics, as well as radiation, to be less effective.[231,232] Tumor vasculature is known to be structurally and functionally abnormal, with tortuous, highly permeable vessels. Proliferating tumor cells compress blood and lymphatic vessels resulting in a microenvironment typified by interstitial hypertension (elevated hydrostatic pressure outside the blood vessels), acidosis, and hypoxia.[233,234] This deficient vascular network impair drug delivery to tumor cells. Moreover, hypoxia renders tumor cells resistant to radiation and several cytotoxic agents and increases genetic instability selecting for tumor cells that have a greater metastatic potential. In addition to the effects on tumor cells, hypoxia leads to vascular abnormalization by signaling via PHD2 in tumor ECs[235] and, along with the low pH within the tumor microenvironment, weakens the cytotoxic functions of tumor-infiltrating immune cells. Collectively, the abnormal vasculature within solid tumors creates a significant barrier to delivery and efficacy of cancer therapeutics.

One potential explanation for the enhancement in efficacy of chemotherapy by antiangiogenic therapy is that these agents may "normalize" tumor vessels. In animal models of cancer, inhibition of VEGF signaling results in a vasculature network that more closely resembles vessels within normal tissue. This "normalized" vasculature is less leaky, less dilated, and has less tortuous vessels with a more normal basement membrane and increased pericyte coverage. Concurrent with these changes, within the tumor there is a decrease in interstitial fluid pressure (IFP), increased oxygenation, and improved delivery of concurrently administered chemotherapeutics (Figure 6).[236–244] Evidence from a Phase I/II clinical trial in locally advanced rectal carcinoma patients receiving bevacizumab and chemotherapy (with radiation) corroborates preclinical findings. Bevacizumab treatment was associated with a decrease in tumor IFP and an increase in mature, pericyte-covered vessels.[245,246]

Table 2 Approved VEGF pathway inhibitors.

Type	Agent	Target	Approval
Monoclonal antibody	Bevacizumab (Avastin)	VEGF-A	FDA approved for CRC, breast cancer, NSCLC, platinum-resistant ovarian carcinoma, and late-stage cervical cancer
	Ramucirumab IMC-1121B	VEGFR-2 extracellular domain	FDA approved for advanced gastric or gastro-esophageal junction adenocarcinoma; metastatic NSCLC
Soluble decoy receptor	VEGF Trap (Aflibercept)	VEGF-A, VEGF-B and PlGF	FDA approved for metastatic colorectal cancer.
RTKIs	Vandetanib	VEGFR-2, EGFR, and RET	FDA approved for progressive medullary thyroid carcinoma
	Sorafenib (BAY 43-9006)	VEGFR-2 and 3, PDGFR-β, Flt-3, c-Kit, and B-Raf	FDA approved for renal cell, hepatocellular cancers, and metastatic differentiated thyroid carcinoma
	Sunitinib (SU11248)	VEGFR-1, 2, PDGFR, c-Kit, RET, and Flt-3	FDA approved for RCC, gastrointestinal stromal tumors, and neuroendocrine tumors of the pancreas
	Axitinib (AG-013736)	VEGFR-1,2,3, and PDGFR	FDA approved for RCC
	Levantinib (E7080)	VEGFR2,3	FDA approved for thyroid cancer
	BIBF 1120 (Nintedanib)	VEGFR-1,2,3, PDGFR, and FGFR-1/3	Approved by FDA and EU for radiopathic pulmonary fibrosis, Approved by EU for NSCLC
	Pazopanib (GW786034)	VEGFR2	FDA approved for RCC, and soft tissue sarcoma
	Regorafenib (BAY 73-4506)	VEGFR1-3, PDGFR-β, FGFR1- 2, c-Kit, RET, and B-Raf	FDA approved for CRC, HCC, liver cancer, and GIST
	Cabozantinib (XL184)	VEGFR2, MET, RET, AXL, Flt-3, and c-Kit	FDA approved for HCC and MTC

Abbreviations: AML, acute myelogenous leukemia; CRC, colorectal cancer; EGFR, epidermal growth factor receptor; FDA, Food and Drug Administration; EU, European Union; GIST, gastrointestinal stromal tumors; GBM, glioblastoma multiforme; HCC, hepatocellular carcinoma; MTC, metastatic medullary thyroid cancer; NSCLC, non-small-cell lung cancer; PlGF, placental growth factor; PDGFR, platelet-derived growth factor receptor; RCC, renal cell carcinoma; RTKI, small-molecule receptor tyrosine kinase inhibitor; VEGF, vascular endothelial growth factor; VEGFR, vascular endothelial growth factor receptor.

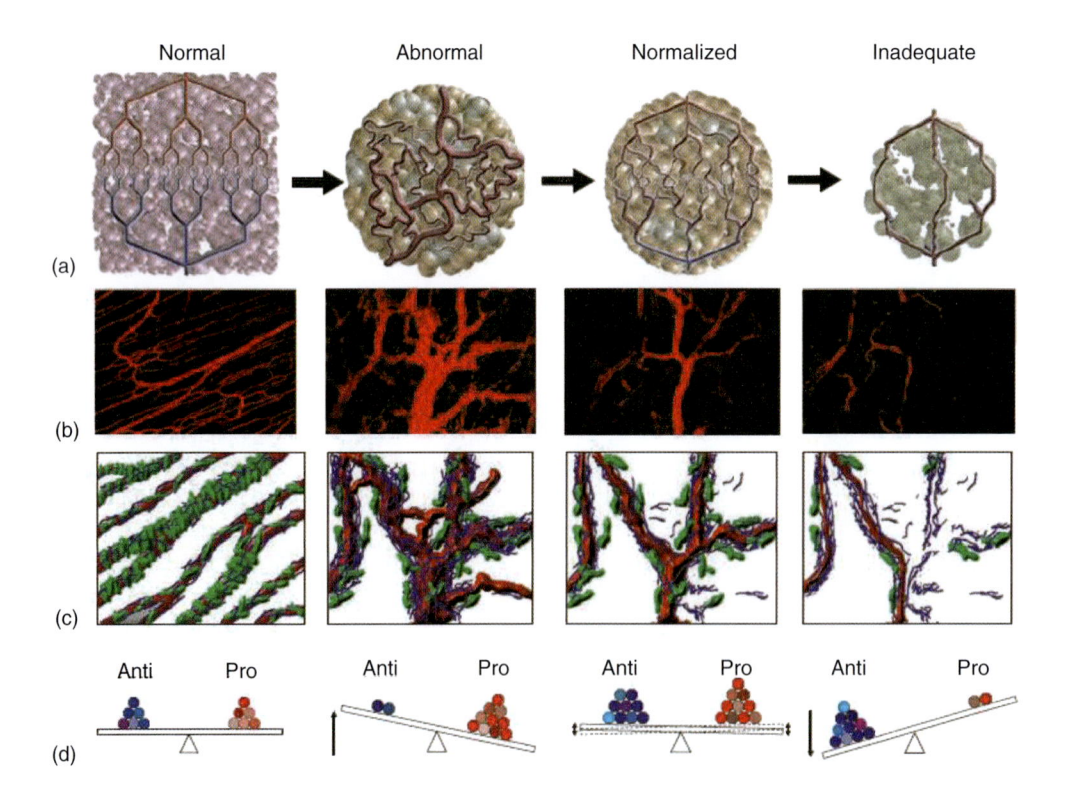

Figure 6 Changes in tumor vasculature during treatment with antiangiogenic agents[231] (a) The tumor vascular network is structurally and functionally abnormal. Antiangiogenic therapies might initially improve both the structure and the function of tumor vessels. Continued or aggressive antiangiogenic regimens may eventually result in a vascular supply that is inadequate to support tumor growth. (b) Vascular normalization due to inhibition of VEGFR2. On the left is a two-photon image depicting normal blood vessels in skeletal muscle; subsequent representative images show human colon carcinoma vasculature in mice at day 0, day 3, and day 5 after treatment with a VEGR2-specific antibody. (c) Diagram illustrating the concomitant changes in basement membrane (blue) and pericyte (red) coverage during vessel normalization. (d) These changes in the vasculature may reflect changes in the balance of pro- and anti-angiogenic factors in the microenvironment. Source: Jain.[231]

Antiangiogenic agents in combination with radiotherapy

Antiangiogenic therapy may enhance the efficacy of radiotherapy for solid tumors. There are several proposed mechanisms through which this enhancement may occur. First, radiotherapy may act by "normalizing" the vasculature as noted above, permitting a more effective delivery of oxygen to tumor tissue, reduction in tumor hypoxia, and augmenting radiation-induced cytotoxicity in part by increasing the formation of oxygen free radicals. This reduction in hypoxia may be transient, however, as prolonged use of antiangiogenic agents may eventually also reduce the "normalized" vessels within tumors resulting in an inadequate vascular supply, such that the tumor would again be hypoxic with reduced radiosensitivity. This concept is supported by mouse xenografts showing the existence of a period of time ("normalization window") during which radiation therapy used in conjunction with an antiangiogenic agent is most effective.[243,247]

While it was initially assumed that the antitumor effect of radiotherapy was due to direct action on tumor cells, more recent evidence has demonstrated that radiotherapy also induces EC apoptosis.[247–250] Thus, the exact mechanism(s) remains unclear. Nevertheless, several preclinical studies demonstrate that antiangiogenic agents can synergize or potentiate the effects of radiotherapy.[251–255] Blockade of VEGF signaling on ECs may render the tumor-associated vasculature more sensitive to radiotherapy. In addition, radiation induces VEGF expression which contributes to radioresistance by blocking radiation-induced EC apoptosis.[256,257]

A cause for concern in testing combinations of antiangiogenic therapy and radiotherapy is the observation from preclinical studies that at least some of the toxicities of radiotherapy such as intestinal radiation damage may also be due to endothelial apoptosis.[258] In lung cancer patients treated with the combination of bevacizumab, chemotherapy, and radiotherapy, trachea-esophageal fistulas have been observed.[259] Additional studies will be needed to assess the feasibility of these combinations.

Antiangiogenic agents in combination with immune checkpoint inhibitors

The development of immune checkpoint blocking strategies to stimulate antitumor immunity has resulted in a major breakthrough in the treatment of multiple solid tumor types. Unfortunately, these therapies are only effective in a proportion of cancer patients, and resistance eventually occurs in the majority of cases. Recent data have shown that a crosstalk exists between the immune system and the vasculature in cancer, whereby tumor angiogenesis blockade can enhance immune effector cell infiltration and decrease immune suppressive signals within the tumor microenvironment, thus improving the efficacy of immunotherapy. Conversely, immune checkpoint inhibitors may also result in an antiangiogenic effect.

Immune checkpoint blockade relies on successful trafficking of antitumor T-lymphocytes into the tumor tissue, which depends on tumor endothelial activation.[260] Such activation generally occurs in response to pro-inflammatory cytokines such as tumor necrosis factor (TNF)α and interleukin (IL)-1, leading to downstream activation of the transcription factor nuclear factor-κB (NF-κB) and upregulation of adhesion molecules, selectins, and chemokines. In cancer, vessels are often poorly activated due to pro-angiogenic signaling in the tumor microenvironment, thus becoming a barrier to efficient leukocyte recruitment.[261]

To illustrate this, it has been shown that VEGF-mediated signaling can directly interfere with TNF-α-induced NF-κB activation.[262] Consistently, VEGFR1 blockade can sensitize ECs to TNF-α.[263] Also related to impaired lymphocyte recruitment is reduced expression of leukocyte adhesion molecules such as E-selectin, intercellular adhesion molecule 1 (ICAM1), ICAM2, and vascular cell adhesion molecule 1 (VCAM1) by tumor ECs, in part as a consequence of upregulation of the NO pathway by angiogenic factors such as VEGFA and fibroblast growth factor 2 (FGF2).[264] T-cell trafficking into the tumor is also dysfunctional owing to the tortuous, structurally altered, and leaky vessels that result from imbalances between pro- and antiangiogenic factors in the tumor microenvironment.

Proangiogenic molecules bind cognate receptors expressed by immune cells and may also affect them directly. Among those molecules, VEGF has been found to inhibit the innate immune system by hampering the differentiation of monocytes into mature dendritic cells and by upregulating PD-L1 expression on dendritic cells.[265,266] Tumor hypoxia, VEGF, and other proangiogenic factors such as IL-8 have additionally been shown to recruit and increase the presence of myeloid-derived immunosuppressive cells and regulatory T cells in the tumor microenvironment, and to block differentiation of progenitor cells into CD8+ and CD4+ T cells, thus maintaining an immunosuppressive context and negatively affecting responses to antiangiogenic and immune checkpoint inhibitor treatments.[267–272] Consistent with these findings, drugs targeting VEGF and Ang2 signaling have been observed to enhance responses to immune checkpoint antibodies in preclinical tumor models.[273,274] Yet only recently it was found that immune cell stimulation can also promote normalization of tumor vessels, as shown by reduced tumor vascular density, improved vessel perfusion, and decreased tumor tissue hypoxia (Figure 7).[275,276]

Together, the increasing evidence supporting a positive reciprocal interaction between the tumor vasculature and immune cells suggests that combining antiangiogenic agents with immune checkpoint inhibitors will result in increased clinical efficacy.[277] It is important to note that most of the promising data regarding these combinations has been generated in RCC, a tumor with both high angiogenic and immunogenic drives.

Clinical advances in the use of antiangiogenic therapy

The hypothesis that tumor angiogenesis could serve as a target for cancer therapy is now strongly supported by results of a number of randomized Phase III clinical trials across multiple different tumor types. Bevacizumab, a monoclonal antibody targeting VEGF, is now a standard therapy for metastatic colorectal, NSCLC, and other tumor types[278,279]; VEGFR TKIs such as sunitinib, pazopanib, axitinib, sorafenib, lenvatinib, cabozantinib, and regorafenib are now approved for RCC or other diseases (Table 2). These advances, coupled with our increased understanding of the biological pathways underlying tumor angiogenesis and the development of improved agents for targeting these pathways, have led to a dramatic increase in the number of clinical trials employing antiangiogenic therapy either alone or in combination with other therapeutic modalities. Currently, the majority of these agents target the VEGF pathway because of its role as a key regulator of tumor angiogenesis.

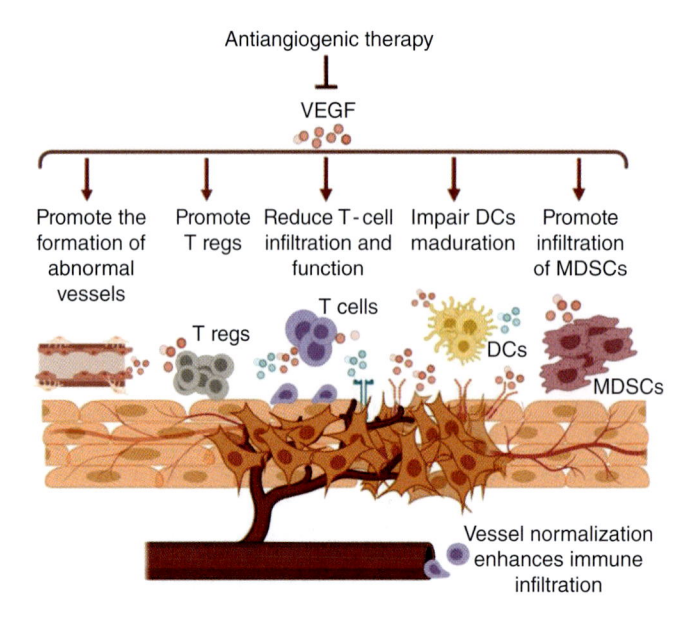

Figure 7 Combination of anti-angiogenic agents and immune checkpoint blockade therapies. Antiangiogenic therapies result in a normalization of tumor vasculature that may enhance the delivery of immunotherapy agents. Also, VEGF is known to be a key regulator of the immunosuppressive microenvironment. VEGF reduces lymphocyte infiltration into tumors and diminishes the proliferation of T-cells while enhancing T regs and myeloid-derived suppressor cells (MDSCs). VEGF also plays a role in impairing dendritic cell maturation. Anti-VEGF therapies may restore immune function and the combination of these agents with immunotherapy is currently under investigation in several clinical studies for different tumor malignancies.

VEGF pathway inhibitors as anticancer therapy: clinical experience

Clinical trials of one of the earliest VEGF pathway inhibitors, bevacizumab, began in 1997. When used as monotherapy for the treatment of advanced solid tumors, the clinical activity of these agents, as judged by objective tumor responses, has generally been low with the exception of RCC. For example, no partial or complete remissions were observed in 25 patients treated in a Phase I trial of bevacizumab.[280] Low response rates have also been reported for VEGFR TKIs when used as single agents as discussed below. For this reason, VEGF pathway inhibitors have often been developed as part of combination regimen with chemotherapy or other targeted therapeutics. Major findings in the clinical development of VEGF pathway inhibitors for several common tumor types are reviewed below.

Renal cell cancer

One tumor type for which VEGF pathway inhibitors are particularly useful, even when used as monotherapy, is metastatic RCC. These tumors are often marked by inactivation of the VHL gene leading to overexpression of VEGF and other angiogenesis mediators (reviewed in Ref. [281]). In randomized studies, bevacizumab, sorafenib, and pazopanib were shown to significantly prolong time to progression compared to placebo controls.[282–284] Sunitinib, axitinib, tivozanib, and cabozantinib also demonstrated substantial antitumor activity in metastatic RCC, with 17–45% objective response rate (ORR) in Phase III testing.[285–289]

After initial Phase II trials suggested the potential for therapeutic activity in renal cell cancers, Phase III trials evaluated anti-VEGF therapies either alone or in combination with other targeted or biological agents. Cytokine therapies (interferon-alfa- and interleukin-2-based therapies) had long been the mainstay of therapy for renal cell cancers, so it was rational to evaluate anti-VEGF therapy in the context of such agents. Phase III trials examining small-molecule TKIs of VEGF receptors as well as monoclonal anti-VEGF therapy were reported, and consistently favored the use of anti-VEGF therapy compared to interferon.[288,290] Based on these findings, VEGFR TKIs became standard frontline and following treatments for advanced RCC as single agents.

More recently, knowledge on the role of the immune system in the progression of specific solid tumors and the development of immune checkpoint inhibitors targeting immune escape mechanisms caused a paradigm shift in the treatment approach for advanced kidney cancer. The combination of immunotherapy with monoclonal antibodies directed against programmed cell death 1 protein (PD-1) and VEGFR TKIs has become standard of care frontline treatment for patients with metastatic RCC.

Trials comparing anti-VEGF therapy for frontline treatment

Three studies compared VEGFR TKIs directly. Motzer and colleagues evaluated the use of sunitinib (at a dose of 50 mg orally daily for 4 weeks, followed by 2 weeks without treatment) versus pazopanib (800 mg oral daily)[289] in a multicenter Phase III trial. Progression-free survival (PFS) (the primary endpoint) data revealed that pazopanib was noninferior to sunitinib (median 8.4 vs 9.5 months, hazard ratio for progression of disease or death from any cause, 1.05; 95% confidence interval 0.90–1.22), but quality of life parameters (a secondary endpoint) favored pazopanib. Hutson et al. performed another randomized Phase III comparing axitinib (5 mg oral twice a day) with sorafenib (400 mg oral twice a day).[291] Treatment with axitinib resulted in no difference in the primary endpoint of PFS (10 vs 6.5 months) but a higher ORR (32 vs 15%). In the Phase II CABOSUN trial, the VEGF receptor, cMET, and AXL tyrosine kinase inhibitor cabozantinib (60 mg oral daily) was compared with sunitinib (50 mg/day oral for 4 weeks on each 6-week cycle) in patients with intermediate- or high-risk metastatic RCC.[286] PFS, the primary endpoint of the trial, was significantly prolonged with cabozantinib (median 8.6 vs 5.3 months, hazard ratio 0.48, 95% confidence interval 0.31–0.74).

Cabozantinib also resulted in higher ORR (20% vs 9%) and longer OS (median 26.6 vs 21.2 months), but the difference did not reach statistical significance (hazard ratio 0.80, 95% confidence interval 0.53–1.21).

Trials comparing anti-VEGF in combination with anti-PD-1 immune checkpoint inhibition for frontline treatment

The combination of axitinib (5 mg oral twice a day) with the monoclonal anti-PD-1 antibody pembrolizumab (200 mg intravenously once every 3 weeks) was compared to sunitinib (50 mg orally once daily for the first 4 weeks of each 6-week cycle) in previously untreated patients in the Phase III KEYNOTE-426 clinical trial.[292] Axitinib plus pembrolizumab resulted in statistically significant improvements in OS (82% vs 72% at 18 months, hazard ratio 0.53, 95% confidence interval 0.38–0.74) and PFS (15.1 months vs 11.1 months, hazard ratio 0.69, 95% confidence interval 0.57–0.84), the two primary endpoints. Treatment-related toxicities were comparable between the two treatment arms. Together with the combination of the immune checkpoint inhibitors ipilimumab and nivolumab,[293] axitinib plus pembrolizumab has become a preferred initial treatment regimen for patients with advanced RCC, regardless of risk stratification (even if in patients with good prognosis sunitinib as single-agent results in similar survival outcomes). Axitinib was also tested in combination with the programmed death-ligand 1 antibody avelumab and compared to sunitinib in the Phase III JAVELIN Renal 101 trial.[294] Axitinib plus avelumab resulted in improved PFS (median 13.8 vs 8.4 months, hazard ratio 0.69, 95% confidence interval 0.56–0.84) and higher overall response rate (51% vs 26%). However, the combination did not show improvement in OS (hazard ratio 0.78, 95% confidence interval 0.55–1.08).

Therapy following initial anti-VEGF treatment

The demonstration of a beneficial effect for anti-VEGF therapy in renal cell cancer fundamentally altered the treatment landscape for this disease. Nevertheless, anti-VEGF therapy is not curative and in general only modestly prolongs survival, leaving room for substantial therapeutic improvement. Patients progressing on one VEGF-targeting agent may still respond to another.[295–297] Whether this cross-sensitivity is a function of the promiscuity of RTKIs, of differential pharmacokinetics, or of varying affinities for VEGF receptors, is unknown.

Antiangiogenic therapy as adjuvant therapy in renal cell cancer

The advent of multiple active antiangiogenic agents led to the development of several adjuvant studies in renal cell cancer at risk for recurrence after surgery. Sunitinib, sorafenib, pazopanib, and axitinib all failed to demonstrate a recurrence-free survival advantage relative to placebo in corresponding Phase III clinical trials[298–300] with the exception of one study, S-TRAC, in which sunitinib (50 mg per day on a 4-weeks-on, 2-weeks-off schedule) for 1 year significantly increased disease-free survival (median 6.8 vs 5.6 years, hazard ratio 0.76, 95% confidence interval 0.59–0.95) at the cost of higher rates of significant side-effects including diarrhea, palmar–plantar erythrodysesthesia, hypertension, fatigue, and nausea.[301] However, sunitinib has not shown an OS benefit in any patient subgroup.

Prediction of therapeutic benefit in renal cell cancer

It has been established that relatively high VEGF levels are associated with worse tumor stage and grade, performance status, and overall prognosis.[302,303] Moreover, in a Phase III trial of sorafenib versus placebo, patients with VEGF in the highest concentration quartile obtained greater relative benefit from sorafenib than those with lower concentrations.[304] However, analyses addressing whether VEGF is a predictive marker for identifying RCC patients who are likely to benefit from VEGF-targeted therapies have yielded inconsistent results.[305] A study in samples from two subsequent Phase II and III studies identified interleukin-6 (IL-6) as predictive of PFS benefit from pazopanib versus placebo.[306] Unfortunately, no biomarkers that are predictive of differential benefit between available and active drugs in RCC have yet to be validated.

Colorectal cancer

Advanced colorectal cancer represented the first human cancer in which a Phase III trial demonstrated clinical benefit, and to this day represents among the best studied of human solid tumors with regard to antiangiogenic therapy. In 2004, results of a Phase III, randomized, placebo-controlled study were reported comparing standard IFL chemotherapy (irinotecan, fluorouracil, and leucovorin) with or without bevacizumab in patients with previously untreated metastatic colorectal cancer.[278] Patients treated with IFL plus bevacizumab had a significantly longer OS and PFS as well a higher ORR. This trial provided definitive evidence that the addition of an angiogenesis inhibitor to chemotherapy could prolong survival and, based on the results of this trial, bevacizumab received approval from the FDA for use in combination with fluorouracil-containing chemotherapy as first-line treatment for metastatic colorectal cancer.

Subsequent studies have built upon this original finding. In a trial of previously treated patients with colorectal cancer, patients treated with bevacizumab combined with FOLFOX4 chemotherapy had a prolonged survival compared to those treated with FOLFOX4 alone,[307] although the magnitude of this benefit (2.1 months) appeared to be smaller than that observed in the first-line trial (4.7 months), presumably related to the more advanced nature of the disease.

First-line studies of bevacizumab or placebo in combination with either FOLFOX or XELOX failed to demonstrate an improvement in OS (21.3 vs 19.9 months) despite improvements in PFS (9.4 vs 8.0 months).[308] The mechanism for the discrepancy between this study and the pivotal IFL study has been attributed to the different cytotoxic backbone or practice patterns of treatment until progression of disease versus regimen interruptions for cumulative oxaliplatin toxicities. Several studies have evaluated the role of bevacizumab after an initial course of oxaliplatin- and fluoropyrimidine-based first-line chemotherapy. These "maintenance" regimens have demonstrated the benefit of bevacizumab when combined with fluoropyrimidines. The CAIRO-3 randomized study demonstrated that continued bevacizumab either alone or in combination with capecitabine provided a survival benefit compared to observation alone.

Cohort studies had suggested a benefit from continued VEGF inhibition after progression on first-line therapy with bevacizumab. The TML study evaluated second-line therapy with FOLFIRI or FOLFOX (as determined by the treating physician) with or without bevacizumab for patients who had previously progressed on first-line bevacizumab-containing regimen. The study demonstrated a modest but statistically significant survival advantage of 1.4 months, resulting in the addition of bevacizumab continuation to treatment guidelines.

A similar study was conducted with ziv-aflibercept, a fusion protein utilizing the extracellular domains of VEGFR1 and VEGFR2, thereby providing inhibition of both VEGF-A and PlGF. Patients who had been previously treated with an oxaliplatin regimen (which may have included bevacizumab) were randomized to FOLFIRI with bevacizumab or placebo.[309] The primary endpoint of OS was met with a 1.4-month improvement (13.5 months vs 12.1 months), with an improvement in PFS and response rate. Grade 3 and 4 diarrhea and stomatitis were substantially higher in the ziv-aflibercept arm, consistent with the established role for PlGF in mucosal lining repair.[310]

An addition agent, ramucirumab, demonstrated activity in second line when combined with FOLFIRI in a Phase III study (RAISE).[311] Ramucirumab, a monoclonal antibody that binds VEGFR2 at the N-terminus and prevents ligand binding and receptor confirmational changes,[312] was identified from phage display library and is notable for its picomolar binding affinity to VEGFR2.[313,314] Median OS was improved by 1.6 months with the addition of ramucirumab, with increased rates of neutropenia, hypertension, and fatigue. As a result of these studies, three antiangiogenic agents are available for use in the second-line setting in combination with chemotherapy for patients who have previously progressed on bevacizumab-based first-line regimens.

Biomarker analyses of colorectal cancer trials have been largely unavailing. Expression levels of VEGF-A, TSP, and microvessel density performed in a subset analysis of the original Hurwitz trial were not associated with clinical outcome.[315] Similarly, analysis of oncogenes known to play a role in colorectal cancer (e.g., K-Ras, b-raf, and p53) failed to demonstrate an association with clinical outcome.[316] VEGF-D has been associated with outcomes from ramucirumab in the RAISE study, although validation is required.[317] As in metastatic breast cancer, the presence of clinically significant hypertension has been associated with clinical outcome in a Phase II trial analysis.[318]

Though monoclonal antibodies are the best-studied antiangiogenic agents in advanced colorectal cancer, TKIs with various selectivity for VEGFRs have also been examined in randomized Phase III trials. A notable initial randomized Phase III trial compared FOLFOX4 chemotherapy alone or in combination with the oral small-molecule RTKI vatalanib (PTK787) as first-line therapy for metastatic colorectal cancer. This study failed to demonstrate improvements in PFS or OS.[319] Similar studies with sunitinib and cediranib, among others, have failed to demonstrate a benefit. The outlier is the approval of regorafenib, a multikinase inhibitor that inhibits VEGFR, which has been shown to improve OS by 1.4 months when compared to placebo in the CORRECT study.[320] Fruquitinib, a potent VEGFR TKI approved in China in refractory disease, is in late-stage studies as a single agent in the United States. While toxicities are generally higher with TKIs, the reason for the general success of large molecule inhibitors and limited success of TKIs in combination with chemotherapy is not known.

Gastric and gastroesophageal junction cancer

Antiangiogenic therapy for advanced gastric cancer was initially evaluated in the AVAGAST study, which evaluated bevacizumab in first-line therapy in combination with cisplatin-capecitabine.[321] Despite improvements in PFS and response rate, there was no difference in OS, and further development of bevacizumab in gastric or gastroesophageal junction (GEJ) cancer has not been pursued.

In contrast, a second line study of 355 patients with gastric or GEJ adenocarcinoma demonstrated benefit of ramucirumab compared to placebo, leading to US FDA approval. A pivotal trial (the REGARD study) demonstrated a survival benefit of second-line ramucirumab when compared to placebo, with median OS of 5.2 months compared to 3.8 months.[322] The agent was well tolerated with modestly higher risk of grade 3 hypertension (8% vs 3%) but no increased risk for thromboembolic events.

Two additional studies were subsequently conducted to further evaluate the role of antiangiogenic therapy in advanced gastroesophageal cancer. As the clinical practice for many oncologists is to provide cytotoxic chemotherapy in second line, the RAINBOW trial was designed to evaluate the addition of ramucirumab or placebo to paclitaxel in patients who had previously progressed on first-line platinum and fluoropyrimidine-based chemotherapy.[323] This 655-patient international study met its primary endpoint with improved OS (9.6 vs 7.3 months). A subgroup analysis found that the survival benefit was notably higher in Caucasian patients than in Asian sites. The same regional differences were seen in the AVAGAST study, suggesting differences in disease biology or treatment patterns between Asian and Caucasian patients. The potential biological mechanism, if any, for this discrepancy is currently awaited.

VEGFR TKIs have likewise been evaluated in gastric cancer. Sunitinib was evaluated in second line in a randomized study of docetaxel with placebo or sunitinib. This smaller Phase II study failed to demonstrate an improvement in time to progression or OS, despite a meaningful increase in response rate (41% vs 14%).[324] In contrast, the VEGFR TKI apatinib, at two different doses, was evaluated in a randomized Phase III study in patients progressing on two or more lines of prior therapy. Both doses of afatinib demonstrated benefit compared to placebo in PFS (1.4 vs 3.7/3.2 months) and OS (2.5 vs 4.8/4.3 months).[325] Toxicities included hypertension and hand-foot syndrome, consistent with the mechanism of action for the agent.

Non-small-cell lung cancer (NSCLC)

Angiogenesis inhibitors as single agents for advanced NSCLC
When tested as monotherapy for advanced NSCLC, inhibitors directed at VEGF have generally led to low rates of objective tumor responses. In a Phase II trial of chemotherapy with or without bevacizumab, 19 patients in the control arm received high-dose, single-agent bevacizumab on progression, and although five had disease stabilization, there were no objective responses.[326] VEGFR TKIs have demonstrated clear evidence of antitumor activity as single agents in NSCLC, although to date there are no studies demonstrating that they prolong OS compared to chemotherapy or other targeted agents.

Vandetanib, a dual VEGFR/EGFR inhibitor, was tested in a Phase III study testing the efficacy of vandetanib compared to standard second-line erlotinib (ZEST). No significant improvement in PFS was detected for patients treated with vandetanib versus erlotinib (median PFS of 2.6 vs 2.0 months). In a noninferiority analysis, both agents showed similar PFS and OS.[327]

Pazopanib, a TKI targeting VEGFRs, PDGFRs, FGFR-1, and FGFR-3, has produced encouraging responses as neoadjuvant therapy in patients with stage I/II NSCLC,[328] with tolerable toxicity profile including hypertension, diarrhea, and fatigue. Other VEGFR TKIs that have demonstrated single-agent activity in advanced NSCLC include sunitinib,[329] vatalanib (PTK787), axitinib (AG-013736),[330] and XL647.[331]

Bevacizumab with chemotherapy for advanced NSCLC
In initial Phase II testing in chemo-naïve, advanced NSCLC patients suggested that bevacizumab improved ORR and time to

progression when added to the standard doublet chemotherapy regimen of carboplatin and paclitaxel (CP).[326] This study also revealed an unanticipated and concerning side effect: severe pulmonary hemorrhage, which was fatal in 4 of 67 patients who received bevacizumab and was associated with central tumor location, proximity to major blood vessels, necrosis and cavitation before or during therapy, and squamous histology. This is discussed in more detail below.

Based on the promising outcomes with bevacizumab in this Phase II trial, a randomized Phase II/III trial was conducted by the Eastern Cooperative Oncology Group (ECOG), E4599, comparing standard CP for six cycles versus CP plus bevacizumab (BCP) in 878 patients with previously untreated, advanced (stage IIIB or IV) nonsquamous NSCLC.[279] Patients receiving BCP had a significantly improved median OS (12.3 vs 10.3 months, HR 0.77, $p = 0.003$) and PFS (6.2 vs 4.5 months, $p < 0.0001$) compared to CP alone. The main grade 3 or higher toxicities associated with bevacizumab were clinically significant bleeding (4.4% vs 0.7% in the standard chemotherapy arm), and hypertension. The overall rate of fatal hemoptysis with bevacizumab when squamous histology was excluded was approximately 1%. This risk can be viewed in light of the absolute improvements in survival of 7% and 8% at 1 and 2 years, respectively.

More recently, the IMPOWER150 randomized Phase III study tested the standard BCP regimen versus BCP plus the PD-L1 inhibitor atezolizumab (ABCP) or ACP in metastatic nonsquamous NSCLC patients with wild-type EGFR and ALK.[332] The median OS was improved in the ABCP group versus the BCP group (19.2 vs 14.7 months; HR for OS, 0.78; $p = 0.02$). Based on these findings, ABCP has been FDA approved for the first-line treatment in this setting.

Ramucirumab with chemotherapy for refractory NSCLC

Ramucirumab is FDA approved for the treatment of relapsed NSCLC patients in combination with second-line docetaxel. In the Phase III REVEL trial of metastatic NSCLC patients who had experienced disease progression after treatment with platinum-based chemotherapy for locally advanced or metastatic disease,[333] an improved median OS was observed in the docetaxel plus ramucirumab arm compared with the placebo plus docetaxel arm (10.5 vs 9.1 months; HR 0.857; $p = 0.0235$). Patients in the ramucirumab group experienced more hypertension and bleeding/hemorrhage events of any grade compared with patients in the placebo group, but the rate of grade 3 or higher bleeding events was similar among the two groups.

VEGFR TKIs with chemotherapy for recurrent NSCLC

Vandetanib has been evaluated in combination with docetaxel for patients previously treated with platinum-containing chemotherapy.[334] About 127 patients were randomized to receive docetaxel with either low dose (100 mg once daily) or high dose (300 mg once daily) vandetanib. This study met its primary endpoint of prolonged median PFS in the vandetanib arm, although a trend toward greater benefit was observed in the low dose arm. In a randomized, Phase III trial of vandetanib 100 mg daily with docetaxel versus docetaxel (ZODIAC), the primary endpoint was achieved, with a prolongation in PFS in the vandetanib arm (PFS HR = 0.79, $p < 0.001$). This did not translate into significantly improved OS.[335] A biomarker analysis from this study suggested that patients with EGFR copy number gains had greater benefit from the addition of vandetanib.[336]

Nintedanib (BIBF1120) was tested in a randomized Phase III trial comparing docetaxel combined with either nintedanib or placebo for platinum-refractory NSCLC patients (LUME-Lung-1) PFS was prolonged in the nintedanib arm compared with the placebo arm, regardless of histology (HR 0.79; $p = 0.0019$; squamous HR 0.77, $p = 0.02$; adeno HR 0.77, $p = 0.0019$). Based on these results, nintedanib has received approval in the European Union (EU) for NSCLC. Furthermore, it is approved by the FDA and in the EU for the treatment of idiopathic pulmonary fibrosis on the basis of two randomized Phase III trials[337,338] and systemic sclerosis-associated interstitial lung disease (SSc-ILD).[339] The efficacy of nintedanib was also under investigation for the treatment of malignant pleural mesothelioma (LUME-Meso) but the Phase III trial did not meet its primary endpoint 2018.[340,341] Similarly, nintedanib has been studied in combination with chemotherapy in the neoadjuvant NSCLC setting but the results of a recent study showed that nintedanib plus chemotherapy did not increase benefit when compared to chemotherapy historical controls in the neoadjuvant setting.[342] Currently, nintedanib is being evaluated for radiotherapy-induced fibrosis and other approaches are being explored, such as the combinations of nintedanib with immunotherapy for NSCLC.

Antiangiogenic VEGF pathway inhibitors agents in combination with other EGFR targeted therapies for EGFR mutant NSCLC

EGFR activating mutations occur in 12–15% of NSCLC cases in the United States and 30–40% in Asia. EGFR tyrosine kinase inhibitors are the mainstay of treatment for these patients. Although EGFR inhibitors are initially effective, resistance inevitably emerges. Dual blockade of the EGFR and VEGF pathways is being studied clinically as these pathways are interrelated. VEGF is downregulated by EGFR inhibition, likely through both HIF-α dependent and independent mechanisms,[197,218,220,221,343–345] and EGFR, like VEGFR-2, may be expressed on tumor-associated endothelium.[346–348] Acquired resistance to the EGFR inhibitor was found to be associated with increased VEGF levels and increased tumor angiogenesis in preclinical studies.[349]

Several clinical trials have evaluated VEGF pathway inhibition in combination with EGFR inhibitors in NSCLC patients in patients with EGFR mutations. The randomized Phase II JO25567 trial evaluated the EGFR inhibitor erlotinib plus bevacizumab versus erlotinib alone as first-line treatment in 154 patients with advanced EGFR-mutant NSCLC.[350] PFS was significantly improved in the combination arm (median PFS 16.0 months) versus erlotinib alone (median PFS 9.7 months) with a HR of 0.54 ($p = 0015$). Similar improvements in PFS for EGFR mutant patients treated with bevacizumab plus erlotinib compared to erlotinib alone were observed in the Phase II NEJ026 trial.[351] The Phase III RELAY study evaluated erlotinib plus ramucirumab versus erlotinib plus placebo in 449 NSCLC patients.[352] A superior PFS was observed for the ramucirumab plus erlotinib arm as compared to the placebo plus erlotinib arm (median PFS 19.4 vs 12.4 months; HR: 0.59; $p < 0.0001$). Moreover, the addition of ramucirumab improved the durability of response (18 vs 11.1 months; $p = 0.0003$). Based on these findings, the combination of ramucirumab plus erlotinib was approved as first-line therapy for EGFR mutant NSCLC. The molecular basis underlying the greater sensitivity of the EGFR-mutant subgroup to VEGF pathway inhibition is not completely understood but may be related to EGFR driving HIF-1α expression resulting in increased VEGF dependence.[221] Together these data support the use of combined VEGF and EGFR inhibition in patients bearing EGFR mutations.

Antiangiogenic therapy for operable NSCLC

The use of angiogenesis inhibitors in the neoadjuvant or adjuvant setting is also being investigated in NSCLC patients with operable disease. In one preoperative trial, the VEGFR TKI pazopanib was found to have significant antitumor activity, with 87% of patients demonstrating a reduction in tumor volume.[353] A Phase III randomized trial testing the addition of bevacizumab to platinum-based chemotherapy in early-stage resected NSCLC (ECOG1505), did not show improved survival in this setting.[354]

Breast cancer

Antiangiogenic agents in breast cancer have failed to reproducibly demonstrate improvements in OS in metastatic disease, and no agents are currently FDA approved. Bevacizumab received accelerated approval in 2008 on the basis of a randomized study of paclitaxel with or without bevacizumab in previously untreated women with metastatic HER2-negative breast cancer.[355] This study demonstrated statistically significant improvements in response rate (37% vs 21%), but no difference in OS. The accelerated approval was conditional on further evidence of improved survival from additional studies. The AVADO study of docetaxel with or without bevacizumab saw similarly improved response rates and PFS, but no improvements in OS in HER-2 negative patients.[356] The RIBBON-1 study of chemotherapy with or without bevacizumab produced similar incremental benefits in response rates and PFS without improved OS.[357] A study in the HER2-positive population of docetaxel, trastuzumab, with or without bevacizumab improved response rates (66% vs 77%) but failed to improve PFS or OS.[358] On the basis of the available data, the FDA revoked the agency's approval of bevacizumab for breast cancer in 2011. Similarly disappointing results were seen in the ROSE study, which evaluated ramucirumab in combination with docetaxel, and failed to demonstrate an improvement in PFS.[359] Analyses of the AVADO study demonstrated that high VEGF-A plasma levels may be predictive of benefit from bevacizumab.[360]

Hepatoma

Hepatoma (hepatocellular carcinoma, HCC) is an important cancer on a global basis and has been characterized by remarkably poor prognosis and few active agents. The advent of antiangiogenic therapy has reinvigorated therapeutic attacks on hepatoma.

In a randomized placebo-controlled Phase III trial, sorafenib prolonged OS compared with control (5.5 vs 2.5 months).[361] The RESORCE study investigated regorafenib for the treatment of patients with HCC who have progressed with the drug sorafenib.[362] They reported median OS for patients taking regorafenib of 10.6 months, compared to 7.8 of the placebo group. Regorafenib was FDA approved for HCC or liver cancer in 2017. More recently cabozantinib (inhibitor of cMET and VEGFR2 tyrosine kinases between others) received also FDA approval for patients with HCC who have been previously treated with sorafenib thanks to the positive results of the CELESTIAL trial.[363]

Other malignancies

Antiangiogenic therapies (particularly anti-VEGF therapies) have been examined in numerous other human malignancies, with initial positive results (and a few signal failures) in several cancers. Many of these approaches are discussed elsewhere in this book and will be summarized only briefly here.

Pancreatic cancer

A large Phase III trial comparing gemcitabine plus bevacizumab versus gemcitabine plus placebo was reported as a negative trial. Pancreatic cancer continues to elude our best therapeutic efforts.

Soft-tissue sarcoma

In 2012, the FDA approved pazopanib for the treatment of metastatic nonadipocytic soft tissue sarcoma following positive results from the Phase III PALETTE clinical study (NCT 00753688).[364]

Ovarian cancer

In the Phase III AURELIA clinical study, the addition of bevacizumab to chemotherapy significantly improved PFS and ORR in platinum-resistant ovarian cancer patients, prompting FDA approval in 2014.[365]

Cervical cancer

Results from a Phase III trial (GOG 240) testing the efficacy of bevacizumab and nonplatinum combination chemotherapy in patients with advanced cervical cancer led to the FDA approval of bevacizumab to treat patients with persistent, recurrent, or late-stage cervical cancer.[366]

Glioblastoma

While early clinical studies testing the efficacy of bevacizumab in patients with glioblastoma appeared promising,[367,368] in further Phase III testing, bevacizumab did not improve OS in patients with newly diagnosed glioblastoma.[369] Based in part on data from the Phase II BRAIN study testing bevacizumab alone and in combination with irinotecan,[367] and the BELOB trial investigating combination of bevacizumab plus lomustine in patients with recurrent glioblastoma[370] bevacizumab was approved by the FDA for use in glioblastoma. Data from the Phase III EORTC 26101 study demonstrated that the treatment with lomustine plus bevacizumab did not confer a survival advantage over lomustine alone in patients with progressive glioblastoma.[371] The Phase III study (REGAL) testing the efficacy of cediranib as monotherapy or in combination with lomustine versus lomustine alone in patients with recurrent glioblastoma was also negative.[372]

Glioma

Several Phase II trials of anti-VEGF therapy as monotherapy have suggested that bevacizumab has therapeutic activity in advanced gliomas. These promising results have led to a submission to the FDA for accelerated approval and to the development of a proof-of-concept Phase III trials. A Phase II trial of aflibercept conducted by the North American Brain Tumor Consortium (NABTC) showed only modest results in recurrent high-grade gliomas (HGG).[373]

Non-Hodgkin's lymphoma

Positive early results for anti-VEGF therapy have been reported from several Phase II trials, and have led to the development of Phase III trials, which are ongoing.

Toxicities of antiangiogenic therapy

Angiogenesis inhibitors have been developed with the hope that they would provide a relatively nontoxic means prevent tumor growth that could be used over long periods of time, toward the goal of converting cancer into a manageable, chronic condition.

To date, it appears that they do have a generally favorable side effect profile that is nonoverlapping with chemotherapy. Certain toxicities have emerged, however, that appear to be specific to entire classes of agents and, in some cases, potentially life-threatening.

Pure VEGF antagonists (e.g., bevacizumab) offer an important window into the physiologic and pathophysiologic effects of VEGF blockade. Agents that combine VEGF blockade with blockade of other kinases (e.g., sorafenib and sunitinib) add side effects specific to the kinases blocked. The availability of multiple Phase III trials allows us to gauge these toxicities across large populations, while smaller studies have focused on individual toxic effects. In this section, we will focus on toxicities that are VEGF-related and mechanistic in nature (i.e., a function of a ligand–receptor interaction in a normal tissue organ).

Hypertension

The most commonly reported toxicity in patients receiving anti-VEGF therapies is hypertension. It is generally mild-to-moderate in nature, though very rarely severe (malignant) hypertension has been reported. Hypertension is thought to be related to alterations in endothelial function related to blockade of the NO pathway downstream from the VEGF receptor.[374] In contrast to anti-VEGF therapy, VEGF infusions are associated with decreases in blood pressure. Management of anti-VEGF-related hypertension appears responsive to standard antihypertensive agents and is reversible upon discontinuation of anti-VEGF therapy. For patients experiencing mild-to-moderate degrees of hypertension, anti-VEGF therapy may be continued in the presence of appropriate antihypertensive therapy. Recent data suggest that the presence of hypertension may be associated with improved outcome, and as such hypertension may represent a type of pharmacokinetic or pharmacodynamic surrogate biomarker of response.[375,376] The E2100 Phase III breast cancer trial demonstrated a relationship between hypertension and particular single nucleotide polymorphisms for VEGF, though this finding awaits and requires confirmation.[377] Analysis of data derived from six Phase II trials evaluating axitinib in patients with various solid tumor types indicated the potential role of diastolic blood pressure >90 mmHg as biomarker of prolonged survival.[378] Prospective studies to validate hypertension as a reliable biomarker of response in clinical practice are warranted.

Arterial thromboembolic events

An increased incidence of thromboembolic and cardiovascular events has been observed in some but not all clinical trials of VEGF inhibitors. These events, while uncommon, may be serious and life threatening. Data pooled from five Phase III trials with bevacizumab (all of which excluded patients with recent history of stroke or heart attack) demonstrated a HR of 2.0 for such events, with an increase in absolute risk from 1.7% in control patients to 3.8% in bevacizumab-treated patients. There was no associated increase in venous thromboembolic events. Cerebrovascular ischemia reported with bevacizumab may involve either transient ischemic attacks or stroke; myocardial infarction and angina have also been reported to occur with increased frequency.[379] These toxicities are more common in the elderly (age >65) and in patients with a prior history of arterial thromboembolic events. Management of these complications is similar to those in patients not receiving anti-VEGF therapy. In contrast to hypertension, which is generally readily managed with antihypertensive therapy, discontinuation of VEGF-targeted therapy in the presence of arterial thromboembolic events seems appropriate.

Reversible posterior leukoencephalopathy syndrome (RPLS)

Reversible posterior leukoencephalopathy syndrome (RPLS) is a rare central nervous system complication of anti-VEGF therapy. RPLS is a subacute neurologic syndrome typically consisting of headache, cortical blindness, and seizures, and has been reported anecdotally in patients receiving VEGF-targeting therapy. The etiology of RPLS is not well understood at present, nor is its relationship to VEGF inhibition; though it has been suggested that vasospasm of the posterior cerebral arteries may be important. Immediate cessation of anti-VEGF therapy and appropriate antihypertensive management (a potential predisposing factor) are indicated.[380,381]

Nephrotoxicity

Nephrotoxicity, in the form of proteinuria, is common in patients receiving prolonged anti-VEGF therapy with as many as 40% of patients having at least some degree of proteinuria. More severe protein loss (e.g., nephrotic syndrome) is rare, occurring in approximately 1–2% of patients. While not well studied, proteinuria is reversible when anti-VEGF therapy is held, and patients may be re-challenged. A standard approach has been to discontinue bevacizumab temporarily if urine protein excretion is $\geq 2\,g/24\,h$ and resume when protein excretion is $<2\,g/24\,h$. Bevacizumab treatment should be discontinued if nephrotic-range proteinuria develops. VEGF is important in renal glomerular homeostasis, so the renal effects of anti-VEGF therapy are perhaps unsurprising.[382] Bevacizumab-induced proteinuria is associated with renal thrombotic microangiopathy, suggesting that VEGF plays a critical role in protection against this condition.[383]

Pulmonary hemorrhage

Pulmonary hemorrhage was reported in the initial Phase II trial of lung cancer patients, where fatal hemorrhagic events were observed.[326] This trial suggested that patients with squamous cell cancer histology were at increased risk for this complication, and were excluded from the Phase III NSCLC trial E4599. Despite these exclusions, the rate of life-threatening pulmonary hemorrhage was 1.9% (with 1.2% fatal events), suggesting that we remain imperfect at predicting which patients will experience this complication.[279] The discussion of pulmonary hemorrhagic events should be part of the informed consent discussion for all lung cancer patients receiving bevacizumab or other VEGF-targeting agents. The relationship with squamous cell lung carcinoma may be related to the tendency of these cancers to undergo central necrosis; central cavitation is common in lung cancers treated with anti-VEGF therapy.

Bowel perforation

Bowel perforation has been seen predominantly in patients with advanced colorectal cancer and ovarian cancer, though it has been reported to occur in virtually every cancer treated with bevacizumab, albeit less commonly in cancers not involving the abdomen or pelvis. One analysis suggested a 30-day mortality of 12.5% for patients undergoing this complication.[384] One review suggested that the incidence of bowel perforation is higher in patients with an intact primary tumor, recent history of sigmoidoscopy or colonoscopy, or previous abdominal or pelvic radiotherapy. A prior history of peptic ulcer disease, diverticulosis, or use of nonsteroidal anti-inflammatory drugs was not obviously associated with an increased risk of bowel perforation.[385] We presently lack any useful exclusion factors that might prevent patients from developing this complication. The etiology of this side effect is uncertain, though preclinical evidence suggests that anti-VEGF therapy may reduce the vascular density of normal intestinal villi.[386] This may be exacerbated when anti-VEGF therapy is combined with radiation.[253]

The management of bowel perforation involves awareness and recognition of symptoms and emergent surgical intervention. Surgical intervention in the face of anti-VEGF therapy may itself be associated with an increased risk of postsurgical complications such as further bowel perforation and abdominal fistulae. These, however, should not prevent a life-saving surgical intervention.[163,387]

Lessons from preclinical and clinical studies of antiangiogenic therapy and future directions

Mechanisms of resistance to VEGF pathway inhibitors

The therapeutic efficacy of conventional chemotherapy for most solid tumors is limited by the emergence of drug resistance in rapidly mutating tumor cells. Because antiangiogenic agents are directed against tumor endothelium, which was presumed to be genetically stable, it was thought that tumors will not develop resistance to antiangiogenic therapy.[163,387] Clinical experience, however, suggests that virtually all tumors do eventually progress despite treatment with a VEGF inhibitor. Studies have suggested several mechanisms by which tumors may initially have or acquire resistance, or decreased sensitivity, to VEGF pathway inhibitors.[122,388]

Incomplete target inhibition
Drugs may not be present at sufficient concentrations at their targets to cause sustained inhibition of VEGF receptor signaling and tumor angiogenesis. In trials of VEGFR inhibitors tumor biopsies revealed that VEGFR phosphorylation was inhibited by <50% in all cases, providing a potential explanation for the lack of significant clinical activity observed.[389,390] For other TKIs such as gefitinib and imatinib, incomplete target inhibition has been shown to result from genetic changes, for example secondary mutations in EGFR or BCR-ABL, or epigenetic changes reducing the intracellular concentrations of the inhibitor.[391–393] It is not yet known whether mutations may be present within VEGFR in tumor endothelium.

Bypass of the VEGF pathway through expression of additional angiogenic factors
Genetic mutations or the activation of pathways such as HIF-1 may lead to the expression of additional angiogenic factors (or the loss of angiogenic inhibitors) by malignant cells.[196,394] These changes may promote the proliferation and survival of ECs even in the presence of VEGF blockade. It has been observed, that advanced-stage breast cancers express a greater number of proangiogenic factors than early-stage cancers[395] which may explain why previously untreated patients with metastatic breast cancer appeared to have a greater benefit from the addition of bevacizumab to standard chemotherapy than previously treated patients.[396,397]

Tumor stroma has been shown to play a role in resistance to anti-VEGF therapy. Cascone et al. demonstrated that gene expression changes associated with acquired resistance to bevacizumab occurred predominantly in stromal cells in murine models of NSCLC.[398] Specifically, the EGFR and FGFR pathways were upregulated in the stroma, and increased expression of activated EGFR was detected on pericytes of xenografts that acquired resistance to VEGF inhibition and on endothelium of tumors with relative primary resistance. Furthermore, different patterns of vascular changes characterize the phenotype of resistance. Murine models of human NSCLC that acquired resistance to bevacizumab were characterized by a pattern of pericyte-covered, normalized revascularization, whereas tortuous, uncovered vessels were observed in models of relative primary resistance.

Other cytokines have been associated with anti-VEGF resistance. In a Phase II trial evaluating the regimen FOLFIRI in combination with bevacizumab for the treatment of patients with colorectal cancer, increased baseline levels of IL-8 correlated with poorer PFS. In the same study, prior to the radiographic development of disease progression, circulating levels of several proangiogenetic cytokines known to be associated with angiogenesis and myeloid recruitment increased compared to baseline, such as FGF, HGF, PlGF, stromal cell-derived factor (SDF), and monocyte chemoattractant protein (MCP).[399]

Tumors may escape VEGFR pathway inhibition by increasing other angiogenic factors. In preclinical models, inhibition of FGFR signaling can restore sensitivity to VEGF targeting agents.[59] Galectin-1 (Gal1) has also been shown to play a role in resistance to antiangiogenic therapies. Gal1 is upregulated in hypoxic conditions, modulates trafficking of EGFR and VEGF, and promotes tumor angiogenesis. Targeting of Gal1 along with anti-VEGF therapy improved antitumor activity.[400]

Several studies have implicated the HGF/c-Met signaling pathway as an important mediator of tumor resistance to anti-VEGFR therapies. Shojaei et al. reported that upregulation of HGF rendered lymphomas and Lewis lung carcinomas refractory to VEGFR TKI sunitinib.[401] In those studies, c-Met expression was found to be significantly higher in ECs than in tumor cells, suggesting that HGF might target the vasculature in resistant tumors. Administration of HGF in the sensitive tumor models conferred resistance to sunitinib, and, conversely, combined therapy using sunitinib and the highly selective c-Met inhibitor PF-04217903 impaired angiogenesis and tumor growth mainly by targeting the vasculature of resistant tumors. More recently, the HGF/MET pathway was shown to be a mediator of resistance to the VEGFR TKIs cediranib and vandetanib in murine models of NSCLC.[402] Ectopic HGF expression in cancer cells reduced tumor sensitivity to VEGFR TKIs and increased blood vessel tortuosity while combined targeting of VEGFR/c-MET signaling pathways delayed the onset of therapeutic resistance and abrogated the vascular morphology alterations. Furthermore, in cancer patients treated with VEGFR TKIs, elevated pretreatment plasma levels of HGF correlated with poorer survival outcomes. These and other preclinical studies[403] support the dual combination of VEGF and the HGF/c-MET pathways as an approach to combat resistance.

Role of myeloid cells in VEGF inhibitor resistance
Increased tumor infiltration of myeloid cells has also been linked to antiangiogenic therapy resistance.[404] Elevated numbers of CD11b+Gr1+ myeloid-derived suppressor cells (MDSCs) have been observed in refractory tumors compared to tumors sensitive to antiangiogenic agents.[121] Tumor-infiltrating neutrophils (Gr1+) have been shown to be critical in the initial angiogenic switch in RIP-Tag murine model of pancreatic β-cell tumorigenesis. In a recent report, IL-17, produced by T helper type 17 (TH17) cells, was shown to facilitate IL-17-dependent but VEGF-independent angiogenesis through upregulation of G-CSF which in turn leads

Table 3 Surrogate markers under investigation for the evaluation of efficacy of antiangiogenic agents.

Marker	Parameter evaluated	Comments/limitations	References
Tumor-based			
Tissue biopsy	Immunohistochemistry: • Protein expression as a marker • Microvascular density • Perivascular cell coverage of tumor vessels • Cell proliferation/apoptosis genomic analyses: identification of genomic alterations by whole-exome or RNA sequencing	Not easily available in some tumors	245, 246, 330, 389, 407, 417–419
Interstitial fluid pressure measurement	Tumor interstitial fluid pressure	Limited accessibility in some tumors	245, 246, 420, 421
Measurements of tissue oxygenation	Tumor oxygen tension	Difficult accessibility in some tumors	422
Skin wound healing	Wound healing time	Investigated as biomarker of efficacy and indicator of side effects	423
Circulating markers in blood or urine			
Blood CECs, CPCs, or CEPs	Concentration of viable CEC/CPCs/CEPs	Unclear origin, viability, and surface phenotype of the circulating cells	245–247, 424–429
Circulating proteins (cytokines, angiogenic factors, etc)	Concentration of levels of cytokines, angiogenic factors, markers of hypoxia, endothelial damage, and other factors in the blood	Can be done using commercially available multiplexed assays, ELISAs	247, 425, 430–435
Protein level in urine	Urine MMPs, VEGF, etc.	Limited to excreted proteins, depends on factors that might be altered by treatment such as renal function (e.g., proteinuria)	436
Radiographic			
CT imaging	Blood flow and volume, permeability-surface area product mean transit time	Resolution, measurement of composite parameters	245, 246, 437
PET imaging	Tracer uptake	Resolution, measurement of composite parameters	245, 246, 424, 437
MRI	Blood flow, permeability	Resolution, measurement of composite parameters	247, 438–440

Abbreviations: CAF, circulating angiogenic factor; CECs, circulating endothelial cells; CEPs circulating endothelial progenitors; CT, computer tomography; MMPs, matrix metalloproteinases; MRI, magnetic resonance imaging; PET, positron emission tomography; VEGF, vascular endothelial growth factor.

to the mobilization and recruitment of MDSCs from the bone marrow and spleen to the tumor.[405] In mice, the efficacy of anti-VEGF therapy in refractory tumors was improved when IL-17 was targeted. More recently, to determine whether TH17 cells have direct impact on ECs, Protopsaltis et al. showed that blockade of IL-22, a key cytokine expressed by TH17 cells, dramatically inhibited tumor growth associated with reduced microvascular density on murine lymphoma and glioblastoma models.[406]

Altered threshold for hypoxia-induced apoptosis
Certain changes within a tumor cell may make it less sensitive to the diminished vascular supply and resulting hypoxia induced by antiangiogenic therapy. For instance, it has been demonstrated in murine xenograft models that tumor cells bearing mutated p53 are less sensitive to hypoxic conditions *in vitro* and respond somewhat less well to VEGFR2 inhibition.[407] Studies performed in tissue biopsies obtained from patients with recurrent HGG treated with bevacizumab and irinotecan revealed that high expression levels of carbonic anhydrase 9 (CAIX), a marker of hypoxia, were significantly associated with poor 1-year survival.[408] Similarly, findings of another tumor tissue study of patients with malignant glioma revealed that low CAIX expression and increased VEGF expression were associated with improved PFS in those patients who received metronomic etoposide and bevacizumab.[409]

Genetic variability in host
Recent studies have suggested that polymorphisms in the VEGF gene are associated with the risk of developing cancer[410–412] and may also influence the response to bevacizumab when given with chemotherapy in breast cancer[377] and glioblastoma patients.[413] Polymorphisms in other genes regulating angiogenesis, such as IL-8 and the HIF family, have also been described. The availability of high throughput methods for analyzing polymorphisms on a genome-wide basis should facilitate the analysis of genetic differences in the host and their impact on response to angiogenesis inhibitors.

Potential biomarkers for VEGF pathway inhibitors

The critical need for biomarkers for VEGF pathway inhibitors
Despite significant progress, the benefits of antiangiogenic therapy to date have been modest, are seen only in subsets of patients, and inevitably yield to therapeutic resistance. There is an urgent need for biomarkers to identify which patients are most likely to respond to treatment or develop therapeutic resistance, select the optimal drug dosage, and determine whether the intended molecular target has been effectively inhibited.[414–416] Ideally such methods should be noninvasive and practical for routine clinical care. There are currently no validated biomarkers for routine clinical use, but a number are under investigation in clinical and preclinical studies (Table 3). These can be divided into invasive markers that assess changes in tissue or vasculature directly, circulating markers detectable in blood or urine, radiographic markers, and genomic markers. Several of these are discussed below.

Invasive markers

Serial biopsies taken prior to and during treatment have the potential to directly demonstrate drug effects on tumors and other tissues at the cellular and molecular level but are typically not practical to obtain outside the setting of a clinical trial. This approach has been used to demonstrate that bevacizumab induces changes in microvessel density, tumor-cell apoptosis, and proliferation in rectal cancer patients.[245,246,441] Changes in tumor IFP, a key parameter impacting vascular function, have also been demonstrated.[424] This approach may also provide insights into the lack of significant clinical activity seen for some agents. For example, in clinical trials of the VEGFR TKIs SU5416 and SU6668, it was observed that VEGFR and other key targets were incompletely inhibited in posttreatment tumor biopsies[389,390] suggesting that higher drug concentrations, or more potent inhibitors, may be required.

Circulating markers in blood and urine

Plasma and serum levels of VEGF and soluble VEGFR-2 have been investigated as pharmacodynamic biomarkers of activity of VEGF inhibitors, prognostic markers, and predictive markers of clinical benefit. In preclinical models, rapid increases of plasma VEGF, and decreases in soluble VEGFR-2, have been observed in both nontumor bearing and tumor-bearing mice.[442–444] These increases were induced in a dose-dependent manner, and correlated with the treatment efficacy, suggesting that they may be useful for selecting the appropriate drug dosage.

These markers have also been evaluated in clinical trials. Bevacizumab (alone and with cytotoxics) has been shown to increase both serum and plasma total VEGF levels.[245,280,282,424] Interestingly, free serum VEGF concentrations decreased to undetectable levels even with low doses of bevacizumab in one of the studies.[280] VEGFR TKIs such as sunitinib have been shown to consistently induce on-therapy increases in VEGF plasma levels and decreases in soluble (s)VEGFR-2, which are rapidly reversible when the therapy is stopped.[247,430,445–449] In one study, changes in sVEGFR-2 correlated with plasma levels of the drug.[425] More recently, an analysis of angiogenesis biomarkers in the ramucirumab RAISE study identified VEGF-D as a potential predictive biomarker for ramucirumab efficacy in second-line metastatic colorectal carcinoma.[317] Collectively, these findings suggest that VEGF and sVEGFR-2 may be useful pharmacodynamic markers. Baseline levels of VEGF may also be predictive of benefit for some drugs although this has not been consistently observed in all studies. NSCLC patients with high VEGF were more likely to respond to the combination of bevacizumab with chemotherapy compared to chemotherapy alone.[431] Interestingly, a trend in the opposite direction was observed for the TKI vandetanib, as patients with low VEGF appeared to derive a greater clinical benefit from the vandetanib-containing arm compared to the control arm in three randomized Phase II studies.[450] It appears that the predictive value of markers such as VEGF will depend on the specific drug and disease setting.

Recent technological advances such as multiplex bead assays have permitted investigators to assess a much wider variety of factors. A signature derived from a profile of 35 cytokines and angiogenic factors was shown to be predictive of vandetanib benefit in a randomized Phase II study.[432] PlGF has been shown to be consistently increased by anti-VEGF therapy in cancer patients regardless of the tumor type or agent used, suggesting that it might be an additional pharmacodynamic biomarker for antiangiogenic therapy.[245,247,424,430,433,451] Future studies will establish if PlGF levels have any predictive value for this therapy. Circulating Tie2 has been also proposed as a vascular response biomarker for bevacizumab-treated ovarian cancer patients and more recently in in metastatic colorectal cancer.[452–454] Distinct patterns of circulating Tie2 were associated with worse progression-free survival suggesting that Tie2 may be also monitored clinically.[453] Finally, this approach may also prove to be useful for identifying potential mechanisms of therapeutic resistance. Several candidates are SDF1α-CXCR4 pathways, bFGF, IL-6, HGF, and IL-8.[246,247,424,434,451]

Circulating endothelial cells (CECs) and precursors (CEPs)

Mature circulating endothelial cells (CECs) (derived from existing vessels) and bone marrow-derived circulating precursor cells (CPCs) or circulating endothelial precursors (CEPs), which can differentiate into mature ECs and contribute to neovascularization, have been investigated as biomarkers for antiangiogenic therapy.[112,113,116,247,425,426,455–457] Consistent with preclinical models,[427,458] increases during treatment in mature CECs, which have a large percentage of apoptotic cells and are thought to represent cells shed from tumor endothelium, may be associated with benefit in patients treated with antiangiogenic or VTAs.[425,428,459,460] In one study evaluating patients with metastatic breast cancer who were treated with low-dose metronomic chemotherapy using cyclophosphamide and methotrexate, the CEC count after 2 months of continuous therapy correlated with DFS and OS at more than 2-year follow-up.[428] CPCs, by contrast, appear to decrease with bevacizumab[245,246,424] or sunitinib treatment.[451] Despite these encouraging results, the clinical application of circulating cells as biomarkers will require standardization and further phenotypic definition of cell populations.[461–463]

Imaging

A number of different techniques are under investigation for assessing parameters related to tumor vasculature such as perfusion, permeability, hypoxia, and metabolic activity. These include dynamic contrast-enhanced MRI (DCE-MRI), CT, and positron emission tomography (reviewed in Refs. 415, 416, 438, 464–469). These methods have the important advantage of permitting longitudinal assessments noninvasively. There are a number of limitations for each of these methods, however. There is significant heterogeneity in blood flow and permeability within tumors, and the currently available methods generally lack the spatial resolution to assess this. Furthermore, most assess composite parameters, which depend on both tumor blood flow and permeability[388]. The cost of these studies may also limit their use, particularly for large randomized clinical trials needed to validate their utility.

Genomic alterations

Somatic genomic alterations in tumor cells may be also play an important role in the response to antiangiogenic therapy. Using preclinical models of colon cancer Yu et al. demonstrated that mutations in the tumor suppressor TP53 reduce the response of anti-VEGFR therapies *in vivo* by modifying the vascular dependence of tumors demonstrating that TP53 mutant tumors may possess a survival advantage under hypoxic conditions.[407] In lung cancer, mutations in EGFR have been associated with improved response to antiangiogenic therapy inhibitors[470] while recent studies suggest that mutations in the tumor suppressor gene *STK11/LKB1* may be associated with worse response to anti-VEGF therapy.[417] A recent retrospective clinical study reported the possible role of *STK11/* LKB1 mutations as biomarkers of sensitivity to bevacizumab and chemotherapy in NSCLC. Although further mechanistic studies are needed, these data highlight the importance of tumor genomic alterations on regulating the dependence of tumors to hypoxic environments and consequently affecting the response to antiangiogenic therapy.

Concluding remarks

Nearly four decades ago, tumor angiogenesis was recognized as a potential therapeutic target for the treatment of cancer.[1] Since that seminal observation, the field has moved from conception to the clinical testing of dozens of new agents. Angiogenesis inhibitors are now part of the standard treatment regimens for lung, colorectal, renal, breast, and several other types of cancers. While these recent advances have validated antiangiogenic therapy as a treatment modality and provided benefit to countless patients, it is also true that the clinical gains thus far have been modest. As the field moves from infancy into adolescence, a number of key issues will need to be addressed in order for antiangiogenic therapy to realize its therapeutic potential for cancer patients. Among these issues are understanding the mechanism(s) by which antiangiogenic therapy enhances the efficacy of chemotherapy, radiotherapy, and immunotherapy and designing combinations appropriately; identifying critical pathways driving angiogenesis other than VEGF, and developing drugs to inhibit them; creating biomarkers to identify which patients will benefit (or experience toxicity) from a given agent; and exploring the application of angiogenesis inhibitors to earlier stages of cancer, with the goal of rendering microscopic tumors dormant.

Acknowledgments

This article is dedicated to Judah Folkman, M.D., for his pioneering work in tumor angiogenesis and for his generous mentorship. We would also like to acknowledge Rakesh Jain, PhD and George Sledge, MD for their contributions to earlier versions of this article.

Key references

The complete reference list can be found on Vital Source version of this title, see inside front cover.

1 Folkman J. Tumor angiogenesis: therapeutic implications. *N Engl J Med*. 1971;**285**(21):1182–1186.
2 Hanahan D, Weinberg RA. The hallmarks of cancer. *Cell*. 2000;**100**(1):57–70.
3 Carmeliet P, Jain RK. Angiogenesis in cancer and other diseases. *Nature*. 2000;**407**(6801):249–257.
7 Gimbrone MA Jr, Leapman SB, Cotran RS, Folkman J. Tumor dormancy in vivo by prevention of neovascularization. *J Exp Med*. 1972;**136**(2):261–276.
8 Folkman J, Watson K, Ingber D, Hanahan D. Induction of angiogenesis during the transition from hyperplasia to neoplasia. *Nature*. 1989;**339**(6219):58–61.
9 Hanahan D, Folkman J. Patterns and emerging mechanisms of the angiogenic switch during tumorigenesis. *Cell*. 1996;**86**(3):353–364.
22 Folkman J. The vascularization of tumors. *Sci Am*. 1976;**234**(5):58–64 70–73.
28 Shing Y, Folkman J, Sullivan R, et al. Heparin affinity: purification of a tumor-derived capillary endothelial cell growth factor. *Science*. 1984;**223**(4642):1296–1299.
32 Jain RK. Vascular and interstitial barriers to delivery of therapeutic agents in tumors. *Cancer Metastasis Rev*. 1990;**9**(3):253–266.
38 Folkman J, Long DM, Becker FF. Tumor behavior in isolated perfused organs: in vitro growth and metastases of biopsy material in rabbit thyroid and canine interstinal segment. *Ann Surg*. 1963;**164**:491–502.
47 Borgstrom P, Hillan KJ, Sriramarao P, Ferrara N. Complete inhibition of angiogenesis and growth of microtumors by anti-vascular endothelial growth factor neutralizing antibody: novel concepts of angiostatic therapy from intravital videomicroscopy. *Cancer Res*. 1996;**56**(17):4032–4039.
68 Ferrara N, Henzel WJ. Pituitary follicular cells secrete a novel heparin-binding growth factor specific for vascular endothelial cells. *Biochem Biophys Res Commun*. 1989;**161**(2):851–858.
79 Inoue M, Hager JH, Ferrara N, et al. VEGF-A has a critical, nonredundant role in angiogenic switching and pancreatic beta cell carcinogenesis. *Cancer Cell*. 2002;**1**(2):193–202.
97 Carmeliet P, Lampugnani MG, Moons L, et al. Targeted deficiency or cytosolic truncation of the VE-cadherin gene in mice impairs VEGF-mediated endothelial survival and angiogenesis. *Cell*. 1999;**98**(2):147–157.
102 Ellis LM, Hicklin DJ. VEGF-targeted therapy: mechanisms of anti-tumour activity. *Nat Rev Cancer*. 2008;**8**(8):579–591.
116 Lyden D, Hattori K, Dias S, et al. Impaired recruitment of bone-marrow-derived endothelial and hematopoietic precursor cells blocks tumor angiogenesis and growth. *Nat Med*. 2001;**7**(11):1194–1201.
118 Kaplan RN, Riba RD, Zacharoulis S, et al. VEGFR1-positive haematopoietic bone marrow progenitors initiate the pre-metastatic niche. *Nature*. 2005;**438**(7069):820–827.
126 Cascone T, Heymach JV. Targeting the angiopoietin/Tie2 pathway: cutting tumor vessels with a double-edged sword? *J Clin Oncol*. 2012;**30**(4):441–444.
135 Koch AE, Polverini PJ, Kunkel SL, et al. Interleukin-8 as a macrophage-derived mediator of angiogenesis. *Science (New York, NY)*. 1992;**258**(5089):1798–1801.
149 O'Reilly MS, Holmgren L, Shing Y, et al. Angiostatin: a novel angiogenesis inhibitor that mediates the suppression of metastases by a Lewis lung carcinoma. *Cell*. 1994;**79**(2):315–328.
196 Semenza GL. Targeting HIF-1 for cancer therapy. *Nat Rev Cancer*. 2003;**3**(10):721–732.
231 Jain RK. Normalization of tumor vasculature: an emerging concept in antiangiogenic therapy. *Science*. 2005;**307**(5706):58–62.
278 Hurwitz H, Fehrenbacher L, Novotny W, et al. Bevacizumab plus irinotecan, fluorouracil, and leucovorin for metastatic colorectal cancer. *N Engl J Med*. 2004;**350**(23):2335–2342.
279 Sandler A, Gray R, Perry MC, et al. Paclitaxel-carboplatin alone or with bevacizumab for non-small-cell lung cancer. *N Engl J Med*. 2006;**355**(24):2542–2550.
282 Yang JC, Haworth L, Sherry RM, et al. A randomized trial of bevacizumab, an anti-vascular endothelial growth factor antibody, for metastatic renal cancer. *N Engl J Med*. 2003;**349**(5):427–434.
292 Rini BI, Plimack ER, Stus V, et al. Pembrolizumab plus axitinib versus sunitinib for advanced renal-cell carcinoma. *N Engl J Med*. 2019;**380**(12):1116–1127.
306 Tran HT, Liu Y, Zurita AJ, et al. Prognostic or predictive plasma cytokines and angiogenic factors for patients treated with pazopanib for metastatic renal-cell cancer: a retrospective analysis of phase 2 and phase 3 trials. *Lancet Oncol*. 2012;**13**(8):827–837.
311 Tabernero J, Yoshino T, Cohn AL, et al. Ramucirumab versus placebo in combination with second-line FOLFIRI in patients with metastatic colorectal carcinoma that progressed during or after first-line therapy with bevacizumab, oxaliplatin, and a fluoropyrimidine (RAISE): a randomised, double-blind, multicentre, phase 3 study. *The Lancet Oncol*. 2015;**16**(5):499–508.
322 Fuchs CS, Tomasek J, Yong CJ, et al. Ramucirumab monotherapy for previously treated advanced gastric or gastro-oesophageal junction adenocarcinoma (REGARD): an international, randomised, multicentre, placebo-controlled, phase 3 trial. *Lancet*. 2014;**383**(9911):31–39.
325 Motzer RJ, Hutson TE, Cella D, et al. Pazopanib versus sunitinib in metastatic renal-cell carcinoma. *N Engl J Med*. 2013;**369**(8):722–731.
333 Garon EB, Ciuleanu TE, Arrieta O, et al. Ramucirumab plus docetaxel versus placebo plus docetaxel for second-line treatment of stage IV non-small-cell lung cancer after disease progression on platinum-based therapy (REVEL): a multicentre, double-blind, randomised phase 3 trial. *Lancet*. 2014;**384**(9944):665–673.
335 Herbst RS, Sun Y, Eberhardt WE, et al. Vandetanib plus docetaxel versus docetaxel as second-line treatment for patients with advanced non-small-cell lung cancer (ZODIAC): a double-blind, randomised, phase 3 trial. *Lancet Oncol*. 2010;**11**(7):619–626.
337 Richeldi L, du Bois RM, Raghu G, et al. Efficacy and safety of nintedanib in idiopathic pulmonary fibrosis. *N Engl J Med*. 2014;**370**(22):2071–2082.
350 Naumov GN, Nilsson MB, Cascone T, et al. Combined vascular endothelial growth factor receptor and epidermal growth factor receptor (EGFR) blockade inhibits tumor growth in xenograft models of EGFR inhibitor resistance. *Clin Cancer Res*. 2009;**15**(10):3484–3494.
352 Nakagawa K, Garon EB, Seto T, et al. Ramucirumab plus erlotinib in patients with untreated, EGFR-mutated, advanced non-small-cell lung cancer (RELAY): a randomised, double-blind, placebo-controlled, phase 3 trial. *The Lancet Oncol*. 2019;**20**(12):1655–1669.

389 Heymach JV, Desai J, Manola J, et al. Phase II study of the antiangiogenic agent SU5416 in patients with advanced soft tissue sarcomas. *Clin Cancer Res.* 2004;**10**(17):5732–5740.

398 Cascone T, Herynk MH, Xu L, et al. Upregulated stromal EGFR and vascular remodeling in mouse xenograft models of angiogenesis inhibitor-resistant human lung adenocarcinoma. *J Clin Invest.* 2011;**121**(4):1313–1328. doi: 10.1172/JCI42405.

399 Kopetz S, Hoff PM, Morris JS, et al. Phase II trial of infusional fluorouracil, irinotecan, and bevacizumab for metastatic colorectal cancer: efficacy and circulating angiogenic biomarkers associated with therapeutic resistance. *J Clin Oncol.* 2010;**28**(3):453–459.

434 Hanrahan EO, Heymach JV. Vascular endothelial growth factor receptor tyrosine kinase inhibitors vandetanib (ZD6474) and AZD2171 in lung cancer. *Clin Cancer Res.* 2007;**13**(15):4617s–4622s.

470 Saito H, Fukuhara T, Furuya N, et al. Erlotinib plus bevacizumab versus erlotinib alone in patients with EGFR-positive advanced non-squamous non-small-cell lung cancer (NEJ026): interim analysis of an open-label, randomised, multicentre, phase 3 trial. *The Lancet Oncol.* 2019;**20**(5):625–635.

PART 3

Quantitative Oncology

17 Cancer bioinformatics

John N. Weinstein, MD, PhD

Overview

Bioinformatics is a rapidly advancing interdisciplinary field in which computational methods are applied to the analysis, interpretation, and visualization of biological and/or medical data, most often at the cell or molecular level and usually in the form of large, multivariate datasets. PubMed citations for "bioinformatics" have risen sharply, increasing 24-fold since the year 2000. Massively parallel sequencing and imaging technologies are now generating a data deluge—many trillions of numbers in all—that strain the capacity of our hardware, software, and personnel infrastructures for bioinformatics; hence, the computational aspect of a sequencing project is often more expensive and time-consuming than the laboratory work. The field of bioinformatics includes "data scientists," for whom useful innovative algorithms, software, and data structures are publishable ends in themselves, and "computational biologists," for whom algorithms, software, and computers are just tools of the trade for answering biological or medical questions. Bioinformatic analysis can be hypothesis-generating or hypothesis-testing, and a large number of statistical and artificial intelligence algorithms, scripts, and software packages are now available for each type of analysis. In fact, the rapidly increasing number of options is almost paralyzing. Computational consortia formed around large-scale, public, molecular profiling projects like The Cancer Genome Atlas project have served as incubators for rapid computational advance, particularly driving major innovations in single-cell informatics, artificial intelligence, and computational immunology. One attractive working arrangement is a stable "dyad" in which the bioinformatician focuses primarily on database management, statistical analysis, and data visualization, whereas the biologist/clinical researcher focuses primarily on interpretation and biomedical application.

I can assure you that data processing is a fad that won't last out the year.
— *Editor for a major publishing house, 1957*

Introduction

Little more than a generation ago, the results of most laboratory studies on cancer could be processed in a simple spreadsheet and the results written into a laboratory notebook. The data were generally analyzed by experimentalists themselves, using very basic statistical algorithms. That landscape shifted progressively with the advent of microarrays in the mid-1990s and then massively parallel next-generation sequencing a decade later. At the turn of the millennium, I predicted—only half in jest—that most biomedical researchers would abandon the wet laboratory within a generation and be hunched over their computers, mining the data produced by "biology factories." That has not happened (yet); of course, small wet laboratories are thriving. But we do see increasing numbers of biology factories, prominent among them the high-throughput sequencing centers.

Overall, the trend toward computation is unmistakable. That trend is largely a result of new, robotically enhanced technologies that make it faster, cheaper, and more reliable to perform the *laboratory portions* of large-scale molecular profiling projects and screening assays. As a result, large centers and also small laboratories can churn out increasingly robust streams of data. Those trends have conspired to produce massive datasets that often contain many billions or even trillions of entries, requiring more complex, larger-scale, often subtler statistical analyses, interactive machine learning/artificial intelligence, semantically informed natural language processing, and "biointerpretive" resources. One picture is worth a thousand data table entries, so complex, interactive visualizations have come to the fore.

The aim of this article is not to provide a comprehensive treatment of the rapidly evolving arena of cancer bioinformatics. That would, in any case, be impossible to do at any depth in the space available. The aim is also not to give due credit to pioneers in the field or to cite all of the contemporary tools and resources that deserve mention. The aims are (1) to illuminate some generic aspects of cancer bioinformatics in its current and likely future states; (2) to highlight a sample of the statistical algorithms, computational tools, and data resources available; and (3) to showcase some issues that should be borne in mind by the nonspecialist who is trying to use bioinformatics in a project, navigate the bioinformatics literature, or comprehend what bioinformatician collaborators are doing and saying.

The definition and scope of bioinformatics

Definition of "bioinformatics"

The term "bioinformatics" is not new. The first PubMed citation was in 1958 (see Figure 1), and in 1970 the term was described with a very broad meaning.[1] Use for the term, and the field itself, has grown dramatically since then in popularity and importance. But the definition and scope, as applied currently, are matters of almost Talmudic debate. Multiple committees, academic surveys, and publications have struggled with the subject, even attempting to distinguish between "bioinformaticians" and "bioinformaticists".[2] For present purposes, an extended definition of bioinformatics attributed to the U.S. National Center for Biotechnology Information (NCBI) will suffice: "Bioinformatics is the field of science in which biology, computer science, and information technology merge into a single discipline. There are three important sub-disciplines within bioinformatics: the development of new algorithms and statistics with which to assess relationships among members of large data sets; the analysis and interpretation

---

Holland-Frei Cancer Medicine, Tenth Edition. Edited by Robert C. Bast, John C. Byrd, Carlo M. Croce, Ernest Hawk, Fadlo R. Khuri, Raphael E. Pollock, Apostolia M. Tsimberidou, Christopher G. Willett, and Cheryl L. Willman.
© 2023 John Wiley & Sons, Inc. Published 2023 by John Wiley & Sons, Inc.

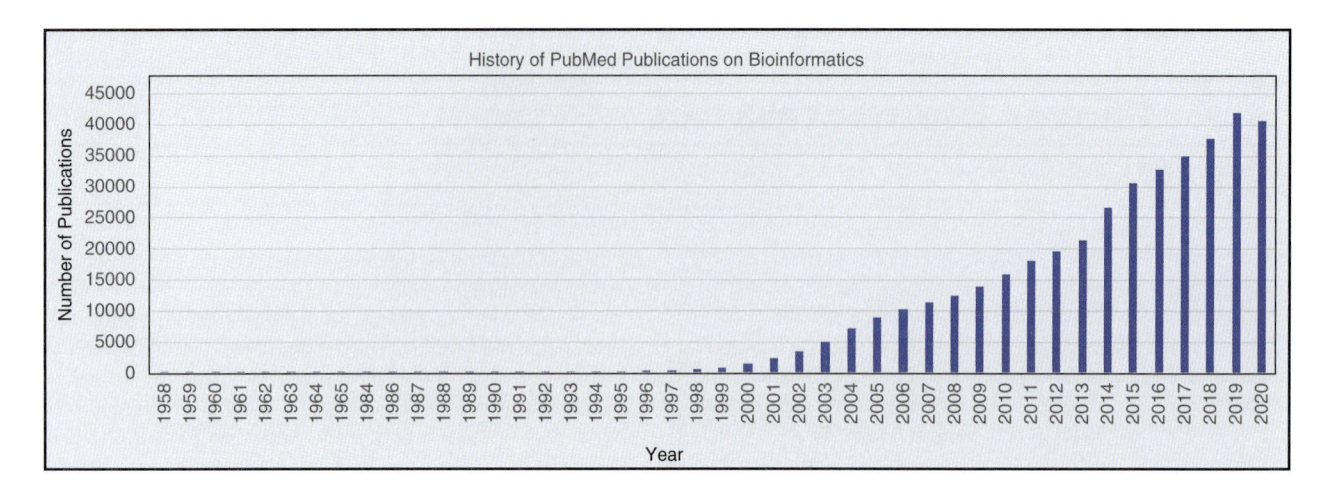

Figure 1 History of PubMed publications for the search term "bioinformatics." There were only a handful prior to 1990. The apparent slight decrease in 2020 may have been due to incomplete data.

of various types of data including nucleotide and amino acid sequences, protein domains, and protein structures; and the development and implementation of tools that enable efficient access and management of different types of information".[3]

In the end, a word means what we collectively choose it to mean. The ingredients of most bioinformatics projects include biological molecules, large databases, multivariate statistical analysis, high-performance computing, graphical visualization of the molecular data, and biological or biomedical interpretation. Typical sources of data for bioinformatic analysis include microarrays, DNA sequencing, RNA sequencing, mass spectrometry of proteins and metabolites, histopathological descriptors, and clinical records. Some of the salient datasets originate within studies being conducted in particular laboratories, but search resources and publicly available "big data" from the biology factories are playing ever-larger roles.

One distinction worth bearing in mind is that between "data scientists" and "computational biologists." For the former type of bioinformatician, databases, algorithms, pipelines, and software are the primary points of focus, even if they are designed to be useful for biology or medicine; for the latter, those entities are simply means to the biological or medical end.

Questions typically addressed by bioinformatic analysis and interpretation

Questions typically addressed by bioinformatic analysis relate to biological mechanisms, pathways, networks, biomarkers, biosignatures, macromolecular structures, subsetting of cancer types, early detection, and prediction of clinical outcome variables such as risk, survival, metastasis, response to therapy, and recurrence. The paradigmatic bioinformatics project—the type that will be cited throughout this article—involves the design, statistical or artificial intelligence analysis, and biological interpretation of molecular profiles. Figure 2 shows a schematic view of the specimen and information flows in a generic sequencing project whose aim is to identify mutational and/or DNA copy number aberrations as possible biomarkers. The data from such studies can also be used to subset cancers or to make direct comparisons such as tumor versus paired normal tissue, tumor type versus tumor type, responder versus nonresponder, metastatic versus nonmetastatic, and primary versus recurrent cancer.

One frequent aim has been the identification of "prognostic" biomarkers for survival, time to recurrence, or metastasis. But the focus has turned largely to "predictive" biomarkers for predicting which subpopulations of patients will respond to a particular therapy. An allied concept is that of the "actionable" biomarker. An actionable, predictive biomarker may be a target for therapy or it may simply be correlated with response. Historically, bioinformatic analysis has identified associations and correlations more often than it has identified causal relationships, but "bioperturbing" technologies such as siRNA, shRNA, CRISPR, and consequent synthetic lethal pharmacological screens are producing large datasets with immediate causal implications. As the technological tools, particularly at the single-cell level, have become sharper, questions impossible even to pose a few years ago are now immediately answerable. The pace of change is breathtaking. That is particularly the case for immunology with the advent of immune checkpoint and T-cell therapies, as well as for newly prominent fields like metabolomics and microbiome research.

The analog (microarray) to digital (sequencing) transition

The digital revolution took hold in computing, then in television, in watches, in cameras and cars, and now in biomedical research. DNA and RNA sequencing provides more precise, incisive, and extensive information about the molecular profiles of cancers than could generally be obtained from microarrays. For example, sequencing the mixture of mRNAs in a tumor (RNA-seq) can yield information on mRNA splicing, mRNA editing, clonal heterogeneity, tumor evolution, viral insertion, fusion gene expression, and allelic components of the overall expression level. In contrast, expression microarrays generally indicate only the relative amounts of the mRNA species present in a sample. Massively parallel ("next-generation sequencing technologies—sometimes combined with immunohistological imaging for spatial information—now dominate and challenge the bioinformatics community at the levels of hardware, software, and "wetware" (i.e., personnel).

Hardware challenges

Moore's law[4] is familiar. It relates to the number of transistors that can be crammed into unit surface area on a very large integrated circuit. That number increased in a remarkably consistent

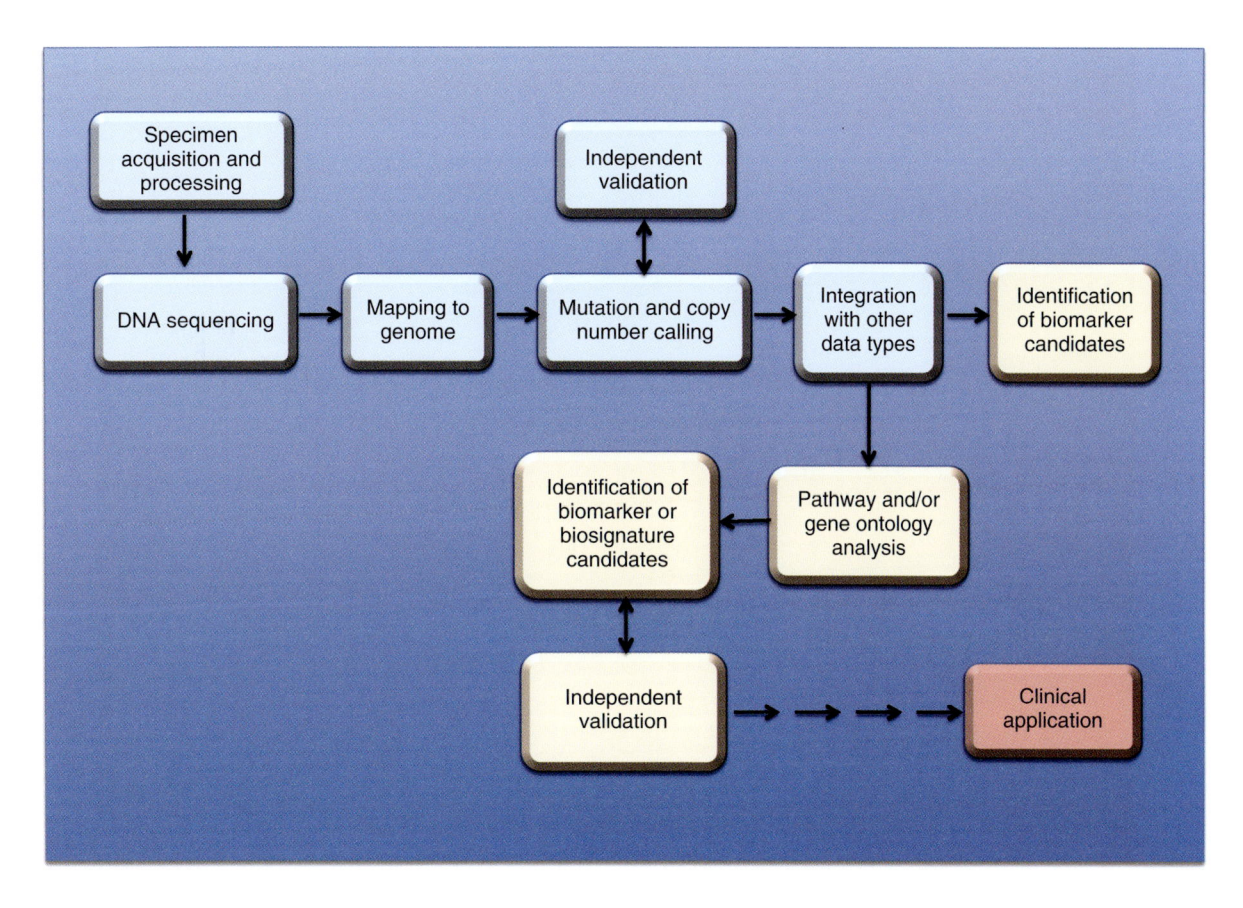

Figure 2 Schematic view of specimen and information flows for sequencing of cancers to identify mutations and/or copy number aberrations as possible biomarkers for clinical application. Amber boxes indicate downstream "biointerpretive" aspects of the pipeline. As indicated by the multiple arrows, many hurdles (scientific, technical, logistical, ethical, and regulatory) must be overcome before possible clinical application. Analogous schematics can be drawn for other data types at the DNA, RNA, protein, and metabolomic levels (including studies based on microarrays, rather than sequencing).

way, about twofold every other year from the 1960s until the growth slowed modestly in about 2008. There was a commensurate decrease in price. How much more the density of transistor elements can increase is in doubt as the size of transistor units has approached molecular size. The Moore's law decrease in price has not kept up with the decline in sequencing cost, which was cut 1000-fold (from about $10 million per human genome to about $10 thousand) in the 4 years from late 2007 to late 2011 as next-generation sequencing became available (Figure 3). Currently, the price for sequencing of a human genome is less than $1000. Even our high-performance computer clusters with large amounts of memory and thousands of CPUs or GPUs operating 24 h a day are often saturated with genomic calculations. The computational demands are so great that heat dissipation and the availability of electricity are often limiting. Some large data centers require their own power stations.

Less familiar but an even more serious problem is Kryder's law,[5] analogous to Moore's law but for the cost of data storage, rather than computing power. The original version of Kryder's law in 2004 predicted that the cost would decrease by about twofold every 6 months. The storage space needed for a standard whole-genome BAM file (binary alignment sequence/map file) with 30-fold average coverage of the genome is "only" about 100 gigabytes, but to identify mutations in minority clones within a tumor can require coverage redundancies in the many hundreds (if they can be identified at all without specialized methods). The storage space required can be reduced by coding only differences from a reference standard, but the reduction is limited by the need to record quality-control information and other types of annotations. Even large institutions are in danger of running out of storage space. It may be less expensive to re-sequence samples than to store sequencing data from them over time.

Another big-data problem is the prohibitively long time it can take to transmit large numbers of sequences and associated annotations from place to place, even along high-speed lines. Cloud computing is sometimes considered the answer to our limitations of power and storage space, but one still has to worry about the time and expense of getting the large amounts of data to and from the cloud. For that reason, computational tools are increasingly being brought to the data, rather than the reverse. Software is also being "containerized" with the Docker of Singularity packages and managed in code repositories like GitHub and GitLab (web-based version-control and collaboration platforms for software developers).

However, there are new possibilities for mass storage on the horizon, paradoxically including DNA itself. DNA and DNA analogs may be the most compact storage media in prospect. A single gram of DNA could encode about 700,000 gigabytes of data (roughly 7000 whole-genome BAM files). One team encoded all of Shakespeare's sonnets in DNA and another encoded an entire book—with an intrinsic error rate of only two per million bits, far better than magnetic hard drives or human proof-readers can achieve.[6] They then replicated the DNA to produce 70 billion

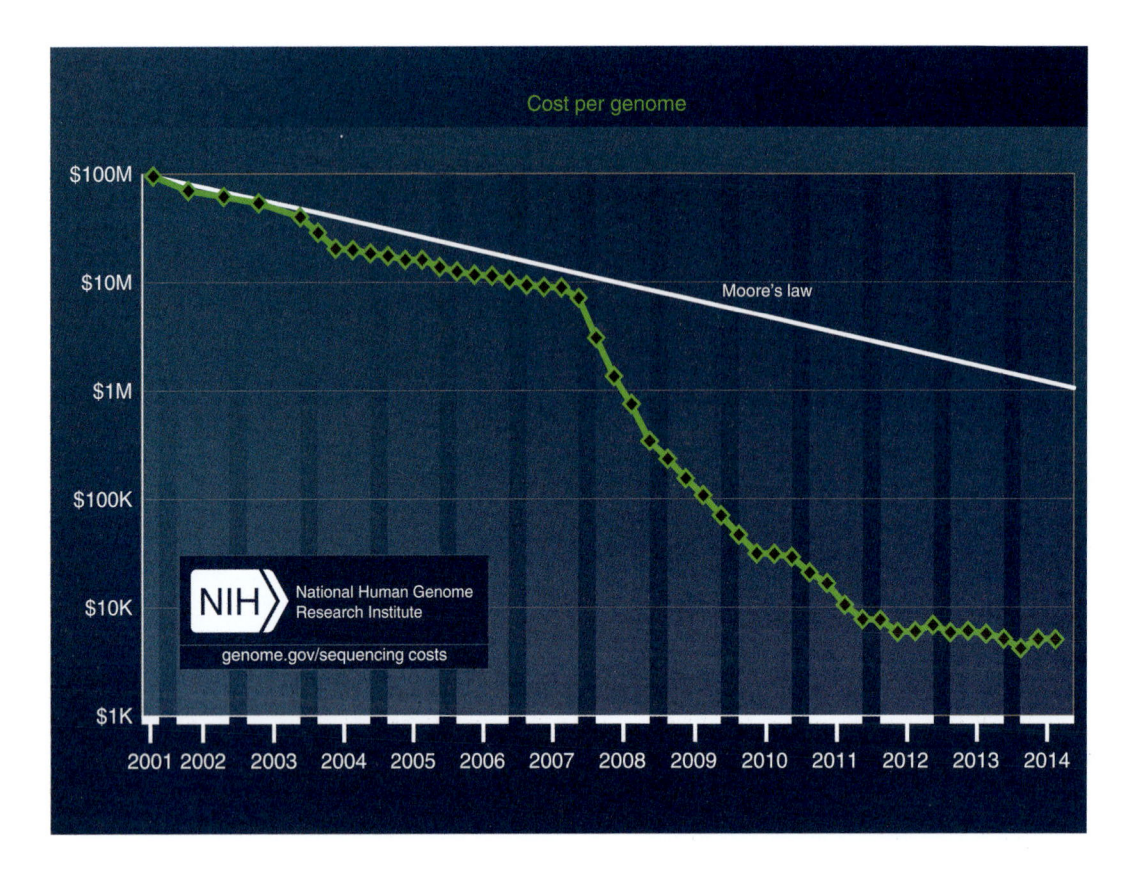

Figure 3 Cost per genome for human whole-genome sequencing. The figure shows an inflection point in late 2007 as second-generation (also known as "next-generation" and "massively parallel" sequencing came into practice), recently reducing the cost to less than $1000 per whole genome. We are awaiting the maturation and cost-effectiveness of "third-generation" technologies, principally based on sequencing of single molecules. Source: From https://www.genome.gov/about-genomics/fact-sheets/DNA-Sequencing-Costs-Data (The National Human Genome Research Institute).

copies of the book—enough for each person in the world to own 9 copies (without taking up space on their bookshelves). Under the right storage conditions, DNA can remain stable, potentially for hundreds of thousands of years, even at room temperature. Sequences can be obtained from frozen mammoths—but not from dinosaurs a la Jurassic Park, it is claimed because nowhere on earth has been frozen for all of the intervening 70 million years. If you were faced with the challenge of passing knowledge down to future civilizations, storage in DNA or an analogue thereof, would be a good bet. Getting the data into and out of the DNA is far too expensive for large-scale use at this time, but the price is decreasing rapidly.

Software challenges

Creative ideas are flowing through the field of bioinformatics software development. Many thousands of capable software packages are being developed and deployed, some of them commercial but most of them academically developed, open-source, and publicly available. The range of choices for any given computational function is almost paralyzing. One result is fragmentation of the community of users, who, for the most part, have only sometimes coalesced around particular algorithms, software, or websites. Among bioinformaticians, the "not-invented-here" syndrome often applies. As a consequence, bioinformatics is a classic Tower of Babel in which software packages may fail to communicate well with each other. One reason for that fragmentation (a serious barrier to progress) is the mutual incompatibility of various annotation schemes and data formats, but there are now major efforts to standardize and harmonize popular datasets.

Particularly in terms of sequencing, there are also algorithmic challenges of major import. If the next-generation sequencing technologies and the data from them were truly digital, one should be able identify with certainty whether there is or is not a mutation at a given DNA base pair. That is not the case, however. One reason is simply probabilistic; if each of two callers were 99.999% accurate in identifying mutation at a given base-pair in a genome of three billion bases, then they would still disagree on tens of thousands of calls. Important calls, for example, calls of driver mutations and other cancer biomarkers, may have to be validated by an independent technology. Two such strategies are (1) validation of DNA and mRNA calls against each other for the same samples; (2) use of a consensus of calls by different sequencing centers or algorithms[7]; or (3) follow-up with a different technology such as polymerase chain reaction focused on particular bases. If one thinks beyond the algorithms used in analysis and includes the idiosyncrasies of biology and of sequencing itself, there are additional possible sources of unexplained variation: clonal heterogeneity at the macroscopic or microscopic levels, low percentage of tumor cells, poor sequencing coverage in some regions of the genome, and/or degradation of the DNA or RNA (Figure 4).

Wetware challenges

At the present time, personnel ("wetware") and expertise are even more seriously limiting than the hardware or software issues. Bioinformatics is highly interdisciplinary and multidisciplinary,

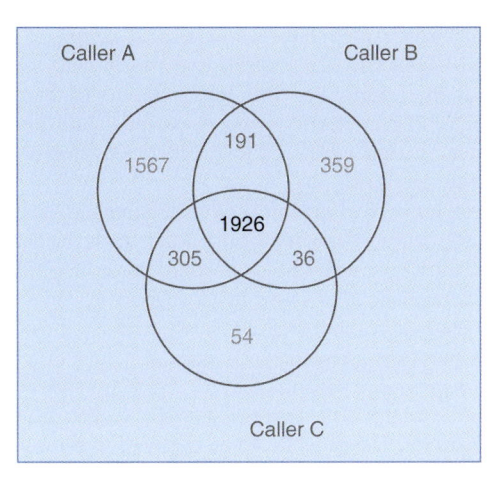

Figure 4 Venn diagram of the somatic point mutations detected as of 2013 in 20 TCGA endometrial tumor-normal exome-seq pairs by three different mutation-calling algorithms. The differences among callers were considerable. Despite substantial progress in the meantime, genomic consortia still use the consensus of several different mutation-calling algorithms as their best estimates of the reality. Source: From Ref. 7.

at the interface of computer science, statistics, artificial intelligence, biology, and medicine. There are not many individuals with expertise in all of those disciplines to operate across the interfaces among them. Despite stereotyped pipelines for some parts of the necessary analyses—generally the steps from raw data to mapped sequence—bioinformatics projects usually require customization of analyses and a multidisciplinary team.

The bioinformatics components of a typical large molecular profiling project can be divided roughly into data management, statistical analysis, and biointerpretation. Data management sounds mundane, but for a project that includes data from multiple molecular technologies and clinical data sources, it can be challenging. When the Hubble telescope was launched in 1990, it was initially crippled by a 1.3-mm error in its mirror because a custom "null corrector" was substituted for the conventional one during final testing. In 1999, the Mars Climate Orbiter was lost because computer software produced output in pound-seconds instead of newton-seconds (metric units); the orbiter's incorrect trajectory brought it too close to Mars, and it disintegrated in the atmosphere. Analogous data mismatch problems are endemic to bioinformatics. Missing or carelessly composed annotations and other metadata often result in puzzlement or wrong conclusions about the exact meaning of a data field.

Roles in the multidisciplinary bioinformatics team: an opinion

Statistical analysis of highly multivariate data, unlike that of the simple laboratory experiment, generally calls for specialist expertise in computational analysis. The biomedical researcher should be *involved in* the statistical analysis, equipped with a basic understand of the methods employed and the potential pitfalls. He or she should be prepared to provide the analyst with (1) questions to be asked of the data, (2) biomedical domain information, and (3) information on idiosyncrasies of the data-generating technologies and experimental design that might affect analysis. If a data analyst is not given those types of information, he or she may generate the right answer to the wrong question or an answer based on incorrect premises. It's dangerous, however, for the untrained to perform the data management tasks and statistical analyses alone or without very close supervision. Experience has shown a remarkable tendency for the untrained to make mistakes, generally mistakes of over-optimism. They often achieve apparently positive, even ground-breaking, results that later prove to be meaningless. "Unnatural selection" plays a role in that phenomenon; there is a human tendency, reinforced by wishful thinking, to do analyses different ways until one of them gives the desired result. And then stop. There is also a remarkable, highly tuned tendency for the human mind to find patterns in data where none exist. The analogy of allowing a statistician to perform brain surgery (or a brain surgeon to perform statistical analyses) may overstate the case, but not dramatically so.

In biointerpretation and medical interpretation, to the contrary, the biomedical researcher should preferably take the lead on the basis of specific domain expertise and general knowledge of cancer biology. Every basic, translational, or clinical cancer researcher should be able to use a selection of the available tools of biointerpretation to explore the genes, pathways, networks, cell biological entities, pathological diagnoses, and clinical correlates that come into focus on the basis of large-scale molecular data sets. Training researchers in the use of such tools can be considered a primary responsibility of the bioinformatician. The bioinformatician should be prepared to explain the essence of statistical or machine-learning algorithms that he or she is using and to do so in visual, nonmathematical terms (i.e., without equations). That is almost *always* possible to do. However, the bioinformatician is likely to have the broader knowledge necessary for selection of the optimal tools and data resources for a project and can do the programming that is usually necessary to customize an algorithm or a graphical visualization of the data.

Bioinformatic analysis, visualization, and interpretation

Table 1 lists some molecular data types and phenomena that can be significant in the analysis of cancers, often for early detection or for prediction of cancer risk, diagnosis, prognosis, response to treatment, recurrence, or metastasis. The "omic" terminology sometimes seems strained, but it's compact, convenient, and etymologically justified. The suffix "-ome" is from the Greek for an "abstract entity, group, or mass," so omics is the study of entities in aggregate.[8] (A curiosity: we use genetics for the single-gene counterpart of genomics but not protetics for the single-gene counterpart of proteomics or metaboletics for the single-compound counterpart of metabolomics.)

Many of the statistical principles, algorithms, and software used in the field are agnostic to the type of data, but each type has its own peculiarities that require customized attention. Issues like background level, normalization, filtering for variation, distributional properties, thresholds, and representation as continuous or dichotomized values all require careful attention. Poor choices of those procedures can lead to fundamentally wrong results in the analysis. In fact, the most important and most challenging, often unresolvable problems in bioinformatics arise from the most mundane, least glamorous task: preprocessing the data to minimize noise without eliminating signal. Also important, there is a tremendous loss of opportunity and a real danger of uncorrected or uncorrectable error if the datasets and analytical procedures used on them cannot be reproduced months or years later for cross-checking and independent analysis.

"Data integration" is a field of intense study. There are many methods for making disparate data types commensurate with each other and therefore able to be integrated, but none of them

Table 1 Some bioinformatic data types, phenomena, and data sources.

Data types	Data sources
Genomic—germline, somatic (DNA level)	Bulk measurement
Single-nucleotide variation (SNV)	Whole exome sequencing (WES)
Insertion/Deletion (Indel)	Whole genome sequencing (WGS)
Copy number variation	Bisulfite sequencing
Loss of heterozygosity (LOH)	Low-coverage copy number sequencing
Translocation	Reverse-phase protein arrays
Repeat element	Mass spectrometry
Functional motif	Antibody arrays
Domain structure	Nucleic acid microarrays
Fusion gene	Single-cell measurement
Viral insertion	Single-cell sequencing (DNA, RNA)
Pseudogene	Flow cytometry (fluorescence, mass-tagging)
Epigenomic	Clinical
DNA methylation (CpG island)	Medical records
DNA methylation (non-CpG island)	Clinical trials
DNA modification (other)	Other
Histone modification (acetylation, methylation, etc.)	siRNA, shRNA
Transcriptomic (RNA level)	CRISPR
mRNA expression	Mass spectrometry
microRNA expression	Microdissection, tumor disaggregation
long non-coding RNA expression	Microscopy
Transcript splice variation	Imaging
RNA editing	Circulating exosomes, tumor cells
Allele-specific indices	
Proteomic	
Protein expression	
Posttranslational modification	
Location in the cell	
Protein complexes and interactions	
Metabolomic	
Metabolite flux	
Metabolite expression level	
Targeted identification (mrm)	
Chromosomic	
Transcription factor target	
Histone modifier target	
Replication start site (and kinetics)	
Transcription start site and kinetics	
Modulation of chromosome accessibility	
Microsatellite instability (MSI)	
Chromosomal instability (CIN)	
3D chromosomal arrangement	
Long-range genomic regulation	
Choreography of mitosis and meiosis	
Pharmacomic	
Response	
Natural and acquired resistance	
Immunomics	
Epitope-mapping	
Immune cell profiling	
Immune regulatory network modeling	
Connectomic	
Co-occurring and mutually exclusive elements	
Hub nodes	
Random versus scale-free properties	
Disassortivity	
Pathological	
Classification, subclassification	
Grade	
Percent tumor cells	
Clonal heterogeneity (microscopic, macroscopic)	
Marker studies (by immunohistochemistry, in situ hybridization, etc.)	
Clinical	
Survival	
Disease-free survival	
Time to Relapse	
Response to therapy	

are totally satisfactory. Table 2 lists a small sample of the many web-based tools that are available and widely used for analysis, visualization, integration, and interpretation of bioinformatic data. According to "FAIR" principles, data should be Findable, Accessible, Interoperable, and Reusable. (Sadly, that is rarely the case in the real world.)

A large number of graphical representations are central tools in bioinformatics. Hierarchical cluster analysis is the data-mining method most frequently used. It builds trees of similarity and difference analogous to those in phylogenetics. For example, a typical gene expression profiling study across a set of patients' samples produces a rectangular matrix of values in which each column represents a patient, each row represents a gene, and each entry in the matrix is the expression level of a gene in a particular patient's tumor. The patients can be clustered to show patterns of similarity and difference in their profiles, and the genes can be clustered to show the similarities and differences in their patterns across the patients' samples.

Clustered heat maps (CHMs)

Clustered heat maps (CHMs) are the most frequently used graphics for summarizing patterns in bioinformatic data. Hierarchical clustering in *both* horizontal and vertical directions serves to illuminate patterns in the data. CHMs were introduced into bioinformatics in the early 1990s,[16a,b] and they then become the ubiquitous graphic for visualizing patterns in omic data. They have appeared in many thousands of publications and in multiple different formats. The first CHM known to have influenced medical practice (in 1993) is shown in Figure 5.[16a] It represents drug activity correlations in a study of platinum-containing compounds in the NCI-60 anticancer cell line screen. It tipped the balance in favor of clinical development of oxaliplatin, still a standard agent for treatment of colorectal cancer. More recently, dynamically interactive "Next-Generation CHMs have been developed for exploration of large data sets.[16c]

Hypothesis-generating and hypothesis-driven research

Throughout most of its history, biology was predominantly an observational science. Darwin formulated his hypothesis about natural selection by unbiased observation of the Galapagos finches and other archipelago species, not by experimenting on them. By the middle of the twentieth century, however, the dominant research paradigm in biology had shifted to tightly focused, hypothesis-driven experiments. Taking a lesson from the concept in physics of a critical experiment, *patterns* of experimental result in biology were relegated to the background. In the 1990s, with the maturation of microarrays and other high-throughput molecular technologies, the balance shifted again—toward a synergistic balance between hypothesis-driven experiments and hypothesis-generating omic research. Announcement in 2001 of the draft human genome sequence solidified that trend, serving as motivation and justification for additional large-scale molecular profiling programs such as The Cancer Genome Atlas (TCGA) and International Cancer Genome Consortium (ICGC) projects.

The multiple hypothesis-testing trap

This has been the most common error in bioinformatic analysis made by those without training in statistics. When mining large molecular or clinical databases for biomarkers, p-values <0.05 are not hard to find. Consider, for example, a database of 20,000 gene expression values generated by microarray or RNA sequencing for

Table 2 A sample of web-based bioinformatics tools and data resources useful in bioinformatics.

The UCSC Genome Browser[9]—Offers interactive online access to a database of genomic sequences and rich annotation data for a wide variety of organisms. Genome sequence is displayed horizontally, accompanied by a set of annotation tracks (which can be user-selected). For example, there are tracks that give the locations of predicted genes, transcription factor targets, DNA repeat elements, microRNAs, and cross-species comparative genomic information. There is an associated Cancer Genomics Browser for displaying and analyzing cancer genomics data along with associated clinical data[10] (http://genome.ucsc.edu/)

The cBioPortal[11]—A resource for intuitive, interactive exploration of multiple cancer genomics data sets and correlative information from many different public molecular profiling project, including TCGA (http://www.cbioportal.org/)

Cytoscape—A flexible open-source software platform for analyzing, visualizing, and annotating complex interaction networks (http://www.cytoscape.org/)

Bioconductor—An extensive open-source, open-development collection of programs (934 of them as of March 2015), mostly written in R, for analysis, graphical visualization, and annotation of bioinformatics data[12] (http://www.bioconductor.org)

Ingenuity Pathway Analysis—Integrated analysis of pathway, regulatory, and disease data (available in public and commercial versions) (http://www.ingenuity.com)

Pathway Studio—A resource of molecular interactions and associated tools, based in part on natural language processing of biological and medical literature (commercial product) (http://www.elsevier.com/solutions/pathway-studio)

Oncomine—An integrated collection of hundreds of public microarray gene expression studies on cancers, with associated tools for meta-analysis of the data, for example to tumor subtypes, biomarkers, and therapeutic targets (available in public and commercial versions)[13] (http://www.lifetechnologies.com/us/en/home/life-science/cancer-research/cancer-genomics/cancer-genomics-data-analysis-compendia-bioscience/oncomine-cancer-genomics-data-analysis-tools/oncomine-gene-browser.html))

The Gene Ontology (GO)[14]—Product of an international initiative to unify the annotations of genes and gene products by imposing a controlled vocabulary and hierarchical structure of categories (or terms). Formally, the structure is an "acyclic graph" in which each category in the hierarchy can have more than one parent category. There are three independent ontologies: biological process, molecular function, and cellular component. GO is frequently used to identify categories that are relatively enriched with overexpressed or under-expressed genes in a comparison of two gene expression profiles. The many tools for statistical assessment of the enrichment include AmiGo, David, GoMiner, and OBO-Edit (http://geneontology.org/)

Compendium of TCGA Next-Generation Clustered Heat Maps (NG-CHMs)—CHMs are the graphical visualizations ubiquitous in bioinformatics for identifying patterns in molecular profile databases. However, they are static images. NG-CHMs are highly interactive versions in which one can zoom and navigate using a Google-Maps-like technology; link out to pertinent public data resources including pathway programs, the UCSC Genome Browser, and the cBio Portal; re-color the map on the fly; access a statistical toolbox for detailed analysis of the data; produce high-resolution graphics; and store all metadata necessary to reproduce the map months or years later (http://bioinformatics.mdanderson.org/main/TCGA/NGCHM)

The Cancer Genome Atlas (TCGA) Data Portal—A primary source for access to nonrestricted TCGA data (http://cancergenome.nih.gov)

The Cancer Proteome Atlas (TCPA) Portal—A collection of proteomic databases and tools for analysis and visualization of proteomic data, principally but not exclusively from TCGA (http://cancergenome.nih.gov)

Firehose—An analysis infrastructure that coordinates the flow of gigabyte- or terabyte-scale datasets through dozens of analysis algorithms for cancer genome projects including TCGA. An add-on, Nozzle, provides user-friendly formats for the results (http://gdac.broadinstitute.org)

Regulome Explorer—A suite of tools for exploration and visualization of large, complex data sets featuring a machine-learning algorithm (random forest) plus a circular ideogram layout, a linear multi-track browser, and 2D plots (http://explorer.cancerregulome.org)

Paradigm—A program that infers patient-specific genetic activities on the basis of curated pathway interactions among genes. It incorporates multiple types of omic data on tumor samples and predicts a pathway's activity level based on probabilistic inference (http://sbenz.github.com/Paradigm).[15] A related program, Paradigm-Shift (http://github.org/paradigmshift) uses a belief-propagation algorithm to infer gene activity from gene expression and copy number data in the context of pathway interactions

NCI Genomic Data Commons—Comprehensive computational infrastructure under development to store and harmonize genomic data on cancer generated through NCI-funded research programs (https://gdc.cancer.gov/)

GenBank: The NIH/NLM genetic sequence database, an annotated collection of all publicly available DNA sequences (http://www.ncbi.nlm.nhi.gov/genbank)

GEO (Gene Expression Omnibus): A functional genomics data repository of curated microarray- and sequence-based gene expression datasets (http://www.ncbi.nlm.nih.gov/geo)

Cancer Genomics Hub (CGHub): A secure repository for storing, cataloging, and accessing cancer genome sequences, alignments, and mutation information (including restricted-access personally identifiable data) from The Cancer Genome Atlas consortium and related projects (https://cghub.ucsc.edu/)

tumors from 50 patients who responded to a particular drug and 50 who did not respond. If the aim is to discover a gene whose expression in the tumor is positively correlated with response to the drug (therefore a potential predictive biomarker), then ~20,000 different hypotheses are being tested in parallel, one for each gene. Since the p-value (for rejection of the null hypothesis that there is *no* difference) will be less than 0.05 about one in 20 times by chance, even if the data are simply random, there will appear to be on the order of 1000 potential biomarkers. More subtle versions of the multiple-hypothesis problem occur, for example, any time multiple statistical algorithms, subsets of genes, or subsets of sample are analyzed. If one tries five different algorithms before finding one that yields p-values less than 0.05, then the p-value is misleading because it was chosen among the five possibilities. Conceptually the simplest remedy is the Bonferroni correction in which the critical p-value (e.g., 0.05) is divided by the number of independent hypotheses to get a corrected critical value. For 20,000 genes, viewed as independent, that would be $p = 0.05/20{,}000 = 2.5 \times 10^{-6}$ before one would accept the p-value as statistically significant. However, the Bonferroni correction is usually too conservative (i.e., it overcorrects) because the hypotheses are generally not independent of each other. Most popular for correction are algorithms based on false discovery rate (FDR), the fraction of apparently positive results (i.e., apparent rejections of the null hypothesis) that are expected actually to be *false* positives. The statistical nuances are complex, and dozens of different algorithms for the correction have been proposed.[17] One popular approach in bioinformatics is the Statistical Analysis of Microarrays (SAM) algorithm, which takes correlation structures in the data into account.[18]

The multiple-hypothesis problem brings into sharp focus the important difference between *hypothesis generation* and *hypothesis testing* in bioinformatics. For the latter, the strict rules of statistical inference must be observed or the results will be incorrect. For example, about 1000 genes in the above case would spuriously be identified as biomarkers if the investigator were simply mining for genes with uncorrected $p < 0.05$. However, if the investigator started, before looking at the data, with a single-minded focus on one particular gene out of the 20,000, then the critical level for that gene would be $p = 0.05$, regardless of how many other genes were present in the dataset. (That may seem paradoxical, but not as paradoxical as an intent-to-treat clinical trial design when an untreated patient is counted as treated.)

Hypothesis generation would consist of asking for each gene whether it is a plausible enough candidate biomarker to merit further study. The FDR provides one metric of that plausibility. One can list the genes in order of their FDR values, from lowest to highest, and keep as candidates all of the genes at the top of

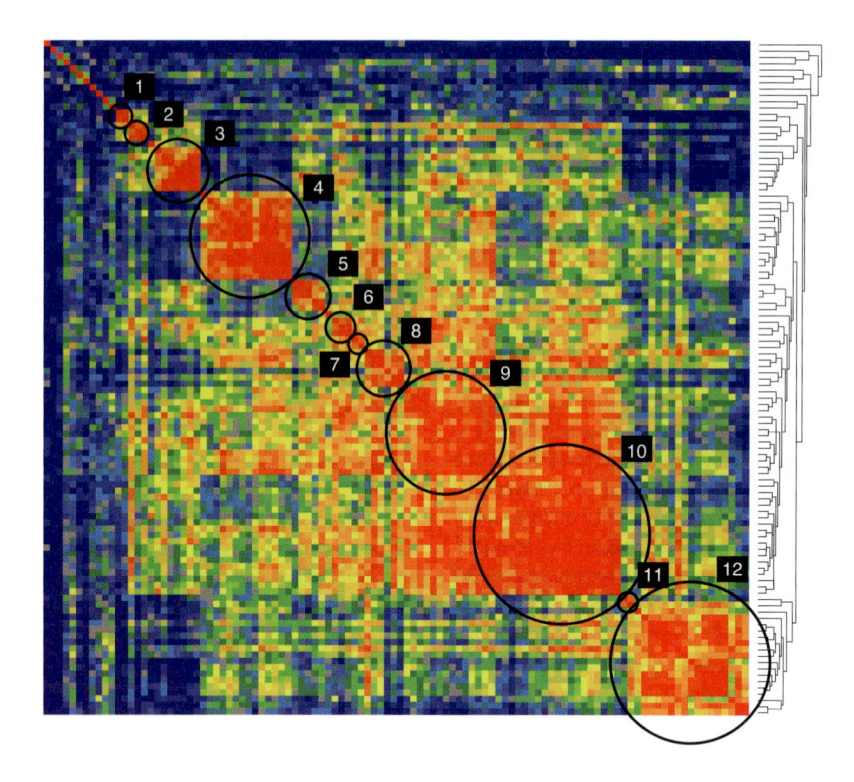

Figure 5 Drug versus drug clustered heat map for the activity of platinum-containing compounds against the NCI-60 panel of human cancer cell lines. Drugs are listed on both axes in the same clustered order, hence the heat map is symmetrical around the diagonal. Red indicates high correlation of activity profiles, blue indicates low correlation. The data define 12 families (which are highly correlated with the chemical structures of the compounds). Cluster #4 drugs, which consisted entirely of diaminocyclohexyl derivatives, including oxaliplatin, were selectively active against colorectal cell lines. That information tipped the balance for clinical development of oxaliplatin, now a standard agent for treatment of colorectal cancers (due to Weinstein, Myers, and Fojo, unpublished).

the list, extending as far down the list as desired. There is a tendency to select an FDR cutoff of 0.05 by analogy with the usual *p*-value criterion, but that may be too conservative. How often in biology or medical science do we expect to be correct 19 out of 20 times? As a practical matter, the number of candidates accepted as positive should depend on a balance between the "cost" of independently validating a candidate and the "cost" of missing a *true* positive. If the validation step is a simple assay, one can afford many false positives; if the next step is major surgery, then few if any false positives can be tolerated. The issues of false positives, true positive, and "positive predictive value" are familiar in many areas of public health and clinical practice, for example in the controversies over prostate-specific antigen (PSA) screening. It is important, therefore, that anyone interpreting a statistical analysis know the question being asked, the reason why it is being asked, and the cost/benefit ratio of follow-up. But even if a *p*-value is validly low, it is important that they consider the magnitude of difference between groups; since the *p*-value toward zero as the sample size gets large, even a tiny, meaningless, extraneous bias in the data can yield a low *p*-value for large samples. Reliance on the *p*-value alone is another frequent mistake of over-optimism; an experiment is almost always more publishable (or patentable) if it is claimed to show a difference between group, rather than no interpretable difference.

Analysis and biointerpretation in major molecular profiling projects

Table 3 lists some of the more prominent public molecular profiling projects. The first waves of large-scale projects focused on cancer cell lines and, later, bulk samples of primary tumors paired with blood or normal tissue controls. However, more recent projects are asking, or will be asking, incisive questions based on microdissection, single-cell sequencing,[36] archived formalin-fixed paraffin-embedded samples, liquid biopsies (e.g., for circulating tumor cells or free nucleic acids), pretreatment/posttreatment pairs, primary tumor/metastasis pairs, comparison of samples from different parts of the same primary tumor, comparison of different metastases from the same patient, primary/recurrent pairs, and samples from responders and nonresponders at different longitudinal time points. Those new waves of projects are making use of many of the same algorithms and programs for data analysis and interpretation, but they also motivate novel bioinformatics tools. For example, single-cell sequencing, particularly at the DNA level, imposes a new set of requirements as well as providing a new set of opportunities for customized analysis. Serial sampling from a patient can clearly yield invaluable information. For example, recurrent tumors can reflect clones that were minor in the primary but important for choice of therapy. Hence, the logistical, financial, and ethical barriers to re-biopsy are rapidly being overcome for more and more tumor types and clinical contexts.

Figure 6 shows schematically the flows of tissue and information in the most prominent molecular profiling project to date, TCGA. Over 50 Tissue Source Sites provided paired tumor samples and normal samples (blood and/or tumor-adjacent "normal" tissue) plus information on the pathology and clinical history for 33 tumor types. The samples were processed in Biospecimen Core Resources to produce DNA, RNA, and protein preparations, which were then profiled (principally by microarray or sequencing) in Genome Sequencing and Genome Characterization Centers. Primary data generation was completed as of 2015, but data analysis and

Table 3 Some major molecular profiling projects on human cancers, normal tissues, and cell lines.

Cultured cancer cells

The NCI-60—A panel of 60 human cell lines used since 1990 by the NCI to screen >100,000 chemical compounds plus large numbers of natural products for anticancer activity.[19] This was the first large public project molecular profiling project on cancers. It linked pharmacology to "integromic" molecular profiling of diverse cancer cells. One byproduct was development of new tools for bioinformatics including the clustered heat map[16a] and other statistical and machine-learning innovations.[20] The NCI-60 provided a template for the design of CCLE, GDSC, and it informed the design of TCGA (see below) (data at http://discover.nci.nih.gov/cellminer/home.do)

The Cancer Cell Line Encyclopedia (CCLE)—Gene expression, DNA copy number, and sequencing data on 1,000 diverse human cancer cell lines, with metabolic inhibition assays of anticancer drugs in many of the 1457 the cell lines profiled as of April 2021. Naïve Bayes and elastic net algorithms, among other approaches, were used to predict response profiles on the basis of cell lineage, genetic defects, and gene expression[21] (http://www.broadinstitute.org/ccle)

The Genomics of Drug Sensitivity in Cancer (GDSC)—Point mutations, indels, microsatellite instability, DNA rearrangements, and gene expression for 1000 diverse human cancer cell lines, with metabolic inhibition assays of 100s of anticancer agents on many of the cell lines. Elastic net regression was used to predict drug sensitivity from the molecular profiles[22] (http://www.cancerrxgene.org/)

Clinical tumors and tissues

The Human Genome Project—Planning began in 1986,[23] draft sequences were published in 2001,[24,25] and a "99%" complete sequence was published in 2004.[26] Surprisingly to many, bioinformatic analysis showed only about 23,000 human genes, not the >50,000 expected. Continuing refinements of the reference sequence are a major pain for bioinformatics algorithms and software (http://www.cancerrxgene.org/)

The International HapMap Project—Initiated in 2002 to define common DNA sequence variations among subsets of the human population and aid in Genome-Wide Association Studies (GWAS). Unrelated individuals are ~99.9% identical in sequence, but the remaining sequence and copy number polymorphisms are both important and a nuisance for bioinformatic analysis[27] (http://hapmap.ncbi.nlm.nih.gov/)

The Cancer Genome Atlas (TCGA)—Initiated in 2005 by the NCI, >10,000 human cancers of 33 different types at the genomic, epigenomic, transcriptomic, proteomic, pathologic, and clinical levels. The first project, published in 2008, was on glioblastoma[28]

The PanCancer Atlas—integrated data from TCGA disease-type projects[29,30] to address (1) occurrence of functional themes (e.g., driver mutations, aberrant pathways, drug resistance) across tumor types, and (2) subdivision of cancer types into finer subcategories with clinical implications. Protein studies by reverse-phase protein array (RPPA) and mass spectrometry were added[31,32] (http://cancergenome.nih.gov/)

The International Cancer Genome Consortium (ICGC)[33]—Launched in 2008 for molecular profiling of 50 diverse human cancer types in a manner similar to the profiling in TCGA (https://icgc.org/)

The PanCancer Analysis of Whole Genomes (PCAWG)—An ICGC/TCGA international collaboration to identify common patterns of mutation in >2600 cancer whole genomes (https://dcc.icgc.org/pcawg)

The Adjuvant Lung Cancer Enrichment Marker Identification and Sequencing Trials (ALCHEMIST)—Launched in 2014 by the NCI's National Clinical Trials Network to identify early-stage lung cancer patients with tumors that have genetic changes (EGFR mutations or ALK rearrangements) to evaluate drug treatments targeted against those changes (http://www.cancer.gov/types/lung/research/alchemist)

The Exceptional Responders Initiative—Launched by the NCI in 2014 to explore the molecular underpinnings of exceptional responses to treatment. The primary technologies used are whole exome- and mRNA sequencing (http://www.nih.gov/news/health/sep2014/nci-24.htm)

The Genotype-Tissue Expression Project (GTEx)—Initiated in 2006 by the NIH/NHGRI to correlate genotype and expression levels in multiple normal tissues—to aid in GSWAS studies and serve as normal background data for studies of many diseases (http://www.gtexportal.org/home/)

1000 Genomes Project—Launched in 2008 as an international effort to establish the most detailed catalog available on human germline genomic variation[34] (http://www.gtexportal.org/home)

The Encyclopedia of DNA Elements (ENCODE)—An international consortium launched by the NHGRI as a follow-up to the Human Genome Project. Its ultimate aim was to identify all functional elements in the human genome, particularly those not located in RNA-coding regions[35] (https://www.encodeproject.org)

The Therapeutically Applicable Research to Generate Effective Treatments (TARGET)—Multi-institutional molecular profiling of genetic changes (gene expression, DNA copy number, DNA methylation, and microRNA expression) that affect the initiation, progression, and response to therapy of pediatric cancers (https://ocg.cancer.gov/programs/target)

The Human Cell Atlas (HCA)—Launched in 2017 as an international consortium to develop comprehensive reference maps of all human cell types based principally on highly multiplexed single-cell omic technologies at the DNA, RNA, and protein levels (https://www.humancellatlas.org/)

The Human Tumor Atlas Network (HTAN)—An NCI-funded Cancer Moonshot initiative to construct 3-dimensional atlases of the dynamic cellular, morphological, and molecular features of human cancers as they evolve from precancerous lesions to advanced disease (https://humantumoratlas.org/#)

---

interpretation are still continuing. The Data Coordinating Center (replaced later by the Genomics Data Commons; GDC) organized and further quality-controlled the data, then made "nonrestricted" datasets publicly available as soon as feasible on the TCGA Data Portal and in the GDC. Re-examination by panels of pathologists with specialist expertise in the particular tumor type proved critical. "Restricted" data containing personally identifiable information were made accessible only to researchers who had gone through a registration and vetting process intended to ensure confidentiality and appropriate use. Raw DNA and RNA sequences, for example, were restricted because they were considered personally identifiable. Central to analysis and interpretation were the seven designated Genome Data Analysis Centers (GDACs). The GDACS matured into a TCGA community of shared, progressively more sophisticated bioinformatic expertise.

A major spin-off of TCGA and Pan Cancer Analysis of Whole Genomes (PCAWG) has been the coalescence of a large bioinformatics community. Each Analysis Working Group (AWG) was a self-assembled aggregate of the multidisciplinary expertise required for data analysis and biological/medical interpretation. At the center were the GDACs, but many other individuals and institutions joined in. Since everyone in an AWG was drilling down into the same datasets and data types, the result was a powerfully creative environment for development of new, innovative tools for analysis, visualization, and interpretation. Figure 7 is based on TCGA's multifaceted Urothelial Bladder Cancer profiling project. Figure 7a shows a compact graphical visualization of the DNA-sequencing data, Figure 7b shows a dynamically interactive "next-generation" CHM for the RNA expression levels,[16c] and Figure 7c shows a particular representation of key pathways. Figure 8 represents the Pan-Cancer Atlas project schematically as a 3D matrix of results.[29]

Statistical methods

Table 4 is a list, by no means comprehensive, of statistical and machine-learning algorithms commonly used in bioinformatics. The descriptions in the table are intended to give the reader a general sense of how the algorithm can be used, rather than to be rigorous or complete for the statistically trained.

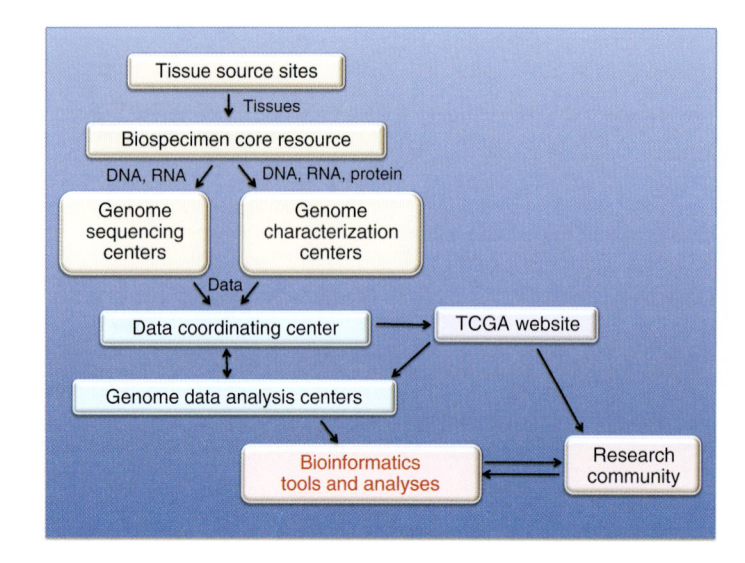

Figure 6 Simplified generic view of the flow of samples and information in The Cancer Genome Atlas program. Tumor plus normal blood and/or "normal tumor-adjacent" tissue specimens were collected with consent by tissue source sites and handled according to defined protocols for submission to the project. The Biospecimen Core Resource vetted the specimens and accompanying clinical data, generated DNA, RNA, and protein samples, quality-controlled the samples, and sent them to the Genome Sequencing and Genome Characterization Centers. Those Centers profiled the samples by sequencing, microarray, or other technologies and sent the data to the Data Coordinating Center. As soon as feasible, nonrestricted forms of the data were made public on TCGA's website for use by the research community, including TCGA's GDACs. For each of the 33 tumor types, an AWG self-assembled under the auspices of TCGA's Program Office to perform and integrate analyses, then write a "marker" manuscript on the project. An analogous PanCancer Working Group did the same to compare and contrast results across the first 12 tumor-type projects. Omitted here for simplicity are many additional components of the information flow such as the Broad Institute's Firehose, which performed and presented large numbers of analyses on the data; Sage Bionetics' Synapse, which provided an environment and tools that facilitated wide collaborative use of the data; Memorial Sloan-Kettering's cBioPortal, which presented the data in a form accessible to nonspecialists; and MD Anderson's compendia of Next Generation Clustered Heat Maps ref for pattern recognition in the DNA, RNA, and protein datasets. Also not shown are reviews of clinical data and pathology by expert specialists in each of the tumor types under study.

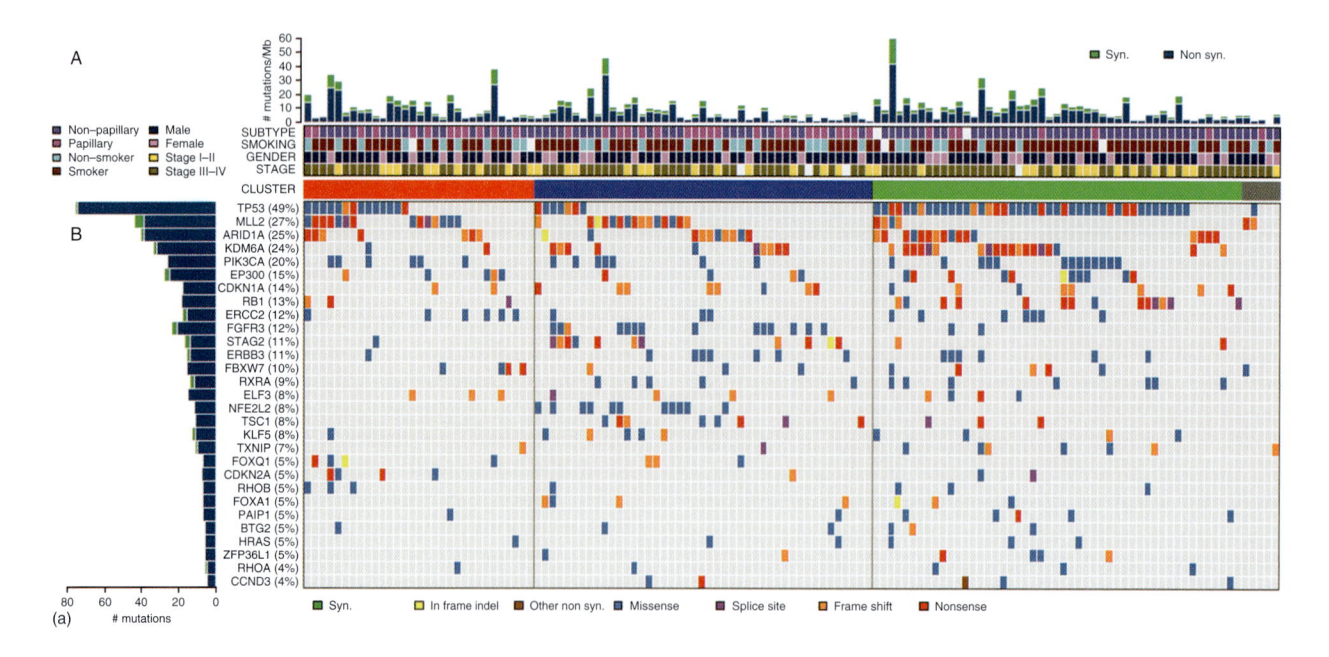

Figure 7 Data visualizations in TCGA's Urothelial Bladder Cancer Project. Modified from Ref. 37. Tumor specimens from 131 patients were included in the analyses. (a) A compact visualization of mutation profiles across the bladder cancer specimens for genes scored by the MutSig 1.5 algorithm as significantly mutated (due to J. Kim, A. Cherniack, D. Kwiatkowski). (b) An interactive Next-Generation Clustered Heat Map representation of the mRNA expression data. Genes are on the vertical axis; patient specimens are on the horizontal axis. (due to B. Broom, R. Akbani, D. Kane, M. Ryan, C. Wakefield, J. Weinstein). (c) Representation of four pathways found to be altered at the DNA level in urothelial bladder cancer. Somatic mutations and copy number alterations (CNAs) were found in the p53/Rb pathway, RTK/RAS/PI(3)K pathway, histone modification system, and SWI/SNF complex. Red, activating genetic alterations; blue, inactivating genetic alterations. Percentages shown denote activation or inactivation of at least one allele. (Due to C. Creighton, D. Kwiatkowski, L Donehower, P Laird.)

(b)

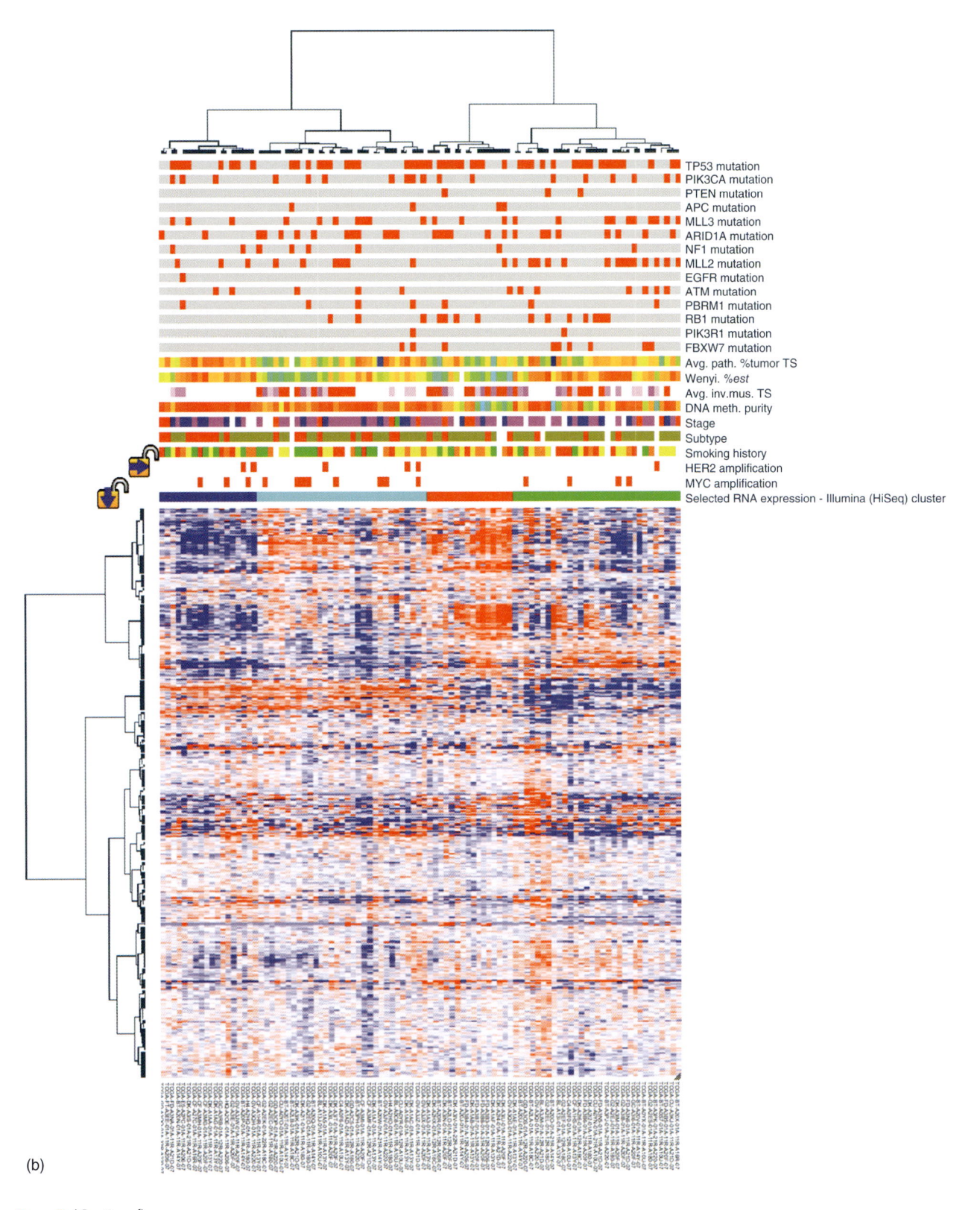

Figure 7 (*Continued*)

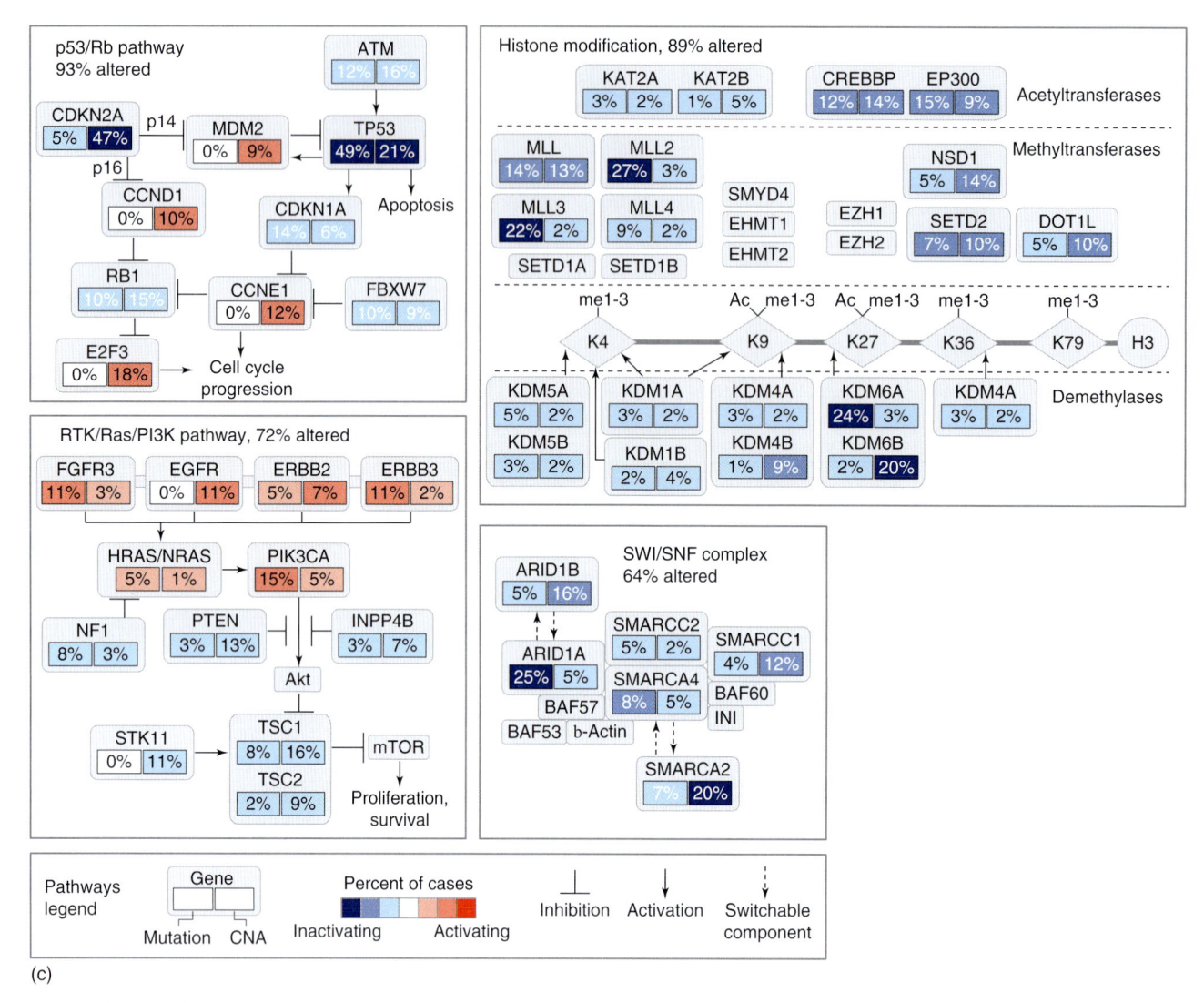

Figure 7 (*Continued*)

Some current trends in bioinformatics

The omic technologies and attendant bioinformatics tools are evolving at an exhilarating pace. It is hard to keep up. Here are some of the trends and increasingly important practical principles:

1. Large molecular profiling databases are becoming more available and becoming the norm, often for hypothesis generation or for hypothesis validation in combination with a researcher's own smaller datasets.
2. In particular, use of highly multiplexed single-cell studies (principally sequencing or flow cytometry), rather than analysis of bulk tumors, is increasing. A single sample may generate data on many hundreds of thousands of individually bar-coded cells, with sequences quantitated for ~20,000 genes.
3. Preexisting algorithm modules are more often being strung together in pipelines or networks, rather than being developed from scratch.
4. The new generation of biologists and clinical research trainees typically has much more competence with computers and mathematics than did their predecessors; they can comfortably do much more of the bioinformatics, coding included.
5. However, over-confidence can be a problem. Large omic databases generally require sophisticated multivariate analysis or artificial intelligence-based methods that can go badly wrong if not performed and assessed with sufficient expertise. The tendency is to get, or at least select, overly optimistic results.
6. Machine learning/artificial intelligence is becoming useful more often, given the large datasets. But many of the methods are only as good as the datasets used to train them, and the possibilities for serious bias or getting definitive answers to the wrong question are rife.
7. Given the size of datasets, fluent graphical visualizations are more important than ever. For human pattern recognition, a picture is usually worth a thousand numerical table entries.
8. Increasingly, bioinformaticians and biologists/clinical researchers should consider dyad relationships with each other to solve computational problems; the bioinformatician to focus on data management and data science, particularly for the statistics and A/I; the clinical researcher to focus on biological and medical interpretation.

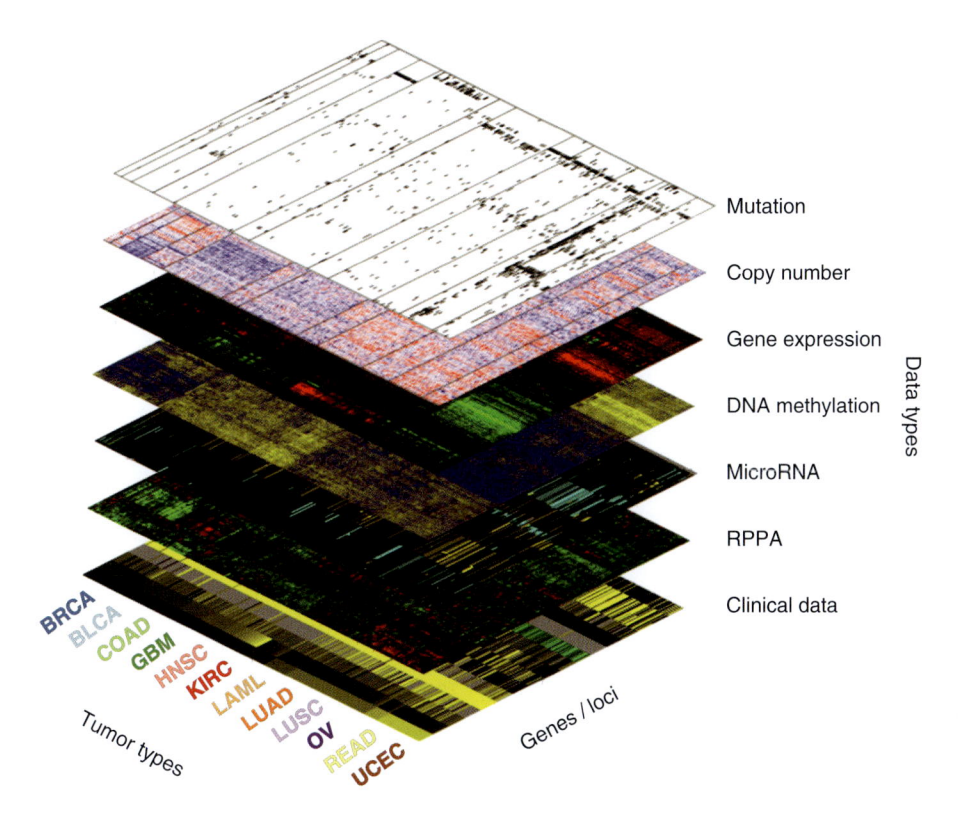

Figure 8 Representation of the Pan-Cancer TCGA project as a three-dimensional matrix in which the axes are tumor type, data type, and gene or locus.

Table 4 A sample of statistical algorithms commonly used in bioinformatics.

Univariate analysis

t-test (unpaired): A two-sample *t*-test examines whether two samples are different and is commonly used when the variances of two normal distributions are unknown and when an experiment uses a small sample size

t-test (paired): A version of the *t*-test in which samples are paired (e.g., with tumor specimens before and after treatment)

Permutation t-test: A version of the t-test applicable without assuming normal distribution (but assuming that the distributions of the two samples are the same). Almost all "parametric" statistical tests (i.e., ones in which the reference distributions are obtained from a theoretical probability distribution, e.g. normal distribution) have nonparametric equivalents in which the *p*-value is obtained by permuting the samples in an appropriate way

Wilcoxon signed-rank test: Nonparametric equivalent of the paired t-test (based on ranks so normality not necessary)

Wilcoxon rank-sum (Mann–Whitney) test: Nonparametric equivalent of unpaired t-test (based on ranks; normality not necessary)

Multivariate analysis

Analysis of variance (ANOVA): Various forms of ANOVA extend the t-test to situations in which multiple variables are involved and normal distribution is assumed (e.g., multiple characteristics of more than two types of tumor specimens are being compared)

Multivariate analysis of variance (MANOVA): Like ANOVA but taking into account the interactions (dependencies) among variables

Cross-validation: Useful in predicting an outcome (e.g., survival) on the basis of expression of one or more genes in a set of samples. A predictive model is trained on, say 90%, of the patients and then tested on the other 10%. Different sets of 10% are then left out iteratively in order to pile up statistics on the model's success on patient samples it has not "seen" during the particular round of training and testing. However, if the model is "tweaked" in any way to optimize it on the basis of the cross-validation, it must then be validated against a separate set of samples to avoid overly optimistic conclusions. Hence, there are generally training, test, and validation data sets. If the validation set is from a different study (e.g., a different institution), then performs two tasks are performed simultaneously: validation of results and extrapolation to a different context as a test of robustness

Bootstrap: Finds statistical confidence limits for a calculated statistic (e.g., a Pearson or Spearman correlation coefficient between two patients' tumors based on similarities and differences in their expression patterns across *N* genes). To proceed, we select *with replacement* a random sample of size *N* from the set of genes to produce a "pseudo-sample" of *N* values, then calculate the Pearson correlation coefficient for that sample. We do that many times, say 10,000 times, to build a histogram of estimates of the Pearson correlation coefficient and pick 95% confidence limits on the basis of that histogram. Because the sampling is done with replacement, any given gene may appear in a given sample 0, 1, 2, 3, or more times (according to the Poisson distribution with a mean of 1)

ROC (Receiver-operator Characteristic): A plot of sensitivity versus 1-specificity that indicates the performance of a binary classifier (e.g., expression of a particular gene as a predictor of recurrence) as the discrimination threshold of expression is varied from low to high. The area under the ROC curve is directly related to the (nonparametric) Wilcoxon signed-rank test

Hierarchical cluster analysis: The clustering brings similar profiles (e.g., across tumor specimens or across genes) together in a tree-like structure to illuminate patterns of similarity and difference among them. Clustering (supervised or nonsupervised) is often used to define subcategories of tumor types

Fisher's exact test: A permutation test for the independence of variables in a contingency table. For example, if each patient in a clinical trial is labeled as a responder or nonresponder to a treatment and labeled as wild-type or mutant with respect to a particular gene, the results of the study can be expressed in a 2 × 2 contingency table. Fisher's exact test (one- or two-tailed) gives a *p*-value for the null hypothesis that the gene's status has no effect on response. The word "exact" indicates that the *p*-value is accurate for even very small sample sizes. The test can be extended to larger (i.e., m × n) contingency tables

Bayesian methods: Statistical methods that assign probabilities or distributions to (a posteriori) outcomes or parameters based on a priori experience or best guesses specified before the data are analyzed. Bayes' theorem is then applied to revise the posterior probabilities. Bayesian methods differ in concept from the more common "frequentist" ones. An example is a multi-arm, biomarker-driven clinical trial in which accumulating experience is used to reassess the likelihood that a particular biomarker predicts response—and then using that information to put more patients on the arm with the most promising biomarker-predicted therapy

9. Generation of omic databases requires especially careful proactive attention to experimental design and quality control. A small, hypothesis-driven experiment can often be re-done the next day or next week if the design proves inadequate or quality control fails; in contrast, when generating a large database that has to be internally consistent or externally consistent with other data, it's often too expensive to start over again.
10. For that reason, it is vital not to skimp on controls and standards simply to put more test samples through the process. The most serious design limitation of TCGA was the lack of cross-over replicates among the 33 tumor types as the technologies and analysis algorithms evolved.
11. Open-source, academically generated (as opposed to commercial), software is occupying a larger share of the bioinformatics market than previously. That trend has been accelerated by consortial projects like TCGA that have encouraged high-quality academic development.
12. Liquid biopsy technologies are becoming more sensitive and selective, offering major possibilities for early diagnosis and the accompanying predictive informatics.
13. Newer methods like ATAC-seq (assay for transposase-accessible chromatin), CITE-seq (cellular indexing of transcriptomes and epitope by sequencing), TCR-seq (T-cell receptor-seq), and Hi-C are proliferating and require customized analysis pipelines.
14. Immunomics, metabolomics, and microbiomics are three fields of increasing bioinformatic activity and sophistication.

References

1. Hesper B, Hogeweg P. Bioinformatica: een werkconcept. *Kameleon*. 1970;**1**:28–29.
2. Luscombe NM, Greenbaum D, Gerstein M. What is bioinformatics? A proposed definition and overview of the field. *Methods Inf Med*. 2001;**40**(4):346–358.
3. Bioinformatics definition – a review. 2015; http://bioinformaticsweb.tk.
4. Moore GE. Cramming more components onto integrated circuits. *Electronics*. 1965:114–117.
5. Kryder MH, Kim CS. After hard drives - what comes next? *IEEE Trans Magn*. 2009;**45**(10):3406–3413.
6. Church GM, Gao Y, Kosuri S. Next-generation digital information storage in DNA. *Science*. 2012;**337**(6102):1628.
7. Kim SY, Speed TP. Comparing somatic mutation-callers: beyond Venn diagrams. *BMC Bioinformatics*. 2013;**14**:189.
8. Weinstein JN. Fishing expeditions. *Science*. 1998;**282**(5389):628–629.
9. Kent WJ, Sugnet CW, Furey TS, et al. The human genome browser at UCSC. *Genome Res*. 2002;**12**(6):996–1006.
10. Goldman M, Craft B, Swatloski T, et al. The UCSC cancer genomics browser: update 2013. *Nucleic Acids Res*. 2013;**41**(Database issue):D949–D954.
11. Cerami E, Gao J, Dogrusoz U, et al. The cBio cancer genomics portal: an open platform for exploring multidimensional cancer genomics data. *Cancer Discov*. 2012;**2**(5):401–404.
12. Huber W, Carey VJ, Gentleman R, et al. Orchestrating high-throughput genomic analysis with Bioconductor. *Nat Methods*. 2015;**12**(2):115–121.
13. Rhodes DR, Kalyana-Sundaram S, Mahavisno V, et al. Oncomine 3.0: genes, pathways, and networks in a collection of 18,000 cancer gene expression profiles. *Neoplasia*. 2007;**9**(2):166–180.
14. Ashburner M, Ball CA, Blake JA, et al. Gene ontology: tool for the unification of biology. The Gene Ontology Consortium. *Nat Genet*. 2000;**25**(1):25–29.
15. Vaske CJ, Benz SC, Sanborn JZ, et al. Inference of patient-specific pathway activities from multi-dimensional cancer genomics data using PARADIGM. *Bioinformatics*. 2010;**26**(12):i237–i245.
16. (a) Weinstein JN, Myers TG, O'Connor PM, et al. An information-intensive approach to the molecular pharmacology of cancer. *Science*. 1997;**275**(5298):343–349. (b) Weinstein JN, Myers T, Buolamwini J, et al. Predictive statistics and artificial intelligence in the U.S. National Cancer Institute's Drug Discovery Program for Cancer and AIDS. *Stem Cells*. 1994;**12**(1):13–22. (c) Broom BM, Ryan MC, Brown RE, et al. A galaxy implementation of next-generation clustered heatmaps for interactive exploration of molecular profiling data. *Cancer Res*. 2017;**77**:e23–e26.
17. Farcomeni A. A review of modern multiple hypothesis testing, with particular attention to the false discovery proportion. *Stat Methods Med Res*. 2008;**17**(4):347–388.
18. Tusher VG, Tibshirani R, Chu G. Significance analysis of microarrays applied to the ionizing radiation response. *Proc Natl Acad Sci U S A*. 2001;**98**(9):5116–5121.
19. Shoemaker RH, Monks A, Alley MC, et al. Development of human tumor cell line panels for use in disease-oriented drug screening. *Prog Clin Biol Res*. 1988;**276**:265–286.
20. Weinstein JN, Kohn KW, Grever MR, et al. Neural computing in cancer drug development: predicting mechanism of action. *Science*. 1992;**258**(5081):447–451.
21. Barretina J, Caponigro G, Stransky N, et al. The cancer cell line encyclopedia enables predictive modelling of anticancer drug sensitivity. *Nature*. 2012;**483**(7391):603–607.
22. Garnett MJ, Edelman EJ, Heidorn SJ, et al. Systematic identification of genomic markers of drug sensitivity in cancer cells. *Nature*. 2012;**483**(7391):570–575.
23. DeLisi C. Meetings that changed the world: Santa Fe 1986: Human genome baby-steps. *Nature*. 2008;**455**(7215):876–877.
24. McPherson JD, Marra M, Hillier L, et al. A physical map of the human genome. *Nature*. 2001;**409**(6822):934–941.
25. Venter JC, Adams MD, Myers EW, et al. The sequence of the human genome. *Science*. 2001;**291**(5507):1304–1351.
26. International Human Genome Sequencing C. Finishing the euchromatic sequence of the human genome. *Nature*. 2004;**431**(7011):931–945.
27. International HapMap C, Altshuler DM, Gibbs RA, et al. Integrating common and rare genetic variation in diverse human populations. *Nature*. 2010;**467**(7311):52–58.
28. Cancer Genome Atlas Research N. Comprehensive genomic characterization defines human glioblastoma genes and core pathways. *Nature*. 2008;**455**(7216):1061–1068.
29. Cancer Genome Atlas Research N, Weinstein JN, Collisson EA, et al. The cancer genome atlas pan-cancer analysis project. *Nat Genet*. 2013;**45**(10):1113–1120.
30. Hoadley KA, Yau C, Wolf DM, et al. Multiplatform analysis of 12 cancer types reveals molecular classification within and across tissues of origin. *Cell*. 2014;**158**(4):929–944.
31. Li J, Lu Y, Akbani R, et al. TCPA: a resource for cancer functional proteomics data. *Nat Methods*. 2013;**10**(11):1046–1047.
32. Akbani R, Ng PKS, Werner HMJ, et al. A pan-cancer proteomic perspective on The Cancer Genome Atlas. *Nat Commun*. 2014;**5**:3887.
33. International Cancer Genome C, Hudson TJ, Anderson W, et al. International network of cancer genome projects. *Nature*. 2010;**464**(7291):993–998.
34. Genomes Project C, Abecasis GR, Altshuler D, et al. A map of human genome variation from population-scale sequencing. *Nature*. 2010;**467**(7319):1061–1073.
35. Consortium EP. The ENCODE (ENCyclopedia Of DNA Elements) project. *Science*. 2004;**306**(5696):636–640.
36. Liberali P, Snijder B, Pelkmans L. Single-cell and multivariate approaches in genetic perturbation screens. *Nat Rev Genet*. 2015;**16**(1):18–32.
37. Cancer Genome Atlas Research N. Comprehensive molecular characterization of urothelial bladder carcinoma. *Nature*. 2014;**507**(7492):315–322.

18 Systems biology and genomics

Saima Hassan, MD, PhD, FRCSC ■ Joe W. Gray, PhD ■ Laura M. Heiser, PhD

Overview

Cancers are complex, adaptive systems comprised of cancer cells that are influenced by supporting cells, immune cells, as well as soluble and insoluble proteins that make up the local physical environment. Features associated with cancer cells are referred to as intrinsic to the cancer and those comprising the proximal and distal microenvironments are referred to as extrinsic to the cancer. Genomics studies seek to develop comprehensive cellular and molecular profiles of cancers while cancer systems biology studies seek to develop the experimental and theoretical methods needed to understand how these diverse components work together to determine cancer function. The overall goal of these efforts is to develop analytical approaches to predict cancer behavior—including progression and response to therapy—from measurements of the intrinsic and extrinsic molecular and cellular components of tumors. Here, we review recent progress in international efforts to measure the genomic, epigenomic, and proteomic features of major tumor types. We summarize work to establish associations between these omic features and cancer behavior including risk of progression and response to therapy. Finally, we summarize the computational and experimental models employed to understand and manipulate the behavior of complex cancer systems.

Introduction

Studies of the behavior of biological systems have traditionally been reductionist, focusing on specific genes or pathways. Systems biology, in contrast, seeks a comprehensive understanding of how the elements of multicomponent biological systems interact together to determine the overall behavior of the system.[1,2] The systems approach is intended to reveal "emergent" aspects of systems behavior that result from component interactions that cannot be predicted from studies of the individual components. Development of a systems level understanding typically proceeds through three phases (1) comprehensive measurement of the collection of molecular features (profiles) that comprise the system, (2) identification of associations between collections of molecular features and biomedical behavior, and (3) development of unifying theories that mechanistically link changes in molecular features to the biomedical behaviors they control. Today, efforts to generate molecular profiles of cancers are well established, momentum is building to establish associations between features and biomedical behavior, and efforts to establish mechanistic theoretical models are beginning. In cancer, systems approaches may focus on the intrinsic behavior of the tumors themselves or may include extrinsic influences from the micro and macroenvironments in which the cancer cells reside (Figure 1).

Intrinsic cancer systems biology, defined here as a comprehensive study of the malignant cells that comprise the tumor mass, has evolved with advancements in genomic and epigenomic profiling technologies. These technologies produce comprehensive measurements of the genomic, transcriptional, and proteomic changes that occur in individual tumors. These studies have identified recurrent events that define cancer subsets, have led to a better understanding of cancer heterogeneity, identified prognostic subgroups and predictors of response to therapy, and have facilitated discovery of novel therapeutic targets.[3,4]

Extrinsic systems biology focuses on external influences that alter the behavior of tumor cells. Extrinsic signals may come from microenvironments that are in close proximity to tumor cells (e.g., invading immune cells, cancer-associated fibroblasts (CAFs), and vascular endothelial cells[5]) and from distal organs, especially the brain.[6,7] The clinical importance of the tumor microenvironment (TME) has been demonstrated in several different ways. For example, tumor stroma has been shown to be a strong prognostic biomarker,[8] the TME has been implicated in mediating therapeutic response and resistance,[9] and the immune microenvironment is increasingly appreciated as a major mediator of cancer genesis, progression,[10] and therapeutic response.[11–13]

Together, intrinsic and extrinsic systems biology approaches strive to enable an all-encompassing understanding of the cancer cell and its interactions with its environments. This article will discuss both intrinsic and extrinsic systems biology. The intrinsic systems biology section will focus on the clinical impact of high-throughput genomics and the use of cancer cell lines as predictive models of therapeutic response in patients. The extrinsic systems biology section will discuss the clinical significance, various components, and approaches to incorporate microenvironmental signals into various preclinical models.

Summary 1: Potential of omics

- Large-scale international studies have used patient samples to identify novel tumor classifications with prognostic significance and to identify novel therapeutic targets
- Panels of cancer cell lines have been used to identify gene signatures that are predictive of therapeutic response and are also present in patient samples
- Data analytical tools are being developed and validated to integrate diverse "omic" data types

Intrinsic systems biology and genomics in cancer

Since the mapping of the human genome, numerous technological advancements have enabled the "omics" era in which high-throughput profiling efforts provide comprehensive assessment of changes in deoxyribonucleic acid (DNA), ribonucleic

---

Holland-Frei Cancer Medicine, Tenth Edition. Edited by Robert C. Bast, John C. Byrd, Carlo M. Croce, Ernest Hawk, Fadlo R. Khuri, Raphael E. Pollock, Apostolia M. Tsimberidou, Christopher G. Willett, and Cheryl L. Willman.
© 2023 John Wiley & Sons, Inc. Published 2023 by John Wiley & Sons, Inc.

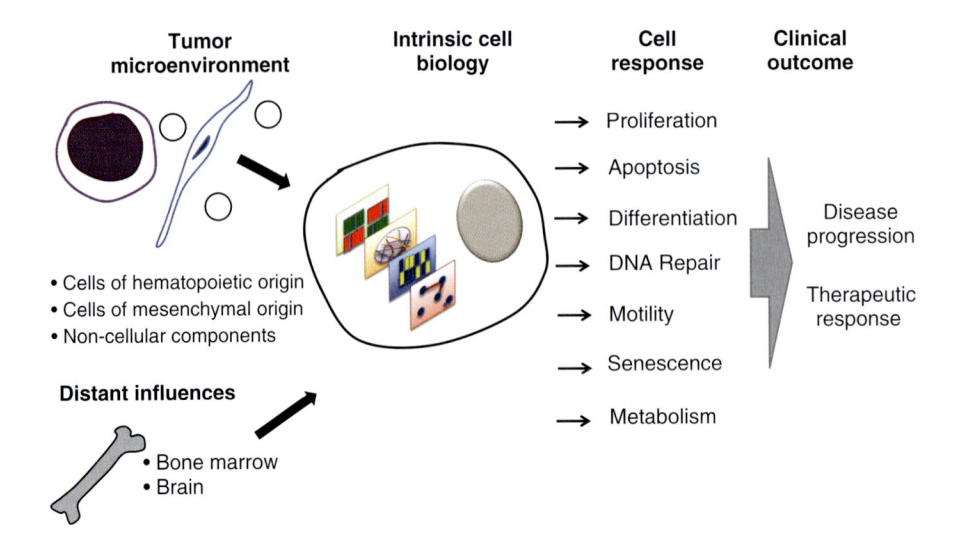

Figure 1 A schematic illustration of the influence of extrinsic and intrinsic systems biology upon cellular function with the potential to identify progression and response to therapy in patients. The extrinsic systems biology component consists of the tumor microenvironment including cells of hematopoietic origin, mesenchymal origin, and noncellular components, in addition to distant influences, from the bone marrow and other multiple organs. Together with a systems biology approach, cellular function can be studied using various endpoints, including cellular proliferation, apoptosis, differentiation, DNA repair, motility, senescence, and metabolism. Many researchers are striving to combine these endpoints to better understand tumor progression and response to therapy in the laboratory and how this may correlate to patients in the clinic.

acid (RNA), and protein levels in tumors and associated stroma that occur during cancer genesis, progression, and response to therapy.[14] Much work today is aimed at developing strategies to use these data to improve the clinical management of cancer. The bottleneck now lies in data processing and interpretation.[15] Removing the bottleneck will require novel bioinformatic approaches that can effectively identify actionable molecular events and druggable therapeutic targets. Although the robustness of platforms and validation of gene signatures are some of the major concerns regarding their clinical utility,[16,17] there are multiple pragmatic issues that must be addressed to better integrate genomic platforms into the clinic. For example, next-generation tumor banks now require greater infrastructure with a larger team of healthcare providers that acquire and manage relevant tissue and the associated clinical metadata.[18] Tissues for study include surgical specimens, tissue biopsies, and blood samples, each requiring different standard operating protocols and sample preparation techniques.[18] Nonetheless, several institutions have been using genomic platforms to guide clinical trials or in clinical contexts, particularly for diseases where there is little evidence supporting current management practices such as tumors of unknown origin.[14,19,20]

High-throughput omic approaches to assess tumor molecular state

High-resolution genome analysis techniques are being used in international cancer genome analysis efforts to catalog aberrations driving the pathophysiology of nearly all major cancer types. Two landmark programs, The Cancer Genome Atlas[21] (TCGA) and the International Cancer Genome Consortium[22,23] (ICGC) have assessed aberrations in over 20,000 samples in 55 tumor lineages.[24] The broad goal of these efforts has been to improve the prevention, diagnosis, and treatment of cancer patients.[21] In these projects, patient samples have been profiled on multiple platforms that examined whole genomes and whole-exomes,[25–28] messenger ribonucleic acid (mRNA), DNA methylation,[29] micro ribonucleic acid (miRNA),[30,31] and protein and phosphoprotein levels.[32] Results for several cancers are publically available[27,33–35] and include integrative analyses of multiple cancer types.[36–38] Genome aberrations[39] found to be important in human cancers include: (1) somatic changes in DNA copy number that increase or decrease the levels of coding and noncoding RNA transcripts; (2) somatic mutations that alter gene expression, protein structure, protein stability, and/or change the way transcripts are spliced, (3) structural changes that modify transcript levels by altering gene-promoter associations or create new fusion genes,[40,41] and (4) epigenomic modifications that alter gene expression.[42,43]

Additionally, analysis of these rich datasets has yielded clinically relevant insights into how we may better treat different cancers. For example, urothelial bladder cancers were found to be enriched in mutations in chromatin regulatory genes, suggesting the potential use of therapeutic agents that target chromatin modifications.[25] Half of the high-grade serous ovarian cancers analyzed were found to be defective in homologous recombination, increasing their likelihood to be more susceptible to poly (ADP-ribose) polymerase (PARP) inhibitors.[27] In fact, PARP inhibition has demonstrated a significant improvement in progression-free survival.[44,45] This has led to the FDA approval of this family of targeted therapeutics in ovarian and breast cancer patients.

Our understanding of the molecular landscape of breast cancer is particularly advanced. A key observation from the TCGA breast cancer study[35] is that there are a few common mutations (e.g., TP53, PIK3CA, CDH1, MLL3, GATA3, MED12) occurring in more than 5% of tumors[45,46] and hundreds of mutations that occur in fewer than 1% of breast cancers. The genomic aberrations in an individual tumor are comprised of a mix of "driver" and "passenger" aberrations. Driver aberrations are selected during tumor progression because they enable one or more aspects of the cancer pathophysiology that allow initiation, progression, and determination of cancer behavior including response to therapy.[47] Passenger aberrations do not contribute to cancer pathophysiology but arise by chance during progression in a genomically unstable tumor.

Recent analyses of glioblastoma have illustrated the strong interplay between the genome and treatment. The initial TCGA studies[33,48] demonstrated a link between O6-methylguanine-deoxyribonucleic acid methyltransferase (MGMT) promoter methylation and a hypermutator phenotype consequent to mismatch repair deficiency in temozolomide-treated glioblastomas. Johnson et al. performed exome sequencing for initial and recurrent low-grade gliomas.[49] Of 10 tumors treated with adjuvant temozolomide, 6 were hypermutated when they recurred and carried driver mutations involving the AKT-mTOR pathways. This suggests a role for therapeutic agents that target the AKT-mTOR pathways in patients with recurrent low-grade gliomas previously treated with temozolomide. In many cases, the genome landscapes of the recurrent tumors were dramatically different than those of the primary tumor, illustrating the need for longitudinal following of patients during treatment.

While initial analyses of the data emerging from the TCGA and ICGC programs focused on identification of lineage-specific changes, a newer program, PanCancer Analysis of Whole Genomes (PCAWG),[50] has focused on identification of molecular patterns that transcend cancer types. Interestingly, the pan-cancer approach to proteomic profiling revealed an elevated expression of HER2 in several cancers, including endometrial cancer, bladder cancer, and lung adenocarcinoma.[32] Although trastuzumab has demonstrated limited efficacy in endometrial cancer, this observation suggests that other anti-HER2 agents, such as TDM1, may play an important role in endometrial cancer.[32] The pan-cancer approach lends itself to basket-style clinical trials, which are guided by specific molecular aberrations across different tumor types, as opposed to the traditional clinical trial designs that use large populations based on histologic classifications.[51] Other studies from the PCAWG consortium have leveraged these large-scale data to identify pan-cancer patterns of genomic rearrangements,[52] mutational signatures,[53] cancer drivers,[54] and mutational processes that distinguish hypoxic and normoxic tumors.[55] Organization of these large-scale data for convenient visual and computational analysis is critical to enable their community-wide use. Several of the most popular tools are listed in Table 1.

Gene signatures: prognostic and predictive biomarkers of response

The limitations of clinicopathologic criteria that are used to stage and predict aspects of cancer progression have long been recognized. Tissue histology and locally invasive properties are still commonly used as surrogate markers for distant metastatic spread and indicators of outcome. In the last decade, conventional classification strategies have been supplemented by omic-based strategies. These efforts began in 1999 with the demonstration that gene expression analysis could be used to distinguish between acute myeloid leukemia and acute lymphoblastic leukemia.[56]

Table 1 Tools for visualization and computational analysis of large-scale genomic data.

Tool	Uniform resource locator (URL)
UCSC Cancer Genome Browser	https://genome-cancer.ucsc.edu
cBioPortal for Cancer Genomics	http://www.cbioportal.org
Sage Synapse	https://www.synapse.org
Catalog of Somatic Mutations in Cancer	http://cancer.sanger.ac.uk/cosmic
The Cancer Proteome Atlas	https://tcpaportal.org
Cancer Dependency Map	https://depmap.org/portal
Genomics of Drug Sensitivity in Cancer	https://www.cancerrxgene.org
Pan Cancer Analysis of Whole Genomes (PCAWG)	https://dcc.icgc.org/pcawg

This was quickly followed by an analysis of gene expression in breast cancer that identified intrinsic breast cancer subtypes, designated as hormone receptor-positive luminal A and luminal B, HER2-enriched, basal-like, and normal-like.[57] The classification of such subtypes was validated in several independent cohorts and was found to have strong prognostic significance.[57] More recent studies have refined these subtypes to identify additional molecularly distinct subpopulations, indicating substantial patient-to-patient variation.[58,59] There have been several proposals for how pancreatic cancers may be subtyped,[60–62] including one that demonstrated a differential prognosis response to therapy[61] and another that considers contributions of the surrounding stroma.[62]

Efforts are now underway to use such information to develop clinically validated prognostic signatures. In breast cancer, for example, Van't veer and colleagues identified a 70-gene signature that could predict recurrence in a select group of younger patients with early breast cancers.[63] This signature, now marketed by Agendia BV as MammaPrint, was validated in independent cohorts and outperformed Adjuvant! Online software in clinicopathologic risk assessment.[64,65] Although smaller retrospective studies have demonstrated the use of MammaPrint as a prognostic marker,[65,66] no prospective data are yet available that demonstrates its benefit in the adjuvant setting. Another test, marketed by Exact Sciences as OncotypeDX, was developed in 2004 using a reverse transcription-polymerase chain reaction (RT-PCR) assay on RNA extracted from formalin-fixed paraffin-embedded (FFPE) tumor blocks. This 21-gene assay was tested retrospectively in two National Surgical Adjuvant Breast and Bowel Project (NSABP) trials, was found to have prognostic significance, and is now currently widely used in the clinic to assess the risk of distant recurrence and potential benefit of chemotherapy.[67,68] Several competing prognostic and predictive gene expression signatures have been published[68–70] including a 17-gene signature for ER+, node-negative breast cancer,[71] a 50-gene PAM50 risk of recurrence signature,[72] and a 44-gene Rotterdam Signature.[73]

Cancer subtype signatures are being developed for a growing number of other cancers. In colon cancer, for example, three unique gene signatures have been identified. Commercial assays include OncotypeDX colon cancer assay (Exact Sciences Corporation), ColoPrint (Agendia), and ColDx (Almac).[74] Although these tests have been shown to be independent prognostic biomarkers, their predictive value is still unknown.[75] In a positive move, academic efforts have sought to reconcile diverse colorectal cancer classification schemes based on gene expression signatures.[76] Gene expression analysis identified basal-like and luminal subtypes that are associated with overall and disease-specific survival.[77] Importantly, several ongoing community-wide classification efforts have begun to integrate genomic and proteomic profiles from across diverse tumor types to identify subtypes that transcend tumor origin.[36,50,78,79] This approach will become more powerful as additional tumor types are added to the analysis.

Mathematical modeling to identify novel treatment strategies

A major goal of cancer systems biology is to develop mathematical models that can be used to predict optimal treatment regimens. Such models can be used to identify the treatment strategies most likely to be beneficial for different patient populations and direct limited resources toward standing up rationally designed clinical trials that test specific drug combinations, doses, and sequencing schedules with the highest chance of success. Here, we highlight two examples in which mathematical models have provided insights that have led to improvements in treatment paradigms. One of the first successes of mathematical modeling of cancer treatment was based on the observation that tumors show Gompertzian patterns in growth—in short, smaller tumors grow faster than larger ones. The so-called Norton-Simon hypothesis showed that because the rate of tumor shrinkage was proportional to the rate of growth, the most effective treatment plans were "dose dense" that is, frequent administration of tolerable, effective doses.[80] Based on mathematical principles, dose dense chemotherapy regimens are now a mainstay of treatment for patients with early breast cancer.[81] More recently, Game Theory has been used to identify optimal treatment strategies for patients with prostate cancer.[82] Game Theory uses mathematical models to describe the interactions and strategic responses between rational decision-making entities; here, the "players" are the tumor and the treating physician.[83] In brief, a physician can make a rational treatment decision based on the fullest set of information about a patient's cancer and the tumor will respond accordingly. Using this approach, Zhang et al. developed an adaptive clinical trial that modified abiraterone treatment based on a patient's response, as assessed by PSA levels in the blood, which serve as a biomarker of tumor burden.[82] Such adaptive approaches to treatment have the potential to improve therapeutic responses and ultimately improve patient outcomes.

Experimental models of patient tumors for pharmacogenomics studies

Identification of molecular features that are causally related to clinical behavior such as cancer progression or response to therapy requires experimental models in which cells carrying aberrant genes and networks can be manipulated. Collections of cell lines derived from patient tumors are widely used as laboratory models of cancer.[84] Cell lines are an attractive model system for studying cell-intrinsic biology for several reasons, including (1) they are a renewable resource; (2) they can be manipulated in the laboratory setting; (3) they are amenable to genomic profiling; and (4) therapeutic responses can be quickly assessed.[84,85] Although the first tumor-derived cell lines were established in the 1950s, their use as an experimental tool gained traction with the development of the National Cancer Institute 60 (NCI60) platform.[86,87] The NCI60 consists of 60 human tumor cell lines, representing 9 cancer types, and has been used to screen over 100,000 compounds for therapeutic efficacy.[88] Analysis of these data with the COMPARE algorithm has provided a quantitative method for identifying associations between molecular features of cells and sensitivity to particular compounds.[88]

Since the demonstration of the utility of the NCI60, several other groups have developed panels of cancer cell lines, including "pan-cancer"[89–92] and tissue-specific collections (e.g., breast,[93] lung,[94,95] and melanoma.[96]) One of the most well-developed panels, comprised of ~70 breast cancer cell lines, has been used to assess gene function and to identify mechanisms of therapeutic response and resistance.[93,97,98] These cell line collections have been used to identify associations between molecular features and response to molecular perturbagens across tumor types.[90,91,99–101] Comparison of the genomic and epigenomic features of cell lines with those measured from primary tumors showed that cell lines mirror many aspects of "omic" diversity in primary tumors that are likely to influence therapeutic response. Cell line and tumor similarities include: (1) recurrent copy number changes and mutations,[92,93,97,102] (2) transcriptional subtypes,[97,102] and (3) pathway activity.[97] However, there are significant exceptions. For example, cell lines grown on plastic have been reported to change epigenomic status[103] and some cell lines fail to retain genomic aberrations that were present in the tumors from which they were derived. Glioblastoma is a notable example of the latter, since cells grown on plastic usually fail to retain a region of amplification involving the epidermal growth factor receptor (EGFR) oncogene that is frequently present in primary tumors.[104]

In breast cancer, analysis of correlations between drug sensitivity and molecular features revealed that approximately 30% of the compounds tested are associated with subtype or genome copy number aberration,[97] and robust integrated predictive signatures of sensitivity can be identified for ~50% of compounds.[97,98] Importantly, many of the *in vitro* signatures can be observed in primary patient samples[89–91,98] suggesting that cell line studies may be used to guide the development of signatures that can be used to stratify patients in the clinic. More recently, there has been a push toward using sophisticated *machine learning* approaches to predict drug response across diverse cancer cell lines[104–106] and also to systematically transfer predictions from cell lines to patient tumors.[107] The latter has the potential to detect signals conserved between cell line models and primary tumors, thereby identifying novel therapeutic targets or biomarkers most likely to succeed in patients.

Evidence from diverse tissue types supports the notion that cell lines are a powerful system for studying the molecular underpinnings of therapeutic response. For example, *in vitro* model systems accurately recapitulated several clinical observations, including that: (1) lung cancers with EGFR mutations respond to gefitinib,[108] (2) breast cancers with HER2/ERBB2 amplification respond to trastuzumab and/or lapatinib,[93,109] and (3) tumors with mutated or amplified BCR-ABL respond to imatinib mesylate.[110]

Principles of integrative analysis

Several computational tools have been developed to identify molecular signatures that are associated with biological behavior. One of the first of these is known as Gene Set Enrichment Analysis (GSEA).[111] The rationale behind GSEA is to analyze the expression gene sets—predefined groups of genes that share a common biological function, chromosomal location, or regulation—and to determine whether they show wholesale differences in gene expression between comparator populations. For example, GSEA analysis identified the RAS, NGF, and IGF1 pathways as differentially expressed in TP53 mutant versus TP53 wildtype cancers.[111]

The network analysis tool PARADIGM[112] was designed to identify pathways whose activities differ between comparator populations. PARADIGM integrates multiple omic data types, including DNA copy number and gene expression, to calculate integrated pathway levels (IPLs) for over 1300 curated signal transduction, transcriptional, and metabolic pathways from publicly available databases (e.g., NCI's PID, KEGG, Reactome, and BioCarta). These IPLs can then be used to identify subnetworks that differ between comparator populations (e.g., responsive vs resistant tumors). The subnetworks are composed of interlinked *pathway features* (genes, proteins, complexes, families, processes, etc.) that take on activities distinctive in one class of tumors compared to another. For example, PARADIGM analysis of TCGA breast cancer samples identified HIF1-α/ARNT pathway activity as high in basal-like breast cancers, which suggests that these malignancies might be susceptible to angiogenesis inhibitors and/or bioreductive drugs that become activated under hypoxic conditions.[35] NetSig is another integrative network approach that has been used to discover novel oncogenic genes, thereby generating a prioritized list of aberrations for more detailed study.[113]

One of the problems associated with tools that rely on the curated literature for pathway structure is the inherent bias due to the fact that some genes and networks have been more extensively studied than others (e.g., TP53, PIK3CA are two very well studied cancer-associated genes). Several algorithms have been developed to overcome this curation bias limitation by employing "heat diffusion," which transfers signal from one gene in a network to neighboring genes, thereby inferring the activity of genes that may be less well studied. This heat diffusion approach has been used to identify frequently mutated networks that affect well-known cancer phenotypes;[113,114] to identify relationships between gene networks;[115] and to infer the functional impact of mutations.[116]

Summary 2: The tumor microenvironment (TME)

- The TMR is comprised of Multiple cellular and noncellular components
- Stromal and immune cells have strong prognostic significance
- Aspects of the TME are implicated in therapeutic response and resistance
- Preclinical modeling of the TME can be used to reveal tumor extrinsic mechanisms of cancer
- Patient-derived xenografts can predict response to therapy and can potentially be used alongside clinical trials

---

Tumor microenvironment

Constituents of the tumor microenvironment

Although there are different ways of categorizing the TME,[9] one simplistic approach divides the TME into three main groups: cells of hematopoietic origin, cells of mesenchymal origin, and noncellular components.[117] Cells of hematopoietic origin populate two cell lymphoid and myeloid lineages. The lymphoid cell lineage consists of T cells, B cells, and natural killer cells, whereas the myeloid cell lineage consists of macrophages, neutrophils, and myeloid-derived suppressor cells. Cells of mesenchymal origin include fibroblasts, myofibroblasts, mesenchymal stem cells, adipocytes, and endothelial cells. The two cancer-related components of this group are cancer-associated fibroblasts (CAFs) and endothelial cells. CAFs are fibroblasts that have been co-opted by the tumor to promote tumor growth, angiogenesis, and distant metastasis.[118,119] Endothelial cells and pericytes have also been shown to play an important role in vessel growth formation needed for tumor progression.[120] The most important player of the noncellular group is the extracellular matrix (ECM). The ECM can be further subdivided into two parts: the basement membrane, which consists of type IV collagen, laminin, and fibronectin; and the interstitial matrix, which is made up of fibrillar collagens, proteoglycans, and glycoproteins. The ECM has been shown to play roles in maintaining tissue architecture, cell invasion, tumor progression, and angiogenesis.[121]

Tumor microenvironment and the hallmarks of cancer

Hanahan and Weinberg defined six capabilities of cancer that are essential for tumor growth.[122] These hallmarks include: (1) evading apoptosis; (2) self-sufficiency in growth signals; (3) insensitivity to antigrowth signals; (4) tissue invasion and metastasis; (5) limitless replicative potential; and (6) sustained angiogenesis. Eleven years later, an update of these six hallmarks was published, with recognition of the TME as an important player in tumor growth, and the addition of two hallmarks: reprogramming of energy metabolism and evading immune destruction. However, it became apparent that categorizing the cancer hallmarks into two distinct categories of origin—tumor cell and TME—is an artificial classification, as most cancer hallmarks are a product of the cross-talk between stromal and cancer cells.[123] A detailed role for TME in mediating the cancer hallmarks has been proposed, which suggests potential therapeutic approaches that target constituents of the TME.[5]

Role of tumor microenvironment in modulating therapeutic response, recurrence, and survival

The TME can serve as a mediator of either response or resistance to therapeutic agents. One classic example is that of vessel normalization, wherein tumor vasculature can be manipulated to improve delivery of chemotherapy.[9,124] Vasculature associated with tumors is abnormal and consists of immature vessels with increased permeability as well as compromised delivery of nutrients and therapeutics. The administration of antiangiogenic therapy leads to pruning of immature vessels, which results in "normalized vasculature" and enhanced delivery of chemotherapy agents.[124]

Resistance to therapy can either be an innate process mediated by intrinsic properties of the TME or an acquired process that results from an adaptive response to therapeutic intervention.[9,125] Several mechanisms have been proposed to explain intrinsic resistance to therapy including survival signals that arise from the TME, impaired drug delivery from vascular impairments and leakage, paracrine signaling with secretion of chemokines from stromal cells, and immunosuppression.[9,126] Immune responses are important factors in mediating acquired therapeutic resistance. For example, resistance to paclitaxel has been shown to result from enhanced expression of IL-34, colony-stimulating factor (CSF)-1, and macrophage infiltration.[127] Indeed, a monoclonal antibody has been identified, RG7155 (Roche), that targets macrophages and CSF-1 receptor activation, and which has demonstrated response in patients with diffuse-type giant cell tumors.[128] Other mechanisms that have been implicated in acquired resistance include the induction of senescence-associated secretory phenotype and changes in cell differentiation.[9]

Studies of the TME have yielded predictive markers of local recurrence in mouse models and prognostic markers in patients. An inflammatory signature has been identified that was associated with recurrence of clinically detectable disease but not advanced recurrent disease. This inflammatory signature was characterized by an increase in serum concentrations of IL-6 and VEGF. The progression of minimal residual disease to a recurrence occurred through an evasion of the immune response by cancer cells.[129,130] Park's group established the importance of the TME as a prognostic marker in breast cancer by employing laser capture microdissection to isolate stromal cells from the primary tumor cells.[8] A gene signature derived from the stroma was found to be a strong prognostic marker of overall survival and relapse-free survival. Immune cells were an important component of this gene signature, with the good-outcome patients demonstrating an enrichment of T cell and NK cell markers, suggesting a T_H1-type immune response. The prognostic significance of the amount of stroma within the primary tumor, termed tumor-stroma ratio, has also been demonstrated in colon cancer and breast cancer.[131] Furthermore, the prognostic value of immune cells has since been demonstrated in breast cancer and colon cancer.[132–135] A stromal lymphocytic infiltrate was found to be an independent prognostic marker associated with overall survival in two randomized

Table 2 Summary of advantages and disadvantages of chemosensitivity models.

Model	Advantages	Disadvantages
Cell lines	• Unlimited source of self-replicating material • Easy to use • Amenable to high-throughput screening	• Typically Generated from more aggressive tumors • Do not model the complex paracrine and endocrine influences associated with tumor growth
2-Dimensional	• Easy to use • Amenable to high-throughput screening	• Differences in cell morphology, polarity, receptor expression, oncogene expression, between 2D monolayers and in vivo[142]
3-Dimensional	• 3D spheroids may better model the hypoxic core and drug diffusion found in solid tumors	• May show variability in cell size and shape • May require more specialized equipment and cost • More labor-intensive • Matrigel shows lot-to-lot variability which may influence experimental results[143]
Microenvironment microarray	• Amenable to high-throughput screening • Can be used to examine the Influence of different microenvironment proteins upon therapeutic response and resistance	• Difficult to model tumor heterogeneity • Requires sophisticated analytical approaches[144] • Requires validation[144]
Mouse models	• Can be used to test therapeutic response upon primary tumor growth and distant metastasis • Both transgenic mice and xenografts can be used to observe response alongside clinical trials[145,146]	• Difficult to use on a larger scale to test multiple therapeutic compounds
Xenografts	• Relatively easy to use, as cancer cell lines can either be easily injected or transplanted	• Use immunodeficient mice and cancer cell lines that often represent more aggressive tumors
Transgenic	• Can model human tumor progression[147]	• Requires substantial time and financial investment
Patient-derived xenografts	• Renewable tissue resource[148] • Similar genomic properties as found in patient tumors[145] • Therapeutic response in PDX models are similar to clinical outcome achieved in patients[145]	• Requires set-up to acquire patient samples and to grow tumors in mice • Requires immunodeficient mice[145] • Engraftment failure can be high and time to treatment long in some tumor types[145]
Humanized patient-derived xenografts	• Can model human systemic and immune response • Can be used to assess immunotherapies	• Expensive • Difficult to use in large-scale experiments

controlled trials with triple-negative breast cancer patients.[134] In colon cancer, a score that measures the presence of certain lymphocyte populations, termed Immunoscore, was shown to be a stronger prognostic marker than current American Joint Committee on Cancer (AJCC) prognostic markers, including T stage (tumor depth) and N stage (nodal involvement).[136] Interestingly, the Immunoscore may have great potential in patients with localized colorectal cancer with no detectable spread or lymph node involvement on pathology of imaging, of which 25% of such patients go on to develop recurrence.[137] In two independent cohorts, Immunoscore was able to identify a group of patients that were at higher risk of developing recurrence and may have otherwise benefited from adjuvant therapy.[137,138] Given the prognostic significance of stromal gene signatures, it is important to consider the proportion of the stroma in tumor samples when tumor-derived gene signatures are being generated.[139]

Modeling the tumor microenvironment

The majority of pharmacologic agents targeting aspects of the microenvironment suggested by laboratory studies have not been successful in clinical trials.[140,141] This may be due to intrinsic tumor factors or limitations associated with preclinical models. A common criticism about preclinical models is that cancer cell lines alone do not encompass the complexity inherent to heterotypic signaling associated with cancer cells and their microenvironment. We will summarize a few of the chemosensitivity models that have been proposed using cell lines, mouse models, and patient-derived tumors to better capture the complex interactions of the tumor and its microenvironment. The advantages and disadvantages of these models are summarized in Table 2.

Two-dimensional (2D) models in which cancer cells are grown as monolayers on plastic tissue culture dishes are commonly used to assess chemosensitivity.[142] As outlined in the previous section, these 2D models have been instrumental in driving the development of many therapeutic agents currently used in the clinic. Several approaches have been developed to include constituents of the microenvironment. For example, cells can be grown on substrates comprised of proteins from the diverse microenvironments to which cancer cells are known to spread. This can be accomplished efficiently by constructing microenvironment microarrays that consist of thousands of unique combinations of soluble and insoluble proteins found in the TME.[149,150] Insoluble proteins are printed on a solid substrate to form pads upon which cells can be grown. Soluble factors are added to the culture medium, yielding thousands of unique combinatorial microenvironments in which cells grow. This platform allows assessment of factors that are secreted by multiple different cell types, including macrophages, infiltrating lymphocytes, stromal fibroblasts, vascular endothelial cells, and tumor cells. Typically, after several days of growth on the microenvironment microarray, cells are immunofluorescently stained to report on cancer-related phenotypes (e.g., proliferation, apoptosis, differentiation status, and senescence) and then quantified using high-content imaging.[144,151] This platform has been used to identify microenvironment-mediated resistance mechanisms in breast cancer and to identify therapeutic strategies to counter them.[152] Alternatively, cancer cells can be co-cultured together with stromal cells. Such 2D co-culture models have identified changes in tumor genotype, phenotype, and response to therapy.[153,154]

Three-dimensional (3D) culture methods establish cells in 3D environments comprised of extracellular proteins and sometimes other cell types.[9,142,155,156] Matrix components such as matrices (e.g., matrigel) or scaffolds (e.g., collagen, laminin, alginate) can be added to 3D models in order to better model tissue architecture. Isolated from mouse sarcoma cells, matrigel is a basement membrane-derived hydrogel that has been commonly used in cancer models and shown to support tumor growth and angiogenesis.[156–158] However, one of the challenges in the use of matrigel is its relatively undefined molecular composition and high lot-to-lot variability therein.[143] The fidelity with which co-culture models mirror *in vivo* microenvironments is increasing as 3D cell printing techniques, which are used to arrange multiple cell types into laboratory cancer "tissues".[159–161] Multi-cell-type bioprinted tissues can recapitulate aspects of *in vivo* neoplastic tissues and provide a manipulable system for the interrogation of multiple tumorigenic endpoints in the context of distinct TMEs.[162]

3D cultures of primary cells are termed "organoids" to reflect their ability to maintain cell types and architecture resembling the organ from which they were derived as well as their ability to regenerate tissue when transplanted orthotopically.[163] Genetic modification of organoids allows disease modeling in a setting that approaches the physiological environment. Additionally, organoids can be grown with high efficiency from patient-derived tumor tissues, which can enable patient-specific drug testing and the development of individualized treatment regimens.[164,165] For example, 3D organoids have been used to successfully model immune checkpoint blockade with anti-PD-1- and/or anti-PD-L1, indicating that organoid-based propagation of primary tumor epithelium with endogenous immune stroma may facilitate personalized immunotherapy testing.[166]

Finally, microfluidic systems, which consist of three connected wells—an inlet reservoir, a cell culture chamber, and an outlet reservoir—have been developed to recapitulate various environmental signals and generate organs-on-chips.[142,167] Organ chips enable experimentalists to vary local cellular, molecular, chemical, and biophysical parameters in a controlled manner, both individually and in precise combinations, which can inform how they contribute to human cancer formation, disease progression, and responses to therapy.

The importance of the TME has also been well established from mouse models. In xenograft mouse models, cancer cell lines are injected into immunocompromised mice. Metastasis develops infrequently when cell lines are injected subcutaneously in ectopic sites. With a favorable microenvironment, tumors grown in orthotopic models tend to grow faster than their ectopic counterparts and have a greater propensity to metastasize.[168] Although xenograft models are useful tools to study tumor growth and metastasis, they are limited by the immunocompromised status of the host mice and the use of cell lines that are derived from more aggressive tumors.[145] Efficacy of therapeutic agents in xenograft models have not been shown to correlate well with efficacy in clinical trials,[169] and as a result, there has been an effort to develop genetically engineered or transgenic mice as more realistic models. The advantage of this model is that the mice are immunocompetent and tumors progress from preinvasive, invasive, to distant metastasis in a manner akin to human tumor progression.[147] Some transgenic mouse models develop tumors with short tumor latency and have been used as chemosensitivity models.[141,146,170] However, these models are difficult to use on a large scale, due to the need to synchronize the generation of pups, onset of tumors, and subsequent administration of therapy.[170]

More recently, patient-derived xenograft (PDX) models have become popular for the study of therapeutic efficacy. PDXs are established from patient biopsies engrafted into immunocompromised mice.[145] The rate of engraftment is variable ranging from 13% to 71%.[171,172] PDX models enable transplantability of human tissue from mouse to mouse and are therefore a renewable tissue resource.[148] Whole-genome sequencing has revealed high similarity between PDX tumors and human tumors in terms of copy number and structural variations. PDXs have been used as a model to understand clonal evolution in the growth of breast cancers.[173] PDXs are being used now to assess chemosensitivity of breast, lung, skin, and pancreatic cancers.[145,174] A recent large-scale profiling study examined the responses of ~1000 PDX samples across diverse cancers to assess responses to 62 anticancer agents, thereby identifying associations between a genotype and drug response, and established mechanisms of resistance.[175] Other studies, albeit with a small number of patients, have identified a good correlation with therapeutic response in PDX models and clinical outcome.[172,174] Therefore, PDX models are gradually being integrated into the later stages of preclinical development of therapeutic agents. PDX models are also being considered in co-clinical trials, in which therapeutic agents are tested on patients in a clinical trial alongside mice in order to better understand how best to strategize against therapeutic resistance.[145]

Humanized NOD scid gamma (hNSG) models have recently emerged to better model patient tumor heterogeneity and influences from the hematopoietic and immune cells.[176] In this model, young mice are irradiated and engrafted with human CD34+ stem cells; subsequently, after the peripheral blood is comprised of 25% hCD45+ cells, the mice are implanted with tumors. Two independent groups have demonstrated that even with a partially HLA-matched hNSG host and PDX tumors, tumors grow rapidly.[176,177] Furthermore, humanized PDX models did not show evidence of graft-versus-host reaction. The fidelity of this model was also demonstrated amongst triple-negative breast cancers, where an inhibition in tumor growth was observed with pembrolizumab, a PD-L1 inhibitor, but not with ipilimumab, a CTLA-4 inhibitor, which is similar to the response profile observed in the clinic. Although expensive, this approach allows for preclinical testing of immune checkpoint inhibitors.

Conclusion

The long-term goal of cancer systems biology is to develop the experimental and theoretical methods needed to understand and manipulate the behavior of the complex and adaptive cancers with which we are confronted. This will require that we be able to measure the molecular composition, cellular organization, and anatomic locations of cancers and that we develop the theoretical framework needed to predict the behavior of cancer cells including the effect of the proximal and distal environmental signals that influence their behavior. International cancer genome efforts are now providing increasingly detailed information about the molecular components of cancers, imaging strategies are emerging that allow assessment of the multiscale organization of cancerous tissues, and increasingly accurate biological models are being developed that enable identification of molecular features that are causally related to cancer cell behavior. It now remains to develop the analytics that can be used to predict the behavior of complex adaptive systems so that this information can be used to more accurately predict cancer behavior and to devise more durable treatment strategies.

> **Summary**
>
> Cancer genomics and systems biology studies seek to describe molecular and cellular features that are intrinsic and extrinsic to cancer cells and to interpret the resulting data in ways that allow prediction of the behavior of individual cancers. These studies guide several aspects of precision medicine including prediction of cancer behavior, identification of optimal therapeutic targets, and development of strategies for durable control of individual cancers. International omic analysis efforts are now yielding comprehensive omic profiles of hundreds to thousands of tumors of most major cancer types and these data have been made available to the scientific community. Computational scientists are mining such data to establish associations between cancer omic profiles and cancer behavior—especially aspects of cancer progression and response to therapy. Systems biologists are now developing experimental and theoretical strategies to understand and predict the behavior of the complex systems. These studies focus both on the behavior of the cancer cells themselves and the influence of distal and proximal environmental signals on the behavior of cancer cells. This article highlights work in all of these areas and provides illustrative examples of recent progress in each.

Acknowledgments

We would like to thank our funding organizations: Saima Hassan is supported by the Fonds de Recherche Santé-Quebec Clinical Research Scholar Award, l'Institut de Cancer de Montréal, Centre de Recherche de Centre Hospitalier de l'Université de Montréal. Joe W. Gray is supported by the Susan G. Komen Foundation.

Laura M. Heiser is supported by the Breast Cancer Research Foundation and The Jayne Koskinas Ted Giovanis Foundation. Joe W. Gray and Laura M. Heiser are supported by grants from the National Institutes of Health and the National Cancer Institute.

Key references

The complete reference list can be found on Vital Source version of this title, see inside front cover.

3 Werner HM, Mills GB, Ram PT. Cancer systems biology: a peek into the future of patient care? *Nat Rev Clin Oncol*. 2014;**11**:167–176.

4 Zou J, Zheng MW, Li G, Su ZG. Advanced systems biology methods in drug discovery and translational biomedicine. *Biomed Res Int*. 2013;**2013**:742835.

5 Hanahan D, Coussens LM. Accessories to the crime: functions of cells recruited to the tumor microenvironment. *Cancer Cell*. 2012;**21**:309–322.

7 Antoni MH, Lutgendorf SK, Cole SW, et al. The influence of bio-behavioural factors on tumour biology: pathways and mechanisms. *Nat Rev Cancer*. 2006;**6**:240–248.

8 Finak G, Bertos N, Pepin F, et al. Stromal gene expression predicts clinical outcome in breast cancer. *Nat Med*. 2008;**14**:518–527.

9 Klemm F, Joyce JA. Microenvironmental regulation of therapeutic response in cancer. *Trends Cell Biol*. 2014. doi: 10.1016/j.tcb.2014.11.006.

14 Tran B, Dancey JE, Kamel-Reid S, et al. Cancer genomics: technology, discovery, and translation. *J Clin Oncol*. 2012;**30**:647–660.

15 Good B, Ainscough B, McMichael J, et al. Organizing knowledge to enable personalization of medicine in cancer. *Genome Biol*. 2014;**15**:438.

16 Chibon F. Cancer gene expression signatures–the rise and fall? *Eur J Cancer*. 2013;**49**:2000–2009.

17 Hatzis C, Bedard PL, Birkbak NJ, et al. Enhancing reproducibility in cancer drug screening: how do we move forward? *Cancer Res*. 2014;**74**:4016–4023.

18 Basik M, Aguilar-Mahecha A, Rousseau C, et al. Biopsies: next-generation biospecimens for tailoring therapy. *Nat Rev Clin Oncol*. 2013;**10**:437–450.

19 Manolio TA, Chisholm RL, Ozenberger B, et al. Implementing genomic medicine in the clinic: the future is here. *Genet Med*. 2013;**15**:258–267.

20 Sameek R, Chinnaiyan AM. Translating genomics for precision cancer medicine. *Annu Rev Genomics Hum Genet*. 2014;**15**:395–415.

36 Hoadley KA, Yau C, Wolf DM, et al. Multiplatform analysis of 12 cancer types reveals molecular classification within and across tissues of origin. *Cell*. 2014;**158**:929–944.

37 Omberg L, Ellrott K, Yuan Y, et al. Enabling transparent and collaborative computational analysis of 12 tumor types within The Cancer Genome Atlas. *Nat Genet*. 2013;**45**:1121–1126.

39 Collisson EA, Cho RJ, Gray JW. What are we learning from the cancer genome? *Nat Rev Clin Oncol*. 2012;**9**:621–630.

135 Pages F, Berger A, Camus M, et al. Effector memory T cells, early metastasis, and survival in colorectal cancer. *N Engl J Med*. 2005;**353**:2654–2666.

19 Statistical innovations in cancer research

J. Jack Lee, PhD, MS, DDS ■ Donald A. Berry, PhD

> **Overview**
>
> Cancer research is rapidly changing, with fast-growing numbers of possible cancer targets and drugs to investigate and no end in sight. Advances in genomics, proteomics, epigenetics, and immune oncology provide remarkably detailed profiles of each patient's tumor and its microenvironment and, as a result, allow science to consider each patient as unique, with the goal of delivering individualized precision medicine. The low success rates of late-phase clinical oncology trials, high costs, and long duration of bringing new drugs to market, however, have necessitated changes in the drug-development process. Statistical innovations can help in the design and conduct of clinical trials to facilitate the discovery and validation of biomarkers and streamline the clinical trial process. The application of Bayesian statistics provides a sound theoretical foundation that can encourage the development of adaptive designs to improve trial flexibility and efficiency, while maintaining desirable statistical-operating characteristics.

The principal goals of the innovations presented in this article are to (1) use information from clinical trials more efficiently in drawing conclusions about treatment effects; (2) use patient resources more efficiently, while treating patients who participate in clinical trials as effectively as possible; and (3) more rapidly identify and develop better drugs and therapeutic strategies. The underlying premise is to exploit all available evidence and incorporate information gleaned from an ongoing clinical trial into the context of what is already known outside the trial for decision making. The innovations considered are intuitively appealing. Some are being used in actual clinical trials, while others are still being developed and evaluated for such use.

This article addresses two types of innovations. One is a natural extension of the traditional practice of frequentist statistics. The other type results in novel designs based on a Bayesian statistical philosophy. The Bayesian approach is tailored to real-time learning (as data accrue), and the frequentist approach is tied to particular experiments and their designs. Despite their differences, there is substantial overlap between these complementary approaches.

There are seven main topics covered in this article. (1) The introduction of basic probability theory and Bayesian approach is explained through examples. Differences between frequentist and Bayesian methods are compared and contrasted. (2) The development of adaptive designs by applying outcome adaptive randomization, predictive probability, interim and extraim analyses are discussed. (3) Model-assisted designs combine the advantages of the easy-to-conduct rule-based designs and the good performance of model-based designs. (4) In addition, hierarchical modeling can be used to synthesize information available from the trial, as well as external to the trial. (5) Seamless Phases I/II and II/III designs can be applied to shorten the drug development period. (6) Platform designs, umbrella trials, and basket trials can be constructed in master protocols to evaluate many drugs simultaneously. The application of these statistical innovations is illustrated in the BATTLE trials, I-SPY 2 trials, GBM-Agile, and other adaptive platform trials. (7) Finally, information on computing resources for the design and implementation of innovative trials is given.

Cancer research (and medical research, in general) is rapidly changing; the number of possible cancer targets and drugs to investigate is growing, with no end in sight. Advances in genomics, proteomics, epigenetics, and immune oncology provide remarkably detailed profiles for each patient's tumor and its microenvironment, allowing researchers to consider each patient as unique. Modern computing has supported these advances, allowing statisticians to simulate trials with more sophisticated adaptive designs and to evaluate design properties, such as statistical power and false-positive rate. The basic requirement is that the design be specified prospectively.

The low success rates of late-phase clinical oncology trials,[1,2] high costs, and long duration of bringing new drugs to market[3] have necessitated changes in the drug-development process. Recognizing the need to modernize, the FDA issued its *Critical Path Opportunities Report* in March 2006, identifying biomarker development and streamlining clinical trials as essential changes to be made in this process.[4] Further guidance was then issued by centers within the FDA: The Center for Devices and Radiological Health (CDRH) published initial guidelines for using Bayesian statistics in medical device clinical trials in 2006, final guidelines in 2010,[5] and a guidance on adaptive designs for medical device clinical studies in 2016.[6] The Center for Biologics Evaluation and Research (CBER) and the Center for Drug Evaluation and Research (CDER) issued a joint guidance document for planning and implementing adaptive designs in clinical trials[7] and encouraging the use of complex innovative trials[8] in 2019 and 2020, respectively.

The principal goals of the innovations presented in this article are to (1) use information from clinical trials more efficiently in drawing conclusions about treatment effects; (2) use patient resources more efficiently, while treating patients who participate in clinical trials as effectively as possible; and (3) more rapidly identify and develop better drugs and therapeutic strategies. The underlying premise is to exploit all available evidence, placing information gleaned from an ongoing clinical trial into the context of what is already known outside the trial for decision making. The innovations considered are intuitively appealing. Some are in use with actual clinical trials, while others are still being developed and evaluated for such use.

This article addresses two types of innovations. One is a natural extension of the traditional practice of frequentist statistics. The other type results in novel designs based on a Bayesian statistical philosophy. Readers who are familiar with Bayesian ideas

Holland-Frei Cancer Medicine, Tenth Edition. Edited by Robert C. Bast, John C. Byrd, Carlo M. Croce, Ernest Hawk, Fadlo R. Khuri, Raphael E. Pollock, Apostolia M. Tsimberidou, Christopher G. Willett, and Cheryl L. Willman.
© 2023 John Wiley & Sons, Inc. Published 2023 by John Wiley & Sons, Inc.

may wish to skip the introductory Bayesian sections. The Bayesian approach is tailored to real-time learning (as data accrue), and the frequentist approach is tied to particular experiments and to their designs. Despite their differences, there is substantial overlap between these complementary approaches. Much of this article's development of clinical trial design employs the Bayesian approach as a tool that tends to treat patients in the clinical trial more effectively and that can identify better drugs more rapidly. However, the frequentist properties (such as the control of false-positive rate and power) of the design are still desirable and can be found in Bayesian trials.

Preliminaries

The basis of all experimentation is comparison. Evaluating an experimental therapy in a clinical trial requires information about the outcomes of the patients had they received some other therapy. The best way to address this issue is to randomize patients to the experimental therapy and to some comparison therapy with equal assignment probabilities to the therapeutic strategies, or "arms," being compared, or with fixed or adaptive ratios that depend on data accumulating in the trial.

Clinical trials are always prospective and conducted under protocols. A protocol describes how the trial is to be conducted, including how patients will be assigned to a therapy, study endpoints, when the trial will end, and how statistical inference will be drawn. Valid inference can only be made based on sound statistical theory in properly conducted trials. In the case of the two types of statistical framework in making inference, the frequentist approach assumes that the unknown quantity of interest (i.e., parameter such as the response rate of a drug) is fixed and the observed data (number of responses) is random, while the Bayesian approach assumes that the data is fixed, because it has been observed and the unknown parameter is random.

Bayesian approach

This section shows how Bayesian learning takes place and how the Bayesian approach relates to the more traditional frequentist approach. It is necessarily superficial. Further reading includes an elementary introduction to Bayesian ideas and methods,[9,10] discussions of their role in medical research and of clinical trials in particular,[11,12] and books describing more advanced Bayesian methods.[13,14]

Bayesian updating

The defining characteristic of any statistical approach is how it deals with uncertainty. In the Bayesian approach, uncertainty is measured by probability. Any event whose occurrence is unknown has a probability. Examples of probabilities in the Bayesian approach that do not have frequentist counterparts include the probability that the response rate of a drug is greater than 30%; the probability that patient Smith will respond to a particular chemotherapy; and the probability that, given the current results, the future results in the trial will show a statistically significant benefit for a particular therapy.

The Bayesian paradigm is one of learning. As information becomes available, one updates one's knowledge about the unknown aspects of the process that are producing the information. The fundamental tool for learning under uncertainty is Bayes' rule. Bayes' rule relates inverse probabilities. An example that will be familiar to many readers is finding the positive predictive value (PPV) of a diagnostic test. For example, in view of a positive CT scan, what is the probability that the individual being tested has lung cancer? It can be considered as the "inverse probability" of a positive test given the presence of the disease, which is called the test's sensitivity. PPV also depends on the test's specificity, which is the probability of a negative test, given that the individual does not have the disease. Moreover, PPV depends on the prevalence of the disease in the population. In applying Bayes' rule, the analog of disease prevalence is the "prior probability" that the person has lung cancer. The outcome of a positive CT scan is the data. Bayes rule synthesizes the prior probability and the data to derive the "posterior probability," which is PPV, that the person has lung cancer given a positive test.

Consider another overly simplified example. Suppose that there are only two possible states of a drug: a drug is either effective ($e=1$) or ineffective ($e=0$). If you are accustomed to thinking about PPV for diagnostic tests, consider one of these to be that the patient has the disease and the other to be that the patient does not have the disease. The question is this: Is e equal to 1 or 0? Before any experimentation, these two possibilities are regarded to be equally likely: $P(e=1) = P(e=0) = 1/2$.

The Bayesian approach allows continuous learning. Probabilities are calculated as new information becomes available and is taken to be "given." Statisticians have a notation that facilitates thinking about and calculating probabilities as new information accrues. They use vertical bars to separate the unknown event of interest from known quantities (or taken to be given): $P(A|B)$ is read "probability of A given B." Assign R for tumor response and N for nonresponse. Using this notation, for example, let us assume that $P(R|e=1) = 0.75$ and $P(R|e=0) = 0.5$. Typically, we are more interested in knowing the probability of $e=1$, given a tumor response: $P(e=1|R)$. These two expressions are reciprocally inverse, with the roles of the event of interest and the event being assumed. Bayes' rule connects the relationship between these two expressions, namely that the updated (posterior) probability of $e=1$ is as follows:

$$P(e = 1 \mid R) = P(R \mid e = 1)P(e = 1)/P(R)$$

The denominator on the right-hand side of the equation follows from the law of total probability:

$$P(R) = P(R|e = 1)P(e = 1) + P(R|e = 0)P(e = 0)$$
$$= (0.75)(1/2) + (0.5)(1/2) = 5/8$$

That is, $P(R)$ is the average of the two response rates under consideration, 0.75 and 0.50, where the average is—with respect to the corresponding prior probabilities—half each in this example. Substituting the numerical values into Bayes' rule, the posterior probability of $e=1$ is as follows:

$$P(e = 1|R) = (0.75)(1/2)/(5/8) = 3/5$$

Therefore, the new evidence boosts the probability of $e=1$ from 1/2 (or 50%) to 60%. As the total probability is 100%, the evidence in a single response lowers the probability of $e=0$ from 50% to 40%.

Consider a second independent observation. The probability of e before this second observation is the posterior probability of the first observation. If the second observation is also a response, then a second application of Bayes' rule applies to give $P(e=1|R, R) = 9/13 = 69\%$, which is a further increase from the previous values of 50% and 60%. On the other hand, if the second observation is a nonresponse, then $P(e=1|R, N) = 3/7 = 43\%$, a decrease from 60%. This process can go on indefinitely, updating either after each observation or all at once on the basis of whatever evidence is available. These updates and real-time learning are important advantages of the Bayesian approach to designing and conducting clinical trials.

The previously mentioned example considered only two possible values of e. More realistically, the response rate of a drug r may be any number between 0 and 1. The left-hand panel in Figure 1a shows a constant or flat curve that is a candidate for prior distribution. The flat curve indicates that the probability spreads equally over this range of values for r. This might be termed an "open-minded prior distribution." because it does not give any preference on a low or high response rate. After a single-tumor response, Bayesian updating serves to change the probability distribution to the one shown in the right-hand panel of Figure 1a—that is, the right-hand panel is the posterior distribution after observing R when the prior distribution is the one shown in the left-hand panel. The shift in the distribution to larger values of r corresponds to the intuitive notion that larger response rates become more likely after observing R. Bayes' rule quantifies this intuition.

There are many candidate prior distributions other than the first one shown in Figure 1a. Three other prior/posterior pairs are shown in Figure 1b–d. The right-hand panel within each pair is the posterior distribution after observing R when the prior distribution is the one shown in the left-hand panel. Moreover, the left-hand curves in Figure 1b–d are themselves posterior distributions for the right-hand curves in Figure 1a–c, respectively, but in the situation when the observation is an N. Intuitively, after a nonresponse, the concentration of probabilities shifts to smaller values of r.

An implication is that moving left to right and top to bottom in Figure 1 corresponds to starting with the prior distribution in the left-hand panel of Figure 1a and observing $RNRNRNR$. The eight curves shown in Figure 1 are proportional to the following respective functional forms: 1, r, $r(1-r)$, $r^2(1-r)$, $r^2(1-r)^2$, $r^3(1-r)^2$, $r^3(1-r)^3$, and $r^4(1-r)^3$. Each observation of response (R) increases the exponent of r by 1, and each observed no response (N) increases the exponent of $(1-r)$ by 1. As is evident in the figure, additional observations lead to narrower distributions. As the number of observations increases, the distribution tends to concentrate about a single point, which is the "true" value of r, the response rate that produces the observations. Free software that provides a visual demonstration of the Bayesian update in the context of the so-called beta-binomial distribution can be accessed at https://trialdesign.org/one-page-shell.html#BU1BB.

Prior probabilities

Bayesian updating requires a starting point: a prior distribution of the parameter of interest. In the example, one must have a probability distribution for response rate r in advance of or separate from the experiment in question. This prior distribution may be subjectively assessed or based explicitly on the results of previous experiments. In some settings, such as some regulatory scenarios, an appropriate default distribution is noninformative or open-minded in the sense that all possible values of the parameters are assigned the same prior probabilities. The left-hand panel of Figure 1a is an example.

Noninformative or flat prior distributions limit the benefits of taking a Bayesian approach because the information available

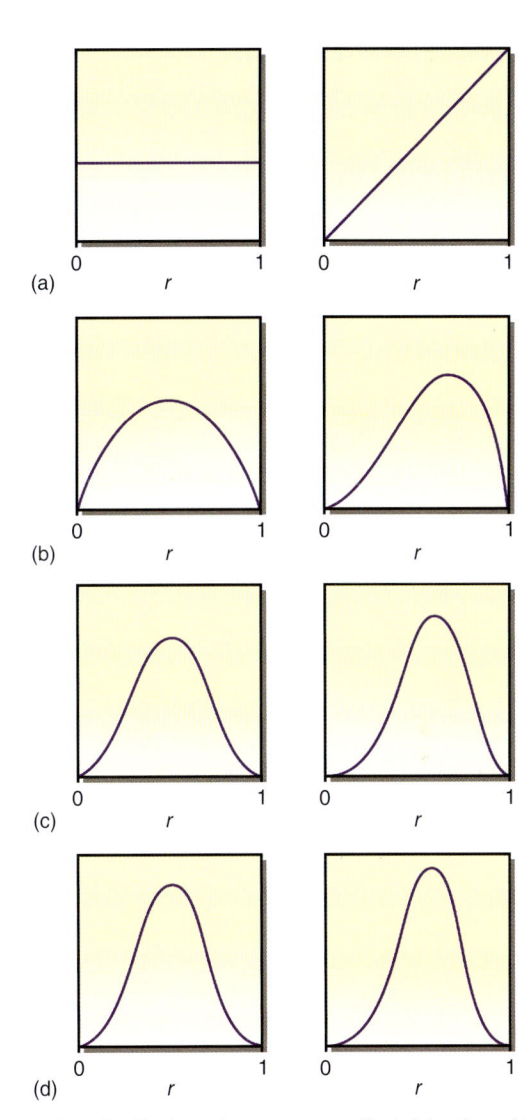

Figure 1 Prior distributions of response rate r. The left-hand panel in each pair is the prior distribution of response rate r. The right-hand panel is the posterior distribution of r after having observed a response in a single patient. The (predictive) probability of a response for each left-hand panel is 0.500, increasing in the right-hand panels to 0.667, 0.600, 0.571, and 0.556 in cases (a), (b), (c), and (d), respectively. Changes are greater and learning is more rapid when the prior distribution reflects greater uncertainty.

from outside the experiment is ignored. Nevertheless, the benefit of employing Bayesian updating may still be meaningful, even if one starts with a flat distribution that does not reflect anyone's assessment of the prior information. Flat prior distributions also serve some important roles. One is that it may be helpful to distinguish the evidence in the data in the experiment under consideration from the information that exists before the experiment. Another is that the Bayesian conclusions that arise from using flat prior distributions are often the same as the corresponding frequentist conclusions.

Prior distributions are usually based on historical data. As a result, informative prior distributions can be constructed. However, given that there may be differences between the historical setting and that of the current trial, we often discount the historical evidence as it applies to the context of the current trial. For example, down-weighing the historical information equivalent of 20–30% of that of a current observation would be reasonable.

Robustness and sensitivity analysis

Even though different prior distributions are used, in the presence of enough data, essentially all posterior distributions are similar; this is robustness. An implication is that the particular prior distribution assumed does not matter much when the sample size is moderate or large. If two prior distributions are markedly different, sensitivity analysis can be conducted to evaluate how different priors affect the posteriors. If the corresponding information contained in the prior distribution is strong, robustness still applies with sufficiently large data to bring two disparate distributions close together.

Frequentist/Bayesian comparison

In the frequentist approach, hypotheses and parameters do not have probabilities. Rather, probability assignments apply only to data, with particular values assumed for given unknown parameters in calculating these probabilities. For example, the ubiquitous p-value is the probability of data as or more extreme than the observed data, assuming that the null hypothesis is true. In symbols:

- Frequentist p-value: $P(\text{observed or more extreme data} | H_0)$
- Bayesian posterior probability: $P(H_0 | \text{observed data})$

It is easy to confuse these two concepts. A p-value is commonly interpreted as the probability of no effect, and 1 minus the p-value as the probability of an effect. This interpretation is wrong, as it assumes a Bayesian posterior probability without a prior probability, which is impossible.

There are two important differences between a frequentist p-value and a Bayesian posterior probability. One is the inversion of the conditions: what is assumed in the former (H_0) has a probability in the latter. The second difference is that p-values include probabilities of "more extreme data" that is not observed in the experiment.

As an example, consider a single-arm Phase II trial for testing H_0: $r = 0.5$ versus H_1: $r = 0.75$. Assuming a type I error rate $\alpha = 5\%$, a sample size of $n = 33$ gives 90% power. Suppose that the final results are of 22 responses of 33 patients, the (frequentist) one-sided p-value is the probability of 22 or more responses of the 33 patients, assuming the null hypothesis, H_0: $r = 0.5$. Under this assumption, the probability of observing 22, 23, 24, ... responses is $0.0225 + 0.0108 + 0.0045 + \cdots = 0.0401$. As this p-value is less than 5%, observing 22 responses is said to be "statistically significant."

The Bayesian measure is the posterior probability of the hypothesis that $r = 0.75$ (or $r = 0.5$) given 22 responses out of 33 patients. As indicated earlier, the Bayesian calculation depends only on the probability of the data actually observed, 22 responses of 33, while the frequentist calculation also includes probabilities of 23, 24, etc., responses. Using Bayes' rule:

$$P(H_1 | 22 \text{ of } 33) = P(22 \text{ of } 33 | H_1) P(H_1) / P(22 \text{ of } 33)$$

As mentioned in the equation, the denominator follows from the law of total probability assuming H_0 and H_1 are equally likely before observing the data:

$$P(22 \text{ of } 33) = P(22 \text{ of } 33 | H_1) P(H_1) + P(22 \text{ of } 33 | H_0) P(H_0)$$
$$= (0.0823)(0.5) + (0.0225)(0.5) = 0.0524$$

Therefore,

$$P(H_1 | 22 \text{ of } 33) = (0.0823)(0.5)/0.0524 = 0.785 \text{ and}$$
$$P(H_0 | 22 \text{ of } 33) = (0.0225)(0.5)/0.0524 = 0.215$$

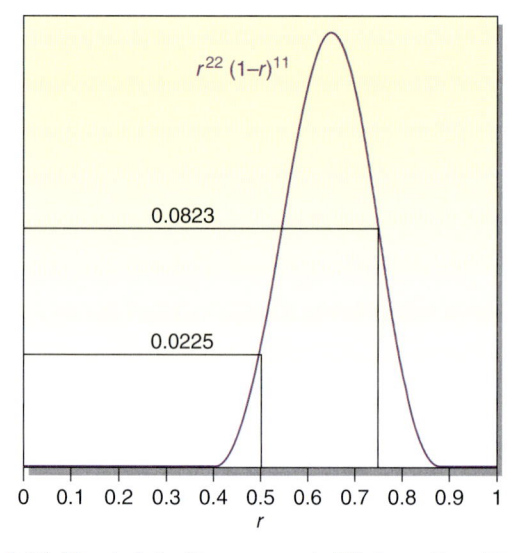

Figure 2 Likelihood of r for 22 responses out of 33 observations. The likelihood is $P(22 \text{ of } 33 | r)$, which is proportional to $r^{22}(1-r)^{11}$.[11] The likelihoods at $r = 0.5$ and 0.75 are highlighted. These values are used in the calculational example in the text.

The calculation considers just two hypotheses, $r = 0.5$ and $r = 0.75$. In considering other values of r, Bayes' rule weighs them by $P(22 \text{ of } 33 | r)$, which is called the likelihood function of r. The likelihood function is pictured in Figure 2. It indicates the degree of support for response rate r provided by the observed data. Values of r having the same likelihood are equally supported by the data. Only relative likelihoods matter. For example, conclusions about $r = 0.5$ versus 0.75 depend only on the ratio of their likelihoods, 0.0823 and 0.0225, values that are highlighted in Figure 2. Because $0.0823/0.0225 = 3.66$, the data lend 3.66 times as much support to $r = 0.75$ as they do to $r = 0.5$.

The conclusions of the two approaches are different conceptually and numerically. In the frequentist approach, the results are statistically significant, with $p = 0.0401$. Some researchers interpret statistical significance to mean that H_0 is unlikely to be true. That is not what it means. It means that the observed data are unlikely when H_0 is true. The Bayesian posterior probability of H_0 directly addresses the question of the probability that H_0 is true. This probability is 0.215. Although smaller than the prior probability of 0.50 (because the data lean somewhat more strongly to H_1 than to H_0), it is five times as large as the p-value.

Interval estimates also have different interpretations in the two approaches. In the Bayesian approach, one can find the probability that a parameter lies in any given credible interval. In the frequentist approach, confidence intervals have a long-run frequency interpretation for fixed and given parameters. So it is not correct to say that a 95% confidence interval has a probability of 95% containing the parameter of interest. Despite the different interpretations, there is a point of agreement between the two approaches. If the prior distribution is flat (e.g., the left-hand panel of Figure 1a), then the Bayesian credible interval is essentially the same as the frequentist confidence interval. For example, if the prior distribution is flat, then the Bayesian posterior probability, indicating that a parameter lies in its 95% credible interval is in fact 95%. For prior distributions that are not flat, the posterior probability of a 95% confidence interval may be greater than or less than 95%. If the historical data upon which the prior distribution is based are consistent with those from the current experiment, then the posterior probability indicating that the parameter is in the 95% confidence interval will be >95%. If the historical data are different from those in the current experiment, then the probability that the 95% confidence interval contains the true parameter will typically be <95%.

Predictive probabilities

The ability to predict the future—with the requisite uncertainty—is important for designing and monitoring trials. The Bayesian approach allows for calculating probabilities of future results without having to assume that any particular hypothesis is true. The process is straightforward. For a specified experimental design, one finds the conditional probabilities of the future data for each parameter value and averages them with respect to the current probabilities of the various parameter values. Predictive probability properly addresses the uncertainty of future data, as well as the uncertainty of the parameter values—a strength of the Bayesian approach in making inference. Predictive probability can be calculated to perform interim analysis. At the time of interim analysis, if the predictive probability of success is very low or very high, the trial can be stopped early due to futility or efficacy, respectively.

A breast cancer trial illustrates some advantages of a Bayesian design.[15] Women with breast cancer who were at least 65 years of age were randomized to receive either standard chemotherapy or capecitabine. The sample size was expected to be 600–1800. After the 600th patient had enrolled in the trial, and following the protocol, predictive probabilities were calculated. Calculations were made of the predictive probability of statistical significance given the present sample size and with additional patient follow-up at the present sample size. If that achieved a predetermined level, patient accrual would stop, but follow-ups of the existing patients would continue. The predictive probability cutoff point was achieved at the first interim analysis, and so accrual stopped (the final sample size was 633). Indeed, the study later showed that the women in this study population who were treated with standard chemotherapy had a lower risk of breast cancer recurrence and death than women treated with capecitabine.[16]

Hierarchical modeling: synthesizing information

When analyzing data from a clinical trial, other information is usually available about the treatment under consideration. This section deals with a method called hierarchical modeling. One of its uses is synthesizing information from different sources. The method applies in many settings, including meta-analysis and incorporating historical information. A hierarchical model is a random-effects model. In a meta-analysis, one level of the experimental unit is the patient (within a trial) and the second level is the trial itself. Hierarchical models also apply for design issues, such as combining results across diseases or disease subtypes, and for seemingly disparate issues, such as cluster randomization. Design issues for hierarchical modeling are considered in the next section.

Consider a Phase II trial in which 21 of 33 patients responded. The one-sided p-value is 0.08 for the null hypothesis H_0: $r = 0.50$, and so the results are not statistically significant at the 5% level. Now consider an earlier Phase I trial using the same treatment in which 15 of 20 patients responded. This information seems relevant, even if the population being treated might have been somewhat different and the trial might have been conducted at a different institution. However, it is not obvious how to incorporate the information into an analysis. The frequentist approach is experiment specific, which requires imagining that the two trials are part of some larger experiment. If one assumes that the entire set of data resulted from a single trial involving 53 patients with 36 responses, then from a frequentist perspective this would lead to a p-value of 0.0063, which is highly statistically significant. However, this conclusion is wrong because the assumption is wrong. Moreover, it is not clear how to make it right.

Any Bayesian analysis that assumes the same response rate applies in both trials would be similarly flawed. Response rate r may be reasonably expected to vary from one trial to another. Two response rates for the same therapy may be different, even if the eligibility criteria in the two trials are the same. For one thing, the eligibility criteria may be applied differently in the two settings. However, even if the patients accrued appear similar, their accruals differ in time and place. Our understanding of cancer and its detection changes over time. Moreover, there could be differences in the use of concomitant therapy and variations in the ability to assess clinical and laboratory variables. A way to mend the analysis is to explicitly consider two values of r, say $r1$ for the first trial and $r2$ for the second.

In the first attempt, there are two extreme assumptions that lead to analyses that are easier to carry out, but both are wrong. One is to assume that $r1$ and $r2$ are unrelated and to base any inferences about $r1$ or $r2$ on the results of the its respective trial alone. The other is to assume that $r1 = r2$ and combine the results in the two trials.

The two r-values may be the same or different. In a Bayesian hierarchical model, both possibilities are allowed, but neither is assumed. In other words, $r1$ and $r2$ are regarded as having come from a population of r-values. Hence, they are related and, without knowing their values, they are exchangeable. The population may have little variability (homogeneity) or substantial variability (heterogeneity). The observed response rates give information concerning the extent of heterogeneity, with disparate rates suggesting greater heterogeneity. When the observed rates are similar, applying the hierarchical model, the precision of estimates of $r1$ and $r2$ will be greater than when the observed rates are disparate. In the former case, there will be greater "borrowing of strength" across the trials. If it happens that the results of the trials are markedly different, then there will be little borrowing and the information from any one trial will not apply much beyond that trial.

More generally, there may be any number of related studies or databases that provide supportive information regarding a particular therapeutic effect. The studies may be heterogeneous and may consider different patient populations. The next example is generic, but it is more complicated than the previous example because it includes nine studies.[17] The only commonality in the studies is that all addressed the efficacy of the same therapy.

The response rates can take any value between 0 and 1. The number S of responses and sample size n are shown for each study in Table 1 and Figure 3. There are nine response rates, $r1$, $r2$, up to $r9$, one for each study. Each of the nine sample response proportions S/n is an estimate of the corresponding r. There were 106 responses among 150 patients. If all nine of the response rates are assumed to be equal, then the posterior distribution of the common response rate r (assuming a flat prior distribution) is that shown in Figure 3, labeled "pooled analysis."

Even though this pooled analysis is wrong, the overall estimate of 106/150 may be quite reasonable. However, the precision associated with this estimate is too great (equivalently, its standard error is too small). In contrast, the "hierarchical analysis" curve in Figure 3 is a Bayesian estimate of the distribution of the response

Table 1 Numbers of responses S, sample size n, observed response proportions (including its standard error), and adjusted estimates of response rates by study applying the Bayesian hierarchical model.

Study number	Responses S	Sample size n	Observed response proportions (standard error)	Bayes estimate (standard deviation)
1	11	16	0.69 (0.116)	0.69 (0.094)
2	20	20	1.00 (0.000)	0.90 (0.064)
3	4	10	0.40 (0.155)	0.53 (0.121)
4	10	19	0.53 (0.115)	0.57 (0.094)
5	5	14	0.36 (0.128)	0.48 (0.109)
6	36	46	0.78 (0.061)	0.77 (0.058)
7	9	10	0.90 (0.095)	0.80 (0.097)
8	7	9	0.78 (0.139)	0.73 (0.110)
9	4	6	0.67 (0.192)	0.68 (0.125)
Total	106	150	0.71 (0.037)	0.68 (0.064)

Note: The Bayes estimate column is described in the text.

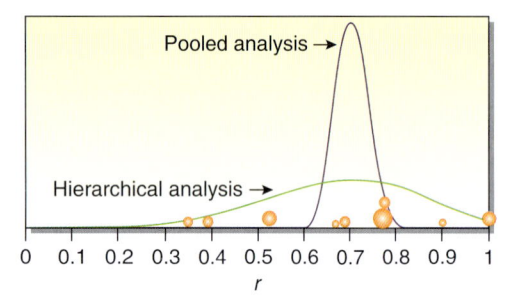

Figure 3 Response comparisons. The dot plot on the r-axis shows the observed response proportions given in Table 1. The areas of the dots are approximately proportional to sample sizes n. The pooled-analysis curve shows the distribution of response rate r assuming no study effect. The hierarchical analysis curve shows the Bayesian estimate of the distribution of response rates allowing for heterogeneity across the various studies.

rates in the population of studies. (This curve is the mean posterior distribution of the response rate across all trials, assuming a noninformative prior for the parameters in a particular class of distributions for r-values, called *beta distributions*.) As is typical of hierarchical analyses, this curve shows greater variability than does the analogous curve under the assumption of homogeneity.

In a hierarchical analysis, an individual study's r has a distribution that depends on the data from that study, but it also depends on the data from the other studies. The rightmost column in Table 1 shows the mean of the distribution of each study's response rate. This is also the predictive probability of the response for a future patient in that study. The individual study probabilities are shrunk toward the overall mean. This shrinkage is greater for smaller studies and for studies with observed proportions further from the overall mean. Hierarchical borrowing is defensible because it does not make the assumption that all studies had the same true response rate, and because the extent of borrowing is determined by the data.

Figure 4 provides a pictorial comparison of the rightmost two columns in Table 1, demonstrating shrinkage. The Bayesian estimates are intermediate between simple pooling (complete borrowing) and each trial standing alone (no borrowing). The amount of shrinkage—including the two extremes mentioned previously—depends on the prior distribution of the population of trials. This aspect of the prior distribution should be set in advance or varied to allow for assessing the sensitivity of the overall conclusion.

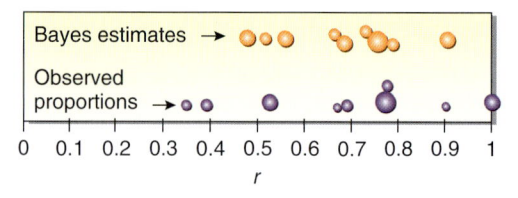

Figure 4 Observed response proportions compared to the adjusted response rate estimates. Values are given in the two rightmost columns in Table 1. The dot plot on the r-axis shows the observed response proportions, just as in Figure 3. The Bayes estimates assume a hierarchical model and show shrinkage toward the overall mean.

Shrinkage is a consequence of hierarchical modeling. The motivation for such modeling is to use the available information appropriately in improving precision or in decreasing the required sample size. Consider study number 1 in Table 1. Simply pooling the data from the other eight studies together would greatly increase the precision of its estimated response rate. For example, the standard error would be reduced from 0.116 to 0.037. However, in view of the possibility of heterogeneity in the studies, such pooling would not be justified. Borrowing hierarchically also strengthens the conclusion, but not as much. The standard deviation of the Bayes estimate is only about 20% smaller, from 0.116 to 0.094. Although smaller than the reduction with unabashed pooling, this reduction implies that >50% savings in sample size is necessary to carry out a clinical trial (in the setting of study number 1 in Table 1) with the same precision: $(0.116/0.094)^2 - 1 = 52\%$. For example, to achieve the same standard error in a stand-alone study would require 25, as opposed to 16 patients in study number 1 of Table 1.

Patient covariates can be incorporated into a hierarchical analysis, thus adjusting for known differences in the studies, but still accounting for unknown heterogeneity. In this example and also in more complicated hierarchical settings,[18] modeling allows for borrowing from other studies and databases. If the results are consistent across studies, then the amount of borrowing will be greater. If the results are sufficiently different (after accounting for covariates), then this suggests heterogeneity among the studies and there is little borrowing.

Hierarchical modeling in trial design

There are many settings in which trials can be set up to borrow strength from related, but not necessarily identical, experimental units. The hierarchical models can serve as a theoretical foundation of the basket trial design to be discussed later. Consider designing a trial for a therapy for a disease that has several subtypes, such as several different histologies that exist for one type of tumor. The response rates will likely differ for the different subtypes. The setting is essentially the same as that of the previous section. The focus is then the tumor response rate within the individual subtype. These have a distribution, just as in the previous section. Recognizing the possibility of borrowing across subtypes means greater precision for estimating each individual response rate, and therefore that the sample size within each subtype can be smaller.

The extent of borrowing depends on the results, just as in the previous section. In the Phase II design setting, the response rate in the subtypes can be classified into low- or high-response clusters; then, more meaningful borrowing occurs within the clusters, but not across clusters to reduce bias and increase efficiency.[19] A more general clustered hierarchical model was introduced to allow the number of clusters to be dynamically determined by the data.[20] In the hierarchical model, the savings in terms of sample size cannot be predicted with certainty. However, this is not a problem if the interim results can be monitored. The interim results can be used to determine the precision associated with the estimates of the various response rates. If the interim results will not be available when the decision to stop the trial must be made, then the uncertainties regarding heterogeneity across subtypes can be assessed at the trial design stage and the sample size chosen accordingly, recognizing that the eventual precisions cannot be predicted perfectly.

Adaptive designs of clinical trials

The focus of this section is a family of designs that are adaptive or dynamic in the sense that observations made during the trial can affect the subsequent course of the trial. The attention here is on clinical trials, but the ideas also apply to other settings.

Designs of clinical trials are usually static in that the sample size and any prescription for assigning treatment, including randomization protocols, are fixed in advance. Results observed during the trial are not used to guide its course. There are exceptions. Some Phase II cancer trials have two stages, with stopping after the first stage possible if the results are not sufficiently promising. Moreover, most Phase III protocols specify interim analyses that determine whether the trial should be stopped early for sufficiently strong evidence of a difference between competing treatment arms. However, traditional early stopping criteria are very conservative, and few trials stop early.

The simplicity of trials with static designs makes them solid inferential tools. Their sample sizes tend to be large, at least in comparison with the alternatives to be discussed in this section. In addition, they usually consider two therapeutic strategies, or arms, thus enabling straightforward treatment comparisons. Despite their virtues, static trials result in slow and unnecessarily costly drug development. The number of cancer drugs available for development is increasing exponentially. It is inefficient to focus on a single drug when a myriad of others are sitting on the sidelines waiting to be evaluated. Pharmaceutical companies and medical researchers generally must be able to consider hundreds or thousands of drugs for development at the same time. Static trials inhibit the simultaneous development of many drugs. Moreover, they cannot efficiently address dose–response questions when many drugs are being considered. Dynamic designs that are integrated with the drug-development process are necessary for reasonable progress in medical research.

Using an adaptive design means examining the accumulating data periodically, or even continually, with the goal of modifying the trial's design. These modifications depend on what the data show about the unknown hypotheses. Among the modifications possible are stopping early, restricting eligibility criteria, expanding accrual to additional sites or inclusion of certain subgroups of patients, extending accrual beyond the trial's original sample size if its conclusion is still not clear, randomizing more patients to more effective treatment arms, dropping arms or doses, and adding arms or doses. All of these possibilities are considered in the light of the accumulating information.[21]

Adaptation is not limited to the data accumulating in the trial. Information that is reported from other ongoing trials can also be used. This is easier to implement if one takes a Bayesian approach, possibly using hierarchical modeling as described in the previous section. Note that the Bayesian approach is innately adaptive but not all adaptive designs are Bayesian.

Bayesian adaptive designs are increasingly being used in cancer trials. This is true for trials sponsored by pharmaceutical companies, and more generally. For example, a variety of trials conducted at The University of Texas MD Anderson Cancer Center are prospectively adaptive.[22,23] Based on their design and conduct, adaptive trials can be broadly classified into three classes: algorithm-based, model-assisted, and model-based. Algorithm-based designs are governed by rules for study conduct. These rules are derived based on empirical and heuristic reasoning without statistical models. They are easy to conduct but have a lack of good statistical properties. On the other hand, model-assisted designs and model-based designs are based on statistical models reflecting the trial settings. Good statistical properties can be achieved by optimizing certain criteria such as maximizing statistical power or minimizing sample size. Model-assisted designs also provide rules to facilitate the study conduct.[24] Model-based designs can be tailored to address the study objectives, but they require special software for the study design and conduct. Examples of commonly used adaptive designs are given in the next sections below.

Adaptive Phase I trials

The purpose of Phase I cancer trials is to identify the maximum-tolerated dose (MTD). Phase I trial designs generally use either a rigid, algorithm-based up-and-down design or an adaptive design that is based on a statistical model. Variants of the so-called 3 + 3 design[25] and the accelerated titration design[26] are forms of the up-and-down design that are commonly used in Phase I trials. On the other hand, variants of the continual reassessment method (CRM) are forms of the model-based dose-finding design. A new class of the model-assisted designs is also described.

The 3 + 3 design enrolls patients in groups of three. If none of the three patients experiences toxicity, the dose is increased one level for the next group of three. If two or three of the three patients experience toxicity, then the next lower dose is the MTD, providing that at least six patients have been treated at that dose. If one of the three experiences toxicity, then three more patients are added at the same dose level. If two or more of the six patients at that dose experience toxicity, then again the next lower dose with at least six patients treated is the MTD. This algorithm-based design is crudely adaptive and is likely to assign low doses and to select an ineffective MTD. Moreover, the decision of the next dose depends on only the result of the current dose and ignores the information accumulating from all other doses administered in the trial.

The CRM and its extensions[27–29] use Bayesian updating, which assumes a particular model of the relationship between dose and toxicity (such as the logistic function). The CRM assigns each patient to the dose that has the probability of toxicity closest to some predetermined target value. This is the Bayesian posterior probability calculated from the data available up to that point. Variations of the CRM include the escalation with overdose control (EWOC) design[30] and the Bayesian model averaging continual reassessment method (BMA-CRM),[31] which provides more flexible ways to specify the dose-toxicity relationship.

The Bayesian optimal interval (BOIN) design[32] is a model-assisted design. Based on the toxicity outcome at a given dose, the next cohort of patients can be treated at the next higher dose (escalate), at the next lower dose (de-escalate), or at the same dose (stay). Table 2 gives the dose decision boundaries for the targeted toxicity rates ranging from 0.15 to 0.40. To determine at which

Table 2 Dose decision boundaries for assigning the dose of the next cohort of patients for the Bayesian optimal interval (BOIN) design.

Boundaries	Target toxicity rate					
	0.15	0.20	0.25	0.30	0.35	0.40
Escalation if the observed toxicity rate is ≤	0.118	0.157	0.197	0.236	0.276	0.316
De-escalation if the observed toxicity rate is ≥	0.179	0.238	0.298	0.358	0.419	0.479

dose the next cohort of patients will be treated, we first calculate the observed toxicity rate at the current dose. For example, when the target toxicity rate is 0.3, the next cohort of patients will be treated at the next higher or the next lower dose if the observed toxicity rate is less than or equal to 0.236 or greater than or equal to 0.358, respectively. Otherwise, the next cohort of patients will be treated at the current dose level. The process continues until the maximum sample size is reached. These decision boundaries are chosen to minimize the decision error of dosing. Upon the specification of the target toxicity rate, the decision boundaries can be calculated and listed in the protocol to guide the dose selection. Thus, the model-assisted design is easy to conduct and also has good statistical properties.

Both the BOIN and the CRM designs can effectively find the MTD with a higher probability of selecting the right dose than that of the 3 + 3 design. These two designs also assign more patients to be treated at the MTD compared to the 3 + 3 design. The 3 + 3 design has poor statistical properties and is not recommended. Several generalizations of the BOIN design have been proposed, including the time-to-event Bayesian optimal interval design (TITE-BOIN)[33] for the delayed toxicity outcome, BOIN design for combination studies (BOIN comb),[34] BOIN design incorporating the historical data (iBOIN),[35] designs that can evaluate toxicity and efficacy simultaneously to find the optimal biological dose (OBD) by the BOIN12 design[36] and the utility-based U-BOIN design.[37] Figure 5 shows the decision tree to help in choosing the proper design among the BOIN design family.

Similarly, the CRM design has been generalized in several ways. For dealing with late-onset toxicity, the TITE-CRM and the data augmentation CRM[38] are able to assign a next dose, even though patients previously treated are not yet fully evaluable.[39,40] The expectation-maximization CRM[41] has been proposed to ease the computation burden. Model-based dose-finding designs have also been developed for trials that evaluate drugs in combination.[42–46]

Additional limitations of a Phase I design are the assumption that toxicity is dichotomous and the exclusion of efficacy from consideration. A better approach would be to account for both the severity of toxicity and the efficacy in a Phase I/II design.[47–50] Along the same line, certain biologics and immune therapies are expected to have low toxicity within the range of therapeutic doses, and the optimal dose is generally defined as the lowest safe dose of the targeted agent that has the highest rate of efficacy. Several other approaches have been proposed for determining the OBD in Phase I dose-finding trials.[51,52] There are books that provide comprehensive discussions of adaptive designs for Phase I and Phase I/II trials.[13,53,54]

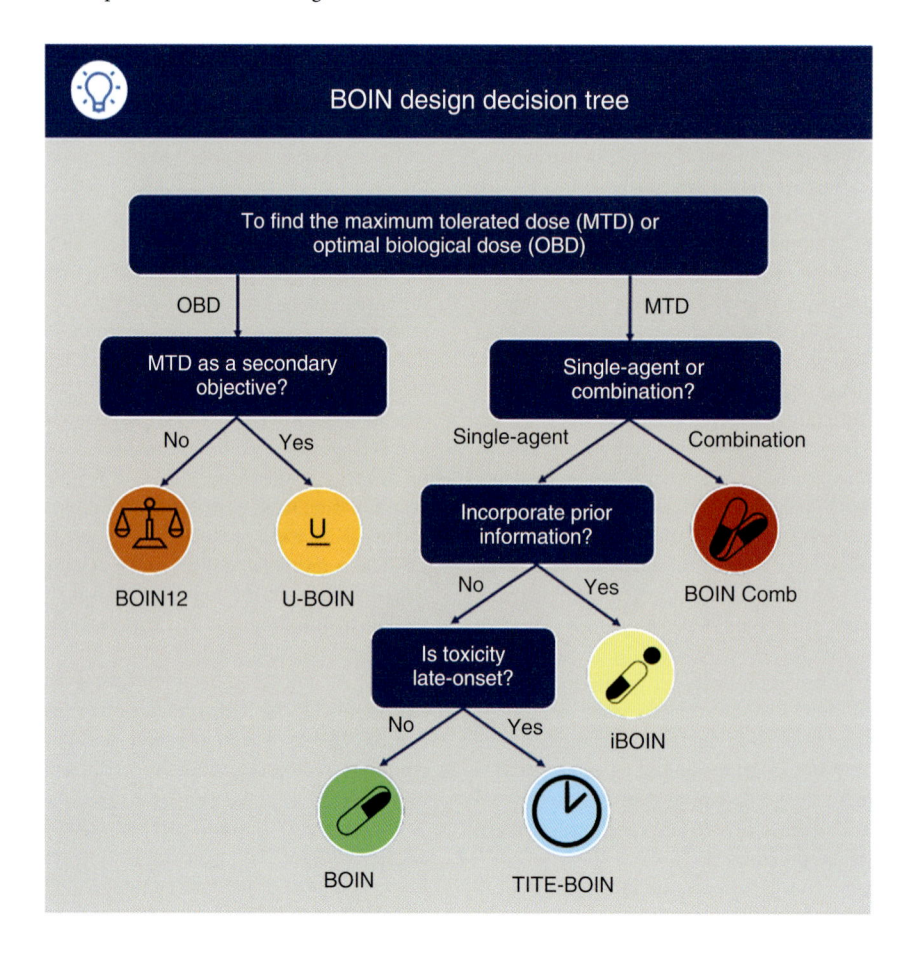

Figure 5 BOIN designs decision tree to help in choosing the proper design.

Adaptive Phase II trials

In many diseases, the standard dose-finding efficacy design allocates a fixed number of patients to each of a number of doses in a grid to study the drug effect. Such questions are of less interest in cancer chemotherapy trials because of the goal of administering as much of the drug as the patient can tolerate. However, with increased use of biological and immune agents, dose evaluation for efficacy while monitoring safety is becoming more important in cancer research.

Upon the identification of MTD or OBD in a Phase I trial, the recommended Phase II dose is selected. Early single-arm designs provide a formal evaluation of the drug's efficacy with a goal to screen out ineffective agents. The most commonly used design, Simon's optimal or minimax designs,[55] are two-stage designs that allow for early futility stopping (lack of efficacy) in the first stage. If the interim result is sufficiently promising, more patients will be enrolled in the second stage. By specifying the null response rate (the rate under the null hypothesis that the drug does not work) and the alternative response rate (the rate under the alternative hypothesis that the drug works), sample size can be calculated by controlling the type I and type II error rates. Bayesian adaptive trial designs for a binary outcome measure have been proposed with efficacy and/or futility-stopping rules.[56,57]

The Bayesian optimal Phase 2 (BOP2) design[58] is an efficient model-assisted design that can handle simple and complex endpoints under a unified framework. The design allows multiple interim monitoring such that the trial can be stopped early if the drug is not efficacious, too toxic, or both. The design can also optimize the statistical power given sample size and control for type I error. Table 3 lists the stopping boundaries for four examples with interim monitoring at 10, 15, 20, 25, 30, and 35 patients and the maximum sample size at 40. The endpoint in Example 1 is the object response rate. Example 2 has two ordinal response endpoints: complete response rate and complete or partial response rates. Example 3 has two efficacy endpoints: objective response rate and 6-month progression-free survival rate. Example 4 monitors the objective response rate and toxicity rate simultaneously. The parameters under the null and alternative hypotheses are given in the footnote of the table. All four examples control type I error rates to 10%. The statistical powers are 88%, 85%, 96%, and 70%, respectively.

Table 3 Stopping boundaries for the Bayesian optimal Phase 2 (BOP2) design in four trial examples.

Trial	Stop the trial if	10	15	20	25	30	35	40
Example 1[a]	Number of OR ≤	1	2	4	5	7	9	10
Example 2[b]	Number of CR ≤	0	1	3	4	5	7	9
	And number of CR/PR ≤	2	3	5	8	10	13	16
Example 3[c]	Number of OR ≤	0	1	2	3	4	5	7
	And number of PFS6m ≤	1	2	4	5	7	9	12
Example 4[d]	Number of OR ≤	2	5	7	10	13	15	18
	And number. of toxicity ≥	4	6	7	8	9	11	12

The maximum sample size is 40. Type I error rates are controlled at 10%. Statistical powers for Examples 1, 2, 3, 4 are 88%, 85%, 96%, and 70%, respectively. The stopping boundaries are optimized based on the following null hypotheses (H_0) and alternative hypotheses (H_1).
[a]H_0: Pr(OR) = 0.2 vs H_1: Pr(OR) = 0.4.
[b]H_0: Pr(CR) = 0.15, Pr(CR or PR) = 0.30 vs H_1: Pr(CR) = 0.25, Pr(CR or PR) = 0.50.
[c]H_0: Pr(OR) = 0.1, Pr(PFS6m) = 0.20, Pr(OR and PFS6m) = 0.05 vs H_1: Pr(OR) = 0.3, Pr(PFS6m) = 0.35, Pr(OR and PFS6m) = 0.15.
[d]H_0: Pr(OR) = 0.45, Pr(Toxicity) = 0.3, Pr(OR and toxicity) = 0.135 vs H_1: Pr(OR) = 0.60, Pr(toxicity) = 0.2, Pr(OR and toxicity) = 0.12.

The BOP2 design can be extended for trials with time-to-event endpoints, for example, in immunotherapy trials in which immune agents often take longer to show the benefit. The Bayesian time-to-event optimal Phase II (TOP) design[59] is a flexible and efficient design for multiple endpoints. It allows a real-time "go/no-go" interim decision to be made in the presence of late-onset responses by using all available data and maximizes statistical power for detecting effective treatments. TOP also allows a number of interim looks. Compared to some existing designs, the TOP design could shorten the trial duration by 4–10 months, and it improves the power to detect effective treatment up to 90% while controlling type I errors.

The BOIN family designs, BOP2, and TOP designs are developed as model-assisted designs to overcome one major barrier for the implementation of novel model-based designs, i.e., these designs often require special software and are complicated to conduct. Model-assisted designs possess the simplicity of algorithm-based designs without sacrificing the superior performance of model-based designs, seizing the best of two worlds.[24] Freely available user-friendly software can be found at http://trialdesign.org to facilitate implementation. This approach establishes a new KISS principle: keep it simple and smart!

Sequential designs for Phase II studies have been developed to evaluate the efficacy of new treatments within a prespecified range of doses. This dose-ranging stage continues until a decision is made that the drug is not sufficiently effective to pursue future development or that the optimal dose for the confirmatory Phase III trial is sufficiently well known. The design of Berry et al.[60] also proceeds sequentially, analyzing the data as they accumulate, as well as applying predictive probability for utility early stopping in the Phase II design.[61] A longitudinal model can be derived based on the current patient data to predict the ultimate endpoint. Hence, the probability distributions of the treatment effect can be updated accordingly. Further discussion of group sequential designs can be found in the work of Jennison and Turnbull.[62]

Finding the right dose is a ubiquitous problem in pharmaceutical development, and it is seldom done well or efficiently. A design with adaptive dosing is more effective than the standard design at identifying the right dose. In addition, it usually identifies the right dose with a smaller sample size than when using fixed-dose assignments. Another advantage is that many more doses can be considered in an adaptive design. (Even though some doses will be little used and some may never be used, these cannot be predicted in advance.) An adaptive design, therefore, has some ability to distinguish responses at adjacent doses and to estimate the nuances of the dose–response curve. Furthermore, the Bayesian adaptive design can be applied to screen efficacious combination therapies in Phase II trials by formulating the selection procedure as a Bayesian hypothesis testing problem and using the current values of the posterior probabilities to adaptively allocate patients to treatment combinations.[63] Finally, the possibility of moving seamlessly from Phase I to Phase II or from Phase II to Phase III, contingent upon promising results, exists for many types of drugs. This issue leads naturally to the subject of the next section.

Seamless Phase I/II and Phase II/III designs

The convention of discretizing drug development into phases is unfortunate. We proceed from one phase to the next when we think we know something: the MTD from Phase I, or that a drug's impact on a Phase II endpoint will translate into a benefit in Phase III, and at the Phase II dose. In the Bayesian approach, one never takes a quantity to be perfectly known. Instead, the Bayesian perspective is to carry along uncertainty with whatever knowledge is available. Phases of drug development are arbitrary labels that describe a process that is, or should be, continuous.

One of the consequences of partitioning drug development into phases is that there are delays between phases. For example, there is a pause between Phases II and III to set up one or more pivotal studies. On the other hand, seamless designs allow for moving from one phase to another without designing a new trial, hence, avoiding a hiatus, or white space between trials. At each time point, say weekly, the algorithm that guides the conduct of the trial carries out a decision analysis and recommends either (1) continue the dose-ranging stage of the trial, (2) stop the trial for lack of efficacy, or (3) shift into a confirmatory trial. This shift can be made seamlessly, with no break in the accrual.

Many trial designs have encompassed both Phases I and II.[36,47] Such designs allow for addressing toxicity and efficacy throughout the trial. Only "admissible" doses or combinations of doses are used, and doses are escalated as others become admissible. All the while, the designs allow for learning about the relationship between dose and efficacy, as well as about dose and toxicity.

Trials designed to encompass both Phases II and III use a seamless switch to Phase III.[64–67] The seamless aspect is as follows: patients are accrued to a trial, which we can think of as Phase II. If the accumulating data are sufficiently strong in suggesting that the drug/treatment has no effect on local control or survival, then the trial stops. If the data suggest that the drug may have an impact on local control and that this impact translates into a survival benefit, then the trial will be expanded and the accrual rate will increase accordingly by adding more sites. During such an expansion, patients continue to accrue at the initial site so that there is no downtime in the local accrual while other sites prepare to join the trial. This is an efficient use of patient resources, because data from the patients who enrolled early contribute to the eventual inferences about survival. These patients are the most informative of all those enrolled, because their follow-up times are the longest.

The trial continues until stopping occurs because (1) continuing would be futile, judged by predictive probabilities, or (2) the maximum sample size is reached, or (3) the predictive probability of eventually achieving statistical significance becomes sufficiently large. If the third event occurs, the accrual ceases and the pharmaceutical company prepares a marketing application.

For example, the sample size of a conventional Phase III trial with the desired operating characteristics is 900. This also is taken to be the maximum sample size in the seamless design. Actual accrual is very likely to be much less than this maximum sample size, particularly, when the experimental treatment is either very promising or not promising at all. On the other hand, incorporating the same number of interim analyses in a conventional design using a conventional type of stopping boundary allows for only a slight decrease in the average sample size. A Bayesian design occasionally leads to a relatively large trial (close to 900 patients). However, a pleasant aspect of the design is that the sample size is large precisely when a large trial is necessary. Conventional trials may well (and sometimes do) come to their predetermined end with an ambiguous conclusion. In a Bayesian approach, one may choose to continue such a trial to resolve the ambiguity, and this option has substantial utility. Within a seamless adaptive design, one can use the data accumulating in the trial to reestimate the sample size, which can result in reduced sample sizes.[68,69]

A conventional drug-development strategy involves running a Phase I trial to identify the MTD, then following that with a Phase II trial to address local control; analyzing the results, if they are positive, development begins on a Phase III trial with survival as the primary endpoint. In comparison with such a strategy, a seamless approach can greatly reduce the sample size. In addition, a seamless design minimizes the pauses between phases, which greatly shortens the total drug development time.

Adaptive randomization

The adaptive designs discussed so far are motivated by the desire to learn efficiently and as rapidly as possible. Another kind of adaptive design aims to assign patients to treatments as effectively as possible. Adaptive randomization encompasses two primary approaches: baseline covariate-adjusted adaptive randomization and outcome-adaptive randomization. A baseline covariate-adjusted adaptive randomization scheme may assign patients to a treatment arm on the basis of measurements of particular characteristics that are associated with prognosis (prognostic markers) before treatment starts. This balances the determinant factors among the treatment arms. In contrast, an outcome-adaptive randomization scheme assigns patients to a treatment arm on the basis of the responses to treatment that are accumulating from patients already enrolled in the trial, which tends to assign more participants to treatments that are achieving better patient responses. Outcome-adaptive randomization increases the likelihood that more patients will receive the more efficacious treatment. This strategy benefits the individuals participating in the trial, which strengthens the "individual ethics" of the trial.[70] Equal randomization, on the other hand, maximizes the statistical power, which emphasizes the "group" or "collective ethics" of the trial, with the goal of identifying effective treatments from the trial and then applying that information to benefit future patients. In addition to making clinical trials more attractive to patients and thereby increasing participation in clinical trials, outcome-adaptive randomization strategies have the important side benefit of being efficient, and so they result in rapid learning.

The purpose of adaptive randomization is to shift the probability weight toward better-performing arms as the trial proceeds and the results accumulate. Several allocation algorithms can be considered, for example, assigning doses in proportion to the success probabilities. Many of these trials have more than two treatment arms. An example is a trial to determine the dose of an additional prophylactic agent that would inhibit acute graft-versus-host disease (GVHD) in leukemia patients who received bone marrow transplants.[71] The trial evaluated five doses (including 0) of a drug (pentostatin) added to the standard prophylaxis regimen. The problem was that the drug might inhibit the successful engraftment of the transplant, which was necessary for survival. Such inhibition might be related to dose. A combination endpoint was used in the trial: survival at 100 days free of GVHD. The conflict between engraftment and freedom from GVHD meant that the dose–response curve might not be monotone. In particular, it might increase for small doses and then decrease. Doses were initially assigned in a graduated manner, slowly climbing the dose ladder. However, as doses became admissible, more patients were assigned to the doses that were performing well.

Consider a patient who qualifies for the trial. To decide which pentostatin dose to assign, one calculates the current (Bayesian) probabilities that each admissible dose is better than the placebo. This calculation uses all the information from the patients treated to date. Doses are allocated randomly, with weights proportional to these probabilities. Doses that are doing sufficiently poorly become inadmissible in the sense that their assignment weight becomes 0. When and if it is learned that the drug is effective, the trial is stopped. When and if it is learned that the drug is ineffective, then again the trial is stopped. Patients in the trial benefit from data collected in the trial. The explicit goal is to treat patients more effectively, as well as to learn more efficiently. Each design's frequentist operating characteristics are evaluated using Monte Carlo simulation, with possible modification of the parameters of the assignment algorithm to achieve desired characteristics.

Outcome-adaptive randomization can be constructed under either a frequentist or a Bayesian framework. A frequentist approach has been used to derive the optimal randomization probability under various criteria,[72,73] and interim data available at the time of patient allocation have been used to estimate the response rates. The "doubly adaptive biased coin" design[74] extends this approach by considering the proportion of patients assigned to each treatment and the current estimate of the desired allocation proportion to compute the randomization probability to achieve optimal design properties with less variability.

The most intuitive approach is standard Bayesian adaptive randomization, which assigns patients to treatment arm 1 with $\phi_1 = \text{Prob}(\theta_1 > \theta_2)$, where θ_i is the posterior probability of p_i for $i = 1, 2$ at the time of randomization. This approach has been extended by applying a power transformation, $\phi_1 = \text{Prob}(\theta_1 > \theta_2)^c / (\text{Prob}(\theta_1 > \theta_2)^c + \text{Prob}(\theta_1 < \theta_2)^c)$, and using $c = n/(2N)$, where n is the number of currently enrolled patients and N the maximum number of patients in the trial, to decrease the variability of the randomization probability.[75] Thus, the randomization probability is approximately 0.5 at the start of the trial and varies as more data accumulate, particularly if the data show a large difference in the response rates between the treatment arms. The randomization probability can be restricted to a range around 0.5 to decrease its variability. Other schemes use the posterior mean (or median) of the treatment effect to determine the randomization probability[76]: $\phi = \hat{\theta}_1 / (\hat{\theta}_1 + \hat{\theta}_2)$, where $\hat{\theta}_i$ is the posterior mean (or median) of θ_i for $i = 1, 2$.

To ensure that the adaptive randomization possess is robust to random variation of the process, three regularization methods were proposed.[77] One can design a clinical trial to begin with an equal randomization scheme and then transition to an adaptive randomization scheme after observing patient responses to the treatment. A minimum randomization probability can be enforced to ensure a reasonable randomization probability for each viable arm. In addition, a power transformation can be used to strengthen or weaken the imbalance of randomization probability. The adaptive randomization strategy can be combined with early stopping rules for futility and/or efficacy based on predictive probability. This format can result in a sensible drug development process. (1) When the trial starts, equal randomization is applied as there is not much information on treatment efficacy. (2) After a reasonable amount of data are accumulated, one can switch to adaptive randomization so more patients can be assigned to the better-performing arms based on the available data. (3) The trial continues to accrue patients toward the maximum sample size but allows for interim monitoring such that the trial can be stopped early when sufficient evidence has accrued that will allow for the inference of treatment efficacy. The flexible format of the trial illustrates the advantages of the Bayesian adaptive clinical trial design.[78]

Using adaptive randomization to evaluate multiple treatments requires the trial statistician to carefully check for population drift to prevent biased comparisons of the various treatments. This is of concern when using an adaptive randomization scheme that tends to assign more patients to the better-performing treatments, because the scheme may cause imbalance in the patient characteristics across the treatment arms.[79] The trial can be designed to partially correct for population drift by including a control arm and placing limits on the randomization probability to achieve a nonnegligible randomization probability for each treatment arm. A marked population drift can invalidate proper inference. This issue can be resolved using regression analysis, for example, to account for the imbalance in prognostic covariates among the treatment arms. Recommendations for monitoring adaptive trials are provided by Marchenko et al.[80]

The advantages and disadvantages of incorporating outcome-adaptive randomization strategies in a clinical trial have prompted numerous discussions and may depend on the specific scenario under which the strategy is applied. Equal randomization has been preferred in a two-arm trial with a binary endpoint because it is easier to implement, and it results in smaller sample sizes and fewer nonresponders.[79] A recent analysis of outcome-adaptive randomization questioned the ethics of using this strategy for two-arm trials.[70] Adaptive randomization strategies can increase the favorable response rate and achieve better statistical power when a large difference exists between the effects of the different treatments tested in a trial. Adding an early stopping rule to the trial design will somewhat decrease this advantage. Compared to equal randomization strategies, adaptive randomization strategies may be advantageous in trials that evaluate a rare disease. Adaptive randomization is advantageous in trials that evaluate multiple treatments and which combine multiple stages of study and are particularly applicable when one treatment is much more beneficial than the others.[81]

Extraim analyses

A common circumstance is that a clinical trial ends without a clear conclusion. For example, a statistical significance level of 5% in the primary endpoint may be required for drug registration, and the p-value may turn out to be 6%. The regulatory agency then suggests that the trial was "underpowered" and that the company should carry out another trial. It would be much more efficient to simply increase the sample size in the present trial. The problem is that the possibility of such an extension increases the type I error rate. The principle is identical to that for interim analyses.

The solution is to build into the design the possibility of continuing the trial depending on the results and suitably adjusting the significance levels. In contrast to the adjustments for interim analyses, the adjustments for "extra-im" (extraim) analyses are reversed, with much of the overall significance level "spent" at the originally planned sample size. For example, taking equal significance levels at each possible termination point is preferable to O'Brien-Fleming stopping boundaries, because the latter are too conservative for extraim analyses. Allowing for extending the trial increases the maximal sample size and also the average sample size. However, a modest increase in the average sample size (such as 20%) comes with a substantial increase in statistical power (such as 80% increasing to 95%). The reason for this beneficial tradeoff is that the trial is extended only when such an extension is worthwhile.

The "penalty" in the significance level can be either partially or fully offset by including futility analyses as part of the design, namely the trial would be stopped for sufficiently negative results at preset interim time points. The reason such analyses offset the penalty for extraim analyses is that the null hypothesis is never rejected when the trial stops for futility. The increment in sample size depends on the available data at the time the decision is made to continue the accrual. It also depends on the number of possible extensions. In trials we have designed, we have based each extension on the predictive power. The usual definition of power assumes a particular value of the parameter of interest, say r. Predictive power considers all possible values of r. The data available at the time of the extraim analysis plays two roles. First, they count in the final results of the trial. Second, they are used to update the (Bayesian) probability distribution of r. Fix the total sample size n and calculate the power for detecting each possible value of r. Average this power with respect to the probability distribution of r to give the predictive power for sample size n. Extend the accrual by the minimum sample size that will achieve a total sample size having a prespecified predictive power. If there is no such value of n, then continuing the accrual may be unwise.

The Bayesian framework is ideally suited for incorporating information from outside the trial to make inference. For example, hierarchically commensurate priors and power priors can be applied to adaptively incorporate historical information into clinical trials.[82,83] Historical data on similar therapies or devices can be readily available in many settings. The efficient and appropriate use of such historical information to strengthen the inference for a new trial has been demonstrated in the development of medical devices.[84]

Decision analysis

Clinical practice and clinical research involve making decisions. A list of the possible results such as efficacy and toxicity, pros and cons, risk, benefit, and cost can be expressed as utilities or loss function to account for the tradeoff among complex value space. Optimal decisions can be made by maximizing the utility or minimizing the loss function, allowing for the choice of one decision over another. Predictive probabilities play a central role in the decision-making process, which makes the Bayesian approach ideal. Choosing the trial design and selecting the optimal sample size are decisions that benefit from the use of decision analysis, which is described in greater detail in other references.[85–87]

Process or trial? Evaluating many drugs simultaneously in platform trials with or without adaptive allocation

The greatest need for innovation in drug development is the process of effectively dealing with the enormous numbers of potential drugs that are available for development. The notion of developing drugs one at a time is changing. Companies that are able to screen many drugs simultaneously and effectively will survive, while others will not.

The platform-based clinical trial design is an example of innovation in the process of developing new agents and therapies.[88,89] A platform is an operational and statistical framework that is specific to a particular disease or condition, rather than being specific to a particular clinical protocol. Each new agent or therapy can be considered as a "module" that can be plugged in and out of the "platform" that targets a particular disease or condition. These new treatments can be simultaneously screened as they are developed as an alternative to conducting several separate Phase II trials to evaluate multiple treatment arms. Bayesian modeling and randomization can be easily incorporated into the platform-based design. It can be shown that the platform design is much more efficient than running multiple, separate trials. Once the appropriate dose of a new agent has been determined in a Phase I trial, that new agent may be added to the platform. An agent may also be dropped from the platform if the data accumulating in the screening process demonstrate that the agent is not producing the desired results. An agent that is dropped from the platform can be returned to a Phase I study to reexamine the optimal treatment dose or schedule of doses. If that Phase I trial determines that an alternative dose or schedule of doses may be beneficial, then the agent previously dropped from the platform may reenter the screening process.

The platform-based design brings important statistical challenges to the conduct of such screening trials. The Bayesian posterior distributions and predictive probabilities are computationally intensive to calculate; however, after the predictive probabilities are calculated, boundaries can be specified for the continuous monitoring of the platform-based designs. Sequential adaptive strategies must be properly implemented to monitor the futility of the many experimental agents while maintaining the predetermined type I error rate. The platform-based design bases its futility stopping rule on the posterior predictive probability of achieving a successful trial. The design uses a Bayesian model to account for the uncertainty emanating from interim estimations of the model parameters and uses simulations to calibrate the design parameters. A Bayesian model is also used to account for the variability resulting from the treatment responses of future patients in the trial.

The concept of a master protocol has been proposed to expedite the development of oncology drugs[90] and devices.[91] A master protocol trial consists of a general protocol that can evaluate several cancer types and/or several treatments or devices simultaneously. Patients are enrolled in the master protocol first, then, depending on the objectives and eligibility, enrolled in specific subprotocols. Subprotocols can be an umbrella trial with a single cancer type but multiple drugs to tackle multiple disease pathways. Alternatively, subprotocols can be a basket trial with a drug for a specific molecular subtype but in multiple cancer types.

Master protocols can also be platform trials in certain settings, e.g., metastatic nonsmall cell lung cancer, with a backbone of a standard double chemotherapy and modules with targeted therapies, immunotherapies, or combinations that can be plugged into or out of the platform. For example, Figure 6 illustrates a conceptual schema of the platform design. The control arm shown in blue is considered as the backbone and is always present in the trial. The experimental arms shown in orange are considered as modules. In Year 1, arms Exp 1 and Exp 2 were added to the trial. In Year 2, Exp 3 was added. In Year 3, Exp 1 was determined as not efficacious, hence, dropped. In Year 4, Exp 4 was added. In Year 5, Exp 2 was determined as efficacious, then, it graduated to further evaluation, but Exp 3 was too toxic, and hence it was dropped. In Year 6, Exp 6 was added. The trial can go on perpetually. The platform-based design and the related umbrella trials and basket trials, with particular application to biomarker studies, are discussed by Berry.[12] The platform-based design has potential advantages that include decreasing the overall duration of the treatment screening process; substantially decreasing the number of patients allocated to the control arm; increasing the number of treatments that can be screened, thereby expanding the treatment options available to patients in the trial; decreasing the bias arising from the heterogeneity of separate trials; improving the control of inherent multiplicities; and better informing decisions about subsequent confirmatory trials.

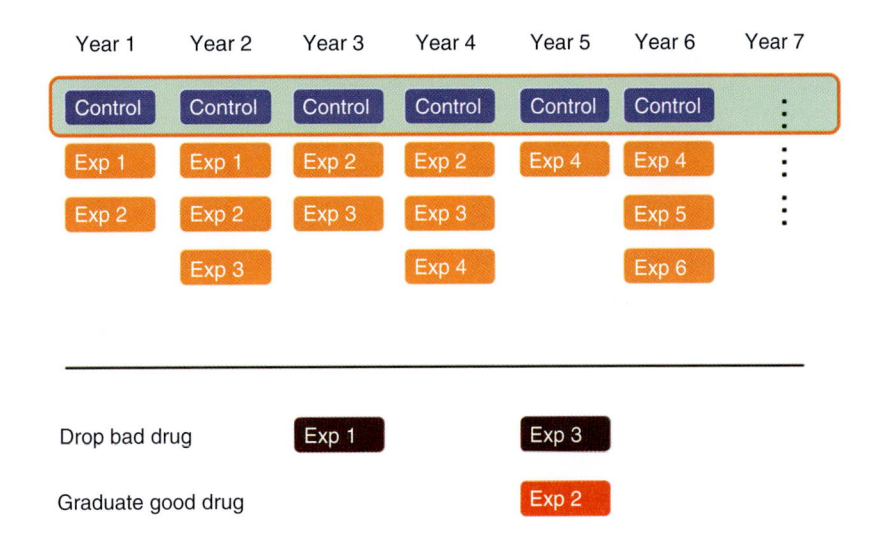

Figure 6 Conceptual schema of the platform design.

Application of statistical innovation in clinical oncology trials

This section briefly describes two clinical oncology trials that employ statistical innovations: the biomarker-integrated approaches of targeted therapy of lung cancer elimination (BATTLE) trial and the Investigation of serial studies to predict your therapeutic response with imaging and molecular analysis (I-SPY 2) trial.

The BATTLE trial[92,93] evaluated four targeted therapies in patients with stage IV recurrent non-small-cell lung cancer, matching each therapy with one of the four biomarker profiles evaluated (defined by expressions of genes, gene mutations, copy numbers, and proteins measured by immunohistochemistry). The outcome was the 8-week disease control rate. The trial incorporates outcome-adaptive randomization and a futility stopping rule under the probit hierarchical model. The stopping rule may exclude specific agents from randomization possibilities for a given patient when that patient's biomarker profile indicates that they will not benefit from that agent. The BATTLE-2 trial uses the results from the first trial to screen patients for 10–15 candidate biomarkers. It incorporates adaptive randomization in a two-stage design to evaluate four treatments for non-small-cell lung cancer. The trial is a process, involving training, testing, and validation procedures to select the most appropriate biomarkers to use in the trial. The design uses group lasso and adaptive lasso methods to identify prognostic and predictive markers.[94,95]

The multicenter I-SPY 2 trial[96] employs adaptive randomization within each biomarker-based patient group and uses a futility or efficacy stopping rule. The I-SPY 2 trial evaluates neoadjuvant treatments in breast cancer in addition to the administration of up to 12 experimental drugs. This trial has randomized more than 950 patients, transferred two experimental agents to confirmatory studies, and successfully demonstrated that this adaptive trial design can reduce drug development costs and improve the efficiency of screening new drugs.

Results in two promising agent-patient groups: veliparib-carboplatin in triple-negative breast cancer and neratinib in HER-2 positive breast cancer have been published.[97,98]

GBM AGILE is a multi-arm, seamless Phase II/III response adaptive randomization platform trial[99] designed to evaluate multiple therapies in newly diagnosed and recurrent glioblastoma with the overall survival as the primary endpoint. The goal is to screen effective treatment and biomarker pairs for glioblastoma. GBM AGILE is composed of two stages under a single master protocol, allowing multiple drugs or drug combinations to be evaluated simultaneously. In the first stage, Bayesian adaptive randomization is used to identify effective drugs within disease subtype. The randomization probabilities to the treatments within subtypes are proportional to the Bayesian posterior probabilities of prolonging overall survival longer than the control. Highly promising treatments will seamlessly graduate to the second stage, which is a Phase III, equally randomized, confirmatory trial in the identified population. The schematic diagram for the GBM-Agile trial is shown in Figure 7. As shown, it is a continuous learning, evaluation, and decision-making trial. The design allows multiple agents to be evaluated in multiple disease subtypes in an efficient and flexible way, such that ineffective treatments can be dropped early and effective treatments can be graduated for further testing.

Clinical trial software

Numerous software programs for use in planning and implementing clinical trials are available online as propriety products or as free offerings.[100] Many useful computer programs for the design, conduct, and analysis of innovative trials can be found at the MD Anderson software download site. (https://biostatistics.mdanderson.org/SoftwareDownload/). In addition, the MD Anderson team also developed many user-friendly R/Shiny web-based applications for novel clinical trial designs (http://trialdesign.org). With more software available for the design and conduct of novel clinical trials, more rapid translation of statistical innovation from theory to practice can be achieved.

Acknowledgments

The authors thank the Cancer and Leukemia Group B for permission to use data from CALGB 8541 and Jessica Swann for editorial assistance. This work was supported in part by Grant CA016672 from the National Cancer Institute.

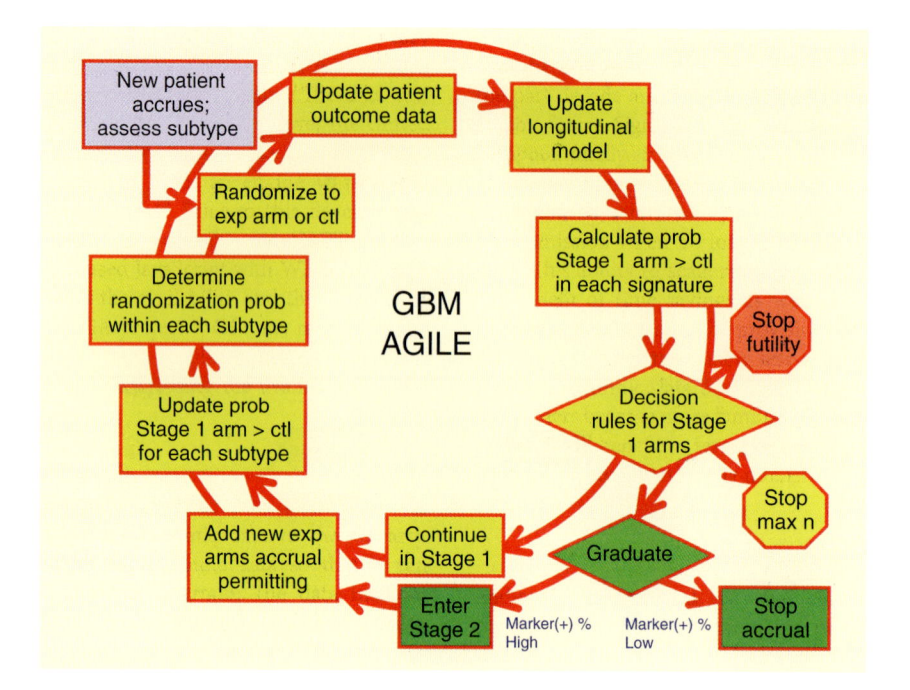

Figure 7 Schematic diagram for the adaptive GBM-Agile trial.

Key references

The complete reference list can be found on Vital Source version of this title, see inside front cover.

2. DiMasi JA, Reichert JM, Feldman L, Malins A. Clinical approval success rates for investigational cancer drugs. *Clin Pharmacol Therapeut*. 2013;**94**:329–335.
4. *Critical Path Reports* (2006) https://www.fda.gov/science-research/critical-path-initiative/critical-path-opportunities-reports (accessed 9 August 2021).
5. *Guidance for the Use of Bayesian Statistics in Medical Device Clinical Trials* (2010) https://www.fda.gov/regulatory-information/search-fda-guidance-documents/guidance-use-bayesian-statistics-medical-device-clinical-trials (accessed 9 August 2021).
6. *Adaptive Designs for Medical Device Clinical Studies* (2016) https://www.fda.gov/regulatory-information/search-fda-guidance-documents/adaptive-designs-medical-device-clinical-studies (accessed 9 August 2021).
7. *Adaptive Designs for Clinical Trials of Drugs and Biologics Guidance for Industry* (2019) https://www.fda.gov/media/78495/download (accessed 9 August 2021).
8. *Complex Innovative Trial Designs* (2020) https://www.fda.gov/media/130897/download (accessed 9 August 2021).
9. Berry DA. Introduction to Bayesian methods III: use and interpretation of Bayesian tools in design and analysis. *Clin Trials: J Soc Clin Trials*. 2005;**2**:295–300.
10. Berry DA. *Statistics: A Bayesian Perspective*. Belmont, CA: Duxbury Press; 1996.
11. Berry DA. Bayesian clinical trials. *Nat Rev Drug Discov*. 2006;**5**:27–36.
12. Berry DA. The Brave New World of clinical cancer research: adaptive biomarker-driven trials integrating clinical practice with clinical research. *Mol Oncol*. 2015;**9**:951–959.
13. Berry SM, Carlin BP, Lee JJ, Mueller P. *Bayesian Adaptive Methods for Clinical Trials*. Chapman & Hall/CRC: Boca Raton; 2011.
14. Gelman A, Carlin J, Stern H, et al. *Bayesian Data Analysis*. Chapman & Hall/CRC: Baton Rouge, LA; 2013.
15. Muss H, Berry D, Cirrincione C, et al. Adjuvant Chemotherapy for Breast Cancer in Older Women. *Women Health*. 2009;**5**:453–457.
16. Klepin HD, Pitcher BN, Ballman KV, et al. Comorbidity, chemotherapy toxicity, and outcomes among older women receiving adjuvant chemotherapy for breast cancer on a clinical trial: CALGB 49907 and CALGB 361004 (alliance). *J Oncol Pract*. 2014;**10**:e285–e292.
17. DuMouchel W. In: Berry DA, ed. *Bayesian Metaanalysis in Statistical Methodology in the Pharmaceutical Sciences*. New York: Dekker; 1990:509–529.
18. Thall PF, Wathen JK, Bekele BN, et al. Hierarchical Bayesian approaches to phase II trials in diseases with multiple subtypes. *Stat Med*. 2003;**22**:763–780.
19. Chen N, Lee JJ. Bayesian hierarchical classification and information sharing for clinical trials with subgroups and binary outcomes. *Biom J*. 2019;**61**:1219–1231.
20. Chen N, Lee JJ. Bayesian cluster hierarchical model for subgroup borrowing in the design and analysis of basket trials with binary endpoints. *Stat Methods Med Res*. 2020;**29**:2717–2732.
21. Berry DA, Fristedt B. *Bandit problems: sequential allocation of experiments*. Heidelberg: Springer; 2013.
22. Biswas S, Liu DD, Lee JJ, Berry DA. Bayesian clinical trials at the University of Texas M. D. Anderson Cancer Center. *Clin Trials*. 2009;**6**:205–216.
23. Tidwell RSS, Peng SA, Chen M, et al. Bayesian clinical trials at The University of Texas MD Anderson Cancer Center: an update. *Clin Trials*. 2019;**16**:645–656.
24. Yuan Y, Lee JJ, Hilsenbeck SG. Model-assisted designs for early-phase clinical trials: simplicity meets superiority. *JCO Precis Oncol*. 2019;**3**:PO.19.00032.
25. Liu S, Yuan Y. Bayesian optimal interval designs for phase I clinical trials. *J R Stat Soc: Ser C: Appl Stat*. 2014;**64**:507–523.
33. Yuan Y, Lin R, Li D, et al. Time-to-event bayesian optimal interval design to accelerate phase I trials. *Clin Cancer Res*. 2018;**24**:4921–4930.
34. Lin R, Yin G. Bayesian optimal interval design for dose finding in drug-combination trials. *Stat Methods Med Res*. 2015;**26**:2155–2167.
53. Yin G. *Clinical Trial Design: Bayesian and Frequentist Adaptive Methods*. Hoboken, NJ: John Wiley & Sons; 2012.
54. Yuan Y, Nguyen H, Thall P. *Bayesian Designs for Phase I-II Clinical Trials*. Boca Raton: Chapman and Hall/CRC; 2017.
58. Zhou H, Lee JJ, Yuan Y. BOP2: Bayesian optimal design for phase II clinical trials with simple and complex endpoints. *Stat Med*. 2017;**36**:3302–3314.
61. Lee JJ, Liu DD. A predictive probability design for phase II cancer clinical trials. *Clin Trials*. 2008;**5**:93–106.
66. Kimani PK, Glimm E, Maurer W, et al. Practical guidelines for adaptive seamless phase II/III clinical trials that use Bayesian methods. *Stat Med*. 2012;**31**:2068–2085.
81. Lee JJ, Chen N, Yin G. Worth adapting? Revisiting the usefulness of outcome-adaptive randomization. *Clin Cancer Res*. 2012;**18**:4498–4507.
82. Hobbs BP, Carlin BP, Mandrekar SJ, Sargent DJ. Hierarchical commensurate and power prior models for adaptive incorporation of historical information in clinical trials. *Biometrics*. 2011;**67**:1047–1056.
85. Lewis RJ, Berry DA. *Decision Theory. Encyclopedia of Biostatistics*. John Wiley & Sons, Ltd; 2005.
88. Hobbs BP, Chen N, Lee JJ. Controlled multi-arm platform design using predictive probability. *Stat Methods Med Res*. 2018;**27**:65–78.
89. Lee JJ, Chu CT. *Novel Statistical Models for NSCLC Clinical Trials. Lung Cancer*. John Wiley & Sons, Inc; 2014:488–504.
90. Woodcock J, LaVange LM. Master protocols to study multiple therapies, multiple diseases, or both. *N Engl J Med*. 2017;**377**:62–70.
93. Kim ES, Herbst RS, Wistuba II, et al. The BATTLE trial: personalizing therapy for lung cancer. *Cancer Discov*. 2011;**1**:44–53.

94 Berry DA, Herbst RS, Rubin EH. Reports from the 2010 Clinical and Translational Cancer Research Think Tank meeting: design strategies for personalized therapy trials. *Clin Cancer Res*. 2012;**18**:638–644.

96 Barker AD, Sigman CC, Kelloff GJ, et al. I-SPY 2: an adaptive breast cancer trial design in the setting of neoadjuvant chemotherapy. *Clin Pharmacol Therapeut*. 2009;**86**:97–100.

100 Lee J, Chen N. *Software for Design and Analysis of Clinical Trials. Handbook of Statistics in Clinical Oncology*, 3rd ed. Boca Raton: Chapman and Hall/CRC; 2012:305–324.

20 Biomarker based clinical trial design in the era of genomic medicine

R. Donald Harvey, PharmD, BCOP, FCCP, FHOPA ■ Yuan Liu, PhD, MS ■ Taofeek K. Owonikoko, MD, PhD, MSCR ■ Suresh S. Ramalingam, MD, FASCO

> **Overview**
>
> The expansion of understanding in genomics and molecular biology of cancer development and progression has led to greater subtyping of tumor types beyond histology alone. Along with improved drug development and medicinal chemistry approaches, this understanding has led to a need for an evolution in clinical trial design and analysis. Multiple groups of smaller populations treated with targeted agents have been employed to improve speed and efficiency of efficacy signals. We review these novel trial designs for the development of biomarker-driven therapeutics and diagnostics to inform their use.

Introduction: the need, current state, and evolution of biomarker-driven clinical trial design and analysis

Oncology clinical trial design and conduct have evolved to meet the continually expanding number and variety of targeted agents. The ability to enrich a population for the presence of a molecular predictor of response has led to smaller and, often, more efficient development pathways which subsequently bring effective therapies to patients more rapidly. These designs are in contrast to the historical but still relevant randomized clinical trial which generally evaluates a new treatment relative to an established one for a broadly defined population characterized by tumor primary site, histology, stage, and other clinical and demographic factors. Molecular medicine has allowed for the continual splitting of common anatomic and histologic cancer types into many distinct subtypes, and, most recently, created a regulatory pathway for agents independent of site of origin, such as the initial tissue-agnostic US Food and Drug Administration approvals of pembrolizumab and larotrectinib. These approvals are just the first of many to come, and are beneficial to patients, physicians, and regulators in their ability to define populations likely to benefit early in the drug development process due to unique genomic and protein-based drivers of cancer progression.[1] In contrast, unselective anticancer agent trials must have broad eligibility criteria and may be severely underpowered for detecting benefit for the subset of patients whose tumors are most susceptible to the action of the new drug. In the broad eligibility clinical trials which are statistically successful because the sample size has been increased to such an extent that even small average treatment effects are significant, only a small proportion of the intent to treat population actually benefits from treatment resulting in toxicity for patients who do not benefit and a large societal economic cost for over-treatment of the population. These two trial paradigms would optimally be merged as much as possible, as overly selective trials may only benefit a relatively small proportion of patients with a given cancer type, while very broad trials with expansive criteria may come to sweeping conclusions that do not apply to all patients enrolled or potentially subsequently treated post-approval.

Today we have implemented powerful tools for characterizing tumor tissue and blood-based genomics for both routine clinical care and in research. By using this characterization to prospectively structure the design and analysis of additional informative clinical trials that result in larger treatment effects for a larger portion of treated patients, we can leverage more efficient development strategies. In this article, we discuss these modern designs and analyses to continue to serve greater numbers of patients through more targeted therapeutics.

Phase I and II trials of molecularly targeted agents with companion diagnostics

Many first, second, and even subsequent generation targeted oncology drugs are being developed for existing and newly defined molecular pathways. Often, targets are well understood from both preclinical and clinical data and compelling biological rationale dictates restricting development to the subset of patients whose tumors are characterized by deregulation of the drug target. For other drug classes, there are multiple targets and more uncertainty about how to measure whether a drug target is driving tumor biology in an individual patient. Novel approaches including dynamic translational modeling and simulation in laboratory assessments as well as early clinical trial data may serve to close the knowledge gap and refine earlier go–no go decisions for multitargeted agents.[2]

The ideal approach in the setting of a novel molecularly or otherwise targeted agent's development is simultaneous evaluation of the drug and a companion diagnostic that measures the deregulation of the drug target or pathway in a robust way.

In the era of molecular oncology, the phase I first-in-human trial must still define the optimal dose of a drug, and there is increasing interest in including biomarker-driven patient selection in the earliest trials.[3] While patient selection will likely improve response rates, potentially even at lower doses than the maximum tolerated one, inherent challenges in phase I trial biomarker selection exist. If there is a strong relationship between the biomarker and target already established, and the assay to detect it is fully validated in patient samples, the likelihood of a successful phase I trial is higher. However, if this relationship is suboptimal and/or the

---

Holland-Frei Cancer Medicine, Tenth Edition. Edited by Robert C. Bast, John C. Byrd, Carlo M. Croce, Ernest Hawk, Fadlo R. Khuri, Raphael E. Pollock, Apostolia M. Tsimberidou, Christopher G. Willett, and Cheryl L. Willman.
© 2023 John Wiley & Sons, Inc. Published 2023 by John Wiley & Sons, Inc.

agent targets additional pathways at higher doses, both response and dose tolerance data may be compromised. Additionally, an early winnowing of a population may prevent efficacy signals from being observed in biomarker-negative patients, and trial enrollment efficiency may suffer if biomarker positivity is required for enrollment and frequency of required expression is low. Even when a biomarker strategy is validated in early phase trials, successful application requires ample and timely tumor tissue or sample collection and established assay validation, performance, validation, and reproducibility. Some recent biomarker strategies utilized in the clinic such as programmed death-ligand 1 (PD-L1) receptor expression are inconsistently predictive across tumor types, were employed in later stages of drug development, and lower cutoffs did not fully exclude responders.

If a biomarker-driven phase II trial is pursued, it determines whether there is activity of the drug overall in a histologic type and must also determine whether the subsequent phase III trial should be restricted based on a candidate companion diagnostic. Freidlin et al. have described a design for use with a single binary candidate biomarker in a randomized phase II design.[4] Their design enables one to determine whether the drug should be (1) developed in a phase III enrichment trial, (2) developed in an analysis stratified all comers' trial, (3) developed in an all comers' trial without measurement of the biomarker, or (4) dropped from further development. This design is shown in Figure 1. The sample size is determined so that the treatment effect on PFS in the marker-positive subset has power 0.9 for detecting a doubling of median progression-free survival at a one-sided significance level of 0.10. This will generally provide at least as many events for evaluating treatment effect in the marker-negative subset. If the treatment effect in the marker-positive subset is not significant, then the overall treatment effect is tested at a one-sided 0.05 significance level. If that treatment effect is not statistically significant, then the drug is not recommended for phase III development.

If the overall treatment effect is significant, then a traditional phase III trial without measurement of the candidate biomarker is recommended. If the treatment effect in the marker-positive subset is significant, then one examines an 80% confidence interval for the hazard ratio of treatment effect in the marker-negative subset. If the upper confidence interval is below 1.3, then one concludes that the treatment is not active in the marker-negative patients and an enrichment phase III trial is recommended. If the lower confidence limit is above 1.5, then one concludes that the treatment works well in the marker-negative patients and a traditional phase III trial in which the biomarker is not even measured is recommended. Otherwise, a biomarker stratified phase III trial is recommended.

Other phase II designs for evaluation of a treatment within marker subsets in single-arm phase II studies have been described by Pusztai and Hess and Jones and Holmgren.[5,6] These designs are focused primarily on ensuring that promising activity of the drug is not missed in cases where its activity is restricted to test-positive patients, and yet excessive numbers of patients are not required in cases where its activity is sufficiently broad that the marker is not needed.

There are more complicated phase II settings, where no natural cut-point of the biomarker is known in advance, or where there are multiple candidate biomarkers. The BATTLE I trial in NSCLC is an example of a phase II clinical trial using a response-adaptive randomization, which is discussed in another article of this encyclopedia.[7] Of note, some statisticians have raised doubts about the effectiveness of such adaptive randomization designs.[8]

Phase IIa master trials—umbrella, basket, and platform trials

The evolution of greater numbers of subsets of cancer types, along with medicinal chemistry advances to design agents that

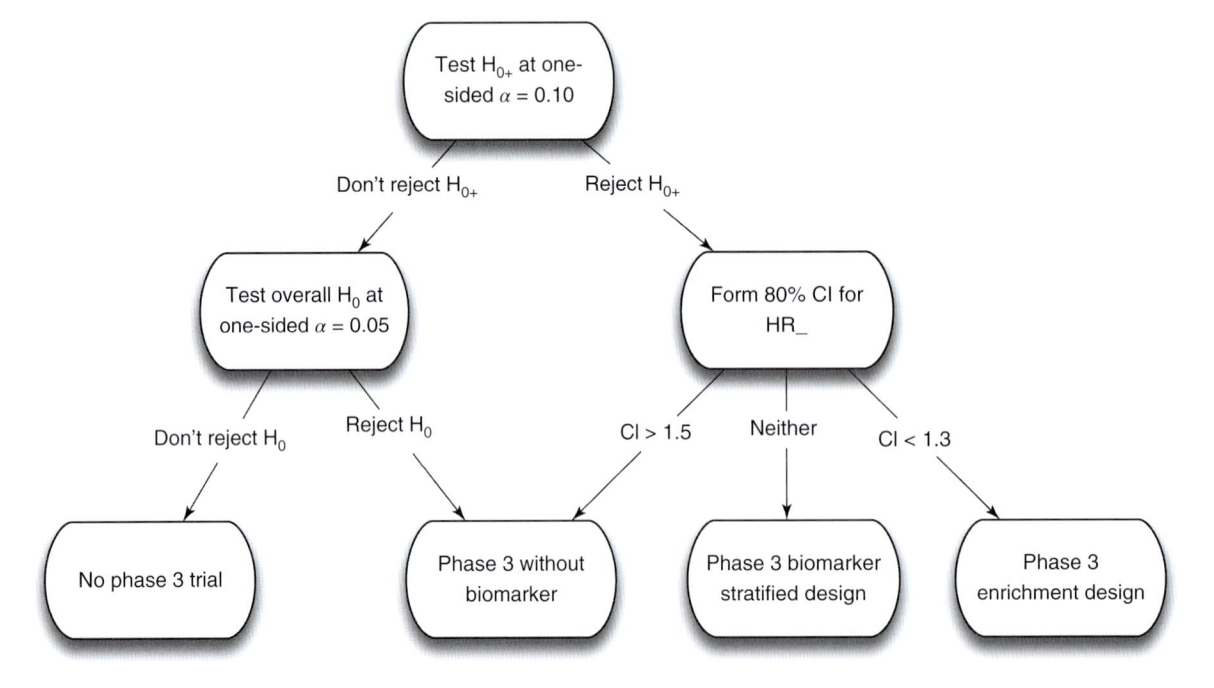

Figure 1 Analysis strategy for randomized phase II design to decide whether phase III trial should be restricted to biomarker-positive population, should include positives and negatives, whether biomarker should not even be measured or whether the conduct of a phase III trial is not supported by phase II results. Data from Ref. 4. HR_+ is hazard ratio in biomarker-positive group. HR_- is hazard ratio for treatment in biomarker-negative group. H_{0+} is null hypothesis that $HR_+ = 1$. H_0 is null hypothesis that overall $HR = 1$.

Table 1 Master protocol designs.

Trial design	Primary objective	Operational characteristics	Example(s)
Umbrella	To investigate multiple biomarker-driven therapies in a single cancer type	Screening of patients at study entry for targets of interest, may be randomized or use external controls, may or may not include treatment arm for those who are biomarker negative	BATTLE-1, Lung-MAP
Basket	To investigate a single biomarker-driven therapy in multiple cancer types	Patients screened at entry, may contain multiple strata.	B2225, multiple industry-sponsored trials
Platform	To investigate multiple biomarker-driven therapies in multiple cancer types or subtypes	Perpetual design, therapies may leave the platform based on predetermined go-no go decisions and can be replaced by other therapies	TAPUR, NCI MATCH

Source: Modified from Woodcock and LaVange.[9]

singularly target drivers, has led to the reality that the classic "one intervention compared to another" trial design is increasingly inefficient to determine anticancer activity in smaller populations.[9] Trial designs that may address questions of biomarker-driven agent(s) in smaller cancer subtypes simultaneously include basket, umbrella, and platform designs described in Table 1. Let us take the example of HER2 mutations that, contrary to HER2 gene amplification, occur at the low frequency of 1–2% in advanced breast cancer. There is evidence that these mutations are actionable using a potent irreversible tyrosine kinase inhibitor.[10] Conducting a "confirmatory" phase II trial of around 40 patients would require the screening of 2000–4000 women with advanced breast cancer (BC). Moreover, at the end of this exercise, the potential value of the new drug versus standard of care or in other tumor types harboring similar mutations would remain unknown. Figure 2 highlights the challenges of a registration path of such a drug in a "small" genomic segment of the BC population. This genomic aberration, therefore, would be best matched with its candidate drug in the context of an "umbrella" discovery trial where a panel of genomic aberrations would be screened and investigated in the context of several breast cancer phase II arms. Alternatively, a basket trial could examine HER2 mutations across several tumor types and investigate the activity of the TKI in each of them with early stopping rules in case of lack of antitumor activity. These increasingly popular forms of clinical trials are described below.

"Basket" discovery trials include patients with advanced cancer of multiple primary sites that are resistant to standard treatment.[11] A sequencing assay is used to evaluate the tumor DNA of a patient and it is determined whether an actionable aberration is present. "Actionable" means that a drug is available whose range of molecular targets overlap with the genomic alterations of the tumor in a way that suggest treatment may result in benefit for that patient. Various kinds of evidence may be used to determine whether a drug is a reasonable candidate for a given mutation. It will include biological understanding of the targets of the drug and the role of those targets in the disease. It may involve using the COSMIC (Catalog of Somatic Mutations in Cancer) database to determine whether the gene is mutated frequently enough in that histologic type to be considered a "driver" mutation. It may involve using algorithms to determine whether mutations

Registration "path" for a HER2-TKI used against breast tumors harboring HER2 mutations

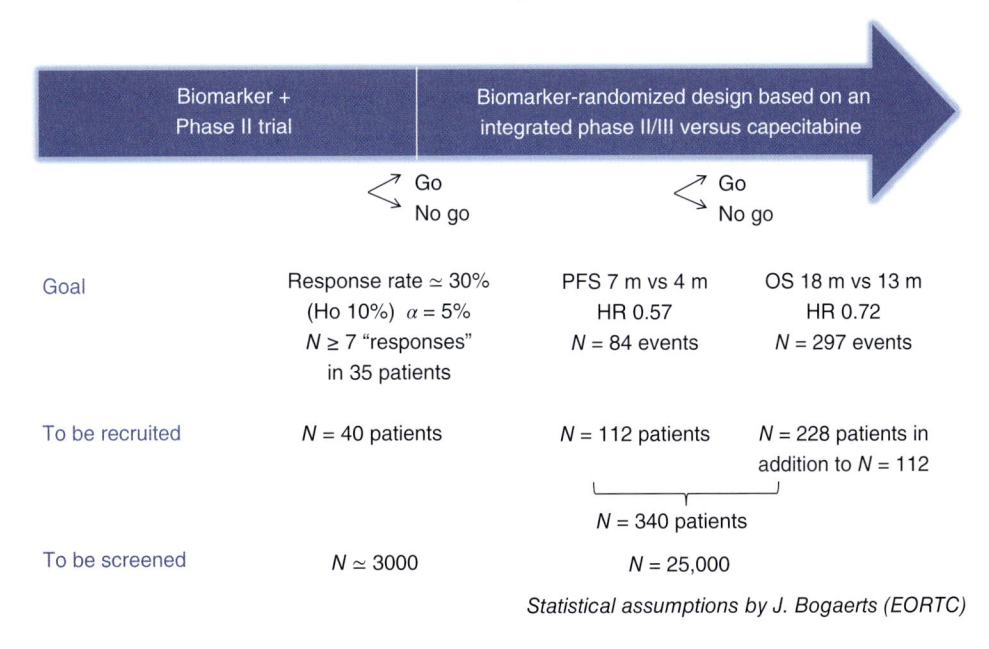

	Biomarker + Phase II trial	Biomarker-randomized design based on an integrated phase II/III versus capecitabine	
	↗ Go ↘ No go	↗ Go ↘ No go	
Goal	Response rate ≃ 30% (Ho 10%) $\alpha = 5\%$ $N \geq 7$ "responses" in 35 patients	PFS 7 m vs 4 m HR 0.57 $N = 84$ events	OS 18 m vs 13 m HR 0.72 $N = 297$ events
To be recruited	$N = 40$ patients	$N = 112$ patients	$N = 228$ patients in addition to $N = 112$
		$N = 340$ patients	
To be screened	$N \simeq 3000$	$N = 25,000$	

Statistical assumptions by J. Bogaerts (EORTC)

Figure 2 Schema for phases II and III clinical trials for developing a drug that inhibits a target, which is mutated in only 1–2% of cases. Although the number of patients required for the clinical trials is reasonable, the number screened is very large. It is more efficient to incorporate development of such a drug in an infrastructure of common national and international screening with regard to multiple targets and then triaging patients to clinical trials for which they are eligible.

found in a gene are predicted to alter protein function. It may also involve using nonclinical data about drug activity in cell lines or tumor grafts bearing that mutation, or clinical data in a different tumor type. The rules of actionability should be prospectively defined. Defining levels of evidence for actionability of a drug and a genomic aberration may help trial organizers resolve difficult binary decisions of whether there is sufficient evidence to warrant considering a drug actionable.

Both basket and umbrella trials are early discovery trials and attempt to identify the genomic characterization of tumors for which there is evidence of substantial anti-cancer activity of a drug. These positive signals should be confirmed in later expanded phase II or II/III trials.

Some umbrella trials are randomized and outcomes for patients who receive drugs based on actionability rules are compared to outcomes on a controlled drug or on drugs selected based on physician's choice without genomic characterization. Both the MPACT clinical trial being conducted by the National Cancer Institute and the Stand-Up-To-Cancer sponsored clinical trial in BRAF^{WT} melanoma use 2:1 randomization plans.[12] The randomized umbrella designs address two distinct questions, first, testing the null hypothesis that the policy of trying to match the drug to the genomics of the tumor is no more effective than a treatment strategy that does not use any tumor characterization beyond that used for standard of care. Whereas most traditional randomized clinical trials evaluate a single drug or regimen, the null hypothesis here relates to a matching policy for a given set of drugs and biomarkers available for the study. This makes it particularly important to obtain a broad enough menu of potent inhibitors of the selected targets. The matching policy is also determined by the type of genomic characterization performed and by the "rules" for matching drug to tumor. If matching is done by a tumor board and is not rule based or if the rules change frequently, the pragmatic value of the clinical trial will be limited. It may also be difficult for regulatory bodies to approve investigational drugs for use as decided by a tumor board rather than in a more rule-based manner. The use of a randomized control group facilitates the use of progression-free survival (PFS) as endpoint. The proof-of-principle embodied by the null hypothesis may be more meaningful, however, in a trial of a single histologic category than in cases where a wide range of primary sites of disease are included.

A second objective of randomized umbrella studies is the screening of individual drugs used in specific genomic and histologic contexts. For some primary sites, a gene such as "RAS" may be mutated sufficiently frequently for the study to provide an adequate phase II evaluation of the drug for that new indication. In many cases, however, the numbers will not be adequate for a proper phase II evaluation. Nevertheless, the trial may serve to screen for drug-mutation matches for which there is a substantial degree of activity, larger than is usually tested for in traditional phase II trials. These leads should be confirmed in an expanded cohort of a follow-up trial.[10] In this discovery mode, assessment of activity of a drug against tumors with a given gene mutation must take into account the possibility that the cell type in which the mutation occurs or the histology of the tumor may modulate activity of the drug against the alteration.

A third type of trial which is effectively an amalgamation of the basket and umbrella trial is the platform design.[13] Conceptually, platform trials attempt to integrate multiple therapies into one or more cancer types on an ongoing basis, and often have predetermined go-no go decisions within each arm such as a two-stage approach. Platform trials also allow for combinations in addition to single agents, with rapid replacement of ineffective treatments. These trials may enroll across many years and have multiple results available.

New statistical designs specifically for master trials have not yet been introduced. Most such trials incorporate a traditional two-stage design for drug-mutation strata that will have sufficient patients to be separately analyzed. A traditional two-stage design for distinguishing a response rate of 10% from one of 35% with 85% power and 10% type I error requires only 5 first-stage patients and has a 60% chance of terminating at the first stage if the true response probability is only 10%.[14] Such designs can be computed online at http://brb.nci.nih.gov

LeBlanc et al. previously introduced a design for multiple histology phase II trials that can be used in some basket or umbrella clinical trials.[15] It combines statistical significance tests of drug activity within histology strata with a combined analysis which borrows information from all the patients in the study. Sequential futility analyses are conducted once each strata or the overall group reaches a specified minimum amount. Thall et al. developed a hierarchical Bayesian method for evaluating treatment effects in discrete strata of a phase II trial while accounting for the relatedness of the strata.[16] This approach has been critiqued by Freidlin and Korn who concluded that "there appears to be insufficient information in the outcome data to determine whether borrowing across subgroups is appropriate."[17]

Phase III designs with a single binary biomarker

Targeted (enrichment) designs

Designs in which eligibility is restricted to those patients considered most likely to benefit from the experimental drug are called "targeted designs" or "enrichment designs" and are illustrated in Figure 3a. With an enrichment design, the analytically validated diagnostic test is used to restrict eligibility for a randomized clinical trial comparing a regimen containing a new drug to a control regimen. This approach has now been used for pivotal trials of many drugs whose molecular targets were well understood in the context of the disease. Recent first-in-class examples include selpercatinib, larotrectinib, and capmatinib.[18–20]

Simon and Maitournam developed general formulas for comparing the enrichment design to the standard design with regard to the number of randomized and screened patients.[21,22] They found the enrichment design very efficient and have made the methods of sample size planning for the design of enrichment trials available online at http://brb.nci.nih.gov. The web-based programs are available for binary and survival/disease-free survival endpoints. The enrichment design is appropriate for contexts where there is a strong biological basis for believing that test-negative patients will **not** benefit from the new drug.

All comers' (stratification) designs

When a predictive biomarker has been developed but there is not compelling biological or phase II data that test-negative patients do not benefit from the new treatment, it is often best to include both classifier positive and classifier negative in the phase III clinical trials comparing the new treatment to the control regimen. This is shown in Figure 3b. The biomarker is measured in all patients at entry to the trial, and then all patients are randomized to the test treatment or the control regimen. In this case, it is essential that an analysis plan be predefined in the protocol

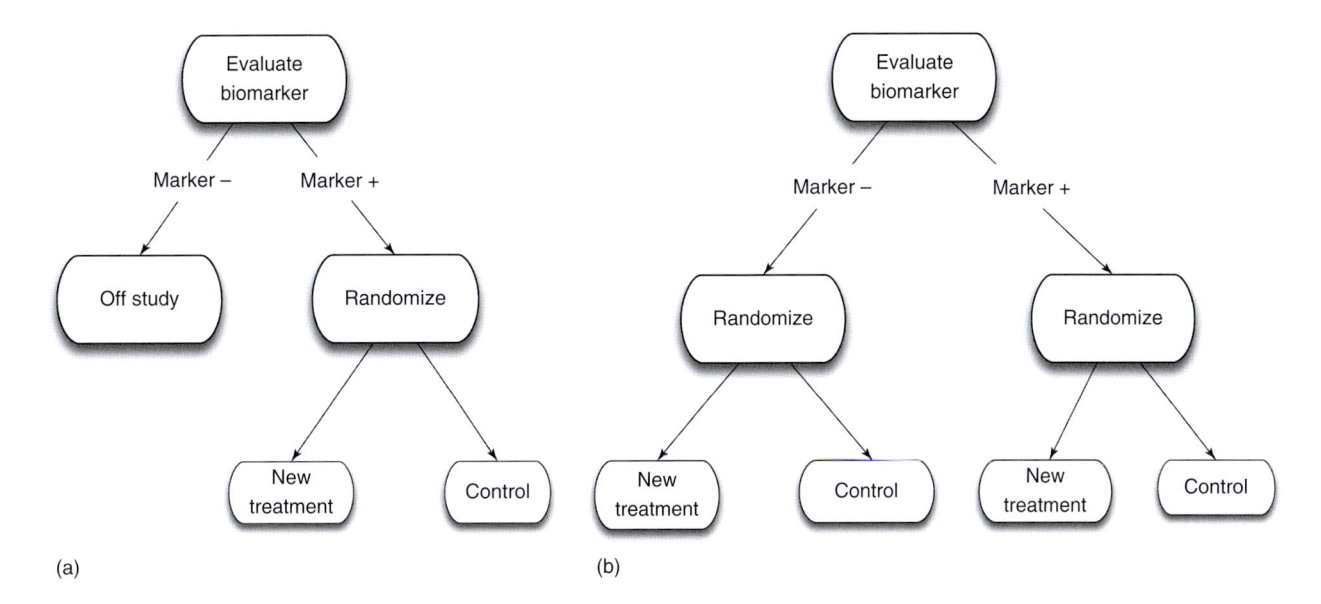

Figure 3 (a) The targeted enrichment design is used for evaluating a new treatment in the population of patients who are identified using a predictive biomarker as best candidates for benefit from the new treatment. It is primarily for settings where there is a compelling basis for believing that "marker-negative" patients will not benefit from the new treatment and an analytically validated test is available. (b) The "all comers' design" or "marker stratification design" is used for evaluating the effectiveness of a new treatment versus a control in a population prospectively characterized by a binary predictive marker. A detailed prospective analysis plan should describe the primary comparison of treatment to control, in the marker-positive, marker-negative, and overall populations. With a focused analysis plan that limits the study-wide type I error to the traditional 5% level, claims of treatment effectiveness in marker-positive patients need not be restricted to cases where the treatment is effective overall or there is a significant interaction.

for how the predictive classifier will be used in the analysis. The analysis plan will generally define the testing strategy for evaluating the new treatment in the test-positive patients, the test-negative patients, and overall.[23] The testing strategy must preserve the overall type I error of the trial. The overall type I error is the probability that a claim for a statistically significant difference is made from any of the comparisons when in fact the treatments are equivalent both overall and within the biomarker-specific subsets. Controlling the overall type I error often requires that a threshold of significance less than 0.05 is used for interpreting the individual significance tests. The clinical trial should also be sized to provide adequate statistical power for these tests. It is not sufficient to just stratify, i.e., balance, the randomization with regard to the classifier without specifying a complete analysis plan. The main value of "stratifying" (i.e., balancing) the randomization is that it assures that only patients with adequate test results will enter the trial. Pre-stratification of the randomization is not necessary for the validity of inferences to be made about treatment effects within the test-positive or test-negative subsets.[24] If an analytically validated test is not available at the start of the trial but will be available by the time of analysis, then it may be preferable not to pre-stratify the randomization process.

Several primary analysis plans have been described for these trials. If one has moderate strength evidence that the treatment, if effective at all, is likely to be more effective in the test-positive cases, one might first compare treatment versus control in test-positive patients using a threshold of significance of 5%. Only if the treatment versus control comparison is significant at the 5% level in test-positive patients will the new treatment be compared to the control among test-negative patients, again using a threshold of statistical significance of 5%. This sequential approach controls the overall type I error at 5%.[25] In the situation where one has limited confidence in the predictive marker, it can be effectively used for a "fall-back" analysis. Outcomes for the new treatment group are first compared to those for the control group overall. If that difference is not significant at a reduced significance level such as 0.03, then the new treatment is compared to the control group just for test-positive patients. The latter comparison uses a threshold of significance of 0.02, or whatever portion of the traditional 0.05 not used by the initial test.[25] In situations where one has an intermediate level of confidence in the candidate biomarker, one can use the MAST analysis plan.[26] At the final analysis one first tests the null hypothesis of no treatment effect for the marker-positive patients. The threshold of significance for this test is prespecified as some value α_+ less than the total type I error 0.05 of the design. For example, α_+ may be 0.04. If that null hypothesis is rejected, then the null hypothesis for the marker-negative patients is tested using a significance threshold of 0.05. If the null hypothesis for the marker-positive patients is not rejected, then the null hypothesis for the pooled overall population is tested using a significance threshold of 0.05-α_+, 0.01 in this example.

Other "real world" experience with stratification and enrichment designs are described by Freidlin et al. and by Mandreakar and Sargent.[27,28] Adaptive forms of the enrichment design in which one starts with "all comers" and adaptively restricts the eligibility are described by Wang et al., Rosenbloom and Van Der Laan, and Simon and Simon.[29–31]

Prospective–retrospective designs

In some cases, a completed randomized clinical trial with archived tumor specimens can be used to evaluate treatment effect in a subset determined by a new candidate biomarker. For example, the hypothesis that the effectiveness of anti-EGFR antibodies in colorectal cancer would be limited to patients whose tumors did not contain *KRAS* mutations was evaluated in randomized clinical trials that had been planned before this hypothesis was suggested by other investigators. Simon, Paik, Hayes described a prospective–retrospective approach to using archived tumor specimens for a focused re-analysis of a randomized phase III trial with regard to a predictive biomarker.[32] The approach requires that archived specimens be available on most patients and that an analysis plan focused on a single marker be developed prior to performing the blinded assays. The finding must also be evaluated in two such prospective–retrospective trials in order to be considered type I evidence. It is not necessary that the randomization should have used the marker as a stratification variable. This is not relevant to the validity of the analysis of treatment effect in marker-positive patients.[24] Simon has also pointed out that there is no critical minimum proportion of the tumors archived necessary for the retrospective–prospective approach. The key factor is that there should be no bias between treatment groups with regard to availability of archived specimens. Lack of such bias can be assured if patient and physician agreement for tissue archival is established prior to randomization.

Run-in designs

Predictive biomarkers are usually thought of as biological measurements that are obtained from the tumor or the patient prior to the start of treatment. Hong and Simon developed a run-in design which permits a pharmacodynamic, immunologic, or intermediate response endpoint measured after a short run-in period on the new treatment or the control to be used as the predictive biomarker.[33] After measuring the biomarker during the run-in period, either all patients are randomized between continuing the new treatment or switching to control, or just the "marker-positive" patients, those showing substantial change in the measurement from the pretreatment baseline measurement are randomized. The biomarker is not used as an endpoint for comparing the treatments and randomization is not performed until after the marker is measured. The marker is used for stratifying the patients for separate analysis as in the all comers' stratified design or for excluding the marker-negative patients as in the enrichment design. The run-in period should be short, because one does not want the survival or disease-free survival of the patients subsequently randomized to the control group to be extended during the run-in period on the test drug. The run-in designs offer substantial opportunity for increasing the efficiency of clinical trials in situations where pretreatment predictive biomarkers cannot be identified.

Phase II/III enrichment designs with multiple biomarkers

The Lung-MAP study is a biomarker-driven clinical trial being used for drug development in patients with refractory lung cancers. The design was developed as a collaboration of FDA, pharmaceutical industry, US National Clinical Trials Network, NCI, and Foundation Medicine under the coordination of Friends of Cancer Research. The goal is to enroll up to 5000 patients at more than 700 medical centers in the United States through randomized phase II/III studies of novel agents.[34] Participants are screened for genomic alterations of their tumors using the Foundation Medicine DNA sequencing platform. Based on the results of the screening, patients are channeled to one of five randomized phase II/III trials. Each of the five randomized trials has a phase II stage and will progress to the phase III stage if results are promising. The primary endpoint is progression-free survival. These trials are all potentially pivotal phase III enrichment clinical trials with companion diagnostics for different patient subsets. As the evaluation of these drugs is completed, an additional five to seven agents will be tested.

The new models of collaboration required by clinical trials of the "genomic era" and the challenges ahead

We are still learning to classify cancers molecularly in a therapeutically relevant manner. It is likely that we will soon be moving from simple classifications relying on aberrations at the DNA level toward more complex classifications also incorporating critical information generated by RNA sequencing and (phospho)protein platforms. It can also be foreseen that pathway-directed treatment strategies will replace single-target-directed strategies, as aiming at the latter is likely to fail in view of the plasticity of the cancer cell. Moving platform genomic results to therapeutics implies dealing with uncertainty and statisticians will continue to play a critical role in this regard.

At the same time, it is clear that achieving the benefits of personalized oncology requires paradigm changes in academic clinical investigation, with the setup of large collaborative teams, in industry drug development, with walls between drug development paths when it comes to combination strategies, and in regulatory evaluation, with more adaptive licensing routes for new compounds or innovative drug combinations.

Conclusion

In oncology, treatment of broad populations with regimens that do not benefit most patients is less economically sustainable with expensive molecularly targeted therapeutics currently in development and less likely to be successful. The established molecular heterogeneity of human diseases requires the development of new design and analysis paradigms for using randomized clinical trials to provide a reliable basis predictive medicine.

References

1. Verweij J, Hendriks HR, Zwierzina H. Cancer drug development forum. Innovation in oncology clinical trial design. *Cancer Treat Rev.* 2019;**74**:15–20.
2. Yamazaki S, Spilker ME, Vicini P. Translational modeling and simulation approaches for molecularly targeted small molecule anticancer agents from bench to bedside. *Expert Opin Drug Metab Toxicol.* 2016;**12**:253–265.
3. Wong KM, Capasso A, Eckhardt SG. The changing landscape of phase I trials in oncology. *Nat Rev Clin Oncol.* 2016;**13**:106–117.
4. Freidlin B, McShane LM, Polley MY, et al. Randomized phase II trial designs with biomarkers. *J Clin Oncol.* 2012;**30**:3304–3309.
5. Pusztai L, Hess KR. Clinical trial design for microarray predictive marker discovery and assessment. *Ann Oncol.* 2004;**15**:1731–1737.
6. Jones CL, Holmgren E. An adaptive Simon two-stage design for phase 2 studies of targeted therapies. *Contemp Clin Trials.* 2007;**28**:654–661.
7. Kim ES, Herbst JJ, Wistuba II, et al. The BATTLE Trial: personalizing therapy for lung cancer. *Cancer Discov.* 2011;**1**:44–53.
8. Korn EL, Freidlin B. Outcome-adaptive randomization: is it useful? *J Clin Oncol.* 2011;**29**:771–776.
9. Woodcock J, LaVange LM. Master protocols to study multiple therapies, multiple diseases or both. *N Engl J Med.* 2017;**377**:62–70.
10. Bose R, Kavuri S, Searleman A, et al. Activating HER2 mutations in HER2 gene amplification negative breast cancer. *Cancer Discov.* 2013;**3**:224–237.
11. Simon R, Roychowdhury S. Implementing personalized cancer genomics in clinical trials. *Nat Rev Drug Discov.* 2013;**12**:358–369.
12. Simon R, Polley E. Clinical trials for precision oncology using next generation sequencing. *Pers Med.* 2013;**10**:485–495.
13. Berry SM, Connor JT, Lewis RJ. The platform trial: an efficient strategy for evaluating multiple treatments. *JAMA.* 2015;**313**:1619–1620.
14. Simon R. Optimal two-stage designs for phase II clinical trials. *Control Clin Trials.* 1989;**10**:1–10.
15. LeBlanc M, Rankin C, Crowley J. Multiple histology phase II trials. *Clin Cancer Res.* 2009;**15**:4356–4262.

16 Thall PF, Wathen JK, Bekele BN, et al. Hierarchical Bayesian approaches to phase II trials in diseases with multiple subtypes. *Stat Med*. 2003;**22**:763–780.
17 Freidlin B, Korn EL. Borrowing information across subgroups in phase II trials: is it useful? *Clin Cancer Res*. 2013;**19**:1326–1334.
18 Drilon A, Oxnard GR, Tan DSW, et al. Efficacy of selpercatinib in RET fusion-positive non-small-cell lung cancer. *N Engl J Med*. 2020;**383**:813–824.
19 Drilon A, Laetsch TW, Kummar S, et al. Efficacy of larotrectinib in TRK fusion-positive cancers in adults and children. *N Engl J Med*. 2018;**378**:731–739.
20 Wolf J, Seto T, Han J-Y, et al. Capmatinib in MET exon 14-mutated or MET-amplified non-small cell lung cancer. *N Engl J Med*. 2020;**383**:944–957.
21 Simon R, Maitournam A. Evaluating the efficiency of targeted designs for randomized clinical trials. *Clin Cancer Res*. 2005;**10**:6759–6763.
22 Maitournam A, Simon R. On the efficiency of targeted clinical trials. *Stat Med*. 2005;**24**:329–339.
23 Simon R. *Genomic Clinical Trials and Predictive Medicine* (Practical Guides to Biostatistics and Epidemiology). Cambridge: Cambridge University Press; 2013. doi: 10.1017/CBO9781139026451.
24 Simon R. Stratification and partial ascertainment of biomarker value in biomarker driven clinical trials. *J Biopharm Stat*. 2014;**24**:1011–1021.
25 Simon R. Using genomics in clinical trial design. *Clin Cancer Res*. 2008;**14**:5984–5993.
26 Freidlin B, Korn EL. Biomarker enrichment strategies: matching trial design to biomarker credentials. *Nat Rev Clin Oncol*. 2014;**11**:81–90.
27 Freidlin B, McShane LM, Korn EL. Randomized clinical trials with biomarkers: Design issues. *J Natl Cancer Inst*. 2010;**102**:152–160.
28 Mandrekar SJ, Sargent DJ. Predictive biomarker validation in practice: lessons from real trials. *Clin Trials*. 2010;**7**:567–573.
29 Wang SJ, Hung HMJ, O'Neill RT. Adaptive patient enrichment designs in therapeutic trials. *Biom J*. 2009;**51**:358–374.
30 Rosenblum M, Van Der Laan MJ. Optimizing randomized trial designs to distinguish which subpopulations benefit from treatment. *Biometrika*. 2011;**98**:845–860.
31 Simon N, Simon R. Adaptive enrichment designs in clinical trials. *Biostatistics*. 2013;**14**:613–625.
32 Simon RM, Paik S, Hayes DF. Use of archived specimens in evaluation of prognostic and predictive biomarkers. *J Natl Cancer Inst*. 2009;**101**:1–7.
33 Hong F, Simon R. Run-in phase III trial designs with pharmacodynamic predictive biomarkers. *J Natl Cancer Inst*. 2013;**105**:1628–1633.
34 Lung-MAP. Master protocol for lung cancer. National Cancer Institute, www.cancer.gov/types/lung/research/lung-map (accessed 15 November 2020).

21 Clinical and research informatics data strategy for precision oncology

Douglas Hartman, MD ■ Uma Chandran, PhD ■ Michael Davis, MS ■ Rajiv Dhir, MD ■ William E. Shirey, MS ■ Jonathan C. Silverstein, MD, MS ■ Michael J. Becich, MD, PhD

Overview

Oncology informatics in the era of precision oncology is challenging because no unified comprehensive system exists linking Health Information Technology (HIT) deployed in clinical settings to the translational needs of researchers. Many advanced informatics solutions have been developed for clinical trials, biobanking, cancer imaging, and high-throughput-omic technologies. These are fundamentally transforming the treatment and management of cancer patients. However, the lack of fully developed interoperable cancer research informatics and HIT technologies to move between the bench and the bedside remains a significant challenge. Oncologists and translational cancer investigators require knowledge of informatics, data science, and advanced machine learning (artificial intelligence) as these are the major change agents influencing the development of new therapies, especially in the era of Precision Medicine and Learning Health Systems for oncology. In addition, cancer care delivery is very dependent on new developments in clinical practice and requires a thorough, systematic reevaluation of the electronic health records (EHRs) in use today. The ability (through mobile computing) to have information "on demand" during daily oncology practice is reshaping our thinking of how we record, document, and share data toward the common purpose of improving cancer outcomes for the patients we serve. This article looks at HIT and clinical, translational, and research informatics for oncologists and cancer researchers and begins to paint a picture of what an "ideal" environment for cancer care delivery would look like to support Precision Oncology and Learning Health Systems.

We describe the key elements of the cancer clinical workspace (e.g., EHRs, cancer registry, Clinical Trials Management, and Imaging (Picture Archiving and Communication Systems, PACS)) to understand how to configure workflows to take full advantage of Health Information Technology (HIT) solutions for oncology that aim to enable precision oncology.[2,4-6] We then discuss how new "clinical" data sources not generally supported by EHRs, but routinely collected as part of a cancer patient's journey (e.g., genomic testing or sequencing, tissue banking, and new emergent areas such as AI applied to computational pathology), are also critical to create an ideal research environment for enabling precision oncology advances and research insights.[2,7-13] Finally, we discuss the critical role of tissue banking information systems and cancer registries in the modern cancer center and how their evolution will be key to precision oncology.[2,7,14,15]

Health information technology (HIT) systems for the clinical workspace

Electronic health records (EHRs) for oncology

As part of the Health Information Technology for Economic and Clinical Health Act (HITECH), EHRs have been adopted in both in- and out-patient settings at a record pace.[16] Further influencing this pace were incentives and penalties from the Affordable Care Act that drove adoption deeply into private practice.[17] Oncology EHR adoption is driven by many factors, and some healthcare systems have specialized systems for oncology. A recent analytics firm KLAS report[18] ranked EHRs in medical oncology and rated Epic, Elekta, Flatiron, Cerner, Varian, and McKesson as the "highest rated" medical oncology vendor solutions in place in January 2020. Another important consideration for EHRs for precision oncology is their interoperability with other systems, and KLAS also ranked Epic, athenahealth, Cerner, MEDITECH, Greenway, NextGen, Allscripts, eClinicalWorks, GE Healthcare, and McKesson in terms of their KLAS "scorecard" system.

No matter which EHR is used in an oncology practice, these patient, provider, and payer facing transactional and billing systems provide limited search and analytic capabilities, thereby requiring a strategy for extracting key information into an RDW (described above in *Infrastructure*). A critical consideration for precision oncology is to architect an RDW in a manner that effectively extracts clinical data of cancer patients and links it with many types of cancer research data. Thus, genomic sequencing, clinical trials, tissue banking, advanced pathology/radiology imaging, and cancer registry data can be extracted and combined to allow for flexible analysis and insights/innovations. With an

Introduction and roadmap

A data warehouse containing a broad spectrum of structured clinical, imaging, and molecular data organized longitudinally at the individual patient level is a key component of any precision oncology initiative for a cancer center.[1,2] The warehouse must be flexible enough to arrange data from multiple disparately organized sources, including the ability to easily add information arising from new sources. The ability to provide broad access to summarized data and to provide deep access for data mining is vital.

We envision an ideal environment for precision oncology (Figure 1) which connects the clinical workspace to the research workspace, allowing application of analytical and machine learning tools. This structure enables the transformation and secure delivery of data to a research data warehouse (RDW) which manages subject ID linkage, deidentification and maximizes research usability via Findable, Accessible Interoperable, and Reproducible or findable, accessible, interoperable and reproducible (FAIR)[3] data practices.

Holland-Frei Cancer Medicine, Tenth Edition. Edited by Robert C. Bast, John C. Byrd, Carlo M. Croce, Ernest Hawk, Fadlo R. Khuri, Raphael E. Pollock, Apostolia M. Tsimberidou, Christopher G. Willett, and Cheryl L. Willman.
© 2023 John Wiley & Sons, Inc. Published 2023 by John Wiley & Sons, Inc.

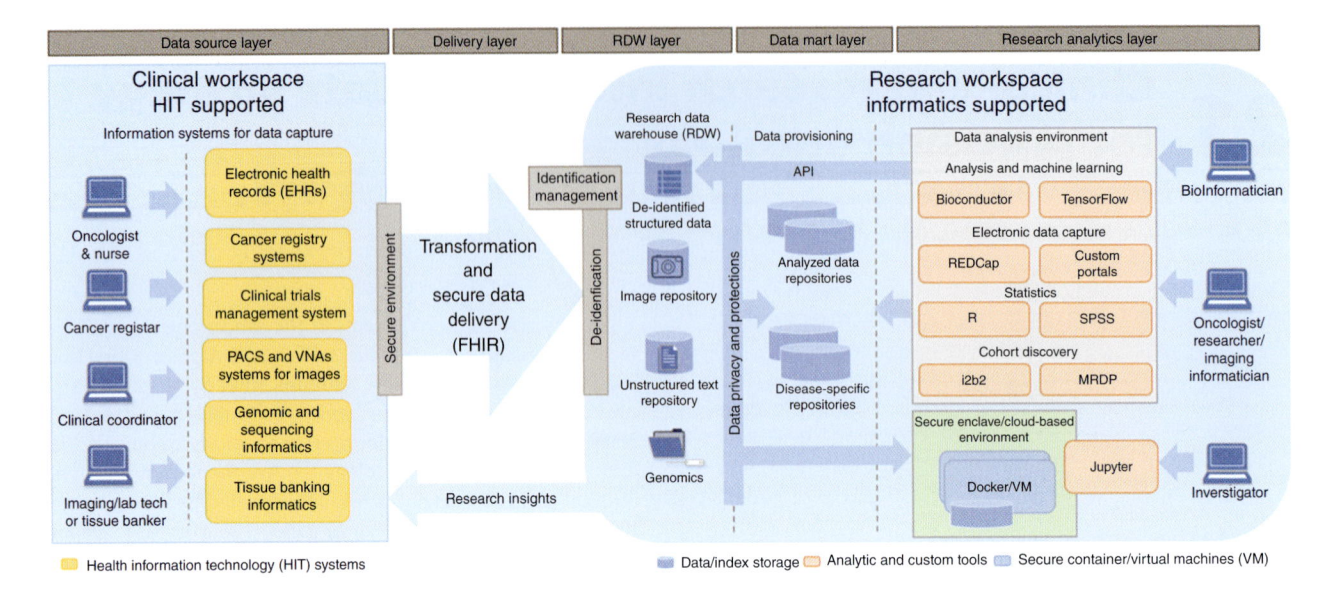

Figure 1 Ideal environment for precision oncology.

appropriately structured RDW, oncologists and cancer researchers can then serve the evolving needs of patient care through precision oncology. Using data extracted and deidentified from the "clinical workspace" and the "research workspace" (Figure 1), the tools for research insights, testing, and implementation of therapeutic agents into clinical trials for precision oncology are greatly enabled.

Cancer registry systems for oncology

One of the most neglected data systems for precision oncology and research insights into cancer outcomes is the cancer registry.[1,2,15] Although hospital and community-based cancer registries are universal, they are often ignored for their research value. A close look shows many unique attributes of this data which if curated by certified cancer registers have great value.[15,19,20] Current commercial cancer registry systems are based on the North American Association for Central Cancer Registries (NAAACR) data standard[21] which is endorsed by pathologists, oncologists, and surgeons. Recent versions of the NAAACR standard have adopted the College of American Pathologists (CAP) synoptic reporting templates for solid tumors[22] after early work in pathology and tissue banking informatics laid the foundation for this CAP effort.[23–26] The current leading cancer registry software vendors include C/Net Solutions (Oakland, CA), Electronic Registry Systems (Cincinnati, OH), Elekta (Stockholm, Sweden), McKesson Corporation (Irving, TX), Onco (Wall Township, NJ), and Rocky Mountain Cancer Data Systems (Salt Lake City, UT).

Cancer registry systems include many critical data types including tumor histology grading, staging, treatment, outcomes, comorbidities, and biomarkers specific to tumor types. There are challenges for the cancer registries to enter, support, and maintain high-quality data (e.g., reporting lag time, incompleteness of records, and quality issues) which may account for uneven implementation of cancer registries across health systems. However, when appropriately managed by certified cancer registrars and supported by the health system leadership to prioritize high-quality curation and follow-up, registries can play a very valuable (and unique) asset to implementation of precision oncology.

Cancer registry systems can play an important role in precision oncology[27,28] because they store valuable and detailed diagnosis, high-level treatment information, and vital status, providing the capacity to efficiently generate key evidence needed to create a learning health system for cancer care. Most clinical domains of medical care do not have registry systems and so are uniformly supported by subspecialty as oncology.[29] Oncology is fortunate to have dedicated curation specialists supported by a professional society with certification examinations to ensure high-quality annotation supported by a data standard[16,29] creating a longitudinal record that chronicles the key elements of the care of cancer patients.

Clinical trials management systems (CTMS) for oncology

Beginning in 1999, the National Cancer Institute (NCI) began an initiative called the Cancer Informatics Infrastructure.[6] The goal of this initiative was fourfold: (1) to host a web-based site to integrate basic and clinical research; (2) employ usable standards increasing interoperability; (3) simplify clinical trials and support protocol development; and (4) host a secure site that could be tailored to individual authorized users.[6] The primary goal of this undertaking was to build a robust resource to catalyze research and efficiently advance it from the "bench to the bedside." Investment into this initiative was a public–private partnership that has effectively streamlined the pathway for translational research. This infrastructure has facilitated the development of http://clinicaltrials.gov, which is an online repository of registered clinical trials within medicine. Together these tools have given rise to more rapid scientific developments and trials as well as new oncologic treatments. The development and implementation of an open interoperability standard for oncology treatment planning and summarization[30] holds great promise for precision oncology.

Despite the many innovations and progress with EHRs for medical oncology, none of the existing systems support the full life cycle of clinical trials. This has resulted in an emergent HIT software segment, Clinical Trials Management Systems (CTMS). Commercial vendors for oncology CTMS include Forte Systems

- 50 CTSA sites have Epic EHR
- 31 CTSA sites have OnCore (including enterprise-wide and cancer centers)
- 24 CTSAs have both Epic EHR and OnCore as CTMS

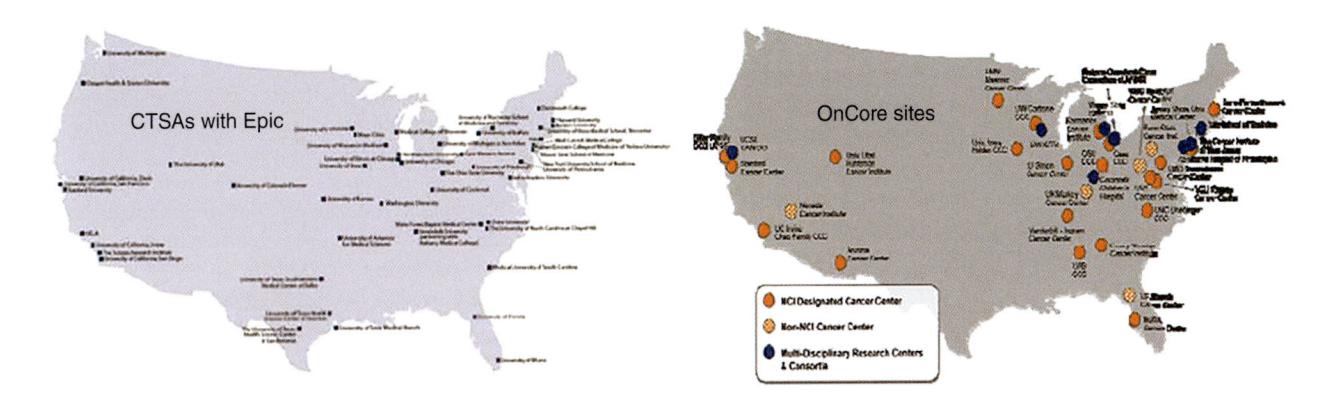

Figure 2 EHR and CTMS systems in CTSA Programs and Cancer Centers (see acknowledgments).

OnCore (recently acquired by Advarra), Medidata Rave (Dassault Systemes), Velos eResearch (recently acquired by WCG), and many others including some installations still with home-grown CTMS.[31] It is clear from the evolution of CTMS systems over the past two decades, driven by the emphasis on clinical trials and clinical research in the Clinical and Translational Science Award (CTSA) program of the National Center for Advancing Translational Science (NCATS),[32,33] that this is now a commercial vendor-dominated space. Cancer Informatics for Cancer Centers (CI4CC)[34] has profiled CTMS installations in cancer center programs and regularly surveys its membership as part of its ongoing service to the cancer informatics community. CI4CC as a not-for-profit (501c3) member organization is illustrative of the maturity of the cancer informatics community, and this effort parallels other emerging informatics subspecialty communities in pathology[35] and radiology.[36]

Lack of EHR interfaces and scalability of CTMS have significantly complicated data sharing[37] for precision oncology. Success factors for implementation of a CTMS "…included organizational commitment to clinical research, a dedicated research information technology unit, integration of research data across disparate systems, and centralized system usage workflows…".[38] The best nationwide effort to address this has come from the OnCore CTMS (Advarra/Forte Systems, Madison, WI) and Epic's EHR (Verona, WI) and has resulted in widespread adoption of their systems at many cancer centers as well as CTSA[32,33] institutions. A recent survey (Figure 2) from Forte Systems/Advarra (parent company of OnCore, Madison, WI) showed that 50 of the CTSA programs had adopted Epic and 31 of the sites had adopted OnCore (for both enterprise-wide clinical trials and for the cancer center). Over one-third of the CTSA sites had both Epic for their EHR and OnCore for their CTMS. Of note, Velos' eResearch is another dominant vendor in the CTSA with 24 installations as well as at 43 NCI-designated cancer centers.[39] The integration of the EHR with CTMS systems holds great promise for precision medicine/oncology, and there is a significant synergy coming from these efforts across CTSA programs in collaboration with the Cancer Center Support Grant (CCSG) program of the NCI.

Picture archiving and communications systems (PACS) for oncology

Oncology medical imaging particularly radiology and pathology have become critically important in both treatment and management of cancer patients. Radiology has always had a central role in oncology, especially with evolution toward radiomics,[4] but recent developments in digital pathology are noteworthy including the FDA approval of whole slide imaging (WSI) systems for anatomic pathology beginning in 2017.[40] The digitization of anatomic pathology slides of cancer patients has catalyzed the launch of computational pathology,[12,13] and pan cancer analysis of the tumor microenvironment has been enabled by large knowledgebases such as The Cancer Genome Atlas (TCGA),[11] which includes whole slide images.[41] Multiplex immunohistochemical analyses of cancer patient biopsies have further fueled computational pathology[42,43] and its impact in precision oncology.

Despite the considerable opportunities radiomics and computational pathology have for precision oncology, it is critical to understand the HIT infrastructure for the clinical capture of radiology images via commercial PACS systems and their relationship to another health care enterprise product called Vendor "Neutral" Archives (VNAs). Both pathology and radiology PACS require specialized systems due to the different digital structures of the images created during a clinical care episode. VNAs combine various medical imaging modalities into one "centralized" image repository for clinical care. For a successful integration of images from the clinical workspace for precision oncology (Figure 1), it is critical for coordination between HIT and informatics (research workspace) to have a strategy for the transformation, deidentification, and secure data delivery with subject ID linkages of these mission critical imaging modalities (pathology and radiology).

The top-rated commercial PACS systems in 2020 from large vendors include Sectra, Intelerad, Change Healthcare, Fujifilm, Agfa Healthcare, Philips, IBM Watson Health, and GE Healthcare.[44] The top-rated VNAs in 2020 are Fujifilm, Philips, Hyland, IBM Watson Health, NTT DATA, and GE Healthcare.[44] The integration of radiology and pathology WSI support and integration is underway as FDA has approved Philips and Leica for WSI,[40,45] with Philips being one of a handful of vendors with solutions in both PACS and VNAs.

Emergent HIT solutions for the clinical workspace

Genomic and sequencing informatics

Genomic and Sequencing Informatics solutions for precision oncology is in its infancy, and its integration into EHRs will be critical to the integration of (1) genomic data types: variant calls, copy number variation, gene rearrangements, polymerase chain reaction (PCR) "hotspots," gene expression "scores," and whole-exome and -genome sequencing results and (2) technologies employed in genomic testing as it evolves: fluorescence *in situ* hybridization, PCR, gene expression panels, next-generation sequencing, single-cell sequencing, and whole-exome and -genome sequencing.[46] Many molecular genetic pathology laboratories in cancer centers utilize a variety of technologies to generate clinical genomic testing, but most are run on free-standing systems that do not integrate into the pathology Laboratory Information Systems (LIS). Some of the major vendors have attempted to integrate PCR and genomic panels into their LIS, but the lack of standards for reporting has significantly hindered progress in this area. As a result, genomic testing done in the clinical workspace is frequently reported in PDF format and stored as images in the EHR.[47] Adding to the complexity, since the majority of genomic testing is currently provided by commercial vendors (e.g., Agendia, Caris, Foundation Medicine, Genomic Health, and Tempus), this data is infrequently digitally "callable" as part of the oncology EHR nor research workspace (via RDWs) fed by clinical systems at a single institution. Warner et al.[46] provide review of the use of "…non-standard integration approaches, "middleware", application programming interfaces (APIs), efforts to create standardized EHR applications, and emerging knowledge bases…" which will be critical to the integration of genomic data into the EHR. Although genomic testing/sequencing as a contributor to the clinical workspace (Figure 1) is still maturing, its impact in precision oncology in the research workspace (Figure 1) is undeniable as evidenced in the TCGA pan cancer efforts.[11,48–50]

Tissue banking informatics

Although biospecimen banking has been a high-priority focus area for both the NCI[51–54] and precision medicine/oncology for years, there has been an increasing realization and focus on high-quality annotating of biospecimens with clinical information (phenotyping).[25,52,53,55] The NCI Cancer Moonshot initiative, launched in 2016,[56,57] served to further emphasize the value and need for synergy between informatics and tissue banking. The initiative has the ambitious goals to encourage annotated biospecimen sharing by catalyzing "…data and technology innovators will help to revolutionize the ways in which cancer related data are shared and used to achieve new breakthroughs, and the federal government may seek ways to facilitate data sharing among researchers who are currently reluctant to disseminate their data and results…".[56] The Moonshot Initiative encouraged team science and engaged large, multidisciplinary teams of researchers, clinicians, policy experts, educators, and staff to mount comprehensive, goal-oriented programs focused on changing the trajectory of advances in prevention, early detection, and treatment options for a variety of tumor types that are responsible for significant morbidity and mortality.[58] Although the Moonshot was announced in the United States, other countries have had similar efforts in place to accrue biospecimens and data.[58] One such focused effort is that of the Seoul National University Prospectively Enrolled Registry for Genitourinary Cancer (SUPER-GUC).[59] This initiative, focused on prostate, urothelial, and renal cancers, is a prospective cohort clinical database and biospecimen repository system. Each cohort consists of several subcohorts based on the treatment or disease status. Detailed longitudinal clinical information and general and disease-specific patient-reported outcomes are captured. A similar large multicenter translational research project focused on newly diagnosed breast and ovarian cancers is the BRandO biology and outcome (BiO) project.[60] Clinical data combined with primary tumor tissue samples and longitudinal repeatedly collected blood samples are being acquired from more than 4000 patients. In addition, standardized questionnaires are given to patients for assessing the life style and cancer risk factors. Concomitantly, storage of paraffin-embedded tumor samples as well as liquid biopsy samples is being done to potentially service a variety of translational research projects. Initiatives such as the International Cancer Genome Consortium (ICGC)[11] project have resulted in the creation of well-annotated cohorts with abundant clinical and molecular data. This in turn has resulted in fruitful attempts aimed at characterization of the landscape of genomics alteration in cancer.[11] Another key development has been the increasing use of formalin fixed paraffin embedded (FFPE) for molecular characterization of cancer biospecimens and its established critical role in downstream translational efforts.[61] Emphasis on the quality control of these specimens, and the annotating data, is an important task for biobanking that can be facilitated and improved by development of appropriate informatics tools. The ability to transfer data from the clinical workspace (EHR and Cancer Registry, Figure 1) to the research workspace via an RDW (Figure 1) is an important step for increasing phenotype annotation, research value, and efficiency of a tissue bank.

Synoptic reporting/standardization of data reporting
The description of cancer characteristics has long been recognized as prognostic factors, and beginning in the late 1980s and early 1990s, formal checklists were generated by the American Cancer Society and CAP.[24] These checklists ensure that complete data is reported for each cancer type and have been incorporated into Anatomic Pathology Laboratory Information Systems. In fact, the National Cancer Center Network mandates compliance with synoptic data reporting for pathology reports during inspection visits. These checklists standardize the individual cancer descriptors and have allowed for the creation of discrete data elements that can more seamlessly integrate with downstream electronic systems.[23] Using computerized checklists, the completeness of the surgical pathology report in relation to the cancer biospecimens can be ensured, thus creating a robust description of relevant cancer characteristics,[23,25,53,55] which then are deployable for automated data entry into cancer registry systems.[62] The utilization of discrete data elements also makes it much simpler to perform searches and case identification for relevant data elements.[23] The NCI has long championed the use of common data elements,[6] and this has fueled the value of biobanks in the NCI specialized program of research excellence (SPORE) and CCSG program, which both require the active banking of tissue/blood samples and curation of data derived from cancer patients involved in translational research and clinical trials.

Biobanks and tissue banking information systems have long been recognized for their valuable contribution to cancer research efforts.[15,25,53,55,59,60,63,64] In the era of precision oncology (and medicine), biobanks and their associated information systems have a more prominent role to play as genomic DNA derived from banked blood samples can be a "callable" information source for clinical decision support and customizing therapeutic choices.

Thus, EHR-linked biobanks and their joint phenotyping/callable biospecimen resources play an important role in facilitating opportunities in translational research in the research workspace as well as "callable" data for the clinical workspace in precision oncology. Unfortunately, commercial vendors supporting the clinical workspace do not integrate nor interoperate well with the laboratory information management systems (LIMS) systems provided by commercial vendors for biobanking, and this is another developmental area needed to move precision oncology forward.

Informatics tools for the research workspace for precision oncology

Research workspace architecture

In order to support deep scientific investigation and learning health systems, the following features of a research workspace are essential and must be highly efficient: (1) policy, procedures, and technologies that enable sensitive data to be available to investigators; (2) data ingestion and linkage in an RDW; (3) supports and tools for cohort discovery and data provisioning; (4) secure and robust data analysis environments; and (5) methods to exchange real-time analytics in clinical care.

Data governance and data stewardship
One of the most critical aspects of any research architecture built upon clinical data is managing the policy, procedures, and technologies to assure secure data liquidity, which refers to data being freely movable (liquid) yet protect the privacy and confidentiality of patients (secure).[27] Choosing the right context of data use for any project is critical, because federal regulations for clinical, quality improvement, and research with clinical data (Health Insurance Portability and Accountability Act, HIPAA) and human protections (Institutional Review Board, IRB) are driven by the use case of a particular project. A successful strategy includes expert consultation with those who understand the regulations and are informed of all intended uses of any data, and consideration of how the two intersect. However, rather than "recreate the wheel" with every project, institutional practices can be developed which appropriately designate purposes of large, sometimes interinstitutional, data collections, including discrete clinical, text, imaging, and -omic data.[65,66] Supporting technologies including federated identity management and data movement can substantially improve the efficiency for authenticating users, subsetting, moving, and authorizing specific datasets.[67]

Data ingestion and linkage in an RDW has been covered in this article from a functional perspective. From an architectural perspective, it is critical that the warehouse be built with extensible policy and technical features that support cohort discovery and data provisioning. For example, at the University of Pittsburgh, we have developed a policy framework and deployed technical systems that enable large databases of discrete clinical data to be augmented with other data types such as text, DICOM data, whole slide images from pathology, and -omics data. These are linked and deidentified at the patient level and down to every atomic transaction, with honest brokers dedicated to extraction and formatting of the data for each research need. These sociotechnical systems provision data to more than 100 different investigator teams per year and are structured to be able to add data sources and data types continuously.[68]

These approaches also include some "direct researcher access" features such as the use of data marts for cohort discovery and for specific large projects (e.g., PCORnet,[69] ACT i2b2,[70] and disease-specific data marts[25]), but as is typical for most institutions, provisioning data into secure analytic environments is rare. Instead, data is typically deidentified and moved to small or large computing environments for investigator analysis as needed. Moving forward, as larger and more sensitive and more complex analyses use artificial intelligence approaches, we expect the use of secure third-party environments to be much more common. Secure and scalable computing environments may include the use of technologies such as Jupyter notebooks to separate the investigator's interactive analytic environment from the data and computation via APIs, secure enclaves by public cloud service providers (e.g., Microsoft Azure Data Science Virtual Machines built into institutional frameworks and Amazon Web Services HIPAA BAA services), or large centers with encrypted data stored locally and coupled with local high-performance computing.

Ultimately, the community needs to marry the research workspace architecture with the clinical transactional architecture to achieve the goal of learning health systems. Producing data for research as a routine part of care, analyzing that data in real-time leveraging large-scale and secure and authorized analytics, and feeding results back into clinical care in real time among multiple institutions require architectures based on standard APIs that have yet to be written. While Fast Healthcare Interoperability Resources (FHIR) provides a stub of bulk research data extraction, and features for data inserts into EHRs,[71] fully operational environments that enable robust and complete bidirectional data among clinical and research environments are essentially experimental to date.

Advanced bioinformatics analysis for precision oncology

Large consortia projects such as TCGA project and the ICGC projects have produced an explosion of genomic data leading to detailed characterization of the molecular landscape of genomics alteration in cancer.[11,48] Such large data require computing infrastructure such as the Genome Data Commons[72] for querying, searching, and analyzing research data; translation of these novel insights and discoveries for precision oncology requires validation in larger cohorts supported by a robust informatics infrastructure for specimen annotation, metadata annotation, and clinical grade sequencing. The informatics needs of precision oncology include methods for biospecimen annotation,[73,74] variant calling,[75,76] building knowledgebases or repository of variants identified from institutional clinical sequencing projects,[77] standards and guidelines for clinical sequencing,[78] and cutting-edge imaging to find correlative markers in tissue specimens.[79] Projects such as AACR's Genie[10] are at the forefront of precision oncology and accelerating the discovery of novel actionable variants by creating the informatics framework for sharing high-quality harmonized clinical sequencing and metadata from 19 participating multinational academic institutions.[80]

The cancer genome atlas
The purpose of TCGA was to research multidimensional molecular alterations in human cancer and provide this data to the broader research community. The first human cancer studied was glioblastoma and was reported in October 2008.[81] This study was composed of 206 glioblastomas and provided new insights into several genes including ERBB2, NF1, TP53, RB, and PIK3R1 and various pathways that might be altered in this disease.[81] Given

the size of the molecular raw data, making it available for easy and broad distribution was a major improvement for research that was facilitated by informatics infrastructure. The data was collected from academic medical centers from all over the United States from preexisting retrospective tissue banks with a minimal 80% tumor cell percentage.[81] In 2013, an engine was created to index and annotate TCGA files.[82] Prior to this development work, the TCGA files were only accessible via HTTP from a public site.[82] This work that used JavaScript with W3C, RDF, and SPARQL markedly increased the availability and the usability of the data files within the TCGA project.[82] Of note, many of these updates make this data more freely available through the use of open-source software—further increasing the availability to the research community.

Genomic data commons
The National Cancer Institute's Genomic Data Commons was launched in 2016 and provides genomic data to the research community.[8] This liberalizes the genomic data so that it can be used by any interested research group. The data includes raw sequencing data and derived results such as mRNA results, whole-exome sequencing, and whole-genome sequencing for over 84,000 patients[8] and can be accessed at https://portal.gdc.cancer.gov/. The underlying data can be accessed via an API which greatly increases the functionality of the underlying data.[8] This API uses Javascript object notation (JSON) for communications and has RESTful API conventions.[8] This API can act in a bidirectional fashion, so that as researchers generate more data it can be sent back into the underlying database to expand the whole database. This expanded availability to genomic data for the research community represents a marked advance in the science community's ability to generate more knowledge, even if a researcher does not have access to expensive sequencing equipment and tissue material.

The generation of large sets of biomedical data has been increasing over the past several decades to the point that we are reaching exascale quantities of biomedical data produced per year.[83] These data include several important types including medical imaging, omics, structured, medical machine generated, and free-text clinical data from both clinical and research settings. There are many existing tools, especially those utilizing deep learning methods on genetic sequence and medical imaging data that are proving to be effective on these large amounts of data. Admittedly, more tools are needed, but with these existing tools, the emergence of new, similar tools and the ever-increasing capacity and cost reductions of high-performance computing (HPC) will drive the future of personalized medicine.[83]

There have been many gains toward personalized medicine using machine learning techniques. However, the wide use and success of AI in nonhealthcare, mainstream applications have created the perception that traditional research can be replaced with data science, which is unquestionably not the case.[84] Data science has, however, had many successes including more than 160 pharmacogenetic biomarkers approved for stratifying patients and biomarkers, from which, for example, comes the rule to administer Herceptin if HER2/neu receptor is overexpressed. Much of the research in this area has produced working models for questions with binary outcomes, but to continue the advance much more effort needs to be concentrated to problems that have more complex outcomes.[84]

The increase in next-generation sequencing (NGS) technologies has driven the need for more compute and storage resources. The recent expansion and accessibility of cloud computing is well positioned to help fill the current and future gaps in this area.[9]

Cloud computing offerings from several commercial vendors have been becoming increasingly affordable, reliable, and secure over the past decade and will likely follow this trajectory for the foreseeable future. Significant cost savings are realized when executing computationally intensive genomic and imaging applications on shared cloud infrastructure. The cost savings are a result of being able to commission resources on-demand, as needed, and decommission when no longer needed, paying only for the time used. This ability to scale resources on-demand at large scale has the benefit of time savings as well in that larger machines and clusters of machines can be provisioned which can be used to finish analyses faster than using less-resourced dedicated hardware. As more genomic data becomes available on cloud services and researchers become more familiar to using these services, genomic research will benefit in terms of both cost and time savings while performing computationally intensive tasks.

Quantitative imaging informatics, radiomics, and computational pathology

Radiomics is emerging as what could become an important component of precision medicine programs.[4] The quantitative, standardized output of a well-designed radiomics pipeline is ideal as inputs for machine learning and other data science algorithms. Analyzed data from radiographic medical images will be available in a quicker, more timely fashion, enabling quicker feedback to clinicians at the time they are called upon to render decisions. More work toward standardizing outputs is needed, and proposed standards such as the "Radiomics Quality Score" (RQS) and Response Criteria In Solid Tumors (RECIST) may help to address these challenges.[4,85]

Following a similar development path computational radiology (radiomics), it is likely that with the increased adoption and implementation of WSI and the digitization of anatomic pathology images, the field of computational pathology will mature sufficiently so that it too will lead to reliable tools and software that can support clinical decisions to fuel the development and optimization of therapeutics for precision oncology. Computational pathology publications are currently doubling every 18 months.[86] Many different concepts are covered by computational pathology including artificial intelligence and various types of machine learning. It can be defined as "the 'omics' or 'big-data' approach to anatomic pathology whole slide images, where multiple sources of patient information including pathology image data and meta-data are combined to extract patterns and analyze features."[87] Several authors have described validations of AI for use with clinical cases. These efforts demonstrate how artificial intelligence can be used to support improved pathologic diagnoses (i.e., identify missed cancer).[88] Several public challenges have been developed to encourage and support further development of artificial intelligence and machine learning through publicly available data sets.[89] Automated image analysis for biomarkers also represents an advancement since the automation is more reproducible than manual assessment by pathologists.[90,91] An example of automated image analysis of a colonic adenocarcinoma is seen in Figure 3.

Although many promising strides have been made toward developing machine learning and artificial intelligence-based computational pathology tools that advance precision oncology, the regulatory path to approvals for such technologies is still immature,[40,87] and this field is just beginning to receive wider acceptance. Future work certainly will accelerate the adoption of computational pathology, particularly in the area of tumor microenvironment and its application to precision immunooncology.[42,43,88,90,91]

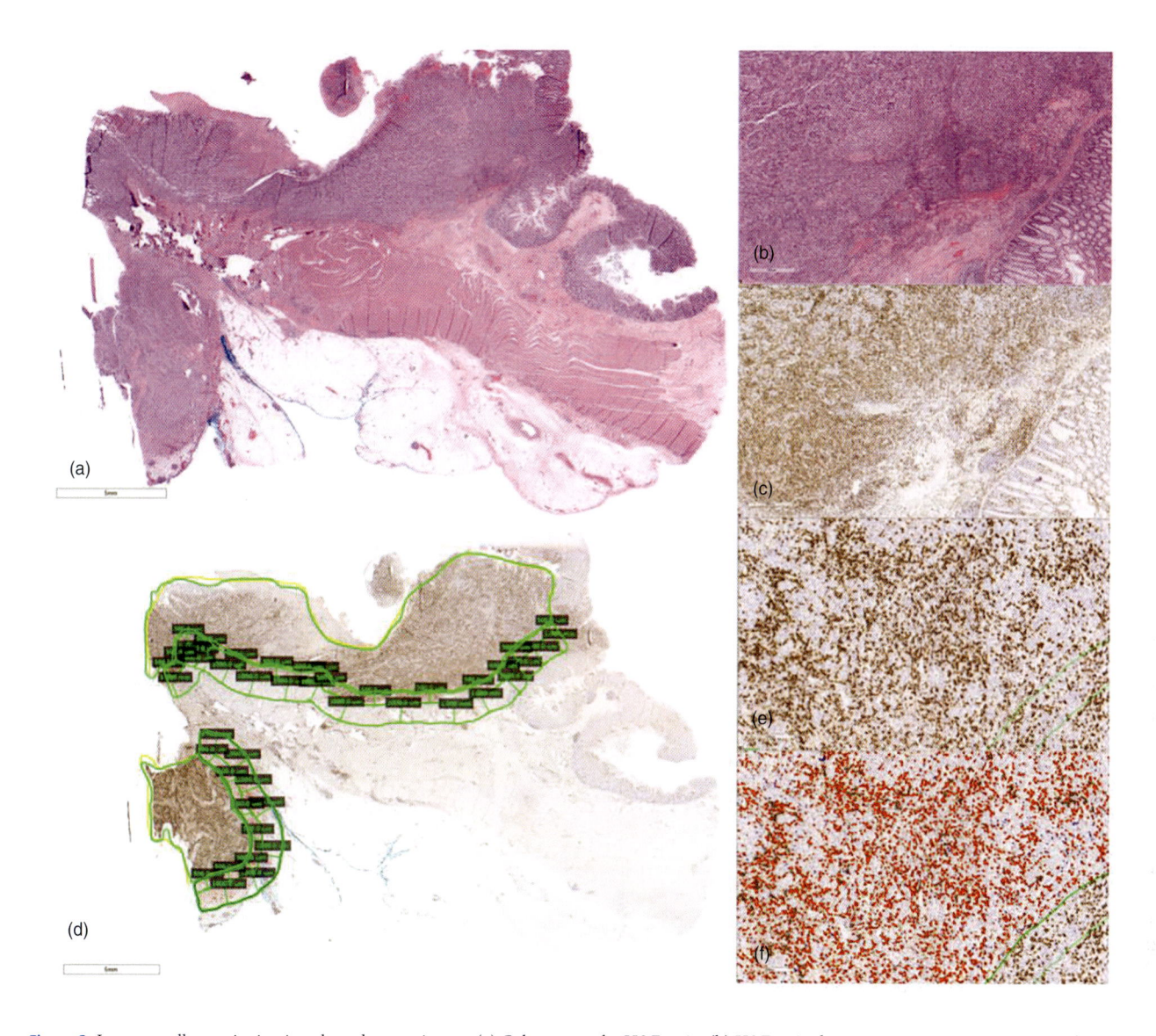

Figure 3 Immune cell quantitation in colon adenocarcinoma: (a) Colon cancer by H&E stain; (b) H&E stain demonstrating prominent intra- and peritumoral lymphocytes; (c) CD8 immunostain from the same field as B; (d) CD8 immunostain with annotations; (e) CD8 immunostain, note annotation line at lower left-hand corner of image; (f) CD8 immunostain showing image analysis results; The image analysis results show various intensities of the CD8 immunostain (3+ = red; 2+ = orange; 1+ = yellow).

Conclusions

A critical need is to help define for oncology-adapted EHRs the critical elements needed to make them useful for precision oncology.[92] The essential elements include access to pathology grading/staging and biomarker studies, chemo- and immunotherapy ordering and dosing modifications, e-Prescribing management encounters, communications between specialists and prescribers, integration of clinical trials data and "standard of care" practices, patient interaction/personal health outcomes and performance standards reported by patient-reported outcomes measures,[92,93] comorbidities, radiation therapy documentation, and quality measurements in face of the increasing adoption of "cancer treatment" pathways.[92,94] Today's clinical workspace systems (see Figure 1) fall far short of this list of ASCO-endorsed improvements to oncology EHRs.[92,95]

Critical to the success of precision oncology spanning, both the clinically supported HIT solutions and the research workspace "open-source" solutions integrated and made interoperable is a fully functioning RDW. The data stored in the research workspace by the RDW must subscribe to FAIR data practices.[3,14] FAIR, Findable, Accessible, Interoperable, and Reusable, is a set of principles that are becoming much more prevalent in research communities.[3] While these principles are normally thought of in the context of openly available data, they still apply to data that has restricted access, like much of the clinical and human genetic sequence data used in oncology research. The FAIR principles are an important part to any data store, such as an oncology data warehouse where ease of entry to using the data is important. Proper use of these principles will greatly shorten the learning curve to use that data for anyone needing to access it and use it for any kind of research or during the creation of tools, such as decision support systems, and would hopefully increase the use of the data and will be particularly critical for implementing precision oncology for cancer research and cancer care.

Precision oncology has many new drivers including the integration of genomic and sequencing data which is unfortunately highly fragmented due to partial support by molecular genetic pathology laboratories and their LIS and the increasing trend to outsource clinical sequencing to commercial laboratories (see section titled "Genomic and sequencing informatics"). The challenge to both the clinical workspace and research workspace (see Figure 1) for genomics data integration and interoperability using FAIR principles is very complex but will be an important challenge for cancer centers and oncology treatment centers to address.

New opportunities in biobanking integration into LIS and EHRs and the value of computational pathology and radiology will drive future innovations in precision oncology. The increasing digitization of medical images and the maturity of PACS and VNAs will be critical to the evolution of cancer treatment as understanding for the tumor microenvironment mapped to intercellular communications will drive therapeutic decision making in the era of immuno-oncology. Many challenges exist, but HIT and informatics innovation hold great promise for the modern cancer center. We are hopeful that the leadership in cancer research and cancer care delivery as well as our government agencies will work aggressively to partner on the necessary investment to make these dreams a reality.

Acknowledgments

The authors would like to acknowledge Tesheia Johnson MBA MHS, Deputy Director, Chief Operating Officer, Yale Center for Clinical Investigation, and Allen Hsiao MD, CMIO of Yale University, for sharing Figure 2, which was presented to the CTSA Informatics Domain Task Force in on 6 January 2017. The authors would also like to acknowledge the following experts who have provided critical feedback and input into this article: Ellen Beckjord PhD MPH, UPMC Health Plan and author of *Oncology Informatics*, Academic Press, 2016; David Foran PhD, Rutgers Cancer Institute of New Jersey, CIO and Executive Director of Biomedical Informatics and Computational Imaging; and S. Joseph Sirintrapun MD, Memorial Sloan Kettering Cancer Center, Director of Pathology Informatics.

Key references

The complete reference list can be found on Vital Source version of this title, see inside front cover.

1. Foran DJ, Chen W, Chu H, et al. Roadmap to a comprehensive clinical data warehouse for precision medicine applications in oncology. *Cancer Informat*. 2017;**16**:1176935117694349.
2. Hesse BW, Ahern D, Beckjord E. *Oncology Informatics: Using Health Information Technology to Improve Processes and Outcomes in Cancer*. Cambridge, MA: Academic Press; 2016.
3. Wilkinson MD, Dumontier M, Aalbersberg IJ, et al. The FAIR Guiding Principles for scientific data management and stewardship. *Sci Data*. 2016;**3**:160018.
4. Lambin P, Leijenaar RTH, Deist TM, et al. Radiomics: the bridge between medical imaging and personalized medicine. *Nat Rev Clin Oncol*. 2017;**14**(12):749–762.
6. Silva, J. and Wittes, R. (1999) *Role of Clinical Trials Informatics in the NCI's Cancer Informatics Infrastructure*. Proceedings of the AMIA Symposium, 950–954.
7. Becich MJ. The role of the pathologist as tissue refiner and data miner: the impact of functional genomics on the modern pathology laboratory and the critical roles of pathology informatics and bioinformatics. *Mol Diagn*. 2000;**5**(4):287–299.
8. Wilson S, Fitzsimons M, Ferguson M, et al. Developing cancer informatics applications and tools using the NCI genomic data commons API. *Cancer Res*. 2017;**77**(21):e15–e18.
10. AACR Project GENIE Consortium. AACR Project GENIE: powering precision medicine through an international consortium. *Cancer Discov*. 2017;**7**(8):818–831.
11. ICGC TCGA Pan-Cancer Analysis of Whole Genomes Consortium. Pan-cancer analysis of whole genomes. *Nature*. 2020;**578**(7793):82–93.
12. Louis DN, Feldman M, Carter AB, et al. Computational pathology: a path ahead. *Arch Pathol Lab Med*. 2016;**140**(1):41–50.
13. Louis DN, Gerber GK, Baron JM, et al. Computational pathology: an emerging definition. *Arch Pathol Lab Med*. 2014;**138**(9):1133–1138.
14. Elbers DC, Fillmore NR, Sung F-C, et al. The veterans affairs precision oncology data repository, a clinical, genomic, and imaging research database. *Patterns*. 2020;**1**(6):100083.
15. Dhir R, Patel AA, Winters S, et al. A multidisciplinary approach to honest broker services for tissue banks and clinical data: a pragmatic and practical model. *Cancer*. 2008;**113**(7):1705–1715.
16. Blumenthal D. Launching HITECH. *N Engl J Med*. 2010;**362**(5):382–385.
19. Hartmann-Johnsen OJ, Kåresen R, Schlichting E, et al. Using clinical cancer registry data for estimation of quality indicators: results from the Norwegian breast cancer registry. *Int J Med Inform*. 2019;**125**:102–109.
21. Blumenthal W, Alimi TO, Jones SF, et al. Using informatics to improve cancer surveillance. *J Am Med Inform Assoc*. 2020;**27**(9):1488–1495.
22. Kwiatkowski A. Enabling quality data reporting: national implementation of standardization pathology reporting. *J Clin Oncol*. 2014;**32**(30_suppl):122.
23. Leslie KO, Rosai J. Standardization of the surgical pathology report: formats, templates, and synoptic reports. *Semin Diagn Pathol*. 1994;**11**(4):253–257.
24. Markel SF, Hirsch SD. Synoptic surgical pathology reporting. *Hum Pathol*. 1991;**22**(8):807–810.
25. Amin W, Parwani AV, Schmandt L, et al. National Mesothelioma Virtual Bank: a standard based biospecimen and clinical data resource to enhance translational research. *BMC Cancer*. 2008;**8**:236.
26. Patel AA, Gilbertson JR, Showe LC, et al. A novel cross-disciplinary multi-institute approach to translational cancer research: lessons learned from Pennsylvania Cancer Alliance Bioinformatics Consortium (PCABC). *Cancer Informat*. 2007;**3**:255–274.
27. Rubin JC, Silverstein JC, Friedman CP, et al. Transforming the future of health together: The Learning Health Systems Consensus Action Plan. *Learn Health Syst*. 2018;**2**(3):e10055.
29. White MC, Babcock F, Hayes NS, et al. The history and use of cancer registry data by public health cancer control programs in the United States. *Cancer*. 2017;**123**(Suppl 24):4969–4976.
30. Warner JL, Maddux SE, Hughes KS, et al. Development, implementation, and initial evaluation of a foundational open interoperability standard for oncology treatment planning and summarization. *J Am Med Inform Assoc*. 2015;**22**(3):577–586.
32. Hayward A. *The CTSA: What They Are and What They Will Accomplish for Whom*. Beverly, MA: American Federation for Medical Research; 2010.
33. Liu G, Chen G, Sinoway LI, Berg A. Assessing the impact of the NIH CTSA program on institutionally sponsored clinical trials. *Clin Transl Sci*. 2013;**6**(3):196–200.
37. Krauss JC, Warner JL, Maddux SE, et al. Data sharing to support the cancer journey in the digital era. *J Oncol Pract*. 2016;**12**(3):201–207.
38. Campion TR Jr, Blau VL, Brown SW, et al. Implementing a clinical research management system: one institution's successful approach following previous failures. *AMIA Jt Summits Trans Sci Proc*. 2014;**2014**:12–17.
40. Abels E, Pantanowitz L. Current state of the regulatory trajectory for whole slide imaging devices in the USA. *J Pathol Inform*. 2017;**8**:23.
41. Saltz J, Gupta R, Hou L, et al. Spatial organization and molecular correlation of tumor-infiltrating lymphocytes using deep learning on pathology images. *Cell Rep*. 2018;**23**(1):181–93.e7.
42. Spagnolo DM, Al-Kofahi Y, Zhu P, et al. Platform for quantitative evaluation of spatial intratumoral heterogeneity in multiplexed fluorescence images. *Cancer Res*. 2017;**77**(21):e71–e74.
43. Uttam S, Stern AM, Sevinsky CJ, et al. Spatial domain analysis predicts risk of colorectal cancer recurrence and infers associated tumor microenvironment networks. *Nat Commun*. 2020;**11**(1):3515.
46. Warner JL, Jain SK, Levy MA. Integrating cancer genomic data into electronic health records. *Genome Med*. 2016;**8**(1):113.
47. Sirintrapun SJ, Artz DR. Health information systems. *Clin Lab Med*. 2016;**36**(1):133–152.
48. Priestley P, Baber J, Lolkema MP, et al. Pan-cancer whole-genome analyses of metastatic solid tumours. *Nature*. 2019;**575**(7781):210–216.
51. McIntosh LD, Sharma MK, Mulvihill D, et al. caTissue Suite to OpenSpecimen: developing an extensible, open source, web-based biobanking management system. *J Biomed Inform*. 2015;**57**:456–464.
52. Jacobson RS, Becich MJ, Bollag RJ, et al. A federated network for translational cancer research using clinical data and biospecimens. *Cancer Res*. 2015;**75**(24):5194–5201.
53. Patel AA, Kajdacsy-Balla A, Berman JJ, et al. The development of common data elements for a multi-institute prostate cancer tissue bank: the Cooperative Prostate Cancer Tissue Resource (CPCTR) experience. *BMC Cancer*. 2005;**5**:108.
54. Eiseman E, Bloom G, Brower J, et al. *Case Studies of Existing Human Tissue Repositories: "Best Practices" for a Biospecimen Resource for the Genomic And Proteomic Era*. Santa Monica, CA: Rand Corporation; 2003.

55. Mohanty SK, Mistry AT, Amin W, et al. The development and deployment of Common Data Elements for tissue banks for translational research in cancer—an emerging standard based approach for the Mesothelioma Virtual Tissue Bank. *BMC Cancer.* 2008;**8**:91.
56. Lowy DR, Collins FS. Aiming high—changing the trajectory for cancer. *N Engl J Med.* 2016;**374**(20):1901–1904.
57. Singer DS, Jacks T, Jaffee E. A US "Cancer Moonshot" to accelerate cancer research. *Science.* 2016;**353**(6304):1105–1106.
58. Lowy D, Singer D, DePinho R, et al. Cancer moonshot countdown. *Nat Biotechnol.* 2016;**34**(6):596–599.
59. Jeong CW, Suh J, Yuk HD, et al. Establishment of the Seoul National University Prospectively Enrolled Registry for Genitourinary Cancer (SUPER-GUC): a prospective, multidisciplinary, bio-bank linked cohort and research platform. *Investig Clin Urol.* 2019;**60**(4):235–243.
60. De Gregorio A, Nagel G, Möller P, et al. Feasibility of a large multi-center translational research project for newly diagnosed breast and ovarian cancer patients with affiliated biobank: the BRandO biology and outcome (BiO)-project. *Arch Gynecol Obstet.* 2020;**301**(1):273–281.
61. Gaffney EF, Riegman PH, Grizzle WE, Watson PH. Factors that drive the increasing use of FFPE tissue in basic and translational cancer research. *Biotec Histochem.* 2018;**93**(5):373–386.
62. Renshaw AA, Mena-Allauca M, Gould EW, Sirintrapun SJ. Synoptic reporting: evidence-based review and future directions. *JCO Clin Cancer Inform.* 2018;**2**:1–9.
63. Amin W, Singh H, Pople AK, et al. A decade of experience in the development and implementation of tissue banking informatics tools for intra and inter-institutional translational research. *J Pathol Inform.* 2010;**1**:12.
64. Patel AA, Gilbertson JR, Parwani AV, et al. An informatics model for tissue banks–lessons learned from the Cooperative Prostate Cancer Tissue Resource. *BMC Cancer.* 2006;**6**:120.
69. Amin W, Tsui FR, Borromeo C, et al. PaTH: towards a learning health system in the Mid-Atlantic region. *J Am Med Inform Assoc.* 2014;**21**(4):633–636.
70. Visweswaran S, Becich MJ, D'Itri VS, et al. Accrual to Clinical Trials (ACT): a clinical and translational science award consortium network. *JAMIA Open.* 2018;**1**(2):147–152.
72. Grossman RL. Data lakes, clouds, and commons: a review of platforms for analyzing and sharing genomic data. *Trends Genet.* 2019;**35**(3):223–234.
77. Chakravarty D, Gao J, Phillips SM, et al. OncoKB: a precision oncology knowledge base. *JCO Precis Oncol.* 2017;**2017**:PO.17.00011.
78. Roy S, Coldren C, Karunamurthy A, et al. Standards and guidelines for validating next-generation sequencing bioinformatics pipelines: a joint recommendation of the Association for Molecular Pathology and the College of American Pathologists. *J Mol Diagn.* 2018;**20**(1):4–27.
79. Fedorov A, Beichel R, Kalpathy-Cramer J, et al. Quantitative imaging informatics for cancer research. *JCO Clin Cancer Inform.* 2020;**4**:444–453.
80. Thomas S, Lichtenberg T, Dang K, et al. Linked entity attribute pair (LEAP): a harmonization framework for data pooling. *JCO Clin Cancer Inform.* 2020;**4**:691–699.
81. Cancer Genome Atlas Research Network. Comprehensive genomic characterization defines human glioblastoma genes and core pathways. *Nature.* 2008;**455**(7216):1061–1068.
82. Robbins DE, Grüneberg A, Deus HF, et al. A self-updating road map of The Cancer Genome Atlas. *Bioinformatics (Oxford, England).* 2013;**29**(10):1333–1340.
83. Cirillo D, Valencia A. Big data analytics for personalized medicine. *Curr Opin Biotechnol.* 2019;**58**:161–167.
84. Fröhlich H, Balling R, Beerenwinkel N, et al. From hype to reality: data science enabling personalized medicine. *BMC Med.* 2018;**16**(1):150.

PART 4

Carcinogenesis

22 Chemical carcinogenesis

Lorne J. Hofseth, PhD ■ Ainsley Weston, PhD ■ Curtis C. Harris, MD

> **Overview**
>
> Human exposure to chemical carcinogens can result in cancer. What dictates this outcome is relatively predictable but highly variable. Factors governing the outcome include type of exposure, amount of exposure, time of exposure, and genetic makeup of the human host. The latter is comprised of variations in single nucleotides within genes (e.g., single nucleotide polymorphisms in DNA repair genes), as well as the metabolomic, proteomic, microbiomic, transcriptomic, and epigenomic background of the individual. It is becoming increasingly clear that these endpoints and signatures can be modified by chemical carcinogens and that the inflammatory load influences outcome. To this end, the past decade has seen an explosion of extremely sensitive and highly accurate technology for measuring the impact of carcinogens. Linking this technology to the rapid development of bioinformatics has enabled us to begin merging the totality of lifetime exposure ("exposome") with the totality of metabolomic, proteomic, microbiomic, transcriptomic, epigenomic, and other "omic" profiles. We feel optimistic that the next decade will bring the development of tools to identify an individual's weighted risk signature as a biomarker for cancer risk and develop a personalized and precise approach to cancer chemoprevention and treatment.

Human chemical carcinogenesis is a multistage process that results from carcinogen exposure, usually in the form of complex chemical mixtures, and often encountered in the environment or through our lifestyle and diet (Tables 1 and 2). A prominent example is tobacco smoke which can cause cancers at multiple sites with the highest risk being that of lung cancer. Although most chemical carcinogens do not react directly with intracellular components, they are activated to carcinogenic and mutagenic electrophiles by metabolic processes evolutionarily designed to clear the body of toxins and to modify endogenous compounds. Electrophilic chemical species are naturally attracted to nucleophiles like deoxyribonucleic acid (DNA) and protein Genetic damage results through covalent bonding of electrophiles to DNA. Once internalized, carcinogens are subject to competing processes of metabolic activation and detoxification, although some chemical species can act directly. There is considerable variation among the human population in these competing metabolic processes, as well as the capacity for repair of DNA damage and cellular growth control. This is the basis for inter-individual variation in cancer risk and is a reflection of gene–environment interactions, which embodies the concept that heritable traits modify the effects of chemical carcinogen exposure.[29,30] Such variations in constitutive metabolism, DNA repair, and cellular growth control contribute to the relative susceptibility of individual members of the population to chemical exposures. For example, only 10% of tobacco smokers develop lung cancer, albeit that tobacco use accounts for other fatal conditions, including cardiovascular disease, emphysema, and chronic obstructive pulmonary disorder. Within the conceptual framework of multistage carcinogenesis, the primary genetic change that results from a chemical–DNA interaction is termed *tumor initiation*.[11,12] Thus, initiated cells are irreversibly altered and are at a greater risk of malignant conversion than are normal cells. The epigenetic effects of tumor promoters facilitate the clonal expansion of the initiated cells.[31,32] Selective, clonal growth advantage causes a focus of preneoplastic cells to form. These cells are more vulnerable to tumorigenesis because they now present a larger, more rapidly proliferating, target population for the further action of chemical carcinogens, oncogenic viruses, and other cofactors. Additional genetic and epigenetic changes continue to accumulate.[31,32] The activation of oncogenes, and the inactivation of tumor suppressor and DNA-repair genes, leads to genomic instability or the *mutator phenotype* and an acceleration in the genetic changes taking place.[33–35] This scenario is followed by malignant conversion, tumor progression, and metastasis. The underlying molecular mechanisms that govern chemical carcinogenesis are becoming increasingly understood, and the insights generated are assisting in the development of better methods to investigate human cancer risk and susceptibility. The results of such studies are intended to mold strategies for prevention and intervention. Moreover, insights into the normal operations of so-called *gatekeeper* genes,[36] like the tumor suppressor *TP53*, have provided an opportunity to develop new, targeted, therapeutic approaches.

Multistage carcinogenesis

Carcinogenesis can be divided conceptually into four steps: tumor initiation, tumor promotion, malignant conversion, and tumor progression (Figure 1, Box 1). The distinction between initiation and promotion was recognized through studies involving both viruses and chemical carcinogens.[11,12,37] This distinction was formally defined in a murine skin carcinogenesis model in which mice were treated topically with a single dose of a polycyclic aromatic hydrocarbon (PAH) (i.e., initiator), followed by repeated topical doses of croton oil (i.e., promoter),[11] and this model has been expanded to a range of other rodent tissues, including bladder, colon, esophagus, liver, lung, mammary gland, stomach, and trachea.[32] During the last 65 years, the sequence of events comprising chemical carcinogenesis has been systematically dissected and the paradigm increasingly refined, and both similarities and differences between rodent and human carcinogenesis have been identified.[38] Carcinogenesis requires the malignant conversion of benign hyperplastic cells to a malignant state, and invasion and metastasis are manifestations of further genetic and epigenetic changes.[39] The study of this process in humans is necessarily

Table 1 Selected examples of human chemical carcinogenesis.

Organ system (specific pathology)	Chemical carcinogen	Co-carcinogen
Lung (small and nonsmall cell)	Tobacco smoke	Asbestos
	Metals: As, Be, Cd, Cr, Ni	—
	BCME	—
	Diesel exhaust	—
Pleural mesothelium	Asbestos	Tobacco smoke
Oral cavity	Smokeless tobacco	—
	Betel quid	Slaked lime [Ca(OH)$_2$]
Esophagus	Tobacco smoke	Alcohol
Nasal sinuses	Snuff	Powdered glass
	Isopropyl alcohol	—
Skin (scrotum)	Cutting oil	—
	Coal soot[a]	—
Liver (angiosarcoma)	Aflatoxin B1	HBV, HCB
	Vinyl chloride	Alcohol
Bladder	Aromatic amines (e.g., 4-ABP and benzidine)	—
	Aromatic amines from tobacco smoke[b]	—
ALL	Benzene	—
Lymphatic and hematopoietic malignancies	Ethylene oxide	—

A comprehensive treatise on the evaluation of the carcinogenic risk of chemicals to humans can be found in the ongoing International Agency for Research on Cancer monograph program initiated in 1971.
4-ABP, 4-aminobiphenyl; ALL, acute lymphoblastic leukemia; BCME, bis-chloromethyl ether; HBV, hepatitis B virus; HCV, hepatitis C virus.
[a]Early report of occupational chemical carcinogenesis from 225 years ago.
[b]Strong circumstantial evidence.[1]

Table 2 Landmark discoveries in environmental carcinogenesis.

Year	Event/discovery/finding	References
3000 BC	First written description of cancer (breast) in the Edwin Smith Papyrus	2
1500 BC	Egyptians treat tumors with chemicals (arsenic)	2
1742	Hermann Boerhaave and Jean Astruc link inflammation to cancer	3–5
1775	Percival Pott describes association between soot exposure and scrotal cancer in chimney sweeps	6
1863	Rudolf Virchow: cancers tend to occur at sites of chronic inflammation	7
1909	First Chemotherapy Drug (an arsenobenzene analogue, compound 606, or Salvarsan) Treats Syphilis	8
1910	Viruses found to cause cancer	9
1932	Female hormones (estrogen) cause breast cancer in mice	10
1941	Two-stage initiation and promotion of cancers by chemical carcinogens proposed	11, 12
1950	Tobacco exposure linked to lung cancer	13, 14
1956	Evidence that enzymes can be activated by chemical carcinogens	15
1973	Ames assay identified to test mutagenicity of chemical carcinogens	16
1974	Evidence that chemical carcinogens are activated to form DNA adducts in human tissues	17
1981	First quantitative estimation of the contribution of the environment and genetics to carcinogenesis	18
1982	Formal structure/model of molecular epidemiology introduced	19
1988	Chemical carcinogens cause site-specific mutagenesis	20
1991	Identification of selective mutations in p53 ("mutational hotspots") associated with specific environmental and chemical carcinogens	21, 22
2005	Concept of the exposome (the entirety of exposure to which an individual is subjected, from conception to death) is introduced	23
2011	National Research Council (US) Committee on A Framework for Developing a New Taxonomy of Disease introduces Precision Medicine	24
2012	Use of integrative Personal Omics Profile to distinguish between healthy and diseased states at an individual level	25
2020	Linking mutation signatures to the exposome	26–28

indirect and uses information from lifestyle or occupational exposures to chemical carcinogens. Measures of age-dependent cancer incidence have shown, however, that the rate of tumor development is proportional to the sixth power of time, suggesting that at least four to six independent steps are necessary.[40] Partial scheduling of specific genetic events in this process has been possible for some cancers. Examples of sequential genetic and epigenetic changes that occur with the highest probability are those found in the development of lung cancer[41] and colon cancer.[42] Recent advances in sequencing technology have allowed us to identify the genomic landscape of many tumors. In common solid tumors such as those derived from the colon, breast, brain, or pancreas, an average of 33–66 genes display subtle somatic mutations that can alter their protein products.[43] Certain tumor types display many more or many fewer mutations than average. Melanomas and lung tumors, for example, contain ~200 nonsynonymous mutations per tumor; a reflection of the involvement of potent mutagens (ultraviolet light and cigarette smoke, respectively) in the pathogenesis of these tumor types.[43]

Tumor initiation

Earlier concepts of tumor initiation indicated that the initial changes in chemical carcinogenesis are irreversible genetic damage. However, recent data from molecular studies of preneoplastic human lung and colon tissues implicate epigenetic changes as an early event in carcinogenesis. DNA methylation of promoter regions of genes can transcriptionally silence tumor suppressor genes.[44] In a broad sense, then, chemical carcinogens can be divided into genotoxic [e.g., Benzo(a)Pyrene or B(a)P; generally considered to act at the initiation stage] and nongenotoxic agents (e.g., 3,7,8-Tetrachlorodibenzo-p-dioxin (TCDD) or 12-O-tetradecanoylphorbol-13-acetate (TPA); generally considered to act in the promotion stages). These nongenotoxic or epigenetic agents (Figure 1) do not induce mutations, nor do they induce direct DNA damage in the target organ. They modulate cell growth and death and exhibit dose–response relationships between exposure and tumor formation. While the exact mechanism(s) of action of these agents on neoplastic cell formation are yet to be determined, changes in gene expression and cell growth parameters appear to be critical and nongenotoxic compounds exhibit temporal and threshold characteristics frequently requiring chronic treatment for carcinogenicity.

Overall, most human cancers are caused by two to eight sequential alterations that develop over the course of 20–30 years.[43] For mutations to accumulate, they must arise in cells that proliferate and survive the lifetime of the organism. A chemical carcinogen causes a genetic error by modifying the molecular structure of DNA that can lead to a mutation during DNA synthesis.

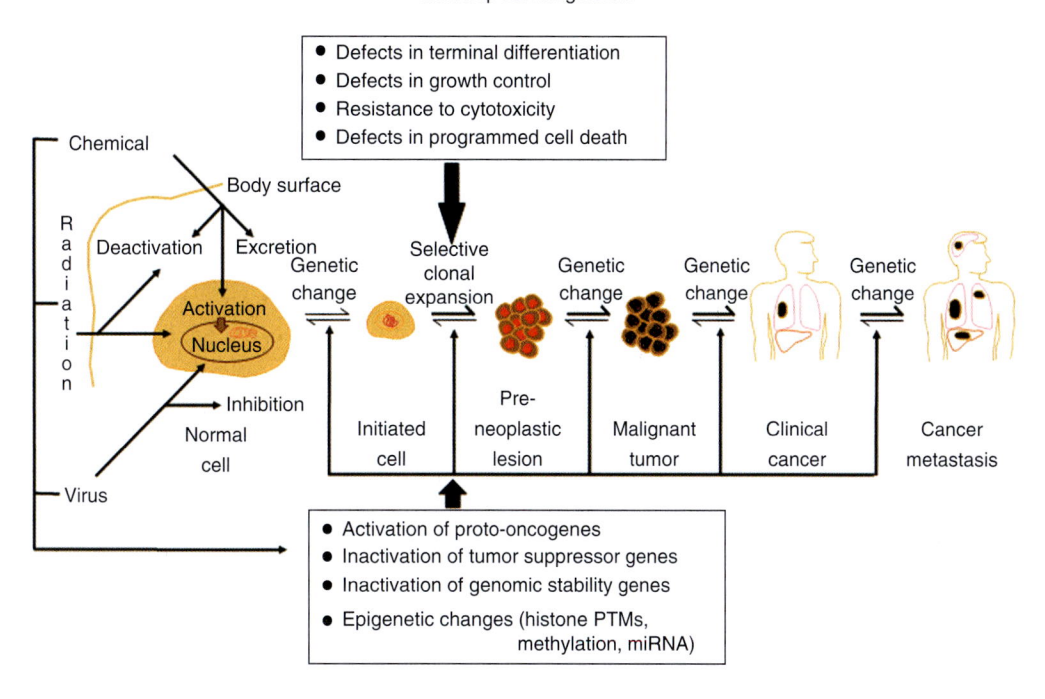

Figure 1 Multistep chemical carcinogenesis can be conceptually divided into four stages: tumor initiation, tumor promotion, malignant conversion, and tumor progression. The activation of proto-oncogenes and the inactivation of tumor suppressor genes are mutational events that result from covalent damage to DNA caused by chemical exposures. The accumulation of mutations, and not necessarily the order in which they occur, constitutes multistage carcinogenesis. During these stages, progressive epigenetic changes are also occurring due to chemical exposure.

Box 1 Multistage Carcinogenesis

Multistage carcinogenesis involves 4 stages:

1. *Tumor Initiation*: The initial changes to normal cells that occur early in chemical carcinogenesis and involve irreversible genetic mutation(s) ("genotoxic initiation") or epigenetic changes ("nongenotoxic initiation") so that they are able to form tumors.
2. *Tumor Promotion*: The selective clonal expansion of a population of initiated cells, causing additional genetic changes with a growth advantage that will then be at risk for malignant conversion. Tumor promoters are generally nongenotoxic, cannot drive tumorigenesis alone, and require repeat exposure over time.
3. *Malignant Conversion*: The transformation of a preneoplastic cell into one that expresses a malignant phenotype. The probability of malignant conversion increases through additional genetic changes, continued exposure of preneoplastic cells to DNA-damaging agents, and may be mediated through the activation of proto-oncogenes and inactivation of tumor suppressor genes.
4. *Tumor Progression*: The expression of the malignant phenotype and the tendency of malignant cells to acquire more aggressive characteristics over time. A prominent characteristic of the malignant phenotype is the propensity for genomic instability and uncontrolled growth. During this process, further genetic and epigenetic changes can occur, again including the activation of proto-oncogenes and the functional loss of tumor suppressor genes.

Most often, this is brought about by forming an adduct between the chemical carcinogen or one of its functional groups and a nucleotide in DNA (the process by which this occurs for the major classes of chemical carcinogens is discussed in detail under the section titled "Carcinogen Metabolism"). In general, a positive correlation is found between the amount of carcinogen–DNA adducts that can be detected in animal models and the number of tumors that develop.[45,46] Thus, tumors rarely develop in tissues that do not form carcinogen–DNA adducts. Carcinogen–DNA adduct formation is central to theories of chemical carcinogenesis, and it may be a necessary, but not a sufficient, prerequisite for tumor initiation (the concept of so-called nongenotoxic carcinogens is also explored under the section titled "Carcinogen Metabolism"). DNA adduct formation that causes either the activation of a proto-oncogene or the inactivation of a tumor suppressor gene can be categorized as a tumor-initiating event (see the sections titled "Tumor Progression" and "Oncogenes and Tumor Suppressor Genes" in this article).

Tumor promotion

Tumor promotion comprises the selective clonal expansion of initiated cells. Because the accumulation rate of mutations is proportional to the rate of cell division, or at least the rate at which stem cells are replaced, clonal expansion of initiated cells, produces a larger population of cells that are at risk of further genetic changes and malignant conversion.[39,43] Tumor promoters are generally nongenotoxic, are not carcinogenic alone, and often (but not always) are able to mediate their biological effects without metabolic activation. These agents are characterized by their ability to reduce the latency period for tumor formation after exposure of a tissue to a tumor initiator or to increase the number of tumors formed in that tissue. In addition, they induce tumor formation in conjunction with a dose of an initiator that is too low to be carcinogenic alone. Croton oil (isolated from *Croton tiglium* seeds) is used widely as a tumor promoter in murine skin carcinogenesis, and the mechanism of action for its most potent constituent, TPA, which occurs via protein kinase C activation, is arguably the best understood among tumor promoters.[47] Chemicals or agents capable of both tumor initiation and promotion are known as complete carcinogens [e.g., B(a)P and 4-aminobiphenyl]. Identification of new tumor promoters in animal models has accelerated with the sophisticated development of model systems designed to assay for tumor promotion. Furthermore, ligand binding properties can be determined in recombinant protein kinase C isozymes that are expressed in cell culture.[48] Chemicals, complex mixtures of chemicals, or other agents that have been shown to have tumor-promoting properties include dioxin, TPA, TCDD, benzoyl peroxide, macrocyclic lactones, bromomethylbenzanthracene, anthralin, phenol, saccharin, tryptophan, dichlorodiphenyl-trichloroethane (DDT), phenobarbital, cigarette-smoke condensate, polychlorinated biphenyls (PCBs), teleocidins, cyclamates, estrogens and other hormones, bile acids, ultraviolet light, wounding, abrasion, and other chronic irritation (i.e., saline lavage).[49]

Malignant conversion

Malignant conversion is the transformation of a preneoplastic cell into one that expresses the malignant phenotype. This process requires further genetic changes. The total dose of a tumor promoter is less significant than frequently repeated administrations, and if the tumor promoter is discontinued before malignant conversion has occurred, premalignant or benign lesions may regress. Tumor promotion contributes to the process of carcinogenesis by the expansion of a population of initiated cells, with a growth advantage, that will then be at risk for malignant conversion. Conversion of a fraction of these cells to malignancy will be accelerated in proportion to the rate of cell division and the quantity of dividing cells in the benign tumor or preneoplastic lesion. In part, these further genetic changes may result from infidelity of DNA synthesis.[50] The relatively low probability of malignant conversion can be increased substantially by the exposure of preneoplastic cells to DNA-damaging agents,[51] and this process may be mediated through the activation of proto-oncogenes and inactivation of tumor suppressor genes.

Tumor progression

Tumor progression comprises the expression of the malignant phenotype and the tendency of malignant cells to acquire more aggressive characteristics over time. Also, metastasis may involve the ability of tumor cells to secrete proteases that allow invasion beyond the immediate primary tumor location. A prominent characteristic of the malignant phenotype is the propensity for genomic instability and uncontrolled growth.[52] During this process, further genetic and epigenetic changes can occur, again including the activation of proto-oncogenes and the functional loss of tumor suppressor genes. Frequently, proto-oncogenes are activated by two major mechanisms: in the case of the *ras* gene family, point mutations are found in highly specific regions of the gene (i.e., the twelfth, thirteenth, fifty-ninth, or sixty-first codons), and members of the *myc*, *raf*, *HER2*, and *jun* multigene families can be overexpressed, sometimes involving amplification of chromosomal segments containing these genes. Some genes are overexpressed if they are translocated and become juxtaposed to a powerful promoter, for example, the relationship of *bcl-2* and immunoglobulin heavy chain gene promoter regions in B-cell malignancies. Loss of function of tumor suppressor genes usually occurs in a bimodal fashion, and most frequently involves point mutations (caused by DNA-adducts, errors in DNA replication, and errors in DNA-repair) in one allele and loss of the second allele by a deletion (caused by a recombinational event, chromosomal nondisjunction, or hypermethylation). These phenomena confer to the cells a growth advantage as well as the capacity for regional invasion, and ultimately, distant metastatic spread. Despite evidence for an apparent scheduling of certain mutational events, it is the accumulation of these mutations, and not the order or the stage of tumorigenesis in which they occur, that appears to be the determining factor.[43] Recent evidence from microarray expression analysis of human cancers supports an alternative, and not mutually exclusive, mode of tumor progression. Gene expression profiles of a primary cancer and its metastases are similar, indicating the molecular progression of a primary cancer is generally retained in its metastases.[53]

Over the last decade, sequencing efforts have identified genomic landscapes of common forms of human cancer. Vogelstein recently defined these landscapes as consisting of a small number of "mountains" (genes altered in a high percentage of tumors) and a much larger number of "hills" (genes altered infrequently).[43] Approximately 140 genes that, when altered by intragenic mutations, can drive tumorigenesis. A typical tumor contains two to eight of these "driver gene" mutations that control cell fate, cell survival, and genomic maintenance. Other "passenger mutations" confer no selective growth advantage. Overall, the identification of specific genes and their function in primary cancers and metastases have clinical implications in molecular diagnosis of primary cancers and targeted therapeutic strategies for personalized medicine.

Epigenetics and chemical carcinogenesis

Epigenetics describes a change in gene activity without a change in the DNA sequence.[54] Well-described mechanisms involved in epigenetics include DNA methylation and histone modification; each of which alters how genes are expressed without altering the underlying DNA sequence. Another mechanism (described in detail below) also falling under the definition of "epigenetic" is the effects of microRNA (miRNA; Figure 2, Box 2) on carcinogenesis. Both nongenotoxic and genotoxic chemical carcinogens impact these epigenetic processes. At the cellular level, exposure to environmental factors may leave an epigenomic signature that can be exploited in discovering new biomarkers for risk assessment and cancer prevention.[55,56]

> **Box 2** Epigenetics
>
> Epigenetics describes a change in gene activity without a change in the DNA sequence. It involves changes in *DNA methylation* [hypomethylation/hypermethylation caused by carcinogens modifying methylation enzymes (e.g., DNMTs)], *histone tail modification* [acetylation, methylation, ubiquitination, sumoylation, and phosphorylation caused by carcinogens modifying enzymes involved in such changes (e.g., HDACs)], and *small noncoding RNAs* (e.g., microRNAs caused by genetic abnormalities, modulation of biogenesis machinery and/or epigenetic mechanisms).

DNA methylation is catalyzed by a family of DNA methyltransferases (DNMTs). In somatic mammalian cells, DNA methylation occurs at cytosine residues of CpG dinucleotides; in embryonic stem cells, DNA methylation occurs at both CpG and non-CpG sequences. DNMT expression, and therefore indirect control of DNA methylation, is controlled by DNMT3L, lymphoid-specific helicase (Lsh), miRNAs, and piwi-interacting RNAs (piRNAs).[57] It is becoming increasingly

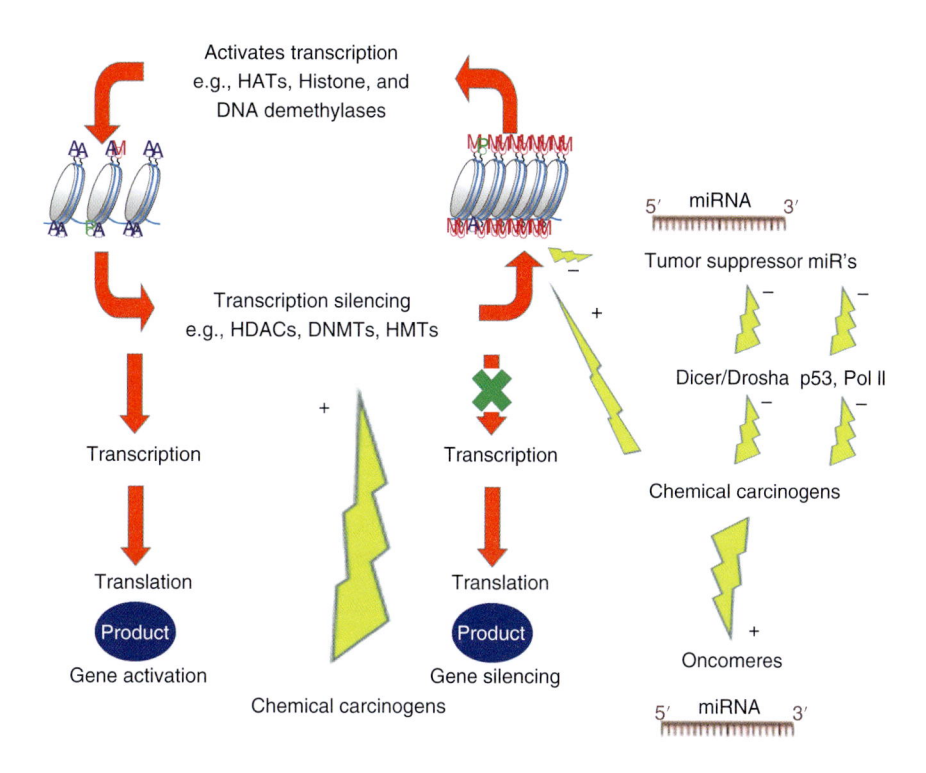

Figure 2 Epigenetic impact of chemical carcinogens. Chemical carcinogens can affect the activity of the different enzymes involved in epigenomics. Ac, acetyl; Me, methyl; DNMT, DNA methyltransferase; HAT, histone acetyltransferase; HDAC, histone aeacetylase; HMT: histone methyltransferase.

clear that many chemical carcinogens are involved in DNA methylation. For example, the tobacco-specific carcinogen, 4-(methylnitrosoamino)-1-(3-pyridyl)-1-butanone (NNK), induces DNMT accumulation and tumor suppressor gene hypermethylation in mice and lung cancer patients.[58] As well, B(a)P and many others; not only genotoxic but also nongenotoxic chemical carcinogens have been shown to induce aberrant methylation patterns.[57,59] Several mechanisms may explain aberrant methylation patterns due to chemical carcinogens. As an example, cigarette smoke may alter DNA methylation by (1) inducing DNA damage, stimulating recruitment of DNMT1; (2) the ability of nicotine to downregulate DNMT1 mRNA and protein expression; (3) modulating expression and activity of DNA-binding factors, such as Sp1; and (4) inducing hypoxia, which increases HIF1α, leading to the upregulation of methionine adenosyltransferase 2A[60] (Figure 2).

Chromatin is the complex of DNA wrapped around histone octamers, consisting of four different histones, H2A, H2B, H3, and H4. Gene expression changes with histone posttranscriptional modification (e.g., acetylation, phosphorylation, and methylation) in the N-terminal tail region. Enzymes that regulate histone modification include histone deacetylases (HDACs), histone acetyltransferases (HATs), and histone methyltransferases (HMTs). Chemical carcinogens can alter the activity of such enzymes. For example, challenging cells with B(a)P induce early enrichment of the transcriptionally active chromatin markers histone H3 trimethylated at lysine 4 (H3K4Me3) and histone H3 acetylated at lysine 9 (H3K9Ac) and reduces association of DNA methyltransferase-1 (DNMT1) with the long interspersed nuclear element-1 (L1) promoter. These changes are followed by proteasome-dependent decreases in cellular DNMT1 expression and sustained reduction of cytosine methylation within the L1 promoter CpG island.[61] Similarly, long-term exposure of immortalized bronchial epithelial cells (HBEC-3KT) to low doses of tobacco-related carcinogens leads to oncogenic transformation, increased HDAC expression, cell-cycle independent increased DNMT1 stability, and DNA hypermethylation.[62]

Another epigenetic signaling mechanism key to carcinogenesis involves microRNAs. The subject of microRNAs and cancer is covered in detail in **Chapter 9**. Of note, however, miRNA expression is regulated by a growing list of factors, including inflammatory cytokines, free radicals, and chemical carcinogens.[63–66] Indeed, because miRNA levels change upon exposure to environmental and endogenous chemicals, it is possible that miRNAs can be used for biomonitoring purposes. This is supported by the understanding that miRNAs are released from the target tissues into the bloodstream; and therefore, their analysis is feasible via noninvasive sampling (e.g., urine, feces).[67–69]

Changes in miRNA levels by environmental carcinogens appear to be reversible at low doses and short periods of exposure, but irreversible with higher doses and long periods of exposure; and that irreversible miRNA changes are predictive of the future appearance of cancer.[66,70] The mechanisms of how chemical carcinogens lead to an imbalance and changes in miRNA expression appear to involve genetic abnormalities, modulation of the biogenesis machinery, and/or epigenetic mechanisms[71–73] (Box 2). Genetic abnormalities include chromosomal rearrangements, genomic amplifications, deletions, and mutations.[73] This was demonstrated in the first studies identifying miRNAs in tumorigenesis. The miRNA-15/16-1 cluster was shown to be deleted in CLL, with subsequent reduced accumulation.[74] Germline mutation was also associated with reduced accumulation of this cluster.[75] The miRNA biogenesis machinery can be altered through multiple mechanism; each resulting in altered miRNA levels. For example, mutations can occur in key biogenesis enzymes (Dicer and Drosha) and/or their complexes,[76] resulting in aberrant miRNA production. Indeed, it has been shown that a series of chemical carcinogens (e.g., PAHs, heterocyclic compounds, nitrosamines, morpholine, ethylnitrosourea, benzene derivatives, hydroxyl amines, alkenes) interfere with miRNA maturation by binding Dicer.[66,76] Although the effects of environmental chemical carcinogens on the miRNA machinery have been described in detail recently,[66] they can be summed up by three mechanisms. First, in response to DNA damage, the p53/miRNA interconnection can modify the expression of miRNA genes in the nucleus. Second, electrophilic metabolites of environmental carcinogens can bind to nucleophilic sites of miRNA precursors thus forming miRNA adducts, which cannot access the catalytic pockets of Dicer in the cytoplasm. Third, metabolites of environmental carcinogens can bind to Dicer in the proximity of miRNA catalytic sites thus blocking maturation of miRNA precursors[66] (Figure 2). It remains, however, unclear to why oncomiRs are upregulated; which will be an important mechanism to delineate for a better understanding of chemical carcinogenesis and chemoprevention. To this end, there are ongoing studies identifying specific small molecule inhibitors of oncomir biogenesis.[77]

Because miRNA expression is also altered by nongenotoxic carcinogens,[66] there are additional mechanisms modulating expression outside of the DNA damage response pathway. Epigenetic mechanisms (e.g., hypermethylation of tumor suppressor miRNA), as well as direct effects on the transcriptional machinery and posttranscriptional modifiers, play a role. For example, hypermethylation of miRNA-124a in colon cancer results in the upregulation of the oncogene, Cdk6 kinase, and the phosphorylation of the tumor suppressor, pRb.[78] CpG island hypermethylation of additional tumor suppressor miRNAs has been shown, and the list is growing.[79-82] miRNAs have also been shown to target and alter the activity of DNMTs and other enzymes involved in epigenetic modulation (HDACs and histone acetyl transferases)[83-86] (Figure 2). Carcinogens, in turn, can play an integral part in this process. For example, nickel sulfide, which is a weak mutagen but strong carcinogen, can downregulate miRNA-152 via promoter-DNA hypermethylation.[84] Similarly, reactive oxygen species (ROS) inhibit miR-199a and miR-125b expression through increasing the promoter methylation of the miR-199a and miR-125b genes by DNMT1.[87]

Since many miRNAs are transcribed by PolII and associated factors,[73,88,89] it stands to reason that miRNA levels are altered by an impact of environmental carcinogens on PolII and other factors with resulting altered transcriptional regulation. miR-34a and miR-34b/c for example, are direct, conserved p53 target genes that mediate induction of apoptosis, cell cycle arrest, and senescence by p53.[90] When p53 is mutated [often by environmental carcinogens[91]], its transcriptional activity is compromised.[92] In a similar way, environmental carcinogens affect the activity of Pol II.[93]

Overall, it is clear that chemical carcinogens alter miRNA expression. As with many biological entities, these changes occur initially due to exposure as an adaptive response to the chemical insult. Such mechanisms that miRNA work include the activation of p53, cell cycle arrest, and apoptotic induction (e.g., by the miR-34 suppressor miRNA family). Proto-oncogene mutation ("initiation") (e.g., k-ras) can induce expression of other suppressor miRs such as the let7 family.[94] With long-term, extensive exposure, miRNA expression changes can become irreversible. This has been shown with the miR-34 and let-7 family members where their inactivation results in the suppression of p53 and activation of k-ras.[66,95] If miRNA replacement therapy becomes mainstream, this will be a powerful tool for changing and perhaps reversing the carcinogenic process induced by chemical carcinogens. Interestingly, recent studies have found that plant miRNAs consumed by mammals are detected in mammals (including humans), have activity in mammals, and have tumor-suppressive properties.[96-98]

Gene–environment interactions and interindividual variation

A cornerstone of human chemical carcinogenesis is the concept of gene–environment interactions (Figure 3, Box 3).[30,99] Potential inter-individual susceptibility to chemical carcinogenesis may well be defined by genetic variations in the host elements of this compound system. Functional polymorphisms in human proteins that have, or may have, a role in chemical carcinogenesis include enzymes that metabolize (i.e., activate and detoxify) xenobiotic substances, enzymes that repair DNA damage, cell surface receptors that activate the phosphorylation cascade, and cell cycle control genes (i.e., oncogenes and tumor suppressor genes that are elements of the signal transduction cascade).

> **Box 3** Gene–Environment Interactions
>
> Genes identified that modify response to chemical carcinogens include those involved in carcinogen metabolism (e.g., p450s), DNA repair (e.g., NER), cell signaling, cell cycle, and hormonal regulation.

When chemicals or xenobiotics encounter biological systems, they become altered by metabolic processes. This is an initial facet of gene–environment interaction. The inter-individual variation in carcinogen metabolism and macromolecular adduct formation arising from such processes was recognized almost 40 years ago.[100] The cytochrome P450 (CYP) multigene family is largely responsible for the metabolic activation and detoxication of many different chemical carcinogens in the human environment.[101] CYPs are Phase I enzymes that act by adding an atom of oxygen onto the substrate; they are induced by PAHs and chlorinated hydrocarbons.[101] Phase II enzymes act on oxidized substrates and also contribute to xenobiotic metabolism. Some Phase II enzymes are methyltransferases; acetyltransferases; glutathione transferases; uridine 5′-diphosphoglucuronosyl transferases; sulfotransferases; nicotinamide adenine dinucleotide (NAD)- and nicotinamide adenine dinucleotide phosphate (NADP)-dependent alcohol dehydrogenases; aldehyde; and steroid dehydrogenases; quinone reductases; NADPH diaphorase; azo reductases; aldoketoreductases; transaminases; esterases; and hydrolases. The pathways of activation and detoxification are often competitive, providing yet further potential for individual differences in propensity for carcinogen metabolism to DNA-damaging species. This scenario is further complicated by a second facet of gene–environment interaction that leads to enzyme induction or inhibition. In this case, environmental exposures alter gene expression, and genes responsible for carcinogen metabolism can be upregulated or repressed by certain chemical exposures.

A third facet of gene–environment interaction occurs when the chemical alters gene structure (environmentally predisposed abnormal DNA). Once a procarcinogen is metabolically activated to an ultimate carcinogenic form, it can bind covalently to cellular macromolecules, including DNA. This DNA damage can be repaired by several mechanisms.[102] Differences in rates and fidelity of DNA repair potentially influence the extent of carcinogen adduct formation (i.e., biologically effective dose) and, consequently, the total amount of genetic damage. The

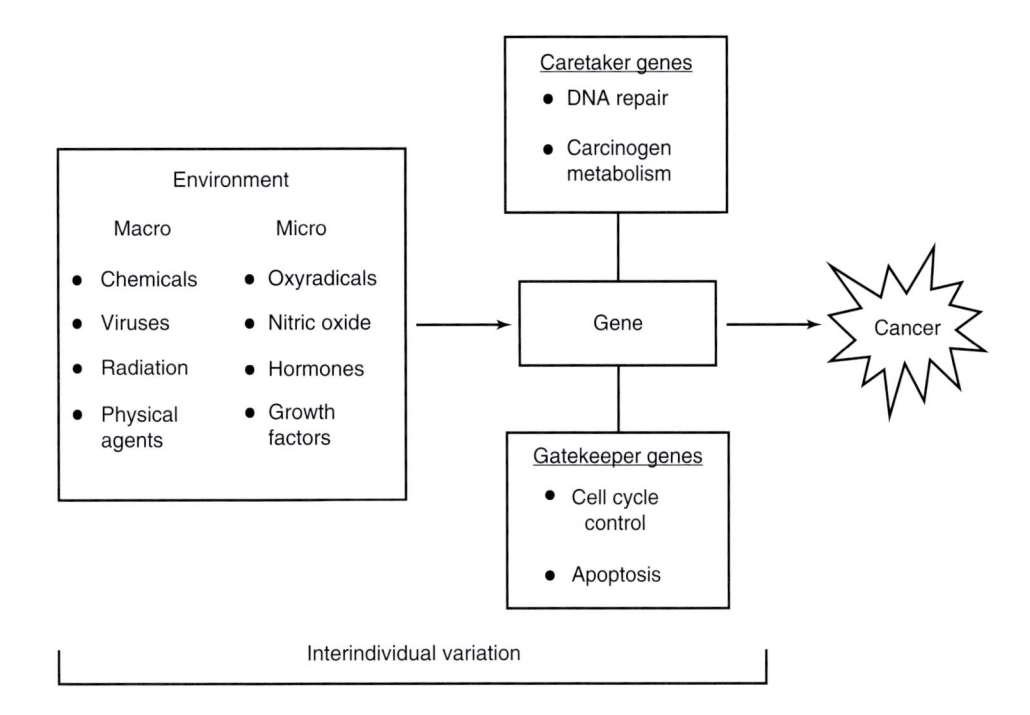

Figure 3 The concept of gene–environment interactions is multifaceted: (1) environmental chemicals are altered by the products of metabolic genes; (2) environmental chemicals disrupt the expression (induce or inhibit) of carcinogen metabolizing genes; and (3) environmental exposures cause changes (mutations) in cancer-related genes. The cancer-related genes have been classified as gatekeeper (e.g., APC) and caretaker (e.g., MSH1 and MLH1) genes. The interaction of these genes with external and internal environmental agents can lead to the derangement of regulatory pathways that maintain genetic stability and cellular proliferation.

consequences of polymorphisms in genes controlling the cell cycle (serine/threonine kinases, transcription factors, cyclins, cyclin-dependent kinase inhibitors, and cell surface receptors) are much less clear. However, molecular epidemiologic evidence suggests that certain common variants of these types of genes have a role in susceptibility to chemical carcinogenesis.[103] The evaluation of polymorphisms as potential biomarkers of susceptibility in the human population is discussed under "Implications for Molecular Epidemiology, Risk Assessment, and Cancer Prevention."

Carcinogen metabolism

Inter-individual variation in cancer susceptibility, and, consequently, meaningful human cancer risk assessment, involve determination of inherited host factors as well as exposure assessment. Metabolic polymorphisms have historically been determined by the use of indicator drugs (e.g., caffeine, debrisoquine, dextromethorphan, dapsone, and isoniazid), however, these assays are being replaced by direct genetic assays. This approach has allowed the investigation of diverse host factors for which indicator drugs were not available, and it has been applied to a wide variety of cancers.[104–108] Such studies have not only made a key impact in the area of pharmacogenomics,[109,110] but genetic indicators of propensity for carcinogen activation and detoxification, DNA-repair capacity, apoptosis, and cell-cycle control are all features of molecular epidemiologic studies that are complementary to adduct studies because of the implications for a biologically effective dose after exposure.

CYP polymorphisms, involved in carcinogen activation, and glutathione-S transferases, uridine diphosphate (UDP) glucuronosyltransferases, sulfotransferases, and N-acyltransferases, involved in both carcinogen activation and detoxification, could explain variations in cancer susceptibility among the human population. Evidence that absent protection of a functionally intact *GSTM1* gene correlates with an increased risk of tobacco-related lung cancer.[111] Similarly, the absence of GSTM1 and GSTT1 genes increases the risk of lung cancer because of radon exposure.[112] There is a substantial reduction in risk of lung adenocarcinoma associated with genetic polymorphism in CYP2A13, the most active CYP for the metabolic activation of tobacco-specific carcinogen NNK.[113] The finding that XRCC1, GSTM1, and COMT polymorphisms were strongly associated with lung cancer risk in smoking women is supportive of an interaction of repair, tobacco smoke metabolism, and estrogen metabolism in this disease and continues the controversy of an increased risk of lung cancer in women.[114] Also, UDP glucuronosyltransferases (e.g., *UGT1A1*, *UGT1A9*, *UGT2B7*) have been implicated in cancers of the head and neck. Persons inheriting reduced activity variants of *NAT1* and *NAT2* genes, resulting in the slow acetylator phenotype, are at a greater risk of aromatic amine-induced bladder cancer. This may include persons exposed through tobacco smoke inhalation.[115,116] Over the past 25 years, there have been advances in the understanding of carcinogen metabolism, interindividual variations, and cancer risk. A good review of the existing literature can be found elsewhere.[117]

PAHs, for example, B(a)P, were the first carcinogens to be chemically isolated.[118] They are composed of variable numbers of fused benzene rings that form incomplete combustion of fossil fuels and vegetable matter, they are common environmental contaminants. PAHs are chemically inert and require metabolism to exert their biological effects.[118] This multistep process involves the following: initial epoxidation (CYP), hydration of the epoxide (epoxide hydrolase), and subsequent epoxidation across the olefinic bond.[101,119] The result is the ultimate carcinogenic metabolite; in the case of B(a)P, it is r7, t8-dihydroxy-c9, 10 epoxy-7,8,9,10-tetrahydroxybenzo[a]pyrene (B[a]P-7,8-diol 9,10-epoxide, BPDE).[120] The biology of CYP (e.g., CYP1A1) metabolism has been elucidated, providing a molecular basis for inducibility and interindividual variation. Variations in cytochrome levels among humans have been documented.[121] The arene ring of BPDE opens spontaneously at the 10 position, revealing a carbonium ion that can form a covalent addition product (adduct) with cellular macromolecules, including DNA. Several DNA-adducts can be formed, the most abundant being at the exocyclic amino group of deoxyguanosine ([7R]-N 2-[10-7 β,8 a,9 a-trihydroxy-7,8,9,10-tetrahydro-benz[a]pyrene}yl]-deoxyguanosine; BPdG). One electron oxidation has been suggested as an alternative pathway of PAH activation, here a radical cation forms at the meso position (L-region). The resulting DNA adducts at the C8 of guanine (B(a)P-6-C8Gua and BP-6-C8dGua), the N7 of guanine and adenine (B(a)P-6-N7Gua and BP-6-N7Ade) likely undergo spontaneous depurination. Firm evidence for the exfoliation of these adducts in urine has been provided.[122]

Aromatic amines are found in cigarette smoke, diesel exhaust, industrial environments, and certain cooked foods. The compound, 4-aminobiphenyl, is thought to be responsible for bladder cancer among tobacco smokers and rubber industry workers.[123] In addition, nitrated PAHs are environmental contaminants that are related to aromatic amines by nitroreduction. Aromatic amines can be converted to an aromatic amide that is catalyzed by an acetyl-coenzyme A-dependent acetylation.[124] The acetylation phenotype varies among the population. Persons with the rapid acetylator phenotype are at a higher risk of colon cancer (especially in smokers),[125] whereas, those who are slow acetylators are at risk of bladder cancer.[125] This latter association may result from the fact that activation of aromatic amines by N-oxidation is a competing pathway for aromatic amine metabolism. The N-hydroxylation products when protonated (e.g., in the urinary bladder) are reactive and can cause DNA damage.

An initial activation step for both aromatic amines and amides is N-oxidation by CYP1A2. The reactions of N-hydroxyarylamines with DNA appear to be acid catalyzed, but they can be further activated by either an acetyl-coenzyme A-dependent O-acetylase or a 3′-phosphoadenosine-5′phosphosulfate-dependent O-sulfotransferase. The N-arylhydroxamic acids arise from the acetylation of N-hydroxyarylamines or N-hydroxylation of aromatic amides; they are not electrophilic and require further activation. The predominant pathway here occurs through acetyltransferase-catalyzed rearrangement to a reactive N-acetoxyarylamine. Sulfotransferase catalysis forms N-sulphonyloxy arylamines. This complex pathway results in two major adduct types, amides (acetylated) and amines (nonacetylated).

Heterocyclic amines form in food cooking from pyrolysis (>150 °C) of amino acids, creatinine, and glucose. They have been recognized as food mutagens, shown to form DNA adducts and cause liver tumors in primates.[126] These compounds are activated by CYP1A2, and their metabolites form DNA adducts in humans. The N-hydroxy metabolites of heterocyclic amines like 2-amino-3-methyl-imidazo-[4,5-f]quinoline (IQ) can react directly with DNA. Enzymic O-esterification of N-hydroxy metabolites plays a key role in activating food mutagens, and because the N-hydroxy metabolites are good substrates for transacetylases these chemicals may be implicated in colorectal cancer.

Aflatoxins (B1, B2, G1, and G2), metabolites of Aspergillus flavus, contaminate cereals, grain, and nuts. A positive correlation exists between dietary aflatoxin exposure and the incidence of liver cancer in developing countries, where grain spoilage is high. Aflatoxins B1 and G1 have an olefinic double bond at the 8,9-position that can be oxidized by several CYP.[101,119] This implies that the olefinic 8,9-bond is the activation site. Further support for this mechanism comes from studies of DNA-adducts and the prevalence of TP53 mutations in liver cancer. In people with liver cancer from parts of China and Africa, where food spoilage caused by molds is high, G : C to T : A transversions in codon 249 are frequent.[21,22,127] This phenomenon is consistent with metabolic activation of aflatoxin B1 and the formation of depurinating carcinogen–deoxyguanosine adducts.

Carcinogenic N-nitrosamines are ubiquitous environmental contaminants and can be found in food, alcoholic beverages, cosmetics, cutting oils, hydraulic fluid, rubber, and tobacco.[128] Tobacco-specific N-nitrosamines (TSNs), for example, NNK, are not formed by pyrolysis, which accounts for the highly carcinogenic nature of snuff and chewing tobacco.[129] TSNs are not symmetric so both small alkyl-adducts and large bulky adducts can be formed; for example, NNK metabolism gives rise to either a positively charged pyridyl-oxobutyl ion or a positively charged methyl ion, both of which are able to alkylate DNA.[45,130] Endogenous nitrosamines form when an amine reacts with nitrate alone or nitrite in the presence of acid. Thus, nitrite (used to cure meats) and L-cysteine, in the presence of acetaldehyde (from alcohol), form N-nitrosothiazolidine-4-carboxylic acid. N-nitrosodimethylamine undergoes a-hydroxylation, catalyzed primarily by the alcohol inducible CYP2E1, to form an unstable a-hydroxynitrosamine. The breakdown products are formaldehyde and methyl diazohydroxide. Methyl diazohydroxide and related compounds are powerful alkylating agents that can add a small functional group at multiple sites in DNA.

Nongenotoxic carcinogens may function at the level of the microenvironment by dysregulation of hormones and growth factors, or indirectly inducing DNA damage and mutations through the action of free radicals. These chemicals are not reactive or poorly reactive and are resistant to activation through metabolism. They are also characterized by their persistence in biological systems and consequently tend to accumulate in the food chain. However, they can stimulate oxyradical formation by at least three mechanisms: organochlorine species interact with the Ah receptor which can lead to CYP induction and associated oxyradical formation; interaction with other receptors, like IFN-γ, can stimulate elements of the primary immune response and again generate oxyradicals; and agents like asbestos can promote oxyradical formation through interaction with ferrous metal. The resulting oxyradicals can then damage DNA. Some of the so-called "nongenotoxic" carcinogens might more appropriately be considered to be "oxyradical triggers." Indeed, chronic inflammatory states, which involve oxyradical formation, can also be cancer risk factors.[131–135]

DNA damage and repair

Another facet of inter-individual variation in risk for cancer from chemical carcinogens is inter-individual differences in the ability to repair damage from chemical carcinogens. DNA damage initiates a complex network of signaling cascades.[136] The chemical structure of DNA can be altered by a carcinogen in several ways: the formation of large bulky aromatic adducts, small alkyl adducts, oxidation, dimerization, and deamination. In addition, double- and single-strand breaks can occur. Chemical carcinogens can cause epigenetic changes, such as altering the DNA methylation status that leads to the silencing of specific gene expression.[44]

A complex pattern of carcinogen–DNA adducts likely results from a variety of environmental exposures, because of the mixture of different chemical carcinogens present.

Many DNA-repair genes have been described recently, and a growing number of polymorphisms have been identified for which molecular epidemiologic studies have provided evidence that genetic variation in these attributes can be a human cancer risk factor; as well as be used to tailor cancer chemotherapy.[137,138] Typically, these types of molecular epidemiological studies initially focus on high exposure groups such as workers, patients taking therapeutic drugs, and tobacco smokers. Several polymorphisms in DNA repair genes have now been implicated in tobacco-related neoplasms.[139] An interesting theory developed recently is a so-called, "hide-then-hit" hypothesis. This describes and importance of DNA repair variants in escaping checkpoint surveillance. Only cells with subtle defects in repair capacity arising from low-penetrance variants of DNA repair genes would have the opportunity to grow and accumulate the genetic changes needed for cancer formation, without triggering cell-cycle checkpoint surveillance.[140]

BPDE reacts with the exocyclic (N2) amino group of deoxyguanosine and resides within the minor groove of the double helix; it is typical of PAHs. This adduct, BPdG, is probably the most common, persistent adduct of B(a)P in mammalian systems, but others are possible. Adducts like BPdG are thought to induce ras gene mutations, which are common in tobacco-related lung cancers.[141,142] Aromatic amine adducts are more complex, because they have both acetylated and nonacetylated metabolic intermediates, and they form covalent bonds at the C8, N2, and sometimes O6 positions of deoxyguanosine as well as deoxyadenosine. The major adducts, however, are C8-deoxyguanosine adducts, which reside predominantly in the major groove of the DNA double helix.[143]

Aflatoxin B1 and G1 activation through hydroxylation of the olefinic 8,9-position results in adduct formation at the N7-position of deoxyguanosine. These are relatively unstable with a half-life of approximately 50 h at neutral pH; depurination products have been detected in urine.[144] The aflatoxin B1–N7-deoxyguanosine adduct also can undergo ring opening to yield two pyrimidine adducts; alternately, aflatoxin B1-8,9-dihydrodiol could result, restoring the DNA molecular structure if hydrolysis of the original adduct occurs.[145]

DNA alkylation can occur at many sites either following the metabolic activation of certain N-nitrosamines, or directly by the action of the N-alkylureas (N-methyl-N-nitrosourea) or the N-nitrosoguanidines. The protonated alkyl-functional groups that become available to form lesions in DNA generally attack the following nucleophilic centers: adenine (N1, N3, and N7), cytosine (N3), guanine (N2, O6, and N7), and thymine (O2, N3, and O4). Some of these lesions are known to be repaired (O6-methyldeoxyguanosine), while others are not (N7-methyldeoxyguanosine), which explains why O6-methyldeoxyguanosine is a promutagenic lesion and N7-methyldeoxyguanosine is not.[146,147]

Another potentially mutagenic cause of DNA damage is the deamination of DNA-methylated cytosine residues. 5-Methylcytosine comprises approximately 3% of deoxynucleotides. In this case, deamination at a CpG dinucleotide gives rise to a TpG mismatch. Repair of this lesion most often restores the CpG; however, repair may cause a mutation (TpA).[148] Deamination of cytosine also can generate a C to T transition if uracil glycosylation and G-T mismatch repair are inefficient.

Oxyradical damage can form thymine glycol or 8-hydroxydeoxyguanosine adducts. Exposure to organic peroxides (catechol, hydroquinone, and 4-nitroquinoline-N-oxide) leads to oxyradical damage; however, oxyradicals and hydrogen peroxide can be generated in lipid peroxidation and the catalytic cycling of some enzymes, as well as environmental sources (e.g., tobacco smoke).[131,149] Certain drugs and plasticizers can stimulate cells to produce peroxisomes, and oxyradical formation is mediated through protein kinase C when inflammatory cells are exposed to tumor promoters like phorbol esters.[150] Oxyradicals can contribute to deamination through induction of NO synthase.[151]

Maintenance of genome integrity requires mitigation of DNA damage. Thus, diminished DNA repair capacity is associated with carcinogenesis, birth defects, premature aging, and foreshortened lifespan. DNA-repair enzymes act at DNA damage sites caused by chemical carcinogens, and six major mechanisms are known: direct DNA repair, nucleotide excision repair, base excision repair, nonhomologous end joining (double-strand break repair), mismatch repair, and homologous recombination (postreplication repair).[152,153]

In the presence of nonlethal DNA damage, cell-cycle progression is postponed for repair mechanisms. This highly coordinated process involves multiple genes. A DNA-damage recognition sensor triggers a signal transduction cascade and downstream factors direct G1 and G2 arrest in concert with the proteins operationally responsible for the repair process. Although there are at least six discrete repair mechanisms, within five of them there are numerous multiprotein complexes comprising all the machinery necessary to accomplish the step-by-step repair function.

Generically, DNA repair requires damage recognition, damage removal or excision, resynthesis or patch synthesis, and ligation. Recent advances have led to the cloning of more than 130 human genes involved in five of these DNA repair pathways. A list of these genes and their specific functions was published elsewhere.[154] These genes are responsible for the fidelity of DNA repair, and when they are defective the mutation rate increases. This is the mutator phenotype.[33–35] Mutations in at least 30 DNA-repair-associated genes have been linked to increased cancer susceptibility or premature aging (Table 3).[154] Moreover, the role of common polymorphisms in some of these genes is associated with increased susceptibility in a gene–environment interaction scenario (this is discussed under "Implications for Molecular Epidemiology, Risk Assessment, and Cancer Prevention"). Indeed, molecular epidemiologic evidence suggests that tobacco-smoking-related lung cancer is associated with a polymorphism in the nucleotide excision repair gene, XPC (ERCC2).[155]

Direct DNA repair is affected by DNA alkyltransferases. These enzymes catalyze translocation of the alkyl moiety from an alkylated base (e.g., O6-methyldeoxyguanosine) to a cysteine residue at their active site in the absence of DNA strand scission. Thus, one molecule of the enzyme is capable of repairing one DNA alkyl lesion, in a suicide mechanism. The inactivation of this mechanism by promoter hypermethylation is associated with Kras G to A mutations in colon cancer.[156]

In DNA nucleotide excision repair, lesion recognition, preincision, incision, gap-filling, and ligation are required, and the so-called excinuclease complex comprises 16 or more different proteins. Large distortions caused by bulky DNA adducts (e.g., BPDE-dG and 4ABP-dC) are recognized (XPA) and removed by endonucleases (XPF, XPG, FEN). A patch is then constructed ($pol\Delta$, $pol\varepsilon$) and the free ends are ligated.

Base excision repair also removes a DNA segment containing an adduct; however, small adducts (e.g., 3-methyladenine) are

Table 3 Examples of disease susceptibility and disease syndromes associated with mutations in DNA-repair genes.

Gene	Function	Pathology or cancer
Cancer susceptibility		
MMRa		
MLH1	Damage recognition	HNPCC2b, glioma
MLH2	DNA binding	HNPCC1, ovarian cancer
MSH3	—	Endometrial cancer
MSH6	Sliding clamp	Endometrial cancer, HNPCC1
PMS1	Damage recognition	HNPCC3
PMS2	Repair initiation	HNPCC4, glioblastoma
NER		
BRCA-1	Directs p53 transcription towards DNA-repair pathways	Breast cancer, ovarian cancer
RB1	Cell-cycle restriction	Retinoblastoma, breast cancer, and progression osteosarcoma
DSB		
BRCA-2	Regulation of RAD51	Breast cancer, pancreatic cancer
HR		
RAD54	Helicase	Colon cancer, breast cancer, NHL
Other		
TP53 (DSB, NER, HR)	Cell-cycle control; exonuclease; apoptosis; DNA binding	Colon cancer, common somatic defect in human cancer in general; inherited in Li-Fraumeni syndrome and some breast cancers
hOgg1 (Various)	Glycosylase	Cancer susceptibility
Xeroderma pigmentosum (XP)		
NER		
XPD	DNA Helicase	Skin and neurologic, but later onset than XPA
XPB	DNA Helicase	Skin lesions
XPG	Endonuclease	Acute sun sensitivity, mild symptoms; late skin cancer
XPC (and BER)	Exonuclease	Mental retardation; skin sensitivity; microcephaly
DDB1 and DDB2	Binds specific DNA damage	XPE—Mild skin sensitivity
XPA	Damage sensor	XPA—Skin and neurologic problems: the most severe XP
XPC	Damage sensor	XPC—Skin, tongue, and lip cancer
XPE	Damage sensor	XPE—Neurologically normal
PRR		
POLH	Polymerase	XPV—Mild to severe skin sensitivity; neurologically normal
Other syndromes		
NER		
Cockaynes		
CSB	ATPase	Cutaneous, ocular, neurologic, and somatic abnormalities; short stature, progressive deafness, mental retardation, neurologic degeneration, early death; sometimes presents together with XPB
Juberg-Marsidi		
ATRX	Putative helicase	Thalassemia/mental retardation
SB		
Nijmegen		
NBS1	Nibrin, cell-cycle regulation	Microencephaly; mental retardation; immunodeficiency; growth retardation; radiation sensitivity; predisposition to malignancy
Ataxia-telangiectasia		
ATM	Phosphorylation	Neurologic deficiencies, manifest by inability to coordinate muscle actions; skin and corneal telangiectases. Leukemia, lymphoma, and other malignancies (breast cancer?)
MRE11 (Ataxia-like)	Exonuclease	DNA damage sensitivity; genomic instability; telomere shortening; aberrant meiosis; severe combined immunodeficiency
PRKDC	Ser/Thr kinase	SCID
Bloom's		
BLM	DNA Helicase	High rate of spontaneous lymphatic and other malignancy; high rate SCEc
Fanconi anemia		
FANCA-G	Protein control	Multiple congenital malformations; chromosome breaks; pancytopenia Telomere shortening
Werner		
WRN	DNA Helicase/Exonuclease	Premature senility, short stature, exonuclease rapidly progressing cataracts, loss of connective tissue and muscle, premature arteriosclerosis, increase risk of malignancy
RecQ4	DNA Helicase	Osteosarcoma; premature aging

BER, base excision; DSB, double-strand break; HR, homologous recombination; MMR, mismatch; NER, nucleotide excision; PRR, postreplication; SB, strand break; HNPCC, hereditary nonpolyposis colon cancer; NHL, non-Hodgkin lymphoma; SCE, sister chromatid exchange; SCID, severe combined immunodeficiency.

generally the target so that there is overlap with direct repair. The adduct is removed by a glycosylase (hOgg1, UDG), an apurinic endonuclease (APE1 or HAP1) degrades a few bases on the damaged strand, and a patch is synthesized (pol β) and ligated (DNA ligases: I, II, IIIα, IIIβ, and IV).

DNA mismatches occasionally occur, because excision repair processes incorporate unmodified or conventional, but noncomplementary, Watson–Crick bases opposite each other in the DNA helix. Transition mispairs (G-T or A-C) are repaired by the mismatch repair process more efficiently than transversion mispairs (G-G, A-A, G-A, C-C, C-T, and T-T). The mechanism for correcting mispairings is similar to that for nucleotide excision repair and resynthesis described earlier, but it generally involves the excision of large pieces of the DNA containing mispairings. Because the mismatch recognition protein is required to bind simultaneously to the mismatch and an unmethylated adenine in a GATC recognition sequence, it removes the whole intervening DNA sequence. The parental template strand is then used by the polymerase to fill the gap.

Double-strand DNA breaks can occur from exposure to ionizing radiation and oxidation. Consequences of double-strand DNA breaks are the inhibition of replication and transcription, and loss of heterozygosity. Double-strand DNA break repair occurs through homologous recombination, where the joining of the free ends is mediated by a DNA–protein kinase in a process that also protects the ends from nucleolytic attack. The free ends of the DNA then undergo ligation by DNA ligase IV. Genes known to code for DNA-repair enzymes that participate in this process include XRCC4, XRCC5, XRCC6, XRCC7, HRAD51B, HRAD52, RPA, and ATM.

Postreplication repair is a damage-tolerance mechanism and it occurs in response to DNA replication on a damaged template. The DNA polymerase stops at the replication fork when DNA damage is detected on the parental strand. Alternately, the polymerase proceeds past the lesion, leaving a gap in the newly synthesized strand. The gap is filled in one of two ways: either by recombination of the homologous parent strand with the daughter strand in a process that is mediated by a helical nucleoprotein (RAD51); or when a single nucleotide gap remains, mammalian DNA polymerases insert an adenine residue. Consequently, this mechanism may lead to recombinational events as well as base-mispairing.

Persistent nonrepaired DNA damage blocks the replication machinery. Cells have evolved translesion synthesis (TLS) DNA polymerases to bypass these blocks.[157] Most of these TLS polymerases belong to the recently discovered Y-family, have much lower stringency than replicative polymerases, and thus are error prone. An increased mutation frequency is an evolutionary trade-off for cellular survival.

Mutator phenotype

Cancer cells contain substantial numbers of genetic abnormalities when compared with normal cells. These abnormalities range from gross changes such as nondiploid number of chromosomes, that is, aneuploidy, and translocations or rearrangements of chromosomes, to much smaller changes in the DNA sequence including deletions, insertions, and single nucleotide substitutions. Therefore, carcinogenesis involves *errors* in (1) chromosomal segregation; (2) repair of DNA damage induced by either endogenous free radicals or environmental carcinogens; and (3) DNA replication. Loeb originally formulated the concept of the mutator phenotype in 1974[33,34] to account for the high numbers of mutations in cancer cells when compared to the rarity of mutations in normal cells. Recent advances in the molecular analysis of carcinogenesis in human cells and animal models have refined the mutator phenotype[35,158] concept that is also linked to the clonal selection theory proposed by Nowell (Figure 4).[159] Generally, the mutator phenotype hypothesis proposes that mutation rates in normal cells are insufficient to account for the large number of mutations found in cancer cells. Consequently, human tumors exhibit an elevated mutation rate that increases the likelihood of a tumor acquiring advantageous mutations. The hypothesis predicts that tumors are composed of cells harboring hundreds of thousands of mutations, as opposed to a small number of specific driver mutations, and that malignant cells within a tumor, therefore, constitute a highly heterogeneous population.[158]

Racial, gender, and socioeconomic disparities in chemical carcinogenesis

Genetic polymorphisms may also partially explain the increased risk of cancer-associated chemical carcinogens amongst different genders, race, and ethnicity. One of the biggest controversies

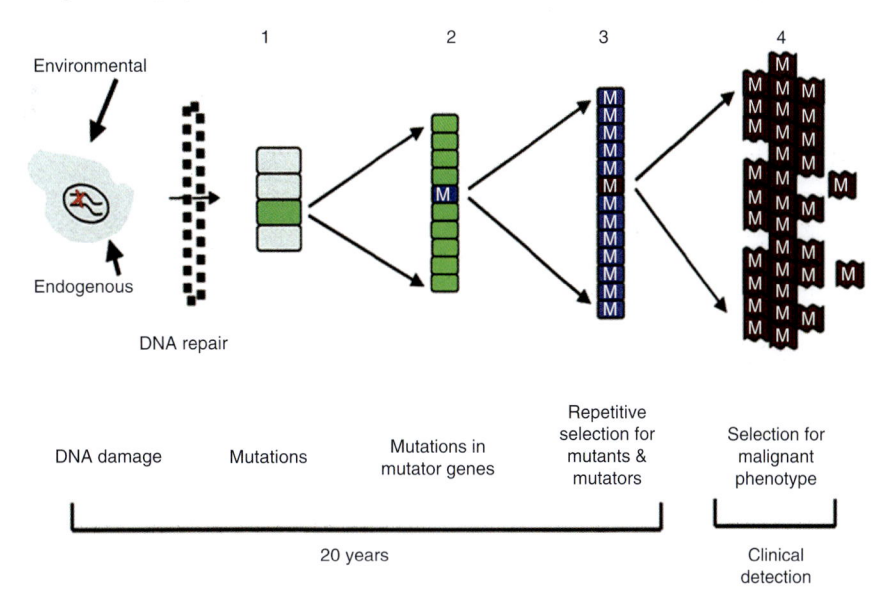

Figure 4 Mutation accumulation during tumor progression. (1) Random mutations result when DNA damage exceeds the cell's capacity for error-free DNA repair. (2) These random mutations can result in clonal expansion and mutations in mutator genes (M). (3) Repetitive rounds of selection for mutants yield co-selection mutants in mutator genes. (4) From this population of mutant cancer cells, there is selection for cells that escape the host's regulatory mechanisms for the control of cell replication, invasion, and metastasis.

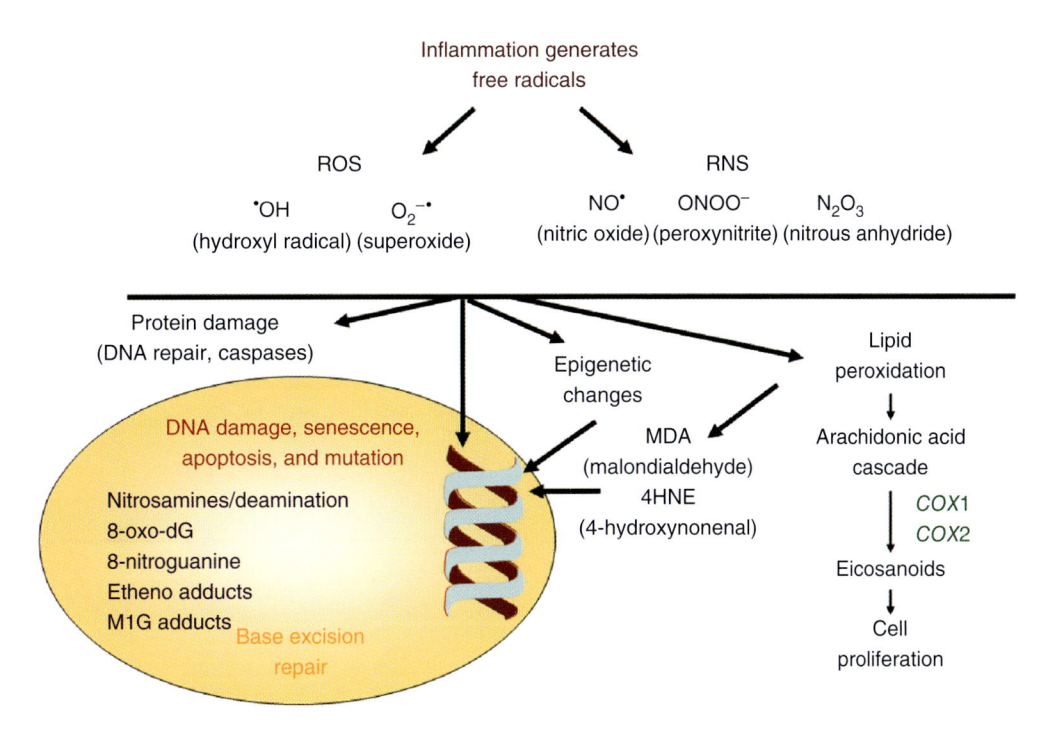

Figure 5 Several reactive oxygen (ROS) and reactive nitrogen species (RNS) are generated during chronic inflammation. The reactive species can induce DNA damage, including point mutations in cancer-related genes, and modifications in essential cellular proteins that are involved in DNA repair, apoptosis, and cell cycle, either directly or indirectly through the activation of lipid peroxidation and generation of reactive aldehydes, for example, malondialdehyde (MDA) and 4-hydroxynonenal (4-HNE).

(e.g., GpX, catalase, MnSOD) free radicals also exist; can modify the effects of drugs; and increase or decrease cancer risk associated with exogenous chemical carcinogens.[186–194] Indeed, many environmental carcinogens, including both conventional cigarettes and e-cigarettes[195] have the capacity to drive inflammation and cause DNA damage[195,196]; and this is a key component of the carcinogenic process associated with lung cancer.

Oncogenes and tumor suppressor genes

Chronic exposures to carcinogens, accumulation of mutations, development of the mutator phenotype, and clonal selection during several decades result in cancer. Although the phenotypic traits of individual cancers are highly variable, commonly acquired capabilities include limitless replicative potential, self-sufficiency in growth signals, insensitivity to antigrowth signals, evading apoptosis, tissue invasion, sustained angiogenesis, and metastasis.[39] These phenotypic traits reflect a complex molecular circuitry of biochemical pathways and protein machines within cancer cells.[197]

The genes encoding the proteins within the cancer-associated molecular circuitry are of many functional classes and, historically, have been conceptually divided into oncogenes and tumor suppressor genes[197,198] (Box 4). Detailed descriptions of oncogenes and tumor suppressor genes are found in *Chapters 4* and *5*. The *ras* oncogene and the *TP53* tumor suppressor gene will be used as examples of molecular targets of chemical carcinogens.

> **Box 4** Oncogenes and Suppressor Genes
>
> Oncogenes and Suppressor genes are targets of chemical carcinogens. Many genes, including K-ras and p53, have specific sequences targeted by chemical carcinogens resulting in mutational "hotspots." These mutations cause a change in expression and activity of the RNA and protein they code for.

Activated *ras* genes predominate as the family of oncogenes to be isolated from solid tumors that are induced by chemicals in laboratory animals. Members of the *ras* gene family code for proteins of molecular weight 21,000 (p21); these proteins are membrane bound, have GTPase activity, and form complexes with other proteins. The *ras* genes encode small G-proteins (guanine nucleotide binding) that exert a powerful proliferative response through the signal transduction cascade. The first direct evidence of proto-oncogene activation by a chemical carcinogen was obtained from in vitro studies.[199] A wild-type recombinant clone of the human *Ha-ras* gene (pEC) was modified with BPDE. The treated plasmid was then used to transfect murine NIH-3T3 cells, with the result that the transformed cell foci contained the same point mutations (in either codon 12 or 61) known to exist in activated *ras* genes isolated from human tumors including the bladder (pEJ). In animal models of chemical carcinogenesis and surveys of different types of human tumors that arise from a variety of environmental exposures, *ras* mutations have been found.[200–203] For example, tobacco smoke can mutate *K-ras* during the molecular pathogenesis of human lung adenocarcinoma.[204] In rodents, PAHs (3-methylcholanthrene, 7,12-dimethylbenz[a]anthracene and B[a]P) have been used repeatedly to produce both benign tumors and malignant carcinomas. A large proportion of these premalignant and malignant lesions have mutations in either the twelfth or sixty-first codons. Similarly, treatment of rats with either 7,12-dimethylbenz[a]anthracene or N-methyl-N-nitrosourea resulted in the development of mammary carcinomas containing *ras* codon 12 or 61 mutations. These types of mutations also have been observed in mouse skin after initiation with 7,12-dimethylbenz[a]anthracene and tumor promotion with TPA. Mutations in *ras* have been found in mouse liver after treatment with vinyl carbamate, hydroxydehydroestragole, or N-hydroxy-2-acetylaminofluorene. The same point mutations have been found in murine thymic lymphomas after treatment with N-methyl-N-nitrosourea or γ-radiation, and in other rodent skin models after treatment with methylmethanesulfonate, α-propiolactone, dimethylcarbamyl chloride, or N-methyl-N9-nitro-N-nitrosoguanidine.

These data indicate that chemical carcinogens may produce site-specific mutations based, in part, on nucleoside selectivity of the ultimate carcinogen. Interestingly, noncovalent binding sites for (+)-anti-BPDE have recently been found on codons 12 and 13 of the K-ras gene.[205] Persistence of a specific mutation, however, also depends on the amino acid substitution in that the function of the mutant protein is altered to confer on the cell a selective clonal growth advantage. The types of mutations that are found in chemically activated ras genes cause conformational changes that alter protein binding (GTPase-activating protein) in such a way that the ras-MAP kinase pathway is permanently activated. Data support the hypothesis that ras activation is associated with malignant conversion as well as tumor initiation. Transfection of activated ras genes into benign papillomas that did not contain a constitutively activated ras gene caused malignant progression.[203,206] These and other results implicate ras mutations in chemical carcinogenesis. Similarly, malignant transformation occurred when immortalized human bronchial epithelial cells were transfected with an activated ras gene.[207,208] Ki-ras gene mutations are also one of many changes that can arise either early or late in the development of colorectal carcinoma.[209] These findings indicate that the accumulation of mutations, and not necessarily the order in which they occur, contributes to multistage carcinogenesis. Furthermore, the stage of carcinogenesis in which each mutation occurs is not necessarily fixed. In the model for human colorectal carcinoma, ras mutations most often occur during malignant conversion but can be an early event (i.e., tumor initiation), but in the rodent skin models, ras mutations appear to be primarily a tumor-initiating event. These differences may reflect the type of exposure, both in terms of chemical class and chronic versus acute exposure, or they may be a function of tissue type.

The TP53 tumor suppressor gene is central in the response pathway to cellular stress.[210] For example, DNA damage caused by chemical carcinogens activates the p53 tumor suppressor protein by posttranslational modification to transduce signals to "guard the genome"[211] by engaging cell cycle checkpoints and enhancing DNA repair, and as a fail-safe mechanism, to cause replicative senescence or apoptotic death.[212,213] Mutations in the TP53 gene or inactivation of its encoded protein by viral oncoproteins generally lead to a loss of these cellular defense functions. Not surprisingly, TP53 mutations are common in human cancer.[214,215]

Molecular analysis of TP53 can give clues to the environmental etiology of cancer (Table 5). It is implicit from the preceding text (see "DNA Damage and Repair") that the covalent binding of activated carcinogens to DNA is not random. Therefore, the formation of a particular DNA lesion to some extent may be deduced from the resulting mutation. A dramatic example of this phenomenon is the previously mentioned TP53 codon 249 mutation, which is detected in almost all aflatoxin-related hepatocellular carcinomas.[217–219] The striking nature of this association could arise by two distinct mechanisms. First, the third base in codon 249 (AGG) may be unusually susceptible to activated aflatoxin B1 mutations. As discussed earlier, aflatoxin B1-8,9-oxide causes a promutagenic lesion by covalently binding to the N7 position of deoxyguanosine. Alternately, cells bearing the codon 249 lesion may have an important selective growth advantage. Evidence that a combination of these factors is responsible has been presented as well.[220] Another prominent example where circumstantial evidence points to specific molecular events is that of TP53 mutations indicative of pyrimidine dimer formation in ultraviolet light-related skin cancers.[221] In the case of tobacco smoking and lung cancer, G : C to T : A transversions indicate the formation of adducts from activated bulky carcinogens (e.g., PAHs).[217,222]

Table 5 Mutational spectra of TP53 in human cancers.[a]

Carcinogen exposure	Neoplasm	Mutation
Aflatoxin B1	Hepatocellular carcinoma	Codon 249 (AGG 6 AGT)
Sunlight	Skin carcinoma	Dipyrimidine mutations (CC 6 TT) on nontranscribed DNA strand
Tobacco smoke	Lung carcinoma	G:C 6 T:A mutations on nontranscribed DNA strand (frequently codons: 157, 248, and 273)
Tobacco and alcohol	Carcinoma of the head and neck	Increased frequency p53 mutations (especially codons 157 and 248)
Radon	Lung carcinoma	Codon 249 (AGG 6 ATG)
Vinyl chloride	Hepatic angiosarcoma	A:T 6 T:A transversions
Aristolochic acid	Urothelial Carcinoma	A to T transversions

[a]For reviews Pfeifer and Besaratinia.[216]

Mutation signatures associated with chemical carcinogenesis

Somatic mutations in cancer genomes are caused by multiple mutational processes, each of which generates a characteristic mutational signature. In line with specific mutation hotspots associated with exposure to chemicals (Table 5), databases, bioinformatics, and technology have evolved such that we can identify somatic mutation signatures and link these to environmental exposure. Recently, the Pan-Cancer Analysis of Whole Genomes (PCAWG), Consortium of the International Cancer Genome Consortium (ICGC), and The Cancer Genome Atlas (TCGA) characterized mutational signatures using >80 million somatic mutations from 4645 whole-genome and 19,184 exome sequences that included most types of cancer. They revealed associations of signatures to exogenous or endogenous exposures (e.g., mutation signatures caused by tobacco mutagens, UV light, aflatoxin, and chemotherapy), as well as to defective DNA-maintenance processes.[26,27] Linking dysbiosis to carcinogenesis, it was found that E. coli releasing colibactin (which alkylates DNA on adenine residues and drives double strand breaks) causes a distinct mutation signature and may be a key driver of CRC in some people.[28] However, many signatures are of unknown cause; and the next steps toward linking specific exposome agents to these signatures require further precise and rigorous study. The next phases will bring the cancer genomics community together with epidemiologists, healthcare providers, pharmaceutical companies, data science, and clinical trials groups to build comprehensive knowledge banks of mutation signatures in otherwise healthy tissue, clinical outcome, and treatment data from patients with a wide variety of cancers, matched with detailed molecular profiling.

Precision medicine, molecular epidemiology, and prevention

Precision medicine is a concept developed by an *ad hoc* committee of the National Research Council in 2011.[24] The four basic premises are (1) the *Information Commons* for cancer has to be populated with a variety of—omic, phenotypic, clinical, and epidemiological data; (2) these data are integrated into a *Knowledge Network* that examines the interconnectivity of each layer of data from the Information Commons; (3) the Knowledge Network is used to develop *Taxonomic Classifiers* with the goal of improving patient diagnosis, decisions on therapeutic strategies and health outcomes; and, finally, the knowledge is used to *guide biomedical, prevention and clinical research* in mechanistic and observational studies (Figure 6). Precision Medicine builds on the—omics revolution in molecular biology advances in bioinformatics, tumor metabolism, tumor immunology, and the gene–environment concept of molecular epidemiology.

One of the biggest challenges in molecular cancer epidemiology associated with exposure to chemical carcinogens is to accurately measure exposure then link this exposure to cancer risk. In this sense, so far, results have been disappointing. Traditionally, the paradigm, first defined by Perera and Weinstein in 1982,[19] has involved the assessment of exposure (what chemical and how much of that chemical; for example, how much tobacco smoke or more specifically, B(a)P; BPDE; TSN, etc.), internal dose (how much of that chemical is in the body fluids, and tissues; e.g., amount of nicotine/cotinine), biologically effective dose (the interaction of the chemical with biological entities; e.g., BPDE adducts), early biological response (e.g., TP53 mutation; k-ras mutation), altered structure/function (e.g., TP53 downstream functions; k-ras overexpression), and clinical disease (cancer). Intertwined with this paradigm are genetic factors and an individual's susceptibility (e.g., polymorphisms in metabolic enzymes such as p450's discussed earlier). A goal, then, of molecular cancer epidemiology is to identify biomarkers (of exposure, effect, and susceptibility) that accurately predict risk of disease. Unfortunately, to date, other than susceptibility markers (e.g., BRCA1/2 for breast cancer risk; APC for familial colon cancer and more), few truly accurate biomarkers exist. Part of the reason, is the money, manpower, and time it takes to identify a biomarker, then follow that ahead in time (decades for the most part) to accurately assess cancer risk.

To this end, over the past decade, with new, highly sensitive, and sophisticated technology, this concept is evolving. The "omics" field, for example, has quickly advanced, with uses in the field of chemical carcinogen exposure and risk of cancer from that exposure. Using genetic information ("genomics"), biomarkers of susceptibility have been identified. In addition to such examples as BRCA1 or APC, polymorphisms in metabolic enzymes and DNA repair pathways have been discussed. Genomics, tied in with other "omics" (adductomics, epigenomics, transcriptomics, proteomics, microbiomics, metabolomics, and cytokinomics) can

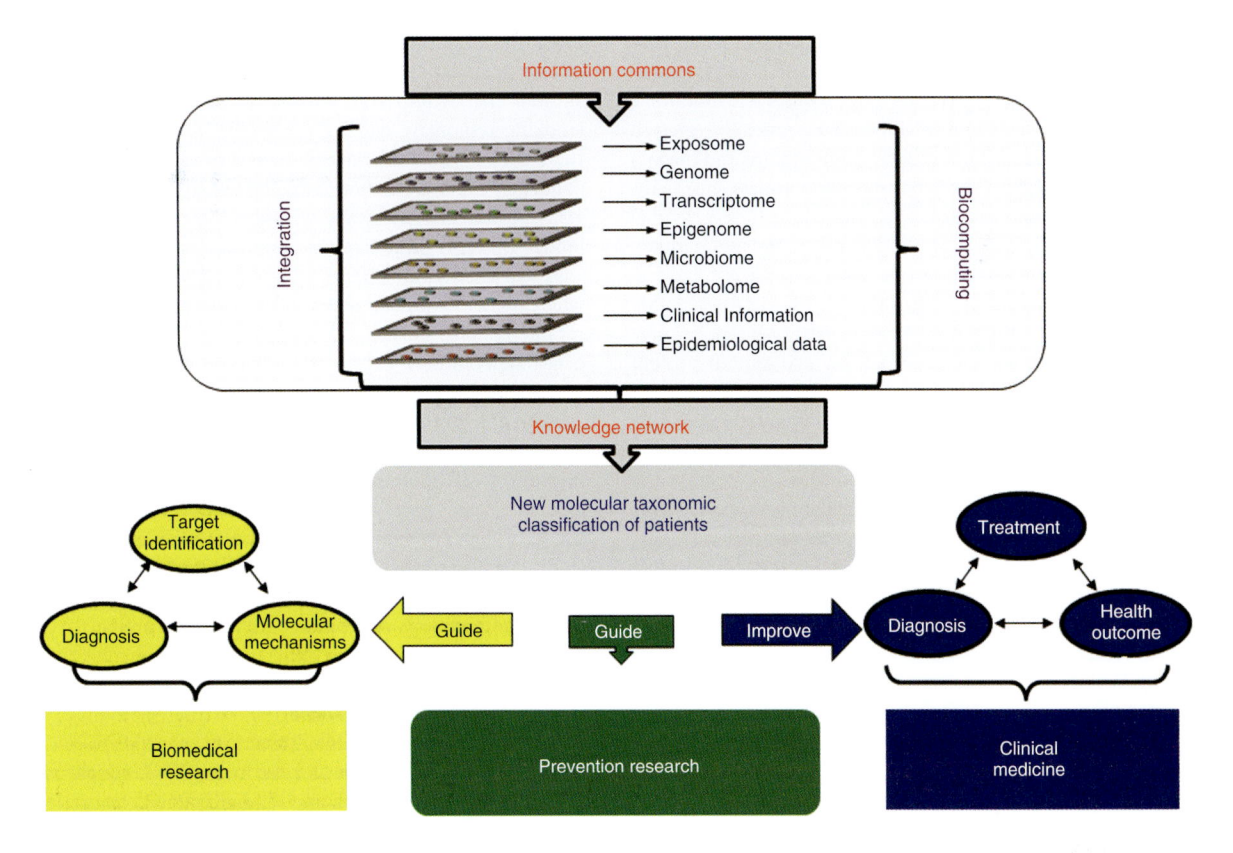

Figure 6 Precision Medicine. In March 2011, at the request of the Director of the National Institutes of Health, an ad hoc Committee of the National Research Council met to discuss the feasibility, need, scope, impact, and consequences of defining a "New Taxonomy" of human diseases based on molecular biology. The concept that developed, that of Precision Medicine, includes four basic premises.[24] First, the Information Commons for each disease type has to be populated with a variety of omic, phenotypic, clinical, and epidemiological data. Second, these data are integrated into a Knowledge Network that examines the interconnectivity of each layer of data from the information commons. Third, the knowledge network is used to develop new Taxonomic Classifiers with the goal of improving patient diagnosis, decisions on therapeutic strategies, and health outcomes. Finally, the knowledge is used to guide biomedical and clinical research in mechanistic and observational studies. If realized, the benefits of precision medicine can be leveraged for most, if not all, disease types including cancer.

be a powerful tool if properly linked to environmental chemical exposure. An evolving concept has been the "exposome".[23,223] In general, the exposome comprises every exposure to which an individual is subjected, from conception to death. Three broad categories of exposure are categorized: (1) internal exposure (metabolism, endogenous circulating hormones, body morphology, physical activity, gut microbiota, inflammation, aging); (2) specific external exposures (radiation, infections, chemical contaminants, diet, tobacco, alcohol, occupation, medical interventions); and (3) more general exposures/social/economic influences (education, financial status, psychological stress, climate). Although the concept has obvious uses in epidemiological studies to establish risk factors at a population level,[223] linking numbers to and quantifying the exposome ("exposomics") will be a necessary step to devise chemopreventive strategies (Figures 6 and 7).

Reconsideration of the dogma is necessary, because an extremely difficult task is to directly link a single genomic change to risk of specific types of cancer. Using genomics for somatic mutations, for example, as discussed above, we have identified specific Kras and TP53 mutational hotspots linked to specific carcinogens. The catalog of somatic mutations in cancer (COSMIC) indicates k-ras is the most frequently mutated isoform of ras isoforms and is present in 22% of all tumors analyzed compared to 8% for N-ras and 3% for H-ras and may prove to be an indicator of prognosis or a guide to treatment. The TP53 tumor suppressor gene is mutated in most types of human cancers and it is the most commonly mutated gene yet known (e.g., mutations in TP53 are found in approximately 50% of lung cancers).[217] Unlike ras gene mutations that are found in highly specific regions (codons 12, 13, 59, and 61), TP53 mutations occur more widely. This is presumably because a positive growth advantage is conveyed only with specific ras mutations and the loss of TP53 tumor suppressor function can occur with less specificity. However, for some malignancies, TP53 mutations have provided clues to cancer etiology with a specific signature ("hotspot") linked to specific carcinogenic exposure (see Table 5).[21,22,29,214,217,224,225] TP53 is further distinguished from other genetic lesions in that several possible mutant phenotypes can exist. Mutations may simply lead to the absence of TP53, an inactive mutant protein may exist, or the mutant might convey a growth advantage. Several studies have investigated TP53 expression, and even though its role in prognosis has not been clearly defined, it may provide a guide to treatment options. To this end, recent advances have led to the decoding the "cancer landscape,"[43] with the identification of driver genes, classified into signaling pathways that regulate cell fate, cell survival, and genome maintenance. Such an understanding of these driver mutations will allow for the synthesis of new drugs focusing in on these molecules/pathways within a specific cancer of a specific individual to allow for specific treatment options in personalized medicine.

With the advent of microarray and other RNA detection technology (e.g., quantitative real-time PCR), transcriptomics has also evolved, and transcription signatures have been identified associated with specific cancer subtypes, as well as with specific chemical carcinogen exposure. For example, papillomavirus infection is associated with the deregulation of genes involved in cell cycle; most of them E2F genes and E2F-regulated genes.[226] Genes upregulated in samples from HCV-related HCC have been shown to be classified in metabolic pathways, and the most represented are the aryl hydrocarbon receptor (AHR) signaling and protein ubiquitination pathways, which have been previously reported to be involved in cancer, and in particular in HCC progression. Genes upregulated in samples from HCV-related non-HCC tissue have been shown to be classified in several pathways involved in inflammation and native/adaptive immunity; and most over-expressed genes belonged to the antigen presentation pathway.[227]

Most studies to date investigating transcriptome changes in response to environmental exposures have relied on peripheral blood. Although details of these studies have been reviewed by Wild et al.,[223] here are a few highlights. Using peripheral blood mononuclear cells (PBMCs), Thomas et al. showed low levels of benzene (at or below 0.1 ppm) were observed in association with altered expression of AML pathway genes and CYP2E1. This is an important finding, because it shows that benzene alters disease-relevant pathways (AML) and genes in a dose-dependent manner, with effects apparent at doses as low as 100 ppb in air.[228] Another study showed leukemia-related chromosomal changes in hematopoietic progenitor cells from workers exposed to benzene.[229] Others have found that telomere length was modestly, but significantly ($p = 0.03$) elevated in workers exposed to >31 ppm of benzene compared with controls.[230] Finally, polymorphisms in the CYP2E1 gene have been shown to be involved in benzene-induction of micronuclei and may contribute to risk of cancer among exposed workers.[231]

Interestingly, many gene expression changes associated with smoking are involved in inflammatory and oxidative stress pathways. Recently, Tilley et al. identified a "chronic obstructive pulmonary disease (COPD)-like" small airway epithelium transcriptome signature and found xenobiotic and oxidant-related categories contained the genes displaying the greatest magnitude of change in expression levels in healthy smokers.[232] Beane et al. showed that while large airway epithelial expression of many smoking-responsive genes is reversible upon smoking cessation, there are a number of smoking-responsive genes with persistently abnormal expression after smoking cessation. In this study, they also showed that pathways related to the metabolism of xenobiotics by CYP, retinol metabolism, and oxidoreductase activity were enriched among genes differentially expressed in smokers; whereas chemokine signaling pathways, cytokine–cytokine receptor interactions, and cell adhesion molecules were enriched among genes differentially expressed in smokers with lung cancer.[233] More recently, the same group showed SIRT1 activity is significantly upregulated in cytologically normal bronchial airway epithelial cells from active smokers compared with nonsmokers.[234] Pierrou et al.[235] found significant changes in the expression of oxidant-related genes in the large airway epithelium of non-smokers, healthy smokers, and COPD smokers, as did other studies[236,237] examining nonsmokers vs healthy smokers. Overall, transcriptomics has shown that it is possible to distinguish individual pathways associated with tobacco smoke, distinguish between individuals exposed and unexposed to tobacco smoke, and distinguish between current and past exposure to tobacco smoke. As reviewed by Wild et al.,[223] transcriptomics has also been able to identify specific signatures associated with dioxin (cell growth/ proliferation, glucose metabolism, apoptosis, DNA replication, repair), metal fumes (inflammation, oxidative stress, phosphate metabolism, cell proliferation, apoptosis), and diesel exhaust (inflammation and oxidative stress). In human lung tissues, a gene expression signature of 599 transcripts consistently segregated never from current smokers. Members of the CYP1 family, including CYP1A1, CYP1A2, and CYP1B1 were among the top genes upregulated by smoking. The gene most strongly upregulated by smoking was the aryl hydrocarbon receptor repressor (AHRR). Interestingly, 6 known genes were still significantly higher than never smokers after 10 years of smoking cessation

(SERPIND1, AHRR, FASN, PI4K2A, ACSL5, and GANC).[238] Together, studies done with transcriptomics have demonstrated specific signatures associated with specific exposures to chemical carcinogens, suggesting potential mechanisms promoting cancer and identification of biomarkers associated with cancer risk.

The epigenome describes the totality of epigenomic changes (epigenetic marks present along the DNA and associated structures (e.g., histones) in a particular cell type). We have already described some of the epigenetic events (mainly DNA methylation, histone modifications, and RNA-mediated gene silencing) associated with specific chemical carcinogen exposure. To this end, there have been a few studies to date attempting to link specific exposures of humans to epigenomic change. Overall, the impact of chemical carcinogens on the epigenome in human populations are limited to tobacco smoking (MTHFR and CDKN2A hypermethylation; GPR15, MSH3, NISCH, CYP1A1; RPS6KA3, ARAF, and especially AHRR hypomethylation), benzene (alu, long interspersed nucleotide elements, PTEN, ERCC3, p15, p16 hypermethylation; STAT3, MAGE-1 hypomethylation), cadmium (long interspersed nucleotide elements hypomethylation), air pollution (long interspersed nucleotide elements, tissue factor, F3, ICAM-1, and TLR-2 hypomethylation, and alu, IFN-γ and IL-6 hypermethylation), smokey coal emissions (p16 hypermethylation), workplace exposures (iNOS hypermethylation; SATα, NBL2 hypomethylation; mgmt hypermethylation), and arsenic (alu, long interspersed nucleotide elements, RHBDF1, p16, and p53 hypermethylation).[239–274] It should be pointed out that AHRR hypomethylation has been found as a common biomarker of smoking in multiple recent studies.[242,245–250,252,275] Also, importantly, recent studies suggest epigenetics is proving useful to the identification of both current, and past smoking history. Past exposures can be detected and possibly even quantified based on the epigenetic footprints they leave on specific genes. Zhang et al.[276] found that coagulation factor II (thrombin) receptor-like (F2RL3) methylation intensity showed a strong association with smoking status, which persisted after controlling for potential confounding factors. Clear inverse dose–response relationships with F2RL3 methylation intensity were seen for both current intensity and lifetime pack-years of smoking. Among former smokers, F2RL3 methylation intensity increased gradually from levels close to those of current smokers for recent quitters to levels close to never smokers for long-term (>20 years) quitters. A recent study coming out of the EPIC and NOWAC studies found 8 of 897 CpG sites differentially methylated in former and current smokers, while compared to never smokers, respectively. The eight candidate markers of former smoking showed a gradual reversion of their methylation levels from those typical of current smokers to those of never smokers. Further analyses using cumulative (over varying time windows) smoking intensities, highlighted three classes of biomarkers: short- and long-term biomarkers (measuring the effect of smoking in the past 10, and in the past 10–30 years respectively), and lifelong biomarkers detected more than 30 years after quitting smoking.[277] Such studies show a promising ability, through epigenetics, to detect short-term to lifelong biomarkers of tobacco smoke exposure and, more generally, to potentially identify time-varying biomarkers of exposure.

Histone marks (posttranslational modifications) in humans have also recently been assessed in association with chemical carcinogen exposure. Smoking is associated with a decrease in HDAC2 protein expression by 54% and activity by 47%, and concomitant enhancement of phosphorylation of Akt1 and HDAC2; workplace exposure to nickel is associated with an increase in H3K4me3 and decrease in H3K9me2; exposure to benzene is associated with reduced histone H4 and H3 acetylation and H3K4 methylation, and increased H3K9 methylation in the Topo IIα promoter; and, finally, exposure to arsenic is associated with an increased H3K4me2 and changes in global H3K9ac and H3K9me2 levels.[278–281]

In human populations, miRNA changes have been associated with exposure to: cigarette smoke (40 upregulated in smokers, including miR-21, miR-16, miR-17, miR-29a, miR-221, miR-223; repression of miR-15a, miR-199b, and miR-125b, miR-218, miR-487, miR-4423), workplace exposure (miR-21 and 222 increased in electric furnace steel plant workers postexposure vs. preexposure), benzene (upregulation of miR-34a, miR-205, miR-10b, let-7d, miR-185 and miR-423-5p-2; downregulation of miR-133a, miR-543, hsa-miR-130a, miR-27b,miR-223, miR-142-5p, and miR-320b), air pollution (upregulation of miR-132, miR-143, miR-145, miR-199a*, miR-199b-5p, miR-222, miR-223, miR-25, miR-424, and miR-582-5p), and arsenic (upregulation of miR-190, miR-29a, miR-9, miR-181b; downregulation of miR-200b).[278,282–290] Interestingly, miRNA levels have been shown to be reversed back to baseline after cessation of smoking.[284] Overall, it is becoming increasingly clear that epigenomics is providing useful and specific biomarkers of chemical carcinogen exposure, and that these changes can be detected in humans. In addition, the observation that some changes are reversible, and some changes are not reversible allow careful monitoring of both present and past exposures and their consequences on clinical outcome.

The impact of environmental carcinogens associated with inflammatory load/cytokinomic, proteomics, metabolics, and microbiomics is still emerging. Moore et al. reviewed the use of "omic" technologies to study arsenic exposure in human populations.[291] The reader is referred to this reference for full details. In brief, though, genomic profiling has revealed long-term arsenic exposure may increase the risk of chromosome alteration prevalence in exposed bladder tissue and that chromosome 17p loss was unique to arsenic-exposed bladder cancer cases independent of p53 inactivation or aberrant protein expression. Additionally, in either human tissues or peripheral cells, arsenic has been shown in many studies to change gene expression (often involved in cell-cycle regulation, apoptosis, and DNA damage response), epigenetic events (e.g., heavily methylated promoter regions of p53 and p16), proteomic profiles (e.g., decreased levels of human b-defensin-1 and ADAM28), and metabolomic profiles.[291] In a few examples, an association with HCV and cirrhotic livers, it was recently found that there was a significant upregulation of IL-1α, IL-1β, IL-2R, IL-6, IL-8, CXCL1, CXCL9, CXCL10, CXCL12, MIF, and β-NGF in serum compared to healthy controls.[292]

Although the concept of personalized medicine has been around for decades (and it can be argued, for centuries as medicine is given largely based on personal symptoms), we have only recently reached a tipping point with technology that has allowed us to be more precise with personalized medicine ("precision medicine").[24] In the broadest sense, precision medicine is the molding of medical treatment to individual patient characteristics and moves beyond the current approach of stratifying patients into treatment groups based on phenotypic biomarkers. Now, with sensitive instrumentation and a capacity to gather large amounts of data regarding chemical carcinogens, we are poised to begin packaging, integrating, and quantifying large datasets for precise measurement of chemical carcinogen exposure. We have already discussed the exposome above, which is a key first step toward this goal. Putting this exposure into numbers remains a challenge, but

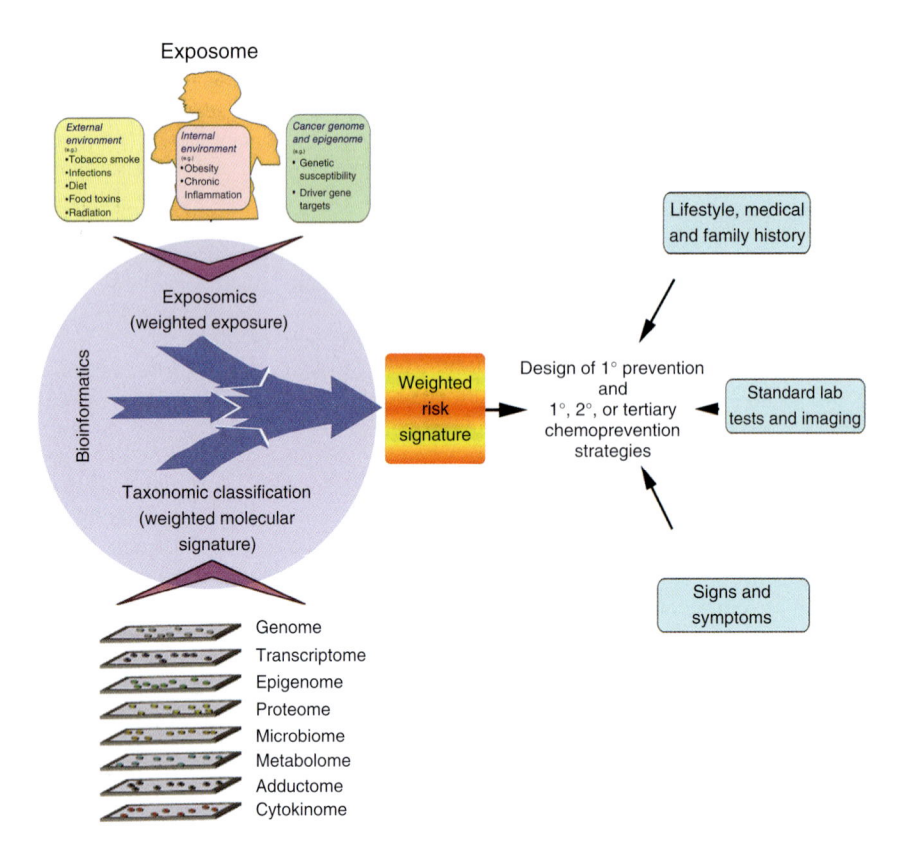

Figure 7 Connecting exposomics to toxonomics to generate a weighted Risk Signature for primary prevention and chemoprevention strategies. With the explosion of technology, extensive, and massive data set generation over the past decade, we are in a position to use bioinformatics to merge the exposome with the various "omics" collected to generate a weighted and precise Risk Signature. Quantifying the internal, specific, and general external exposure of an individual or population ("exposomics") then linking this to the molecular profile of an individual or population can generate a Risk Signature for an individual or population. Additional and continued consideration of signs/symptoms, standard lab tests, and family history will bring together a targeted primary and chemo-prevention strategy to reduce the risk of carcinogenesis in an individual or high-risk population of individuals.

meeting this challenge will bring real and precise numbers that can be linked to a quantified taxonomic profile which is a compilation of the massive data sets acquired through the different "omic" endpoints.[24] In this context, then, a precise risk signature might be realized for precision medicine and chemopreventive purposes (Box 5 and Figure 7).

Box 5 The Exposome

The exposome comprises every exposure to which an individual is subjected, from conception to death. It takes into consideration: (1) internal exposure (metabolism, endogenous circulating hormones, body morphology, physical activity, gut microbiota, inflammation, aging); (2) specific external exposures (radiation, infections, chemical contaminants, diet, tobacco, alcohol, occupation, medical interventions); and (3) more general exposures/social/economic influences (education, financial status, psychological stress, climate). Linking the exposome to metabolomic, proteomic, microbiomic, transcriptomic, and epigenomic profiles will allow us to identify an individual's risk signature as a biomarker for cancer risk and develop a precision medicine approach to cancer chemoprevention and treatment.

Acknowledgments

We thank Karen Yarrick for editorial assistance. This research was supported [in part] by the Intramural Research Program of the NIH, National Cancer Institute, Center for Cancer Research.

Key references

The complete reference list can be found on Vital Source version of this title, see inside front cover.

1 Poirier MC. DNA adducts as exposure biomarkers and indicators of cancer risk. *Environ Health Perspect*. 1997;**105**(Suppl 4):907–912.
2 Hajdu SI. A note from history: landmarks in history of cancer, part 1. *Cancer*. 2011;**117**(5):1097–1102.
3 Hajdu SI. A note from history: landmarks in history of cancer, part 2. *Cancer*. 2011;**117**(12):2811–2820.
4 Astruc J. *Traite de Tumeurs et des Ulceres*. Paris: P. Guillaume Cavelier; 1759.
5 Pott P. *Cancer Scroti. Chirurgical Observations Relative to the Cataract, the Polypus of the Nose, the Cancer of the Scrotum, the Different Kinds of Ruptures, and the Mortification of the Toes and Feet*. London: Hawes, Clarke and Collins; 1775:63–65.
7 Balkwill F, Mantovani A. Inflammation and cancer: back to Virchow? *Lancet (London, England)*. 2001;**357**(9255):539–545.
8 Lenoir T. A magic bullet: research for profit and the growth of knowledge in Germany around 1900. *Minerva*. 1988;**26**:66–88.
9 Rous P. A transmissible avian neoplasm. (Sarcoma of the common fowl.). *J Exp Med*. 1910;**12**(5):696–705.
10 Lacassagne AM. Apparition de cancers de la mamelle chez la souris male, etc. *C R Acad Sci*. 1932;**195**:630–632.
11 Berenblum I, Shubik P. A new, quantitative, approach to the study of the stages of chemical carcinogenesis in the mouse's skin. *Br J Cancer*. 1947;**1**(4):383–391.
12 Berenblum I. The mechanism of carcinogenesis. A study of the significance of cocarcinogenic action and related phenomena. *Cancer Res*. 1941;**1**:807.
13 Doll R, Hill AB. Smoking and carcinoma of the lung; preliminary report. *Br Med J*. 1950;**2**(4682):739–748.
14 Wynder EL, Graham EA. Tobacco smoking as a possible etiologic factor in bronchiogenic carcinoma; a study of 684 proved cases. *J Am Med Assoc*. 1950;**143**(4):329–336.

15 Conney AH, Miller EC, Miller JA. The metabolism of methylated aminoazo dyes. V. Evidence for induction of enzyme synthesis in the rat by 3-methylcholanthrene. *Cancer Res.* 1956;**16**(5):450–459.

16 Ames BN, Durston WE, Yamasaki E, Lee FD. Carcinogens are mutagens: a simple test system combining liver homogenates for activation and bacteria for detection. *Proc Natl Acad Sci U S A.* 1973;**70**(8):2281–2285.

17 Harris CC, Genta VM, Frank AL, et al. Carcinogenic polynuclear hydrocarbons bind to macromolecules in cultured human bronchi. *Nature.* 1974;**252**(5478): 68–69.

18 Doll R, Peto R. The causes of cancer: quantitative estimates of avoidable risks of cancer in the United States today. *J Natl Cancer Inst.* 1981;**66**(6):1191–1308.

19 Perera FP, Weinstein IB. Molecular epidemiology and carcinogen-DNA adduct detection: new approaches to studies of human cancer causation. *J Chronic Dis.* 1982;**35**(7):581–600.

20 Basu AK, Essigmann JM. Site-specifically modified oligodeoxynucleotides as probes for the structural and biological effects of DNA-damaging agents. *Chem Res Toxicol.* 1988;**1**(1):1–18.

21 Hsu IC, Metcalf RA, Sun T, et al. Mutational hotspot in the p53 gene in human hepatocellular carcinomas. *Nature.* 1991;**350**(6317):427–428.

23 Wild CP. Complementing the genome with an "exposome": the outstanding challenge of environmental exposure measurement in molecular epidemiology. *Cancer Epidemiol Biomark Prevent.* 2005;**14**(8):1847–1850.

24 National Research Council Committee on AFfDaNToD. *The National Academies Collection: Reports funded by National Institutes of Health. Toward Precision Medicine: Building a Knowledge Network for Biomedical Research and a New Taxonomy of Disease*. Washington (DC): National Academies Press (US). National Academy of Sciences; 2011.

25 Chen R, Mias GI, Li-Pook-Than J, et al. Personal omics profiling reveals dynamic molecular and medical phenotypes. *Cell.* 2012;**148**(6):1293–1307.

26 Alexandrov LB, Kim J, Haradhvala NJ, et al. The repertoire of mutational signatures in human cancer. *Nature.* 2020;**578**(7793):94–101.

27 ICGC/TCGA Pan-Cancer Analysis of Whole Genomes Consortium. Pan-cancer analysis of whole genomes. *Nature.* 2020;**578**(7793):82–93.

28 Pleguezuelos-Manzano C, Puschhof J, Huber AR, van Hoeck A, Wood HM, Nomburg J, et al. Mutational signature in colorectal cancer caused by genotoxic pks(+) *E. coli. Nature.* 2020, **580**, 269–273.

29 Loeb LA, Harris CC. Advances in chemical carcinogenesis: a historical review and prospective. *Cancer Res.* 2008;**68**(17):6863–6872.

31 Vineis P, Schatzkin A, Potter JD. Models of carcinogenesis: an overview. *Carcinogenesis.* 2010;**31**(10):1703–1709.

35 Loeb LA. Human cancers express mutator phenotypes: origin, consequences and targeting. *Nat Rev Cancer.* 2011;**11**(6):450–457. doi: 10.1038/nrc3063. Epub 2011.

36 Kinzler KW, Vogelstein B. Cancer-susceptibility genes. Gatekeepers and caretakers. *Nature.* 1997;**386**(6627):761–763.

37 Friedewald WF, Rous P. The initiating and promoting elements in tumor production: an analysis of the effects of tar, benzpyrene, and methylcholanthrene on rabbit skin. *J Exp Med.* 1944;**80**(2):101–126.

39 Hanahan D, Weinberg RA. Hallmarks of cancer: the next generation. *Cell.* 2011;**144**(5):646–674.

43 Vogelstein B, Papadopoulos N, Velculescu VE, et al. Cancer genome landscapes. *Science (New York, NY).* 2013;**339**(6127):1546–1558.

45 Hecht SS. Lung carcinogenesis by tobacco smoke. *Int J Cancer.* 2012;**131**(12):2724–2732.

51 Lengauer C, Kinzler KW, Vogelstein B. Genetic instabilities in human cancers. *Nature.* 1998;**396**(6712):643–649.

52 Wogan GN, Hecht SS, Felton JS, et al. Environmental and chemical carcinogenesis. *Semin Cancer Biol.* 2004;**14**(6):473–486.

54 Goldberg AD, Allis CD, Bernstein E. Epigenetics: a landscape takes shape. *Cell.* 2007;**128**(4):635–638.

64 Schetter AJ, Heegaard NH, Harris CC. Inflammation and cancer: interweaving microRNA, free radical, cytokine and p53 pathways. *Carcinogenesis.* 2009;**31**(1):37–49.

68 Xiao YF, Yong X, Fan YH, et al. microRNA detection in feces, sputum, pleural effusion and urine: novel tools for cancer screening (review). *Oncol Rep.* 2013;**30**(2):535–544.

73 Di Leva G, Garofalo M, Croce CM. MicroRNAs in cancer. *Annu Rev Pathol.* 2014;**9**:287–314. doi: 10.1146/annurev-pathol-012513-104715.

84 Ji W, Yang L, Yuan J, et al. MicroRNA-152 targets DNA methyltransferase 1 in NiS-transformed cells via a feedback mechanism. *Carcinogenesis.* 2013;**34**(2):446–453. doi: 10.1093/carcin/bgs343. Epub 2012.

99 Taioli E. Gene-environment interaction in tobacco-related cancers. *Carcinogenesis.* 2008;**29**(8):1467–1474.

119 Guengerich FP. Metabolism of chemical carcinogens. *Carcinogenesis.* 2000;**21**:345–351.

131 Hussain SP, Hofseth LJ, Harris CC. Radical causes of cancer. *Nat Rev Cancer.* 2003;**3**(4):276–285.

147 Staretz ME, Foiles PG, Miglietta LM, Hecht SS. Evidence for an important role of DNA pyridyloxobutylation in rat lung carcinogenesis by 4-(methylnitrosamino)-1-(3-pyridyl)-1-butanone: effects of dose and phenethyl isothiocyanate. *Cancer Res.* 1997;**57**(2):259–266.

154 Ronen A, Glickman BW. Human DNA repair genes. *Environ Mol Mutagen.* 2001;**37**(3):241–283.

165 Fontham ET, Correa P, Reynolds P, et al. Environmental tobacco smoke and lung cancer in nonsmoking women. A multicenter study. *JAMA.* 1994;**271**(22):1752–1759.

192 Fujita Y, Masago K, Hatachi Y, et al. Genetic polymorphisms in the endothelial nitric oxide synthase gene correlate with overall survival in advanced non-small-cell lung cancer patients treated with platinum-based doublet chemotherapy. *BMC Med Genet.* 2010;**11**:167.

194 Ahsan H, Chen Y, Kibriya MG, et al. Susceptibility to arsenic-induced hyperkeratosis and oxidative stress genes myeloperoxidase and catalase. *Cancer Lett.* 2003;**201**(1):57–65.

197 Boehm JS, Hahn WC. Towards systematic functional characterization of cancer genomes. *Nat Rev Genet.* 2011;**12**(7):487–498.

202 Vogelstein B, Kinzler KW. Cancer genes and the pathways they control. *Nat Med.* 2004;**10**(8):789–799.

204 Slebos RJ, Rodenhuis S. The ras gene family in human non-small-cell lung cancer. *J Natl Cancer Inst Monogr.* 1992;**13**:23–29.

211 Lane DP. Cancer. p53, guardian of the genome. *Nature.* 1992;**358**(6381):15–16.

216 Pfeifer GP, Besaratinia A. Mutational spectra of human cancer. *Hum Genet.* 2009;**125**(5–6):493–506.

217 Hollstein M, Sidransky D, Vogelstein B, Harris CC. p53 mutations in human cancers. *Science.* 1991;**253**(5015):49–53.

223 Wild CP, Scalbert A, Herceg Z. Measuring the exposome: a powerful basis for evaluating environmental exposures and cancer risk. *Environ Mol Mutagen.* 2013;**54**(7):480–499.

238 Bosse Y, Postma DS, Sin DD, et al. Molecular signature of smoking in human lung tissues. *Cancer Res.* 2012;**72**(15):3753–3763.

242 Dogan MV, Shields B, Cutrona C, et al. The effect of smoking on DNA methylation of peripheral blood mononuclear cells from African American women. *BMC Genomics.* 2014;**15**:151.

291 Moore LE, Karami S, Steinmaus C, Cantor KP. Use of OMIC technologies to study arsenic exposure in human populations. *Environ Mol Mutagen.* 2013;**54**(7):589–595.

23 Ionizing radiation

David J. Grdina, PhD

> **Overview**
>
> Many experimental and epidemiologic studies have since confirmed the oncogenic effects of radiation. This chapter reviews briefly the effects of ionizing radiation on biological systems, adaptive and bystander effects, cellular and molecular mechanisms for radiation carcinogenesis, and pharmacologic countermeasures that can mitigate against these processes.

Development of radiation injury

The hazards of exposure to ionizing radiation were recognized shortly after Roentgen's discovery of the X-ray in 1895. Acute skin reactions were observed in many individuals working with early X-ray generators, and by 1902, the first radiation-induced cancer was reported arising in an ulcerated area of the skin. Within a few years, a large number of such skin cancers had been observed, and the first report of leukemia in five radiation workers appeared in 1911.[1] Figure 1 describes the interaction of ionizing radiation with biologic tissues and the development of radiation injury. The ionizing event involves the ejection of an orbital electron from a molecule, producing a positively charged or "ionized" molecule. These molecules are highly unstable and rapidly undergo chemical change. This change results in the production of free radicals. The most common products of this process are the result of the decomposition of water giving rise to both superoxide anion (O_2^-) and hydrogen peroxide (H_2O_2) and the highly reactive hydroxyl radical, which has as a result a very short life span and can diffuse only on the average about 4 nm before reacting with other molecules.[2] Reactive oxygen species (ROS) production can be amplified by inter-mitochondrial communication that results in a subsequent magnification of the ROS damage signal.[3] The process of "ROS-induced ROS release," or RIRR is one potential mechanism for this. Under conditions of an excessive oxygen stress burden, the increase in ROS within the mitochondria reaches a threshold that triggers the opening of either the mitochondrial permeability transition (MPT) pore or the inner membrane anion channel (IMAC), which in turn leads to the simultaneous collapse of mitochondrial membrane potential and a transient increase in ROS generation by the electron transfer chain. Release of this ROS burst into the cytosol functions as a second messenger to activate RIRR in neighboring mitochondria.[4,5] Radiation can produce a transient generation of reactive oxygen or nitrogen within minutes accompanied by a reversible depolarization of mitochondrial membrane potential.[3] Radiation damage in a single mitochondrium can be transmitted via a reversible Ca^{2+}-dependent MPT to adjacent mitochondria resulting in the amplification of ROS generation. ROS amplification and propagation resulting from such a cascade can then damage important biological targets such as DNA, the nuclear matrix, cytoplasmic transport mechanisms, and both mitochondrial and cellular membranes resulting in cell death. The ROS amplification process may also be interfered by endogenous antioxidants such as superoxide dismutases (SODs) or exogenously added antioxidants.

Principal cellular and tissue effects of radiation

Cell killing

Radiation can kill cells by apoptosis and interphase death.[6–8] Cells undergoing apoptosis usually die in interphase within a few hours of irradiation. Apoptotic cell death can be induced by exposure to relatively low doses of radiation[6] and be a significant cause of death in hematopoietic or lymphoid cells exposed to higher radiation doses.

Radiation-induced apoptosis is dependent upon both the functional activity of the *p53* gene as well as p53-independent pathways[9] all of which converge on the activation of proteases called caspases.[10] It has been proposed that p53-dependent apoptosis involves the transcriptional induction of redox-related genes with the formation of ROS, leading to cell death by oxidative stress.[11]

The second mechanism for cell killing is radiation-induced reproductive failure. The inhibition of cellular proliferation is the mechanism by which radiation kills most mammalian cells. Symptoms of acute exposure to whole-body irradiation in human beings are usually observed only following doses of 100 cGy or greater.

Mutagenesis

Studies of the induction of single-gene mutations in human cells have been limited to several genetic loci. Of particular note is the X-chromosomal gene for hypoxanthine-guanine phosphoribosyl transferase (HPRT).[12,13] The induction of mutations in human cells is a linear function of dose down to doses as low as 10 cGy, and perhaps as low as 1 cGy, and the dose-rate effect appears to be relatively small.[14,15] DNA structural analyses show that the majority of radiation-induced mutations in human cells result from large-scale genetic events involving loss of the entire active gene and often extending to other loci on the same chromosome.[16]

The major potential consequence of radiation-induced mutations in human populations is heritable genetic effects resulting from mutations induced in germinal cells. For high dose-rate exposure, the induced mutation rate per gamete generally falls in the range of 10^{-4}–10^{-5} per cGy. The rates per locus are in the range of 10^{-7}–10^{-8} per cGy. Protraction of exposure appears to decrease the mutation rate in rodent systems by a factor of 2 or

Holland-Frei Cancer Medicine, Tenth Edition. Edited by Robert C. Bast, John C. Byrd, Carlo M. Croce, Ernest Hawk, Fadlo R. Khuri, Raphael E. Pollock, Apostolia M. Tsimberidou, Christopher G. Willett, and Cheryl L. Willman.
© 2023 John Wiley & Sons, Inc. Published 2023 by John Wiley & Sons, Inc.

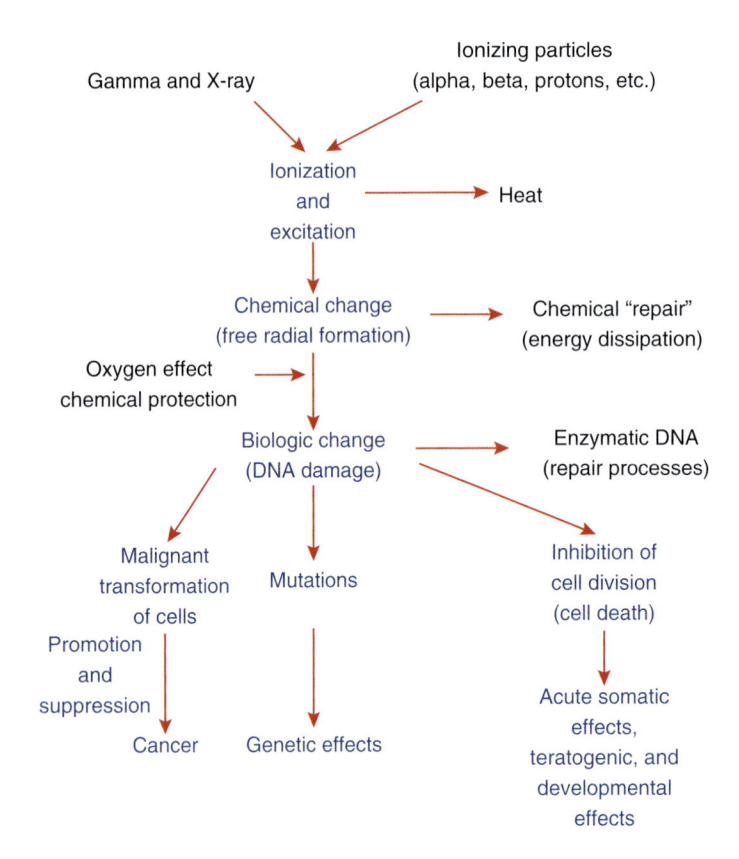

Figure 1 Development of radiation injury.

greater. When all of the experimental data for the various genetic end points are considered, the genetic doubling dose (radiation dose necessary to double the spontaneous mutation rate) for low dose-rate exposure appears to be in the range of 100 cGy.

Chromosomal aberrations

Radiation can induce two types of chromosomal aberrations in mammalian cells. The first have been termed "unstable" aberrations in that they are usually lethal to dividing cells. They include such changes as dicentrics, ring chromosomes, large deletions, and fragments. The frequency of such aberrations correlates well with the cytotoxic effects of radiation.

The second type has been termed "stable" aberrations. These include changes such as small deletions, reciprocal translocations, and aneuploidy changes that do not preclude the cell from dividing and proliferating. Radiation-induced reciprocal translocations may be passed on through many generations of cell replication and emerge in clonal cell populations.[17,18]

Such deletions and translocations can result in gene mutations. Specific chromosomal abnormalities are associated with specific tumor types such as the chromosome 8 : 14 translocation in Burkitt lymphoma. The chromosomal change can result in the activation of a specific oncogene such as a chromosome 13q14 deletion in retinoblastoma (RB).

Radiation-induced genomic instability

Radiation exposure can induce a type of transmissible genetic instability in individual cells that is transmitted to their progeny, leading to a persistent enhancement in the rate at which genetic changes arise in the descendants of the irradiated cell after many generations of replication. This is a nontargeted effect of radiation. The end points include malignant transformation, specific gene mutations, and chromosomal aberrations.

Early evidence was derived from an examination of the kinetics of radiation-induced malignant transformation of cells *in vitro*.[19,20] Transformed foci did not arise from a single, radiation-damaged cell. Rather, radiation appeared to induce a type of instability in 20–30% of the irradiated cell population; this instability enhanced the probability of the occurrence of a second, neoplastic transforming event, which is rare occurring with the frequency of ~10^{-6}. This second event occurs with a constant frequency per cell per generation and has the characteristics of a mutagenic event.[21]

This phenomenon was subsequently demonstrated in a number of experiment systems for various genetic end points.[22–25] In terms of mutagenesis, ~10% of clonal populations derived from single cells surviving radiation exposure showed a significant elevation in the frequency of spontaneously arising mutations compared with clonal populations derived from nonirradiated cells.[26,27] This increased mutation rate persisted for ~30 to 50 generations postirradiation. An enhancement of both minisatellite[28] and microsatellite[29] instability has also been observed in the progeny of irradiated cells selected for mutations at the *thymidine kinase* locus. Transmission of chromosomal instability has been shown to occur *in vivo*,[30,31] but susceptibility to radiation-induced chromosomal instability differed significantly among different strains of mice.[32,33] A persistent increase in the rate of cell death has been shown to occur in cell populations many generations after radiation exposure.[34–36] Delayed reproductive failure has been linked to chromosomal instability[37] and malignant transformation,[38,39] and evidence presented to suggest that DNA is at least one of the critical targets in the initiation of this phenomenon.[40]

A recent novel phenomenon has been identified and coined "the delayed radioprotective effect." It is manifested by an enhanced resistance to ionizing radiation hours to days following exposure of cells to thiol-containing drugs such as N-acetylcysteine and captopril that have the ability to elevate intracellular antioxidant enzymes such as manganese superoxide dismutase (MnSOD).[41,42] The underlying mechanism of action responsible for this effect is the activation of the redox-sensitive nuclear transcription factor κB (NFκB) by thiol-reducing agents that subsequently results in the elevated transcription of MnSOD. The resulting 10- to 20-fold elevation of intracellular MnSOD facilitates the prevention and removal of radiation-induced oxidative damage and can enhance survival of cells by 10–30%.

Bystander effects in irradiated cell populations

It has long been thought that the cell nucleus is the target for the important biologic effects of radiation. However, recent evidence shows that targeted cytoplasmic radiation is significantly mutagenic. Damage signals may be transmitted from irradiated to nonirradiated cells in the population, leading to biologic effects in cells that received no radiation exposure,[43] for example, the "bystander" effect.

Following the exposure of monolayer cultures of cells to very low fluences of α particles, an enhanced frequency of sister chromatid exchanges (SCE) was observed in 20–40% of cells exposed to fluences by which only 1/1000 to 1/100 cells were traversed by an α particle.[44] This effect involves the secretion of cytokines or other factors by irradiated cells that leads to an upregulation of oxidative metabolism in bystander cells.[45,46] Incubation with conditioned medium from irradiated cells has cytotoxic effects on nonirradiated cells, which may be related to the release of a factor(s) into the medium.[47] An enhanced frequency of specific gene mutations[48,49] as well as chromosomal aberrations[50,51] are observed to occur in bystander cells in populations exposed to very low fluences of α particles.

DNA damage in bystander cells appears to differ from that occurring in directly irradiated cells; whereas the mutations induced in directly irradiated cells were primarily partial and total gene deletions, >90% of those arising in bystander cells were point mutations.[52] Suggesting that oxidative metabolism is upregulated in bystander cells.[45,46] Bystander effects indicate clearly that damage signals can be transmitted from irradiated to nonirradiated cells.

Adaptive responses

The original description of an adaptive response was made by investigators working with human lymphocytes in which they observed that following exposure to a very low dose of ionizing radiation in the range of 1–10 cGy cells acquired an enhanced resistance to a second but much larger dose of 2 Gy or more.[53] The expression of an adaptive response was linked to the requirement of de novo protein synthesis since inhibitors of protein synthesis such as cycloheximide were found to be inhibitory to this inductive effect.[54] Adaptive responses can be looked upon as the result of intercellular stress responses. The most studied such response has been identified as being mediated by MnSOD, an antioxidant enzyme localized in the mitochondria of cells, in both normal and malignant cells. As an example, it has been demonstrated that mouse skin JB6P+ epithelial cells exposed to 10 cGy exhibited an enhanced resistance to a subsequent dose of 2 Gy during which time a number of NFκB-regulated genes including MnSOD, p65, phosphorylated extracellular signal-related kinase, cyclin B1, and 14-3-3Z were elevated.[55] The importance of elevated MnSOD synthesis in the adaptive response process has been observed in cells following exposure to not only a low dose of ionizing radiation[55] but also the cytokine tumor necrosis factor α (TNFα)[56] and numerous reductive agents such as amifostine and N-acetylcysteine.[42,57] Treatment of cells with NFκB inhibitors and/or antisense MnSOD oligomers or siRNA MnSOD completely inhibited the adaptive response induced by these agents.[55,56] Three generalized examples of the MnSOD-mediated adaptive responses are presented in Figure 2. Both the radiation and cytokine-induced adaptive responses are the result of oxidative damage-initiated processes in contrast to the thiol-induced reductive response in which NFκB is activated following the reduction of cysteine residues on its p50 and p65 subunits,[58,59] a process that can be maintained in a persistent manner with chronic thiol exposure.[60]

It is now recognized that there are multiple mediators of adaptive responses, each associated with either normal and/or neoplastic cells and different radiation protocols. Under conditions of multifractionated high-dose radiation exposures, each preceded by very low imaging doses, a survivin-mediated adaptive response is expressed in tumor cells.[61] Survivin, a member of the inhibitor of apoptosis protein (IAP) group, is primarily found in neoplastic cells and has been identified as an important factor in tumor cell resistance.[62,63] Its overexpression results in elevated tumor cell resistance to radiation- and chemotherapy-induced cell killing and reduced frequencies of apoptosis.[64-66] The survivin mediated adaptive response is initiated through NFκB activation and affected by redox associated modifying agents, TP53 mutational status of cells, and NADPH oxidase 4 (NOX 4) activity.[67-70] In contrast to the generalization that adaptive responses always result in increased radiation resistance, the survivin mediated adaptive response only results in elevated radiation resistance in TP53 wild type (WT) cells with TP53 mutant cells (TP53 mut) being sensitized. TP53 mutational status determines whether survivin is exported from the nucleus to the cytoplasm resulting in an anti-apoptotic effect in TP53 WT or migration from the cytoplasm to the nucleus in TP53 mut resulting in a pro-apoptotic effect.[69] Cell to cell communication is also an important factor with TP53 mut comprising as little as 10% of the total population being sufficient to control the overall expression of the remaining 90% WT cells resulting in an overall pro-apoptotic effect and reduced survival effect as shown in Figure 3.[70] A model of the redox sensitive radio-adaptive response is presented in Figure 4.[70] An additional adaptive response has also been identified in normal cells where low-dose radiation exposure results in the induction of a metabolic shift from oxidative phosphorylation to aerobic glycolysis in cells and is mediated by the hypoxia-inducible factor HIF-1α.[71]

DNA damage

Track analysis studies of X-ray interactions in DNA have provided evidence for clustered damage, which results in complex DSB (double-strand break).[72] Certain types of DNA base damage such as 8-hydroxydeoxyguanosine and thymine glycols have significant potential biologic importance, but the available data suggest that such isolated base damage by itself probably plays a minor role in radiation mutagenesis. Clustered DNA damage may include abasic sites, oxidized purines, or oxidized pyrimidines.[73] The increased efficiency of DNA breaks induced by high-LET radiation appears to result primarily from their greater complexity.[74]

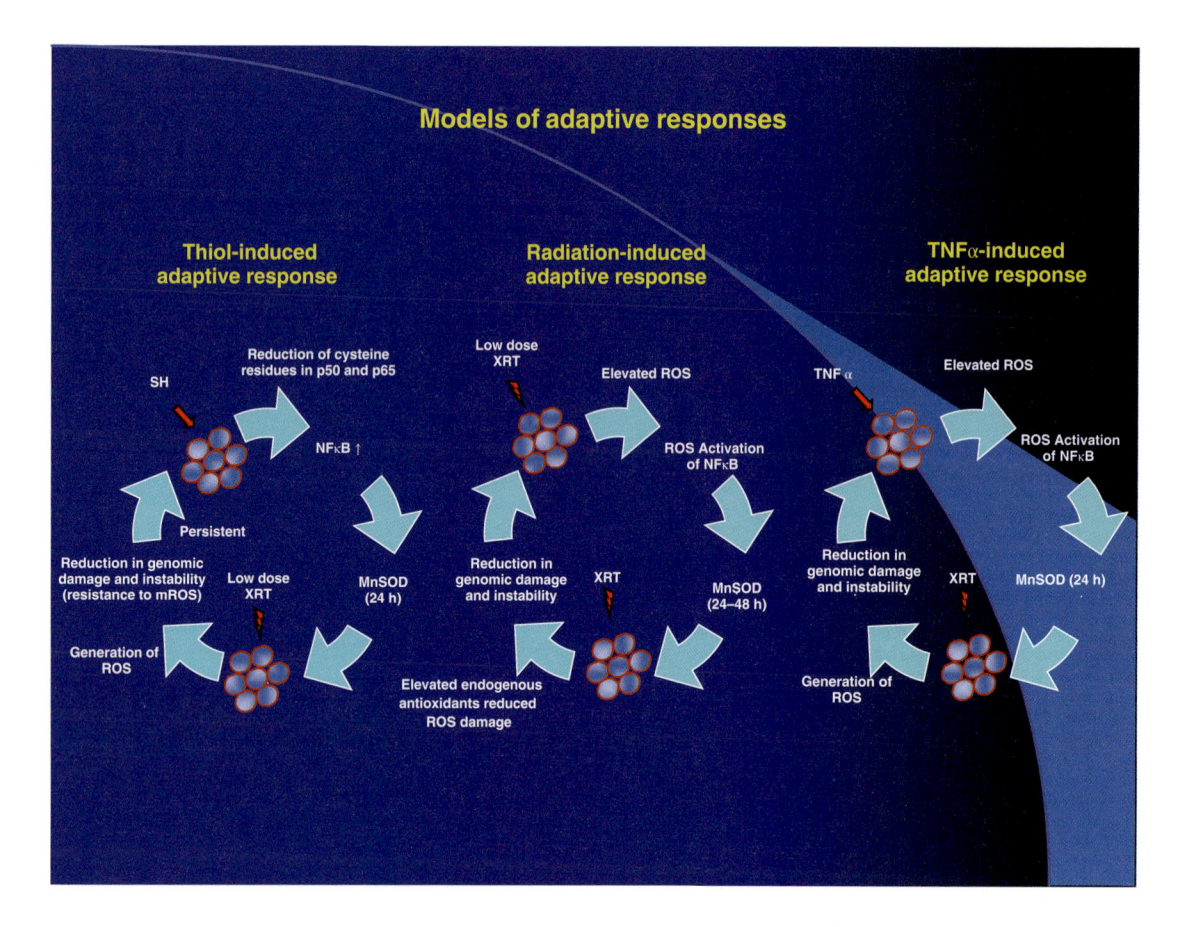

Figure 2 Models of adaptive responses: a non-oxidative damage-mediated event induced through the reducing action of free thiols as contrasted to oxidative damage-initiating events induced through the oxidizing action of ionizing radiation and selected cytokines such as tumor necrosis factor α (TNFα). Adaptive responses in general refer to an altered damaging effect of a relatively high dose of a deleterious agent when induced following exposure to a previous low-dose or non-toxic priming agent.

Cells possess a complex set of signaling pathways for recognizing such DNA damage and initiating its repair. The *ATM* gene is a sensor of DNA damage, which activates by phosphorylation a variety of proteins involved in cell cycle control and DNA repair. Two mechanistically distinct pathways that function in complementary ways are involved in the repair of DSB: nonhomologous end joining (NHEJ), which requires little sequence homology between the DNA ends and is error prone, and homologous recombination (HR), which uses extensive homology and is generally error-free.[75] NHEJ involves a complex of proteins, including Ku70, Ku80, the DNA-PK catalytic subunit DNA-PKcs, XRCC4, and ligase IV. The NBS1/MRE11/RAD50 complex[76] is also involved in the nucleolytic processing stages of NHEJ; this complex also contributes to HR. HR also involves a complex of proteins, notably RAD51 and other factors in the RAD50 epistasis group.[77] Strong links have been established between recombinational repair and the breast cancer susceptibility proteins BRCA1 and BRCA2,[78–80] as well as the Fanconi anemia family of proteins.[81] Un-repaired or mis-repaired DSB led primarily to large-scale genetic changes that are frequently manifested by chromosomal aberrations. However, no genetic alterations unique to radiation have been found in radiation-induced tumors.

General characteristics of radiation carcinogenesis

Ionizing radiation can induce cancer in most tissues of most species at all ages, including the fetus. It is carcinogenic to humans. It is, however, a relatively weak carcinogen and mutagen. The cancers induced by radiation are of the same histologic types as occur naturally, but the distribution of types may differ. There is a distinct latent period between exposure to radiation and the clinical appearance of a tumor.

Radiation carcinogenesis is a stochastic process; that is, the probability of the occurrence of the effect increases with dose with no threshold, but the severity of the effect is not influenced by dose. Radiation-induced cancer appears to be an all-or-none effect. The dose–response relationships for the induction of cancers in specific tissues of small animals vary with site, sex, and species.[82–84] For low LET radiation, the frequency of induced cancers generally rises with dose in the range of 0–300 cGy. In some cases, tumor incidence levels off at higher doses and may even decline. This phenomenon is thought to reflect cell killing. In the dose range up to 200–300 cGy, the dose–response curves for individual tumor types vary but generally assume a linear-quadratic to near-linear relationship. For high LET radiation, the rise in cancer incidence with dose is much steeper. The dose–response curves are approximately linear within the range of 0–20 cGy.[82,85]

The induction of carcinogenesis in experimental animals can be suppressed by treatment with certain agents that are known to inhibit radiation-induced transformation *in vitro*. An example of this includes amifostine, which is the only drug currently approved for clinical use as a radioprotector by the Food and Drug Administration.[86] As described by Kaplan–Meier plots in Figure 5, inoculation of B6CF1 hybrid mice with a single dose of 400 mg/kg

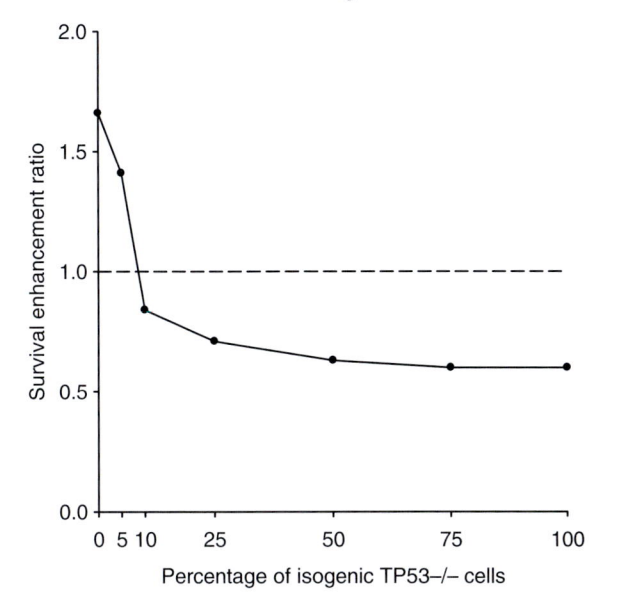

Figure 3 Expression of the survivin-associated radio-adaptive response as a function of the relative composition of Human Colon Carcinoma, HCT116, TP53 WT, and corresponding null Mut cells in mixed cultures. Ratios of integrated survival of mixed cultures following two 2 Gy doses to that following two 5 mGy plus 2 Gy irradiations are plotted as a function of the percentage of isogenic TP53 Mut cells. The survival enhancement ratio of 1 represents a null effect, with values <1 indicating radio-sensitization and those >1 radioprotection. Source: Murley et al.[70]

of amifostine 30 min before whole-body irradiation with 2 Gy of low LET radiation significantly protected against carcinogenesis in both male and female animals. The reduction in cancer deaths due to lymphoreticular tumors by amifostine is reflected by a shift in the Kaplan–Meier survival curves for drug-treated irradiated animals to those describing the survival of nonirradiated control animals.[87–89] Causes of death due to lymphoreticular tumors that included leukemias and lymphomas were determined by both gross and microscopic analysis of individual animals by veterinarian pathologists.[87] Likewise, certain protease inhibitors have also been shown to suppress the induction of cancer in several different tumor systems.[90] It is well known that the hormonal environment is important in certain radiation-induced rodent cancers, particularly ovarian and mammary tumors.

Genetic susceptibility to radiation-induced cancer

There is little evidence to suggest that genetic factors are involved in most human cancers, but they do appear to play a role in some rare hereditary disorders that may serve as models for radiation–genetic interactions. For example, patients with hereditary RB whose somatic cells are heterozygous for the *RB* gene are at markedly increased risk for the development of radiation-induced bone sarcomas,[91] whereas patients with the nevoid basal cell carcinoma syndrome are at high risk for the development of basal cell cancers in irradiated areas. Radiation has also been associated with an enhanced incidence of early onset breast cancer. Transgenic mice heterozygous for either the *p53*[92] or *ATM*[93] tumor suppressor genes show an increased sensitivity to radiation-induced cancer; ATM and p53 heterozygosity are associated, respectively, with the human cancer-prone disorders ataxia telangiectasia and the Li–Fraumeni syndrome.

Human epidemiologic studies

There is now a large body of data on radiation-induced cancer derived from epidemiologic studies in irradiated human populations. They are derived primarily from two sources: (1) the long-term follow-up of survivors of the nuclear bombings of Hiroshima and Nagasaki[94,95] and (2) populations exposed to medical X-rays.[96,97] The results of these studies have yielded significant dose–response data for the induction of cancer in at least five tissue sites. Unfortunately, the epidemiologic studies yielding useful dose–response data generally involve relatively high-dose exposures (>10 cGy). Thus, risk estimates in the low-dose range must be derived from an extrapolation from the high-dose data. The shape of the dose–response relationship becomes of critical importance in making such extrapolations.

The observed dose–response curves from the human epidemiologic studies appear to be either linear or linear-quadratic in form (i.e., a linear component at low doses with a quadratic component at higher doses); although a threshold (dose below which there is no effect) cannot be formally excluded at very low doses.[98,99] A linear curve implies a constant risk per cGy at all doses, whereas the linear-quadratic model implies a smaller risk per cGy in the low-dose range. The assumption of a linear model simplifies the extrapolation from high to low doses and the corresponding estimation of risks. A final parameter of importance in determining the hazards of a given dose of radiation is the choice of risk models. For many years, risks were estimated on the basis of an absolute risk model. This model assumed that a specific number of excess cancers was induced by a given radiation dose. Radiation-induced cancers occurred in addition to the natural incidence. Increased risk could be expressed as the number of excess cancer cases (or cancer deaths) per 10^6 exposed people per year per cGy (the rate per year) or as the total number of excess cancers per 10^6 exposed people per cGy (the total risk or lifetime yield of cancers to be expected from a given radiation dose). The absolute risk model generally assumes a linear dose–response relationship, although with certain corrections it can be applied to a linear-quadratic relationship. Because the radiation exposure in Hiroshima included a small fraction of neutrons, the doses in the atom bomb survivor studies are expressed in Sieverts (Sv) rather than gray, a term that takes into account the RBE (relative biological effectiveness) of neutrons.

An analysis of the recent data from the atom bomb survivors suggests that some types of radiation-induced cancer more likely follow a relative-risk model.[94] The relative-risk model implies that radiation increases the natural incidence of cancer at all ages by a dose-dependent factor. As the excess cancer risk is proportional to the natural incidence, radiation-induced cancers would occur primarily at the times when natural tumors arose, independent of the age at irradiation. Thus, the largest cohort of radiation-induced cancers would occur in older individuals. The relative-risk model appears to fit the epidemiologic data for several solid tumors, although it does not appear to be valid for leukemia or bone and lung cancers. Risk estimates derived from the studies involving medical exposures are similar to those of the atom bomb survivors[97,100,101]; differences in the case of high-dose radiation therapy exposures can be ascribed to cell killing and the effect of dose fractionation.[96] A significantly reduced effect with fractionation for high-dose exposure was observed for lung cancer.[102] This was not the case for breast cancer, although a reduced effect was associated with low dose-rate protracted exposure.[101]

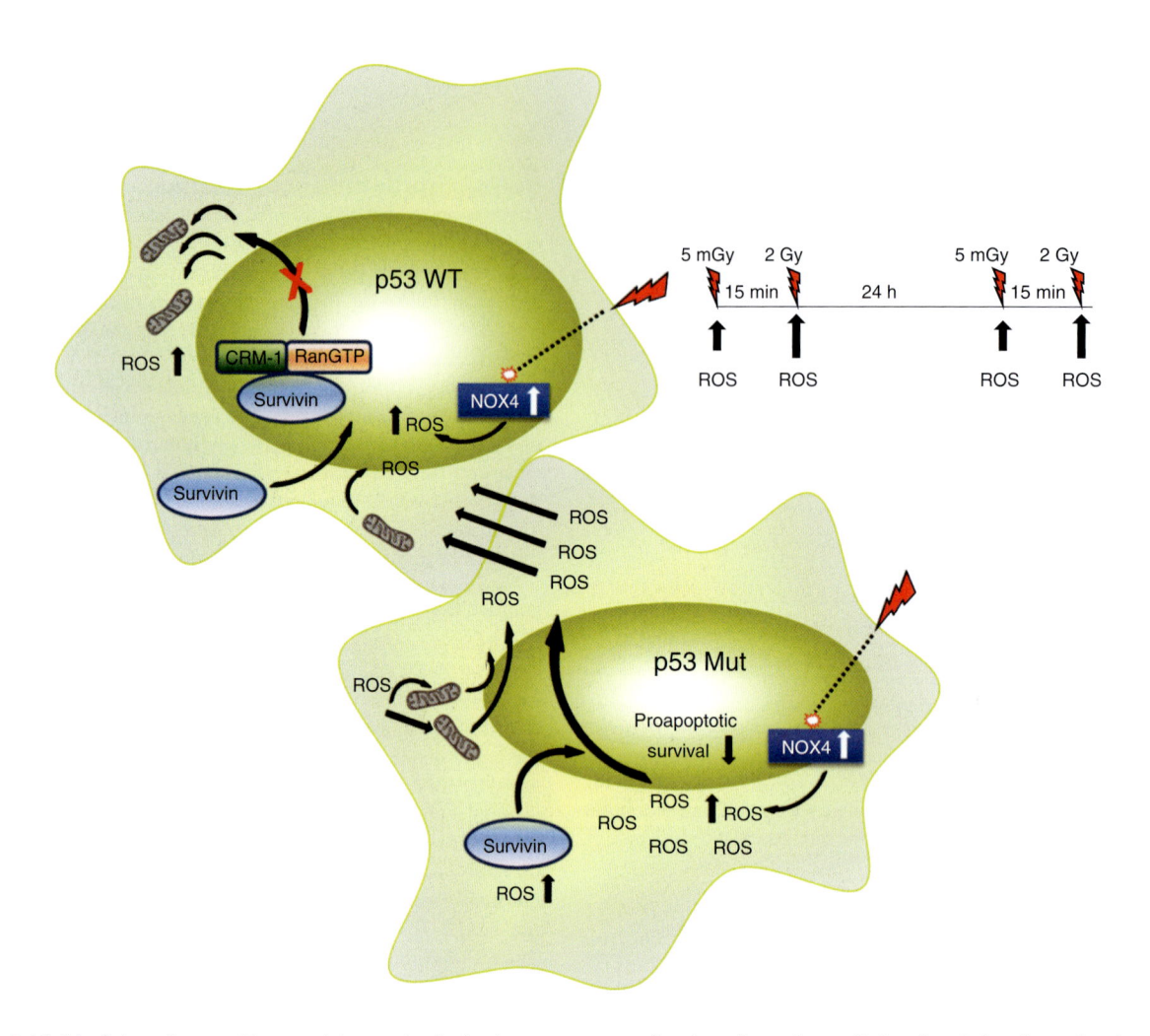

Figure 4 Model of the redox sensitive, survivin-associated adaptive response as a function of very low radiation dose-induced translocation of the bi-functional inhibitor of apoptosis protein survivin and activation of NOX4 in Human Colon Carcinoma, HCT116, tumor cells differing in TP53 mutational status. TP53 plays an important role in survivin localization through the regulation of a number of redox effectors that affect the intracellular ROS environment, with TP53 WT suppressing and TP53 Mut enhancing ROS production. Stimulation of NOX4 by very low dose radiation exposure amplifies ROS levels. Diffusion of ROS from TP53 Mut cells to TP53 WT cells blocks translocation of survivin from the nucleus to the cytoplasm and as a result sensitizing them to subsequent higher dose radiation exposure. Source: Murley et al.[70]

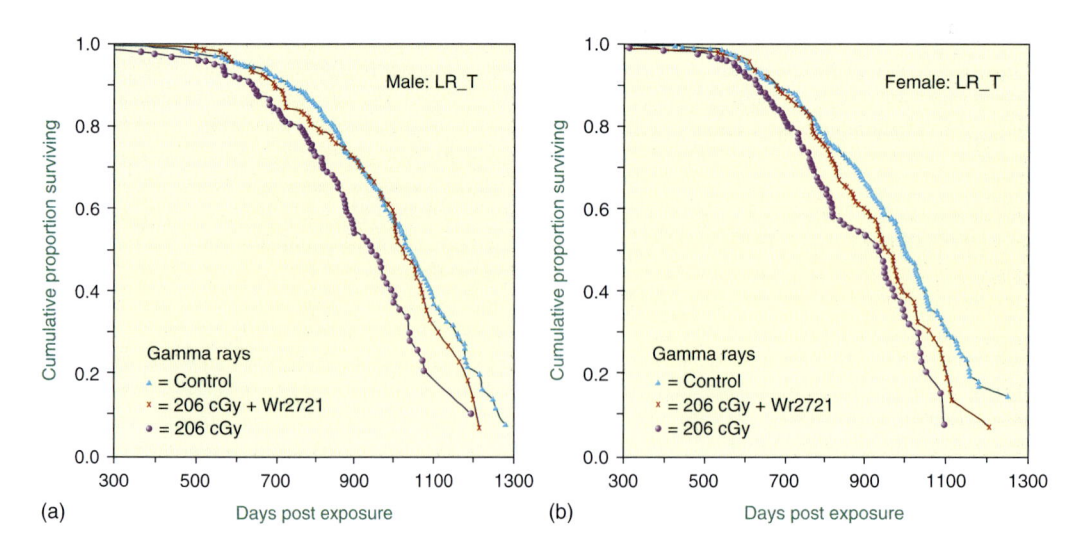

Figure 5 (a, b) Survival curves resulting from lymphoreticular cancers (LR-T), as determined by histopathological analysis of tissues taken from deceased animals that had been irradiated (206 cGy) either with or without amifostine. LR-T includes histiocytic leukemia and lymphoma, lymphocytic–lymphoblastic leukemia and lymphoma, myelogenous leukemia, undifferentiated leukemia and lymphoma, and mixed histiocytic leukemia and lymphoma.

Radiation-induced secondary tumors

Radiation alone used in conventional treatment regimens may not be a very potent inducer of secondary tumors. This prediction arises from the localized nature of the exposure during clinical radiotherapy, in which the dose to normal tissues is minimized, and from the fact that ionizing radiation tends to be cytotoxic rather than mutagenic. The high radiation doses employed may thus kill potentially transformed cells in the treatment field. Exceptions may be the treatment of Hodgkin disease in which lower radiation doses are delivered to a relatively large volume of tissue, and in the use of intensity-modulated radiation therapy (IMRT). IMRT involves the use of more fields with a larger normal tissue volume exposed to lower doses.[103] It has been estimated that IMRT is likely to almost double the incidence of second malignancies compared with conventional radiotherapy from about 1% to 1.75% for patients surviving 10 years.[104] The risk may be even higher for pediatric patients.

Low-dose exposures

Sufficient data are now available from the atomic bomb survivors to allow an analysis of those survivors who received <0.5 Sv; these data are providing preliminary estimates of risk for doses as low as 5–10 cGy.[99] They indicate a statistically significant risk in this range consistent with a linear dose–response relationship, with an upper confidence limit on any possible threshold of 6 cGy.

A careful analysis of nearly all low-dose studies indicates no significant increase in the incidence of all cancers or of cancers at specific sites. Analyses of a large number of radiation workers from the United Kingdom[105] and Canada[106] indicate that the risk estimates for leukemia and all cancers were consistent with an extrapolation from the atom bomb survivor data, providing no evidence for an unexpected increase in sensitivity at low doses such as to suggest that the current radiation protection standards might be appreciably in error.

Acknowledgments

I acknowledge past support of research grant DE-FG02-05ER64086 from the US Department of Energy (DJG), RO1 CA99005 from the National Cancer Institute (DJG) and the Department of Radiation and Cellular Oncology, The University of Chicago.

Key references

The complete reference list can be found on Vital Source version of this title, see inside front cover.

1. Upton AC. Historical perspectives on radiation carcinogenesis. In: Upton AC, Albert RE, Burns FJ, Shore RE, eds. *Radiation Carcinogenesis*. New York: Elsevier; 1986:1–10.
3. Leach JK, Van Tuyle G, Lin PS, et al. Ionizing radiation-induced mitochondria-dependent generation of reactive oxygen/nitrogen. *Cancer Res*. 2001;**61**:3894–3901.
5. Brady NR, Hamacher-Brady A, Westerhoff HV, Gottlieb RA. A wave of reactive oxygen species (ROS)-induced ROS release in a sea of excitable mitochondria. *Antioxid Redox Signal*. 2006;**8**(9,10):1651–1665.
12. Albertini RJ. Validated biomarker responses influence medical surveillance of individuals exposed to genotoxic agents. *Radiat Prot Dosim*. 2001;**97**:47–54.
14. Grosovsky AJ, Little JB. Evidence for linear response for the induction of mutations in human cells by X-ray exposures below 10 rads. *Proc Natl Acad Sci U S A*. 1985;**82**:2092–2095.
17. Kano Y, Little JB. Mechanisms of human cell neoplastic transformation: X-ray–induced abnormal clone formation in long-term cultures of human diploid fibroblasts. *Cancer Res*. 1985;**45**:2550–2555.
20. Kennedy AR, Little JB. Evidence that a second event in X-ray–induced oncogenic transformation *in vitro* occurs during cellular proliferation. *Radiat Res*. 1984;**99**:228–248.
25. Romney CA, Paulauskis JD, Nagasawa H, Little JB. Multiple manifestations of X-ray–induced genomic instability in Chinese hamster ovary (CHO) cells. *Mol Carcinog*. 2001;**32**:118–127.
41. Murley JS, Kataoka Y, Weydert CJ, et al. Delayed cytoprotection after enhancement of $Sod2$ ($MnSOD$) gene expression in SA-NH mouse sarcoma cells exposed to WR-1065, the active metabolite of amifostine. *Radiat Res*. 2002;**158**:101–109.
42. Murley JS, Kataoka Y, Cao D, et al. Delayed radioprotection by NFκB-mediated induction of Sod2 (MnSOD) in SA-NH tumor cells after exposure to clinically used thiol-containing drugs. *Radiat Res*. 2004;**162**:536–546.
50. Little JB, Nagasawa H, Li GC, Chen DJ. Involvement of the nonhomologous end joining DNA repair pathway in the bystander effect for chromosomal aberrations. *Radiat Res*. 2003;**59**:262–267.
51. Azzam EI, de Toledo SM, Gooding T, Little JB. Intercellular communication is involved in the bystander regulation of gene expression in human cells exposed to very low fluences of alpha particles. *Radiat Res*. 1998;**150**:497–504.
53. Olivieri G, Bodycote J, Wolff S. Adaptive response of human lymphocytes to low concentrations of radioactive thymidine. *Science*. 1984;**223**:594–597.
56. Murley JS, Kataoka Y, Baker LL, et al. Manganese superoxide dismutase (SOD2)-mediated delayed radioprotection induced by the free thiol form of amifostine and tumor necrosis factor κB. *Radiat Res*. 2007;**167**:465–474.
57. Murley JS, Kataoka Y, Weydert CJ, et al. Delayed radioprotection by nuclear transcription factor κB- mediated induction of manganese superoxide dismutase in human microvascular endothelial cells after exposure to the free radical scavenger WR1065. *Free Radic Biol Med*. 2006;**40**:1004–1016.
59. Murley JS, Kataoka Y, Hallahan DE, et al. Activation of NFκB and $MnSOD$ gene expression by free radical scavengers in human microvascular endothelial cells. *Free Radic Biol Med*. 2001;**30**:1426–1439.
60. Murley JS, Nantajit D, Baker KL, et al. Maintenance of manganese superoxide dismutase (SOD2)-mediated delayed radioprotection induced by repeated administration of the free thiol form of amifostine. *Radiat Res*. 2008;**169**:495–505.
61. Grdina DJ, Murley JS, Miller RC, et al. A survivin-associated adaptive response in radiation therapy. *Cancer Res*. 2013;**73**(14):4418–4428.
63. Marivin A, Berthelet J, Plenchette S, Dubrez L. The inhibitor of apoptosis (IAPs) in adaptive response to cellular stress. *Cells*. 2012;**1**:711–737.
65. Capalbo G, Rodel C, Stauber RH, et al. The role of survivin for radiation therapy: prognostic and predictive factor and therapeutic target. *Strahlenther Onkol*. 2007;(11):593–599.
67. Grdina DJ, Murley JS, Miller RC, et al. NFκB and survivin-mediated radio-adaptive response. *Radiat Res*. 2015;**183**:391–397.
68. Miller RC, Murley JS, Rademaker AW, et al. Very low doses of ionizing radiation and redoex associated modifiers affect survivin-associated changes in radiation sensitivity. *Free Radic Biol Med*. 2016;**99**:110–119.
69. Murley JS, Miller RC, Weichselbaum RR, Grdina DJ. TP53 mutational status and ROS effect the expression of the survivin-associated radio-adaptive response. *Radiat Res*. 2017;**188**:579–590.
70. Murley JS, Arbiser JL, Weichselbaum RR, Grdina DJ. ROS modifiers and NOX4 affect the expression of the survivin-associated radio-adaptive response. *Free Radic Biol Med*. 2018;**123**:39–52.
71. Lall R, Ganapathy S, Yang M, et al. Low-dose radiation exposure induces a HIF-1-mediated adaptive and protective metabolic response. *Cell Death Diff*. 2014;**21**:836–844.
72. Goodhead DT. Initial events in the cellular effects of ionizing radiations: clustered damage in DNA. *Int J Radiat Biol*. 1994;**65**:7–17.
78. Moynahan ME, Chiu JW, Koller BH, Jasin M. Brca1 controls homology-directed DNA repair. *Mol Cell*. 1999;**4**:511–518.
79. Moynahan ME, Pierce AJ, Jasin M. BRCA2 is required for homology-directed repair of chromosomal breaks. *Mol Cell*. 2001;**7**:263–272.
82. Fry R, Storer JB. External radiation carcinogenesis. In: Lett J, ed. *Advances in Radiation Biology*, Vol. **13**. New York: Academic Press; 1987:31–90.
83. Ullrich RL, Storer JB. Influence of gamma irradiation on the development of neoplastic disease in mice. I. Reticular tissue tumors. *Radiat Res*. 1979;**80**:303–316.
84. Ullrich RL, Storer JB. Influence of gamma irradiation on the development of neoplastic disease in mice. II. Solid tumors. *Radiat Res*. 1979;**80**:317–324.
86. Grdina DJ, Murley JS, Kataoka Y. Radioprotectants: current status and new directions. *Oncology*. 2002;**63**:2–10.
87. Grdina DJ, Carnes BA, Grahn D, Sigdestad CP. Protection against late effects of radiation by S-2-(3-aminopropylamino)- ethylphosphorothioic acid. *Cancer Res*. 1991;**51**:4125–4130.
88. Carnes BA, Grdina DJ. *In vivo* protection by the aminothiol WR-2721 against neutron-induced carcinogenesis. *Int J Radiat Biol*. 1992;**61**:567–576.
89. Grdina DJ, Carnes BA, Nagy B. Protection by WR-2721 and WR-151327 against late effects of gamma rays and neutrons. *Adv Space Res*. 1992;**12**:257–263.

95. Amy Berrington de González AB, Darby S. Risk of cancer from diagnostic X-rays: estimates for the UK and 14 other countries. *Lancet*. 2004;**363**:345–351.
96. Little MP. Comparison of the risks of cancer incidence and mortality following radiation therapy for benign and malignant disease with the cancer risks observed in the Japanese A-bomb survivors. *Int J Radiat Biol*. 2001;**77**:431–464.
98. Hoel D, Li P. Threshold models in radiation carcinogenesis. *Health Phys*. 1998;**75**:241–250.
101. Preston DL, Mattsson A, Holmberg E, et al. Radiation effects on breast cancer risk: a pooled analysis of eight cohorts. *Radiat Res*. 2002;**158**:220–235.
104. Hall EJ, Wuu C-S. Radiation-induced second cancers: the impact of 3D-CRT and IMRT. *Int J Radiat Oncol Biol Phys*. 2003;**56**:83–88.

24 Ultraviolet radiation carcinogenesis

James E. Cleaver, PhD ■ Susana Ortiz-Urda, MD, PhD ■ Sarah Arron, MD, PhD

Overview

Skin carcinogenesis from solar UV exposure is initiated by UV photoproducts formed in the DNA of precursor cells that give rise to squamous cell carcinomas (SCC), basal cell carcinomas (BCC), and cutaneous malignant melanomas (CMM). SCC and BCC are caused by UVB but CMM by reactive oxygen generated through UVA absorption in melanin. The UVB photoproducts consist of dimers between adjacent pyrimidines that are repaired by nucleotide excision repair (NER). Two branches of NER differ in mechanisms of damage recognition: in global genome repair (GGR) damage is recognized in nontranscribed DNA by the DDB2 and XPC proteins; in transcription-coupled repair (TCR) damage is recognized by arrest of the transcribing RNA polymerase at damaged sites. The T=C photoproduct is the predominant mutagenic product which, if unrepaired, gives rise to C to T or CC to TT mutations through replication by the low fidelity polymerase Pol H. TCR reduces the mutation frequency in regions of transcription. Deficiencies in GGR in the human disease xeroderma pigmentosum cause earlier onset and increased rates of skin cancer. Deficiencies in TCR in the human disease Cockayne syndrome are associated with photosensitivity, developmental and neurological disorders, but no cancer has been reported.

Epidemiology of skin cancer

Skin cancer frequency and age of onset

NMSCs are the most common cancers that occur in the United States each year,[1,2] comprising 30–40% of all cancers and have been increasing steadily for a century.[3,4] Skin cancer risks are associated with geographical location, skin type, various photosensitizing, enhancing, and protective applications and vitamin D.[4–10] There is also a possibility of greater risk when the exposure is received during childhood and adolescence.[5,11] NMSC is, therefore, one of the few human malignancies for which there is clear evidence for the initiating agent. The relationship of melanoma to sun exposure and the possible action spectrum is less clear[12,13] but may be related to acute burns rather than accumulated dose.[5,14]

The importance of DNA as a target for UV radiation is highlighted by the autosomal recessive disease XP. In this disease, a failure of DNA repair causes a large increase in NMSC and melanoma.[12,13] Median age for first diagnosis of NMSC in the general United States population occurs after 60 years of age; in XP patients, carcinogenesis is accelerated and median age at first diagnosis is within the first decade (Figure 1).[12,13] Melanoma is also increased in XP patients, but the acceleration is less. Consequently, in XP patients the onset of NMSC precedes melanoma, whereas in non-XP patients melanomas generally occur earlier than NMSC.[13]

Sunlight spectrum and wavelengths responsible for skin cancer

UV is divided into three wavelength ranges UVA, UVB, UVC. UVA (320–400 nm) is photocarcinogenic and involved in photoaging but is weakly absorbed in DNA and protein and may involve reactive oxygen species (ROS), which secondarily cause damage to DNA.[16–19] Recent evidence however suggests that UVA may also induce DNA damage directly in human cells.[20] UVB (290–320 nm) overlaps the upper end of the DNA and protein absorption spectra and is the range mainly responsible for skin cancer through direct photochemical damage to DNA. UVC (240–290 nm) is not present in ambient sunlight but is readily produced by low-pressure mercury sterilizing lamps (254 nm). UVC coincides with the peak of DNA absorption (260 nm) and is extensively used in experimental studies. Absorption of UV by stratospheric ozone greatly attenuates these wavelengths, so that negligible radiation shorter than 300 nm reaches the earth's surface. Hence, although UVA and UVB light constitute a minute portion of the emitted solar wavelengths (10^{-9}) they are primarily responsible for the sun's pathological effects.

Sunlight induced photoproducts in DNA

The absorption spectrum of DNA correlates well with photoproduct formation, lethality, and mutation.[21–25] The absorbed energy produces molecular changes which involve single bases, interactions between adjacent and nonadjacent bases, and between DNA and proteins. The relative proportion of DNA photoproducts varies across the UV spectrum.

Dimerizations between adjacent pyrimidines are the most prevalent DNA photoproducts. Two major photoproducts are the cyclobutane pyrimidine dimer (CPD) and, at about 25% the frequency, the [6-4] pyrimidine dimer ([6-4]PD). [6-4]PDs cause a 47° helical bend in DNA, compared to 7° for CPDs. The [6-4]PD can further undergo a UVB-dependent conversion to its valence photoisomer, the Dewar pyrimidinone.[26]

The distribution of photoproducts in chromatin depends on base sequence, secondary DNA structure, and DNA–protein interactions.[25,27,28] Because cytosine more efficiently absorbs longer wavelengths of UVR than thymine, CPDs containing this base are formed more readily after UVB irradiation.[29] Cytosine CPDs, and [6-4]PDs which are preferentially induced at thymine-cytosine dipyrimidines, may play a major role in UVB (solar) mutagenesis.[30] Cytosine methylation increases the formation of CPDs by UVB, but not UVC, by 1.7-fold.[31] Methylation at PyrCG sequences in the *p53* gene enhances formation of CPDs and [6-4]PDs at sites that are hotspots for mutations.[32,33] Other less common lesions include purine–purine and purine–pyrimidine photoadducts, photohydrates, and photooxidations.[34] The total

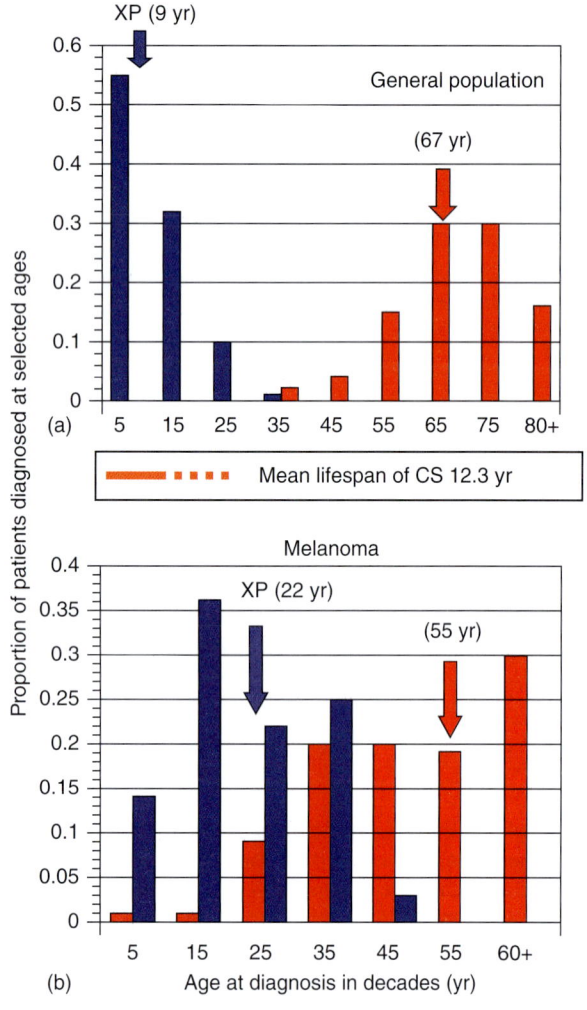

Figure 1 Diagnosis of first cancer by age and type in XP patients compared to the US general population. (a) Proportion of NMSC patients diagnosed at selected ages. (b) Proportion of melanoma patients diagnosed at selected ages. Individuals with both NMSC and melanoma were used in both panels. Ages shown are at the midpoint of each decade. XP, blue bars; general population, red bars. Colored arrows designate median ages of diagnosis for each population. The age span of Cockayne syndrome patients is also shown (orange): solid bar ends at mean age at death (12.25 years), with dashed line extending to maximum reported ages. Source: Bradford et al.[13]; Nance and Berry.[15]

yield of these photoproducts is only 3–4% of the yield of CPDs, but a minor biological role as premutagenic lesions at specific sites cannot be excluded.

Genetic factors in skin carcinogenesis

Recognition of UV photoproducts in DNA
The repair of UV photoproducts in DNA (nucleotide excision repair [NER]) involves sequential steps of photoproduct recognition, assembly of the excision complex, displacement of the excised fragment, and polymerization of the replacement patch.[35] The importance of NER arose from the discovery that cells from patients suffering from XP were deficient in NER.[36,37] Two major pathways of NER are known (Figure 2): transcription-coupled repair (TCR) and global genome repair (GGR) which differ in their mechanisms of damage recognition.[35,38–40] TCR removes damage more rapidly from the transcribed strands of transcriptionally active genes, whereas GGR acts more slowly on nontranscribed regions[41,42] The half-life of [6-4]PDs is 2–6 h whereas for CPDs it is 12–24 h, and much longer in rodent cells.[43,44]

GGR involves initial binding by the DDB1/DDB2(XPE) complex,[45,46] followed by recruitment of XPC/HR23B/centrin via ubiquitylation by the E3 ligase activity of DDB1/DDB2.[47–50] The XPC protein binds to the undamaged strand opposite a pyrimidine dimer, inserting a peptide chain within the helix to displace the dimer to an extra-helical position.[51,52]

TCR is initiated by the arrest of RNA polymerase II at a damaged base, after which specific TCR factors CSA, CSB, UVSSA, USP7, and XABP, a binding partner of XPA, facilitate removal or degradation of arrested RNA polymerase II to permit access of NER proteins to damaged sites.[53,54] TCR is closely involved with the chromatin remodeling function of CSB that is a member of the SWI2/SNF2 chromatin remodeling protein family.[55,56] RNA polymerase II elongation is associated with cycles of ubiquitylation and deubiquitylation of histone H2B (H2Bub); arrest by UV damage tips the balance toward deubiquitylation and acetylation of histone H3.[57] Transcription is restored along with H2Bub after excision of the arresting photoproducts.[57]

The mechanism of nucleotide excision repair
Subsequent to damage recognition, the open helix is stabilized by XPA/RPA which binds with a higher affinity for the [6-4]PDs than CPDs and interacts with the unwinding activity of the 10 component transcription factor TFIIH, and the 3-5′ (XPB) and 5′-3′ (XPD) nucleases.[58,59] The opened helix is cleaved first by the ERCC1/XPF nuclease presenting a 3′OH terminus for chain elongation by the DNA Pol D, proliferating cell nuclear antigen (PCNA), and single strand binding protein.[60,61] XPG is a cryptic nuclease that cuts 3′ to the lesion after the ERCC1/XPF nuclease has cut 5′ to the CPD and polymerization.[61] A 27–29nt oligonucleotide containing the photoproduct is subsequently released and the patch sealed by ligase I.[62]

Mutagenicity of UV photoproducts and low fidelity DNA polymerases
Most photoproducts act as blocks to the replicative class B polymerases, Pol A, D, and E but can be bypassed by damage-specific class Y DNA polymerases.[63–65] The class Y polymerases, Pol H, I, and K, have low fidelity due to expanded active sites which allow the polymerases to read through noninformative sequence information.[66] Pol H has the greatest capacity to replicate a large variety of DNA lesions,[67] and preferentially inserts adenine in the nascent strand opposite the lesion (called the "A rule").[68] Hence, Pol H replicates a thymine-containing CPD faithfully.[69–72] Pol I preferentially inserts guanines and is capable of replicating C-containing photoproducts.[73,74] Pol H or I, therefore, can insert bases opposite dipyrimidine photoproducts, but the 3′ complementary base can be mismatched by an erroneous insertion or the distortion caused by the photoproduct. Pol K or Pol Z can complete the replicative bypass by extension from the mismatched 3′ terminus.[75–77] The absence of Pol H results in increased mutagenesis in the xeroderma pigmentosum variant (XPV) group,[78,79] but the absence of Pol Z has the converse effect of reducing mutation rates.[80]

The replication by-pass mechanism has two important implications for UV mutagenicity. First, mutations will most often occur where cytosine is a component of the photoproduct since insertion

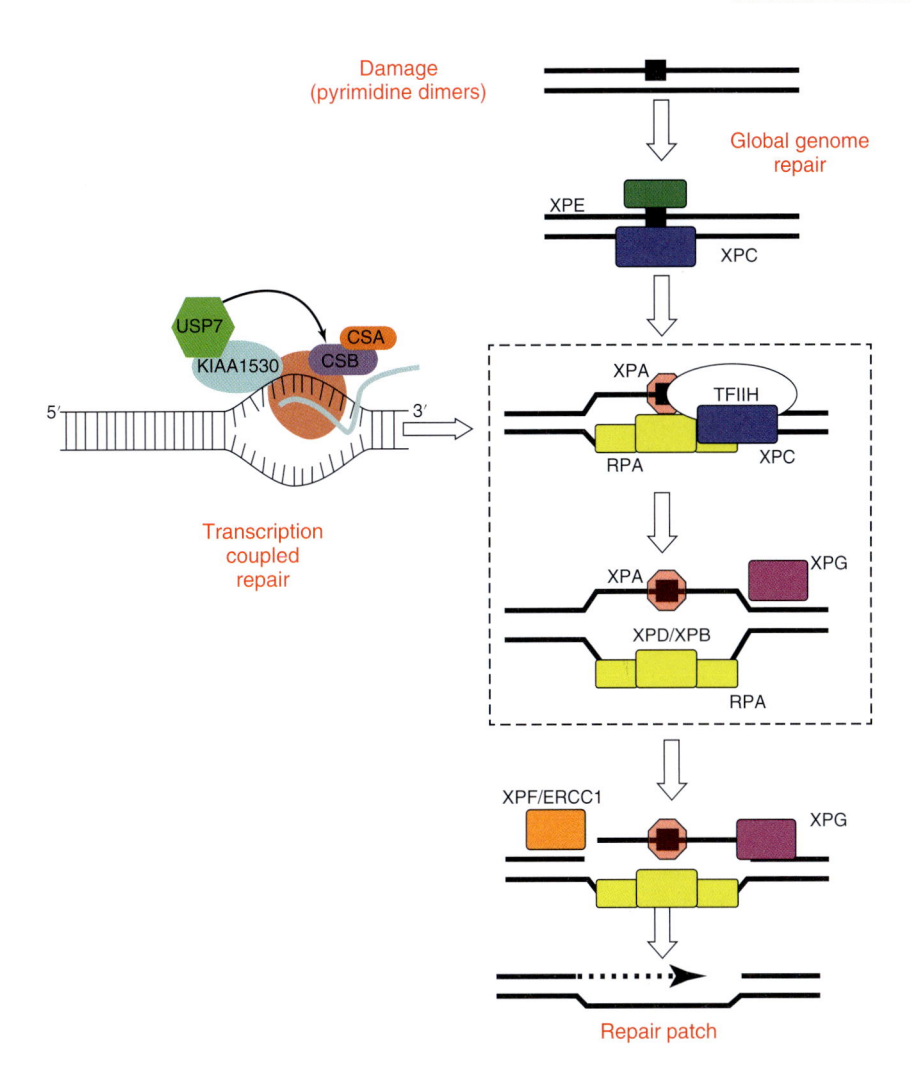

Figure 2 Biochemical steps for nucleotide excision repair of CPDs and [6-4]PDs by global genome repair or transcription-coupled repair. Initial recognition of damage by GGR involves the *DDB2* and *XPC* gene products; initial recognition by TCR involves RNA Polymerase II arrest and disengagement of the transcription complex from damage by CSA, CSB, and UVSSA. Subsequent steps involve XPA and RPA that bind to photoproducts and download the helicases XPB and XPD for local unwinding. Excision occurs when UV-specific endonucleases (XPF/ERCC1 and XPG) make incisions on the 5′ and 3′ sides. Excision and subsequent polymerization release a 29 base oligonucleotide containing the CPD and activates the cryptic XPG endonuclease for the final cut.

of adenine opposite thymine is a correct and nonmutagenic event. Hence CPDs that form between two thymine bases are not mutagenic. Second, the larger distortion of [6-4]PDs is more likely to be lethal than mutagenic.

Diseases of DNA repair

Xeroderma pigmentosum

XP is a rare autosomal recessive disease that occurs at a frequency of about 1 : 250,000 in the United States.[12] Affected patients (homozygotes) have sun sensitivity resulting in progressive degenerative changes of sun-exposed portions of the skin and eyes, often leading to neoplasia. Some XP patients also have progressive neurologic degeneration. Obligate heterozygotes (parents) are asymptomatic. The median age of onset of symptoms is 1–2 years of age and the median age of first diagnosis of NMSC is 9 years of age (Figure 1).[12,13] The skin rapidly takes on the appearance of that seen in individuals with many years of sun exposure. Pigmentation is patchy and skin shows atrophy and telangiectasia with development of NMSC and melanoma. The frequency of NMSC is about 2000 times that seen in the general population less than 20 years of age, with an approximate 30-year reduction in life span. Some patients develop myelodysplasia and leukemia in later life.

Among patients who are deficient in NER, there are eight complementation groups that correspond to components of NER, XPA through G, and the exceedingly rare ERCC1.[81] An additional group, the XP variant, has mutations in the low fidelity polymerase Pol H (Table 1). UV damaged plasmids passaged through XP cells show increased mutagenesis due to defective repair of CPDs and nondimer photoproducts.[82] Carcinogenesis from UV damage in XP patients arises, therefore, from the loss of either NER capacity or Pol H; both lead to an increase in the amount of persistent genetic damage (mutations, gene rearrangements, deletions, and genomic instability).

Cockayne syndrome

CS is an autosomal recessive disease characterized by photosensitivity, cachectic dwarfism, retinal abnormalities, microcephaly, deafness, neural defects, and retardation of growth and development after birth.[15,83] A major symptom is cerebellar degeneration and Purkinje cell loss causing difficulties in walking

Table 1 Genes involved in repair of UV damage in humans.[a]

Group (gene)	Chromosome location	Central nervous system and developmental disorders	Relative DNA repair[b] (%)
Xeroderma pigmentosum			
A	9q34.1	Yes	2–5
B[c]	2q21	Yes	3–7
C	3q25	No	5–20
D[c]	19q13.2	Yes	25–50
E	11p11–12	No	50
F	16q13.1	No	18
G	13q32.3	Yes	<2
V (pol H)	6p21	No	100
ERCC1[d]	19q13.32	Yes	15
Cockayne syndrome			
A (ERCC8)	5q12.1	Yes	100[b]
B (ERCC6)	10q11.23	Yes	100[b]
UVSSA	4p16.3	No	100[b]

[a]Further details can be found in the websites http://www.photobiology.info/ and http://www.cgal.icnet.uk/DNA_Repair_Genes.html
[b]Measurement of relative DNA repair represent mainly global genome repair. Cockayne syndrome is defective in transcription-coupled repair, and has normal levels of global genome repair.
[c]Patients also exhibit symptoms commonly associated with Cockayne syndrome: dwarfism, cutaneous features, and mental retardation. Group B is designated ERCC3 and Group D is designated ERCC2, F is designated ERCC4, G is designated ERCC5. Some patients also have symptoms of trichothiodystrophy.
[d]ERCC1 is rare and causes a neonatal fatal disorder, Cerebro-Oculo-Facio-Skeletal Syndrome.

and balance.[84] Solar carcinogenesis is not seen in patients with CS, setting this disease apart from XP, even though their lifespan encompasses ages at which skin cancers are seen in XP (Figure 1).[15] Mutations in either of two genes, CSA and CSB, are associated with CS.[83,85] Similar symptoms occur in XP groups B, D, and G.[86] The CS proteins facilitate removal of RNA polymerase II from damaged sites permitting access for the NER machinery (Figure 2). An additional gene product UVSSA also contributes to TCR but mutations in the UVSSA gene only give rise to mild photosensitivity.[87,88]

CSA and CSB proteins also contribute to the redox balance of cells by interaction with oxidative phosphorylation in the mitochondria and mitophagy.[89] Conceivably, their mitochondrial role may be more important in the developmental and neurological pathology of CS than their nuclear TCR function.[90]

Trichothiodystrophy

TTD is a rare autosomal recessive disorder characterized by sulfur-deficient brittle hair that splits longitudinally into small fibers and ichthyosis. The levels of cysteine/cystine in hair proteins are 15–50% of those in normal individuals. Patients show physical and mental retardation of varying severity and often have an unusual facial appearance, with protruding ears and a receding chin. Mental abilities range from low normal to severe retardation.[91] Several categories of the disease can be recognized on the basis of UV sensitivity and DNA repair deficiencies.[92,93] The most severe cases with repair deficiencies have mutations in XPB and XPD.[92] Several other TTD genes are known that are not involved in DNA repair.

Mutations in XPD that give rise to XP symptoms correspond to missense mutations in the DNA helicase motifs whereas those that give rise to TTD are missense mutations in the RNA helicase motifs and the C-terminal end of the protein.[94] Some TTD cases do not have mutations in XPB or XPD and are due to mutations in a small 8 kDa component of TFIIH that appears to regulate the overall level of the transcription factor.[95]

Carcinogenesis

Mutations and skin cancer types

Loeb was the first to recognize the high frequency of mutations in cancer cells and invoked the concept of a mutator phenotype.[96] In triple-negative breast cancer, for example, the mutation frequency is 13.3 times that of the normal rate of 0.6 mutations per cell division.[97] NMSC and melanoma have among the highest mutation frequencies, most of which are C to T or CC to TT transitions resulting from sun exposure.[98,99] The frequency of mutations in normal and cancer genomes is reduced in transcribed regions, compared to the rest of the genome, and shows the strand bias of TCR.[97,98,100] Patients with reduced TCR, that is CS patients, should therefore have higher frequencies of mutations in transcribed regions of the genome and hence more cancers. But they do not, unlike Cs-a or Cs-b mice that do develop skin cancer from carcinogen exposure.[101] Mutant cells in CS must therefore be prevented or delayed from progressing to cancers.

Nonmelanoma skin cancer

SCCs and BCCs both have UV-type mutations in genes that drive development of these tumors. Actinic keratoses, precursors to SCCs, share many mutational spectrum and global gene expression profiles.[102–104] The initiating molecular changes in SCC are UV-type mutations in p53 that result in expanding clones in the sun-exposed areas of the skin that are initially confined within the proliferating units.[105] In normal skin 50% of SCCs have p53 mutations; in XP patients the frequency is 90%.[106–110] Loss of p53 function causes genomic instability during DNA replication when subjected to further UV irradiation.[111–113] Many of these are likely passenger mutations that do not confer a growth advantage; mutated p53 being the more potent driver of SCC.

SCC mutations have been identified in Notch, KNSTRN, a kinetochore gene, EGF, RAS, NFkb, JNK2, and MMP9[114–118] Activating mutations in H-RAS and N-RAS oncogenes at codon 61, have been associated with solar UV exposure even though they involve transversions at a TT site.[119–122]

BCCs and BCNS involve the Sonic Hedgehog (HH) pathway in which a transmembrane receptor, Patched (PTC), and the membrane protein Smoothened (SMO), regulate signal transduction by the extracellular protein HH that binds to PTC.[123] In the general population, most UV-type BCC mutations are in the PTC gene or less frequently SMO, and rarely HH.[109,124–126] In XP patients, however, a significant number of mutations occur in SMO and HH.[127,128]

Melanoma

Melanomas involve a series of mutations, deletions, and amplifications (copy number changes) along the MAP kinase pathway, a phosphorylation cascade that regulates cell proliferations and differentiation[129–135] (Figure 3). A common mutation occurs in BRAF (V600E), but this sequence change is not a UV-type.[136,137] but associated with ROS. In contrast, 10 of 11 mutations in BRAF from XP melanomas were UV-type and different from V600E.[136] Mutations of UV-type have been identified in the promoter region of hTERT resulting in gene activation.[138,139] In addition to point mutations, melanomas have a significant frequency of translocations involving protein kinases.[140] Nevi and melanomas in XP patients are generally lentiginous and have a high incidence (53–61%) of UV-type inactivating mutations in PTEN.[136] These frequencies are much higher than those in BRAF, NRAS, and KIT, unlike the general population where PTEN mutations are lower.

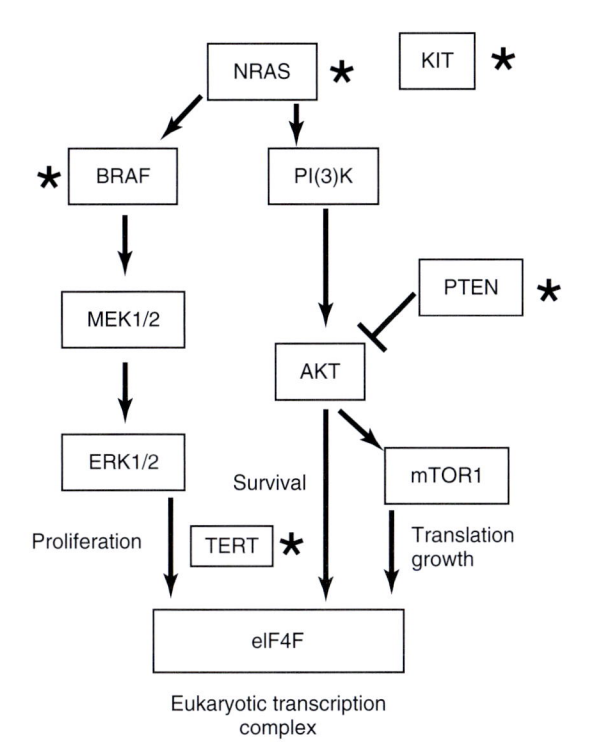

Figure 3 Pathways involved in melanoma. Proteins mutated by UV light in XP patients or the general population are designated by a star. Mutations in TERT are UV type but have yet to be reported in XP patients. Note the common *BRAF* melanoma mutation V600E is not induced by UV as it does not occur at a dipyrimidine site, but other mutations are formed by UV light in *BRAF*.[136] The most common mutated gene in XP patients is *PTEN*, in contrast to the MAPK pathway in the general population.[136] Source: Based on Masaki et al.[136]

Relative importance of UVA and UVB in melanoma and SCC in XP patients

In XP patients the age of peak incidence for SCCs is earlier in life than for melanoma, which is the reverse of that for the general population, and the relative risk for SCCs is much larger. These two features suggest that NER of solar UVB-induced photoproducts is more important for SCCs. A large fraction of melanoma patients in the general population exhibit a characteristic mutation, V600E, which is a site for mutations arising from ROS generated by UVA acting on melanin.[141]

Acknowledgments

This work was support by the E.A. Dickson Emeritus Professorship of the University of California San Francisco (JEC) and the Simon Memorial Fund of the UCSF Academic Senate (JEC).

Summary

Skin tumors in man account for about 30% of all new cancers reported annually.[1,142] Epidemiological and laboratory studies provide evidence for a direct causal role of sunlight exposure in the induction of most forms of skin cancer,[5,143] and the high rate of skin carcinogenesis is a direct result of the high dose rate from the ultraviolet (UV) light component. Nonmelanoma skin cancers (NMSC), basal cell carcinomas (BCC), and squamous cell carcinomas (SCC) and melanomas are found on sun-exposed parts of the body (e.g., the face and trunk in men, face, and legs in women) and their incidence is correlated with cumulative or acute sunlight exposure. Tumor incidence and mortality increase with occupational exposure, such as in ranchers fishermen and even flight crew members.[6,144–146] There is also an increased risk of melanoma for people using tanning parlors,[146,147] PUVA or UVA therapy[148] or sildenafil (Viagra).[149] The use of sunscreens can also contribute to melanoma if their use results in persons staying in the sun for increased times.[150] Melanomas are additionally found on protected sites, so other factors contribute to the incidence as well as sun exposure.[12,151,152]

Human skin can be classified into types I–IV, ranging from individuals who always burn and never tan, to those who tan but never burn; skin cancer susceptibility varies accordingly.[153] The most dramatic examples of variations in human susceptibility to sunburn and skin cancer are the human genetic disorders: xeroderma pigmentosum (XP), Cockayne syndrome (CS), trichothiodystrophy (TTD), basal cell nevus syndrome (BCNS), the porphyrias, albinism, and phenylketonuria.[12] XP, CS, and TTD involve genes with major roles in repair of UV damage to DNA. Other disorders associated with acquired sun sensitivity include polymorphous light eruption, actinic reticuloid and prurigo, solar urticaria, lupus erythematosus, and Darier's disease as well as medication and immunological status. Sunlight exposure can have an immunosuppressive effect leading to loss of antigen-presenting Langerhans cells and the appearance of dyskeratotic keratinocytes (apoptotic sunburn cells) in the upper epidermis. The erythemal response is also associated with vasodilation caused by a release of prostaglandins.[154] Immunosuppression in organ transplant and HIV patients also increases skin cancer incidence.[155]

"Mad Dogs and Englishmen Go Out in the Mid-Day Sun" – Noel Coward

Key references

The complete reference list can be found on Vital Source version of this title, see inside front cover.

12 Kraemer KH, Lee MM, Andrews AD, Lambert WC. The role of sunlight and DNA repair in melanoma and nonmelanoma skin cancer. The xeroderma pigmentosum paradigm. *Arch Dermatol.* 1994;**130**:1018–1021.

13 Bradford PT, Goldstein AM, Tamura DT, et al. Cancer and neurologic degeneration in xeroderma pigmentosum: long term follow-up characterises the role of DNA repair. *J Med Genet.* 2011;**48**:168–176.

15 Nance MA, Berry SA. Cockayne syndrome: review of 140 cases. *Am J Med Genet.* 1992;**42**:68–84.

26 Taylor JS, Cohrs MP. DNA, light, and Dewar pyrimidinones: the structure and significance of TpT3. *J Am Chem Soc.* 1987;**109**:2834–2835.

27 Mitchell DL, Jen J, Cleaver JE. Relative induction of cyclobutane dimers and cytosine photohydrates in DNA irradiated *in vitro* and *in vivo* with ultraviolet C and ultraviolet B light. *Photochem Photobiol.* 1991;**54**:741–746.

28 Mitchell DL, Jen J, Cleaver JE. Sequence specificity of cyclobutane pyrimidine dimers in DNA treated with solar (ultraviolet B) radiation. *Nucleic Acids Res.* 1992;**20**:225–229.

30 Mitchell DL, Cleaver JE. Photochemical alterations of cytosine account for most biological effects after ultraviolet irradiation. *Trends Photochem. Photobiol.* 1990;**1**:107–119.

35 Hoeijmakers JH. Genome maintenance mechanisms for preventing cancer. *Nature.* 2001;**411**:366–374.

36 Cleaver JE. Defective repair replication in xeroderma pigmentosum. *Nature.* 1968;**218**:652–656.

37 Cleaver JE. Xeroderma pigmentosum: a human disease in which an initial stage of DNA repair is defective. *Proc Natl Acad Sci USA.* 1969;**63**:428–435.

38 Cleaver JE, Lam ET, Revet I. Disorders of nucleotide excision repair: the genetic and molecular basis of heterogeneity. *Nat Rev Genet.* 2009;**10**:756–768.

39 Sancar A, Lindsey-Boltz LA, Unsal-Kacmaz K, Linn S. Molecular mechanisms of mammalian DNA repair and the DNA damage checkpoints. *Annu Rev Biochem.* 2004;**73**:39–85.

41 Hanawalt PC. Transcription-coupled repair and human disease. *Science.* 1994;**266**:1957–1958.

47 Fitch ME, Nakajima S, Yasui A, Ford JM. *In vivo* recruitment of XPC to UV-induced cyclobutane pyrimidine dimers by the *DDB2* gene product. *J Biol Chem.* 2003;**276**:46909–46910.

50. Groisman R, Polanowska J, Kuraoka I, et al. The ubiquitin ligase activity in the DDB2 and CSA complexes is differentially regulated by the COP9 signalosome in response to DNA damage. *Cell*. 2003;**113**:357–367.
52. Maillard O, Solyom S, Naegeli H. An aromatic sensor with aversion to damaged strands confers versatility to DNA repair. *PLoS Biol*. 2007;**5**:e79.
53. Lindsey-Boltz LA, Sancar A. RNA poymerase: the most specific damage recognition protein in cellular responses to DNA damage. *Proc Natl Acad Sci U S A*. 2007;**104**:13213–13214.
54. Schwertman P, Lagarou A, Dekkers DHW, et al. UV-sensitive syndrome protein UVSSA recruits USP7 to regulate transcription-coupled repair. *Nat Genet*. 2012;**44**:598–602.
56. Newman JC, Bailey AD, Weiner AM. Cockayne syndrome group B protein (CSB) plays a general role in chromatin maintenance and remodeling. *Proc Natl Acad Sci U S A*. 2006;**103**:9613–9618.
57. Mao P, Meas R, Dorgan KM, Smerdon MJ. UV damage-induced RNA polymerase II stalling stimulates H2B deubiquitylation. *Proc Natl Acad Sci U S A*. 2014;**111**:12811–12816.
59. Wood RD. DNA damage recognition during nucleotide excision repair in mammalian cells. *Biochimie*. 1999;**81**:39–44.
61. Fagbemi AF, Orelli B, Scharer OD. Regulation of endonuclease activity in human nucleotide excision repair. *DNA Repair*. 2011;**10**:722–729.
65. Ohmori H, Friedberg EC, Fuchs RPP, et al. The Y-family of DNA polymerases. *Mol Cell*. 2001;**8**:7–8.
66. Trincao J, Johnson RE, Escalante CR, et al. Structure of the catalytic core of S. cerevisiae DNA polymerase eta: implications for translesion synthesis. *Mol Cell*. 2001;**8**:417–426.
69. Johnson RE, Prakash S, Prakash L. Efficient bypass of a thymine-thymine dimer by yeast DNA polymerase eta. *Science*. 1999;**283**:1001–1004.
87. Nakazawa Y, Sasaki K, Mitsutake N, et al. KIAA1530/UVSSA is responsible for UV-sensitive syndrome that facilitates damage-dependent processing of stalled RNA polymerase IIo in TC-NER. *Nat Genet*. 2012;**44**:586–592.
88. Zhang X, Horibata K, Saijo M, et al. Mutations in KIAA1530/UVSSA cause UV-sensitive syndrome destabilizing ERCC6 in transcription-coupled DNA repair. *Nat Genet*. 2012;**44**:593–597.
89. Scheibye-Knudsen M, Croteau DL, Bohr VA. Mitochondrial deficiency in Cockayne syndrome. *Mech Aging Develop*. 2013;**134**:275–283.
90. Cleaver JE, Brennan-Minnella AM, Swanson RA, et al. Mitochondrial reactive oxygen species are scavenged by Cockayne syndrome B protein in human fibroblasts without nuclear DNA damage. *Proc Natl Acad Sci U S A*. 2014;**111**:13487–13492.
96. Loeb L. Mutator phenotype may be required for multistage carcinogenesis. *Cancer Res*. 1991;**51**:3075–3079.
97. Wang Y, Waters J, Leung ML, et al. Clonal evolution in breast cancer revealed by single nucleus genome sequencing. *Nature*. 2014;**512**:155–160.
98. Lawrence MS, Stojanov P, Polak P, et al. Mutational heterogeneity in cancer and the search for new cancer-associated genes. *Nature*. 2013;**499**:214–218.
99. Pleasance ED, Cheetham RK, Stephens PJ, et al. A comprehensive catalogue of somatic mutations from a human cancer genome. *Nature*. 2010;**463**:191–196.
113. Laposa RR, Huang EJ, Cleaver JE. Increased apoptosis, p53 up-regulation, and cerebellar neuronal degeneration in repair-deficient Cockayne syndrome mice. *Proc Natl Acad Sci U S A*. 2007;**104**:1389–1394.
124. Epstein EH. Basal cell carcinomas: attack of the hedgehog. *Nat Rev Cancer*. 2008;**8**:743–754.
136. Masaki T, Wang Y, DiGiovanna JJ, et al. High frequency of PTEN mutations in nevi and melanomas from xeroderma pigmentosum patients. *Pigment Cell Melanoma Res*. 2014;**27**:454–464.
137. Davies H, Bignell GR, Cox C, et al. Mutations of the *BRAF* gene in human cancer. *Nature*. 2002;**417**:949–954.
141. Noonan FP, Zaidi MR, Wolnicka-Glubisz A, et al. Melanoma induction by ultraviolet A but not ultraviolet B radiation requires melanin pigment. *Nat Commun*. 2012;**3**:884.
142. Scotto J, Fears TR, Fraumeni JF. *Incidence of Nonmelanoma Skin Cancer in the United States*. U.S. Department of Health and Human Services, NIH Publication; 1983, No. 83-2433.
154. Kripke ML. Immunological effects of ultraviolet radiation. *J Dermatol*. 1991;**18**:429–433.

25 Inflammation and cancer

Jelena Todoric, MD, PhD ■ *Atsushi Umemura, MD, PhD* ■ *Koji Taniguchi, MD, PhD* ■ *Michael Karin, PhD**

Overview

Epidemiological studies and experimental evidence have provided strong support to the long-standing notion that chronic inflammation stimulates the development and progression of malignant neoplasms. It is now clear that preexisting inflammation caused by persistent viral and microbial infections, autoimmune diseases, environmental irritants, and even obesity promote tumor development and may account for up to 20% of all cancer deaths. Inflammation also appears subsequent to cancer development and such "tumor-elicited inflammation" plays a key role in the malignant progression and metastatic dissemination of most cancers. Although some common anti-inflammatory drugs, such as aspirin, substantially reduce cancer risk, there is still an unmet need for the clinical development of new therapeutics that target cancer-associated inflammation.

Chronic inflammation and cancer

A potential link between inflammation and cancer was first proposed by the German pathologist, Rudolf Virchow, in the nineteenth century. Virchow supposedly detected immune cell infiltrates in solid tumors, leading him to suggest that inflammation could be a cause of tumorigenesis. Although largely forgotten for more than a century, the interest in the link between inflammation and cancer was rekindled by epidemiological studies suggesting that underlying chronic inflammation is associated with nearly 20% of all cancer deaths. More recently, solid evidence has accumulated pointing to inflammation as a critical hallmark of cancer, and some of the key underlying molecular mechanisms were elucidated.[1] Furthermore, it is well established that an inflammatory microenvironment is an important component of most cancers, including certain hematopoietic malignancies, even in tumors where a direct causal relationship is yet to be established.[2] Notably, only 10% of all cancers are linked to germ line mutations, whereas the vast majority (90%) are caused by acquired somatic mutations, many of which may be caused by environmental factors that are often associated with chronic inflammation. However, in most cases, chronic inflammation caused by persistent infections and autoimmune disease acts as a tumor promoter.[3] One of the most notable examples is inflammatory bowel disease (IBD), such as ulcerative colitis, which greatly increases the risk of colorectal cancer (CRC).[3] Similarly, persistent *Helicobacter pylori* infection causes chronic gastritis and can lead to gastric cancer. Infections with hepatitis B virus (HBV) or hepatitis C virus (HCV) give rise to hepatitis (chronic liver inflammation), eventually culminating in liver cancer (hepatocellular carcinoma or HCC). About 85% of the current HCC cases, one of the leading causes of cancer death worldwide, are derived from chronic liver damage caused by either HBV or HCV infections (Table 1).

In the past generation, obesity and excessive sugar consumption became major public health problem in most developed countries, increasing the risk of numerous diseases, including cancer. Obesity induces low-grade, sustained inflammation that influences many organ systems and is currently one of the most common risk factors for almost all types of cancer. Likewise, excessive consumption of fructose can result in gastrointestinal (GI) and hepatic inflammation and increased cancer risk at these sites. Inversely, long-term use of anti-inflammatory drugs, such as aspirin or selective cyclooxygenase-2 (COX-2) inhibitors, results in a substantial reduction in the risk of cancer development. Even the most common antidiabetic and anti-lipidemic drugs, metformin, and statins have anti-inflammatory properties and their use also prevents cancer onset. Antimicrobial and antiviral drugs that reduce stomach and liver inflammation (gastritis and hepatitis, respectively) also decrease cancer burden. These results further underscore the importance of inflammation as one of the major causes of cancer and a driver of malignant progression and metastatic dissemination.

It is important to note that only in some types of cancer is chronic inflammation present before malignant transformation or tumor initiation, but in the majority of cancers, oncogenic, and neoplastic changes induce a localized inflammatory microenvironment that further enhances tumor development and progression. Understanding the links between inflammation and cancer is essential for the development of better preventative and therapeutic strategies.

Inflammatory cells, the microenvironment, and cancer

Macrophages

Macrophages are the most abundant immune cells in the tumor microenvironment (TME). Tumor-associated macrophages (TAMs) acquire protumorigenic properties in both primary and metastatic sites[5] and play several supportive roles in cancer development and progression. The tumor-promoting functions of TAMs affect cancer cell proliferation and survival, angiogenesis, invasion, motility, intravasation, and extravasation, as well as suppression of cytotoxic T-cell responses.[6,7] During tumor initiation/early promotion, TAMs secrete cytokines and growth factors that stimulate the proliferation and survival of initiated epithelial cells bearing oncogenic mutations.[8] It is not clear whether, at this early stage of tumor development, macrophages can eliminate abnormal cells before they undergo polarization to acquire tumor-promoting properties. Two major subsets of macrophages were described: classically activated (M1) and alternatively activated (M2).[9]

*Corresponding author

Table 1 Major cancer sites and types associated with infectious agents.[a]

Infectious agent	Cancer site and type
Helicobacter pylori	Gastric cancer
Hepatitis B virus (HBV), hepatitis C virus (HCV)	Liver cancer
Human papillomavirus (HPV)	Cervical cancer, anogenital cancer, oropharynx cancer
Epstein–Barr virus (EBV)	Nasopharynx cancer
Schistosoma haematobium	Bladder cancer
Human immunodeficiency virus (HIV)	Non-Hodgkin lymphoma, Kaposi sarcoma, cervical cancer

As of 2008, around 16% of cancer cases worldwide are attributed to infectious agents. The most important players are *Helicobacter pylori*, HBV and HCV, and HPV.
[a]Source: de Martel.[4] Reproduced with permission of Elsevier.

M1 macrophages express and secrete a variety of proinflammatory cytokines, chemokines, and effector molecules, including IL-12, IL-23, tumor necrosis factor (TNF), and iNOS, whereas M2 macrophages release anti-inflammatory mediators, such as IL-10, TGF-β, and arginase-1. During early tumor progression, several factors cause a phenotypic switch from the M1 to the M2 phenotype, thereby providing an immunosuppressive microenvironment that is permissive for tumor growth. Exposure of macrophages to IL-4 produced by $CD4^+$ T cells and/or cancer cells,[6,10] growth factors such as colony-stimulating factor-1 (CSF1),[11] GM-CSF,[12] and TGF-β secreted by cancer cells induces the tumor-promoting M2 phenotype, but the actual origin of TAMs is still a matter of debate. Most TAMs may be derived from $Ly6C^+$ circulating monocytes,[13–15] but the classical view of the bone marrow (BM) as the major site of monocyte production has been challenged by recent studies suggesting that extramedullary hematopoiesis sustains a reservoir of tumor-infiltrating monocytes.[16] However, lineage-tracing experiments demonstrated that the splenic contribution is minor and that the BM is still the major source of monocytes that give rise to TAMs, at least in some tumor models.[17] In addition to its ability to support TAM proliferation and activation, CSF1 is the major lineage regulator and a chemotactic factor for macrophages.[18] Blood vessels that provide oxygenation and nutrition dramatically increase in most tumors during malignant conversion, a process often referred to as the "angiogenic switch." TAMs that express TIE2 regulate this process mostly via production of vascular endothelial growth factor (VEGF).[19] $TIE2^+$ macrophages also promote cancer cell migration and intravasation into the circulation.[20] Furthermore, immunosuppression in the tumor bed is partially mediated by macrophages, monocytes, and granulocytes, collectively known as myeloid-derived suppressor cells (MDSC) that contribute to the inhibition of cytotoxic $CD8^+$ cells.[21] Other immunosuppressive cell types are IgA-producing plasma cells and plasmablasts, referred to as immunosuppressive plasmocytes.[22,23]

T and B lymphocytes

Many tumors express antigens that can be recognized by T lymphocytes, and analysis of the TME in a variety of solid tumors has revealed the presence of T-cell infiltrates. However, despite an active immune response in a subset of patients, including infiltration with cytotoxic $CD8^+$ T cells, tumors that progress are obviously not rejected. This indicates the existence of immunosuppressive mechanisms that counteract anticancer immunity. One such mechanism depends on accumulation of $CD4^+Foxp3^+$ regulatory T cells (Treg) that play a pivotal role in maintenance of immunological self-tolerance.[24] Furthermore, Treg can also produce cytokines, such as RANK ligand (RANKL) that promote tumor progression, as first demonstrated in breast cancer.[25] Another important immunosuppressive mechanism first revealed in HCC involves the accumulation of IL-10 and PD-L1 producing IgA-expressing plasmocytes.[22] Productive $CD8^+$ T-cell priming in tumors involves the participation of stress-associated or damage-associated molecular patterns (DAMP), through which tissue injury or cancer cell death can promote antitumor immunity. Production of type I interferon by $CD8α^+$ dendritic cells (DCs) also favors the activation of anticancer immunity.[26] DCs and macrophages express major histocompatibility complex (MHC) class I molecules or human leukocyte antigens (HLA) that inhibit activation of natural killer (NK) cells but promote activation of $CD8^+$ T-cells[27] HLA-G and HLA-E also inhibit NK-cell secretion of IFN-γ, an important mediator of $CD8^+$ T-cell activation.[28] Activation of the inhibitory receptors programmed cell death protein 1 (PD-1) and cytotoxic T lymphocyte antigen 4 (CTLA-4) by ligands that are expressed on either cancer cells or immune cells controls the intensity of immune response and inhibits T-cell receptor (TCR) and B-cell receptor (BCR) signaling.[29] TAMs have been shown to upregulate PD-1 ligand expression in response to hypoxia-inducible factor 1α (HIF-1α) in hypoxic tumor regions, leading to T-cell suppression.[30] Furthermore, TAMs secrete a variety of cytokines and chemokines that can directly suppress T-cell activation and recruit immunosuppressive Treg cells. Th17 cells are T cells that produce the inflammatory cytokines IL-17A and IL-17F. These cells are recruited into early colon cancers and play an important role in accelerating tumor progression.[31] B lymphocytes are also present in the TME. In mouse models of skin cancer or squamous cell carcinoma, B cells promote tumor progression by activating cells and other myeloid cells.[32,33] In prostate cancer, newly recruited B cells promote the development of aggressive castration-resistant tumors by producing the pro-inflammatory cytokine lymphotoxin.[34] Tumor-infiltrating B cells can also respond to the high local concentration of TGF-β present within certain tumors and assume an immunosuppressive phenotype that prevents the activation of cytotoxic T cells. This mechanism is of particular relevance to IgA-expressing B cells, whose differentiation is TGF-β dependent, which suppresses CTL activation through the production of PD-L1 and IL-10.[22,35]

Cancer-associated fibroblasts (CAFs)

Cancer-associated fibroblasts (CAFs) are fibroblastic cells that reside within the TME CAFs promote tumorigenesis by stimulating cancer cell proliferation, enhancing angiogenesis, and modifying the architecture of the extracellular matrix (ECM).[36–41] In normal tissues, fibroblasts prevent initiation of neoplastic growth through negative regulation of epithelial proliferation by TGF-β-mediated signaling. In contrast, CAFs show pro-inflammatory and tumor-promoting properties[42] and produce a wide variety of chemokines and cytokines including osteopontin (OPN), CXCL1, CXCL2, IL-6, IL1-β, CCL-5, stromal-derived factor (SDF-1α), and TNF.[43,44] In the early stages of the tumorigenic process, fibroblasts "sense" changes in tissue architecture that result from increased proliferation of neighboring epithelial cells. This results in activation of proinflammatory signaling in fibroblasts.[45–47] Furthermore, the pro-inflammatory properties of CAFs are enhanced by mediators secreted by resident immune cells.[44] For example, B cells produce antibodies that are deposited in the tumor bed owing to small amounts of blood seeping out of leaky blood vessels and can induce secretion of IL-1 by resident immune cells. This, in turn, drives fibroblasts into a proinflammatory phenotype.[48,49] CAFs can also be affected by tumor hypoxia, which upregulates their ability to produce TGF-β and certain chemokines.[50] The major mechanism of tumor promotion by CAFs involves the secretion of cytokines and chemokines that recruit immune cells into the TME and alter their function. For example, CAF-secreted CCL2 recruits macrophages to the tumor, whereas CAF-derived immunosuppressive cytokine TGF-β inhibits the function of NK and CD8+ T cells[51] while inducing differentiation of Treg cells.[52] CAF-derived CXCL13 mediates recruitment of B cells into androgen-deprived prostate cancer, leading to development of castration resistance.[50]

Pro- and anti-inflammatory cytokines in cancer

Cytokines are small proteins produced and released by many types of cells, especially immune cells, that function as mediators of cell–cell communication via specific membrane receptors.[8] Cytokines are usually induced in response to inflammation and provide an important link between inflammation and cancer through cancer-intrinsic (cancer cell proliferation, survival, and invasive properties) and cancer-extrinsic (TME-specific) effects (Figure 1).[53] TNF and IL-6 are the best-studied protumorigenic cytokines linking inflammation to cancer and are overexpressed in most cancers (Table 2).[54] Several transcription factors, NF-κB, signal transducer and activator of transcription 3 (STAT3), and AP-1, are the major downstream effectors of cytokine signaling and are activated in the majority of cancers, where they cooperate to regulate many cancer-related pathophysiological processes, including cell proliferation and survival, differentiation, immunity, metabolism, and metastatic behavior.[55]

Tumor necrosis factor

TNF is the founding member of a large cytokine family and major activator of inflammatory and immune responses to a variety of pathogens.[56,57] TNF is an important mediator of cachexia and several acute and chronic inflammatory diseases, such as sepsis, rheumatoid arthritis (RA), and IBD. TNF is mainly produced by macrophages, which are activated by pathogen-associated molecular patterns (PAMPs), such as lipopolysaccharide (LPS), via toll-like receptors (TLRs). TNF activates several signaling pathways by binding to TNF receptor (TNFR)1 and/or TNFR2.

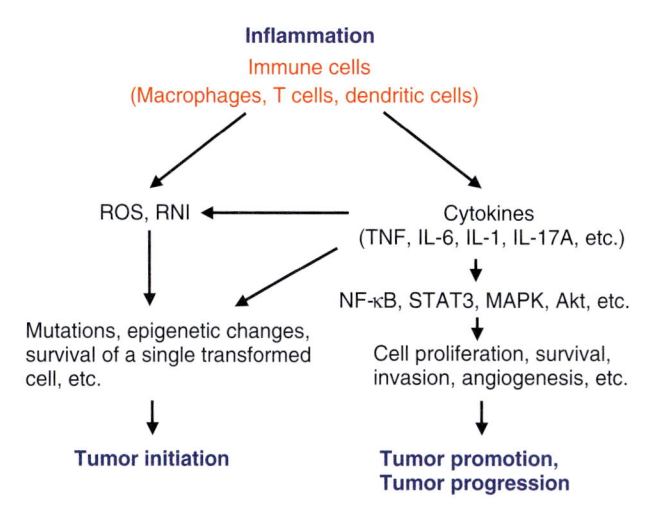

Figure 1 The role of inflammation in tumor initiation, promotion, and progression.

Table 2 Cytokines in inflammation and cancer.

Cytokine	Functions in cancer and immune cells	Pathways
TNF	Proinflammatory, cell survival or death	NF-κB, MAPK
IL-6	Proinflammatory, cell proliferation, and survival	JAK/STAT3, ERK, Akt
IL-11	Tissue-protective, cell proliferation, and survival	JAK/STAT3, ERK, Akt
IL-1	Proinflammatory, activates immune cells	NF-κB, MAPK
IL-17A	Proinflammatory, increases inflammation	NF-κB, MAPK
IL-12	Proinflammatory, Th1 differentiation	JAK/STAT4
IL-23	Proinflammatory, Th17 differentiation	JAK/STAT3, STAT4
IL-10	Anti-inflammatory, inhibits NF-κB	JAK/STAT3
IL-22	Tissue-protective, cell proliferation, and survival	JAK/STAT3
TGF-β	Anti-inflammatory, dual role in tumorigenesis	Smad, MAPK

Activation of these pathways induces production of other inflammatory cytokines, such as IL-6 and IL-1 and, depending on cellular context, modulates cell survival, and death. Elevated TNF expression promotes tumorigenesis and metastasis at multiple steps, including cellular transformation, survival, proliferation, invasion, and angiogenesis.[56,57] TNF-induced NF-κB activation enhances β-catenin activation, which leads to dedifferentiation of nonstem cells that acquire tumor-initiating capacity in a mouse model of CRC.[58] Several TNF inhibitors are clinically available and are approved for the treatment of RA and IBD. Although high doses of TNF have been used in the treatment of sarcomas of the extremities, localized production of TNF is associated with tumor promotion. Despite the obvious protumorigenic effects of TNF it was suspected that TNF inhibitors used in IBD and rheumatology may increase cancer risk. These suspicions have been diffused through extensive meta-analysis of available clinical data.[59] Recent data suggest that TNF contributes to the evolution of checkpoint inhibitor resistance, suggesting that its inhibition synergizes with cancer immunotherapy.[60]

The IL-6 family of cytokines

IL-6 is another proinflammatory cytokine that activates the acute phase response characterized by expression of C-reactive protein (CRP) and serum amyloid A (SAA).[61] IL-6 is also a mediator of cancer cachexia and is one of the best-characterized protumorigenic cytokines.[62,63] The IL-6 family also includes IL-11, IL-27, IL-31, leukemia inhibitory factor (LIF), oncostatin M (OSM), ciliary neurotrophic factor (CNTF), cardiotrophin-1 (CT-1), and cardiotrophin-like cytokine (CLC), all of which control cell proliferation, survival, migration, invasion, metastasis, angiogenesis, and inflammation. IL-6 family members activate the Janus kinase (JAK)-STAT3 pathway, the Src homology 2 (SH2)-containing protein tyrosine phosphatase-2 (SHP-2)-Ras-Raf-MEK-extracellular signal-regulated kinase (ERK) pathway, and the phosphoinositide 3-kinase (PI3K)-Akt-mammalian target of rapamycin (mTOR) pathway through engagement of their unique receptor(s) that associate with the common signaling subunit gp130. Among these effectors, STAT3 is considered an oncogene and a major downstream mediator of gp130 signaling in cancer.[64,65] IL-6 and IL-11 are produced by many different types of cells, including immune cells, fibroblasts, and epithelial cells, and IL-6, IL-11, and STAT3 are highly expressed in many solid tumors. IL-6 and other family members can also lead to activation of the regeneration inducing transcription factor YAP and thereby contributes to colorectal tumorigenesis.[66,67] A recent report described IL-11 as the dominant IL-6 family member during GI tumorigenesis in mice.[68] IL-6 antagonists originally approved for the treatment of RA and related diseases were found useful for suppressing the cytokine storm that often accompanies CAR T cell therapy.[69] Recent clinical data suggest that IL-6 antagonists may also be active as monotherapies.[70]

Interleukin 1

IL-1 is another major proinflammatory and protumorigenic cytokine produced by a variety of cell types.[71] IL-1 induces fever and plays an important role in sepsis. There are two isoforms of IL-1: IL-1α and IL-1β, both of which activate NF-κB, JNK, p38, and ERK via IL-1 receptor (IL-1R) and can induce expression of other cytokines. IL-1α and IL-1β have similar functions although they are only 26% similar at the protein level. Several IL-1 antagonists have been developed and are used for the treatment of auto-inflammatory conditions. Interestingly a recent clinical trial of an IL-1β blocking antibody in cardiovascular disease revealed a dramatic decrease in the incidence of lung cancer.[72] These results suggest that IL-1 antagonism can be used both for the prevention and the treatment of lung cancer, the most common inflammation-related malignancy.

Interleukin 17A

IL-17A is a member of the IL-17 family and is mainly produced by IL-17-producing T-helper (Th17) cells, γδ T cells, and innate lymphoid cells (ILCs).[73,74] IL-17A normally provides protection against extracellular bacteria and fungi and is associated with autoimmune diseases, such as psoriasis. IL-17A activates NF-κB, JNK, p38, and ERK via IL-17 receptor A (IL-17RA) in many cell types and promotes tumorigenesis, metastasis, angiogenesis, and chemotherapy resistance.[75] IL-17A induces production of many proinflammatory cytokines, including TNF, IL-6, and IL-1β, suggesting an important role of IL-17A in amplifying inflammation. IL-17A also signals within transformed enterocytes and promotes growth and progression of aberrant crypt foci in a mouse model of CRC.[75] IL-17 also plays an important role in several other GI malignancies including gastric cancer and alcohol-related liver cancer, where it was found to signal both in hepatocytes and macrophages.[76] In breast cancer, IL-17A signaling contributes to chemoresistance.[77] IL-17 can also promote generation of an immunosuppressive TME.[78] However, in some cases, IL-17 was described to have antitumor activity mainly via enhancement of cytotoxicity.[79] These Janus-like features have hampered the clinical development of IL-17 antagonists in cancer.

IL-12 and IL-23

IL-12 and IL-23 are related heterodimeric proinflammatory cytokines that share a p40 subunit, whose receptors contain a common IL-12 receptor (IL-12R) β1 subunit.[80] They are mainly produced by antigen-presenting (AP) cells and are key players in the regulation of T-cell responses. IL-12 stimulates the development of Th1 cells (typically antitumorigenic) that produce IFN-γ, whereas IL-23 promotes the development of Th17 cells (often protumorigenic) together with IL-6 and TGF-β. By enhancing IL-17A production, IL-23 signaling contributes to colorectal tumorigenesis.[31]

IL-10 and IL-22

IL-10, the founding member of the IL-10 family, is an anti-inflammatory cytokine that activates the JAK-STAT3 pathway via IL-10 receptor 1 (IL-10R1), which is mainly expressed in immune cells.[81] IL-10 exerts its anti-inflammatory activity in part through NF-κB inhibition. IL-10 knockout mice spontaneously develop chronic colitis that resembles human IBD. In contrast, IL-22, another member of the IL-10 family of cytokines, is a proinflammatory cytokine that is produced by Th17- and IL-22-producing T-helper (Th22) cells and ILC. IL-22 also activates the JAK-STAT3 pathway via IL-22 receptor 1 (IL-22R1), which is exclusively expressed on epithelial cells and not on immune cells. IL-22 regulates innate responses related to host defense and autoimmune disease, promotes cell proliferation, survival, tissue regeneration, metastasis, and angiogenesis in a similar way to the IL-6 family of cytokines.[82]

Transforming growth factor-beta

TGF-β is the prototypical member of the TGF-β superfamily of anti-inflammatory cytokines.[83] TGF-β activates the Smad pathway and non-Smad signaling via the JNK, p38, and ERK MAPKs, through binding to heterodimeric type I and II TGF-β receptors (TGF-RI and -RII). TGF-β also inhibits cell proliferation and regulates Treg and Th17 differentiation. TGF-β plays a dual role in the progression of cancer;[84] exerting suppressive effects in normal cells and early carcinomas, and promoting malignant progression, invasion, and metastasis in advanced tumors. TGF-β antagonists were found to potentiate the response to PD-1 inhibitors.[85,86]

Inflammation and tumorigenesis

The tumorigenic process is composed of several steps: initiation, promotion, and metastasis. These progressive steps are accompanied by tumor angiogenesis, formation of new blood, and lymph vessels that supply the growing tumor with essential nutrients and oxygen. These vessels also provide routes for metastatic dissemination. Through the release of inflammatory mediators, chronically activated TAM and CAF in the TME control malignant progression and tumor angiogenesis.

Tumor initiation

The initiation phase involves induction of oncogenic mutations that lead to oncogene activation and/or loss of tumor suppressors. These mutations change the behavior of normal cells to become malignant by providing them with growth and survival advantages over their neighbors. Mediators such as reactive oxygen species (ROS) and reactive nitrogen intermediates (RNI) produced by inflammatory cells can lead to DNA damage and acquisition of oncogenic mutations. These reactive intermediates also cause genomic instability and can accelerate cell proliferation, but their over-production leads to cell death. Another mechanism through which inflammation may enhance tumor initiation is the production of growth factors and cytokines that confer a stem-cell-like phenotype upon tumor progenitors or stimulate stem cell expansion, thereby enlarging the cell pool that is targeted by environmental mutagens. However, this mechanism is more akin to early tumor promotion, which is discussed in the following sections.

In most cases, a single mutation is insufficient to cause cancer and at least 4–5 mutations are needed.[87,88] Thus, tumor initiation requires continuous exposure to ROS and RNI resulting in irreversible and persistent DNA damage and accumulation of numerous mutations in dividing cells. Chronic inflammation also leads to epigenetic alterations, including DNA methylation and histone modifications, that may further contribute to tumor initiation.

Tumor promotion

Tumor promotion is the process of tumor growth from a single initiated cell into a clonal population giving rise to a primary tumor. Tumor-promoting cytokines and growth factors produced by immune/inflammatory cells are central to this process. For instance, TNF and IL-6 activate AP-1, NF-κB, and STAT3 to induce genes that stimulate cell proliferation and survival. Cytokines that stimulate angiogenesis provide the growing primary tumor with blood vessels that increase oxygen and nutrient availability, altogether resulting in net tumor growth. Most, inflammatory cytokines act as strong tumor promoters, not only by stimulating cancer cell proliferation but also through suppression of cancer cell death. The general transcriptional activator YAP, a master regulator of tissue regeneration is also a key mediator of tumor promotion, acting downstream to members of the IL-6 receptor family and gp130.[67]

Inflammation and angiogenesis

As mentioned earlier, the demand for blood supply increases during the course of tumor growth. Inflammatory cells are an important source of angiogenic cytokines, including VEGF. Tumor hypoxia can lead to activation of CAF and increased production of chemokines that recruit more inflammatory and immune cells into the hypoxic tumor.[50]

Metastasis

The final stage in tumor progression is metastasis, which eventually causes over 90% of cancer deaths. Metastasis is a complex process that requires close collaboration among cancer cells, immune/inflammatory cells, and stromal elements. Initially, cancer cells acquire mesenchymal characteristics through the loss of cell polarity and adhesive properties, resulting in increased motility and ability to invade epithelial linings/basal membranes and enter efferent blood vessels or lymphatics.[89] This process is called epithelial-mesenchymal transition (EMT) and it is characterized by loss of E-cadherin expression. NF-kB activation plays an important role in the stimulation of EMT.[90] Next, cancer cells intravasate into blood vessels and lymphatics. Inflammation promotes both EMT and intravasation through production of mediators that activate NF-κB in cancer cells and increase vascular permeability, respectively. This is followed by the third step in which metastasis-initiating cells survive and travel throughout the circulation. It is estimated that only about 0.01% of cancer cells that enter the circulation will eventually survive and give rise to micrometastases.[91] Integrin-mediated attachment allows the extravasation of circulating cancer cells, and this process is governed by neutrophil-dependent upregulation of adhesion molecules.[92] Finally, single metastatic progenitors interact with immune, inflammatory, and stromal cells and start to proliferate.[93] Systemic inflammation enhances attachment of circulating cancer cells to target organs and stimulates neutrophil mobilization. Several proinflammatory cytokines present in the circulation of cancer patients upregulate expression of adhesion molecules on the endothelium or target organs, thereby enhancing metastatic cell attachment.[2]

Inflammation-dependent cancers—examples and treatment

Colorectal cancer

IBD and colorectal cancer
IBD patients are at an elevated risk for CRC, which when present in such patients is referred to as colitis-associated cancer (CAC). Although IBD contributes to only 2–3% of all cases of CRC,[94,95] up to 20% of IBD patients develop CAC within 30 years after disease onset. In mice, CAC-like disease can be induced by combining the chemical procarcinogen azoxymethane (AOM) with the mucosal irritant dextran sulfate sodium (DSS) salt, which elicits colitis-like pathology.[96] Using this model, the IL-6/IL11-STAT3 axis and NF-κB were proven to be required for the proliferation and survival of premalignant intestinal epithelial cells and CAC development.[8,97]

Sporadic colorectal cancer and inflammation
Even sporadic CRC that does not develop as a consequence of apparent colonic inflammation exhibits extensive inflammatory infiltrates, referred to as "tumor-elicited inflammation," with high levels of cytokine expression in the TME.[8] Long-term intake of nonsteroidal anti-inflammatory drugs (NSAIDs), such as aspirin, that inhibit the enzymatic activity of COX-2, reduces the relative risk of sporadic CRC and hereditary CRC, suggesting that inflammation also plays an important role in spontaneous CRC development.[94] The *Adenomatous polyposis coli* (*APC*) tumor suppressor gene, encoding a negative regulator of Wnt-β catenin signaling, is the most frequently mutated gene in sporadic CRC (60%), and germ line *APC* mutations cause familial adenomatous polyposis (FAP). Accordingly, *Apc*^{min} mutant mice and *Apc* intestinal epithelial-specific knockout mice provide good models for sporadic CRC and FAP.[96,98,99] In these mouse models, colorectal adenomas, which develop upon loss of the normal *Apc* allele, exhibit defective expression of several epithelial barrier proteins, resulting in entry of microbial products into the tumors but not the adjacent tissue.[31] These microbial products activate macrophages associated with early adenomas to produce IL-23 and expand the population of IL-17 producing cells that drive tumor progression through activation of IL-17RA.[75]

Gut microbiota and colorectal cancer
The GI tract is the largest reservoir of commensal bacteria in the human body.[100] Commensal bacteria affect various physiological functions in the gut via host–microbe interactions, and dysbiosis of the microbiota can lead to or promote various GI diseases including IBD and CRC.[101] A correlation between gut microbiota composition and GI cancers has been investigated in experimental animal models and clinical and epidemiological studies. Certain commensal microbes, such as *Bacteriodes fragilis*, *Escherichia coli*, *Streptococcus gallolycticus*, *Enterococcus faecalis*, and *Fusobacterium nucleatum* were found to promote CRC development in various models,[102] although none of them is considered a verified carcinogen, as is *H. pylori*, which induces gastritis and gastric cancer.[94] Pathogenic and commensal microbes may promote intestinal tumorigenesis through chronic activation of inflammation, alteration of TME, induction of genotoxic responses, and metabolism. Alternatively, tumor-promoting alterations could be caused by loss of protective or beneficial microbes. Recently, a microbial metabolite was shown to switch p53 from being a tumor suppressor to a tumor promoter.[103]

Cancer prevention, therapy, and side effects

Conventional therapy for CRC includes surgery, chemotherapy, and radiation therapy. Given the growing body of evidence that inflammation triggers and promotes CAC and sporadic CRC, there is room for drugs that reduce inflammation in the prevention or treatment of CRC and other GI cancers. As mentioned earlier, NSAIDs and selective COX-2 inhibitors were proven effective for CRC prevention. Inhibitors of proinflammatory cytokines, such as neutralizing antibodies or decoy receptors to TNF, IL-6, IL-1, IL-17A, and IL-23 or inhibitors of cytokine signaling, including JAK, STAT3, IKK, and NF-κB, might also be useful for the treatment of CAC and spontaneous CRC.[94] However, it is unlikely that such drugs would be effective as monotherapies, and thus, they should be tested in combination with chemo- or radiotherapy. Notably, JAK inhibitors were found effective for the treatment of IBD, but their side effects include mucositis, anemia, thrombocytopenia, liver dysfunction, and infection. Importantly, mucositis is the major dose-limiting factor in cytotoxic chemotherapy, and therefore, caution should be exercised when drugs that inhibit the activity of cytokines, such as IL-6, IL-17A, and IL-23 that promote mucosal healing, are combined with chemotherapeutic agents. Some chemotherapeutics may be more amenable to such combinations, as recently shown for 5-FU in an *Apc* mutant mouse, where it was found to be much more effective in combination with an IL-17A neutralizing antibody.[75]

Another approach to control GI inflammation is to use prebiotics or probiotics, with the aim of normalizing or skewing the host–microbiome to influence cancer development.[101] Bacteriophages were recently found to be useful in eliminating certain gut bacteria (Duan et al. 2019). Although first demonstrated as a potential treatment for alcoholic hepatitis, the same approach may also be applied to the prevention of CRC and HCC. Several dietary compounds were found to reduce inflammation and CRC risk, including carbohydrates, fiber, unsaturated n-3 fatty acids, vitamins, minerals, and phytochemicals (resveratrol and curcumin) although the underlying molecular mechanisms are unknown.[94] Aryl aromatic hydrocarbon receptor (AhR) agonists represent another interesting group of potential chemopreventive agents, acting through their ability to suppress colitis and restore barrier integrity.[104] However, the ability of such compounds to induce IL-22 requires more careful evaluation of their cancer preventive ability.

Pancreatic cancer

Inflammation and pancreatic ductal adenocarcinoma (PDAC)

Pancreatic ductal adenocarcinoma (PDAC) is an aggressive malignancy with an overall 5-year survival rate of <5%.[105] One of the major features of PDAC is remarkable desmoplasia that is composed of ECM, fibroblasts, vascular, and immune cells.[106] This cellular milieu is rich in inflammatory cytokines, growth factors, and proteinases that stimulate the proliferation and survival of malignant cells.[107,108] Increased levels of proinflammatory cytokines including IL-6, IL-8, and TNF, as well as the anti-inflammatory cytokines IL-10 and TGF-β were found to correlate with cachexia and poor prognosis in PDAC patients.[109–112] The progression of early PanIN lesions into PDAC in pancreatic *KRAS*-mutated mice has been shown to depend on activation of the STAT3 pathway by JAK tyrosine kinases in response to IL-6.[113] In addition, IL-6 induces expression of VEGF in pancreatic cancer cells, thereby stimulating angiogenesis.[114] Although high-dose TNF was shown to have toxic effects on cancer cells, in the PDAC microenvironment, binding of TNF to TNFR2 results in upregulation of EGF receptor and its ligand TGF-α, leading to increased cancer cell proliferation.[115] IL-10 and TGF-β facilitate the shift from the Th1 immunophenotype, which has antitumor activity, to the Th2 immunophenotype, which has protumor activity.[116]

Anti-inflammatory strategies for PDAC therapy

Major strategies to activate antitumor immune responses that were found to be effective in highly immunogenic cancers, such as cutaneous melanoma and bladder cancer, include adoptive transfer of cancer-reactive T cells and the use of immune checkpoint inhibitors.[117] For instance, blockade of the inhibitory receptors CTLA-4 and PD-1 with specific monoclonal antibodies or depletion of Treg cells with antibodies against CD25 can result in activation of anticancer immunity.[118,119] Such strategies, so far, have not been too effective against PDAC, perhaps due to the existence of additional, yet-to-be-discovered, immunosuppressive mechanisms. IL-6 monoclonal antibodies, Siltuximab and Tocilizumab, that bind to the soluble form of the IL-6 receptor are currently under evaluation in ovarian cancer patients (clinicaltrials.gov) and should be tested in PDAC as well. Ruxolitinib is a selective JAK1/JAK2 inhibitor that was approved by the U.S. Food and Drug Administration (FDA) in 2011 for the treatment of myelofibrosis. Ruxolitinib can block STAT3 activation by IL-6 and was found to significantly improve the survival rate of a subgroup of patients with recurrent or treatment-refractory PDAC (clinicaltrial.gov). Testing whether IL-6 neutralizing antibodies or JAK inhibitors may also potentiate the activation of cytotoxic T cells targeting PDAC would be of interest.

Liver cancer

Etiology and pathogenesis

HCC is the fifth most common cancer worldwide and the third leading cause of cancer deaths. More than 90% of HCC develops in the context of chronic liver disease and persistent inflammation, with HBV or HCV infections being the main causes. Additional risk factors for HCC include fatty liver disease, aflatoxin, alcohol, and hereditary conditions such as hemochromatosis. HCC is characterized by phenotypic and molecular heterogeneity reflecting diverse pathological origin. Because of that, no clear evidence for oncogene addiction has been proved, even though hTERT, β-catenin, and *p53* gene alterations are relatively common. As HCC develops in a liver with extensive inflammation and fibrosis, the role of inflammation in HCC development is particularly important.

Therapy

Early-stage HCC may be eligible for surgical resection (total or partial hepatectomy), liver transplantation, or local ablation therapy. However, 70% of HCC cases recur at 5 years after these curative therapies. If the tumor is already at advanced stages at the time of diagnosis or recurs after curative treatment, systemic chemotherapy using molecular targeted drugs is considered besides chemoembolization. However, the 5-year survival rate for recurrent HCC has remained very low (<8%).

The protein kinase inhibitor sorafenib is currently the only approved systemic drug for advanced HCC and median survival was only 2.8 months longer for patients treated with sorafenib than control group (10.7 months vs 7.9 months, respectively). Although drugs that target signaling pathways involved in HCC-tumorigenesis have been the subject of many clinical trials after the approval of sorafenib, no other drug demonstrated clear survival benefits or positive results in first-line (brivanib, sunitinib, erlotinib, and linifanib) or second-line (brivanib, everolimus) HCC therapy. Currently, clinical trials testing the MET inhibitor tivantinib and MEK inhibitor refametinib in RAS(+) HCC patients are ongoing. However, these drugs may be beneficial only for a subset of HCC patients because *RAS*-mutated cases represent no more than 5% of HCC patients.[120]

These failures may be due to the heterogeneous and complex molecular features of HCC, which remains a poorly understood malignancy. Liver toxicity was also seen frequently during clinical trials and is a main cause of their failure. Of note, coexistence of liver cirrhosis frequently limits treatment options for HCC patients. For instance, the rapalog everolimus did not extend overall survival compared to placebo and its use resulted in increased incidence of liver injury. Interestingly, either rapamycin treatment or hepatocyte-specific ablation of the raptor subunit of mTORC1, the molecular target for rapalogs, increased IL-6 production and activated the protumorigenic transcription factor STAT3 in a mouse model. Furthermore, loss of mTORC1 activity resulted in low-grade liver inflammation leading to enhancement of HCC development.[121]

Obesity, inflammation, and putative therapeutic options
Many HCC patients in Western countries do not exhibit viral infections.[122] Most of these patients are obese with manifestations of the metabolic syndrome and suffer from nonalcoholic steatohepatitis (NASH), a severe form of nonalcoholic fatty liver disease (NAFLD).[123] Indeed, obesity increases male HCC risk by up to 4.5-fold.[124] Because the prevalence of obesity has been increasing rapidly worldwide, its association with liver tumorigenesis has attracted much attention. Importantly, obesity strongly enhances HCC development in mice, allowing mechanistic studies, which revealed that obesity increases HCC risk by triggering low-grade liver inflammation associated with elevated expression of TNF and IL-6.[125] IL-6 signaling is also important to HCC development in nonobese settings, and HCC progenitor/stem cell expansion and malignant progression depend on autocrine IL-6 signaling.[126,127] In addition, obesity[128,129] and HBV/HCV infections[130] induce endoplasmic reticulum (ER) stress in hepatocytes and this may promote hepatosteatosis in humans.[131] Furthermore, ER stress contributes to NASH-like disease development and progression to HCC in mice.[132] Interestingly, HCC development in this model can be blunted through attenuation of ER stress or inhibition of TNF signaling in hepatocytes. These findings suggest that NASH and its progression to HCC may be prevented or ameliorated by anti-TNF drugs and molecules termed "chemical chaperons" that are capable of relieving ER stress. In addition to obesity and consumption of energy-dense diets, it has been suggested that much of the recent increase in NASH incidence is due to excessive intake of sugars, in particular fructose which stimulates hepatic steatosis. Recent studies in mice indicate that fructose consumption can stimulate both NASH and HCC development by causing barrier disruption and endotoxemia.[133] If verified in humans, these findings may lead to the development of new cancer preventive strategies based on restoration of barrier integrity.

Key references

The complete reference list can be found on Vital Source version of this title, see inside front cover.

1 Karin M. Nuclear factor-kappaB in cancer development and progression. *Nature*. 2006;**441**(7092):431–436.
2 Mantovani A, Allavena P, Sica A, Balkwill F. Cancer-related inflammation. *Nature*. 2008;**454**(7203):436–444.
3 Aggarwal BB, Vijayalekshmi RV, Sung B. Targeting inflammatory pathways for prevention and therapy of cancer: short-term friend, long-term foe. *Clin Cancer Res*. 2009;**15**(2):425–430.
5 Biswas SK, Allavena P, Mantovani A. Tumor-associated macrophages: functional diversity, clinical significance, and open questions. *Semin Immunopathol*. 2013;**35**(5):585–600.
6 Coussens LM, Zitvogel L, Palucka AK. Neutralizing tumor-promoting chronic inflammation: a magic bullet? *Science*. 2013;**339**(6117):286–291.
8 Grivennikov SI, Greten FR, Karin M. Immunity, inflammation, and cancer. *Cell*. 2010;**140**(6):883–899.
19 Lin EY, Pollard JW. Tumor-associated macrophages press the angiogenic switch in breast cancer. *Cancer Res*. 2007;**67**(11):5064–5066.
21 Gabrilovich DI, Nagaraj S. Myeloid-derived suppressor cells as regulators of the immune system. *Nat Rev Immunol*. 2009;**3**:162–174.
22 Shalapour S, Lin XJ, Bastian IN, et al. Inflammation-induced IgA$^+$ cells dismantle anti-liver cancer immunity. *Nature*. 2017;**551**:340–345.
24 Spranger S, Spaapen RM, Zha Y, et al. Up-regulation of PD-L1, IDO, and T(regs) in the melanoma tumor microenvironment is driven by CD8(+)T cells. *Sci Transl Med*. 2013;**5**(200):200ra116.
25 Tan W, Zhang W, Strasner A, et al. Tumour-infiltrating regulatory T cells stimulate mammary cancer metastasis through RANKL-RANK signalling. *Nature*. 2011;**470**(7335):548–553.
26 Fuertes MB, Kacha AK, Kline J, et al. Host type I IFN signals are required for antitumor CD8+ T cell responses through CD8{alpha}+ dendritic cells. *J Exp Med*. 2011;**208**(10):2005–2016.
30 Noman MZ, Desantis G, Janji B, et al. PD-L1 is a novel direct target of HIF-1alpha, and its blockade under hypoxia enhanced MDSC-mediated T cell activation. *J Exp Med*. 2014;**211**(5):781–790.
31 Grivennikov SI, Wang K, Mucida D, et al. Adenoma-linked barrier defects and microbial products drive IL-23/IL-17-mediated tumour growth. *Nature*. 2012;**491**(7423):254–258.
34 Ammirante M, Luo JL, Grivennikov S, et al. B-cell-derived lymphotoxin promotes castration-resistant prostate cancer. *Nature*. 2010;**464**(7286):302–305.
36 Allinen M, Beroukhim R, Cai L, et al. Molecular characterization of the tumor microenvironment in breast cancer. *Cancer Cell*. 2004;**6**(1):17–32.
38 Bhowmick NA, Neilson EG, Moses HL. Stromal fibroblasts in cancer initiation and progression. *Nature*. 2004;**432**(7015):332–337.
42 Neumann E, Lefèvre S, Zimmermann B, et al. Rheumatoid arthritis progression mediated by activated synovial fibroblasts. *Trends Mol Med*. 2010;**16**(10):458–468.
44 Erez N, Truitt M, Olson P, et al. Cancer-associated fibroblasts are activated in incipient neoplasia to orchestrate tumor-promoting inflammation in an NF-kappaB-dependent manner. *Cancer Cell*. 2010;**17**(2):135–147.
45 Chiquet M, Gelman L, Lutz R, Maier S. From mechanotransduction to extracellular matrix gene expression in fibroblasts. *Biochim Biophys Acta*. 2009;**1793**(5):911–920.
49 Mantovani A. La mala educación of tumor-associated macrophages: diverse path-ways and new players. *Cancer Cell*. 2010;**17**(2):111–112.
50 Ammirante M, Shalapour S, Kang Y, et al. Tissue injury and hypoxia promote malignant progression of prostate cancer by inducing CXCL13 expression in tumor myofibroblasts. *Proc Natl Acad Sci U S A*. 2014;**111**(41):14776–14781.
51 Ksiazkiewicz M, Gottfried E, Kreutz M, et al. Importance of CCL2-CCR2A/2B signaling for monocyte migration into spheroids of breast cancer-derived fibroblasts. *Immunobiology*. 2010;**215**(9–10):737–747.
52 Yang L, Pang Y, Moses HL. TGF-beta and immune cells: an important regulatory axis in the tumor microenvironment and progression. *Trends Immunol*. 2010;**31**(6):220–227.
53 Hanahan D, Weinberg RA. Hallmarks of cancer: the next generation. *Cell*. 2011;**144**(5):646–674.
54 Grivennikov SI, Karin M. Inflammatory cytokines in cancer: tumour necrosis factor and interleukin 6 take the stage. *Ann Rheum Dis*. 2011;**70**(Suppl 1):i104–i108.
57 Balkwill F. Tumour necrosis factor and cancer. *Nat Rev Cancer*. 2009;**9**(5):361–371.
62 Taniguchi K, Karin M. IL-6 and related cytokines as the critical lynchpins between inflammation and cancer. *Semin Immunol*. 2014;**26**(1):54–74.
63 Chang Q, Daly L, Bromberg J. The IL-6 feed-forward loop: a driver of tumorigenesis. *Semin Immunol*. 2014;**26**(1):48–53.

64. Yu H, Pardoll D, Jove R. STATs in cancer inflammation and immunity: a leading role for STAT3. *Nat Rev Cancer*. 2009;9(11):798–809.
66. Taniguchi K, Wu LW, Grivennikov SI, et al. A gp130-Src-YAP module links inflammation to epithelial regeneration. *Nature*. 2015;519:57–62.
71. Garlanda C, Dinarello CA, Mantovani A. The interleukin-1 family: back to the future. *Immunity*. 2013;39(6):1003–1018.
75. Wang K, Kim MK, Di Caro G, et al. Interleukin-17 receptor a signaling in transformed enterocytes promotes early colorectal tumorigenesis. *Immunity*. 2014;41:1052–1063.
76. Ma HY, Yamamoto G, Xu J, et al. IL-17 signaling in steatotic hepatocytes and macrophages promotes hepatocellular carcinoma in alcohol-related liver disease. *J Hepatol*. 2020;72:946–959.
77. Cochaud S, Giustiniani J, Thomas C, et al. IL-17A is produced by breast cancer TILs and promotes chemoresistance and proliferation through ERK1/2. *Sci Rep*. 2013;3:3456.
84. Meulmeester E, Ten Dijke P. The dynamic roles of TGF-beta in cancer. *J Pathol*. 2011;223(2):205–218.
90. Huber MA, Azoitei N, Baumann B, et al. NF-kappaB is essential for epithelial-mesenchymal transition and metastasis in a model of breast cancer progression. *J Clin Invest*. 2004;114:569–581.
94. Terzic J, Grivennikov S, Karin E, Karin M. Inflammation and colon cancer. *Gastroenterology*. 2010;138(6):2101.e5–2114.e5.
97. Greten FR, Eckmann L, Greten TF, et al. IKKbeta links inflammation and tumori-genesis in a mouse model of colitis-associated cancer. *Cell*. 2004;118(3):285–296.
102. Alhinai EA, Walton GE, Commane DM. The role of the gut microbiota in colorectal cancer causation. *Int J Mol Sci*. 2019;20:5295.
103. Kadosh E, Snir-Alkalay I, Venkatachalam A, et al. The gut microbiome switches mutant p53 from tumour-suppressive to oncogenic. *Nature*. 2020;586:133–138.
104. Metidji A, Omenetti S, Crotta S, et al. The environmental sensor AHR protects from inflammatory damage by maintaining intestinal stem cell homeostasis and barrier integrity. *Immunity*. 2018;49:353–362.
106. Gukovsky I, Li N, Todoric J, et al. Inflammation, autophagy, and obesity: common features in the pathogenesis of pancreatitis and pancreatic cancer. *Gastroenterology*. 2013;144(6):1199.e4–1209.e4.
107. Feig C, Gopinathan A, Neesse A, et al. The pancreas cancer microenvironment. *Clin Cancer Res*. 2012;18(16):4266–4276.
109. Ebrahimi B, Tucker SL, Li D, et al. Cytokines in pancreatic carcinoma: correlation with phenotypic characteristics and prognosis. *Cancer*. 2004;101(12):2727–2736.
113. Lesina M, Kurkowski MU, Ludes K, et al. Stat3/Socs3 activation by IL-6 transsignaling promotes progression of pancreatic intraepithelial neoplasia and development of pancreatic cancer. *Cancer Cell*. 2011;19(4):456–469.
117. Dougan M, Dranoff G. Immune therapy for cancer. *Annu Rev Immunol*. 2009;27:83–117.
121. Umemura A, Park EJ, Taniguchi K, et al. Liver damage, inflammation, and enhanced tumorigenesis after persistent mTORC1 inhibition. *Cell Metab*. 2014;20(1):133–144.
122. El-Serag HB. Hepatocellular carcinoma. *N Engl J Med*. 2011;365(12):1118–1127.
123. Cohen JC, Horton JD, Hobbs HH. Human fatty liver disease: old questions and new insights. *Science*. 2011;332(6037):1519–1523.
125. Park EJ, Lee JH, Yu GY, et al. Dietary and genetic obesity promote liver inflammation and tumorigenesis by enhancing IL-6 and TNF expression. *Cell*. 2010;140(2):197–208.
126. He G, Dhar D, Nakagawa H, et al. Identification of liver cancer progenitors whose malignant progression depends on autocrine IL-6 signaling. *Cell*. 2013;155(2):384–396.
131. Rutkowski DT, Wu J, Back SH, et al. UPR pathways combine to prevent hepatic steatosis caused by ER stress-mediated suppression of transcriptional master regulators. *Dev Cell*. 2008;15(6):829–840.
132. Nakagawa H, Umemura A, Taniguchi K, et al. ER stress cooperates with hyper-nutrition to trigger TNF-dependent spontaneous HCC development. *Cancer Cell*. 2014;26(3):331–343.

26 RNA tumor viruses*

Robert C. Gallo, MD ■ Marvin S. Reitz, PhD

> **Overview**
>
> Retroviruses are enveloped viruses that contain a diploid RNA genome and are defined by the presence of reverse transcriptase (RT), a DNA polymerase that transcribes RNA into DNA, which is then inserted into the host cell chromosome. These processes often lead to the capture and/or alteration of genetic material and the transfer of information between cells, with neoplastic transformation of the infected cell being an occasional outcome of infection. Retroviruses are also associated with immunodeficiencies and with neurologic diseases, although infection is often asymptomatic. Retroviruses can also enter the germ line and be present as a part of the genetic complement of some or all members of a species. These viruses are called endogenous retroviruses. Although most retroviral malignancies occur as leukemia/lymphomas in nonhuman species, human T-cell leukemia virus type I (HTLV-I) causes adult T cell leukemia/lymphoma in a minority of infected humans, as well as a neurologic disease and a variety of other pathologies. Human immunodeficiency virus type 1 (HIV-1), although not considered a true tumor virus, is associated with an increased incidence of several types of tumors, especially those caused by viruses such as human papillomavirus and Epstein–Barr virus.

Retroviruses were discovered early in the twentieth century. Ellerman and Bang showed the transmission of leukemia in chickens by a cell-free filtrate[1] and Rous was similarly able to transmit sarcomas in chickens.[2] These findings were extended to mammals by Bittner in the case of breast tumors in mice[3] and by Gross for murine leukemias.[4] Gross recognized the importance of inoculating newborn mice for development of leukemia, and in many respects, his work heralded the beginning of modern studies of retroviruses. Jarrett showed that a similar virus was responsible for leukemia in cats, which was the first demonstration of naturally transmitted leukemia in an outbred species.[5,6] Kawakami and Theilen and colleagues first showed that retroviruses could cause leukemia in primates, specifically in gibbon apes and new world monkeys.[7–9]

Biologic assays for these viruses were in use from the 1950s, but a more fundamental understanding of their life cycle was considerably advanced in the early 1970s by the discovery that they contained reverse transcriptase (RT).[10,11] This provided a far simpler, quicker, and more sensitive assay for retroviruses. Another important finding in the 1970s was that some retroviruses (e.g., Rous sarcoma virus [RSV]) contained genes for cell transformation and tumorigenesis (oncogenes) that represented captured cellular genes (proto-oncogenes).[12] This led to the identification of many similar genes and to an appreciation of their roles in cell growth and neoplastic transformation.

Despite this work and the interest that it engendered, it was widely believed during the 1970s that retroviruses did not play a role in human disease and were likely not even present in the human population. Several discoveries made it clear that this was not the case. Human T-cell leukemia virus type I (HTLV-I) was the first infectious human retrovirus identified; it was discovered and shown to be a unique virus by Gallo and his colleagues.[13–16] HTLV-I was soon established as the etiologic agent of adult T-cell leukemia (ATL), a type of leukemia endemic to various locales, including southern Japan and the Caribbean.[17–21] This was quickly followed by the discovery of HTLV-II,[22] a related virus that (although widespread) has not been compellingly associated with any disease. HTLV-I was shown to be able to neoplastically transform cord blood T cells.[23] Subsequently, HTLV-3 and -4 have been reported in primate hunters in Central Africa,[24] but as with HTLV-II, have not been associated with disease. HTLV-4 appears to have been recently acquired through the bushmeat trade from gorillas.[25]

Several years later, an epidemic of immunodeficiency and malignancies appeared within gay communities, especially in the United States. The first member of another group of human retroviruses was isolated from people with this disease, called acquired immunodeficiency syndrome (AIDS).[26] When it became possible to culture the virus on a large scale,[27] it was proven to be the etiologic agent of AIDS.[28,29] This virus, now called human immunodeficiency virus type 1 (HIV-1), has become established over much of the world, and AIDS represents a current global medical and economic catastrophe. As with HTLV-I, a related virus, HIV-2, was discovered[30] that also appears to be far less pathogenic than HIV-1.[31]

Classification

The retroviridae are a large family of viruses that have been classified using a variety of criteria,[32] originally according to their biologic effects. The subfamilies included oncoviruses, which cause leukemias or other malignancies in their hosts; lentiviruses, or "slow" viruses, which cause slow degenerative diseases; and spumaviruses, or foamy viruses, which produce a "foamy" cytopathic effect in infected cultures. The subfamilies have been divided further based on their genomic structures (Table 1). They have been historically classified based on the morphology of budding and mature virions in electron micrographs (Table 2). Retroviruses can also be classified as exogenous or endogenous depending upon whether they are transmitted by infection or genetically within the germ line of a species.

Structure

Retrovirus particles are composed of a core structure or capsid, which encloses two copies of the single stranded genomic RNA,

*The authors thank Elissa Miller for administrative support.

Table 1 Retrovirus groups.

Oncornaviruses
Avian leukosis-sarcoma viruses (ALSV)
Avian reticuloendotheliosis virus
Mammalian leukemia and sarcoma viruses (mouse/cat type C viruses)
Mouse mammary tumor virus
Primate type D viruses (Mason-Pfizer monkey virus/simian AIDS virus)
Human T-cell leukemia virus/bovine leukemia virus/simian T-cell leukemia virus
Lentiviruses (including immunodeficiency viruses)
Spumaviruses

Table 2 Retrovirus morphology.

A-type particles
Intracellular core formation and budding
Intracisternal A-type particles (IAP) are products of endogenous proviruses
Noninfectious
B-type particles (MMTV)
Core formation occurs in the cytoplasm
After budding at the plasma membrane, maturation to an eccentric core occurs
Prominent surface spikes
C-type particles
Most oncornaviruses
Initially form electron-dense patches at the plasma membrane
Budding at plasma membrane
Maturation of core to yield centrally located cores
Spikes may or may not be prominent
D-type particles
Mason-Pfizer monkey virus, simian AIDS virus
Intracellular nucleocapsid formation, budding at plasma membrane
Eccentric core
Less prominent spikes
Lentiviruses
Visna-maedi, EIAV, CAEV, SIV, HIV, FIV, BIV
Core formation and budding as for C-type particles
Condensed mature core forms pyramidal shape
Spumaviruses
IAP-like cores

surrounded by an envelope containing a lipid bilayer. The entire virion, or extracellular viral particle, is 100 nm in diameter. The genomic RNA is generally 8-9500 nucleotides long, and the simplest retroviruses contain three major genes (*gag*, *pol*, and *env*), all of which are contained in the virion (Figure 1). The genomic RNA contains repeat regions at both ends, called the R region. The DNA form of the genome integrated into the host cell genome contains the R region and other regulatory sequences in structures called the long terminal repeat (LTR) (Figure 1). Retroviruses often become replication-defective by loss of large regions of their genomes, which are sometimes replaced by oncogenes derived from the host cell. We now describe the genome and proteins of replication-competent retroviruses.

Viral genome and gene products

Space precludes a detailed description of retroviral genome structure and the viral proteins. Interested readers are referred to for details. However, these are presented schematically in Figures 2 and 3.

Genomic structure

The genomic structure described earlier is representative of the simplest retroviruses; other retroviruses, especially lentiviruses, and members of the HTLV group (including the related bovine leukemia virus, BLV, and the closely related simian viruses, STLV), contain extra genes and have a more complex genomic structure. HIV-1 and -2 (and the closely related SIV nonhuman primate viruses) encode at least six regulatory proteins that include a protein that activates viral RNA expression, another that regulates viral RNA splicing patterns, and proteins that interfere with host immune functions. The extra genes also result in a more complicated RNA splicing pattern, including multiple splicing for many of the regulatory genes. Similarly, HTLV-I encodes at least five additional proteins, including (like HIV) a protein that activates viral RNA expression and another that regulates viral RNA splicing patterns. Recently, evidence has been presented[33–35] that a protein called HTLV-I bZIP protein (HBZ) is transcribed from the 3′ LTR, translated from minus-strand viral RNA, and expressed in infected T cells and in uncultured ATL cells as a 31-kDa protein. The HBZ protein binds to cellular bZIP transcription factors including members of the CREB and Jun families[36,37] to repress Tax-mediated viral transcription and support ATL cell proliferation. HIV-1 also encodes a protein ASP that is transcribed in an antisense manner and is thought to be involved in autophagy and negative regulation of viral transcription.[38] MMTV and the spumaviruses also encode additional proteins, including those that activate viral RNA expression. Other retroviruses, especially those that are acutely transforming (such as the avian and mammalian sarcoma viruses), are generally replication-defective and have parts of their genomes deleted and replaced with captured cellular genes that confer transforming capability. These viruses require a replication-competent helper virus for transmission and replication.

Replication cycle

Space precludes a detailed description of the viral replication cycle. Details of the pertinent steps are covered in detail in.[39–42] Some of the steps are presented schematically in an abbreviated form in Figures 4–6. A few important points concerning the retroviral replication cycle should be noted. First, formation of the provirus, by the integration reaction, results in a stable genetic copy of the virus that cannot be removed from the infected cell except by targeted gene editing. Infected cells can and do persist for the life of the host, and whenever the cell divides, the provirus is passed on to both daughter cells. Furthermore, when germ line cells are infected, the proviruses become part of the genome of subsequent offspring. In fact, >5% of the human genome consists of proviruses from past retroviral infections. Integration, however, is not always accurate, and deletions and rearrangements can occur. Integrated proviruses can also occasionally become deleted or rearranged. Reflecting this, most endogenous proviruses are defective and not usually expressed, although expression of some does occur. It is likely, however, that this massive insertion of foreign DNA has had a profound impact on evolutionary processes. Second, after proviral formation, transcription and translation of viral gene products depend almost entirely on cellular factors. Thus, a retrovirus generally persists silently in quiescent cells. Activation of infected cells, such as occurs when cells of the immune system are stimulated by antigen or cells are activated by hormones, can activate viral expression, although this is modulated by the suite of transcriptional factor binding sites in the viral LTR. Also, complex retroviruses such as HTLV and HIV encode transcriptional activators that can profoundly affect the activity of the viral RNA polymerase promoter.[43–48]

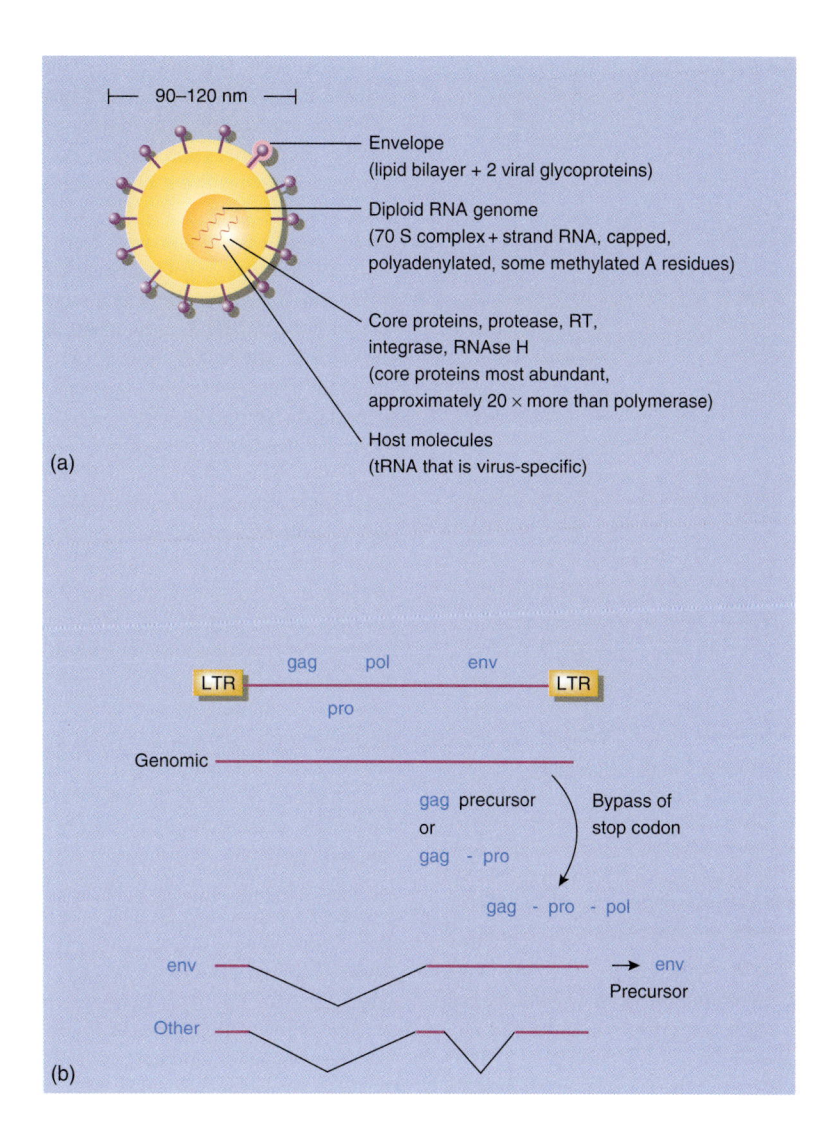

Figure 1 (a) Structure of typical retrovirus virion. (b) Structure of typical retroviral genome. All replication-competent retroviruses generate a full-length genomic ribonucleic acid (RNA) that encodes the gag and pol products and a singly spliced RNA that encodes the env product. Some retroviruses also generate smaller multiply spliced messages. *Abbreviations*: env, envelope; gag, core proteins; pol, polymerase; pro, protease.

Mechanisms of oncogenesis

Some retroviruses are acutely transforming; they can transform cells directly. Retroviral induction of neoplasias *in vivo* in the infected host, however, involves a variety of mechanisms in addition to cell transformation by acutely transforming viruses. These are summarized in Figure 7.

Oncogene capture

Acutely transforming viruses are usually generated when a cellular proto-oncogene is captured by insertion into the viral genome during viral replication. This process usually causes genetic changes in the proto-oncogene, resulting in an oncogene, or dominant transforming gene. The same process usually also results in a replication-defective virus that requires a helper virus for its replication. The helper virus provides viral proteins to form the virion in which the RNA of the defective virus is packaged. These mixed particles are called pseudotypes.

The first discovered oncogenic virus was RSV, which was shown to be a transmissible agent causing sarcomas in chickens.[2] RSV was the first acutely transforming virus of many shown to have acquired its oncogenicity by the capture of a cellular gene, in this case, *src*.[12] This was made possible in part because RSV, unlike most acutely transforming viruses, is replication competent and does not require a helper virus, thus making it simpler to study. The *src* gene in RSV is inserted as a separate gene immediately 3′ of the other viral genes.[49,50] The transforming potential could be assigned to the viral *src* gene (v-*src*) because transformation-defective RSV was shown to have mutations specifically in v-*src* and because it conferred transforming ability to recombinant viruses that contained it.[51–53] These findings led to the recognition that normal cellular genes when modified and in the appropriate setting could cause malignant transformation.

Acutely transforming retroviruses produce tumors in susceptible hosts within days to weeks after infection. Because their transforming ability is so potent, a large fraction of infected cells become transformed; hence, the tumors that arise tend to be polyclonal. RSV infection of young chickens induces a variety of related tumor types, notably fibrosarcomas and histiocytic sarcomas. The younger the animal, the more sensitive it is to tumor formation. Tumor formation can occur within days in chicks younger than 1 month,

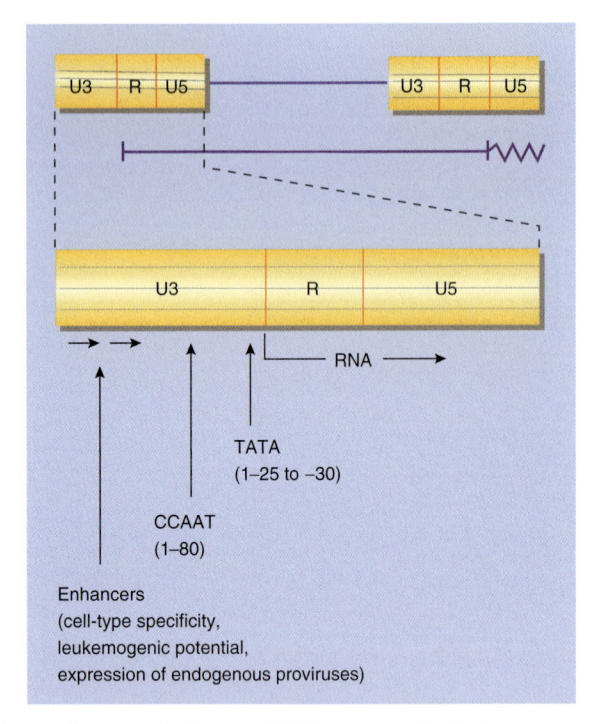

Figure 2 Long terminal repeat (LTR) structure. Replication-competent retroviruses contain identical LTRs at the 5′ and 3′ ends. The U3 portion of the 5′ LTR contains all the enhancer and promoter elements necessary for efficient initiation of transcription of either retroviral or cellular genes. *Abbreviations*: CA, capsid; FeLV, feline leukemia virus; IN, integrase; MA, matrix protein; MMTV, Maloney mammary tumor virus; MuLV, murine leukemia virus; NC, nuclear capsid; PR, protease; RT, reverse transcriptase.

the tumors progress rapidly, occur at many sites, and kill the animal. In the presence of an immune response, as in older chickens, the tumors tend to regress and disappear. Injection of v-*src* DNA into young birds can also induce tumors, further implicating v-*src* as causing the tumors.[54] Tumor formation with DNA is less efficient, probably reflecting the inefficiency of functional DNA uptake compared with retroviral infection. RSV can also cause tumors in baby rodents, although inefficiently and the tumors are restricted to the site of inoculation and tend to regress as the animal becomes older and presumably more immunocompetent. The lower tumorigenic potential probably reflects the reduced replication rate of RSV in rodent cells.[55,56]

A more typical acutely transforming oncogene-containing retrovirus is typified by Abelson murine leukemia virus (A-MuLV). Infection of a nude mouse with a replication-competent MuLV[57,58] resulted in the replacement of most of the MuLV genes with a modified copy of the proto-oncogene c-*abl*,[59] a tyrosine kinase that is the target of the anticancer drug imatinib. Like most viral oncogenes and their cellular counterparts (summarized in Table 3), the *abl* portion of v-*abl* differs genetically from c-*abl*. The recombinant A-MuLV is unable to synthesis any of the viral genes, and only codes for a fusion protein containing part of Gag and Abl (v-Abl). The presence of the amino-terminal portion of Gag on v-Abl causes it to be myristoylated and transported to the cell membrane, and this is critical for transformation by A-MuLV. The lack of functional viral genes means that A-MuLV is replication-defective and can infect and transform target cells only with the assistance of a helper virus. A-MuLV induces B-cell lymphomas in young mice, but adult animals are generally resistant.[60]

Several models have been put forth for how cellular sequences are acquired by retroviral genomes, summarized in Figure 7.

In one scenario (Figure 7a), a retrovirus integrates into the host cell genome just upstream from a proto-oncogene.[61] A subsequent deletion removes the 3′ portion of the provirus and the 5′ portion of the proto-oncogene, fusing the viral genome with cellular sequences and resulting in a reading frame for a fusion protein, generally including part of the *gag* gene. This gene is transcribed under regulation of the viral LTR, processed, and co-packaged into a pseudotype retroviral particle with the helper virus genome. When the pseudotype infects a target cell, RT mediates recombination between the 3′ ends of the two viral RNAs, which places a 3′ LTR on the end of the transduced cellular gene, allowing the resultant double-stranded DNA to be integrated into the host cell DNA. In a second model (Figure 7b), a replication-competent virus again integrates upstream from a proto-oncogene. On rare occasions, the termination signal in the 3′ LTR is not recognized, and transcription proceeds through the downstream gene. The large combined transcript then undergoes splicing or recombination that deletes the 3′ portion of the viral region and the 5′ portion of the cellular region and creates the open reading frame for the viral-proto-oncogene fusion, which is then pseudotyped for subsequent infection and generation of an integratable DNA. This requires either homologous regions between the viral and cellular genes to facilitate recombination or splice signals in the appropriate area for forming the fused open reading frame. Although examples of such homologies are found between the *pol* gene of the avian retrovirus MC29 and the chicken c-*myc* in the area of the fusion,[61,62] such homologies are not obvious in most retroviruses, suggesting that the first scenario is probably more common.

Insertional mutagenesis

Most retroviruses that cause neoplasms in their hosts are not acutely transforming, contain the minimum complement of *gag*, *pol*, and *env* genes, and are replication competent. Because many of these viruses induce leukemias and are genetically somewhat related, they are collectively referred to as leukemia viruses. Representatives include avian, murine, feline, and gibbon ape leukemia viruses. The kinds of leukemias induced vary with the viral strain; thus, some strains of GaLV are associated with lymphocytic leukemia,[7,63] whereas another strain is associated with myeloid leukemia.[64] Their lack of acutely transforming oncogenes means that they are not competent for direct transformation and do not transform target cells *in vitro*. The leukemias and other tumors that result from infection of the host are clonal in origin, as is evident from the insertion site of the provirus being identical in all of the neoplastic cells from a given tumor. This reflects the rarity of infection leading to malignant transformation and indicates that infection with the retrovirus preceded (and, by implication, resulted in) transformation. It also suggests that the specific insertion site is important, and it leads to the concept of insertional mutagenesis. In these kinds of viral neoplasias, the provirus is often integrated into the vicinity of known cellular proto-oncogenes. The proximity of the viral LTR (or the insertion of the provirus into regulatory regions of the proto-oncogene) causes a dysregulation of its expression, leading in turn to dysregulated cell growth or differentiation. Alternatively, insertion may disrupt genes whose expression tends to prevent transformation. This mechanism of insertional mutagenesis obviously requires high levels of viral replication, since integration occurs somewhat at random, and as a result, leukemia may only occur in a minority of infected animals. Latency phases (the time between infection and leukemia onset) can be quite lengthy.

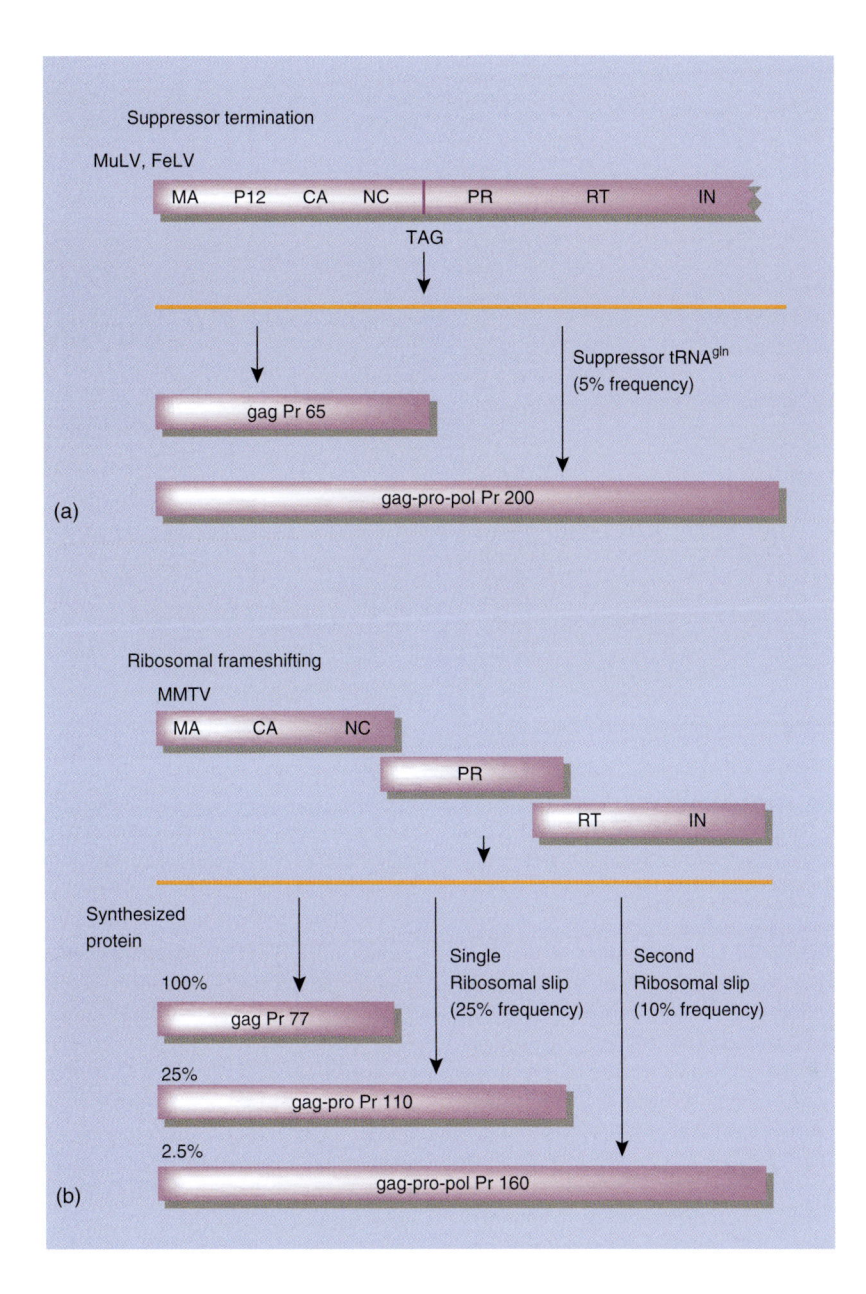

Figure 3 Alternative methods different retroviruses use to bypass the gag stop codon to generate the pro-pol products from the full-length genomic transcripts.

Avian leukosis virus (ALV) is the prototypical simple leukemia virus. ALV is transmitted in birds both horizontally and vertically. Within several months, B-cell lymphoblasts begin to accumulate in the bursa of Fabricius.[65] With involution of the bursa, many of the enlarged follicles regress, but some tumor nodules persist and grow, eventually giving rise to metastatic lymphomas. These tumors generally have a predominant provirus integrated near c-*myc*, a cellular proto-oncogene,[66–68] and c-myc RNA expression in these tumors is significantly higher than in the normal cell counterparts. Transcription is often initiated from the 3′ LTR,[69] resulting in a chimeric viral-cellular transcript, but continued expression of viral genes and viral replication is no longer needed.

Insertional mutagenesis also appears to play a critical role in MMTV and murine mammary tumors. As with ALV, MMTV can be transmitted either horizontally or vertically, and there is generally a predominant provirus in the mammary tumor cells, with similar implications. Integration was found to often occur around but not within a 30 kbp sequence containing the *int*-1 proto-oncogene.[70–72] *Int*-1 expression generally only occurs in the neural tube of mid-gestational embryos and in testicular postmeiotic cells, suggesting that inappropriate expression in cells in the breast contributes to tumorigenesis by MMTV. Transgenic mice in which an int-1 transgene is regulated by the MMTV LTR develop mammary tumors, but this is also the case when any of several other genes (including c-*myc*) are substituted for *int*-1,[73–76] suggesting that tumorigenesis simply depends on the delivery of a breast-specific promoter to dysregulate the expression of any of several proto-oncogenes.

Growth stimulation and two-step oncogenesis

The polycythemic strain of Friend MuLV (F-MuLV) represents another type of transforming replication-defective retroviruses.

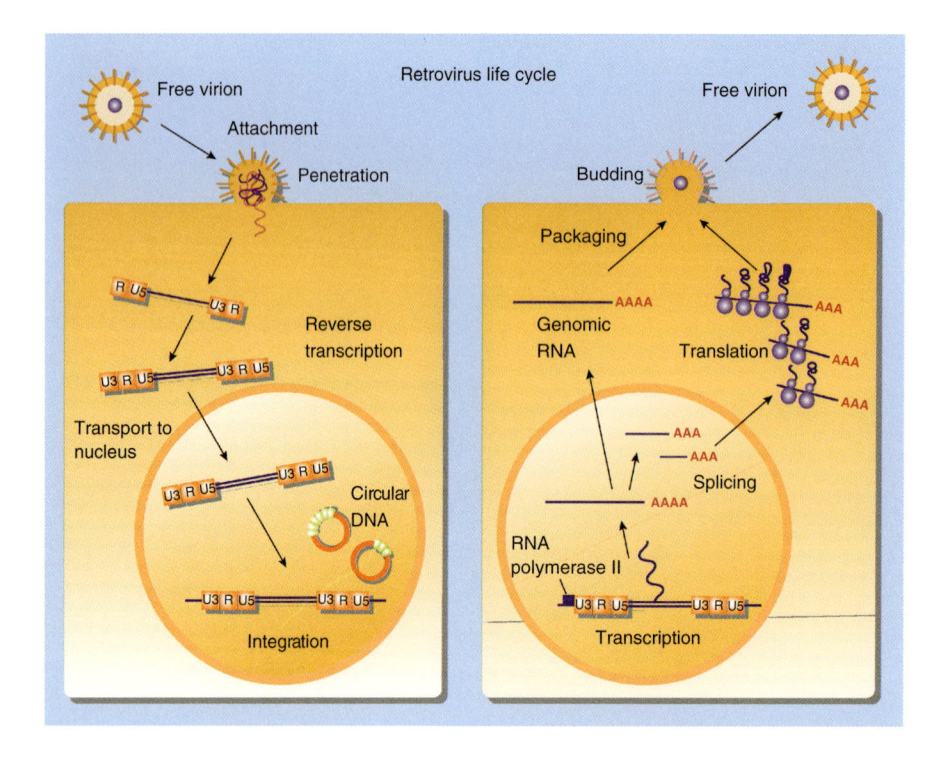

Figure 4 Life cycle of retrovirus. Following binding of the retrovirus to its specific cell membrane receptor, the viral and cellular membranes fuse, and the core virion is internalized into the cell. Reverse transcriptase-directed double-stranded retroviral genomic deoxyribonucleic acid (DNA) is then generated, followed by integrase-directed integration into host cell DNA. Retroviral transcripts using host transcriptional machinery then proceed, with the eventual formation of new retroviral virions that bud from the cell surface, allowing a new round of infection to occur.

Unlike other viruses of these types, F-MuLV does not encode a cell-derived oncogene. An internal deletion of the *env* gene encompassing portions of the TM and SU proteins results in a nonfunctional Env, which can serve as a mimic of erythropoietin (Epo) and activate the growth of erythroid precursor cells through interaction with the Epo receptor.[77] This results in erythroleukemia and pronounced splenomegaly in infected mice,[78] which is more properly a hyperplasia than a transformation, since the resultant erythrocytes do not form tumors in nude mice and are not immortalized. However, if erythrocytosis is maintained, subsequent genetic alterations will occasionally transform one of the replicating cells after a long latent period, leading to a monoclonal erythroid leukemia. These events are summarized in Figure 7c.

Transactivation

Insertional mutagenesis leading to the activation of expression of proto-oncogenes by the proximity of the viral LTR or the interruption of negative regulatory sequences by the integration event is referred to as *cis* activation. The genomes of some leukemia viruses are more complex than the simple leukemia viruses such as ALV and MuLV and contain extra genes that perform regulatory functions. The two prototypical examples are HTLV and BLV. These viruses (like the simple leukemia viruses) are replication competent, do not contain transduced proto-oncogenes in their genomes, and induce monoclonal hematopoietic malignancies only in the minority of infected hosts. However, they are like the acutely transforming viruses in that they transform cells in culture and do not appear to require a specific integration site for oncogenesis (Figure 7d). HTLV is the causative agent for ATL, a monoclonal T-cell lymphoma/leukemia with frequent cutaneous manifestations that is endemic to several areas including southern Japan and the Caribbean,[17–19,21,79] and is also the cause of a neurologic disease resembling multiple sclerosis, called tropical spastic paraparesis or HTLV-associated myelopathy.[80]

HTLV and BLV code for proteins, respectively, called Tax[44–47] and p34 Tax,[81] that activate expression by binding to the viral LTR in cooperation with transcription factors. This type of activation by a protein product rather than a DNA regulatory region is called *trans* activation, and these viral proteins are called transactivators. HTLV-I codes for several other proteins as well, including Rex, a protein that regulates the complex splicing pattern of HTLV-I mRNAs.[82,83] Three proteins of unknown function are encoded by HTLV-I: p30(II), another transactivator that binds to CREB binding protein/p300 (CBP/p300),[84] a transcriptional factor; p12(I), which activates the transcriptional factor NFAT and binds to the cytoplasmic domain of the IL-2 receptor[85,86]; and p13(II), which localizes to mitochondria and interacts with farnesyl pyrophosphate synthetase, an enzyme involved in activation of the proto-oncogene *ras*.[87,88] Most interest has focused on Tax since it is clearly critical to the viral replication cycle through transactivation of the viral LTR, and because its transactivation extends to cellular genes, including those for the IL-2 receptor, lymphotoxin, and granulocyte-macrophage stimulating factor.[89–93] The cross-transactivation of cellular genes leads to the idea that dysregulation of growth regulatory genes by Tax may play an important role in its pathogenesis.

A body of experimental evidence suggests that Tax could indeed play a role in leukemogenesis. The HTLV-I provirus in T cells transformed by HTLV-I infection or in leukemic ATL cells often has extensive deletions, but the Tax open reading frame is almost always preserved. Mice that are transgenic for Tax develop tumors,

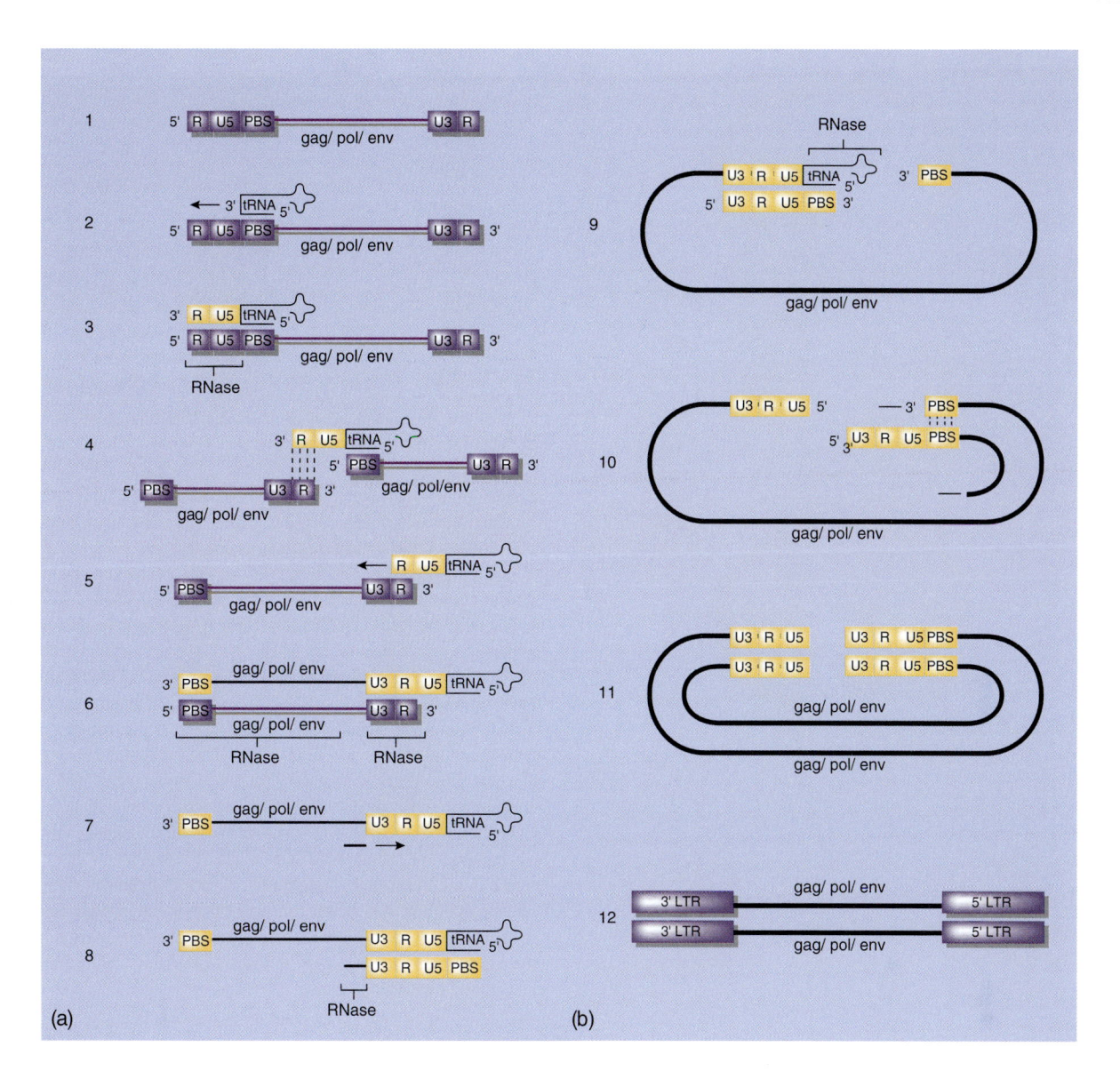

Figure 5 Reverse transcription. From a single-stranded ribonucleic acid genomic precursor (a), reverse transcriptase synthesizes a double-stranded deoxyribonucleic acid (DNA) provirus ready for integration into host cell DNA (b).

including lymphocytic leukemia, when the transgene is regulated by the viral LTR or a T-cell-specific promoter.[94–97] These T-cell lymphomas, however, differ phenotypically from ATL cells.[94,95] Tax directly transforms a rat fibroblast cell line and transforms primary rat embryo cells in cooperation with *ras in vitro*,[98,99] showing that Tax indeed has oncogenic properties. When Tax was inserted into the genome of a replication competent but transformation-defective herpesvirus saimiri mutant, human hematopoietic cells infected *in vitro* by the chimeric virus were transformed, and resembled ATL cells in morphology and cell surface phenotype,[100] suggesting that Tax is indeed important in ATL pathogenesis. It is likely that, as with F-MuLV leukemogenesis, subsequent steps are required for ATL to occur. The rarity of ATL as an outcome of HTLV-I infection and the lag time before leukemia onset (which can be 60 years or greater) indicates that a simple infection is not sufficient, and the lack of a common set of integration sites supports the idea that insertional mutagenesis does not play a role. Most tellingly, the leukemic cells do not express viral plus-strand RNA until after they are cultured,[101] indicating that by the time the cells are leukemic, they no longer require viral expression, and suggesting there must be subsequent genetic steps in ATL leukemogenesis.

A better understanding has emerged of the signaling pathways used by Tax for transactivation and transformation. Tax associates with members of the ATF/CREB family of transcriptional factors,[65,102–105] and the HTLV-I LTR have three ATF/CREB binding sites. Several cellular genes, such as serum responsive factor (SRF) and NFkB/Rel, are transactivated by Tax through the same pathway. Tax also transactivates its LTR, as well as some cellular gene promoters such as those for IL-2 and the IL-2 receptor, directly through NFkB.[106–108] This depends upon an interaction of Tax and MEKK1, which leads to phosphorylation of the NFkB inhibitor IkB. Phosphorylation of IkB targets its removal by ubiquitination and degradation in the proteasome, which unmasks the nuclear localization signal of NFkB. This allows it to be transported to the nucleus, where it activates gene expression by binding to NFkB enhancer elements present in the viral LTR. Tax also appears to directly affect the cell cycle. Tax can bind to the cell cycle inhibitor p16/INK4a and interfere with its ability to inhibit the activity of CDK4, a cyclin kinase important for G1-S progression.[109,110] Tax

Table 3 Differences between v-onc and c-onc genes.

Often only a portion of the cellular oncogene is present in v-onc
v-onc is derived from processed mRNA, which is devoid of introns and flanking sequences
Loss of cellular control elements (promoters/repressors as well as RNA destabilizers) for some oncogenes (myc and mos) elevated level of expression in itself may be transforming
Deletions/rearrangements may affect the structure of the protein itself: • Loss of C-terminal Tyr-containing region of c-src causes loss of phosphorylation-mediated control by host cell kinases   • v-erb B differs from EGF receptor by deletion of the extracellular domain
v-onc genes are often fused to viral sequences important for transforming function: • gag-abl acquires a myristoylation signal for membrane localization important for transforming activity   • v-fms is the CSF-1 receptor fused to the gag gene product, the latter providing a signal sequence for placement into the cell membrane

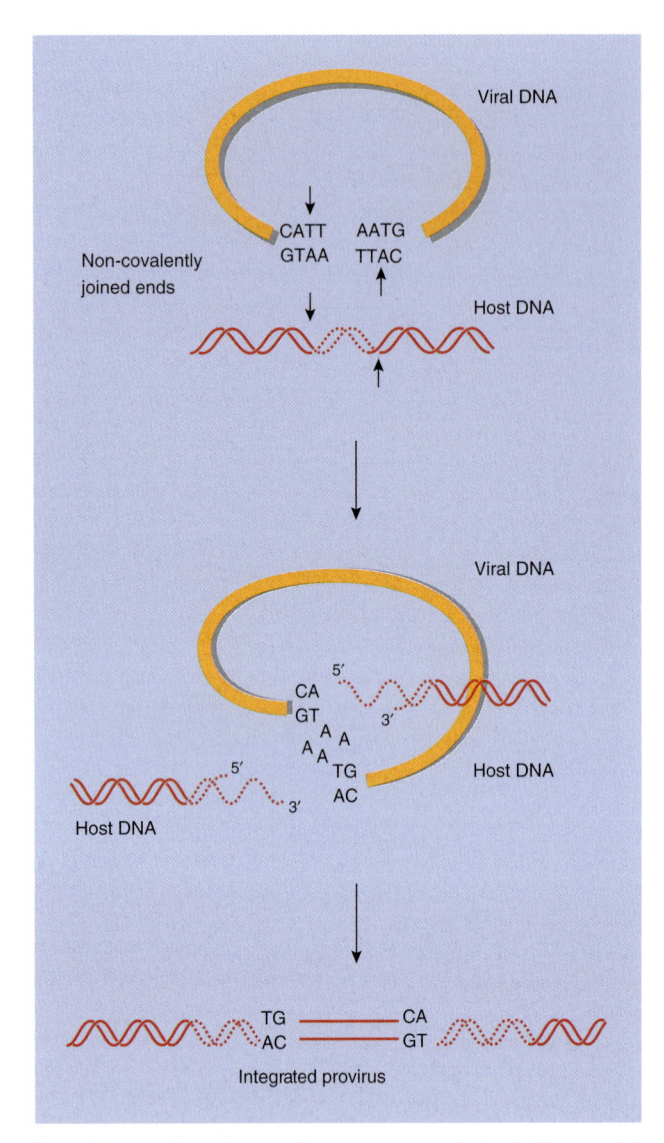

Figure 6 Integration. The newly reverse-transcribed double-stranded retroviral deoxyribonucleic acid (DNA) genome and a piece of chromosomal DNA are specifically cleaved by the retroviral integrase protein. This is accompanied by a deletion of two base pairs from the retroviral genome and a duplication of four to six base pairs from the host DNA. Following retroviral genomic insertion into the cleaved host DNA, the DNA is re-ligated.

also mediates the phosphorylation of cyclin D3[111] and upregulates the expression of E2F[110,112] through ATF/CREB signaling, both of which likely contribute to dysregulation of the cell cycle. Cell cycle dysregulation often leads to p53-mediated apoptosis.[113] Tax also dysregulates activities of p53 required for cell cycle arrest and apoptosis,[114–116] which allows unregulated hyperproliferation and immortalization of cells expressing Tax. Tax appears to inhibit p53 functions in part by an NFκB-dependent mechanism and in part by competing with p53 for binding to CBP/p300. Tax also has been reported to inhibit MAD1, a protein involved in G2/M transition.[117] It is interesting that Tax interferes with the p16/INK4a and p53 pathways, as alteration of these genes or their activities is quite common in naturally occurring cancers.

The HBZ protein, translated from the minus strand of viral RNA, could also be a determinant of HTLV-I leukemogenesis. HBZ appears to be the only viral gene product consistently expressed in ATL cells.[118] HBZ heterodimerizes with members of the CREB and Jun families[33] and supports proliferation of ATL cells.[118] HBZ transgenic mice developed skin lesions and T-cell lymphomas resembling ATL.[119] The phenotype of Tax/HBZ double transgenic mice did not differ appreciably from HBZ single transgenic mice.[120] HBZ protein and transcripts appear to have nonoverlapping functions. HBZ mRNA supports proliferation of ATL cells in the absence of HBZ protein.[118] HBZ transcripts have splice variants called SP1, the shorter of the two, and SP2.[34] The SP1 isoform negatively regulates Tax- and c-Jun-dependent transcription. Thus, one function of HBZ protein appears to be to inhibit expression of viral proteins. Conversely, HBZ protein cooperates with JunD to upregulate expression of telomerase (hTERT).[121] To add to the complexity of regulation of viral gene expression, Tax upregulates expression of HBZ.[122]

HTLV-II, although originally isolated from a hairy cell leukemia,[22] has not been consistently associated with any disease. HTLV-3 and -4 have been identified as other members of the HTLV family,[24] but appear to be quite rare, and are also not associated with any diseases.

HIV

Infection with HIV, although not considered a tumor virus, results in a greatly increased incidence of several types of tumors, most of which are linked to coinfection with other viruses such as human papilloma virus (HPV), Kaposi sarcoma herpesvirus, or Epstein–Barr virus (EBV),[123,124] suggesting immune deficiency as a cofactor. Retroviruses are also associated with immunodeficiency in infected animals, as in the case of FeLV. The best example of an immunopathogenic virus is, of course, HIV-1, which is the cause of AIDS. Since HIV-1 is not found in tumor cells, the mechanism of increased tumorigenesis must be indirect. One of the clearest examples is its effect on pathogenesis by human herpesvirus 8 (HHV-8) (also known as Kaposi sarcoma herpesvirus [KSHV]).[125] HHV-8 is clearly the cause of Kaposi's sarcoma (KS) and a B-cell lymphoma called peripheral effusion lymphoma (PEL).[126] In the absence of HIV-1 or other immunosuppressive conditions, HHV-8 appears to cause these diseases only rarely. HIV-1 infection raises the risk of these diseases by many orders of magnitude,[123,124] but is not found in the tumor cells. Since the advent of effective viral suppressive therapies, the incidence of KS has decreased precipitously, further confirming the role of HIV infection as a cofactor. A greatly elevated incidence of non-Hodgkin lymphoma (NHL) is also seen in a setting of HIV infection,[123,124] and a substantial

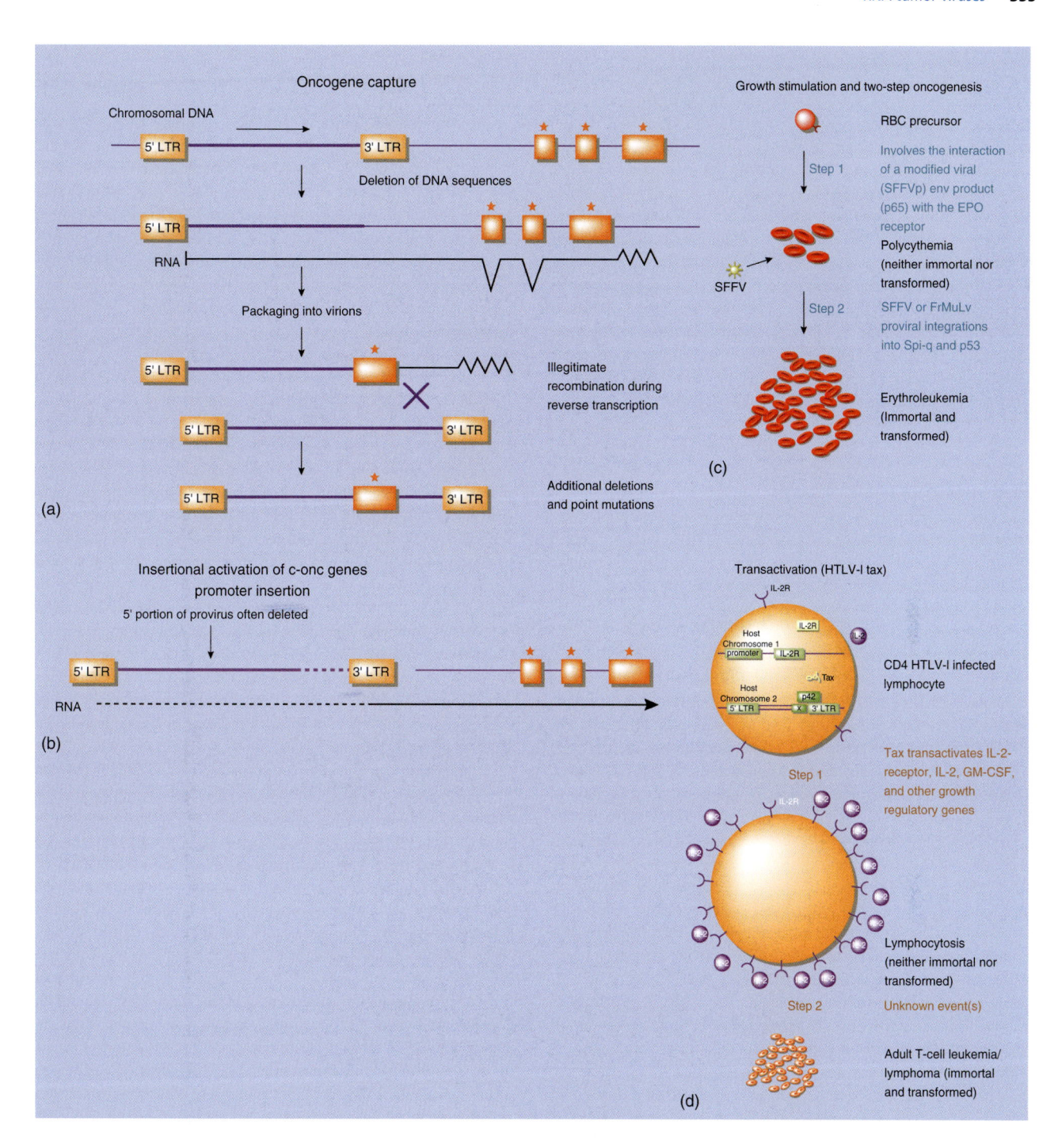

Figure 7 Four mechanisms of retrovirus-induced oncogenesis. (a) Oncogene capture. A mutated form of a cellular proto-oncogene (v-onc) is transferred (transduced) to a normal cell, thus inducing transformation (*c-oncogene). (b) Insertional activation. There is a significant increase in the rate of proto-oncogene expression secondary to LTR-directed transcriptional enhancement (*c-oncogene). (c) Growth stimulation plus two-step oncogenesis. A mutated env protein from the defective spleen focus-forming virus (SFFV) binds to the erythropoietin (EPO) receptor, causing an erythrocyte hyperplasia. This increases the target population susceptible to the actual transforming event, a retroviral insertional disruption of the Spi-I or TP53 gene. *Abbreviation*: FrMuLV, Friend murine leukemia virus. (d) Transactivation. The viral transactivating protein (tax in the case of human T-cell leukemia virus type I) causes expansion of the potential target population through transactivation of growth regulatory genes. An unknown second event then induces the actual transformation of a clone of these cells.

portion of these AIDS-NHL cases is associated with EBV infection. Infection with HIV-1 also appears to increase the risk of childhood leiomyosarcomas[124] (associated with EBV) and of cervical cancer and hepatocarcinoma (associated with HPV and hepatitis B and C virus infections, respectively). Infection with these viruses tends to be higher in HIV-infected people, but there also appears to be a higher risk of cancer in people who are coinfected with HIV and one of these viruses. As with KS, the tumor cells are not infected with HIV-1, indicating an indirect role.

Immunodeficiency likely plays an important role in elevated cancer rates in the setting of HIV infection, most clearly in the case of cancers with a viral etiology. It is also possible, however, that

HIV may play a more direct role in tumorigenesis. Mice that are transgenic for Tat, the HIV transactivator protein that is functionally homologous to HTLV-I Tax, develop KS-like lesions.[127] Also, Tat accelerates tumorigenesis in a murine xenotransplant model of KS in a paracrine manner.[128] A subset of AIDS-NHL is not associated with EBV, and the reasons for its increased incidence are not clear. Some suggestive evidence has pointed to a role for HIV viral proteins, perhaps especially the p17 matrix protein. Viral proteins persist for extended time periods in lymph nodes of infected people, even in the absence of detectable viral RNA or replication.[129] HIV transgenic mice have a significantly elevated incidence of B cell lymphoma.[130] The viral transgene, although deleted for parts of the *gag* and *pol* genes, expresses many viral proteins, including p17. Recently, p17 was shown to promote lymphangiogenesis *in vitro*, reportedly through binding to and activation of the chemokine receptors CXCR1 and 2.[131]

Endogenous retroviruses

Endogenous retroviruses are part of the normal genetic complement of species and make up an extremely large fraction (up to 5%) of various mammalian genomes. Many of these appear to have emerged after speciation, based on differences in their type and number among species. Since retroviruses insert at random and since there are so many present, it is clear that they have played a profound if unclear role in evolution. It is less clear whether any endogenous retroviruses play a role in human cancer or other diseases. First, they are for the most part defective because of large deletions, although some only have a few point mutations and a very few may be replication competent. Second, endogenous retroviruses are generally not expressed even at the RNA level. This may be because of mutations in the regulatory regions of their LTRs, because of their location in transcriptionally inactive areas of the chromatin, or because of methylation of promoter sequences in the LTR. When endogenous viruses are expressed as RNA, protein, or virions, it is usually in normal placentas or in teratomas, which may reflect the presence of hormone-responsive elements in the LTRs of many endogenous retroviruses. It is possible that integration of endogenous retroviruses may result in recessive mutations. The Hr (hairless) and D (dilute brown) recessive phenotypes in mice are associated with the presence of endogenous retroviruses at the affected loci,[132–134] and reversion of the mutation is associated with proviral deletion, raising the possibility that there may be analogous situations in humans. Indeed, insertion of a GaLV-related provirus upstream from a duplicated pancreatic amylase gene appears to have allowed its expression in saliva,[135–137] and may have led to the inclusion of starch-rich foods in the human diet. One specific endogenous retroviral RNA is highly expressed in placenta. Its protein product, syncytin, may be important in human placental morphogenesis, and dysregulation of its expression is associated with preeclampsia.[138,139] In general, expression or the lack of expression of endogenous retroviral genes has not been associated with human diseases, although the AKR strain of mice develops leukemia by a complex process that involves expression and recombination of endogenous MuLVs.[140–142]

Recently, koala retrovirus (KoRV) has attracted interest. Discovered in 1988,[143,144] it has apparently occurred in koala populations for several centuries[145] and has become endogenous in north Australia, while it is primarily exogenous in the south. KoRV causes immunodeficiencies and lymphomas in infected koalas[146–148] (to the point of endangering koala populations), and appears to be invading the koala germ line in real time.[147,149] It is most closely related to GaLV,[144] and apparently originated as a cross-species transmission from an Asian mouse species,[150] as did GaLV itself.

The integration pattern and the content of endogenous retroviruses can differ among members of the same species, suggesting that they are not entirely stable and that many are not currently essential to their hosts. Their existence as fixed genetic elements, however, suggests that they were important at one time. Retroviruses that use the same receptor exhibit interference, because infection either blocks or downregulates the cell surface expression of the receptor, rendering the cell refractory to superinfection. It may be that endogenous retroviruses provided protection by interference against pathogenic retroviruses that no longer exist and are therefore no longer important.

Retroviral vectors and gene therapy

As the understanding of the roles of specific genes in different diseases has evolved, treatment of diseases by gene therapy, or the delivery of desired genes, has become more of a possibility. One of the main obstacles has been efficient and specific delivery of a gene to the appropriate tissue and cell type. Delivery by transfection of DNA, or introduction into cells in which the membrane has been partially permeabilized by chemicals or an electrical charge, is relatively inefficient, not very specific, and not generally suitable for delivery *in vivo*. Delivery by gene gun, which shoots DNA on the surface of gold microparticles into skin and muscle, and direct injection of DNA result in expression of proteins *in vivo*, but these methods are not very specific and may be best suited for the delivery of DNA vaccines.

An alternative is to use a recombinant virus to deliver the gene of interest into the appropriate tissue. This method of gene delivery is called transduction. Viruses can be highly tissue-specific and, in principle, transduction of cells with a recombinant virus may be the best approach to gene delivery. Different viruses have been used for gene delivery, including adenovirus, which has disadvantages of a lack of persistence and the likelihood of immune responses against viral proteins upon repeated administration. Retroviral vectors are perhaps the best-studied and most promising transducing vectors.[151–154] They integrate, so they theoretically only need to be administered once. In addition, as seen with the acutely transforming replication-defective retroviruses, the vector genome does not need to be able to code for any viral proteins to be integrated. The only requirements for transduction of the gene of interest are that the vector RNA contains the proper packaging signal and has LTRs at both its ends. Tissue and cell tropisms can be altered by pseudotyping with different envelope proteins.[155] The proteins required to form virions are provided by cell lines that express all the viral proteins from genes that cannot themselves be packaged. When the vector RNA containing the gene of interest is transfected into a packaging cell line, only the vector RNA is packaged into the virion. Since the pseudotyped RNA does not encode viral proteins, the virions are only capable of a single round of infection and integration. This allows the stable expression of the gene of interest in the absence of any retroviral proteins, which would be likely to elicit an immune response that would eliminate the genetically altered cells. The majority of retroviral vectors in the past have been based on the Moloney strain of MuLV (Mo-MuLV).[151–154] Mo-MuLV vectors efficiently infect a wide variety of cell types, including those of human origin. More recently, retroviral vectors based on lentiviruses have shown promise. These have the advantage of being able to transduce nondividing cells by the same mechanisms that allow natural lentiviruses to infect resting cells.[156,157]

There are several potential problems with retroviral vectors. One is the possible generation of replication competent helper viruses during the packaging of the vector, which can occur by homologous recombination. Two approaches have been used to minimize this possibility. One is to place the viral structural genes on different genetic units, so that multiple recombination events must occur before a replication-competent helper virus is generated. A second approach, not mutually exclusive with the first, is to minimize areas of homology among the units expressing the helper virus proteins and the vector by, for example, using heterologous promoters for helper virus RNA transcription. Another potential problem derives from the risk that integration in the vicinity of a proto-oncogene could lead to tumorigenesis. Although the risk appears small, it is not zero. This was the apparent reason for three of seven monkeys developing lymphomas in one gene therapy study.[158] Mo-MuLV does not replicate well in human cells, but this is not the case for other potential retroviral vectors. Minimizing integration events by rigorously excluding the presence of replication competent helper viruses somewhat avoids this problem, but does not completely eliminate it. Indeed, treatment of young severe combined immunotherapy X1 patients with a lentiviral vector devoid of replicating helper virus resulted in insertion near the LMO2 proto-oncogene promoter followed by a leukemia-like clonal T-cell outgrowth in several of the patients.[159] Another problem is that expression is not maintained indefinitely; retroviral promoters tend to become inactivated over time by methylation. A further limitation is that the genetic capacity of retroviruses is only about 8–9 kb, which restricts their capacity to only a single gene or two.

Conclusions

The study of retroviruses has led to much of today's techniques and understanding of molecular biology. This is obviously especially true in the case of cell transformation and tumorigenesis, since many retroviruses either cause cancers or (in the case of acutely transforming viruses) capture cellular genes that have the potential to contribute to neoplastic transformation. Retroviruses were the first example of a reversal of the normal order of the flow of genetic information, that is, from RNA to DNA. The identification and elucidation of reverse transcription provided the means for cloning and characterizing mRNA, which greatly facilitated understanding gene expression and function. Furthermore, studies of the regulation of viral transcription, retroviral RNA processing, viral entry mechanisms, viral protein processing, and virion assembly have greatly increased our knowledge in the areas of transcriptional regulation, RNA splicing and translational regulation, membrane biochemistry and fusion, and protein processing and protein–protein interactions, respectively. An understanding of how retroviruses package and deliver genetic material holds promise that these viruses will be successfully used in the clinic to deliver therapeutic genes to appropriate cells and tissues in human diseases. New generations of vectors currently being developed are bringing us closer to realizing this goal.

Perhaps among the most important contributions of retroviral research to human health were the discovery of HTLV-I and HIV-1, two pathogenic human retroviruses. During the 1970s, much of the research carried out with retroviruses came under the aegis of the virus cancer program (VCP) as part of President Richard Nixon's War on Cancer. The VCP was ended because of a lack of discovery of human cancer viruses and the growing feeling that human retroviruses did not exist. Shortly thereafter, however, HTLV-I was discovered and linked to ATL. Although this discovery has not led so far to better treatment for ATL, it has led to better prevention of infection by, for example, screening blood samples and by avoiding transmission by breastfeeding, a common route of infection of babies. Ironically, the most important consequence of the VCP and retroviral research was the relatively rapid discovery and characterization of a virus not directly linked with cancer, but with immunodeficiency. HIV-1 was discovered and shown to be the cause of AIDS and a blood test was developed in a relatively short span of time, and therapies based on structural determinations of its reverse transcriptase and protease were developed and successfully used. This rapid progress would have been far slower had the means for isolating, culturing, and characterizing retroviruses not already been in place.

Key references

The complete reference list can be found on Vital Source version of this title, see inside front cover.

10 Baltimore D. RNA-dependent DNA polymerase in virions of RNA tumour viruses. *Nature*. 1970;**226**(5252):1209–1211.

11 Temin HM, Mizutani S. RNA-dependent DNA polymerase in virions of Rous sarcoma virus. *Nature*. 1970;**226**(5252):1211–1213.

12 Stehelin D, Varmus HE, Bishop JM. Detection of nucleotide sequences associated with transformation by avian sarcoma viruses. *Bibl Haematol*. 1975;**43**:539–541.

13 Kalyanaraman VS, Sarngadharan MG, Poiesz B, et al. Immunological properties of a type C retrovirus isolated from cultured human T-lymphoma cells and comparison to other mammalian retroviruses. *J Virol*. 1981;**38**(3):906–915.

14 Poiesz BJ, Ruscetti FW, Gazdar AF, et al. Detection and isolation of type C retrovirus particles from fresh and cultured lymphocytes of a patient with cutaneous T-cell lymphoma. *Proc Natl Acad Sci U S A*. 1980;**77**(12):7415–7419.

15 Poiesz BJ, Ruscetti FW, Reitz MS, et al. Isolation of a new type C retrovirus (HTLV) in primary uncultured cells of a patient with Sezary T-cell leukaemia. *Nature*. 1981;**294**(5838):268–271.

16 Reitz MS, Poiesz BJ, Ruscetti FW, Gallo RC. Characterization and distribution of nucleic acid sequences of a novel type C retrovirus isolated from neoplastic human T lymphocytes. *Proc Natl Acad Sci U S A*. 1981;**78**(3):1887–1891.

17 Catovsky D, Greaves MF, Rose M, et al. Adult T-cell lymphoma-leukaemia in Blacks from the West Indies. *Lancet*. 1982;**1**(8273):639–643.

19 Kalyanaraman VS, Sarngadharan MG, Nakao Y, et al. Natural antibodies to the structural core protein (p24) of the human T-cell leukemia (lymphoma) retrovirus found in sera of leukemia patients in Japan. *Proc Natl Acad Sci U S A*. 1982;**79**(5):1653–1657.

20 Robert-Guroff M, Ruscetti FW, Posner LE, et al. Detection of the human T cell lymphoma virus p19 in cells of some patients with cutaneous T cell lymphoma and leukemia using a monoclonal antibody. *J Exp Med*. 1981;**154**(6):1957–1964.

21 Yoshida M, Miyoshi I, Hinuma Y. Isolation and characterization of retrovirus from cell lines of human adult T-cell leukemia and its implication in the disease. *Proc Natl Acad Sci U S A*. 1982;**79**(6):2031–2035.

22 Kalyanaraman VS, Sarngadharan MG, Robert-Guroff M, et al. A new subtype of human T-cell leukemia virus (HTLV-II) associated with a T-cell variant of hairy cell leukemia. *Science*. 1982;**218**(4572):571–573.

26 Barre-Sinoussi F, Chermann JC, Rey F, et al. Isolation of a T-lymphotropic retrovirus from a patient at risk for acquired immune deficiency syndrome (AIDS). *Science*. 1983;**220**(4599):868–871.

27 Popovic M, Sarngadharan MG, Read E, Gallo RC. Detection, isolation, and continuous production of cytopathic retroviruses (HTLV-III) from patients with AIDS and pre-AIDS. *Science*. 1984;**224**(4648):497–500.

28 Gallo RC, Salahuddin SZ, Popovic M, et al. Frequent detection and isolation of cytopathic retroviruses (HTLV-III) from patients with AIDS and at risk for AIDS. *Science*. 1984;**224**:500–503.

29 Sarngadharan MG, Popovic M, Bruch L, et al. Antibodies reactive with human T-lymphotropic retroviruses (HTLV-III) in the serum of patients with AIDS. *Science*. 1984;**224**(4648):506–508.

30 Clavel F, Guetard D, Brun-Vezinet F, et al. Isolation of a new human retrovirus from West African patients with AIDS. *Science*. 1986;**233**(4761):343–346.

31 Kanki PJ, M'Boup S, Ricard D, et al. Human T-lymphotropic virus type 4 and the human immunodeficiency virus in West Africa. *Science*. 1987;**236**(4803):827–831.

32. Teich N, Weiss R, Varmus HE, Coffin J. *Taxonomy of Retroviruses. RNA Tumor Viruses*. Cold Spring Harbor, NY: Cold Spring Harbor Laboratory; 1984:509.
33. Mesnard JM, Barbeau B, Devaux C. HBZ, a new important player in the mystery of adult T-cell leukemia. *Blood*. 2006;**108**(13):3979–3982.
34. Cavanagh MH, Landry S, Audet B, et al. HTLV-I antisense transcripts initiating in the 3′LTR are alternatively spliced and polyadenylated. *Retrovirology*. 2006;**3**:15.
35. Ludwig LB, Ambrus JL Jr, Krawczyk KA, et al. Human Immunodeficiency Virus-Type 1 LTR DNA contains an intrinsic gene producing antisense RNA and protein products. *Retrovirology*. 2006;**3**:80.
36. Gaudray G, Gachon F, Basbous J, et al. The complementary strand of the human T-cell leukemia virus type 1 RNA genome encodes a bZIP transcription factor that down-regulates viral transcription. *J Virol*. 2002;**76**(24):12813–12822.
37. Lemasson I, Lewis MR, Polakowski N, et al. Human T-cell leukemia virus type 1 (HTLV-1) bZIP protein interacts with the cellular transcription factor CREB to inhibit HTLV-1 transcription. *J Virol*. 2007;**81**(4):1543–1553.
38. Torresilla C, Mesnard JM, Barbeau B. Reviving an old HIV-1 gene: the HIV-1 antisense protein. *Curr HIV Res*. 2015;**13**(2):117–124.
43. Arya SK, Guo C, Josephs SF, Wong-Staal F. Trans-activator gene of human T-lymphotropic virus type III (HTLV-III). *Science*. 1985;**229**(4708):69–73.
44. Felber BK, Paskalis H, Kleinman-Ewing C, et al. The pX protein of HTLV-I is a transcriptional activator of its long terminal repeats. *Science*. 1985;**229**(4714):675–679.
47. Sodroski J, Rosen C, Goh WC, Haseltine W. A transcriptional activator protein encoded by the x-lor region of the human T-cell leukemia virus. *Science*. 1985;**228**(4706):1430–1434.
59. Reddy EP, Smith MJ, Srinivasan A. Nucleotide sequence of Abelson murine leukemia virus genome: structural similarity of its transforming gene product to other onc gene products with tyrosine-specific kinase activity. *Proc Natl Acad Sci U S A*. 1983;**80**(12):3623–3627.
63. Gallo RC, Gallagher RE, Wong-Staal F, et al. Isolation and tissue distribution of type-C virus and viral components from a gibbon ape (*Hylobates lar*) with lymphocytic leukemia. *Virology*. 1978;**84**(2):359–373.
64. Kawakami TG, Kollias GV Jr, Holmberg C. Oncogenicity of gibbon type-C myelogenous leukemia virus. *Int J Cancer*. 1980;**25**(5):641–646.
67. Hayward WS, Neel BG, Astrin SM. Activation of a cellular onc gene by promoter insertion in ALV-induced lymphoid leukosis. *Nature*. 1981;**290**(5806):475–480.
79. Robert-Guroff M, Nakao Y, Notake K, et al. Natural antibodies to human retrovirus HTLV in a cluster of Japanese patients with adult T cell leukemia. *Science*. 1982;**215**(4535):975–978.
123. Goedert JJ. The epidemiology of acquired immunodeficiency syndrome malignancies. *Semin Oncol*. 2000;**27**(4):390–401.
124. Rabkin CS. Epidemiology of AIDS-related malignancies. *Curr Opin Oncol*. 1994;**6**(5):492–496.
128. Guo HG, Pati S, Sadowska M, et al. Tumorigenesis by human herpesvirus 8 vGPCR is accelerated by human immunodeficiency virus type 1 Tat. *J Virol*. 2004;**78**(17):9336–9342.
136. Samuelson LC, Wiebauer K, Snow CM, Meisler MH. Retroviral and pseudogene insertion sites reveal the lineage of human salivary and pancreatic amylase genes from a single gene during primate evolution. *Mol Cell Biol*. 1990;**10**(6):2513–2520.
139. Mi S, Lee X, Li X, et al. Syncytin is a captive retroviral envelope protein involved in human placental morphogenesis. *Nature*. 2000;**403**(6771):785–789.
146. Denner J, Young PR. Koala retroviruses: characterization and impact on the life of koalas. *Retrovirology*. 2013;**10**:108.
158. Donahue RE, Kessler SW, Bodine D, et al. Helper virus induced T cell lymphoma in nonhuman primates after retroviral mediated gene transfer. *J Exp Med*. 1992;**176**(4):1125–1135.

27 Herpesviruses

Jeffrey I. Cohen, MD

Overview

Eight herpesviruses have been isolated from humans: two of these, Epstein–Barr virus (EBV), and Kaposi sarcoma-associated herpesvirus (KSHV), are associated with human tumors. EBV has been detected in lesions from patients with posttransplant lymphoproliferative disease, nasopharyngeal and some types of gastric carcinoma, Burkitt lymphoma, Hodgkin lymphoma, and certain other lymphoid tumors. KSHV is associated with Kaposi sarcoma, primary effusion lymphoma, and Castleman disease. Each of these viruses encodes proteins important for establishment of latency, transforming cells, and evading the immune system.

Properties of herpesviruses

Herpesviruses are enveloped DNA viruses that have the capacity to establish latent infection as well as to undergo lytic infection. The ability to establish latent infection *in vivo* and to reactivate from latency ensures a source of virus to infect previously uninfected individuals. Most adults latently harbor herpes simplex 1, varicella-zoster virus, human herpesvirus 6 and 7, and Epstein–Barr virus (EBV). Several features of herpesvirus replication are important for the maintenance of latency and for oncogenicity; EBV will serve as an example to illustrate the principles of herpesvirus infection relevant to oncogenicity.

First, viral DNA must be maintained in the cell. The EBV genome is usually maintained in latently infected B cells as a multicopy circular episome in the host cell. Second, a cell transformed by a virus must avoid immune clearance. Replication of EBV requires up to 100 viral proteins; however, latent infection of B cells with EBV results in expression of 12 or fewer genes as well as multiple miRNAs.[1-3] This limited repertoire of gene products prevents frequent virus replication, avoiding death of the infected cell, and restricts the ability of the immune system to recognize and destroy cells latently infected with the virus. Third, specific viral proteins interact with other cell proteins or directly transactivate other cell genes to provide additional functions necessary for cell proliferation and immortalization. Several EBV proteins interact with cellular proteins to activate transcription of viral and cellular genes or to engage signal transduction pathways in the cell. Viral miRNAs regulate viral gene expression during latency and inhibit immune responses.

EBV: an oncogenic human herpesvirus

EBV gene expression in transformed lymphocytes

Infection of primary B cells with EBV *in vitro* results in transformation of the cells which can then proliferate indefinitely. Eight EBV proteins and several nontranslated RNAs are expressed in latently infected B lymphocytes that have been growth transformed by EBV *in vitro* (Table 1). The EBV nuclear proteins EBNA-1, EBNA-2, EBNA-LP, EBNA-3A, EBNA-3B, and EBNA-3C comprise the EBV nuclear antigen complex. EBNA-1 binds to the oriP sequence (origin of viral DNA replication) on EBV DNA and allows the virus genome to be maintained as an episome in transformed B cells.[4,5] EBNA-1 also transactivates its own expression. EBNA-1 inhibits its own protein degradation by proteasomes[6] and limits its own translation,[7] both of which may reduce its presentation to CD8+ cytotoxic T cells; however, EBNA-1 remains a target for CD4+ cells.[8-11] EBNA-1 inhibits apoptosis induced by expression of p53.[12]

EBNA-2 transactivates expression of EBV LMP1[13] and LMP2,[14] and the cellular genes CD23, CD21, and c-*myc*, and c-*fgr*.[15,16] EBNA-2 is targeted to the LMP1, LMP2, Cp EBNA, and CD23 promoters by the GTGGGAA-binding protein Jκ, and thereby activates these promoters.[17] EBNA-2 is a functional homolog of the Notch receptor, which uses Jκ to regulate gene expression during development.[18] EBNA-2 also interacts with the DNA-binding protein PU-1 to transactivate the LMP1 promoter[19] and with AUF to transactivate the EBNA Cp promoter.[20] The transactivation domain of EBNA-2 is essential for B-lymphocyte transformation.[21] This domain interacts with transcription factors TFIIB and the TATA-binding protein-associated factor TAF40.[22] EBNA-2 inhibits apoptosis mediated by Nur77.[23]

EBNA-LP interacts with and enhances the ability of EBNA-2 to transactivate LMP1 and LMP2.[24] Although EBNA-LP binds to Rb and p53 *in vitro*,[25] the significance of these interactions is uncertain. EBNA-LP is required for transforming naive B cells and for recruitment of transcription factors to the EBV genome.[26]

EBNA-3A, EBNA-3B, and EBNA-3C are distantly related to each other. The EBNA-3 proteins bind to Jκ preventing it from binding DNA, thereby inhibiting transactivation by EBNA-2.[27] EBNA-3C upregulates expression of LMP1 and CD21. EBNA-3C binds to Nm23-HI, a human metastasis suppressor protein, and inhibits the protein's ability to suppress migration of Burkitt lymphoma cells.[28] EBNA-3C degrades Rb and enhances kinase activity by disrupting p27.[29,30] EBNA-3A and EBNA-3C are essential for B-lymphocyte transformation *in vitro*, while EBNA-3B is dispensable.[31,32]

LMP1 functions as a transforming oncogene in nude mice.[33] Expression of LMP1 in EBV-negative Burkitt lymphoma cells results in B-cell clumping and increased villous projections. Upregulation of bcl-2, bfl-1, and A20, and inhibition of Bax, by LMP1 in B cells protects the cells from apoptosis.[34,35] Expression of LMP1 in epithelial cells inhibits differentiation of the cells.[36]

LMP1 is a functional homolog of CD40, a member of the tumor necrosis factor receptor (TNFR) family.[37] The carboxy terminus of LMP1 interacts with the TNFR-associated factors (TRAFs) 1, 2, 3, and 5, TRADD, RIP, and JAK3 *in vitro*.[38] LMP1 functions as a constitutively active form of CD40 resulting in activation of NF-κB,

---

Holland-Frei Cancer Medicine, Tenth Edition. Edited by Robert C. Bast, John C. Byrd, Carlo M. Croce, Ernest Hawk, Fadlo R. Khuri, Raphael E. Pollock, Apostolia M. Tsimberidou, Christopher G. Willett, and Cheryl L. Willman.
© 2023 John Wiley & Sons, Inc. Published 2023 by John Wiley & Sons, Inc.

Table 1 Selected EBV genes and their cellular homologs and activities.

Gene	Expression class	Cellular homolog	Activity
EBNA-1	Latent, lytic	None	Episome maintenance, transactivates viral genes, inhibits apoptosis
EBNA-2	Latent	Notch	Transactivates viral and cellular genes, inhibits apoptosis
EBNA-3A,B,C	Latent	None	Regulates EBNA-2 activity, transactivates cellular genes
EBNA-LP	Latent	None	Increases EBNA-2 activity
LMP1	Latent, lytic	CD40	Transactivates cellular genes, inhibits apoptosis
LMP2	Latent	None	Prevents EBV reactivation, transactivates Akt
EBERs	Latent	None	Upregulates cellular genes
BARF-1	Lytic	CSF-1R	Inhibits interferon-α
BCFR1	Lytic	IL-10	Inhibits interferon-γ and IL-12
BNLF2a	Lytic	None	Blocks antigen-specific CD8 T-cell recognition
BHRF1	Lytic	Bcl-2	Inhibits apoptosis
BALF1	Lytic	Bcl-2	Regulates BHRF1 activity
BGFL5	Lytic	None	Blocks synthesis of MHC class I, II
BILF1	Lytic	GPCR	Removes MHC class I from cell surface
BLLF3	Lytic	None	Up-regulates IL-10, TNF-α, IL-1β
BPLFI	Lytic	None	Inhibits toll-like receptor signaling
BZLF1	Lytic	None	Inhibits interferon-γ effects, inhibits function of p53, inhibits TNF-α, initiates lytic infection

stress-activated protein kinases, STATs, adhesion molecules, the B7 co-stimulatory molecule, JNK, and B-cell proliferation.[39] LMP1 upregulates expression of intracellular adhesion molecules, Fas, CD40, and MMP-9[40] in B cells and EGF in epithelial cells.[41] LMP1 inhibits phosphorylation of Tyk2 resulting in inhibition of IFN-α signaling.[42] LMP1 is essential for transformation of B lymphocytes by EBV.[43] Analysis of EBV-containing human lymphomas shows that LMP1 localizes with TRAF-1, TRAF-3, and that activated NF-κB is present.[44]

LMP2 is dispensable for transformation of B cells[45] but induces a transforming phenotype in epithelial cells and promotes their motility.[46,47] LMP2 prevents lytic reactivation of EBV-infected primary B cells in response to activation of the B-cell receptor complex by cross-linking of surface immunoglobulin. LMP2 associates with the *src* family and *syk* protein-tyrosine kinases that are coupled to the B-cell receptor complex.[48] Binding of LMP2 to these proteins results in their constitutive phosphorylation, which inhibits their ability to mediate signaling for virus reactivation.[48,49] B cells from transgenic mice expressing LMP2 survive even without normal B-cell receptor signaling activity.[50] LMP2 activates β-catenin and Ras/PI3K/Akt signaling pathways in epithelial cells resulting in transformation of the cells.[51,52] LMP2 also activates mTOR and increases c-myc expression.[53]

The two EBV-encoded RNAs, EBER-1 and EBER-2, are the most abundant EBV RNAs in latently infected B cells; however, they are not required for latent or lytic EBV infection but may contribute to B-cell transformation.[54,55] The EBERs upregulate expression of bcl-2 and IL-10,[56] interact with the double-stranded RNA-activated protein kinase, interferon-inducible oligoadenylate synthetase, and with PAX5.[57,58]

EBV encodes at least 44 miRNAs from the BART and BHRF1 regions of the genome; BART microRNAs are expressed during latency and regulate viral gene expression, downregulate cellular genes, inhibit apoptosis, enhance B cell proliferation, and inhibit the activity of antiviral T cells.[59,60] Both EBV microRNAs and LMP1 are secreted from infected cells in exosomes which may enhance tumorigenicity.[61,62]

EBV genes expressed during productive infection

Infection of epithelial cells with EBV results in productive infection, with replication of virus and lysis of infected cells. Immediate-early genes encode regulators of virus gene expression, including the BZLF1 and BRLF1 proteins, which act as switches to initiate lytic infection. The BZLF1 protein inhibits TNF-α signaling[63] and helps the virus evade T cell responses.[64] BZLF1 protein also inhibits the expression of the IFN-γ receptor,[65] and inhibits the function of p53.[66] Early genes encode proteins involved in viral DNA synthesis, while late genes encode structural proteins.

Three viral genes expressed during productive infection are functional homologs of cellular genes and are important for the survival of EBV-infected B cells.[67,68] The EBV BCRF-1 protein is homologous to IL-10 and has IL-10 activity.[69] BCRF-1 is a B-cell growth factor and inhibits IFN-γ release from activated peripheral blood mononuclear cells and secretion of IL-12 from macrophages.

The EBV BARF-1 protein acts as a soluble receptor for CSF-1.[70] BARF-1 inhibits IFN-α secretion by human monocytes. The EBV BNLF2a protein interacts with the TAP complex to block antigen-specific CD8 T-cell recognition.[71] The EBV BHRF1 protein is homologous to bcl-2 and protects cells from apoptosis.[72] EBV BALF1 is also homologous to bcl-2 and antagonizes the antiapoptotic effect of BHRF1.[73]

Clinical aspects

EBV infection is usually spread by saliva. The virus infects B cells directly, or oropharyngeal epithelial cells and then spreads to subepithelial B cells.[74] During primary infection, up to a few percent of the peripheral blood B lymphocytes are infected with EBV and have the capacity to proliferate indefinitely *in vitro*. Natural killer (NK) cells, CD4 T cells, and HLA- and EBNA- or LMP-restricted cytotoxic T cells control the latently infected B lymphocytes.[8] T- and B-cell interactions release lymphokines and cytokines, giving rise to many of the clinical manifestations of acute infectious mononucleosis. After recovery, the fraction of B cells latently infected with EBV in the peripheral blood remains at 1 in 10^5 to 1 in 10^6. These lymphocytes are the primary site of EBV persistence and a source of virus for persistent infection of epithelial surfaces.

B-cell tumors that occur early after EBV infection are usually lymphoproliferative processes, in which latent virus infection in B cells is the principal cause of proliferation. In contrast, Burkitt lymphoma and nasopharyngeal carcinoma occur long after primary EBV infection and viral gene expression is less important to the growth of the malignant cells.

Lymphoproliferative disease

EBV is associated with B-cell lymphoproliferative disease in patients with congenital or acquired immunodeficiency. X-linked lymphoproliferative syndrome is an inherited immunodeficiency of males; if untreated most patients die of a fatal lymphoproliferative disorder or fulminant hepatitis, but some survive with hypogammaglobulinemia or develop EBV-positive lymphomas. The gene mutated in X-linked lymphoproliferative syndrome has been identified as SLAM associated protein (SAP),[75] which encodes an SH2-containing protein that interacts with SLAM on B and T cells, and with 2B4 on NK and T cells. Anti-CD20 antibody (rituximab) has been effective in treating some patients with X-linked lymphoproliferative disease and acute EBV infection.[76] Mutations in additional cellular proteins including XIAP, ITK, CD27, CD70, CD137, MagT1, CTP synthase 1, GATA2, RASGRP1, and PI3K 110δ predispose to severe EBV infections.

EBV lymphoproliferative disease occurs in patients who are immunosuppressed as a result of transplantation or AIDS.[77-79] Risk factors for development of lymphoproliferative disease include EBV-seronegativity prior to transplant and receipt of T-cell-depleted bone marrow or antilymphocyte antibody. Lymphoproliferative lesions are most commonly seen in the lymph nodes, liver, lungs, kidney, bone marrow, or small intestine. Tumors in transplant patients are usually classified as lymphomas; some patients have hyperplastic lesions. The proliferating lymphocytes in these tumors generally do not have chromosomal translocations.

AIDS-related lymphomas may be systemic (nodal or extranodal) lymphomas or primary central nervous system lymphomas. While most B-cell tumors in transplant recipients and central nervous system lymphomas in AIDS patients contain EBV, about 50% of other lymphomas in AIDS patients contain EBV. Tumors in patients with AIDS are usually either immunoblastic lymphomas or Burkitt lymphomas; most of the latter have c-myc translocations.

Tissues from transplant recipients or AIDS patients with EBV lymphoproliferative disease show expression of EBERs, EBNA-1, EBNA-2, and LMP1 (Table 2). The EBV viral load in the peripheral blood has been used to predict development of disease and to follow patients after therapy. The expression of EBV genes, which are targets for cytotoxic T cells, has important implications for therapy. Infusion of EBV-specific cytotoxic T cells, nonirradiated donor leukocytes, or HLA-matched allogeneic cytotoxic T cells have been effective in many cases for treatment of EBV lymphoproliferative disease.[80-86] Anti-CD20 antibody (rituximab) has induced remissions in some patients and has been used in some studies as preemptive therapy when EBV viral DNA in the blood is rising in transplant recipients at risk of lymphoproliferative disease,[87] although other studies suggest that preemptive therapy may be unnecessary.[88]

Burkitt lymphoma

Seroepidemiologic studies show a strong association between Burkitt lymphoma and EBV in Africa.[89,90] More than 90% of African Burkitt lymphomas are associated with EBV, whereas only ~20% of Burkitt lymphomas in the United States are associated with the virus. African patients with Burkitt lymphoma often have high levels of antibody to EBV antigens, and the virus can be recovered from the tissue.

Burkitt lymphomas contain chromosomal translocations that result in c-myc dysregulation. The most common chromosomal translocation, t(8;14), places a portion of the c-myc oncogene adjacent to an immunoglobulin heavy chain gene. Less common translocations involve the c-myc oncogene and the κ or λ immunoglobulin light chain genes t(2;8) and t(8;22), respectively. These translocations result in high constitutive expression of c-myc. Burkitt lymphomas may also have somatic mutations as a result of activation of AID or defective mismatch DNA repair in the cell.[91]

EBV-associated endemic Burkitt lymphoma is thought to develop in steps. First, EBV infection may expand the pool of differentiating and proliferating B cells. Second, chronic endemic malaria may cause T-cell suppression and B-cell proliferation. Third, enhanced proliferation of differentiating B cells may favor the chance occurrence of a reciprocal c-myc (t[8;14] or t[8;22]) translocation placing c-myc partially under the control of immunoglobulin-related transcriptional enhancers, with development of a monoclonal tumor.

Nasopharyngeal carcinoma

The nonkeratinizing nasopharyngeal carcinomas are uniformly associated with EBV. Patients with nasopharyngeal carcinoma have high levels of antibodies to EBV antigens. A prospective study of Taiwanese men showed that those with IgA antibodies to EBV viral capsid antigen (VCA) and anti-EBV deoxyribonuclease antibodies had an increased risk for developing nasopharyngeal carcinoma when compared to men without these antibodies.[92] These antibodies are useful in screening patients for early detection of nasopharyngeal carcinoma and are prognostic for patients after treatment. Other studies showed that quantifying the level of EBV DNA in plasma is useful for screening and monitoring patients with nasopharyngeal carcinoma and predicting outcomes.[93,94] Nasopharyngeal carcinoma tissue contains EBV genomes in every cell. These tumors are monoclonal with regard to EBV infection, indicating that EBV infection precedes malignant cell outgrowth at the cellular level. Unlike Burkitt lymphoma, the association of EBV with nasopharyngeal carcinoma is uniform and universal. Infusions of EBV-specific cytotoxic T cells resulted in remissions in some patients with refractory nasopharyngeal carcinoma.

Hodgkin lymphoma

Persons with a history of infectious mononucleosis are at a greater risk of developing Hodgkin lymphoma.[95] Patients with Hodgkin lymphoma generally have higher titers of antibody to EBV VCA than does the general population. Tissues from ~40% to 60% of patients with Hodgkin lymphoma contain EBV genomes.[96] Cases of Hodgkin lymphoma in patients with HIV or from developing countries are more likely to contain EBV genomes than persons without HIV or from developed countries.[97] The EBV genome is monoclonal and present in Reed–Sternberg cells. EBV is more often associated with aggressive subtypes (especially mixed cellularity) of Hodgkin lymphoma. Tumors from patients with EBV+ Hodgkin lymphoma and some from patients with lymphoproliferative disease arise from postgerminal center cells.[98] Infusion of cytotoxic T cells generated from 11 patients with relapsed Hodgkin lymphoma and measurable disease resulted in complete remissions in two patients, partial remission in one patient, stable disease in five patients, and no response in three patients.[99]

Table 2 Diseases associated with EBV latent gene expression.

Disease	BART miRNAs	EBERs	EBNA-1	EBNA-2	LMP1	LMP2
Burkitt lymphoma	+	+	+	−	−	−
Nasopharyngeal carcinoma	+	+	+	−	+	+
Hodgkin lymphoma	+	+	+	−	+	+
Peripheral T-cell lymphoma	+	+	+	−	+	+
Lymphoproliferative disease	+	+	+	+	+	+

Other tumors associated with EBV

EBV has also been detected in non-Hodgkin's lymphomas. EBV-positive diffuse large B-cell lymphoma has a poorer prognosis than EBV-negative lymphoma.[100] Treatment of patients with EBV+ non-Hodgkin's lymphoma in remission with autologous antigen-presenting cells transduced with LMP2 resulted in increased frequencies of LMP2-specific cytotoxic T cells and tumor responses in several patients with relapsed disease.[99] EBV DNA and latency proteins have been detected in tissues from patients with peripheral T-cell lymphoma, extranodal NK/T lymphoma, aggressive NK cell leukemia, central nervous system B cell lymphoma, T cells in patients with virus-associated hemophagocytic syndrome, carcinoma of the palatine tonsil, laryngeal carcinoma, angioimmunoblastic T cell lymphoma, and lymphomatoid granulomatosis.[101]

EBV DNA has been found in leiomyosarcomas in AIDS patients,[102] and viral RNA and EBNA-2 have been detected in smooth muscle tumors in organ transplant recipients.[103] About 7% of primary gastric carcinomas are EBV+, especially in undifferentiated lymphoepithelioma-like carcinomas.

KSHV and malignancies

In 1994, Chang et al.[104] detected sequences of a new human herpesvirus Kaposi sarcoma-associated herpesvirus (KSHV) in Kaposi sarcoma tissues from patients with AIDS. KSHV is present in B cells in asymptomatic persons. B-cell lines derived from primary effusion lymphomas maintain KSHV in a latent state and can be induced to undergo lytic virus replication by the addition of phorbol ester or butyrate. Infection of dermal microvascular endothelial cells *in vitro* with KSHV results in transformation of the cells with maintenance of long-term infection. The cells become spindle-shaped and show loss of contact inhibition with anchorage-independent growth.[105] While KSHV transforms bone marrow-derived endothelial cells, virus is present in only a small fraction of the cells.[106]

Viral proteins

Several KSHV proteins are important for transformation, establishing latency, and modulating the immune response to the virus.[107–109] KSHV encodes a large number of cellular homologs (Table 3) that have been grouped into different classes, depending on when they are expressed in primary effusion lymphoma cell lines.[110] Expression of the KSHV K1 gene in rodent fibroblasts results in transformation of the cells.[111] The K1 protein induces tyrosine phosphorylation in cells[112] and activates the Akt signaling pathway.[113] The K1 protein inhibits apoptosis[114] and results in constitutive calcium-dependent signal activation in B cells.[115]

The KSHV K2 gene encodes an IL-6 homolog (vIL-6). IL-6 is a B-cell growth factor and acts as an autocrine growth factor for lymphoid tumors resulting in proliferation.[116] vIL-6 prevents death of IL-6-dependent B9 cells *in vitro*,[117] promotes hematopoiesis, and induces VEGF to promote angiogenesis.[118] The K3 (modulator of immune recognition 1 [MIR1]) and K5 (MIR2) proteins induce rapid endocytosis of MHC class I molecules and IFN-γ receptor 1 from the surface of cells by ubiquitination of these proteins.[119–121] The K5 protein also downregulates ICAM-1 and B7.2, which results in inhibition of NK cell-mediated cytotoxicity[122] and removes CD31 from the surface of endothelial cells.[123]

The KSHV K4, K4.1, and K6 genes encode three chemokines: the viral macrophage inflammatory proteins (MIPs)-II, -III, and -I, respectively. vMIP-I inhibits replication of HIV strains dependent on CCR5.[117] vMIP-I and vMIP-III are chemokine receptor

Table 3 Selected KSHV genes and their cellular homologs and activities.

Gene	Expression class	Cellular homolog	Activity
K1	II	ITAM motif	Transformation, activates signaling pathways
K2	II	IL-6	B-cell growth factor, angiogenesis, hematopoiesis
K3	III	None	Reduces surface MHC class I
K4	II	MIP-1α	Chemokine receptor antagonist; angiogenesis; chemotaxis
K4.1	II	MIP-1α	Chemokine receptor agonist; angiogenesis; chemotaxis
K5	II	None	Inhibits NK-cell activity; reduces surface MHC class I; increases monocyte proliferation
K6	II	MIP-1α	Chemokine receptor agonist; angiogenesis; chemotaxis
K8	III	None	Inhibits p53
K9	II	IRF	Represses interferon activity, transformation, inhibits p53
K10.5 (LANA-2)	II	IRF	Represses interferon activity; inhibits apoptosis; inhibits p53
K11.1	I	IRF	Represses interferon activity
K12 (Kaposin A)	II	None	Transformation
K12 (Kaposin B)	II	None	Increases cytokine mRNA stability
K14	II	OX-2	Induces proinflammatory cytokines
K15 (LAMP)	III	None	Binds TRAFs, inhibits B-cell receptor signaling
ORF4	II	CR2	Complement-binding protein
ORF16	II/III	Bcl-2	Inhibits apoptosis
ORF45	III	None	Inhibits IRF7
ORF50	III	None	Increases CD21 and CD23 expression, degrades IRF7
ORF63	III	NLR proteins	Inhibits NLRP1
ORF71	I	FLIP	Inhibits apoptosis; activates NF-κB
ORF72	I	Cyclin D	Cell-cycle progression, inhibits Rb
ORF73 (LANA-1)	I	None	Episome maintenance, inhibits p53 and Rb
ORF74	II	GPCR	Angiogenesis, transformation, and proliferation

Expression class I, latent gene, expressed in uninduced primary effusion lymphoma cells, not induced by phorbol ester; class II, expressed in uninduced cells, induced by TPA; class III, lytic gene, expressed only after induction by TPA (includes many structural proteins and DNA replication enzymes). *Abbreviations*: FLIP, FLICE inhibitory protein; GPCR, G protein-coupled receptor; IRF, interferon regulatory factor; ITAM, immunoreceptor tyrosine-based activation motif; MHC, major histocompatibility complex; MIP, macrophage inflammatory protein; NK, natural killer; Rb, retinoblastoma protein; TRAFs, TNFR-associated factors.

agonists for CCR8[124] and CCR4,[125] respectively, while vMIP-II is a broad-spectrum chemokine receptor antagonist. vMIP-II is a chemoattractant for eosinophils,[126] binds to both CC and CXC chemokines, and blocks calcium mobilization induced by chemokines.[127]

The KSHV K9, K11.1, and K10.5 proteins are referred to as viral interferon regulatory factor (vIRF)-1, -2, and -3, respectively. Each of these proteins inhibits virus-mediated activation of the IFN-α promoter.[128] vIRF1 inhibits MHC-1 transcription and surface expression.[129] vIRF1 and vIRF3 inhibit p53-mediated apoptosis[130,131] and transform NIH 3T3 cells.[132] vIRF3 (also called LANA2) protects cells from p53-induced apoptosis.[131,133] KSHV ORF45 blocks the activity of IRF7 and inhibits the activation of IFN-α and -β.[134]

The KSHV K12 locus encodes several proteins termed kaposins. Kaposin A induces transformation of cells.[109,135] Kaposin B increases expression of cytokines by activating MAP kinase-associated protein kinase 2 and inhibiting the degradation of cytokine mRNA.[136,137] The KSHV K14 protein, a homolog of the cellular OX2 protein, stimulates monocytes to produce proinflammatory cytokines such as TNF-α, IL-1β, and IL-6.[138] KSHV ORF4 protein inhibits the complement system.[139] KSHV ORF16 encodes a homolog of bcl-2 and inhibits bax-induced apoptosis.[140] The ORF71 gene encodes a homolog of cellular FLIP that blocks apoptosis. ORF71 binds to Atg3 and protects cells from autophagy. KSHV ORF71 activates NF-κB, promotes tumor growth, and is required for survival of KSHV-infected lymphoma cells.[141–145] KSHV ORF72 encodes a cyclin D homolog that binds to and activates cdk6 and phosphorylates p27 and stimulates cell-cycle progression in normally quiescent fibroblasts resulting in constitutive cellular proliferation.[146,147] The viral cyclin protein phosphorylates and thereby inactivates Rb.[109,148]

KSHV ORF73 encodes LANA1 that localizes with viral DNA episomes and tethers them to chromosomes during cell division.[149] KSHV LANA1 is required for persistence of the episome in dividing cells and transactivates its own promoter. In addition, LANA1 inhibits the activity of both p53 and Rb,[150,151] upregulates expression and stabilizes β-catenin,[152] upregulates and activates survivin,[153] protects the cell from hypoxia,[154] and activates c-myc.[155] Expression of LANA in transgenic mice results in development of lymphomas.[156] LANA inhibits TGF-β signaling.[157] KSHV ORF74 encodes a G protein-coupled receptor that is homologous to the cellular IL-8 receptor; unlike the latter protein, however, the KSHV receptor is constitutively active and induces cellular proliferation.[158] ORF74 protein induces angiogenesis,[159] activates the Akt signaling pathway,[160] and induces proliferation and vascular permeability of endothelial cells.[161–163] ORF74 activates NF-κB and JNK, and upregulates IL-1, IL-8, TNF-α, FGF, and inhibits viral lytic gene expression.[164]

KSHV K15 encodes the latency-associated membrane protein (LAMP) and interacts with TRAFs 1, 2, and 3.[165] K15 suppresses tyrosine phosphorylation and intracellular calcium mobilization, inhibiting B-cell receptor signaling.[166] KSHV encodes several microRNAs located between K12 and ORF71 or within K12 that are expressed during latency and in patient plasma.[167] These microRNAs are important for NF-κB activation and blocking cell cycle arrest of latently infected cells.[108,168] KSHV microRNAs also target cellular genes.[169]

Clinical aspects

Seroprevalence rates for KSHV vary from <5% in normal blood donors in the United States or the United Kingdom to 30–35%

Table 4 Diseases associated with KSHV gene expression.

Gene	Kaposi Sarcoma	Primary effusion lymphoma	Castleman disease
LANA (ORF73)	+	+	+
K12 (Kaposin)	+	+	−
ORF72 (v-cyclin)	+	+	−
ORF71 (v-FLIP)	+	+	+
ORF74 (GPCR)	+	−	−
K10.5 (vIRF3)	−	+	+
K9 (vIRF1)	−	−	+
K2 (vIL-6)	−	±	+

in HIV-positive homosexual men.[170] Antibody to KSHV is more common in African and Mediterranean populations. At least 85% of patients with Kaposi sarcoma have antibodies to KSHV.[171] The prevalence of Kaposi sarcoma is lower in women than in men, and HIV-seropositive women have a much lower incidence of antibody to KSHV than do seropositive men. KSHV seropositivity in HIV-positive homosexual men is predictive of subsequent development of Kaposi sarcoma.[172] Levels of KSHV DNA are higher in patients with active Kaposi sarcoma or multicentric Castleman disease, than in those in remission, and are also elevated in patients with primary effusion lymphoma.[173] The virus is not thought to be pathogenic in most healthy individuals and can persist in a latent phase for life; however, in immunocompromised persons, it is strongly associated with Kaposi sarcoma. Thus, while infection with KSHV appears to be required for development of Kaposi sarcoma, it is probably not sufficient by itself and other cofactors, such as HIV and impaired cellular immunity, are important. KSHV is thought to be sexually transmitted in homosexual men[170] and has been associated with sexual transmission and intravenous drug use in women.[174] In endemic populations (e.g., Africa), KSHV may be transmitted vertically from mother to child and between siblings and has been transmitted by renal allografts.[175,176]

Kaposi sarcoma

KSHV has been found in nearly all biopsies of classic Kaposi sarcoma, African endemic Kaposi sarcoma, Kaposi sarcoma in HIV-seronegative transplant recipients and homosexual men, and Kaposi sarcoma in patients with AIDS.[177,178] KSHV is present in the endothelial and spindle cells of the tumor but not in normal endothelium.[179] Most of the tumor cells are latently infected with the virus, but 1–5% of the spindle cells in HIV-positive Kaposi sarcoma show lytic KSHV infection. Kaposi sarcoma can be polyclonal, oligoclonal, or monoclonal. KSHV is also present in the peripheral blood mononuclear cells of ∼50% of patients with Kaposi sarcoma, and its presence is predictive of development of the malignancy.[170] KSHV has also been detected in the saliva of patients with Kaposi sarcoma, and, infrequently, in semen. Several KSHV proteins are expressed in Kaposi's tissues (Table 4). Foscarnet and ganciclovir reportedly reduce the frequency of new Kaposi sarcoma lesions in some, but not all, studies.[180,181] Cidofovir had no effect on treatment of established lesions.[182] In contrast, HIV protease inhibitors have been reported to induce regression of Kaposi sarcoma lesions.[183] IL-12, in combination with liposomal doxorubicin, resulted in tumor responses in AIDS patients with Kaposi sarcoma receiving HAART; responses were maintained with IL-12 therapy.[184] Sirolimus,[185] imatinib,[186] bevacizumab,[187] and paclitaxel[188] have all been reported to have activity against Kaposi sarcoma.

Primary effusion lymphoma

KSHV has also been found in primary effusion lymphomas in patients with AIDS.[178,179,189] These body cavity-based lymphomas of B-cell lineage are located in the pleural, peritoneal, or pericardial space and usually contain EBV as well as KHSV genomes. Some KSHV-positive lymphomas have been found in patients without AIDS. Primary effusion lymphoma is treated with antiretroviral therapy if the patient has HIV and cytotoxic chemotherapy.

Multicentric castleman disease

KSHV has also been detected in biopsies from some patients with multicentric Castleman disease, especially in the variant known as the plasma cell type.[178,179,190–192] This disease is usually polyclonal and presents as generalized lymphadenopathy, fever, and hypergammaglobulinemia. Symptoms are thought to be due to increased levels of IL-6 and vIL-6.[193] KSHV is detected more frequently in biopsies from HIV-positive patients than in biopsies from those patients without HIV. KSHV is present in the immunoblastic B cells of the mantle zone of the lesions. In the absence of concurrent Kaposi sarcoma, multicentric Castleman disease if is usually treated with rituximab and antiantiretroviral therapy if the patient has HIV; if there is evidence of organ disease liposomal doxorubicin or etoposide are added.

Summary

- Two herpesviruses, Epstein–Barr virus (EBV) and Kaposi sarcoma-associated herpesvirus (KSHV), are associated with human tumors.
- EBV is associated with Burkitt lymphoma, Hodgkin and non-Hodgkin lymphoma, posttransplant lymphoproliferative disease, T cell lymphoma, nasopharyngeal carcinoma, and certain types of gastric carcinoma.
- EBV transformed B cells and EBV posttransplant lymphoproliferative lesions express EBNA-1, -2, -3s, and -LP and LMP1 and LMP2 and RNAs including EBERs and BART miRNAs in culture. Burkitt lymphomas express only EBNA-1, EBERs, and BART miRNAs. Hodgkin lymphomas and nasopharyngeal carcinomas express EBNA-1, LMP1, LMP2, EBERs, and BART miRNAs.
- EBV EBNA-1 is important for maintaining the viral episome during replication of the cells. EBNA-2 transactivates several virus and cellular promoters and is a functional homolog of the Notch receptor. EBNA-3's regulate the activity of EBNA-2 and also transactivate viral genes. LMP1 is a functional homolog of CD40 and binds to TNFR-associated factors to upregulate NF-κB, STATs, JNK, and stress-activated protein kinases.
- KSHV is associated with primary effusion lymphoma, Kaposi sarcoma, and Castleman disease.
- Each of the three KSHV-associated tumors expresses LANA (ORF73) and v-FLIP (ORF71). Other KSHV proteins, including Kaposin (K12), v-cyclin (ORF72), a G-protein coupled receptor (GPCR, ORF74), v-IRF3 (K10.5), v-IRF1 (K9), and v-IL-6 (K2) and miRNAs are expressed in some, both not all virus-associated malignancies.
- LANA maintains the viral episome during replication, inhibits the activity of Rb and p53, and upregulates survivin and β-catenin. KSHV v-FLIP is a homolog of cellular FLIP and inhibits apoptosis and autophagy and activates NF-κB. Kaposin increases the activity of cytokines, and v-cyclin inhibits Rb and helps virus-infected cells to progress through the cell cycle. The viral GPCR activates NF-κB and Akt and contributes to proliferation of KSHV-infected cells. v-IRF1 and v-IRF3 inhibit the activity of interferon and p53 and block apoptosis. v-IL-6 functions as a B cell growth factor, inhibits apoptosis, and upregulates VGEF.

Key references

The complete reference list can be found on Vital Source version of this title, see inside front cover.

1. Longnecker R, Kieff E, Cohen JI. Epstein-Barr virus. In: Knipe DM, Howley PM, Cohen JI, et al., eds. *Fields Virology*. Philadelphia, PA: Lippincott Williams & Wilkins; 2013:1898–1959.
2. Cohen JI. Herpesvirus latency. *J Clin Invest*. 2020;**130**:3361–3369.
3. Price AM, Luftig MA. Dynamic Epstein-Barr virus gene expression on the path to B-cell transformation. *Adv Virus Res*. 2014;**88**:279–313.
8. Hislop AD, Taylor GS, Sauce D, Rickinson AB. Cellular responses to viral infection in humans: lessons from Epstein-Barr virus. *Annu Rev Immunol*. 2007;**25**:587–617.
26. Szymula A, Palermo RD, Bayoumy A, et al. Epstein-Barr virus nuclear antigen EBNA-LP is essential for transforming naïve B cells, and facilitates recruitment of transcription factors to the viral genome. *PLoS Pathog*. 2018;**14**(2):e1006890.
37. Uchida J, Yasui T, Takaoka-Shichijo Y, et al. Mimicry of CD40 signals by Epstein-Barr virus LMP-1 in B lymphocyte responses. *Science*. 1999;**286**:300–303.
44. Liebowitz D. Epstein-Barr virus and a cellular signaling pathway in lymphomas from immunosuppressed patients. *N Engl J Med*. 1998;**338**:1413–1421.
57. Lee N, Yario TA, Gao JS, Steitz JA. EBV noncoding RNA EBER2 interacts with host RNA-binding proteins to regulate viral gene expression. *Proc Natl Acad Sci U S A*. 2016;**113**:3221–3226.
67. Horst D, Verweij MC, Davison AJ, et al. Viral evasion of T cell immunity: ancient mechanisms offering new applications. *Curr Opin Immunol*. 2011;**23**:96–103.
68. Jochum S, Moosmann A, Lang S, et al. The EBV immunoevasins vIL-10 and BNLF2a protect newly infected B cells from immune recognition and elimination. *PLoS Pathog*. 2012;**8**:e1002704.
77. Dierickx D, Habermann TM. Post-transplantation lymphoproliferative disorders in adults. *N Engl J Med*. 2018;**378**(6):549–562.
78. Dharnidharka VR, Webster AC, Martinez OM, et al. Post-transplant lymphoproliferative disorders. *Nat Rev Dis Primers*. 2016;**2**:1508879.
79. Nourse JP, Jones K, Gandhi MK. Epstein-Barr Virus-related post-transplant lymphoproliferative disorders: pathogenetic insights for targeted therapy. *Am J Transplant*. 2011;**11**(5):888–895.
85. Leen AM, Bollard CM, Mendizabal AM, et al. Multicenter study of banked third-party virus-specific T cells to treat severe viral infections after hematopoietic stem cell transplantation. *Blood*. 2013;**121**:5113–5123.
86. Bollard CM, Rooney CM, Heslop HE. T-cell therapy in the treatment of post-transplant lymphoproliferative disease. *Nat Rev Clin Oncol*. 2012;**9**:510–519.
90. Molyneux EM, Rochford R, Griffin B, et al. Burkitt's lymphoma. *Lancet*. 2012;**379**:1234–1244.
91. Grande BM, Gerhard DS, Jiang A, et al. Genome-wide discovery of somatic coding and noncoding mutations in pediatric endemic and sporadic Burkitt lymphoma. *Blood*. 2019;**133**:1313–1324.
92. Chien Y-C, Chen J-Y, Liu M-Y, et al. Serological markers of Epstein-Barr virus infection and nasopharyngeal carcinoma in Taiwanese men. *N Engl J Med*. 2001;**345**:1877–1882.
93. Lin JC, Wang WY, Chen KY, et al. Quantification of plasma Epstein-Barr virus DNA in patients with advanced nasopharyngeal carcinoma. *N Engl J Med*. 2004;**350**:2461–2470.
94. Chan KCA, Woo JKS, King A, et al. Analysis of plasma Epstein-Barr virus DNA to screen for nasopharyngeal cancer. *N Engl J Med*. 2017;**377**:513–522.
96. Murray PG, Young LS. An etiological role for the Epstein-Barr virus in the pathogenesis of classical Hodgkin lymphoma. *Blood*. 2019;**134**(7):591–596.97.
101. Cohen JI, Iwatsuki K, Ko H-Y, et al. Epstein-Barr virus NK and T cell lymphoproliferative disease: report of a 2018 international meeting. *Leuk Lymphoma*. 2020;**61**:808–819.
102. McClain KL, Leach CT, Jensen HB, et al. Association of Epstein-Barr virus with leiomyosarcomas in young people with AIDS. *N Engl J Med*. 1995;**332**:12–18.
106. Flore O, Rafii S, Ely S, et al. Transformation of primary human endothelial cells by Kaposi's sarcoma-associated herpesvirus. *Nature*. 1998;**394**:588–592.
107. Damania B, Cesarman E. Kaposi's sarcoma-associated herpesvirus. In: Knipe DM, Howley PM, Cohen JI, et al., eds. *Fields Virology*. Philadelphia, PA: Lippincott Williams & Wilkins; 2013:2080–2128.
108. Giffin L, Damania B. KSHV: pathways to tumorigenesis and persistent infection. *Adv Virus Res*. 2014;**88**:111–159.
109. Ueda K. KSHV genome replication and maintenance in latency. *Adv Exp Med Biol*. 2018;**1045**:299–320.
137. Yoo J, Kang J, Lee HN, et al. Kaposin-B enhances the PROX1 mRNA stability during lymphatic reprogramming of vascular endothelial cells by Kaposi's sarcoma herpes virus. *PLoS Pathog*. 2010;**6**:e1001046.
147. DiMaio TA, Vogt DT, Lagunoff M. KSHV requires vCyclin to overcome replicative senescence in primary human lymphatic endothelial cells. *PLoS Pathog*. 2020;**16**(6):e1008634.

150. Friborg J, Kong W, Hottiger MO, et al. p53 inhibition by the LANA protein of KSHV protects against cell death. *Nature*. 1999;**402**:889–894.
151. Radkov SA, Kellam P, Boshoff C. The latent nuclear antigen of Kaposi sarcoma-associated herpesvirus targets the retinoblastoma-E2F pathway and with the oncogene *h-ras* transforms primary rat cells. *Nat Med*. 2000;**6**:1121–1127.
152. Fujimuro M, Wu FY, ApRhys C, et al. A novel viral mechanism for dysregulation of beta-catenin in Kaposi's sarcoma-associated herpesvirus latency. *Nat Med*. 2003;**9**:300–306.
159. Bais C, Santomasso B, Coso O, et al. G-protein–coupled receptor of Kaposi's sarcoma-associated herpesvirus is a viral oncogene and angiogenesis activator. *Nature*. 1998;**391**:86–89.
167. Qin J, Li W, Gao SJ, Lu C. KSHV microRNAs: tricks of the devil. *Trends Microbiol*. 2017;**25**:648–661.
176. Cesarman E, Damania B, Krown SE, et al. Kaposi sarcoma. *Nat Rev Dis Primers*. 2019;**5**:9.
186. Koon HB, Krown SE, Lee JY, et al. Phase II trial of imatinib in AIDS-associated Kaposi's sarcoma: AIDS malignancy consortium protocol 042. *J Clin Oncol*. 2014;**32**:402–408.
187. Uldrick TS, Wyvill KM, Kumar P, et al. Phase II study of bevacizumab in patients with HIV-associated Kaposi's sarcoma receiving antiretroviral therapy. *J Clin Oncol*. 2012;**30**:1476–1483.
188. Cianfrocca M, Lee S, Von Roenn J, et al. Randomized trial of paclitaxel versus pegylated liposomal doxorubicin for advanced human immunodeficiency virus-associated Kaposi sarcoma: evidence of symptom palliation from chemotherapy. *Cancer*. 2010;**116**:3969–3977.
192. Uldrick TS, Polizzotto MN, Yarchoan R. Recent advances in Kaposi sarcoma herpesvirus-associated multicentric Castleman disease. *Curr Opin Oncol*. 2012;**24**(5):495–505.
193. Polizzotto MN, Uldrick TS, Wang V, et al. Human and viral interleukin-6 and other cytokines in Kaposi sarcoma herpesvirus-associated multicentric Castleman disease. *Blood*. 2013;**122**:4189–4198.

28 Papillomaviruses and cervical neoplasia

Michael F. Herfs, PhD ■ Christopher P. Crum, MD ■ Karl Munger, PhD

> **Overview**
>
> Even after the 2008 Nobel prize awarded to Prof. Harald zur Hausen, the field of HPV continues to advance rapidly with new insights into pathogenesis, the discovery of novel genotypes/variants, refined screening approaches using HPV testing, and the recent commercialization of vaccines covering several carcinogenic HPV types. The squamocolumnar junction, which is involved in approximately 90% of (pre)neoplastic lesions, has been more precisely characterized, and its potential as a target for prevention in women beyond optimal age for vaccination is being discussed. HPV testing is assuming a major role in screening women over the age of 30, at the expense of the Papanicolaou smear, which will be largely limited to women between age 20 and 30, with a reduction or the elimination of cervical screening for women under the age of 20. For prevention of cervical neoplasia, new broader spectrum vaccines (such as a 9-valent vaccine) were introduced allowing for targeting of extended range of high-risk HPVs.

Introduction

The causal relationship between human papillomavirus (HPV) infections and cervical neoplasia has been an accepted fact for over three decades, and this virus has been the focus of strategies designed to elucidate mechanisms of virus-induced tumorigenesis, to improve the diagnosis and screening of uterine cervical neoplasms, and to exploit the host immune response to prevent HPV-associated diseases and cancers. Technological advances have dictated both the tempo and the direction of this research, which began with descriptive and experimental pathology in the early 1980s, progressed to molecular biology, and finally involved molecular immunology and genomics in order to determine how the virus enters target cells and produces neoplasia as well as to unravel the mechanisms that underlie viral clearance and long-term prevention of infections by host's immune system.

Definitions, HPV-target cells, mechanisms of infection, and transformation

Definitions

Genital HPV infections were originally defined as clinically or colposcopically identifiable flat or raised lesions that contain HPV deoxyribonucleic acid (DNA). Genital warts are the prototype of such lesions. Given that such lesions produce infectious viruses, viral particles/virions can often be identified within the apical layers of the epithelium (Figure 1). Later, the term "HPV-infection" has been expanded to include precancerous lesions and even invasive cancers (Figure 2), the term being used loosely to denote the presence of viral DNA. Depending on lesion grade, HPV genomes may be detected in infected epithelia in two different physical states, extrachromosomal (episomal) *versus* integrated (Figure 3). Advanced lesions typically contain viral DNA sequences that are integrated within the host cell genome.[1] As detailed subsequently (see the section titled "Risk Factors"), HPV infections may be associated with no visible abnormalities; active, clinically, or morphologically conspicuous lesions; and advanced neoplasia (Tables 1 and 2). The hallmark of a clinically significant HPV infection is a morphologic transformation of the target tissue. Of note, this is not synonymous with the term "transformation" as classically applied to changes in cultured cells that arise after introduction of nucleic acid sequences encoding HPV E6/E7 or other oncoproteins. Rather, the term defines the morphologic alterations that are most consistently associated with the presence of HPV in a human tissue. Depending on host factors and HPV genotype(s) involved in the infection, these alterations may define a low- or a high-grade cervical precancerous lesion, either of which is distinct from the normal squamous epithelium (Figures 1 and 2).

HPV-target cells and mechanism of infection/viral entry

The cells initially infected by HPV have traditionally been presumed to be in the basal layer of the squamous epithelium lining both the ectocervix and the region of the cervix where the columnar epithelium has been replaced by squamous mucosa (transformation zone). According to this theory, it is presumed that the virus gains access to the basal proliferating epithelial cells through microtraumas or abrasions in the stratified mucosa that expose these latter cells to viral particles.[2] This model is supported by the presence of HPV DNA and mRNAs in basal cells, and the observation that experimental infection of the squamous mucosa by pseudovirions is enhanced by disturbing the epithelial surface and hence exposing the basal cells before exposure.[3] Although infection of basal keratinocytes likely results in productive infections and subsequent (pre)neoplastic lesions developing in the outer part of the cervix and other mucosal sites (vagina, vulva), this hypothesis is inconsistent with the long-standing observation that approximately 90% of high-grade precancerous lesions and invasive carcinomas develop within or in close proximity to the squamocolumnar junction (SCJ).[4,5] For several decades, this specific microenvironment has been speculated to contain multipotent cells that, by virtue of their biology or location, may render them uniquely vulnerable to HPV infection. In 2012, a discrete population of immature columnar/cuboidal cells has been discovered in the cervical SCJ microenvironment.[6] In addition to being involved in adult cervical remodeling (metaplasia, hyperplasia),[7] these so-called "junctional" cells have been shown to harbor both HPV mRNAs and early viral proteins, supporting the possibility that these cuboidal cells may be the progenitors

---

Holland-Frei Cancer Medicine, Tenth Edition. Edited by Robert C. Bast, John C. Byrd, Carlo M. Croce, Ernest Hawk, Fadlo R. Khuri, Raphael E. Pollock, Apostolia M. Tsimberidou, Christopher G. Willett, and Cheryl L. Willman.
© 2023 John Wiley & Sons, Inc. Published 2023 by John Wiley & Sons, Inc.

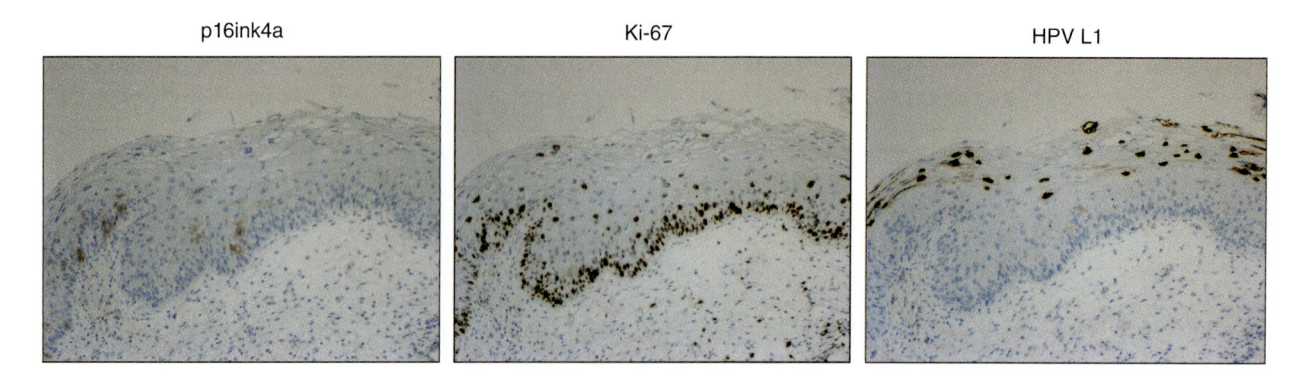

Figure 1 Histopathology of a classic HPV infection (condyloma or low-grade dysplasia) of the cervix associated with low-risk HPV types (most often HPV6 or 11). Morphologic features of HPV infection include nuclear atypia in the superficial epithelial cells with prominent cytoplasmic halos. The lower cell layers contain minimal cytologic atypia. A negative or patchy p16^{INK4A} immunoreactivity associated with some proliferative cells within the suprabasal/apical layers of infected epithelium is usually observed. In parallel, an immunoperoxidase stain for HPV capsid protein L1 highlights several dark-staining nuclei in the superficial epithelium, in keeping with a "productive" HPV infection.

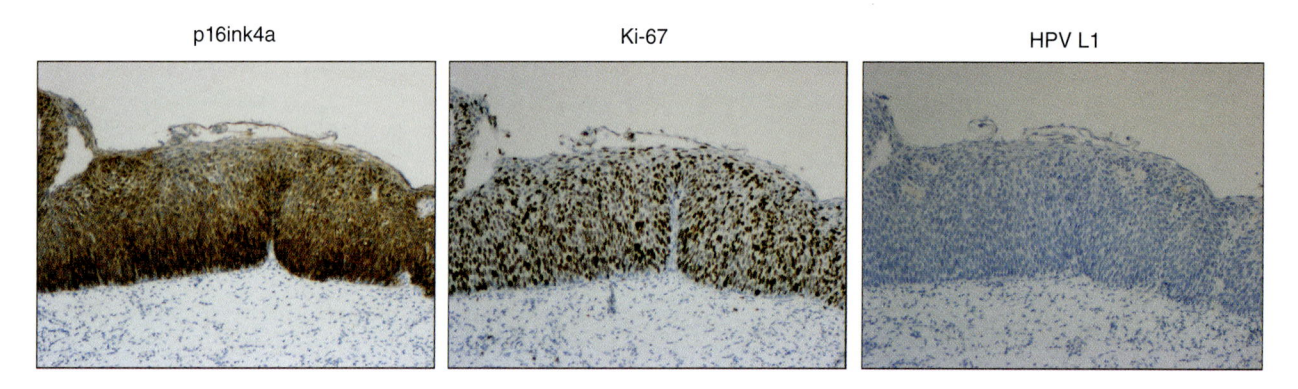

Figure 2 Histopathology of cervical intraepithelial neoplasm associated with high-risk HPV types (i.e., HPV16 and 18). Koilocytotic atypia is present but rare. In contrast, nuclear atypia is conspicuous in the lower cell layers. A strong (full-thickness) p16^{INK4A} staining and a marked increase of the proliferative index are always observed. Regarding capsid proteins (L1/L2), they are infrequently detected by immunostaining, with extremely rare positive nuclei observed.

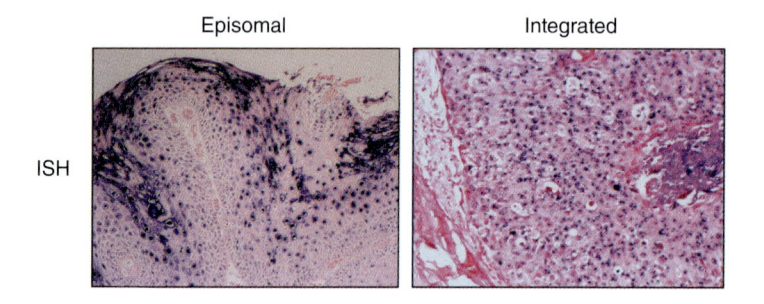

Figure 3 Appearance following *in situ* hybridization of episomal/integrated HPV infections. (a) (episomal infection): the dark staining in the superficial cell nuclei and cytoplasm represents viral DNA produced during viral replication. (b) In high-grade preneoplastic lesions and invasive cancers, viral DNA is frequently integrated into the host genome and dark dots in the nuclei are detected.

Table 1 Definitions.

- **HPV**: human papillomavirus
- **CIN**: cervical intraepithelial neoplasia (synonymous with HPV-related squamous intraepithelial lesion)
- **Low-grade CIN or CIN I**: first step in cervical carcinogenesis, usually synonymous with flat or exophytic condyloma. CIN I lesion exhibits nuclear atypia (principally in the upper epithelial layers) and most often disappear spontaneously within a few months
- **High-grade CIN or CIN II/III**: second/third step in cervical carcinogenesis. CIN II/III is characterized by atypia in all epithelial layers and is usually excised surgically
- **Occult or latent HPV**: presence of HPV DNA in the absence of morphologic evidence of HPV infection (i.e., no lesion is present)
- **High-risk HPV**: HPV with documented association with cancer (this is not an assessment of cancer risk and will vary between high-risk HPV genotypes)
- **Low-risk HPV**: HPV with no association with cancer
- **VLP**: viral-like particle, pertains to papillomavirus-like particles generated *in vitro* and used for vaccination

Table 2 Mucosal HPV genotypes and relationship to disease.

HPV types	Associated diseases
16	More than 50% of high-grade CIN and carcinomas (both squamous and adenocarcinoma)
18	10–15% of squamous carcinomas, 50% of adenocarcinomas, and 90% of neuroendocrine carcinomas
31, 45	3–5% of high-grade CIN and squamous carcinomas
33, 35, 39, 51, 52, 56, 58, 68	Less than 3% (each) of CIN and squamous carcinomas
6, 11, 40, 42, 53, 54, 57, 66, 84	Low-risk HPVs, essentially never detected in high-grade CIN and carcinomas

to most cervical neoplasia.[8] In agreement with an instrumental role of junctional cells in cervical carcinogenesis, several recent studies reported the expression of SCJ-specific/overexpressed biomarkers [e.g., cytokeratin (CK) 7] in the vast majority of cervical (pre)neoplastic lesions.[9–11] According to this model, the basal keratinocytes are still susceptible to HPV infection, but less so relative to the SCJ cells. Endocervical reserve cells have also been proposed to serve as potential HPV target cells.[12,13] However, the broad distribution of these cells in the cervical canal argues against a key involvement in HPV-related carcinogenesis.

Whatever the cell initially infected, host cell entry of HPV is initiated by binding of the mature viral capsid to heparan sulfate proteoglycans on the basement membrane. The HPV entry receptor remains controversial, but cleavage of the HPV minor capsid protein L2 at a furin (convertase) consensus site induces conformational change allowing for HPV capsid internalization and transport to the nucleus through endocytosis and retrograde transport through the trans-Golgi network.[14,15] Interestingly, the HPV virion remains in a transport vesicle when it enters to cell and requires cellular mitosis for nuclear entry.[16–18]

Mechanisms of neoplastic transformation

The mechanisms by which HPV infection induces neoplastic transformation are diverse but have been progressively elucidated over the years. The HPV E6 and E7 proteins encode potent, multifunctional oncoproteins that are consistently expressed in HPV-associated cancers. E6 and E7 expression is necessary for induction as well as maintenance of the transformed state and they have been shown to activate multiple cancer hallmarks (Figure 4).[19] Although about 550,000 cervical cancers are diagnosed every year worldwide,[20] it is important to note that only a minority (<2%) of infected patients ultimately develop cancer, most often years or decades after the initial infection. These observations support both the multistep nature of HPV-related carcinogenesis and the assumption that the main goal of the virus is to assure its replication and not to harm and kill its host. By interacting with and targeting the p53 and retinoblastoma (RB) tumor suppressors for degradation, the E6 and E7 oncoproteins of cancer-associated (high-risk) HPVs simultaneously cause hyperproliferation and block apoptosis of infected cells.[21,22] In addition to p53 and RB, a large number of other cellular targets have also been identified for E6 and E7.[23,24] HPV E7 expression causes expression of the cyclin-dependent kinase inhibitor p16^{INK4A} through an epigenetic mechanism as a result of a cellular defense response.[25,26] In normal cells, p16^{INK4A} signals RB-dependent cell cycle arrest and senescence, but this response is abrogated by E7-mediated RB degradation.[27] The HPV E6 and E7 proteins also induce a variety of mitotic abnormalities including alterations in centrosome synthesis that cause multipolar mitoses and aneuploidy.[28,29] In addition, HPV E6 and E7 expression trigger expression of members of the APOBEC family of deaminases, which cause accumulation of point mutations in the viral and host cellular genomes.[30] By inducing the transcriptional activation of the telomerase hTERT gene, E6 counteracts telomere shortening thereby bypassing replicative senescence.[31] HPV E6 and E7 expression also cause a variety of epigenetic alterations that lead to transcriptional silencing of tumor suppressor genes or increased expression of cellular proto-oncogenes. For example, the epigenetic repression of E-cadherin by HPV16 E7 protein has been shown to increase the migratory properties of HPV-infected cells.[32] Last but not least, HPV oncoproteins also inhibit innate immune signaling pathways (e.g., type I interferon signaling pathway) to establish and maintain long-term persistent HPV infections.[33–35] As a consequence, adaptive antitumor immune responses are altered, leading ultimately to immune tolerance.

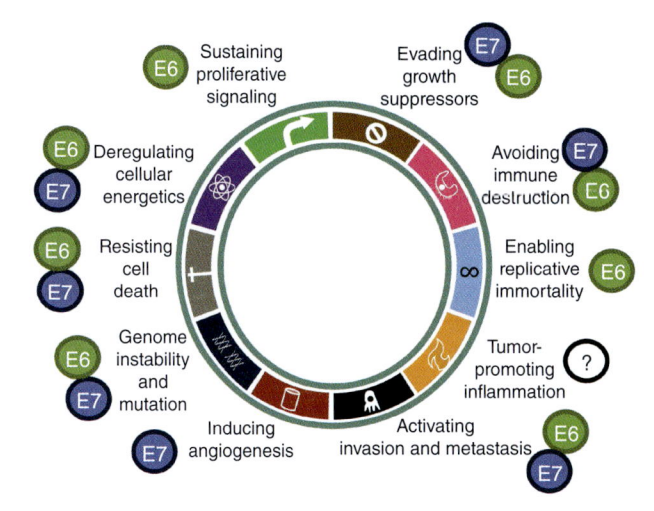

Figure 4 High-risk HPV E6 and E7 encode multifunctional oncoproteins that drive cancer initiation and progression by subverting a variety of cellular processes that lead to the acquisition of cellular abnormalities that have been referred to as hallmarks of cancer. See text for details. Source: Adapted from Mesri et al.[19]

HPV and human genital neoplasia

Risk factors

HPV infection is ubiquitous in the young, sexually active population, peaks in the early reproductive years, is often transient, and becomes increasingly less prevalent with increasing age.[36] As mentioned above, persistent infection by one or several HPV type(s) is strongly associated with the risk of a current or subsequent neoplasm, given that virtually all cervical (pre)cancers are HPV-positive.[37] At least 30 HPV types can cause cervical neoplasia development, with a broad gradient of risk imposed by these HPV types. Types 6 and 11 are prototypical "low-risk" HPVs associated with genital warts (condylomata).[38] In contrast, HPV16 is the prototypical "high-risk" HPV, detected in more than 50% of invasive cervical squamous cell carcinomas.[39] As for HPV18, for still unknown reasons, it predominates in glandular (adenocarcinomas) and neuroendocrine cancers.[40,41] However, complicating the situation, all of these HPV strains may also be detected in women with normal cytology. In addition to HPV16 and 18, several other genotypes (e.g., HPV31, 33, 35, 39, 45, 51, 52, 56, 58, 59) have been designated as carcinogenic agents by the International Agency for Research on Cancer (IARC/WHO) and are associated with cancers, albeit at a lower frequency. The presence of any HPV, high- or low-risk, does not exclude the subsequent emergence of another HPV infection of different risk in a given individual.

If a woman is found to harbor a high-risk HPV in her genital tract, what is her risk of developing a high-grade squamous intraepithelial lesion (HSIL)? In general, approximately 15% of reproductive-age women will score positive for high-risk HPVs. The risk of a HSIL ranges from less than 5% to over 70%, depending on whether the Pap smear is normal, contains a minor or nondiagnostic atypia (atypical squamous cells of undetermined significance [ASCUS]), or whether it already reveals (pre)neoplastic cells. Repeated detection of the same HPV genotype, even in the presence of a normal Pap smear, increases the risk of developing an HSIL to nearly 20%.[42] There is a strong basis, especially with HPV16, for assuming that minor intra-typic sequence variations may influence disease outcome.[43,44] However, the use of such information in patient management awaits greater consistency in study design and outcome analysis. It also requires a clearer understanding of the mechanisms influencing the relationship between HPV variants and the risk of developing high-grade cervical intraepithelial neoplasia (CIN) or cancer. Furthermore, systematic sequencing of all HPV infections is still hardly feasible routinely.

Young, sexually active women are at greatest risk of HPV infection and subsequent (pre)invasive cervical neoplasia and this risk drops significantly with increasing age. As many as 39% of adolescents may score HPV positive at a single visit.[36] The frequency of HPV detection drops with the approach of menopause, presumably linked to the higher sexual activity and possible exposure to HPV early in life.

The risk of HPV infection and related anogenital malignancies in immunosuppressed individuals is well documented, particularly in organ transplant patients or in individuals with untreated human immunodeficiency virus (HIV) infection.[45] The risk of HPV positivity and persistent infection is increased in women who are HIV positive.[46] As an example, persistence was shown to be 1.9 (95% confidence interval [CI] 1.5–2.3) times greater if the subjects had a CD4+ cell count <200 cells/μL compared to patients with >500 CD4+cells/μL.[46] Similarly, the risk of a subsequent squamous intraepithelial lesion is also significantly higher in HIV-infected women.[47] Although an increased risk of invasive carcinoma in HIV-infected women is controversial (because requires a long-term follow-up which is limited to 2–3 years in most studies), we may reasonably think that this latter risk may be influenced by both the level and duration of immunosuppression.[48]

In addition to HPV strain/variant, sexual activity, and immune status, other risk factors have also been proposed such as cigarette smoking, bacterial vaginosis, or the concomitant infection with other sexually transmitted pathogens (e.g., *Candida albicans*, *Chlamydia trachomatis*).[49–51] However, the mechanisms of action are still largely speculative and there are conflicting reports in the literature.

In summary, a multitude of factors, virus- and host-related, influence the risk of cervical neoplasia before, during, and/or following viral exposure.

Applications to clinical medicine

The prevention of cervical cancer has been based on the Pap test for several decades. Because cervical cancers are always preceded by a cervical precursor (CIN) lesion, often by many years, the detection of these precursors is fundamental to cancer prevention. The Pap test recommendations have recently been revised, in concert with recommendations for the use of HPV testing in screening. They are discussed in the next segment. Precursor lesions are recognized clinically on colposcopy, where HPV-related lesions can be identified following the application of acetic acid. The use of colposcopy has maximized the targeting of lesions for biopsy, and outpatient removal is the usual approach, including cryotherapy, laser, and loop electrical excision.[52] The latter procedures target the entire transformation zone, removing the lesion and replacing the process of chronic repair with a brief period of re-epithelialization. Recurrence after removal or ablation is linked to either inadequate excision or infection by another HPV following therapy. The former is increased when margins are positive. Infection with new HPV types appears to explain why so many "recurrences" following ablation for high-grade precursors are low grade in nature.[53] Reinfection with the same HPV type is uncommon except in immunosuppressed women. The potential significance of these findings in cancer prevention is discussed at the end of this article.

HPV testing in management of the abnormal Pap smear and primary screening

After years of discussion and evaluation, HPV testing has emerged as a viable management tool for a subset of women with abnormal cervical cytology. Because HPV is necessary for cervical neoplasia development and because high-risk HPV types predominate in the cervix, a substantial proportion of women with a cytologic diagnosis of low- or high-grade precancerous changes will score high-risk HPV positive. For this reason, HPV testing is of limited value in this population. However, women with nondiagnostic squamous atypias (ASCUS) present a management dilemma in which the clinician must decide between colposcopy and Pap smear follow-up. HPV testing offers the additional opportunity to triage the patient into colposcopy and follow-up groups by immediately testing the cytologic sample, which is possible with the newer liquid-based technologies. HPV testing, such as the Hybrid Capture II or PCR-based tests, is extremely sensitive and will detect more than 95% of women with histologically proven preinvasive disease.[54] Women with ASCUS who are HPV negative have a <1% risk of high-grade CIN, in contrast to a 20% risk if they are high-risk HPV positive.[54] Similar results have been seen with the management of abnormal glandular cells on the smear.[55] The HPV test has been approved as an adjunct to the Pap smear for screening women over age 30 for a several years, now. The basis for this approach lies in the high negative predictive value of both a normal smear and negative HPV assay, which may permit a longer cytology screening interval. In 2012, the American Cancer Society and the United States Preventative Task Force have made the following recommendations that will impact on reimbursement.[56] First screening of women under age 21 and over age 65 will not be recommended unless there is a history of cervical neoplasia. Second, screening interval of women age 21–65 will be lengthened to 3 years. Third, screening of women over age 30 can be lengthened to 5 years if accompanied by HPV testing (for further information, see https://www.cancer.org/cancer/cervical-cancer/detection-diagnosis-staging/cervical-cancer-screening-guidelines.html). Of note, these latter recommendations may vary from one country to another. As an example, primary screening using high-risk HPV detection was recently introduced in Australia and the Netherlands.[57]

Surrogate biomarkers of HPV infections for diagnosis

The distinction of HPV-positive preinvasive lesions (LSIL and HSIL) from benign inflammatory processes may be difficult and can significantly influence management decisions. Improving the precision of these diagnoses has been the focus of many studies designed to identify biomarkers that may simplify the distinction of HPV-related neoplasia from its mimics. Because HPV disrupts several cell functions (see the section titled "Mechanisms of neoplastic transformation"), it is logical to presume that alterations in host genes may serve as "surrogate markers" for HPV infection. Host genes reported to be upregulated in cervical neoplasia include telomerase, $p16^{INK4A}$, cyclin E, Ki-67, stathmin-1, and others.[58–60] Some of these, particularly the combination of Ki-67 and $p16^{INK4A}$ have practical value in triaging histologic abnormalities. Full-thickness immunostaining for CK7, a marker for SCJ cells, which are targets for high-risk HPV infections, was also strongly correlated to disease progression.[9–11] The lower anogenital tract task force has recently recommended $p16^{INK4A}$ staining as an adjunct to histologic evaluation, a positive test being continuous horizontal linear (or block) staining.[61] The most appropriate use of this biomarker is to solidify a CIN2 or CIN3 diagnosis on histologic exam by inferring the presence of a carcinogenic HPV. However, because up to 70% of CIN1 lesions stain also positive for this marker, $p16^{INK4A}$ immunostaining alone cannot be used to make a diagnosis of CIN2 or CIN3. Moreover, strong/full-thickness $p16^{INK4A}$ staining, while predictive for a high-risk HPV-associated high-grade lesion, is not a predictor of lesion progression. Indeed, up to 67% of histologically verified, $p16^{INK4A}$-positive CIN2 lesions regress within a 3-year period.[62]

Clinical management

Management of HPV-related cervical neoplasms continues to be defined and redefined, in step with the methods used for lesion removal. Most women with low- or high-grade CIN on Pap smear or an atypical smear that is HPV positive will be referred to colposcopic examination. Of those who have a negative examination or a low-grade CIN on biopsy, 10–13% will develop a biopsy-proven high-grade CIN within 2 years. Many practitioners will follow patients with low-grade abnormalities and negative colposcopy by repeat cytology in 6–12 months, with attention to this risk. Biopsy-proven high-grade CIN is typically managed by the loop electrical excision procedure or cone biopsy. Thus, the outcome of a given case will be dependent on the application of the histologic criteria for distinguishing low- from high-grade squamous intraepithelial lesions. Long-term follow-up of all women with cervical abnormalities, treated or otherwise, customarily includes Pap smear evaluations but may eventually include periodic HPV testing as well.

Prevention

Efforts to elucidate the anti-HPV immune responses have evolved from studies of fusion proteins and linear epitopes to the *in vitro* production of virus-like particles (VLPs) (Figure 5).[63,64] VLPs are produced by expressing the entire late region (or L1 gene) of one HPV genome in eukaryotic systems. Such VLPs contain conformational epitopes that can generate strong host immunity.[65] This avenue of investigation was by far the most

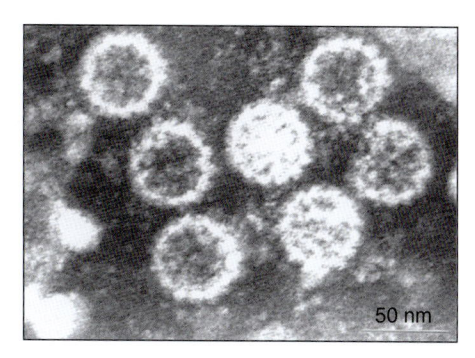

Figure 5 Electron micrograph depicting papillomavirus-like particles generated *in vitro*. Source: Courtesy of Ian Frazer, MD, Princess Alexandra Hospital, Queensland, Australia.

promising because it offered the advantage of intact particles that were highly immunogenic.[66] In the early 2000s, large-scale trials have validated the merits of VLP-based vaccination, demonstrating high efficacy (95% or higher) for both preventing infection and subsequent lesions attributed to the HPV types targeted by the vaccines.[67] Based on these seminal results, 2-valent (Cervarix, GlaxoSmithKline, targeting both HPV16 and 18) and 4-valent [Gardasil 4, Merck & Co, targeting not only HPV16 and 18 but also HPV6 and 11 (involved in the development of >90% condylomata] HPV vaccines were introduced in the market in 2007 and 2006, respectively. Predictably, lower efficacies in women who have been previously exposed were reported, highlighting the necessity to vaccinate prior to the onset of sexual activity. Moreover, it is important to note that the current HPV vaccines are prophylactic and not therapeutic (do not cure already developed HPV-related disease). Given that the incidence and level of cross-protection against nontargeted genotypes have been shown to be relatively low[68], a 9-valent vaccine (Gardasil 9, Merck & Co, targeting HPV6, 11, 16, 18, 31, 33, 45, 52, 58) was developed and approved by the FDA. This newer, more broad-based vaccine should address the regional variations in prevalence of certain high-risk HPV genotypes.

The strong association between the SCJ and cervical carcinoma as well as the discovery of a putative cell of origin in this site have raised the possibility that prophylactic (cryo)ablation of this small region might significantly reduce the risk of cervical cancer.[69] The annual incidence of cervical cancer worldwide exceeds that of vaginal/vulvar carcinoma by nearly 20-fold, further evidence of the potential influence of this peculiar microenvironment on cancer risk.[39] Anecdotic studies of HPV infection following cryoablation, topographic recurrence patterns, and differences in CIN grade following SCJ excision or ablation have all pointed to the possibility of a profound change in precancer risk imposed by removal of the SCJ.[53,70] Whether this information can be translated into a viable cancer prevention program in underserved populations that are still facing to HPV epidemic is unclear and awaits further study.

Key references

The complete reference list can be found on Vital Source version of this title, see inside front cover.

2 Doorbar J, Quint W, Banks L, et al. The biology and life-cycle of human papillomaviruses. *Vaccine*. 2012;**30**(Suppl 5):F55–F70.

3 Roberts JN, Buck CB, Thompson CD, et al. Genital transmission of HPV in a mouse model is potentiated by nonoxynol-9 and inhibited by carrageenan. *Nat Med*. 2007;**13**(7):857–861.

4. Marsh M. Original site of cervical carcinoma; topographical relationship of carcinoma of the cervix to the external os and to the squamocolumnar junction. *Obstet Gynecol.* 1956;**7**(4):444–452.
5. Richart RM. Cervical intraepithelial neoplasia. *Pathol Annu.* 1973;**8**:301–328.
6. Herfs M, Yamamoto Y, Laury A, et al. A discrete population of squamocolumnar junction cells implicated in the pathogenesis of cervical cancer. *Proc Natl Acad Sci U S A.* 2012;**109**(26):10516–10521.
8. Mirkovic J, Howitt BE, Roncarati P, et al. Carcinogenic HPV infection in the cervical squamo-columnar junction. *J Pathol.* 2015;**236**(3):265–271.
12. Martens JE, Smedts F, van Muyden RC, et al. Reserve cells in human uterine cervical epithelium are derived from mullerian epithelium at midgestational age. *Int J Gynecol Pathol.* 2007;**26**(4):463–468.
16. DiGiuseppe S, Luszczek W, Keiffer TR, et al. Incoming human papillomavirus type 16 genome resides in a vesicular compartment throughout mitosis. *Proc Natl Acad Sci U S A.* 2016;**113**(22):6289–6294.
17. Day PM, Weisberg AS, Thompson CD, et al. Human papillomavirus 16 capsids mediate nuclear entry during infection. *J Virol.* 2019;**93**(15). doi: 10.1128/JVI.00454-19.
19. Mesri EA, Feitelson MA, Munger K. Human viral oncogenesis: a cancer hallmarks analysis. *Cell Host Microbe.* 2014;**15**(3):266–282.
20. Bray F, Ferlay J, Soerjomataram I, et al. Global cancer statistics 2018: GLOBOCAN estimates of incidence and mortality worldwide for 36 cancers in 185 countries. *CA Cancer J Clin.* 2018;**68**(6):394–424.
21. Scheffner M, Werness BA, Huibregtse JM, et al. The E6 oncoprotein encoded by human papillomavirus types 16 and 18 promotes the degradation of p53. *Cell.* 1990;**63**(6):1129–1136.
22. Heck DV, Yee CL, Howley PM, Munger K. Efficiency of binding the retinoblastoma protein correlates with the transforming capacity of the E7 oncoproteins of the human papillomaviruses. *Proc Natl Acad Sci U S A.* 1992;**89**(10):4442–4446.
23. Vande Pol SB, Klingelhutz AJ. Papillomavirus E6 oncoproteins. *Virology.* 2013;**445**(1–2):115–137.
24. Roman A, Munger K. The papillomavirus E7 proteins. *Virology.* 2013;**445**(1–2):138–168.
25. McLaughlin-Drubin ME, Crum CP, Munger K. Human papillomavirus E7 oncoprotein induces KDM6A and KDM6B histone demethylase expression and causes epigenetic reprogramming. *Proc Natl Acad Sci U S A.* 2011;**108**(5):2130–2135.
26. McLaughlin-Drubin ME, Park D, Munger K. Tumor suppressor p16INK4A is necessary for survival of cervical carcinoma cell lines. *Proc Natl Acad Sci U S A.* 2013;**110**(40):16175–16180.
28. Duensing S, Duensing A, Crum CP, Munger K. Human papillomavirus type 16 E7 oncoprotein-induced abnormal centrosome synthesis is an early event in the evolving malignant phenotype. *Cancer Res.* 2001;**61**(6):2356–2360.
30. Warren CJ, Westrich JA, Doorslaer KV, Pyeon D. Roles of APOBEC3A and APOBEC3B in human papillomavirus infection and disease progression. *Viruses.* 2017;**9**(8). doi: 10.3390/v9080233.
31. Veldman T, Horikawa I, Barrett JC, Schlegel R. Transcriptional activation of the telomerase hTERT gene by human papillomavirus type 16 E6 oncoprotein. *J Virol.* 2001;**75**(9):4467–4472.
33. Beglin M, Melar-New M, Laimins L. Human papillomaviruses and the interferon response. *J Interferon Cytokine Res.* 2009;**29**(9):629–635.
34. Lau L, Gray EE, Brunette RL, Stetson DB. DNA tumor virus oncogenes antagonize the cGAS-STING DNA-sensing pathway. *Science.* 2015;**350**(6260):568–571.
37. Walboomers JM, Jacobs MV, Manos MM, et al. Human papillomavirus is a necessary cause of invasive cervical cancer worldwide. *J Pathol.* 1999;**189**(1):12–19.
39. de Martel C, Plummer M, Vignat J, Franceschi S. Worldwide burden of cancer attributable to HPV by site, country and HPV type. *Int J Cancer.* 2017;**141**(4):664–670.
40. Pirog EC, Lloveras B, Molijn A, et al. HPV prevalence and genotypes in different histological subtypes of cervical adenocarcinoma, a worldwide analysis of 760 cases. *Mod Pathol.* 2014;**27**(12):1559–1567.
41. Stoler MH, Mills SE, Gersell DJ, Walker AN. Small-cell neuroendocrine carcinoma of the cervix. A human papillomavirus type 18-associated cancer. *Am J Surg Pathol.* 1991;**15**(1):28–32.
44. Mirabello L, Yeager M, Cullen M, et al. HPV16 sublineage associations with histology-specific cancer risk using HPV whole-genome sequences in 3200 women. *J Natl Cancer Inst.* 2016;**108**(9):djw100.
45. Fairley CK, Sheil AG, McNeil JJ, et al. The risk of ano-genital malignancies in dialysis and transplant patients. *Clin Nephrol.* 1994;**41**(2):101–105.
47. Ellerbrock TV, Chiasson MA, Bush TJ, et al. Incidence of cervical squamous intraepithelial lesions in HIV-infected women. *JAMA.* 2000;**283**(8):1031–1037.
49. Collins S, Rollason TP, Young LS, Woodman CB. Cigarette smoking is an independent risk factor for cervical intraepithelial neoplasia in young women: a longitudinal study. *Eur J Cancer.* 2010;**46**(2):405–411.
50. Gillet E, Meys JF, Verstraelen H, et al. Bacterial vaginosis is associated with uterine cervical human papillomavirus infection: a meta-analysis. *BMC Infect Dis.* 2011;**11**:10.
56. Saslow D, Solomon D, Lawson HW, et al. American Cancer Society, American Society for Colposcopy and Cervical Pathology, and American Society for Clinical Pathology screening guidelines for the prevention and early detection of cervical cancer. *CA: Cancer J Clin.* 2012;**62**(3):147–172.
58. Sano T, Oyama T, Kashiwabara K, et al. Expression status of p16 protein is associated with human papillomavirus oncogenic potential in cervical and genital lesions. *Am J Pathol.* 1998;**153**(6):1741–1748.
62. Moscicki AB, Ma Y, Wibbelsman C, et al. Rate of and risks for regression of cervical intraepithelial neoplasia 2 in adolescents and young women. *Obstet Gynecol.* 2010;**116**(6):1373–1380.
63. Zhou J, Sun XY, Stenzel DJ, Frazer IH. Expression of vaccinia recombinant HPV 16 L1 and L2 ORF proteins in epithelial cells is sufficient for assembly of HPV virion-like particles. *Virology.* 1991;**185**(1):251–257.
64. Kirnbauer R, Taub J, Greenstone H, et al. Efficient self-assembly of human papillomavirus type 16 L1 and L1-L2 into virus-like particles. *J Virol.* 1993;**67**(12):6929–6936.
66. Kirnbauer R, Booy F, Cheng N, et al. Papillomavirus L1 major capsid protein self-assembles into virus-like particles that are highly immunogenic. *Proc Natl Acad Sci U S A.* 1992;**89**(24):12180–12184.
67. Schiller JT, Castellsague X, Garland SM. A review of clinical trials of human papillomavirus prophylactic vaccines. *Vaccine.* 2012;**30**(Suppl 5):F123–F138.
68. Malagon T, Drolet M, Boily MC, et al. Cross-protective efficacy of two human papillomavirus vaccines: a systematic review and meta-analysis. *Lancet. Infect Dis.* 2012;**12**(10):781–789.
70. Franceschi S. Past and future of prophylactic ablation of the cervical squamocolumnar junction. *Ecancermedicalscience.* 2015;**9**:527.

29 Hepatitis viruses and hepatoma

Hongyang Wang

Overview

Hepatitis is inflammation of the liver, typically the result of virus infections or the exposure of the liver to toxic substances such as alcohol or aflatoxin B. Hepatitis B virus (HBV) and hepatitis C virus (HCV) are the most common causes of transient and persistent liver infections, frequently resulting in hepatitis and, in the context of chronic infections, liver cirrhosis, and hepatocellular carcinoma (HCC). Hepatitis B may be worsened by super or co-infection with hepatitis delta virus, a subviral satellite.

HBV belongs to the genus *Orthohepadnavirus* of the *Hepadnaviridae* with a circular incomplete double-stranded DNA genome, containing four overlapping open reading frames (ORFs) which encode the three viral envelope proteins (HBsAg), the core protein (HBcAg), and a secreted version of the core protein called e-antigen (HBeAg), a polymerase, and a multifunctional nonstructural protein termed X (HBx). In China, where HBV is endemic, up to 80% of HCC cases are attributable to chronic HBV infection. Besides the possible oncogenic functions of HBV-encoded proteins and random HBV DNA integrations into host DNA, hepatitis B-associated host mutations have been reported to contribute to HCC development.

HCV belongs to the genus *Hepacivirus* of the Flaviviridae family, with a single-stranded positive-sense RNA genome. There is no host genome integration. Proposed mechanisms of HCV-induced hepatocarcinogenesis include oncogenic effects of HCV viral proteins, steatosis and insulin resistance, chronic inflammation and fibrosis, oxidative stress, and chromosomal instability.

This article focuses on hepatitis and HCC caused by HBV and HCV infections, discussing epidemiologic considerations, the role of virus in progression to HCC, and early HCC diagnosis and prophylaxis. A reduction in the morbidity of viral hepatitis and HCC would be of great importance in public health.

Hepatitis and hepatoma

Chronic liver diseases, including hepatitis B and hepatitis C, alcoholic liver disease (ALD), and nonalcoholic fatty liver disease (NAFLD), with associated emergence of cirrhosis and hepatocellular carcinoma (HCC), are major causes of illness and death.[1] HBV chronically infects ~300 million people worldwide; if untreated, the lifetime risk of death from cirrhosis or HCC is about 40%, with a two to threefold higher risk in males. Chronic HCV infection is about fourfold less prevalent worldwide but also has a high risk of progressing to cirrhosis and liver cancer. Fortunately, most HCV infections can now be cured via antiviral therapy.[2,3]

Human hepatitis viruses

Human viruses that selectively infect hepatocytes and cause liver diseases include hepatitis A virus (HAV), hepatitis B virus (HBV), hepatitis C virus (HCV), hepatitis D virus (HDV), and hepatitis E virus (HEV). Following fecal–oral transmission, HAV or HEV causes transient infection of the liver, which can vary in intensity from asymptomatic to fulminant disease leading to liver failure and death. Rarely, HEV can also cause chronic infection.[4] HAV, a single-stranded RNA virus, is a major cause of acute viral hepatitis worldwide.[4] HEV, a single-stranded, nonenveloped RNA virus, is endemic in several Asian and African countries.[4] Pregnant women and patients with preexisting chronic liver diseases are at a high risk of fulminant liver failure upon HEV infection.[4,5] Of relevance to any discussion focused on clinical aspects of HBV and HCV infection, super-infection by HAV or HEV may be a cause of acute hepatitis on a background of chronic hepatitis caused by HBV or HCV. This may also be true following super-infection of HBV carriers by hepatitis delta virus.

Hepatitis B virus

HBV belongs to the genus *Orthohepadnavirus* of the *Hepadnaviridae* with a circular incomplete double-stranded DNA genome, ~3.2 kb in length. The HBV genome contains four overlapping open reading frames (ORFs) that encode, respectively, the three surface envelope proteins (HBsAg), the two core proteins (HBcAg, the nucleocapsid protein, and HBeAg, a secretory protein), a DNA polymerase/reverse transcriptase, and a multifunctional nonstructural protein termed X (HBx). The ORF encoding the polymerase/reverse transcriptase partially overlaps the core and HBx ORFs and completely overlaps the HBsAg gene and a transcriptional enhancer, EhnI. HBx also overlaps transcriptional enhancer II (EnhII) and the basal core (BCP) and core promoters. The BCP controls the transcription of precore mRNA, which is translated to produce HBeAg, while the core promoter controls transcription of the mRNA of the nucleocapsid protein and DNA polymerase/reverse-transcriptase. This latter mRNA, known as the pregenome (pgRNA), is also the template for reverse transcription to produce minus-strand viral DNA, which is then copied into the partially double-stranded DNA found in mature virus. Following entry into hepatocytes, the viral nucleocapsid is uncoated and transported to the nucleus, where the partially double-stranded viral DNA genome is released and processed into a covalently closed circular DNA (cccDNA). cccDNA is transcribed by host RNA polymerase II to produce all viral RNAs including the pregenome. The pgRNA, viral core, and polymerase proteins are assembled into nucleocapsids in the cytoplasm, where all viral DNA synthesis takes place, with completion of the minus strand by reverse transcription and at least partially completion of the plus strand by DNA directed DNA synthesis. Nucleocapsids with a partially double-stranded DNA genome then acquire envelope

---

Holland-Frei Cancer Medicine, Tenth Edition. Edited by Robert C. Bast, John C. Byrd, Carlo M. Croce, Ernest Hawk, Fadlo R. Khuri, Raphael E. Pollock, Apostolia M. Tsimberidou, Christopher G. Willett, and Cheryl L. Willman.
© 2023 John Wiley & Sons, Inc. Published 2023 by John Wiley & Sons, Inc.

proteins via budding into the endoplasmic reticulum. During the so-called immune tolerant phase of infection, which can last for years or decades, approximately 10^{11} virions are released into the circulation of individuals with chronic HBV infection per day and HBV particles are cleared from the plasma with a half-life of approximately 1.2 days. Active hepatitis causes a slow but major drop in virus replication in the liver and virus titers in serum over time, by mechanisms that are still unclear. This decline is often associated with a loss of HBeAg from the circulation, typically due to mutations in the BCP or the leader sequence specifying HBeAg secretion.

Interestingly, HBV reverse transcriptase lacks proofreading capacity, resulting in mutation rates of 1.5×10^{-5} to 5×10^{-5} nucleotide substitutions/site/year, as shown during studies of the HBeAg-positive stage of chronic infection, when virus replication is most active.[6,7] Due to the overlapping ORFs, HBV is probably constrained to maintain protein functions required for viral replication.[8] Mutation of the HBV genome allows the emergence of mutants that can escape the host response; it is thought that this selection is primarily against viral epitopes expressed on infected hepatocytes. While these immune escape mutants likely facilitate virus survival in a given patient, they do not efficiently transmit to new hosts; instead, wild-type virus generally re-emerges following spread. For instance, mutants that become prevalent during chronic infection often lack the ability to make HBeAg, which appears to be necessary to create a new infection leading to chronicity. HBeAg appears to have an essential role in modifying the host immune response to facilitate virus survival at the start of an infection; a possible explanation has been suggested by studies in mice.[9]

Ten HBV genotypes (genotypes A-J) have been identified according to sequence divergence greater than 8% in the entire HBV genome or greater than 4% in the S region.[10] Genotypes have further been classified into subgenotypes if the divergence in the entire genome is between 4% and 8%. For instance, subgenotypes 1–5 of genotype A, subgenotypes 1–8 of genotype B, subgenotypes 1–8 of genotype C, and subgenotypes 1–7 of genotype D. HBV genotypes and subgenotypes have distinct geographical distributions.[6,11,12] HBV genotype A1, A3, A4, and A5 are endemic in Africa, especially in West Africa, whereas genotype A2 is endemic in Europe. Genotypes B and C are endemic in Asia. Of HBV genotypes B and C, subgenotypes B2 and C2 are endemic in most parts of Asia. Subgenotype C4 is encountered in Aborigines from Australia. Subgenotypes B3–B8, C1, C3, and C5–C8 are present in Indonesia and the Philippines. Genotype D is endemic in the entire Old World including Northern Africa, Northern and South Asia, the Mediterranean area, and most European countries. Subgenotype D1 is predominant in areas with Moslem ethnicity. Subgenotype D2 is endemic in Russia and the Baltic region. Subgenotypes D4 and D6 are endemic in Oceania and Indonesia, respectively. HBV genotype E is endemic in Western and Central Africa. HBV genotypes F, G, and H are endemic in Middle and Southern America. Genotype H is common in Central and South America, genotype I in Laos and Vietnam, and genotype J in Japan.[10] HBV genotype and subgenotype may not only correlate with the clinical outcomes but also with the response to interferon-α treatment.[12,13] In East Asia where HBV genotypes B and C are endemic, genotype B is more apt to cause acute infection in young people and to be more easily cleared than genotype C, whereas genotype C leads to higher persistence following infection and is more apt to cause cirrhosis and HCC.[13–16] In addition, genotype B infections are more responsive to antiviral therapy with interferon-alpha. Thus, HBV genotyping is not only important in reconstructing the evolutionary history of HBV and humans but also helpful in indicating clinical outcomes of HBV infection and responses to antiviral treatments.

Chronic HBV infection is most frequently encountered in individuals infected perinatally or during early childhood.[10] HBV infection in adults is mostly asymptomatic or experiences a clinically acute course, followed in either case by recovery. Because HBV is transmitted by parenteral routes, invasive medical procedures, household contact with HBV carriers, body care and beauty treatments, and, of course, lack of HBV vaccination are the major risk factors of acute hepatitis B in adults. About 8.5% of adult patients with acute hepatitis B in mainland China will develop a chronic infection.[14] HBV genotype C (vs genotype B) and genotype D (vs other HBV genotypes) are more apt to cause persistent infection following an acute course.[14,16] Genetic polymorphisms of human leukocyte antigen (HLA) in the *HLA-DP* and *HLA-DQ* regions contribute to immune imbalance (such as Th1/Th2 cells or Th17/Treg cells, neutrophil/lymphocyte, neutrophil/CD8$^+$ T cell, and Th1/Th2 cytokines balances) upon HBV infection, resulting in HBV persistence and possible chronic liver inflammation.[17–19] Allelic frequencies of the *HLA-DP* polymorphisms differ greatly among races. According to the NCBI database (http://www.ncbi.nlm.nih.gov/projects/SNP/), the *HLA-DP* (or *HLA-DQ*) alleles that facilitate chronic HBV infection are the major alleles in the Asian population,[18,19] while they are the variant alleles in the European population. This might be one of the reasons why HBV persistence is more frequent in Asians than in Europeans. These *HLA-II* genetic polymorphisms may predispose the host to maintaining chronic HBV infection, facilitate the immune selection of the disease-related HBV mutants, and affect the risks of cirrhosis and HCC contributed by the HBV mutations.

HBV: cirrhosis and HCC

In general, without efficient treatment, all types of chronic hepatitis will finally progress into ESLDs (end-stage liver diseases), such as cirrhosis and HCC. Most ESLDs displays a poor clinical outcome. Cirrhosis and HCC are major causes of mortality worldwide, and any regional differences in incidence may be explained by differences in HCV and HBV prevalence.[1] In 2015, the World Health Organization reported that primary liver cancer caused 745,517 deaths worldwide and that HCC represented the major histological type of these liver cancers.[20] While HBV is the primary cause of HCC, in a review of global mortality, the importance of HCV was also revealed: deaths from HCV-related HCC were estimated at 195,700 in 2010.

In China, HCC is the second-leading cause of cancer mortality.[21] Approximately 383,203 persons die from liver cancer every year in China, which accounts for 51% of the deaths from liver cancer worldwide.[21] Up to 80% of HCC cases in China are attributable to HBV, and approximately 20% of HCC patients test positive for HCV-RNA.[22]

Epidemiologic considerations

Worldwide, ~2 billion people now alive have been exposed to HBV as assessed by assaying for anti-HBV immunoglobulins, and the majority have recovered. However, ~300 million people are chronically infected with HBV. It has been estimated that 57% of cirrhosis cases are attributable to either HBV (30%) or HCV (27%) and 78% of HCC are attributable to HBV (53%) or HCV (25%).[23] A prospective study conducted in Taiwan on individuals over 30 years of age found that the cumulative lifetime (age 30 to 75 years) incidences of HCC for men and women positive for both HBsAg and antibodies against HCV was 38.35% and 27.40%; for those positive for HBsAg only, 27.38% and 7.99%; and for those positive for neither, 1.55% and 1.03%, respectively.[24] Prospective epidemiological studies have proven that male gender, increasing age, cirrhosis, high viral load, HBeAg positivity, HBV genotype C (vs genotype B), low albumin, alanine aminotransferase (ALT) elevation, and viral mutation A1762T/G1764A independently increase HCC risk in chronic HBV-infected patients.[16,24–28] (The A1762T/G1764A mutation in the BCP, for example, reduces expression of HBeAg, which apparently facilitates HBV survival in the host). These and other HBV mutations are considered HCC-risk mutations.[29–31] A1762T/G1764A, for instance, can predict HCC prospectively, possibly because it reflects the intensity of the host response to infected hepatocytes that produce HBeAg.[32] Similar demographic, clinical, and viral factors arising prior to HCC occurrence should be prognostic and even predictive for HCC development in HBV-infected patients, which as already noted, only affects about 40% of HBV carriers.

Role of HBV mutations in HCC development
Only the HBV strains/variants best adapted to the immune system will survive and thrive in liver. Whether any HBV mutations arising during the course of a chronic infection are more procarcinogenic, or just facilitate virus survival, thereby prolonging chronic liver damage by the host immune system, remains uncertain. While genetic predispositions of HLA-II antigens and other inflammatory factors such as NF-κB and STAT3 may facilitate outgrowth of mutant HBVs during chronic infection (e.g., by activating cytidine deaminases that lead to HBV mutations), the fact that these mutations are prognostic of HCC does not distinguish whether they are risk factors or act directly in the process.[8,18,33,34]

Host somatic mutations
Cytidine deaminases and their analogs, whose expressions and activities can be activated by proinflammatory cytokines generated during the inflammation, not only promote HBV mutagenesis but may also facilitate somatic mutations in the host.[8] Possibly HCC-related somatic mutations are found in critical genes including RNA editing genes (*ADAR1, ADAR2, KHDRBS2,* and *RTL1*), chromatin remodeling genes (*ARID1A, ARID1B,* and *ARID2*), DNA-binding genes (*HOXA1*), growth factor signaling pathway genes (*CDH8, CDK14, CNTN2, ERRFI1, RPS6KA3, P62,* and *PROKR2*), transcriptional regulation genes (*AXIN1, CCNG1, CTNNB1, IRF2, NFE2L2, PARP4, PAX5, ST18, TP53, TRRAP,* and *ZNF717*), cell structure modification genes (*FLNA* and *VCAM1*), and epigenetic modification genes (*MLL3*), and JAK/STAT pathway genes (*JAK1* and *JAK2*).[35] These somatic mutations may affect major signaling pathways that in turn facilitate HCC development.

In addition, random integration of HBV into the host genome, which occurs throughout the course of a chronic infection,[36,37] may also alter expression of genes that promote development of HBV, for example, TERT.[38] In this instance, a significant fraction of HBV integrations found in HCCs have occurred in the promoter region of the human telomerase reverse transcriptase (TERT), where HBV EnhI appears to play a key role in transcriptional activation.[38] Transcription of other genes thought to have a role in HCC also appears to be affected by nearby HBV integration, including MLL4, CCNE1, etc. However, it remains unclear if these integrations or indeed many of the observed somatic mutations are primarily carcinogenic or promote carcinogenesis by facilitating the response of the affected hepatocyte to signals for cell division during chronic liver damage, leading to their clonal expansion and, thereby, indirectly promoting carcinogenesis.[39–41]

The roles of HBV-encoding proteins in HCC
(1) Excess production of the HBV envelope proteins, or truncated forms of the middle (preS2/S) and large (preS1/preS2/S) envelope protein can, at least in model systems, activate cellular signal transduction pathways, or endoplasmic reticulum (ER) stress pathways, induce cell proliferation by upregulating cyclin A expression, and activate c-Raf-1 and extracellular regulated kinase (ERK) signaling to stimulate cell proliferation. In addition, accumulation of the S proteins in the ER can activate the unfolded protein response and cause oxidative stress. Epidermal growth factor receptor (EGFR) overexpression, which occurs in 40–70% of human HCCs, has also been linked with tumorigenesis.[42] Aberrant activation of Raf-MEKERK and PI3K-Akt pathways driven by EGFR is commonly observed and implicated in the tumor growth and progression of many human cancer types, including HCC.[43] Moreover, activation of EGFR signaling pathways via the high expression of either its cognate ligands or itself is strongly associated with the poor prognosis of HCC (2). It has been found in model systems that HBx is a transactivator of several cellular signaling pathways including Wnt which may contribute to HBV-related HCC and that HBx also interacts with tumor suppressor adenomatous polyposis coli (APC) to activate Wnt/β-catenin signaling. HBx has also been suggested to promote the invasive ability and metastatic potential of HCC. These studies may shed light on the possible role of HBx in chronic hepatitis infection and liver cancer.[44]

It has also been reported that carboxy-truncated HBx protein (Ct-HBx), a common consequence of HBV DNA integration into the host genome, can enhance HCC cell invasiveness and metastasis in a manner that is more potent than that evoked by full-length HBx. While a great number of reports from model system suggest that HBx may alter transcription of host genes that are either carcinogenic or pro-carcinogenic, its role in the human liver is less clear.

Finally, a recent study found that HBx is essential for transcription of cccDNA because it induces degradation of the host smc5/smc6 complex which otherwise binds to and inactivates transcription of episomal DNAs.[45] The smc5/smc6 complex is also involved in host DNA repair, and the effect of HBx on this process and, therefore, the potential for HBx mediated damage to this pathway in the development of HCC remains to be determined. This may become clarified through the use of drugs that block this effect of HBx on smc5/smc6.[46]

Early diagnosis and prophylaxis of HCC
Across all countries, 5-year overall survival of HCC is approximately 10%. This poor outcome is due partly to the lack of an effective method for timely diagnosis, which leads to only 30–40% of patients with HCC being suitable for potentially curative treatments at the time of diagnosis, such as surgical removal or chemo-ablation of small tumor nodules. α-Fetoprotein (AFP) has been used as a biomarker for diagnosis of HCC, but its sensitivity is low (25–65%) at the commonly used cutoff of 20 ng/mL, particularly in detection of early-stage HCC.[47] In addition, many patients with nonmalignant chronic liver disease have elevated AFP concentrations in serum, including 15–58% of patients with acute exacerbations of chronic hepatitis, and 11–47% with liver cirrhosis.[47] More reliable diagnostic tools are needed for early diagnosis of HCC. Some newer approaches are discussed below.

Glypican-3 (GPC3) is a heparan sulfate glycoprotein that is highly expressed in approximately 70% of HCC cases[48] but poorly expressed in preneoplastic lesions and in normal liver tissue.[49] GPC3 is considered a potential biomarker for HCC diagnosis.

Multiple studies, including preclinical investigations,[50] have suggested that GPC3 is a liver cancer-specific marker.[51] Recent work suggests that GPC3 has improved sensitivity as compared to AFP for detecting early stages HCCs.[52]

Dickkopf-1 (DKK1), a secretory antagonist of the canonical Wnt signaling pathway is overexpressed in HCC tissue but is not detectable in corresponding noncancerous liver tissue. DKK1 could complement measurements of AFP in the diagnosis of HCC, improve identification of patients with AFP-negative HCC, and distinguish HCC from nonmalignant chronic liver diseases.[50,53,54]

A plasma microRNA panel (plasma miR-122, miR-192, miR-21, miR-223, miR-26a, miR-27a, and miR-801) of potential circulating markers of HCC also demonstrated good diagnostic accuracy, especially for patients with early BCLC stages 0-A (i.e., up to three nodules, none larger than 3 cm) who can benefit from the optimal therapy.[55]

While the above assays might improve the odds of tumor detection and effective therapy at early stages of HCC emergence, there is no highly effective treatment for those with advanced HCC. This has motivated considerable effort on antiviral therapies with the hope of ablating active hepatitis and the progression to cirrhosis and HCC. Antiviral treatments with, for example, nucleoside/nucleotide inhibitors of HBV DNA synthesis or IFN-α, have been found to slow the progression to HCC. Older patients that have high circulating virus titers, over 10^5 per mL, are at higher short-term risk of HCC than patients with lower (<10^4 per mL) or undetectable virus titers[56,57] and are generally considered to have immunologically active disease. For reasons not entirely clear, antiviral treatment with IFN-α and/or nucleos(t)ide analogs can greatly decrease hepatic inflammation and improve liver function and, most importantly, reduce progression of cirrhosis and HCC risk. Antiviral therapy may also increase the survival of patients following surgical removal of tumors.[57–59]

A major question in patients with chronic hepatitis B is why only ~30% of males and ~10% of females develop HCC during their lifetime. Some efforts have been made to identify host genetic markers determining HCC risk on the assumption that patients that develop HCC have stable genetic or epigenetic traits that distinguish them from those who remain tumor free[60]; however, this work is still at early stages.

Worldwide, surgical resection is still the first-line treatment for HCC patients with well-preserved liver function, but the rate of postoperative recurrence within 5 years is as high as 70%. Some prognostic factors indicating postoperative recurrence of HCC can be detected in removed tumor tissues, adjacent liver tissues, and peripheral blood. In tumors, high ratios of neutrophil-to-CD8+ T cell and Treg-to-CD8+ T cell, high expression of pro-angiogenic factors such as hypoxia-inducible factor-1-α and cell growth/survival factors such as CD24 and activation of inflammatory signaling pathways such as Wnt/β-catenin, NF-κB, and STAT3 predict early recurrence. In peri-tumoral hepatic tissues, high HBV DNA, HBV mutations, high densities of macrophages, activated stellate and mast cells, high expression of macrophage colony-stimulating factor receptor and placental growth factor, Th1/Th2-like cytokine shift, inflammation-related signature, and activation of carcinogenesis-related pathways predict late recurrence. In preoperative peripheral blood, high HBV DNA titers, genotype, and BCP mutations, high neutrophil-to-lymphocyte ratio, and high concentrations of macrophage migration inhibitory factor and osteopontin predict poor prognosis.[61] As a chemotherapeutic agent, at least working in part by the targeted inhibition of the hyperactivated extracellular signal-regulated kinase (ERK) pathway which is associated with postoperative liver regeneration, sorafenib is the first systemic therapy to significantly prolong the survival of HCC patients with advanced-stage disease. Recently, it has been shown that use of sorafenib after surgical resection for early-stage HCC was a promising approach for preventing recurrence and improving postoperative outcomes. Thus, sorafenib is currently used as a standard treatment for patients with HCC in spite of its shortcoming in specificity.[62]

A crucial role of EGFR signaling in Kupffer cells or macrophages during inflammation-driven HCC formation has been reported.[63] EGFR is required in liver macrophages to transcriptionally induce interleukin-6, which triggers hepatocyte proliferation and HCC. The presence of EGFR-positive liver macrophages in HCC patients is associated with poor survival.[63] Whether this will become therapeutically useful is unclear.

Hepatitis C virus

HCV is the type species of the genus *Hepacivirus* of the Flaviviridae family. It is a small, enveloped virus with a single-stranded, positive-sense RNA genome of 9.6 kb. It circulates as a highly lipidated viral particle. There are seven major genotypes and many more subtypes of HCV.[64] HCV has a high rate of mutation *in vivo*, which facilitates viral persistence via generation of immune escape variants. So far, emergence of viral resistance to combination therapy with direct-acting antiviral agents, including sofosbuvir, a polymerase inhibitor, and either a drug targeting the viral protease or NS5A, does not seem to be a problem in curing HCV infections.

Once the virus enters the cell, the viral RNA genome is uncoated and translated within the cytoplasm into a single, long polypeptide of 3011 amino acids.[65] The cleavage of the HCV polypeptide, mediated by host and viral proteases, yields 10 viral proteins. These are subclassified as structural proteins (C, E1, E2) and nonstructural (NS) proteins (p7, NS2, NS3, NS4A, NS4B, NS5A, and NS5B). The structural proteins serve the assembly of progeny virions and comprise two envelope glycoproteins (E1 and E2) and a nucleocapsid protein (core protein).[65,66] Core protein is essential for virus particle assembly but has also been claimed to have several regulatory functions, including cellular transcription, virus-induced transformation, and signal transduction.[67] (The importance of these claims, as with those about HBx, is difficult to verify because of the many decades that typically elapse between infection and tumor emergence). The NS proteins are responsible for executing viral replication and propagation.[68,69] The HCV genome undergoes rapid mutation in a hypervariable region coding for the envelope proteins to escape immune surveillance, which has so far impeded vaccine development. Most HCV-infected subjects develop chronic infection and eventually liver cirrhosis.

In 2005, more than 185 million people were estimated to be HCV-specific antibody positive, representing 2.8% of the world population. There are marked differences in HCV prevalence among different countries and regional age and risk groups, ranging from 0.1% to 5%. The most affected regions are Central and East Asia and North Africa. In the United States, it was estimated that 3.9 million individuals (or 1.8% of the general population) are infected with HCV. China has been considered a relatively high endemic area for HCV infection in the past. The prevalence of anti-HCV was estimated to average 3.2% in the general population, according to a national epidemiological survey carried out in most regions of China in 1992, with blood or blood product transfusion as the major route of infection. Since 1993, mandatory screening for anti-HCV and other precautions to prevent blood-borne disease transmission have been implemented extensively. New cases of HCV infection have declined dramatically. As shown by a recent national survey in 2006, the prevalence of anti-HCV in China is now only 0.43%.[70]

HCV genotypes also display substantial differences worldwide.[1] HCV variants are classified into seven genotypes. HCV-1b is the commonest worldwide and more prevalent in patients with HCC than in those with cirrhosis and chronic hepatitis. In the United States, genotype 1a predominates, whereas the predominant genotype in Europe and China is 1b. In China, genotype 1b accounts for 68.4%, followed by 2a at 19.5%.[71] Interestingly, subtype 1b strains are more likely to be associated with transmission by blood transfusion and medical procedures, whereas subtype 6a strains are more likely to be linked to intravenous drug use (IDU) and sexual transmissions.[72] This genotypic difference in HCV between Western countries and China may be, to some extent, associated with each population's responsiveness to Peg-IFN-a and ribavirin (RBV) treatment,[73] which was the only treatment option until the recent development of direct-acting antivirals.[74]

Hepatitis C virus and hepatocellular carcinoma
As of 2015, it was estimated that there are ~70 million individuals chronically infected with HCV worldwide.[75] Only a minority of those infected spontaneously clear the virus; while about 55–85% develop chronic HCV infection, chronically infected individuals are at increased risk of developing cirrhosis and HCC.[76–78] The risk of liver cirrhosis is 15–30% within 20 years. Elevated HCV loads also significantly increase HCC risk, up to 17-fold.[79] The average time from HCV infection to the onset of cirrhosis is 13–25 years, and the time to onset of HCC is 17–32 years.[80] The annual incidence of HCC in HCV-infected subjects with cirrhosis is approximately 3–5%.[81] Successful clearance of HCV infection reduces overall liver-related mortality and HCC incidence.[82]

HCV is an RNA virus with an exclusively cytoplasmic life cycle. The mechanisms of HCV-induced hepatocarcinogenesis are unclear. Several have been proposed, including an oncogenic effect of HCV viral proteins, steatosis and insulin resistance, chronic inflammation and fibrosis, oxidative stress, and chromosomal instability. In experimental animal models, it has been reported that HCV-encoded proteins, core, E2, NS3, and NS5A, are directly involved in the tumorigenic process through interaction with a number of host factors and signaling pathways that affect cell survival, proliferation, migration, and transformation.[83–86] The HCV core protein is suggested to influence or interact with several molecules that play important roles in fatty acid transport and catabolism.[87–89] This makes sense if HCV-associated hepatic steatosis, with insulin resistance and oxidative stress, leads to chronic liver inflammation, apoptosis, and fibrogenesis. These mechanisms may be contributors to the development of liver cirrhosis and HCC in patients with chronic HCV.

Prevention and treatment
Since there is no vaccine for hepatitis C, the primary prevention of HCV infection mainly depends upon reducing the risk of exposure to the virus in higher-risk populations. Among HCV-infected persons, about 15–45% spontaneously clear the virus within 6 months without any treatment. When treatment is necessary, the best current option is therapy with direct-acting antivirals, which are effective against all the genotypes of HCV.[74] Direct-acting antiviral therapies also simplify HCV treatment by significantly decreasing monitoring requirements and by increasing cure rates.

Key references

The complete reference list can be found on Vital Source version of this title, see inside front cover.

1 Wang FS, Fan JG, Zhang Z, et al. The global burden of liver disease: the major impact of China. *Hepatology (Baltimore, MD)*. 2014;**60**(6). doi: 10.1002/hep.27406.
3 Manns MP, Buti M, Gane E, et al. Hepatitis C virus infection. *Nat Rev Dis Primers*. 2017;**3**:17006.
7 Orito E, Mizokami M, Ina Y, et al. Host-independent evolution and a genetic classification of the hepadnavirus family based on nucleotide sequences. *Proc Natl Acad Sci U S A*. 1989;**86**(18):7059–7062.
14 Zhang HW, Yin JH, Li YT, et al. Risk factors for acute hepatitis B and its progression to chronic hepatitis in Shanghai, China. *Gut*. 2008;**57**(12):1713–1720.
16 Chan HL, Tse CH, Mo F, et al. High viral load and hepatitis B virus subgenotype ce are associated with increased risk of hepatocellular carcinoma. *J Clin Oncol*. 2008;**26**(2):177–182.
17 Kamatani Y, Wattanapokayakit S, Ochi H, et al. A genome-wide association study identifies variants in the HLA-DP locus associated with chronic hepatitis B in Asians. *Nat Genet*. 2009;**41**(5):591–595.
18 Zhang Q, Yin J, Zhang Y, et al. HLA-DP polymorphisms affect the outcomes of chronic hepatitis B virus infections, possibly through interacting with viral mutations. *J Virol*. 2013;**87**(22):12176–12186.
23 Perz JF, Armstrong GL, Farrington LA, et al. The contributions of hepatitis B virus and hepatitis C virus infections to cirrhosis and primary liver cancer worldwide. *J Hepatol*. 2006;**45**(4):529–538.
26 Lee MH, Yang HI, Liu J, et al. Prediction models of long-term Cirrhosis and hepatocellular carcinoma risk in chronic hepatitis B patients: risk scores integrating host and virus profiles. *Hepatology (Baltimore, MD)*. 2013;**58**(2):546–554.
27 Yuen MF, Tanaka Y, Fong DY, et al. Independent risk factors and predictive score for the development of hepatocellular carcinoma in chronic hepatitis B. *J Hepatol*. 2009;**50**(1):80–88.
32 Li Z, Xie Z, Ni H, et al. Mother-to-child transmission of hepatitis B virus: evolution of hepatocellular carcinoma-related viral mutations in the post-immunization era. *J Clin Virol Off Publication Pan Am Soc Clin Virol*. 2014;**61**(1):47–54.
33 Xie J, Zhang Y, Zhang Q, et al. Interaction of signal transducer and activator of transcription 3 polymorphisms with hepatitis B virus mutations in hepatocellular carcinoma. *Hepatology (Baltimore, MD)*. 2013;**57**(6):2369–2377.
34 Zhang Q, Ji XW, Hou XM, et al. Effect of functional nuclear factor-kappaB genetic polymorphisms on hepatitis B virus persistence and their interactions with viral mutations on the risk of hepatocellular carcinoma. *Ann Oncol Off J Eur Soc Med Oncol*. 2014;**25**(12):2413–2419.
36 Mason WS, Gill US, Litwin S, et al. HBV DNA integration and clonal hepatocyte expansion in chronic hepatitis B patients considered immune tolerant. *Gastroenterology*. 2016;**151**(5):986–998.e4.
38 Sze KM, Ho DW, Chung CYT, et al. HBV-TERT promoter integration harnesses host ELF4 resulting in TERT gene transcription in hepatocellular carcinoma. *Hepatology (Baltimore, MD)*. 2020;**73**(1). doi: 10.1002/hep.31231.
39 Li W, Zeng X, Lee NP, et al. HIVID: an efficient method to detect HBV integration using low coverage sequencing. *Genomics*. 2013;**102**(4):338–344.
40 Zhao LH, Liu X, Yan HX, et al. Genomic and oncogenic preference of HBV integration in hepatocellular carcinoma. *Nat Commun*. 2016;**7**:12992.
41 Zhu M, Lu T, Jia Y, et al. Somatic mutations increase hepatic clonal fitness and regeneration in chronic liver disease. *Cell*. 2019;**177**(3):608–621.e12.
43 Berasain C, Perugorria MJ, Latasa MU, et al. The epidermal growth factor receptor: a link between inflammation and liver cancer. *Exp Biol Med (Maywood, NJ)*. 2009;**234**(7):713–725.
44 Wang C, Yang W, Yan HX, et al. Hepatitis B virus X (HBx) induces tumorigenicity of hepatic progenitor cells in 3,5-diethoxycarbonyl-1,4-dihydrocollidine-treated HBx transgenic mice. *Hepatology (Baltimore, Md)*. 2012;**55**(1):108–120.
45 Abdul F, Filleton F, Gerossier L, et al. Smc5/6 antagonism by HBx is an evolutionarily conserved function of hepatitis B virus infection in mammals. *J Virol*. 2018;**92**(16). doi: 10.1128/JVI.00769-18.
46 Sekiba K, Otsuka M, Ohno M, et al. Inhibition of HBV transcription from cccDNA with nitazoxanide by targeting the HBx-DDB1 interaction. *Cell Mol Gastroenterol Hepatol*. 2019;**7**(2):297–312.
48 Marrero JA, Lok AS. Newer markers for hepatocellular carcinoma. *Gastroenterology*. 2004;**127**(5 Suppl 1):S113–S119.
49 Shen Q, Fan J, Yang XR, et al. Serum DKK1 as a protein biomarker for the diagnosis of hepatocellular carcinoma: a large-scale, multicentre study. *Lancet Oncol*. 2012;**13**(8):817–826.
51 Zhou J, Yu L, Gao X, et al. Plasma microRNA panel to diagnose hepatitis B virus-related hepatocellular carcinoma. *J Clin Oncol*. 2011;**29**(36):4781–4788.
52 Liu S, Wang M, Zheng C, et al. Diagnostic value of serum glypican-3 alone and in combination with AFP as an aid in the diagnosis of liver cancer. *Clin Biochem*. 2020;**79**:54–60.

54 Inoue T, Tanaka Y. Novel biomarkers for the management of chronic hepatitis B. *Clin Mol Hepatol*. 2020;**26**(3). doi: 10.3350/cmh.2020.0032.

56 Chen CJ, Yang HI, Su J, et al. Risk of hepatocellular carcinoma across a biological gradient of serum hepatitis B virus DNA level. *JAMA*. 2006;**295**(1):65–73.

57 Cho JY, Paik YH, Sohn W, et al. Patients with chronic hepatitis B treated with oral antiviral therapy retain a higher risk for HCC compared with patients with inactive stage disease. *Gut*. 2014;**63**(12):1943–1950.

59 Yin J, Li N, Han Y, et al. Effect of antiviral treatment with nucleotide/nucleoside analogs on postoperative prognosis of hepatitis B virus-related hepatocellular carcinoma: a two-stage longitudinal clinical study. *J Clin Oncol Off J Am Soc Clin Oncol*. 2013;**31**(29). doi: 10.1200/JCO.2012.48.5896.

60 Lin X, Xiaoqin H, Jiayu C, et al. Long non-coding RNA miR143HG predicts good prognosis and inhibits tumor multiplication and metastasis by suppressing mitogen-activated protein kinase and Wnt signaling pathways in hepatocellular carcinoma. *Hepatol Res Off J Jpn Soc Hepatol*. 2019;**49**(8):902–918.

61 Chen L, Zhang Q, Chang W, et al. Viral and host inflammation-related factors that can predict the prognosis of hepatocellular carcinoma. *Eur J Cancer (Oxford, England: 1990)*. 2012;**48**(13):1977–1987.

63 Lanaya H, Natarajan A, Komposch K, et al. EGFR has a tumour-promoting role in liver macrophages during hepatocellular carcinoma formation. *Nat Cell Biol*. 2014;**16**(10):972–977.

66 Pawlotsky JM, Chevaliez S, McHutchison JG. The hepatitis C virus life cycle as a target for new antiviral therapies. *Gastroenterology*. 2007;**132**(5):1979–1998.

69 Gouttenoire J, Castet V, Montserret R, et al. Identification of a novel determinant for membrane association in hepatitis C virus nonstructural protein 4B. *J Virol*. 2009;**83**(12):6257–6268.

72 Fu Y, Wang Y, Xia W, et al. New trends of HCV infection in China revealed by genetic analysis of viral sequences determined from first-time volunteer blood donors. *J Viral Hepat*. 2011;**18**(1):42–52.

75 The Polaris Observatory HCV Collaborators. Global prevalence and genotype distribution of hepatitis C virus infection in 2015: a modelling study. *Lancet Gastroenterol Hepatol*. 2017;**2**(3):161–176.

85 Li XD, Sun L, Seth RB, et al. Hepatitis C virus protease NS3/4A cleaves mitochondrial antiviral signaling protein off the mitochondria to evade innate immunity. *Proc Natl Acad Sci U S A*. 2005;**102**(49):17717–17722.

87 Shintani Y, Fujie H, Miyoshi H, et al. Hepatitis C virus infection and diabetes: direct involvement of the virus in the development of insulin resistance. *Gastroenterology*. 2004;**126**(3):840–848.

88 Tsutsumi T, Suzuki T, Shimoike T, et al. Interaction of hepatitis C virus core protein with retinoid X receptor alpha modulates its transcriptional activity. *Hepatology (Baltimore, MD)*. 2002;**35**(4):937–946.

30 Parasites

Mervat El Azzouni, MD, PhD ∎ Charbel F. Matar, MD ∎ Radwa Galal, MD, MBBCH, PhD ∎ Elio Jabra, MD
∎ Ali Shamseddine, MD, FRCP, ESCO

> **Overview**
>
> Several parasites were investigated for a possible role in oncogenesis. Among the well-known parasitic infections, *Schistosoma haematobium* was proved to play an important role in developing urinary bladder cancer. Moreover, *Schistosoma japonicum* is classified as a colorectal carcinogen especially in the Far East. Other class of parasites, such as helminths *Clonorchis* and *Opisthorchis* are proved to induce hepatobiliary cancer. In Africa, a strong correlation between Ebstein-Barr virus infection and Burkitt lymphoma is present, with an evident enhancing role for *Plasmodium falciparum*. Chronic inflammation was incriminated to be the most accepted mechanism for parasite-induced cancer; however, the roles of certain carcinogens, oncogenes, DNA mutations, and others were all approved as mechanisms enhancing carcinogenesis in parasitic infections. Strikingly, despite the above-mentioned data, it seemed that certain parasites could modulate the host immune response in a manner that would lead to cancer regression or prevention. This is in the prospect of revaluation of the clinical importance of infectious agents; an issue that requires future concern.

Introduction—parasites

The prevalence of parasitic infection can indicate its intensity.[1] Hence, the question of the role of parasites in relation to neoplasms arise when an uncommon cancer becomes prevalent in area with high parasitic disease. In this respect, the two most intriguing examples are probably the relationships of schistosomiasis to bladder cancer (BC) and that of malaria to Burkitt lymphoma (BL). Classic references have been presented before (Table 1).

Schistosomiasis and cancer of the bladder

Bilharzia, or commonly known as schistosomiasis, is named after the German physician doctor Theodor Bilharz who first described it back in 1851 following an autopsy in Egypt.[2,3] It is a chronic entero-pathogenic disease caused by blood flukes of the genus Schistosoma. The first assumption for a possible link between cancer of the urinary bladder and *Schistosoma haematobium* infection was set by Goebel in 1905. This was followed by a confirmatory study done by Fergusson in 1911, who justified the association between urogenital schistosomiasis and primary bladder malignancy in 40 studied biopsy specimens.[4] By 1994, the International Agency of Research on Cancer (IARC) reported the parasite as group I carcinogen.[5,6] Schistosomiasis infection is highly associated with poverty and commonly seen in tropical rural areas. Bilharzial bladder cancer (BBC) can be a preventable malignancy once effective strategies, such as proper screening, treating, and eradicating, are implemented.[7]

Geographical distribution of schistosoma

The main schistosomal species that causes the most morbidity are the *S. haematobium, Schistosoma mansoni*, and *Schistosoma japonicum*. The estimated number of infected humans is over 250 million distributed in over 74 countries, with 201.5 million of them living in Africa.[8-10] Among the infected people, around 60% are symptomatic and 10% have severe illness.[11] According to the Global Burden of Disease Study 2016, an estimation of 1.9 million disability-adjusted life years (DALYs) has been attributed to the global burden of schistosomiasis.[12] Transmission of the parasite occurs by contact with fresh water that contains the intermediate host snails and that enter the venous blood system by percutaneous penetration.[13] Poor hygiene, lack of access to clean water, and the direct contact with infested water are the main causes of infection.[14]

The geographical distribution of Schistosoma is not the same for all type of species. *S. haematobium* is the most common type described in more than 54 countries spread over sub-Saharan and North Africa in addition to the Middle East[9] (Figure 1).

The clinical presentation of a schistosomal infection compromises three phases. The acute infection occurs predominantly in travelers to endemic areas and presents as a fever, myalgia, fatigue, abdominal pain, and possible hematuria—known as Katayama syndrome.[15] On the other hand, the established active and late chronic disease are almost exclusive to the habitants of the poor rural areas due to long-standing infections.[16]

Epidemiology of the bilharzial bladder cancer (BBC)

Recent morbidity and mortality rates

Urinary BC represents a global health problem. Its frequency changes from region to another depending on multiple risk factors. Currently, BC ranks the seventh most common malignancy in men and is three times more common than in women.[17] The main risk factors that contribute to BC onset in developed countries are smoking and occupational chemical exposure.[18] However, in low and middle-income countries (LMIC) such in Africa, the main factor is chronic irritation mostly due to *S. haematobium*.[19]

Histopathological type

Morphologically, we have two main histopathological types of BC. The most common one is transitional cell carcinoma (TCC). It occurs for around 90% of the cases and is predominant in

---

Holland-Frei Cancer Medicine, Tenth Edition. Edited by Robert C. Bast, John C. Byrd, Carlo M. Croce, Ernest Hawk, Fadlo R. Khuri, Raphael E. Pollock, Apostolia M. Tsimberidou, Christopher G. Willett, and Cheryl L. Willman.
© 2023 John Wiley & Sons, Inc. Published 2023 by John Wiley & Sons, Inc.

Table 1 Table representing the different types of parasite species and geographical distribution of schistosomiasis.

Location	Species	Geographical distribution
Intestinal schistosomiasis	*Schistosoma mansoni*	Africa, the Middle East, the Caribbean, Brazil, Venezuela, and Suriname
	Schistosoma japonicum	China, Indonesia, the Philippines
	Schistosoma mekongi	Several districts of Cambodia and the Lao People's Democratic Republic
	Schistosoma guineensis and related *S. intercalatum*	Rain forest areas of central Africa
Urogenital schistosomiasis	*Schistosoma haematobium*	Africa, the Middle East, Corsica (France)

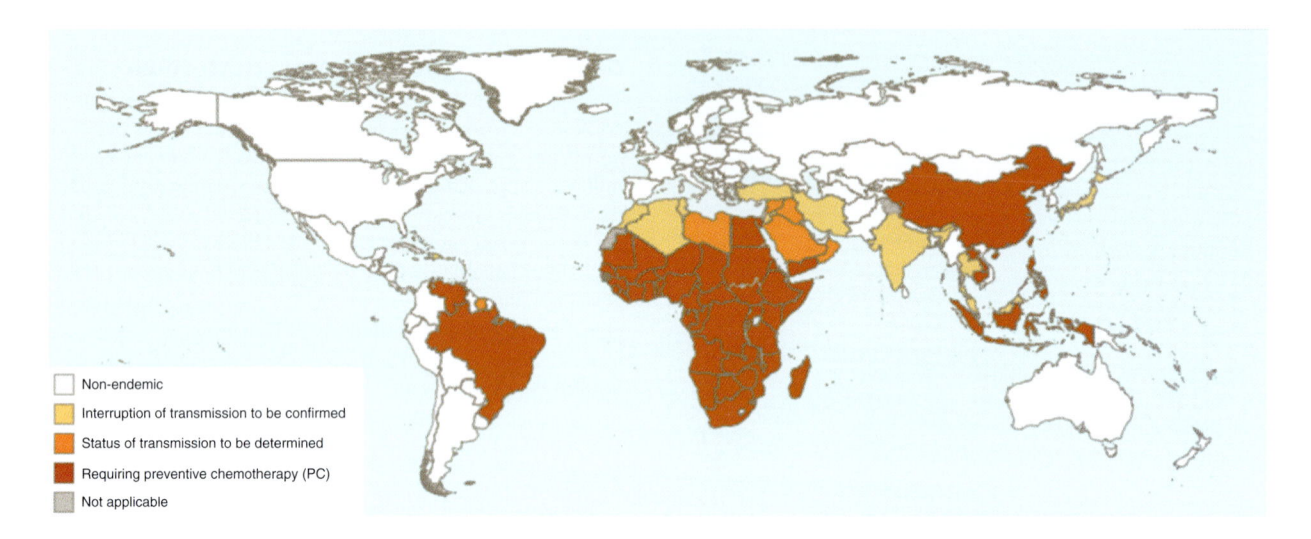

Figure 1 WHO map describing the distribution of Schistosomiasis around the world. Source: http://apps.who.int/neglected_diseases/ntddata/sch/sch.html

high-income countries.[17,20] This latter is witnessing a steady decrease in its rate of morbidity and mortality due to the controls on cigarette smoking. In Africa, squamous cell carcinoma (SCC) is more prevalent specifically in schistosoma endemic areas, which makes it widespread among the fellaheen of Egypt and the Africans of Mozambique, Zimbabwe, and Zambia.[21] However, due to the increased urbanization and industrialization, which is modifying the risk factors in developing countries, there is a noticeable shift toward the TCC subtype.[17]

In Egypt, starting 1960s, the rate of *S. haematobium* infection was gradually replaced by *S. mansoni* due to the construction of the High Dam which caused changes in water flow with a direct impact on the intermediate snail host.[22] Moreover, effective campaigns on eradication and prophylaxis since 1977 led to the decrease in belharizial urinary infections.[23] Earlier reports in Egypt showed that BC rate was around 27% of all cancers in the mid-1970s.[24] In the early 2000s, the rate dropped to 18% and more recently to 13%.[25]

Strikingly, despite the decrease in BBC, the prevalence of TCC type of BC is growing due to the increase in cigarette smoking.[26] This caused BC to remain on the top list of the most common cancer among males in Egypt. This is demonstrated by the shift in the incidence of SCC in Egypt from 78% in the 1980s to 27% in 2005 with a shift to TCC.[27]

Salem et al., conducted a retrospective study on all BC cases in one of the main hospitals in Cairo from 2001 to 2010. The authors compared the cases diagnosed from 2001 until 2005 (group 1) to 2005 until 2010 (group 2) and discovered a decrease from 73% to 25% in the proportion of SCC and an increase from 20% to 60% in TCC. Additionally, the proportion of smokers in group 2, either active smoking or second-hand smoking, was reported to be almost three times that of group 1.[25] Climate changes in Egypt and the rise in temperatures (exceeding 45 °C) along with the increased number of hot days over the year are effecting the schistosomal lifecycle and thus BBC rates.[28] The abundance of schistosomiasis is correlated with the presence of snails, the intermediate hosts of the parasite. Snail populations are affected by seasons, water temperature, and water flow. In Egypt, the construction of new dams, such as the Aswan Dams, is affecting the snail populations, causing a visible increase in numbers. This, in turn, is leading to a wider spread of schistosomiasis in the country.[29]

In developed countries, where bilharzial infection is uncommon, the incidence of BC peaks at the sixth or seventh decade of life[30]; while the mean age of BBC at presentation is 46 years which makes it 10–20 years earlier than that of nonbilharzial BC.[31] The ratio of BBC in males compared to females is 2.2 : 1 in nonendemic areas, with an increased rate of 5 : 1 in countries with infection.[32,33] This higher incidence in males versus females can be explained by the concept of prolonged exposure to contaminated water. In Egypt, most of the men in rural areas work in agriculture, which largely depends on irrigation through canals. These drainage canals create a favorable environment for the snail intermediate host to develop, rendering Egyptian farmers at a continuous risk of reinfection throughout the year.[34]

Diagnosis

The association of BC with schistosomal infection is largely based on observational studies and case series. No prospective study comparing the incidence of BC in infected versus uninfected persons is available due to its unfeasibility.[35] No clear diagnostic criteria exist for bilharzial infection. Detection of schistosomal eggs in urine has low sensitivity and the absence of ova does not exclude a diagnosis of schistosomiasis. In advanced cases, severe bilharzial fibrosis and scar tissue of the inner mucosal bladder wall prevent ova from shedding in urine.[36] In this situation, anamnestic information such as exposure to contaminated water, living in endemic area, and working in agriculture should raise suspicion of infection in case of negative urine tests. In such cases, radiological imaging or cystoscopy may be helpful in detecting tissue scarring and confirm infection.[26,35] Thus, by expanding the criteria for diagnosis of bilharzial bladder, the epidemiological rates of BBC are expected to be more representative.

Late chronic infection—urogenital schistosomiasis

In most patients who are chronically exposed to bilharzial infection, late chronic infection will establish. Interaction between the Schistosoma and the host's immune system will lead to multiple immune responses.[37] Immunomodulation of the human host immune system during schistosomal infection will cause a switch from a T helper cell type 1 (Th1) response during the early stages of infection to a Th2 response following the granuloma formation.[38]

S. haematobium worms infiltrate the pelvic venous plexus resulting in various symptoms.[39] The eggs secreted by the schistosome actively produce antigenic glycoproteins that facilitate the passage of the eggs from the venous system to the urinary system.[40] These eggs will deposit in the bladder epithelial wall and genital organs. Both adult and egg stage parasites secrete molecules, inducing changes in the host microenvironment that may be pro-carcinogenic. In fact, the presence of eggs antigen in the urothelial wall will cause intense inflammatory reaction along with the aggregation of immune cells forming granulomas.[41] The presence of granulomas will activate endothelial cells and increase vascularization, by promoting angiogenesis and upregulation of the vascular endothelial growth factor (VEGF) suggesting its role as a mediator to carcinogenic formation.[42] Eventually, chronic infection will lead to immunological downregulation and replacement of granulomas by fibrotic tissue. Due to the chronic irritation and inflammation, the bladder wall will undergo sloughing, ulceration, bleeding, and thickening—facilitating the formation of pseudo-polyps and masses.[43]

Carcinogenic mechanism

Following an infection with *S. haematobium*, the host bladder undergoes different levels of adaptation and alteration not only at the morphological level but also at the molecular level, which in turn might link to the carcinogenic mechanism. Chronic inflammation and mucosal damage will enable bacterial overgrowth and recurrent urinary tract infection with liberation of N-nitroso compounds.[44] Immune cells such as macrophages, once activated will generate carcinogenic N-nitrosamines and reactive oxygen radicals.[45] Urinary excretion of nitrite increases in individuals with *S. haematobium* infection.[44] When compared to nonbilharzial urinary tract infections, patients with Schistosomal infection will have three times higher concentration of Nitrate in their urine.[45,46]

As with modulation of transcript expression, epigenetic changes in the host genome may also take part in schistosomal BC. At the molecular level, N-nitroso compounds are implicated in tumorigenic alkylation of specific bases and deoxyribonucleic acid (DNA) sequences, along with an increase in their methylation.[47–49] This leads to mutations in oncogenes, tumor suppressor genes, and genes for cell cycle control.[7] Molecular events associated with BBC include the activation of H-ras gene,[50] inactivation of p53, and inactivation of retinoblastoma (Rb) gene.[51]

Alteration of the function of specific genes involved in the control of cell regulation and death, such as the *p53* gene, represents the backbone of cancer development.[52] Any alteration or mutation that leads to inactivation of p53 will contribute to neoplastic changes.

The association between bilharzial infection and alteration of *p53* genes in urothelial cells reinforces the notion that the infection downregulates cell apoptotic pathways and contributes to alteration in bladder cells leading to cancer development. Hence, it is obvious that urogenital schistosomiasis leads to increased expression of *p53* gene that leads to cancer development, and the release of catechol estrogens with the eventual release of reactive oxygen species (ROS) compounds and the formation of DNA adducts, consequently; DNA damage and cancer development.[53,54]

It was detected that overrepresentation of the protein encoded by the *MDM2* gene found in the majority of the studied cases, may account for the frequent inactivation of the gene coding for p53 control pathway observed in BBC, thereby underlining the accumulation of DNA damage and the aggressive clinical course of BBC.[55]

Role of microbiome

More recently, dysbiosis in the urine microbiome during urogenital schistosomiasis has been proposed to be a risk factor for BC following schistosomal infection. Microbiomes represent a group of bacteria that inhabit the body and do not cause disease, but their presence or absence influences organs function. Newly published data reveal that patients with bladder pathologies due to urogenital schistosomiasis share some unique microbial species when compared to other BC.[56] Adebayo et al.[56] reported that several urinary taxa such as Fusobacterium, Sphingobacterium, and Enterococcus have been found in higher concentration, which distinguished urogenital schistosomiasis-induced bladder pathologies. This raises the question on the role of microbiome in mediating the inflammation and in contributing to the recurrent infections seen in bilharziasis. These findings demonstrate another possible mechanism of carcinogenic effect related to *S. haematobium* infection. Therefore, the factor that needs to be determined next is whether this unique urinary microbiome promotes progression of BC or whether the BBC affects the composition of bladder microorganisms.[57]

Human papilloma virus

The possibility of association between human papilloma virus (HPV) and BBC remained open for long. A study done by Khaled et al., 2001 showed that the virus was present in 23 out of 40 cases of BBC.[58] Recently, the use of Mass ARRAY technology in one study showed all 27 BBC blood tested samples to be associated with HPV-16 DNA.[59]

Metabolic observations during schistosomiasis

It is thought that tryptophan metabolism plays a role in the development of bladder neoplasm. In reality, individuals with bilharzial cancer metabolize tryptophan in a manner reminiscent of the pattern seen in many patients with spontaneous BC, with increased excretion of 3-hydroxyanthranilic acid, anthranilic acid, 5-hydroxyindoleacetic acid, and kynurenine.[60] The significance of tryptophan metabolism in the production of BBC was first suggested back in 1950. Following that, many early studies have investigated the disorder of tryptophan metabolism and the role of the intermediate carcinogenic metabolites encountered in bilharzial cases. The results draw attention to the importance of parasitic infection in inducing disordered tryptophan metabolism.[60] Tryptophan is an essential aromatic amino acid and is present in all kinds of food especially milk, cheese, yogurt, eggs, chicken, turkey, pork, salmon, potatoes, and bananas.[60]

The urinary excretion of free 3-hydroxykynurenine, 3-hydroxyanthranilic acid, and 2-amino-3-hydroxyacetophenone seen in some patients with BC, have been documented to be related to the carcinogenic metabolites of β-naphthylamine and are themselves carcinogenic to experimental mice.[34] A marked increase by four to eightfolds from baseline were seen in the schistosomal BC.[61]

Our understanding of the role played by *Schistosoma* infection in disturbed tryptophan metabolism is complicated by geographic variations of dietary habits. Serotonin metabolites such as 5-hydroxyindoleacetic acid, which are excreted in large amounts by plantain-eating Africans, are low in Africans who are on other diets.[62] Similar differences attributable to dietary habits have been found between bilharzial patients in Mozambique and in South Africa. Egyptian peasants are not plantain eaters but subsist mostly on beans, lentils, and rice. Those with bilharzial cancer metabolize tryptophan in a manner reminiscent of the pattern seen in many patients with spontaneous BC, with increased excretion of 3-hydroxyanthranilic acid, anthranilic acid, 5-hydroxyindoleacetic acid, and kynurenine. The excretion of these metabolites is enhanced by a loading dose of tryptophan.[34] Therefore, schistosomiasis should not be considered the only causal factor in the associated excretion of abnormal tryptophan metabolites because, with or without cancer, urinary schistosomiasis is almost universally accompanied by urinary tract infection. The bacterial flora may, thus, contribute to a spurious accumulation of some metabolites of tryptophan. Moreover, untreated pellagra is associated with increased urinary excretion of anthranilic acid, acetylkynurenine, and 5-hydroxyindoleacetic acid.[34]

It seems likely that the carcinogen dose is a determining factor in the aggressiveness of a bladder tumor, and that a low-grade carcinoma can be converted into a high-grade one if exposed continuously to low doses of *N*-nitroso compounds. This would explain, at least in part, the overrepresentation of deeply invasive SCC in the bilharzial urinary bladder.[63] The significant excess of transitions at CpG dinucleotides in the *p53* gene in BBC has been attributed to the endogenous production of nitric oxide provoked by the inflammatory response to schistosomal ova.[63]

Pathology of benign and paraneoplastic schistosomal bladder lesions

Cancer progression
Bladder epithelial cells require the acquisition of specific characteristics before being able to progress into malignant cells and invade surrounding structures. Such properties include the ability of growing and proliferating without control. During chronic schistosomal infection, several cytogenetic changes take place causing a reduction in cell apoptosis and thus enhancing oncogenesis.[64]

In 2009, Botelho et al. demonstrated that cells exposed to *S. haematobium* total antigen (worm extract) were found to divide faster than those not exposed to the antigen, and died much less. This was explained by increased level of Bcl-2,[65] which is one gene that can contribute to oncogenesis by suppressing apoptosis.[7] The overexpression of the Bcl-2 gene in BBC patients was found to be up-regulated in SCC but not TCC.[66]

In addition to Bcl-2, other proteins related to apoptosis were also identified, such as Bcl-x, Bax and Bak, p53, E-cadherin, epidermal growth factor receptor (EGFR) and cerbB-2, OCNA, and Ki-67. These proteins correlated with the clinical outcome of BBC patients and with tumor progression.[67]

During schistosomal infection, urinary bladder wall undergoes various metaplastic, proliferative, and atypical changes.[68] These changes are related to the intense delayed-sensitivity reaction, which is elicited by viable *Schistosoma* eggs plugging the vesical venules leading to tubercules, nodules, or polyps. Thus, BBC arises on top of epithelial metaplasia. In bilharzial bladder, two atypical finds can be identified in infected bladders, dysplasia, and carcinoma *in situ*. Dysplasia is a low-grade neoplasia known as preneoplastic epithelial lesion. In the presence of chronic inflammation, dysplasia can progress into more invasive features in around 15% of cases.[69] On the other hand, carcinoma *in situ* is a more aggressive and more advanced stage and can become invasive in around 35% of cases.[70]

It is important to distinguish simple hyperplasia of the urothelium from atypical lesions. In bilharzial cystitis, the papilloma is essentially a granuloma and not a precancerous lesion. With recurrent inflammation and fibrosis, some transitional epithelial cells become sequestered in the vesical submucosa and acquire a globular arrangement around a central cavity. When they open into the bladder cavity, the cystic formations become pseudoglandular. These structures, as part of cystitis glandularis, are at times precancerous; an adenocarcinoma may arise from the columnar epithelium, into which their lining has differentiated. In patients with schistosomiasis, squamous metaplasia is frequently encountered because it is a common concomitant of chronic inflammation. This type of metaplasia is a nearly consistent precursor of BC, and for this reason, leukoplakia acquires clinical importance as a precancerous condition.[34]

Site of origin
The tumor usually appears as a single, bulky, large nodular mass. In the majority of cases, the gross appearance is nodular fungating type and less commonly the ulcerative types. BBC is histopathologically distinct from BC in western countries. In patients in Western countries, BC frequently arises in the trigone; in patients in Egypt, it usually develops in areas remote from the ureters, mostly in the anterior and posterior bladder walls. This peculiarity tends to strengthen its association with schistosomal infection because the scanty or altogether absent submucosal tissue of the trigone discourages significant deposition of ova.[34]

Histologic classification
Significant variation in the occurrence of the pathological types of schistosomiases associated bladder tumors exists depending on the region. In schistosomal endemic areas of Africa such as rural areas, the prevalence of SCC is high compared to TCC.[71,72] In Egypt, the majority of BC cases are SCC and are related to schistosomal infection. This is similar to other African countries, such as Sudan, Kenya, Uganda, Nigeria, and Senegal.[73–75]

However, over the past decades, some changes have occurred. Comparing the periods 1962 to 1967 and 1987 to 1992, there was a decrease in the incidence of nodular tumors (83.4–58.7%) and of SCC (65.8–54.0%) but an increase in the incidence of papillary tumors (4.3–34.8%) and TCC (31.0–42.0%).[76] Similar results were proved by comparing the periods 2001–2005 and 2006–2010 as was fore-mentioned.[25]

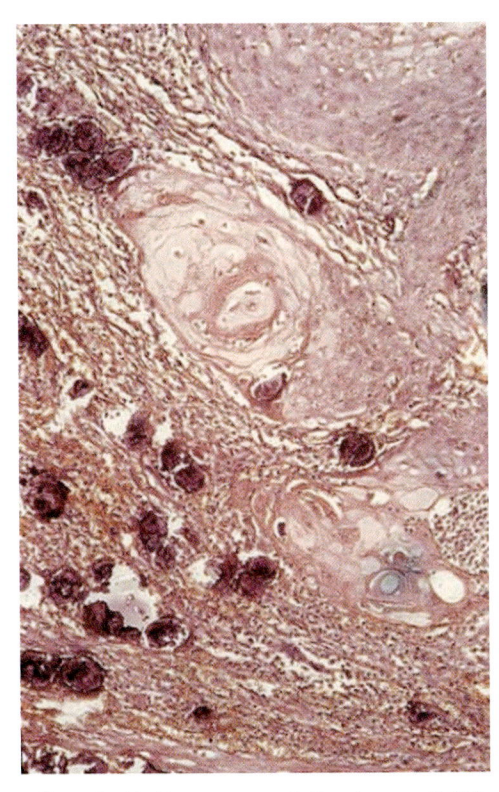

Figure 2 Bilharzial bladder cancer. Infiltrating, well-differentiated squamous cell carcinoma with adjacent calcified S. hematobium eggs (H&E × 100). Source: Courtesy of Drs M.R. Mahran and M. El-Baz, Mansoura University, Egypt.

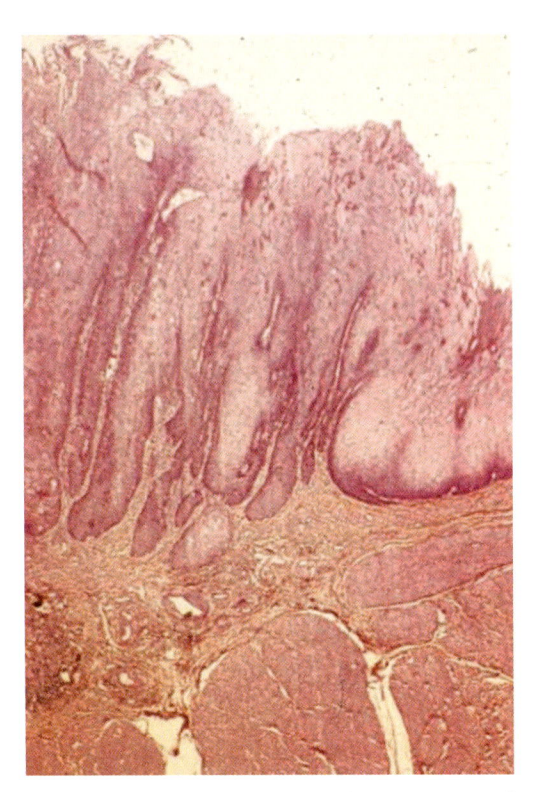

Figure 3 Verrucous carcinoma (noninvasive) of bladder with superficial filamentous elongated surface projections (H&E × 40). Source: Courtesy of Drs M.R. Mahran and M. El-Baz, Mansoura University, Egypt.

The extent of Schistosoma infection apparently plays a significant role in the induction of different types of carcinoma, since SCC is usually associated with moderate and/or high worm burdens whereas TCC occurs more commonly in areas associated with lower degrees of infection[77] (Figure 2). Thus, within the same country, SCC of the bladder is markedly overrepresented only in areas where schistosomiasis is highly endemic.[78,79] Adenocarcinoma of the bilharzial bladder is particularly aggressive: This may be explained by its proneness to develop gross chromosomal aberrations combined with high cell proliferation.[80] Another rare, though distinct, variant of squamous cell cancer is verrucous carcinoma of the bilharzial bladder (Figure 3). Despite reports to the contrary, a large proportion develop into invasive SCC, with which they share the same adverse prognosis.[81]

Experimental data for BBC
In a number of nonhuman primates, infection with S. haematobium resulted in epithelial proliferation, squamous metaplasia, and TCC of the urinary bladder.[82] The American opossum has also been found experimentally suitable for infection with S. haematobium.[83] These early experimental observations were important because eggs of S. haematobium, lyophilized worms, and urine from bilharzia patients have not been found to be carcinogenic to mice.[84,85] Noninvasive papillary and nodular TCC of the urinary bladder were observed in a talapoin monkey (Cercopithecus talapoin), a capuchin monkey (Cebus appella), gibbons (Hylobates lar), and opossums (Didelphys marsupialis),[82,83,86] when infected with S. haematobium. These types of carcinoma were morphologically similar to those observed in human bladders,[87] and such observations suggest that there is an association between S. haematobium and BC.

Schistosomiasis and cancer of other sites
According to accepted international criteria, infection with S. haematobium is carcinogenic to humans (group 1); infection with S. mansoni is not classifiable as to its carcinogenicity to humans (group 3); infection with S. japonicum is possibly carcinogenic to humans (group 2B).[88]

Large intestine
After thorough observation and research, scientists in Asia were able to draw out conclusions regarding the correlation between S. japonicum infestation in the intestine and its contribution to colorectal cancer (CRC). The latter is endemic in China and was classified as a probable human carcinogen by the IARC (Class 2B).[89] S. japonicum is known to lay numerous eggs known as "oviposition" (2000/day/pair) compared to S. mansoni species that lay way less. The number of eggs laid per species is directly associated with its pathogenicity, marking S. japonicum as the most problematic among all schistosome infections.[90]

The epidemiologic link between Schistosomiasis japonica endemicity and the dispersal of CRC was highlighted in Eastern China, providing a strong geographical association between the two. S. japonicum infestations in that region have been shown to increase CRC incidence and mortality.[91] In Shanghai, patients with intestinal schistosomiasis and cancer of the large intestine are, on average, 6 years younger than patients with spontaneous intestinal cancer.[92,93] Furthermore, the male to female ratio of schistosomal CRC is consistently higher than in nonschistosomal cancer.[93] The reasons behind this noticeable difference in the sex ratio could be the occupational (agricultural) exposure to the parasite and also might be related to the influence of male hormones on the pathogenicity of schistosomes.[94]

A recent study by Madbouly et al. has shown that *S. mansoni*-associated CRC and colitis-induced carcinoma are similar in their individual pathological findings. These include high percentage of multicentric tumors and mucinous adenocarcinoma, with strong predilection to the rectum and the tendency of the tumor to present at an advanced stage with a high risk of malignant lymph node invasion.[93] A case of a 35-year-old man with chronic schistosomiasis showed that there were more *S. mansoni* ova in the ulcerated cancerous tumor and the colonic submucosa compared to normal tissue.[95]

S. mansoni-associated CRC has been highly linked to microsatellite instability, a sign of defective DNA repair. Microsatellite instability high (MSI-H) tumor frequency in Western countries was 13% when compared to the 37% of those in Egypt ($p = 0.002$). This causes DNA replication errors which affect target genes such as transforming growth factor (TGF)bRII and insulin-like growth factor (IGF)2R. Once these target genes are altered, the normal colonocyte is rendered incapable of normal homeostasis, leading to malignant growth.[96,97] The expression of hMLH1 and hMSH2 protein, part of the mismatch repair (MMR) protein, in CRC was lower in patients with schistosomiasis when compared to sporadic forms. This could suggest that deletion of these *MMR* genes maybe trigger schistosomiasis-associated CRC.[93,98] Zalata et al., developed a more comprehensive study of the expression pattern of *p53*, Bcl-2, and *C-Myc* in 75 CRC cases, 24 of these had pathological evidence of *S. mansoni* infection. Although they did not find a significant association between parasitism and *p53* and *C-Myc* expression, the results showed that *S. mansoni*-associated colorectal tumors are characterized by Bcl-2 overexpression and less apoptotic activity than ordinary colorectal tumors.[99] This supports the contention that evasion of apoptosis through change in the expression of Bcl-2 may be an alternative molecular pathway through which genotoxic agents can induce carcinogenesis in intestinal schistosomiasis.[95]

Inflammatory cells triggered by schistosomiasis release many genotoxic intermediaries, such as cytokines, reactive oxygen, and nitrogen. These intermediaries lead to the dysregulation of protooncogenes and tumor suppressor genes, promoting tumorigenesis.[100,101] It had been shown that after an infection with *S. mansoni*, cytokines involved in eosinophilia and immunoglobulin E (IgE) secretion, along with T-helper 2 cells, are stimulated. On the other hand, after studying mice postinfected with *S. mansoni*, it was shown that cytokines of T-helper 1 cells and cytotoxic CD8+ T-cells were markedly decreased.[102]

Liver and the gallbladder
A study of liver and colon cancers and their association with a previous diagnosis of schistosomiasis was performed in rural Sichuan, China. Previous schistosomal infection was found to be significantly associated with both liver cancer (odds ratio = 3.7; 95% confidence interval = 1.0–13) and colon cancer (odds ratio = 3.3; 95% confidence interval = 1.8–6.1). The results indicate a fraction of the disease attributable to schistosomiasis (24% for colon cancer, and 27% for liver cancer among hepatitis-negative population).[103] In a study conducted by Toda et al., it was shown that there is no definite and direct relation between schistosomes and liver cancer. Schistosomiasis, in the presence of HBV and HCV infections, could be a possible cofactor for liver damage and failure.[104] The co-infection of schistosoma with HBV extends the carriage state and increases morbidity and liver decompensation. Similarly, co-infection with HCV decreases the capability of the virus to self-resolve, leading to quick liver fibrosis.[105] Previous studies showed that people with chronic schistosomiasis or liver fluke infection have an 8–10% risk of developing cholangiocarcinoma (CCA), hence physicians should check for an underlying parasitic contamination once the patient has been diagnosed with CCA.[106]

c-Jun and STAT3 are protooncogenes, the former is a cancer initiator and apoptosis inhibitor while the latter is a signal transducer and activator of transcription, which is a marker for poor prognosis of HCC.[104,107,108] Experimental data and studies on liver biopsies from humans infected with *S. mansoni* showed that c-Jun and STAT3 were activated in hepatocytes around trapped eggs or when challenged with schistosomal surface egg antigen (SEA).[109]

Lymphoma
There is no clear association between schistosomiasis and lymphoma, making it more infrequent when compared to other cancers.[110] In a Nigerian series, lymphoreticular tumors were overrepresented in infected individuals (16%) as compared with uninfected ones.[111] The occurrence of an isolated, primary T-cell lymphoma of the bladder may represent an unusual immune response to schistosomiasis.[112] In a group of 254 individuals with *S. mansoni*, six developed a documented lymphoma.[113]

Case reports had pointed out two types of lymphomas in patients with chronic hepatosplenic or intestinal schistosomiasis: histiocytic lymphoma[114] and large B cell lymphoma.[115] In another article reporting a case of malignant lymphoma coexisting with *S. japonica*, lymphoma cells thrived around egg emboli in Glisson's capsule and portal vein branches, suggesting a strong relationship between the infection and the lymphoma.[116] A case report on a 19-year-old Nigerian female presenting with a week-long history of abdominal swelling and vomiting showed a colonic tumor. After histopathological examination of that tumor, schistosomal ova and the adult worm in-copula were discovered. Immunohistochemistry showed that the mass was not just a granuloma, but a diffuse B-lymphocyte non-Hodgkins lymphocytic lymphoma. Adisa et al.,[110] after conducting this case report, emphasize that people with chronic infections should be screened for tumors, especially in prone countries where infections, such as schistosomiasis, are common.

Other organs
Immunohistochemical studies confirmed invasive SCC of the prostate in three prostatic schistosomiasis patients coming from a population where prostatic cancer is uncommon.[116] Mazigo et al.[117] reported three cases of prostatic adenocarcinoma in people with chronic schistosomiasis in Tanzania, but the relationship between the parasite and the cancer remains vague and unclear.

In another case of a 34-year-old woman with cervical schistosomiasis, a cervical pap smear showed inflammatory changes and dysplasia of the transitional zone. *S. haematobium* eggs were found inside the chorion, surrounded by granulomatous inflammation without evidence of malignancy. After proper treatment with praziquantel, a follow-up smear showed spectacular response and the previous cytologic changes normalized. This points out that by treating the underlying schistosomal infection, transformation from cervical dysplasia to malignancy can be prevented.[118] Moubayed and others stated that in all studied cases of cervical cancer in patients presenting with schistosomiasis, the lesions were also co-infected with HPV.[119] This leaves the parallelism between schistosomes and cervical cancer uncertain.

On the other hand, the Egyptian cases indicate no relationship between bilharziasis and cancer of the lungs, pancreas, prostate, seminal vesicles, urethra, vulva, vagina, cervix uteri, body of the uterus, or ovaries.[21] Physicians should be cautious in countries which are endemic for schistosomal infections, because severe and progressive infections could be clinically misguided and diagnosed as cancer in the large intestine,[120] or the cervix.[121]

Liver fluke

Liver and pancreas

Three species of flukes, *Clonorchis sinensis*, *Opisthorchis viverrini*, and *Opisthorchis felineus*, share their life cycles, pathology, and infectivity in the human body, specifically the biliary tract. Two things that make these flukes different are their geographical dispersal and morphology. Liver flukes are highly endemic to Asia and Eastern Europe, along with some minor distribution of infected people worldwide.[122] In total, it is estimated that there are around 35 million infected people with *C. sinensis* globally, having 15 million of them residing in China.[123] Out of all 35 million, only around 1.5–2 million people show symptoms or complications secondary to the infection.[124] On another note, *O. viverrini*, is more common in Thailand.[122] CCA is a cancer of the bile ducts that is considered as the most severe complication of liver fluke infection. This made *C. sinensis* and *O. viverrini* infections classified as "carcinogenic to humans" by the IARC in 2009.[125,126] In a hospital-based series in Thailand, the ratio of hepatocellular carcinoma to CCA was 8 : 1 in patients without opisthorchiasis, but the ratio was upturned in patients who were infected with the parasite. This targets the hypothesis that *Opisthorchis* is associated with CCA, along with the *C. sinensis*, which is studied to have more parallelism with the cancer now.[122]

Moreover, intraductal papillary neoplasm of the bile duct is known to be a premalignant condition and it is often associated with mucin overproduction. Chronic inflammatory process that leads to mucin over-production and subsequently intraductal papillary neoplasm progressing to CCA is the key factor for distomiasis-related carcinogenesis. In *O. viverrini*, this underlies genetic alterations involving mainly the tumor suppressor genes; *Tp*53 and *SMAD*4.[127] The chronic inflammatory process associating distomiasis leads to downregulation of retinoblastoma *RB1* gene expression and Cyclin-dependent kinase inhibitor-4 P16^{INK4}, with upregulation of cyclin D1 and CDK4, P13/AKT, and Wnt/β-catenin signaling pathways involved in tumorigenesis.[128] The upregulation of 14-3-3 eta protein which regulates cell cycle signaling and tumor suppressor genes was demonstrated in *O. viverrini*-associated CCA.[129,130] Other parasite-derived molecules contribute to the carcinogenic progression as dimethyl nitrosamine,[131] granulin which promotes proliferation, and the antiapoptotic proteins: thioredoxin and thioredoxin peroxidase.[132,133] However, parasite-derived oxysterols are considered one of the most potentially carcinogenic molecules that can form host DNA adducts with subsequent mutations.[134,135] Another hypothesis for the development of *O. viverrini*-derived CCA is the chronic inflammatory process induced by exotic microbiota associating distomiasis.[136]

There have been a few recent articles revealing that the disease was related with *C. sinensis* infection. Suh et al. reported that five of 16 (31%) of intraductal papillary tumors of the bile duct were associated with *C. sinensis* infection.[137] Jang et al.[138] reported that when CCA was associated with *C. sinensis* infection, intraductal papillary neoplasm was much more common than the usual adenocarcinoma.

Liver flukes enter the human body through eating raw or undercooked freshwater fish. The parasites travel to the duodenum, encyst, then travel through the bile ducts into the gallbladder. Once in the gallbladder, these parasites cause hyperplasia of the biliary epithelial cells and fibrosis. In an experiment done on mice, a carcinogen, dimethylnitrosamine, was given to all specimens for 10 weeks. After 10 weeks, it was shown that all mice previously infected with *Opisthorchis* developed mucin-secreting CCA, whereas the noninfected mice failed to develop tumors.[139,140]

Infection with either *O. viverrini* or *C. sinensis* is carcinogenic to humans (group 1); infection with *O. felineus* is not classifiable as to its carcinogenicity to humans (group 3).[125,126]

There has been a recent study performed on Syrian hamsters infected with the liver fluke *O. viverrini* to observe if there are any changes in the microbiome. Microbial analyses revealed that the fluke-infected hamsters did in fact show changes: Lachnospiraceae, Ruminococcaceae, and Lactobacillaceae were increased, while Porphyromonadaceae, Erysipelotrichaceae, and Eubacteriaceae were decreased when compared to controls ($p \leq 0.05$). Opisthorchiasis is distinguished from other fluke infections because of its noticeably elevated interleukin 6 (IL-6) immune response in the biliary system, leading to periductal fibrosis, a common precursor of CCA. This draws a leading hypothesis that liver flukes and their microbiota may parallelly drive this specific immune response.[141]

Malaria

After noting the number of BL cases in common malarial areas, it had been suggested to study the parallelism between the arthropod vector and cancer.[142,143] BL, a B-cell non-Hodgkin lymphoma, is known to be one of the most aggressive lymphomas in adults and children.[144] Two major epidemiological clues to the pathogenesis of BL are the geographical association with malaria and early infection by Epstein–Barr virus (EBV). Pathogenesis of malaria leading to BL was linked to high retinoic acid exposure to lymphatic tissue after the infection, leading to EBV activation and an increase in retinoic acid-responsive gene expression. Currently, three clinic-epidemiological variants of the disease have been defined according to the 2008-WHO classification; endemic Burkitt lymphoma "African" (eBL), sporadic Burkitt lymphoma (sBL), and acquired immunodeficiency syndrome (AIDS)-related BL. The activation of these genes induces activation-induced cytidine deaminase (AID), triggering C-myc translocation, which finally causes BL.[145] Both agents cause B cell hyperplasia, which is almost certainly an essential component of lymphomagenesis in BL. Recent figures suggest that the incidence in equatorial Africa is similar, in children, to that of acute lymphoblastic lymphoma (ALL) in high-income countries—probably of the order of 3–6 per 100,000 in children aged 0–14 per year, accounting for 30–50% of all childhood cancers in equatorial Africa. This correlates with the high frequency and intensity of malaria in young children.[146] There was a decrease in BL incidences in areas where malaria had been eradicated, hinting at the communal association between the two variables. The distribution of BL cases was more prominent in equatorial Africa when compared to the rest of the world. These studies coined the name eBL to the cases that are specific for Africa.[147]

Researchers have been interested in the sickle-cell trait in eBL patients and control. Sick-cell trait does not help protect against mosquito bites or the infection itself, but it is proven to protect against the lethal effect of *Plasmodium falciparum* in childhood and against from the intense reticuloendothelial stimulation that sometimes progresses to hyper-reactive malarial splenomegaly.[148] Sickle cells exposed to low oxygen tension do not support the growth of parasites *in vitro*. Hemoglobin AS patients with a malarial infection also have a lower mortality rate, and reduced lymphoproliferation (as measured by spleen size). Most of the studies attempting to draw a relation between AS hemoglobinopathy and eBL showed no statistical significance.[149,150] Other hemoglobinopathies, such as ovalocytosis, also protect against malaria. If data show that the frequency of eBL is lower in areas where these hemoglobinopathies prevail, such as Papua and New Guinea,[151] then this supports the fact that malaria could be a risk factor for the genesis of eBL.[149]

One way of explaining the observation that the malaria patient harboring a multitude of parasite-derived antigens becomes a host susceptible to eBL is the suggestion that malaria patients produce so many nonspecific and "useless" antibodies that they are unable to recognize and respond to the threat posed by a small clone of malignant lymphoid cells.[152]

Malaria and EBV

There has been an epidemiological link between eBL and the combined effect of malaria and EBV.[153] Endemic BL is only found in areas where malaria is holoendemic or hyperendemic; and within these areas, it is absent in malaria-free pockets, such as urban centers. Vigorous cellular and serologic responses occur during malarial infection.[154]

B-cell hyperplasia is the mechanism adopted by malaria to induce BL. A cysteine-rich-inter-domain-region1alpha (CIDR1a) of the *P. falciparum* erythrocyte membrane protein 1 (PfEMP1) is expressed on the surface of infected erythrocytes. This protein was shown to cause an increase in the number of circulating B cells carrying the EBV in acute malaria.[155,156] This was explained by two mechanisms; first, the protein stimulates B memory cell replication, including the B cell compartment where EBV resides.[157] Second, CIDR1a can induce virus production from infected B cells, which in turn leads to infection of other B cells.[157–159] Acute malaria not only increases B-cell proliferation, but it also impairs EBV-specific T-cell responses.[142,149] This impairment leads to a large pool of EBV-infected cells, resulting in more frequent chromosomal translocations and lymphomagenesis.[160] In a study conducted by Mulama et al., studied malaria-exposed children from western Kenya to investigate the presence of qualitative differences in EBNA-1 (Epstein–Barr nuclear antigen-1) specific T cells. The authors proposed that malaria-induced exhaustion leads to the deletion of T-cell populations, resulting in EBNA1-specific deficiencies.[161]

Chromosomal aberrations and lymphomagenesis

Whether malaria is an initiator and EBV a promoter in the genesis of eBL, or vice versa, is not fully understood. Either hypotheses still do not account for the fact that *in vitro* infection of B-cells with EBV and stimulation with malaria antigens have yet to produce a cell that carries the chromosomal tumorigenic translocations found in both, sporadic and eBL.[160] Even though *c-myc* overexpression is common in all types of BL, it is specifically central to the pathogenesis of endemic BL, highlighting some important translocation patterns. Typically, sporadic BL has translocations involving sequences within or immediately 5′ to *myc* on chromosome 8 and sequences within or near the immunoglobulin heavy chain S region on chromosome 14. In contrast, eBL tends to be characterized by a translocation involving sequences on chromosome 8 further upstream from *myc* and sequences within or near the JH region on chromosome 14.[162] This shows that the tumorigenesis might be multifactorial in this case, having other unidentified factors (genetic, nutritional, or environmental) play an important role.

During the course of malaria, *P. falciparum*-infected red blood cells adhere to and activate B-cells through *PfEMP1* domains increasing the expression of Toll-like receptors (TLR), especially TLR7 and TLR 10, consequently, B-cells become permanently activated by TLR9 signaling.[159] This will transform the EBV in latently infected B-cells into its lytic state. In addition, malaria directly interacts with TLRs, producing chromosomal translocations associated with BL.[146] These receptors are located on various cells in the innate immune system. They are stimulated in malaria infection by certain agonists such as hemozoin and CpG-enriched DNA which is highly present in micro-organisms. Once bound to the TLRs, the adaptive immune system is activated, inducing cytidine deaminase (AID) in B cells. The AID enzyme triggers hypervariable region mutations and class switch recombination as well as activating B lymphocytes.[163–165] Finally, Derkach and colleagues have assessed role of the cysteine-rich interdomain region α1 (CIDRα1) in (*pfEMP1*) surface antigen in the attenuated humoral immunity in malaria, which could contribute to uncontrollable virus load with the frequent occurrence of eBL in tropical Africa.[158,166]

American Burkitt lymphoma

By the early 1970s, approximately 100 cases of BL had been confirmed by the American BL Registry.[167] Space–time clustering is suggested by the American data.[168] Although malaria is associated with BL in Africa, the relative rarity of the tumor in relation to the holoendemic nature of malaria indicates that a combination of genetic factors plus specific environmental factors may be operative. Host and environmental factors other than malaria are probably important in North American cases.[167]

Giardia lamblia

A direct correlation between *Giardia lamblia* and oncogenesis has not been drawn yet, but there have been a few case reports that make this topic interesting. In a study by Menon et al.,[169] 50 Malaysian children with cancer had their stools tested for parasites. Six out of the 50 children were positive for *G. lamblia*, indicating a prevalence of 6% in this small sample. In another case report by Kurita et al., there has been one case of pancreatic cancer associated with asymptomatic giardiasis. This parasite infection could be associated with the cancer, or it could just be secondary to a low immunity due to chemotherapy.[170] There are no specific reports between the coexistence of giardiasis and pancreatic cancer, but the diagnosis of this precise condition may increase in the forthcoming years.[171] Even though giardiasis, after its cysts had been ingested through contaminated food or water, mainly colonize the proximal small bowel and stomach, some rare cases did report having it infect the pancreas. Pancreatic cancer could be secondary to chronic pancreatitis caused by *G. lamblia*.[172] In a different case reported from a hospital in Japan, a 72-year-old man diagnosed with gallbladder cancer also did have concomitant giardiasis. After intraoperative cytological examination of the bile juice in the patient, several *G. lamblia* trophozoites were present.[173]

Recent evidence

Several studies demonstrated the relationship between several parasites and oncogenesis, for example, the relation between cryptosporidiosis and intestinal cancer.[174,175] The study done by Certad

Table 2 Table representing different types of cancers, their associated parasites, and epidemiology.

Cancer	Associated parasite	Epidemiology	Other notes
BBC	S. haematobium	Africa	Squamous cell carcinoma
CRC	S. japonicum; S. mansoni	Eastern Asia	MSI-high
Histiocytic lymphoma; large B-cell lymphoma	S. mansoni	Africa	No clear association
Burkitt lymphoma	Malaria; EBV	Africa	c-myc overexpression
CCA	C. sinensis; O. viverrini; O. felineus; Schistosomas	Asia and Eastern Europe	Schistosomes should be co-infected with either HBV or HCV for oncogenesis to occur

et al.,[174] was the first to record that a human-derived *Cryptosporidium parvum* isolate can induce cancer in mice. Another protozoan, *Trichomonas vaginalis* was incriminated. Although the latter has an evident role in cancer cervix, its role in prostatic cancer is still arguable.[176] Neurocysticercosis was also incriminated in hematological malignancies.[177] Parasite-induced immunomodulation, DNA damage nitric oxide release due to chronic inflammation were the mechanisms proposed.[178]

The possible role of other parasites and cancer development was investigated. For instance, the relationship of the nematode, *Strongyloides stercoralis*, to hepatobiliary cancer[179] and Kaposi sarcoma[180] was also studied as well as the role of *Toxoplasma gondii* in brain cancer[181,182] and lymphoma.[183] These parasites and others were incriminated in cancer development, however, clues are not yet available to include them in IARC roster.[176]

In view of recent revaluation of the clinical importance of parasites, it was found that infectious agents and their products can orchestrate a wide range of host immune responses, through which they may positively or negatively modulate cancer development and/or progression. Interestingly, certain types of pathogens can decrease the risk of tumorigenesis or lead to cancer regression. The same can be applied to parasitic infections.[184] *Trypanosoma cruzi* was found to decrease the incidence of experimentally induced rodent colon cancer.[185] Another example is the helminth *Trichuris suis* which was investigated clinically and experimentally for its ability to alleviate diseases, such as inflammatory bowel disease (ulcerative colitis, Crohn's disease), multiple sclerosis, and allergy.[186,187] Its applicability to cancer pathology, and more specifically to tumors of the gastrointestinal system, is a question open to future investigations.[184]

Summary

When uncommon neoplasms are noted with undue frequency in countries with a high prevalence of parasitic diseases, parasites become incriminated. Many parasites were studied for a possible role in oncogenesis, however, not all of them were registered as true carcinogens by the IARC. Chronic inflammation, immunomodulation, overexpression of certain carcinogens, DNA mutations, and suppression of apoptosis are the frequent well common mechanisms for parasite-induced oncogenesis. Besides, concomitant presence of other infectious agents is proved to be an enhancing factor in many situations. Epidemiological, cytogenetic, and animal studies were used to prove the relationship between parasites and cancer. In this view, *S. haematobium* was proved to play an important role in developing urinary BC due to chronic irritation by submucosal egg deposition, constant high levels of N-nitroso compounds that lead to DNA mutations, suppression of apoptosis, and hence, histopathological changes in the urinary epithelium. Human papillomavirus is still suspected to play an assistant role in this sequence.

Among *Schistosoma* species, *S. japonicum* is classified as a colorectal carcinogen especially in the Far East. When it comes to helminths, *Clonorchis* and *Opisthorchis* are proven to induce hepatobiliary cancer. In Africa, a strong correlation between *P. falciparum* infection and BL is present, with an evident enhancing role for Epstein–Barr virus. A few case reports did prove the presence of Giardiasis with some cancers, but a direct correlation is not drawn yet, requiring further research. These and more can be viewed as possible human carcinogens in respect of chronic inflammatory process associating several parasitic infections. However, strong evidence, especially cytogenetic, is usually required. Strikingly, despite the abovementioned data, it seems that certain parasites can modulate the host immune response in a manner that could lead to cancer regression or prevention. This is in the prospect of revaluation of the clinical importance of infectious agents; an issue that requires future concern (Table 2).

Key references

The complete reference list can be found on Vital Source version of this title, see inside front cover.

1. Jordan P. Egg-output in bilharziasis in relation to epidemiology, pathology, treatment and control. In: Mostofi FK, ed. *Bilharziasis*. Springer; 1967:93–103.
3. Ross AG, Bartley PB, Sleigh AC, et al. Schistosomiasis. *N Engl J Med*. 2002;346(16):1212–1220.
8. Steinmann P, Keiser J, Bos R, et al. Schistosomiasis and water resources development: systematic review, meta-analysis, and estimates of people at risk. *Lancet Infect Dis*. 2006;6(7):411–425.
11. Chitsulo L, Engels D, Montresor A, Savioli L. The global status of schistosomiasis and its control. *Acta Trop*. 2000;77(1):41–51.
17. Ploeg M, Aben KK, Kiemeney LA. The present and future burden of urinary bladder cancer in the world. *World J Urol*. 2009;27(3):289–293.
22. El-Khoby T, Galal N, Fenwick A, et al. The epidemiology of schistosomiasis in Egypt: summary findings in nine governorates. *Am J Trop Med Hyg*. 2000;62(2_suppl):88–99.
23. Gouda I, Mokhtar N, Bilal D, et al. Bilharziasis and bladder cancer: a time trend analysis of 9843 patients. *J Egypt Natl Canc Inst*. 2007;19(2):158–162.
39. Gray DJ, Ross AG, Li YS, McManus DP. Diagnosis and management of schistosomiasis. *BMJ*. 2011;342:d2651.
44. Tricker AR, Mostafa MH, Spiegelhalder B, Preussmann R. Urinary nitrate, nitrite and N-nitroso compounds in bladder cancer patients with schistosomiasis (bilharzia). *IARC Sci Publ*. 1991;105:178–181.
62. Fripp PJ. Bilharziasis and bladder cancer. *Br J Cancer*. 1965;19:292–296.
63. Badawi AF, Mostafa MH, O'Connor PJ. Involvement of alkylating agents in schistosome-associated bladder cancer: the possible basic mechanisms of induction. *Cancer Lett*. 1992;63(3):171–188.
68. Khafagy M, El-Bolkainy M, Mansour M. Carcinoma of the bilharzial urinary bladder. A study of the associated mucosal lesions in 86 cases. *Cancer*. 1972;30(1):150–159.
69. Cheng L, Cheville JC, Neumann RM, Bostwick DG. Flat intraepithelial lesions of the urinary bladder. *Cancer*. 2000;88(3):625–631.
70. Cheng L, Cheville JC, Neumann RM, Bostwick DG. Natural history of urothelial dysplasia of the bladder. *Am J Surg Pathol*. 1999;23(4):443–447.
74. Fedewa SA, Soliman AS, Ismail K, et al. Incidence analyses of bladder cancer in the Nile delta region of Egypt. *Cancer Epidemiol*. 2009;33(3–4):176–181.

77. Koraitim MM, Metwalli NE, Atta MA, el-Sadr AA. Changing age incidence and pathological types of schistosoma-associated bladder carcinoma. *J Urol.* 1995;**154**(5):1714–1716.
87. Cheever AW. *Schistosomiasis and Neoplasia.* Oxford University Press; 1978.
88. Hutt M, Burkitt D. Aetiology of Burkitt's lymphoma. *Lancet.* 1973;**1**(7800):439.
89. Plummer M, de Martel C, Vignat J, et al. Global burden of cancers attributable to infections in 2012: a synthetic analysis. *Lancet Glob Health.* 2016;**4**(9):e609–e616.
91. Xu Z. *Schistosoma japonicum* and colorectal cancer: an epidemiological study in the people's republic of China. *Int J Cancer.* 1984;**34**(3):315–318.
93. Madbouly KM, Senagore AJ, Mukerjee A, et al. Colorectal cancer in a population with endemic *Schistosoma mansoni*: is this an at-risk population? *Int J Color Dis.* 2007;**22**(2):175–181.
98. Chen Y, Liu Z, Qian J, et al. Expression difference of DNA mismatch repair gene hMLH1 and hMSH2 between schistosomiasis-associated colorectal cancer and sporadic colorectal cancer. *Zhonghua Wei Chang Wai Ke Za Zhi.* 2016;**19**(1):75–79.
104. Toda KS, Kikuchi L, Chagas AL, et al. Hepatocellular carcinoma related to *Schistosoma mansoni* infection: case series and literature review. *J Clin Transl Hepatol.* 2015;**3**(4):260–264.
105. Omar HH. Impact of chronic schistosomiasis and HBV/HCV co-infection on the liver: current perspectives. *Hepat Med.* 2019;**11**:131–136.
111. Edington GM, von Lichtenberg F, Nwabuebo I, et al. Pathologic effects of schistosomiasis in Ibadan, Western State of Nigeria. I. Incidence and intensity of infection; distribution and severity of lesions. *Am J Trop Med Hyg.* 1970;**19**(6):982–995.
117. Mazigo HD, Zinga M, Heukelbach J, Rambau P. Case series of adenocarcinoma of the prostate associated with *Schistosoma haematobium* infection in Tanzania. *J Glob Infect Dis.* 2010;**2**(3):307–309.
125. Bouvard V, Baan R, Straif K, et al. A review of human carcinogens—part B: biological agents. *Lancet Oncol.* 2009;**10**(4):321–322.
128. Yothaisong S, Thanee M, Namwat N, et al. *Opisthorchis viverrini* infection activates the PI3K/AKT/PTEN and Wnt/beta-catenin signaling pathways in a Cholangiocarcinogenesis model. *Asian Pac J Cancer Prev.* 2014;**15**(23):10463–10468.
133. Sripa B, Brindley PJ, Mulvenna J, et al. The tumorigenic liver fluke *Opisthorchis viverrini*—multiple pathways to cancer. *Trends Parasitol.* 2012;**28**(10):395–407.
138. Jang KT, Hong SM, Lee KT, et al. Intraductal papillary neoplasm of the bile duct associated with *Clonorchis sinensis* infection. *Virchows Arch.* 2008;**453**(6):589–598.
143. Burchenal JH. Geographic chemotherapy—Burkitt's tumor as a stalking horse for leukemia: presidential address. *Cancer Res.* 1966;**26**(12):2393–2405.
147. Orem J, Mbidde EK, Lambert B, et al. Burkitt's lymphoma in Africa, a review of the epidemiology and etiology. *Afr Health Sci.* 2007;**7**(3):166–175.
153. Facer CA, Playfair JH. Malaria, Epstein-Barr virus, and the genesis of lymphomas. *Adv Cancer Res.* 1989;**53**:33–72.
156. Njie R, Bell AI, Jia H, et al. The effects of acute malaria on Epstein-Barr virus (EBV) load and EBV-specific T cell immunity in Gambian children. *J Infect Dis.* 2009;**199**(1):31–38.
161. Mulama D, Chelimo K, Collins O, et al. EBNA-1 specific effector T cell deletion associated with holoendemic malaria exposure in the etiology of endemic Burkitt's lymphoma (P3063). *J Immunol.* 2013;**190**(1 Supplement):187.7.
167. Levine PH, Cho BR. Burkitt's lymphoma: clinical features of North American cases. *Cancer Res.* 1974;**34**(5):1219–1221.
168. Patton LL, McMillan CW, Webster WP. American Burkitt's lymphoma: a 10-year review and case study. *Oral Surg Oral Med Oral Pathol.* 1990;**69**(3):307–316.
178. Del Brutto OH, Dolezal M, Castillo PR, Garcia HH. Neurocysticercosis and oncogenesis. *Arch Med Res.* 2000;**31**(2):151–155.
179. Hirata T, Kishimoto K, Kinjo N, et al. Association between *Strongyloides stercoralis* infection and biliary tract cancer. *Parasitol Res.* 2007;**101**(5):1345.
186. Summers RW, Elliott DE, Urban JF Jr, et al. *Trichuris suis* therapy for active ulcerative colitis: a randomized controlled trial. *Gastroenterology.* 2005;**128**(4):825–832.

PART 5

Epidemiology, Prevention, and Detection

31 Cancer epidemiology

Veronika Fedirko, PhD, MPH ■ Kevin T. Nead, MD, MPhil ■ Carrie Daniel, PhD, MPH ■ Paul Scheet, PhD

> **Overview**
>
> This article gives a straightforward introduction to cancer epidemiology and is organized as follows. We first provide US data on cancer cases, deaths, and survival. These data, typically derived from national registries and surveys from scientific organizations devoted to the cause, for example, surveillance by the National Cancer Institute's Surveillance, Epidemiology, and End Results Program (SEER) and the International Agency for Research on Cancer (IARC), form the basis for policies centered around cancer control. We then discuss epidemiological methods the practicing oncologist may encounter in research or literature, followed by a tour of common (e.g., tobacco) and emerging (e.g., energy balance) causes of cancer. We follow this by describing molecular epidemiology, a subfield rejuvenated by molecular technologies to inform components of environmental factors and risks associated with the host, such as genetics, transcriptomics, metabolomics, and the microbiome. Finally, we discuss future directions, the potential and current importance of epidemiology.

The first question a patient asks when diagnosed with a cancer is likely, "Why me?" While this may encompass the metaphysical, it often represents the more basic interpretation of *What caused this to happen?* The field of epidemiology is centered around addressing this question.

Epidemiology identifies the factors underlying health or social phenomena, including diseases such as cancer. As it is designed to identify phenomena affecting potentially many individuals, as in an epidemic, Epidemiology (literally "the study of what befalls a population") has been referred to as "population medicine" or a branch of population health sciences.[1] The role of a medical oncologist is critical in the epidemiology of cancer. The oncologist may be the first to confront data, in the form of clinical observations, that suggest root causes of disease initiation or drivers of progression. Indeed, the practice of epidemiology not only identifies determinants of disease and quantifies their risk to individuals and the population but also forms hypotheses which can be tested experimentally.

In this vein, the field of epidemiology synthesizes contributions from a number of disciplines, spanning biology, toxicology, virology, medicine, and genetics. To draw conclusions that would inform and aid translation, such as the prevention of cancer, an epidemiologist is ultimately motivated to infer causality, rather than merely association. Broadly, to do this, the aforementioned disciplines support knowledge of the host and supporting or parasitic organisms, the physical environment, and human behavior or the societal (or "built") environment. Population research is inherently empirical, and the field of biostatistics is integrated into the practice of epidemiology at nearly every level.

Ultimately, an objective within epidemiology is the quantification of exposures, such as those attributed to tobacco, asbestos, lifestyle, diet/nutrition, and occupation.[2,3] This could stem from classical observation to technology-enabled assessment. An example of the former is John Snow's tracing of a cholera outbreak in London, in 1854, to the water source from the Broad Street pump.[4] Far more recently, tobacco use has been observed to be associated with a large number of cancers, especially of the lung, dominating the landscape of preventable cancers. Across all forms of disease, including cancer and cardiovascular, tobacco causes approximately 480,000 deaths per year, including 41,000 attributable to second-hand smoke. These were striking observations that have led to implementation of a variety of public health strategies to reduce smoking, including key tobacco control demand-reduction measures (e.g., tobacco taxation, packaging and labeling provisions, marketing bans, and cessation programs), creating smoke-free environments via enactment of smoke-free legislation, development of effective media campaigns, and regulation of novel tobacco products (https://tobaccoatlas.org/). This resulted in decreases in smoking prevalence, from 42% in 1964 to approximately 15% today in the United States.[5] In contrast, and as an example of technology-enabled assessment, modern genomic technologies allow for the efficient and cost-effective survey of over a half-million sites along the genome to inform of inherited genetic variation—something that would have been science fiction 20 years ago and vastly more expensive 10 years ago.[6] While genetic susceptibility resulting from specific inherited genetic variants may contribute to the development of cancer, it is not typically thought of as a sole cause but rather acting in unison or combination with environmental exposures. We will see the theme of exposure quantification throughout this article.

Cancer statistics

Population-based cancer registries collect information on newly diagnosed cancer cases, deaths, and survival in geographically well-defined populations. The first cancer registries were established in the United States in 1935, and in Nordic countries in the 1940s.[7] Currently, 291 registries in 68 countries provide high-quality data to a network of registries, the International Association of Cancer Registries (IACR)[8]. Over the last 30 years, cancer registries have become the foundation of cancer surveillance and control. Surveillance data are used to monitor trends, generate hypotheses about emerging risk factors, guide resource allocation, predict future burden and needs, and evaluate the impact of population-based preventive interventions. In some countries, the data can be linked to other administrative databases and registries (e.g., SEER-Medicare), thereby expanding the scope of research to cancer etiology and outcomes, pharmacoepidemiology, access to cancer care, quality of care, quality of life, and cost of care.[7]

Holland-Frei Cancer Medicine, Tenth Edition. Edited by Robert C. Bast, John C. Byrd, Carlo M. Croce, Ernest Hawk, Fadlo R. Khuri, Raphael E. Pollock, Apostolia M. Tsimberidou, Christopher G. Willett, and Cheryl L. Willman.
© 2023 John Wiley & Sons, Inc. Published 2023 by John Wiley & Sons, Inc.

US cancer statistics

In 2020, more than 1.8 million new cancer cases were expected to be diagnosed in the United States with nearly 606,520 estimated cancer deaths.[9] Cancer is the second most common cause of death in the United States, surpassed only by heart disease. However, in individuals younger than 65, it is the leading cause of death (https://www.cdc.gov/nchs/nvss/mortality_tables.htm). The financial burden associated with early mortality and cancer itself is enormous, with approximately $88.3 billion per year for direct medical costs alone in 2011 (https://meps.ahrq.gov/mepsweb/).

According to the projections by the American Cancer Society (ACS) for 2020,[9] the top incident cancers in the United States (excluding nonmelanoma skin cancers) are the following: cancers of the prostate (21%), lung (13%), colorectum (9%), bladder (7%), and melanoma of the skin (7%) in men; and cancers of the breast (30%), lung (12%), colorectum (8%), endometrium (7%), and thyroid (4%) in women (Figure 1). The lifetime risk of being diagnosed with cancer is slightly higher for men (40.1%) than for women (38.7%).[9] While the exact reasons for the excess risk in men are not well understood, differences in environmental exposures and endogenous hormones and their complex interactions may be major factors.

- The overall cancer incidence rate in men declined rapidly from 2007 to 2014, and remained relatively stable through 2017, mirroring stabilizing rates for prostate cancer, which may be an artifact of changes in US Preventive Services Task Force (USPSTF) screening recommendations,[10] and declines in rates for lung and colorectal cancers. In women, the overall cancer incidence rate has remained stable over the past few decades, reflecting slow declines in rates for lung and colorectal cancers being offset by increasing rates of other common cancers (Figure 2). Interestingly, the decrease in colorectal cancer incidence rate has been driven by people aged 50 or older, in large part due to screening. At the same time, incidence rates have been increasing for adults under age 50, the age at which individuals at average risk are recommended to begin screening, and younger adults presented with more advanced disease.[11] Taking into consideration these data, the ACS new colorectal cancer screening guidelines recommend that men and women at average risk for colorectal cancer be regularly screened beginning at 45 years of age.[12] The slight increase in female breast cancer incidence in recent years has been attributed to higher body mass index (BMI) and lower number of births.[13]

Incidence rates continue to increase for cancers of the kidney, liver, pancreas, melanoma of the skin, and oral cavity and pharynx (among non-Hispanic whites). Liver cancer incidence is increasing most rapidly, by 2–3% annually between 2007 and 2016,[9,14] reflecting changes in the leading causes of liver cancer in the United States—obesity, chronic hepatitis C virus (HCV) infection, excessive alcohol consumption, and tobacco use.[14] Socioeconomic development has had a profound influence on the risk and burden of cancer. Improvements in sanitation, vaccination, treatment, and development of biomarkers of risk all had an effect on reducing the incidence of stomach and cervical cancers known to be caused by infectious agents (*Helicobacter pylori* and human papillomavirus [HPV], respectively).

Cancer mortality rates are less affected by changes in detection practices than is cancer incidence, and therefore are considered to better reflect progress against the disease.[15] The overall cancer death rate rose during most of the twentieth century, largely driven by increases in lung cancer deaths among men due to tobacco smoking. However, the death rate started to decline in 1991 due to improvements in cancer early detection and treatment, and decreases in tobacco use occurred and attributed to policies and regulations (Figure 3). The most recent data from 2016 to 2017 demonstrated the largest single-year decline of 2.2% in cancer mortality rate since rates began declining in 1992. This progress reflects large drops in mortality for the four major cancers (lung,

	Male				Female		
Estimated new cases	Prostate	191,930	21%		Breast	276,480	30%
	Lung and bronchus	116,300	13%		Lung and bronchus	112,520	12%
	Colon and rectum	78,300	9%		Colon and rectum	69,650	8%
	Urinary bladder	62,100	7%		Uterine corpus	65,620	7%
	Melanoma of the skin	60,190	7%		Thyroid	40,170	4%
	Kidney and renal pelvis	45,520	5%		Melanoma of the skin	40,160	4%
	Non-Hodgkin lymphoma	42,380	5%		Non-Hodgkin lymphoma	34,860	4%
	Oral cavity and pharynx	38,380	4%		Kidney and renal pelvis	28,230	3%
	Leukemia	35,470	4%		Pancreas	27,200	3%
	Pancreas	30,400	3%		Leukemia	25,060	3%
	All sites	893,660			All sites	912,930	
	Male				Female		
Estimated deaths	Lung and bronchus	72,500	23%		Lung and bronchus	63,220	22%
	Prostate	33,300	10%		Breast	42,170	15%
	Colon and rectum	28,630	9%		Colon and rectum	24,570	9%
	Pancreas	24,640	8%		Pancreas	22,410	8%
	Liver and intrahepatic bile duct	20,020	6%		Ovary	13,940	5%
	Leukemia	13,420	4%		Uterine corpus	12,590	4%
	Esophagus	13,100	4%		Liver and intrahepatic bile duct	10,140	4%
	Urinary bladder	13,050	4%		Leukemia	9680	3%
	Non-Hodgkin lymphoma	11,460	4%		Non-Hodgkin lymphoma	8480	3%
	Brain and other nervous system	10,190	3%		Brain and other nervous system	7830	3%
	All sites	321,160			All sites	285,360	

Estimates are rounded to the nearest 10, and cases exclude basal cell and squamous cell skin cancers and in situ carcinoma except urinary bladder. Estimates do not include Puerto Rico or other US territories. Ranking is based on modeled projections and may differ from the most recent observed data.

© 2020, American Cancer Society. Inc., Surveillance Research

Figure 1 Top incident cancer and leading causes of cancer deaths among men and women in the United States—2020 estimates.[9] Source: Siegel et al.[9]

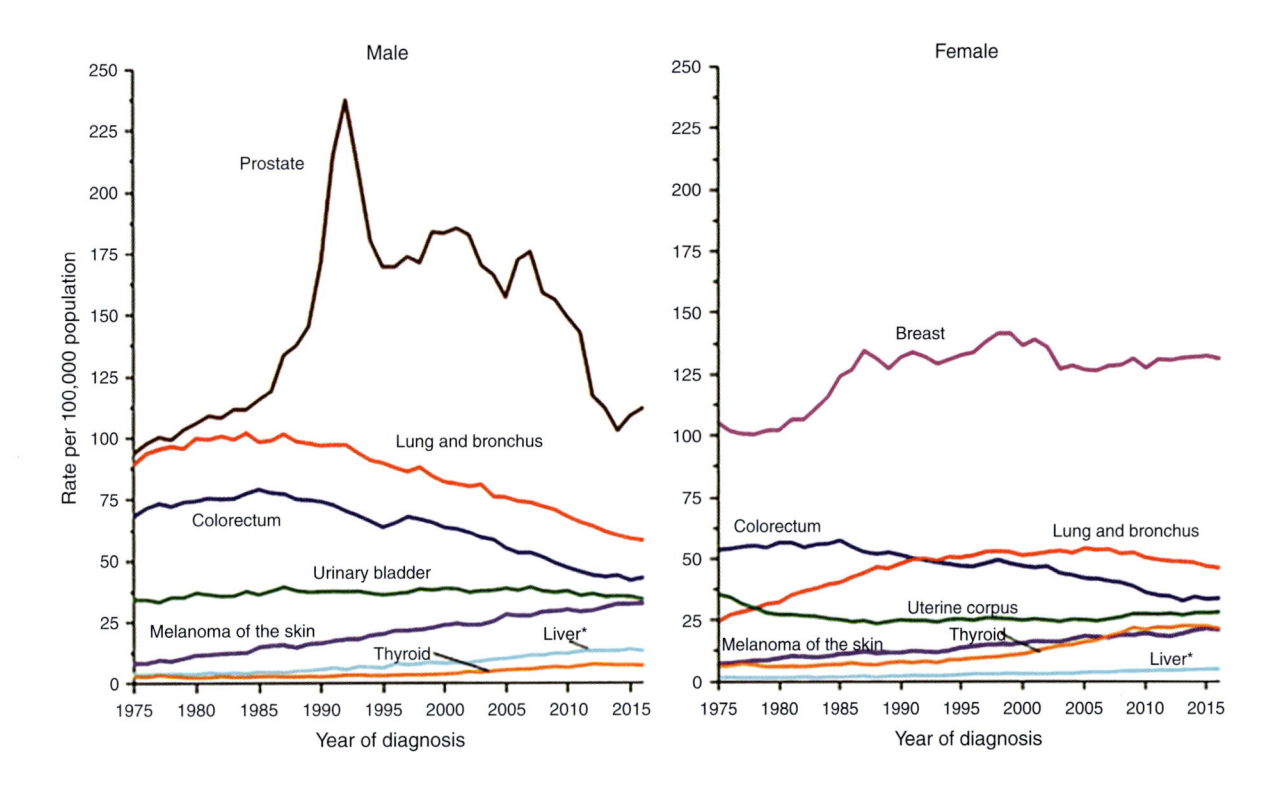

Figure 2 Trends in incidence for selected cancers by sex, United States, 1975–2016.[9] Source: Siegel et al.[9]

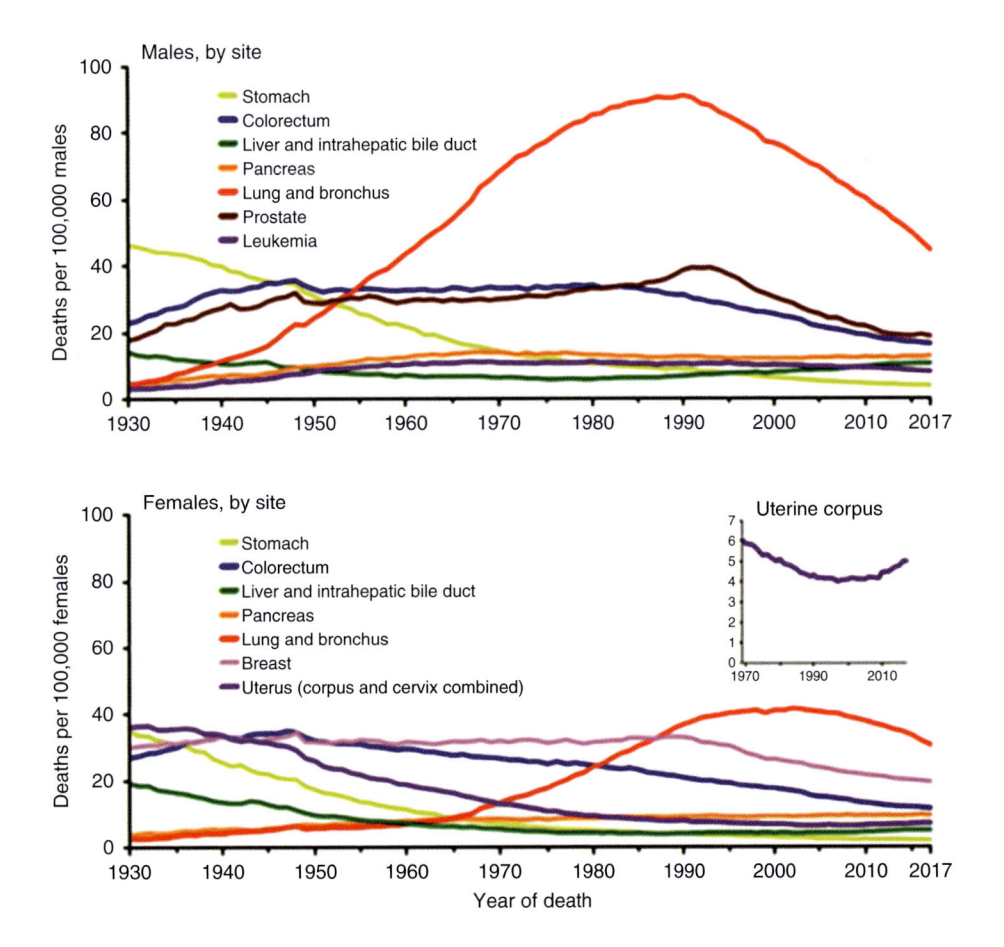

Figure 3 Trends in cancer mortality rates by sex and select cancer sites, United States, 1920–2017.[9] Source: Siegel et al.[9]

breast, prostate, and colorectum) (Figure 3) mostly because of improvements in early detection (e.g., population-based screening for breast and colorectal cancers), development of promising new cancer treatments (e.g., immune checkpoint inhibitors), and the steep drop in smoking prevalence. However, improvement is needed for multiple cancers including cancers of the liver, pancreas, uterine corpus, small intestine, and sites within the oral cavity and pharynx associated with the HPV as the death rates for these cancers rose over the past decade.

Causes of cancer

Many cancers are causally related to potentially modifiable risk factors. In a 1981 review, Doll and Peto[2] estimated the major causes of cancer deaths in the United States to be tobacco smoking (30%), diet and lifestyle (about 35%), infections (10%), reproductive and sexual behavior (7%), and occupation (4%). Their estimates generally continue to hold even after 35 years after they were first calculated[3] and do not include an estimate of genetic contributions to cancer risk.[16] In the United States in 2014, an estimated 42% of all incident cancers and 45% of cancer deaths were attributable to cigarette smoking, secondhand smoke, excess body weight, alcohol intake, consumption of red and processed meat, low consumption of fruits/vegetables, dietary fiber, and dietary calcium, physical inactivity, ultraviolet radiation, and six cancer-associated infections.[17] These estimates, however, may underestimate the overall proportion of cancers attributable to modifiable risk factors, because the impact of all established factors and their interactions could not be easily quantified, and many likely modifiable factors are not yet confirmed as causal.[17]

The impact of two well-established carcinogens, tobacco and alcohol, has been reviewed extensively elsewhere.[18,19] Tobacco causes almost nine of every 10 cases of lung cancer, and significantly contributes to cancers of the head and neck, bladder, kidney, blood (acute myeloid leukemia), cervix, and digestive cancers. Less is known about the long-term effects of electronic cigarettes, which contain nicotine (addictive component) and several other potentially toxic aerosols.[20–22] Drinking alcohol increases the risk of cancers of the breast, colorectum, esophagus (squamous cell), liver, mouth, pharynx, larynx, and stomach. The extent to which alcoholic drinks are a cause of various cancers depends on the amount and frequency of alcohol consumed, but epidemiologic studies show a consistent link with increased cancer risk and alcohol (ethanol), regardless of whether it is beer, wine, or distilled liquor. A comprehensive report ("Third Expert Report") on exposures and cancer risk was assembled in 2018 by the American Institute for Cancer Research, which also maintains the Continuous Update Project.[23]

With obesity being the lead cause of cancer in nonsmokers, evidence-based public health guidelines and diet and lifestyle recommendations to help people make informed choices to manage weight are of growing importance to cancer prevention and survival. Clear examples of rapidly increasing cancers largely attributed to obesity-related risk include renal cell carcinoma and hepatocellular carcinoma.[23] Notably, obesity may play a critical role in the rising incidence of several cancers among younger adults (<50 years).[24]

- More than half of all cancers diagnosed in women and a quarter of those diagnosed in men are associated with being overweight and obese.
- The following 13 cancers are associated with being overweight and obese: meningioma, multiple myeloma, adenocarcinoma of the esophagus, and cancers of the thyroid, postmenopausal breast, gallbladder, stomach, liver, pancreas, kidney, ovaries, uterus, colon, and rectum (colorectal). Poor diet and/or physical inactivity are similarly associated with risk of many (most) of these cancers.[23]

Evidence linking cancer to sustained energy imbalance (energy-dense diet, physical inactivity, and other biological factors), obesity, and obesity-related co-morbidities mainly comes from prospective observational studies. Although observational studies cannot prove a causal relationship, when studies in different populations have similar results and when a possible mechanism for a causal relationship exists from preclinical studies and clinical trials leveraging biological markers, this provides evidence of a causal connection or at the least, very strong evidence that diet and lifestyle improvements may be required to lower risk of several types of cancer through modulation of obesity and other mechanisms. Nonintentional/cancer and treatment-related weight loss (reverse causality) and the imprecision of BMI to differentiate between muscle and fat mass (critical markers for cancer patients) has led to controversial and/or inconsistent findings in obesity and cancer survival.[25,26] Interestingly, obesity is emerging as a potential protective factor in response and survival among immunotherapy patients with mechanistic backing from preclinical models.[27–29]

Cancer disparities in the United States

Rates of cancer incidence and mortality vary significantly between racial and ethnic groups, mostly because of socioeconomic inequalities that lead to differences in risk factor exposures, and barriers to healthcare access (prevention, early detection/screening, and treatment).[30] Biological differences also appear to play a role in some cancer disparities (e.g., in the incidence and/or aggressiveness of the triple-negative breast, colorectal, and prostate cancers). The key cancer incidence and mortality disparities among US racial and ethnic groups identified by the National Cancer Institute include the following (https://www.cancer.gov/about-cancer/understanding/disparities):

> **Breast cancer**
>
> Overweight/obesity and physical inactivity are associated with increased risk of breast cancer and poor prognosis with differences by menopausal status and by tumor subtype. The epidemiologic evidence is most prolific in postmenopausal women with a history of mid-life weight gain.[31] Menopause represents a critical time when energy balance, circulating hormones, chemokines and cytokines, and body fat distribution are in flux, and is also a time when the tumor-promoting effects of obesity emerge. The loss of ovarian production of estrogens with menopause is associated with weight gain, increased adiposity, and decreased physical activity, predisposing women to insulin resistance, diabetes, dyslipidemia, and cardiovascular disease. All of these conditions have also been associated with increased risk for breast cancer and/or poorer outcomes for patients with breast cancer. Exercise is thought to have additional beneficial effects beyond its role in weight control that could significantly impact breast tumors.[31–33] Multiple epidemiological studies have shown a dose–response relationship between exercise and breast cancer with 10–40% reductions in risk, recurrence, and mortality, leading to the initiation of several trials[34–36] (https://www.cancer.gov/about-cancer/causes-prevention/risk/obesity/physical-activity-fact-sheet).

- African Americans have higher death rates than all other groups for many, although not all, cancer types.
- African American women are much more likely than white women to die of breast cancer.

- African Americans are more than twice as likely as whites to die of prostate cancer and nearly twice as likely to die of stomach cancer.
- Colorectal cancer incidence is higher in African Americans than in whites.
- Hispanic and American Indian/Alaska Native women have higher rates of cervical cancer than women of other racial/ethnic groups; African American women have the highest rates of death from the disease.
- American Indians/Alaska Natives have the highest rates of liver and intrahepatic bile duct cancer, followed by Asian/Pacific Islanders and Hispanics.
- American Indians/Alaska Natives have higher death rates from kidney cancer than people of other racial/ethnic groups.

These variations, both in the United States and worldwide, contribute to a growing concern regarding cancer health disparities.

Methods

A critical aspect of understanding cancer epidemiology is grasping the design and interpretation of the various study designs used to examine the association of exposures and outcomes. Clinicians are typically very familiar with clinical trials, but observational studies are critical for inference of phenomena where it would be unethical, or even impossible, to conduct a trial (e.g., the observation that parity is inversely associated with breast cancer risk[13,37]).

Clinical trials

As new interventions are developed, they typically follow a phased process of clinical evaluation. Phase I studies typically include less than 100 healthy volunteers or individuals with a given disease and are designed to examine safety and dosage. Phase II studies can include up to several hundred people and are designed to examine efficacy and common side effects. Phase III studies are often randomized, include hundreds to thousands of individuals, and determine efficacy and side effects of an intervention relative to a standard of care. Here, we will focus on randomized trials.

A *randomized trial* is a prospective study where a defined population is randomly allocated to one of two groups: the experimental group receiving the intervention (e.g., exposure, drug, treatment procedure) and a comparison group (controls) which receives the existing standard of care treatment or placebo. The population is then followed to ascertain an outcome. For example, individuals with early-stage prostate cancer randomly assigned to undergo radiation therapy versus surgery as definitive therapy who are then followed to ascertain mortality risk. Critically, those observing outcomes and administering the intervention or care, as well as the participants, are often blinded to the intervention. The purpose of randomization is to randomly assign trial participants into groups that are similar in all respects other than those being specifically tested under the trial (e.g., radiation therapy vs surgery). Randomization, assuming a large enough sample size that the probability of chance differences between groups is small relative to an assumed effect of intervention, accounts for both known, unknown, measured, and unmeasured confounding factors. Additionally, properly randomized and blinded studies can prevent bias, such as selection bias. Thus, any differences in an outcome observed between randomized groups can be inferred to be cause and effect of the intervention. Accordingly, any analysis that does not examine the groups as initially randomized, such as subgroup analyses or an analysis based on how individuals were actually treated (*per protocol analysis*) rather than as randomized (*intention to treat analysis*), breaks the randomization and inferences regarding causality should be approached cautiously.

While randomized trials provide the highest level of evidence for causality, not all research questions can feasibly or ethically be answered using a randomized study design. A randomized trial is ethical to conduct when we do not know if treatment A is better than treatment B. Additionally, it may not always be feasible, nor ethical, to conduct a randomized trial. Consider a researcher interested in determining whether the vitamin supplementation in early childhood decreases dementia risk. As dementia is a relatively rare outcome, and the latency period between exposure and outcome would be expected to be many decades, a randomized trial would require many thousands of children followed for many decades, creating massive economical and logistical barriers. Therefore, alternative study designs, that is, forms of observational studies, must often be considered for different research questions and different stages of investigation.

Cohort studies

Like randomized studies, *cohort studies* also start with individuals free of outcomes of interest (e.g., they may include individuals with past exposures or incident exposures) who are then followed over time to assess a given outcome. Cohort studies are designed as prospective or retrospective. In a *prospective cohort study*, also known as a longitudinal study, the investigator identifies a nonrandomized exposed and nonexposed population at the start of the study and moves forward in time concurrently with the study population to examine a given outcome. For example, an investigator initiates a study in 2020, identifies a cohort from 2020, and examines outcomes in 2020 or beyond. In a *retrospective cohort study*, the investigator looks back in time to identify an exposed and nonexposed population and then looks forward from that time point to ascertain the presence or absence of the outcome. For example, an investigator initiates a study in 2020, identifies a cohort from 2010, and examines outcomes through 2018. If that investigator followed the cohort for outcomes beyond 2020, this would be an example of a mixed study design. Prospective and retrospective cohort studies have the same design in that they both start with a disease-free (or outcome-agnostic) population and assess exposure status prior to onset of the outcome. The difference in the study design is based on the period in time that the cohort is identified, and that the outcome is ascertained, relative to when the investigator initiates the study. Advantages of cohort studies include establishing a temporal relationship and the ability to study rare exposures as the study is designed around cohort exposure status. Further, in contrast to an experimental study (e.g., trial), an investigator observes, rather than determines, participants' exposure status. These advantages aside, cohort studies often require large numbers of individuals to be followed for a long period of time and are particularly challenging for diseases that are rare or have long latency periods. In these situations, an alternative study design, such as a case-control study, may be appropriate.

Case-control studies

The distinguishing characteristic of a *case-control study* is that it starts by identifying individuals with the disease (cases) and compares them to individuals without the disease (controls). Cases and controls are then compared with respect to their previous exposure to a given risk factor. An example of a case-control study would be to first identify individuals with and without colorectal cancer and to second determine whether they were or were not previously exposed to tobacco products. This is in contrast to prospective and retrospective cohort studies, which start by identifying individuals without colorectal cancer and determining their exposure to tobacco products before colorectal cancer diagnosis. Case-control studies are generally more time- and cost-efficient than cohort studies and are advantageous when a disease is rare or there is a long interval between exposure and development of disease. Disadvantages of case-control studies include the following: recall bias, where individuals who developed a given disease may be more likely to recall past exposures; inefficiency for rare exposures; they generally do not allow straightforward calculation of incidence; and finally, challenges abound when selecting controls, which must be representative of the source population from which the cases were diagnosed.

Case-control studies can also be carried out within an existing cohort using a *nested case-control* or *case-cohort* study design. In a *nested case-control* study design, the investigator starts with a defined, disease-free cohort. As individuals develop the outcome (cases), controls matched on calendar time and length of follow-up are selected. In a *case-cohort* study design, the investigator starts with a defined disease-free cohort and as individuals develop the outcome, controls are randomly selected, creating a sub-cohort. Compared to a *nested case-control* study, the *case-cohort* design allows examination of different outcomes since controls are not individually matched to each case. Case-control studies carried out within an existing cohort do not suffer from recall bias, as exposure is evaluated prior to diagnosis, while still being more economical than full cohort studies as, for example, laboratory evaluations would need to be evaluated on selected cases and controls only rather than the full cohort. These studies are effectively hybrids of cohort and (prospective) case-control studies.

Cross-sectional and ecological studies

An additional economical and efficient study design is the *cross-sectional study*. Cross-sectional studies are those that ascertain exposure and outcome at a single time point. For example, a study that surveys a population and collects information regarding current blood glucose levels and presence of hypertension as determined by a blood pressure measurement. Because cross-sectional studies are a snapshot in time, they are able to measure prevalence (burden of disease at a particular point in time), but not incidence of disease (number of new cases during a period of time), and inferences regarding causality are challenging. Therefore, a higher level of evidence (e.g., utilizing a prospective cohort study design) is warranted to better define the relationship of the association.

Alternatively, the first exploratory step in determining whether an association exists may be to conduct an *ecological study*. In an ecological study, the unit of observation is a group, such as a given population or community. Exposures and disease outcomes are measured at the level of the population and their associations then examined. For example, examination of the incidence of colon cancer by country relative to that country's per capita intake of dietary fiber. While this study design can be useful to indicate a potential association worthy of further study or generate hypotheses, only population-level data are known. Therefore, from the data in the above example alone, it would be unknown whether *individuals* in whom colon cancer developed actually had lower intake of dietary fiber. Indeed, the phenomenon of this not being the case (i.e., that individuals with higher levels of dietary fiber could exhibit higher risk of colon cancer, or that there is no relationship at the individual level) is known as ecological fallacy.

Interpreting epidemiologic evidence

A challenge in the interpretation of observational epidemiological studies is determining whether an association is causal. A spurious association occurs when no association exists, causal or otherwise, but we observe an association in a study. These associations are usually secondary to a bias, which results from an error in how the study was conducted. For example, if we designed a case-control study to determine whether living near a chemical plant conferred an increased risk of developing cancer and we selected cases from areas *with* chemical plants and controls from areas *without* chemical plants. In this study, we would likely find that cases would be more likely to have exposure to chemical plants than controls simply based on how we selected our groups unrelated to whether that exposure is actually associated with the outcome. This is an example of a selection bias and a spurious association.

Where an association is real, a subsequent question is whether it is causal. A fundamental reason that a real association is not a causal association is that it is secondary to confounding. In general, confounding occurs when an exposure and outcome are associated not because of a direct impact of the exposure on the outcome, but rather because a third variable is associated with both the exposure and the outcome variable. In the example above, location was a confounding variable. In another example, a study that shows that increased ice cream consumption is associated with increased drownings. This may be a real association in that increased ice cream consumption is actually associated with more drownings. However, ice cream consumption does not cause drownings, rather warm weather confounds this association as it is associated with both increased ice cream consumption and increased drownings secondary to greater pool use. It is worth noting that a confounding variable can also obfuscate a *bona fide* relationship, so that a lack of association may be spurious as well. Thus, it is critical to identify or be aware of confounding factors in observational studies. This notwithstanding, although bias is a systematic error, confounding effects may be inextricably tied to an environment and must be understood and accounted for in any analyses. Therefore, confounded associations may still be beneficial as they may facilitate prediction and motivate additional inquiry.

When a causal association exists, the possibility of reverse causality should be considered, particularly when considering clinical applications. Reverse causality occurs when the examined outcome actually causes the examined exposure. For example, an epidemiologic study may be designed to examine whether low blood pressure is associated with higher mortality in the elderly. However, another plausible explanation is that frailty at end-of-life may, for a variety of reasons, result in lower blood pressure. If so, intervention to raise blood pressure among elderly individuals with very low blood pressure would not be expected to improve outcomes—and may even cause harm. Study designs that establish temporal relationships may be more appropriate for research questions where reverse causation is a concern.

A final key aspect of the interpretation of epidemiological studies is the interpretation of the results. Results from the various study designs described above can be reported in a number of different ways. *Absolute risk* refers to the incidence of disease in a given population. For example, 30% of individuals who were exposed to tobacco products in a given population developed lung cancer. To determine whether tobacco products confer an excess risk, we compare the risk of lung cancer in those exposed to tobacco products to those unexposed to tobacco products. This can be accomplished by examining the difference in risk or by examining the ratio of the risks. If in this same cohort, individuals not exposed to tobacco products had a 5% risk of developing lung cancer, we would conclude that the *risk difference*, or *absolute increased risk*, of lung cancer from tobacco products in our population was 25% (30% − 5%). The ratio of risks, or *relative risk*, refers to the risk in the exposed relative the risk in the unexposed. Here, the disease risk in the exposed is 30%, while the disease risk in the unexposed is 5%, leading to a ratio of risks, or relative risk, of 6 (30%/5%). These same concepts can be applied to measures of odds when incidence rates cannot be calculated, such as in a case-control study design. Understanding absolute versus relative risk is critical to the successful interpretation of the results of a study. For example, a study may conclude that there is a twofold increased risk of disease from a given exposure. However, if the baseline risk in the unexposed group is 1%, a twofold increased risk of disease indicates only a 2% risk in the exposed group, or a 1% absolute increased risk. Therefore, while the twofold increased risk may be *statistically* significant and of a relatively large magnitude, the modest absolute increased risk may relegate it as a *clinically* insignificant finding. A complete discussion of how to empirically assess significance of findings, that is, statistical significance, is beyond the scope of this article. The practicing oncologist may access classical references in epidemiology or biostatistics,[38,39] or collaborate with a biostatistician. At the least, the oncologist should familiarize oneself with the question, "Is the effect something that is unlikely to be explained by chance?" Findings from observational studies need to be considered for generalizability (application outside the setting of the original study, i.e., "external validity") and bias (or other sources of explanation for cause and effect, i.e., "internal validity"). Further, for findings from observational studies to endure, they need to be replicated in appropriate populations or settings.

Molecular epidemiology

Molecular epidemiology and genetics

Understanding the genetic factors that predispose to cancer is useful for two reasons. The first is that understanding the genes involved in cancer initiation offers insights into cancer etiology and suggests hypotheses to the cancer biologist. Insights gleaned from etiology may suggest targets for cancer treatment[40] or insights into prevention.[41] It is confirming, though perhaps not surprising, that recent findings of genetic variants that are inherited often reflect those found from studies of the tumor with somatic, or postzygotic, noninherited, mutations.[42] The second reason is that knowledge of inherited forms of variation would in principle allow for the identification of individuals at highest risk of developing cancer and thus those who would benefit the most from forms of secondary prevention, such as enhanced screening, chemoprevention, or other tailored interventions for hereditary breast or colon cancers.[43,44]

Molecular epidemiology and genetic epidemiology are no longer clearly distinct fields. While genetic epidemiology primarily concerns the discovery and quantification of inherited genetic factors that predispose to disease, historically, molecular epidemiology could be broader, considering the "molecular level" of genetic or environmental risk factors. They have also been linked via chronology of approach. Traditionally, genetic epidemiology sought to identify alleles (specific nucleotide variation in inherited DNA) as cancer-causing via familial or population studies of cancer cases and suitably matched cancer-free controls. Family-based studies were based on segregation analyses or linkage studies of large, loaded pedigrees.[45] By contrast, a population-based approach is a case-control association study.[46] To follow up on localized genes from such studies, molecular epidemiology techniques such as positional gene cloning would be applied to understand protein and function. With the mapping of the human genome, medical resequencing projects, and the subsequent field of genome biology, this aspect of molecular epidemiology is either less necessary or conducted within the field of genetics using high-throughput techniques.[47] Approaches in molecular epidemiology have mushroomed to include studies of the epigenome, metabolome and microbiome, tumor molecular phenotypes, or other subfields of biology.

Genetic epidemiology

Family-based studies, such as analyses of large pedigrees, have helped elucidate the genetics of cancers of the breast,[48] pancreas,[49] and colon,[50] among others, in addition to Li–Fraumeni Syndrome, which is driven by mutations in P53 that confer risk of cancer in multiple organs.[51] These examples are of penetrant forms of DNA variation, that is, those with strong genetic effects where the probability of disease manifestation, given that the genetic variant is inherited, is relatively high. Such "simple" or Mendelian forms of variation were well studied historically for two reasons: (1) they presented in families and thus were inherently more tractable to analysis, and (2) they were amenable to analysis with data from merely hundreds of positions in the genome (loci). While classical pedigree studies of this variety remain useful, and linkage is a powerful tool in their analyses, modern genetic epidemiology has largely migrated to large-scale genetic surveys that were made possible by advances in molecular biotechnologies such as the DNA microarray and massively parallel ("next-generation") sequencing. These advances also complement the "postlinkage" strategies of genetic epidemiology, that is, those suited to study more "complex" forms of disease such as those with a larger number of causal genetic risk factors, each with a more modest effects, as well as being useful to conduct fine-mapping of signals found from linkage analysis.[52]

Modern, large-scale genetic epidemiological studies of cancer are comprised broadly of two forms of studies, or data types, namely genome-wide association studies (GWAS) using DNA single-nucleotide polymorphism (SNP) microarrays and next-generation sequencing[21] studies. Since nonfamilial cancers are relatively rare in the population, these studies are typically case-control studies, so that a large enough sample of cases can be obtained for analysis. In these studies, as opposed to other epidemiological studies, we can precisely measure the forms of variation (e.g., SNPs) and these sources of risk are thus not subject to recall bias. GWAS have a certain similarity to family-based studies in that in a GWAS one is looking for regions of the genome where cases (cancer patients) are more genetically similar to each other than they are to controls (cancer-free individuals). The simplest way to do this is to conduct a count of allele types among cases and controls at every measured position along the genome, which is typically 300K–5M SNP loci. Even if the causal variant is not measured directly, so long as it is frequent enough in the population it will be similar in distribution to genotypes at one of the measured loci nearby, since recombination events over generations of chromosomes in a population are infrequent in any one interval. In such cases, measuring one locus (e.g., a site measured directly via a SNP array) is a fine surrogate for a nearby unmeasured, potentially causal, locus. Thus, GWAS are well suited to settings where the causal variants are tagged well (of similar frequency, near a measured locus).

Typically, GWAS are conducted on a very large number of subjects (many hundreds to tens of thousands of participants), agnostically examining the entire genome, which is required to find variants with statistically significant but small effect sizes (relative risks of 1.05–1.2), that is, those sufficiently common to be measured well by a surrogate marker but would be missed by studies of loaded pedigrees with strong genetic effects. Indeed, variants found by these methods are expected to be of lower effect size for the following reasons: (1) if they had large effects, and were common, they would dominate the population and disease would be of high prevalence, which they are not; (2) in reality large effect sizes for an outcome such as cancer would likely be selected against in the population. Thus, effect sizes too small to be discovered by family studies of loaded pedigrees and yet too large to be amenable to discovery by GWAS require next-generation sequencing (NGS) studies capable of measuring rare variation directly. Rare variants require careful analysis since they will be too infrequent for standard statistical comparisons alone. Instead, what has emerged with the advent of NGS technologies are methods that intelligently group variants together and assess their aggregation by cases versus controls in these groups. The group, or unit of interest, that is commonly used for such discoveries is the gene, and a milieu of statistical methods have been developed for these studies.[53,54]

> **Gene X environment**
>
> In the age-old debate of Nature versus Nurture the two factors are presented as one or the other. In reality, the vast majority, if not all, human phenotypes are a product of contributions from both our genes and the environment (with "environment" here capturing a milieu of factors including nongenetic host factors including the microbiome). While these factors may contribute marginally (*BRCA* variations, mutations; time; tobacco exposure) to risk, it is possible that the specific combination of factors matters, that is, an interaction, or epistasis. Here, we examine differential risk for bladder cancer conferred by tobacco smoke, as a function of underlying genotype in the gene *NAT2*.[55] Variants in the *NAT2* gene determine whether individuals demonstrate fast or slow activity for *N*-acetyltransferase. This enzyme happens to act on arylamines, which include well-known bladder carcinogens, transforming them to arylamides. *N*-acetyltransferase competes in this step with N-oxidation, which transforms arylamines into active carcinogens. Thus, *NAT2* polymorphisms, which slow down *N*-acetylation, confer a risk for bladder cancer. Looking across multiple studies of individuals of European descent, investigators found heterogeneity in the effect of the *NAT2* polymorphism on cancer risk, with an overall effect of an odds ratio (OR) of 1.42. However, this heterogeneity went away when smokers were classified as "current" and "former." In fact, the risk of *NAT2* was solely in the group of current smokers with an OR of 1.74. Thus, *NAT2* does not confer risk *per se* but does so in the presence of an additional environmental factor, that is, active tobacco smoke.[56] That the effect is mitigated or null in ex-smokers suggests that the damage from this interaction is repairable, starting after cessation of tobacco use.

Gene expression
Gene expression or transcriptomics can be thought of as both phenotype (outcome of variation in primary sequence in DNA) and genotype (from a biologist's viewpoint: the on/off nature of a gene and its impact on traits in model organisms). In epidemiology, it serves as an *endo*-phenotype, downstream of gene and upstream of ultimate phenotype. Messenger RNA (mRNA) is less stable than DNA, and greater care must be taken to procure these nucleic acids for research analysis from samples. Yet, given it is often measured in clinical assays in studies from which other sources of "omics" may not exist, levels of mRNA for specific genes may provide a unique opportunity to study host genetics and epidemiological outcomes.[57] In contrast to mRNA, noncoding RNA is relatively stable. Noncoding RNA molecules are broadly categorized as long (>200 nucleotides) and short (<200 nucleotides), the latter of which include microRNA and short interfering RNA. Given their relative stability, these molecules serve as a rich and promising class of biomarkers.[58,59] The dynamics and forces of gene expression, including the impact of primary DNA variation, are expansive and consume the field of biology. However, one additional source of genetic variation that can be interpreted both as a regulator of expression and thus as genotype, as well as impacted by environment and thus as phenotype, is methylation and the field of epigenetics. Levels of methylation impact gene expression through interference with transcription factors and regulatory elements. Epigenetics and RNA are covered in detail elsewhere in this text.

Exposome
The development, improvement, and commercialization of high-throughput DNA sequencing technologies as well as large-scale initiatives such as the Human Genome Project led to accurate and cost-efficient detection of human genome variation; meanwhile, in this same period, there has been relatively little progress in developing new approaches to measuring environmental, occupational, and lifestyle exposures. Valid and reliable exposure assessment is a crucial element in epidemiologic studies. However, it is a challenging task because the researchers may not always know when to measure (timing of exposure relative to cancer development or progression), how many times to measure (for detecting exposure pattern), and may not have the best measurement tools (questionnaires or biomarkers). Furthermore, the health effects of an exposure may depend on many other factors. To address this problem, Christopher Wild in 2005[60] proposed the concept of the exposome (Figure 4), a model involving the study of the health effects of cumulative environmental exposures and simultaneous biological responses from conception until death.[61] Measuring the breadth of exposures that encompass the exposome requires the integration of information from multiple sources and -omics platforms. Recent developments in analytical instruments and tools, bioinformatics, and high-throughput -omics techniques like epigenomics, transcriptomics, proteomics, metabolomics, and lipidomics, are rapidly advancing the field; but not without the challenges that come with big data.

Metabolomics
The metabolome consists of all low molecular weight (<2000 Da) molecules present in a living system and represents a functional output of genes, epigenetic modifications, environmental and occupational exposures, lifestyle, diet, medications, and other external exposures including the microbiome.[62] It was recently estimated that the human metabolome may include more than one million compounds.[63] High-resolution mass spectrometry with advanced data extraction and annotation algorithms have been used to measure more than 20,000 chemicals in biological samples based upon mass resolution and mass accuracy. These chemicals provide an integrated measurement not only of exposure, but also of internal dose, biological response, altered function, and clinical disease, and include endogenous metabolites, environmental chemicals, dietary components, microbiome-produced metabolites, commercial products, and drugs.[61] Metabolomics is a promising tool for understanding tumor biology, development of biomarkers of exposure, and identifying new biomarkers of cancer risk and cancer progression.

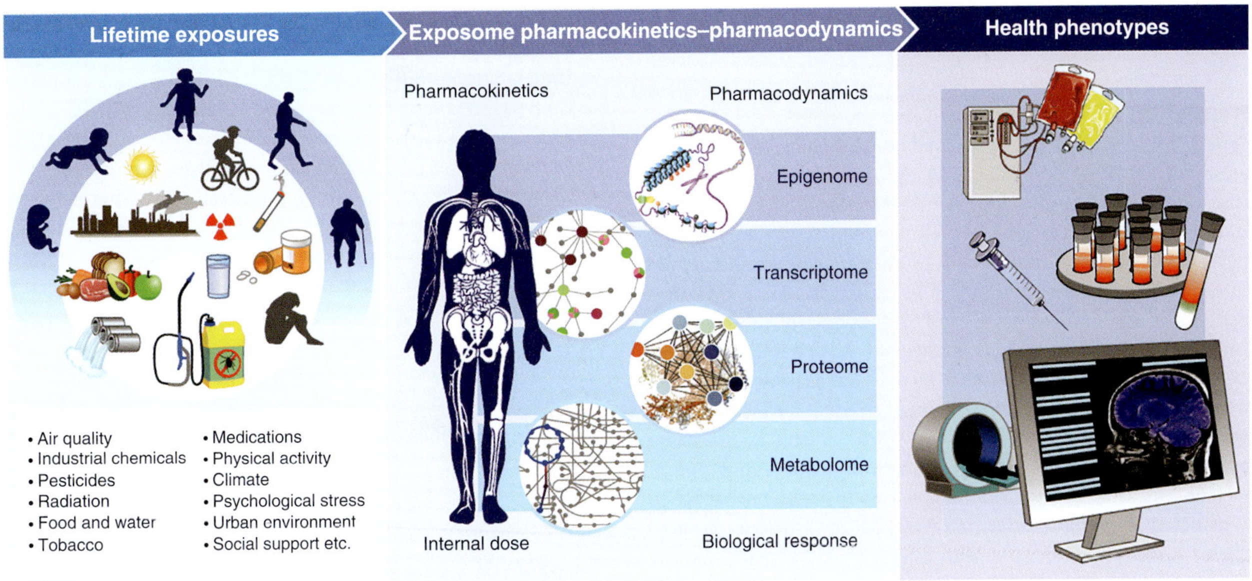

Figure 4 The exposome as an analytical framework linking exposures to health outcomes. Source: Niedzwiecki et al.[61]

Microbiome

The role of the microbiome in cancer, and how to modulate this process, is an area of intense and growing interest with estimates suggesting that microbial agents may cause ~20% of the global cancer burden.[64] The relationship between the microbiome and cancer is multifactorial and, likely, bidirectional. Cancer-associated changes in the microbiome may occur as a result of the emergence or presence of a tumor and may also contribute to cancer progression—both early and over the course of treatment. With microbial mechanisms reaching into several hallmarks of cancer risk (host metabolism, cellular proliferation, inflammation, and immunity), researchers are finding the microbiome to be a critical tool in investigations of cancer initiation, progression, response to therapy, and survival.[65]

The human gut harbors diverse and abundant microbes, creating a complex ecological system that interfaces with both the host and the environment and facilitates biologically relevant interactions between the two. The gut microbiome (collective genome of microorganisms in an environment) or microbiota (a community of microorganisms) comprise the "hidden" organ supporting host immunity, energy homeostasis, and nutrient metabolism. The breadth of the gut microbiome's capacity is reflected in the over three million genes it encodes, as well as the thousands of functional metabolites it produces (if not more, yet unknown). Although the gut microbiome has been most extensively studied, microorganisms also inhabit all of the barrier surfaces of the human, body including the skin, the oral cavity, the nasopharynx, the esophagus and stomach, and also the vagina, the urinary tract, the lungs.

Although the list of bacteria with established causal links to cancer remains relatively short, the hunt is on for any and all potential links between the microbiome and cancer risk with hopes that it may also be a useful early biomarker or tool for screening and diagnosis. A recent review and meta-analysis of 124 human epidemiologic studies identified the most consistent findings for *Fusobacterium, Porphyromonas,* and *Peptostreptococcus,* as being significantly enriched in fecal and mucosal samples of colorectal cancer patients. For the oral microbiome, higher and lower *Fusobacterium* and *Streptococcus*, respectively, were observed in oral cancer patients, as compared to controls.[66]

Fortunately for the host, the gut microbiome is redundant, adaptable, and resilient, such that an encounter with pathogenic bacteria is often not sufficient to cause cancer (with rare exceptions); and can be modulated by a range of different exogenous or endogenous exposures. In healthy individuals, medications (e.g., antibiotics, proton pump inhibitors, nonsteroidal anti-inflammatory drugs, metformin, statins) and diet are the primary culprits (or defense) with the greatest influence and relevance to cancer prevention.

Some of the most well-developed evidence and human prospective data suggesting that the microbiome is not only central to cancer prevention but also readily modifiable, relates to diet and gastrointestinal cancers, namely colorectal cancer. In prospective studies using tissue samples and data from the Nurses' Health Study and Health Professionals Follow-Up Study, Mehta et al.[67] found that a prudent diet rich in plant food sources of dietary fiber, as compared to a typical Western diet, is associated with lower risk of *Fusobacterium nucleatum (F. nucleatum)*-positive colorectal tumors but no association was observed with cancer arising from *F. nucleatum*-negative tumors. The presence of *F. nucleatum* has also been linked to a microenvironment that promotes the progression of colorectal neoplasia by inhibiting T-cell-mediated immune responses against colorectal tumors.[68,69] This is consistent with prior findings in small human feeding trials, where O'Keefe et al.[70] found that reciprocal changes in traditional diets (modulating both fiber and fat) in African Americans and native Africans over just 2 weeks resulted in dramatic changes in the composition and structure of the gut microbiome with parallel changes in an early marker of cancer risk within the colorectal epithelium. While extreme changes in diet can induce rapid alterations in the relative abundance of different bacteria with the gut, predominant phyla and overall structure of the microbial community are largely determined by inter-individual variation and long-term diet.[71,72] Epidemiologic studies have shed light on long-ingrained dietary patterns, for example, Western, Mediterranean, prudent, animal-based, and plant-based diet patterns that significantly contribute to variability in the diversity, composition, and function of the gut microbial community.[73–78]

Mendelian randomization
Genetic epidemiology can additionally provide tools to ask clinical questions that may be challenging or impractical to investigate using traditional study designs. A *Mendelian randomization* analysis is an example of a genetic epidemiology study design that utilizes genetic information to investigate causality of an exposure-outcome association.[79] This study design is akin to a "genetically randomized trial" and is particularly useful where confounding is suspected in traditional epidemiological studies and a randomized controlled trial is not feasible or ethical. Mendel's law of independent assortment states that alleles of genes are sorted independently. In other words, alleles contributing to different traits (such as an exposure of interest and potential confounders) are passed independently from one another. Consider a study interested in investigating whether elevated insulin levels are associated with endometrial cancer.[80] As elevated insulin levels may be associated with a variety of lifestyle factors that are also associated with increased endometrial cancer risk (e.g., obesity), nonrandomized studies are unlikely to fully account for confounding and randomization is not feasible or ethical. Under the above-mentioned Mendel's law of independent assortment, individuals are randomly assigned to varying insulin levels via inherited alleles, independent of alleles impacting confounders, such as obesity. Using this design, a genetically conferred elevation in insulin levels should only be associated with increased endometrial cancer risk if a causal relationship exists. This approach is dependent on three primary assumptions: first, that the genetic variants utilized are associated with the risk factor (e.g., insulin levels); second, that the variants are not associated with other confounders (e.g., obesity); and third, that the variants impact the outcome (e.g., endometrial cancer) only through the exposure-outcome pathway being investigated. In addition to the exposition here, the interested reader may investigate the applications to colon cancer, as well.[81] When appropriately designed, Mendelian randomization offers a powerful strategy from genetic epidemiology to investigate causality.

Future directions
Cancer epidemiology as a field exhibits some maturity. Modifiable behaviors have been identified that could prevent ~40% of cancers and cancer deaths in the United States.[17] Yet, writ broadly, the field still possesses significant untapped potential. We still know only the major contributors to disease initiation. A continued explosion in available data—generated by advances in biotechnologies, imaging, computing, and data science—offers a heretofore unparalleled opportunity to measure our physical, built, and innate environments. Quantification of exposures from these environments, linked to cancer incidence and outcomes, offers us the chance to quantify the risk and inform strategies for personal prevention and policy.

As we look forward to the next 5–10 years in the field of cancer epidemiology, we should not be surprised to observe the following trends in technique, discovery, and innovation:

- Integration of multiple exposures using improved exposure assessment through both "asking the right and complete questions," as in classical epidemiology, but also in molecular epidemiology from informative biological correlates through technology (e.g., metabolomics, microbiomics, tumor markers, wearable "smart" devices);
- Understanding differences in risk factors for cancer molecular subtypes, strengthening our knowledge about cancer etiology, which will lead to development of precision-based, personalized primary and secondary prevention strategies;
- Discovery of genetic variants of moderate effect, rare in the population but discoverable by sequencing, identifying individuals most at risk and who would benefit from enhanced screening or personalized prevention;
- "Big data" from medical claims and machine learning (e.g., for detecting cancer features in pathology slides or inference of features from electronic health records); and
- An aspirational collaborative enrollment in studies, with broad and inclusive participation from communities of diverse racial, ethnic, and economic backgrounds.

COVID-19
As of publication, "epidemiology" has perhaps never been so popularly examined—by scientists and the lay public alike—due to the novel coronavirus disease of 2019 (COVID-19). The discipline, in general, including methods of testing and surveillance, analysis of data, and interpretation of risk has been roundly examined and the importance of population health and its communication to the public has seeped into a collective consciousness. The effects of COVID-19 on cancer are still being determined, although there is little doubt that the immune-suppressed, such as for cancer patients undergoing therapy, represent a vulnerable population. It is even possible that lessons from oncologists treating patients with immune therapies may port to the setting of treating cytokine storms in patients with COVID-19 with interleukin 6 (IL-6) inhibitors, though the efficacy of this is still very much unknown.[82,83] Regardless, due to COVID-19 as a comorbidity, cancer epidemiologists may need to note this era in particular when modeling clinical outcomes. In addition to effects on cancer treatment, delays of screenings or initiation of risk-inducing behaviors may impact the cancer burden in the United States.

Acknowledgments
The authors would like to thank and acknowledge Dr. David Chang for his assistance in identifying the key references and managing the article's bibliography.

Key references
The complete reference list can be found on Vital Source version of this title, see inside front cover.

2. Doll R, Peto R. The causes of cancer: quantitative estimates of avoidable risks of cancer in the United States today. *J Natl Cancer Inst*. 1981;**66**(6):1191–1308.
3. Blot WJ, Tarone RE. Doll and Peto's quantitative estimates of cancer risks: holding generally true for 35 years. *J Natl Cancer Inst*. 2015;**107**(4):djv044.
5. Gallaway MS, Henley SJ, Steele CB, et al. Surveillance for cancers associated with tobacco use - United States, 2010-2014. *MMWR Surveill Summ*. 2018;**67**(12):1–42.
7. Jensen OM, Parkin DM, MacLennan R, et al. (eds). *Cancer Registration: Principles and Methods; IARC Scientific Publication No. 95*. Lyon, France: IARC Publications; 1991.
8. Bray F, Ferlay J, Soerjomataram I, et al. Global cancer statistics 2018: GLOBOCAN estimates of incidence and mortality worldwide for 36 cancers in 185 countries. *CA Cancer J Clin*. 2018;**68**(6):394–424.
9. Siegel RL, Miller KD, Jemal A. Cancer statistics, 2020. *CA Cancer J Clin*. 2020;**70**(1):7–30.

10. Negoita S, Feuer EJ, Mariotto A, et al. Annual Report to the Nation on the Status of Cancer, part II: recent changes in prostate cancer trends and disease characteristics. *Cancer*. 2018;**124**(13):2801–2814.
11. Virostko J, Capasso A, Yankeelov TE, Goodgame B. Recent trends in the age at diagnosis of colorectal cancer in the US National Cancer Data Base, 2004-2015. *Cancer*. 2019;**125**(21):3828–3835.
12. American Cancer Society. *Cancer Facts & Figures 2020*. Atlanta, GA: American Cancer Society; 2020.
13. Pfeiffer RM, Webb-Vargas Y, Wheeler W, Gail MH. Proportion of U.S. trends in breast cancer incidence attributable to long-term changes in risk factor distributions. *Cancer Epidemiol Biomark Prev*. 2018;**27**(10):1214–1222.
17. Islami F, Goding Sauer A, Miller KD, et al. Proportion and number of cancer cases and deaths attributable to potentially modifiable risk factors in the United States. *CA Cancer J Clin*. 2018;**68**(1):31–54.
18. IARC Monograph. *Alcohol Consumption and Ethyl Carbamate*. Lyon, France: World Health Organization; 2010:1440.
19. IARC Monograph. *Personal Habits and Indoor Combustions*. Lyon, France: World Health Organization; 2012:598.
23. World Cancer Research Fund/American Institute for Cancer Research. Diet, nutrition, physical activity and cancer: a global perspective. Continuous update Project Expert Report. WCRF International; 2018.
24. Sung H, Siegel RL, Rosenberg PS, Jemal A. Emerging cancer trends among young adults in the USA: analysis of a population-based cancer registry. *Lancet Public Health*. 2019;**4**(3):e137–e147.
30. Ward E, Jemal A, Cokkinides V, et al. Cancer disparities by race/ethnicity and socioeconomic status. *CA Cancer J Clin*. 2004;**54**(2):78–93.
34. Hardefeldt PJ, Penninkilampi R, Edirimanne S, Eslick GD. Physical activity and weight loss reduce the risk of breast cancer: a meta-analysis of 139 prospective and retrospective studies. *Clin Breast Cancer*. 2018;**18**(4):e601–e612.
35. Friedenreich CM, Stone CR, Cheung WY, Hayes SC. Physical activity and mortality in cancer survivors: a systematic review and meta-analysis. *JNCI Cancer Spectr*. 2020;**4**(1):pkz080.
36. Patel AV, Friedenreich CM, Moore SC, et al. American college of sports medicine roundtable report on physical activity, sedentary behavior, and cancer prevention and control. *Med Sci Sports Exerc*. 2019;**51**(11):2391–2402.
38. Weiss NS, Koepsell TD. *Epidemiology Methods: Studying the Occurrence of Illness*, 2nd ed. New York: Oxford University Press; 2014:480.
39. Rosner B. *Fundamental of Biostatistics*, 7th ed. Cengage Learning: Boston, MA; 2010:888.
42. Carter H, Marty R, Hofree M, et al. Interaction landscape of inherited polymorphisms with somatic events in cancer. *Cancer Discov*. 2017;**7**(4):410–423.
45. Ott J. *Analysis of Human Genetic Linkage*. Baltimore, MD: Johns Hopkins University Press; 1999:416.
46. Tam V, Patel N, Turcotte M, et al. Benefits and limitations of genome-wide association studies. *Nat Rev Genet*. 2019;**20**(8):467–484.
52. Duggal P, Ladd-Acosta C, Ray D, Beaty TH. The evolving field of genetic epidemiology: from familial aggregation to genomic sequencing. *Am J Epidemiol*. 2019;**188**(12):2069–2077.
53. Li B, Leal SM. Methods for detecting associations with rare variants for common diseases: application to analysis of sequence data. *Am J Hum Genet*. 2008;**83**(3):311–321.
54. Yandell M, Huff C, Hu H, et al. A probabilistic disease-gene finder for personal genomes. *Genome Res*. 2011;**21**(9):1529–1542.
58. Sarfi M, Abbastabar M, Khalili E. Long noncoding RNAs biomarker-based cancer assessment. *J Cell Physiol*. 2019;**234**(10):16971–16986.
59. Anfossi S, Babayan A, Pantel K, Calin GA. Clinical utility of circulating non-coding RNAs – an update. *Nat Rev Clin Oncol*. 2018;**15**(9):541–563.
60. Wild CP. Complementing the genome with an "exposome": the outstanding challenge of environmental exposure measurement in molecular epidemiology. *Cancer Epidemiol Biomark Prev*. 2005;**14**(8):1847–1850.
61. Niedzwiecki MM, Walker DI, Vermeulen R, et al. The exposome: molecules to populations. *Annu Rev Pharmacol Toxicol*. 2019;**59**:107–127.
62. Jones DP, Park Y, Ziegler TR. Nutritional metabolomics: progress in addressing complexity in diet and health. *Annu Rev Nutr*. 2012;**32**:183–202.
63. Uppal K, Walker DI, Liu K, et al. Computational metabolomics: a framework for the million metabolome. *Chem Res Toxicol*. 2016;**29**(12):1956–1975.
64. De Flora S, La Maestra S. Epidemiology of cancers of infectious origin and prevention strategies. *J Prev Med Hyg*. 2015;**56**(1):E15–E20.
65. McQuade JL, Daniel CR, Helmink BA, Wargo JA. Modulating the microbiome to improve therapeutic response in cancer. *Lancet Oncol*. 2019;**20**(2):e77–e91.
66. Huybrechts I, Zouiouich S, Loobuyck A, et al. The human microbiome in relation to cancer risk: a systematic review of epidemiologic studies. *Cancer Epidemiol Biomark Prev*. 2020;**29**(10):1856–1868.
79. Davies NM, Holmes MV, Davey SG. Reading Mendelian randomisation studies: a guide, glossary, and checklist for clinicians. *BMJ*. 2018;**362**:k601.
80. Nead KT, Sharp SJ, Thompson DJ, et al. Evidence of a causal association between insulinemia and endometrial cancer: a Mendelian randomization analysis. *J Natl Cancer Inst*. 2015;**107**(9):djv178.
81. Cornish AJ, Law PJ, Timofeeva M, et al. Modifiable pathways for colorectal cancer: a mendelian randomisation analysis. *Lancet Gastroenterol Hepatol*. 2020;**5**(1):55–62.

32 Hereditary cancer syndromes: risk assessment and genetic counseling

Rachel Bluebond, MS ■ Sarah A. Bannon, MS ■ Samuel M. Hyde, MS ■ Ashley H. Woodson, MS ■ Nancy Y.-Q. You, MD ■ Karen H. Lu, MD ■ Banu Arun, MD

Overview

Understanding the etiology of cancer combines a multitude of factors including genetic, environmental, health, and lifestyle influences on the pathway to malignancy. While single-gene inherited causes for cancer account for only 5–10% of cancer cases, identifying these individuals and their family members can provide insight into tumorigenesis, improvement in therapeutic outcomes, prevention of new primary cancers, and identifying family members that may carry the same germline mutation. The process of evaluating an individual's cancer history as well as his or her family history is key in ascertaining those at risk for hereditary cancer. Indeed, several professional organizations recognize the importance of systematic and proficient hereditary cancer assessment. The American Society of Clinical Oncology has attested to the importance of identifying and managing of individuals with inherited susceptibility to cancer as a key aspect to oncology care with specific attention to the following areas: germline implications of somatic mutation profiling, multigene panel testing for cancer susceptibility, quality assurance in genetic testing, education of oncology professionals, and access to cancer genetic services.[1] Genetic counseling is the process of helping individuals recognize and interpret the medical, psychological, and familial implications of the genetic contributions of disease.[2] Given the complicated nature of understanding genetic risks and implications for patient and family members, pretest genetic counseling aid in both accurate hereditary cancer assessment and facilitating patient understanding. The genetic counseling interaction includes information gathering, establishing or verifying diagnosis, risk assessment, information giving, and psychological support.[3] Given the established expertise required to assess hereditary cancer risks, genetic counseling is rapidly becoming a standard of care for patients. While not all institutions have access to genetic counseling services, the Commission on Cancer (CoC) suggests programs without immediate access to formal genetic counseling services identify resources for referral to patients needing assessment.[4]

Risk assessment and risk models

The process of risk assessment includes thorough evaluation of an individual's personal history of cancer, family history of cancer, consideration of potential hereditary cancer syndromes present with likelihood of a germline mutation, and calculation of both hereditary and empiric risks of developing cancer. The importance of these aspects in hereditary cancer risk assessment has been acknowledged by several organizations: the United States Preventative Services Task Force (USPSTF), the National Comprehensive Cancer Network (NCCN), and the CoC.[4–6] Factors significant in an individual's medical history include cancer diagnoses, pathology of the tumor, age of diagnosis, environmental and lifestyle exposures, and preventative surgeries or cancer screening that help assess potential cancer risks.[7] Similar information should be extended to the family history assessment which includes a three-generation collection of all first-, second-, and often third-degree relatives with the purpose of evaluating cancer history patterns. General strategies for obtaining and evaluating the cancer family history include confirmation on tumor diagnoses, evaluating nonmalignant findings (i.e., macrocephaly with Cowden syndrome (CS), dermatologic features associated with several hereditary cancer syndromes), consideration of the accuracy of the historian, and utilizing established standardized pedigree nomenclature.[8] Features suggestive of a hereditary cancer syndrome may be present in an individual alone or in combination with the information gathered in a family history. Typical patterns of hereditary cancer include an individual diagnosed at an earlier than general population age for presenting cancer, multiple primary tumors with the same or different organ sites, rare or suggestive histology, associated genetic traits or congenital defects, and associated cutaneous lesions known to be related to a particular disorder.[9] Within a family history, features of an inherited cancer pattern include three generations of the same or related cancer histories (i.e., breast and/or ovarian cancer, colon and/or uterine cancer) and one or more family members diagnosed at an earlier ages than the general population as defined by a particular cancer syndrome.[6,9] In addition to personal and family cancer history assessments performed by the clinician, several models have been developed to quantify the effect of these risk factors to predict either risk of developing a particular cancer or risk of carrying a high-risk germline genetic mutation. Models such as Gail, also known as NCI model or Breast Cancer Risk Assessment Tool, the Care model specifically for African American, and Claus model based on family history of breast cancer women predict risk of a woman to develop breast cancer.[10–12] Clinicians may utilize the Myriad I and II, Couch model, or BRCAPRO model to predict likelihood of a genetic carrier status for hereditary breast and ovarian cancer.[13–16] There are varying strengths and limitations of each model and identifying an appropriate model for assessment involves expertise in understanding the study demographics used in validating the models.[17] Models predicting risk for germline DNA mismatch repair (MMR) gene mutations, such as MMRpro, PREMM$_{1,2,6}$, and MMRpredict, are also available and useful in determine individuals who may benefit from genetic testing along with clinical assessment.[18–20] If genetic testing and a pathogenic germline mutation identified, Braun et al. created a tool to help clinicians interpret age-related cancer risks based on patient individual age and patient information. The tool, ASK2ME (all syndromes known to man evaluator), delivers absolute cancer risk estimates for various hereditary cancer susceptibility genes.[21]

Given hereditary cancer is rare, it is important to recognize other multifactorial genetic risks that may explain family histories of cancer. Considering population-based registries is critical in assessing magnitude of familial risk, as most individuals with a family history of cancer will utilize this data in cancer risk management decisions. Based on the Utah Population Database, the majority of cancer sites have a familial relative risk (RR) between 2.0 and 3.0, this risk may be higher for certain cancers, such as prostate, breast, and colorectal, when the family history consists of earlier ages of onset.[22] This highlights the multiple contributing factors that cause familial clustering of certain cancers. It is still pertinent to understand these RRs as they may still guide individuals to pursue additional high-risk screening options or more frequent exams in recognition of the higher risk for cancer.

Hereditary breast cancer and gynecologic cancer syndromes

The National Cancer Institute Surveillance, Epidemiology, and End Results Program estimates that approximately 12.4% of American women will be diagnosed with breast cancer in their lifetime, and 1.3% will be diagnosed with ovarian cancer.[23] An estimated 5–10% of breast cancer and 10–15% of ovarian cancer diagnoses are due to an underlying hereditary predisposition.[24] Factors indicative of heritable cancer risk include young age at diagnosis, family history indicative an autosomal dominant hereditary cancer syndrome, certain pathological findings, and bilateral disease.[25] Since the identification of *BRCA1* and *BRCA2* in 1994 and 1995 respectively, the understanding of hereditary breast and ovarian cancers has grown exponentially with predictive testing allowing for tailored cancer treatment, screening, and prevention.[26,27] Mutations in a number of other genes are now recognized to also confer a heightened risk for breast and/or gynecologic cancer. This section will review these hereditary syndromes and moderate penetrance genetic risk factors.

Hereditary breast and ovarian cancer syndrome

Pathogenic germline mutations in *BRCA1* and *BRCA2* are best known for their association with hereditary breast and ovarian cancer syndrome (HBOC). Mutation prevalence in the general population is believed to be up to 0.406% with higher prevalence in individuals of Ashkenazi Jewish descent at a rate of 2.74%.[28,29] Early-onset breast cancer, triple-negative breast cancer, personal and/or family history of ovarian cancer, Ashkenazi Jewish ancestry, and family history of breast cancer are all known to be predictors of *BRCA1/BRCA2* carrier status.[29–31] While the female breast cancer risk to age 70 is widely quoted as up to 87%, more comprehensive studies have estimated the risk as 57–65% and 45–55% for *BRCA1* and *BRCA2*, respectively.[32–36] Ovarian cancer risks are estimated at 39–59% in *BRCA1* and 11–18% in *BRCA2*.[34–36] Men with pathogenic mutations in *BRCA1* and *BRCA2* are known to be at an 1.2–6.8% risk of male breast cancer and an elevated risk for prostate cancer, with higher cancer rates associated with *BRCA2* mutations.[37] Both male and female *BRCA2* mutation carriers are shown to be at a 3.5-fold-risk of pancreatic cancer.[38] There is some evidence showing an association between melanoma and *BRCA2* mutation status, although specific risk estimates are unavailable.[39] More details on HBOC-related pancreatic and prostate cancers can be found in later sections of this article.

Due to the associated cancer risks, tailored management recommendations for individuals with HBOC include enhanced surveillance and prophylactic surgical options. While specific guidelines vary slightly from one professional organization to another, guidelines generally include the following:

1. Clinical breast examination and education on breast awareness annually starting at age 25 or 10 years prior to the earliest breast cancer in the family,
2. Annual breast MRI from age 25 to 29,
3. Annual breast MRI and annual mammography screening starting at age 30, often staggered to shorten the interval between exam and every 6 months,
4. Consider bilateral risk-reducing mastectomy, with discussion on the impact of gene mutation, residual cancer risk, life expectancy, and risks/benefits,
5. Consider risk-reducing bilateral salpingo-oophorectomy in women typically between ages 35 and 40; individualized based on childbearing, comorbidities, family history, and gene mutation,
6. While data has not shown reduction in mortality, biannual transvaginal ultrasound and serum CA-125 screening beginning at age 30 are appropriate until time of risk-reducing bilateral salpingo-oophorectomy,
7. Discussion of lifestyle modifications to reduce cancer risk,
8. Consideration of pancreatic cancer screening depending on gene mutation and family history of cancer risk (see Hereditary pancreatic cancer section),
9. Consideration of annual dermatology exam depending on other risk factors and gene mutation, and
10. Annual breast and prostate cancer exams may be indicated for male carriers, particularly for those with *BRCA1* mutations.[40,41]

In addition to the screening and prevention guidelines tailored to *BRCA1* and *BRCA2* status, recently there have been major changes in implication for treatment recommendations of HBOC related ovarian and breast cancers, using PARP inhibitors.[42–44] These are developing rapidly and up-to-date data should be considered at the time of interest.

HBOC is inherited in an autosomal dominant pattern. Sequence analysis of *BRCA1* and *BRCA2* identifies approximately 90% of mutations with the remaining alterations requiring large rearrangement analysis (deletion/duplication).[45,46] Three founder mutations (*BRCA1* 185delAG, *BRCA1* 5382insC, and *BRCA2* 6174delT) are common in the Ashkenazi Jewish population.[28,47,48] Due to the highly likelihood of identifying one of these founder mutations in individuals of Ashkenazi descent undergoing genetic testing, common practice dictates beginning genetic testing with targeted founder mutation analysis prior to undergoing more comprehensive testing. Additionally, data suggests that proceeding to comprehensive analysis may only be indicated in individuals with personal and family cancer histories highly indicative of HBOC.[48] Since the introduction of next-generation sequencing (NGS) and the invalidation of a patent on *BRCA1* and *BRCA2*, the cost of genetic testing has decreased dramatically. This, along with the improved understanding of other hereditary predispositions to breast cancer, has led to beginning testing with hereditary cancer panel tests examining multiple genes at once.[49,50]

Li–Fraumeni syndrome

Li–Fraumeni syndrome is caused by germline mutations in *TP53*.[51,52] This is a rare condition with a general population prevalence estimated to be as high as 1 in 5000 to 1 in 20,000.[53,54] Li–Fraumeni syndrome was first described in families with high rates of cancers, particularly soft-tissue sarcomas and breast cancers.[55,56] This led to the classic criteria of the syndrome, defining Li–Fraumeni syndrome as a combination of an individual diagnosed at less than 45 years old with a sarcoma with a first-degree relative (FDR) diagnosed with cancer before age 45 and an additional first or second degree relative with cancer prior to age 45 or a sarcoma at any age.[56]

The tumor spectrum in this condition now includes breast cancer, soft tissue sarcoma, osteosarcoma, CNS tumors, and adrenocortical carcinoma, although many other types of cancer have been seen in individuals with Li–Fraumeni syndrome.[57] While research is still required to determine specific cancer risks, one cohort found breast cancer in 60% of affected individuals, soft tissue sarcoma in 27%, osteosarcoma in 16%, CNS tumors in 13%, and adrenocortical carcinomas in 13%.[58] Women are estimated to have a 93% risk of cancer by age 50 whereas men have a 68% with women also experiencing higher rates of cancers at young ages.[59] Multiple primary tumors have been described at high rates, 43% of mutation carriers in one study.[57,58]

To account for the variable cancer rates and the wide spectrum of cancers, the Chompret criteria for testing are often used to determine which patients may benefit from germline *TP53* testing, with an estimated 20% of individuals meeting the criteria having a detectable *TP53* mutation.[60] These include the following:

- A proband with a Li–Fraumeni associated tumor such as a soft tissue sarcoma, osteosarcoma, brain tumor, breast cancer, or adrenocortical carcinoma before age 46 with at least one first or second degree relative with a Li–Fraumeni associated tumor (with the exception of breast cancer if the proband has breast cancer) before age 56,
- A proband with multiple tumors (except multiple breast tumors) with at least one Li–Fraumeni associated tumor and the first tumor occurring before age 46, or
- A proband with an adrenocortical carcinoma or a choroid plexus tumor, regardless of family history.[60]

Testing for women with breast cancer prior to age 31 is also advised as there is a 6% likelihood of a pathogenic *TP53* mutation.[58,61] This is likely due in part to the 7–20% *de novo* rate.[62] While sequencing of the entire coding region is believed to identify approximately 95% of mutations, deletion/duplication analysis is still necessary as deletions involving the promoter region and exon 1 have been described.[54,63,64]

Cancer screening and risk reduction are of utmost importance for individuals with Li–Fraumeni Syndrome. As significant radiation sensitivity with a risk for radiation-induced cancers is noted, special care must be given to reduce radiation exposure to mutation carriers in planning screening protocols and treatment.[65] A screening protocol introduced in 2011 including pediatric and adult recommendations was introduced for asymptomatic individuals.[66] In 2016, this was expanded to include the use of whole-body MRI in addition to the existing recommendations for biochemical tests, targeted brain and breast MRI, physical exam, abdominal ultrasound, colonoscopy, and consideration of risk-reducing bilateral mastectomy.[67] The inclusion of whole-body MRI has been noted to identify a significant number of asymptomatic tumors, particularly because individuals Li–Fraumeni syndrome have a propensity to develop many types of cancers including those beyond the classing Li–Fraumeni spectrum.[68] Professional guidelines, including the NCCN, have supported this screening protocol with recommendations for whole-body MRI.[41] As outcomes data and low-radiation screening technologies develop, these screening protocols will likely continue to develop.

Other high-risk breast cancer syndromes (CDH1, PTEN, STK11)

In addition to the hereditary breast cancer syndromes already discussed in this article, there are a number of well-described hereditary cancer syndromes that with a lesser association with breast cancer. These conditions confer a high cancer risk, but breast cancer is not necessarily the key feature. These include CS, hereditary diffuse gastric cancer (HDGC), and Peutz–Jeghers syndrome (PJS). These conditions are summarized in this section but are further discussed in the section titled "Hereditary gastrointestinal cancers".

Cowden syndrome

CS, also known as *PTEN*-Hamartoma-Tumor syndrome, is associated with pathogenic mutations in the *PTEN* gene.[69] CS is associated with a wide spectrum of benign and malignant tumors, including a 22–85% risk for female breast cancer, 35.2% risk for epithelial thyroid cancer, 28.2% risk for endometrial cancer, 9% risk for colorectal cancer (CRC), 33.6% risk for kidney cancer, and a 6% risk for melanoma.[70,71] The risks for melanoma and kidney cancer are controversial, as there are limitations in available data.[72] The following nonmalignant features are also found in CS: macrocephaly, trichilemmomas, papillomatous papules, acral keratoses, lipomas, palmoplantar keratoses, arteriovenous malformations (AVM), hemangiomas, Lhermitte–Duclos disease, fibrocystic breast disease, gastrointestinal hamartomas, uterine fibroids, multinodular goiter, autism, and macular pigmentations of the glans penis.[72–75] Given the wide spectrum of cancers and nonmalignant associations, diagnostic and testing guidelines exist. Testing of the *PTEN* gene should be considered in an individual with a known familial *PTEN* mutation or meeting the clinical diagnostic criteria summarized in the following table.[72–76] Management of individuals with CS should be tailored to the cancer risks seen, often including various screening and consideration of prophylactic surgeries.[75] Consider up-to-date professional guidelines for screening.

An individual with a personal history of:	Major criteria	Minor criteria
Bannayan–Riley–Ruvalcaba syndrome	Breast cancer	Autism spectrum disorder
Adult Lhermitte–Duclos disease	Endometrial cancer	Colon cancer
Autism spectrum disorder and macrocephaly	Follicular thyroid cancer	Esophageal glycogenic acanthosis (≥3)
Two or more biopsy-proven trichilemmomas	Multiple gastrointestinal hamartomas or ganglioneuromas	Lipomas
Two or more major criteria with one being macrocephaly	Macrocephaly (≥97th percentile)	Mental retardation (IQ ≤75)
Three major criteria without macrocephaly	Macular pigmentation of glans penis	Papillary or follicular variant of papillary thyroid cancer
One major and three minor criteria	Mucocutaneous lesions along if: one biopsy-proven trichilemmoma, multiple palmoplantar keratoses, multifocal or extensive oral mucosal papillomatosis, or multiple cutaneous facial papules	Thyroid structural lesions
Four minor criteria		Renal cell carcinoma Single gastrointestinal hamartoma or ganglioneuroma Testicular lipomatosis Vascular anomalies

Hereditary diffuse gastric cancer

HDGC is associated with germline mutations in the E-cadherin gene (*CDH1*).[77,78] Individuals with mutation in *CDH1* are primarily predisposed to diffuse-type gastric cancer, but women with this condition are also shown to be at an approximately 40% lifetime risk for lobular breast cancer.[79] In addition to management recommendations tailored to the gastric cancer risk, annual breast MRI and mammography screening are recommended for women 35 years and older.[80] Surgical considerations are made based on family history and personal risk factors. For additional details on HDGC, please see the details in the section titled "Hereditary gastric cancer".

Peutz–Jeghers syndrome

PJS is caused by mutations in *STK11* found in 1 in 25,000 to 1 in 280,000 individuals.[81] PJS is best known for the common presenting symptom of mucocutaneous macules on the mouth, eyes, nostrils, perianal area, and/or buccal mucosa.[82,83] Cancer risks are further described in the section titled "Hereditary gastrointestinal cancers," but generally include gastrointestinal cancers (including small bowel, gastroesophageal, pancreatic, and colorectal), breast cancer, and gynecologic cancers (uterine, ovarian, and cervical).[75,84] Specific pathologies and cancer risks of gynecologic cancers are reported as 10% lifetime likelihood of adenoma malignum of the cervix, 21% likelihood of mucinous and sex cord-stromal tumors of the ovary, 9% likelihood of uterine cancer, and 32–50% likelihood of breast cancer.[84–88] The Dutch breast and gynecologic surveillance recommendations include annual breast exam and breast MRI starting at age 25, annual mammography and breast MRI starting at age 30, and annual pelvic exam, cervical smear, transvaginal ultrasonography, and CA-125 starting between ages 25 and 30.[89] Further recommendations pertaining to the risk of gastrointestinal and pancreatic cancers exist and are further described in the corresponding sections.

Lynch syndrome

Lynch syndrome is associated with a 16–54% risk for endometrial cancer and a 1–24% risk for ovarian cancer, depending on the gene affected.[90,91] These substantially increased risks warrant medical intervention. Details on the cancer risks, genetic testing protocols, and medical interventions associated with Lynch syndrome can be found in the section titled "Hereditary CRC syndromes".

Moderate risk breast and ovarian cancer predispositions

In addition to available testing for a myriad of high-risk hereditary predispositions to breast and gynecologic cancers, the advances of NGS have allowed for fast, high-quality, low-cost genetic testing options for several genes at once. The risks associated with the genes now included on these panels are not consistent and individually require evaluation when considering clinical implications. The professional guidelines and clinical management recommendations of individuals carrying a pathogenic mutation in one of these genes are quickly evolving and will likely change in the future.

Moderate risks for developing breast cancer have been described in women with mutations in *ATM, CHEK2, NBN,* and *PALB2*.[92–96] Lifetime breast cancer risks are described as 30%, 32%, 30%, and 44% for *ATM, CHEK2, NBN* (657del5 founder mutation only), and *PALB2* respectively, although limitations are noted for each gene.[97] *ATM*, with a general population carrier frequency believed to be as high as 1%, is also involved in the autosomal recessive condition of Ataxia-Telangiectasia, requiring reproductive counseling on risks for children.[98] The vast majority of data available on *CHEK2* comes from the 1100delC founder mutation; other mutations, the I157T variant, in particular, have not shown the same level of cancer risk with estimated breast cancer risks only mildly elevated.[97,99,100] The founder mutation in *NBN* has been found to be associated with breast cancer rates similar to that of *ATM*, yet the association with breast cancer does not seem to generalize to the rest of mutations in that gene.[94,97,101,102] Many genetic testing panels offer comprehensive analysis of *NBN*, so mutation-specific risks are warranted. Lastly, while *PALB2* is noted to have a breast cancer association bordering on high risk, the breast cancer risk appears to be significantly impacted by family history of cancers in addition to the presence of a mutation.[92] Given the moderately elevated risks for breast cancer, high-risk breast cancer screening with annual mammography and breast-MRI with initiation based on age-related risk and family history.[41,97]

In parallel to the breast cancer genes discussed above, moderate risk for developing ovarian cancer has been described in women with mutations in *BRIP1, RAD51C,* and *RAD51D*.[103–105] The lifetime ovarian cancer risks are reported to be 3.4–11.2%, 5.2%, and 12% for *BRIP1, RAD51C,* and *RAD51D*, respectively.[103–105] Risks vary depending on study design, study population, and family history, but all show a significantly elevated ovarian cancer risk with mutation status. In contrast to the moderate risk breast cancer genes above, ovarian cancer screening is not considered effective. Prophylactic risk-reducing salpingo-oophorectomy is indicated for carriers around menopause, though the specific age at surgical intervention is still debated.[41,97,106]

Hereditary colorectal cancer syndromes

CRC is the third most common cancer diagnosed in the United States, with an estimated 135,430 new cases per year, and the second leading cause of cancer death. The lifetime risk to develop CRC in both men and women in the general population is 4.3%.[97] Familial and hereditary predispositions to CRC have been well-characterized and a family history of CRC is known to increase the risk in close relatives. Approximately 5–10% of CRCs are due to an inherited predisposition, accounted for by up to 17 associated predisposition genes.[107]

Lynch syndrome (hereditary nonpolyposis colorectal cancer)

Lynch syndrome, also known as hereditary nonpolyposis colorectal cancer (HNPCC), is the most common inherited predisposition syndrome for CRC. It affects approximately 1 in 300 people[108,109] and accounts for 1–3% of CRCs and 0.8–1.4% of endometrial cancers.[18,110–112] Lynch syndrome is caused by inherited mutations in the DNA MMR genes, *MLH1*, *MSH2*, *MSH6*, and *PMS2*, or by deletions in the 5′ untranslated region (UTR) of the gene *EPCAM*, upstream of *MSH2*.[113,114] Individuals with germline mutations in the MMR genes are at increased lifetime risks for CRC (ranging from 20% to 80%), as well as for extracolonic cancers including endometrial, gastric, small bowel, hepatobiliary tract, upper urinary tract, sebaceous neoplasms, and malignant brain tumors.[115,116] Gene-specific cancer risks are well characterized. Mutations in *MLH1* and *MSH2* confer the highest lifetime risks for CRC. The lifetime risk for Lynch syndrome-associated CRC ranges between 27% and 74% for men, and 22–53% for women, and that for endometrial cancer ranges between 14% and 54%. Patients are at risk for additional Lynch syndrome-associated malignancies including: gastric (up to 13%), small intestine (up to 12%), upper urinary tract (25%), sebaceous neoplasms (1–9%), pancreas (0.4–4%), hepatobiliary tract (0.2–4%), and brain (1–4%).[115,117] *MSH6* mutations display lower penetrance for CRC and endometrial cancer, with up to 44% lifetime risk respectively, and with less than 5% lifetime risk for other extracolonic cancers.[118,119] *PMS2* mutation carriers have the lowest lifetime cancer risks of ~20% for CRC, 15–120% for endometrial cancer, and less than 5% for additional extracolonic cancers.[120] Given the comparatively low penetrance of *MSH6* and *PMS2* mutations as compared to *MLH1* and *MSH2*, these patients may often present without an appreciable family history of cancer.

Individuals with Lynch syndrome are at increased lifetime risk for cancer and therefore surveillance management guidelines have been proposed by the NCCN. Current surveillance guidelines for MMR mutation carriers include[121]:

1. Colonoscopy every 1–2 years, beginning between ages 20 and 25, or 2–5 years prior to the earliest CRC in the family if it is diagnosed before age 25.
2. There are no clear data to support surveillance for gastric, duodenal and small bowel cancer; however, select individuals with a family history of upper GI cancers or those of Asian descent may have increased risk and may benefit from surveillance including upper endoscopy with visualization of the duodenum every 3–5 years, beginning at age 30–35, as well as testing and treating Helicobacter pylori infection.
3. Though there is insufficient evidence to recommend a particular screening strategy, an option may include annual urinalysis starting at age 30–35 in individuals with a family history of urothelial cancers and/or individuals with MSH2 mutations, particularly males.
4. Consider annual physical/neurologic exam beginning at age 25–30.
5. Consider risk-reducing hysterectomy with bilateral salpingo-oophorectomy in women; timing should be individualized based on childbearing, comorbidities, family history, and gene mutation
6. In the absence of risk-reducing TAH/BSO, considering endometrial biopsy every 1–2 years, transvaginal ultrasound, serum CA-125 at the physician's discretion[122,123]

Lynch syndrome is inherited in an autosomal dominant pattern. The majority of mutations are inherited from a parent, as the *de novo*, or sporadic mutation, rate in Lynch syndrome is very low.

Germline genetic testing for Lynch syndrome has historically been performed as a follow-up confirmatory test after initial screening for evidence of microsatellite instability (MSI) in the tumor. Indeed, a deficiency in MMR system can be detected by PCR and immunohistochemical staining of the MMR enzymes.[124] Tumors caused by germline MMR mutations are hallmarked by high levels of MSI and loss of expression of the implicated gene.[125,126] Personal and family history criteria laid out by the revised Bethesda and Amsterdam I/II criteria have long indicated which individuals should undergo tumor MSI analysis.[127] Over the past decade, universal testing of tumor for MSI has been advocated.

However, direct germline genetic analysis of the MMR genes has become increasingly feasible and accessible, with the advent of NGS-based panels.[128] Sequence mutations and deletion/duplication mutations of the MMR genes have been reported. An inversion of exons 1–7 of the *MSH2* gene has recently been described and accounts for patients with loss of *MSH2* and *MSH6* immunohistochemical expression that were previously negative on genetic testing.[129] Genetic testing for individuals suspected to have Lynch syndrome should always be performed in a laboratory that can detect the *MSH2* inversion, also known as the "Boland Inversion." Additionally, the *PMS2* gene poses difficulty in the technical assay of molecular analysis due to its pseudogene, *PMS2CL*, which if not particularly addressed, can result in spurious findings. Given the highly homologous pseudogene, typical Sanger and NGS sequencing cannot differentiate whether a mutation is found in the *PMS2* gene (causative of Lynch syndrome) or in the pseudogene (not causative of Lynch syndrome).[130] Specialized techniques including long-range PCR are needed to differentiate the true *PMS2* gene from pseudogenes and it is critical that genetic testing laboratories testing individuals for Lynch syndrome are prepared to address this issue.

In a subset of cases, individuals with MMR-deficient tumors will fail to have a germline MMR mutation identified by molecular analysis. Germline mutations in the gene *MUTYH*, associated with a recessive adenomatous polyposis syndrome, can cause tumors that display MSI and should be considered in the absence of a germline MMR mutation.[131] Biallelic somatic mutations in the same MMR gene have been shown to cause MSI and loss of immunohistochemical staining, mimicking possible Lynch syndrome.[132] These individuals tend to be diagnosed at older ages than individuals with germline mutations and also tend to have less family history of Lynch syndrome-related cancers; however, they are often younger and have a stronger family history of cancer than individuals with truly sporadic, MSI-stable CRC.[133] Paired analysis of the tumor and germline can help distinguish which individuals have biallelic somatic mutations accounting for the MSI of their tumor. The etiology and personal and familial consequences of biallelic somatic mutations are not yet clear and much remains undefined regarding this small but interesting population of CRC patients.

Lastly, some families may present with a strong family history of CRC but with no underlying genetic mutation identified. These families have yet unexplained risk for inherited CRC. These families have been termed "Familial Colorectal Cancer Type X" and are defined by three generations of CRC, at least one diagnosed <50 years, and at least 1 is a FDR to the other two (Amsterdam I criteria), and the tumors are MSI-stable.[134] Comprehensive genetic testing for all described CRC genes are recommended in these families to rule out conditions such as attenuated familial adenomatous polyposis (AFAP). In the absence of an identified gene mutations, close colonoscopic surveillance is recommended in FDRs, often beginning at age 40 or 10 years earlier than the youngest diagnosis in the family, every 3–5 years.[121]

Familial adenomatous polyposis

Familial adenomatous polyposis (FAP) is a rare, well-described, autosomal dominant predisposition to CRC and multiple adenomatous polyps caused by mutations in the *APC* gene.[135,136] Estimates of the prevalence of FAP vary from 1:6000 to 1 in 31,000 and historic terms to describe individuals with *APC* mutations include Gardner syndrome and Turcot syndrome.[137] Approximately 1% of CRCs are due to pathogenic *APC* gene mutations.[107] FAP is characterized by the development of numerous adenomas of the colon, typically numbering in the hundreds to thousands in individuals with classic FAP.[138] Extracolonic manifestations of FAP include dental anomalies (supernumerary teeth or missing teeth), jaw and skull osteomas, epidermoid cysts, soft tissue tumors, desmoid tumors (3′ of codon 1399), and congenital hypertrophy of the retinal pigment epithelium (CHRPE).[139,140]

Without colonoscopic or surgical intervention, the risk of CRC approaches 100% in patients with FAP. The mean age of colon cancer in untreated individuals is 39 years.[141] Adenomatous polyps typically develop at age 16 on average, and genetic testing and colonoscopy screening are recommended starting between the ages of 10 and 12. Nearly all patients with FAP will require surgical intervention, either prophylactically or for the treatment of a CRC.[142] Rectal involvement by polyps is often an important factor in determining surgical options which include total abdominal colectomy with ileorectal anastomosis (IRA), total proctocolectomy with either end ileostomy or with restorative ileal pouch-anal anastomosis (IPAA).[143–145] Individuals with classic FAP are also at increased risk to develop tubular adenomas of the periampullary region of the duodenum and fundic gland polyps of the stomach.[146–148] Upper endoscopy with side viewing duodenoscopy is recommended for upper GI tract and small bowel surveillance.[149,150] Individuals with FAP face elevated risks for extracolonic cancers including those of the small bowel, pancreas, thyroid, CNS, liver, bile duct, and stomach.[151,152]

Cancer type	Lifetime risk (%)
Duodenum (periampullary)	4–12[153]
Pancreatic adenocarcinoma	~1[154]
Papillary thyroid cancer	1–12[155]
Hepatoblastoma	1.6[156]
Gastric adenocarcinoma	<1[157]

An attenuated phenotype of FAP, known as AFAP, is phenotypically denoted by a lower overall adenoma burden (average of 30) and later onset of polyps. It is associated with mutations in the 5′ region of the *APC* gene.[158,159] Depending on the polyp burden and the presence or absence of dysplasia, individuals with AFAP may never require colectomy for management of colorectal polyps and may maintain surveillance through frequent colonoscopies.

Sequence analysis of the *APC* gene identifies a mutation approximately 90% of the time in individuals with classic FAP and deletion/duplication analysis detects an additional 8–12% of mutations.[160] In individuals with clinical AFAP or oligopolyposis, mutation detection is lower.[161] Genetic testing should be sure to include analysis of the promoter 1B region of the APC gene, because mutations in this region were recently identified to account for additional individuals with FAP.[162] In individuals with phenotypical AFAP and negative *APC* gene analysis, genetic testing should be considered for *MUTYH*.[163] Approximately 20–25% of individuals with FAP have a *de novo*, or sporadic mutation, that is not inherited from a parent; the remaining are inherited from a parent.[164]

MUTYH-associated polyposis

MUTYH-associated polyposis (MAP) is an inherited predisposition to colorectal polyposis that, clinically, is nearly indistinguishable from FAP and/or AFAP. However, MAP is an autosomal recessive disorder that is due to biallelic (two) mutations in the gene *MUTYH*, one inherited from each parent.[165] MAP presents similarly to FAP/AFAP with a greatly increased risk of CRC (43–100%) due to an increased risk of tubular adenomas, ranging from 10 to hundreds.[163] In contrast to individuals with FAP, individuals with MAP typically begin developing polyposis at a mean age of about 50 years and CRC can occur in the absence of significant polyposis.[166,167] Like FAP, MAP is associated with duodenal adenomas in 17–25% of affected individuals, conferring an increased lifetime risk of 4% to develop duodenal cancer.[168] While FAP is associated with development of tubular adenomas predominantly, serrated adenomas, hyperplastic/sessile serrated polyps, and mixed polyps can occur in individuals with MAP but are typically outweighed by tubular adenomas in the overall polyp burden.[163] Interestingly, the CRCs associated with biallelic *MUTYH* mutations can sometimes display MSI.[169]

Individuals with MAP are recommended to begin screening colonoscopy beginning at age 25–30 repeating every 1–2 years if adenomas are found with surgical intervention as needed for risk reduction and/or CRC treatment.[123] Upper endoscopy with side viewing duodenoscopy is recommended for duodenal surveillance beginning at age 30–35 years.

Approximately 1–2% of the general population are heterozygous carriers of a single mutation in the *MUTYH* gene.[170] There are conflicting reports regarding increased risk of CRC in single mutation carriers. Evidence suggests that heterozygous carriers are at slightly increased lifetime risk of CRC, approaching a similar risk level as that of having a FDR with CRC (~10% lifetime).[166,171] Sequencing of the *MUTYH* gene identifies mutations in ~99% of affected individuals. There are two common Northern European founder mutations, c.536A>G (p.Tyr179C) and c.1187G>A (p.Gly396Asp), which account for at least 90% of all pathogenic mutations in that population.[170] However, given the increasing complexity of ancestry and ethnicity, genetic sequencing of the entire gene is preferred over founder mutation analysis in all individuals regardless of reported ancestry.

Oligopolyposis syndromes

Oligopolyposis is an emerging clinical entity characterized by low to moderate colorectal adenoma burden, ranging from 10 to less than 100 adenomas. Individuals who are negative for mutations in *APC* and *MUTYH*, or those with young-onset MSI stable CRC, may have one of the newer described oligopolyposis genes which can account for modest adenoma development and young-onset CRC risk in a very small percentage of individuals with CRC and/or adenomas.

Oligopolyposis syndrome (Genes)	Inheritance	Clinical manifestations
Polymerase proofreading-associated polyposis (PPAP) *POLD1, POLE*	Autosomal dominant	Oligopolyposis, young-onset MSI-stable CRC, endometrial cancer[172-176]
NTHL1-associated polyposis	Autosomal recessive	Oligopolyposis, CRC[177]
Hereditary mixed polyposis syndrome—*GREM1*	Autosomal dominant	Mixed polyposis, CRC[178]
MSH3-related polyposis	Autosomal recessive	Oligopolyposis, early-onset CRC[179]

Hamartomatous polyposis syndromes

The presence of hamartomatous polyps in the GI tract can indicate a possible inherited predisposition, known as hamartomatous polyposis syndromes. Associated with a lower risk of malignancy than tubular adenomas, hamartomatous polyps can often be further specified based on histopathology as Peutz–Jeghers type polyps or juvenile polyps; this distinction can indicate the potential underlying syndrome.[180]

Peutz–Jeghers syndrome

PJS is caused by mutations in the gene *STK11*. The rare syndrome confers autosomal dominant predisposition to cancer and hamartomatous polyps.[181] The syndrome is characterized by PJS-type polyps in the small bowel (jejunum > ileum > duodenum), colon, and stomach.[136] Intussusception is a common clinical manifestation of children and young adults with PJS, along with chronic anemia and partial obstruction.[182] A distinctive pattern of mucocutaneous hyperpigmented lesions on the lips, buccal mucosa, fingers, and perianal area of affected individuals is pathognomonic for PJS. These may be obvious in childhood but can fade in adulthood.[83] Individuals with PJS are at significantly increased risk for cancers including colorectal, gastric, pancreatic, breast, and ovarian cancers.[88,183] Women are at increased risk for sex cord tumors with annular tubules (SCTAT) and a rare, aggressive cervical malignancy, adenoma malignum.[184] Men with PJS can develop large calcifying Sertoli cell tumors (LCST) of the testes.[185,186] A clinical diagnosis of PJS can be made by the presence of two or more histologically confirmed PJS-type polyps.[187] Surveillance guidelines for the numerous affected organ systems are outlined by professional societies and the NCCN and include endoscopy and imaging-based protocols beginning in childhood.[187] Genetic testing of *STK11* will identify a mutation in 94–96% of affected individuals, most of which are sequence mutations but about 15% are large deletions, duplications, or whole gene deletions.[188,189]

Cancer type	Lifetime risk (%)	Average age at diagnosis (years)
Colorectal	39	42–46
Stomach	29	30–40
Small bowel	13	37–42
Breast	32–54	37–59 years
Ovarian (SCTAT)	21	28
Cervix (adenoma malignum)	10	34–40
Uterus	9	43
Pancreas	11–36	41–52
Sertoli cell testicular tumor	9	6–9
Lung	7–17	47

Juvenile polyposis syndrome (JPS)

Juvenile polyposis syndrome (JPS) is characterized by juvenile polyps in the stomach, small intestine, colon, and rectum.[136,190] The term "juvenile" refers to the subtype of the hamartomatous polyp and not to the age of onset of polyps, although JPS-related polyps can occur in young individuals. The majority of juvenile polyps are benign but there is a low risk of malignant transformation.[191] The diagnosis of JPS is established by >5 histologically confirmed juvenile polyps of the colorectum, multiple JPS-type polyps through the GI tract, or any number of juvenile polyps and a family history of JPS.[192] Mutations in the *SMAD4* and *BMPR1A* genes are causative of JPS and can be identified in approximately 50% of individuals suspected to have JPS.[193,194] Interestingly, there is a phenotypic overlap with hereditary hemorrhagic telangiectasia (HHT) which is also caused by *SMAD4* mutations, characterized by cutaneous and mucosal/intestinal telangiectasia, epistaxis, and AVM.[195]

Individuals with JPS are at increased risk to develop cancers of the stomach and colorectum. The risk of CRC is 68% by age 60, with a median age at diagnosis is 42 years.[196] The incidence of gastric cancer is 21% in those with gastric polyps and prophylactic partial and total gastrectomies have been performed in individuals with JPS both to avoid the development of gastric cancer and/or to treat symptomatic chronic anemia.[197]

Cowden syndrome

CS, also known as *PTEN* hamartoma tumor syndrome, is the third syndrome characterized by hamartomatous polyps.[190] A rare autosomal dominant cancer predisposition syndrome, CS is most often recognized for its association with breast, endometrial, and thyroid cancers.[72] Associated with mutations in the *PTEN* gene, CS is characterized by macrocephaly, trichilemmomas, and papillomatous papules.[198] The GI tract polyps in individuals with CS are not exclusively hamartomatous, although that is a common finding. Ganglioneuromatous polyps, juvenile, and adenomatous polyps have also been reported in individuals with CS contributing to the modest, but still increased, lifetime risk for CRC (9%).[199] Clinical diagnostic criteria, comprised of major and minor criteria, are published and will not be discussed further herein.[73,76]

Hereditary predispositions to gastric cancer

Gastric cancer, also referred to as stomach cancer, is the fifteenth most common cancer occurring in the United States, representing 1.5% of new cancer diagnoses. Gastric cancer incidence is increased in men and among certain race/ethnicities including Black, Asian, American Indian, and Hispanic. The median age of onset for gastric cancer in the general population is 68 years.[200] Gastric cancer is comprised primarily of two main types: intestinal type and diffuse type. Intestinal type gastric cancer, which includes papillary, tubular, and mucinous adenocarcinoma, accounts for the majority of cases and is associated with dietary and other risk factors, notably *Helicobacter pylori* infection. About 10% of gastric cancers have a family history of the disease, but only 1–3% arise from an inherited predisposition.[183] Lynch syndrome, familial adenomatous polyposis, juvenile polyposis, PJS, and Li–Fraumeni syndrome all confer a slightly increased risk for intestinal-type gastric cancer.[152,183,197,201,202] However, diffuse-type gastric cancer, while a less common histologic subtype, is more likely to be associated with an underlying genetic etiology. Diffuse gastric cancer is defined by poorly differentiated carcinoma with high proportion of signet ring cells.[203]

Hereditary diffuse gastric cancer (HDGC)

HDGC caused by inherited mutations in the *CDH1* gene (E-cadherin) is a highly penetrant autosomal dominant cause of diffuse-type gastric cancer.[78,204] Individuals with *CDH1* mutations are at significantly increased risk to develop diffuse gastric cancer in their lifetime due to inactivation of the second *CDH1* allele leading to cancer development.[205] The lifetime risks to develop diffuse gastric cancer is high, as high as 70–80% in men and up to 70% in women.[206] The International Gastric Cancer Consortium (IGCC) has suggested *CDH1* genetic testing in individuals meeting the following criteria: two family members with gastric cancer, at least one of which is confirmed diffuse type; three family members with gastric cancer in first- or second-degree relatives including one with diffuse type; individual diagnosed with diffuse type gastric cancer under age 40' and/or personal or family history of diffuse gastric cancer and lobular breast cancer including one diagnosed before age 50.[207] *CDH1* gene mutations account for approximately 50% of patients whose personal and/or family histories raise concern for HDGC.[208] Genetic testing should include both sequencing and deletion/duplication analysis of the *CDH1* in order to be comprehensive.

Diffuse gastric cancer is characterized clinicopathologically by linitis plastica, a thickening of the stomach lining indicative of the diffuse tumor. In the setting of germline *CDH1* mutations, multifocal microscopic foci of signet ring cell carcinoma arise independently throughout the stomach lining presenting multiple opportunities for tumor growth. Early-stage diffuse gastric cancer growing in the lining of the stomach rarely presents with clinical symptoms. Symptoms often present as the cancer becomes more advanced and even then are mostly nonspecific: bloating, early satiety, decreased appetite, nausea, vomiting, and unintentional weight loss.[209] This presents challenges in early detection and effective screening for individuals with *CDH1*. Endoscopy with multiple biopsies and mapping has been suggested as a screening modality for diffuse gastric cancer in *CDH1* mutation carriers; however, it has not been proven to significantly reduce mortality from diffuse gastric cancer.[210,211] Therefore, prophylactic total gastrectomy (PTG) is currently recommended to prevent the diagnosis of diffuse gastric cancer.[212–214] Timing of PTG is highly personalized and should be considered based on the ages of gastric cancer diagnosis in the family and patient preference.[80,215]

Women with *CDH1* mutations face an approximately 40% lifetime risk of lobular-type breast cancer, similar to those with other highly penetrant hereditary breast cancer susceptibility genes.[79] The NCCN Guidelines for breast cancer surveillance and management include consideration of risk-reducing mastectomies, similar to those the recommendations made for women carrying pathogenic *BRCA1/BRCA2* mutations. Both men and women with *CDH1* mutations are at slightly increased lifetime risk for CRC, specifically signet ring cell histology.[80] Screening colonoscopy is recommended beginning at age 40.

Hereditary predispositions to pancreatic cancer

The majority of pancreatic adenocarcinomas (PC) are sporadic; however, inherited risk factors contribute to at least 5–10% of all PC.[216] Pancreatic neuroendocrine tumors/islet cell tumors (PNET) account for 3–5% of pancreatic malignancies. Most PNETs are sporadic, but a small proportion is due to inherited genetic susceptibility syndromes. The multiple endocrine neoplasia type 1 (MEN1) and Von Hippel–Lindau (VHL) syndromes are discussed elsewhere in this article.

Germline mutations in a growing number of genes have been associated with significantly increased risk of PC: *ATM*, *APC*, *BRCA1*, *BRCA2*, *CDKN2A/CDK4* (*p16*), *MLH1*, *MSH2*, *MSH6*, *PMS2*, *PALB2*, *STK11*, and *PRSS1*.[217,218] Despite identifying genetic mutations in many families with multiple cases of PC, not all cases of inherited pancreatic cancer can be linked to a known gene.[219] Typically germline mutations associated with PC are suggested by kindreds with multiple generations of pancreatic or related cancers (breast, ovarian, colon, etc.), cancer diagnoses under the age of 50, individuals with multiple primary tumors, and/or families with ethnicities that confer an increased mutation carrier frequency, such as Ashkenazi Jewish ethnicity.[38] Thus, a thorough family history is critical to the management of pancreatic cancer risk.

Familial pancreatic cancer (FPC)

Because not all kindreds with multiple cases of PC will have an identified gene mutation, two general categories exist to discuss such families: hereditary pancreatic cancer and familial pancreatic cancer (FPC).[219] Hereditary pancreatic cancer is defined as a genetic syndrome with an identifiable gene mutation associated with an increased risk for PC. FPC is defined as a family with at least two FDRs with PC, without an identifiable syndrome in the family (Brand et al.). Relatives meeting the FPC criteria have an empirically increased risk to develop PC over the general population; these individuals can be even further stratified depending on their degree of relationship to the affected relatives.[220,221]

Number of first-degree relatives (FDR) with PC	Relative risk to develop PC
None	1.5
1 FDR	3–4
2 FDR	5–7
3+ FDR	17–32

Pancreatic cancer risk in FPC families

An individual with three or more FDRs with PC carries up to a 17-fold RR for pancreatic cancer.[221] Nongenetic risk factors, primarily smoking tobacco, increase the risk for PC in families meeting FPC criteria and reduces the age of PC diagnosis by up to a decade.[222–225] In general, individuals with two or more FDRs can consider discussing the risks vs. benefits of pancreatic cancer screening/surveillance with their physician. Individuals with three or more FDRs are highly likely to carry a known hereditary susceptibility gene, and even in the absence of an identifiable mutation, could consider pancreatic cancer screening given the significantly increased empiric risk. What comprises pancreatic screening for individuals at increased risk is not well-defined, but consensus guidelines recommend a multimodality approach including blood work, imaging (magnetic resonance cholangiopancreatography, CT with pancreas protocol), and endoscopic evaluation (EUS).[226] Given the complexity of pancreatic screening and lack of guidelines, targeted surveillance for pancreatic cancer is often reserved for those with clearly increased risk due to a known gene mutation and/or strong family history of PC.

Hereditary breast and ovarian cancer syndrome (HBOC) and moderate penetrance genes

Hereditary breast and ovarian cancer syndrome is an autosomal dominant disorder characterized by increased risks for breast cancer, ovarian cancer, prostate, male breast, melanoma, and pancreatic cancer. The risk for PC in *BRCA1* carriers is only moderate, estimated to be 2.8-fold RR compared to the general population risk of 1.3%.[227] Other reported series have documented no increased risk for PC in *BRCA1* mutation carriers.[39] In general, the PC risk associated with *BRCA1* mutation carriers is small and, alone, does not typically warrant increased surveillance for PC in unaffected individuals. Conversely, *BRCA2* mutations are associated with a 3.5-fold increased risk of pancreatic cancer.[38] *BRCA2* mutations account for 12–16% of families with FPC, making it the most common hereditary susceptibility gene to PC and FPC.[38]

Germline mutations in other moderate penetrance breast cancer genes including *PALB2* and *ATM* have been associated with increased risks of pancreatic cancer; however, the exact risks have not yet been defined.[218,228]

Familial atypical multiple-mole/melanoma syndrome (FAMMM)

Germline mutations in the *p16/CDKN2A* gene are most commonly associated with familial melanoma. Individuals who carry *p16* germline mutations are at substantially increased risk for pancreatic cancer, estimated 17% lifetime risk by age 75.[229]

Peutz–Jeghers syndrome

PJS is a rare hereditary susceptibility primarily to hamartomatous polyps of the GI tract, specifically the small bowel. The lifetime risk of pancreatic cancer within PJS is as high as 36%, one of the highest hereditary risks for pancreatic cancer.[230] These individuals can benefit from a discussion of pancreatic cancer screening as part of their cancer surveillance.[226] As discussed above, individuals with PJS are also at increased risks for breast cancer, cervical cancer (adenoma malignum), sex-cord tumors, gastric, and colon cancers. PJS is characterized by a pathognomonic dark freckling of the lips, tongue, and oral/buccal mucosa.

Hereditary pancreatitis

Hereditary pancreatitis (HP) is a rare hereditary predisposition to both acute and chronic episodes of pancreatitis, typically beginning in childhood. Individuals with HP often experience multiple episodes of acute pancreatitis beginning at a young age and eventually develop chronic pancreatitis. The risk for PC in these individuals arises from the pancreatitis-related PC risk as opposed to a genetic mechanism increasing the independent development of PC. The gene *PRSS1* is associated with the autosomal dominant form of HP, while *SPINK1* and *CTFR* cause an autosomal recessive form of the disease.[231] Screening for pancreatic cancer in these patients with chronic pancreatitis must be considered carefully in light of the procedure-related risk of pancreatitis with ERCP.[226]

Syndrome	Lifetime risk of PC	Other cancers/ symptoms	Gene
Hereditary pancreatitis	40%	Pancreatitis	PRSS1, SPINK1, CFTR
Peutz–Jeghers	36%	Hamartomatous polyps of the small bowel, breast cancer, sex cord tumors, skin freckling	STK11
Familial atypical multiple-mole/ melanoma	17%	Melanoma, multiple atypical moles	P16/CDKN2A
Hereditary breast and ovarian cancer	3–7%	Breast, ovarian, male breast cancer	BRCA1, BRCA2
Lynch syndrome	<10%	Colon, endometrial, gastric, ovarian cancer	MLH1, MSH2, MSH6, PMS2, EPCAM
Familial adenomatous polyposis (FAP)	2%	Colon polyposis, colon cancer	APC
PALB2	Unknown	Breast cancer	PALB2
ATM	Unknown	Breast cancer	ATM
Multiple endocrine neoplasia type 1	40–70% (PNET)	Primary hyperparathyroidism, pituitary adenoma	MEN1
Von Hippel–Lindau	5–17% (PNET)	Clear cell renal cell carcinoma, spine, retinal hemangioblastoma	VHL

Hereditary genitourinary syndromes

Hereditary predispositions to prostate cancer

The lifetime risk of prostate cancer for men is approximately 11% with average age of onset at 66.[232] Familial patterns of prostate cancer have long been observed with heritability estimated between 40% and 50%.[233,234] Heritable genetic factors associated with prostate cancer include rare variants with high- or moderate-penetrance, such as *BRCA1* and *BRCA2* genes, as well as common low-penetrance genes identified by genome wide associated studies (GWAS). Most often, familial clustering of prostate cancer is attributed to shared inherited genetic factors and environmental exposures. RRs of prostate cancer are elevated based on the degree of family history estimated at 2.35 (2.02–2.72), 3.14 (2.37–4.15), or up to 4.39 (2.61–7.39) based on having a father, brother, or two or more FDRs with prostate cancer, respectively.[235] Risk for high-grade or aggressive (Gleason score ≥7) prostate cancer and metastatic prostate cancer is associated with high- and moderate-penetrance syndromes.[236–238] A recent study identified approximately 12% risk of a DNA-repair gene mutation among men with metastatic prostate cancer; approximately 50% of mutations identified were in *BRCA1* and *BRCA2* genes.[238] This finding has significantly altered the landscape of genetic testing among men with prostate cancer as guidelines now recommend genetic analysis of *BRCA1* and *BRCA2* genes for men with metastatic prostate cancer regardless of family history.[239] The indication for ordering genetic testing of other DNA damage repair genes, such as *ATM* or *CHEK2*, for men with prostate cancer has yet to be determined but with the availability of NGS panels, genetic testing of multiple DNA damage repair genes is often performed at the time of genetic analysis.[240]

Hereditary breast and ovarian cancer syndrome

Pathogenic germline mutations in *BRCA1* and *BRCA2* genes a widely known for the associated risks of breast and ovarian cancer. The elevated risks and medical management guidelines are reviewed in detail within the section for inherited breast and ovarian cancer syndromes. Studies have shown these genes confer an elevated risk for prostate cancer among male *BRCA2* mutation carriers (4.7- to 8.6-fold) and possibly *BRCA1* mutation carriers (1.1- to 3.8-fold).[241–245] Further investigation has shown that *BRCA2*-associated prostate cancer is often associated with more aggressive disease and earlier ages of onset.[246–249] While the clinical utility of *BRCA1*/*BRCA2* genetic testing and cancer screening guidelines are well established for breast and ovarian cancer-related risks, a lack of consensus for prostate cancer screening procedures remains among high-risk individuals.[250–252] Proposed screening guidelines for men with pathogenic variants in high-penetrance genes (i.e., BRCA1/BRCA2) include baseline prostate-specific antigen (PSA) and digital rectal exam (DRE) beginning at age 40 or 5 years earlier than the youngest age of metastatic prostate cancer diagnosis among a first- or second-degree, whichever occurs first. If DRE is abnormal, prostate biopsy is suggested, regardless of PSA result. If DRE is normal further follow-up is based on PSA thresholds and age group.[253] Future studies are needed to establish if this same proposal may work among all DNA repair gene mutation carriers.

HOXB13

Among the rare, high-penetrance variants associated with hereditary prostate cancer is the *HOXB13* G84E mutation.[254] This founder allele has been identified in approximately 5% of all hereditary prostate cancer cases in men of European descent and confers an elevated risk for prostate cancer between 2.8- and 8.5-fold with significant contribution to risk of early-onset prostate cancer.[254–258] Further studies to evaluate other cancer risks associated with *HOXB13* and any other risk alleles are needed.

Other potential genetic risks

While other mutations in hereditary cancer-associated genes have been reported to confer a moderately elevated risk for prostate cancer, these studies have shown less consistency in reproducibility. Substantially elevated risks for colorectal and endometrial cancer in DNA MMR genes are well known but risks for prostate cancer have been proposed ranging from 2- to 3.7-fold above the general population.[259,260] Similarly, moderately penetrant genes including *CHEK2* and *NBN* have been found to confer an approximately two- to four-fold risk for prostate cancer but risks may be higher with family history.[261,262]

Hereditary endocrine syndromes

Hereditary endocrine syndromes confer an increased risk for both benign and malignant neoplasms throughout the endocrine system. In addition, some of these syndromes increase the risk for cancers or tumors outside of the endocrine system. Altogether, they represent a heterogeneous group of diseases that typically require multidisciplinary evaluation, management, and treatment. Many endocrine tumors exhibit high rates of heritability and the diagnosis alone of several should prompt genetic evaluation as standard of care. Here, the most commonly encountered hereditary endocrine syndromes are reviewed in detail; other, and in some cases more newly recognized, syndromes and/or predispositions are also introduced, with references for further reading.

Multiple endocrine neoplasia type 1

MEN1 is one of the most well-known hereditary endocrine syndromes, characterized by a classic triad of endocrine tumors involving the parathyroid glands, anterior pituitary gland, and endocrine pancreas. However, more than 20 benign and malignant tumors have been reported in the phenotype.[263] It is caused by germline mutations in the *MEN1* gene and inherited in an autosomal dominant manner.

MEN1 is a highly penetrant condition and affected individuals typically develop numerous endocrine tumors throughout their lives. The estimated lifetime risks for tumors in MEN1 vary in the literature. Almost all individuals will develop primary hyperparathyroidism (PHPT) (90–95%), most often caused by multigland parathyroid hyperplasia and this is often the presenting feature. The overall risk for pituitary tumors has been estimated at 30–40%; MEN1-associated pituitary tumors are typically functional but can in rare cases be nonfunctional. Of functional pituitary tumors, prolactinomas are most common, followed by somatotropinomas and then corticotropinomas. Pancreatic neuroendocrine tumors (pNETs), or islet cell tumors, occur in up to 70% of individuals and confer an increased risk for malignant transformation. Functional pNETs found in patients with MEN1 are often gastrinomas and insulinomas, or less commonly PPomas, glucagonomas, and VIPomas. Other tumors seen in MEN1 include adrenal cortical tumors, pheochromocytoma (PCC), and bronchopulmonary/thymic/gastric neuroendocrine tumors (NETs). Affected individuals often have characteristic dermatological manifestations as well, namely lipomas, angiofibromas, and collagenomas.[263–266]

The diagnosis of MEN1 has historically been made in one of three ways: (1) genetic, (2) clinical, or (3) familial.[266–268] A genetic diagnosis of MEN1 is made when an individual is found to have a pathogenic variant in MEN1 with or without the expected phenotype (the latter being most common in predictive genetic testing scenarios). A clinical diagnosis is most commonly made when an apparently simplex case presents with 2 of the 3 primary MEN1-associated tumors (parathyroid, pituitary, endocrine pancreas). Lastly, a familial diagnosis is made when an individual presents with at least one of the primary tumors and when that individual has a FDR with MEN1 (diagnosed either clinically or through genetic testing).[263] With the increased sensitivity of genetic testing for all hereditary cancer syndromes, a genetic diagnosis of MEN1 is typically considered the gold standard. However, in approximately 5–10% of cases, an MEN1 gene mutation cannot be identified, in which case the patient's phenotype and family history must be carefully considered by the clinician to determine MEN1 status.[267]

To date, there are no clinically relevant or reliable genotype–phenotype correlations in MEN1, and pathogenic variants are found throughout the coding region of the MEN1 gene, although there are several mutation hotspots and there has been work to elucidate possible genotype–phenotype correlations.[267,269–271] Predictive genetic testing in at-risk family members after the familial mutation has been identified is recommended starting in childhood, typically between ages 5 and 10; once a child has been diagnosed with MEN1 through genetic testing, he or she would begin regular biochemical surveillance for MEN1-associated tumors, and imaging tests would be added to his or her surveillance protocol as they age.[263] There is currently no way to prevent tumors in MEN1 from developing; however, close surveillance allows for the earlier detection and diagnosis of tumors, with the goal of mitigating their medical consequences and improving treatment outcomes. Both surgical procedures and medical therapies are used in the treatment and management of MEN1-associated tumors, the discussion of which is beyond the scope of this article.

Multiple endocrine neoplasia type 2

Multiple endocrine neoplasia type 2 (MEN2) is another well-known hereditary endocrine syndrome. It is associated with a very high risk for medullary thyroid carcinoma (MTC) and other features of MEN2, including PHPT, PCC, and Hirschsprung disease (HD), vary by syndrome subtype. All phenotypic variants of MEN2, including those of MEN2A and MEN2B, are caused by activating germline mutations in the RET proto-oncogene and are autosomal dominant.[272] Understanding the genotype-phenotype correlations that exist in MEN2 is critical for appropriate management and treatment of patients with MEN2. Approximately 25% of all MTC is hereditary, and approximately 7% of even apparently sporadic MTC is hereditary.[273,274] Thus, all patients with a diagnosis of MTC are currently recommended to have germline RET testing for MEN2, regardless of family history, age of diagnosis, or presence/absence of other endocrine tumors.[275]

MEN2 syndromes are classified as either MEN2A or MEN2B, depending on the genotype. Historically, there was a third entity called familial medullary thyroid carcinoma (FNMTC); however, the most recent American Thyroid Association (ATA) guidelines for the treatment and management of MTC advise against using this classification and have instead recommended collapsing it into MEN2A.[266,275] Disease-causing RET mutations are further risk-stratified by the ATA as moderate, high, and highest risk. The only highest risk RET mutation is the canonical p.M918T, which causes the classic MEN2B phenotype. High-risk mutations include the very rare p.A883F mutation, which can confer a MEN2B-like phenotype but with a lower MTC risk compared to M918T and the classic MEN2A mutations that alter codon position 634 (p.C634F/G/R/S/W/Y). The remaining MEN2-associated mutations are located at other codons throughout the gene and approximately 95% of these mutations are located within exons 10, 11, 13–16 (the entire gene is comprised of 20 coding exons).[272,274,276,277]

MEN2A is the most common MEN2 syndrome and predisposes to MTC, PCC, and PHPT. The vast majority of cases are inherited from an affected parent.[278] The overall lifetime risk for MTC approaches 95% and the risk for PCC and PHPT varies by genotype. For 634 mutations, the lifetime risk for PCC is greater than 50% with bilateral disease often occurring and the risk for PHPT approaches 20–30%; for moderate risk mutations, the risk for PCC and PHPT varies but is almost always lower than that of mutations at codon 634.[279–281] Certain exon 10 mutations at codon positions 609, 611, 618, and 620 also predispose to HD, typically presenting in infancy. Cutaneous lichen amyloidosis (CLA), a benign skin condition, is common amongst individuals with a 634 mutation especially on the upper back between the shoulders. Papillary thyroid carcinoma (PTC) can also be seen in certain families with MEN2A.[275,282] Obtaining a detailed personal and family history can sometimes help predict mutation status in individuals with MTC; however, there is phenotypic overlap particularly in the moderate risk mutation group.

MEN2B typically presents as a distinct syndrome and is caused by a de novo RET mutation in 75% of cases. Approximately 95% of MEN2B cases are caused by mutation M918T, and less than 5% are caused by mutations at codon 883.[275,283,284] Most of the data on MEN2B from the literature is from cases with the M918T mutation. The risk for MTC in MEN2B is extremely high even from within the first few years of life. In cases of hereditary MEN2B, prophylactic thyroidectomy is typically recommended within the first year of life.[275] Individuals with MEN2B have a 50% risk to develop PCC and there is no increased risk for PHPT. A distinctive facies, oral mucosal neuromas, absent tear production in infancy, everted eyelids, ganglioneuromatosis of the gastrointestinal tract, marfanoid habitus, pes cavus, and other skeletal features are also common amongst individuals with MEN2B. The presence of one or more of these features in infancy or childhood may prompt an evaluation for MEN2B including germline *RET* testing, which, if the child does have MEN2B, could help prevent or diagnose MTC at an early stage.[275,285,286]

Once a familial *RET* mutation has been identified, at-risk family members are typically recommended to have predictive genetic testing in childhood. In the case of MEN2B with M918T, predictive genetic testing is recommended within the first year of life so that prophylactic thyroidectomy can be performed within the first year for those who test positive. In cases of a familial A883F or codon 634 mutation, genetic testing is recommended within the first few years of life so that calcitonin levels can be monitored and prophylactic thyroidectomy can be performed by age 5 years. For family members at risk for a moderate risk mutation, genetic testing is typically recommended starting at age 5, and thyroidectomy should be performed when the serum calcitonin level rises or earlier if the parents do not wish to pursue annual surveillance. Annual biochemical screening for PHPT and PCC differs by genotype. Patients with MEN2 are often treated both medically and surgically; surgery is typically indicated for MTC, PHPT, and PCC, whereas medical therapy is most commonly used in the management of metastatic MTC (recommendations reviewed in Wells et al., "Revised American Thyroid Association guidelines for the management of medullary thyroid carcinoma").[275]

Other hereditary parathyroid diseases

Aside from MEN1 and MEN2A, there are other, rarer causes of hereditary PHPT. Approximately 5–10% of PHPT has an underlying hereditary or familial etiology and certain accompanying features can make a hereditary cause more likely.[287] For example, the combination of PHPT and other endocrine tumors associated with MEN1 or MEN2 should prompt evaluation for the respective syndrome. In addition, those individuals with PHPT diagnosed before age 40, with multiglandular PHPT, with recurrent PHPT, with family histories of PHPT, or with parathyroid carcinoma may benefit from genetic evaluation and/or testing.[288–290] The following offers a brief overview of other hereditary diseases with parathyroid manifestations, but it is not exhaustive and does not include genetic syndromes that can cause hypoparathyroidism (e.g., 22q11.2 deletion syndrome, Barakat syndrome, Kenney-Caffey disease, or certain mitochondrial diseases).

Multiple endocrine neoplasia type 4 (MEN4)

MEN4 is a newly described hereditary endocrine disease that predisposes to the same types of endocrine tumors as seen in MEN1 (parathyroid, pituitary, pNETs); however, the risks for these tumors seem to be lower and overall cause a less aggressive phenotype relative to MEN1. MEN4 is caused by heterozygous pathogenic variants in the *CDKN1B* gene. A relatively small number of patients with MEN4 are reported in the literature, so at present, it is difficult to estimate the true prevalence and penetrance of the disease. This has also made it difficult to optimize surveillance, management, and treatment recommendations for the manifestations of MEN4. Recommendations for the genetic evaluation of MEN4 have been published.[92,291,292]

Hyperparathyroidism-jaw tumor syndrome (HPT-JT)

HPT-JT syndrome is autosomal dominant and caused by pathogenic variants in the *CDC73* gene. It is associated with a 70–80% risk for PHPT and approximately 15–20% of individuals with HPT-JT syndrome have parathyroid carcinoma causing PHPT. As the name suggests, individuals with HPT-JT syndrome are also at increased risk for jaw tumors, specifically ossifying fibromas, kidney tumors (including cysts, hamartomas, and rarely Wilms tumor), and uterine fibroids in women. Parathyroid neoplasms can be evaluated for an underlying *CDC73* germline mutation through immunohistochemistry (IHC) for the gene's protein product, parafibromin.[289,293–295]

Familial hypocalciuric-hypercalcemia (FHH)

FHH can mimic PHPT by increasing serum calcium levels, but the cause of hypercalcemia in these patients is not a parathyroid adenoma or hyperplasia. FHH is most commonly caused by inactivating, heterozygous pathogenic variants in the *CASR* gene, known as FHH type 1; FHH types 2 and 3 are caused by pathogenic variants in the *GNA11* and *AP2S1* genes, respectively. FHH type 1 is caused by a defect in the calcium-sensing receptor which ultimately causes hypocalciuria and hypercalcemia, but in most cases, patients remain asymptomatic and parathyroid surgery is not indicated for these patients.[296,297]

Familial isolated primary hyperparathyroidism (FIHP)

FIHP is considered a diagnosis of exclusion. In families where multiple close relatives are affected with PHPT and no known hereditary disease can be identified, a diagnosis of FIHP may be considered. In these families, affected individuals may present with earlier-onset PHPT, multiglandular PHPT, or recurrent PHPT. The overall risk for PHPT is difficult to quantify in these families and PHPT seems to be inherited in an autosomal dominant manner.[298,299]

Hereditary paraganglioma/pheochromocytoma syndromes

The hereditary paraganglioma/pheochromocytoma (PGL/PCC) syndromes represent a diverse group by both genotype and phenotype that are conventionally divided into two groups. In the first group are those syndromes caused by pathogenic variants in the classic PGL/PCC predisposition genes (e.g., SDHx genes) and in the second are those well-characterized hereditary syndromes that predispose to several types of benign and malignant tumors including PGL/PCC (e.g., MEN2A/B). Like MTC, the diagnosis of PGL/PCC alone should prompt an evaluation for an underlying hereditary disease, regardless of age of diagnosis, family history, or presence/absence of other endocrine tumors. Several professional groups recommended germline genetic testing for all patients with PGL/PCC, as approximately 30–40% of all cases have an identifiable germline pathogenic variant in a PGL/PCC predisposition gene.[300–304] Several decisional algorithms have been published to aid the clinician in ordering germline genetic testing in these cases; with the advancement and availability of NGS technology; however, it has become possible to test all of these genes at once.[304-307]

SDHx

The SDHx genes include *SDHA, SDHAF2, SDHB, SDHC,* and *SDHD*. The most data are currently available for *SDHB* and *SDHD* due to their prevalence among families with hereditary PGL/PCC syndromes. Between all of the SDHx genes, there can be significant phenotypic overlap; however, for some, there are distinct tumor characteristics that would prompt suspicion for one gene over another. All of the associated syndromes are inherited in an autosomal dominant manner, but there are unique parent-of-origin effects to consider for *SDHD* and *SDHAF2* in which high risk for tumors is only conferred when a mutation is paternally inherited.

Germline pathogenic variants in *SDHD* cause hereditary PGL/PCC syndrome type 1. Individuals with this syndrome often present with bilateral carotid body tumors with an overall high propensity for multifocal head & neck paraganglioma (HNPGL). There is a low risk of malignant PGL associated with *SDHD* mutations. Abdominal PGL and PCC have been reported, but are less common compared to HNPGL.[308-310] This is an autosomal dominant syndrome but the high risk for PGL is associated with paternally-inherited mutations due to a proposed three-hit hypothesis (the exact genetic mechanisms of which is quite complicated and continues to be elucidated[311,312]), so paternal inheritance of a mutation should be confirmed whenever possible. Individuals who inherit a pathogenic *SDHD* variant from their mother are not considered to have a high risk for PGL, but the risk is also not zero and there are several reports in the literature of maternally inherited *SDHD* mutations causing PGL.[313-315] Considerations for individuals with a maternally inherited mutation were recently published.[316] Careful genetic counseling and pedigree analysis are a very important part of diagnosing and testing for hereditary PGL syndrome type 1.

Germline pathogenic variants in *SDHB* cause hereditary PGL/PCC syndrome type 4. Individuals with this syndrome often present with abdominal PGL and/or PCC, but HNPGL can also be seen. *SDHB*-associated PCC/PGL have historically been associated with a high risk for malignancy (30–40% of all tumors), but newer data suggests that the incidence of malignant disease may be lower than initially thought, as well as the overall penetrance. The overall lifetime risk for PCC/PGL in hereditary PGL/PCC syndrome type 4 has historically been regarded as quite high, nearing 80% and it is not uncommon for affected individuals to develop multiple tumors throughout their lifetime.[309,310,317,318]

Hereditary PGL/PCC syndrome type 3 is caused by germline pathogenic variants in *SDHC*, and affected individuals may present with single HNPGL; however, tumors in other locations and PCC have been reported. The estimated penetrance associated with this syndrome is not well-characterized.[309,319,320] Hereditary PGL/PCC syndrome type 2 is caused by germline pathogenic variants in *SDHAF2*, in which paternally inherited mutations are associated with high risk for disease. However, this syndrome is rare and most of the published data comes from several large Dutch families. Typically multiple HNPGL are seen with this syndrome and it is considered highly penetrant.[309,321-324] Lastly, germline pathogenic variants in *SDHA* cause the very rare hereditary PGL/PCC syndrome type 5. Affected individuals appear to present typically with HNPGL; however, other PGL and PCC have been reported. The penetrance is not known.[309,321,325]

Carney-Stratakis syndrome (CSS) is characterized by the combination of PGL/PCC, renal cell carcinoma (RCC), gastrointestinal stromal tumors (GISTs), and possibly pituitary adenomas and thyroid cancer.[326-328] The association of RCC with SDHx mutations is described in the section titled "Hereditary RCC". CSS-associated GISTs are almost always gastric in origin, can be multifocal, and are almost always wildtype with regards to somatic *KIT/PDGFRA* mutation status.[329] Germline mutations in *SDHA, SDHB, SDHC,* and *SDHD* have been associated with CSS, which is largely a phenotypic distinction amongst the hereditary PGL/PCC syndromes.[326,330-332]

There are reports of biallelic *SDHx* gene mutations causing mitochondrial diseases in infants and children. The phenotype and severity of disease in affected individuals can vary greatly, which is common for mitochondrial disease.[333-335] Reproductive risk and family planning counseling should be provided to patients of childbearing age who are identified to have a germline mutation in one of these genes, which may include obtaining a family history for the patient's spouse.

MAX, TMEM127

Germline mutations in *MAX* are often associated with bilateral PCC with an increased risk for malignant PCC that is higher than most hereditary PGL/PCC syndromes but does not seem to be as high as the risk for malignancy with *SDHB*. Studies of families with *MAX* mutations suggest a similar parent-of-origin effect to *SDHD* and *SDHAF2*.[336,337] Germline mutations in *TMEM127* are associated primarily with PCC, but PGL have been reported, as has RCC.[321,338,339]

Multiple endocrine neoplasia type 2, Von Hippel–Lindau, and neurofibromatosis type 1

Well-characterized hereditary syndromes that significantly increase the risk for PCC include MEN2A/B, VHL disease, and Neurofibromatosis type 1 (NF1). MEN2A/B both increase the risk for PCC, which can be bilateral or multifocal but have a low risk of malignancy. Risk for PCC is highest with *RET* codon 918 and 634 mutations, nearing 50% or greater. The risk for PCC in moderate risk *RET* mutations can vary widely, and some have not been associated with PCC at all. Apparently sporadic PCC can be the presenting feature of MEN2A in young people particularly when associated with a codon 634 *RET* mutation, so it may be important to include MEN2 syndromes on the differential when evaluating a patient with PCC even if there is no personal or family history of MTC.[275,340,341] There are reports of extra-adrenal PGL in individuals with MEN2.[342]

VHL is reviewed in detail under the section titled "Hereditary RCC". VHL is the most common cause of hereditary RCC, but it also increases the risk for a number of benign and malignant tumors, including PCC/PGL. VHL has important genotype–phenotype correlations which are based primarily on the risk for PCC and RCC. VHL type 1 is characterized by a high risk for RCC but a low risk for PCC; VHL type 2 is characterized by a high risk for PCC and varying levels of risk for RCC depending on the type 2 subtype (detailed in the section titled "Hereditary RCC"). The risk for PCC is higher than the risk for PGL.[343,344]

NF1 is a very well-characterized hereditary syndrome with a high de novo rate. Affected individuals are often diagnosed based on the presence of classic NF1 features including but not limited to café au lait spots, inguinal and axial freckling, Lisch nodules, optic gliomas, and cutaneous neurofibromas.[345] Individuals with NF1 do have an increased risk to develop PCC, which can be bilateral and associated with metastases.[346,347]

Other hereditary syndromes associated with PCC/PGL

There are other hereditary syndromes not classically considered as PCC/PGL predisposition syndromes that increase the risk for these tumors, including MEN1 and hereditary leiomyomatosis and renal cell cancer (HLRCC). MEN1 is reviewed earlier in this section, and individuals with MEN1 are at an increased risk to develop PCC and other functional adrenal cortical tumors; however, the overall incidence is low.[263,266] HLRCC is reviewed in detail in the section titled "Hereditary RCC," and primarily increases the risk for cutaneous and uterine leiomyoma and RCC, specifically type 2 papillary. Recently, malignant PGL have been associated with HLRCC, caused by mutations in the *FH* gene.[348]

There have been case reports of individuals with germline mutations in *KIF1B* and *EGLN1* developing PCC/PGL.[349,350] Understanding of the phenotypes associated with mutations in these two genes is based on a small number of individuals, but their recognition as new PCC/PGL predisposition genes demonstrates that the number of genes associated with hereditary PCC/PGL is likely to increase in the future.

Carney triad

Carney triad (CTr) is recognized as the combination of PCC/PGL, GISTs (often gastric in origin), and pulmonary chondromas.[326] CTr is almost never inherited; however, rare cases of individuals with the diagnosis have been reported to have germline mutations in *SDHB*, *SDHC*, and *SDHD*. Affected individuals are most commonly women and are often diagnosed in their 20s–30s.[329,351,352] CTr-associated PCC/PGL show SDHB complex deficiency by IHC, as do CTr-associated GISTs; somatic mutations in *KIT* and *PDGFRA* are not expected in CTr-associated GISTs.[329] Certain recurrent somatic changes have been identified in CTr-associated tumors, including chromosomal losses involving *SDHC* on chromosome 1 and *SDHC* locus-specific methylation.[353,354]

Hereditary renal cell carcinoma syndromes

Approximately 5–8% of RCC cases are due to inherited genetic risks. RCC refers to kidney cancer involving the renal pelvis or renal medulla. Hereditary renal cancer syndromes are often characterized by both benign and malignant tumors of the kidney and other organs.

Table 1 Clinical criteria for Cowden's syndrome.

Tumor type and/or location	Typical age of diagnosis (years)	Frequency (%)
Retinal hemangioblastoma	12–25	25–60
Cerebellum hemangioblastoma	18–25	44–72
Brainstem hemangioblastoma	24–35	10–25
Spinal cord hemangioblastoma	24–35	13–50
Endolymphatic sac tumor	24–35	10–25
Renal cysts and RCC	25–50	25–60 (RCC 70% by age 60y)
Pheochromocytoma	12–25	10–20
Pancreatic cysts and PNET	24–35	35–70

Von Hippel–Lindau syndrome

The most common hereditary explanation of RCC is VHL disease occurring in 1 in 36,000 individuals.[355,356] VHL is caused by mutations in the tumor suppressor gene *VHL* and characterized by benign and malignant tumors including hemangioblastomas of the brain (cerebellum) and spine, retinal capillary hemangioblastomas, renal cysts and clear cell RCCs, PCCs, endolymphatic sac tumors of the middle ear, serous cystadenomas, pancreatic cysts and pancreatic neuroendocrine tumors (PNET), papillary cystadenomas of the epididymis and broad ligament.[356] Typical age of onset of tumors and frequency are outlined in Table 1.[355–358]

VHL is inherited in an autosomal dominant manner. Genetic testing of the VHL gene consists of sequencing and deletion/duplication analysis of the three coding exons. Genetic analysis of the *VHL* gene has a very high clinical specificity at nearly 100%. Consequently, the absence of an identified *VHL* gene mutation essentially eliminates a diagnosis of VHL in an individual.[359] Mosaicism has been described infrequently but may complicate the interpretation of results particularly in cases of atypical VHL disease in a family in which case a diagnosis of VHL cannot be excluded.[360] Approximately 72% of pathogenic mutations in *VHL* are identified by sequence analysis and 28% by deletion/duplication analysis.[361–363] Genotype–phenotype correlations have been identified on the basis of likelihood of PCC and RCC among individuals with VHL. VHL type 1, due to truncating and missense mutations disrupting the folding of the VHL protein, is characterized by a high risk of RCC but low risk of PCC.[364] VHL type 2 is often due to missense pathogenic mutations and a high risk for PCC with subgroups including type 2A (risk for PCC but low risk for RCC), 2B (risk for PCC and high risk for RCC), and 2C (risk for PCC only).[365–367] Additional studies have found exceptions to these patterns and suggested further investigation into correlations at the mutation type level, mutation region level, and mutation codon level to aid in directed surveillance and management of VHL patients accordingly.[368] As with most hereditary cancer syndromes, early detection through surveillance is key in removing tumors to prevent or minimize the impact on an individual. Surveillance for individuals with VHL begins at age on year with annual evaluation for neurologic symptoms, vision problems, hearing disturbance as well as blood pressure monitoring and progresses with more targeted screening modalities through early childhood through adulthood.[344] Among individuals with an active VHL-related diagnosis, systemic therapy options are being studied. Several antiangiogenic agents have been developed for patients with metastatic RCC with or without a VHL syndrome diagnosis including sunitinib and pazopanib.[369,370] Clinical trials to evaluate these chemotherapeutic agents among individuals with VHL and VHL-related tumors were performed with effectiveness seen in VHL-associated RCC but not hemangioblastomas.[285]

Hereditary leiomyomatosis and renal cell cancer syndrome

HLRCC is an autosomal dominant syndrome (*FH* gene) characterized by cutaneous and uterine leiomyomas and risk for papillary type 2 renal cancer.[371,372] Cutaneous leiomyomas are the most common HLRCC manifestation found in 76–100% of individuals.[371,373] The majority of women with HLRCC develop uterine leiomyomas at an early age; tumors are often frequent and large in size necessitating hysterectomy before the age of 40 in many cases.[374] While the lifetime risk for renal tumors among HLRCC patients is between 10% and 18%, tumors are often unilateral, solitary, and highly aggressive and can metastasize even when small.[371,373–375] Given the aggressive nature of HLRCC-associated renal tumors, at-risk individuals are screened annually by abdominal MRI. Screening begins in childhood with suggested guidelines ranging from ages 8 to 11 years of age.[376,377] The gene fumarate hydratase (*FH*), encodes the enzyme which converts fumarate to malate in the Kreb's cycle.[374] Biallelic mutations in *FH* gene cause individuals to develop FH Deficiency described by rapidly progressive neurologic impairment, progressive encephalopathy, hypotonia, failure to thrive, and seizures.[378] Although family members could undergo FH enzymatic activity screening to determine potential carrier status by reduced levels, genetic testing remains a more effectual method to identify at-risk individuals.[379] Gene sequencing identifies approximately 70–90% of pathogenic mutations and a smaller proportion are identified by deletion/duplication analysis.[371,373,374] The incidence of HLRCC in the population is unknown given HLRCC is a rare and relatively new genetic condition, but it is likely underdiagnosed due to often mild presentation in the absence of RCC.

Birt–Hogg–Dubé syndrome

Birt–Hogg–Dubé syndrome (BHD) has pathogenic mutations in the *FLCN* gene inherited in an autosomal dominant manner. BHD is thought to occur in approximately 1 of 200,000 people, but like many hereditary RCC syndromes, it is likely underdiagnosed due to its variable presentation. BHD is characterized by cutaneous lesions including fibrofolliculomas and trichodiscomas, lung cysts, and risk for spontaneous pneumothorax, and renal cancer.[380–382] The most frequent manifestations of BHD are fibrofolliculomas and lung cysts, while the risk of at least one pneumothorax is up to 30%.[383,384] It is estimated that the risk of an individual with BHD to develop renal tumors is 33% and often presents as bilateral multifocal tumors of chromophobe RCC, oncocytoma, or hybrid oncocytoma but clear cell RCC has also been reported.[385] Renal oncocytosis describes individuals with microscopic scattering of multiple oncocytic tumors often seen among individuals with BHD.[385] Genetic testing can be used to confirm a diagnosis of BHD among individuals with suspected features. Sequence analysis identifies 88% of pathogenic variants in *FLCN* while partial- or whole-gene deletions account for 3–5% of germline mutations.[384,386] Seven to nine percent of individuals with a clinical diagnosis of BHD will not have an identifiable *FLCN* pathogenic mutation. Individuals with a pathogenic mutation in *FLCN* should undergo recommended screening recommendations primarily for the detection and management of renal tumors. Surveillance by annual or biannual CT or MRI is recommended beginning at age 20 years.[387] Annual dermatologic evaluation is recommended along with thoracic and abdominal imaging to screen for lung cysts and indication of pneumothorax.[387,388]

Hereditary papillary renal cancer syndrome

Hereditary papillary renal cancer (HPRC) is a rare inherited renal cancer syndrome due to mutations in the *MET* proto-oncogene notable for elevated risks of papillary type 1 RCC which are often multifocal and bilateral.[389,390] While there have been families with early-onset presentation of papillary type 1 RCC characteristic of inherited cancer syndromes, the typical presentation of renal tumors is often in the 6th and 7th decades of life.[389,391]

BAP1

More recently discovered is the association of germline *BAP1* mutations among individuals with familial clear cell renal cell cancer.[392,393] *BAP1*-associated renal tumors tend to be more aggressive with decreased overall survival.[394,395] *BAP1* mutations have been identified in families with early-onset, bilateral, and multifocal clear cell RCCs as well as risks for atypical spitz tumors, uveal and cutaneous melanoma, and mesothelioma.[392,393,396]

MiTF-associated cancer syndrome

Microphthalmia-associated transcription factor (MiTF) is considered a moderately penetrant hereditary renal cancer gene. MiTF is a member of the MiTF family of transcription factors.[397] A single germline missense variant, c.952G>A or p.E318K, has been reported among individuals with family history of cutaneous malignant melanoma and renal cancer with risks approximately fivefold above noncarriers.[398,399] No specific renal tumor histology or age of onset has been characterized at this time. More research is needed to understand the cancer risks and phenotype of MiTF pathogenic mutations.

Succinate dehydrogenase-deficient renal cancer

Autosomal dominant inheritance of succinate dehydrogenase (SDH) genes are associated primarily with hereditary paraganglioma and PCC syndromes as discussed in detail in the inherited endocrine section of this article. Along with significantly elevated risks for paraganglioma, individuals with germline mutations in SDH subunits (*SDHA, SDHB, SDHC, SDHD*) may also be at an increased risk for kidney cancer. SDH–RCC is defined by loss of IHC staining for *SDHB* and highly associated with a germline mutation in one of the SDH subunits.[400] SDH–RCC is often characterized by multifocal, early-onset renal tumors and bilateral disease is seen in as many as 26% of cases.[400–402] Tumor pathology continues to be characterized but has been reported to consist primarily of clear cell, chromophobe, and oncoytic neoplasms.[403]

Tuberous sclerosis complex

Tuberous sclerosis complex (TSC) is characterized by autosomal dominant inheritance of germline mutations in *TSC1* or *TSC2* that encode hamartin and tuberin proteins, respectively.[404,405] Individuals with TSC have varying presentations of both major and minor features of the neurocutaneous condition including cerebral cortical tubers, facial angiofibromas, lymphangioleiomyomatosis (LAM) of the lung, and renal angiomyolipomas (AML).[406] The presenting renal phenotypes of TSC include AMLs (85%), renal cysts (45%), and RCC (4%).[407] There is a higher frequency of the renal manifestations among individuals with *TSC2* mutations than *TSC1* mutations.[407] While risk for renal cancer is not particularly elevated above that of the general population, there appears to be a high risk of multifocal, bilateral, and earlier age of onset than seen in the general population.[407–409] Less frequently, renal oncocytoma tumors have been reported.[410] Associated renal condition with *TSC2* may also be polycystic kidney disease given the proximity to autosomal dominant polycystic kidney disease, *PKD1*, gene. The presence of a contiguous gene deletion leads to *TSC2/PKD1* disorder that is often diagnosed in the first year of life or early childhood.[411,412]

Cowden syndrome

Pathogenic mutations in *PTEN* gene are associated with autosomal dominant CS. The incidence of CS is estimated between 1 in 200,000 and 250,000.[413] CS is characterized by multiple benign and malignant tumors of multiple organ systems as well as mucocutaneous lesions (trichilemmomas, acral keratosis, and/or facial/oral papules) in nearly 100% of individuals.[71,414] Elevated risks of cancer include breast, thyroid, endometrial, colorectal, and renal cancers.[70,72,415] CS is also often associated with macrocephaly.[71,416] The risk of RCC among individuals with CS is estimated between 2% and 5% but some reports have reported as high as a 34% lifetime risk.[76,417,418]

Chromosome 3 translocations

In a subset of familial clear cell RCC cases, constitutional chromosome 3 translocations co-segregate with disease. Several families have been reported with varying translocations involving chromosome 3.[419–421] The exact mechanism constitutional chromosome 3 translocations have in RCC development is not known, but a multi-step model has been proposed due to the presence of a nonhomologs chromatid exchange involving chromosome 3 resulting in a germline balanced chromosome 3 translocation. The nondisjunctional loss of the derivative chromosome containing the 3p segment occurs in the cell resulting in the presence of only one chromosome 3 allele. A somatic mutation may then occur in a tumor suppressor gene, such as VHL, on the remaining chromosome 3 allele followed by RCC tumorigenesis.[419,421] Other possibilities for the underlying explanation of this risk have not been excluded but the presence of chromosome 3 translocations among families with familial RCC warrants consideration of cytogenetic analysis.[420]

Upper urinary tract cancer

Cancer of the upper urinary tract, particularly the ureter and renal pelvis, is seen at a higher frequency among individuals with Lynch syndrome due to mutations in the DNA MMR genes.[115,422,423] As discussed in more detail within the section titled "Hereditary gastrointestinal cancers," Lynch syndrome is primarily associated with elevated risks for colorectal and endometrial cancers. An elevated risk for upper tract urothelial carcinoma (UTUC) has been estimated at 8% by age 70 among individuals with Lynch syndrome.[423] MSI testing to demonstrate MSI and IHC to show loss of staining among the MMR proteins is commonly used to assess tumors likely due to Lynch syndrome; however, the use of MSI and IHC in other Lynch syndrome tumors has not been as thoroughly evaluated. The efficacy of tumor studies in a UTUC population is unknown; therefore, germline testing of MMR genes associated with Lynch syndrome may still be the most appropriate when personal and family history is suggestive of Lynch syndrome.

Testicular cancer

Among men ages 15–35, testicular cancer remains the most common solid malignancy, predominantly testicular germ cell tumor (TGCT).[424] TGCTs have a high heritable component and family history is the strongest known risk factor for development of these tumors. First-degree male relatives of men with TGCT are at a significantly elevated risk to develop TGCT themselves including a four- to six-fold risk for sons and eight- to ten-fold risk for brothers of an affected individual.[425] Several genome wide association studies have been conducted in efforts to locate genetic risks for TGCT with success.[426,427] Efforts to create polygenic risk scoring among men to stratify TGCT risk based on GWAS findings may better establish screening recommendations in the future.[428] While there has been limited evidence of single-gene hereditary explanations for TGCTs, a case-control study involving men with pathogenic variants in CHEK2 were significantly more likely to develop TGCTs and at younger ages providing some insight into potential management strategies and treatment for men at high-risk (PMID: 30676620).

Hereditary predispositions to hematologic malignancies

Hematologic malignancies comprise a large group of malignancies of the hematopoietic system. Chronic and acute leukemia can arise from either lymphoid or myeloid lineage precursor cells resulting in aberrations to the circulating blood cells and decreased immune function. Myelodysplastic syndromes (MDS) are clonal blood disorders characterized by ineffective hematopoiesis, cytopenias, bone marrow dysplasia, and an increased risk to develop AML. Aplastic anemia (AA), also called bone marrow failure, is a drastic decrease in bone marrow cellularity and the production of red blood cells, white blood cells, and platelets. Within the past 10 years, nearly a dozen adult-onset inherited leukemia and MDS predisposition syndromes have been identified. While previously considered quite rare, increased awareness of and testing for these syndromes has resulted in increased detection. In patients with hematologic malignancies referred for clinical testing, germline predisposition mutations have been identified in 12–19% of patients, similar to the rate in solid tumor populations.[429,430]

Acute myeloid leukemia (AML) and myelodysplastic syndrome (MDS) predisposition syndromes

To date, there are several well-defined syndromes that confer an increased lifetime risk of MDS and AML. They are characterized by predisposition to myeloid neoplasm, with or without concomitant or precedent cytopenias (often thrombocytopenia) or other phenotypic characteristics. The known predisposition syndromes are summarized in the table below.

Syndrome	Gene	Inheritance	Heme malignancy	Other characteristics	Reference(s)
Familial platelet disorder with propensity to myeloid neoplasms	RUNX1	Autosomal dominant	MDS/AML, T-cell ALL	Thrombocytopenia, bleeding propensity, aspirin-like platelet dysfunction	431, 432
Thrombocytopenia 2	ANKRD26	Autosomal dominant	MDS/AML	Thrombocytopenia, bleeding propensity	433
Thrombocytopenia 5	ETV6	Autosomal dominant	MDS/AML, CMML, B-cell ALL, multiple myeloma, aplastic anemia	Thrombocytopenia	434
SAMD9-related disorders	SAMD9, SAMD9L	Autosomal dominant	Monosomy 7 MDS/AML	MIRAGE syndrome, ataxia	435
Familial AML with mutated CEBPA	CEBPA	Autosomal dominant	AML	None	436
Familial AML with mutation DDX41	DDX41	Autosomal dominant	MDS/AML, CMML	None	437
GATA2 deficiency	GATA2	Autosomal dominant	MDS/AML, CMML	None, or neutropenia, monocytopenia (MonoMac), lymphedema, extragenital warts, immunodeficiency	438
Myeloid neoplasms with duplications of ATG2B and GSKIP	ATG2B/GSKIP	Autosomal dominant	AML, ET, CMML, myelofibrosis, CML, aCML	None	439
Telomere biology disorders (dyskeratosis congenita)	TERC, TERT Telomere length <1%	Autosomal dominant, autosomal recessive, X-linked	MDS/AML, aplastic anemia	Macrocytosis, hypocellular bone marrow, squamous cell carcinoma, chemo/XRT toxicity	440
Familial aplastic anemia with SRP72 mutation	SRP72	Autosomal dominant	MDS, aplastic anemia	None	441
Fanconi anemia	Complementation groups DEB or MMC assay	Autosomal recessive	MDS/AML, aplastic anemia	Short stature, café-au-lait macules, skeletal malformations, microcephaly	442

Genetic testing is clinically available for the newly described leukemia predisposition syndromes but is underutilized, likely due to lack of awareness in both the hematologist/oncologist and genetic counseling communities.[429] These syndromes overlap substantially in their associated risks of both MDS and AML making them difficult to distinguish based on clinical phenotype alone.

Familial platelet disorder with propensity to myeloid malignancy (FPD-AML)

Familial platelet disorder with propensity to myeloid malignancy is an autosomal dominant familial MDS/AML syndrome caused by inherited mutations in the hematopoietic transcription factor RUNX1. Most germline mutations in RUNX1 lead to protein loss-of-function or confer dominant-negative effects to the remaining RUNX1 allele.[432] Clinically, patients with FPD/AML typically present with life-long thrombocytopenia and aspirin-like functional platelet defects.[443] The degree of thrombocytopenia in individuals with RUNX1 mutations is typically mild to moderate and can vary widely even within the same family. The lifetime risk of MDS or acute leukemia is estimated to be 35–40%, with an average age at diagnosis of 33 years (range: 6–76 years).[431] Hematologic malignancies described in FPD/AML patients include MDS, AML, and T-cell ALL. No clinical or laboratory markers are currently available to predict when a patient with FPD/AML will develop an overt malignancy; however, recent data suggests clonal hematopoiesis can be detected in >80% of asymptomatic FPD/AML individuals by age 50 and may provide a future means of disease surveillance.[444] For individuals without hematologic malignancy who harbor germline RUNX1 mutations, current recommendations include a bone marrow biopsy at baseline with cytogenetic analysis, followed by CBC and clinical exams at regular intervals. In the event that a RUNX1 mutation carrier develops acute leukemia or MDS requiring allogeneic stem cell transplantation (SCT), genetic testing should be performed urgently on HLA-matched related and those who also carry the mutation should not be used as donors. Adverse outcomes including donor-derived leukemia and failure to engraft have been reported.[445]

Thrombocytopenia 2

Associated with germline mutations in the 5' UTR of the gene Ankyrin Repeat Domain 26 (ANKRD26), Thrombocytopenia 2 is an autosomal dominant disorder that is characterized by moderate thrombocytopenia with or without bleeding propensity, similar to FPD/AML. In a recent study of 78 affected individuals from 21 families with familial Thrombocytopenia 2, the average platelet count was 48,000/microL.[446] In affected individuals, bone marrow morphology can demonstrate dyskmegakaryopoeisis with hypolobulated micromegakaryocytes at baseline, presenting a diagnostic challenge for hematopathologists to appropriately distinguish individuals with germline ANKRD26 mutations versus dysmegakaryopoiesis related to development of MDS.[446] The prevalence of Thrombocytopenia 2 is not well described; an inherited thrombocytopenia registry identified ANKRD26 mutations in 23 cases out of 215 individuals (11%).[447] Individuals with

ANKRD26 are clinically difficult to distinguish from those with FPD/AML.[445]

Familial AML with mutated DDX41

One of the most recently described inherited susceptibility loci for myeloid neoplasms, DDX41 germline mutations are associated with autosomal dominant familial MDS/AML. A recurrent mutation, p.D140Gfs*2, appears to account for the majority of germline mutations.[448] DDX41 mutations result in an increased lifetime risk of myeloid neoplasms including MDS, AML, and CML, although notably after a long latency, with an average age of disease onset of 61 years.[449] This average age at diagnosis falls within the expected age range of MDS/AML in the general population, thus it may be clinically difficult to distinguish patients with *de novo* MDS/AML from those with a germline predisposition due to a germline mutation in DDX41 and this syndrome may be particularly under diagnosed. Myeloid malignancies in patients with DDX41 mutations often demonstrate an acquired somatic mutation in the wild-type DDX41 allele, suggesting that it may act as a tumor suppressor.[448] The prevalence of DDX41 germline mutations is not known; however, in a study screening 1000 myeloid neoplasm cases, DDX41 was identified in 1.5%, half of which were germline, suggesting that identification of a somatic DDX41 mutation should prompt consideration of germline analysis.[437]

Unlike the majority of syndromes predisposing to MDS, DDX41-related malignancies have no preceding clinical signs or symptoms as harbingers of the increased risk for hematologic malignancy. In families with known DDX41 mutations, like other predisposition syndromes, a bone marrow biopsy is recommended at diagnosis with cytogenetic analysis and CBC at regular intervals.[445] Several cases of DDX41 donor-derived leukemia in the post-SCT setting have been reported in the last few years.[450,451] This heightens the importance of increasing detection of DDX41 mutations in affected probands and their potential related donors to optimize SCT planning and improve outcomes.

Thrombocytopenia 5

Thrombocytopenia 5 is an inherited autosomal dominant MDS/AML predisposition syndrome associated with moderate thrombocytopenia, with or without a clinical bleeding propensity.[452] Similar to RUNX1 and ANKRD26 mutation carriers, individuals with mutations in ETV6—associated with Thrombocytopenia 5—present with a variable degree of thrombocytopenia and mild-to-moderate bleeding tendencies.[453] Individuals with germline ETV6 mutations are at increased risk for several hematologic malignancies, including MDS, AML, CMML, B-lymphoblastic leukemia, and plasma cell myeloma.[454] Early-onset CRC has also been reported in a small number of individuals to date.[434] As with other hereditary familial platelet disorders, individuals carrying germline ETV6 mutations are recommended to undergo bone marrow biopsy with cytogenetic analysis at diagnosis with CBC screening at regular intervals; care should be taken to avoid using family members who also carry the mutation for SCT due to adverse outcomes.[445]

Familial MDS/AML with mutated *GATA2* (*GATA2* deficiency)

GATA2 deficiency is a clinically heterogenous predisposition to myeloid malignancies. Individuals with germline *GATA2* mutations can present without any hematopoietic or organ system involvement prior to the development of MDS or AML. There are two distinct syndromic presentations which can be seen clinically. Emberger syndrome describes *GATA2* deficiency characterized by primary lymphedema, sensorineural hearing loss, cutaneous/extragenital warts, and a low CD4/CD8 T-cell ratio with a predisposition to MDS/AML.[455] MonoMac syndrome is characterized by dendritic cell, monocyte, and B/NK cell deficiencies, atypical mycobacterial or fungal infections, pulmonary alveolar proteinosis, and MDS/AML predisposition.[438] Individuals with *GATA2* germline mutations are at significantly increased lifetime risk of MDS/AML of approximately 70% by a median age of onset of 29 years (range 0.4–78).[456] Management and surveillance of individuals with *GATA2* deficiency often involve a multidisciplinary care team given multi-organ involvement. The high incidence of MDS/AML in these individuals beginning in childhood and adolescence also warrants close evaluation. A bone marrow biopsy, like with most hereditary MDS/AML syndromes, is recommended at baseline with cytogenetic analysis and repeated with any changes trending on complete blood count that portends a developing MDS or AML.[445,456]

Familial aplastic anemia/MDS with SRP72 mutation

Germline mutations in gene *SRP72* have been identified as a rare cause of familial MDS and bone marrow failure. Two pedigrees with autosomal dominant MDS and AA have been reported. In both families, MDS developed in adulthood. Given the rarity of these germline mutations, little is known regarding the incidence, lifetime risk for AA/MDS, and/or targeted clinical management guidelines of these families.[457]

Inherited bone marrow failure syndromes

Bone marrow failure syndromes are typically associated with onset of MDS, AA, and/or AML in childhood or adolescence. While the majority of individuals with bone marrow failure syndromes will have syndromic phenotypic abnormalities, there may be subtle or absent phenotypic presentations resulting in a delayed diagnosis in adulthood.[458] Individuals with Fanconi anemia (FA) and dyskeratosis congenita (DC) are at significantly increased risk for treatment-related toxicities when treated with cytotoxic therapies, particularly in the context of SCT, and also at risk for treatment-induced malignancies.[459]

Fanconi anemia

FA is a rare autosomal recessive or X-linked inherited predisposition to bone marrow failure. Accompanied by congenital limb anomalies including absent thumbs and other radial ray defects, FA is characterized by increased chromosomal fragility and breakage when treated with cross-linking agents diepoxybutane (DEB) or mitomycin C (MMC).[460] Bone marrow failure with pancytopenia typically appears in the first decade and by age 50 the incidence of bone marrow failure is estimated to be 90%. The incidence of hematologic malignancies is 10–30% and there is also an increased risk of solid tumors, particularly squamous cell carcinomas of the head and neck and anogenital tract.[461] Up to 40% of individuals with FA lack the physical abnormalities associated with the disease and are also less likely to develop early-onset bone marrow failure.[442] FA is caused by homozygous or compound heterozygous mutations in the 19 FA complementation groups, *FANCA–FANCP*.[460] Mutations in *FANCA* are the most common, accounting for 60–70% of cases of FA, followed by *FANCC*, accounting for 14%. The remaining 13 complementation groups account for 1–3% of cases each.[462]

Dyskeratosis congenita/telomeropathies

DC is a telomere biology disorder originally characterized by the diagnostic triad of dysplastic nails, lacy reticular skin pigmentation, and oral leukoplakia. These features, however, are not present in all individuals with DC.[440] Individuals with DC are at increased risk for BMF, MDS, or AML, solid tumors (typically squamous cell carcinomas of the head, neck, anogenital tract), and pulmonary fibrosis. The median age of onset of MDS is 35 years (range 19–61).[463] DC is characterized by very short telomeres defined as less than 1% of age-matched normal controls. Eleven genes have been identified to cause DC: *ACD, CTC1, DKC1, RTEL1, PARN, TERC, TERT, TINF2, NHP2, NOP10,* and *WRAP53*; however, germline mutations are detected in ~50% of individuals meeting clinical diagnostic criteria.[464] *TERT* and *TERC* germline mutations have been associated with MDS, AA, idiopathic pulmonary fibrosis, and adult-onset disease.[465] Telomere length by flow-FISH is recommended in these patients to detect an underlying diagnosis of DC.[466]

Hereditary predispositions to acute lymphoblastic leukemia (ALL)

Inherited predisposition to lymphoid malignancies and chronic leukemia are still rare. Acute lymphoblastic leukemia is the most common leukemia in childhood. Hereditary predispositions to ALL were first described within the spectrum of Li–Fraumeni syndrome in 1988 by Li et al.[56] Since that time, *TP53* germline mutations have remained in the differential for rare cases of familial pediatric ALL. In 2013, Holmfeldt et al. described the unique association of *TP53* mutations with the characteristic genotype of hypodiploid/masked hypodiploid ALL.[467] Constitutional mismatch repair deficiency syndrome (CMMRD) was described first in 1999 in patients from consanguineous marriages in families with known Lynch syndrome. These individuals that have biallelic germline mutations (homozygous or compound heterozygous) in the MMR genes are predisposed to childhood hematological malignancies in contrast to patients whom have Lynch syndrome and inherit as monoallelic (autosomal dominant heterozygote) mutation that predisposes to solid tumors during adulthood.[468]

Autosomal dominant germline mutations in *ETV6* were first described is 2015 in three separate publications. Affected individuals in these families present clinically with a mild bleeding propensity with an associated mild to moderate thrombocytopenia, with or without macrocytosis, and an inherited predisposition to hematologic malignancies, most commonly ALL.[434] Topka et al. identified a novel germline mutation in *ETV6* in two families; in one kindred affected individuals had thrombocytopenia and childhood pre-B ALL, and in a second kindred patients with an *ETV6* mutation had thrombocytopenia, ALL, and therapy-related MDS.[454]

Inherited mutations in *PAX5* were described by Shah et al. in 2013. This was the first published report of a dominantly inherited susceptibility to pre-B cell ALL caused by germline *PAX5* mutations and described two unrelated families with familial pre-B cell ALL.[469] Auer et al. described a third family; all three cases described the same *PAX5* mutation, c.547G>A segregating with development of pre-B ALL.[470] While germline *PAX5* mutations have been described in only three families to date, an emerging association with the specific subtype of pre-B cell ALL is seen. The clinical phenotype of germline *PAX5* mutations will likely be further refined as additional families are discovered.

Biallelic mutations in the gene *SH2B3* cause a recessive predisposition to ALL that has been described in only a single family.[471] This autosomal recessive syndrome should be considered, with *ETV6, TP53, PAX5*, and constitutional mismatch repair syndrome in families with affected siblings with ALL, especially pre-B cell ALL, with or without syndromic features of developmental delay and autoimmune disease or personal or family history of thrombocytopenia or other hematologic malignancies.

Familial lymphoproliferative disorders

Lymphoproliferative disorders, the class of diseases encompassing chronic lymphocytic leukemia (CLL), Hodgkin's and non-Hodgkin's lymphoma, and multiple myeloma among others, have long shown a trend towards increased familial incidence but very few single gene etiologies have been elucidated.[472] This is likely due to the multifactorial nature of lymphoproliferative neoplasms including both environmental risks and immune dysregulation due to viral infections. In families with lymphoproliferative disorders, a slightly increased incidence of nearly all lymphoproliferative disorders is seen in FDRs, not simply limited to the diagnosis in the index patient.[473] For example, individuals with a family history of CLL are at slightly increased risk for CLL (2.3–8 RR) but also for non-Hodgkin's lymphoma (1.9 RR), Hodgkin's lymphoma (1.3–1.5 RR), Waldenstrom's macroglobulinemia (4.0 RR), and multiple myeloma (1.2 RR).[472] *POT1* is one of the only single gene predispositions to familial CLL and lymphoproliferative disorders, but mutations only account for a very small number of affected families.[474] In the absence of a *POT1* gene mutation, recurrence risk estimates for family members via RRs is the most appropriate way to counsel family members. The relatively low incidence of lymphoma and lymphoproliferative disorders, modest familial risk, and the lack of effective screening and intervention argue against active clinical surveillance for lymphoproliferative disorders in unaffected FDRs.[472]

Special considerations for genetic counseling and testing

Genetic counseling and genetic testing for leukemia patients present several unique challenges. Identification of individuals with underlying germline mutations, however, difficult, is also of paramount importance. Hematopoietic stem cell transplant (HSCT) is the only curative option for severe BMF or MDS/leukemia; however, care must be taken given an increased rate of HSCT-related complications including increased risk of graft failure, graft-versus-host disease, sepsis, pulmonary fibrosis, hepatic cirrhosis, and veno-occlusive disease caused in part by the underlying pulmonary and liver disease particularly in patients with DC or other inherited bone marrow failure syndromes. Long-term survival of individuals with DC or FA following standard SCT regimens has been poor.[475] Reduced-intensity conditioning regimens are recommended to decrease toxicity and reduce the risk of posttransplant toxicity and graft-versus-host disease.[476,477]

Additionally, HLA-matched related siblings are the optimal donors for allogeneic SCT in patients with MDS/AML. In families with germline mutations, careful familial evaluation and avoidance of SCT with a sibling who shares the same germline mutation is crucial. Poor outcomes from SCT in recipients of stem cells from a related donor who carries the same germline mutation are well documented and include increased risk for slow engraftment or failure to graft, and donor-derived leukemia.[445] Donor-derived leukemia is a rare posttransplant complication in which a new leukemia arises from the donor marrow and is an increased risk in individuals with germline MDS/AML predisposition syndromes if careful attention to use a mutation-negative donor is not paid.[451]

Genetic testing is complicated in hematologic malignancy patients by the nature of the malignancy. Genetic testing laboratories obtain DNA from the lymphocytes in peripheral blood, found in the buffy coat of a blood sample, or contained within saliva/buccal swabs. Saliva contains a significant amount of peripheral blood-derived elements, particularly in the setting of patients with leukemia and thrombocytopenia due to gum bleeding. Leukemia and lymphomas are malignancies of the bone marrow and of the lymphocyte-producing stem cells. In addition to acquiring somatic drive mutations, there are often numerous chromosomal aberrations within the malignant white blood cells of leukemia patients. Therefore, genetic testing of the peripheral blood in patients with blood cancers provides a somatic analysis of the leukemia and does not reflect the true inherited (germline) status of the patient. A nonhematologic sample is required for accurate genetic testing. Saliva and buccal swabs in leukemia patients are also significantly contaminated with malignant cells and are not suitable samples. Germline DNA can be obtained from multiple nonhematologic sources in leukemia patients including fingernails and eyebrows; however, skin fibroblasts obtained from skin punch biopsy are the gold standard. A relatively easy outpatient clinical procedure, 3–4 mm standard skin punch biopsy of normal skin yields enough fibroblasts for culture and analysis. This sample, after culture, is not contaminated by malignancy and is an accurate sample for genetic testing.

Key references

The complete reference list can be found on Vital Source version of this title, see inside front cover.

1. Robson ME, Bradbury AR, Arun B, et al. American Society of Clinical Oncology policy statement update: genetic and genomic testing for cancer susceptibility. *J Clin Oncol.* 2015;**33**(31):3660–3667.
11. Adams-Campbell LL, Makambi KH, Palmer JR, et al. Diagnostic accuracy of the Gail model in the Black Women's Health Study. *Breast J.* 2007;**13**(4):332–336.
12. Claus EB, Risch N, Thompson WD. Autosomal dominant inheritance of early-onset breast cancer. Implications for risk prediction. *Cancer.* 1994;**73**(3):643–651.
13. Shattuck-Eidens, D., Oliphant A, McClure M et al., BRCA1 sequence analysis in women at high risk for susceptibility mutations. Risk factor analysis and implications for genetic testing. *JAMA,* 1997. **278**(15): p. 1242-50.
15. Couch FJ, ML DS, Blackwood MA, et al. BRCA1 mutations in women attending clinics that evaluate the risk of breast cancer. *N Engl J Med.* 1997;**336**(20):1409–1415.
16. Parmigiani G, Berry D, Aguilar O. Determining carrier probabilities for breast cancer-susceptibility genes BRCA1 and BRCA2. *Am J Hum Genet.* 1998;**62**(1):145–158.
22. Goldgar DE, Easton DF, Cannon-Albright LA, et al. Systematic population-based assessment of cancer risk in first-degree relatives of cancer probands. *J Natl Cancer Inst.* 1994;**86**(21):1600–1608.
24. Claus EB, Schildkraut JM, Thompson WD, et al. The genetic attributable risk of breast and ovarian cancer. *Cancer.* 1996;**77**(11):2318–2324.
31. Kwon JS, Gutierrez-Barrera AM, Young D, et al. Expanding the criteria for BRCA mutation testing in breast cancer survivors. *J Clin Oncol.* 2010;**28**(27):4214–4220.
32. Ford D, Easton DF, Bishop DT, et al. Risks of cancer in BRCA1-mutation carriers. *The Lancet.* 1994;**343**(8899):692–695.
33. Easton DF, Steele L, Fields P, et al. Cancer risks in two large breast cancer families linked to BRCA2 on chromosome 13q12-13. *Am J Hum Genet.* 1997;**61**(1):120–128.
34. Antoniou A, PDP P, Narod S, et al. Average risks of breast and ovarian cancer associated with BRCA1 or BRCA2 mutations detected in case series unselected for family history: a combined analysis of 22 studies. *Am J Hum Genet.* 2003;**72**(5):1117–1130.
43. Somlo G, Frankel PH, Arun BK, et al. Efficacy of the PARP inhibitor veliparib with carboplatin or as a single agent in patients with germline BRCA1- or BRCA2-associated metastatic breast cancer: California Cancer Consortium Trial NCT01149083. *Clin Cancer Res.* 2017;**23**(15):4066–4076.
44. Robson M, Im SA, Senkus E, et al. Olaparib for metastatic breast cancer in patients with a germline BRCA mutation. *N Engl J Med.* 2017;**377**(6):523–533.
59. Hwang S-J, Lozano G, Amos CI, et al. Germline p53 mutations in a cohort with childhood sarcoma: sex differences in cancer risk. *Am J Human Genet.* 2003;**72**(4):975–983.
63. Malkin D. Li-fraumeni syndrome. *Genes Cancer.* 2011;**2**(4):475–484.
72. Pilarski R. Cowden syndrome: a critical review of the clinical literature. *J Genet Counsel.* 2009;**18**(1):13–27.
77. Masciari S, Larsson N, Senz J, et al. Germline E-cadherin mutations in familial lobular breast cancer. *J Med Genet.* 2007;**44**(11):726–731.
84. Lim W, Olschwang S, Keller JJ, et al. Relative frequency and morphology of cancers in STK11 mutation carriers. *Gastroenterology.* 2004;**126**(7):1788–1794.
87. Lancaster JM, Powell CB, Chen LM, et al. Society of Gynecologic Oncology statement on risk assessment for inherited gynecologic cancer predispositions. *Gynecol Oncol.* 2015;**136**(1):3–7.
90. Bonadona V, Bonaiti B, Olschwang S, et al. Cancer risks associated with germline mutations in MLH1, MSH2, and MSH6 genes in Lynch syndrome. *J Am Med Assoc.* 2011;**305**(22):2304–2310.
92. Antoniou AC, Casadei S, Heikkinen T, et al. Breast-cancer risk in families with mutations in PALB2. *N Engl J Med.* 2014;**371**(6):497–506.
94. Couch FJ, Shimelis H, Hu C, et al. Associations between cancer predisposition testing panel genes and breast cancer. *JAMA Oncol.* 2017;**3**(9):1190–1196.
97. Tung N, Domchek SM, Stadler Z, et al. Counselling framework for moderate-penetrance cancer-susceptibility mutations. *Nat Rev Clin Oncol.* 2016;**13**(9):581–588.
99. CHEK2 Breast Cancer Case-Control Consortium. CHEK2*1100delC and susceptibility to breast cancer: a collaborative analysis involving 10,860 breast cancer cases and 9,065 controls from 10 studies. *Am J Human Genet.* 2004;**74**(6):1175–1182.
103. Ramus SJ, Song H, Dickes E, et al. Germline mutations in the BRIP1, BARD1, PALB2, and NBN genes in women with ovarian cancer. *J Natl Cancer Inst.* 2015;**107**(11):djv214.
107. Lynch HT, de la Chapelle A. Hereditary colorectal cancer. *N Engl J Med.* 2003;**348**(10):919–932.
111. Chadwick RB, Pyatt RE, Niemann TH, et al. Hereditary and somatic DNA mismatch repair gene mutations in sporadic endometrial carcinoma. *J Med Genet.* 2001;**38**(7):461–466.
112. Cunningham JM, Kim CY, Christensen ER, et al. The frequency of hereditary defective mismatch repair in a prospective series of unselected colorectal carcinomas. *Am J Hum Genet.* 2001;**69**(4):780–790.
113. Kovacs ME, Papp J, Szentirmay Z, et al. Deletions removing the last exon of TACSTD1 constitute a distinct class of mutations predisposing to Lynch syndrome. *Hum Mutat.* 2009;**30**(2):197–203.
122. Schmeler KM, Lynch HT, Chen LM, et al. Prophylactic surgery to reduce the risk of gynecologic cancers in the Lynch syndrome. *N Engl J Med.* 2006;**354**(3):261–269.
124. Deng G, Bell I, Crawley S, et al. BRAF mutation is frequently present in sporadic colorectal cancer with methylated hMLH1, but not in hereditary nonpolyposis colorectal cancer. *Clin Cancer Res.* 2004;**10**(1 Pt 1):191–195.
126. Ribic CM, Sargent DJ, Moore MJ, et al. Tumor microsatellite-instability status as a predictor of benefit from fluorouracil-based adjuvant chemotherapy for colon cancer. *N Engl J Med.* 2003;**349**(3):247–257.
134. Lindor NM, Rabe K, Petersen GM, et al. Lower cancer incidence in Amsterdam-I criteria families without mismatch repair deficiency: familial colorectal cancer type X. *JAMA.* 2005;**293**(16):1979–1985.
148. Bianchi LK, Burke CA, Bennett AE, et al. Fundic gland polyp dysplasia is common in familial adenomatous polyposis. *Clin Gastroenterol Hepatol.* 2008;**6**(2):180–185.
155. Cetta F, Ugolini G, Martellucci J, et al. Screening for thyroid cancer in patients with familial adenomatous polyposis. *Ann Surg.* 2015;**261**(1):e13–e14.
160. Aretz S, Stienen D, Uhlhaas S, et al. Large submicroscopic genomic APC deletions are a common cause of typical familial adenomatous polyposis. *J Med Genet.* 2005;**42**(2):185–192.
163. Sieber OM, Lipton L, Crabtree M, et al. Multiple colorectal adenomas, classic adenomatous polyposis, and germ-line mutations in MYH. *N Engl J Med.* 2003;**348**(9):791–799.
172. Palles C, Cazier JB, Howarth KM, et al. Germline mutations affecting the proof-reading domains of POLE and POLD1 predispose to colorectal adenomas and carcinomas. *Nat Genet.* 2013;**45**(2):136–144.

178 Jaeger EE, Woodford-Richens KL, Lockett M, et al. An ancestral Ashkenazi haplotype at the HMPS/CRAC1 locus on 15q13-q14 is associated with hereditary mixed polyposis syndrome. *Am J Hum Genet*. 2003;**72**(5):1261–1267.

193 Howe JR, Ringold JC, Summers RW, et al. A gene for familial juvenile polyposis maps to chromosome 18q21.1. *Am J Hum Genet*. 1998;**62**(5):1129–1136.

205 Hansford S, Kaurah P, Li-Chang H, et al. Hereditary diffuse gastric cancer syndrome: CDH1 mutations and beyond. *JAMA Oncol*. 2015;**1**(1):23–32.

214 Lynch HT, Lynch JF. Hereditary diffuse gastric cancer: lifesaving total gastrectomy for CDH1 mutation carriers. *J Med Genet*. 2010;**47**(7):433–435.

221 Brune KA, Lau B, Palmisano E, et al. Importance of age of onset in pancreatic cancer kindreds. *J Natl Cancer Inst*. 2010;**102**(2):119–126.

227 Brose MS, Rebbeck TR, Calzone KA, et al. Cancer risk estimates for BRCA1 mutation carriers identified in a risk evaluation program. *J Natl Cancer Inst*. 2002;**94**(18):1365–1372.

238 Pritchard CC, Mateo J, Walsh MF, et al. Inherited DNA-Repair Gene Mutations in Men with Metastatic Prostate Cancer. *N Engl J Med*. 2016;**375**(5):443–453.

247 Castro E, Goh C, Olmos D, et al. Germline BRCA mutations are associated with higher risk of nodal involvement, distant metastasis, and poor survival outcomes in prostate cancer. *J Clin Oncol*. 2013;**31**(14):1748–1757.

254 Ewing CM, Ray AM, Lange EM, et al. Germline mutations in HOXB13 and prostate-cancer risk. *N Engl J Med*. 2012;**366**(2):141–149.

266 Brandi ML, Gagel RF, Angeli A, et al. Guidelines for diagnosis and therapy of MEN type 1 and type 2. *J Clin Endocrinol Metab*. 2001;**86**(12):5658–5671.

288 Wilhelm SM, Wang TS, Ruan DT, et al. The American Association of Endocrine Surgeons guidelines for definitive management of primary hyperparathyroidism. *JAMA Surg*. 2016;**151**(10):959–968.

291 Alrezk R, Hannah-Shmouni F, Stratakis CA. MEN4 and CDKN1B mutations: the latest of the MEN syndromes. *Endocr Relat Cancer*. 2017;**24**(10):T195–T208.

299 Warner J, Epstein M, Sweet A, et al. Genetic testing in familial isolated hyperparathyroidism: unexpected results and their implications. *J Med Genet*. 2004;**41**(3):155–160.

310 Andrews KA, Ascher DB, Pires DEV, et al. Tumour risks and genotype-phenotype correlations associated with germline variants in succinate dehydrogenase subunit genes SDHB, SDHC and SDHD. *J Med Genet*. 2018;**55**(6):384–394.

321 Bausch B, Schiavi F, Ni Y, et al. Clinical characterization of the pheochromocytoma and paraganglioma susceptibility genes SDHA, TMEM127, MAX, and SDHAF2 for gene-informed prevention. *JAMA Oncol*. 2017;**3**(9):1204–1212.

332 McWhinney SR, Pasini B, Stratakis CA, et al. Familial gastrointestinal stromal tumors and germ-line mutations. *N Engl J Med*. 2007;**357**(10):1054–1056.

349 Yeh IT, Lenci RE, Qin Y, et al. A germline mutation of the KIF1B beta gene on 1p36 in a family with neural and nonneural tumors. *Hum Genet*. 2008;**124**(3):279–285.

356 Lonser RR, Glenn GM, Walther M, et al. von Hippel-Lindau disease. *Lancet*. 2003;**361**(9374):2059–2067.

369 Motzer RJ, Hutson TE, Tomczak P, et al. Sunitinib versus interferon alfa in metastatic renal-cell carcinoma. *N Engl J Med*. 2007;**356**(2):115–124.

388 Menko FH, van Steensel MAM, Giraud S, et al. Birt-Hogg-Dube syndrome: diagnosis and management. *Lancet Oncol*. 2009;**10**(12):1199–1206.

395 Kapur P, Pena-Llopis S, Christie A, et al. Effects on survival of BAP1 and PBRM1 mutations in sporadic clear-cell renal-cell carcinoma: a retrospective analysis with independent validation. *Lancet Oncol*. 2013;**14**(2):159–167.

33 Behavioral approaches to cancer prevention

Roberto Gonzalez, MD ■ Maher Karam-Hage, MD

> **Overview**
>
> Various behaviors are well known to increase the risk of developing cancer. Between 30% and 50% of all cancer-related deaths worldwide can be prevented by following healthier behaviors that relate to food intake, substance use, sun exposure, and physical activity. This article will summarize the available literature on the overall effects of modifiable behaviors as risk factors of chronic disease, in particular cancer, as well as describe behavioral changes and/or interventions that could lead to cancer prevention.

Tobacco use

In the United States, tobacco use remains the leading preventable cause of disease, disability, and death, accounting for approximately 480,000 deaths—roughly 20% of yearly deaths from all causes.[1] Cigarette smoking accounts for approximately 30% of all cancers diagnosed and cancer deaths and over 80% of all lung cancer deaths annually.[2] In addition to lung cancer, smoking cigarettes increases the risk of at least 12 different types of cancer, including cancers of the oral cavity, larynx, pharynx, esophagus, stomach, liver, pancreas, kidney, bladder, cervix, colon, rectum, and blood cells (acute myeloid leukemia).[2] Secondhand tobacco smoke exposure is also considered a risk factor for lung cancer, and it is responsible for the death of approximately 7330 adults each year.[3] In addition to cigarettes, cigar smoking is known to cause cancers of the lung, mouth, throat, larynx, and esophagus.[4] While smokeless tobacco use spares users from lung cancer, it is still associated with an increased risk for other cancers such as mouth, throat, esophagus, bladder, and pancreas.[5]

Tobacco policies such as taxation and the promotion of clean-air laws, public health awareness campaigns, and increased provisions of tobacco treatment have led to a significant decline in cigarette smoking. This started with the release of the first US Surgeon General's Report on Smoking and Health in 1964; currently, about 14% of American adults continue to smoke cigarettes, and 11% smoke daily.[6] The incorporation of various flavorings in tobacco products in more recent years, in particular with electronic cigarettes (e-cigs), is believed to have led to an unfortunate increase in overall use of tobacco products among American youth. In 2019, about 12.5% of middle school students and 31.2% of high school students reported using a tobacco product in the last 30 days, mostly due to e-cig popularity within these age groups.[7] This growing concern led Congress to modify federal laws, as of January 2020, giving the Food and Drug Administration (FDA) the authority to make illegal the sale of all tobacco products (including e-cigs) to anyone under the age of 21. The very high nicotine levels in the later generations of e-cigs (JUUL and JUUL-like pod devices) thought of by youth as "water-based devices with flavors" have led to a dangerous combination of acceptance and use by teenagers while containing a highly addictive substance, nicotine.[7] Newer threats are emerging on the horizon as new tobacco products are released on the US market; the FDA published a news release on 30 April 2019 authorizing the marketing and sale of a new "heat not burn (HnB)" tobacco product manufactured by Philip Morris. This HnB tobacco product uses the proprietary tobacco heating system, called "iQOS" (I Quit Ordinary Smoking). It is essentially a modified cigarette that can be heated electronically to lower temperatures instead of burning it as in traditionally combustible cigarettes. In July 2020 the FDA approved iQOS as a modified risk tobacco product (MRTP) with "exposure modification" orders, permitting its marketing as "containing reduced level or exposure to substances", with mandated postmarket surveillance.[8]

Tobacco treatment in healthcare settings

The second half of the 1990s saw a significant emergence of published research regarding the treatment of nicotine dependence, as well as the publication of multiple practice standards and guidelines from various government health agencies and medical professional organizations describing general approaches to tobacco treatment. The United States Public Health Service (PHS) published the first clinical practice guideline for the treatment of tobacco use and dependence in 1996, with updates in 2000[9,10] and 2008. It represents the basis of current best practices, in particular, establishing the standard of care in tobacco treatment as the combination of counseling and pharmacotherapy.[11] The US Preventive Services Task Force (USPTF) published a review in 2015 concluding that treating tobacco with a combination of behavioral intervention and pharmacotherapy is effective and gave it the highest score for level of evidence "A".[12] In January 2021, the USPTF reviewed the newer evidence in the field and their conclusions were consistent with their prior 2015 review.[13] In early 2020, the last Surgeon General's report focused on summarizing the evidence for tobacco treatment, reaching similar conclusions, while adding newer studies.[1]

Brief counseling

The PHS Guideline recommends the use of brief counseling and the "5 A's Model" for the treatment of tobacco use and dependence in a clinical setting. As outlined in Table 1, it is recommended that health care providers to "Ask, Assess, Advise, Assist, and Arrange" in service to their tobacco using patients at every clinical encounter.[14] These steps encourage providers to: (1) "Ask" their patients about their smoking status at every encounter, at least every 30 days; (2) once a tobacco user is identified, "Assess" their

---

Holland-Frei Cancer Medicine, Tenth Edition. Edited by Robert C. Bast, John C. Byrd, Carlo M. Croce, Ernest Hawk, Fadlo R. Khuri, Raphael E. Pollock, Apostolia M. Tsimberidou, Christopher G. Willett, and Cheryl L. Willman.
© 2023 John Wiley & Sons, Inc. Published 2023 by John Wiley & Sons, Inc.

Table 1 The 5As: a model for treating tobacco use and dependence.

Ask about tobacco use	Inquire and document tobacco use status for every patient at each visit
Advise to quit	In a personalized, yet strong and clear manner, urge every patient to quit
Asses willingness to make quit attempt	Is patient willing to make quit attempt at present time?
Assist with quit attempt	For patient willing to make attempt, provide or refer for medication management and counseling to assist with cessation
	For those unwilling to quit at present, provide interventions to facilitate future attempts
Arrange follow-up	For patient willing to make quit attempt, arrange follow-up contacts, beginning within first week after quit date
	For those unwilling to quit at present, address tobacco dependence and willingness to quit at next visit

readiness to quit in order to inform the respective treatment plan; (3) then "Advise" them against smoking, and personalize the risk of cancer and risks of respiratory and cardiovascular diseases from persistent smoking and the benefits of cessation in relation to their patients' disease and treatment; (4) most importantly, "Assist", which involves providing education, addressing barriers to quitting by suggesting behavioral strategies that may overcome these barriers, developing a quit plan, and prescribing pharmacotherapy as indicated (and for patients who are reluctant to quit, clinicians would provide motivational counseling in an effort to encourage them to reduce their daily cigarette consumption in preparation for eventually quitting); (5) and finally, "Arrange" for follow-up support with them or referral to outside resources, such as to the Quit-line number or onsite tobacco treatment specialists where available. Other briefer interventions have since emerged for busy practitioners to make it more feasible to screen and intervene, such as Ask, Advise, and Refer (AAR) or Ask, Advise, and Connect (AAC).[15]

Pharmacotherapy

The 2008 guidelines and the recent USPTF 2021 review recommend use of pharmacotherapy along with counseling to optimize cessation outcomes and significantly increase smoking abstinence, by 83% versus usual care or minimal support control groups not using medication (risk ratio [RR] 1.83 [95% confidence interval [CI], 1.68–1.98].[13] In fact, when comprehensive strategies are provided, almost half of cancer patients quit smoking.[16] To date, the FDA has approved seven pharmacotherapies for smoking cessation: nicotine replacement therapies (NRTs) in various forms (i.e., patches, gum, lozenges, nasal spray, and inhaler), bupropion (Wellbutrin), and varenicline (Chantix). See Table 2 for a list of medications for tobacco cessation treatment including dose, duration, potential contraindications, and side effects. Current research is focusing on developing newer methods for personalized treatments, including the tailoring of interventions to the smoker's readiness to quit, sociocultural factors, genetic profile, gender, age, and health status. Of particular importance is neuroscience research focusing on the biologic and genetic basis of nicotine addiction in the hopes of developing precision and personalized interventions, particularly for high-risk groups and recalcitrant smokers.[17–23]

Electronic cigarettes

E-cigs have been proposed as an alternative solution in harm reduction and possibly cancer prevention, for those highly addicted to nicotine, if not able to or uninterested in quitting tobacco. That is to provide them nicotine in high enough levels without the toxins and carcinogens of combustible tobacco. Hence, the idea that e-cigs could be a less harmful alternative.[24] Initial studies on first generation e-cigs reported similar quit rates as NRTs, concluding that they are not worth the long-term risk of "unknown consequences" of consuming them.[25] Yet, newer data from a British study comparing tank device e-cigs to the nicotine patch showed those randomized to the former to be twice as likely to switch from cigarettes (28% vs 10%; RR=1.8 95% CI 1.30–2.58). However, the study also demonstrated that 80% of those in the tank device arm were still using the device at one year of follow-up, versus only 10% of those in the patch arm still using the patch.[26] This important and remarkable difference highlights the risk of remaining addicted to nicotine by switching to the tank device e-cigs; and unfortunately, the long-term impact/hazards of using them remains a major unanswered question. Newer third and fourth generation devices (pod devices such as JUUL or JUUL-like) can deliver even higher levels of nicotine[27,28] and arguably have an improved safety profile,[29–31] therefore, widening the dilemma of benefit versus risk of using e-cigs in general over the long run. This conflict is even more accentuated, in particular, for cancer patients and survivors who are not able to or not motivated to quit smoking. At the present time, there is much debate as to whether e-cigs will facilitate or impede smoking cessation and around the potential magnitude of harm reduction from e-cigs compared to the well-known hazards of traditional cigarettes and other combustible tobacco products.[32] The American Cancer Society (ACS) position (November 2019) was updated as follows: No youth or young adult should begin using any tobacco product, including e-cigs. The ACS also believes e-cigs should not be used to quit smoking. Additionally, current e-cig users should not also smoke cigarettes or switch to smoking cigarettes, and former smokers now using e-cigs should not revert to smoking.[33]

Prevention of tobacco use

The development and implementation of effective multi-pronged tobacco use prevention programs are crucial for preventing tobacco-related cancers. The Centers for Disease Control and Prevention's (CDC) most recent Best Practices for *Comprehensive Tobacco Control Programs* recommends statewide programs combining community-based interventions. The CDC recommendations focus on (1) preventing initiation of tobacco use among youth and young adults through tobacco control policies (i.e., taxation, tobacco-free laws); (2) promoting quitting among adults and youth; (3) eliminating exposure to secondhand smoke; and (4) identifying and eliminating tobacco-related disparities among various population groups.[34] Tobacco prevention programs should also consider targeting children and young adults with the highest genetic and sociocultural risk factors that would increase the risk for initiating regular smoking.[35]

While tobacco industry-sponsored programs have been deemed ineffective by CDC, the FDA and CDC have developed specific action plans to assist states and localities to prevent and reduce youth and adult tobacco use. Among them are several tobacco education, prevention, and treatment programs developed for teens and youth; and many are free of charge for anyone to use or implement. Examples include:

Table 2 Pharmacotherapy guidelines for tobacco treatment.

Medication	Dose	Duration	Side effects	Possible contraindications
Nicoderm patches	21 mg/24 h	4 wk	Local skin irritation	Eczema, psoriasis, unstable angina
	14 mg/24 h	2 wk	Insomnia	
	7 mg/24 h	2 wk	Headaches	
Gum	Time to 1st	Up to 12 wk	Nausea	Dentures
2 mg	cig > 30 min		Heartburn/Dyspepsia	
4 mg	Time to 1st			
	cig ≤ 30 min			
	between 6 and 24 gum/day			
Lozenges	Time to 1st	Up to 12 wk	Nausea	Mouth sores
2 mg	cig >30 min		Heartburn/Dyspepsia	
4 mg	Time to 1st			
	cig≤30 min			
	between 6 and 24 loz/day			
Nasal spray	8–40 doses/day	3–6 mo	Nasal irritation	Sinus irritation/infection
Inhaler	6–16 cartridges per day	Up to 6 mo	Local mouth/throat irritation	Mouth sores
Bupropion (Wellbutrin)	150 mg QAM ×3 d, Then 150 mg BID	3 mo, maintenance up to 6 mo	Insomnia Dry mouth	History of: seizure eating disorder
Varenicline (Chantix)	0.5 mg daily ×3 d, then BID ×4 d, then 1 mg BID	3–6 mo	Nausea/insomnia Vivid dreams	Acute or chronic renal failure, dialysis

1. A Smoking Prevention Interactive Experience (ASPIRE), an interactive, online program developed by faculty at MD Anderson Cancer Center that targets tobacco prevention and cessation messages to middle and high school students.[36]
2. Intervention for Nicotine Dependence: Education, Prevention, Tobacco and Health (INDEPTH), developed by the American Lung Association to target tobacco use and vaping, it consists of four 50-minute sessions taught by a trained adult.[37]
3. Catch my Breath, a program developed by CATCH® in collaboration with The University of Texas Health Science Center at Houston to address vaping and e-cig use by teens.[38]
4. The Tobacco Prevention Toolkit a program of Stanford University: A theory-based and evidence-informed resources created by educators, parents, and researchers aimed at preventing middle and high school students' use of tobacco and nicotine.[39]
5. Smoke-Free Text to quit by CDC: A free smoking assistance by text program sponsored by CDC. Participants receive 3–5 messages per day for about 6–8 weeks, depending on their selected quit date.[40]

Secondary and tertiary prevention

For individuals diagnosed with cancer, smoking has been associated with various adverse outcomes: increased complications from surgery, increased treatment-related toxicity, decreased treatment efficacy, poorer quality of life, increased risk of cancer recurrence, increased risk of a second primary tumor, increased comorbidity and mortality unrelated to cancer, and decreased survival.[41–45] Despite these risks, about 15.1% of adult cancer survivors still report current cigarette smoking.[46] Continued tobacco use after diagnosis and resumption of smoking after initial quit attempt need to be considered as a modifiable risk factor and a clinical problem. There is a growing consensus among oncology treatment leadership, facilities, and organizations that tobacco use assessment and treatment is one of the qualities of care metrics to focus on in order to maximize the benefit/value of care received by cancer patients.[47–50] While most National Cancer Institute (NCI)-designated Comprehensive Cancer Centers (CCC) offer some form of tobacco treatment services to cancer patients, very few have comprehensive programs with reported results[51]; this lead the NCI to launch in 2017 a special funding program to stimulate development of tobacco treatment program in all CCCs.[52,53] Barriers to addressing tobacco use may include patient factors (addiction, feelings of shame or helplessness), physician barriers (beliefs about patients' lack of interest or ability to quit, lack of training and referral sources), and system-level factors (inability to adequately identify smokers, associate costs) that may inhibit the delivery of effective tobacco treatment or treatment programs.[54,55] In an attempt to bridge these barriers CDC has specific recommendations for the level of treatment and funding for the national quitline 800-QUIT-NOW that routes the callers seeking help to quit smoking to their state own program additional research examining these issues is crucial for improving engagement and retention of smokers in evidence-based tobacco treatment.[56]

Energy balance: diet, physical activity, and body weight

Diet, physical activity, and body weight have each been demonstrated to contribute to the global burden of cancer. The relationship between these three risk factors is currently[56] referred to as energy-balance. While research continues to elucidate how these factors interplay and relate to cancer and cancer outcomes, current evidence supports the association between the disruption in energy balance, cancer development and progression, treatment complications, impaired quality of life, and poorer disease outcomes.[57]

In the United States, physical inactivity, dietary factors, and obesity are estimated to account for nearly 35% of all cancer cases.[58] Excess body weight and obesity, critical modifiable risk factors, are associated with an increased risk of 13 common cancer types, according to the CDC, see Table 3. Broader dietary patterns with prudent plant-based diets limiting meat and dairy intake are generally associated with a reduced cancer risk. Performing physical activity has consistently been shown to confer a protective effect across common types of cancer.[59]

An expansive literature is available, providing a foundation for lifestyle-based cancer prevention and control guidelines that all patients and survivors are or should be encouraged to adopt. Classic and universally accepted recommendations include consuming a plant-based diet, maintaining a normal body weight, and engaging in regular physical activity, all of which are considered to be essential in the prevention of cancer and the pursuit of long-term health.[60,61]

Table 3 Obesity-related cancers U.S. data (2001–2017).

Type of cancer	Frequency	Percentage (%)
Esophageal adenocarcinoma	135,969	1.5
Gastric cardia	93,295	1.1
Colon and rectum	1,965,832	22.2
Liver	300,226	3.4
Gallbladder	51,353	0.6
Pancreas	543,822	6.2
Kidney	688,321	7.8
Meningioma	371,690	4.2
Thyroid	572,050	6.5
Multiple myeloma	272,819	3.1
Post-menopausal female breast cancer	2,926,080	33.1
Corpus and uterus NOS	641,740	7.3
Ovary	277,932	3.1

Content source: Division of Cancer Prevention and Control, Centers for Disease Control and Prevention.
Source: Adapted from CDC at https://www.cdc.gov/cancer/uscs/public-use/dictionary/obesity-related-cancers.htm Page last accessed 12-20-2021, it was last reviewed by CDC on June 8, 2021.

Table 4 American Cancer Society (ACS).

Energy Balance Guidelines for Cancer Prevention and Control	
Maintain a healthy weight	Maintain a balance of energy intake and expenditure via portion control, an emphasis on a plant-based diet and the limitation of high caloric foods and beverages
Regular physical activity	Limit sedentary activity and engage in either 2 h of moderate or 75 min of vigorous physical activity weekly, (e.g., brisk walking or jogging, respectively)
Maintain a healthy diet	Consume a plant-based diet that includes whole grains and 2.5 cups of fruits and vegetables daily, while limiting the intake of red and processed meat. Men and women should limit the consumption of alcohol to 2 and 1 standard drinks per day, respectively

Various national organizations have published guidelines regarding lifestyle behaviors. The ACS highlights the importance of maintaining a healthy body weight, consuming a healthy diet, and regularly engaging in exercise.[59,62] See Table 4 for a summary of these recommendations. The broad nature of these recommendations aligns with disease prevention guidelines beyond cancer, and adherence would also serve to reduce the risk of other chronic conditions such as cardiovascular disease, diabetes, and hypertension. Unfortunately, adherence to these recommendations among the general population and cancer survivors' alike remains low, despite a variety of efforts made to raise awareness.[63–65] Calls for the promotion and use of the term "energy-balance" in clinical practice and oncology have been made to reinforce the interdependent nature of diet, exercise, and weight, with the hope of getting patients to think of these factors as a whole, rather than thinking of each one in isolation.[66] In 2011, a study of nearly 112,000 nonsmoking individuals examined the relationship between adherence to ACS health guidelines and disease outcomes across a 14-year period. Results demonstrated that greater adherence to these health recommendations were associated with a reduced risk of both cancer (men, RR = 0.70, 95% CI: 0.61–0.80; women, RR = 0.76, 95% CI: 0.65–0.89) and all-cause mortality (men, RR = 0.58, 95% CI: 0.53–0.62; women, RR = 0.58, 95% CI: 0.52–0.64).[67] The following section will provide an overview of select research findings concerning the relationship between energy balance and cancer. While acknowledging the synergistic and interrelated nature of diet, weight, and physical activity, we addressed each separately with a focus on the four most common cancers diagnosed in the United States.

Diet and cancer

Certain foods such as green leafy vegetables and fruits contain high levels of fiber and are thought to be protective, while other foods such as meat, are considered a risk factor for cancer development. The International Agency for Research on Cancer recently re-classified processed meat as Group 1 (carcinogenic) and red meat as Group 2A (probably carcinogenic) cancer risks.[68]

Breast cancer

Over the past three decades, there has been significant attention given to the possible link between diet and breast cancer. Based on several observational studies, the World Cancer Research Fund (WCRF) reported that certain dietary patterns including high fruit and vegetable consumption, along with fish, poultry, and low-fat dairy products, were associated with a reduced risk.[69] A systematic review and meta-analysis of 39 case-control and cohort studies by Brennan et al. demonstrated similar findings regarding dietary patterns.[70] Limited evidence exists supporting the isolated protective effect of fruit and vegetable intake alone, despite their inclusion in prudent dietary patterns.[71] In a randomized clinical trial involving nearly 50,000 postmenopausal women, The Women's Health Initiative Trial sought to determine whether reduced fat intake could affect the risk of cancer. Reduced fat intake was associated with only a marginal reduction in risk of disease, and there was no difference in the number of cases of invasive breast cancer during the eight-year follow-up period.[72,73] Regarding alcohol, evidence suggests that consumption may increase the risk of breast cancer with a dose–dependent effect for both pre- and postmenopausal women.[69,71] Finally, a prior meta-analysis from 2010 suggested there was no evidence linking red and processed meat to breast cancer risk across the lifespan.[74]

Prostate cancer

Studies examining the relationship between diet and prostate cancer suggest that their association may differ based on aggressiveness of the disease process. A systematic review by Ma and Chapman suggested additional work is needed to examine this possible influence and that there is not sufficient evidence to provide solid recommendations on the effect of diet on prostate cancer.[75] Despite the above, there is suggestive evidence supporting a protective effect of vegetable and soy consumption, while dairy products increase the risk of disease.[76] Further analysis in the prostate, lung, colorectal, and ovarian cancer screening (PLCO) trial with nearly 30,000 men established a modest increase in risk of nonaggressive cancers among those reporting higher consumption of dairy products, with no association shown for more aggressive forms of disease.[77] Kirsh et al. reported a decreased risk of aggressive prostate cancer in men who had a high intake of cruciferous vegetables, such as cabbage and broccoli.[78] Others have found a positive effect of comprehensive lifestyle changes on low-risk prostate cancer at 5-year follow-up.[79]

Colorectal cancer

Great effort has been given to studying the potential effect of nutrition on the development and progression of colorectal cancer. Several international reports and meta-analyses have shown convincing evidence of an association between the consumption of red and processed meat products with an increased risk of colon, colorectal, and rectal cancers.[80] A meta-analysis from Chan et al. noted a dose–dependent relationship between meat consumption and cancer risk, including a 21% increased risk with 50 g/day consumed and a 29% increased risk with 100 g/day consumed.[81] For reference purposes, the recommended serving size of a portion of lean meat is about 85 g. More recent reviews confirm this negative association between red meat intake and cancer, in particular colorectal cancer.[82]

Considerable attention has been given to dietary fiber and its relationship to disease risk. Despite plausible biological mechanisms, early reports found little evidence of an association between the consumption of fiber and colorectal cancer.[83–85] More recent studies, however, have indeed noted a relationship.[86,87] A systematic review of 25 prospective studies reported a dose-dependent inverse relationship between cereal fiber and whole grains and risk of colorectal cancer.[88] The authors reported a statistically significant 10% decrease in cancer risk with 10 g of daily fiber intake. For reference, the U.S. recommended daily fiber intake for adults is 25 g.

The consumption of alcohol has been associated with an increased risk of colorectal cancer.[80] In reviewing 103 cohort studies, Huxley et al. found that those reporting the highest levels of alcohol consumption had a 60% increased risk of colorectal cancer, compared to light or nondrinkers; this relationship was significant especially among male participants.[89,90]

Lung cancer
The American Institute for Cancer Research (WRCF/AICR) report demonstrated that consuming more fruits and vegetables is consistently associated with a reduced risk of lung cancer among smokers and nonsmokers alike.[80] Despite this consistency, however, the protective effect of a healthy diet pales in comparison to the risk associated with tobacco use. Therefore, quitting smoking is by far the most robust strategy for lung cancer risk reduction that any smoker can pursue.

Obesity and cancer
Over the past 30 years, rates of obesity have continued to increase dramatically, with 42.4% of US adults considered obese.[91] Rodriguez et al. estimated that 14–20% of all cancer deaths were attributable to excess weight, and when combined with diet, accounts for nearly one in three cancers.[80,92,93] A report published by the WCRF/AICR, along with a systematic review and meta-analysis by Renehan in 2008, noted evidence of a link between excess body weight and many common types of cancer.[80,94] Examples include colon, kidney, and pancreatic cancers as well as esophageal adenocarcinoma among both sexes, along with thyroid cancer for men, and gallbladder, endometrial, ovarian, and postmenopausal breast cancers among women.

Breast and prostate cancer
Both excess body weight and weight gain during the period of adulthood have been consistently linked to risk of breast cancer.[95,96] More specifically, a meta-analysis by Vrieling et al. noted a stronger association between weight gain and estrogen-/progesterone-positive breast cancers among postmenopausal women.[97]

As the impact of obesity on prostate cancer appears to be moderated by disease severity, more recent studies have emphasized the need to examine this relationship more rigorously. Obesity has been associated with greater risk of being diagnosed with advanced disease, increased risk of recurrence, and poorer prognosis.[98–100] In contrast to the above, Wright et al. reported an inverse relationship between body mass index (BMI) and risk of early-stage disease among a large population of men enrolled in the National Institutes of Health–AARP Diet and Health Study.[101] Though research continues, this complexity in relationship is believed to be due in part to challenges inherent to the screening and diagnosis of prostate cancer in men with obesity.

Colorectal cancer and other notable findings
The majority of studies available, including a meta-analysis of 56 observational studies, support a positive relationship between weight and risk of colorectal cancer, most notably among men.[80,92,102] This association was more consistent among studies that examined measures of body fat distribution beyond BMI alone, with excess weight in the abdominal region being most predictive of increased risk of cancer.[80] With an estimated 60% of new cases being attributed to obesity, endometrial cancer is considered as the type of cancer most consistently linked to excess weight.[103] Women with obesity are 2–3.5 times more likely to be diagnosed with endometrial cancer, as demonstrated by a large-scale European study that followed one million women for approximately 40 years; this study also reported that obese women were 2.5 times more likely to be diagnosed with cancer of the uterine corpus, compared to women of normal weight.[104]

Physical activity and cancer
Performing regular physical activity is an important component of health recommendations and has been associated with reduced risk across a number of common cancer types.[62] Unfortunately, most cancer survivors do not meet the minimal physical activity recommendations, but those who are active seem to have improved health-related quality of life. Therefore, targeted interventions to improve adherence to physical activity among cancer survivors are needed.[105]

Breast and prostate cancer
The relationship between physical activity and the risk of breast cancer has been researched extensively and is regarded as convincing.[106] Such research has included a review of more than 70 observational reports that established an absolute risk reduction of between 20% and 30% in breast cancer risk when comparing those who were most active to those who were least active.[107,108] Regarding prostate cancer, Liu et al. reported that engagement in physical activity was associated with an overall risk reduction of 10% via systematic review and meta-analysis of over 40 reports, including over 2 million men and nearly 90,000 cases of cancer.[109]

Colorectal and lung cancer
Considerable empirical attention has also been given to the association between physical activity and colorectal cancer. A meta-analysis by Wolin et al. examined over 50 studies and reported an overall reduction in risk of 24%, with greater risk reduction reported in case-control studies.[110] Regarding colon cancer, Harris and Thune reported similar findings, including evidence of a dose–response relationship between physical activity and cancer risk among both genders; but no evidence of a relationship was noted among seven studies of rectal cancer.[111,112]

In a review of predominantly cohort studies, Emaus and Thune reported a 23% reduction in risk of lung cancer among those engaged in physical activity, with a greater rate of 38% once again reported among case-control studies.[113] Although risk reduction varied based on intensity of activity, a meta-analysis by Tardon et al. reported similar results, showing that moderate engagement was associated with a 13% risk reduction and rigorous activity was associated with a 30% risk reduction.[114] In a recent systematic review, Koutsokera et al. called for the need of additional research in this area, especially among women, as 10 studies reported an inverse association between physical activity and lung cancer and nearly as many reported a null association.[115]

Energy balance and cancer survivorship

With the increasing rates of survival over the years across many common types of cancer, emerging research has started to address the role of lifestyle in cancer prognosis and survivorship. Research and clinical programs in this area have sought to build upon the potential of a cancer diagnosis to serve as a teachable moment, seizing this critical period in which both patients and survivors may be more motivated to implement healthier lifestyle changes.[116-119] A systematic review of 27 published studies reported sufficient evidence to support an association between physical activity and a reduction in all-cause mortality, as well as breast and colon-specific cancer mortality.[120] A review by Davies et al. suggested that a healthy diet with low fat and high fiber may be broadly associated with a reduced risk of cancer recurrence and progression, though additional research is needed.[121] This is particularly true in regard to establishing whether the protective effects of a healthy diet and/or physical activity may be due to their promotion of a healthy body weight. Finally, a systematic review by Parekh et al. reported that the majority of studies available suggest a negative effect of excess weight on cancer survival outcomes, specifically with breast, colon, and prostate cancers.[122] Of note, the authors pointed out that there is an over-representation of breast cancer in this literature, and many of the studies examining obesity and cancer survival were not initially designed to examine such outcomes. The American Society of Clinical Oncology has, therefore, created a toolkit to help oncologists counsel their patients about the importance of weight management for cancer survivors.[123]

Promoting behavioral change in diet and physical activity

While the positive impact of exercise on cancer and cancer survivorship is becoming evident, there are many barriers to accepting it as an effective component of cancer treatment and to implement it as such. A recent review found persistent treatment-related side effects was the most commonly reported barrier to initiating or maintaining exercise, followed by lack of time and fatigue. The review also found that the most common facilitators of exercise were gaining a feeling of control over one's health and managing emotions and mental well-being; and the preferred method of exercise was walking.[124] A recommendation from a physician or healthcare provider may play an important role in promoting energy balance and lifestyle change, but some individuals may require a more intense intervention.[57] Referrals to evidence-based behavioral lifestyle programs are recommended for those requiring additional support. These programs usually last anywhere from 6 to 12 months, adopt a group-based format, and include counseling on diet and reduction of caloric intake, as well as the promotion of physical activity. Such programs routinely result in weight loss of 5–10% of initial body weight and may provide clinically relevant improvements in many disease markers with plausible downstream benefits for reducing cancer risk. However, as the maintenance of weight loss remains a challenge, providers should remain supportive of patients seeking to sustain these changes.[125-128] Evidence regarding the impact of behavioral changes on cancer-related outcomes continues to grow, with evidence suggesting that bariatric surgery is associated with a reduced cancer risk, and that behavioral changes related to diet and physical activity may improve biological markers among survivors.[129,130]

Risk behaviors for skin cancer

Cancers of the skin are commonly grouped into melanomas and nonmelanomas, and while melanomas are less common, they are more aggressive than other types and affect roughly 100,350 Americans each year.[2] Ultraviolet radiation (UVR), whether from the sun or indoor tanning devices, is a significant risk factor for skin cancer, and there are well-established behavioral strategies for skin cancer prevention.[131] Recommendations for the prevention of skin cancer include avoidance of UVR tanning beds and devices, as well as limiting unprotected sun exposure, especially at midday when sunlight is strongest. This is of particular importance for children and adolescents. Researchers have found that it is feasible to promote sunscreen use and skin self-examination in the context of an adolescent school-based education.[132] When the avoidance of sunlight is not possible, one should liberally apply a broad-spectrum sunscreen 30 minutes before exposure to sunlight, reapplying every 2 hours or after any exposure to water. Of note, sunscreen should be effective against both UVA and UVB radiation with a sun protection factor (SPF) of 30 or greater.[133] Individuals should be advised that sunscreens only offer partial protection from UVR and they should be used in combination with protective clothing (i.e., hats, long-sleeved garments) and avoidance of exposure to strong sunlight when at all possible. Unfortunately, only 30% of US adults report using sunscreen and/or sun-protective clothing routinely.[134] Furthermore, surveys show that even cancer survivors do not consistently protect themselves from UV light, especially those who are younger and more likely to be exposed to UVR.[135-137]

Sleep and cancer

Sleep problems to include insomnia, sleep apnea, and others which have not been sufficiently evaluated regarding their impact on health and cancer prevention. The Healthy People 2030 goals have identified sleep as one of the objectives to improve upon. About 1 in 3 adults—and even more adolescents—do not get enough sleep, which can affect individuals' health and well-being.[138] Healthy People 2030 focuses on helping people get enough sleep, treating sleep disorders, and decreasing drowsy driving. People who do not get enough sleep are more likely to have a variety of health problems including obesity, diabetes, heart disease, stroke, dementia, and cancer.[139,140]

Summary

The positive impact and significance of behavioral risk reduction on cancer prevention are well-established in the scientific literature.[141] Goals emphasized by Healthy People 2030 include the promotion of the following health behaviors: abstinence from drug and tobacco use, nutrition and healthy eating, physical activity, adequate sleep, and minimization of exposure to UVR.[140]

Key references

The complete reference list can be found on Vital Source version of this title, see inside front cover.

1. US Department of Health and Human Services. *Smoking Cessation: A Report of the Surgeon General*. Washington, DC: US Department of Health and Human Services; 2020.
2. American Cancer Society. *Cancer Facts & Figures 2020*. Atlanta: American Cancer Society; 2020.
3. U.S. Department of Health and Human Services. *The Health Consequences of Smoking - 50 Years of Progress: A Report of the Surgeon General*. U.S. Department of Health and Human Services; 2014.
5. IARC Working Group on the Evaluation of Carcinogenic Risks to Humans. Smokeless tobacco and some tobacco-specific N-nitrosamines. *IARC Monogr Eval Carcinog Risks Hum*. 2007;**89**:1–592.
6. Creamer MR, Wang TW, Babb S, et al. Tobacco product use and cessation indicators among adults—United States, 2018. *MMWR Morb Mortal Wkly Rep*. 2019;**68**(45):1013–1019.
7. Wang TW, Gentzke AS, Creamer MR, et al. Tobacco product use and associated factors among middle and high school students – United States, 2019. *MMWR Surveill Summ*. 2019;**68**(12):1–22.
11. Clinical Practice Guideline Treating Tobacco Use and Dependence 2008 Update Panel, Liaisons, and Staff. A clinical practice guideline for treating tobacco use and dependence: 2008 update. A U.S. Public Health Service report. *Am J Prev Med*. 2008;**35**(2):158–176.
13. Patnode CD, Henderson JT, Melnikow J, et al. *Interventions for Tobacco Cessation in Adults, Including Pregnant Women: An Evidence Update for the U.S. Preventive Services Task Force: Evidence Synthesis, No. 196*. AHRQ Publication; 2021.
16. Cinciripini PM, Karam-Hage M, Kypriotakis G, et al. Association of a comprehensive smoking cessation program with smoking abstinence among patients with cancer. *JAMA Netw Open*. 2019;**2**(9):e1912251.
21. Chen L-S, Baker T, Hung RJ, et al. Genetic risk can be decreased: quitting smoking decreases and delays lung cancer for smokers with high and low CHRNA5 risk genotypes—a meta-analysis. *EBioMedicine*. 2016;**11**:219–226.
24. Warner KE, Mendez D. E-cigarettes: comparing the possible risks of increasing smoking initiation with the potential benefits of increasing smoking cessation. *Nicotine Tob Res*. 2019;**21**(1):41–47.
26. Hajek P, Phillips-Waller A, Przulj D, et al. A randomized trial of E-cigarettes versus nicotine-replacement therapy. *N Engl J Med*. 2019;**380**(7):629–637.
28. Yingst JM, Hrabovsky S, Hobkirk A, et al. Nicotine absorption profile among regular users of a pod-based electronic nicotine delivery system. *JAMA Netw Open*. 2019;**2**(11):e1915494–e1915494.
41. Warren GW, Kasza KA, Reid ME, et al. Smoking at diagnosis and survival in cancer patients. *Int J Cancer*. 2013;**132**(2):401–410.
42. Toll BA, Brandon TH, Gritz ER, et al. Assessing tobacco use by cancer patients and facilitating cessation: an American Association for Cancer Research policy statement. *Clin Cancer Res*. 2013;**19**(8):1941–1948.
45. Enyioha C, Warren GW, Morgan GD, Goldstein AO. Tobacco use and treatment among cancer survivors. *Int J Environ Res Public Health*. 2020;**17**(23):9109.
51. Day AT, Tang L, Karam-Hage M, Fakhry C. Tobacco treatment programs at National Cancer Institute-designated Cancer Centers: a systematic review and online audit. *Am J Clin Oncol*. 2019;**42**(4):407–410.
53. Croyle RT, Morgan GD, Fiore MC. Addressing a core gap in cancer care - the NCI moonshot program to help oncology patients stop smoking. *N Engl J Med*. 2019;**380**(6):512–515.
55. Rojewski AM, Bailey SR, Bernstein SL, et al. Considering systemic barriers to treating tobacco use in clinical settings in the United States. *Nicotine Tob Res*. 2019;**21**(11):1453–1461.
58. Danaei G, Vander Hoorn S, Lopez AD, et al. Causes of cancer in the world: comparative risk assessment of nine behavioural and environmental risk factors. *Lancet (London, England)*. 2005;**366**(9499):1784–1793.
59. Rock CL, Doyle C, Demark-Wahnefried W, et al. Nutrition and physical activity guidelines for cancer survivors. *CA Cancer J Clin*. 2012;**62**(4):243–274.
60. Ford ES, Bergmann MM, Kröger J, et al. Healthy living is the best revenge: findings from the European Prospective Investigation Into Cancer and Nutrition-Potsdam study. *Arch Intern Med*. 2009;**169**(15):1355–1362.
62. Kushi LH, Doyle C, McCullough M, et al. American Cancer Society Guidelines on nutrition and physical activity for cancer prevention: reducing the risk of cancer with healthy food choices and physical activity. *CA Cancer J Clin*. 2012;**62**(1):30–67.
65. Basen-Engquist, K., Alfano, C.M., Maitin-Shepard, M. et al. (2018) *Moving Research into Practice: Physical Activity, Nutrition, and Weight Management for Cancer Patients and Survivors*. NAM Perspectives. Discussion Paper. National Academy of Medicine, Washington, DC. https://doi.org/10.31478/201810g
66. Sparling PB, Franklin BA, Hill JO. Energy balance: the key to a unified message on diet and physical activity. *J Cardiopulm Rehabil Prev*. 2013;**33**(1):12–15.
67. McCullough ML, Patel AV, Kushi LH, et al. Following cancer prevention guidelines reduces risk of cancer, cardiovascular disease, and all-cause mortality. *Cancer Epidemiol Biomark Prev*. 2011;**20**(6):1089–1097.
68. The International Agency for Research on Cancer(IARC) (2020) *Monographs on the Evaluation of Carcinogenic Risks to Humans; Volume 114. IARC Working Group on the Evaluation of Carcinogenic Risks to Humans, Meeting in Lyon, 6–13 October 2015, Lyon, France – 2018*, https://publications.iarc.fr/Book-And-Report-Series/Iarc-Monographs-On-The-Identification-Of-Carcinogenic-Hazards-To-Humans/Red-Meat-And-Processed-Meat-2018 (accessed 31 August 2021).
69. Chan DSM, Abar L, Cariolou M, et al. World Cancer Research Fund International: Continuous Update Project-systematic literature review and meta-analysis of observational cohort studies on physical activity, sedentary behavior, adiposity, and weight change and breast cancer risk. *Cancer Causes & Control*. 2019;**30**(11):1183–1200.
71. Heath AK, Muller DC, van den Brandt PA, et al. Nutrient-wide association study of 92 foods and nutrients and breast cancer risk. *Breast Cancer Res*. 2020;**22**(1):5.
73. Chlebowski RT, Aragaki AK, Anderson GL, et al. Association of low-fat dietary pattern with breast cancer overall survival: a secondary analysis of the women's health initiative randomized clinical trial. *JAMA Oncol*. 2018;**4**(10):e181212.
79. Ornish D, Lin J, Chan JM, et al. Effect of comprehensive lifestyle changes on telomerase activity and telomere length in men with biopsy-proven low-risk prostate cancer: 5-year follow-up of a descriptive pilot study. *Lancet Oncol*. 2013;**14**(11):1112–1120.
80. World Cancer Research Fund / American Institute for Cancer Research (2018) *Diet, Nutrition, Physical Activity and Cancer: A Global Perspective. Continuous Update Project Expert Report*, https://www.wcrf.org/diet-and-cancer/ (accessed 31 August 2021).
82. Yip CSC, Lam W, Fielding R. A summary of meat intakes and health burdens. *Eur J Clin Nutr*. 2018;**72**(1):18.
90. Blount BC, Karwowski MP, Shields PG, et al. Vitamin E acetate in bronchoalveolar-lavage fluid associated with EVALI. *N Engl J Med*. 2019;**382**(8):697–705.
91. Hales CM, Carroll MD, Fryar CD, Ogden CL. *Prevalence of Obesity and Severe Obesity Among Adults: United States, 2017–2018. NCHS Data Brief, No 360*. Hyattsville, MD: National Center for Health Statistics; 2020.
93. Wolin KY, Carson K, Colditz GA. Obesity and cancer. *Oncologist*. 2010;**15**(6):556–565.
112. Thune I, Furberg AS. Physical activity and cancer risk: dose-response and cancer, all sites and site-specific. *Med Sci Sports Exerc*. 2001;**33**(6 Suppl):S530–S550; discussion S609-10.
132. Hubbard G, Kyle RG, Neal RD, et al. Promoting sunscreen use and skin self-examination to improve early detection and prevent skin cancer: quasi-experimental trial of an adolescent psycho-educational intervention. *BMC Public Health*. 2018;**18**(1):666.
140. health.gov (2021) *Office of Disease Prevention and Health Promotion Healthy People 2030 | health.gov*, https://health.gov/healthypeople (accesed 1 April 2021).

34 Diet and nutrition in the etiology and prevention of cancer

Steven K. Clinton, MD, PhD ■ Edward L. Giovannucci, MD, ScD ■ Fred K. Tabung, MSPH, PhD ■ Elizabeth M. Grainger, RD, PhD

> **Overview**
>
> Over the last two centuries, improvements in food production, processing, storage, and distribution have led to major changes in diet composition throughout the world. During this period, life expectancy also dramatically increased within economically developed nations because of a combination of factors, including public health measures, improved occupational safety, and major reductions in nutrient deficiency syndromes. As the population has aged, there has been a shift in the major causes of morbidity and mortality toward chronic diseases, such as cancer and cardiovascular disease. In the United States, recent decades are characterized by an increasingly sedentary population with an epidemic of obesity, a trend that is emerging worldwide. Although nutritional deficiencies still plague subpopulations in developed nations amongst the poor, aged, chronically ill, and alcoholics, we now recognize that the affluent dietary pattern contributes to the pathogenesis of many chronic diseases, including cancer, that afflict the vast majority of the population. Efforts to understand the often complex etiologies of various cancers have led to laboratory, clinical, and epidemiologic studies that strongly implicate specific nutrients and certain dietary patterns in human carcinogenesis. The objective of this article is to provide an overview of efforts to define public health guidelines that impact policy for global health organizations and nations, while also providing a foundation for individuals seeking to consume healthy dietary patterns.

It is important to establish a conceptual framework for organizing data regarding diet, nutrition, and cancer that will help readers provide guidance to the public and patients. We arbitrarily divide the topic into the realms of prevention, therapy, and survivorship. Organizations such as the World Cancer Research Fund/American Institute for Cancer Research (WCRF/AICR), the American Cancer Society (ACS), as well as the US Department of Health and Human Services (HHS)/US Department of Agriculture (USDA) through its Dietary Guidelines for Americans, have published recommendations defining achievable dietary and nutritional goals that can promote health and reduce the overall cancer burden through primary prevention (Table 1).[1,2,4,5] These goals are evidence-based and increasingly utilize a rigorous systematic review process. These efforts contribute to government policies in many nations surrounding food and agriculture to promote health, yet much remains to be accomplished.

Such public health guidelines are also employed by individuals as a foundation for health. In addition, those deemed to be at higher risk of specific types of cancer as a result of environmental exposures, family history, or the presence of premalignant conditions seek guidance and pursue dietary and lifestyle interventions that may be designed to lower their chances of developing a specific cancer. Patients actively undergoing cancer therapy represent another group profoundly interested in the role of dietary and nutritional interventions to enhance the efficacy of treatment while reducing the frequency and severity of side effects. These issues are complex and best addressed in medical clinics with a therapeutic team which includes registered dietitians (RD). Finally, as cancers are detected earlier and treatment interventions become more successful, the number of cancer survivors is increasing rapidly. Those completing cancer therapy are seeking guidance regarding diet and lifestyle interventions that will lower their risk of recurrence (secondary prevention) and reduce the severity of long-term complications of their cancer treatment, including therapy-related second malignancies and long-term organ dysfunction. Thus, clinicians involved in cancer therapy and management of long-term health are increasingly being asked to provide evidence-based guidance for survivorship, where scientific studies are few. Thus, vulnerable survivors frequently fall prey to purveyors of alternative diet- or nutrient-based interventions marketed in the absence of scientific data regarding efficacy and safety. Although this article focuses upon prevention, we briefly review the therapeutic and survivorship phases and provide information that will assist in counseling individuals and groups interested in dietary and nutritional interventions. The vast majority of research conducted in the field of diet, nutrition, and cancer focuses on etiology and prevention. Accordingly, this article emphasizes the public health model and focuses on the interventions that may reduce the overall cancer burden of large populations. We then consider the evidence for prevention of the most commonly occurring cancers involving specific organs. Rather than detailing the complex, often incomplete, and occasionally contradictory literature concerning the role of dietary components in the etiology of specific cancers, this article provides a general guide with an emphasis on the major emerging concepts in the area. We conclude with a brief overview of the role of diet and nutrition to enhance therapy and survivorship.

Methodologic issues in diet, nutrition, and cancer studies

It is valuable to briefly consider how evidence-based dietary recommendations are established. The unbiased detection and quantification of risks are associated with variations in diet and nutrient intake would ideally be achieved through randomized, prospective trials. Unfortunately, the enormous costs of long-term nutrition studies and the scientific difficulties in controlling or measuring dietary patterns and nutrient intake limit feasibility. Therefore, current nutritional guidelines for disease prevention are

---

Holland-Frei Cancer Medicine, Tenth Edition. Edited by Robert C. Bast, John C. Byrd, Carlo M. Croce, Ernest Hawk, Fadlo R. Khuri, Raphael E. Pollock, Apostolia M. Tsimberidou, Christopher G. Willett, and Cheryl L. Willman.
© 2023 John Wiley & Sons, Inc. Published 2023 by John Wiley & Sons, Inc.

Table 1 A summary of public health guidelines for diet, nutrition, and health outcomes including the prevention of cancer.[a]

Body weight	Be a healthy weight. Maintain appropriate energy balance through diet and exercise during each stage of life so as to keep your weight within the healthy range and avoid weight gain during adulthood. If overweight, limit high calorie-dense and nutrient-poor foods and beverages. For people who struggle to obtain a healthy weight, weight maintenance should be encouraged
Physical activity	Be physically active and limit sedentary habits. Meet or exceed the national guidelines which include engaging in at least 150 min per week of moderate intensity or 75 min per week of vigorous-intensity physical activity. This amount represents the minimum for cardiometabolic health. Including strength training exercises at least 2 days per week is also recommended
Dietary pattern	Eat a diet rich in whole grains, fruits, vegetables, and beans/legumes. Consume a diet that provides at least 25–30 g of fiber each day
Vegetable and fruit	Eat at least 400 g (15 ounces or about 4.5 cup equivalents) of fruits and vegetables each day. Choose a variety of green, red, and orange vegetables. Include nonstarchy vegetables and legumes regularly
Breads, grains, and cereals	Choose whole-grain breads, cereals, and pasta. Adults should consume at least 3–5 ounce equivalents of whole grains per day. Where possible, substitute refined grains with whole-grain foods
Animal products	People who choose to eat red meat should consume less than 500 g (18 ounces) per week. Processed meats should be limited, if consumed at all. Choose lean meat, poultry, fish, and eggs
Dietary fat	It is beneficial to replace saturated fat with mono- and polyunsaturated fats. For cardiovascular health, minimize intake of *trans* fats
Added sugar	Added sugars should be limited to no more than 5–10% of total calories. Do not consume sugar-sweetened drinks
Sodium	Sodium should be limited to no more than 2300 mg/day
Alcohol	For people who choose to drink alcoholic beverages, limit intake to two drinks per day or less for men and one drink per day or less for women. For cancer prevention, it is best not to consume alcohol
Miscellaneous	Nutritional needs should be met primarily through foods and consumption of a healthy dietary pattern. When consuming a healthy dietary pattern there is no role for nutritional supplements to meet recommended requirements

[a]Source: World Cancer Research Fund/American Institute for Cancer Research[1]; Arnett et al.[2]; Rock et al.[3]; Dietary Guidelines Advisory Committee.[4]

based on the integration of information derived from a variety of different epidemiologic approaches and laboratory investigations, so most guidelines are developed by expert committees convened by organizations such as the National Institutes of Health (NIH), the ACS, the AICR/WCRF, and the World Health Organization (WHO), among others.[1,3,5–8] The evidence derived from epidemiologic studies, clinical investigations, and laboratory studies are reviewed and discussed relative to criteria of causality, defined as a specific occurrence or outcome that is consistently preceded by a known set of circumstances or conditions.[9] In nutritional sciences, clear representations of causality have been the demonstration of single-nutrient deficiency syndromes and their complete reversal by exposure to the nutrient. For example, the lack of fruits and vegetables in the diet leads to scurvy, which is readily reversed by vitamin C. Unfortunately, relationships between diet and cancer are much more complex than simple nutrient deficiency syndromes. To establish causality, conclusions about the occurrence of an event and its etiologic factors are based on consensus criteria. These criteria have evolved over many years and include consistency, strength of association, biologic gradient, temporality, specificity, biologic plausibility, biologic mechanism, coherence, and experimental evidence.[10] Precisely quantitating risk due to a dietary variable has been difficult because the etiologies of most cancers are multifactorial and the interactions poorly understood. Human cancers show striking variations based on factors such as age, sex, race, socioeconomic status, and host genetics, as well as many environmental, occupational, and lifestyle variables. The potential for complex interactions between these factors and diet is enormous, and this emphasizes the difficulties in demonstrating causal associations with the same clarity as is demonstrable for high-risk environmental exposures, such as the impact of cigarette smoking on lung cancer.

Assessment of the human diet

Nutritional epidemiology possesses some unique obstacles in that food is a universal exposure, in stark contrast to many cancer-causing environmental exposures, such as cigarette smoke. Table 2 details the strengths and limitations of various types of study designs used in nutrition research. The exposures of interest in epidemiology include nutrients, nonnutrient bioactive components, and dietary patterns. Nutrients are dietary components where known deficiency syndromes have been characterized. These include the energy-supplying macronutrients, which are lipids, carbohydrates, and proteins, and the various constituents, such as essential fatty acids and amino acids, as well as vitamins and minerals. Nonnutrient components include thousands of potential bioactives, such as fiber, polyphenols, and carotenoids, all of which are particularly rich in fruits and vegetables. Currently, strategies to define dietary patterns, such as a Mediterranean-style, vegetarian, or affluent (western) dietary pattern, may provide greater insight into combined effects of multiple variables; nevertheless, standardized approaches for studying the effects of complex dietary patterns across regions are lacking.

The critical limiting feature of most human studies is the imprecision of quantifying dietary intake. Estimating the usual intake of foods or nutrients, as well as accounting for intra-individual variation over time, is a critical area of research.[11–13] An estimate of human nutrient intake is derived from a two-step process. First, interviews, questionnaires, or food diaries must determine the amounts and types of foods that are consumed.[14] This information is then used to calculate nutrient intake if an accurate database has been established that quantifies the amount of each nutrient contained in the foods consumed by the population under investigation. Each step can be associated with significant error and contributes to the challenges in defining nutrient and cancer associations. The human diet is a complex array of foods that exhibits significant day-to-day and seasonal variations in composition. The complexity of diet also differs widely among populations, cultures, and geographic areas. This often requires the development of different assessment methods for each population or subgroup. Future progress will depend, in part, on identifying biomarkers of nutrient exposure. Development of valid and reliable biomarkers of nutrient intake or dietary patterns offers the promise of improved precision in epidemiologic studies because of reduced misclassification of participants according to intake estimates.[15] In addition, for many of the bioactive compounds in foods that may impact cancer risk, including the vast array of nonnutrient phytochemicals derived from plants, our ability to estimate exposure remains a challenge, as databases regarding content in foods often do not exist.[16] Current research efforts integrating omics technologies (e.g., metabolomics and microbiome) with dietary pattern data, are promising.[17–23]

Table 2 Types of studies used to assess diet and disease relationships.

Study type	Methods	Strengths	Limitations
Ecologic/correlational studies	The unit of observation is a population defined by a discriminator location (Japan vs the United States, northern Europe vs southern Europe). Mortality or incidence among groups is compared with estimates of nutrient or food intake	Large differences in cancer incidence and dietary patterns are often identified, and hypotheses can be generated	There are often many diet and lifestyle differences between populations; therefore, correlations between disease incidence and dietary factors are confounded or biased by known or unknown variables Cancer incidence data and diet patterns may not be similarly and accurately quantitated among nations
Case-control studies	Individuals experiencing a disease are identified, and a similar group of matched subjects without the disease are identified. Information about past diet and nutrients is obtained from both the cases and controls for comparison	Studies can be conducted over a relatively short period of time	Selection bias can occur if a nonrepresentative control group is selected Recall bias can occur when subjects with a disease alter their perceptions and recall of past dietary habits. This often occurs when participants are familiar with a particular diet/disease hypothesis
Prospective/cohort studies	A study population is identified and diet patterns assessed. The population is followed over time for disease outcome and changes in exposure to dietary risk factors	Dietary intake can be monitored periodically over time Diet assessment does not rely on long-term memory and is less affected by recall bias Biochemical measures can be obtained periodically	Long periods of time may be necessary for a disease to be diagnosed, so cohort studies often require many years of follow-up A large number of subjects are required to compensate for subjects who drop out, subjects lost to follow-up, and/or the possibility that the frequency of the outcome of interest is low Long-term, large prospective studies are expensive
Randomized controlled trials	Individuals are screened, and, based on specific characteristics, a proper target population is identified and randomized to a control arm (standard of care) or an intervention arm. The subjects are followed for disease outcome or other biomarkers	Especially useful for testing compounds (vitamins and minerals) that can be incorporated into pills or capsules and provided in a double-blind fashion over a period of years	Difficult to implement for many nutrition and cancer hypotheses (weight loss, exercise, dietary fat, fiber, fruits, and vegetables), because trials of dietary change cannot be blinded Manipulation of single dietary components in large-scale intervention studies is difficult, since foods are complex and contain many compounds Compliance with food changes may be difficult to determine. Randomized, controlled trials can take a long time to complete and can be very expensive

Laboratory models

The effects of nutrients or food components and their interactions on carcinogenesis can be rigorously tested in a growing array of animal models. Although the information derived from animal models must be extrapolated to humans with caution, the literature does provide important evidence for the biologic plausibility of relationships suggested by epidemiologic studies. The nutrient requirements of most laboratory animals have been precisely defined, and purified ingredients can be used to formulate diets for cancer studies. The rapid emergence of new animal models based upon transgenic and knockout technology has provided new opportunities to examine interactions between specific genetic targets and dietary variables.[24]

Public health guidelines for nutrition and cancer prevention

We begin this section with a synthesis of public health dietary guidelines for cancer prevention and health published by several organizations, including the WCRF/AICR/ACS, The American Heart Association (AHA), and the US Departments of Agriculture and HHS.[1,3–6,25,26] The public health approach is a preventive strategy to decrease overall disease incidence by reducing the adverse dietary habits of the entire population. To achieve success, dietary recommendations must be clear, as well as feasible and minimal risk, bearing low cost to society and the potential to benefit many people.[1,3,4,25] Implementation of dietary recommendations requires not only individual action, but also cooperation among the media, food industry, public health workers, medical practitioners, educators, and government agencies.[1,3,4,25] Though such implementation is often attenuated by economic concerns of the food and agricultural industry, past efforts in nutrition have been successful. For example, iron fortification of cereals benefits a large number of children and adult women through prevention of anemia, while risk is limited to a small number of individuals with hemochromatosis. The current evidence-based dietary recommendations are made with a reasonable degree of certainty with minimal risk and the potential for significant public health benefits.[1,3,8,27–29] Table 1 summarizes current population-based dietary recommendations that together may lower the risk of chronic diseases, including cancer.[1,3–6] In late 2020, a revision of Dietary Guidelines for Americans will be available.[30]

Maintain a healthy weight

Increasingly, studies document that sedentary behavior, weight gain during adulthood, overweight, and obesity are major risk factors for human cancer.[1,3,5–7,31–35] Multiple systematic reviews, meta-analyses, and published public health guidelines indicate that adiposity and sedentary behavior significantly increase the risk of at least 20 different cancer subtypes, including esophageal adenocarcinoma, colon cancer, endometrial cancer, postmenopausal breast cancer, and kidney cancer, among others.[1,3,35,36] Enhancing our understanding regarding the complex dynamics of how energy balance, physical activity, and body weight and composition over the life cycle impacts cancer risk, response to therapy, and survivorship are critical.[37] Currently, widespread use of tools to measure body composition, including computed tomography and dual-energy X-ray absorptiometry are not routinely used in public health and cancer prevention screenings, so calculated body mass index (BMI, weight in kg/height in m^2), which can be augmented with measurement of waist circumference and other measures, remains the most important surrogate for obesity.[38,39] Women with a BMI of greater than 25 kg/m^2 and men with a BMI greater than 27 kg/m^2 should make weight loss a priority. Weight loss of just 5–10% is associated with improved health and can reduce the incidence or severity of several cancers.[5,40–43] Weight loss is best achieved by reducing total calorie consumption and increasing calorie expenditure to create a negative energy balance resulting in a modest, but consistent weight loss over time. Maximum weight loss of 1–2 pounds per week is appropriate for most people. Rapid weight loss achieved through fad diets does not encourage individuals to establish healthy eating and physical activity patterns, and weight loss is typically not maintained with these regimens.[33] It is increasingly clear that maintaining a healthy weight throughout life may be one of the most critical approaches to protect against many common malignancies, as well as cardiovascular and metabolic diseases.[5–7,31]

Participate in physical activity daily and reduce time spent in sedentary activities

The energy expenditure associated with physical activity is a critical component of maintaining a healthy body weight, preserving lean body mass, and preventing adult weight gain, all of which are associated with reduced cancer risk.[1,3,5,6,44] Additionally, a combination of daily physical activity and regular bouts of moderate-to-vigorous intensity exercise has been shown in many studies to promote improved health and reduce cancer risk, independent of weight and diet.[45–47] Public health guidelines for physical activity were recently updated to recommend adults engage in 150–300 min of moderate-intensity aerobic activity, or 75–150 min of vigorous-intensity activity, or an equivalent combination, each week, plus some anaerobic muscle-strengthening activity at least 2 days each week.[4] The inverse relationship between physical activity and cancer risk is particularly strong for colon, endometrial, and postmenopausal breast cancers, but reductions in risk have been reported for many other cancer subtypes, including esophageal adenocarcinoma and renal cancer.[1,44,47] In addition to increasing physical activity, reducing sedentary time (defined as an activity with an energy expenditure of 1.5 metabolic equivalents while in a sitting or lying down position) is an important way to decrease cancer risk.[48] Fewer than 25% of Americans are meeting physical activity guidelines, while time spent in sedentary activities, which includes time spent sitting, has increased over time.[4] Importantly, for individuals who do not participate in moderate-to-vigorous activity, replacing sedentary time with light-intensity physical activity (i.e., walking slowly, light household chores) may reduce all-cause mortality and may also decrease cancer risk, although including periods of more intense physical activity should be encouraged.[49]

Consume a plant-based diet that is rich in fruits, vegetables, and a variety of whole grains and beans

Several hundred studies have examined the relationships between fruit and vegetable intake and cancer risk.[1,49–51] The vast majority suggest a significant protective effect of a plant-based diet relative to cancer risk at many sites, in addition to other healthy outcomes.[30] Fruits and vegetables not only contain a diverse array of vitamins, minerals, and fiber, as well as potentially bioactive phytochemicals, but also they are lower in calories and fat than most other foods. A variety of nonstarchy fruits and vegetables should be included at every meal with a goal of consuming at least five servings (or at least 400 g, or 15 ounces, in total) of fruits and vegetables per day. Additionally, emphasis should be placed on consumption of beans and legumes, which provide protein, fiber, B vitamins, and iron, as along with whole-grain breads, cereals, and pastas, which provide fiber, B vitamins, and a vast array of phytochemicals. Fruits, vegetables, nuts, and whole-grain foods should provide at least 25–30 g of dietary fiber per day.[1] Dietary fiber consumption from food sources is well below these recommendations for both children and adults (approximately 13–16 g/day, respectively) in the United States.[52] Increasing plant foods in the diet represents an important mechanism to improve dietary quality while reducing caloric intake. Since a plant-based diet is compatible with modest lean meat consumption, it should not be interpreted as a strictly vegetarian dietary pattern.

Minimize consumption of energy-dense "fast" foods and processed foods that are rich in fat, starches, or sugars, and limit sugar-sweetened drinks

This recommendation has emerged as vital to the overall prevention of weight gain, obesity, and their metabolic complications. Diets that are rich in processed foods and ultra-processed foods (including sugar-sweetened and artificially sweetened beverages, sweetened cereals, packaged snacks, confections, desserts, and reconstituted meats) are typically high in refined sugars and/or fats that contribute excess calories to the diet. In parallel, these foods do not provide a concentrated source of vitamins, minerals, fiber, and bioactive phytochemicals. Higher frequency of consumption of such foods is associated with excess weight and an increased risk of all-cause mortality.[53,54] Consumption of processed foods with added salt, sugars, and fat has significantly increased in recent decades and currently contributes over half of total calorie consumption.[55,56] The majority of this increase comes from the consumption of sugary beverages, especially soda.[1] The Dietary Guidelines Scientific Advisory Committee recommended a reduction in consumption of added sugars to 6% or less. Drinks containing added sugars are associated with an increased risk of overweight and obesity across the life course for children, adolescents, and adults. The consumption of sugary beverages should be minimized.

For people who enjoy red meat, moderate portion sizes, and reduced intake of highly processed red meats are advisable

Populations consuming plant-based diets exhibit lower risk for various diseases, including several types of cancer; however, a specific role for meat in promoting cancer independent of other variables is not causally established. In addition, meat is an important source of many nutrients, such as protein, iron, and vitamin B12. Thus, modest meat consumption is recommended.

Experts debate the level of intake where it begins to increase risk. In general, the data suggests that 18 ounces or less of red meat (beef, lamb, and pork) per week likely does not significantly increase cancer risk, especially if meat does not displace consumption of fruits, vegetables, and whole grains.[1] The impact of different cooking methods which lead to the production of carcinogens, thus impacting cancer risk, continues to be examined.[57] Modest exposure to meats cooked for long periods of time and over flames is prudent.[58] Historically, populations consuming diets rich in various forms of processed meat, including smoked, cured, or salted meats, have experienced greater risk of various cancers; therefore, limiting consumption of these meat products is advised.[1,3] For those choosing meat, it is sensible to select a variety of sources, including fresh chicken, fish, and turkey.[1,3]

Alcohol, if consumed at all, should be limited

The risks and potential benefits of modest alcohol consumption remain a subject of debate. Although the health effects of alcohol or specific types of alcoholic beverages is an active area of research, chronic consumption of alcohol is strongly associated with cancers of the oropharynx, larynx, esophagus, and breast (both pre- and postmenopausal).[1,3,5,6] Additionally, smoking tobacco acts synergistically with alcohol in the pathogenesis of oral and upper aerodigestive cancers.[59,60] Even a moderate amount of daily alcohol consumption may slightly, but significantly, increase the risk of breast cancer, and no amount of alcohol consumption is defined as safe with regards to breast cancer risk.[1,3,61] Significant consumption of alcoholic beverages also contributes to liver cancer and perhaps colon cancer.[1,3] Because there is some evidence that alcohol in moderation may reduce the risk of heart disease, individuals need to consider their personal health history and risk profile when deciding whether or not to consume alcohol. For those who choose to drink, alcohol intake should be limited to one drink per day for women and two drinks per day for men, however, nondrinkers should not be encouraged to begin consuming alcohol.[1,3,5-7]

Optimal food preservation, processing, and preparation

Salt is vital for human health, but adequate amounts are achieved at levels much lower than that typically found in the American diet.[62] Salt-preserved foods are associated with gastric cancer, a major malignancy worldwide, particularly in developing nations. Although relationships remain uncertain, diets containing high amounts of salt-rich processed meats are associated with risk of several cancers and, consequently, should be consumed in moderation.[1,3,63] Meat that is cooked at very high temperatures, grilled, and charred favors the formation of certain types of chemical carcinogens and should be consumed in moderation.[1,3] Microbial contamination of the food supply is a major problem globally. For example, the contamination of grains and legumes with fungal aflatoxins contributes significantly to the risk of liver cancer, and public heath approaches by government agencies to limit exposures are necessary.

Dietary supplements are probably unnecessary in the context of a healthy diet

An increasing proportion of the American population consumes some type of self-prescribed nutrient or dietary supplement on a regular basis. The public increasingly perceives heavily marketed supplements and alternative medications as an important form of self-therapy for the prevention and treatment of many ailments, including cancer.[1,3,64] Multivitamin and mineral supplements are usually inexpensive, easy to consume, obtained without a prescription, and relatively free of side effects when taken at the dosages approximating the recommended dietary allowance (RDA). There has been very little evidence in support of routine dietary supplements for population-wide cancer prevention.[6,65,66] Although it is clear that Americans can achieve adequate nutrient intake by consuming a diverse diet based upon the published recommendations, a standard multivitamin/mineral supplement providing the RDA may be beneficial to some and entails minimal risk. Increasingly, supplements that contain high concentrations of specific nutrients combined with other components, such as herbals, extracts, and concentrates, are being aggressively marketed. Consumers should be aware that regulations regarding implied health claims and requirements that products contain the stated ingredients and have demonstrated safety and efficacy are minimal, and the buyer should maintain skepticism and caution. The Office of Dietary Supplements of the NIH provides web-based information for interested consumers (https://ods.od.nih.gov).

For mothers: breastfeed your baby if you can

The WHO recommends that women breastfeed exclusively for the first 6 months and continue as complementary foods are introduces up to two years of age and beyond[67] In addition to providing important immune benefits, breastfed babies also have a lower risk of excess body fatness as children. Additionally, there is strong evidence that mothers who breastfeed have a lower risk of breast cancer.[1]

Summary of research efforts focusing on specific cancers

It is unlikely that any food, nutrient, or dietary pattern will influence all cancers uniformly.[6,26,64] Thus, in reviewing the relationships between nutrition and cancer risk, it is important to examine the data for each tissue or organ separately. It is clear that research will continue to improve our ability to identify individuals at high risk of specific cancers based upon genetic testing, family history, exposure to carcinogenic agents, and the presence of premalignant conditions. Thus, individuals and clinicians will be particularly interested in recommendations that are more refined than general public health guidelines. A future goal is to provide tailored dietary recommendations and chemopreventive strategies for individuals at risk. Additional research will define unique preventive strategies for various cancers. The following is a brief summary of the current understanding of relationships between diet, nutrition, and the risk of specific, commonly occurring cancers. For additional information, please refer to Table 3.

Colon and rectum

According to the International Agency for Research on Cancer in 2018, colorectal cancer accounted for approximately 1.8 million new cases and 900,000 deaths annually in the world.[68] Colorectal cancer is the third most common cancer, the second leading cause of cancer deaths worldwide, and the third leading cause of cancer death in the United States. Genetic factors and premalignant conditions are being characterized that will define high-risk groups for chemoprevention and diet intervention studies. The international variation in colorectal cancer is large. Although screening differences may contribute to some of the international variation, it is unlikely to account for the greater than tenfold

Table 3 Summary of strong evidence on diet, nutrition, physical activity, and cancer prevention.[a]

	Mouth, pharynx, larynx	Naso-pharynx	Esophagus (adeno-carcinoma)	Esophagus (squamous cell)	Lung	Stomach	Pancreas	Gallbladder	Liver	Colorectum	Breast pre-menopause	Breast post-menopause	Ovary	Endo-metrium	Prostate	Kidney	Risk of weight gain, overweight, or obesity
Adult body fatness[b]	↑		↑↑			↑↑[c]	↑↑	↑	↑↑	↑↑			↑	↑↑	↑[d]	↑↑	
Adult weight gain												↑↑					
Physical activity (moderate and vigorous)										↓↓[e]		↓		↓			↓[f]
Physical activity (vigorous)											↓						
Alcoholic drinks[g]	↑↑			↑↑		↑			↑↑	↑↑	↑	↑↑					
Whole grains										↓							
Foods containing dietary fiber										↓							↓
Red meat										↑							
Processed meat										↑↑							
Sugar-sweetened drinks																	↑↑
Dairy products										↓[h]							
Calcium supplements										↓[i]							
Foods preserved by salting						↑											
Cantonese-style salted fish		↑															
Glycemic load														↑			
Arsenic in drinking water					↑↑												
Mate				↑													
Aflatoxins									↑↑								
Coffee									↓								
High dose beta-carotene supplements					↑↑[j]												
Adult attained height[k]							↑			↑↑	↑	↑↑	↑↑	↑	↑	↑	
Mediterranean dietary pattern																	↓
Western dietary pattern[l]												↑					↑
Fast food consumption																	↑
Breastfeeding/having been breastfed[m]											↓						↓

[a]Source: Modified from World Cancer Research Fund International/American Institute for Cancer Research.[35]
[b]Body fatness is marked by body mass index (BMI) and where possible waist circumference and waist-hip ratio.
[c]Stomach cardia only.
[d]Advanced prostate cancer only.
[e]Colon cancer only.
[f]Aerobic physical activity only.
[g]Stomach and liver: based on ethanol intake >45 g/day (about three drinks); Colorectal and Kidney: based on ethanol intake of 30 g/day (approximately two drinks); Breast cancer (postmenopausal): Based on intakes of up to 30 g/day (about two drinks)-there is insufficient data for higher levels of alcohol.
[h]Includes evidence on total dairy, milk, cheese, and dietary calcium intakes.
[i]Calcium supplements: evidence derived from studies of supplements >200 mg/day.
[j]Evidence is from high-dose supplementation in smokers.
[k]Adult height is unlikely to directly influence the risk of cancer. It is a marker for genetic, environmental, hormonal, and nutritional factors affecting growth during the period from preconception to completion of growth in length.
[l]Characterized by high intakes of free sugars, meat, and dietary fat; the overall conclusion includes all these factors.
[m]For breast cancer (pre and postmenopausal) evidence related to the mother who is breastfeeding and not to the child who is breastfed. For obesity, evidence relates to the child who has been breastfed.

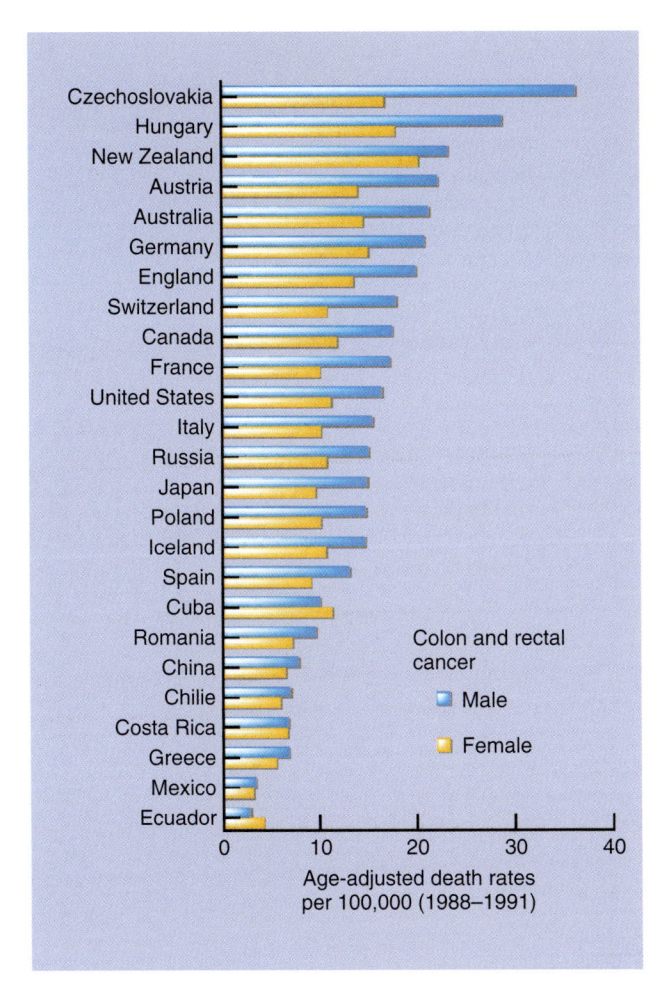

Figure 1 Age-standardized colon and rectal cancer incidence per 100,000 men in Japan from 1960 through 1977, a period of dramatic social and economic change associated with profound changes in diet.

variation in risk that is observed between nations.[69] The lower rates in Asian nations suggest that cultural and lifestyle variables, rather than modernization, are the critical factors.[26,70,71] Dramatic increases in incidence among Japanese and Chinese migrants to the United States[72] further indicate that international variations primarily result from environmental influences rather than genetic background.[73,74] Examination of time trends in colorectal cancer incidence, particularly in Japan since the 1940s, strongly suggests major contributions from diet and lifestyle factors associated with the Westernization of cultures (Figure 1).[26]

Energy balance, body mass, and physical activity
Energy intake, physical activity, and various measures of body size or obesity are all intimately interrelated and associated with colorectal cancer risk (Figure 2). The associations have generally been stronger for colon compared to rectal cancer. It is difficult to quantitate or ascertain the role of each component without considering them as a group.[75] An association between BMI or other adiposity measures, such as waist circumference, and elevated risk of colon cancer has been consistently reported.[1,74,76–78] Associations, though typically stronger in men, have been observed for both men and women. A convincing inverse association between physical activity and risk of colon cancer has been consistently reported.[1,69,79,80] The associations between obesity and physical inactivity with colon cancer risk have been observed in multiple countries (United States, China, Sweden, and Japan), among men and women, and for both occupational and recreational physical activity.[69] Obesity and physical inactivity, also, have been associated with risk of colon adenoma.[81] Taller adult attained height is related to a higher risk of colorectal cancer.[82–84] Studies in rodent models of colorectal carcinogenesis have reported enhanced carcinogenesis with greater *ad libitum* intake[85] and reduced risk with restricted intake.[86] Overall, the evidence is convincing that physical activity, appropriate energy balance, and ideal BMI maintenance will decrease risk of colon cancer.[1]

Dietary pattern
Across studies conducted in different populations worldwide, two dietary patterns have been identified with reasonable consistency.[87] One of these patterns is the so-called "healthy" or "prudent" pattern and is characterized by greater intake of fruits and vegetables, coupled with that of whole grains, nuts or legumes, fish or other seafood, and low-fat milk or dairy products. In parallel, an "unhealthy" or "western" dietary pattern is characterized by higher intakes of red and processed meat, sugar-sweetened beverages, refined grains, desserts, and potatoes. In general, the unhealthy dietary pattern has been associated with an increased risk of colorectal cancer, whereas the prudent dietary pattern has been associated with a decreased risk.[1,88,89] Dietary patterns research is emerging rapidly and may contribute to the understanding of colorectal cancer risk due to the additive and synergistic impact of specific components (e.g., saturated fat, fiber), but may also contribute to that of broad patterns of diet and exercise impacting critical processes, such as inflammation or insulinemia.[75,90,91]

Fats and meats
The relationship between total fat intake, fat saturation, or different sources of fat and risk of colon cancer remains an active area of research, but definitive conclusions regarding fat *per se* have not emerged.[1,3,5,6,87,92–94] Some cohort studies suggest that fat from red meats rather than total fat may increase colon cancer risk, suggesting that it may not be fat in isolation but related components in red meat, as well.[78,95–98] Consumption of processed meats in particular has emerged as a convincing risk factor for colorectal cancer.[69] Potential mediators include carcinogenic compounds such as heme iron, exogenous N-nitroso compounds, ionized fatty acids, and heterocyclic amines and polycyclic aromatic hydrocarbons formed when meats are cooked at high temperatures. Thus, moderation in consumption of red meats and processed meats should be considered for those at risk of colorectal cancer (Figure 3).

Fruits, vegetables, and fiber
Dietary patterns rich in plant products, particularly grains and vegetables, are often associated with a lower risk of colorectal cancer, and many have postulated that the fiber content is one major mediating factor.[27,69,80,92,95,99–102] The chemistry of dietary fiber is exceptionally complex, and the quantitative and qualitative assessment of fiber intake in human epidemiologic studies is very difficult. However, the majority of studies suggest a diet rich in diverse fiber-containing foods, particularly from whole-grain sources, may be beneficial. The large European Prospective Investigation into Cancer (EPIC) study involving over 500,000 men and women reported a 13% reduction in colon cancer risk for each 10 g/day increase in dietary fiber derived from cereals, fruit, or vegetables.[103,104] A few intervention trials have evaluated interventions focusing upon specific types of dietary fiber and colorectal adenoma risk, and, to date, the results are equivocal.[105–109]

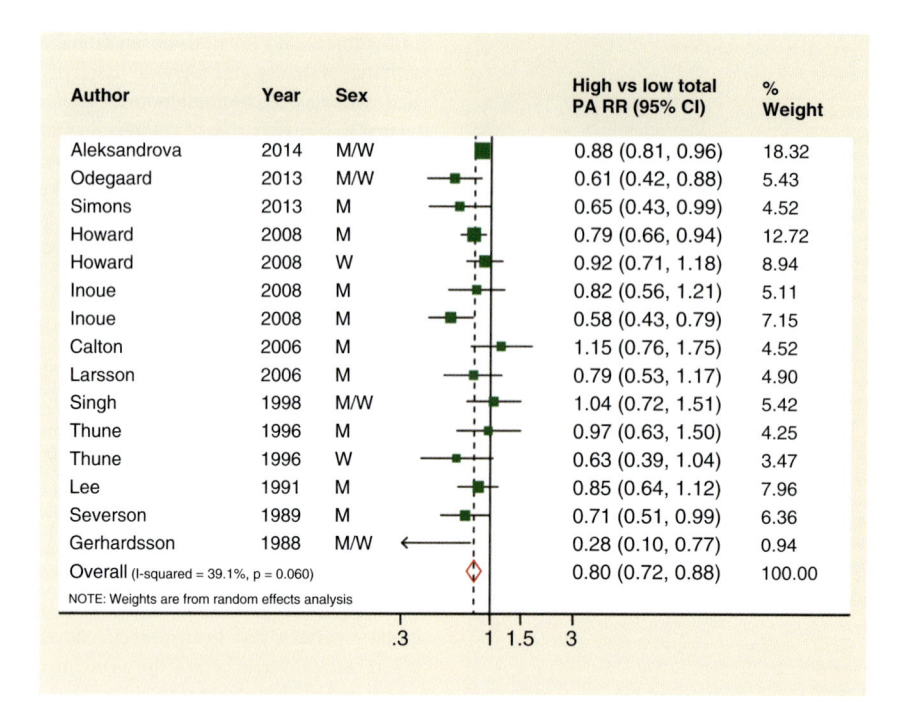

Figure 2 Highest versus lowest analysis of total physical activity and colon cancer. Source: This material has been reproduced from the World Cancer Research Fund/American Institute for Cancer Research.[69] Available at dietandcancerreport.org.

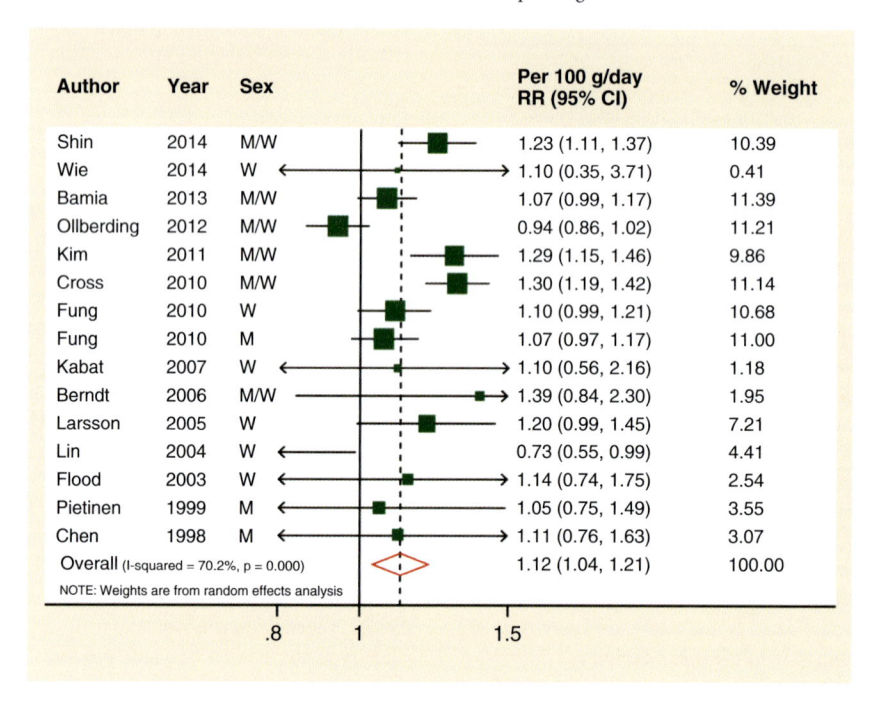

Figure 3 Dose–response meta-analysis of red and processed meat and colorectal cancer per 100 g/day. Source: This material has been reproduced from the World Cancer Research Fund/American Institute for Cancer Research.[69] Available at dietandcancerreport.org.

Reflecting the uncertainty, the WCRF/AICR demoted the level of evidence supporting a protective role of dietary fiber from 'convincing' in 2011[69] to "probable" in 2017, and added whole grain as a probable protective factor.[69]

Alcohol

A positive association between alcohol intake and risk of colorectal cancer is consistent among many studies across diverse populations in both men and women.[5,6,69,110–112] Alcohol is also related to higher risk of colorectal adenoma.[1,3,5,6,69] Overall, the association is related more closely to total alcohol intake rather than to the specific source of alcohol.[1,3,5,6] In a meta-analysis of 14 cohort studies from North America, Europe, and Asia published in 2018, even light drinking (≤1 alcoholic drink per day) was associated with a slightly increased risk of colorectal cancer compared with no or occasional drinking of alcohol,[113] but typically the increased risk is seen more clearly at intakes exceeding two drinks per day.[114] Acetaldehyde, a key metabolite of ethanol, has been established as carcinogenic to humans by the International Agency for Research.[115] After alcohol is ingested, it reaches the large bowel through circulation and then the luminal ethanol is metabolized by microbial alcohol dehydrogenase into acetaldehyde.[116] High concentrations of acetaldehyde might account for the susceptibility of the colorectum to alcohol intake.

Dairy products and calcium
Although a western dietary pattern has been associated with a higher risk of colorectal cancer, greater intake of dairy products and milk has typically been associated with lower risk. Intake of calcium from the diet has also been associated with lower risk of colorectal cancer. However, dietary calcium is largely from dairy products and strongly correlated to other items in dairy. Nonetheless, calcium supplements have also been associated with lower risk of colorectal cancer, and in randomized trials, lower risk of colorectal adenoma.[117] The World Cancer Research Fund/American Institute for Cancer Research considers dairy products and calcium supplements as probable protective factors for colorectal cancer.[69] The mechanisms are unclear, but calcium precipitates secondary bile acids, ionized fatty acids, and heme iron in the colorectal lumen and may influence proliferation, differentiation, and apoptosis through binding to the calcium-sensing receptor, which is expressed in colorectal tissue.[69] Some evidence also suggests that maintaining adequate vitamin D status may help protect against colorectal cancer.[118]

In summary, increased risk of colorectal cancer is strongly associated with a physically inactive lifestyle, a higher BMI, and greater alcohol intake. In addition, an affluent or western dietary pattern, which is especially rich in red and processed meats and highly processed carbohydrates and sugars and low in whole-grain products, plant fiber, and calcium, is associated with an increased risk. The potential interactions among these components and other factors contributing to risk, such as early life dietary exposures, exercise, the colonic microbiome, and genetics, are numerous. At present, it is sensible to consider the combined influence of the total dietary pattern and physical activity when making recommendations for colon cancer prevention, rather than focusing on a single factor. More than half of colorectal cancers are likely preventable by adhering to a healthy diet and lifestyle.

Breast cancer
Cancer of the breast is most common in the affluent nations of North America and Western Europe and much less common in many parts of Asia and Africa,[1,3,5,6,119] and, like colorectal cancer, we observe that migrants from low-risk nations show increasing risk after moving to a high-risk nation,[1,3,5,6,73,119] particularly in succeeding generations. This observation suggests that nutritional or other environmental factors active during youth and adolescence may have a long-term and major impact on subsequent risk of breast cancer.[1,3,5,6,119] The risk of breast cancer is reduced by early age of pregnancy and lactation.[1,3,40,120] A number of dietary and nutritional factors characteristic of an affluent culture have also been proposed to enhance risk of breast cancer[1,3,5,6] and are briefly summarized.

Alcohol use
The accumulated evidence concerning alcohol intake and risk of breast cancer shows a positive association.[1,3,5,6,40] The relative risk (RR) from the consumption of one typical serving of beer, wine, or liquor (~12 g of ethanol) per day is estimated to be 1.4, whereas three drinks per day approximately doubles the risk, compared to those who drink lower amounts or do not drink. Studies have reported a linear relationship between breast cancer risk and each 10 g increase in daily alcohol consumption, even across different estrogen/progesterone hormone subtypes.[61,121–123]

Energy balance, body weight, and obesity
Evidence is accumulating that body fatness, adult weight gain, and a lack of physical activity are important risk factors for breast cancer.[1,3,5,6,69,124,125] The role of energy intake as a stimulator of mammary carcinogenesis has been well established by rodent studies using diet or energy restriction[126,127] and regression analysis of ad libitum feeding.[128,129] Overall, higher levels of adult physical activity seem to provide a modest protection (~25% risk reduction) against breast cancer, and the protective effect may be independent of BMI or weight gain as an adult.[125,130–132] However, the precise relationships between energy intake, energy expenditure, anthropometrics, and risk of breast cancer must be examined for different critical periods in a woman's life cycle. The effects of these factors may vary during adolescence, the reproductive years, and the postmenopausal period.

Dietary fat
The controversy concerning the contribution of dietary fat concentrations or sources, independent of energy intake, to risk of breast cancer can best be appreciated through examination of the representative data presented in Figure 4. Geographic studies show strong correlations between national rates of breast cancer and the estimated per capita fat consumption.[93,133] There are wide international variations in breast cancer rates as well as per capita fat consumption, or the percentage of calories derived from fat. Breast cancer rates have been observed to increase significantly in populations migrating from low-risk areas, such as Japan, where diets were traditionally low in fat, to high-risk areas, such as the United States, where populations consume diets rich in fat.[73,134] Time-trend studies also support a dietary fat and breast cancer association. Within Japan, estimates of per capita daily fat intake have risen over the decades following World War II. During this period, breast cancer mortality increased in Japan by >30%. Despite these correlations, many investigators argue that fat intake may be an indicator of other unidentified combinations of diet and environmental components that are the truly critical risk factors. The relationship between fat intake and risk of breast cancer has been examined in many case-control and cohort studies with inconsistent results.[135–138] The large EPIC study followed over 33,000 women for 11.5 years and found that diets high in total and saturated fat were associated with a significantly increased risk of ER(+)PR(+) disease but not with ER(−)PR(−) breast cancer.[139] However, findings from randomized controlled trials have not provided definitive results. One randomized intervention study of women who had been treated for breast cancer suggested a 24% risk reduction in breast cancer recurrence among women who were able reduce their dietary fat consumption to ~33 g/day (vs 51 g/day for the control group).[140] Although not statistically significant, similar trends were observed in the very large, randomized Women's Health Initiative study.[135] Long-term follow-up (~20 years) of these women has revealed a 20% reduction in breast cancer-related death for women who reduced fat intake in their diets compared to those in the comparison group,[141] though it is not known how the women in the intervention group changed their dietary pattern in other ways during the long observational follow-up period. Although the data from epidemiologic studies and randomized controlled trials have not provided definitive results concerning dietary fat and

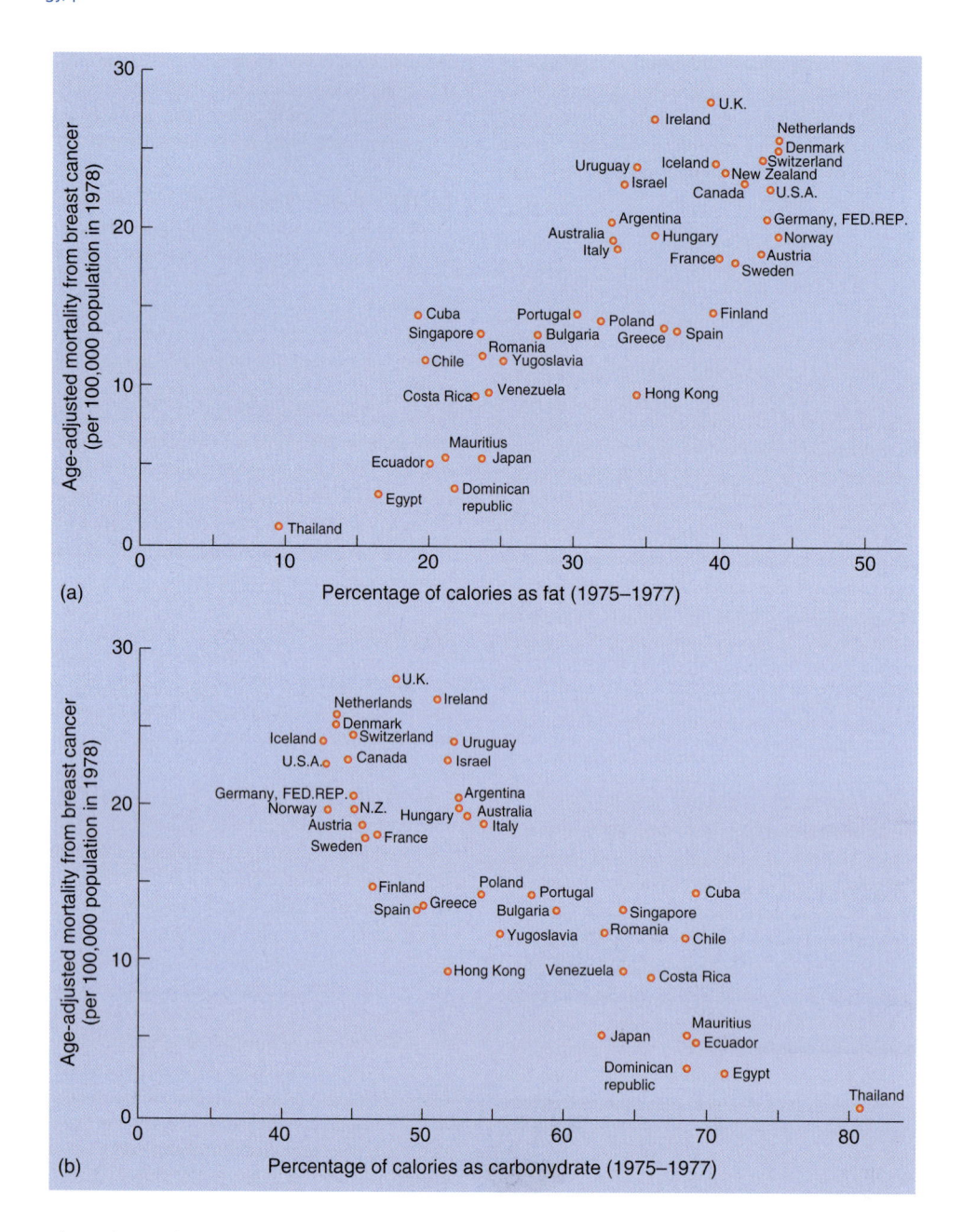

Figure 4 International correlation of (a) estimated dietary fat intake (percentage of calories as fat) and (b) estimated carbohydrate intake (percentage of calories as carbohydrate) and age-adjusted breast cancer mortality. Source: Carroll.[93]

breast cancer, accumulated evidence from >100 animal studies using chemical carcinogens, hormones, irradiation, or viruses to induce breast cancer indicate that, as a single variable, fat enhances mammary carcinogenesis.[1,3,85,128,129] Overall, the possibility that achievable reductions in fat intake during adulthood will cause an appreciable reduction in breast cancer risk remains uncertain, and dietary patterns during adolescence and reproductive years may prove to be more critical to future breast cancer risk.[1,3]

Other dietary factors
Overall, a plant-based dietary pattern rich in vegetables, fruits, and grains may have a role in decreasing the risk of breast cancer, but a conclusive and specific role for selected plant components has not been demonstrated.[1,3,5,6,69,138,142] There are no consistent relationships for the consumption of specific vitamins or minerals and breast cancer risk, and recommendations regarding supplement use for prevention remain to be defined.[1,3,5,6] Other bioactive compounds found in the diet, such as soy isoflavones, lignans, and fiber, may play a role in breast cancer, but evidence remains insufficient for recommendations.[1,3,5,6,138] In summary, the most well-established recommendations for breast cancer prevention are to engage in vigorous physical activity on a regular basis, avoid or limit intake of alcoholic beverages, and minimize lifetime weight gain and body fatness through the combination of physical activity and energy restriction.

Prostate cancer

Cancer of the prostate is one of the most frequently diagnosed malignancies in the United States and many developed nations, and it is especially common among men of African descent.[1,3,119] Prostate cancer is a disease of aging men; in the United States, over 95% of cases are diagnosed in men age 50 and older. The international distribution of prostate cancer is similar to that of colon and breast cancer; therefore, it correlates with affluent dietary patterns.[143,144] Relationships between specific dietary variables and prostate cancer have not been clearly elucidated, and specific recommendations to prevent the disease remain speculative. A role for weight gain and obesity resulting from excess energy intake and a lack of physical activity is accumulating in human studies and is clearly demonstrated in rodent studies.[31,144–147] The evidence is most compelling for the increase in the risk of advanced prostate cancer.[143] International and intra-country correlational studies suggest associations between prostate cancer mortality and the per capita intake of total fat.[1,3,144] There is inconsistent data from cohort studies regarding the relationship between different sources of animal fat and protein and risk of prostate cancer.[143] There is limited and inconclusive evidence that dairy products, possibly related to calcium, is associated with an increased risk of prostate cancer.[143,148–152]

Several studies have suggested that specific nutrients such as vitamin E and selenium may influence prostate cancer risk.[153] A lower risk of prostate cancer was noted among men randomized to vitamin E supplementation in a trial of smokers in Finland.[153] The possible role of selenium in the prevention of prostate cancer has been hypothesized based upon various lines of indirect evidence.[1,3,154–156] The largest prostate cancer chemoprevention trial to date, the Selenium and Vitamin E Chemoprevention Trial (SELECT), randomized 33,000 men beginning in 2001. The study design was a 2 × 2 factorial of vitamin E, selenium, and a placebo. After a median follow-up of 5.4 years, selenium, vitamin E, or a combination of the two were not found to be protective for prostate cancer in this group of healthy men.[157]

Prostate cells express vitamin D receptors, and exposure to a ligand tends to induce differentiation pathways. These complex relationships have spurred many cell culture, animal, and cohort studies, with several suggesting an inverse relationship between vitamin D and prostate cancer risk, although benefits beyond correction of deficient or marginal intake are unknown.[123,158–161] The evidence to date is insufficient to support vitamin D supplementation for prostate cancer prevention.[121]

The overall consumption of fruits and vegetables has not been shown a consistent reduction in risk of prostate cancer.[1,3,143,144] However, a reduced risk of prostate cancer associated with the consumption of tomatoes and processed tomato products has been observed repeatedly in the prospectively evaluated Health Professionals Follow-up Study.[81,162,163] On the basis of these findings, it has been hypothesized that the carotenoid lycopene may account for some of the anticancer properties of tomato products, although other compounds found in tomato foods may also be important.[89,144,163–168] However, the World Cancer Research Fund/American Institute for Cancer Research downgraded initially strong evidence for tomatoes and lycopene-rich foods and lower risk of prostate cancer in 2007[3] to limited evidence in the most recent 2014 report.[143] Yet, subsequently, the largest pooling study of serum and plasma levels showed high prediagnostic concentrations of lycopene were associated with a lower risk of advanced prostate cancer,[169] and a meta-analysis supported an inverse association with dietary lycopene.[170] A recent prospective cohort study has shown higher consumption of canned and cooked tomato product to be associated with a lower risk of prostate cancer in Seventh-Day Adventists.[171] Interestingly, several interventions where subjects have been fed either tomato products or a lycopene supplement have reported modulation of both blood and prostate tissue biomarkers of prostate cancer.[167,172–174]

In summary, epidemiologic studies and a limited number of laboratory investigations suggest a role for an affluent dietary pattern in prostate cancer risk. Rates of prostate cancer are higher in nations consuming an affluent dietary pattern coupled with adult obesity and a sedentary lifestyle, although the contributions of specific components are not well-defined and are being actively investigated. Tomato products, possibly related to their content of the carotenoid lycopene, remain among the most promising foods with a potentially protective association.

Lung cancer

Lung cancer is one of the most common cancers worldwide and the leading cause of cancer-related death.[175] Cigarette smoking accounts for the vast majority of cases, and incidence rates continue to climb globally in parallel with the globalization of cigarette manufacturing, marketing, and advertising. In some countries, with initially high rates, incidence has come down with reductions in cigarette use. Certain occupational exposures, such as asbestos or radiation, may act synergistically with cigarette smoking to increase the risk.[175] Compared with the role of tobacco, the potential contribution of diet and nutrition appears relatively modest.[175] An inverse relationship between the greater intake of fruits and vegetables and lung cancer incidence has been a frequent finding in human nutritional epidemiology.[175–178] However, because smokers tend to have poor dietary patterns, it has been difficult to conclusively link low intakes of fruits and vegetables, to lower lung cancer risk, independent of smoking. It was initially hypothesized that beta-carotene found in fruits and vegetables or vitamin A derived from cleavage of beta-carotene may be the critical active agents in these foods lowering cancer risk.[1,3,179] However, two randomized controlled intervention trials in high-risk populations found no reduction, and perhaps an increase, in the incidence of lung cancer among male smokers after several years of supplementation with beta-carotene at 20 or 30 mg/day.[180] In a study of over 72,000 Chinese women, among those who were exposed to side-stream smoke, dietary intake of foods rich in tocopherols was inversely related to lung cancer incidence. In contrast, supplemental vitamin E significantly increased risk of total lung cancers and, in particular, increased lung adenocarcinoma.[181] These reports emphasize that potential protective benefits of diets rich in fruits and vegetables may involve many interacting phytochemicals or nutrients and may not be reproduced by providing a single agent.[122,175] Overall, elimination of cigarette smoking and occupational risk factors will have the greatest impact on decreasing the incidence of lung cancer. Among high-risk individuals, the frequent consumption of a diverse array of fruits, vegetables, and other plant foods may provide some degree of protection against lung cancer.

Oral cavity, larynx, and oropharynx cancers

Over 600,00 cancers of the oral cavity (including cancers of the lips and salivary glands), pharynx, and larynx are diagnosed worldwide yearly, making this group the seventh most frequent type of cancer worldwide. As for lung cancer, these malignancies are strongly related to the use of tobacco products.[7,64,182] Historically, studies have documented strong associations between the consumption of alcoholic beverages and cancers in these tissues. A dose–response relationship of alcohol and oral cancer, independent of tobacco usage, has been observed in a number of studies (Figure 5).[184,185] Additional evidence is derived from studies of populations who exhibit increased risk, such as alcoholics, and from Seventh-Day Adventists and Mormons in the United

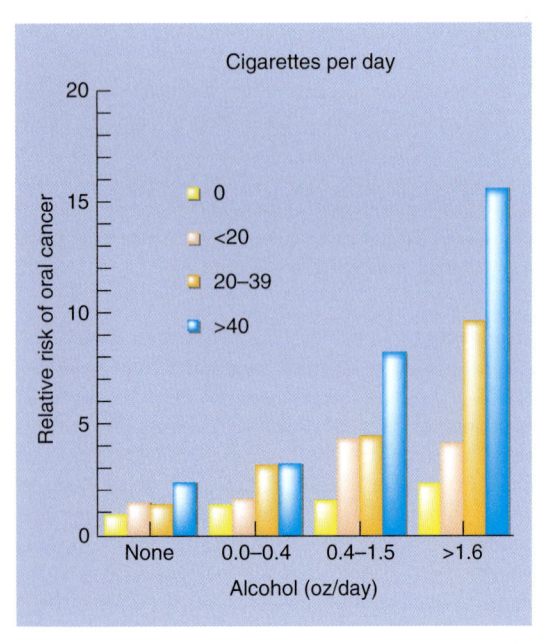

Figure 5 The interactions between alcohol intake and cigarette smoking on the relative risk of oral cancer. Source: Based on Rothman and Keller.[183]

States, who refrain from alcohol and have a much lower risk.[186,187] Although much of the evidence is from case-control studies, the strength and consistency of the evidence, plus strong biologic plausibility, led the World Cancer Research Fund to consider alcohol as a convincing cause of oropharyngeal cancers.[182] In fact, tobacco and alcohol account for approximately 90% of all these cancers. Of note, feeding pure alcohol as part of a nutritionally sound diet does not produce oral cancers in experimental animals. The extent that this represents biochemical differences between man and rodents, the lack of a direct carcinogenic effect of ethanol, the presence of carcinogens in alcoholic beverages consumed by man, the passive inhalation of ambient tobacco smoke in the places where ethanol is consumed, and the importance of other interacting carcinogens and nutritional deficits must be further evaluated. According to the World Cancer Research Fund, excess body fatness (as determined by BMI, waist circumference, and waist-to-hip ratio) is a probable contributor to cancers of the mouth, pharynx, and larynx.[182] There is some evidence from both epidemiologic and laboratory studies that high intake of nonstarchy vegetables is associated with a lower risk of these cancers, but the evidence is not considered convincing to date.[77,182] In addition, clinical and laboratory investigation has suggested that vitamin A and analogs or metabolites, as well as certain carotenoids, may serve as inhibitors of carcinogenesis in the oral and respiratory epithelia.[188] In summary, tobacco products are major contributors to cancers of the mouth and pharynx, especially in conjunction with the consumption of alcoholic beverages.[1,3] Further efforts to better define the roles of vitamin A and derivatives, other phytochemicals, and a diverse plant-based diet for prevention in high-risk groups are warranted.

Squamous cell esophageal cancer

Squamous cell cancer of the esophagus is the eighth most common cancer worldwide, with almost a half a million cases reported annually; this malignancy varies several hundredfold between nations and between geographic regions within nations.[189,190] In most developed nations, correlational analyses between countries and case-control studies indicate that the major risk factors for squamous cell esophageal cancer are alcohol and cigarette smoking.[190] In addition, between 10% and 30% of worldwide incidence is attributable to human papillomavirus (HPV).[190] Risk increases in proportion to the amount of alcohol consumed.[1,3,191,192] A number of studies show an alcohol dose–response relationship after controlling for cigarette smoking, and risk is particularly high in those who both smoke and consume alcohol.[190] Increasing consumption of alcohol is often associated with the marginal intake of many nutrients, which may predispose individuals to greater risk. For example, alcohol may interact with folate, vitamin B12, and methyl group metabolism to modulate risk.[193] A number of studies suggest an inverse relationship between risk of esophageal cancer and diets marginal in fresh fruits and vegetables, although the association is not considered convincing by the World Cancer Research Fund.[177,190,194] In certain parts of Asia where alcohol consumption does not explain the high risk for esophageal cancer, there may be a relationship between esophageal cancer and the indigenous diet, which is low in fresh fruits, vegetables, and animal products, and the estimated intakes of vitamin A, vitamin C, riboflavin, zinc, and several trace elements, such as molybdenum, are low.[195,196] In summary, cigarette smoking and alcohol consumption are the most important etiologic factors for squamous cell carcinoma of the esophagus. The possibility that marginal intakes of one or more nutrients may contribute to risk in affluent populations has been suggested but is not firmly established.[190] It is possible that the deleterious effects of smoking and alcohol are amplified when the diet is of low quality and modest in fruits and vegetables.

Adenocarcinoma of the esophagus and gastric cardia

In recent years, investigators have identified a divergent incidence pattern for cancers of the gastric cardia and noncardia stomach (all other sites), which suggests different etiologies. Adenocarcinoma of the cardia, although technically part of the stomach, is typically grouped etiologically with those arising from the metaplastic distal esophagus (esophageal adenocarcinoma), which show a similar histology, epidemiology, and risk factors. The incidence of adenocarcinoma of the distal esophagus and gastric cardia has been increasing rapidly over the last two decades in the United States and Western Europe, while that of the distal stomach has been declining.[197,198] Current or past cigarette smoking may be one of the contributing factors.[198,199] However, one of the most consistent observations has been a positive association between BMI and/or abdominal obesity and risk of adenocarcinoma of the esophagus.[200–203] In parallel, strong evidence supports a role of obesity in an increased risk of cancers of the cardia.[204] As the prevalence of obesity has increased in the United States, a parallel trend is observed in the incidence of adenocarcinoma of the esophagus and gastric cardia.[205] Cohort studies consistently link various measures of excess adiposity with increased risk of adenocarcinoma of the stomach cardia esophagus.[204] The mechanism remains under investigation; however, it has been speculated that obesity may predispose to gastroesophageal reflux disease, leading to histological changes (e.g., Barrett's esophagus, metaplasia), which predisposes to cancer. Other nutritional factors that have been investigated relative to the increased adenocarcinoma risk include affluent dietary patterns, characterized as rich in animal sources of fat, low in fiber, and low in fruits and vegetables, though none are established as definitive.[206] Additional efforts are needed to clarify the risk factors in addition to obesity that are responsible for the dramatic increases in the incidence of adenocarcinoma of the esophagus and to devise effective intervention strategies.

Stomach cancer (noncardia)

Gastric cancer (also known as stomach cancer) is the fifth most common cancer worldwide, accounting for almost a million cases a year.[207] The incidence varies dramatically among countries and is highest in parts of Asia (e.g., Japan) and South America. A dramatic decrease in the incidence of noncardia stomach cancer in many affluent nations has been documented over the last century. In the United States, the current rate is among the lowest in the world, whereas, in 1930, gastric cancer was the most frequently diagnosed malignancy in Americans. Alcohol has been established as a probable factor for stomach cancer; the association is observed primarily at higher levels of alcohol (e.g., >45 g/day) and appears stronger in smokers.[204] According to the World Cancer Research Fund, the evidence is consistent for a causal effect of salt-preserved vegetables, salt-preserved fish, and salt-preserved foods for risk of stomach cancer.[204] It is believed that high salt intake can damage the mucosa of the stomach, leading to inflammation and atrophy, and possibly predisposing the stomach to *Helicobacter pylori* colonization.[208] Several variables under study are considered to be likely related to stomach cancer, including the following: (1) the potential protective role of diets rich in fruit[209,210]; (2) the protective effects of modern food processing and storage reducing spoilage; (3) increased risk due to high exposure to foods with salt curing, pickling, and nitrates for preservation[211]; (4) the role of *H. pylori* infection and interactions with dietary factors[212–214]; (5) identification of natural carcinogens or precursors, such as nitrates, found in foods[215]; (6) the production of carcinogens during food storage and preparation; and (7) the synthesis of carcinogens from dietary precursors, such as nitrates, in the acid environment of the stomach.[1,3,199,212,213] Recent evidence supports an association between processed meat intake and noncardia gastric cancer, warranting further investigation.[204]

Liver cancer

Historically, primary hepatocellular carcinoma has been relatively uncommon in the United States and Northern Europe. However, in the United States, liver cancer incidence has tripled since the 1980s and by 2030 is projected to be the third leading cause of cancer-related death.[216,217] Liver cancer is one of the most frequent malignancies in the developing nations of sub-Saharan Africa and Asia and is now ranked as the sixth most common cancer worldwide.[1,3] Hepatitis B and C infections are the major etiologic factors in many high-risk areas, where the carrier state imparts an increased risk of ~200-fold.[218] Contamination of foods with carcinogenic fungal products, such as certain aflatoxins, also likely contribute to risk in some populations.[219] Aflatoxins are found in geographic areas where food processing and storage are not optimal. Countries with high aflatoxin exposure often have high rates of hepatitis B infection, parasitic infections, and nutritional deficiencies, which may interact to determine risk. In low-risk nations, obesity, overweight, the syndrome of nonalcoholic steatohepatitis (NASH), and the consumption of alcohol are the relevant dietary factors in the pathogenesis of liver cancer.[1,3,92,101,220,221] Obesity is the strongest risk factor for nonalcoholic fatty liver disease and its progression to NASH, which may ultimately progress to cirrhosis and the greater risk of liver cancer.[219] The data also suggest that risk factors may act in an additive or synergistic fashion.[222] Chronic consumption of 3 or more alcoholic beverages daily increases risk of liver cancer. Chronic high alcohol consumption causes liver damage, associated with activation of inflammatory cascades promoting fibrosis and ultimately cirrhosis.[219] It has been hypothesized that liver cancer is most common in those who have the greatest cumulative experiences with alcohol, viral hepatitis, and toxin exposure. Increasing evidence indicates that coffee intake is associated with a decreased risk of liver cancer. The mechanism is not known but coffee components appear to reduce inflammation in the liver.[219] There is limited suggestive evidence that consumption of fish, possibly related to omega-3 fatty acids, and regular physical activity may also reduce the risk of liver cancer.[223–226] Although liver cancer has been relatively rare in affluent nations, its rates are rising sharply, largely due to nonviral causes, especially obesity and diet.

Pancreatic cancer

Pancreatic cancer is frequently detected at an advanced stage and, thus, is highly lethal. It is the thirteenth most common cancer worldwide, but eighth ranked in cause of cancer death because of its high lethality[227] Cigarette smoking has been firmly established as one etiologic factor, accounting for approximately 25% of the cases.[64,228] The risk of pancreatic cancer in those who smoke at least a pack per day is approximately fourfold, compared with that of nonsmokers.[1,3] Body fatness, as measured by BMI, waist circumference, and waist-to-hip ratio, is positively associated with pancreatic cancer risk and is an established cause of this malignancy.[227,229] The causality of this association is consistently supported by studies in animal models.[230] Insulin resistance and type 2 diabetes mellitus are risk factors for pancreatic cancer and may in part mediate some of the effects of excess adiposity on pancreatic cancer risk.[227] There is limited but not definitive evidence that diets rich in red and processed meats, alcohol, fructose-containing foods, and saturated fat may increase pancreatic cancer risk.[227] There is no clear linear association between alcohol and pancreatic cancer risk, but there is a suggested increased risk at higher levels of intake, generally exceeding 3 alcoholic beverages daily.[231,232] Smoking and obesity account for less than half of the cases of pancreatic cancer, so additional causes need to be established.

Endometrial cancer

In general, endometrial cancer shows an international distribution similar to that of other cancers of affluence, such as breast, colon, and prostate cancers. Evidence for association between higher endometrial cancer risk and excess energy intake, lack of physical activity, obesity, and high glycemic load continues to accumulate.[1,3,31,41,134,146,228] Coffee consumption has emerged as a likely protective factor in the development of endometrial cancer, with several studies suggesting a 7–8% reduction in risk for each cup consumed on a daily basis.[41,233] A role for fruits and vegetables in decreasing the risk of endometrial cancer is suggested by some studies, but the evidence is not conclusive.[1,3,234] At the present time, the most appropriate guidance is to avoid obesity through reduced energy consumption and regular physical exercise, coupled with a dietary pattern rich in fruits, vegetables, and grains (Figure 6).

Ovarian cancer

There is considerable international and geographic variation in the incidence and mortality rates of ovarian cancer. The disease is more common in nations exhibiting Western culture, especially among the higher socioeconomic groups.[1,3,228] At present, no conclusive role for dietary components in the pathogenesis of ovarian cancer has been established, although there is some evidence that body fatness increases risk and limited evidence that lactation

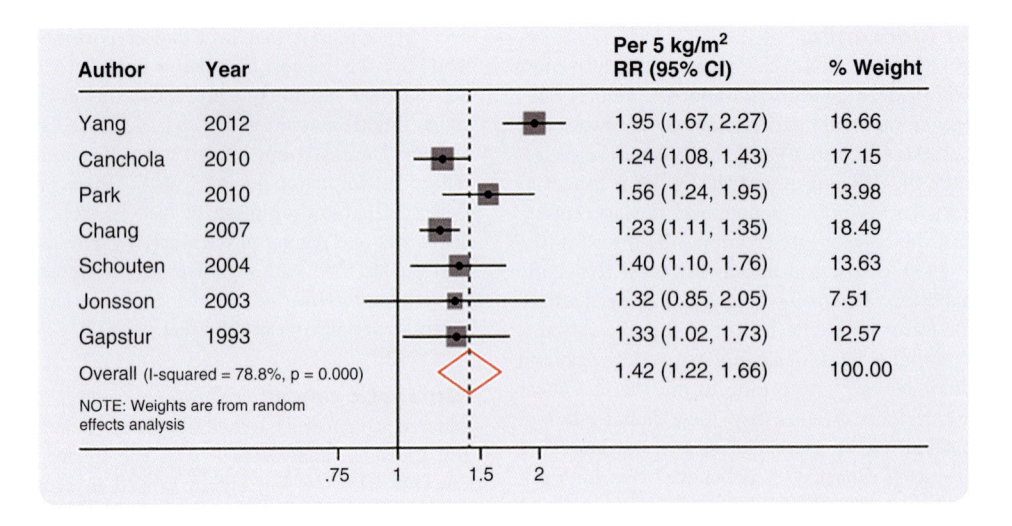

Figure 6 CUP dose–response meta-analysis for the risk of endometrial cancer, per 5 kg/m² increase in body mass index at age 18–25 years. Source: Based on World Cancer Research Fund/American Institute for, Cancer Research.[41]

may decrease risk.[42] Additional studies are needed, particularly in conjunction with known risk factors of low parity and specific inherited genetic abnormalities.[1,3]

Urinary bladder cancer

Bladder cancer is more frequent in industrialized nations, especially among smokers and those in urban areas and of lower socioeconomic status.[1,3,92,177,235,236] Smokers have two to six times the risk of bladder cancer compared to nonsmokers.[237,238] There is suggestive evidence that a diet rich in fruits and vegetables lower risk of bladder cancer, but the data are not convincing to date.[177,235,238,239] In some studies, cruciferous vegetables, such as broccoli, but not other classes of fruits and vegetables, are more strongly associated with a reduced bladder cancer risk.[240] The role of total fluid intake in diluting exposure to carcinogens in the bladder has frequently been proposed,[240] although results for bladder cancer risk have not been conclusive to date.[238] Among specific types of beverages, the data have been most suggestive of a protective association in high tea consumers.[241] Beyond providing fluid, tea provides a source of novel bioactive phytochemicals that may target multiple aspects of the carcinogenic cascade in laboratory studies.[242] Several recent studies have reported that diets rich in red and processed meats may be a contributor to bladder cancer risk.[243–245] However, the evidence is stronger from case-control studies, which are more prone to bias, than from cohort studies.[171] More study is warranted, as processed meats are a source of nitrosamines, known bladder carcinogens.[246] There is strong evidence that arsenic, a genotoxic compound, in drinking water is a cause of bladder cancer.[238] This issue is especially important in specific countries, including Bangladesh, India, Cambodia, Argentina, Chile, and Mexico.

Current research

Specific foods, nutrients, dietary components, and dietary patterns frequently associated with cancer risk and prevention

Many people at risk of cancer focus their attention upon specific foods, nutrients, or bioactives, in part because of the extensive marketing of products and publicity generated by the popular press. This tendency is facilitated by the news media when science reporters publicize results of single studies or preliminary findings, often confusing readers with contradictory and conflicting results over time. Indeed, the scientific approach, favored by funding agencies, is often very reductionist rather than examining complex foods or dietary patterns. Although findings from single foods and single nutrients or bioactives are important, recommendations for cancer prevention are best presented as an achievable dietary pattern that meets all known nutrient requirements and emphasizing the quantity, variety, and proportion of different foods or food groups and beverages, as well as the frequency with which they should be consumed. The following section briefly summarizes data regarding selected food components or nutrients and dietary patterns and might assist the medical practitioner in responding to specific inquiries from individuals.

Dietary patterns

The study of diet and cancer is increasingly benefiting from advances in dietary pattern analysis for many reasons. Estimating the impact of an individual dietary component is challenging, given that foods vary in composition over time and place, are generally eaten in combination, and changes in the intake of one food or nutrient is likely associated with changes in the intake of other foods and nutrients. Major strategies for defining dietary patterns include the use of dietary guidelines or hypotheses (based on prevailing evidence) regarding a diet-disease relation to define a pattern, *a priori*, such as the Healthy Eating Index (HEI) that measures adherence to the Dietary Guidelines for Americans. Another strategy is purely empirical (data-driven) and employs statistical approaches to group dietary variables into patterns, *a posteriori*, based on the explained variation in the diet (e.g., western or prudent dietary patterns). Yet a third and more recent strategy uses a hybrid approach to define empirical hypothesis-oriented dietary patterns that are data-driven but based on a specific hypothesis (e.g., hyperinsulinemia, chronic systemic inflammation, etc.) relating diet with disease outcomes.

Higher adherence to healthy dietary patterns as recommended by the World Cancer Research Fund/American Institute for Cancer Research, Dietary Guidelines for Americans, and American Cancer Society have been generally associated with lower risk for cancer or cancer mortality.[247–251] Associations have been most consistent for gastrointestinal tract cancers, especially colorectal cancer. For example, recent review[87] synthesized food group components into multiple dietary patterns and found two distinct global dietary patterns associated with colorectal cancer risk: an unhealthy dietary pattern characterized by high intakes of red and processed meat, sugar-sweetened beverages, refined grains, desserts, and potatoes associated with higher risk and, conversely, a healthy pattern, characterized by higher intake of fruits, vegetables, whole grains, nuts and legumes, fish and other seafood, milk, and other dairy products, associated with lower colorectal cancer risk.[87] In addition, dietary patterns that stimulate higher systemic inflammation or insulin hypersecretion have been associated with higher risk of several cancer sites.[90,91,252–254]

Vitamins

Vitamin A
Vitamin A is essential for the normal growth and development of epithelial tissues. Vitamin A deficiency is common in many parts of the developing world but is extremely rare in Americans. Vitamin A is provided in the diet as retinol and its esters, primarily from milk and organ meats, and as beta-carotene and a few other provitamin A carotenoids in yellow and leafy green vegetables. A protective effect of consuming foods rich in vitamin A has been hypothesized for several types of cancer.[1,3,5,6,177] However, there is no clear evidence that vitamin A supplementation will decrease the risk of cancer in populations or individuals consuming a healthy diet meeting the vitamin A requirement. Although many studies in laboratory models indicate that vitamin A deficiency increases the susceptibility of tissues to chemical carcinogenesis, these observations do not support the concept that a lower risk will be observed by supplementation in persons with adequate vitamin A status. The use of vitamin A and synthetic retinoids as pharmacologic agents in chemoprevention trials or oral and other cancers to determine their efficacy in specific high-risk populations is an important area of translational research, but the anticancer benefits must be balanced by risks for toxicity when provided a pharmacologic dose.[255]

Vitamin D
Vitamin D is a hormone-like nutrient that is endogenously produced in the skin with exposure to sunlight and naturally provided in the diet from oily fish, dairy products, some mushrooms, and eggs. Recent studies indicate that a vitamin D insufficiency may be much more common than previously recognized and may contribute to cancer risk.[256] Cancer cells derived from many tissues express the receptor for 1,25-dihydroxy vitamin D3 and respond to this agent *in vitro*, and some carefully controlled rodent studies suggest suppression of the carcinogenesis cascade, but the translation to human cancer remains uncertain, particularly beyond dosages considered adequate to correct risk of deficiency.[5,6,257] The human epidemiology is complex and studies of estimated intake, blood concentrations, and Mendelian randomization evaluating relationships for vitamin D and cancer incidence are inconclusive.[258] Still, stronger data is suggestive in reducing overall cancer mortality.[258] Clear dose–response relationships and a benefit beyond the recommended daily allowances is uncertain.[1,3,149] Recent randomized trials have not generally supported a benefit of vitamin D supplementation on cancer incidence, but intriguingly, individuals randomized to vitamin D appear to have a reduction in cancer mortality.[121,259]

Vitamin E
Vitamin E is a family of eight compounds that are collectively referred to as *tocopherols*. Vegetable oil, eggs, and whole grains are the major sources of dietary vitamin E. The antioxidant and free radical scavenger properties of vitamin E suggest a possible role in the inhibition of carcinogenesis.[257,260] However, the totality of rodent, epidemiologic, or randomized controlled studies does not provide strong evidence supporting the consumption of vitamin E supplements, particularly beyond the requirement, to prevent cancer and other chronic disease.[1,3,261,262]

Vitamin C
Vitamin C, which includes ascorbic acid and dehydroascorbic acid, functions as a water-soluble antioxidant and a component of several enzymatic reactions in intermediary metabolism. Citrus fruits, leafy vegetables, tomatoes, and potatoes are rich sources of vitamin C, which prevents the deficiency syndrome known as scurvy. Despite a large volume of publications, very little evidence supports a critical role for dietary or supplemental vitamin C beyond that required to prevent deficiency in the etiology of human cancers, except that diets rich in fruits and vegetables containing vitamin C may be cancer protective.[5,6] Supplement studies, although few in number, have failed to show a reduced risk of cancer.[262] Some provocative evidence concerns the ability of vitamin C to inhibit the formation of carcinogenic nitrosamines, which ultimately may reduce the incidence of cancers that are thought to be associated with nitrosamines, such as gastric cancer.[263] At present, there is no evidence to suggest that consumption of vitamin C supplements at levels higher than that which can be achieved in a well-balanced diet containing ample fresh fruits and vegetables is useful in the prevention or treatment of human cancer.[1,3,5,6]

Folate
Folate is an essential, water-soluble B vitamin required for the normal metabolism of amino acids, methyl groups, and nucleotides. It is found in many vegetables, fruits, beans, nuts, and whole grains, and folic acid is also found in fortified grain products in the United States.[264] Folate plays a role in the methylation of DNA, which may be critical for the normal regulation of gene expression and tissue differentiation. Epidemiologic and laboratory studies are beginning to accumulate evidence suggesting that deficient intake of folate may relate to the risk of several malignancies.[265] Cancer risk may also be higher among persons who consume alcohol regularly, often in association with a low-folate diet.[5,6,28,266,267] However, caution should be advised, as folate is critical for DNA metabolism and cell proliferation, and the potential for high folate to enhance progression of established cancers has been raised.[268,269]

Minerals

Calcium
Calcium and dairy products are linked to a reduced the risk of colon cancer but there is some evidence for enhancing the risk of prostate cancer.[1,3,5,6] For example, several prospective cohort studies have found that those who develop colon cancer had a significantly lower intake of calcium and vitamin D.[1,3,5,6,270] Calcium supplementation of 1.2 g/day reduced the proliferative rate of colonic cells in patients who are considered to be at an increased risk of colon cancer.[69,271] Several clinical trials to determine the effects of calcium supplementation on polyp formation are currently ongoing, with initial reports suggesting a modest benefit.

Conversely, calcium from dietary sources and from supplements has been demonstrated in some prospective studies to be associated with an increased risk of prostate cancer,[148,151,272] particularly cancers with more aggressive characteristics. At this time, it is appropriate to target calcium intake at RDA levels from a variety of food sources. The RDA is currently 1000 mg/day for those ages 19–50 years and 1200 mg/day for people older than age 50 years.

Selenium

Selenium is a mineral required in the diet at very small concentrations, with an RDA of 55 µg/day for both men and women. Grains, cereals, seafood, and meat are good sources of selenium, an essential constituent of glutathione peroxidase. Selenium participates in the destruction of hydrogen peroxide and organic hydroperoxides using reducing equivalents from glutathione and thus, participates in cellular and tissue defense against oxidative damage. A major obstacle for epidemiologic studies is that estimates of dietary selenium intake are unreliable, especially in the developed nations where foods are extensively processed and shipped for long distances, because the selenium content of food is very sensitive to soil concentrations. An inverse association between the selenium levels in forage crops from different geographic areas or tissue selenium and mortality rates from certain cancers has been suggested.[1,3,5,6,154] A landmark human intervention trial reported that selenium supplements might reduce the risk of lung, colon, and prostate cancers.[154] However, larger randomized controlled trials are required to confirm and expand upon these findings. Overall, individuals choosing to consume a selenium supplement should be advised to consume the requirement of 55 µg/day and not more than 200 µg/day, because there is a narrow margin between safe and potentially toxic dosages.[1,3,5,6]

Foods and food components

Soy products

People living in East Asian countries such as Japan and China, where soy foods are regularly consumed, have a lower risk of breast, colon, and prostate cancer than do people living in the United States, where soy foods are not commonly consumed. However, many other variables in addition to soy undoubtedly contribute to the geographic variations. Soy foods contain several components, including soy protein, isoflavones, lignans, and saponins, which have been investigated for their anticancer effects in laboratory models.[273,274] Although investigations continue, there is no convincing evidence from intervention studies demonstrating that the use of soy supplements, soy extracts, pure soy concentrates, or other soy components will significantly impact human cancer risk. Some concerns have been raised about the risks and benefits for soy consumption relative to breast or endometrial cancer. Several soy isoflavones have a chemical structure similar to estrogen and may bind to the estrogen receptor and act as weak estrogen. It is plausible that high amounts of phytoestrogens may actually increase cancer risk, although this remains controversial. At this time, it is probably best for women at high risk of breast cancer to avoid concentrated isoflavone supplements, but it is unlikely that moderate amounts of soy foods as part of a plant-based diet will increase cancer risk.[65,275–279]

Beta-carotene

Foods rich in beta-carotene, including many fruits and vegetables, are associated with a lower risk of cancer. However, intervention trials with pharmacologic doses of beta-carotene clearly question the hypothesis that the benefits of a plant-based diet can be reproduced through beta-carotene supplements. Two large intervention studies of beta-carotene, utilizing doses beyond that achieved from dietary sources, demonstrated a higher risk of lung cancer in smokers.[180,280,281] Although beta-carotene is a potential antioxidant and source of vitamin A, supplements should be discouraged for cancer prevention, and diets rich in carotenoids should be encouraged.

Lycopene

The bright red color of tomato products is due to the carotenoid lycopene. Interest in lycopene has emerged based upon studies demonstrating that the consumption of tomato products is associated with a lower risk of several cancers, particularly aggressive prostate cancer.[164,282–284] However, the relationship between lycopene and prostate cancer in humans is too limited to draw a conclusion.[1,3] At the present time, it is sensible to consume tomatoes and tomato products as one component of a carotenoid-rich dietary pattern based upon fruit and vegetable intake.

Omega-3 fatty acids, fish oil, and olive oil

Diets rich in total fat have a high caloric density and may contribute to excess energy intake, obesity, and cancer risk. However, differing types of lipids also may have varying impacts upon cancer. Fish, as well as some nuts and plant oils, are sources of omega-3 fatty acids that modulate the production of specific bioactive prostaglandins and leukotrienes, suppressing inflammatory cascades and cellular pathways involved in carcinogenesis. Animal models suggest some benefits for cancers, such as those of the prostate and breast, however, studies in humans have been less clear.[285,286] Olive oil is rich in medium-chain lipids and has generated interest because of its lack of association with cancer risk in studies, where total lipids, saturated fats, and other measures of lipid intake demonstrate positive associations. Like other lipids, olive oil contributes to caloric intake and risk of obesity but can be used in certain recipes to replace other types of lipid that may have a greater association with cancer and cardiovascular disease. Overall, precise recommendations regarding lipid sources or fatty acid profiles and human cancer risk are not clear; it is yet under study, and diets limited in saturated fats due to risk of cardiovascular disease are recommended.[1,3,5,6]

Contemporary topics in nutrition and cancer

Organic foods

Government regulators will continue to evaluate information and provide updated standards and recommendations to consumers regarding expectations when the term "organic" is used in food labeling. In general, the term refers to foods grown without the use of synthesized pesticides or herbicides, and it has been expanded to include nongenetically manipulated foods. Certainly, exposures to high concentrations of such compounds through industrial and agricultural exposures are associated with health concerns, including cancer risk. At the present time, there are very few studies suggesting that consuming organic foods will substantially lower cancer risk when compared to the same foods produced by standard farming practices.[1,4–6] A recent large cohort study from France reported a significantly reduced cancer risk among adults consuming the highest quartile of organic foods compared with adults in the lowest quartile of organic food consumption.[285] Another notable prospective study evaluating intake of organic foods and cancer risk in over 600,000 women followed for 9.3 years found that consumption of organic foods was not associated with total cancer incidence or cancer subtype incidence, with the exception of non-Hodgkin lymphoma.[286] Studies of organic versus conventional foods and cancer risk are often difficult to interpret because of the multitude of variables that may impact the outcome, including other health behaviors and nutrient intake. At this time encouraging diets rich in fruits, vegetables, and whole grains, whether conventionally or organically produced, continues to be the foundation of a cancer prevention dietary pattern.

Artificial sweeteners (aspartame and saccharin)
Artificial sweeteners are the basis of many low-calorie foods currently marketed. No links between aspartame and cancer have been identified. Saccharin has been shown to slightly enhance the risk of bladder cancer in rodent studies when provided concentrations that would greatly exceed that consumed by humans. Human epidemiologic studies have not identified saccharin or aspartame consumption as a risk factor for human cancer.[1,4–6,287]

Sugar
Highly refined simple sugars provide calories but without the nutrients associated with whole foods. Diets containing large amounts of simple sugars are frequently nutrient poor and contribute to obesity, metabolic syndrome, and potentially increase cancer risk. However, sugars *per se* are not carcinogens, and a diet with a modest amount of sweets should not be a concern in the context of a healthy dietary pattern.[1,3,5,6] Public health guidelines among many nations recommend limiting consumption of added sugars to less than 10% of total calories, significantly lower than many Americans currently consume.[4] Nearly 70% of added sugars come from the following food categories: sugar-sweetened beverages, desserts, and sweet snacks, additions to coffee and tea, candy, breakfast cereals, and bars. Reducing added sugars in the diet should focus on reducing intake of these foods.[4,288,289]

Coffee and tea
Coffee and tea are the most commonly consumed beverages in the world and are rich sources of polyphenols and other phytochemicals, some of which have demonstrated anticancer activity in preclinical investigations.[290–293] Observational and epidemiologic studies suggest that tea may reduce the risk of oral,[294,295] liver,[296] and gastric cancers,[297] although the dose and duration of consumption vary between studies, and some large cohort studies have not reported a protective effect.[298–300] Moderate coffee consumption (both caffeinated and decaffeinated) has been strongly linked to a reduced risk of endometrial and liver cancers.[1,301–303] Beverage temperature is an important consideration with coffee and tea, and several studies suggest that consuming beverages at a high temperature (> 60 °C or 140 °F) increase cancer risk, in particular esophageal cancer.[1,297,304]

Survivorship: diet and nutritional guidance during and following cancer treatment

Although the focus of this article is diet and nutrition in the etiology and prevention of cancer from a public health perspective, we briefly introduce the emerging field of diet and nutrition during cancer survivorship. "Survivorship" is now accepted as beginning at the time of cancer diagnosis and continuing throughout the life of the individual. Diet and nutrition may have a role in several components of cancer survivorship, including the following: (1) enhancing the benefits of treatment and reducing the frequency or severity of acute treatment-related toxicities; (2) promoting recovery during the immediate posttreatment phase; (3) supporting patients suffering from cancer cachexia and during terminal phases of incurable or advanced cancers; and (4) promoting long-term survivorship by reducing the chance of recurrent disease, preventing secondary cancers, reducing the frequency and severity of late complications of therapy, and enhancing overall health and longevity. At current rates, well over a million Americans are diagnosed with cancer each year, and >10 million are categorized as survivors. The need for scientifically-based recommendations is now acute and has not kept pace with the desire of medical practitioners, patients, and survivors to obtain information on diet, nutrition, and physical activity that is relevant to their unique situation. The American Cancer Society published a review of the field summarizing the state of nutrition and physical activity research and providing guidelines for communicating with survivors (Table 4),[65] and the World Cancer Research Fund is currently revising their recommendations.[1]

Diet and nutrition represent, for many cancer patients, an opportunity to counteract the profound sense of loss of control that accompanies cancer treatment. Quality of life is improved when patients feel that they are active participants in the course of their care. Unfortunately, scientific evidence to help a patient choose optimal diet and nutritional information is insufficient in most areas. Cancer survivors are faced with a bewildering array of sources of dietary information, ranging from well-intended family and friends to alternative healthcare providers and those marketing products or selling publications touting dietary approaches. Coupled with the limited training and knowledge of nutrition by many healthcare providers, including physicians and nurses, a survivor is frequently confused or easily misled. Although definitive and detailed guidelines are not possible at the present, the following provides a framework for communicating with patients and directing future survivorship research.

Active treatment phase

Cancer treatment often includes surgery, radiation, chemotherapy, or biologic treatments, as well as combinations of approaches as multimodality interventions are established for a greater number of clinical scenarios. The key to guiding a patient undergoing therapy is to individualize the nutritional support. The care team should monitor individual needs through assessment of body weight, lean body mass, and the presence of eating or digestive impairments. Treatments for some cancers may compromise nutritional status as a result of impairment of food intake, digestion, absorption, and metabolism of nutrients. For example, loss of appetite, nausea, vomiting, altered taste and smell perception, constipation, and diarrhea may transiently occur during care. Individually tailored interventions to nutritionally support a patient during these periods will enhance quality of life and compliance with therapeutic goals. In some patients, maintaining adequate energy intake is an obstacle, and specific, commercially prepared, and tested nutritional products can easily be incorporated into a diet plan. Early referrals of patients at high risk for nutritional complications to a RD can prevent the development of more severe malnutrition that may limit the ability of the medical team to provide the optimal treatment intensity.[65]

The use of vitamin or mineral supplements during cancer therapy is controversial, and few studies have been conducted to provide detailed guidance. For example, vitamin supplements with high doses of antioxidants (vitamins C or E, selenium, etc.) during chemotherapy or radiation therapy are considered by some clinicians to potentially reduce the efficacy of treatments that may

Table 4 Guidelines for cancer survivorship.

	American Cancer Society[5]	National Comprehensive Cancer Network[305]
Bodyweight	Achieve and maintain a healthy body weight throughout life. Keep body weight within the healthy range and avoid weight gain in adult life	Maintain a healthy weight. Weight gain and being overweight during survivorship may increase risk of cancer recurrence and lower odds for survival
Physical activity	Be physically active. Adults should engage in 150–300 min of moderate-intensity physical activity per wk, or 75–10 min of vigorous-intensity physical activity, or an equivalent combination; achieving or exceeding of 300 min is optimal	Engage in at least 30 min of moderate-intensity activity on 5 days per week or more, or at least 20 min of vigorous-intensity activity on 3 days or more. In addition, perform strength training at least 2 days per week
	Limit sedentary activities such as sitting, lying down, watching television, and other forms of screen-based entertainment	
Physical activity	Follow a healthy eating pattern at all ages. A healthy eating pattern includes: foods high in nutrients in amounts that help to achieve and maintain a healthy body weight; a variety of fruits and vegetables	Aim for a variety of foods. Create a balanced plate that is one-half cooked or raw vegetables, one-fourth lean protein (chicken, fish, lean meat, or dairy), and one-fourth whole grains
Vegetable and fruit	Eat a variety of vegetables - dark green, red, and orange, fiber-rich legumes (beans and peas), and others. Eat a variety of fruits, especially whole fruits. Consume at least 2.5–3 cups of vegetables and 1.5–2 cups of fruit daily	Eat a minimum of five servings of fruits and vegetables per day. Use plant-based seasonings, such as herbs and spices
Breads, grains, and cereals	Choose whole grains instead of refined grain products. Eat plenty of high-fiber foods	Choose whole grains. Opt for high-fiber breads and cereals. Avoid refined foods and those high in sugar
Animal products	Choose protein foods such as fish, poultry, and beans more than red meat. For individuals who consume processed meat products, do so sparingly, if at all	Choose lean protein such as fish, poultry, and tofu. Limit red meat and processed meats
Dietary fat	Limit consumption of highly processed foods high in saturated fats	Eat fatty fish twice a week. Choose low-fat dairy products. Eat fatty fish, such as salmon, sardines, and canned tuna, at least twice a week. Walnuts, canola oil, and flaxseeds are additional sources of heart-healthy omega-3 fats
Processed foods and refined sugar	Limit the consumption of sugar-sweetened beverages, "fast foods" and other highly processed foods high in saturated fat, starches, or added sugars because of their association with body weight	Avoid refined foods and those high in sugar
Alcohol	People who do choose to drink alcohol should limit their consumption to no more than one drink per day for women and two drinks per day for men	Limit alcohol consumption. Alcohol has been linked to cancer risk. Men should have no more than two drinks per day and women no more than one drink per day
Supplements	If a dietary supplement is used for general health purposes, the best choice is a balanced multivitamin/mineral supplement with no more than 100% of the "daily value" of nutrients. The ACS does not recommend the use of dietary supplements for cancer prevention	Foods—not supplements—are the best source of vitamins and minerals. There is no evidence that dietary supplements alone provide the same anticancer benefits as a healthy dietary pattern. Some high-dose supplements may actually increase cancer risk

depend upon oxidative stress in the cancer cell as the mechanism of action. However, others suggest that antioxidant supplements may provide a benefit to patients by limiting damage to normal tissues, such as bone marrow. In general, it is judicious for clinicians to advise patients undergoing chemotherapy or radiation therapy to limit supplemental antioxidants to levels that do not exceed the RDAs and avoid other products that contain herbals or extracts enriched in antioxidant components. Folic acid is one nutrient where large dosages exceeding the RDA could influence the outcome of chemotherapy with agents such as methotrexate or 5-fluorouracil (5-FU) that target metabolic pathways involving folate. Daily supplements containing folate above the RDA should be discouraged for these patients.[65]

Recovery following treatment

The days and weeks following completion of intensive treatment are points in the cancer care continuum where many patients explore dietary and nutritional interventions to enhance survivorship. During this period, the frequency of contact with healthcare providers lessens, and the patient is concerned about the potential for cancer recurrence and recovery from therapy. Diet and physical activity should be a component of the treatment plan with the goal of restoring muscle mass and functional status. Health-care providers must continue to question patients regarding supplements and alternative medical treatments and provide counseling as needed. Continuing individualized nutritional evaluation will identify those with more serious long-term nutritional complications of therapy, such as dysphagia, malabsorption, and bowel changes common in those treated for cancers of the oral pharynx, esophagus, stomach, pancreas, bowel, and others. A focus on energy balance and ensuring adequate intake of essential nutrients is critical. For example, gastric surgery or resection of the terminal ileum may lead to a vitamin B12 deficiency unless parenteral administration is initiated.[65] Consultation with a RD can provide each individual with a risk assessment and personalized counseling.

Advanced cancer

In general, progressive cancer is associated with a loss of appetite, and, if a patient does not succumb quickly to a complication of the disease or co-morbid condition, progressive weight loss and other features of malnutrition will become evident. Unfortunately, many families and caretakers have the impression that reversal of the nutritional deficits will significantly prolong meaningful life. In reality, the failure to control the growth of the cancer, rather than malnutrition, has proven to be the critical issue in most studies. Frequently, the patient and caregivers experience conflict based upon loss of appetite and food consumption. The medical team should be alert in order to identify conflicts between caregivers and patients centering on food, help establish understanding, and provide guidance to families. In the setting of advanced disease, dietary and nutritional interventions can contribute to a sense of well-being and quality of life. Dietitians and the medical team can assist the patient in altering food choices and eating patterns and help maintain nutritional status in the setting of advanced disease often complicated by pain control issues and the resulting constipation caused by side effects of narcotic analgesics. Some medications can be coupled with limited physical activity to enhance appetite and improve bowel function. In some cases, additional nutritional support may be indicated.[65]

Prevention of cancer recurrence and long-term complication of therapy

The patient who achieves a complete remission from cancer is concerned about the reappearance of the primary cancer. Additionally, survivors of certain cancers are at greater risk of second primaries. Indeed, survivors of oral or lung cancer may experience a ~10% chance of a second tobacco-related primary cancer yearly. Many cancer survivors are also at risk for cancers of other sites, which can be related to treatment; for instance, patients cured of testis cancer via treatment with etoposide-based chemotherapy are at a higher risk for secondary leukemia, and survivors of adolescent lymphoma treated with mediastinal radiation have a higher risk of secondary breast cancer. Very little research has been undertaken to establish optimal dietary patterns to prevent recurrent disease or second primaries at the same or different sites. In general, most experts will focus on the public health dietary recommendations summarized at the beginning of this article and by various groups for the prevention of an initial cancer.[1,3,5,6,65]

As the population of cancer survivors expands and physicians continue to monitor them over longer periods, long-term complications of treatments that are potential targets of dietary interventions are becoming apparent. For example, premature menopause in women treated with chemotherapy for breast cancer may contribute to accelerated osteoporosis[306] that may require specific assessments and recommendations for dietary calcium and physical activity. Mediastinal radiation in young adults and children may contribute to premature coronary atherosclerosis that can be accelerated by poor dietary and lifestyle choices. Medical caregivers should emphasize early interventions with dietary and exercise patterns that will maintain healthy blood cholesterol and triglyceride profiles. Although thus far very little research concerning diet and nutrition has been accumulated to provide clear guidance to cancer survivors, we anticipate that future efforts in this area will expand rapidly as a result of patient demands and the response of the NIH through their support of survivorship research.

Key references

The complete reference list can be found on Vital Source version of this title, see inside front cover.

8   World Health Organization. *Diet Nutrition and the Prevention of Chronic Diseases.* Geneva, Switzerland: WHO; 1990.
17 Maruvada P, Lampe JW, Wishart DS, et al. Perspective: dietary biomarkers of intake and exposure-exploration with omics approaches. *Adv Nutr.* 2020;**11**:200–215.
26 World Cancer Research Fund/American Institute for Cancer Research (2018) *Diet, Nutrition, Physical Activity and Colorectal Cancer: Continuous Update Project Expert Report 2018. Whole Grains, Vegetables and Fruit and the Risk of Cancer.*
30 Dietary Guidelines Advisory Committee (2020) *Dietary Guidelines for Americans 2020-2025: Government Printing Office.*
40 World Cancer Research Fund/American Institute for, Cancer Research (2017) *Continuous Update Project Report. Food, Nutrition, Physical Activity, and the Prevention of Breast Cancer.*
43 Chlebowski RT, Luo J, Anderson GL, et al. Weight loss and breast cancer incidence in postmenopausal women. *Cancer.* 2019;**125**:205–212.
60 Kabat GC, Chang CJ, Wynder EL. The role of tobacco, alcohol use, and body mass index in oral and pharyngeal cancer. *Int J Epidemiol.* 1994;**23**:1137–1144.
92 Armstrong B, Doll R. Environmental factors and cancer incidence and mortality in different countries, with special reference to dietary practices. *Int J Cancer.* 1975;**15**:617–631.
143 World Cancer Research Fund/American Institute for, Cancer Research (2018) *Continuous Update Project Report. Food, Nutrition, Physical Activity, and the Prevention of Prostate Cancer.*
177 Cancer Research World Cancer Research Fund/American Institute for Cancer Research (2017) *Continuous Update Project Report. Food, Nutrition, Physical Activity, and the Prevention of Lung Cancer.*

35 Chemoprevention of cancer

Ernest Hawk, MD, MPH ■ Karen C. Maresso, MPH ■ Powel Brown, MD, PhD ■ Michelle I. Savage, BA ■ Scott M. Lippman, MD

> **Overview**
>
> The field of cancer chemoprevention is underpinned by two phenomena of neoplasia: field carcinogenesis and multistep carcinogenesis. Accurate cancer risk models are critical to chemoprevention, and may accelerate drug development in this setting. The Food and Drug Administration has approved several chemoprevention agents. This article describes cancer risk modeling and phase II/III chemoprevention clinical trials focused on the four major cancer sites in Western populations (lung, colon and rectum, prostate, and breast), as well as broader, site-agnostic chemoprevention studies. Immunoprevention strategies, including vaccines, are highlighted.

Biology of chemoprevention

The field of cancer chemoprevention is underpinned by two phenomena of neoplasia: (1) field carcinogenesis, which is the multifocal development of intraepithelial neoplasia (IEN, or precancer) or the clonal spread of one or more IENs, and (2) multistep carcinogenesis, which is driven by genetic instability and accumulates progressive genetic and epigenetic changes.[1–5] These processes spur evasion of apoptosis, strong replicative potential, and sustained angiogenesis leading to IEN and cancer development. Multistep carcinogenesis allows chemopreventive interventions at step(s) of neoplasia that precede invasive cancer. Drugs developed for cancer therapy can be examined for cancer chemoprevention because of important commonalities—including genetic and epigenetic abnormalities, loss of cellular control, and certain phenotypic characteristics—between cancer and multistep IEN.[6] Field carcinogenesis makes approaches such as systemic agents attractive for controlling the neoplastic results of diffuse exposure to carcinogens throughout an epithelial field. Several agents have been approved by the Food and Drug Administration (FDA) for the treatment of IEN or cancer risk reduction (Table 1).[7] Ongoing efforts to better understand the premalignant genome and immune profile may lead to the identification of additional chemopreventive agents.[8] This article provides a review of chemoprevention trials targeted to the four most common cancers in the United States—lung, colorectal, breast, and prostate—as well as site-agnostic chemoprevention trials. A separate section highlights immunopreventive strategies, given the success of vaccines in viral-induced cancers and immunotherapies in advanced cancers with data suggesting their promise at earlier disease stages.[9,10] Cancer risk modeling is first briefly discussed as it relates to chemoprevention.

Cancer risk modeling

Accurate cancer risk models are critical to chemoprevention, in order to identify individuals who are most likely to benefit from an agent and least likely to be harmed by it. Models premised on familial and germline risks due to inheritance of major tumor suppressor mutations place carriers at very high risk of cancer development (i.e., often >40–100% lifetime risk of cancer development) and have been successfully used to target both surgical[11] and chemopreventive interventions.[12] Models based on combinations of clinical/demographic factors have been developed for breast cancer risk (Gail model or the Breast Cancer Risk Assessment Tool (BCRAT)) and lung cancer risk (Spitz model), and established identifiers of increased risk include precursor clinical/histologic lesions.[13,14] The Gail model/BCRAT is used to identify women for preventive therapy with the anti-estrogen (AE) drugs tamoxifen and raloxifene, while the Spitz model can be useful in counseling individuals in tobacco cessation. While these risk models and lesions are useful on a population-wide basis, they are less helpful in identifying individual or personalized risk. The Breast Cancer Surveillance Consortium (BCSC) model is similar to the Gail model/BCRAT but takes into account mammographic breast density and has been shown to have greater discriminatory accuracy than the BCRAT.[15] Work is ongoing to refine this model further with single nucleotide polymorphisms and other breast cancer risk factors such as benign breast disease and serum hormone levels.[16,17] In lung cancer risk models, the addition of pulmonary function has been shown to improve risk prediction as has the incorporation of genomic (somatic gene expression arrays and host DNA-repair capacity) and metabolomic markers.[18–20] Most recently, pro-surfactant protein B and diacetylspermine have been shown to increase the predictive power of lung cancer models.[21,22] For colon cancer risk prediction, the Freedman/NCI's Colorectal Cancer Risk Assessment tool is one of the few colorectal cancer (CRC) models that has been validated in an independent cohort and is generalizable to a large portion of the US population that is eligible for CRC screening.[23] It predicts both current and future risk of CRC.[24] Numerous risk prediction models have also been developed for prostate cancer, but as with CRC, only a few have been validated through replication in independent populations. Two of the most commonly used and externally validated models are the Prostate Cancer Risk Calculator, derived from the Prostate Cancer Prevention Trial (PCPT), and the model based on the European Randomized Study of Screening for Prostate Cancer (ERSPC). In a comparison of these two models, the ERSPC model was found to significantly outperform the PCPT 2.0 model.[25]

In summary, risk prediction is most advanced for breast cancer, where it is used to help determine who receives preventive AE

Holland-Frei Cancer Medicine, Tenth Edition. Edited by Robert C. Bast, John C. Byrd, Carlo M. Croce, Ernest Hawk, Fadlo R. Khuri, Raphael E. Pollock, Apostolia M. Tsimberidou, Christopher G. Willett, and Cheryl L. Willman.
© 2023 John Wiley & Sons, Inc. Published 2023 by John Wiley & Sons, Inc.

Table 1 FDA-approved agents for the treatment of intraepithelial neoplasia or cancer risk reduction.[a]

Cancer site	Intervention
Anal cancer	HPV vaccine (Gardasil-9; for cancer caused by infection with HPV 16, 18, 31, 33, 45, 52, and 58 and for precancerous or dysplastic lesions caused by infection with HPV 6, 11, 16, 18, 31, 33, 45, 52, and 58)
Bladder cancer (dysplasia)	Bacillus Calmette–Guérin Valrubicin
Breast cancer	Tamoxifen Raloxifene
Cervical cancer	HPV vaccine (Cervarix; for cancer caused by infection with HPV 16 and 18) HPV vaccine (Gardasil; for cancer caused by infection with HPV 16 and 18) HPV vaccine (Gardasil-9; for cancer caused by infection with HPV 16, 18, 31, 33, 45, 52, and 58 and for precancerous or dysplastic lesions caused by infection with HPV 6, 11, 16, 18, 31, 33, 45, 52, and 58)
Colonic adenomas	Celecoxib[b]
Esophageal cancer (dysplasia)	Photofrin + photodynamic therapy (PTD)
Oropharyngeal/head and neck	HPV vaccine (Gardasil-9; for cancer caused by infection with HPV 16, 18, 31, 33, 45, 52, and 58)
Skin cancer (actinic keratosis)	5-aminolevulinic acid + photodynamic therapy (PTD) Diclofenac sodium Fluorouracil Imiquimod Ingenol mebutate Masoprocol
Vulvar cancer	HPV vaccine (Gardasil-9; for cancer caused by infection with HPV 16, 18, 31, 33, 45, 52, and 58 and for precancerous or dysplastic lesions caused by infection with HPV 6, 11, 16, 18, 31, 33, 45, 52, and 58)
Vaginal cancer	HPV vaccine (Gardasil-9; for cancer caused by infection with HPV 16, 18, 31, 33, 45, 52, and 58 and for precancerous or dysplastic lesions caused by infection with HPV 6, 11, 16, 18, 31, 33, 45, 52, and 58)

[a]Source: Based on Maresso et al.[7]
[b]FDA labeling voluntarily withdrawn by Pfizer, February 2011.

therapy. There are no currently recommended risk prediction models with high discriminatory power for lung, colorectal, or prostate cancers. All current cancer risk models suffer from limitations, including suboptimal model discrimination, lack of external validation, and a lack of clear generalizability to relevant populations. Moreover, the clinical utility and uptake of many of these models are uncertain. In the future, the addition of molecular markers and/or as yet undiscovered risk factors to current risk prediction models may help improve their discriminatory power. Selection of high-risk individuals for chemoprevention based on cancer risk modeling is considered a key factor to increase the therapeutic index of any given intervention, leading to successful drug development in this area.

Chemoprevention trials

The lung

Premalignancy
Clinical and translational chemoprevention trials, including five negative randomized trials of retinoids in smokers with metaplasia, have had little to no effect in reversing lung premalignancy.[26] Phase II trials of the nonsteroidal anti-inflammatory agent (NSAID) sulindac[27] and the serine-threonine-kinase inhibitor enzastaurin[28] failed to meet their primary endpoints of change in histologic grade and Ki-67 labeling index, respectively, in current and former smokers with bronchial dysplasia. A phase II trial of aspirin showed no effect on changes in lung cancer–related gene expression profiles from nasal brushings of heavy smokers.[29] Results from another phase II trial of aspirin (NCT02169271), examining its effects on changes in the size of CT-detected lung nodules in current or former smokers, are awaited. In contrast to these null results of phase II trials, encouraging phase IIb data have emerged from studies of 9-*cis*-retinoic acid modulation of RAR-β and Ki-6,[30,31] *myo*-inositol modulation of PI3 kinase gene-expression pathway,[32,33] budesonide modulation of CT-detected peripheral nodules,[34,35] anethole dithiolthione[36] and iloprost[37] modulation of bronchial dysplasia, and combination zileuton (a 5-lipooxygenase inhibitor) and celecoxib (a selective COX-2 inhibitor) modulation of urinary prostaglandin E metabolite (PGE-M) and leukotriene E4 (LTE4) levels in healthy smokers.[38] Phase III trials of one or more of these agents await further confirmation of efficacy with acceptable safety in additional phase II trials, as well as the identification of appropriately defined at-risk cohorts in whom to optimally test them.

Prevention of primary lung cancer
The NCI-sponsored Alpha-Tocopherol, Beta-Carotene (ATBC) Cancer Prevention Study was a phase III trial of α-tocopherol and β-carotene to prevent primary lung cancer. The ATBC study involved 29,133 male smokers between 50 and 69 years of age who had smoked an average of one pack of cigarettes a day for approximately 36 years.[39] This trial's 2 × 2 factorial design called for α-tocopherol (50 mg/day) and β-carotene (20 mg/day) to be given in a randomized, double-blind, placebo-controlled fashion. The factorial design allowed the study scientists to assess the individual effects of each agent. Significant increases in lung cancer incidence (18% increase; $p = 0.01$) and total mortality (8%; $p = 0.02$) occurred in the β-carotene-treated subjects after 6.1 years median follow-up. α-Tocopherol had no significant impact on the lung cancer mortality rate, and there was no evidence of an interaction between α-tocopherol and β-carotene.[40]

The Beta-Carotene and Retinol Efficacy Trial (CARET) tested the combination of β-carotene (30 mg/day) plus retinyl palmitate

(25,000 IU/day) in 17,000 smokers and asbestos workers.[41] It confirmed the major finding of the ATBC study with its primary finding that the β-carotene combination increased lung cancer risk in this high-risk population. There was no evidence from either the ATBC study or the CARET that β-carotene increased lung cancer risk in nonsmokers, or former or moderate (less than one pack a day) smokers.

Both the Nutritional Prevention Cancer Trial (NCP) and the Selenium and Vitamin E Cancer Prevention Trial (SELECT) examined lung cancer incidence as a secondary endpoint. While the NCP showed an initial statistically significant reduction in lung cancer incidence after 4.5 years of follow-up in those randomized to the selenium treatment arm (RR: 0.54; 95% confidence interval (CI): 0.30–0.98; $p = 0.04$),[42] results were no longer significant after almost 8 years of follow-up (RR: 0.70; 95% CI: 0.40–1.21; $p = 0.18$).[43] Treatment with selenium was not associated with decreased incidence of lung cancer in the SELECT trial after 5 years of treatment[44] or after extended follow-up.[45]

Most recently, a combined analysis of individual patient-level data from eight randomized controlled trials (RCTs) of aspirin versus no aspirin for a treatment period of at least 4 years found a nonsignificant 32% reduction in risk of lung cancer death (hormone receptor (HR): 0.68; 95% CI: 0.42–1.10; $p = 0.11$).[46] When the analysis was limited to those trials with a treatment period of five or more years with long-term follow-up data available, the 20-year risk of death from lung cancer was significantly reduced by 29% (HR: 0.71; 95% CI: 0.58–0.89; $p = 0.002$). Further, when analyzed by histologic subtype, aspirin nearly halved the risk of death from lung adenocarcinoma (HR: 0.55; 95% CI: 0.33–0.94; $p = 0.04$) but had no effect on small-cell (HR 0.85, 0.52–1.39; $p = 0.56$) or squamous-cell (1.26, 0.73–2.18; $p = 0.49$) carcinomas. Subsequently, the effect of aspirin on lung-cancer-related biomarkers has been tested in phase II trials (described above) of smokers with disappointing results.

SPT prevention
Based on encouraging high-dose retinoid data in the head and neck and lung,[47] two large-scale, phase III retinoid trials have been completed in the setting of second primary tumor (SPT) prevention; one in Europe (investigating retinyl palmitate and/or N-acetyl-L-cysteine),[48] the other in the United States (investigating low-dose 13cRA).[49] Neither demonstrated a reduction in SPT in the population overall. Selenium also failed to prevent SPTs compared to placebo in an RCT of 1151 patients with resected stage I non-small-cell lung cancers (NSCLCs).[50]

In the future, drugs that have recently been shown to be effective in the treatment of lung cancer, such as PARP inhibitors,[51,52] may be tested in lung cancer prevention trials. The section titled "Immunoprevention" later in the article discusses immune-based strategies that show promise in lung cancer prevention.

The colon and rectum
Colorectal trial designs have primarily employed the intermediate endpoints of adenomatous polyp development and response as well as hyperproliferation markers. Chemoprevention trials in CRC have principally focused on NSAIDs, although vitamins, dietary patterns and agents, and hormone replacement therapy have also been examined.

Hereditary syndromes
Sulindac and celecoxib can effectively treat and inhibit adenoma development in familial adenomatous polyposis (FAP).[12,53] High-dose celecoxib (800 mg/day) reduced large-bowel polyposis by 28% and duodenal polyposis, which is difficult to resect, by 14% (vs placebo).[54] These studies led to the interim FDA approval of celecoxib as an adjunct to endoscopic and surgical treatment of FAP patients. However, the labeled indication for polyp management in FAP patients was sacrificed due to challenges in conducting confirmatory trials in this high-risk setting. A phase I dose–escalation study in children with FAP demonstrated that short-term treatment with celecoxib (16 mg/kg/day) was safe, well-tolerated, and significantly reduced the number of polyps.[55] Subsequently, the CAPP-1 and CAPP-2 trials examined aspirin (600 mg QD) in subjects with FAP and Lynch syndrome, respectively. CAPP-1 identified a nonsignificant reduction (23%) in polyp count and a trend toward reduced largest polyp size within the aspirin-treated group, after a median of 17 months of intervention. CAPP-2 found a significant reduction in risk of CRC (59%) only in subjects completing at least 2 years of intervention after a mean of 55.7 months of follow-up.[56,57] The ongoing CAPP-3 study (NCT02497820) is examining the overall Lynch syndrome cancer incidence rate at 5 years according to different doses of aspirin (100, 300, 600 mg/day) taken for at least 2 years. A prespecified, secondary outcome of this trial will compare the incidence of primary CRCs among the three treatment groups.

More recently, three trials have tested difluoromethylornithine (DFMO) and sulindac in combination with other agents in the setting of FAP. A phase II RCT of celecoxib with and without DFMO in 112 individuals with FAP did not find a significant difference in colorectal polyp count between the DFMO–celecoxib treatment group and the celecoxib-only treatment group (mean reduction in the number of polyps of at least 2 mm: 13% (SE = 10%) vs 1% (SE = 14%); $p = 0.69$).[58] However, a secondary measure of polyp burden based on global video assessments suggested a significant difference following treatment with the combination regimen. (Change in polyp burden based on video assessment: −0.80 (SE = 0.14) vs −0.33 (SE = 0.15); $p = 0.03$.) In another phase II trial, the NSAID sulindac was tested in combination with the epidermal growth factor receptor (EGFR) inhibitor erlotinib in 92 patients with FAP. The combination treatment resulted in a significant 71.2% reduction in duodenal polyp burden compared to placebo (95% CI, −100.2% to −45.3%, $p < 0.001$).[59] In secondary data analysis of this trial, the sulindac–erlotinib combination was also shown to significantly reduce the polyp number by 69.4% in the colon compared to placebo (95% CI, 28.8–109.2%; $p = 0.04$).[60] However, 68% of patients suffered from an acneiform cutaneous eruption and another 32% suffered from oral mucositis, which are common side effects of treatment with erlotinib. The authors suggest a need for more dose-ranging studies to determine if a lower or less frequent dose of erlotinib could reduce the occurrence of these side effects but maintain efficacy.[60] Finally, a phase III trial comparing DFMO and sulindac in combination to each agent alone is ongoing.[61] Combinations of chemopreventive agents continue to hold promise for clinical use in patients with hereditary CRC syndromes.

In addition to NSAIDs, some dietary agents have been recently tested in phase II trials of FAP patients. A regime of 12 months of curcumin (1500 mg orally twice a day (BID)) was tested in 50 FAP patients, but no significant differences in mean number of polyps or mean polyp size were found between the treatment and placebo groups.[62] However, an enteric-coated formulation of eicosapentaenoic acid (EPA; 2 g daily) for 6 months significantly reduced the polyp number and the sum of polyp diameters in 55 FAP patients.[63]

Sporadic colorectal cancer

Four RCTs have tested the efficacy of aspirin in preventing sporadic adenomas, showing significant reductions in recurrent adenomas among patients treated for one or more years.[64–67] However, results of the APACC trial no longer showed a preventive benefit of aspirin on adenoma recurrence after 4 years of follow-up.[68] While there was no protective effect of aspirin on CRC risk in men and women in either the Physician's Health Study (PHS)[69] or the Women's Health Study (WHS) initially,[70] the WHS reported a significantly reduced risk for CRC in healthy women after an overall follow-up time of 18 years.[44] Long-term follow-up results of the PHS remained null.[71] A pooled analysis of the British Doctors Aspirin Trial and the United Kingdom Transient Ischaemic Attack Aspirin Trial found that aspirin was associated with a significant 26% reduction in CRC risk; and the effect was greatest with at least 5 years treatment and did not appear for at least 10 years.[72] Most recently, the Systematic Evaluation of Aspirin and Fish Oil (seAFOod) Polyp Prevention Trial tested the chemoprevention efficacy of aspirin and EPA, alone and in combination, in individuals with high-risk colorectal adenoma features at screening (as part of the English Bowel Cancer Screening Program). While aspirin did not result in a reduction in the proportion of individuals with at least one colorectal adenoma (primary outcome of the trial), it did reduce the total number of adenomas per participant and those randomized to aspirin had a reduced number of adenomas in the right colon, especially for serrated adenomas, as well as a reduced risk of conventional adenomas.[73]

Systematic reviews and meta-analyses of randomized trials show significant protective effects of aspirin on CRC incidence and mortality as well as adenoma recurrence.[74,75] In 2016, the U.S. Preventive Services Task Force updated their recommendation for the use of aspirin in those at high risk of cardiovascular disease to include the benefit of CRC prevention.[76] Nevertheless, there remain significant risks associated with aspirin use and it is unclear who may derive the most benefit from aspirin with minimal harm.[77,78] The ongoing ASPirin Intervention for the REDuction of Colorectal Cancer Risk (ASPIRED; NCT02394769) trial is a prospective, double-blind, multi-dose, placebo-controlled, biomarker clinical trial of aspirin use in individuals previously diagnosed with colorectal adenoma that will help determine those individuals in whom the benefits of aspirin outweigh the risks.[79]

Three RCTs assessed coxibs (vs placebo) in preventing sporadic adenomas in patients with a prior history of colorectal polyps. The Adenomatous Polyp Prevention on Vioxx (APPROVe) trial tested rofecoxib, and various doses of celecoxib were tested in the Adenoma Prevention with Celecoxib (APC) and Prevention of Colorectal Sporadic Adenomatous Polyps (PreSAP) trials. Interim cardiovascular event rates were unexpectedly higher in APPROVe and APC but not PreSAP.[80–82] The relevant data and safety monitoring committees stopped all three RCTs early because of these safety issues, despite significant activity against colorectal adenomas, and rofecoxib was withdrawn from the world market by the manufacturer. In APPROVe (2587 randomized subjects), rofecoxib reduced adenomas by 24%.[83] In the APC (2035 randomized patients), adenoma rates were significantly reduced by celecoxib treatment at 37.5% (celecoxib, 400 mg twice daily), 43% (celecoxib, 200 mg twice daily), and 60% (placebo) ($p<0.001$).[84] However, serious cardiovascular adverse event rates were also significantly increased in a dose-dependent manner. The PreSAP trial, with 1561 randomized patients, found incidences of adenomas of 33.6% (celecoxib, 400 mg once daily) and 49.3% (placebo) ($p<0.001$).[80] The risk of cardiovascular events did not increase in the PreSAP trial. In a recent extension analysis of APC patients, it appeared that the serious cardiovascular event rate wore off 2 years after stopping the drug and that a repression of adenomas persisted (albeit diminished), particularly for advanced adenomas. Results of a 2008 pooled analysis of the major celecoxib placebo-controlled trials (double-blind and planned follow-up of at least 3 years in nonarthritis disease settings) suggested that there was no increase in serious cardiovascular events at any studied dose (up to 400 mg BID) in people with a low-baseline cardiovascular risk (about 15–20% of people on these trials).[85] These results strongly suggest that low baseline cardiovascular risk can improve risk-benefit and help in selecting patients for future COX-2-specific NSAID trials.

Preclinical studies of low doses of the NSAID sulindac and the ornithine decarboxylase inhibitor DFMO or eflornithine supported an RCT of combined oral sulindac (150 mg) and DFMO (500 mg; vs placebo) for 36 months in 375 patients with a history of resected (≥3 mm) adenomas (stratified by use of low-dose aspirin [81 mg] at baseline and clinical adenoma site).[86] Colorectal adenoma recurrence rates were as follows: one or more adenomas—41.1% placebo versus 12.3% (combination; RR 0.30; 95% CI, 0.18–0.49; $p<0.001$); one or more advanced adenomas—8.5% (placebo) versus 0.7% (combination; RR 0.085; 0.011–0.65; $p<0.001$); multiple adenomas—13.2% (placebo) versus 0.7% (combination; RR 0.055; 0.0074–0.41; $p<0.001$). These results have led to additional trials of DFMO combinations in those at high risk of CRC. A phase II RCT of DFMO and aspirin in individuals with current or previous adenomas did not find a significant difference in polyp burden between treatment and placebo arms, but did demonstrate a significant reduction in total rectal aberrant crypt foci burden (74% vs 45%; $p=0.020$) after 1 year of treatment.[87] The phase III Preventing Adenomas of the Colon with Eflornithine (DFMO) and Sulindac (PACES) trial (NCT01349881) in patients previously treated for Stages 0–III CRC is ongoing with an estimated completion date in 2029. Combination chemoprevention has been long believed to have great potential for enhancing the activity and reducing the toxicity of active single agents, a belief that is reinforced by recent results of phase II and III trials of combinations in both sporadic and hereditary (see above) populations.

In addition to NSAIDs, which continue to be actively investigated, trials of vitamins, minerals, and dietary patterns (e.g., low-fat, high in fruits, vegetables, and fiber) for reducing colorectal adenoma risk have had largely null results. Results from a trial of a low-fat, high-fiber diet on the recurrence of colorectal adenomas were null, as were results from a trial of supplementation with wheat-bran fiber (13.5 g/day).[88,89] Calcium (1200 mg/day) reduced the risk of sporadic adenomas by a significant 15–25% in the Calcium Polyp Prevention trial,[90] and this effect persisted in long-term follow-up.[91] While results from the European Cancer Prevention Organization Study Group also suggested a protective effect of calcium on recurrent adenomas, they were not statistically significant (RR: 0.66; 95% CI: 0.38–1.17; $p=0.16$).[92] Further, this trial documented a significantly increased risk of adenomas due to fiber supplementation (RR: 1.67; 95% CI: 1.01–2.76; $p=0.042$), particularly in those with elevated calcium levels.[92] Results from the Women's Health Initiative RCT of the combination of calcium (500 mg BID) and vitamin D3 (200 IU BID) in 36,282 postmenopausal women suggested no effect on incidence on CRC.[93] Long-term follow-up confirmed these results.[94] A more recent trial of calcium (1200 mg), vitamin D3 (1000 IU), and their combination in 2259 participants with previous colorectal adenomas showed no protective effect of either agent alone or in combination.[95] However, a subsequent analysis of this trial suggested variable effects of vitamin D3 on advanced adenomas according to vitamin D receptor genotypes.[96] Two RCTs of folate showed no reduction in adenoma risk with a 0.5 or 1 mg/day dose; a subset analysis of one study suggested that folate (1 mg/day) may even increase the risk of advanced or multiple adenomas.[67,97] The mineral selenium has also been tested in several large RCTs with largely equivocal results.[42,44,45,98,99] Results are anticipated for a recently completed phase III trial (NCT00078897) of 5 years of selenium (200 mcg daily (quaque die) (QD)) versus placebo in approximately 1800 participants stratified by daily aspirin use. The seAFOod Polyp Prevention Trial (mentioned above) tested EPA, alone and in combination with aspirin, in individuals with high-risk colorectal adenoma features at screening colonoscopy. EPA was not associated with a reduction in the proportion of patients with at least one adenoma, but those randomized to the EPA-only treatment group had a reduced total number of and adenoma detection rate of conventional adenomas in the left colorectal than did those in the placebo group.[73] Unfortunately, results for dietary patterns and vitamins and minerals have largely been disappointing in their ability to prevent colorectal adenomas.

Hormone replacement therapy (HRT) has also been examined for its ability to prevent CRC in women, although largely in observational studies, in which findings vary by population and HRT formulation. Findings from the Women's Health Initiative RCT, where CRC incidence was a secondary outcome, suggested a significant protective effect from combined estrogen plus progestin (HR: 0.63; 95% CI: 0.43–0.92), but this formulation was shown to have a poor risk–benefit balance overall, as it increased risk of CVD, stroke, pulmonary embolism, and breast cancer.[100] The estrogen-only formulation showed no protective benefit on CRC incidence (HR: 1.08; 95% CI: 0.75–1.55).[101] A recent follow-up report of this trial confirmed the estrogen-only findings and also suggested a nonstatistically significant increase in CRC deaths in the estrogen-only group (HR: 1.46; 95% CI: 0.86–2.46; $p = 0.16$).[102] CRC incidence was also examined as a secondary outcome in the Heart and Estrogen/progestin Replacement Study (HERS) RCT and in the HERSII observational follow-up component but no protective effect was seen for combined HRT.[103]

The biguanide drug metformin/glucophage used to lower blood sugar in diabetics has shown preventive efficacy in suppressing colorectal aberrant crypt foci in a short-term clinical trial[104] and has since been actively investigated as a potential CRC chemopreventive agent. In a phase III trial of 151 nondiabetic patients with colorectal polyps, 1 year of metformin (250 mg/day) significantly reduced the incidence of total polyps (hyperplastic and adenomas combined, RR: 0.67; 95% CI: 0.47–0.97) and of adenomas only (RR: 0.60; 95% CI: 0.39–0.92) with minimal adverse events.[105] However, a more recent phase IIa trial examining 12 weeks of metformin (1000 mg BID) in nondiabetic, obese subjects showed no effect on colonic mucosal biomarkers.[106] There are currently phase II (NCT03047837) and phase III (NCT02614339) trials ongoing testing metformin in the secondary/tertiary prevention of CRC.

Finally, as discussed in the section titled "Immunoprevention", various vaccines and immune modulatory agents are being tested in early-phase trials for their ability to prevent colorectal adenomas from progressing to CRC.

The breast
The positive results of therapeutic clinical trials designed to assess the efficacy and safety of AE drugs as an adjuvant therapy for women with early-stage breast cancer led to the development of numerous phase III clinical trials testing AE drugs (e.g., tamoxifen, which was associated with a 50% reduction in the development of contralateral primary breast tumors vs placebo for cancer prevention) (Table 2).[128–130] Based on highly significant positive results of the Breast Cancer Prevention Trial (BCPT), the selective estrogen-receptor (ER) modulator (SERM) tamoxifen became the first chemopreventive agent to earn FDA approval. Conducted by the National Surgical Adjuvant Breast and Bowel Project (NSABP), the BCPT compared tamoxifen with placebo in preventing breast cancer in 13,388 women at high risk of this disease.[110] The major high-risk eligibility criteria were age >60 years and history of lobular carcinoma in situ (LCIS), or women from 35 to 59 years old with 5-year breast cancer risk of 1.66% based on the Gail model. The actual overall average, 5-year baseline, breast cancer risk was 3.2%. At a median follow-up of 55 months, primary invasive breast cancer findings for the tamoxifen and placebo groups were 89 versus 175, respectively, for a 49% relative reduction ($p < 0.00001$). The relative breast cancer risk reduction was similar for all age and risk groups and was limited to ER-positive tumors. Tamoxifen nonsignificantly reduced overall and breast cancer mortality. Beneficial secondary findings included 19% fewer fractures in the tamoxifen group. Secondary adverse findings associated with tamoxifen were increased endometrial cancers, vascular events, and cataracts.

Although the BCPT successfully completed testing its primary hypothesis, it also raised several key unresolved issues, such as effects on mortality, optimal tamoxifen duration, generalizability of results, and the issue of prevention versus treatment. The FDA subsequently approved tamoxifen for breast cancer risk reduction in high-risk women. The FDA recommendation is 20 mg/day for 5 years for high-risk women and warns of tamoxifen-associated risks. The FDA also approved tamoxifen for reducing the incidence of contralateral breast cancers, based on consistent secondary adjuvant data.[131]

The NSABP B-24 study tested 5 years of tamoxifen (20 mg/day) versus placebo after resection and radiation in 1804 patients with ductal carcinoma in situ (DCIS).[132] At 74 months median follow-up, 5-year incidences of all breast cancer events (invasive and noninvasive) were 8.2% and 13.4% in the tamoxifen and placebo groups, respectively, representing a 43% relative risk reduction ($p = 0.0009$). The cumulative incidence at 5 years of all invasive breast cancer events in the tamoxifen group was 4.1% versus 7.2% in the placebo group ($p = 0.004$). The FDA approved tamoxifen for risk reduction in the setting of locally treated (resection and radiation) breast DCIS.

The International Breast Cancer Intervention Study (IBIS-I) randomized 7410 women and showed a 32% reduction in breast cancer risk with tamoxifen.[114] The positive results in this trial and the BCPT (the two stronger RCTs in this setting) were limited to ER-positive cancers. A report of the long-term follow-up of IBIS-I suggests that the beneficial tamoxifen effects on breast cancer risk reduction persist for at least 10 years, but most side effects resolve after the 5-year treatment period, including all serious adverse events (e.g., thrombotic events and endometrial cancer).[115] The long-term follow-up (16.0 years; IQR 14.1–17.6) results of this trial showed that tamoxifen provided long-term prevention of ER-positive but not ER-negative breast cancer after treatment cessation.[116] These long-term findings have important implications for the risk/benefit profile of tamoxifen for prevention.

Currently ongoing is a clinical trial investigating the effectiveness of a topical tamoxifen gel for the prevention of breast cancer (NCT03063619). This phase II trial is currently accruing 152 women with mammographically dense breast to receive afimoxifene (4-hydroxytamoxifen (4-OHT)) or placebo daily for 52 weeks.

Table 2 Breast cancer prevention clinical trials of select estrogen-receptor modulators (SERMs).[a]

Trial and phase	Patient population	Study design	Results	Reference
Tamoxifen				
Royal Marsden Phase III	2494 high-risk women 30–70 yr of age	Tamoxifen (20 mg QD) or placebo for 8 yr	No difference initially; longer follow-up showed reduced incidence of invasive and ER-positive breast cancer; no significant change in incidence of ER-negative or overall breast cancer; 25-yr follow-up showed reduced ER expression in posttreatment ER-positive breast cancers and reduced ER-positive but not ER-negative breast cancers (largely posttreatment)	Powles et al.[107] Powles et al.[108] Detre et al.[109] ISRCTN07027313
NSABP-P1 (BCPT) Phase III	13,388 high-risk women >35 yr of age	Tamoxifen (20 mg QD) or placebo for 5 yr	Reduced incidence of invasive, noninvasive, and ER-positive breast cancer; no significant change in incidence of ER-negative breast cancer	Fisher et al.[110] Fisher et al.[111]
Italian Phase III	5408 normal-risk women with a hysterectomy 35–70 yr of age	Tamoxifen (20 mg QD) or placebo for 5 yr	Reduced incidence of invasive and ER-positive breast cancer; no significant change in incidence of ER-negative breast cancer	Veronesi et al.[112] Veronesi et al.[113]
IBIS-I Phase III	7154 high-risk women 35–70 yr of age	Tamoxifen (20 mg QD) or placebo for 5 yr	Reduced incidence of invasive, noninvasive (DCIS), ER-positive, and overall breast cancer; no significant change in incidence of ER-negative breast cancer; long-term follow-up (16 yr) showed long-term reduction in incidence of ER-positive but not ER-negative breast cancer	Cuzick et al.[114] Cuzick et al.[115] Cuzick et al.[116]
NSABP-P2 (STAR) Phase III	19,747 high-risk, postmenopausal women >35 yr of age	Tamoxifen (20 mg QD) or raloxifene (60 mg QD) for 5 yr	Reduced incidence of invasive and noninvasive ER-positive breast cancer; raloxifene was less effective but had less toxicity than tamoxifen	Vogel et al.[117] Vogel et al.[118] NCT00003906
Phase III	500 women ≤75 yr of age Operated on for breast LIN 2 and 3 or ER-positive or unknown DIN 1–3 (excluded DIN 1a)	Low-dose tamoxifen (5 mg) or placebo PO QD for 3 yr	Reduced recurrence of breast intraepithelial neoplasia with limited toxicity	DeCensi et al.[119] NCT01357772
Phase II	152 women 40–69 yr, or less than 40 yr if 5-yr breast cancer Gail risk is ≥1.66% Mammographically dense breast	Topical OHT gel (4 mg) or placebo QD for 52 wk	Primary endpoint: percent change in mammographic density (trial is currently ongoing)	NCT03063619
Raloxifene				
MORE Phase III	7705 postmenopausal women with low BMD <80 yr of age	Raloxifene (60 or 120 mg/d) or placebo for 4 yr	Reduced incidence of invasive, ER-positive, and overall breast cancer; no significant change in incidence of ER-negative breast cancer	Cummings et al.[120] Ettinger et al.[121]
CORE Phase III	4011 postmenopausal women with low BMD (reconsented from MORE trial) <80 yr of age	Raloxifene (60 mg QD) or placebo for an additional 4 yr after 4 yr of raloxifene on the MORE trial	Reduced incidence of invasive, ER-positive, and overall breast cancer incidence; no significant change in incidence of noninvasive of ER-negative breast cancer	Martino et al.[122]
RUTH Phase III	10,101 postmenopausal women with CHD >35 yr of age	Raloxifene (60 mg QD) or placebo for a median of 5.6 yr	Reduced incidence of invasive ER-positive breast cancer	Barrett-Connor et al.[123] NCT00190593
Lasofoxifene				
PEARL Phase III	8556 women with low BMD 59–80 yr of age	Lasofoxifene (0.25 or 0.5 mg QD) or placebo for 5 yr	Reduced incidence of invasive ER-positive breast cancer	Cummings et al.[124] LaCroix et al.[125] NCT00141323
Arzoxifene				
Generations Phase III	9369 women with low BMD 60–85 yr of age	Arzoxifene (20 mg QD) or placebo for 4 yr	Reduced incidence of invasive ER-positive breast cancer	Cummings et al.[126] Powles et al.[127] NCT00088010

Abbreviations: OHT, 4-hydroxytamoxifen (afimoxifene); BMD, bone mineral density; CORE, continued outcomes of raloxifene evaluation; CHD, coronary heart disease; QD, daily (quaque die); DCIS, ductal carcinoma *in situ*; DIN, ductal intraepithelial neoplasia; ER, estrogen receptor; IBIS-I, International Breast Intervention Study; Italian, Italian Randomized Tamoxifen Prevention Trial; LIN, lobular intraepithelial neoplasia; MORE, multiple outcomes of raloxifene evaluation; NSABP-P1, National Surgical Adjuvant Breast and Bowel Project Breast Cancer Prevention Trial (BCPT) P1; NSABP-P2, National Surgical Adjuvant Breast and Bowel Project Study of Tamoxifen and Raloxifene (STAR) P2; PEARL, Postmenopausal Evaluation and Risk-Reduction with Lasofoxifene Trial; RUTH, Raloxifene Use for the Heart Trial; Royal Marsden, Royal Marsden Tamoxifen Prevention Trial.
[a]Source: Based on Steering Committee[128]; Cuzick and Baum[129]; Early Breast Cancer Trialists Collaborative Group.[130]

Table 3 Breast cancer prevention clinical trials of select aromatase inhibitors (AIs).

Trial and phase	Patient population	Study design	Primary endpoint	Reference
DCIS trials				
NSABP B-35 Phase III	3104 postmenopausal women ER-positive/PR-positive DCIS	Anastrozole (1 mg QD) or tamoxifen (20 mg QD) for 5 yr	Reduced incidence of invasive and ER-positive DCIS with anastrozole versus tamoxifen; longer follow-up showed anastrozole was only more effective in women under 60 yr of age	NCT00053898 Margolese et al.[136] Ganz et al.[137]
IBIS-II (DCIS) Phase III	2980 postmenopausal women DCIS	Anastrozole (1 mg QD) or tamoxifen (20 mg QD) for 5 yr	No statistically significant difference in incidence of invasive breast cancer or DCIS with anastrozole versus tamoxifen	Cuzick[138] Cuzick[139] Forbes et al.[140] Sestak et al.[141] NCT00072462
Prevention trials				
NCIC-MAP.3 ExCel Phase III	4560 postmenopausal women High-risk	Exemestane (25 mg QD) or placebo for 5 yr	Reduced incidence of invasive ER-positive breast cancer; no significant change in incidence of noninvasive of ER-negative breast cancer	Richardson et al.[142] Goss et al.[143] NCT 00083174
IBIS-II Phase III	3864 postmenopausal women High-risk	Anastrozole (1 mg QD) or placebo for 5 yr	Reduced incidence of invasive ER-positive breast cancer; no significant change in incidence of noninvasive of ER-negative breast cancer	Cuzick[138] Cuzick[139] Cuzick et al.[144] Sestak et al.[141] Cuzick et al.[145] NCT00072462

Abbreviations: QD, daily (quaque die); DCIS, ductal carcinoma *in situ*; ER, estrogen receptor; NSABP B-35, National Surgical Adjuvant Breast and Bowel Project B-35; NCIC CTG MAP.3, or NCIC-MAP.3, NCIC Clinical Trials Group Mammary Prevention.3 trial; PR, progesterone receptor; IBIS-II, The Second International Breast Cancer Intervention Study.

The primary endpoint of this study is the change in mammographic density, the results of which could provide the rationale for further study of tamoxifen gel for the prevention of breast cancer.

The Study of Tamoxifen and Raloxifene (STAR) tested the SERM raloxifene against its fellow SERM tamoxifen for better efficacy and lesser toxicity in breast cancer prevention.[117] 19,747 postmenopausal women with an increased risk of breast cancer were randomized to tamoxifen (20 mg/day) or raloxifene (60 mg/day) for 5 years. On long-term follow-up, raloxifene had slightly higher rates of invasive breast cancer (RR 1.24; 95% CI 1.05–1.47), but produced fewer cases of uterine cancer than tamoxifen (RR 0.55; 95% CI 0.36–0.83). Furthermore, the risks of thromboembolic events and cataracts were statistically significantly lower with raloxifene than with tamoxifen. Tamoxifen and raloxifene had similar effects in reducing noninvasive breast cancer.[118] Raloxifene was approved by the FDA for invasive breast cancer risk reduction in postmenopausal women at a high such risk or with osteoporosis.

Following these seminal trials, the chemopreventive effect of third-generation SERMs were investigated. The Postmenopausal Evaluation and Risk-Reduction with Lasofoxifene (PEARL) Trial studied the effects of lasofoxifene in postmenopausal women with low bone mineral density (BMD),[124,125] showing a 79% reduction of invasive breast cancer and an 83% reduction in ER-positive breast cancer. A similar phase III prevention trial, known as the Generations Trial, reported a 56% decrease in invasive breast cancers in postmenopausal women with low BMD treated with arzoxifene.[126,127] These trials found that both lasofoxifene and arzoxifene reduce risk of nonvertebral and vertebral fractures; however, these third-generation SERMs, like raloxifene and tamoxifen, still increase risk of venous thromboembolic events.

A 2013 meta-analysis that included all nine of the large-scale phase III SERM prevention trials found that both overall and ER-positive breast cancer incidence is decreased by SERMs, and that DCIS incidence is decreased by all SERMs analyzed except raloxifene.[133]

Based largely on results of the Anastrozole, Tamoxifen Alone or in Combination (ATAC) trial,[134] there has been great interest in aromatase inhibitors (AIs) for breast cancer prevention in postmenopausal women. The increased focus on AIs was due to the initial findings of the ATAC, which showed a reduction of 58% in contralateral primary breast cancers in women treated with anastrozole versus tamoxifen (OR = 0.42; $p = 0.007$). With the report of the 10-year follow-up data, the results showed that women with early-stage breast cancer who were treated with anastrozole developed 32% fewer contralateral breast cancers than those taking tamoxifen (HR = 0.68; $p = 0.01$ for all breast cancers), and 38% fewer ER-positive contralateral breast cancers (HR = 0.62; $p = 0.003$).[135] These findings led to the development of a series of clinical trials investigating the efficacy of AIs for the prevention of breast cancer in women at high risk of breast cancer or with previous DCIS breast cancer (Table 3).

The NSABP B35 trial accrued 3104 postmenopausal women with DCIS breast cancer, who were treated with anastrozole (1 mg) or tamoxifen (25 mg) daily for 5 years (NCT00053898). Anastrozole was found to be more effective than tamoxifen at reducing breast cancer events (HR, 0.73; 95% CI, 0.56–0.96; $p = 0.0234$), invasive breast cancers (HR, 0.62; 95% CI, 0.42–0.90; $p = 0.0123$), contralateral breast cancers (HR, 0.64; 95% CI, 0.43–0.96; $p = 0.0322$), and DCIS recurrence (HR, 0.88; 95% CI, 0.59–1.30; $p = 0.52$) in women with ER-positive DCIS. However, results reported after 9 years of follow-up showed that anastrozole was only more effective in women under 60 years of age ($p = 0.0379$), but did result in decreased grade 4 thrombosis or embolism events (tamoxifen: 17; anastrozole: 4).[136]

The efficacy and safety of anastrozole and tamoxifen in the prevention of invasive and contralateral breast cancer in 2980 postmenopausal women were also compared in the IBIS-II DCIS trial.[138] Anastrozole and tamoxifen were found to similarly prevent DCIS recurrence. Similarly, no statistically significant difference was observed in the prevention of breast cancer events (HR 0.89; 95% CI, 0.64–0.123; $p = 0.49$), invasive breast cancers (HR 0.80;

95% CI, 0.52–1.24; $p = 0.32$), or DCIS recurrences (HR 0.99; 95% CI, 0.60–1.65; $p = 0.98$) in women treated with anastrozole versus tamoxifen.[140] However, women treated with tamoxifen experienced increased incidence of hot flushes, deep vein thrombosis, muscle spasms, and uterine cancers. Conversely, women treated with anastrozole experienced increased incidence of bone fractures, musculoskeletal events, hypercholesterolemia, and strokes with anastrozole.

The mammary prevention (MAP) 3 trial randomized 4560 high-risk postmenopausal women to receive exemestane 25 mg or placebo for 5 years.[142] There was a 65% reduction in the annual incidence of invasive breast cancer in favor of exemestane (HR 0.35; 95% CI 0.18–0.70).[143] There were no differences between the groups in bone fractures, cardiovascular events, or other cancers. The IBIS-II trial evaluated anastrozole 1 mg daily versus placebo for 5 years in 3864 high-risk postmenopausal women, and also demonstrated a reduction in the incidence in invasive breast cancer in favor of the AI (HR 0.47; 95% CI 0.32–0.68).[144] Anastrozole also reduced the incidence of skin, gynecologic, gastrointestinal, and other cancers. More aches and pains, joint stiffness, vasomotor symptoms, dry eyes, and hypertension were seen in the anastrozole group, but there were no statistically significant difference in the incidence of fractures between the arms. Early patient-reported symptoms published in 2018 outlined that symptoms associated with treatment in both the DICS and prevention studies were primarily mild or moderately severe, and that greater adherence in the anastrozole treatment group was associated with hot flashes ($p = 0.02$).[141] Follow-up after an additional 5 years showed significant, but reduced, preventive efficacy over time versus that observed in the first 5 years.[145] While AIs provide a promising strategy for the prevention of ER-positive breast cancer, these drugs still are not being frequently used by high-risk women because of concerns about side effects.

Given the cancer preventive activity of AE drugs, and the concerns about toxicities, new strategies are being tested to prevent ER-positive breast cancer. One of these strategies is to use topical AE drugs that are applied directly to the skin of the breast. This strategy was tested in a phase II trial in patients with ER-positive DCIS breast cancer,[146] and is now being tested in a phase I trial in women at high risk of breast cancer (who have high mammographic density) (NCT03063619). Other agents are being tested to prevent hormone-dependent breast cancer. Some of the most promising drugs are progesterone antagonists. The progesterone antagonist mifepristone has been shown to prevent mammary tumors in BRCA1-mutant mice,[147] and the progesterone antagonist, onapristone, has been tested in women with breast cancer and was shown to cause tumor regressions.[148] These promising results led to the development of an ongoing clinical trial of the anti-progesterone drug, telapristone, which is being tested in a phase II trial in women with early breast cancer (stages 0–2) (NCT01800422).

Other forms of AEs are being tested in at-risk women. One of the most promising is low-dose oral tamoxifen. This low-dose form of tamoxifen (at 5 mg/day) has reduced side effects, but still has cancer preventive activity, similar to that of the standard dose of tamoxifen (20 mg/day).[119] In this phase III trial in women at high risk of breast cancer, low-dose tamoxifen (5 mg/day given for 3 years) was compared to placebo and was found to significantly reduce breast cancer development,[119] with all breast cancer events being reduced at 5 years by 41%, and contralateral breast cancers being reduced at 5 years by 74%. Despite the cancer preventive activity of AE drugs, no agent investigated thus far has proven efficacy in the prevention of ER-negative breast cancer, which accounts for 30–40% of all breast cancer diagnoses, a number of drugs are currently under investigation. Among these chemopreventive agents are the RXR-selective retinoids (rexinoids) bexarotene,[149–152] which have demonstrated preventive efficacy for the development of ER-negative and "triple-negative" breast cancer in the preclinical setting. Based on positive results from these animal studies, an early-phase biomarker modulation trial testing the rexinoid bexarotene was conducted in women at risk of breast cancer (NCT00055991).[149] This trial demonstrated an anti-proliferative effect on breast tissue, but was associated with unacceptable toxicity. Therefore, topical bexarotene is now being tested in another clinical trial (NCT03323658) to determine whether the toxicity of this drug cancer can be reduced while retaining its cancer preventive activity. Another rexinoid, UAB30, which has reduced toxicity compared to bexarotene, is now being tested in women with breast cancer (NCT02876640) (Table 4).

Epidemiologic studies that suggested increased risk of breast cancer was associated with low vitamin D provided the rational to design studies of the efficacy of vitamin D for the prevention of breast cancer.[164–167] While these studies have shown that treatment with high doses of vitamin D has minimal side effects, first reports from these clinical trials have not demonstrated that treatment with vitamin D affects mammographic density in premenopausal women.[154,155]

Another drug that has previously been shown to be safe is metformin, an anti-diabetic agent that has been repurposed due to its ability to inhibit epithelial cell growth. As with vitamin D, a number of studies are currently underway investigating the efficacy of metformin in preventing breast cancer, the results of which are expected in the upcoming years. Among these is the phase III National Cancer Institute of Canada trial (NCT01101438), which has defined endpoints of disease-free survival, overall survival, and incidence of contralateral breast cancer. While this trial is currently ongoing, results at 6 months of the first 492 patients with paired blood samples showed that highly sensitive C-reactive protein (hs-CRP), insulin, glucose, leptin, and weight were significantly improved with treatment with metformin versus placebo.[157]

Epidemiologic studies showing an inverse association of the active ingredient of green tea, epigallocatechin gallate (EGCG), and cancer incidence[168–170] led to preclinical and early-phase clinical trials of EGCG for the prevention of breast cancer. Preclinical studies have now shown that treatment with EGCG suppresses mammary tumor development.[171–175] More recently, early-phase clinical trials have shown liver enzymes and GI toxicity to be the primary negative effects of treatment with the maximum tolerated dose of 600 mg twice daily (equivalent to 8–10 cups of green tea).[158] A phase II clinical trial being conducted by the University of Minnesota is currently ongoing,[159] but has released preliminary results. Treatment with EGCG (843 mg) was generally well tolerated and was associated with primarily mild and transient adverse events, with only 6.7% and 1.3% of participants treated with EGCG experiencing elevated ALT levels or ALT-related serious adverse events, respectively, versus placebo.[160] Most recently, results from this study suggested that treatment with EGCG versus placebo for 12 months did not reduce sex-steroid hormones, but did increase circulating estradiol concentrations in high-risk postmenopausal women.[161]

Clinical trials of anti-human epidermal growth factor receptor 2 (HER2) drugs have also been conducted to determine the efficacy of these agents for the prevention of breast cancer. While trastuzumab has not been shown to have a significant impact on anti-proliferation or apoptosis, it significantly augmented

Table 4 Breast cancer prevention clinical trials of select novel agents.

Agent and phase	Patient population	Study design	Primary endpoint (PE) or results (R)	Reference
Rexinoid				
Bexarotene Phase II	87 high-risk, postmenopausal women	Bexarotene (200 mg/m^2) or placebo for 28 d	PE: Reduction in cyclin D1 RNA (results not yet reported)	Brown et al.[149] NCT00055991
Bexarotene Phase I	40 high-risk women	Bexarotene (1% weight by weight gel): 10 mg QOD for 4 wk; 10 mg QOD for 1 wk and then QD for 3 wk; or 10 mg QOD for 1 wk and then QD for 1 wk and then 20 mg QD for 2 wk	PE: Determination of the recommended phase II dose of topical bexarotene 1% gel (results not yet reported)	NCT03323658
9cUAB30 IB	40 women ≥18 yr of age Invasive breast cancer	9cUAB30 (PO QD for 14–28 d before surgery)	PE: Changes in Ki67 expression (results not yet reported)	NCT02876640
Vitamin D				
Phase II	20 high-risk premenopausal women ≥21 yr of age LCIS or DCIS	Vitamin D (20,000 or 30,000 IU/wk) for 1 yr	R: Increased vitamin D levels and decreased IGF-1/IGFBP-3 ratio	Crew et al.[153] NCT00976339
Phase II	20 high-risk postmenopausal women ≥21 yr of age	Vitamin D (20,000 or 30,000 IU/wk) for 1 yr	R: Increased vitamin D levels and decreased IGF-1/IGFBP-3 ratio	Crew et al.[153] NCT00859651
SWOG S0812 Phase IIB	200 high-risk, premenopausal women 18–74 yr of age	Vitamin D (weekly and daily), or placebo (week) and vitamin D (daily) for 1 yr	R: No significant change in mammographic density at 12 mo	Crew et al.[154] NCT01097278
CALGB 70806 Phase III	300 premenopausal women ≤55 yr of age Breast density ≥25% (scattered fibroglandular densities or greater)	Vitamin D (2000 IU QD) or placebo for 1 yr	R: No significant change in mammographic density at 12 mo	Wood et al.[155] NCT01224678
Phase II	30 premenopausal women at increased risk ≤55 yr of age	Vitamin D (10,000 IU/wk) for 6 mo	PE: Change in mammographic density at 6 mo (results not yet reported)	NCT01166763
Metformin				
Phase I	5 women ≥18 yr of age Operable stage I or II breast cancer	Metformin (850 mg, BID) for 7–21 d	PE: Changes in Ki67 and cleaved caspase-3 expression; trial closed early due to slow accrual	NCT00984490 (results on clinicaltrials.gov)
Phase II	200 nondiabetic women with breast cancer	Metformin (850 mg, BID) or placebo for 28 d	R: No difference in Ki67, but different insulin-resistance-based effects (in luminal B tumors)	Bonanni et al.[156]
Phase II	151 premenopausal women 21–54 yr of age BMI ≥25 kg/m^2	Metformin (850 mg PO QD for 4 wk, then 850 mg PO BID or placebo for 48 wk)	PE: Change in mammographic density at 12 mo (results not yet reported)	NCT02028221
NCIC CTG MA.32 Phase III	3649 women with ER- and/or PR-positive invasive breast cancer 18–74 yr of age	Metformin (850 mg PO QD or placebo in weeks 1–4, then 850 mg PO BID or placebo for 4 yr and 11 mo)	PE: Invasive disease-free survival (results not yet reported; preliminary results included in text)	NCT01101438 Goodwin et al.[157]
Phase I	40 women with newly diagnosed invasive breast cancer or DCIS ≥21 yr of age	Metformin (1500 mg: 500 QAM and 1000 QHS) plus atorvastatin (80 mg QHS) for 2 wk prior to surgery	PE: Changes in Ki67 expression (results not yet reported)	NCT01980823
Phase I	24 overweight or obese women at elevated risk for breast cancer 18–75 yr of age	Metformin (850 mg PO QD or placebo for 30 d, and then 850 mg PO BID or placebo for 30 d, to repeat for 12 courses)	PE: Changes in the signal pathway profile of breast tissue (results not yet reported)	NCT01793948
Phase III	128 premenopausal women at elevated risk for breast cancer 25–55 yr of age	Metformin (850 mg PO QD or BID or placebo for 24 mo, and then 850 mg PO BID or placebo for 24 mo)	PE: Cytological atypia in unilateral or bilateral RPFNA aspirates (suspended due to placebo supply availability)	NCT01905046
EGCG (active agent of green tea)				
Phase I/IB	40 women 21–65 yr of age with prior hormone receptor-negative stage I–III breast cancer	Poly E (200, 600, 800 mg, BID) or placebo for 6 mo	R: The maximum tolerated dose for Poly E is 600 mg BID	Crew et al.[158] NCT00516243
Phase II	1075 postmenopausal women with high risk of breast cancer due to dense breast tissue with differing COMT genotypes	EGCG (800 mg QD) or placebo for 12 mo	R: Elevated liver enzymes (6.7%), mammographic density not yet reported)	NCT00917735 Samavat et al.[159] Dostal et al.[160] Samavat et al.[161]

(continued overleaf)

Table 4 (Continued)

Agent and phase	Patient population	Study design	Primary endpoint (PE) or results (R)	Reference
Trastuzumab Phase pilot	69 women with DCIS	Single dose of trastuzumab (8 mg/kg)	R: Augmented antibody-dependent cell-mediated cytotoxicity	Kuerer et al.[162] NCT00496808
Lapatinib Phase II	20 women with HER2-postitive DCIS	Lapatinib (1500 mg) versus placebo for 4 wk	R: Decreased expression of pHER2 and pERK; no change in Ki67 or p27 expression	Estévez et al.[163]
Phase II	40 women with EGFR-positive or HER-positive DCIS	Lapatinib (1000 mg PO QD) versus placebo for 6 wk	PE: Changes in Ki67 expression, safety (results not yet reported)	NCT00555152

Abbreviations: BMI, body mass index; CALGB, cancer and leukemia group B; COMT, catechol-*O*-methyltransferase; QD, daily (quaque die); DCIS, ductal carcinoma *in situ*; EGCG, epigallocatechin gallate; ER, estrogen receptor; QAM, every morning (quaque ante meridiem); QHS, every night at bedtime (before hours of sleep, quaque hora somni); QOD, every other day (quaque altera die); HER2, human epidermal growth factor receptor 2; IGF-1, insulin-like growth factor-1; IGFBP-3, insulin-like growth factor-binding protein-3; LCIS, lobular carcinoma *in situ*; PO, orally (per os); pERK, phosphorylated extracellular signal-regulated kinase; pHER2, phosphorylated human epidermal growth factor receptor 2; Poly E, polyphenon E; PE, primary endpoint; PR, progesterone receptor; RPFNA, random periareolar fine-needle aspiration; R, results; SWOG, previously known as the Southwest Oncology Group (SWOG); BID, twice a day.

antibody-dependent cell-mediated cytotoxicity in 100% of study participants.[162] Similarly, while no effect was seen on cell proliferation (assessed by Ki67 levels), lapatinib was well-tolerated and significantly decreased phosphorylated human epidermal growth factor receptor 2 (pHER2) and pERK1 expression, thereby modulating the HER2 signaling pathway.[163]

Vaccines showing promise for breast cancer risk reduction and prevention are discussed in the section titled "Immunoprevention" later in the article.

The prostate

Prostate carcinogenesis is an androgen-driven process, and a large-scale RCT, the PCPT, tested finasteride (5 mg/day), which inhibits five-alpha-reductase from converting testosterone into the more potent androgen dihydrotestosterone, versus placebo for 7 years in 18,882 men 55 years of age or older who had normal digital rectal exam (DRE) and prostate-specific antigen (PSA) level. Finasteride reduced the 7-year prostate cancer prevalence by 24.8%[176] but also appeared to increase high-grade disease (defined as a Gleason score of 8–10)—6.4% (finasteride) versus 5.1% (placebo). Finasteride also reduced the risk of high-grade prostatic IEN.[177] PCPT analyses also indicated a reduction in benign prostatic hypertrophy symptoms and an increase in sexual side effects, although a detailed analysis found that the effect of finasteride on sexual functioning was minimal.[178] Secondary PCPT findings indicated a high risk of prostate cancer, including high-grade disease, among men with normal PSA levels[179] and differences in PSA screening performance in men taking or not taking finasteride.[180,181] The adverse high-grade disease finding has sharply limited public interest in finasteride for prostate cancer prevention, and another major concern is that intensive PSA/DRE screening and early detection of prostate cancer in the PCPT could mean that finasteride may have prevented more clinically "insignificant" than "significant" prostate cancer. Several analyses, however, challenge these concerns.[177,181–186] The 18-year follow-up report attempted to address the significance of the high-grade finding (e.g., finasteride-driven artifact vs new finasteride-induced high-grade cancers) and found no significant between-group difference in the rates of overall survival or survival after the diagnosis of prostate cancer.[187] In 2019, mortality results were published showing that there was a 25% lower risk of death from prostate cancer in those in the finasteride group than in those who were in the placebo group (HR:0.75; 95% CI: 0.50–1.12).[188] Because of the small number of prostate cancer deaths (finasteride = 42; placebo = 56), the mortality difference between the groups was not statistically significant.[188]

Nested cohort and case-control studies within the PCPT have tested the preventive efficacy of statins and vitamin D in prostate cancer.[189–191] No association was found for statins with risk of total, low-grade or high-grade prostate cancer.[189] However, higher vitamin D levels were found to be associated with a slight increase in the risk of low-grade disease (defined as a Gleason score of 2–6),[190] a reduction in risk of high-grade disease, and an increased risk of prostate cancer in men with higher circulating levels of insulin-like growth factor-2 (IGF-2).[191]

The Reduction by Dutasteride of Prostate Cancer Events (REDUCE) study compared dutasteride 0.5 mg/day versus placebo in 8231 men 50–75 years of age, with a PSA level between 2.5 and 10 ng/mL and a negative prostate biopsy within 6 months. Participants underwent ultrasound-guided biopsies at years 2 and 4 of treatment. There was a 22.8% relative risk reduction in prostate cancer favoring dutasteride (95% CI 15.2–29.8, $p < 0.001$). There were 29 and 19 cancers with Gleason scores of 8–10 in the dutasteride and placebo groups, respectively ($p = 0.15$), over years 1–4; however, during years 3 and 4, there were 12 tumors with Gleason scores of 8–10 in the dutasteride group, and only one in the placebo group ($p = 0.003$). Acute urinary retention was less frequent, but the composite endpoint of cardiac failure, as well as erectile dysfunction and loss of libido were more common in the dutasteride group.[192] A 2013 follow-up study of prostate cancers diagnosed in the 2 years following the REDUCE trial in a subset of the men did not find additional high-grade cancers and demonstrated a similar low rate of new prostate cancers in the former dutasteride and placebo arms.[193] And a *post hoc* analysis in a subset of 1617 men from REDUCE showed that dutasteride significantly reduced the clinical progression of benign prostatic hyperplasia.[194]

Another very large RCT, the SELECT, recently discontinued supplements and reported results demonstrating that selenium or vitamin E, alone or in combination, did not prevent prostate cancer at the doses and formulations used in a heterogeneous population of 35,533 relatively healthy men. A harmful trend for increased risk of prostate cancer in the vitamin E arm ($p = 0.06$; RR 1.13; 99% CI: 0.195–1.35)[44] became statistically significant on further follow-up.[45] A recent follow-on analysis of SELECT investigated whether Se or vitamin E might benefit men with low baseline Se. Contrary to this hypothesis, there was no evidence of benefit of the intervention in the low baseline Se group, in fact vitamin E supplementation actually increased risk of total prostate cancer by 63% in men with low baseline toenail Se, and this effect was even stronger for high grade.[195] A case-cohort study nested within SELECT examined plasma vitamin D levels in relation to prostate cancer risk and found that both low and high vitamin D concentrations were associated with an increased risk of prostate cancer, and associations were stronger for high-grade disease.[196]

More recently, aspirin is being tested alone or in combination for the prevention of prostate cancer progression or recurrence in the PROVENT (NCT03103152) and Add-Aspirin (NCT2804815) trials.

Overall cancer

Two important large US trials have tested the ability of β-carotene to reduce overall cancer incidence. The PHS was a 12-year test of β-carotene effects on overall cancer incidence.[197] β-Carotene produced no significant differences in overall incidence of cancer (including lung cancer). Only 11% of this population were current smokers. Similar β-carotene results of the WHS were reported.[198] Results of the PHS II trial ($N = 14{,}641$ men) demonstrated that daily low-dose multivitamin led to a statistically significant reduction in the incidence of total cancer compared with placebo (17.0 and 18.3 events, respectively, per 1000 person-years, HR 0.92, 95% CI: 0.86–0.998; $p = 0.04$), primarily in individuals with a prior cancer history. There were no reductions in the incidence of site-specific cancers.[199] Two very recent RCTs have examined the impact of aspirin on cancer incidence and mortality as secondary endpoints. The ASCEND trial (A Study of Cardiovascular Events in Diabetes) compared 100 mg of daily aspirin to placebo in 15,480 men and women with Type II diabetes but no CVD. While the trial documented a significant cardioprotective effect of aspirin, there was no significant difference in cancer incidence between the trial groups (HR: 1.01; 95% CI: 0.92–1.11) and minimal nonsignificant decreases in cancer mortality (HR: 0.98; 95% CI: 0.84–1.15) and all-cause mortality (HR: 0.94; 95% CI: 0.85–1.04) at a mean follow-up of 7.4 years.[200] The ASPREE trial (Aspirin in Reducing Events in the Elderly) examined 100 mg of daily aspirin in 19,114 individuals aged 70+ (aged 65+ among blacks and Hispanics) who did not have CVD, dementia, or physical disability. Results of ASPREE showed a significantly increased risk of all-cause mortality in the aspirin group compared to placebo (HR: 1.14; 95% CI: 1.01–1.29).[201] This increase was largely driven by deaths due to cancer, as aspirin treatment resulted in a 31% (HR: 1.31; 95% CI: 1.10–1.56) increase in cancer mortality over an median of 4.7 years of follow-up.[201] These results are concerning, although they do not align with other published data. The ARRIVE trial (Aspirin to Reduce the Risk of Initial Vascular Events) enrolled 12,546 participants free of Type II diabetes but with low-to-moderate risk of CVD to test 100 mg daily aspirin versus placebo. While results have been reported for its primary composite outcome of time to first CV death, myocardial infarction, unstable angina, stroke, or transient ischemic attack, secondary results related to cancer outcomes have yet to be published and are eagerly awaited.[202]

Immunoprevention

Immunoprevention is the use of both vaccines and immune-modulating agents, such as checkpoint inhibitors, to prevent cancer. The success of vaccines in treating virally induced cancers (e.g., hepatitis B virus (HBV)- and human papillomavirus (HPV)-related cancers) and the more recently demonstrated efficacy of anti-programmed cell death protein-1 (PD-1) immunotherapy in treating mismatch-repair-deficient tumors provide a strong rationale for the pursuit of immunoprevention strategies against several types of cancers. Recent study identified chromosome copy-number driven immune escape in the oral precancer-invasive cancer transition in HPV-negative head and neck cancer; and identified chromosome 9p loss as the culprit genomic biomarker of anti-PD-1 resistance in this cancer interception setting.[203] The latter finding has important implications on immune oncology in chemoprevention trial designs testing immune-checkpoint inhibitors, such as the Immune Prevention of Oral Cancer, or IPOC, trial. The use of vaccines for prevention is perhaps most advanced in breast and colon cancer, and the use of immunotherapy agents is being actively explored in early stages of lung, head and neck and colon cancers.

Vaccines

The efficacy of the HBV vaccine in reducing infection, chronic liver disease (CLD), and hepatocellular carcinoma (HCC) mortality has been demonstrated by Taiwan's National Hepatitis B Immunization Program[204] as well as the Qidong Hepatitis B Intervention Study.[205] Thirty-year outcomes of each of these programs have documented the effectiveness of infant HBV vaccination in reducing the incidence and mortality of HCC.[206,207] These studies have laid the foundation for vaccination against infection-related cancer. Several other studies have further established the efficacy of the HBV vaccine and a dual hepatitis A virus (HAV)/HBV vaccine administered alone or in combination with bivalent or quadrivalent HPV vaccines (Table 5).

A range of other studies have developed and are currently developing and testing vaccines for hepatitis C virus (HCV)-related cancer. The antiviral/antineoplastic drug, interferon alpha-2b (IFNα-2b), was used in a study of 150 HCC patients who were HCV-positive and were to have early-intermediate stage HCC resection (NCT00273247). While there was no difference in recurrence-free survival between patients treated with IFNα-2b versus control (24.3% vs 5.8%; $p = 0.49$), the primary study endpoint, there was a significant reduction in late recurrence in HCV-pure patients adherent to treatment (HR: 0.3; 95% CI: 0.09–0.9; $p = 0.04$).[213] Phase II/III studies that have been conducted and are currently in progress for vaccine strategies for the prevention of HCC include those focused on IFNα-2b, cytokine induced killer cells, gp-96 peptide complex, and alpha-hepcortespenlisimut-L (Hepko-V5; Table 6).

HPV infection increases risk of cervical cancer, and positive results from many clinical trials of HPV vaccines in female participants (both girls and young women) led to the approval of HPV vaccination by the FDA. Multiple types of HPV vaccines have been developed and assessed for cancer prevention, including monovalent (HPV-16), bivalent (HPV-16/18), quadrivalent (HPV-6/11/16/18), and nanovalent (HPV-6/11/16/18/31/33/45/52/58) vaccines (Table 7).

Two phase III studies that focused on the bivalent HPV vaccine are the Papilloma Trial Against Cancer In Young Adults (PATRICIA; NCT00122681) and Costa Rica Vaccine Trial (CVT; NCT00128661). PATRICIA assessed the efficacy of the bivalent HPV vaccine in preventing HPV-16/18 infection in 18,644 females 15–25 years of age with no evidence of prior HPV infection. This study showed no difference in safety between the vaccine and placebo, and 90.4% vaccine efficacy against cervical intraepithelial neoplasia (CIN)2+ containing HPV-16/18

Table 5 Select phase III HBV clinical trials of vaccines.

Agent and phase	Patient population	Study design	Primary endpoint (PE) or results (R)	Reference
Phase III	744 girls 9–15 yr of age	2vHPV VLP/AS04 and ENGERIX-B vaccination (administered together or individually for three study arms) at months 0, 1, and 6	R: Concomitant administration of 2vHPV and ENGERIX-B was well-tolerated, and delivered high antibody response to HBV and HPV-16/18	Schmeink et al.[208] NCT00652938
FUTURE Phase III	1877 participants 16–23 yr of age Agree to refrain from vaginal/anal sexual activity for 48 h prior to all scheduled visits	4vHPV V501 and HBV vaccination (administered together or individually for three study arms) at months 0, 1, and 6	R: Coadministration of 4vHPV V501 and HBV vaccines was well-tolerated, and maintained antibody response associated with individual administration of V501, and high anti-HBV antibody response although lower than that associated with HBV vaccine alone	Wheeler et al.[209] NCT00517309
Phase IIIb	152 participants 20–25 yr of age	ENGERIX-B vaccination with or without 2vHPV VLP/AS04 vaccination administered at months 0, 1, 2, and 12	R: Coadministration of ENGERIX-B and VLP/AS04 at an accelerated schedule (potentially required by women at high risk) was well-tolerated, and maintained antibody response associated with individual administration of each vaccine	Leroux-Roels et al.[210] NCT00637195
Phase III	814 girls 9–15 yr of age	2vHPV VLP/AS04 and TWINRIX vaccination (administered together or individually for three study arms) at months 0, 1, and 6	R: Coadministration of VLP/AS04 and TWINRIX was well-tolerated, and maintained antibody response associated with individual administration of each vaccine	Pedersen et al.[211] NCT00578227
Phase III	75 girls ≥16 yr of age Presence of vulvo vaginal genital warts HIV-negative or HIV-infected and CD4 ≥ 300 cells/mm³ OR viral load controlled OR ARV compliant >6 mo	4vHPV V501 or HBV vaccination administered at months 0, 2, and 6	PE: Change in the maximum size of the genital wart lesion over the trial period (as measured in mm; time frame: baseline, weeks 8, 16, 24, 36, 48, 60, 72)	NCT02750202
Phase III	1260 participants ≥18 yr of age Using cocaine/heroin in last 7 d From 1 of 2 target communities known with high rate of drug use and STDs	HBV vaccine (5 μg) administered at months 0, 1, and 2 (accelerated schedule) or at months 0, 1, and 6 (normal schedule), both with standard or enhanced behavioral intervention (four arms)	R: Accelerated HBV vaccination enhanced adherence among IDUs independently of behavioral intervention	Hwang et al.[212] NCT00841477
Nationwide hepatitis B vaccination program phase III	5,188,929 newborns (July 1984–December 2002) 1984–1986: all newborns with high-risk mothers ser-positive for HBsAg July 1986: all newborns July 1987: all preschool children 1988–1990: all primary school children	Plasma-derived HBV vaccine (5 μg) administered at 0, 5, and 9 wk, and 12 mo; infants of highly infectious carrier mothers also received the vaccine within 24 h of birth; 1 November 1992 changed to recombinant yeast HBV vaccine administered at months 0, 1, and 6	R: HBV vaccination in children significantly reduced risk of CLD, HCC, and IFH	Chen et al.[204] Sun et al.[205] Chiang et al.[206]

Abbreviations: ARV, anti-retro-viral; CLD, chronic liver disease; TWINRIX, hepatitis A and hepatitis B (recombinant) vaccine; ENGERIX-B, GSK Biologicals' hepatitis B vaccine (recombinant; 103860); FUTURE, females united to unilaterally reduce endo/ectocervical disease; GARDASIL; qHPV, V501, GARDASIL quadrivalent HPV-6/11/16/18 vaccine; CERVARIX; VLP/AS04, GSK Biologicals' HPV 16/18 bivalent L1 virus-like particle (580299); HBsAg, hepatitis B surface antigen; HBV, hepatitis B virus; HCC, hepatocellular carcinoma; HPV, human papillomavirus; IFH, infant fulminant hepatitis; IDU, injection drug user; PE, primary endpoint; R, results; STD, sexually transmitted disease.

DNA (97.9% CI: 53.4–99.3; p, 0.0001).[215] Follow-up results at 39 months showed improved efficacy of the virus in participants with no evidence of high-risk HPV infection at baseline versus those with HPV-16/18 infection.[216] Vaccine efficacy against HPV-16/18-related CIN1+/CIN2+/CIN3+ in the total vaccinated cohort (which included 26% HPV-16/18-positive women) was 55.5, 52.8, and 33.6, respectively, and against CIN1+/CIN2+/CIN3+ irrespective of HPV DNA was 21.7, 30.4, and 33.4, respectively. Conversely, vaccine efficacy against HPV-16/18-related CIN1+/CIN2+/CIN3+ in HPV-16/18 disease-free women 96.5, 98.4, and 100%, respectively, and against CIN1+/CIN2+/CIN3+ irrespective of HPV DNA was 50.1, 70.2, and 87.0%, respectively.

The CVT evaluated the bivalent vaccine versus hepatitis A vaccine in 7466 Costa Rican women 18–25 years of age. One of the initial reports from this study showed that HPV-16/18 vaccination

Table 6 Select phase II/III HCV and HCC clinical trials of vaccines.

Agent and phase	Patient population	Study design	Primary endpoint (PE) or results (R)	Reference
HCV				
Phase III	150 participants 18–75 yr of age HCV-RNA-positive HBsAg-negative HCC undergoing potentially curative resection	IFNα-2b (three million units three times per week; for adverse events other than anemia the dose was reduced to 1.5 million units three times per week until the event resolved) or control for 48 wk	R: 28 adherent patients (37%); 45-mo follow-up: OS was 58.5%; no significant difference in RFS; significantly reduced late recurrence in HCV-pure patients who were adherent to treatment	Mazzaferro et al.[213] NCT00273247
Vaccines for hepatocellular cancer (HCC)				
Phase III	150 participants 18–75 yr of age HCV-RNA-positive HBsAg-negative HCC undergoing potentially curative resection	IFNα-2b (three million units three times per week; for adverse events other than anemia the dose was reduced to 1.5 million units three times per week until the event resolved) or control for 48 wk	R: 28 adherent patients (37%); 45-mo follow-up: OS was 58.5%; no significant difference in RFS; however, significantly reduced late recurrence in HCV-pure patients who were adherent to treatment was demonstrated	Mazzaferro et al.[213] NCT00273247
Phase III	100 patients 18–100 yr of age Life expectancy >12 wk Previously resected HCC	CIK vaccine versus no intervention for four cycles	PE: Time to recurrence	NCT01749865; 2007043-HCC012
Phase II/III	80 men and women 18–75 yr of age Previously undergone radical resection; AJCC TNM II, III, IV	Autologous gp96 vaccination (25 µg via subcutaneous injection) or no anti-tumor treatment for six injections QW within 8 wk after surgery)	PE: 2-yr RFS rate	NCT04206254
Phase II	75 men and women HCC diagnosis and SFP serum test ≥30 IU/mL 23 were HBV-positive, 34 were HCV-positive, 9 were HBV- and HCV-positive, 4 were HBV- and HCV-negative, 5 were without established viral diagnosis	Hepko-V5 vaccine (850 mg pill administered PO QD) versus placebo	R: AFP was reduced (baseline 245.2 IU/mL, 95% CI: 1186–7280; posttreatment 102.3 IU/mL, 98% CI 503–4575); median OS time not established as 70 of 75 patients survive at 90-mo follow-up	Tarakanovskaya et al.[214] NCT02256514
Phase III	120 men and nonpregnant women ≥18 yr of age Prior HCC diagnosis	Hepko-V5 vaccine (850 mg pill administered PO QD) versus placebo	PE: Change in plasma AFP levels at monthly intervals (recruiting participants at the time this was written)	NCT02232490

Abbreviations: AFP, alpha-fetoprotein; AJCC, American Joint Committee on Cancer; CI, confidence interval; CIK, cytokine-induced killer cell; QD, daily (quaque die); gp96, gp96-peptide complex; HBsAg, hepatitis B surface antigen; HBV, hepatitis B virus; HCV, hepatitis C virus; HCV-positive, anti-HBc-negative, HCV-pure; Hepko-V5, alpha-hepcortespenlisimut-L; HCC, hepatocellular cancer; IFNα-2b, interferon alpha-2b; QW, once per week; OS, overall survival; PO, orally (*per os*); PE, primary endpoint; RFS, recurrence-free survival; R, results; SFP, soluble fibrin polymer; TNM, tumor, node, metastasis (classification of tumors).

does not accelerate clearance of the virus.[236] This study also showed highest vaccine efficacy in compliant HPV-negative women, with results against: HPV-16/18 infections: 90.9% (95% CI: 82.0–95.9); HPV-31/33/45 infections: 44.5% (95% CI: 17.5–63.1); any oncogenic infection: 12.4% (95% CI: −3.2–25.6).[217] While these rates were lower in the intention-to-treat (ITT) cohort of all randomized women, vaccine efficacy remained highest in virgins (79.8%) and younger women (18–19 years of age: 68.9%; 24–25 years of age: 21.8%). Follow-up results 4 years after vaccination showed an estimated vaccine efficacy against oral HPV-16/18 infections of 93.3% (95% CI: 63–100%), and against HPV-16/18-related cervical infections of 72.0% (95% CI: 63–79%).[218] This study reported no statistically significant protection of the vaccine against other oral HPV infections. Overall, vaccine efficacy 4 years after vaccination against HPV-16/18-associated CIN2+ was 89.9% (95% CI: 39.5–99.5), against other non-HPV-16/18 oncogenic HPVs CIN2+ was 59.9% (95% CI: 20.7–80.8), and against CIN2+ regardless of HOV type was 61.4% (95% CI: 29.5–79.8).[219]

The Phase III Females United to Unilaterally Reduce Endo/Ectocervical Disease (FUTURE I; NCT00092521) clinical trial studied the efficacy of the quadrivalent HPV vaccine in 5455 females 16–24 years of age. This study showed 100% efficacy of the vaccine in reducing incidence of genital warts, vulvar/vaginal IEN or cancer, cervical IEN, adenocarcinoma *in situ*, and HPV-6/11/16/18-related cancer in women vaccinated without prior HPV infection.[220] In addition, the quadrivalent vaccine reduced the incidence of both vulvar/vaginal perianal lesions (34%; 95% CI: 15–49) and cervical lesions (20%; 95% CI: 8–31) regardless of the causal HPV type. These findings led to the FUTURE II (NCT00092534) study, which tested the quadrivalent vaccine in 12,167 females 15–26 years of age. This study showed 98% efficacy of the vaccine in preventing adenocarcinoma *in situ*, cervical IEN grade 2 or 3, or HPV-16/18-related cancer versus placebo. As with FUTURE I, this study showed prevention of high-grade cervical lesions independent of HPV type (17%; 95% CI: 1–31).

The quadrivalent HPV vaccine has also been tested in 4065 males 16–26 years of age from 18 countries (NCT00090285). The qudrivalent HPV vaccine decreased external genital lesions by 60.2% (95% CI: 40.8–73.8), and HPV-6/11/16/18-related lesions by 65.5% (95% CI: 45.8–78.6) versus placebo in the ITT analysis, but increased efficacy in the per-protocol analysis to a 90.4% decrease (95% CI: 69.2–98.1) in HPV-6/11/16/18-related lesions.[222] The quadrivalent vaccine was also shown to reduce incidence of HPV-6/11/16/18-related anal IEN by 50.5% (95% CI: 25.7–67.2) in the ITT analysis and by 77.5% (95% CI: 39.6–93.3) in the per-protocol analysis.[223] A lower reduction was observed for anal IEN associated with any type of HPV (ITT: 25.7%; per-protocol: 54.9%). In addition, the quadrivalent HPV vaccine was well

Table 7 Select phase III HPV clinical trials of vaccines.

Agent and phase	Patient population	Study design	Primary endpoint (PE) or results (R)	Reference
HPV—bivalent vaccine				
PATRICIA Phase III	18,644 female participants 15–25 yr of age Intact cervix Lifetime history of ≤4 sexual partners	VLP/AS04 or HAV vaccine administered at months 0, 1, and 6	R: Adjuvanted HPV 16/18 vaccination reduced incidence of HPV16- or HPV18-related CIN 2+; 39-mo follow-up: VLP/AS04 vaccination of adolescents prior to sexual debut significantly reduced the incidence of high-grade cervical abnormalities, and catch-up vaccination up to 18 yr of age is most likely effective	Paavonen et al.[215] Apter et al.[216] NCT00122681
CVT Phase III	7466 female participants 18–25 yr of age Resident of Guanacaste Province, Costa Rica, and surrounding area	VLP/AS04 or HAV vaccine administered at months 0, 1, and 6	R: VLP/AS04 vaccination is highly effective against HPV 16/18, partially effective against HPV 31/33/45, and is most effective prior to initiation in sexual activity; 4-yr follow-up: HPV prevalence was significantly lower 4 yr after vaccination with VLP/AS04 versus HAV; additional 4-yr follow-up: high efficacy and immunogenicity of VLP/AS04 against HPV infections and cervical disease associated with HPV 16/18 and other oncogenic HPV types, and the safety profile was sound	Herrero et al.[217] Herrero et al.[218] Hildesheim et al.[219] NCT00128661
HPV—quadrivalent vaccine				
FUTURE I Phase III	5455 female participants 16–24 yr of age Intact uterus Lifetime history of 0–4 sexual partners	V501 vaccine or placebo or HPV 16 monovalent vaccine administered at day 1 and months 2 and 6	R: V501 significantly reduced the incidence of HPV-related anogenital diseases, including cervical, vulvar, and vaginal perianal lesions, versus placebo	Garland et al.[220] NCT00092521
FUTURE II Phase III	12,167 female participants 15–26 yr of age No abnormal Papanicolaou smear Lifetime history of ≤4 sexual partners	V501 vaccine or placebo administered at day 1 and months 2 and 6	R: V501 significantly reduced the incidence of high-grade intraepithelial HPV16 or HPV18-related neoplasia versus placebo	The FUTURE II Study Group[221] NCT00092534
Phase III	4065 male participants 16–26 yr of age Healthy heterosexual males or MSMs	V501 vaccine or placebo administered at day 1 and months 2 and 6	R: V501 vaccination reduced incidence of HPV-6, 11, 16, and 18, and development of HPV-type related anogenital disease	Giuliano et al.[222] Palefsky et al.[223] NCT00090285
HPV—nanovalent vaccine				
Phase III	924 female participants 12–26 yr of age Previously received GARDASIL V503-006 (three-dose regimen) Lifetime history of ≤4 sexual partners	9vHPV V503-006 vaccine (0.5 mL intramuscular injection) or placebo at day 1 and months 2 and 6	R: V503-006 vaccination after vaccination with quadrivalent HPV vaccine is well tolerated and highly immunogenic for HPV types 31,33, 45, 52, and 58	Garland et al.[224] Moreira et al.[225] Moreira et al.[226] NCT01047345
Phase III	1212 female participants 16–45 yr of age No abnormal Papanicolaou smear	9vHPV V503-004 (0.5 mL) vaccine at day 1 and months 2 and 6 in women 27–45 yr of age versus women 16–26 yr of age	PE: Anti-HPV GMTs for each anti-HPV type	NCT03158220
Phase III	14,840 female participants 16–26 yr of age No abnormal Papanicolaou smear	9vHPV V503-001 (0.5 mL) or V501 vaccine in a three dose regimen (a subset of participants received a fourth vaccination in the extension study)	R: 9vHPV vaccination was well-tolerated, prevented HPV-31/33/45/52/58-related infection and disease, generated an antibody response to HPV-6/11/16/18 comparable to the quadrivalent HPV vaccine, but did not impact infection/disease related to other HPV types; 6-yr follow-up: showed vaccine efficacy was sustained for up to 6 yr	Joura et al.[227] Huh et al.[228] NCT00543543
Phase III	3066 male and female participants Boys and girls 9–15 yr of age Women 16–26 yr of age No abnormal Papanicolaou smear	9vHPV V503-002 vaccine at day 1 and months 2 and 6 in boys and girls 9–15 yr of age versus women 16–26 yr of age	R: 9vHPV vaccination was better tolerated in girls and boys than young women, vaccine response was comparable in both groups, anti-HPV response was sustained through 2.5 yr after the final dose	Van Damme et al.[229] NCT00943722

(continued overleaf)

Table 7 (Continued)

Agent and phase	Patient population	Study design	Primary endpoint (PE) or results (R)	Reference
Phase III	201 male and female participants 9–26 yr of age 9–15: has not had coitarche 16–26: no abnormal Papanicolaou smear	9vHPV V503-017 (0.5 mL) vaccine at day 1 and months 2 and 6	PE: Seroconversion percentages to HPV-6/11/16/18/31/33/45/52/58 at month 7	NCT03546842
Phase III	100 female Japanese participants 9–15 yr of age Not sexually active	9vHPV V503-008 (0.5 mL) vaccine at day 1 and months 2 and 6	R: 9vHPV vaccination was well-tolerated, 100% of participants exhibited seroconversion for each HPV type, anti-HPV response was sustained for 2 yr after the final dose, increased the geometric mean of the titers for anti-HPV 6/11/16/18/31/33/45/52/58 comparably to the Phase III Japanese study of women 16–26 yr of age (NCT00543543)	Iwata et al.[230] NCT01254643
Phase III	3074 male and female participants Boys and girls 9–15 yr of age Women 16–26 yr of age 9–15: has not had coitarche 16–26: no abnormal Papanicolaou smear, 0–4 sexual partners	9vHPV V503-002 (0.5 mL) intramuscular vaccination at day 1 and months 2 and 6	R: Three lots of 9vHPV vaccine-elicited equivalent antibody response for all nine vaccine types.	Luxembourg et al.[231] NCT00943722
Phase III	2520 male and female participants Men and women 16–26 yr of age 9–15: has not had coitarche 16–26: no abnormal Papanicolaou smear, 0–4 sexual partners	9vHPV V503-003 (0.5 mL) intramuscular vaccination at day 1 and months 2 and 6 in women, heterosexual males, or MSMs	R: 9vHPV vaccination was well-tolerated, led to 99.5% seropositivity in all subjects, and generated comparable results in heterosexual males and women, but lower GMTs in MSMs	Castellsagué et al.[232] NCT01651949
Phase III	1241 boys and girls 11–15 yr of age	9vHPV V503-005 (0.5 mL) intramuscular vaccination at day 1 and months 2 and 6 with MCV4 and Tdap each given as a 0.5 mL intramuscular injection on day 1 versus at month 1	R: Concomitant administration of 9vHPV and MCV4/Tdap was well-tolerated, and maintained antibody response associated with individual administration of each vaccine	Schilling et al.[233] NCT00988884
Phase III	1054 boys and girls 11–15 yr of age Not sexually active	9vHPV V503-007 (0.5 mL) intramuscular vaccination at day 1 and months 2 and 6 and REPEVAX (0.5 mL) intramuscular vaccination at day 1 or month 1	R: Concomitant administration of 9vHPV and REPEVAX was well-tolerated, and maintained antibody response associated with individual administration of each vaccine	Kosalaraksa et al.[234] NCT01073293
Phase III	600 girls 9–15 yr of age	9vHPV V503-009 (0.5 mL) or V501 intramuscular vaccination at day 1 and months 2 and 6	R: 9vHPV vaccination was well-tolerated and elicited a strong immune response to HPV-6/11/16/18/31/33/45/52/58 that was comparable to the immune response of V501 for HPV-6/11/16/18	Vesikari et al.[235] NCT01304498

Abbreviations: CIN, cervical intraepithelial neoplasia; CVT, Costa Rica Vaccine Trial; Adacel; Tdap, diphtheria/tetanus/acellular pertussis; REPEVAX, diphtheria/tetanus/pertussis/poliomyelitis vaccine; FUTURE, females united to unilaterally reduce endo/ectocervical disease; GARDASIL; qHPV, V501, GARDASIL quadrivalent HPV-6/11/16/18 vaccine; GMTs, geometric mean titers; Havrix; HAV, GSK Biologicals hepatitis A vaccine; CERVARIX, VLP/AS04, GSK Biologicals HPV 16/18 bivalent L1 virus-like particle (580299); HPV, human papillomavirus; MSM, men having sex with men; 9vHPV; V503, nonavalent HPV-6/11/16/18/31/33/45/52/58 V503-006 vaccine; Menactra; MCV4, Neisseria meningitides serotypes A/C/Y/W-135; PATRICIA, Papilloma Trial Against Cancer In Young Adults; PE, primary endpoint; R, results.

tolerated, and reduced the risk of persistent anal infection with HPV-6/11/16/18 by 59.4% and 94.9% in the ITT and per-protocol population analyses, respectively.

More recently, the nanovalent HPV vaccine was the focus of a phase III study in 924 females 12–26 years of age (NCT01047345). The vaccine was found to be well-tolerated, and to provide over 98% seropositivity for HPV-31/33/45/52/58 at 4 weeks after the final dose.[224] Across seven phase III studies of the nanovalent HPV vaccine in over 15,000 subjects 9–26 years of age, it was found to be generally well-tolerated.[225] Similarly, the vaccine has shown to be well-tolerated in young men.[226] The nine-valent HPV vaccine has been shown to be well-tolerated, effective, and immunogenic in studies of Asian participants (including girls, boys, and young women from Hong Kong, India, Japan, South Korea, Taiwan, and Thailand; NCT00543543 and NCT00943722).[237] This vaccine has also been proven to have the same impact on Latin American participants (NCT00543543 and NCT00943722).[238]

Given the success of vaccines in reducing the risk of viral-associated cancers, and given the enhanced understanding of the immune system's role in cancer development and treatment that has come with checkpoint inhibitors, vaccines for non-viral-associated cancers are being tested in clinical studies. These studies are most advanced in breast and colon cancers. With the identification of several breast cancer–specific antigens, clinical trials are now investigating the potential of vaccines for the prevention of breast cancer. Breast cancer prevention vaccines fall into three primary categories: peptide vaccines, pulsed dendritic-cell vaccines, and DNA-based vaccines (Table 8).

Vaccines against the HER2 oncoprotein (HER2/Neu peptide vaccines) have been conducted, the results of which have shown it to be safe, as well as capable of inducing an anti-HER2 immune response.[251–254] Similarly, anti-HER2 immunity has been shown to be induced by DNA-based anti-HER2 vaccines,[255–257] and an antigen-specific immune response has been shown in patients with stage IV breast cancer following vaccination with a HER2/neu T-helper peptide-based vaccine (NCT00194714).[239] Several phase I/II clinical trials are currently ongoing, examining the efficacy of anti-HER2 vaccines in patients with stage III–IV breast cancer. While the majority of breast cancer vaccines target HER2, STEMVac is novel in that is comprised of DNA fragments of three different antigens in triple-negative breast cancer that have been combined into a complex DNA-based vaccine (NCT02157051). The Phase I STEMVac clinical trial is currently ongoing, the results of which could be significant for the prevention of triple-negative breast cancer in the future.

More recently, HER2 peptide E75, GP2, and AE37 vaccines have been brought to clinical trial in high-risk patients. Results of a clinical trial using the HER2 peptide nelipepimut-S (NeuVax; E75) vaccine showed minimal toxicities, and 5-year DFS of 89.7% versus 80.2% in vaccine versus control (no vaccination) groups ($p = 0.08$; NCT00841399/NCT00584789).[240] However, as 65% of participants received suboptimal dosing of the vaccine (due to the study design), the 5-year DFS of optimally (94.6%) versus suboptimally (87.1%) dosed patients was also reported ($p = 0.05$). In addition, 21 patients who elected to participate in a voluntary booster program had a DFS of 95.2% with only one recurrence. Based on these results, a phase III trial of the E75 vaccine in women at high risk of breast cancer has been initiated. While the 25.7-month follow-up results of another phase II study of E75 vaccination combined with Herceptin (trastuzumab) treatment (NCT01570036) did not show efficacy of the E75 vaccine versus control for improving the estimated DFS (HR: 0.62; 95% CI: 0.31–1.25; $p = 0.18$), improved DFS was shown for patients with triple-negative breast cancer who received the E75 vaccine versus control (HR: 0.26; 95% CI: 0.08–0.81; $p = 0.01$).[241] These results support the translation of these findings to a phase III clinical trial, perhaps particularly for those with triple-negative breast cancer. In addition, the Nelipepimut-S Peptide Vaccine in Women with DCIS of the Breast (VADIS) trial is currently ongoing, and is investigating the efficacy of the E75 vaccine in women with HLA-A2 positive DCIS (NCT02636582).

GP2 is derived from the transmembrane portion of HER2/neu, and has binding characteristics that differ from E75. The first results of a clinical trial of the GP2 vaccine in disease-free breast cancer patients showed minimal toxicity, and HER-2/Neu immunogenic responses to both GP2-specific CD8+ T-cells (prevaccination: 0.4% (0.0–2.9%); maximum: 1.1% (0.4–3.6%), $p < 0.001$) and E75-specific CD8+ T-cells (prevaccination: 0.8% (0.0–2.41%); maximum: 1.6% (0.86–3.72%), $p < 0.001$).[242] Hence, GP2 elicited a HER-2/neu-specific immune response that involved epitope spreading in these high-risk patients. These results have led to a phase I trial testing combined treatment with GP2 and trastuzumab (NCT03014076), and a phase II trial of GP2 and granulocyte colony-stimulating factor (GM-CSF) in disease-free breast cancer patients who are lymph node-positive or high-risk lymph-node negative.

A phase II clinical trial investigated the efficacy of the GP2 plus GM-CSF vaccine and the AE37 plus GM-CSF vaccine versus GM-CSF alone in disease-free node-positive and high-risk node-negative breast cancer patients (NCT00524277). After 34 months of follow-up, the GP2 vaccine was shown to have minimal toxicities, and the estimated 5-year DFS in immunohistochemical (IHC)3+/FISH+ patients was 94% in vaccinated patients ($n = 51$) versus 89% in control patients ($n = 50$; $p = 0.86$) in the ITT analysis, and was 100% in vaccinated patients versus 89% in control patients in the per-treatment analysis ($p = 0.08$).[244] The preliminary results of this trial for the HER2 peptide AE37 vaccine have also shown it to be safe and well-tolerated, and were shown to provide an estimated 5-year DFS in patients with IHC1+/2+ HER2-positive tumors of 77.2% with AE37 versus 65.7% with control, which increased to 77.7% with AE37 versus 49% with control in patients with triple-negative breast cancer.[243] The 55-month follow-up results showed a trend for improved DFS in patients with stage IIB/III breast cancer (vaccine, $n = 73$, 82% vs control, $n = 61$, 67%; HR 0.48; $p = 0.06$) and low HER2 expression patients (vaccine, $n = 68$, 89% vs control, $n = 66$, 51%; HR 0.47; $p = 0.1$), and improved DFS in patients with both stage IIB/III breast cancer and low HER2 expression (vaccine, $n = 39$, 90% vs control, $n = 39$, 32%; HR 0.3; $p = 0.02$) and in patients with triple-negative breast cancer (vaccine, $n = 21$, 89% vs control, $n = 21$, 0%; HR 0.26; $p = 0.05$). As with the E75 vaccine, these results provide the rationale for further evaluation of the HER2 peptide AE37 vaccine in a phase III clinical trial for patients with triple-negative breast cancer, but also those ineligible for treatment with trastuzumab.

Combination therapy of the GP2 vaccine with standard-of-care trastuzumab has also been investigated in a phase IB trial in disease-free, HLA-A2+/A3+, HER2-positive breast cancer patients (NCT03014076). Combined treatment with the GP2 vaccine and trastuzumab was shown to be safe, and to stimulate an immunologic response to GP2 (ELISPOT: baseline 47 ± 19; after vaccination 144 ± 60; $p = 13$); the appropriate dose was identified as GP2 1000 μg with GM-CSF 250 μg.[246]

HER2/Neu pulsed dendritic-cell vaccines, in which dendritic cells are pulsed with HER2 peptides, then subsequently injected (e.g., in an intranodal or intralesion manner) have now been developed and brought to clinical trial in women with DCIS. These HER2/Neu pulsed dendritic cell vaccines have proved to be safe and capable of inducing an anti-HER2 immune response (NCT00107211).[247] This study identified no residual DCIS in 40% of vaccinated patients with ER-negative DCIS and 5.9% of vaccinated patients with ER-positive breast cancer ($p = 0.04$). In addition, phenotypes shifted postvaccination: 43.8% of patients who initially presented as ER-positive, HER2/neu-positive, luminal B DCIS shifting to ER-positive, HER2/neu-negative, luminal A, and 50% of patients who initially presented as ER-negative, HER2/neu-positive shifting to ER-negative, HER2-negative. This study also showed that the anti-HER2/neu immune response endured 52 months postimmunization.[249] Because the DC1 vaccine was shown to be more effective in ER-negative patients, the phase I/II study (NCT02061332) was amended to treat all subsequent ER-positive patients with hormone-dependent (ER-positive) tumors with concurrent AE therapy (which began with ER-positive patient 8, and affected the remaining 21 ER-positive patients enrolled to the study). The addition of AE therapy improved the pathologic complete response (pCR) of ER-positive patients (28.6%) versus no AE therapy (4.0%; $p = 0.03$); the pCR for ER-negative patients was 31.4%.[250] Results from the phase I/II study also showed that the pCR was higher in patients with DCIS (28.6%) versus invasive breast cancer (8.3%), and an anti-HER2 CD4 immune response was observed in the sentinel lymph node of all patients who achieved a pCR.[258] A phase I/II trial investigating

Table 8 Breast cancer prevention clinical trials of select vaccines.

Agent and phase	Patient population	Study design	Primary endpoint (PE) or results (R)	Reference
HER2/NEU peptide vaccines in patients with stage III–IV breast cancer				
Phase I	26 patients Stage IV breast cancer Receiving trastuzumab	HER2/neu T-helper peptide-based vaccine administered ID QM for 6 mo	R: Minimal toxicity; prolonged, robust, antigen-specific immune response (median follow-up of 36 mo from first vaccine)	Disis et al.[239]
Phase II	56 patients Stage III/IV breast cancer Completed chemotherapy Are receiving trastuzumab Completed HER2 ICD plasmid-based vaccine trial	HER2 ICD protein mixture or sterile water administered ID 6 mo postvaccination with pNGVL3-hICD vaccine	PE: Determine generation of immunologic memory to the HER2 ICD protein	NCT00363012
Phase I/II	23 patients ≥18 yr of age with HER-2-positive stage IV breast cancer	HER2/Neu peptide vaccine admixed with GM-CSF (ID on days 1, 8, and 15) plus cyclophosphamide (once on day 1) and *ex vivo*-expanded HER2-specific T cell (IV 30 min once on day 1); Rx repeated every 3–10 d for ≤3 immunizations; one booster HER2/Neu vaccine at 1 mo, followed by two at 2-mo intervals	PE: Toxicity of infusing HER2-specific T-cells (results not yet reported)	NCT00791037
Phase I	30 HER2-negative stage III–IV breast cancer patients	STEMVac with rhuGM-CSF ID Q 28 d for 3 mo, and booster vaccines at 6 and 12 mo	PE: Immunology efficacy (increased Th1 cell immunity) and incidence of toxicity per cancer therapy evaluation (results not yet reported)	NCT02157051
HER2 E75, AE37, and GP2 peptide vaccines in high-risk disease-free patients				
Phase I/II	195 high-risk node-negative patients HER2-positive breast cancer	E75 (100, 500, or 1000 µg) peptide + 250 µg GM-CSF vaccine QM for 6 mo) versus no vaccination	R: Minimal toxicity; improved DFS with vaccine versus control, particularly in optimally dosed patients	Mittendorf et al.[240] NCT00841399; NCT00584789
Phase II	275 disease-free node-positive and ER-/PR-node-negative HLA-A2, A3, A24, and/or A26+ positive HER2 IHC 1+/2+ FISH nonamplified breast cancer patients node positive and/or HR-negative (TNBC)	Herceptin (6 mg/kg Q 3 wk for 1 yr) + E75 vaccine (1.5 mg/mL, six vaccinations administered Q 3 wk, four boosters administered Q 6 mo for a total duration of 30 mo)	R: 25.7-mo follow-up: estimated DFS did not significantly differ between E75 and control; however, DFS was improved for patients with TNBC treated with E75 versus control	Clifton et al.[241] NCT01570036
VADIS Phase II	13 women >18 yr of age DCIS diagnosis by core needle biopsy HLA-A2 positive	E75 plus GM-CSF vaccine ID or GM-CSF alone on days 0 and 14, and surgery on day 28	PE: Change in E75-cytotoxic T lymphocyte count detected by dextramer assay	NCT02636582
Phase I	18 disease-free women HLA-A2 positive HER2/Neu positive (IHC 1-3+) High-risk, lymph node-negative breast cancer	GP2 (100, 500, or 1000 µg) plus GM-CSF (250 µg) vaccine versus GM-CSF alone QM for 6 mo	R: Minimal toxicity; GP2 vaccine-elicited HER2/Neu-specific immune responses for both GP2-specific and E75-specific CD8+ T-cells	Carmichael et al.[242]
Phase II	456 total (180 GP2 analysis (89 GP2, 91 GM-CSF); 298 (AE37 analysis: 153 AE37, GM-CSF 145)) disease-free breast cancer patients Node-positive or high-risk node-negative	GP2 plus GM-CSF vaccine or AE37 plus GM-CSF vaccine or GM-CSF alone (ID vaccination Q 3–4 wk to total six vaccinations, followed by four boosters at months 12, 18, 24, and 30)	*R for GP2:* Interim report (34-mo follow-up): Minimal toxicity; overall ITT analysis did not demonstrate benefit of GP2 vaccine versus control *R for AE37:* Minimal toxicity; estimated 5-yr DFS is improved in patients with IHC 1+/2+ HER2-positive tumors or TNBC treated with vaccine versus control; 55-mo follow-up results: trend for improved DFS in stage IIB/III patients and HER2 LE patients, and an improved DFS in patient with both stage IIB/III and HER2 LE and patients with TNBC patients	Mittendorf et al.[243] Mittendorf et al.[244] Peace et al.[245] NCT00524277
Phase IB	17 in results disease-free breast cancer patients HLA-A2+/A3+, HER2-positive breast cancer	GP2 plus GM-CSF vaccine (six 1.0 mL inoculations given every 21 d) with standard-of-care trastuzumab infusion or trastuzumab alone	R: No dose-limiting or grade 3–5 local or systemic toxicities; appropriate dose was 1000 µg of GP2 + 250 µg of GM-CSF	Clifton et al.[246] NCT03014076

(*continued overleaf*)

Table 8 (Continued)

Agent and phase	Patient population	Study design	Primary endpoint (PE) or results (R)	Reference
HER2/NEU pulsed dendritic cell vaccines in women with DCIS				
Phase I	29 (30) women ≥18 yr of age HER2/neu-positive DCIS or DCIS with microinvasion (<1 mm)	HER2/Neu DC1 vaccine by intranodal, intralesional, or both, vaccination QW for 4 wk	R: Minimal toxicity; vaccine-induced decline and/or eradication of HER-2/neu expression; no DCIS remained in 40% ER− and 5.9% ER+ patients; phenotypes shifted postvaccination; sensitization of Th cells to ≥1 class II peptides and HER2/neu peptide responses endured 52-mo postimmunization	Sharma et al.[247] Datta et al.[248] Koski et al.[249] NCT00107211
Phase I/II	58 women ≥18 yr of age HER-2/neu-positive DCIS, DCIS with microinvasion, DCIS with invasive disease (<5 mm), or Paget's disease of the nipple	HER2/Neu (1.0–2.0 × 107 cells per dose) DC1 vaccine by intranodal, intralesional, or both, QW for 6 wk	R: Vaccination was well tolerated; pCR was highest in ER-negative patients; AE therapy improved pCR of ER-positive patients; vaccination route did not affect immune response rate; pCR rate was higher in DCIS versus IBC patients; all pCR patients had anti-HER2 CD4 immune response in sentinel lymph node	Lowenfeld et al.[250] NCT02061332
Phase I/II	Five (58) women ≥18 yr of age HER-2/3-positive DCIS	HER2/Neu DC1 vaccine (QW for 6 wk) plus trastuzumab (loading dose 8 mg/kg, maintenance dose 6 mg/kg at week 4) and pertuzumab (420 mg IV given concurrently with trastuzumab)	PE: Related adverse events (results not yet reported)	NCT02336984

Abbreviations: CDH-3, cadherin 3; STEMVac, CD105/Yb-1/SOX2/CDH3/ MDM2-polyepitope plasmid DNA vaccine; DFS, disease-free survival; DCIS, ductal carcinoma *in situ*; CD105, endoglin; ER, estrogen receptor; Q, every; FISH, fluorescence *in situ* hybridization; GP2, HER2/Neu-derived epitope GP2 (amino acids 654–662); AE37, HER2 peptide AE37; GM-CSF, granulocyte colony-stimulating factor (sargramostim); HR, hormone receptor; HER2, human epidermal growth factor receptor 2; NeuVax; E75, HER2 peptide nelipepimut-S; HLA, human leukocyte antigen; IHC, immunohistochemistry; ITT, intention-to-treat; ICD, intracellular domain; ID, intradermal; IV, intravenous; IBC, invasive breast cancer; LE, low expression; lum, luminal; MDM2, MDM2 proto-oncogene; QM, once per month (quaque mensis); QW, once per week; VADIS, Nelipepimut-S Peptide Vaccine in Women with DCIS of the Breast; pCR, pathologic complete response; DC1, pulsed dendritic cell; SOX-2, SRY-box transcription factor 2; Th1, T helper type 1 cell; TNBC, triple-negative breast cancer; Yb-1, Y-box 1.

the DC1 vaccine with trastuzumab and pertuzumab is currently ongoing in women with HER-positive DCIS (NCT02336984).

The results from these, and future, ongoing clinical trials investigating vaccines for the prevention of breast cancer will determine the effectiveness of vaccines in this setting. However, cross-sectional combination therapy (e.g., strategies that fuse behavioral and dietary changes, chemotherapeutic drug(s) and vaccine(s)) will likely be necessary for the prevention of all breast cancers.

In addition to preventing breast cancer, vaccines are showing promise for preventing CRC prevention. Mucin 1 (MUC1) is a promising target for vaccination efforts in this cancer. It is overexpressed and hypo-glycosylated in different stages of CRC, including in premalignant lesions.[259] In animal models using MUC1 transgenic *APC* Min+ and IL10-knock-out mice, vaccination with a MUC1 peptide resulted in a reduced number of polyps, amelioration of inflammation and prevented progression to colitis-associated colon cancer.[260,261] In a subsequent phase I/II open-label trial of 39 evaluable patients with a history of adenomas, MUC1 vaccination resulted in a strong anti-MUC1 IgG antibody response among 44% of participants and induced a long-term memory response among 75% of those receiving the booster at 52 weeks.[262] No toxicities were observed among responders to the vaccine. A phase II trial is currently ongoing (NCT02134925).

Therapeutic vaccines targeting carcinoembryonic antigen (CEA), KRAS, and TP53 have been tested in animal models and in early-phase clinical trials for advanced cancers, including CRC, but have yet to be examined in earlier and premalignant disease stages.

The future of vaccine strategies for the prevention of cancer is extremely promising. Vaccines to prevent virally induced cancers have made a significant public health impact. Going forward, vaccines for nonvirally induced cancers may become a critical public health strategy to reduce the burden of cancer further.

Immune checkpoint inhibitors

Immune checkpoint inhibitors (ICIs) are monoclonal antibodies that target key regulatory proteins in the immune response. By binding to their cognate receptors, ICIs prevent suppression of the immune system in the tumor microenvironment, therefore allowing a selected immune response against the tumor. Several of these ICIs have been approved for the treatment of various advanced cancers. Pembrolizumab, which targets the PD-1 on activated T-cells, has been approved for treating mismatch repair deficient (dMMR) and microsatellite instability-high (MSI-H) tumors, irrespective of tissue of origin.[263] This tumor-agnostic approval was based upon five clinical trials (KEYNOTE-012, 016, 028, 158, and 164) totaling 149 patients, more than half of which had dMMR/MSI-H CRC.[263] These findings suggest that individuals at risk of CRC due to Lynch syndrome, defined by mutations in the dMMR genes, may benefit from PD-1 inhibition. Work is presently ongoing to better understand the immune profile of the earliest stages of CRC development to advance the use of ICIs for CRC immunoprevention in a subset of high-risk individuals.[264] A phase II clinical trial is currently testing if nivolumab, another PD-1 inhibitor, can decrease the incidence of colonic adenomas in patients with genetic predisposition to CRC and a history of hemicolectomy due to colon cancer or advanced colon adenoma (NCT03631641).

Along with showing promise in CRC, ICIs have significantly altered the treatment of NSCLC in the last several years. Numerous seminal phase III clinical trials have established the use of PD-1 inhibitors in various treatment settings for both squamous and nonsquamous NSCLC.[265] While clinical responses are correlated with the expression level of PD-1 on both tumor cells and tumor-infiltrating immune cells, PD-1 is not a perfect biomarker of response in lung cancer treatment and tumor mutational burden has also been shown to play a role.[265] Recent preclinical work in lung squamous cell carcinoma has shown that immune activation and escape occur before tumor invasion,[266] revealed relevant immune biomarkers of the preinvasive stages of lung carcinogenesis,[266] and identified four molecular subtypes of premalignant lesions with distinct differences in epithelial and immune processes that may guide immunopreventive therapy.[267]

While ICIs are now being used to treat advanced cancers, ongoing preclinical and clinical studies will determine if and how they might be used at earlier stages of neoplasia, particularly for early colorectal and lung neoplasia. The current body of evidence suggests that the immune system plays a pivotal role in modulating the biology of premalignant lesions, providing a strong premise for investigation of immunotherapies at earlier disease stages.[9,10] Recent study identified chromosome copy-number driven immune escape in the oral precancer-invasive cancer transition,[203] which has important implications for immune oncology in chemoprevention trial designs testing immune-checkpoint inhibitors. It is likely that in the near future, ICIs and/or other related immune-modulatory agents will be harnessed to prevent cancer. With immunomodulatory agents, cancer preventive vaccines, and traditional chemopreventive agents, the prospect of safely preventing most cancers is highly likely.

Conclusions

Clinical cancer chemoprevention has matured with the FDA approvals of at least 14 agents to prevent cancer or to treat or prevent IEN. For the most common malignancies, agents have been approved for breast and CRCs, but lung and prostate cancers have yet to see approvals for preventive agents. Personalized approaches to identify patients most likely to benefit and least likely to be harmed by particular interventions are evolving from continued study of aspirin and celecoxib in colorectal neoplasia. Aspirin, alone and in combination, has been and continues to be actively investigated for its preventive effects in CRC. In the future, a comprehensive, long-term assessment of all of aspirin's benefits and harms—taking into account CVD risk reduction, cancer risk reduction, GI bleeding risks, and overall mortality—will be needed given the important and wide-ranging data that continue to accrue regarding its effects in most "healthy" or asymptomatic populations, except the elderly. The recent approvals of the HPV vaccines for cervical cancer prevention provide hope for the creation and approval of additional preventive vaccines for other cancer types. Two of the most promising current directions of cancer chemoprevention are agent combinations and immunoprevention. The concept that combinations can increase the ratio of benefit (activity) to risk (toxicity) for effective single agents received strong support from the stunning colorectal adenoma results of the DFMO–sulindac trial discussed earlier. Based on this and subsequent trials of agent combinations, this approach may be at the threshold of becoming a standard clinical reality, and other active combinations should be moved into clinical trials.[268] Immune-based preventive strategies are just coming into clinical investigations, premised on their efficacy in later stages of cancer and the documented suppression of immunosurveillance in early carcinogenesis.

Summary

Cancer chemoprevention has added impressive data to the long list of advances resulting from cancer therapy. There have been several exciting developments in clinical chemoprevention, including, for example, the FDA approval of agents for breast and CRC prevention, followed by subsequent FDA approvals of the HPV vaccines for reducing cervical neoplasia risk, and, most recently, for oropharyngeal and head and neck cancers. More recently, AIs have been shown to prevent breast cancers in postmenopausal women, with a favorable side-effect profile. A RCT of combined sulindac and DFMO achieved an extraordinary 70% reduction in colorectal adenomas (>90% in advanced adenomas) highlighting the potential of combined agents and signaling, perhaps, the near realization of this approach in standard clinical practice. Chemopreventive agents have yet to be approved for lung or prostate cancers, although recent advances in the treatment of advanced lung cancers with molecularly targeted agents including PARP inhibitors and immune-checkpoint inhibitors suggest these approaches as possible strategies to be tested at earlier stages of the disease. Immunoprevention strategies, including vaccines, show great promise.

Key references

The complete reference list can be found on Vital Source version of this title, see inside front cover.

2 Lippman SM, Benner SE, Hong WK. Cancer chemoprevention. *J Clin Oncol.* 1994;**12**(4):851–873. doi: 10.1200/JCO.1994.12.4.851.

5 Kensler TW, Spira A, Garber JE, et al. Transforming cancer prevention through precision medicine and immune-oncology. *Cancer Prev Res (Phila).* 2016;**9**(1):2–10. doi: 10.1158/1940-6207.CAPR-15-0406.

8 Spira A, Yurgelun MB, Alexandrov L, et al. Precancer atlas to drive precision prevention trials. *Cancer Res.* 2017;**77**(7):1510–1541. doi: 10.1158/0008-5472.CAN-16-2346.

13 Gail MH, Brinton LA, Byar DP, et al. Projecting individualized probabilities of developing breast cancer for white females who are being examined annually. *J Natl Cancer Inst.* 1989;**81**(24):1879–1886.

39 The Alpha-Tocopherol, Beta-Carotene Cancer Prevention Study Group. The effect of vitamin E and beta carotene on the incidence of lung cancer and other cancers in male smokers. *N Engl J Med.* 1994;**330**(15):1029–1035. doi: 10.1056/NEJM199404143301501.

41 Omenn GS, Goodman GE, Thornquist MD, et al. Effects of a combination of beta carotene and vitamin A on lung cancer and cardiovascular disease. *N Engl J Med.* 1996;**334**(18):1150–1155.

45 Klein EA, Thompson IM Jr, Tangen CM, et al. Vitamin E and the risk of prostate cancer: the Selenium and Vitamin E Cancer Prevention Trial (SELECT). *JAMA.* 2011;**306**(14):1549–1556. doi: 10.1001/jama.2011.1437.

53 Steinbach G, Lynch PM, Phillips RK, et al. The effect of celecoxib, a cyclooxygenase-2 inhibitor, in familial adenomatous polyposis. *N Engl J Med.* 2000;**342**(26):1946–1952.

57 Burn J, Gerdes A-M, Macrae F, et al. Long-term effect of aspirin on cancer risk in carriers of hereditary colorectal cancer: an analysis from the CAPP2 randomised controlled trial. *Lancet.* 2011;**378**(9809):2081–2087.

59 Samadder NJ, Neklason DW, Boucher KM, et al. Effect of sulindac and erlotinib vs placebo on duodenal neoplasia in familial adenomatous polyposis: a randomized clinical trial. *JAMA.* 2016;**315**(12):1266–1275. doi: 10.1001/jama.2016.2522.

64 Sandler RS, Halabi S, Baron JA, et al. A randomized trial of aspirin to prevent colorectal adenomas in patients with previous colorectal cancer. *N Engl J Med.* 2003;**348**(10):883–890.

65 Baron JA, Cole BF, Sandler RS, et al. A randomized trial of aspirin to prevent colorectal adenomas. *N Engl J Med.* 2003;**348**(10):891–899.

70. Cook NR, Lee IM, Gaziano JM, et al. Low-dose aspirin in the primary prevention of cancer: the Women's Health Study: a randomized controlled trial. *JAMA*. 2005;**294**(1):47–55. doi: 10.1001/jama.294.1.47.
76. Bibbins-Domingo K. Force USPST. Aspirin use for the primary prevention of cardiovascular disease and colorectal cancer: U.S. preventive services task force recommendation statement. *Ann Intern Med*. 2016;**164**(12):836–845. doi: 10.7326/M16-0577.
81. Bresalier RS, Sandler RS, Quan H, et al. Cardiovascular events associated with rofecoxib in a colorectal adenoma chemoprevention trial. *N Engl J Med*. 2005;**352**(11):1092–1102. doi: 10.1056/NEJMoa050493.
84. Bertagnolli MM, Eagle CJ, Zauber AG, et al. Celecoxib for the prevention of sporadic colorectal adenomas. *N Engl J Med*. 2006;**355**(9):873–884.
85. Solomon SD, Wittes J, Finn PV, et al. Cardiovascular risk of celecoxib in 6 randomized placebo-controlled trials: the cross trial safety analysis. *Circulation*. 2008;**117**(16):2104–2113.
86. Meyskens FL, McLaren CE, Pelot D, et al. Difluoromethylornithine plus sulindac for the prevention of sporadic colorectal adenomas: a randomized placebo-controlled, double-blind trial. *Cancer Prev Res (Phila)*. 2008;**1**(1):32–38. doi: 10.1158/1940-6207.CAPR-08-0042.
93. Wactawski-Wende J, Kotchen JM, Anderson GL, et al. Calcium plus vitamin D supplementation and the risk of colorectal cancer. *N Engl J Med*. 2006;**354**(7):684–696.
95. Baron JA, Barry EL, Mott LA, et al. A trial of calcium and vitamin D for the prevention of colorectal adenomas. *N Engl J Med*. 2015;**373**(16):1519–1530. doi: 10.1056/NEJMoa1500409.
108. Powles TJ, Ashley S, Tidy A, et al. Twenty-year follow-up of the Royal Marsden randomized, double-blinded tamoxifen breast cancer prevention trial. *J Natl Cancer Inst*. 2007;**99**(4):283–290.
110. Fisher B, Costantino JP, Wickerham DL, et al. Tamoxifen for prevention of breast cancer: report of the National Surgical Adjuvant Breast and Bowel Project P-1 Study. *J Natl Cancer Inst*. 1998;**90**(18):1371–1388.
113. Veronesi U, Maisonneuve P, Rotmensz N, et al. Tamoxifen for the prevention of breast cancer: late results of the Italian Randomized Tamoxifen Prevention Trial among women with hysterectomy. *J Natl Cancer Inst*. 2007;**99**(9):727–737.
116. Cuzick J, Sestak I, Cawthorn S, et al. Tamoxifen for prevention of breast cancer: extended long-term follow-up of the IBIS-I breast cancer prevention trial. *Lancet Oncol*. 2015;**16**(1):67–75. doi: 10.1016/s1470-2045(14)71171-4.
117. Vogel VG, Costantino JP, Wickerham DL, et al. Effects of tamoxifen vs raloxifene on the risk of developing invasive breast cancer and other disease outcomes: the NSABP Study of Tamoxifen and Raloxifene (STAR) P-2 trial. *JAMA*. 2006;**295**(23):2727–2741. doi: 10.1001/jama.295.23.joc60074.
119. DeCensi A, Puntoni M, Guerrieri-Gonzaga A, et al. Randomized placebo controlled trial of low-dose tamoxifen to prevent local and contralateral recurrence in breast intraepithelial neoplasia. *J Clin Oncol*. 2019;**37**(19):1629–1637. doi: 10.1200/JCO.18.01779.
130. Early Breast Cancer Trialists Collaborative Group. Effects of adjuvant tamoxifen and of cytotoxic therapy on mortality in early breast cancer. An overview of 61 randomized trials among 28,896 women. *N Engl J Med*. 1988;**319**(26):1681–1692. doi: 10.1056/NEJM198812293192601.
143. Goss PE, Ingle JN, Ales-Martinez JE, et al. Exemestane for breast-cancer prevention in postmenopausal women. *N Engl J Med*. 2011;**364**(25):2381–2391.
145. Cuzick J, Sestak I, Forbes JF, et al. Use of anastrozole for breast cancer prevention (IBIS-II): long-term results of a randomised controlled trial. *Lancet*. 2020;**395**(10218):117–122. doi: 10.1016/S0140-6736(19)32955-1.
176. Thompson IM, Goodman PJ, Tangen CM, et al. The influence of finasteride on the development of prostate cancer. *N Engl J Med*. 2003;**349**(3):215–224.
187. Thompson IM Jr, Goodman PJ, Tangen CM, et al. Long-term survival of participants in the prostate cancer prevention trial. *N Engl J Med*. 2013;**369**(7):603–610. doi: 10.1056/NEJMoa1215932.
188. Goodman PJ, Tangen CM, Darke AK, et al. Long-term effects of finasteride on prostate cancer mortality. *N Engl J Med*. 2019;**380**(4):393–394. doi: 10.1056/NEJMc1809961.
199. Gaziano JM, Sesso HD, Christen WG, et al. Multivitamins in the prevention of cancer in men: the Physicians' Health Study II randomized controlled trial. *JAMA*. 2012;**308**(18):1871–1880. doi: 10.1001/jama.2012.14641.
206. Chiang CJ, Yang YW, You SL, et al. Thirty-year outcomes of the national hepatitis B immunization program in Taiwan. *JAMA*. 2013;**310**(9):974–976. doi: 10.1001/jama.2013.276701.
215. Paavonen J, Jenkins D, Bosch FX, et al. Efficacy of a prophylactic adjuvanted bivalent L1 virus-like-particle vaccine against infection with human papillomavirus types 16 and 18 in young women: an interim analysis of a phase III double-blind, randomised controlled trial. *Lancet*. 2007;**369**(9580):2161–2170. doi: 10.1016/S0140-6736(07)60946-5.
219. Hildesheim A, Wacholder S, Catteau G, et al. Efficacy of the HPV-16/18 vaccine: final according to protocol results from the blinded phase of the randomized Costa Rica HPV-16/18 vaccine trial. *Vaccine*. 2014;**32**(39):5087–5097. doi: 10.1016/j.vaccine.2014.06.038.
223. Palefsky JM, Giuliano AR, Goldstone S, et al. HPV vaccine against anal HPV infection and anal intraepithelial neoplasia. *N Engl J Med*. 2011;**365**(17):1576–1585. doi: 10.1056/NEJMoa1010971.
228. Huh WK, Joura EA, Giuliano AR, et al. Final efficacy, immunogenicity, and safety analyses of a nine-valent human papillomavirus vaccine in women aged 16-26 years: a randomised, double-blind trial. *Lancet*. 2017;**390**(10108):2143–2159. doi: 10.1016/S0140-6736(17)31821-4.
262. Kimura T, McKolanis JR, Dzubinski LA, et al. MUC1 vaccine for individuals with advanced adenoma of the colon: a cancer immunoprevention feasibility study. *Cancer Prev Res (Phila)*. 2013;**6**(1):18–26. doi: 10.1158/1940-6207.CAPR-12-0275.
266. Mascaux C, Angelova M, Vasaturo A, et al. Immune evasion before tumour invasion in early lung squamous carcinogenesis. *Nature*. 2019;**571**(7766):570–575. doi: 10.1038/s41586-019-1330-0.

36 Cancer screening and early detection

Otis W. Brawley, MD, MACP

> **Overview**
>
> Cancer screening is a means of early detection of malignancy in an asymptomatic individual at risk for the disease. A positive screening test calls for additional diagnostic tests. The purpose of screening is to find a small, localized tumor that is destined to grow, metastasize, and kill before it spreads. Effective treatment can then lead to prevention of death. Simply finding disease is not adequate proof of benefit. Proper evaluation of a screening *test* involves demonstration that it leads to reduced risk of death. Screening is a population-based intervention; appropriate individuals should be in a program of routine screening. Screening and treatment involve interventions which are often invasive. Proper evaluation of a screening *program* involves assessment of outcomes and a comparison of the benefits and risks.

Cancer screening is a means of early detection of malignancy in an asymptomatic individual at risk for that disease. A positive test indicates that disease may be present and additional "diagnostic" testing is necessary to confirm the presence and extent of disease. In a symptomatic person, the same test is often considered "diagnostic" rather than screening.[1]

The purpose of screening is not simply to find disease but to reduce the incidence of advanced disease and find disease at a point in its natural history where treatment will prevent death. Early detection is desired because prognosis is usually better when treating lower stage versus metastatic cancers. Some screening efforts now focus on identifying and treating precursor lesions to prevent malignancy. Secondarily, a screening test may decrease morbidity associated with treatment and/or improve quality of life. In clinical study, prevention of death is demonstrated by reduction in cancer mortality rates.[2]

Key criteria for screening

Cancer screening is most effective and efficient if performed for diseases with high prevalence and significant population impact. The *sojourn time* is the period in which an occult tumor can be detected by screening before metastasis or the onset of symptoms.[2] For successful screening, the sojourn time should be sufficiently long to allow periodic screening to detect many cancers in the target population before disease has spread; treatment of disease should have greater benefit when given before, compared with after, symptom onset; and the screening test should meet acceptable levels of accuracy and cost.[1]

Evaluation of early detection programs

Evaluation of a screening test should assess whether the test finds cancer or increases survival time and whether subjects have a lower risk of dying from the disease as a result of screening. Evaluations of screening tests outside the context of a rigorous research design are subject to many biases that can invalidate the conclusions drawn.

Potential biases in the evaluation of screening

Lead-time bias: the time from an occult condition being detected by screening and the moment that condition would have become known through development of symptoms is known as the *lead time*. A bias toward better survival always exists in a screened group, because screening moves the point of diagnosis to an earlier time point. True lead-time bias occurs when earlier detection only advances the time of a patient's diagnosis, without prolonging life (Figure 1). Because of the effect of lead-time bias, an increase in survival or improved 5-year survival rates cannot be used alone to assess a screening test.

Length bias is the bias toward detection of less-threatening cancers (Figure 2). Cancers that grow more slowly and have a long sojourn time are more likely to be detected in screening. Faster growing, more aggressive cancers with a short sojourn time are more apt to escape detection and be diagnosed due to symptoms in between scheduled screens. A cohort of cancer patients with screen-detected tumors will have a higher proportion with slow-growing tumors compared to a population diagnosed without screening, and thus will appear to have better survival.

Overdiagnosis is the concept that some tumors fulfill all histologic criteria of malignancy but are not destined to cause death and would not have become known to the patient without screening (Figure 3).[3] Overdiagnosis is an extreme form of length bias. There are two kinds of overdiagnosis. First is the disease that histologically is indistinguishable from precancer or cancer but has no biological propensity to progress.[4] This is common among screen-detected premalignant lesions of the uterine cervix and cancers of the prostate and thyroid. Second are tumors that can be lethal but not in the specific patient because s/he would have died from another cause during the sojourn time.[4] A persistently higher incidence rate within a population can be due to lead time, the introduction of previously unscreened cohorts into the screening program, and overdiagnosis.

Selection bias is the concept that individuals who participate in screening may differ from those who do not, that is, they may be more health conscious, more likely to control risk factors, more disease aware, more adherent to treatment, and generally healthier.[5] Selection bias can give the appearance of better screening outcomes than expected and may even limit the generalizability of results from studies designed to overcome the influence of selection bias. For example, current and former smokers who entered the National Lung Screening Trial (NLST) had substantially less emphysema, cardiac disease, and diabetes compared to a representative sample of Americans.[5]

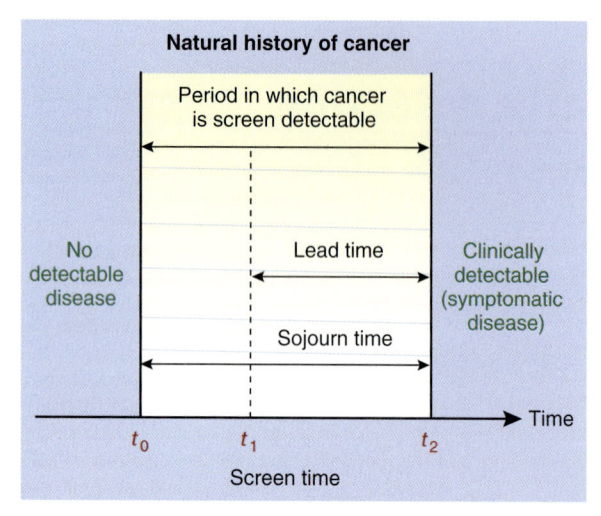

Figure 1 The natural history of cancer. In this figure, $t_2 - t_0$ is the duration of the preclinical screen-detectable period, known as the "sojourn time"; $t_2 - t_1$ is the amount of time by which the diagnosis is advanced by screening, known as the "lead time." Under the assumption of an exponential distribution of sojourn time, the expected lead time of an individual screen-detected case is equal to the mean of the distribution of the sojourn time.

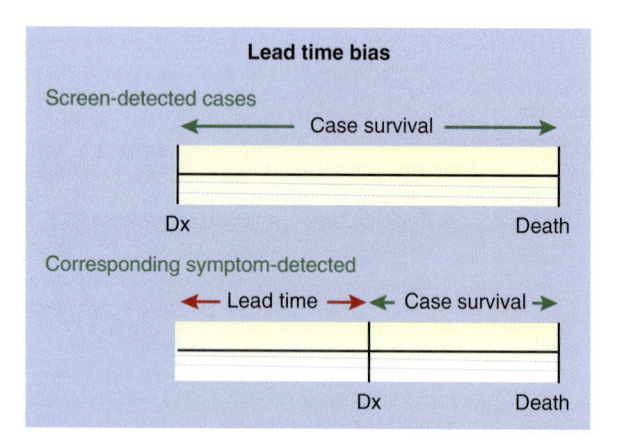

Figure 2 Lead-time bias. In this figure, Dx is the time of diagnosis. Note that the screen-detected cases and the cases diagnosed with symptoms each die at the same time, but the survival time looks greater in the screen-detected case because of lead-time bias. Source: Adapted from www.3.cancer.gov/prevention/lss/vaslides.html.

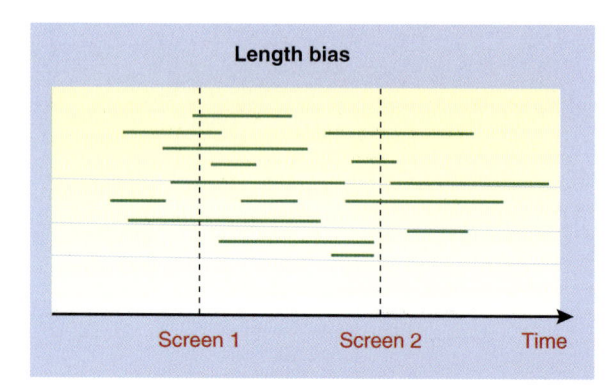

Figure 3 Length bias. In this figure, the horizontal lines represent the sojourn times of individual tumors detected in a screening program. The two screening examinations detect six out of eight long sojourn-time tumors, but only two out of six short sojourn-time tumors.

Table 1 Measures of screening performance.

	Disease	Status
Screening test results	Yes	No
Positive	a	b
Negative	c	d

Sensitivity = $a/(a+c)$; specificity = $d/(b+d)$; positive predictive value (PPV) = $a/(a+b)$; negative predictive value (NPV) = $c/(c+d)$.

A unique form of selection bias can occur in a randomized trial in which subjects in the intervention arm are consented, while those in the control arm are not aware that they are being followed in the study. Less-healthy individuals in the intervention arm may refuse participation, while those in the control arm cannot.[6,7]

Characteristics of a screening test

Sensitivity and specificity: sensitivity, or the positive rate, is the probability of a positive result when applied to a person who truly has the disease. Specificity, or the true negative rate, is the probability of a negative result in a person who does not have the disease (Table 1). Both high sensitivity and high specificity are desirable in a screening test. Unfortunately, they tend to be negatively correlated. While tests with high sensitivity succeed at detecting most occult disease, a test with low specificity will lead to many false positives and additional workup.

Positive and negative predictive values: the positive predictive value (PPV) is the probability that a subject with a positive screening result actually has the disease (Table 1). The negative predictive value (NPV) is the probability that a subject who screens negative is truly free of disease; this provides some quantification of the reassurance value of a negative test. It is arguably more important to have a high NPV, as this will mean that few disease subjects are missed and potentially have delayed diagnosis and treatment.

Efficacy versus effectiveness: screening studies usually assess the *efficacy* of an intervention, that is, whether the test saves lives among the population enrolled in the trial. An additional question is the *effectiveness* of the intervention when it is widely used. A few large clinical trials come close to assessing effectiveness, although these studies may be influenced by healthy volunteer effects due to the consent process.[1] Ultimately, the effectiveness of a screening intervention should be assessed through program evaluation in real-world situations rather than experimental studies in order to consider factors such as provider experience, improvements in screening technology over time, acceptability to the population, and cost-effectiveness, which must encompass downstream considerations such as recall rate and the costs of treating overdiagnosis.

Research designs to evaluate a screening intervention

Descriptive studies are the easiest screening studies to perform and often provide the first evidence that screening may contribute to disease control. These are uncontrolled observations based on the experience of physicians, clinics, or cancer registries. Descriptive studies that examine populations, or groups, as the unit of observation are known as ecological studies. Descriptive studies can yield useful information but provide the weakest evidence due to inherent biases and cannot establish efficacy because of the absence of a control group.

Case-control studies are typically retrospective studies comparing a group of patients (cases) who have an outcome of interest (disease, death, interval cancer, etc.) with a group (controls) who do not, in order to examine factors that may have contributed to the outcome. Cases and controls are matched for key characteristics, such as age, gender, socio-economic status, etc. Case-control studies are generally inexpensive and provide evidence more quickly than prospective studies. These studies are challenging due to the need to avoid biases, and results can be easily confounded by uncontrolled factors.

Prospective randomized clinical trials (RCTs) are the most rigorous assessment of screening, in that they typically compare disease-specific mortality in a group randomized to receive a screening invitation with a group that receives usual care. The distorting effects of self-selection and other biases are minimized through randomization. The mortality endpoint is not subject to the effects of lead time, length bias, or overdiagnosis. RCTs should be analyzed by intention-to-treat analysis, meaning that end results are based on comparisons between invited and uninvited groups rather than screened and unscreened groups. An analysis that includes only those who are screened interjects bias.

The large sample size required, the expense, and the long study duration has limited the number of prospective RCTs conducted. Some have argued that all-cause mortality is preferred to disease-specific mortality as the primary endpoint, as it avoids potential biases in allocation of cause of death and avoids failure to measure other causes of death that may be an outcome of diagnostic and treatment interventions. The greater size and cost of an RCT measuring all-cause mortality makes them highly impractical.[8]

Meta-analyses—statistical analyses combining the results of multiple studies addressing the same question—are often used in the screening literature. A meta-analysis usually assesses prospective randomized studies and can assess evidence-based trends. Statistical modeling of screening interventions is also becoming popular and is used to predict screening effects in certain circumstances.[9] While modeling studies can be useful, limitations exist and caution in interpretation is merited. Modeling studies require assumptions and are often idealizations or simplifications of reality.[10]

A number of medical and professional organizations review the scientific literature and develop screening recommendations or guidelines.[11] The US Preventive Services Task Force (USPSTF) is known for using a very conservative process designed to minimize the influence of conflicts of interest and financial-, intellectual-, and emotional factors.[12,13] These recommendations are updated continuously and available at www.uspreventiveservicestaskforce.org. The American Cancer Society (ACS) also publishes guidelines (Table 2) and numerous medical specialty societies publish either guidelines or screening recommendations for their represented disease.

Organized versus opportunistic screening: screening can be offered in a regimented program in which subjects are tracked for compliance with screening recommendations and quality of screening is measured through systematic audit. Breast screening is done in this way in many European countries. In the United States, most screening is opportunistic, with limited tracking of compliance or quality. Some American mammography facilities meet European standards for organized screening programs. In both the United States and Europe, very few broad standards exist for screening for other diseases.

Breast cancer screening

Among women worldwide, breast cancer is the most commonly diagnosed cancer and the leading cause of cancer death. In the United States, the median age at diagnosis is 61, and the median age of death is 68.[14]

Screening methods for breast cancer

Mammography is an X-ray examination of the breasts that produces high-quality craniocaudal and mediolateral oblique images of each breast with minimal X-ray dose. Evidence suggests that digital imaging provides more accurate interpretation, improved diagnosis in women with dense breasts, and equivalence to traditional film mammography for postmenopausal women.[15]

The rate of abnormal interpretations is higher for first screening (5–10%) than for later mammograms.[16] Most abnormalities are resolved through additional imaging with other mammographic views or by ultrasonography. Abnormalities that cannot be resolved are biopsied with ultrasonographic- or radiographically directed fine-needle aspiration, core-needle biopsy, or surgical excision.

Nine RCTs for breast cancer screening have been published to date (Table 3). The trials vary in the age range of women enrolled, the screening tests used (mammography alone or with clinical breast examination [CBE]), the screening intervals, and even the years of follow-up. All RCTs were started and most completed before the modern era of adjuvant chemotherapy, and several were prior to the advent of hormonal therapy. Screening and diagnostic equipment have also improved.[28] There is consensus that a well-run screening program has the potential to reduce risk of breast cancer-specific death.[29,30]

There has been tremendous debate about whether screening of normal risk women should begin at age 40 or 50.[28] The dispute is largely based on the lack of clear RCT-based evidence that mammography screening for women aged 40–49 years is effective. Some studies show a statistically significant advantage to screening women in their forties and others do not.[31]

The most recent RCT is the UK AGE Study, in which some patients may have received modern adjuvant therapy.[27] In all, 53,884 women of ages 39–41 were invited to screening. The control group was unaware of their participation and received "usual medical care." As discussed earlier, this presents a bias. After 10.7 years of follow-up, a statistically nonsignificant, 17% lower, relative risk (RR) of breast cancer death was found in the screening versus control groups (RR = 0.83, 0.66–1.04).[27]

An analysis of the nine large randomized trials of screening suggests that screening leads to an 8% relative risk reduction in mortality (RR 0.92; 95% confidence interval [CI] 0.75–1.02) for mammography screening in women of ages 39–49 after up to 20 years of follow-up. Of note, about half of all women between ages 40 and 49 who are screened annually will have a false-positive mammogram necessitating further evaluation, which can include biopsy.

The USPSTF meta-analysis of large RCTs (Table 4), including the AGE study, found a 15% relative risk reduction in mortality (RR = 0.85; 95% CI, 0.75–0.96) for women of ages 40–49 who were invited to 2–9 rounds of screening after 11–20 years of follow-up.[36,37] This translates into 1904 women being invited to screening to prevent or delay one breast cancer death.[38] More than half of these women are estimated to have had a false-positive scan during the 10 years of screening. Changing the screening interval to every 2 years marginally decreases the number of lives saved while nearly halving the false-positive rate.[39]

Table 2 American Cancer Society screening guidelines for the early detection of cancer in average-risk asymptomatic people.

Breast	Women aged 40–54 yr	Mammography	Women should have the choice to start annual screening mammography starting at ages 40–44 yr; women aged 45–54 yr should be screened annually
	Women aged ≥55 yr	Mammography	Women aged ≥55 yr should switch to screening every 2 yr can continue annual screening annually. Screening should continue as long as the woman is in good health and is expected to live at least 10 more years
Cervix	Women aged 25–65 yr	Primary HPV testing or a HPV test plus a Pap test	Cervical cancer screening should begin at age 25 and should continue every 5 yr. If HPV testing is not available, individuals should be screened with co-testing (an HPV test and a Pap test) every 5 yr or a Pap test every 3 yr (acceptable).
	Women aged >65 yr		Women who had regular cervical cancer testing in the past 10 yr with normal results should not be tested for cervical cancer. Once testing is stopped, it should not be resumed. Those with a history of a serious cervical precancer should continue to be tested for at least 25 yr after that diagnosis, even if testing goes past 65
	Women who have had a total hysterectomy		Women whose cervix has been removed by surgery for reasons not related to cervical cancer or serious precancer should not be tested
Colorectal	Men and women, aged 45–75 yr, for all tests listed	Fecal immunochemical test (annual), or high-sensitivity guaiac-based fecal occult blood test (annual), or multitarget stool DNA test (every 3 yr, per manufacturer's recommendation), or colonoscopy (every 10 yr), or CT colonography (every 5 yr), or flexible sigmoidoscopy (every 5 yr).	Adults aged 45 yr and older should undergo regular screening with either a high-sensitivity, stool-based test or a structural (visual) examination, depending on patient preference and test availability. As part of the screening process, all positive results on noncolonoscopy screening tests should be followed with timely colonoscopy; adults in good health should continue screening through the age of 75 yr
	Men and women aged 76–85 yr		Screening decisions should be discussed with a health care provider based on the patient's preferences, health status, and prior screening history
	Men and women aged >85 yr		These individuals should no longer get colorectal cancer screening
Endometrial	Women, at menopause		At the time of menopause, women should be informed about risks and symptoms of endometrial cancer and strongly encouraged to report any unexpected vaginal bleeding or spotting to their physicians
Lung	Current or former smokers aged 50–80 yr in fairly good health with at least a 20-pack-year history of smoking	Low-dose CT scan	Annual screening in adults who currently smoke or have quit within the past 15 yr AND have at least a 20 pack-year smoking history. Those who will be screened should also (1) receive counseling to quit smoking if they currently smoke (2) be told by their doctor about the possible benefits, limits, and harms of screening with LDCT scans, and (3) that they can go to a center that has experience in lung cancer screening and treatment
Prostate	Men aged ≥50 yr	Prostate-specific antigen (PSA) test with or without digital rectal examination	Men should talk to a health care provider about the pros and cons of testing so they can decide if testing is the right choice for them. Men who are African American or who have a father or brother who had prostate cancer before age 65 should talk with their health care provider about the pros and cons of testing starting at age 45. Men who decide to be tested should get a PSA blood test with or without a rectal exam. How often you get tested will depend on your PSA level

The higher prevalence of mammographic density among women in their forties compared to their fifties complicates interpretation of mammograms in the younger group. Studies show that the accuracy, sensitivity, and specificity of a given mammogram varies by radiologist, but in general, improves with increasing patient age.[40,41] Among women screened regularly, interval cancers are more prevalent in those aged 40–49 years.[42]

Clinical breast examination (CBE) and breast self-examination (BSE)

A competent CBE involves physical palpation of the breast—in small segments, from the nipple to the periphery of the breast including the axilla—by a trained healthcare provider. In some settings (especially in developing countries), this may be the only method of breast cancer screening available.[37]

Table 3 Breast cancer screening randomized trials.

Study	Randomization	Sample size	Intervention	Follow up	Finding
Health Insurance Plan, United States 1963[a]	Individual	60,565–60,857	MMG and CBE for 3 yr	18 yr	RR 0.77 (0.61–0.97)
Malmo, Sweden 1976[b,c]	Individual	42,283	Two-view MMG every 18–24 mo × 5	12 yr	RR 0.81 (95% CI, 0.62–1.07)
Ostergotland (County E of Two-County Trial) Sweden 1977[d,e]	Geographic cluster	38,405–39,034 study 37,145–37,936 control	Three single-view MMG Every 2 yr women-50 Every 33 mo women 50+	12 yr	RR 0.82 (95% CI, 0.64–1.05) Ostergotland
Kopparberg (County W of Two-County Trial) Sweden 1977[d,e]	Geographic cluster	38,562–39,051 intervention 18,478–18,846 control	Three single-view MMG Every 2 yr women-50 Every 33 mo women 50+	12 yr	RR 0.68 (95% CI, 0.52–0.89)
Edinburgh, United Kingdom[f]	Cluster by physician practice	23,266 study 21,904 control	Initially, two-view MMG and CBE Then annual CBE with single-view MMG years 3, 5, and 7	10 yr	RR 0.84 (95% CI, 0.63–1.12)
NBSS-1, Canada 1980[g]	Individual	25,214 study (100% screened after entry CBE) 25,216 control	Annual two-view MMG and CBE for 4–5 yr	13 yr	RR 0.97 (95% CI, 0.74–1.27)
NBSS-2, Canada 1980[h]	Individual	19,711 study (100% screened after entry CBE) 19,694 control	Annual two-view MMG and CBE	11–16 yr (mean 13 yr)	RR 1.02 (95% CI, 0.78–1.33)
Stockholm, Sweden 1981[i]	Cluster by birth date	Declined from 40,318 to 38,525 intervention group Rose from 19,943 to 20,978 control group	Single view MMG every 28 mo × 2	8 yr	RR 0.80 (95% CI, 0.53–1.22)
Gothenberg, Sweden 1982[j]	Complex	21,650 invited 29,961 control	Initial two-view MMG. Then single-view MMG every 18 mo × 4. Single read first three rounds, then double-read	12–14 yr	RR 0.79 (95% CI, 0.58–1.08)
AGE Trial[h,k]	Individuals	160,921 (53,884 invited; 106,956 not invited)	Invited group aged 48 and younger offered annual screening by MMG (double-view first screen, then single mediolateral oblique view thereafter); 68% accepted screening on the first screen and 69% and 70% were reinvited (81% attended at least one screen).	10.7 yr	RR 0.83 (95% CI, 0.66–1.04)

[a] Shapiro et al.[17]
[b] Andersson et al.[18]
[c] Nystrom et al.[19]
[d] Tabar et al.[20]
[e] Tabar et al.[21]
[f] Roberts et al.[22]
[g] Miller et al.[23]
[h] Miller et al.[24]
[i] Frisell et al.[25]
[j] Bjurstam et al.[26]
[k] Moss et al.[27]

No RCT has adequately evaluated CBE as a single screening modality. A small proportion of palpable masses are not seen on mammography, leading to screening guidelines that include routine CBE, ideally just prior to mammography. Some data suggest that CBE contributes very little in a setting of high adherence with regularly scheduled high-quality mammography.[37]

Breast self-examination (BSE) has appeal as a screening test because it is simple, convenient, and noninvasive. Having a monthly BSE was once widely advocated.[43] However, two prospective RCTs have reported a lack of evidence of efficacy and even some evidence of harm with this regimen, although both studies had some methodological issues.[33,44] Monthly BSE promotion distracts from the importance of mammography, can provide false reassurance, can heighten anxiety about breast cancer, and creates false positives. Today, no professional organization encourages monthly BSE and instead advocates for breast awareness and the consultation of a healthcare provider if a possible abnormality is found.[28]

Evaluation of the effectiveness of screening

Whereas the RCTs of breast cancer screening suggest a benefit, estimating the effectiveness of routine screening programs in the

Table 4 Pooled RRs for breast cancer mortality from mammography screening trials for all ages.[a]

Age (yr)	Trials included, n	RR for breast cancer mortality (95% CrI)	NNI to prevent 1 breast cancer death (95% CrI)
39–49	8[b]	0.85 (0.75–0.96)	1904 (929–6378)
50–59	6[c]	0.86 (0.75–0.99)	1339 (322–7455)
60–69	2[d]	0.68 (0.54–0.87)	377 (230–1050)
70–74	1[e]	1.12 (0.73–1.72)	Not available

CrI, credible interval; NNI, number needed to invite to screening; RR, relative risk.
[a]Source: Taken from Nelson et al.[32]
[b]Health Insurance Plan of Greater New York,[f] Canadian National Breast Screening Study-1,[g] Stockholm,[h] Malmö,[h] Swedish Two-County trial (two trials),[h,i] Gothenburg trial,[j] and Age trial.[k]
[c]Canadian National Breast Screening Study-1,[g] Stockholm,[h] Malmö,[h] Swedish Two-County trial (2 trials),[1,33] and Gothenburg trial.[j]
[d]Malmö[h] and Swedish Two-County trial (Östergötland).[h]
[e]Swedish Two-County trial (Östergötland).[h]
[f]Habbema et al.[34]
[g]Miller et al.[23]
[h]Nyström et al.[19]
[i]Tabar et al.[35]
[j]Bjurstam et al.[26]
[k]Moss et al.[27]

community is not straightforward. The United States experienced a 40% decline in age-adjusted breast cancer mortality from 1989 to 2018.[45] Mathematical modeling estimates that screening and improvements in breast cancer therapy, especially hormonal therapy, are each responsible for about half of the mortality decline.[46] Other models suggest that failure to receive systemic treatment is a greater contributor to breast cancer mortality compared to failure to get screened.[47] While screening in the United States is associated with a reduction in the incidence of metastatic cancer diagnosis, a disproportionately large increase in early-stage disease has occurred, suggesting a substantial amount of overdiagnosis.

The harms of breast cancer screening

Every screening test has associated harms. Slightly more than half of women screened in a 10-year period will have a false positive requiring, at minimum, additional imaging.[16,48] Surveys show about a quarter of these women suffered distress and anxiety 3 months after cancer had been ruled out.[49] False negatives lead to a false sense of security. Overdiagnosis estimates in breast cancer screening range from 0% to 54% of cancers diagnosed with the aid of mammography, with most estimates suggesting overdiagnosis is 10–30%.[50,51]

Mammography screening has also caused a dramatic rise in the diagnosis of ductal carcinoma *in situ* (DCIS). Previously a rare, incidental finding after mastectomy, >70,000 DCIS cases are now diagnosed annually in the US Study has yet to show that early detection and treatment of DCIS reduces mortality, while most DCIS lesions do not progress to invasive cancer.[52,53] Indeed, there is increasing interest in reducing overtreatment.[54,55] Renaming DCIS has been suggested to remove the word *carcinoma*.[56] In the future, genomic medicine may allow us to distinguish between the DCIS that should be observed and the DCIS cancer that needs aggressive therapy.

New technologies

Digital breast tomosynthesis or 3D mammography is a newer technology that appears to offer increased sensitivity and a reduction in recall rates.[57] The Tomosynthesis Mammographic Imaging Screening Trial (TMIST) trial is one of several ongoing trials globally to assess the worth of 3D mammography.[58] TMIST is a US National Cancer Institute (NCI)-sponsored, randomized breast cancer-screening trial to assess the effectiveness of digital two-dimensional mammography versus 3D or tomosynthesis mammography. The concern is that tomosynthesis or 3D mammography may result in more overdiagnosis of breast cancer without reducing the breast cancer death rate.[59]

Magnetic resonance imaging (MRI) is more sensitive but less specific than mammography in detecting breast cancer.[60] MRIs are associated with a high number of false-positive results but are useful for screening women with significant breast density and those who may be at elevated risk due to mutations in breast cancer susceptibility genes.[61]

Ultrasound imaging has been used for many years as a diagnostic tool. The limitations of mammography in screening dense breasts have led to ongoing interest in using ultrasound for primary screening or as an adjunct to mammography.[62,63]

In 2003, the American College of Radiology Imaging Network (ACRIN) initiated a multicenter trial in women at increased risk for breast cancer due to family history and significant breast density.[64,65] The breast cancer detection rate was increased by 4.2 cancers per 1000 women screened with mammography and ultrasound versus mammography alone (11.8 vs 7.6 per 1000). However, the false-positive and -negative biopsy rates were also very high. While a significant improvement was seen in the diagnostic yield of small, node-negative cancers in this higher-risk population, questions remain about the potential for screening ultrasound for some subpopulations.[63] Routine ultrasound screening is not advocated at this time.

An interesting technology that is gaining use is 3D automated breast ultrasound. It offers more standardized imaging compared to conventional ultrasound and can be performed by a technologist instead of a radiologist. While still used as a diagnostic tool, interest persists in its use as an initial screening test with mammography and CBE.

Screening recommendations

As of 2015, the ACS guidelines recommend that women aged 40–45 have the opportunity to begin annual screening, if they choose, and that women aged 45–54 should be screened annually with mammography. Women aged 55 and older should transition to screening every 2 years but have the opportunity to continue every year if they choose. Women should continue screening as long as their overall health is good and they have a life expectancy of 10 years or longer. The ACS no longer recommends a CBE except when mammography is not available.

The 2016 USPSTF recommends that women aged 40–49 should make an individual decision about screening after a physician–patient discussion about individual risks and concerns.[36] Those who place a higher value on screening's potential benefit may choose to begin biennial screening between ages 40 and 49. Those more concerned with harms may choose not to begin screening. The USPSTF recommends biennial screening for women between 50 and 74 years of age.

The American College of Physicians, and the Canadian Task Force on the Periodic Health Examination recommend routine screening beginning at age 50.[66] An advisory committee on cancer prevention in the European Union recommends that screening be offered to women aged 50–69 in an organized screening program.[67]

Based on the accumulation of data, but no RCTs, the ACS now recommends that women at very high risk of breast cancer begin annual mammography and MRI at age 30, or perhaps earlier, if she and her physician believe it is prudent.[60] Performing a prospective RCT in this population is impossible. *High risk* is defined as having a known mutation, a 20–25% or greater lifetime risk based on family history, a high-risk genetic syndrome such as Li–Fraumeni syndrome or Cowden disease, or having received high-dose mantle radiation to the chest.

Colorectal cancer screening

Worldwide, colorectal cancer (CRC) is the third most commonly diagnosed cancer in men and the second in women and accounts for 8% of all deaths. In the United States, CRC is the third most commonly diagnosed cancer and the third leading cause of cancer death among men and women, individually. While most cases are diagnosed among individuals aged 60–80, there is increasing concern about CRC in those aged 40–50.

The goals of colorectal screening include both the detection of early-stage adenocarcinomas and the detection and removal of adenomatous polyps, given the significant evidence that adenomatous polyps are precancerous lesions. Colorectal polyps are common in adults over age 50. One-half to two-thirds of all colorectal polyps are adenomatous, which can progress to cancer, although the majority never will. It is estimated that it takes 10 years for an adenomatous polyp <1 cm to become an invasive lesion.[68] Other polyps, including incidental hyperplastic polyps and mucosal tags, are not significant in the development of CRC.[69]

Screening methods for colorectal cancer

Evidence suggests that numerous tests, applied in a program of regular surveillance, have the potential to reduce deaths from CRC.

(1) *Fecal occult blood tests (FOBTs)* aim to discover occult blood in stool often caused by polyps (especially >2 cm). Common FOBTs include the *guaiac-based test (gFOBT)* and the *fecal immunochemical test (FIT)*.

The guaiac Fecal occult blood test (gFOBT) detects blood in the stool through the pseudoperoxidase activity of heme. This test requires diet modification, as it can positively react with red meat, cruciferous vegetables, and some fruits that have been eaten. Rehydration of gFOBT slides in the laboratory improves sensitivity but also increases the false-positive rate.[70] The gFOBT can be performed in the physician's office but it is preferred that patients collect specimens at home for processing in a laboratory. Any blood-positive stool test requires follow-up diagnostic colonoscopy.

Limitations of gFOBT have led to a decrease in usage but some high-sensitivity tests are still available. The gFOBT performed with stool collected during a digital rectal examination (DRE) is not recommended.

The FIT reacts to human globin. Unlike the gFOBT, the FIT is not reactive to consumed foods and will not react to digested human blood from upper gastrointestinal bleeding. The threshold for fecal hemoglobin can be altered to balance sensitivity and specificity based on individual risk or programmatic requirements. FITs are usually processed in a laboratory. Sensitivity declines with delay in sample processing—a 5-day delay is significant.[71]

In 1000 ambulatory patients (with and without symptoms of CRC), the sensitivity for cancer with three FIT samples with a hemoglobin threshold of 75 ng/mL was 94.1%, and specificity was 87.5%.[72] In a screening study with one FIT evaluation of stool followed by colonoscopy, FIT had higher sensitivity for detection of advanced neoplasms in patients taking low-dose aspirin compared to those not taking aspirin. There was a minor decrease in specificity.[73]

In a systematic review of gFOBT and FIT, no clear evidence was shown for superiority of either test.[74] Bleeding from cancers or large polyps may be intermittent. Generally, FIT requires two tests over a week or so, while gFOBT generally requires three. In practice, FIT is replacing gFOBT.

(2) *Stool DNA (sDNA)* testing detects relatively well-defined DNA markers associated with colorectal neoplasia in cells exfoliated by colorectal polyps and malignancies into the colonic lumen. Available sDNA tests focus on >21 separate point mutations in the K-*RAS* oncogene, a probe for BAT-26 (a marker of microsatellite instability), and a marker of DNA integrity analysis to achieve high sensitivity.[75] The currently marketed sDNA kit also includes a FIT test. As with stool-blood testing, any positive stool blood or DNA test must be followed up with colonoscopy to rule out the presence of polyps or cancer.

(3) *Flexible sigmoidoscopy* (FSIG) with a 60-cm scope is a relatively simple procedure, requires minimal preparation, and allows for examination of about half of the average colon.[76] The test is generally performed without sedation. The presence of polyps in the distal bowel signals an elevated risk for polyps or cancer in the proximal bowel. If FSIG is positive, the patient is referred for colonoscopy.

Quality indicators for FSIG have been published[10] and emphasize appropriate training, satisfactory examination rates to >40 cm, expected adenoma detection rates based on age and gender, and ability to biopsy suspected adenomas.

(4) *Colonoscopy* has a unique advantage among CRC screening tests in that direct visualization of the entire bowel is possible, with >90% of examinations terminating at the cecum, and clinically significant adenomas can be identified and removed during the examination.[77,78] Colonoscopy is commonly done in an outpatient setting. While conscious sedation is standard, some patients receive general anesthesia. Proper bowel preparation is critical to ensure adequate visualization of the bowel.

The examination is more complicated than sigmoidoscopy, with higher risk of complications, mostly due to sedation, biopsy, or polypectomy. Blood loss can be seen with polyps of any size but is more common when removing large polyps, or polyps in the proximal colon. Risk of bowel perforation increases with age and is higher in individuals with diverticular disease. Perforation occurs in about 1 in 500 Medicare beneficiaries, and 1 in 1000 patients in the general population.

In 1256 adults rescreened about 5 years after negative colonoscopy, no cancers were detected, but 201 adults (16%) had one or more adenomas, of which 16 were advanced.[79] The findings support the conclusion that among individuals with no evidence of cancer or advanced adenomas at screening, the 5-year risk of CRC is extremely low.

In a study of 35,000 asymptomatic patients in Manitoba who had undergone negative colonoscopy and were followed for 10 years, 45% and 72% reductions in the expected CRC incidence were observed at 5 and 10 years, respectively.[80] These findings suggest some detection failures during the initial, apparently normal, colonoscopy.

The long duration of reduced risk of CRC after colonoscopy depends on quality of the examination and complete removal of polyps. Quality assurance recommendations emphasize training and experience, proper risk assessment and documentation, complete examination to the cecum with adequate mucosal visualization and bowel preparation, ability to detect and remove polyps safely, documentation of polypoid lesions and removal, timely and appropriate management of adverse events, appropriate follow-up of histopathology findings, appropriate recommendation for surveillance or repeat screening based on published guidelines, and continuous assessment and evaluation of performance with corrective action when necessary.

(5) *Computed-tomography (CT) colonography* or virtual colonoscopy is an imaging procedure that computationally combines multiple, helical, CT scans to create two- or three-dimensional images of the colon interior. These images can be rotated for different views and even combined for a complete, virtual view.[81]

Evaluations of CT colonography have typically involved CT examination followed by optical colonoscopy, with the colonoscopist blinded to the CT results. Although early results with 2D imaging were disappointing, recent back-to-back evaluations of CT colonography using faster scanners, updated 3D luminal displays, and oral stool tagging with digital subtraction have demonstrated sensitivities for large adenomas equivalent to colonoscopy. Using these advances, one study of back-to-back CT and optical colonoscopy in asymptomatic adults reported CT colonography had a 94% sensitivity for large adenomas, with per-patient sensitivity for adenomas ≥6 mm of 89%.[82]

In a collaborative ACRIN/NCI trial,[83] CT colonography detected 90% of patients with large (≥10 mm) adenomas and cancers, with 86% specificity and 84% per-polyp sensitivity. Thirty large lesions were detected by CT colonography that were not detected by optical colonoscopy. Five of 18 lesions ≥10 mm were confirmed by colonoscopy as true positives. Although the sensitivity of CT colonography is lower for lesions ≤6 mm, these lesions generally are regarded as clinically insignificant. For lesions of ≥1 cm in size, CT colonography has performance very similar to optical colonoscopy.[82]

CT colonography requires the same full bowel preparation and restricted diet as optical colonoscopy, and as an imaging-only evaluation, patients with polyps ≥6 mm in size must be referred to therapeutic colonoscopy and polypectomy.[83] The test is most appropriate for those who hope to avoid anesthesia or manipulation of the hips and legs required for colonoscopy.

Colorectal screening trials

The initial evidence that colorectal screening saves lives was based on studies showing that gFOBT found lesions at earlier stages than in cases diagnosed with symptoms. This led to prospective trials in Europe and the United States evaluating the efficacy of FOBT. In the Minnesota trial, 46,551 asymptomatic participants aged 50–80 were randomized to invitation to annual screening, biennial screening, or usual care.[84] Participants with positive gFOBT received colonoscopy. The 13-year cumulative mortality was 5.33, 8.33, and 8.83 per 1000 in the annual screening-, biennial screening-, and usual care (control) groups, respectively. After 18 years of follow-up, both annual and biennial gFOBT were associated with a 20% and 18% reduction in cancer incidence, respectively, and with a statistically significant reduction in deaths.[70] Cancer prevention was attributed to detection and removal of adenomatous polyps.[70] Similar results with gFOBT every 2 years have been observed in two other trials.[85]

Sigmoidoscopy. In the early 1990s, two case-control studies that evaluated the efficacy of screening sigmoidoscopy reported a 70% or more reduction in risk of CRC death.[86,87] Five sigmoidoscopy screening RCTs have reported incidence and mortality results. In a meta-analysis, a 28% relative risk reduction in CRC mortality (RR = 0.72; 95% CI, 0.65–0.80) was found. Incidence was reduced by 18% (RR = 0.82; 95% CI, 0.73–0.91). Left-sided cancer was reduced by 33% (RR = 0.67; 95% CI, 0.59–0.76).[88,89]

Combined stool-blood testing and FSIG every 5 years is superior to FOBT or FSIG alone. FOBT provides some surveillance in the proximal colon (outside the reach of FSIG), and FSIG has higher sensitivity and specificity than FOBT in the distal colon. In an RCT in asymptomatic individuals aged ≥40, there were fewer CRC deaths in patients receiving annual FOBT and sigmoidoscopy than in those receiving sigmoidoscopy alone (0.36 vs 0.63 per 1000; $P = 0.53$) after 5–11 years of follow-up.[88] Based on modeling, the USPSTF concluded that combining FSIG every 5 years with high-sensitivity FOBT every 3 years is approximately equivalent, in terms of life-years gained, to colonoscopy every 10 years.[89]

Colonoscopy. No prospective RCTs with mortality endpoints have been conducted to evaluate whether colonoscopy screening prevents CRC death. Perhaps the strongest evidence of efficacy is that more than 40% of those receiving annual FOBT in the Minnesota trial ultimately received at least one colonoscopy. In addition, several case-control studies suggest that screening with colonoscopy and polypectomy has significant impact on CRC incidence and by extension, mortality.[90,91]

Screening recommendations

As shown in Table 2, the ACS recommendations for average-risk individuals include seven options for regular surveillance for CRC beginning at age 45,[92,93] including annual high-sensitivity FOBT (gFOBT or FIT); sDNA every 3 years; FSIG every 5 years; total colonic examination with CT Colonoscopy every 5 years; or total colonic examination with colonoscopy every 10 years. Nevertheless, most adults who undergo screening have stool testing with gFOBT, FIT, sDNA, or colonoscopy. Annual DRE is no longer recommended, due to low sensitivity, but DRE should be done prior to FSIG or colonoscopy. Strong consensus exists among US organizations about the value of CRC screening in adults ≥50 years of age, and many are considering recommendations starting at age 45.[94]

Guidelines for higher-risk individuals recommend earlier onset of surveillance and more thorough examinations of the colon (Table 5). Higher-risk individuals include those with a family history of adenomatous polyps, CRC, familial adenomatous polyposis, hereditary nonpolyposis CRC (HNPCC), or inflammatory bowel disease.[95]

Table 5 Guidelines for screening and surveillance for early detection of colorectal polyps and cancer for individuals at greater than average risk.

Risk category and description	Recommendation	Age to begin	Screening interval and recommendation
Moderate risk			
People with single, small (<1 cm) adenomatous polyps	Colonoscopy	At the initial polyp diagnosis	TCE within 3 yr after initial polyp removal; if normal, follow recommendations for average-risk individuals
People with large (≥1 cm) or multiple adenomatous polyps of any size	Colonoscopy	At the time of initial polyp diagnosis	TCE within 3 yr after initial polyp removal; if normal TCE every 5 yr
Personal history of curative-intent resection of colorectal cancer	TCE[a]	Within 1 yr after resection	If normal, TCE in 3 yr; If second TCE is normal, TCE in 5 yr
Colorectal cancer or adenomatous polyps, in first-degree relative younger than age 60 or in two or more first-degree relatives of any ages	TCE[a]	40 yr or 10 yr before the youngest case in the family, whichever is earlier	Every 5 yr
Colorectal cancer in other relatives (not first degree)	Follow recommendations for age-risk individuals	—	—
High risk			
Family history of FAP	Early surveillance with endoscopy, counseling to consider genetic testing, and referral for specialty care	Puberty	If genetic test is positive or polyposis is confirmed, consider colectomy; otherwise, continue endoscopy every 1–2 yr
Family history of HNPCC	Colonoscopy and counseling to consider genetic testing	21 yr	If untested, or if genetic test is positive, colonoscopy every 2 yr until age 40; after age 40, colonoscopy every year
Inflammatory bowel disease	Colonoscopy with biopsies for dysplasia	8 yr after the start of pancolitis; 12–15 yr after the start of left-sided colitis	Colonoscopy every 1–2 yr

Abbreviations: FAP, familial adenomatous polyposis; HNPCC, hereditary nonpolyposis colorectal cancer; TCE, total colon examination.
[a]TCE includes either colonoscopy, DCBE, or CT colonography. CT colonography or DCBE should be added to the colonoscopy examination in those instances when the entire colon cannot be visualized by colonoscopy.

Cervical cancer screening

Cervical cancer is the third most commonly diagnosed cancer in women, fourth leading cause of cancer death worldwide[14,96] and is still the leading cause of cancer death among women in some areas of Africa and Asia. A dramatic decline in mortality due to improvements in both treatment and early detection has occurred particularly in the United States and western Europe, where the mortality rates in 1980 were >70% lower than in 1930.[97]

The improvement in early detection was due to the Pap test (or smear) developed by Dr. George Papanicolaou in the 1920s. In many Western countries, the test gained widespread adoption in the late 1940s–1950s.[98] It diagnoses early cancers and precursor lesions (dysplasia or cervical intraepithelial neoplasia), for which a variety of treatment options are available. The diagnosis of *treatable precursor lesions* is considerably more common than the diagnosis of *invasive disease*. The finding and treatment of early precursor lesions through screening has caused a drop in cervical cancer incidence.[99]

Screening and diagnostic methods

In many respects, the Pap test is not very technical. It involves the collection of exfoliated epithelial cells from the cervical squamocolumnar junction (or transformation zone). Both the ectocervix and endocervix are sampled. Two samples are applied to one side of a glass slide and quickly fixed to prevent air drying. The slide is stained and examined under a microscope by a cytotechnologist. Although simple to conduct, its accuracy is highly dependent upon obtaining a high-quality specimen, good slide preparation, and expert microscopic examination and interpretation.[93,100]

The Pap smear has a significant error rate. Sampling error is estimated to account for about two-thirds of false-negative tests while errors in interpretation account for the remaining third. Pap-smear screening is estimated to have specificity of 98% and sensitivity of 51%.[101] The NCI's Bethesda System (Table 6), released in 1988, provides "… a uniform format for cytopathology reports (and) is intended to communicate clinically relevant information using standardized terminology."[102]

Clinical studies of efficacy

Screening with the Pap smear is comparatively inexpensive and is widely accepted, although no RCTs of its efficacy have been conducted. Perhaps the most widely cited evidence for its effect on mortality is the long-term decline in cervical cancer death rate in the United States coincident with the introduction of the Pap smear.[43] While death rates had begun to decline prior to widespread use of the test, due to factors such as an increase in the hysterectomy rate and improved treatment of cervical cancer, the decline in incidence and mortality was so significant that improvements in treatment could not account for all of it. Furthermore, from the 1950s to the 1970s, cervical cancer mortality remained comparatively unchanged in Norway, a late adopter of cervical screening, whereas it dropped by more than 70% in Iceland, an early adopter.[97] Numerous case-control studies also found a benefit from cervical cancer screening. Evidence that screening reduces incidence is best shown by the fact that the majority of American women diagnosed with cervical cancer today have no history of cervical screening in the 3 years before diagnosis.[103]

Precursor lesions usually take years to progress to cancer. Overdiagnosis and overtreatment are a significant concern as observational studies show that untreated lesions such as atypical squamous cells of undetermined significance (ASCUS) often regress.[104] Strategies of triage, observation, and repeat testing are

Table 6 Bethesda system 2001.

Specimen type	Indicate conventional smear (Pap smear) versus liquid-based versus other
Specimen adequacy	
Satisfactory for evaluation	Describe presence or absence of endocervical/transformation zone component and any other quality indicators, for example, partially obscuring blood and inflammation
Unsatisfactory for evaluation	Specimen rejected/not processed (specify reason), or specimen processed and examined, but unsatisfactory for evaluation of epithelial abnormality because of (specify reason)
General categorization (optional)	Negative for intraepithelial lesion or malignancy Epithelial cell abnormality: see interpretation/result (specify "squamous" or "glandular" as appropriate) Other: see interpretation/result (e.g., endometrial cells in a woman >40 yr of age)
Automated review	If case examined by automated device, specify device and result
Ancillary testing	Provide a brief description of the test methods and report the result so that it is easily understood by the clinician
Interpretation/result negative for intraepithelial lesion or malignancy	When there is no cellular evidence of neoplasia, state this in the general categorization above and/or in the interpretation/result section of the report, whether or not there are organisms or other nonneoplastic findings)
Organisms	*Trichomonas vaginalis* Fungal organisms morphologically consistent with *Candida* spp. Shift in flora suggestive of bacterial vaginosis Bacteria morphologically consistent with *Actinomyces* spp. Cellular changes consistent with herpes simplex virus
Other nonneoplastic findings (Optional to report; list not inclusive)	Reactive cellular changes associated with inflammation (includes typical repair) radiation intrauterine contraceptive device (IUD) Glandular cells status post hysterectomy Atrophy
Other	Endometrial cells (in a woman ≥40 yr of age) (specify if "negative for squamous intraepithelial lesion")
Epithelial cell abnormalities	
Squamous cell	Atypical squamous cells of undetermined significance (ASC-US) cannot exclude HSIL (ASC-H) Low grade squamous intraepithelial lesion (LSIL) encompassing: HPV/mild dysplasia/CIN 1 High grade squamous intraepithelial lesion (HSIL) encompassing: moderate and severe dysplasia, CIS/CIN 2, and CIN 3 with features suspicious for invasion (if invasion is suspected) Squamous cell carcinoma
Glandular cell	Atypical Endocervical cells (NOS or specify in comments) Endometrial cells (NOS or specify in comments) Glandular cells (NOS or specify in comments) Endocervical cells, favor neoplastic Glandular cells, favor neoplastic Endocervical adenocarcinoma *in situ* Adenocarcinoma Endocervical Endometrial Extrauterine Not otherwise specified
Other malignant neoplasms	Specify
Educational notes and suggestions (optional)	Suggestions should be concise and consistent with clinical follow-up guidelines published by professional organizations (references to relevant publications may be included)

being used to avoid overtreatment.[105] Recommendations note that screening normal risk women every 5 years or more is safe.[106]

New technologies

Liquid-based cytology uses specimen-collection techniques similar to those of the conventional Pap smear. Equally dependent on collecting an adequate sample, the liquid-based cytology sample is suspended in a fixative solution, dispersed, filtered, and distributed on a glass slide to achieve a monolayer of cells. Computer-aided diagnosis of the test is common, and abnormal smears are referred to a cytotechnologist.[107,108]

Because there are fewer artifacts (blood, mucus, etc.) and because cells are not overlapping, accuracy is increased. Studies have shown liquid-based cytology, compared to the Pap smear, to have higher sensitivity in populations with lower prevalence of cytologic abnormalities.[108] Reviews applying rigorous evidence-based criteria found no significant advantage in sensitivity or specificity for liquid-based over conventional Pap testing. The number of inadequate specimens is considerably reduced, however, with liquid-based cytology.

A strong association between persistent infection exists with certain subtypes of human papillomavirus (HPV) and cervical cancer.[109] The ability to test for HPV DNA or HPV RNA has allowed for better diagnosis of cervical dysplasia. HPV testing is increasingly used as a co-test to triage women with abnormal cytologic tests and atypical glandular cells of undetermined significance (AGUS).

Many now prefer the use of HPV screening instead of the Pap smear in women age ≥25.[110] A prospective-cluster randomized trial in India demonstrated that HPV testing detected high-grade cervical dysplasia and early cervical cancer and that treatment led to a decrease in mortality.[111] The US Food and Drug Administration (FDA) has approved an HPV DNA test that can be used alone for primary screening. This screen is not used in women under age 25, because active and transient HPV infections in this age group are common. Because of the reduced complexity of the sample collection and its lack of reliance on trained cytopathologic expertise, HPV testing may represent a lower resource-intense strategy for screening.[112]

In a cluster-randomized trial in India, some clusters (women age 35–64) were randomized to one-time cervical visual inspection with acetic acid followed by immediate colposcopy, biopsy, and/or cryotherapy (when indicated) versus counseling to reduce cervical cancer deaths. The age-standardized rate of death due to cervical cancer was 39.6 versus 56.7 per 100,000 person-years in the intervention- and control groups, respectively—a 31% reduction in cervical cancer mortality.[113]

Screening recommendations

In 2012, the ACS, the American Society for Colposcopy and Cervical Pathology, and the American Society for Clinical Pathology issued joint guidelines for cervical cancer screening based on a systematic and collaborative review of evidence among 25 professional organizations.[114] Similar recommendations were released in 2012 by the USPSTF.[112] These recommendations encouraged less frequent cervical cancer screening realizing that many women get screened too often and a subset of women who need screening and do not receive it.[106] These were the first guidelines that examined evidence of HPV infection.[100]

In 2018, the American College of Obstetrics and Gynecology issued new screening guidelines[115] as follows:

- Women under age 21 years should not be screened regardless of their age of sexual initiation.
- Women aged 21–29 years should have a Pap test in isolation every 3 years. HPV testing is not recommended in this age group.
- Women aged 30–65 years should preferably have a Pap test and an HPV test (co-testing) every 5 years. It is also is acceptable to have only a Pap test every 3 years.
- Women should stop having cervical cancer screening after age 65 years if:
  ○ They do not have a history of moderate or severe abnormal cervical cells or cervical cancer, and
  ○ They have had either three negative Pap test results in a row or two negative co-test results in a row within the past 10 years, with the most recent test performed within the past 5 years.

The USPSTF recommends screening for cervical cancer in:

- Women aged 21–29 years every 3 years with cervical cytology alone.
- Women aged 30–65 years
  ○ every 3 years with cervical cytology alone
  ○ every 5 years with high-risk HPV testing alone, or
  ○ every 5 years with high-risk HPV testing in combination with cytology (co-testing)

The USPSTF recommends against screening for cervical cancer in:

- Women younger than 21 years and
- Women older than 65 years who have had adequate prior screening and are not otherwise at high risk for cervical cancer.
- Women who have had a hysterectomy with removal of the cervix and do not have a history of a high-grade precancerous lesion or cervical cancer.[100,101]

In 2020, the ACS began recommending high-risk HPV testing as the preferred method of cervical cancer screening.[116] They recommend to start at age 25 and have the test every 5 years until age 65. The recommendation states that cytology (the Pap smear) should be used every 3 years if HPV testing is not available.

All groups recommend that screening practices should not change based on a patient's HPV vaccination status.

Prostate cancer screening

Worldwide, prostate cancer is the second most common cancer diagnosed and the sixth most common cause of cancer death among men.[14,117] Incidence and mortality rates vary considerably. Among American males, prostate cancer is the most commonly diagnosed nonskin cancer and the second leading cause of cancer death. Mortality rates are higher in men of African ancestry, in Caucasian men in the Americas, and in Scandinavia; rates are lowest in Asia.

A subset of prostate cancers is aggressive and poses a significant risk of death. Unfortunately, they often do not produce symptoms until locally advanced or metastatic. Prostate cancer among older men is more often slow-growing or indolent. Efforts to distinguish clinically significant versus nonsignificant localized prostate cancer have included pathologic grading and genomic testing.[118]

Screening and diagnostic methods

DRE aims to find hard nodular areas that sometimes indicate the presence of prostate cancer. Three principal limitations of DRE must be considered: the test is highly operator dependent, the majority of palpable cancers are not early cancers, and many clinically important cancers are located in regions of the prostate inaccessible to palpation. DRE is often recommended as a screening component because it can detect prostate cancers missed by other tests, may predict high-grade disease, is a low-cost procedure, and can detect other abnormalities such as benign prostatic hyperplasia. As well, in the early phases of the European Randomized Study of Prostate Cancer (ERSPC), DRE appeared to have limited value as a stand-alone test even though one-quarter to one-third of all prostate cancers were detected by DRE in the normal prostate-specific antigen (PSA) range (<4.0 ng/mL).[119]

PSA is a glycoprotein secreted by the epithelial component of the prostate. Progression of prostate cancer is correlated with a rise in serum PSA. Serum PSA measurement was first used to monitor metastatic disease in the early 1980s. By 1992, the ACS recommended annual serum PSA screening for men at ages 40 and above[120] and the test quickly became widely used for screening in the United States. Unfortunately, how to best use the test was determined much later.[121] Today, we know that serum PSA can be elevated in a variety of conditions besides cancer, such as benign prostatic hyperplasia, inflammation of the prostate, and following trauma to the gland. PSA screening both finds and misses a lot of cancer. Whether PSA screening results in a decline in mortality rate is one of the most pressing questions in cancer medicine today.[122]

Accumulating evidence supports the efficacy (vs effectiveness) of PSA testing, alone or in combination with DRE, in finding localized disease.[119,123] Approximately one in four men at ages ≥50 with a PSA >4 ng/mL have cancer after prostate biopsy. Reducing the PSA cut point makes the test more sensitive but reduces specificity.

The Prostate Cancer Prevention Trial (PCPT) randomized more than 19,000 men age ≥55 with an initial PSA of 3.0 ng/mL to receive either finasteride or placebo.[124] Subjects were screened every year for 7 years (eight total screens) with serum PSA and DRE and 14% were diagnosed with prostate cancer. Among men with normal PSAs and DREs, an additional 14% were diagnosed with prostate cancer based on an end-of-study biopsy.[124] That >25% of men completing this trial were diagnosed with prostate cancer suggests some overdiagnosis. As well, a PSA cut off of 4 or a 1 ng/mL increase in 1 year missed as much cancer as it found. No natural cut point exists for PSA screening. Indeed, men were diagnosed with prostate cancer with serum PSAs <0.6 ng/mL.[121]

Transrectal ultrasonography (TRUS) uses a small rectal probe placed against the prostate to image the entire gland. Unfortunately, cancer within the prostate has no unique or reliably assessed ultrasonic signature. TRUS as a sole screening modality has poor sensitivity and specificity; however, it can be used to accurately measure gland dimensions and volume and to direct prostate needle biopsies.

Endorectal MRI is not used in screening but its role is evolving in prostate diagnostic evaluation and following men with confirmed disease.[125]

Clinical trials of prostate cancer treatment

In a study started before the PSA era, 767 men with localized prostate cancer were treated only with observation or androgen-withdrawal therapy, but only a small proportion died of prostate cancer, suggesting significant overdiagnosis. After 20 years of follow-up, 4–7%, 6–11%, and 18–30% of men with Gleason 2–6 disease, respectively, had died of prostate cancer.[118] This raised the question whether treatment of localized or locally advanced prostate cancer was beneficial or saved lives. Prospective RCTs published in the late 1990s were the first to demonstrate a positive treatment effect for men with locally advanced disease. These studies demonstrated an advantage using radiation and hormonal therapy in men over radiation therapy alone.[126,127]

In 2002, the Scandinavian Prostate Cancer Group-4 (SPCG-4) study researchers were the first to show that treatment of localized disease saved lives. They randomized 695 men with clinically localized prostate cancer to either radical prostatectomy or watchful waiting, with hormonal therapy if symptoms dictated. At a median follow-up of 12.8 years, 14.6% of the prostatectomy group had died versus 20.7% of the watchful-waiting group (RR = 0.75; $P = 0.007$). The number needed to treat to prevent one death was 15. Less than 15% of participants had PSA-detected disease.[128] One would predict that number in a screened population to be much higher.

The Prostate Intervention Versus Observation Trial (PIVOT) trial randomized 731 men with PSA screen-detected disease to either radical prostatectomy or watchful waiting.[129] At a median follow-up of 12 years, prostatectomy was associated with a statistically insignificant 2.9% absolute- and a 2.6% prostate cancer-specific reduction in mortality. Subgroup analyses suggested a small, but statistically significant, mortality benefit for men diagnosed with PSA >10 ng/mL and for those with intermediate- and high-risk disease.[129]

In the ProtecT trial, Hamdy and colleagues[130] randomized 1643 men with screen-detected, apparently localized disease to active surveillance- (545 men), radical prostatectomy- (553 men), or external-beam radiotherapy groups (545 men). At 10 years, the number of deaths was low and not statistically significant in all three groups. A higher rate of disease progression was found in the active-surveillance group (112 men), compared to the surgery- (46 men), or radiotherapy groups (46 men). About 20% of the surveilled men had progressive disease, but nearly half had received treatment; the other half were still being observed at 10 years.

Taken together, results from the SPCG-4, PIVOT, and ProtecT trials suggest that our therapeutic interventions save lives in a small minority of those diagnosed and that a substantial proportion of men diagnosed with localized prostate cancer are overdiagnosed and do not need treatment. Substantial efforts are being made to identify these patients. Several commercial gene-expression tests are available to assess the potential of localized, low-Gleason-stage disease to progress.[131]

The effects of prostate cancer screening

Prostate cancer screening rates increased dramatically after the 1989 FDA approval of PSA for following men with diagnosed disease. The FDA has since approved PSA to diagnose suspected disease but not for screening. The simplicity of a blood test had enabled mass PSA screening at health fairs and community events and American prostate cancer incidence rates to rise.

Prostate cancer mortality rates were rising for 20 years prior to the approval of PSA testing. While rates peaked in 1993, the United States has experienced a 50% decline in age-adjusted prostate cancer death rates.[132] How much of the decline is due to screening is unknown.[133] Prostate cancer mortality rates have declined in 21 countries;[134] screening is common in the United States and very few other countries.

Possible explanations for the decline in prostate cancer mortality seen in all countries include a shift in the tendency to classify prostate cancer as the underlying cause of death and the significant improvements in prostate cancer treatment at all stages.[135] Supporting the first theory, the World Health Organization algorithm for adjudicating cause of death was changed as mortality rates began to rise in the late 1970s, and the older algorithm came back into favor in 1991—about the time when prostate cancer mortality began declining.[136] Supporting the second theory is the fact that prostate cancer is overwhelmingly a disease of older men. Even a two to three-month increase in median survival due to more effective treatment could cause a decline in prostate cancer mortality as competing causes of death become more significant. Others have speculated that aggressive use of newer hormonal therapies may have increased cardiovascular deaths and thereby prevented prostate deaths.[137] All three could contribute to the decline in prostate cancer death rates in the United States in addition to the possibility that screening could have had a positive effect.

Epidemiological studies showed a significant decrease in the incidence of distant disease at diagnosis by the year 2000. Based on the assumption that screening results in a shift from distant to local or regional disease, modeling efforts within the NCI's Cancer Intervention Surveillance Modeling Network estimate that 45–70% of the observed prostate cancer mortality decline in the United States could plausibly be attributed to screening-induced stage shifts.[133]

Ultimately, the strongest assessment of screening efficacy requires long-term large, prospective, RCTs having a mortality endpoint. Five of these studies have been reported, all of which are judged to have some limitations. The two trials considered of higher quality are the multicenter US NCI Prostate, Lung, Colorectal, and Ovarian trial (PLCO) and the multicenter ERSPC.[119,123]

The PLCO was initiated in 1992.[123] Nearly 77,000 men age 55–74 years were randomized to receive either annual PSA testing for 6 years or usual care. At 13 years of follow-up, a statistically insignificant increase in prostate cancer mortality was observed among men randomized to annual screening (RR = 1.09; 95% CI, 0.87–1.36).[123] At a 15-year median follow-up, no reduction was seen in prostate cancer in the intervention arm versus the control arm.[138] The trial was limited due to the high rate of PSA testing in the control arm, which reduced statistical power. Rather than focusing on screening versus no screening, PLCO is best viewed as comparing routine to opportunistic screening.

The ERSPC was initiated in 1991[107] and seven countries reported results. In the initial analysis of 182,160 men, aged 50–74, prostate cancer-specific mortality was not reduced by screening but was significantly decreased in a subset of men age 55–69 years. A 21% relative reduction of prostate cancer death (RR = 0.79; 95% CI, 0.68–0.91) was observed after a median follow-up of 11 years and was maintained at 13 years. One prostate cancer death was averted per 781 men invited and per 27 excess cases detected.[139] In a 16-year follow-up, PSA screening reduced prostate cancer mortality with a larger absolute benefit. One prostate cancer death was averted per 570 men invited to screening and per 18 excess cases detected.[140]

The ERSPC trial would have been negative if not for the Swedish component. In that country, screening was very effective, while it was marginally effective in the Netherlands and showed a statistically insignificant trend toward benefit in four countries. The Finnish component of ERSPC was the largest and did not show benefit at 12 years.[141] Screening may have been more effective in Sweden because of the higher risk of prostate cancer death in that country. Another very important factor to consider is the randomization scheme in Sweden which might also have created a "healthy volunteer" selection bias among those in the screening arm not seen in the control group—those in the screening arm were consented while those in the control arm did not know they were in a clinical trial.[135]

Screening recommendations

Numerous professional organizations in the United States, Europe, and Canada have issued prostate cancer screening guidelines. All acknowledge legitimate concerns regarding the risk-to-benefit ratio of screening. Most agree that screening should only be done in the context of fully informed consent with a shared decision being made between the man and his doctor.[142–144] All recommend against mass screening in public places. The investigators of ERSPC also concluded that available data do not support widespread screening.[139]

The 2010 ACS guidelines state that the balance of benefits and harms related to early detection of prostate cancer are uncertain and the existing evidence is insufficient to support a recommendation for or against routine PSA screening.[143] The ACS calls for discussion and shared decision-making within the physician–patient relationship.

The 2012 USPSTF guideline recommends against the routine use of PSA screening based on moderate certainty that the harms of PSA testing outweigh the benefits.[13] The task force acknowledged that some men will continue to request screening and some physicians will continue to offer it. Like the ACS and the American Urological Association (AUA), they state that screening under such circumstances should respect an informed patient's preferences.[13]

In 2013, the AUA conducted a systematic review of over 300 studies and[144] concluded that the greatest benefit of screening appears to be in men of ages 55–69 years although "the quality of evidence for benefits associated with screening was moderate, whereas the quality of the evidence for harm was high." The AUA places primacy on shared decision-making versus physician judgments about the balance of benefits and harms at the population level even for men of ages 55–69.[145] It also recommends screening every 2 years instead of every year; and recommend *against* screening men <40 years of age, average-risk men aged 40–54 years, most men >70 years of age, and men with a life expectancy of <10–15 years. Finally, the committee recommends that screening decisions be individualized for higher-risk men of ages 40–54 years and men >70 years of age in excellent health.

The American Society of Clinical Oncology has published a guideline for men considering prostate screening (https://www.asco.org/sites/new-www.asco.org/files/content-files/practice-and-guidelines/documents/2012-psa-pco-decision-aid.pdf). They identified the following from current prostate-screening trials:

- From 1000 men who had screening for 11 years, 96 cases of prostate cancer were found.
- From 1000 men who did not have screening, approximately 60 cases of prostate cancer were found.
- From 1000 men in their 50s getting regular PSA testing for 11 years, four died of prostate cancer; from 1000 men who did not get screening, five died of prostate cancer. Therefore, there is a 20% reduction in RR of death from screening for prostate cancer.
- Men should be fully informed of the potential benefits and documented harms associated with screening, especially the risk of overdiagnosis. Observation-only is an appropriate treatment for many. The decision to screen should include a commitment not to rush into aggressive therapy, if diagnosed.

Lung cancer screening

As in the United States, lung cancer is the most commonly diagnosed nonskin cancer worldwide and is the leading cause of cancer death in men and the second leading cause of cancer death in women.[14,96]

Screening and diagnostic methods

Chest X-ray screening was first advocated in the early 1950s, and by 1960, several lung cancer screening campaigns began. The Mayo Lung Project, initiated in 1971, enrolled more than 9200 male smokers and randomized them to receive chest X-ray and sputum cytology either every 4 months or every year, for 6 years. Follow-up continues to this day.[146,147] After 13 and 20 years of follow-up, the intensively screened arm had an increased number of lung cancers diagnosed and a significant increase in disease-specific survival.[147,148] Lung cancer mortality was not reduced, demonstrating that screening can increase survival rates without decreasing mortality. An estimated 18% of cancers diagnosed in the intensive group were overdiagnosed cancers.[149] Three other large, randomized studies of chest X-ray and sputum cytology using different screening schedules confirmed the findings of the Mayo Lung Project.[150,151]

These chest X-ray studies had important limitations, that is, they did not randomize to an unscreened control group and they used X-ray and treatment technology from the 1960s and 1970s. Whether lung cancer screening was ineffective was readdressed in the US PLCO.[152] Participants were randomized to receive either annual postero-anterior-view chest radiograph for 4 years or usual care (without screening). With a median of 12 years of follow-up, PLCO found no mortality advantage to using chest X-ray screening.[153]

Spiral CT is more sensitive than chest X-ray in detecting small lung nodules. Low-dose CT (LDCT) uses an average of 1.5 mSv of radiation during 15 s to perform a lung scan. This led to the launch of the NLST in 2002.[154] Approximately 53,000 persons at high risk for lung cancer were randomized to receive either three annual LDCT scans or three single-view postero-anterior chest X-rays. With a median follow-up of 6.5 years, a 20% relative reduction in lung cancer mortality (95% CI, 6.8–26.7; $P = 0.004$) was found when compared to the chest X-ray arm[154] corresponding to lung cancer death rates of 247 and 309 per 100,000 person-years in the LDCT-scan versus single-view X-ray groups, respectively. A 6.7% decrease in death from any cause was seen in the LDCT group (95% CI, 1.2–13.6; $P = 0.02$), a rare finding in a prospective RCT. Screening prevented the most lung cancer deaths among participants who were at highest risk and very few deaths among those at lowest risk. These findings provide empirical support for risk-based screening.[155]

The NLST showed the promise of LDCT screening but also has limitations. In the trial, 96.4% of positive findings were false.[154,156] Positive results require additional diagnostic procedures—mostly conventional CT scans but in some cases needle biopsy, bronchoscopy, mediastinoscopy, or thoracotomy—which are associated with anxiety, expense, and complications (e.g., pneumo- or hemothorax after lung biopsy). The NLST reported 16 deaths within 60 days of an invasive diagnostic procedure; whether the procedure was causative is unknown. Of these participants, six did not have cancer. Interest has increased in evaluating algorithms to decrease the number of invasive diagnostic procedures.[157,158] Overdiagnosis was estimated to be 18.5% (95% CI, 5.4–30.6%) in the NLST.[159]

The Dutch-Belgian Randomized Lung Cancer Screening Trial (NELSON study) randomized 13,195 people aged 50–74 at high risk for lung cancer to receive either screening approximately every 3 years or no screening.[160] The no-screening group was followed through a registry. After 10 years of follow-up, the screening arm had a referral rate for suspicious nodules of 2.1%. The incidence of lung cancer was 5.58 cases per 1000 person-years in the screening group and 4.91 cases per 1000 person-years in the control group; lung cancer mortality was 2.50 deaths per 1000 person-years and 3.30 deaths per 1000 person-years in the two groups, respectively. Screening was associated with a 24% reduction in RR of lung cancer death at 10 years, RR = 0.76 (95% CI, 0.61–0.94; P = 0.01). In a subset analysis, women had a 33% reduction in risk of death (rate ratio, 0.67; 95% CI, 0.38–1.14) at 10 years of follow-up. Harms were not reported.

Screening recommendations

The ACS, the American College of Chest Physicians, and the American Society of Clinical Oncology recommend that clinicians discuss lung cancer screening with patients who would have qualified for the NLST: those between the ages of 55–74 years, with a ≥30 pack-year smoking history, who currently smoke or have quit within the past 15 years, and who are in relatively good health. In 2021, the Task Force began recommending lung screening for those aged 50–80 who qualify and want this screening after informed decision making.[161]

This discussion should include the benefits, uncertainties, and harms associated with LDCT screening for lung cancer. Adults who choose to be screened should enter an organized screening program at an institution with access to a multidisciplinary team with expertise in LDCT who are skilled in the evaluation, diagnosis, and treatment of abnormal lung lesions. If a high-quality program is not available, the risks of harm associated with screening may be greater than the benefits.[162,163] Recommendations state that an annual LDCT should be performed as long as subjects would benefit from treatment, if diagnosed. All screening guidelines also stress that current smokers should be offered help with smoking cessation.

Testicular cancer screening

Testicular cancer is relatively uncommon, and its treatment is often successful.[14,96] Over 70% of patients with this cancer and metastatic disease have prolonged complete remissions.

Screening and diagnostic methods

Most diagnoses are made when the patient or physician recognizes an abnormality. Suspicious masses are further evaluated through ultrasonography and biopsy.

While self-palpation of the testes is simple, available data suggest this is of low specificity and predictive value and is done infrequently.[164] Self-examinations result in false alarms that burden the healthcare system and can be costly. A useful intervention may be health education to encourage men to seek medical care if they notice a lump or nodule or any change in the size, shape, or consistency of the testes. Patient delay after becoming aware of a testicular abnormality is clearly associated with poorer survival.

Screening recommendations

No organization recommends routine screening for testicular cancer in average-risk men. The American Academy of Family Physicians recommends palpation of testicles for men aged 13–39 at higher risk for the disease due to a history of cryptorchidism, orchiopexy, or testicular atrophy.[164]

Hepatocellular cancer screening

Hepatocellular cancer (HCC) is the fourth most common cancer worldwide.[165] Age-standardized incidence rates vary 40-fold between populations of China and North America, although rates are rising in the United States.[96]

Chronic hepatitis B and C are major risk factors. Other risk factors include alcoholic cirrhosis, hemochromatosis, alpha-l-antitrypsin deficiency, glycogen storage disease, porphyria cutanea tarda, tyrosinemia, nonalcoholic fatty liver disease, and Wilson disease.[165,166] In parts of Africa, the high incidence of HCC may be related to ingestion of aflatoxin-contaminated foods.

Four types of tumor markers are currently being used or studied as screening tests: oncofetal antigens and glycoprotein antigens, enzymes and isoenzymes, genes, and cytokines.[167] A test for serum alpha-fetoprotein (AFP), a fetal-specific glycoprotein antigen, is the most widely used. In high-risk populations, sensitivity of 39–97%, specificity of 76–95%, and PPVs of 9–32% have been reported. An AFP increase is not specific to HCC; it also rises due to hepatitis, pregnancy, and germ-cell tumors.[165]

Ultrasound and CT imaging have been studied as adjuncts to AFP.[168] These tests have limited sensitivity and specificity. A prospective randomized study in China using AFP and ultrasound found HCC mortality to be lower in the screened group (83.2 vs 131.5 per 100,000 with a mortality rate ratio of 0.63 [95% CI, 0.41–0.98]). Whether these data were from an intention-to-screen analysis is unclear: these results differ from those in other publications.[169,170]

Screening recommendations for HCC

Screening for HCC is not advocated in the general population; its benefit among those with HCC risk factors is questioned.

Endometrial cancer screening

Endometrial cancer is the most commonly diagnosed gynecologic malignancy among women in the United States and western Europe[14,96] where approximately one in four endometrial cancers is advanced at the time of diagnosis.

Screening and diagnostic methods

The efficacy of screening for endometrial cancer has never been evaluated in a prospective RCT. The Pap test, which occasionally identifies endometrial abnormalities, is insensitive for endometrial cancer screening and should not be used. While endometrial biopsy is the gold standard screening test, interest in transvaginal ultrasound (TVU) screening has recently increased.[171] However, two well-designed studies of endometrial screening with TVU and biopsy have reported both disappointing results and significant harms, including some cases of uterine perforation.[172,173]

Screening recommendations

Currently, no organization recommends routine screening for endometrial cancer in average-risk women. The ACS recommends women be informed of the risk and symptoms of endometrial cancer at the time of menopause and be strongly encouraged to report unexpected bleeding or spotting to their physician.[174]

The ACS recommends a risk-based approach for women at high risk for endometrial cancer including those known to carry HNPCC-associated mutations (Lynch syndrome), those likely to be a mutation carrier based on relatives known to be mutation carriers, and those from families appearing to have an autosomal dominant predisposition to colon cancer in the absence of genetic testing results.[175] Women known or suspected to have Lynch syndrome should be offered annual endometrial screening beginning at age 35 following discussion of testing benefits, risks, and limitations.

Ovarian cancer screening

Ovarian cancer has the highest mortality rate of all gynecologic cancers and accounts for 6% of all cancer deaths among women in the United States.[14] Recent evidence shows that many so-called ovarian cancers are actually primary fallopian-tube cancers, while a few starts as primary abdominal-wall tumors. Most women are diagnosed as having ovarian cancer after symptoms develop, while only 19% have disease truly localized to the ovary.[176]

Screening and diagnostic methods

Pelvic examination has low sensitivity and specificity for the detection of ovarian cancer, and thus cannot be recommended as a sole screening method. However, recent studies suggest that a more favorable diagnosis may be possible if early symptoms are evaluated.[177]

CA-125, a tumor-associated antigen, is the most extensively studied ovarian cancer serum marker and is mainly used for surveillance after surgical removal of an epithelial ovarian cancer. The currently available assay, CA-125 II, uses both OC125 and MC11 antibodies.[178] CA-125 levels >30–35 U/mL are considered abnormal. Although CA-125 is elevated in most advanced ovarian cancers, only half of early ovarian cancers yield a positive test. Moreover, CA-125 levels can be elevated in noncancerous diseases of the ovaries[179] and are influenced by the presence of other cancers, a history of hormone use, and current smoking.

Ultrasonography: abdominal ultrasonography has been used in ovarian cancer screening with poor results, owing to low specificity.[180] TVU is capable of detecting small masses but is poor at indicating malignancy. Color Doppler ultrasonography was believed to hold promise for differentiating benign from malignant masses, but studies have not shown that it improves diagnostic accuracy. Current data are insufficient to support TVU or other imaging modalities as stand-alone screening tools in average-risk asymptomatic women.

Combination CA-125 and ultrasound: nonrandomized cohort studies and pilot RCTs in average- and high-risk women have shown both the limited sensitivity of CA-125 or ultrasound (abdominal or transvaginal) alone at an acceptable level of specificity and the poor predictive value of a positive test. High specificity is especially important because laparoscopy and/or laparotomy is required to rule out the presence of ovarian cancer when screening is positive. The PLCO, a prospective RCT, enrolled 78,237 women of ages 55–74; 39,115 were randomized to either ovarian cancer screening with baseline CA-125 and TVU tests, followed by three additional annual rounds of TVU and five of CA-125, or usual care (were not offered annual screening). There were 3.1 deaths in the intervention arm versus 2.6 ovarian cancer deaths in the control group per 10,000 person-years (RR = 1.18; 95% CI, 0.82–1.71).[176]

The UK Collaborative Trial of Ovarian Cancer Screening (UKCTOCS) is a randomized trial assessing the efficacy of CA-125 and TVU in more than 200,000 postmenopausal women. In this trial, CA-125 is being used as a first-line test with TVU as a follow-up test.[181,182] The study measures changes in CA-125 over time rather than using a predefined cut-point.[183] In this study, the risk of ovarian cancer algorithm (ROCA)—believed to improve sensitivity for smaller tumors without measurably increasing the false-positive rate[184]—was initially shown to be associated with a nonsignificant mortality reduction after 14 years (95% CI, −3% to 30%; $P = 0.10$) In follow-up analysis, no significant reduction in ovarian and tubal cancer deaths was observed.[185]

Serum proteomic pattern recognition algorithms are being developed to identify a key subset of peptides that discriminate ovarian cancer cases from control subjects. The potential for either a stand-alone or adjunctive proteomic test for ovarian cancer screening is regarded as promising but remains unrealized.

Screening recommendations

No major guideline-making organization recommends ovarian cancer screening in average-risk women, and the USPSTF specifically recommends against it.[186] In 1994, a NIH Consensus Panel concluded that all women should have a comprehensive family history taken, and women having two or more first-degree relatives with a history of ovarian cancer should be offered counseling by a gynecologic oncologist (or other qualified specialist), since these women have a 3% chance of being positive for an ovarian cancer hereditary syndrome.[187] Women with known hereditary ovarian cancer syndrome—including mutations in *BRCA1* and *BRCA2*, breast-ovarian cancer syndrome, site-specific ovarian cancer syndrome, and HNPCC—should receive annual recto-vaginal pelvic examinations, CA-125 determinations, and TVU until childbearing is completed or at least until age 35, at which time prophylactic bilateral oophorectomy is recommended. While women with these hereditary syndromes represent only about 0.05% of the female population, they have a 40% estimated lifetime risk of ovarian cancer.

Melanoma and nonmelanoma skin cancer screening

Skin cancers—the most common cancers diagnosed in the United States and worldwide—account for nearly half of all malignancies.[14,96] The most common forms are basal cell- and squamous-cell skin cancer, which are jointly referred to as nonmelanoma skin cancer (NMSC). NMSC is highly curable, although significant morbidity can result from delayed diagnosis and treatment. Melanoma, however, is a significant cause of cancer death. In the United States, melanoma accounts for only 2% of all skin cancer cases but the vast majority of skin cancer deaths.

Screening and diagnostic methods

Interest in screening for melanoma has increased in recent years because mortality rates are increasing. Screening involves a visual skin examination by a clinician or a self-examination. A 2–3-min total examination of the skin is preferable because skin cancers can occur at anatomic sites that are not directly exposed to sunlight. Skin examinations by a healthcare provider, while uncommon in the United States, are more common among dermatologists than primary-care physicians. Basal-cell skin cancer may appear as a flat growth or a small, raised, pink or red, translucent, shiny area that may bleed following a minor injury. Squamous-cell skin cancer may appear as a growing lump, often with a rough surface, or as a flat, reddish patch that grows slowly. Signs of melanoma include changes in size, shape, or color of a mole or other skin lesion over time, as is summarized by the ABCD algorithm that emphasizes asymmetry [A] of the lesion, uneven borders [B], changes in color [C], and changes in diameter [D]. A Cochrane review endorsed the addition of an "E" category *evolving* to emphasize the importance of changes in the lesion's appearance over time.[188] However, most dermatologists rely on the overall pattern of appearance (ugly-duckling sign) versus a stepwise assessment of features.

Case-control studies have suggested that increased awareness of melanoma and its symptoms lead to earlier presentation and thinner lesions at presentation.[189] High-risk patients routinely screened by dermatologists have thinner lesions at diagnosis than do historical- or population-based controls.

The American Academy of Dermatology program of skin cancer screening has examined >600,000 people of various risk categories since 1985.[190] In addition to detecting >35,000 NMSCs, melanomas diagnosed by screening were more likely, compared to historical controls, to be <1.5 mm. Skin cancer screening may be more effective if targeted to high-risk persons such as Caucasian patients age >20 with atypical mole syndrome or congenital melanocytic nevi, those with specific phenotypic traits, or those with a history of NMSC.[190]

No RCT has assessed whether skin cancer screening decreases mortality. Some large observational studies suggest its efficacy. A Scottish campaign to promote melanoma awareness and early detection may be associated with a decline in mortality.[191,192] The Skin Cancer Research to Provide Evidence for Effectiveness of Screening project launched an intensive screening program among 360,000 participants in one area of Germany. Although many false positives were found, melanoma incidence increased 16% in men and 38% in women over a 2-year time period and returned to baseline after conclusion of the intervention period. Five years after the end of the intervention period, melanoma death rates in those participants were halved compared to the rest of Germany.[193,194] A community-based, randomized population trial of self- versus clinician skin examination is underway in Australia, with a primary outcome of melanoma mortality after 15 years of follow-up.[93,195]

Screening recommendations

The ACS recommends skin examination during periodic preventive health examinations. The American College of Preventive Medicine recommends periodic total cutaneous examinations for high-risk populations, including those of Caucasian race, or with fair complexion, presence of pigmented lesions (dysplastic or atypical nevus), several large nondysplastic nevi, many small nevi, moderate freckling, or familial dysplastic nevus syndrome.

The USPSTF recommends that individuals, especially those at high-risk, be alert to skin abnormalities. The taskforce concluded that evidence was insufficient to recommend or not recommend routine screening using total-body skin examination for the early detection of cutaneous melanoma, basal-, or squamous-cell skin cancer.

Oral cancer screening

Oral cancer is more common in men than women.[14] Approximately one-third of oral cancers are diagnosed at a localized stage.[196]

Screening and diagnostic methods

Oral cancer is generally accessible to physical examination by the patient and healthcare providers, especially the dentist. Screening can be made more efficient by inspecting high-risk sites where 90% of squamous-cell cancers arise: in the floor of the mouth, the ventrolateral aspect of the tongue, and the soft-palate complex. Leukoplakia and erythroplastic lesions are the earliest and most serious signs of squamous cell carcinoma.[197] Although new technological approaches to screening are being evaluated—such as toluidine blue, brush cytology, tissue reflectance, and autofluorescence—none has been reliably shown to be superior to conventional oral examination.

Using a cluster-RCT design, high-risk men and women of ages ≥35 years in Kerala, India, were randomized to receive either four rounds of oral visual inspection by trained health workers at 3-year intervals or usual care and one round of visual screening.[198] There were 21% fewer oral cancer deaths in the 96,517 participants in the intervention group compared with the control group (RR = 0.79; 95% CI, 0.51–1.22), which rose to 34% fewer among tobacco and alcohol users.

While some have advocated oral-cavity inspection as part of every dental- and physician physical examination, the absence of a general recommendation means that this occurs infrequently. The USPSTF evaluated related data in 2014 and declared them to be insufficient to recommend screening.[199] Ironically, those at highest risk for oral cancer (smokers and heavy alcohol drinkers) are less likely to see a physician or dentist than those at lower risk. Common symptoms leading to diagnostic evaluation include sores on the lip or mouth, oral bleeding, persistent white or red patches in the mouth or on the gums, oral swelling and/or pain, sore throat, and difficulty swallowing.

The future of cancer screening

Newer screening technologies are using molecular medicine. Blood tests are in development that will ultimately be used to screen for cancer. These tests search for circulating DNA segments, changes in methylation, or other molecular signatures. The serum-based DNA fragments or cells come from dying or viable cancer cells. Several large clinical trials are underway in the United States and Europe; some may eventually be used for cancer screening if they reach the sensitivity and specificity required of a screening test.[200–202]

Conclusion

In the near term, the greatest potential for reducing deaths from cancer is through early detection followed by appropriate treatment. Complete benefit of early detection strategies remains unfulfilled globally due to limitations in access, insufficient resources, uneven quality, and lack of organized systems. Screening opportunistically, rather than systematically, is inefficient at both the individual and population level. A comprehensive system of early detection and intervention can potentially lead to high levels of participation, can provide the readiness to implement any new early detection technology that could improve disease control, and can ensure that all program elements are highly competent, interrelated, and interdependent. A systematic approach has the potential not only to increase quality but also to reduce the volume of small errors that contribute to incremental erosion of efficiency, as well as the volume of gross failures that result in avoidable mortality. While many practical barriers must be overcome to establish true population-based screening programs, a system of organized screening holds the greatest potential to reduce the incidence rate of advanced cancers and subsequently to avoid premature mortality.

Key references

The complete reference list can be found on Vital Source version of this title, see inside front cover.

1. Croswell JM, Ransohoff DF, Kramer BS. Principles of cancer screening: lessons from history and study design issues. *Semin Oncol.* 2010;**37**:202–215.
3. Welch HG, Black WC. Overdiagnosis in cancer. *J Natl Cancer Inst.* 2010;**102**:605–613.
4. Baker SG, Prorok PC, Kramer BS. Lead time and overdiagnosis. *J Natl Cancer Inst.* 2014;**106**:dju346.
5. Pinsky PF, Miller A, Kramer BS, et al. Evidence of a healthy volunteer effect in the prostate, lung, colorectal, and ovarian cancer screening trial. *Am J Epidemiol.* 2007;**165**:874–881.
6. Boyle P, Autier P. Colorectal cancer screening: health policy or a continuing research issue? *Ann Oncol.* 1998;**9**:581–584.
10. Xie Y. Values and limitations of statistical models. *Res Soc Stratif Mobil.* 2011;**29**:343–349.
12. Krist AH, Wolff TA, Jonas DE, et al. Update on the methods of the U.S. Preventive Services Task Force: methods for understanding certainty and net benefit when making recommendations. *Am J Prev Med.* 2018;**54**:S11–S18.
27. Moss SM, Cuckle H, Evans A, et al. Effect of mammographic screening from age 40 years on breast cancer mortality at 10 years' follow-up: a randomised controlled trial. *Lancet.* 2006;**368**:2053–2060.
28. Brawley OW, O'Regan RM. Breast cancer screening: time for rational discourse. *Cancer.* 2014;**120**:2800–2802.
30. Nelson HD, Fu R, Cantor A, et al. Effectiveness of breast cancer screening: systematic review and meta-analysis to update the 2009 U.S. Preventive Services Task Force recommendation. *Ann Intern Med.* 2016;**164**:244–255.
31. Nelson HD, Zakher B, Cantor A, et al. Risk factors for breast cancer for women aged 40 to 49 years: a systematic review and meta-analysis. *Ann Intern Med.* 2012;**156**:635–648. doi: 10.7326/0003-4819-156-9-201205010-00006.
33. Semiglazov VF, Manikhas AG, Moiseenko VM, et al. Results of a prospective randomized investigation [Russia (St.Petersburg)/WHO] to evaluate the significance of self-examination for the early detection of breast cancer. *Vopr Onkol.* 2003;**49**:434–441.
36. Siu AL. Screening for breast cancer: U.S. Preventive Services Task Force recommendation statement. *Ann Intern Med.* 2016;**164**:279–296.
44. Gao DL, Thomas DB, Ray RM, et al. Randomized trial of breast self-examination in 266,064 women in Shanghai. *Zhonghua Zhong Liu Za Zhi [Chin J Oncol].* 2005;**27**:350–354.
45. Siegel RL, Miller KD, Jemal A. Cancer statistics, 2020. *CA Cancer J Clin.* 2020;**70**:7–30.
55. Merrill AL, Esserman L, Morrow M. Clinical decisions. Ductal carcinoma *in situ*. *N Engl J Med.* 2016;**374**:390–392.
56. Esserman LJ, Thompson IM Jr, Reid B. Overdiagnosis and overtreatment in cancer: an opportunity for improvement. *JAMA.* 2013;**310**:797–798.
57. Kerlikowske K, Hubbard RA, Miglioretti DL, et al. Comparative effectiveness of digital versus film-screen mammography in community practice in the United States: a cohort study. *Ann Intern Med.* 2011;**155**:493–502.
58. Hofvind S, Holen AS, Aase HS, et al. Two-view digital breast tomosynthesis versus digital mammography in a population-based breast cancer screening programme (To-Be): a randomised, controlled trial. *Lancet Oncol.* 2019;**20**:795–805.
60. Saslow D, Boates C, Burke W, et al. American Cancer Society guidelines for breast screening with MRI as an adjunct to mammography. *CA Cancer J Clin.* 2007;**57**:90–104 http://caonline.amcancersoc.org.
61. Saadatmand S, Geuzinge HA, Rutgers EJT, et al. MRI versus mammography for breast cancer screening in women with familial risk (FaMRIsc): a multicentre, randomised, controlled trial. *Lancet Oncol.* 2019;**20**:1136–1147.
65. Tonelli M, Connor Gorber S, Joffres M, et al. Recommendations on screening for breast cancer in average-risk women aged 40-74 years. *CMAJ.* 2011;**183**:1991–2001.
69. Shaukat A, Mongin SJ, Geisser MS, et al. Long-term mortality after screening for colorectal cancer. *N Engl J Med.* 2013;**369**:1106–1114.
70. Mandel JS, Church TR, Bond JH, et al. The effect of fecal occult-blood screening on the incidence of colorectal cancer. *N Engl J Med.* 2000;**343**:1603–1607.
75. Imperiale TF, Ransohoff DF, Itzkowitz SH, et al. Multitarget stool DNA testing for colorectal-cancer screening. *N Engl J Med.* 2014;**370**:1287–1297.
85. Lou S, Shaukat A. Noninvasive strategies for colorectal cancer screening: opportunities and limitations. *Curr Opin Gastroenterol.* 2021;**37**:44–51.
92. Levin B, Lieberman DA, McFarland B, et al. Screening and surveillance for the early detection of colorectal cancer and adenomatous polyps, 2008: a joint guideline from the American Cancer Society, the US Multi-Society Task Force on Colorectal Cancer, and the American College of Radiology. *CA Cancer J Clin.* 2008;**58**:130–160.
95. Lin JS, Piper MA, Perdue LA, et al. *U.S. Preventive Services Task Force Evidence Syntheses, formerly Systematic Evidence Reviews. Screening for Colorectal Cancer: A Systematic Review for the US Preventive Services Task Force.* Rockville, MD: Agency for Healthcare Research and Quality (US); 2016.
100. Melnikow J, Henderson JT, Burda BU, et al. *U.S. Preventive Services Task Force Evidence Syntheses, formerly Systematic Evidence Reviews. Screening for Cervical Cancer With High-Risk Human Papillomavirus Testing: A Systematic Evidence Review for the US Preventive Services Task Force.* Rockville, MD: Agency for Healthcare Research and Quality (US); 2018.
101. Curry SJ, Krist AH, Owens DK, et al. Screening for cervical cancer: US Preventive Services Task Force Recommendation Statement. *JAMA.* 2018;**320**:674–686.
111. Sankaranarayanan R, Nene BM, Shastri SS, et al. HPV screening for cervical cancer in rural India. *N Engl J Med.* 2009;**360**:1385–1394.
112. Moyer VA. Screening for cervical cancer: U.S. Preventive Services Task Force recommendation statement. *Ann Intern Med.* 2012;**156**:880–891 W312.
113. Shastri SS, Mittra I, Mishra GA, et al. Effect of VIA screening by primary health workers: randomized controlled study in Mumbai, India. *J Natl Cancer Inst.* 2014;**106**:dju009.
116. Fontham ETH, Wolf AMD, Church TR, et al. Cervical cancer screening for individuals at average risk: 2020 guideline update from the American Cancer Society. *CA Cancer J Clin.* 2020;**70**:321–346.
117. Bray F, Ferlay J, Soerjomataram I, et al. Global cancer statistics 2018: GLOBOCAN estimates of incidence and mortality worldwide for 36 cancers in 185 countries. *CA Cancer J Clin.* 2018;**68**:394–424.
118. Albertsen PC, Hanley JA, Fine J. 20-year outcomes following conservative management of clinically localized prostate cancer. *JAMA.* 2005;**293**:2095–2101.
119. Schroder FH, Hugosson J, Roobol MJ, et al. Screening and prostate-cancer mortality in a randomized European study. *N Engl J Med.* 2009;**360**:1320–1328.
121. Thompson IM, Ankerst DP, Chi C, et al. Operating characteristics of prostate-specific antigen in men with an initial PSA level of 3.0 ng/ml or lower. *JAMA.* 2005;**294**:66–70.
123. Andriole GL, Crawford ED, Grubb RL 3rd, et al. Mortality results from a randomized prostate-cancer screening trial. *N Engl J Med.* 2009;**360**:1310–1319.
128. Holmberg L, Bill-Axelson A, Helgesen F, et al. A randomized trial comparing radical prostatectomy with watchful waiting in early prostate cancer. *N Engl J Med.* 2002;**347**:781–789.
130. Hamdy FC, Donovan JL, Lane JA, et al. 10-year outcomes after monitoring, surgery, or radiotherapy for localized prostate cancer. *N Engl J Med.* 2016;**375**:1415–1424.
140. Hugosson J, Roobol MJ, Månsson M, et al. A 16-yr follow-up of the European Randomized study of Screening for Prostate Cancer. *Eur Urol.* 2019;**76**:43–51.
145. Carter HB. American Urological Association (AUA) guideline on prostate cancer detection: process and rationale. *BJU Int.* 2013;**112**:543–547.
146. Marcus PM, Bergstralh EJ, Zweig MH, et al. Extended lung cancer incidence follow-up in the Mayo Lung Project and overdiagnosis. *J Natl Cancer Inst.* 2006;**98**:748–756.
148. Fontana RS, Sanderson DR, Taylor WF, et al. Early lung cancer detection: results of the initial (prevalence) radiologic and cytologic screening in the Mayo Clinic study. *Am Rev Respir Dis.* 1984;**130**:561–565.
149. Marcus PM. Estimating overdiagnosis in lung cancer screening. *JAMA Intern Med.* 2014;**174**:1198.
159. Patz EF Jr, Pinsky P, Gatsonis C, et al. Overdiagnosis in low-dose computed tomography screening for lung cancer. *JAMA Intern Med.* 2014;**174**:269–274.
161. Krist AH, Davidson KW, Mangione CM, et al. Screening for lung cancer: US Preventive Services Task Force Recommendation Statement. *JAMA.* 2021;**325**:962–970.
163. Bach PB, Mirkin JN, Oliver TK, et al. Benefits and harms of CT screening for lung cancer: a systematic review. *JAMA.* 2012;**307**:2418–2429.
164. Lin K, Sharangpani R. Screening for testicular cancer: an evidence review for the U.S. Preventive Services Task Force. *Ann Intern Med.* 2010;**153**:396–399.
171. Cuzick J, Forbes JF, Sestak I, et al. Long-term results of tamoxifen prophylaxis for breast cancer–96-month follow-up of the randomized IBIS-I trial. *J Natl Cancer Inst.* 2007;**99**:272–282.
174. Smith RA, Brawley OW. The National Breast and Cervical Cancer Early Detection Program: toward a system of cancer screening in the United States. *Cancer.* 2014;**120**(Suppl 16):2617–2619.
175. Smith RA, Andrews KS, Brooks D, et al. Cancer screening in the United States, 2019: a review of current American Cancer Society guidelines and current issues in cancer screening. *CA Cancer J Clin.* 2019;**69**:184–210.
177. Dilley J, Burnell M, Gentry-Maharaj A, et al. Ovarian cancer symptoms, routes to diagnosis and survival – population cohort study in the 'no screen' arm of the UK Collaborative Trial of Ovarian Cancer Screening (UKCTOCS). *Gynecol Oncol.* 2020;**158**:316–322.
179. Johnson CC, Kessel B, Riley TL, et al. The epidemiology of CA-125 in women without evidence of ovarian cancer in the Prostate, Lung, Colorectal and Ovarian Cancer (PLCO) Screening Trial. *Gynecol Oncol.* 2008;**110**:383–389.
185. Menon U, Gentry-Maharaj A, Burnell M, et al. Ovarian cancer population screening and mortality after long-term follow-up in the UK Collaborative

Trial of Ovarian Cancer Screening (UKCTOCS): a randomised controlled trial. *Lancet*. 2021;**397**:2182–2193.
186 Moyer VA. Screening for ovarian cancer: U.S. Preventive Services Task Force reaffirmation recommendation statement. *Ann Intern Med*. 2012;**157**:900–904. doi: 10.7326/0003-4819-157-11-201212040-00539.
187 NIH Consensus Conference. Ovarian cancer. Screening, treatment, and follow-up. NIH Consensus Development Panel on Ovarian Cancer. *JAMA*. 1995;**273**:491–497.
194 Katalinic A, Waldmann A, Weinstock MA, et al. Does skin cancer screening save lives?: an observational study comparing trends in melanoma mortality in regions with and without screening. *Cancer*. 2012;**118**:5395–5402.
202 Mattox AK, Bettegowda C, Zhou S, et al. Applications of liquid biopsies for cancer. *Sci Transl Med*. 2019;**11**:eaay1984.

PART 6

Clinical Disciplines

37 Clinical cancer genomic diagnostics and modern diagnostic pathology

Katherine Roth, MD ■ *Stephen B. Gruber, MD, PhD, MPH* ■ *Kevin McDonnell, MD, PhD*

> **Overview**
>
> New techniques in next-generation sequencing, digital pathology, and artificial intelligence have emerged as important tools to inform early detection, clinical and pathologic diagnoses as well as therapeutic decision-making. This chapter focuses on multiple types of tests that take advantage of next-generation sequencing for current applications in clinical practice. Genome-wide mutational signatures are informative at a number of levels, not only linking specific exposures to cancer, but also providing prognostic and predictive information. Digital pathology and analytic approaches with artificial intelligence are also highlighted. Finally, the potential of liquid biopsy is discussed across the spectrum from early detection to monitoring for residual disease, surveillance, and recurrence and treatment planning.

Introduction

Precision oncology holds the promise that cancer patients, based on the results of clinical genomic sequencing tests, may benefit from therapies targeted to specific cancer-promoting mutations or perturbed cellular pathways. Such therapeutic targeting seeks to optimize the therapeutic index, with a higher potential for effective therapy, while minimizing unacceptable adverse events and avoiding drugs and other therapeutic interventions that are not likely to be effective. Precision oncology additionally offers the potential for pathologists to offer greater diagnostic sensitivity and specificity and for clinicians to predict a patient's response to therapy or anticipate mechanisms of treatment resistance. Most commonly this involves evaluating DNA extracted from a patient's tumor tissue for somatic changes. In addition to somatic testing, by also evaluating a patient's germline DNA, identified germline alterations can potentially expand a patient's therapeutic options and inform cancer screening and prevention strategies. This information is relevant not only for the patient but also potentially for the patient's family members. Clinical germline genetic testing is also increasingly being used for cancer risk assessment, as prospective identification of individuals identified to be at significant risk for developing cancer based on germline test results may facilitate their navigation to appropriate screening, earlier interception, and precision prevention of cancer. Compared to current clinical genomic tests using targeted panels of known cancer-associated genes, newer and more comprehensive "next-generation sequencing" (NGS) technologies which simultaneously interrogate the somatic and constitutional genomes (or exomes) are particularly informative, especially when supplemented to take advantage of RNA transcriptome profiling to detect fusions and other pathogenetic and allele-specific variants. Such NGS approaches are likely to be essential for detection of the spectrum of cancer-promoting mutations in the study of more diverse and understudied populations and in understudied and rarer forms of cancer.

Clinical cancer genomic testing encompasses the domains of tumor profiling and germline cancer genetics to not only understand the pathogenetic drivers of cancer cells but also to understand and quantify the underlying familial predisposition to cancer that can be understood through germline genetic testing for highly penetrant cancer genes and measuring polygenic variation that cumulatively contributes to cancer. The premise for evaluating a patient's tumor and germline genome is that changes in chromosomes are a critical step in tumorigenesis,[1] and that cancer is driven by changes in the genome.[2] To link molecular biology to cancer physiology and treatment, technologies for molecular profiling have been developed to help diagnose, risk-stratify, prognosticate, inform treatment, and prevent cancer. Molecular profiling has already emerged as the standard of care for several types of cancer and is rapidly becoming an essential element of a cancer diagnostic workup for therapeutic decision-making.

An increasing number of cancer therapeutics have been US Food and Drug Administration (FDA)-approved based on biomarkers identified through genomic and transcriptomic sequencing, and companion diagnostic tests have been developed (Figure 1). While the richness and complexity of the history of biomarker-driven FDA approvals are difficult to encapsulate, selective highlights identify themes that continue to advance the precision oncology field (Figure 1). Arguably, one of the first pioneering biomarker-based therapies was tamoxifen, a selective estrogen receptor modulator. Originally intended as a contraceptive therapy, tamoxifen was approved in 1977 for patients with advanced breast cancer. Now tamoxifen is used as a treatment for all stages of hormone receptor-positive breast cancer as well as for chemoprevention, with receptor status being determined by immunohistochemistry.

The recognition that specific, expressed biomarkers can be measured with standard immunohistochemistry continues to drive much of the field of clinical cancer genomics and modern pathology. A landmark discovery that drove the expansion of the field of precision oncology, which established the paradigm for therapeutic targeting specific cancer-associated genomic mutations, was the identification of imatinib, one of the first targeted tyrosine kinase inhibitor therapeutics found to be highly effective for the treatment of chronic myelogenous leukemia (CML). The diagnostic and pathogenetic hallmark of CML is the *BCR-ABL1* fusion gene, resulting from a reciprocal translocation between chromosomes 9 and 22 commonly known as the Philadelphia chromosome translocation, t(9;22)(q34;q11). This novel genomic fusion protein results in the persistent ABL1-mediated activation of tyrosine kinase signaling which is a necessary driver for leukemogenesis. In elegant work that led to the identification and optimization of tyrosine kinase inhibitors that block tyrosine phosphorylation

---

Holland-Frei Cancer Medicine, Tenth Edition. Edited by Robert C. Bast, John C. Byrd, Carlo M. Croce, Ernest Hawk, Fadlo R. Khuri, Raphael E. Pollock, Apostolia M. Tsimberidou, Christopher G. Willett, and Cheryl L. Willman.
© 2023 John Wiley & Sons, Inc. Published 2023 by John Wiley & Sons, Inc.

FDA biomarker-based therapeutic approvals by year

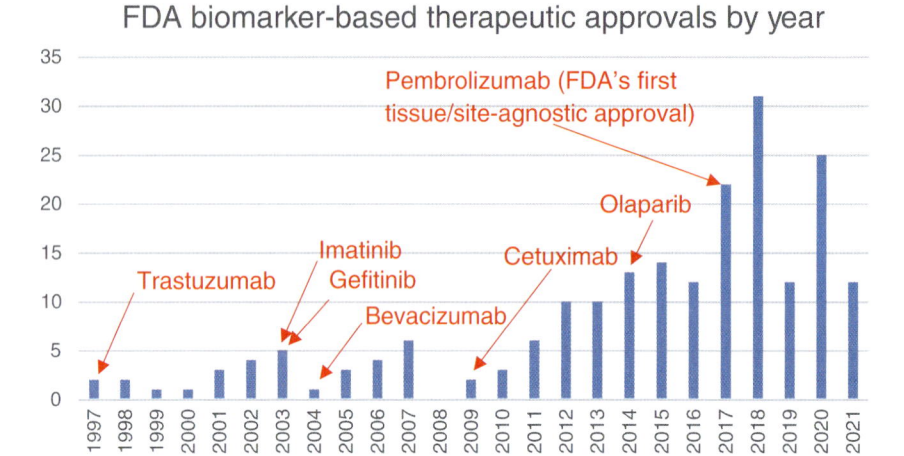

Figure 1 Number of FDA biomarker-based therapeutic approvals per year since 1997. Selected milestones in the history of precision oncology are featured along the timeline: *Trastuzumab*, FDA-approved in 1997, is the first monoclonal antibody (designated by the "-ab" suffix) used to treat cancer, specifically HER2 receptor-positive breast cancer. *Imatinib* and *gefitinib*, both approved in 2003, represent the first in class of small molecule inhibitors (designated by the "-ib" suffix) targeted against the BCR-ABL tyrosine kinase driver mutation of chronic myelogenous leukemia, and the first selective inhibitor of epidermal growth factor receptor's (EGFR) tyrosine kinase domain of non-small-cell lung cancer, respectively. *Bevacizumab* was the first angiogenesis inhibitor approved by FDA in 2004. *Cetuximab* is an EGFR inhibitor approved in 2009 for wild-type KRAS colon cancer but not mutant KRAS, representing the first drug approval linked to a specific somatic mutation. *Olaparib* is an inhibitor of poly ADP ribose polymerase (PARP), the first drug approved for the treatment of advanced cancer on the basis of a germline mutation, initially approved for advanced ovarian cancer in patients with germline BRCA1/2 pathogenic variants having received three or more prior lines of chemotherapy. *Pembrolizumab*, a checkpoint inhibitor form of immunotherapy, is the first drug receiving tissue/site agnostic approval for unresectable or metastatic, microsatellite instability-high or mismatch repair deficient solid tumors. Each approved therapy (not shown) represents a major advance in precision oncology and improvement in outcomes for patients. The rate of approvals continues to impress at the time of this writing (2022).

of proteins involved in BCR-ABL signal transduction, a highly specific compound, STI571, was synthesized that competitively inhibited the ATP-binding site of the enzyme. Imatinib is this drug; it inhibits BCR-ABL and became the first targeted therapy in the era of precision oncology, revolutionizing the care of patients with CML.[3] While the landmark Philadelphia chromosome translocation is traditionally detected using cytogenetic or fluorescence *in situ* hybridization (FISH) techniques, more recent studies have revealed that the use of next-generation genomic sequencing technologies not only results in more sensitive detection of this alteration in CML and other forms of acute leukemia but also importantly identify additional *BCR-ABL* mutations that may confer resistance to imatinib.[4,5]

Beyond the seminal advances in targeted therapy for leukemia, precision oncology has also made parallel strides in solid tumors, perhaps best illustrated in the early application of molecular testing and targeted therapy in non-small-cell lung cancer (NSCLC). The tyrosine kinase inhibitors gefitinib and erlotinib both play an important role in the treatment of NSCLC cancer patients with a sensitizing mutation of *EGFR* (Figure 1). Another NSCLC-associated cancer mutation, the *EML4-ALK* fusion oncogene which arises from an inversion of the short arm of chromosome 2 that leads to exons 1–13 of *EML4* with exons 20–29 of *ALK*, is targeted by crizotinib. Crizotinib was FDA-approved for the treatment of advanced NSCLC patients in 2011 (Figure 1). The exceptional cumulative progress that has been made in the Precision Oncology field is also represented by the recognition by the FDA of a partial listing of a tumor mutation database from The Memorial Sloan Kettering Cancer Center's Oncology Knowledge Base (oncoKB) as a source of valid scientific evidence for Level 2 (clinical significance) and Level 3 (potential clinical significance) biomarkers. This recognition has opened the door for test developers to use these data to support the clinical validity of tumor profiling tests.

Large-scale studies like The Cancer Genome Atlas (TCGA) supported by The National Institutes of Health, the National Cancer Institute (NCI), and the International Cancer Genomics Consortium (ICGC) have been undertaken with a goal of creating a comprehensive set of driver mutations related to cancer from tissue samples from cancer patients. However, the results of these studies demonstrate how complex and challenging the cancer genome can be to interpret.[6] Furthermore, these studies were initiated before newer computational biology and bioinformatics tools were developed which continue to yield new insights.

The emergence of NGS or massively parallel sequencing technologies are rapidly accelerating the incorporation of precision medicine into cancer research and clinical care. This technology has been applied with a variety of methods ranging from targeted cancer gene panels to whole-exome sequencing (WES), RNA or transcriptomic sequencing, and now whole genome sequencing (WGS) assays and tests. These tests, in comparison to their predecessors, are fast, accurate, and able to use formalin-fixed paraffin-embedded (FFPE) samples as well as frozen tissues and are becoming increasingly more affordable. While this section discusses the utility of NGS in molecular pathology and cancer care, with a particular focus on paired tumor-normal testing, NGS has wide-reaching potential benefits for other fields, including pharmacogenetics, microbiology, and the study of other human diseases beyond cancer. Tests that employ NGS are currently being used as tools to complement clinical diagnosis and therapeutic decision-making.

Current applications in clinical practice

One challenge of implementing NGS tests into clinical practice is that there is currently significant heterogeneity among the tests in terms of the technology employed and the bioinformatic methods used to adjudicate somatic variants. Additionally, the benefit of utilizing these tests has not been consistently demonstrated, mostly owing to lags in understanding the data compared to the availability of the data.

To date, the only randomized controlled trial specifically testing the impact of precision medicine, the SHIVA trial, showed no clinical benefit.[7] This trial enrolled patients with metastatic solid tumors who were refractory to standard therapies, and patients were assigned to targeted therapies based on their tumor molecular profiling.[7] Some large nonrandomized studies also did not show statistically significant clinical benefits to this approach, but like the SHIVA trial, these trials were performed on patients with advanced cancer or whose disease was heavily pretreated.[8] In contrast, several studies have shown improved survival for patients,[9–13] including meta-analyses of phase I and phase II precision medicine trials.[14,15]

The inconsistent lack of clinical benefit can be attributed to several factors. For one, these studies often include patients with a variety of cancer types who have advanced disease, thus introducing heterogeneity into the cohort. Each cancer type is not only a unique disease but there is heterogeneity within a particular tumor, which can sometimes acquire alterations as the disease progresses or have revertant mutations after therapy.[16,17] Additionally, patients with advanced disease might be more refractory to a single, targeted therapy compared to a patient whose disease is treatment-naïve, but also there is a paucity of available targeted therapies to offer patients in comparison to the genomic data available regarding their tumors.

A large, comprehensive study of 203 patients with multiple myeloma is worth highlighting as it demonstrates this complexity well, as well as the types of hypothesis-generating data that NGS provides.[18] Using paired tumor-normal testing, significantly mutated genes were identified by either WES or WGS, but when identified, these mutations were not significantly associated with clinical features of the patient's disease or if the patient had previously received treatment. Additional analysis demonstrated significant patterns of multiple gene mutations that were involved in either the same pathway or had similar functions such that while each of these mutations might not have been statistically significant individually, their combination was statistically significant for a patient. This shows that low clonality might not be associated with a low likelihood of disease causality and these patterns of mutations should be explored, as a particular pathway could be implicated in causing disease and targeted therapeutically. Finally, the complexity of each cancer diagnosis was also shown by illustrating the clonal heterogeneity of a patient's disease. Interestingly, some driver mutations were found to be subclonal within patients' tumors and multiple mutations within patients' tumors which were clonal and functionally redundant were also seen. Differences were observed in pretreated patients, whose tumors had significantly recurrent mutations that were found to be more clonal, than those found in untreated patients, thus providing insight into how treatment might lead to the selection pressure of particular clones. This information could help guide therapeutic decision-making with regards to the order of therapy, the use of combination therapy, or avoiding targeted therapy if the clone is not present in a high percentage of cells. The approach also offers justification for re-testing patients upon disease progression or recurrence.

Despite having advanced testing technologies, relying on DNA testing alone might not be sufficient; rather, a multiomics approach incorporating additional technologies offers advantages. While all the details of these multiomics approaches are beyond the scope of this chapter, proteomics and epigenomics are powerful fields that are yielding new insights that are likely to further inform clinical cancer genomics and precision oncology approaches to patient care in the near future.

Types of tests

As introduced above, NGS technology has been applied with a variety of methods to generally three types of genomic tests: targeted cancer gene panels, WES, and WGS.

Targeted gene panels

Targeted gene panels were the first application of NGS used in the clinical diagnostic setting and can be executed with different techniques. In general, these tests evaluate specific regions known to harbor oncogenic drivers or that are therapeutic targets. While gene panels are limited in their utility as they rely on the disease-causing gene being included in the panel, they do have higher coverage depth and a lower false-positive rate of the genes of interest compared to broader tests. However, for large panels, targeted regions that do not receive sufficient coverage sometimes need to be supplemented or confirmed with additional testing by other methods, like Sanger sequencing. As such, targeted gene panels have proven to be particularly useful when researchers want to create a customized panel that can look with greater depth at regions of interest identified on whole-exome sequencing (discussed next). One benefit of greater coverage depth is the potential to identify variants with greater sensitivity in FFPE with poorer tissue quality, in circulating tumor DNA (ctDNA) which often has a lower DNA quantity, and to identify variants more reliably with low frequency in the targeted regions. However, this testing may not capture structural variations unless they are specifically searched. One method used for targeted gene panels is *amplicon-based hotspot panels*, where targeted regions are amplified through primers with multiplex polymerase chain reaction (PCR). While this method can identify single nucleotide variants and large insertion/deletion (indel) variants less than 10 bp, it usually cannot capture large deletions or duplications, or structural rearrangements. A second method applied to targeted gene panels is the *hybridization-based enrichment*. In this method, DNA is fragmented, and regions of interest are targeted with probes that are then sequenced, mapped on a reference genome, and then reconstructed. This technique preserves gene dosage, meaning that it maintains the copy number of a variant, which is often not preserved with amplicon-based panels. In comparison to the amplicon-based panels, hybridization-based enrichment can identify single nucleotide variants, large indel variants, large deletions/duplications, and structural rearrangements.

One type of targeted gene panel worth highlighting is *the multigene prognostic test* used for therapeutic decision-making for a subset of patients with breast cancer. The most widely used of these assays in the United States at the time of this writing is Oncotype DX, which both provides prognostic information as well as predicts the likely benefits of specific therapeutic interventions. Using FFPE specimens, the expression of 16 cancer-related genes and five reference genes is measured using quantitative reverse transcriptase polymerase chain reaction (RT-PCR) technology, and after employing a computational algorithm, the result is a score that determines the risk of disease recurrence for the patient.[19] Oncotype DX is the only genomic assay currently recommended in formal treatment guidelines.

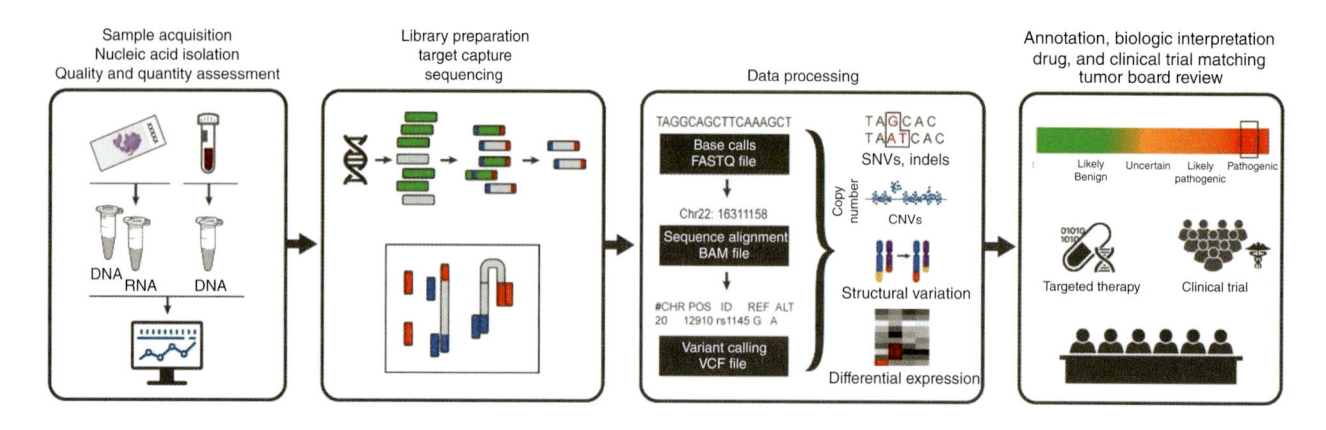

Figure 2 Paired tumor-normal genomic profiling by next-generation sequencing. Sample acquisition requires a source of tumor DNA and germline (constitutional) DNA. These DNA samples are usually derived from formalin-fixed, paraffin-embedded (FFPE) tissue and a blood sample but can alternatively be derived from fresh or snap-frozen tissue for tumor and saliva, buccal cells, or cultured skin fibroblasts for normal germline DNA. Ideally, DNA and RNA are extracted from tumor, whereas RNA is usually not required from normal cells. Next-generation sequencing (also known as massively parallel sequencing), shown in the second panel, is characterized by fragmentation of DNA, ligation of DNA to adaptors that allow DNA to be sequenced and hybridized into a flow cell. This step is called library preparation. DNA is then amplified by PCR, denatured, washed, "bridge-amplified," and repeated many times. One DNA fragment generates multiple copies by PCR, yielding both forward and reverse single-stranded DNA. Sequencing is performed by a technique called sequencing by synthesis, using fluorescently labeled nucleotides. Light is captured to identify the sequence of each fragment. The data analysis then proceeds as shown in the third panel, where the raw data are assembled into base calls in files called FASTQ files. The data are then aligned to a reference human genome, generating BAM files. Variant calling examines whether each nucleotide matches the expected nucleotide of the reference genome or identifies a known variant or other previously unrecognized alteration. The final panel illustrates that annotation and curation, and biological interpretation of the information. This step typically involves both high-powered computational comparisons, as well as human expert interpretation, especially with respect to how the information is used to identify patient eligibility for a targeted therapy or clinical trial. Multidisciplinary tumor boards are usually involved in this final process.

Whole exome sequencing

WES sequences the entire exome, not specific genes, and is therefore more comprehensive, allowing the detection of known variants as well as novel variants, which will be particularly important as these clinical assays are applied to more diverse populations and in expansive studies of different types of cancer. The boundaries between introns and exons are also evaluated, thus making it possible to detect splice variants and key regulatory elements. Compared to targeted gene panels, WES has lesser coverage depth. However, there are several benefits to WES. First, WES allows for the identification of any cancer-causing genes, and therefore the test does not need to be reinterpreted or performed again for a patient who previously had targeted gene panels.[20] Additionally, evaluating all protein-coding regions allows for diagnosing complex phenotypes, as many diseases, particularly cancers, are not caused by a single alteration. At this time, the clinical application of WES is largely limited to academic centers but there are a rapidly growing number of commercially available tests.

Whole-genome sequencing

WGS theoretically provides the optimal tool for evaluating disease-causing alterations. A landmark study demonstrated the potential utility of NGS WGS.[21] Paired tumor-normal tissue from a patient with acute myelogenous leukemia (AML), FAB Classification M1 with "normal" cytogenetics, underwent WGS. This comprehensive sequencing method revealed two known cancer genes with acquired mutations that have been shown to promote leukemogenesis and tumor progression, and eight newly described or novel mutations which were present in all tumor cells. This study demonstrates the feasibility of such testing and the clinical value of discovering novel alterations that can elucidate cancer pathogenesis and identify potential therapeutic targets.[21] However, the requirement for significant computational and bioinformatics analysis and interpretation of WGS and the relatively high cost compared to other forms of NGS, currently limits the clinical utility of WGS. However, as WGS and NGS costs continue to decline and bioinformatic methodologies continue to be developed that can be adapted to the clinical diagnostic setting, it seems highly likely that WGS may replace WES in the near future.

Paired tumor-normal samples for somatic testing

One method to identify somatic mutations is to detect the differences between a patient's tumor tissue and the patient's normal tissue, called "paired tumor-normal testing (Figure 2)." If normal tissue is not available for comparison or not utilized by a particular somatic panel test, then unanticipated germline variants can be inferred or they can be identified *in silico* using data from large population and clinical mutation databases, or analytical methodologies.[22,23] Population databases are useful in filtering out benign germline variants seen in different populations, but the utility of using such a database is limited by the available data from specific populations.[24] Thus, it is possible that benign variants might be overcalled as pathogenic or likely pathogenic. Additionally, filtering germline variants using population databases might overestimate tumor mutational burden (TMB) as compared to germline subtraction, as shown with a retrospective cohort of 50 tumor samples of 10 different tumor types.[25] While submitting one sample derived from only tumor is easier for the patient and logistically simpler for the ordering provider, this testing is far less accurate than paired tumor-normal testing, often leading to an increased rate of "false positive" and "false negative" classifications.

By comparing a patient's normal genome to their tumor genome, one can more accurately identify the mutations that are specific to that patient's cancer cells and distinguish them from any germline variants or somatic mutations derived from clonal hematopoiesis secondary to previous cancer therapy. When only the tumor DNA is sequenced to look for somatic variants, it is possible that germline variants can be incidentally identified, particularly with larger panels. However, somatic testing should not be relied upon to comprehensively identify germline pathogenic variants.[26] The classification system for tumor variants as cancer drivers is quite distinct from the criteria that are used to assess whether germline variants are pathogenic. Most somatic panel tests now include at least a limited scope of clinically significant pathogenic germline variants and paired testing contributes to making these findings more accurate. Therefore, it is important for clinicians and pathologists to be aware that somatic sequencing from the DNA obtained from tumor tissue can give insights into germline alterations, but tumor profiling alone is not sufficient to deduce germline alterations.[27]

Annotation and curation of somatic alterations

The thousands to millions of variants identified by whole exome and WGS respectively result in large quantities of complex data that are difficult to interpret (Figure 2). Computational filtering strategies are applied to variant calling and to variant annotation in order to identify and prioritize the desired types of causative variants with high specificity and sensitivity. Variant calling is the identification of variants from the sequencing data. The nucleotide sequencing data are formatted in a text file called FASTQ (Figure 2). These sequences are then aligned to a reference genome and formatted into a binary alignment map (BAM) file, or its compressed format referred to as a compressed reference-oriented alignment map (CRAM) file. The differences between the sequence data and the reference genome are identified and formatted into a variant call format (VCF) file. Variant annotation adds information about the variant location, the associated amino acid change, and any associated clinically significant information. Germline and somatic variants may occur in known genes which have been associated with cancer risk, causation, or progression, or they may occur in coding and noncoding regions where their significance is unknown or undetermined. A "variant of uncertain significance" (VUS) is a genetic change whose impact on the individual's cancer risk is not yet known.

While standards for germline variant interpretation have been established,[28,29] there is not currently a shared standard for genomic testing technologies. Definitions of pathogenicity for somatic alterations continue to be further refined and it will be essential to develop standards for reporting these variants.[30] Germline variant interpretation is further complicated by the inherent heterogeneity of most types of cancer. Similar or identical variants may behave differently in different patients or in different tissue contexts, but there can also be different cell types within a tumor that have different mutation profiles, differences in the spectrum of mutations, and variants between the primary site of disease and metastatic sites, and finally, significant epigenetic heterogeneity.[31] Thus, it is possible that a broader, multimodal approach and repeat testing throughout a patient's disease course will provide the most informative data to understand mechanisms of tumor progression and heterogeneity and selection of the most important therapeutic targets for intervention.

RNA sequencing

Two limitations of WES are the inability to detect translocations and fusions, and these alterations have been shown to be major drivers of tumorigenesis, although not always sufficient for it.[32] While these types of genomic alterations are often characteristically seen in hematologic malignancies, they also are increasingly detected as hallmarks and pathogenetic changes in solid tumors. In this context, targeted RNA sequencing (RNA-Seq) is a highly useful technology that is used to detect known clinically significant chromosomal rearrangements, which are often sub-microscopic and not necessarily detectable using standard cytogenetic technologies.

In addition to identifying translocations and fusion genes, RNA-Seq has been increasingly used to evaluate gene expression patterns, which can help localize the genetic origin of the cancer-causing pathway, thus potentially identifying therapeutic targets. There are several types of RNA-Seq including total RNA Seq, targeted RNA Seq, and mRNA Seq. Generally, RNA is first isolated from tissue and fragmented. It then undergoes reverse transcription to form complementary DNA (cDNA). Sequencing adaptors or probes are added to identify each unique sample, but they can also be applied to specific exons known to be fused in cancer. PCR amplification is performed, and then NGS is applied. Probes are designed to target exons of genes known to be fused in cancer, which then hybridize with the patient's RNA sample.

Not only have the identification of somatic variants of tumor DNA benefitted from paired testing, but complementing this with transcriptional profiles of paired tumor-normal samples can improve our understanding of a patient's cancer and prognosis as well as identify therapeutic opportunities.[33-35] As described earlier, not all DNA alterations are good therapeutic targets. The WINTHER trial prospectively assigned therapeutic recommendations to patients with treatment-refractory cancer based on either NGS testing of tumor tissue DNA or RNA evaluation that incorporated paired tumor-normal testing, and the addition of RNA profiling was found to expand the number of patients eligible for targeted therapies.[8]

RNA-Seq is a technology of immense interest and is beginning to be added as a component of clinical genomic testing in cancer patients by several academic institutions and companies that offer clinical grade and research grade testing. It has been shown to be a valuable supplement to DNA testing.[36,37] The paradigm of identifying a mutation in the DNA of a patient's tumor and treating them with a single therapy designed to target that mutation is rapidly evolving. As described, the integration of germline data provides meaningful context to somatic events, and RNA-Seq not only identifies fusions but also helps discern the clinical significance of alterations. Integrating additional "second-order" features such as tumor mutation burden, microsatellite instability, and genome-wide mutational signatures can provide even greater clinical significance for the patient by increasing the number of potentially actionable variants and increases the number of patients with clinically actionable events.[38]

Genome-wide mutational signatures

At the risk of over-simplification, cancer is a genetic disease.[39] Somatic mutations that drive cancer etiology and progression can be studied in ways that offer insight into genome-wide mutational signatures associated with specific pathogenetic contributions to the development of cancer. This type of information is useful to pathologists, epidemiologists, and oncologists, who leverage these mutational "fingerprints" for diagnostic, etiologic, and therapeutic purposes. One of the most valuable uses of mutational signatures lies within its application for therapeutic decision-making and selection of targeted therapies. This next section will highlight the historical significance of mutational signatures, describe the methods for determining mutational signatures, and illustrate examples of their use in practice.

Historical significance

Following a long and productive history of growth in the field of chemical carcinogenesis and environmental toxicology, one of the earliest and most important examples of a mutational signature directly to linked to a specific chemical exposure associated with cancer development was published in 1996. Denissenko et al.[40] conducted a seminal series of experiments mapping the distribution of benzo[*a*]pyrene diol epoxide (BPDE) adducts to selective guanine positions in the tumor suppressor TP53. Specifically, guanine positions within codons 157, 248, and 273 were the preferred targets for BPDE adduct formation in three different cell lines, corresponding to major mutational hotspots observed within lung cancer. While the association between tobacco smoke and risk of lung cancer was clearly established and quantified by the 1990s, cigarette manufacturers had successfully avoided legal liability until definitive, reproducible evidence linked specific components of cigarette smoke to lung cancer mutational hotspots at nucleotide resolution. The *Science* paper published by Denissenko et al.[40,41] serves as a landmark in the history of mutational signatures and tobacco policy. New methods to characterize mutational signatures, described below in detail, continue to illustrate mutational signatures that are highly specific to tobacco smoke.[42]

Another mutational signature of historical significance is microsatellite instability, characterized by the expansion or contraction of microsatellite repeats across the genome that arise as the consequence of deficient mismatch repair. First described in 1993 in colorectal cancer, the somatic changes in repeat lengths of mononucleotide or dinucleotide microsatellite repeats were observed in proximal, right-sided tumors, where they were associated with a better prognosis and linked to the phenotype of what was then known as hereditary nonpolyposis colorectal cancer, now referred to as Lynch syndrome.[43–45] The microsatellite instability-high (MSI-H) phenotype of colorectal cancer not only facilitated the positional cloning of the mismatch repair genes, but the discovery of this biomarker also ultimately led to the development of FDA-approved therapeutic strategies that specifically target MSI-H tumors and those that are mismatch repair deficient.[46–48] Another frequently used biomarker that can be used to predict the efficacy of immune checkpoint blockade is tumor mutational burden (TMB), which is the number of mutations per million bases (Mb) of sequenced data.[49,50]

Unsupervised mutational signatures

The most widely used genome-wide mutational signatures are derived from unsupervised patterns recognized in association with specific features of cancer. First described in 2013 by Ludmil Alexandrov, Michael Stratton, and colleagues, their study of 4,938,362 mutations in 7042 cancers led to the recognition of 20 specific genome-wide mutational signatures associated with either known exposures like tobacco smoke or phenotypic signatures like microsatellite instability.[51] The statistical technique used to reduce the dimensionality of these machine learning data was called "nonnegative matrix factorization." To oversimplify, this technique is a computer algorithm that uses no prior information to group data that share similar features.

Powerful in its capacity to distinguish subsets of cancer that share etiologic or pathogenetic features, mutational signatures are essentially pathognomonic for profoundly apparent tumors driven by mutations in polymerase epsilon (Polε), more commonly designated as *POLE*. For example, tumors that are associated with *POLE* have an extraordinarily high TMB that we like to call "Vesuvian" due to its metaphorical resemblance to a volcanic eruption of mutations. Within the framework of the mutation signature numbering system proposed by Alexandrov et al., Polε tumors are uniquely associated with Signature 10. Tumors arising in individuals who have a germline pathogenic variant in *POLE* have a cancer genetic syndrome called polymerase proofreading-associated polyposis syndrome (PPAP), with an exceptionally high lifetime risk of colorectal cancer. Similarly, tumors associated with mutations in polymerase delta (POLδ or POLD) are also part of PPAP and are recognized by Signature 10d. In contrast, cancers arising in patients with Lynch Syndrome, which is due to a different, mismatch-repair type of DNA repair defect is associated with Signature 6.

Mutational signatures are of particular interest to cancer epidemiologists and environmental toxicologists, since etiologic studies of measured exposures in their mutational sequelae may offer insights that were previously hidden from view. WGS provides far better resolution for identifying mutational signatures than exome sequencing, and those studies that have completed WGS have been especially informative. Hearkening back to the early days of BPDE studies in cell lines to link smoking to lung cancer[40] and the ultraviolet (UV) light-induced pyrimidine dimers that are observed in UV-associated squamous and basal cell skin cancers,[52] new studies of known environmental carcinogens are now able to identify a panoply of associated mutational signatures with distinct carcinogens.[53]

Supervised mutational signatures

Supervised machine learning techniques have also been applied to mutational signatures to derive further insights into cancer etiology and classification. One of the hallmark examples of the utility of supervised mutational signatures, called SuperSigs, is the identification of mutational signatures associated with obesity, among other well-known exposures.[54] Using prior information to inform and derive mutational signatures seems to offer advantages over unsupervised mutational signatures in specific circumstances, although the signatures are not as universally interpretable. However, by not requiring an assumption that the same mutational factors operate in the same way in all tissues, tissue-specific signatures may be revealed by supervised analysis. For example, SuperSigs associated with *BRCA* gene mutations differ between breast and ovarian cancers. Similarly, SuperSigs associated with smoking differ in bladder, head and neck, and lung cancers. Obesity SuperSigs were readily identifiable in uterine cancer and kidney cancers, with test performance characteristics as measured by AUCs (AUC is area under the curve, from receiver-operator curves) that appear to exceed those from unsupervised mutational signatures. While this field is still developing, one of the interesting considerations is that supervised and unsupervised mutational signature techniques may be used together, perhaps more powerfully than in isolation. Specifically, a "partially supervised" approach uses SuperSigs to subtract the effects of the mutational load of patients with known annotated factors, to then allow unsupervised mutational signatures to find new mutational patterns.

Digital pathology and artificial intelligence

Machine learning and a variety of statistical techniques are making a major impact on the interpretation of digital images in anatomic pathology. Broadly considered "artificial intelligence," some pathologists prefer to consider the addition of supplemental machine learning approaches to pathologic interpretation of images as "augmented intelligence." Either way, it is clear that powerful computational tools can perform well for the recognition

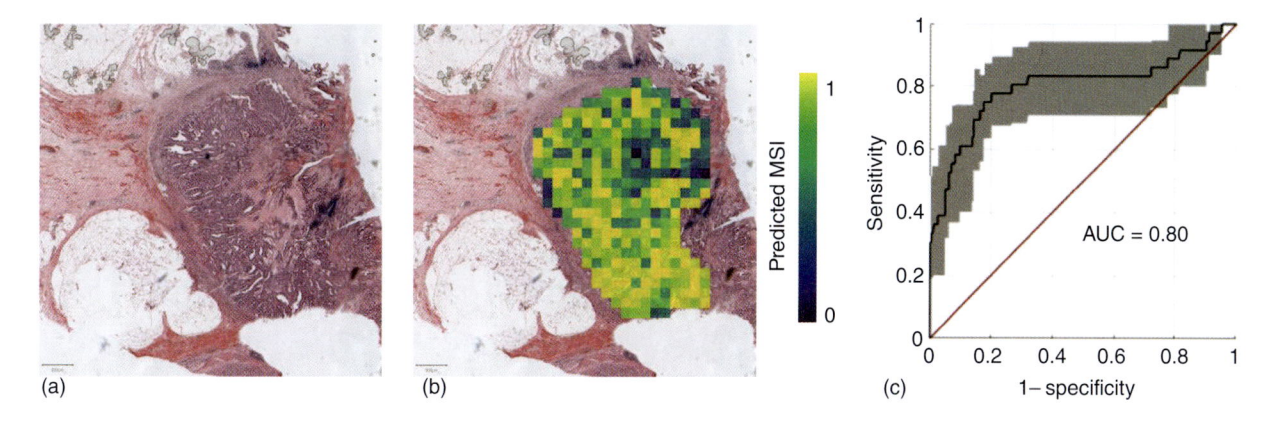

Figure 3 Digital pathology and machine learning to predict microsatellite instability. (a) High resolution scanned image from FFPE recut H&E stained slide from an MSI-H colorectal cancer shown at low power magnification. (b) Spatial patterns of predicted MSI score from MSIDetect network algorithm. (c) Example of a Receiver-operator curve predicting MSI among 279 colorectal cancer cases, yielding AUC = 0.80, (95% confidence interval, 0.74–0.89).

of specific histopathologic features, and even some phenotypically characterized underlying molecular drivers. In a study of tissue slides from 5000 patients with a variety of solid cancers, a single deep learning algorithm was trained to predict a wide range of molecular alterations from FFPE slides stained with hematoxylin and eosin.[55] Gene expression signatures such as the TCGA molecular subtype and homologous repair deficiency were reproducibly and accurately identified by machine learning.

A number of histopathologic features that are readily observed by expert pathologists are strong predictors of survival, including measures of tumor-infiltrating lymphocytes (TILs) and Crohn's-like lymphoid reaction (CLR) in colorectal cancer.[56] Therefore, it is highly desirable to develop algorithms that can help pathologists and clinicians identify known (and unknown) prognostic factors within a pathology image. One specific example with prognostic, predictive, and therapeutic implications is microsatellite instability, first observed in colorectal cancers as noted earlier in this chapter.[43,45] Several papers have now been published illustrating that MSI-H phenotype can be identified by deep learning algorithms (Figure 3).[57–59]

There are at least two statistical analytic strategies that can be effectively leveraged to bring machine learning to digital pathology: ensemble methods and regularized regression methods. Other simpler strategies like discriminant analysis, logistic regression, or support vector machines may work well with few predictors, but machine learning for digital pathology takes advantage of thousands of potential predictors (each possible digital pathology feature, and potentially each clinical or molecular annotation) as well as the complex relationships among them. The data also may suffer from category sparseness in the situation where conditions are rare. Learning algorithms require very large sample sizes to train the identification of relevant patterns, but once trained can lead to highly accurate classification.

Ensemble methods

Random forests and gradient boosting
These strategies build many predictors (1–10 thousand) with subsets of the candidate informative variables and combine them to provide a more robust "ensemble" predictor. Both random forests and gradient boosting usually arrange candidate variables in the models in a conditional hierarchical structure – a tree. Each additional feature improves predictions in only a subset of the patients, dependent on previous features in the model. Random forests train multiple trees, selecting at random a small subset of the candidate variables each time and growing large trees, possibly with pruning. Gradient boosting builds multiple weak classifiers, small trees which on their own cannot provide a good prediction, but weights them in a sequential manner so that each subsequent tree gives more weight to observations that were not correctly classified in the previous tree. The ensemble of many small weighted parallel trees usually provides the best classification accuracy in contexts with complex variables.

Regularized regression methods

Elastic nets
These techniques are based on multivariate regression using a penalized likelihood function. The penalty parameters fix a maximum value on the sum of the regression coefficients, producing a shrinkage of them, that results in more conservative estimates or variable selection. The elastic net is a family of models that range from ridge regression, in which all candidate variables are considered in the model, but with shrunk parameters, to lasso regression, in which some of the parameters are forced to zero and this accounts for variable selection. The optimal predictive parameters for the models are selected using cross-validation.

Overfitting is the major challenge of learning algorithms. Given a big enough dataset, regarding the number of candidate variables, it is usually easy to perfectly classify any outcome in that dataset. The problem arises when the classifier is applied to other datasets with slightly different characteristics. Then the predictions often fail, because the learning was too tailored to the initial dataset. To avoid overfitting, optimal learning algorithms use penalization strategies such that it will be preferable not to reach perfect classification of the training data but have high accuracy in any data that needs classification. To properly estimate the predictive accuracy of the learning algorithm, internal validation strategies such as cross-validation are effective.

Liquid biopsy

Introduction
Presently, tissue-based biopsy serves as the mainstay for cancer diagnosis, genomic profiling, and guiding precision oncology therapeutics. Ancillary to tissue-based biopsy and acquiring

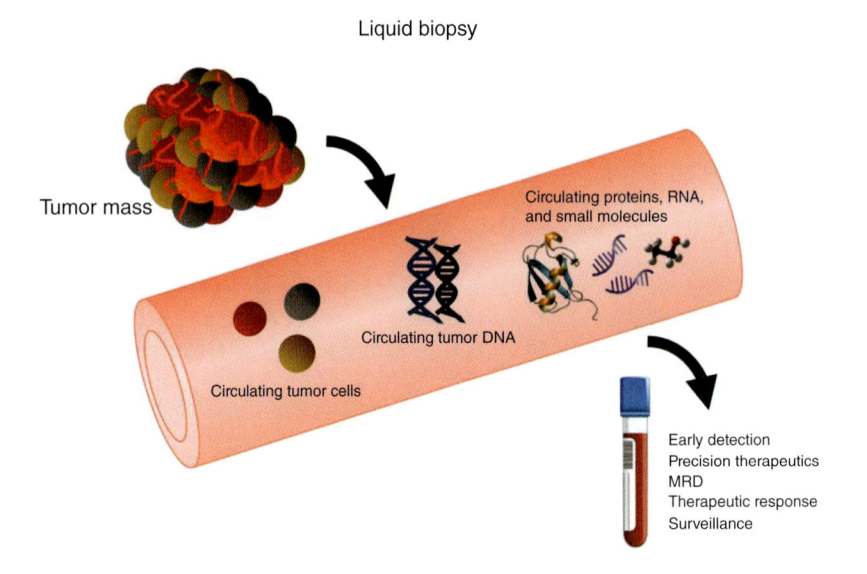

Figure 4 Liquid biopsy enables comprehensive cancer genomic analyses. Solid tumors release into the blood circulation numerous clinically informative assayable elements that include circulating tumor cells, DNA, RNA, proteins, and small molecules. Laboratory assessment of these elements enables early detection of cancer, identification of precision therapeutics, quantification of minimal residual disease, determination of therapeutic response, and surveillance of disease recurrence.

accelerated clinical currency, liquid biopsy (Figure 4) promises to complement or potentially substitute the current mainstay. Liquid biopsy utilizes biofluid rather than solid tissue as analyte for clinical assessment. In the context of cancer medicine, liquid biopsy most frequently makes use of blood as assay biofluid and for analysis, circulating tumor cells (CTCs), and ctDNA (Figure 4).

Circulating tumor cells (CTCs)

Tumors release cells into the circulation (i.e., CTCs) through active intravasation as a step in the metastatic program; alternatively, CTCs enter the circulation due to passive, degradative tumor cell shedding.[60] Subsequently, CTCs may extravasate into distant tissue sites to form metastatic nidi. As such, CTCs potentially provide important biologic, molecular, and genomic information relating to both the primary tumor and metastatic disease. Liquid biopsy, used in tandem with detection of transcriptome signatures and protein expression patterns, antibody-based selection, and physical sequestration, facilitates the identification and collection of CTCs.[61]

Circulating cell-free DNA (cfDNA) and circulating tumor DNA (ctDNA)

Micro- and macro-molecular blood component fractionation studies, together with DNA fragment size analyses indicate that cell-free DNA (cfDNA) exists primarily in blood as constituents of nucleosomes or within exosomes.[62–64] The absolute amounts and relative fractions of nucleosomal versus exosomal cfDNA vary according to the state of a patient's overall general health and cancer course. In the case of a healthy individual, cfDNA derives primarily from hematopoietic cells and localizes within nucleosomes following cell necrosis and apoptosis.[65] In contrast, in patients with active cancer, cfDNA derives not only from healthy cells but from tumor cells as well. In the cancer patient, the quantity of cfDNA may rise significantly, as much as an order of magnitude above what is normally observed in the healthy patient[66]; furthermore, cfDNA from the patient with cancer originates not only from hematopoietic cells but additionally from the tumor cells themselves, so-called ctDNA. ctDNA may be found outside the nucleosomal fraction of cfDNA, making up a major constituent of exosomal cfDNA.[67,68] Unlike nucleosomal cfDNA that results from cell death and turnover, exosomal ctDNA comes from the biologically active processes of exosome formation and DNA shedding. These cellular processes occur not only after cell death but, also reflect conditions of active cellular metabolism, histologic stage, cancer aggressiveness, tumor histology, and treatment response.[69,70]

Advantages of liquid biopsy

Liquid biopsy may offer a number of advantages compared to solid tissue-based sampling. Liquid biopsy requires solely a routine blood sample versus the invasive acquisition of a tissue sample that may entail local or general anesthesia, cause significant bleeding, result in discomfort, inflict organ injury, incur procedural expense or simply not be feasible given the anatomic location of a tumor. Liquid biopsy permits real-time serial sampling of the cancer that theoretically provides an accounting of molecular genomic states across tumor evolutionary time. Also, as liquid biopsy assesses the entirety of a tumor and all metastatic lesions simultaneously, liquid biopsy conceivably overcomes the problem of intra- and metastatic tumor heterogeneity thus offering the possibility of a panoptic perspective of the tumor genomic landscape.

Challenges

Liquid biopsy faces a number of challenges that balance its ostensible advantages and moderate enthusiasm for wide-scale clinical adoption.

In order to achieve the substantial sequencing depths required to detect low-level genetic variants found in tumor clonal populations, liquid biopsy assays often utilize panel-based gene testing restricted to resequencing of a select subset of canonical driver mutations. Such restrictions miss detection of potentially clinically important noncanonical driver mutations and therefore may deprive the patient of opportunities for targeted therapies and clinical trial enrollment.

Unlike liquid biopsy, tissue-based biopsy permits assessments of cell histology, cell surface receptor presence, and protein expression together with the full repertoire of genomic analysis. These assessments provide important prognostic and predictive information having critical implications for therapeutic decision-making, for example, the presence of hormone receptor positivity in breast cancer or mismatch repair protein absence in colorectal cancer. Liquid biopsy platforms generally remain agnostic as to tumor receptor states or protein expression; however, innovations in the molecular analysis of circulating tumor cells may ameliorate these information voids.[71]

Previous studies have highlighted discordance between tissue-based biopsy and liquid biopsy results; this discordance raises questions relating to the sensitivity and analytic validity of liquid biopsy.[72] In liquid biopsy, ctDNA levels may fall below lower levels of detection. Low ctDNA amounts may result from nonshedding of DNA by tumors, overall low tumor burden or the occurrence of nonassayable DNA due to tumors residing in an anatomically privileged site such as the central nervous system; assay limiting levels of ctDNA may contribute to liquid biopsy-associated false-negative variant calls. It is important to recognize, however, that not all discordance between liquid biopsy and tissue-based genomic sequencing reflects deficiencies in the liquid biopsy assay. As noted previously, liquid biopsy has the ability to assess tumor heterogeneity as well as primary and metastatic tumor sites simultaneously, thus potentially generating variant calls not detected with single site, anatomically discrete solid tissue biopsy samples.

Early detection and diagnosis

The ability to detect and diagnose an incipient cancer at its earliest stages has paramount clinical importance. Early detection facilitates improved treatment response and optimizes health outcomes. Health care providers have employed a variety of strategies to achieve effective cancer surveillance including interval imaging and direct visualization protocols. Liquid biopsy represents an additional, potentially more effective surveillance tool.

The detection and isolation of CTCs offer unique advantages with regard to cancer detection as it permits not only genomic assessment of tumor DNA, RNA, and protein but also cellular diagnosis and tumor biologic characterization. Investigators have successfully implemented CTC-based multicancer early detection approaches for breast, colon, and lung cancers.[73] Optimism remains high for the use of CTC assessment in the detection of early-stage cancers, albeit with the recognition of inherent limitations. These limitations include suboptimal sensitivity and potential genomic mischaracterization of the primary tumor due to acquired genetic changes of the CTCs, for example, epithelial to mesenchymal transition of the CTCs.[74] These limitations associated with the use of CTCs risk incomplete or inaccurate genomic accounting of the primary tumor.

Alongside the use of CTCs, analysis of ctDNA has provided an additional means to detect early cancer occurrence. One ctDNA-based early cancer detection approach analyses the methylation status of the cell polarity SEPT9 gene. Scientists have demonstrated that SEPT9 undergoes methylation during neoplastic transformation in colorectal cancer.[75] When assessed in peripheral blood, levels of methylated SEPT9 demonstrate clinically acceptable sensitivity and specificity for the early detection of colorectal cancer.[76] The FDA granted approval for this assay as a screening test for colon cancer in 2016.[77] Since then, other genomic tests that identify tumor-associated pathogenic variants have been granted breakthrough status by the FDA as early cancer detection devices. In clinical studies, these newer tests have demonstrated the ability to reliably detect early occurrence of pancreatic, ovarian, gastric, lung, colorectal, and breast cancers.[78,79] Ongoing efforts to expand the use of liquid biopsy for the early cancer detection of cancer continue.[61]

Therapeutic decision making

The number of FDA-approved targeted and immunotherapeutic agents continues to increase; over the past decade, approvals have accelerated driven by a number of factors that include intensified drug discovery, establishment of rapid drug review pathways, and more substantive financial support from the FDA.[80] Along with increased therapeutic options, growing clinical adoption of precision tumor genotyping and expanded immunological biomarker assessment identifies an ever-growing set of patients eligible for precision treatments and clinical trials. In one large institutional genomic sequencing initiative, nearly 40% and 11% of patients qualified for a targeted therapeutic agent and clinical trial, respectively.[81] The expanding implementation of precision oncology underscores the potential utility and clinical value of liquid biopsy as a means to accommodate intensified precision therapeutic demand.

Multiple studies provide compelling evidence for feasible and effective liquid biopsy-enabled precision cancer care. The ENSURE study, a randomized, Phase III trial, compared the clinical effectiveness of erlotinib to conventional chemotherapy in advanced stage NSCLC.[82] Investigators assessed *EGFR* mutations (*EGFR* Exon19 deletion and *EGFR* Exon21 L858R alterations) by PCR genotyping DNA obtained from either tumor tissue or ctDNA from liquid biopsy samples. Of patients who tested positive for an *EGFR* mutation by tumor testing, 76.7% were found to have the same mutation with liquid biopsy; for patients testing negative for an *EGFR* mutation by tumor testing, 98.2% were negative by liquid biopsy assessment. The SOLAR-1 trial, another randomized, Phase III trial, evaluated the ability of the targeted agent alpelisib plus fulvestrant to prolong progression-free survival versus fulvestrant alone in hormone receptor-positive, HER2-negative advanced stage breast cancer.[83] Investigators assessed *PIK3CA* mutation status by PCR genotyping of both DNA from tumor tissue tumor and ctDNA from liquid biopsy specimens. They observed a 35% reduction in risk for disease progression in patients who demonstrated an alteration in *PIK3CA* by tumor tissue testing; in comparison, the investigators observed a 45% reduction in patients testing positive for *PIK3CA* alterations with liquid biopsy. The ENSURE and SOLAR-1 trials provided compelling evidence for the clinical utility and benefit of liquid biopsy. Referencing these 2 landmark trials the FDA issued inaugural approvals for liquid biopsy-based single gene PCR genotyping to guide precision oncology therapeutic management.[84]

Building upon the insights from the ENSURE and SOLAR-1 trials, subsequent investigations have reinforced the versatility of liquid biopsy-informed precision oncology. The TRITON2 trial, a multicenter, open-label Phase II trial, evaluated whether patients with metastatic castration-resistant prostate cancer (mCRPC) and evidence of homologous recombination gene deficiency responded to treatment with the poly ADP ribose polymerase (PARP) inhibitor, rucaparib.[85] In this study investigators employed a NGS 311 multigene panel to assess alterations in homologous recombination genes in tumor tissue in order to qualify patients for targeted treatment; in a companion bridging study investigators demonstrated the ability of the same multigene panel to identify alterations in *BRCA1* and *BRCA2* in ctDNA obtained from liquid biopsy. The bridging study demonstrated an objective response rate of 46.3% in *BRCA*-mutated patients assessed by liquid biopsy compared to 43.5% in *BRCA*-mutated patients assessed by tumor tissue or conventional germline testing of peripheral blood mononuclear cells. These data led to FDA approval for liquid biopsy as a companion diagnostic to assess *BRCA1* and *BRCA2* mutations in mCRPC. Subsequently, additional bridging and concordance studies established the ability of the multigene panel to successfully identify targetable mutations in *EGFR, BRCA1, BRCA2, ALK,* and *PIK3CA* using liquid biopsy samples from patients with NSCLC, epithelial ovarian, and breast cancers.[77]

Another FDA-approved liquid biopsy-based NGS multigene panel assay demonstrated the ability to assess 55 cancer-related genes. The FDA granted initial approval to this panel assay as a liquid biopsy companion diagnostic to detect *EGFR* exon19, L858R, and T90M alterations. The approval took account of bridging studies that used blood samples from the FLAURA[86] and AURA3[87] clinical trials; these trials examined response to osimertinib in advanced stage, *EGFR*-mutated NSCLC.[88] Subsequently, the FDA expanded approval of this liquid biopsy assay for the identification of *KRAS* G12C mutations in advanced stage NSCLC. This approval considered bridging studies utilizing blood samples collected in the CodeBreak100 clinical trial[89] that examined response to sotorasib in advanced-stage solid tumors.[77]

The multigene capability of these NGS liquid biopsy assays holds enormous promise for continued expansion of FDA approvals to include the entirety of genes assayed on these panels. Sensitivity issues of the liquid biopsy-based assays, however, limit their adoption as stand-alone assays to replace tumor tissue-based assays. The FDA acknowledges this limitation, noting on their approvals; "A negative result from a plasma specimen does not mean that the patient's tumor is negative for genomic findings. Patients who are negative for the mutation should be reflexed to routine biopsy and their tumor mutation status confirmed using an FDA-approved tumor tissue test, if feasible."[77] Continued optimization of existing liquid biopsy platforms and the advent of emerging technologies hold promise to overcome current limitations.

Minimal residual disease and response to therapy

Once the cancer patient completes treatment the question arises as to whether the treatment has worked. Determinations of minimal residual disease (MRD) and therapeutic response can address this question; liquid biopsy analysis of CTCs and ctDNA can assist in making these determinations.[90]

The FDA first approved an assay system for the physical detection of CTCs in 2004. Since approval, seminal studies employing this system following surgical resection or medical therapy validated the clinical value of liquid biopsy to assess treatment response. CTC analysis successfully predicted recurrence[78,91] and survival[92,93] in multiple subgroups of posttreatment cancer patients.

Resequencing of ctDNA represents an alternative approach to assess MRD and response to therapy. Clinicians have available to them two methods of ctDNA assessment: a comprehensive ctDNA genotyping method and a custom, bespoke method that relies on knowledge of a patient's previously determined personal tumor molecular profile. Comprehensive ctDNA genotyping permits a full genomic understanding of a patient's residual cancer including detection of new, potentially therapeutically targetable clonal entities. In contrast, bespoke ctDNA genotyping limits assessment to previously identified genetic variants; these variants, however, typically undergo high fidelity deep amplification allowing for more sensitive detection of MRD. Liquid biopsy-based assays allow more sensitive detection of residual cancer relative to other modalities such as radiographic imaging or biochemical analysis. Earlier detection affords the opportunity for earlier treatment and, theoretically, mitigates the risk of developing therapy-resistant disease if the cancer recurrence is not detected early (Figure 5).

ctDNA liquid biopsy assessment has proven its importance as a tool to detect MRD and evaluate therapeutic response. Monitoring of ctDNA in early-stage breast cancer patients following treatment accurately predicts recurrence.[94] As well, bespoke resequencing of ctDNA in early- and late-stage breast cancer patients has demonstrated its dependability to assess molecular response and detect residual disease.[95]

Developing liquid biopsy technologies and emerging opportunities

A concern that arises with regard to practical implementation of liquid biopsy centers on whether CTC assays and ctDNA genotyping have the ability to detect the extremely limited numbers of neoplastic cells and low-level tumor-associated genetic

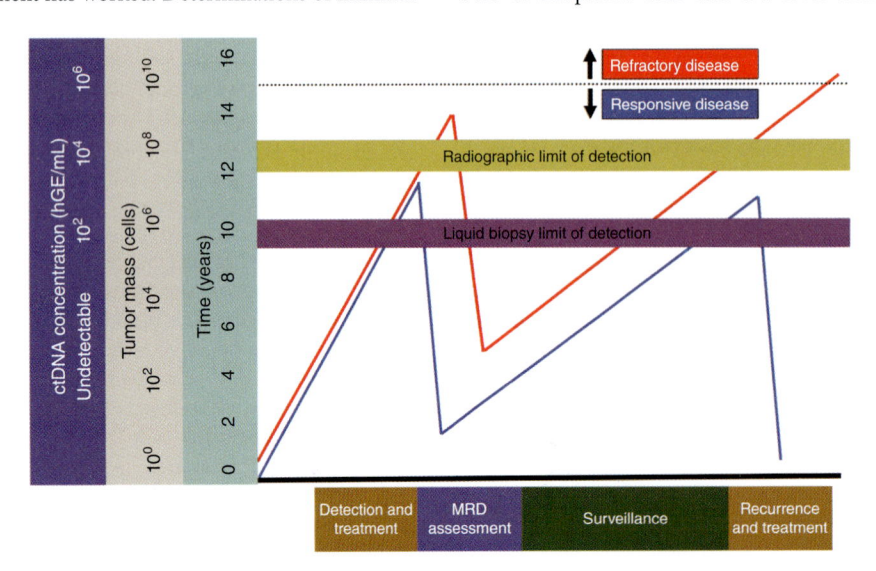

Figure 5 Liquid biopsy enhances detection of minimal residual disease and cancer recurrence. Optimized liquid biopsy protocols afford more sensitive detection of MRD and cancer recurrence relative to existing biochemical and radiographic approaches. Increased sensitivity meaningly impacts clinical care as it facilitates identification of disease at a therapeutically responsive stage.

alterations. Tumor cells present in the circulation may be as low as less than 100 cells per 10 mL of blood[96]; ctDNA may be disproportionately lower secondary to multiple factors including low burden of disease, sequestering of the tumor within an anatomically privileged site such as the central nervous system and inherently low shedding of DNA by the tumor. Technical innovations have helped to overcome limitations in assay performance and enhance the clinical utility of liquid biopsy.

One innovation that boosts sensitivity and accuracy of the CTC assay employs immunomagnetic depletion of contaminating cells in the blood analyte. This technique together with flow cytometric cell sorting has led to the development of an integrated analytic platform that permits tandem genotypic and transcriptomic assessment of CTCs as well as the isolation of rare live cells for downstream biologic analyses.[97] Additional physical isolation approaches such as nanomaterial-enabled microfluidic strategies promise more efficient detection and capture of CTCs; the FDA has granted breakthrough device status to a number of CTC isolation platforms.[98,99]

In parallel to CTC-focused innovations, breakthrough analytic approaches have boosted abilities to efficiently isolate and reliably resequence often limitingly scarce ctDNA. Techniques such as integrated digital error suppression now permit exquisitely sensitive detection and assessment of genotypes associated with ultra-low variant allele frequencies.[100] Additional innovations such as cancer gene mutation multiamplicon and multiplex-PCR in combination with assessment of circulating cancer proteins allow consistent detection of multiple cancer types for which no established screening test previously existed.[78] Investigators recently employed this approach to screen more than 10,000 patients for the occurrence of early undiagnosed cancer. This study demonstrated a specificity of 98.9% and positive predictive value of 19.4% for the detection of cancer.[101]

Other innovations in liquid biopsy have advanced our capabilities to assess ctDNA originating from anatomically sequestered sites (e.g., central nervous system tumors) and tumors that shed minimal DNA (e.g., renal carcinomas). For example, laboratory examination of ctDNA methylomes has facilitated the epigenetic detection and identification of both intracranial and renal tumors.[102,103] Ongoing innovations and emerging technologies provide assurance of continued improvement in assay performance and growing affirmation of the utility and reliability of liquid biopsy in the oncology clinic.

Conclusion

Clinical cancer genomics, next-generation genomic sequencing methods, modern diagnostic pathology, digital pathology, and blood-based genomic detection and monitoring techniques are rapidly evolving, allowing greater precision in the diagnosis, targeted therapeutic intervention, management, and outcome prediction in cancer patients. New techniques in the laboratory, complemented by advances in computational biology, bioinformatics, predictive modeling, and artificial intelligence, and other analytic advances are creating new opportunities to drive precision prediction and intervention. The future is likely to hold exceptional insight into early detection of cancer using techniques that leverage highly sensitive detection of mutations and multiomic signatures, leading to precision prevention, and early intervention. Rigorous studies and clinical trials will be required to understand the performance of these tests, not only on the basis of their analytic validation, but how these tests may be optimized for clinical use and patient acceptability. Clearly, clinical cancer genomics and paired tumor-normal profiling will continue to have a powerful impact on patient management. Complemented by germline genetic testing that is critical to the recognition of cancer genetic syndromes and offers cost-effective prevention to at-risk family members,[104] germline genetic testing is also increasingly driving therapeutic decision making. One can only anticipate how the waves of information will be managed by expert clinicians and understood by patients; tools that facilitate clinical decision support throughout a patient's disease course will be essential to help navigate this ocean of valuable data.

Key references

The complete reference list can be found on Vital Source version of this title, see inside front cover.

1. Hansford S, Huntsman DG. Boveri at 100: Theodor Boveri and genetic predisposition to cancer. *J Pathol.* 2014;**234**:142–145.
2. Vogelstein B, Papadopoulos N, Velculescu VE, et al. Cancer genome landscapes. *Science.* 2013;**339**:1546–1558.
3. Druker BJ, Talpaz M, Resta DJ, et al. Efficacy and safety of a specific inhibitor of the BCR-ABL tyrosine kinase in chronic myeloid leukemia. *N Engl J Med.* 2001;**344**:1031–1037.
4. Soverini S, De Benedittis C, Polakova KM, et al. Next-generation sequencing for sensitive detection of BCR-ABL1 mutations relevant to tyrosine kinase inhibitor choice in imatinib-resistant patients. *Oncotarget.* 2016;**7**:21982–21990.
6. Futreal PA, Coin L, Marshall M, et al. A census of human cancer genes. *Nat Rev Cancer.* 2004;**4**:177–183.
7. Le Tourneau C, Delord JP, Gonçalves A, et al. Molecularly targeted therapy based on tumour molecular profiling versus conventional therapy for advanced cancer (SHIVA): a multicentre, open-label, proof-of-concept, randomised, controlled phase 2 trial. *Lancet Oncol.* 2015;**16**:1324–1334.
8. Rodon J, Soria JC, Berger R, et al. Genomic and transcriptomic profiling expands precision cancer medicine: the WINTHER trial. *Nat Med.* 2019;**25**:751–758.
11. Stockley TL, Oza AM, Berman HK, et al. Molecular profiling of advanced solid tumors and patient outcomes with genotype-matched clinical trials: the Princess Margaret IMPACT/COMPACT trial. *Genome Med.* 2016;**8**:109.
13. Schwaederle M, Parker BA, Schwab RB, et al. Precision oncology: the UC San Diego Moores Cancer Center PREDICT experience. *Mol Cancer Ther.* 2016;**15**:743–752.
14. Schwaederle M, Zhao M, Lee JJ, et al. Association of biomarker-based treatment strategies with response rates and progression-free survival in refractory malignant neoplasms: a meta-analysis. *JAMA Oncol.* 2016;**2**:1452–1459.
15. Schwaederle M, Zhao M, Lee JJ, et al. Impact of precision medicine in diverse cancers: a meta-analysis of phase II clinical trials. *J Clin Oncol.* 2015;**33**:3817–3825.
16. Bertucci F, Ng CKY, Patsouris A, et al. Genomic characterization of metastatic breast cancers. *Nature.* 2019;**569**:560–564.
18. Lohr JG, Stojanov P, Carter SL, et al. Widespread genetic heterogeneity in multiple myeloma: implications for targeted therapy. *Cancer Cell.* 2014;**25**:91–101.
19. Paik S, Shak S, Tang G, et al. A multigene assay to predict recurrence of tamoxifen-treated, node-negative breast cancer. *N Engl J Med.* 2004;**351**:2817–2826.
21. Ley TJ, Mardis ER, Ding L, et al. DNA sequencing of a cytogenetically normal acute myeloid leukaemia genome. *Nature.* 2008;**456**:66–72.
23. Lawrence MS, Stojanov P, Polak P, et al. Mutational heterogeneity in cancer and the search for new cancer-associated genes. *Nature.* 2013;**499**:214–218.
25. Parikh K, Huether R, White K, et al. Tumor mutational burden from tumor-only sequencing compared with germline subtraction from paired tumor and normal specimens. *JAMA Netw Open.* 2020;**3**:e200202.
26. Lincoln SE, Nussbaum RL, Kurian AW, et al. Yield and utility of germline testing following tumor sequencing in patients with cancer. *JAMA Netw Open.* 2020;**3**:e2019452.
27. Yap TA, Ashok A, Stoll J, et al. Rate of incidental germline findings detected by tumor-normal matched sequencing in cancer types lacking hereditary cancer testing guidelines. *J Clin Oncol.* 2021;**39**:10582.
28. Rehm HL, Bale SJ, Bayrak-Toydemir P, et al. ACMG clinical laboratory standards for next-generation sequencing. *Genet Med.* 2013;**15**:733–747.
29. Richards S, Aziz N, Bale S, et al. Standards and guidelines for the interpretation of sequence variants: a joint consensus recommendation of the American College of Medical Genetics and Genomics and the Association for Molecular Pathology. *Genet Med.* 2015;**17**:405–424.

30 Nykamp K, Anderson M, Powers M, et al. Sherloc: a comprehensive refinement of the ACMG-AMP variant classification criteria. *Genet Med*. 2017;**19**: 1105–1117.

34 Román-Pérez E, Casbas-Hernández P, Pirone JR, et al. Gene expression in extratumoral microenvironment predicts clinical outcome in breast cancer patients. *Breast Cancer Res*. 2012;**14**:R51.

35 Huang X, Stern DF, Zhao H. Transcriptional profiles from paired normal samples offer complementary information on cancer patient survival--evidence from TCGA pan-cancer data. *Sci Rep*. 2016;**6**:20567.

37 Abraham J, Heimberger AB, Marshall J, et al. Machine learning analysis using 77,044 genomic and transcriptomic profiles to accurately predict tumor type. *Transl Oncol*. 2021;**14**:101016.

38 Reardon B, Moore ND, Moore NS. et al., Integrating molecular profiles into clinical frameworks through the Molecular Oncology Almanac to prospectively guide precision oncology. *Nat Cancer*. 2021;**2**(10):1102–1112.

39 Vogelstein B, Kinzler KW. Cancer genes and the pathways they control. *Nat Med*. 2004;**10**:789–799.

40 Denissenko MF, Pao A, Tang M, Pfeifer GP. Preferential formation of benzo[*a*]pyrene adducts at lung cancer mutational hotspots in P53. *Science (New York, NY)*. 1996;**274**:430–432.

42 Alexandrov LB, Ju YS, Haase K, et al. Mutational signatures associated with tobacco smoking in human cancer. *Science (New York, NY)*. 2016;**354**:618–622.

43 Thibodeau SN, Bren G, Schaid D. Microsatellite instability in cancer of the proximal colon. *Science (New York, NY)*. 1993;**260**:816–819.

46 Le DT, Uram JN, Wang H, et al. PD-1 blockade in tumors with mismatch-repair deficiency. *N Engl J Med*. 2015;**372**:2509–2520.

47 Le DT, Durham JN, Smith KN, et al. Mismatch repair deficiency predicts response of solid tumors to PD-1 blockade. *Science (New York, NY)*. 2017;**357**:409–413.

48 Le DT, Kim TW, Van Cutsem E, et al. Phase II open-label study of pembrolizumab in treatment-refractory, microsatellite instability-high/mismatch repair-deficient metastatic colorectal cancer: KEYNOTE-164. *J Clin Oncol*. 2020;**38**:11–19.

51 Alexandrov LB, Nik-Zainal S, Wedge DC, et al. Signatures of mutational processes in human cancer. *Nature*. 2013;**500**:415–421.

54 Afsari B, Kuo A, Zhang Y, et al. Supervised mutational signatures for obesity and other tissue-specific etiological factors in cancer. *elife*. 2021;**10**:e61082.

58 Kather JN, Krisam J, Charoentong P, et al. Predicting survival from colorectal cancer histology slides using deep learning: a retrospective multicenter study. *PLoS Med*. 2019;**16**:e1002730.

61 Ignatiadis M, Sledge GW, Jeffrey SS. Liquid biopsy enters the clinic - implementation issues and future challenges. *Nat Rev Clin Oncol*. 2021;**18**:297–312.

63 Snyder MW, Kircher M, Hill AJ, et al. Cell-free DNA comprises an *in vivo* nucleosome footprint that informs its tissues-of-origin. *Cell*. 2016;**164**:57–68.

67 Fernando MR, Jiang C, Krzyzanowski GD, Ryan WL. New evidence that a large proportion of human blood plasma cell-free DNA is localized in exosomes. *PLoS One*. 2017;**12**:e0183915.

71 Heitzer E, Haque IS, Roberts CES, Speicher MR. Current and future perspectives of liquid biopsies in genomics-driven oncology. *Nat Rev Genet*. 2019;**20**:71–88.

72 Merker JD, Oxnard GR, Compton C, et al. Circulating tumor DNA analysis in patients with cancer: American Society of Clinical Oncology and College of American Pathologists Joint Review. *J Clin Oncol*. 2018;**36**:1631–1641.

75 Lofton-Day C, Model F, Devos T, et al. DNA methylation biomarkers for blood-based colorectal cancer screening. *Clin Chem*. 2008;**54**:414–423.

78 Cohen JD, Li L, Wang Y, et al. Detection and localization of surgically resectable cancers with a multi-analyte blood test. *Science*. 2018;**359**:926–930.

80 Brown DG, Wobst HJ. A decade of FDA-approved drugs (2010–2019): trends and future directions. *J Med Chem*. 2021;**64**:2312–2338.

81 Zehir A, Benayed R, Shah RH, et al. Mutational landscape of metastatic cancer revealed from prospective clinical sequencing of 10,000 patients. *Nat Med*. 2017;**23**:703–713.

86 Soria JC, Ohe Y, Vansteenkiste J, et al. Osimertinib in untreated EGFR-mutated advanced non-small-cell lung cancer. *N Engl J Med*. 2018;**378**:113–125.

87 Mok TS, Wu YL, Ahn MJ, et al. Osimertinib or platinum-pemetrexed in EGFR T790M-positive lung cancer. *N Engl J Med*. 2017;**376**:629–640.

89 Hong DS, Fakih MG, Strickler JH, et al. KRAS(G12C) inhibition with sotorasib in advanced solid tumors. *N Engl J Med*. 2020;**383**:1207–1217.

90 Pantel K, Alix-Panabieres C. Liquid biopsy and minimal residual disease - latest advances and implications for cure. *Nat Rev Clin Oncol*. 2019;**16**:409–424.

91 Sparano J, O'Neill A, Alpaugh K, et al. Association of circulating tumor cells with late recurrence of estrogen receptor-positive breast cancer: a secondary analysis of a randomized clinical trial. *JAMA Oncol*. 2018;**4**:1700–1706.

92 Rack B, Schindlbeck C, Juckstock J, et al. Circulating tumor cells predict survival in early average-to-high risk breast cancer patients. *J Natl Cancer Inst*. 2014;**106**:dju066.

98 Tsai WS, You JF, Hung HY, et al. Novel circulating tumor cell assay for detection of colorectal adenomas and cancer. *Clin Transl Gastroenterol*. 2019;**10**:e00088.

99 Ranade A, Bhatt A, Page R, et al. Hallmark circulating tumor-associated cell clusters signify 230 times higher one-year cancer risk. *Cancer Prev Res (Phila)*. 2021;**14**:11–16.

101 Lennon AM, Buchanan AH, Kinde I, et al. Feasibility of blood testing combined with PET-CT to screen for cancer and guide intervention. *Science*. 2020;**369**:eabb9601.

102 Nuzzo PV, Berchuck JE, Korthauer K, et al. Detection of renal cell carcinoma using plasma and urine cell-free DNA methylomes. *Nat Med*. 2020;**26**: 1041–1043.

103 Nassiri F, Chakravarthy A, Feng S, et al. Detection and discrimination of intracranial tumors using plasma cell-free DNA methylomes. *Nat Med*. 2020;**26**: 1044–1047.

104 Dinh TA, Rosner BI, Atwood JC, et al. Health benefits and cost-effectiveness of primary genetic screening for Lynch syndrome in the general population. *Cancer Prev Res (Phila)*. 2011;**4**:9–22.

38 Molecular diagnostics in cancer

Zachary L. Coyne, BMBS, BSc ■ Roshni D. Kalachand, MBBCh ■ Robert C. Bast, Jr., MD ■ Gordon B. Mills, MD, PhD ■ Bryan T. Hennessy, MD

Overview

Molecular diagnostics refers to the use of molecular alterations that are associated with cancers to facilitate detection, diagnosis, monitoring, and/or treatment selection. Molecular biomarkers have primarily been studied in cancer tissue but can potentially be assayed in readily available patient samples (saliva, sputum, blood, urine, feces), thereby minimizing the need for invasive biopsies. Traditional blood biomarkers—CEA, PSA, hCG, AFP, CA125, and CA15-3—have been used to monitor response to treatment and to detect disease recurrence. Their clinical utility often depends upon the availability of effective treatment for residual or recurrent disease. Early detection requires biomarkers with high sensitivity to detect preclinical and ideally premetastatic disease, as well as high specificity to permit efficient, cost-effective screening. Two-stage strategies are often most promising where rising biomarkers trigger imaging or results of imaging are combined with biomarkers to improve positive predictive value. Cancer-specific genomic aberrations have been identified which guide therapy and predict outcomes in subgroups of patients. Targeting HER2 has dramatically altered the outcomes of patients with *HER2* amplified breast cancers, as have EGFR inhibitors in the treatment of metastatic *EGFR* mutation-positive non-small-cell lung cancer. As single driver gene aberrations are frequently not sufficient to predict therapeutic responses, gene signatures, and multi-marker panels incorporating DNA, RNA, and/or protein aberrations are being evaluated as potential effective biomarkers. A panel of multiple biomarkers (Onco-Type Dx®) has proven useful in predicting the need for chemotherapy in addition to hormonal therapy in hormone receptor-positive breast cancer. As targeted therapies are becoming a reality, so is the predictable emergence of resistance to these therapies, often occurring through gene amplification, secondary mutations, or re-activation of signaling mechanisms downstream from the targeted molecular aberration. The search for molecular biomarkers, so-called companion diagnostics, predictive of first-line therapy resistance and of second-line therapy response is now inherent to targeted drug development. However, these emerging integrative technologies have yet to benefit the majority of patients with cancer. Progress is being made in particular with liquid biopsies that sequence ctDNA in peripheral blood-seeking evolving resistance mechanisms or germline mutations. Interpretation of the extensive number of aberrations identified by high-throughput technologies, availability of adequate high-quality tissue, integrative analysis across different analytics including DNA, RNA and protein, intra- and intertumoral heterogeneity, cost, and clinical validation remain significant challenges to developing and implementing effective biomarkers. Strategic use of bioinformatics, international collaboration, development of prospectively collected clinically annotated biobanks containing fresh frozen tissue, and clinical validation in large prospective datasets are key to bringing useful molecular biomarkers into clinical practice.

Introduction

Molecular diagnostics involves the use of molecular biomarkers (Box 1) to detect, diagnose, or monitor cancer, as well as to estimate patient prognosis or to predict therapeutic interventions likely to benefit the individual patient. Ultimately, the development of molecular diagnostics is expected to facilitate the individualization of cancer treatment with the goal of maximizing treatment benefit for specific cancer patients, while minimizing toxicity. Important progress has already been made in developing and applying molecular diagnostics to clinical management. This article provides an overview of the current status of molecular diagnostics for cancer. It will also review potential approaches to the integration of biomarker-driven approaches into the future development of individualized cancer therapies, as well as new techniques and likely problems and hurdles that will need to be addressed and overcome.

Box 1 Cancer biomarkers

A cancer biomarker includes any characteristic of tumor cells, stroma, normal tissues, or body fluids that aid in detecting, diagnosing, monitoring, defining prognosis, or predicting response or toxicity from treatment. Thus, biomarkers include alterations in DNA, RNA, protein, carbohydrate, lipid, or metabolites as well as biophysical characteristics of tumor cells, the tumor microenvironment, or the host genome and response. Pathologic examination and imaging techniques have provided conventional tumor histologic and staging information that have guided patient management to date. However, these approaches do not take into account the full inter- and intra-tumoral heterogeneity of cancers at the molecular level. Individualization of screening, prevention, and treatment should be substantially improved by considering the profile of multiple molecular biomarkers across different platforms.

Molecular biomarkers for screening and early detection of cancer

Early detection implies the diagnosis of cancer at its earliest stage of development. It is essential that early diagnosis occurs at a stage of tumor development where cure can be achieved with currently available therapy. Screening strategies generally require high sensitivity and specificity. Selectivity is important to determine the location of a screen-detected cancer. Early detection could be facilitated by identifying individuals at high risk for developing specific cancers, decreasing the hurdle of specificity by assessing higher-risk individuals.[1–4] Screening is a term used for approaches that facilitate detection of tumors at an early curable stage. Effective cancer screening strategies must be cost-effective, acceptable to patients, and associated with limited morbidity from both the intervention and from false-positive results. Further, it is important to distinguish indolent lesions that would not alter the individual's life span from aggressive, lethal tumors that require intervention. Since screening of the entire population is seldom practicable, guidelines for patient risk assessment are often necessary to appropriately target approaches to prevent and diagnose cancer early. As our understanding of cancer's molecular heterogeneity advances, novel criteria can be added to the conventional criteria that describe an ideal screening biomarker (Box 2). Thus, as most cancer treatments are effective in only a minority of cancer patients, future useful screening biomarkers could also guide appropriate therapies in individual patients.

> **Box 2** An optimal screening test
>
> Five critical terms describe the criteria for a screening test: *sensitivity, specificity, selectivity*, and *positive* and *negative predictive values*. Sensitivity is the fraction of cases of the disease that are detected by the test (number of true positives/numbers of true positives plus false negatives). Specificity is the fraction of cases without cancer that are detected as negative by the test (number of true negatives/numbers of true negatives plus false positives). Selectivity represents the ability of a screening test to differentiate between different types of cancer. When a test result is a continuous variable, sensitivity and specificity are inversely related and a cutoff for the presence of disease is placed in an arbitrary fashion that indicates the clinical consequences of an incorrect result. In most effective screening approaches, a two-stage strategy has proven optimal with a primary diagnostic test followed by a secondary test that optimizes sensitivity and/or specificity beyond that achievable with only a primary test alone (e.g., colposcopy following PAP smear). This approach can help control the consequences of false-positive results, invasive approaches, and cost. The prevalence of the disease in a population also affects screening test performance: in low-prevalence settings, even very good tests have poor positive predictive values (the proportion of patients with positive test results who are correctly diagnosed, that is, number of true positives/numbers of true positives plus false positives). Hence, knowing the prevalence of the disease is a critical prerequisite to interpreting screening test results. Screening for relatively uncommon cancers (e.g., ovarian and pancreatic) requires much greater specificity than screening for more common cancers (e.g., breast or prostate).

Emerging radiologic and endoscopic techniques afford increasingly more sensitive noninvasive procedures for early detection of small tumors. Despite some controversy, low-dose computed tomography appears to detect early lung cancer and decrease lung cancer-related mortality in people at high risk from cigarette smoking, in contrast to routine chest films[5]. Similarly, the addition of annual bilateral breast magnetic resonance imaging to annual mammography as an early breast cancer detection strategy for *BRCA1/2* gene mutation carriers could decrease bilateral prophylactic mastectomies to reduce the risk of breast cancer in these patients.[6,7] In colon cancer, the ability of colonoscopy to visualize small lesions and to remove polyps as a preventative approach throughout the entire colon has made this the screening method of choice over double-contrast barium enemas. Nonetheless, such tools depend on a tumor's anatomical features for detection, whereas molecular markers could identify cancer at an early and perhaps premalignant stage, prior to anatomical detection. Moreover, biomarkers can be detected in bodily fluids (urine, feces, blood), avoiding potential patient discomfort from endoscopy preparation as well as potentially harmful ionizing radiation from radiologic imaging.

Screening is generally applied to those populations where there is conclusive evidence of an associated survival benefit and, to assure cost-effectiveness, where the cancer is a common cause of mortality. As an example, although controversial, most regulatory agencies in the United States recommend annual mammography for women aged 40 years and older.[8] Alternatively, risk assessment can be used to stratify select patients to screening or, if the risk is high enough, prevention. This way, the exposure of large numbers of individuals to false-positive screening tests and unnecessary biopsies is avoided whilst maintaining a high cancer detection rate in at-risk patients. Risk assessment is currently largely based on patient-specific factors, including age, family history, and social factors (e.g., tobacco use), as is the case in lung cancer screening. However, some molecular markers such as mutations in cancer predisposition genes (e.g., BRCA1, BRCA2, p53) have demonstrated utility in the identification of at-risk populations.

Molecular biomarkers in current clinical practice for screening, prevention, and early detection

Progress has been made over the last two decades in early detection of multiple cancers.[9]

Lung cancer

Development of spiral low dose computerized tomography (LDCT) has detected early-stage lung cancer and improved survival by as much as 20% in individuals with a heavy smoking history. False positives are, however, frequently observed with indeterminate nodules up to 30 mm in diameter.[10] Two blood biomarker panels based on a proteomic mass spectroscopic signature[11] and on 7 autoantibodies[12,13] exhibit high negative predictive value, as does a gene expression signature from bronchial epithelial cells.[13] These tests can identify patients with indeterminate nodules that are unlikely to have lung cancer. Methylome-based DNA sequencing has exhibited impressive positive predictive value with 75% sensitivity for stage Ia and 86% sensitivity for Ib lung cancer, assaying plasma from patients with indeterminate nodules.[14]

Prostate cancer

Prostate-specific antigen (PSA) is normally present in the blood at very low levels ranging between 0 and 4.0 ng/mL. Increased PSA levels can be associated with an underlying prostate cancer but can also relate to benign conditions. Serum PSA measurement for prostate cancer screening is controversial, despite widespread use.[15] Up to 15% of prostate cancers can occur in the absence of an elevated PSA. Further, PSA levels can be elevated due to prostate infection, irritation, benign prostatic hypertrophy, or recent ejaculation. Thus, PSA is not an adequately sensitive or specific marker for prostate cancer screening. PSA screening can lead to a high rate of unnecessary biopsies, over-diagnosis, and overtreatment resulting in morbidity. Both prostatectomy and radiotherapy can be associated with impotence and incontinence. Patients diagnosed with less aggressive (Gleason score less than 7) prostate cancer can survive decades with their cancer, often dying from co-morbid diseases. PSA screening in men over the age of 50 years can confer up to a 20% decrease in prostate-cancer specific mortality, although this may or may not translate into a decrease in overall mortality, judging from large multi-center trials.[16,17] In the past, PSA screening has been recommended for men older than 50 years with an expected life expectancy of 10 years or more, following discussion with the patient about screening-associated risks.[18] The United States Preventive Health Task Force now recommends against using PSA for screening.[19] The American Urological Association (AUA) has more nuanced age-dependent guidelines.[20] The AUA recommends against PSA screening for men under age 40. Between age 40 and 54, PSA screening is recommended only for African American men or men with a positive family history conferring increased risk. For men ages 55–69, the benefits of preventing prostate cancer mortality in 1 man for every 1000 men screened over a decade must be weighed against the known harms associated with screening and overtreatment. In an effort to reduce this unintentional harm an interval of at least two years is preferred over annual screening. PSA screening is not recommended for men over 70 years.

Most PSA in the blood is bound to serum proteins. A small amount is not protein bound and is called free PSA, an isoform of which, [-2] proPSA, is highly associated with prostate cancer. The combination of PSA, free PSA and [-2] proPSA in a single score, the Prostate Health Index (PHI), shows increased sensitivity over PSA screening alone in men with PSA levels between 4 and 10 ng/mL and has been used to identify men with elevated PSA who would benefit from biopsies.[21,22] PCA3 is a noncoding RNA transcript associated with prostate cancer that can be detected in urine after digital rectal examination.[23] A PCA3 assay has been approved by the United States Food and Drug Administration (FDA) to identify men with suspected prostate cancer who should undergo repeat biopsy.

Ovarian cancer

The relatively low prevalence of ovarian cancer—1:2500 in the United States in postmenopausal women—means strategies for early ovarian cancer detection must have relatively high sensitivity (>75%) for asymptomatic preclinical disease and an extremely high specificity (99.6%) to attain a positive predictive value of at least 10%, that is, 10 operations for each case of ovarian cancer detected. Serum CA125 has received the most attention, but single values lack the sensitivity or specificity to function as a stand-alone screening test. Two-stage screening strategies promise to be more effective, where increasing levels of serum biomarkers over time prompt transvaginal sonography (TVS) to detect lesions that require laparotomy.[24] With annual determination of CA125 in women at average risk for ovarian cancer, a Bayesian computer algorithm has been developed to determine deviations from each woman's own baseline. If CA125 increases significantly, TVS is performed, and if imaging is abnormal, laparotomy is undertaken. If the CA125 is unchanged, a woman returns in one year and if CA125 is mildly elevated, biomarker levels are obtained in 3 months. Two large trials have been conducted to assess this strategy and both have shown adequate 99.6% specificity with 3–4 operations per case of ovarian cancer detected.[25,26] The largest randomized trial involving 200,000 postmenopausal women in the United Kingdom is powered to test the impact of this strategy on survival and mortality. In the initial report of the study, overall mortality was not significantly reduced, but a prespecified subset of incident patients who developed ovarian cancer while on the study had a 20% reduction in mortality ($P = 0.021$), although there were wide bounds around this estimate, discouraging its acceptance.[26] Final results of the study will be reported in 2021. Currently, there is insufficient evidence to recommend ovarian cancer screening with CA125 in the general population. This has been reinforced by recommendations from UK national screening committee[27] and the U.S. Prevention Task Force.[28] A greater impact might be achieved by increasing the sensitivity of serum biomarkers and of imaging.[24] As only 80% of ovarian cancers express CA125, other markers will be required to detect a greater fraction of ovarian cancer at an early stage. Autoantibodies against TP53 that is mutated in most high-grade ovarian cancers, can be elevated 8 months before increases in CA125 and 22 months before clinical diagnosis in patients whose CA125 does not rise.[29] A variety of biomarkers are being evaluated to provide a more sensitive panel including ctDNA mutations and copy number abnormalities, methylated DNA, miRNAs, glycopeptides, and polyamines.[24]

Cervical cancer

The establishment of national cervical cancer screening programs involving the detection and treatment of the premalignant stage of cervical intra-epithelial neoplasia (CIN) through cervical Pap smear cytology has reduced incidence and mortality from cervical cancer by 80%. Isolated Pap smears have false-negative rates of 20–40%, which are partly overcome by regular screening (every 3 years). The human papilloma virus (HPV), in particular strains 16 and 18, is critical to cervical carcinogenesis. Testing for HPV DNA in cervical smears increases the cervical cancer detection by 30% over cytology-based screening and could lengthen the screening interval to 5 years.[30] HPV-based screening has now been incorporated in to the screening guidelines.[31]

Colorectal cancer

In the United State, optical colonoscopy has been the primary method for screening for colorectal cancer (CRC), although in many countries two-stage strategies have been used where stool tests prompt colonoscopy in a subset of individuals screened.[32] Detection of blood in stool with a fecal immunochemical test (FIT) has generally provided the initial stage. In recent years, other biomarkers including DNA-based tests have been added to increase the sensitivity for CRC and precancerous polyps.[33] Cologuard™ (FIT-DNA) supplements FIT with detection of aberrantly methylated *BMP3* and *NDRG4* DNA, mutant *K-RAS* DNA, and beta-actin in stool. While FIT detected 73.8% of all CRC and 70% of early-stage cancers, FIT-DNA detected 92.3% and 94%, respectively.[34] FIT-DNA also detected a greater fraction of precancerous lesions, 42.4% versus 23.8%. Epi proColon™ measures methylated *SEPT9* DNA in plasma and in a meta-analysis has detected 71% of CRC at 92% specificity and 23% of adenomas and polyps >1 cm at 92% specificity.[35] As blood tests may prove more convenient than stool-based assays, panels of blood biomarkers are currently being evaluated to improve sensitivity.[32]

Esophageal cancer

Adenocarcinomas of the esophagus can arise from metaplastic small intestinal epithelial cells at the gastro-esophageal junction, termed Barrett's esophagus.[36] Upper endoscopy is generally used to detect and monitor Barrett's esophagus. In brushings obtained at endoscopy, a combination of methylated *VIM* and methylated *CCNA/A1* DNA can detect 95% of Barret's esophagus, dysplasia, and adenocarcinoma at 91% specificity.[37] A balloon-based device has been developed that can be swallowed and return cells within 5 min from the gastro-esophageal junction for DNA analysis without endoscopy. The two methylated DNA biomarkers detected nondysplastic Barrett esophagus with a sensitivity of 90% and specificity of 92% prompting US FDA approval.

Hepatocellular cancer (HCC)

Incidence of hepatocellular cancer (HCC) has been rising in the United States in the context of chronic liver disease caused by nonalcoholic fatty liver disease, alcoholic liver disease, and hepatitis C and B. Screening with abdominal ultrasound has been recommended at 6-month intervals, which can detect early stage, potentially curable, HCC in 45% of cases.[38] Addition of alpha-fetoprotein (AFP) to ultrasound can increase early detection of HCC to 63%.[39] Additional biomarkers can improve sensitivity, including des-gamma carboxyprothrombin (DCP), and lectin-bound α-fetoprotein (AFPL3).[40] Using a score that incorporates gender, AFP, AFPL3, and DCP, early-stage disease could be detected with a sensitivity of 80–91% at a specificity of 81–90% across multiple cohorts.[41]

Individuals at elevated risk
Specific guidelines exist for patients with strong family histories of cancer, particularly for carriers of genomic biomarkers of high cancer risk. When the cancer risk associated with the specific (usually hereditary) biomarker is high enough, recommendations focus on prevention rather than early detection. Since prevention strategies generally impact quality of life to a greater degree than does screening, the identification of inherited mutations associated with a very high cancer risk necessitates patient education and careful shared decision making. Furthermore, hereditary biomarkers testing has significant implications for family members. Prophylactic surgery and chemoprevention are particularly effective risk reduction techniques that are reserved for people at highest risk. Prophylactic oophorectomy and/or mastectomy has the greatest protective effect for *BRCA1/BRCA2* mutation carriers, reducing the risk of ovarian and breast cancer by more than 90%.[42,43] However, some patients prefer mammography, MRI, or other screening approaches to delay surgical intervention either for personal preference or to allow childbearing. There are many factors (e.g., ethics, cost) to consider in discussing options for early detection and prevention with very high-risk patients and this area of medicine is a rapidly evolving specialty.[44–46]

Breast and ovarian cancer
In families with a significant history of breast and/or ovarian cancer, key cancer risk biomarkers (usually hereditary mutations) can now be identified in a minority of cases, using clinical prediction models (e.g., BRCAPRO model).[47] Such models can be useful in guiding specific molecular tests that further stratify risk and guide subsequent screening or prevention. Inherited mutations in *BRCA1* and *BRCA2* account for 5–10% and 10–15% of all breast cancers and ovarian cancers respectively.[48,49] Furthermore, approximately 15% of patients with triple-negative breast cancers or with high-grade serous ovarian cancer will carry deleterious germline mutations in BRCA1/2 in the absence of a significant family history. Moreover, *BRCA1/2* mutations guide therapy in ovarian cancer, as outlined in the following section. Approximately 12% of women at high risk do not carry *BRCA1/2* mutations are estimated to have another cancer-predisposing genomic alteration,[50] suggesting a need for improved testing approaches that identify additional risk biomarkers. Less well-studied breast cancer susceptibility genes include *CHEK2, ATM, RAD51C, BRIP1, PALB2, NBS1, LKB1, PTEN, p53, XRCC1,* and *STK11*, but these are not commonly assessed due to the rarity of inherited mutations.[51–54] Recently, these genes have been integrated into multiplex sequencing assays both providing more information and greater challenges into patient decision-making for genes associated with a lower frequency of cancer development.

Colon cancer
Familial adenomatous polyposis (FAP) and hereditary non-polyposis colon cancer (HNPCC) predispose to early-onset familial/hereditary colon cancer. They are characterized by germline mutations in the adenomatous polyposis coli (*APC*) and DNA mismatch repair genes, respectively. In HNPCC, routine tumor molecular screening using antibodies to mismatch repair proteins has superseded clinical risk models to guide screening (e.g., revised Bethesda guidelines). Tumor molecular screening, however, results in excessive genetic testing for HNPCC, as 10–15% of cases represent sporadic disease.[55] Combining the clinical risk prediction models with tumor molecular screening, or testing the tumor for molecular markers of sporadic disease (*MLH1* promoter methylation and/or *BRAF* V600E gene mutation) could improve screening for HNPCC while maintaining high detection rates.[56] Management guidelines entail surgical cancer prevention (colectomy) with FAP and intensive colonoscopic screening with HNPCC.

In a recent study, fecal hemoglobin detection was combined with fecal DNA tests for mutant K-Ras, aberrant *NDRG4* and *BMP3* methylation, and B-actin.[34] When compared to a standard FIT in 9989 evaluable participants at average risk, the composite Cologuard® test demonstrated greater sensitivity for detecting CRC (92.3% vs. 73.8%, $P = 0.002$), greater sensitivity for detecting advanced precancerous lesions (42.4% vs. 23.8%, $P < 0.001$), a higher rate of detection of high-grade dysplastic polyps (69.2% vs. 46.2%, $P = 0.004$), greater detection of serrated sessile polyps measuring 1 cm or more (42.4% and 5.1%, $P < 0.001$). Specificity, however, was somewhat lower with DNA testing than with FIT (86.6% vs. 94.9%). Based on these results, the test was approved in 2014 by the United States FDA for individuals greater than 50 years old.

Future approaches to early detection and screening

While current approaches to early detection have impacted mortality from certain forms of malignancy such as cervical cancer, low sensitivity, unnecessary use of invasive diagnostic procedures due to false positives and over-diagnosis/treatment remain significant issues. Moreover, many tumor types, such as ovarian and pancreatic cancer, do not yet benefit from these approaches. Patients continue to present with advanced disease and thus have poor outcomes. Elevation of circulating tumor biomarkers may require a substantial tumor volume. Autoantibodies could be evoked by small volumes of cancer at an earlier interval. Novel molecular screening techniques including circulating DNA, RNA, and exosomes have the potential to complement current protein-based screening markers and revolutionize early cancer detection, whilst facilitating accurate risk assessment and individual treatment planning. Multi-cancer early detection (MCED) approaches based on changes in circulating DNA, methylation, and other analytes have the advantage of a higher prevalence of cases but have the disadvantage of a potential lack of specificity.[57,58] However, MCED can in some cases provide an indication of the tissue of origin of a screened cancer. Large-scale MCED studies are underway with results expected in 2021.

Current molecular biomarkers for predicting outcomes and therapy responsiveness

Although molecular biomarkers that predict outcomes in cancer patients are useful, greater clinical utility lies in biomarkers that predict benefit from specific cancer therapies. There is considerable overlap between both types, since those biomarkers that predict benefit for particular patients from specific cancer therapies will, therefore, predict improved outcomes.

Breast cancer

Hormone receptors (HR)
HR-positive breast cancer comprises approximately 70% of all breast cancers and is marked by the expression of estrogen receptor (ER) α and/or progesterone receptor (PR). The HR biomarkers identify breast tumors that are sensitive to growth

Table 1 The panel of 21 genes in *Oncotype Dx* and their subdivision based on function.

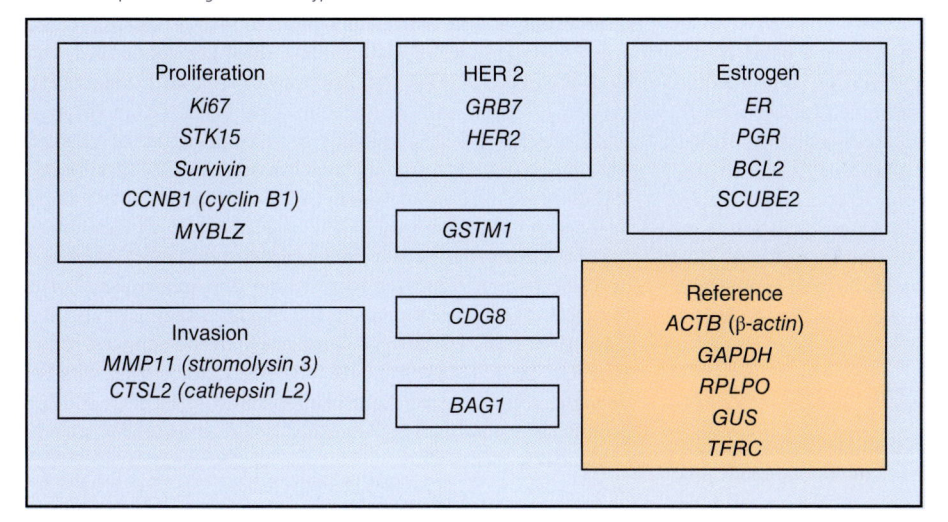

Proliferation	HER 2	Estrogen
Ki67	GRB7	ER
STK15	HER2	PGR
Survivin		BCL2
CCNB1 (cyclin B1)		SCUBE2
MYBLZ	GSTM1	
	CDG8	Reference
Invasion		ACTB (β-actin)
MMP11 (stromolysin 3)		GAPDH
CTSL2 (cathepsin L2)	BAG1	RPLPO
		GUS
		TFRC

inhibition by antihormonal treatments, including ER partial agonists/antagonists (e.g., tamoxifen), ER downregulators (SERDs e.g., fulvestrant), and aromatase inhibitors (e.g., letrozole).[59,60] A suite of oral SERDs are in clinical trials and have the potential to replace fulvestrant and due to greater efficacy, further improve patient outcomes. In clinical practice, HR protein expression is routinely assessed in all breast cancers using immunohistochemistry. Despite 5 years of adjuvant antihormonal therapy, however, a significant fraction of women with early-stage HR-positive breast cancer relapse, and the majority of women with metastatic HR-positive breast cancer develop resistance to antihormonal manipulation. Indeed, ER mutations are acquired in a number of patients following antihormonal treatments leading to acquired resistance. Thus, in the United States, over 25,000 women with HR-positive breast tumors die each year, more annual deaths than are caused by all other types of breast cancer combined.

In advanced HR-positive breast cancer cyclin D overexpression is common making the G1-toS checkpoint an ideal therapeutic target. CDK 4/6 inhibitors prevent progression through this checkpoint leading to cell cycle arrest.[61] Recent approval of CDK 4/6 inhibitors through Paloma,[62] Monaleessa,[63] and Monarch[64] trials have markedly improved overall survival resulting in a major sea change in the treatment of metastatic HR-positive breast cancer.

Multiparameter gene expression profiles
Our ability to predict the likelihood of cure for patients with HR-positive breast cancer after treatment with antihormonal drugs has improved dramatically. *Oncotype Dx* (Table 1), based on the expression of 21 genes, predicts the benefit for individual node-negative HR-positive breast tumor patients from adjuvant tamoxifen and selects patients for cytotoxic chemotherapy based on features associated with tamoxifen resistance.[65] However, despite this approach's clinical utility, this and similar assays such as PAM50 and Mammoprint do not increase our understanding of antihormone resistance mechanisms in HR-positive breast cancer beyond the known roles of tumor grade, HER2, and HR levels.[34,36,66] The phosphatidylinositol-3-kinase (PI3K)/AKT/mTOR and mitogen-activated protein kinase (MAPK) pathways are major mediators of the effects of membrane receptor tyrosine kinases (RTKs) such as HER2 and mediate resistance to antihormonal therapies.[67] The mTOR inhibitor everolimus improves progression-free survival for approximately 60% of women with HR-positive breast cancers resistant to antihormonal therapies.[68] A predictive molecular biomarker of response to this drug is however lacking.

Further understanding of PI3K mutations has led to development of PI3K inhibitors. Approximately 40% of HR-positive breast cancers have activating mutations in PIK3CA gene. This mutation is thought to lead to a resistance mechanism to hormonal therapy. SOLAR-1 a Phase 3 randomized control trial showed an increase in progression free survival (PFS) of 11 months in alpelisib (PI3K-inhibitor) and fulvestrant arm compared to 5.7 months in the placebo and fulvestrant arm in PIK3CA mutated tumors.[69]

HER2
The oncogene encoding *HER2* is amplified and the protein overexpressed in 15–20% of invasive breast cancers. *HER2* overexpression dictates an aggressive breast tumor phenotype and poor prognosis.[70] Combining trastuzumab (Herceptin), a recombinant humanized monoclonal antibody targeting *HER2*, with cytotoxic chemotherapy to treat patients with metastatic and early-stage *HER2* oncogene-amplified breast cancer resulted in increased response rates and improved survival.[71] Following the initial success of trastuzumab in this disease, *HER2* has served as a biomarker for breast tumor responsiveness multiple other *HER2*-targeted therapies (e.g., pertuzumab, lapatinib, TDM1, Neratinib, Tucatinib, and trastuzumab–deruxtecan) resulting in a marked improvement in outcomes for this population of patients.[72-74] Indeed, while in the past HER2-positive breast cancer had the worst outcome, the long-term outcome for patients with this disease is not amongst the best in breast cancer. More recently, HER2 has also been validated as a biomarker predictive of response to trastuzumab-based chemotherapy in 15–20% of advanced gastric cancer patients with HER2-driven oncogenesis.[75]

A significant fraction of *HER2*-amplified breast and gastric cancers do not initially respond to trastuzumab or acquire resistance to trastuzumab. This could be mediated by a cleaved form of *HER2* that does not bind trastuzumab (p95-HER2), by upregulation of other membrane RTKs such as IGF1R or MET, or by upregulation of the PI3K/AKT pathway.[76-79] The latter can occur through inactivating mutations of PTEN (a negative PI3K/AKT regulator), PTEN loss, or by PIK3CA mutations, the oncogene that encodes the p110α subunit of PI3K.[80] Indeed, PI3K pathway activation and mutations in PIK3CA and PTEN are negative prognostic markers in HER2-positive breast cancers treated with anti-HER2 targeted therapies.[81]

Based on the efficacy of HER targeted therapy, a panel of the American Society of Clinical Oncology (ASCO) thus recommended that *HER2* status should be determined for all invasive breast cancers.[82] This panel has proposed a testing algorithm that relies on accurate, reproducible assay performance, including newly available types of bright-field *in situ* hybridization (ISH), and has specified elements to reliably reduce assay variation (e.g., specimen handling, assay exclusion, and reporting criteria). This emphasizes the need for quality control and validation approaches for all predictive markers both in terms of reliability and clinical utility.

Ovarian cancer: BRCA1/2

Approximately 20% of high-grade serous ovarian cancers have an underlying inherited or somatic *BRCA1/2* mutation, rendering them deficient in homologous recombination, a pathway essential for high-fidelity repair of double-stranded DNA breaks.[83] These tumors rely on alternative DNA repair mechanisms low fidelity mutation prone nonhomologous end joining (NHEJ). Inhibitors of PARP exploit vulnerability of *BRCA1/2* mutated ovarian cancers to DNA damage. This was originally thought to be due to the role of the PARP enzyme in base excision repair with single-strand breaks being converted into double strand breaks during DNA replication. However, more recently, PARP enzymes have been demonstrated to play a role in multiple other processes such as replication fork protection that leads to double strand DNA breaks. A number of PARP inhibitors trap PARP on DNA preventing efficient DNA repair and further exacerbating the effects of PARP inhibitors. In a randomized Phase III trial, SOLO1, the PARP inhibitor olaparib showed a 70% reduction in disease progression or death compared to placebo when used as maintenance therapy in platinum-sensitive recurrent *BRCA1/2*-mutated ovarian tumors.[84,85] Based on similar trials, several PARP inhibitors have been approved for use in ovarian cancer. Across the studies, patients with germline or somatic BRCA1/2 mutations (and mutations in select members of the HR pathway) demonstrate the greatest benefit, which those with evidence for HR deficiency having lower levels of benefit and with the remaining population of ovarian cancers showing modest but statistically significant benefit. Resistance mechanisms include function restoring *BRCA1/2* mutations, loss of 53BP1 (a protein involved in an alternative DNA repair mechanism), and upregulation of the PI3K/AKT/mTOR pathway.[86] The combination of olaparib and BKM120, a PI3K inhibitor, has shown activity in early clinical studies of high-grade serous ovarian and triple-negative breast cancer.[87]

Lung cancer

Epidermal growth factor receptor (EGFR)
Tumor molecular testing is standard of care for advanced adenocarcinoma non-small-cell lung cancer (NSCLC). Epidermal growth factor receptor (EGFR) mutations are commonly found in NSCLC and can be seen in up to 28% of lung adenocarcinomas. The most common mutations location on exon 19 and exon 21.[88] Female, nonsmokers of Asian origin with adenocarcinoma represent the typical phenotype, although EGFR mutations are also observed in men and (ex)smokers. EGFR-mutant lung cancer has undergone rapid drug development in recent years, with five approved EGFR tyrosine kinase inhibitors (TKI) developed. First-generation TKI's (erlotinib and gefitinib) are reversible EGFR TKI's. Second-generation EGFR TKI included afatinib and dacomitinib which irreversibly bind to EGFR mutant, HER2, and wild-type EGFR. Osimertinib, a third-generation TKI, with evidence from FLUARA trial has shown increased median overall survival (38.6 months) compared to other EGFR TKI in advanced EGFR-mutant NSCLC, making it first-line agent of choice.[89] Multiple acquired resistance mechanisms to EGFR inhibitors including secondary mutation in *EGFR* (T790M) and MET amplification limit the efficacy of EGFR targeted therapy.[90] Osimertinib has also shown efficacy in overcoming resistance mechanism such as T790M when compared to platinum plus pemetrexed.[91] Due to success of these treatments in the advanced setting (Stage IB to Stage IIA), trials are currently underway in the adjuvant setting (resected Stage IB to Stage IIA). The ADUARA trial, which is ongoing, comparing adjuvant osimertinib to placebo is showing promising results with significantly longer disease-free survival compared to placebo.[92]

ALK and ROS-1
Two targetable chromosomal gene rearrangements leading to oncogenic gene fusions guide novel therapies in advanced adenocarcinoma of the lung.[93,94] Anaplastic lymphoma kinase (ALK) and ROS-1 gene translocations are present in 4–6% and 1–2% of advanced lung adenocarcinomas, respectively, rendering them markedly sensitive to the ALK, ROS-1 and MET inhibitor, crizotinib, and newer generation inhibitors. The short period between the identification of these targets and crizotinib's approval engenders excitement for an evolution away from the prolonged time period traditionally required for drug discovery and implementation. Crizotinib is associated with response rates of over 70% and a median progression-free survival of 11 and 19 months for ALK and ROS-1 rearranged tumors, respectively. Gene overexpression, bypass mechanisms, and secondary mutations commonly cause acquired resistance, though unlike EGFR-mutated NSCLC, multiple mutation types are observed in a single tumor at disease progression. Second-generation ALK-inhibitors include ceritinib, brigatinib, and alectinib. Alectinib was compared to crizotinib in the Phase III randomized ALEX trial which showed impressive median PFS of 34.8 months, compared with 10.9 months.[95] Most recently, Lorlatinib a third-generation ALK TKI has shown efficacy against resistance mutations and is approved in first-line or in patients who have progressed on previous ALK TKI.[96]

ROS-1 gene rearrangements are oncogenic drivers seen in approximately 1–2% of NSCLC.[97] These tumors are commonly seen in young nonsmokers with lung adenocarcinoma. Crizotinib is an effective treatment in ROS-1 fusion NSCLC showing a high response rate of 72% and a median PFS of 19.2 months.[98] Newer agents such as entrectinib have shown durable disease control in ROS-1 fusion-positive NSCLC in an integrated analysis of three Phase 1–2 trials.[99]

BRAF
BRAF mutations, frequently seen in melanoma, are also observed in lung adenocarcinoma with a prevalence in the region of 2–4%, making this a potential treatment option for lung cancer. In a recent Phase II trial of previously treated BRAF V600E mutant lung cancer were given dabrafenib plus trametinib (BRAF inhibitor and MEK inhibitor combo) showing response rate of over 60% and PFS of 9.7 months.[100]

Other molecular driver alterations that may lead to promising treatments include RET, MET, HER2, and NTRK which have been granted approval for larotrectinib and entrectinib as tumor agnostic therapies for individuals with NTRK fusion genes independent of the tumor lineage. This joins immune checkpoint blockade for microsatellite instable (MSI) as a tumor agnostic therapy.

Based on these results, routine molecular testing is recommended for EGFR, ALK, ROS1, and BRAF in all advanced-stage lung adenocarcinomas (or lung tumors with an adenocarcinoma component), regardless of clinical characteristics. Tumors that do not contain an adenocarcinoma component perhaps due to a sampling error but are suspected as such due to clinical characteristics (young, never smoker) may also be tested.[101]

Colon cancer

Microsatellite instability

Current guidelines recommend adjuvant 5-fluorouracil-based chemotherapy in stage II colon cancer in "high-risk" patients, defined by the presence of high-grade tumors with lymphovascular space invasion, evidence of tumor perforation, and/or less than 12 nodes extracted at surgery. Approximately 11% of stage II colon cancers have a deficiency in mismatch DNA repair, manifested as microsatellite instability.[102] Such tumors have good outcomes in the absence of adjuvant chemotherapy particularly when treated with immune checkpoint inhibitors. Therefore, guidelines advise routine immunohistochemical testing of stage II colon cancers for mismatch repair proteins, the absence of which obviates the need for adjuvant chemotherapy.

With regards to microsatellite instability-high (MSI-H) or MMR in CRC, numerous trials have shown the benefit of immunotherapy in these tumors. This has led to the approval of tumor agnostic therapy with PDL1 inhibitor pembrolizumab and other immune checkpoint inhibitors in advanced disease previously treated with first-line treatment. Keynote-177 a Phase III study demonstrate that front line pdl-1 inhibitor pembrolizumab doubled PFS versus standard of care chemotherapy in MSI-H or mismatch repair deficient (dMMR) metastatic colon cancer.[103]

KRAS, BRAF, and NRAS

KRAS is a proto-oncogene downstream of EGFR, that initiates signaling through the Ras-Raf-MAPK pathway. Approximately 60% of metastatic CRCs have the favorable wild-type KRAS profile, predicting sensitivity to the anti-EGFR monoclonal antibodies, cetuximab, and panitumumab. KRAS mutations, found mainly at codons 12 and 13 of exon 2, predict resistance to these therapies, as do the rarer NRAS mutations.[104–107] Downstream BRAF mutations occur in about 5–9% of cases and correlate with poor prognosis, although recent data have shown an increase in PFS with triplet therapy (encorafenib, cetuximab, and binemetinib targeting BRAF, EGFR, and MEK, respectively) compared to standard therapy in patients with BRAF mutant metastatic CRC.[108] KRAS alterations, a prevalent oncogenic driver mutation which has long been considered undruggable is no longer true. The discovery of KRAS inhibitors has shown promising early evidence in anticancer activity and safety profile in treating KRAS mutant tumors, in particular, for the KRAS G12C inhibitor Adagarasib.

Gastrointestinal stromal tumors (GIST): KIT and PDGFRA

Gastrointestinal stromal tumors (GIST) are associated with primary activating mutations in the KIT (80% of GISTs) or platelet-derived growth factor receptor A (PDGFRA; 5–10% of GISTs) genes that result in constitutive RTK activation.[109] Imatinib mesylate (Gleevec) which inhibits both KIT and PDGFRA results in clinical benefit in approximately 85% of patients with unresectable or metastatic disease, with a median progression-free survival of 20–24 months, though patients with exon 11 mutations fare better than exon 9 mutations. In the latter case, a higher dose of imatinib confers a greater benefit. The mechanisms of acquired resistance to imatinib are heterogeneous, involving mostly the emergence of secondary mutations in KIT exons 13, 14, or 17. In patients with imatinib-resistant GIST, novel kinase inhibitors such as sunitinib, nilotinib, dasatinib, and regorafenib can inhibit the mutant protein's function and restore antitumor activity.

Bladder cancer

Muscle invasive urothelial cancer has limited treatment options and poor prognosis making its more effective treatment for a high unmet medical need. Fibroblast growth factor receptor (FGFR) alterations are frequently seen in advanced urothelial carcinoma. FGFR signaling plays a role in cell proliferation, survival, migration, and differentiation. Mutation and fusions in FGFR are common in advanced urothelial carcinomas and it is believed they contribute to carcinogenesis.[110] Erdafitinib a potent FGFR inhibitor has exhibited an objective response rate of 40% in an open-label Phase 2 study leading to accelerated approval by the FDA in this cohort of patients.[73,111]

Another novel molecular target in urothelial carcinoma is Nectin-4 which is highly overexpressed in advanced urothelial carcinomas. Nectin-4 is a transmembrane protein involved in cell adhesion. Due to its high expression in advanced urothelial carcinoma, it makes for an interesting and potentially effective target for an antibody–drug conjugate. Enfortamab-vedotin binds to nectin-4 expressing cells followed by internalization and release of the cytotoxic payload, monomethyl auristatin E, which results in cell cycle arrest and apoptosis. Early-stage clinical trials have seen good response rates, with the potential for additional much-needed treatment option in bladder cancer.[112]

Melanoma

BRAF

About half of all melanomas carry the BRAF V600E gene mutation, leading to constitutive downstream activation of the MAPK pathway engendering sensitivity to BRAF inhibitors (e.g., vemurafenib, dabrafenib).[113,114] Clinically, the duration of response to these drugs is short, with progression occurring at a median of 6–7 months. Novel approaches to overcome resistance resulting from compensatory overactivation of the MAPK pathway involve the upfront combination of BRAF and MEK inhibitors (such as trametinib), which increases the efficacy and decreases the toxicity of therapy.[115]

NRAS

MEK inhibitors will likely play a significant role in treating NRAS-mutated melanoma, which involves approximately 15–20% of all melanomas and dictates a particularly aggressive biology. Interestingly, MEK inhibitors may demonstrate activity in combination with immune therapies.[116]

KIT

A small number (3%) of BRAF/NRAS-negative melanomas carry KIT proto-oncogene mutations, particularly in mucosal and acral melanomas. Targeted therapies with imatinib or sunitinib are viable therapeutic options that can provide durable responses, with evidence of nilotinib activity at progression post imatinib therapy.[117,118]

Melanomas without mutations in the RAS pathway, due to the high mutation burden associated with UV radiation have amongst the best response to immune checkpoint blockade.

Chronic myeloid leukemia (CML)

Bcr-Abl translocation
Most chronic myeloid leukemia (CML) cases are driven by constitutive activation of the Abl kinase as a result of the breakpoint cluster region (Bcr) to the Abl kinase translocation (Philadelphia chromosome). Imatinib targeted therapy, which inhibits the kinase activity of Abl, has markedly improved the outlook for patients with CML. Indeed real-world data from multiple countries have now indicated that the life span of individuals with CML is not shortened by having the disease representing over 20 years of life gained for many patients. Further, about half of patients who stop imatinib do not have a recurrence of their disease indicating that they are "cured" by a single oral drug, a paradigm-shifting process for cancer therapy. However, imatinib resistance can emerge despite initial benefit. Furthermore, efficacy of imatinib is limited in advanced "blast-crisis" CML.[119] Resistance is predominantly due to novel mutations in the Abl kinase domain, interfering with drug binding. Thus, new Abl kinase inhibitors (AKIs) were developed, among which nilotinib, dasatinib, and bosutinib have gained regulatory approval. Unfortunately, all available AKIs exhibit inactivity to certain kinase domain mutations, the cross-resistant *Bcr-Abl (T315I)* mutant being the most common. The third-generation AKI ponatinib demonstrates clinical benefit in *Bcr-Abl (T315l)* mutant CML and some other multidrug-resistant mutations. However, cardiovascular toxicity concerns, potentially related to the choice of a high drug dose during clinical development, precluded regulatory approval. Trials investigating dose-optimized ponatinib are underway.[120]

Lymphoma

CD20 and other biomarkers
Biomarker-targeted therapeutics have significantly impacted the treatment of non-Hodgkin lymphoma (NHL).[121,122] The development of the chimeric anti-CD20 antibody rituximab heralded a new era in NHL treatment approaches. Rituximab is now standard monotherapy for front-line treatment of follicular lymphoma and is used in conjunction with chemotherapy for other CD20-positive B-cell lymphomas. The subsequent development and approval of radio-immunoconjugates of rituximab (^{90}Y-ibritumomab tiuxetan and ^{131}I-tositumomab) have further improved outcomes.

Clinical evaluation of antibodies has been based largely on knowledge of antigen expression on the lymphoma cells' surface, leading to the development of antibodies against CD22 (e.g., unconjugated epratuzumab), CD80 (galiximab), CD52 (alemtuzumab), CD2 (siplizumab), CD40 (SGN-40), and CD30.[123] The anti-CD30 antibody brentuximab has been conjugated with a drug, vedotin, to target cytotoxic drug delivery to CD30-positive Hodgkin's or anaplastic large-cell lymphoma, producing significant clinical benefit with acceptable toxicity. This represents a key member of a class of antibody–drug conjugates that are showing activating across a number of diseases. Brentuximab was recently approved for use in relapsed Hodgkin's lymphoma following autologous stem cell transplant and relapsed anaplastic large-cell lymphoma. It is currently being investigated for use upfront with chemotherapy.

Oropharyngeal cancer (OPC)

Human papilloma virus (HPV)
The epidemiology of oropharyngeal cancer (OPC) has changed over the last two decades with studies reporting the presence of HPV p16 subtype in 60–70% of all OPC in western countries. Molecular tumor testing is easily done using p16 immunohistochemistry, which has a high concordance with HPV FISH. Retrospective analyses of large clinical trials demonstrate superior response rates and survival with chemoradiotherapy in HPV-related OPCs, as compared to HPV-negative OPCs.[124] HPV is, therefore, an important stratification tool for future therapeutic investigations in OPCs and may dictate a different therapeutic approach. Suggestions that HPV-associated OPCs may benefit from less intensive chemoradiotherapy require further evaluation.

Tumor agnostic therapies

The development of tumor agnostic therapies is an exciting area in cancer care. Classically oncologists determine their treatment for solid cancers based on the organ from which the cancer arises. In the era of precision medicine and targeted therapies, treatments have been adopted that are directed against individual targets shared by cancers that arise from multiple sites. Tumor agnostic therapies identify a molecular target or genomic anomaly regardless of tumor site of origin. To date, there are three approved tumor agnostic therapies. Trials often referred to as basket studies have guided the development of tumor agnostic therapies. A basket trial is a trial that tests how well a specific drug works across cancers from different sites that have a specific genomic or molecular alteration in common. In 2017, we saw the first approval with MSI-High or MMR tumors with progression on first-line treatment then saw a benefit in immunotherapy pembrolizumab. The approval of pembrolizumab was based on multiple single-arm Phase 1 or Phase 2 trials (Keynote-012,016, -158, and -164) which saw good response rates and progression-free survival compared to other therapies.[125,126]

Focusing on immunotherapy, tumor mutational burden (TMB) is a measure of the number of gene mutations within a tumor. A high TMB is likely to respond to immunotherapy, a retrospective analysis showed increase in ORR and PFS in patient with high TMB >10 this has led to further tumor agnostic approval of pembrolizumab across all solid organ malignancies with a high TMB.[127]

Finally, NTRK fusion cancers were studied in multiple Phase 1 and 2 trials. Larotrectinib is licensed for all solid organ malignancies with NTRK fusion-detected cancers.[128]

Tumor agnostic therapy is an expanding area and will likely see increasing pan-cancer tumor agnostic therapies. Ongoing work in potential molecular targets include RET, BRAK ALK, and ROS1.

Molecular biomarkers for monitoring of cancer

Multiple serum and imaging biomarkers have been used for monitoring response to therapy and providing evidence for early recurrence. These approaches provide the potential for an early intervention on progression which has the theoretical benefit of changing to a new effective therapy when the tumor burden is low.

Alpha-fetoprotein (AFP) and human chorionic gonadotropin (hCG)

Many germ cell tumors [most male testicular cancers, gestational trophoblastic disease (choriocarcinoma), and rare ovarian cancers] produce circulating tumor markers [AFP, chorionic gonadotropin (hCG), lactate dehydrogenase (LDH)].[78] These biomarkers are useful in diagnosing, staging, monitoring therapeutic response, and detecting early tumor recurrence. Since recurrent germ cell tumors can be cured with cytotoxic chemotherapy, particularly when the recurrence is detected early, increasing tumor marker levels during patient follow-up is an indication for initiating therapy, despite absence of evident disease. The markers' half-lives must be considered when evaluating therapeutic responses.

AFP is a glycoprotein normally produced by the fetal yolk sac, liver, and gastrointestinal tract but not by normal adult tissues. It is re-expressed in germ cell tumors, including yolk sac tumors and embryonal carcinomas. hCG is a glycoprotein produced by syncytiotrophoblastic cells consisting of two subunits, α and β. The α-subunit is common to three pituitary trophic hormones: FSH, LH, and TSH; the β-subunit makes hCG enzymatically and immunologically distinct. Assays measure only the β subunit (β-hCG). In males, it is highly specific for testicular cancer, in particular choriocarcinomas cells and 5–10% of pure seminomas. LDH reflects "tumor burden," growth rate, and cellular proliferation, and has independent prognostic significance. LDH is increased in about 80% of advanced seminomas and about 60% of advanced nonseminomatous germ cell tumors. The LDH isoenzyme 1 seems to be more specific and sensitive for germ cell tumors than isoenzymes 2–5.[129]

AFP, HCG, and LDH have been used as GCT biomarkers since the 1970s but their major drawback is their low sensitivity and specificity.[130] New biomarkers are under development such as serum level of microRNA-371a-3p (M371 test). A prospective, multicentric study comparing microRNA to AFP, BHCG, and LDH in 637 patients with GCT showed both a sensitivity and specificity of over 90% compared to 50%, this may be a novel GCT biomarker pending FDA approval.[131]

CA125

CA125 is a mucinous transmembrane glycoprotein product of the *MUC16* gene that ranges up to 5 mD. CA125 is best known as an ovarian cancer marker, though elevations in endometrial, fallopian tube, lung, breast, and gastrointestinal cancers, as well as relatively benign conditions including endometriosis, are observed. As described above, CA125 alone is not sufficient for cancer screening, serum CA125 is very useful for following treatment response, for predicting posttherapy prognosis, and for detecting recurrence in women with ovarian cancer. During first-line platinum-based ovarian cancer chemotherapy, CA125 levels should be followed regularly (e.g., every 3 weeks). The CA125 level at nadir, 3-month normalization of CA125, and CA125 half-life are strong predictors of progression-free and overall survival times.[132–134] The failure of serum CA125 normalization after initial treatment with surgery and platinum-based chemotherapy is a particularly ominous indication of poor prognosis in women with ovarian cancer.

In women in clinical remission following previously treated ovarian cancer, the National Comprehensive Cancer Network (NCCN-www.nccn.org) recommends evaluation of serum CA125 level at each follow-up visit if the CA125 level was elevated at the initial diagnosis. After a documented CA125 elevation, the median time to clinical disease relapse is over 4 months, although increases within the normal range can produce much longer lead times.

One large, randomized study in the United Kingdom concluded a lack of overall survival benefit when women with recurrent disease were treated at the time of CA125 elevation, although only 25% of women on the control and experimental arms were treated promptly with optimal combination chemotherapy.[135] At a minimum, earlier recurrence detection with CA125 provides time to receive known and novel agents, given the relatively short interval between symptomatic recurrence and death. With such controversy, however, using CA125 to monitor recurrence should be discussed with each patient.

CA15-3 and CA27.29

CA15-3 and CA 27.29 are well-characterized assays that detect circulating MUC1 antigen in peripheral blood.[136] Several studies support the prognostic relevance of this circulating marker in early-stage breast cancer though monitoring MUC1-based serum markers have not demonstrated definitive utility in making treatment decisions.[137,138] However, ASCO regards available data as insufficient to recommend using CA15-3 or CA 27.29 for breast cancer screening, diagnosis, staging, or for monitoring patients for recurrence, as conclusive evidence that early detection of recurrence improves survival is lacking.[113] Although present data cannot recommend the use of CA15-3 or CA 27.29 alone for monitoring treatment response, rising CA15-3 or CA27.29 may be used to indicate treatment failure in the absence of readily measurable disease. However, caution should be used when interpreting a rising CA27.29 or CA15-3 level during the first 4–6 weeks of a new therapy, as spurious early rises may occur and indeed may indicate response to therapy.

CA19-9

Carbohydrate antigen 19-9 is elevated primarily in the serum of patients with gastrointestinal carcinomas. The greatest utility of serum CA19-9 is in monitoring treatment response in pancreatic cancer. For patients with locally advanced or metastatic pancreatic cancer undergoing active therapy, ASCO recommends measurement of serum CA19-9 levels every 1–3 months.[139] Serial CA19-9 elevations suggest progressive disease in the face of treatment but confirmatory studies (e.g., CT scanning) should be sought before a therapy change is initiated.

Carcinoembryonic antigen (CEA)

Carcinoembryonic antigen (CEA) is a cell adhesion glycoprotein.[140] It is normally produced during fetal development and is not usually present in healthy adults' blood, although levels are raised in heavy smokers. Serum CEA may be elevated in patients with colorectal, gastric, pancreatic, lung, breast, and medullary thyroid carcinomas. ASCO has developed clinical practice guidelines to monitor serum CEA levels in patients with CRC, in whom serum CEA should be ordered preoperatively, if it would assist in staging and surgical planning. Postoperative CEA levels should be performed every 3 months for patients with stages II and III CRC for at least 3 years if the patient is a potential candidate for surgery (e.g., liver resection) or chemotherapy for metastatic disease. CEA is also the marker of choice for monitoring systemic therapy response in metastatic CRC.

Prostate-specific antigen (PSA)

Measuring serum PSA is important in men with an established diagnosis of prostate cancer. The rate of PSA rise can predict prostate cancer prognosis. Men with prostate cancer whose PSA level increased by more than 2.0 ng/mL during the year before the diagnosis of prostate cancer have a higher risk of death from prostate cancer after radical prostatectomy. PSA level along with clinical stage and Gleason tumor grade are components of most nomograms and predictive models used for prostate cancer risk assessment.[141] Further, serum PSA provides an indicator of disease response to treatment.

For prostate cancer, patients initially treated with curative intent, serum PSA level should be assessed every 6–12 months for 5 years and annually thereafter. A rising PSA level indicates biochemical failure and often precedes a clinically detectable recurrence by several years. Since biochemical failure may represent an isolated local recurrence, it is important to identify those patients as they may be candidates for salvage therapy.

Novel molecular biomarkers and platforms for their detection

Malignant tumors are characterized by multiple molecular anomalies responsible for the behavior of individual cancers. The driving aberrations can be in the germline genome or may occur in a somatic or acquired fashion in the cancer genome and/or proteome. Novel cancer biomarkers may not only be detectable in the tumor or its microenvironment but may be present in the circulation, either as circulating tumor cells (CTCs) or circulating nucleotides, proteins, or metabolites.

Novel high-throughput molecular technologies that comprehensively characterize the cancer genome and proteome are creating many new possibilities for the identification of biomarkers and particularly the development of multi-marker (e.g., multigene) panels that integrate information across many markers and across multiple levels (i.e., DNA, RNA, protein). Many of the earlier high throughput approaches such as gene methylation analysis, gene microarrays, comparative genomic hybridization, mass spectrometry/spectroscopy, and bead-based analysis methods are being replaced by next-generation sequencing. Gene expression profiles have been extensively explored in identifying good and poor prognosis subsets of various human tumors.[142] The ability of methylation analysis to detect early cancer cell DNA methylation aberrations is being investigated currently as an early diagnostic approach. The high-throughput reverse-phase protein lysate array (RPPA) proteomic technology allows concurrent analysis of the expression and activation of multiple specific kinases and other proteins.[143-147] This platform is particularly suited to investigate kinase signaling in cancer and the molecular effects of novel agents (e.g., TKIs) during treatment and in high-risk tissue during chemoprevention. Emerging mass spectrometry approaches such as MRM (multiple reaction monitoring) and SWATH could provide additional information on candidate genes when high-quality antibodies are not available and mass spectrometry is particularly useful for biomarker discovery. Together, genomic and proteomic platforms provide information that can be incorporated to develop meta-signatures reflecting global DNA, RNA, and protein abnormalities. These may be capable of outperforming data derived from a single technology examining only one of these platforms.[148] For example, proteomic studies can augment genomic panels by providing information on posttranslational modifications and on proteins' relative levels and activation. As such, data sets, systems for effective data management, integrated analysis of pathways, and "meta-analysis" are critical components of successful development of molecular markers.[149-151]

Novel germline biomarkers

The germline genome likely contains an underexplored trove of novel cancer risk biomarkers as well as biomarkers for toxicity and efficacy of specific anticancer treatments. For example, germline polymorphisms have been associated with toxicity and efficacy of the EGFR inhibitor erlotinib in lung cancer.[152] Recent large scale studies of the germline genome have also begun to uncover a large set of cancer susceptibility markers, many with low penetrance, thereby improving our ability to predict high cancer risk as well as response to therapy utilizing novel germline biomarkers.[153-155]

Tissue-specific biomarkers of high risk and for early detection of cancer

Early malignant change may be an indicator of high cancer risk in specific tissues. With availability of less invasive ways to obtain cells likely to be at risk of or to harbor early neoplastic change in tissue at risk of cancer (e.g., in sputum, bronchial washings, blood, feces, urine, or nipple aspirate), the study of tissue markers for screening of carcinogenesis risk and of early malignant transformation becomes more feasible. To date, the cost, invasiveness, lack of large prospective outcome validation studies, and absence of standardized guidelines have confined most of these potentially useful approaches to small clinical studies.

Although screening to detect lung cancer at an early stage using routine cytological examination of sputum did not decrease cancer-specific mortality, the application of molecular detection methods to sputum and bronchial washings is now being studied in an attempt to detect molecular changes associated with premalignant and early malignant bronchial epithelial cells.[156] For example, FISH with locus-specific probes to chromosomal regions 5p15, 7p12 (EGFR), 8q24 (C-Myc), and the centromere of chromosome 6 may significantly improve the sensitivity for detection of malignancy in sputum and bronchial washing specimens.[157]

Cancer-specific biomarkers

As discussed above, progress has already been made in identifying single biomarkers and multimarker panels (e.g., *Oncotype Dx*) to predict responses and overcome resistance to targeted therapy. However, progress in this regard has been more limited in other cancer types. Emerging basket clinical trials may in part address this deficiency. Basket trials are based on the observation that common molecular aberrations occur across different cancer types. These trials evaluate the role of targeted therapies against specific molecular aberration(s), regardless of cancer type, within the same trial.[158]

In the future, pharmacodynamic biomarkers of early drug activity must also be defined in preclinical tumor models and then confirmed in patient samples to assure that patients are receiving a biologically relevant dose of the drug. In this regard, optimal target inhibition by the drug in the tumor may be a more important endpoint than maximum tolerated dose of the drug. However, it is not yet known for most drugs whether optimal drug activity is dependent on maximal target inhibition, area under the curve, or trough values. Precepts derived from Systems Biology such as sensitivity analysis may provide guidelines as to the optimal inhibition pattern required. This approach may optimize drug efficacy, decrease toxicity, in particular off-target toxicity, and facilitate early identification of nonresponders for triage to alternative therapies. For example, perifosine-induced inhibition of AKT in the tumor correlates remarkably well with tumor growth inhibition using multiple dosing schedules of perifosine. Furthermore, the integrated assessment of the activation status of multiple PI3K/AKT pathway members in the tumor soon after initiation of therapies using proteomics assays such as RPPA may prove superior to single markers for prediction of tumor response to PI3K pathway inhibitors.

Serum and urine biomarkers

Novel serum biomarkers have potential utility in cancer screening, in prediction of tumor responsiveness to specific therapies, and in monitoring tumor responses to therapy. As discussed above, while conventional serum cancer biomarkers are used routinely for cancer monitoring, their application to screening is limited by suboptimal sensitivity and specificity.[159–161] Specificity can be improved by monitoring increases in individual marker levels over time, but marker panels will almost certainly be required to increase sensitivity for screening. The conventional concept concerning the screening utility of serum biomarkers is that their detection should trigger clinical assessment by imaging and biopsy, or increased surveillance if appropriate. Alternatively, novel serum markers might be used following screening by other means to increase the specificity of the latter approach. Thus, a novel biomarker may allow definition of an equivocal mammographic lesion as appropriate for serial monitoring or immediate biopsy.

Mass Spectrometry-based unbiased approaches to identify novel serum biomarkers from the proteome or metabolome present in blood or urine have the potential to identify biomarker panels could identify tumors at an early stage of development. Ovarian cancer has been the subject of several such studies because of diagnosis in advanced stages, poor patient outcomes, and the absence of a well-established screening method. Two general approaches have been utilized: identification of distinctive signatures and discovery of discrete markers that might be assembled into panels. However, none of the mass spectrometry-based approaches have validated in large prospectively based sample sets.[162]

In the urine, the sensitivity of FISH or of cytokeratin (e.g., keratin 19, 20) detection using IHC or reverse transcriptase (RT) PCR may be higher than that of conventional cytology for bladder and urothelial cancer screening.[163] A commercial kit (UroVysion) containing hybridization probes for chromosomes 3, 7, 9p21, and 17 is used for FISH analysis of urine. The sensitivity and specificity associated with this analysis were 60% and 82.6%, respectively, for detection of bladder cancer. In contrast, the sensitivity and specificity associated with urine cytology were 24.1% and 90.5%, respectively. Thus, a FISH assay for chromosomes 3, 7, 9, and 17 may have a higher sensitivity than cytology and a similar specificity for the detection of urothelial cancers. Table 2 summarizes the various approaches that have been investigated as potential tools to facilitate bladder cancer screening.[164]

Liquid biopsy

The National Cancer Institute (NCI) defines a liquid biopsy as "A test done on a sample of blood to look for cancer cells from a tumor that are circulating in the blood or for a piece of DNA from tumor cells that are in the blood" that is, CTCs or circulating tumor nucleotides/DNA (CTDNA) as defined below.[165] Research into liquid biopsies across all solid tumor malignancies is ongoing.

Circulating tumor cells

CTCs have potential utility in cancer screening, target identification, response prediction, and in monitoring response to treatment. Indeed, the predictive and prognostic utility of CTCs, and more recently circulating tumor DNA, have already been demonstrated in metastatic breast cancer.[166,167] Initial studies of the utility of CTCs in breast cancer screening are proceeding.[168] In ovarian cancer, peripheral blood CTC-specific *p53* sequences are detectable in some FIGO stage III/IV ovarian cancer patients, suggesting that this approach may be useful as a building block toward early detection.[169]

The use of CTCs to study molecular biomarkers is limited currently to gene expression signatures because of the need for substrate amplification. However, CTCs have the potential to replace invasive tumor biopsies with "liquid" biopsies and facilitate early access to the tumor genome and proteome for molecular biomarkers predictive of therapy response and resistance, as demonstrated in lung and prostate cancers.[170,171] A major challenge is the difficulty in harvesting CTCs and exploring molecular markers in a limited number of cells. Methods of CTCs enrichment are being explored and include the enhanced density gradient system.[172] We are currently investigating novel methods of DNA and protein extraction to allow detection of mutations and protein expression/activation changes in CTCs, the latter utilizing RPPA.[173,174]

Circulating nucleotides

DNA, RNA, microRNA, and proteins are released from tumor cells and can be found in the circulation. Circulating biomarkers have the potential to reflect processes occurring across all tumor sites in the body that cannot be detected by analysis of the primary tumor and/or metastatic sites. Thus, there is great excitement in the potential for "liquid" biopsies to provide information not accessible from tumor biopsies. Moreover, they would obviate the need for tumor biopsy and in particular repeat tumor biopsies to determine tumor response and molecular evolution following therapy. Tumors can release large amounts of nucleotides into the circulation with up to 20% of circulating DNA being derived from a patient tumor.

Table 2 Sensitivity, specificity, and positive predictive value of urine cytology, bladder tumor antigen (BTA) immunoassay, nuclear matrix protein-22 (NMP22) detection, immunoCyt, and urine FISH for early detection of bladder cancer.[a]

	Sensitivity (%)	Specificity (%)	PPV (%)
PSA	72	93	25
Urine cytology	48–73	48–100	48–69
BTA	53	77	63
NMP22	71	66	21
ImmunoCyt	78–81	74–100	26
FISH	69–71	78–95	68

Serum prostate-specific antigen (PSA) in prostate cancer screening is shown only as a point of reference. ImmunoCyt is currently approved by the US Food and Drug Administration for the monitoring of recurrent bladder cancer. ImmunoCyt uses a cocktail of three monoclonal antibodies to detect bladder cancer cells in the urine. One antibody is directed against a high molecular-weight form of glycosylated carcinoembryonic antigen, 19A211. The other two antibodies, LDQ10 and M344, are directed against mucins that are specific for bladder cancer and are labeled with fluorescein.
[a] Source: Based on Shaw et al.[98]

Thus, any aberration such as mutation, rearrangement, increased copy number, increased microRNA or RNA level could be detected in the circulation, as is the case with *KRAS* and *p53* mutations. However, the amount of DNA in the circulation and the ability to detect tumor-related aberrations varies markedly across tumor types. Nevertheless, commercial tests based on circulating DNA are becoming available.

New practical uses of liquid biopsy are now available. For example, the detection of EGFR T790M resistance mutations in NSCLC. Liquid biopsy can now detect specific EGFR mutations which can determine TKI treatment change. This is currently FDA approved for this use under Guardant health and foundation medicine liquid biopsy.

FoundationOne Liquid CDx is an FDA-approved companion diagnostic.[175] It is a blood-based test that analyses over 300 genes including TMB and MSI from circulating free DNA (cfDNA). As already discussed, this is of clinical use now due to the approval of tumor agnostic therapies. It can also detect PIK3CA mutations, BRCA1, BRCA 2, ALK, and EGFR mutations all from one single blood test. This is far less invasive in comparison to a core biopsy and will hopefully significantly improve patient care.

Challenges in validation of novel molecular biomarkers

The novel unbiased technologies being used to profile the cancer genome or proteome to define new biomarker panels are susceptible to challenges in reproducibility that can be attributed to the simultaneous assay of many gene or protein markers with a limited number of cancer specimens. The large number of potential biomarker combinations introduces a significant likelihood that uncovered associations are simply the result of chance. It is critical to adopt a rigorous training, test, and validation approach to novel biomarker studies to meaningfully impact patient management. Most studies presenting novel biomarker panels have not impacted patient management to date, either because they did not rigorously deal with this multiple parameter problem or because they did not adopt sufficiently robust statistical approaches to validation. The importance of bioinformatic and biostatistical support for the development of novel molecular diagnostics cannot be overemphasized.

Rigorous validation of molecular marker panels in large numbers of well-documented cases is required to test their clinical utility before routine use in patient management. The applicability of several preliminary panels is still being validated.[176,177] A major hindrance to designing novel molecular studies for biomarker discovery and validation is the frequent lack of availability of adequately preserved and annotated tissue or blood samples in large numbers to correlate with outcome using emerging technologies. In particular, novel high-throughput approaches are often limited in their utility to fresh frozen specimens (paraffin-embedded samples are more plentiful). Thus, a popular model for biomarker development involves discovery using novel high-throughput profiling technologies (e.g., transcriptional profiling) in frozen tissue, followed by validation using moderate-throughput technologies (e.g., RT-PCR) applied to paraffin-embedded tissue. It is critical to define the specific tissue type in which a molecular marker will be validated for clinical use.[178,179] Novel comprehensive approaches to biomarker discovery using proteome- or genome-wide expression profiling have now redefined ways tumor banks collect and store tumor samples, with a major emphasis placed on fresh frozen specimens.[180,181]

Presently, it is not possible to apply all available investigative technologies to every person, or even every patient at high risk for the development of cancer. Putting cost issues aside, one challenge is to obtain adequate material from biopsy, cellular, or serum specimens. Indeed, for comprehensive analysis of genomic *DNA* or *RNA,* several hundred nanograms are required, but the amount of DNA and RNA available from a fine needle aspirate is in picograms. Furthermore, biopsies frequently have relatively low tumor content thereby complicating analysis. In the case of CTCs and circulating nucleotides, the DNA and RNA yield can be even smaller. Amplification by PCR can increase mRNA yield, but PCR-generated errors are not uncommon. Approaches to deal with low amounts of protein are minimal. As noted above, MRM and other mass spectrometry approaches may complement antibody-based approaches. We are currently exploring "barcoding" antibodies with DNA sequences to allow use of amplification approaches that have been applied to DNA detection. These major difficulties need to be addressed to facilitate the routine application of novel molecular technologies to cancer diagnostics.

Recommendations

The effective discovery of novel cancer biomarkers requires the integration of multiple critical factors, including collaborative studies, availability of appropriate human tissue sample sets, standardized reagents, and technologies for analyzing, identifying, and quantitating candidate biomarkers in tissue and fluid, mouse models of disease, integrated bioinformatics platforms, and implementation of automation, all of which were key to achieving the Human Genome Project, for example. Standard operating procedures (SOPs) regarding tumor specimen biobanking, specimen processing, and quality control, validation, performance, and interpretation of analytical assays should be developed at a national or ideally international level, to allay concerns regarding potentially unreliable study results and permit accurate pooling and comparison of cross-study results. The American Association for Cancer Research (AACR)—FDA—NCI Cancer Biomarker Collaborative and the European Group on Tumor Markers have defined these key procedures for effective biomarker development. These strategies can be facilitated by the creation of national biospecimen repositories such as the Cancer Human Biobank, which retrieves highly clinically annotated tumor specimens across centers in the United States and processes them according to SOPs prior to being made available for analysis.

As biomarker discovery programs characterize tissues using high-throughput genomic, transcriptional, and proteomic approaches, it is critical that adequate and centralized computational infrastructure be developed to allow storage, utilization, and integration of the vast and heterogeneous data derived from novel "omics" technologies. Such a computational resource should be made available to all investigators in a manner that is easy to use, that protects confidentiality, and avoids duplication of efforts. These resources should facilitate data mining, retrieval, and automated analysis, thus facilitating data integration across molecular platforms and between datasets, and the association of specific aberrations with clinical endpoints. Repeated updating should be facilitated as novel "omics" technologies are introduced and upgraded. Access would also allow novel biostatistical approaches that further our ability to effectively select clinically useful cancer biomarkers. Further, approaches are being implemented to facilitate both sample and data sharing across the community, given that the amount of data available far exceeds the ability of any group to adequately mine and interpret the data. The Biospecimen and Biorepositories Research Branch of the NCI provides effective tools and resources to establish high-quality biobanking. A significant number of online data repositories, such as The Cancer Genome Atlas Portal and The Clinical Proteomic Tumor Analysis Consortium, are now publicly available, thereby facilitating the interrogation of biomarkers by different research groups.

The selection of novel biomarkers from data derived using novel high-throughput technologies needs careful consideration, to discern chance associations from true biological relationships. False biomarker discovery can result from selection bias, overfitting, multiplicity, multiple clinical endpoints, and intrapatient correlation, which must be eliminated from research designs using accurate statistical methods and study designs including sample sizes that enable markers meeting prespecified performance characteristics for well-defined clinical applications to be identified. New biomarkers should be validated prior to potential introduction into clinical management by measuring the biomarker's impact on costs and carefully chosen clinical outcomes in a prospective, randomized study.[182] However, study costs and regulatory and healthcare market constraints often make such clinical trials impractical. Improved study designs involving retrospective samples, such as the ProBE method, have been developed as alternatives. Alternatively, retrospective analysis of archived prospectively collected samples or pooled analyses of published and unpublished cohorts with a systematic review can also provide a high level of evidence, as long as specific requirements ensuring high quality within these study designs are met. Moreover, researchers and policymakers turn to simulation modeling to predict the effects of new biomarkers on outcomes. The latter approach can optimize sensitivity, specificity, and cost in addition to identifying leverage points where more definitive biomarkers may be needed. This approach has already been used to assess the cost-effectiveness of flexible sigmoidoscopy for CRC screening.

A Committee on Developing Biomarker-Based Tools for Cancer Screening, Diagnosis, and Treatment of the Institute of Medicine of the National Academies has put forth a formal set of recommendations for development of biomarker-based tools for cancer (Box 3).

Conclusion

In summary, significant progress has already been made in the developing molecular diagnostics in certain forms of cancer such as breast cancer. Recent molecular studies have revealed the biologic heterogeneity and complexity of cancer and this necessitates the application of more global studies of the cancer genome and proteome to identify novel biomarkers that facilitate further advances in the understanding, treatment, and early detection of cancer. Indeed, the application of high-throughput technologies is already significantly advancing the ability to identify patients who will benefit from specific cancer treatments. Improving understanding of the molecular heterogeneity of cancer along with rapid improvements in molecular technologies that can profile this heterogeneity have also unearthed further possibilities for the development of molecular diagnostics in cancer. It is expected that these approaches will eventually not only advance our ability to diagnose cancer at an early stage but will also allow simultaneous profiling of molecular targets that will facilitate individualization of patient care. The achievement of these goals necessitates overcoming many challenges that lie in the way of the successful implementation of both traditional and novel molecular technologies to cancer diagnostics. As high-throughput technologies acquire an increasing foothold in the development of novel molecular cancer diagnostics, the establishment of robust collaborations and bioinformatics approaches to high-throughput data storage, integration, analysis, and validation will be critical.

Box 3 Summary of recommendations to develop biomarker-based tools for cancer

Methods, tools, and resources needed to discover and develop biomarkers

1. Federal agencies should develop an organized, comprehensive approach to biomarker discovery, and foster development of novel technologies.
2. Industry and other funders should establish international consortia to generate and share precompetitive biomarker data.
3. Funders should place a major emphasis on developing pathway biomarkers to broaden applicability.
4. Funders should sponsor demonstration projects to develop biomarkers that can predict efficacy and safety in patients for drugs already on the market.
5. Government agencies and other funders should sustain support for high-quality biorepositories of prospectively collected samples.
6. Biomarkers should be developed and validated with high negative predictive value for prediction of response to ne targeted therapies, particularly those with high cost.

Guidelines, standards, oversight, and incentives needed for biomarker development

7. Government agencies and other stakeholders should develop a transparent process to create well-defined consensus standards and guidelines for biomarker development, qualification, validation, and use.
8. The FDA and industry should work together to facilitate the codevelopment and approval of diagnostic-therapeutic combinations.
9. The FDA should clearly delineate and standardize its oversight of biomarker tests used in clinical decision-making.
10. The Centers for Medicare and Medicaid Services should develop a specialty area for molecular diagnostics under the CLIA.

Methods and processes needed for clinical evaluation and adoption

11. The Centers for Medicare & Medicaid Services should revise and modernize its coding and pricing system for diagnostic tests.
12. The Centers for Medicare and Medicaid Services, as well as other payors, should develop criteria for conditional coverage of new biomarker tests.

As a component of conditional coverage, procedures for high-quality population-based assessments of efficacy and cost-effectiveness of biomarker tests should be established.

Source: Institute of Medicine of the National Academies.

Key references

The complete reference list can be found on Vital Source version of this title, see inside front cover.

1 Fisher B, Costantino JP, Wickerham DL, et al. Tamoxifen for the prevention of breast cancer: current status of the National Surgical Adjuvant Breast and Bowel Project P-1 study. *J Natl Cancer Inst*. 2005;**97**:1652–1662.

6 Kriege M, Brekelmans CT, Boetes C, et al. Efficacy of MRI and mammography for breast cancer screening in women with a familial or genetic predisposition. *N Engl J Med*. 2004;**351**:427–437.

13 Edelsberg J, Weycker D, Atwood M, et al. Cost-effectiveness of an autoantibody test (EarlyCDT-Lung) as an aid to early diagnosis of lung cancer in patients with incidentally detected pulmonary nodules. *PLoS One*. 2018;**13**(5):e0197826. doi: 10.1371/journal.pone.0197826.

15 Amling CL. Prostate-specific antigen and detection of prostate cancer: what have we learned and what should we recommend for screening? *Curr Treat Options in Oncol*. 2006;7:337–345.

18 Basch E, Oliver TK, Vickers A, et al. Screening for prostate cancer with prostate-specific antigen testing: American Society of Clinical Oncology Provisional Clinical Opinion. *J Clin Oncol*. 2012;**30**(24):3020–3025.

28 Force, U.S.P.S.T. *Ovarian cancer: screening*, 2018; https://www.uspreventiveservicestaskforce.org/uspstf/document/RecommendationStatementFinal/ovarian-cancer-screening (accessed 28 May 2020).

30 Ronco G, Dillner J, Elfström KM. Efficacy of HPV-based screening for prevention of invasive cervical cancer: follow-up of four European randomised controlled trials. *Lancet*. 2014;**383**(9916):524–532.

31 U.S. Preventive Services Task Force. *Cervical Cancer: Screening*, 2018. https://www.uspreventiveservicestaskforce.org/uspstf/recommendation/cervical-cancer-screening (accessed 28 May 2020).

34 Imperiale TF, Ransohoff DF, Itzkowitz SH, et al. Multitarget stool DNA testing for colorectal-cancer screening. *N Engl J Med*. 2014;**370**:1287–1297.

35 Nian J, Sun X, Ming SY, et al. Diagnostic accuracy of methylated SEPT9 for blood-based colorectal cancer detection: a systematic review and meta-analysis. *Clin Transl Gastroenterol*. 2017;**8**:e216. doi: 10.1038/ctg.2016.66.

37 Moinova HR, LaFramboise T, Lutterbaugh JD, et al. Identifying DNA methylation biomarkers for non-endoscopic detection of Barrett's esophagus. *Sci Transl Med*. 2018;**10**:4.

38 Parikh ND, Mehta AS, Singal AG, et al. Biomarkers for the diagnosis of hepatocellular carcinoma. *Cancer Epidemiol Biomark Prev*. 2020;**29**:2495–2503.

42 Meijers-Heijboer H, van Geel B, van Putten WL, et al. Breast cancer after prophylactic bilateral mastectomy in women with a BRCA1 or BRCA2 mutation. *N Engl J Med*. 2001;**345**:159–164.

47 Berry DA, Iversen ES Jr, Gudbjartsson DF, et al. BRCAPRO validation, sensitivity of genetic testing of BRCA1/BRCA2, and prevalence of other breast cancer susceptibility genes. *J Clin Oncol*. 2002;**20**:2701–2712.

55 Pérez-Carbonell L, Ruiz-Ponte C, Guarinos C. Comparison between universal molecular screening for Lynch syndrome and revised Bethesda guidelines in a large population-based cohort of patients with colorectal cancer. *Gut*. 2012;**61**(6):865–872.

61 O'Leary B, Finn RS, Turner NC. Treating cancer with selective CDK4/6 inhibitors. *Nat Rev Clin Oncol*. 2016;**13**:417–430.

69 André F, Ciruelos E, Rubovszky G, et al. Alpelisib for PIK3CA-mutated, hormone receptor–positive advanced breast cancer. *N Engl J Med*. 2019;**380**:1929–1940.

88 Jordan EJ, Kim HR, Arcila ME, et al. Prospective comprehensive molecular characterization of lung adenocarcinomas for efficient patient matching to approved and emerging therapies. *Cancer Discov*. 2017;**7**:596–609.

90 Engelman JA, Jänne PA. Mechanisms of acquired resistance to epidermal growth factor receptor tyrosine kinase inhibitors in non-small cell lung cancer. *Clin Cancer Res*. 2008;**14**:2895–2899.

91 Mok TS, Wu Y-L, Ahn M-J, et al. Osimertinib or platinum–pemetrexed in EGFR T790M–positive lung cancer. *N Engl J Med*. 2016;**376**:629–640.

95 Peters S, Camidge DR, Shaw AT, et al. Alectinib versus crizotinib in untreated ALK-positive non–small-cell lung cancer. *N Engl J Med*. 2017;**377**:829–838.

97 Bergethon K, Shaw AT, Ou S-HI, et al. ROS1 rearrangements define a unique molecular class of lung cancers. *J Clin Oncol*. 2012;**30**:863–870.

100 Planchard D, Besse B, Groen HJM, et al. Dabrafenib plus trametinib in patients with previously treated BRAF(V600E)-mutant metastatic non-small cell lung cancer: an open-label, multicentre phase 2 trial. *Lancet Oncol*. 2016;**17**:984–993.

103 Andre T, Shiu K-K, Kim TW, et al. Pembrolizumab versus chemotherapy for microsatellite instability-high/mismatch repair deficient metastatic colorectal cancer: the phase 3 KEYNOTE-177 study. *ASCO*. 2020;**2020**.

104 Douillard JY, Oliner KS, Siena S, et al. Panitumumab-FOLFOX4 treatment and RAS mutations in colorectal cancer. *N Engl J Med*. 2013;**369**:1023–1034.

109 Cioffi A, Maki RG. GI stromal tumors: 15 years of lessons from a rare cancer. *J Clin Oncol*. 2015:27. doi: 10.1200/JCO.2014.59.7344.

111 Loriot Y, Necchi A, Park SH, et al. Erdafitinib in locally advanced or metastatic urothelial carcinoma. *N Engl J Med*. 2019;**381**:338–348.

119 O'Hare T, Eide CA, Deininger MW. New Bcr-Abl inhibitors in chronic myeloid leukemia: keeping resistance in check. *Expert Opin Investig Drugs*. 2008;**17**:865–878.

121 McLaughlin P, Grillo-López AJ, Link BK, et al. Rituximab chimeric anti-CD20 monoclonal antibody therapy for relapsed indolent lymphoma: half of patients respond to a four-dose treatment program. *J Clin Oncol*. 1998;**16**:2825–2833.

124 Rischin D, Young RJ, Fisher R. Prognostic significance of p16INK4A and human papillomavirus in patients with oropharyngeal cancer treated on TROG 02.02 phase III trial. *J Clin Oncol*. 2010;**28**(27):4142–4148.

125 Marcus L, Lemery SJ, Keegan P, Pazdur R. FDA approval summary: pembrolizumab for the treatment of microsatellite instability-high solid tumors. *Clin Cancer Res*. 2019;**25**:3753–3758.

129 von Eyben FE, Skude G, Fossa SD, et al. Serum lactate dehydrogenase (S-LDH) and S-LDH isoenzymes in patients with testicular germ cell tumors. *Mol Gen Genet*. 1983;**189**:326–333.

132 Prat A, Parera M, Peralta S, et al. Nadir CA-125 concentration in the normal range as an independent prognostic factor for optimally treated advanced epithelial ovarian cancer. *Ann Oncol*. 2008;**19**:327–331.

141 Partin AW, Mangold LA, Lamm DM, et al. Contemporary update of prostate cancer staging nomograms (Partin Tables) for the new millennium. *Urology*. 2001;**58**:843–848.

142 Chibon F. Cancer gene expression signatures - the rise and fall? *Eur J Cancer*. 2013;**49**(8):2000–2009.

156 Baryshnikova E, Destro A, Infante MV. Molecular alterations in spontaneous sputum of cancer-free heavy smokers: results from a large screening program. *Clin Cancer Res*. 2008;**14**(6):1913–1919.

158 Sleijfer S, Bogaerts J, Siu LL. Designing transformative clinical trials in the cancer genome era. *J Clin Oncol*. 2013;**31**(15):1834–1841.

162 Kozak KR, Su F, Whitelegge JP, et al. Characterization of serum biomarkers for detection of early stage ovarian cancer. *Proteomics*. 2005;**5**:4589–4596.

168 Reinholz MM, Nibbe A, Jonart LM, et al. Evaluation of a panel of tumor markers for molecular detection of circulating cancer cells in women with suspected breast cancer. *Clin Cancer Res*. 2005;**11**:3722–3732.

39 Principles of imaging

Lawrence H. Schwartz, MD

> **Overview**
>
> Radiological studies offer vital information about tumor detection, characterization, staging, and therapeutic response monitoring. There are a myriad of imaging modalities available for each of these tasks and their use is dependent upon both the primary tumor type and the clinical need. Increasingly, integration of other diagnostic tools including genomic and proteomic assays. Other techniques including AI enhancements to imaging diagnostics aid in diagnostic potential.

Imaging plays a major and fundamental role in every aspect of oncology. Radiological studies provide invaluable information about tumor detection, characterization, staging, and therapeutic response monitoring. Increasingly, imaging in oncology is being used as a both prognostic and predictive biomarkers either alone or in combination with other tissue and serum biomarkers. Screening examinations such as mammography, low-dose CT for lung cancer, and virtual colonoscopy are yet another example of the use imaging in oncology. Finally, image-guided intervention has significantly evolved over the past few years and has tremendous potential for minimizing the invasiveness of many cancer therapies.

Cross-sectional imaging studies, including computed tomography (CT) and positron emission tomography scans using ionizing radiation as well as nonionizing magnetic resonance (MR) imaging, are the mainstay of care in the oncology patient and typically complement more traditional radiographs (X-ray) studies of the chest and abdomen. While conventional radiological studies such as plain diagnostic X-ray examinations films are easy to perform, deliver a low dose of radiation, are relatively inexpensive, their utility in the care of cancer patients is limited.

The type and frequency of radiological evaluation of the cancer patient depend on the tumor, the stage of the patient, and the specific clinical indication for the scan. There is a wide spectrum of indications that includes screening, workup of the symptomatic patient, further evaluation of an abnormality found on another imaging study, assessing response or progression of a patient's disease after a therapy or intervention, and evaluating complications of therapy. Before each radiology study is ordered, it is imperative to understand the clinical scenario, the disease that is suspected, the type of information that is required, whether the test can provide the necessary evidence, and importantly, what can and will be done with the results to change the treatment of the patient and potentially the patient's outcome.

Integration of imaging with other diagnostic tools, including genomic and proteomic assays are enabling complimentary and even more valuable information to be obtained for the cancer patient. However, there is growing need for these imaging studies to provide more information that simple anatomic visualization and localization of tumors. Contemporary oncology requires that these tests evaluate these basic molecular events which would increase our understanding of malignancies, and eventually could be used to influence clinical practice.

The growth of molecular imaging began in the early 1990s, with the use of positron emission tomography (PET) imaging and the glucose analog probe, $[^{18}F]$-2-fluoro-2-deoxy-D-glucose (FDG). Over the last several years, FDG–PET imaging has become one of the most important tools to evaluate cancer patients for characterization of primary tumors and their metastases as well as for monitoring treatment response to cancer therapy. PET images are less detailed anatomically, but it has been recognized at there is a potential for fusion of morphologic, detailed anatomic information from a CT scan with a PET scan. Hybrid, dual PET/CT scanners as well as PET/MRI became available providing combination imaging which is of higher diagnostic value than separate PET or CT or MRI scans in many cancers and clinical indications As a move toward molecular imaging continues, the development of new targets, techniques, and tumor-specific imaging probes should provide more accurate diagnostic information. There is an increased use of imaging with PET and other molecular imaging techniques, including with MRI to evaluate cell metabolism, cell proliferation, hypoxia, apoptosis, receptor expression, gene expression, angiogenesis, signal transduction. In the future, molecular imaging may be able to address many current, unresolved diagnostic issues in oncology. Although the technology is undergoing a dramatic expansion, it is also incumbent upon the radiologic community to carefully study new molecular imaging techniques and determine if they are truly useful and cost-effective. The ability to create ever more spectacular images does not necessarily improve patient management and outcomes.

Artificial intelligence in cancer imaging has a potential to assist clinicians in the tasks of cancer care by automating the interpretation of imaging studies, but more importantly by deriving more information from imaging studies, especially in a quantitative manner. This includes, but is not limited to total tumor burden assessment of tumors over time, extrapolation of the tumor genotype information, and biological and therapeutic course from the imaging features including phenotype, prediction of outcome, and assessment of the impact of disease and treatment on organs. AI has the potential to automate tasks that are repetitive for the Radiologist and change the function and workflow from detection to aid in management decisions.

Hypothesis-driven, evidence-based studies are essential if non-invasive anatomic and molecular imaging is to have an impact on patient care. Because imaging is a fundamental part of diagnostic evaluation, understanding the utility of particular tests will guide a more efficient patient evaluation. This section's collection of chapters provides an overview of imaging principles, with a focus on the cancer patient. Imaging plays a central role in clinical management, and the information presented here provides general guidelines for using radiologic studies in everyday clinical practice.

Holland-Frei Cancer Medicine, Tenth Edition. Edited by Robert C. Bast, John C. Byrd, Carlo M. Croce, Ernest Hawk, Fadlo R. Khuri, Raphael E. Pollock, Apostolia M. Tsimberidou, Christopher G. Willett, and Cheryl L. Willman.
© 2023 John Wiley & Sons, Inc. Published 2023 by John Wiley & Sons, Inc.

Further reading

Apolo AB, Pandit-Taskar N, Morris MJ. Novel tracers and their development for the imaging of metastatic prostate cancer. *J Nucl Med*. 2008;**49**:2031–2041.

Bi WL, Hosny A, Schabath MB, et al. Artificial intelligence in cancer imaging: clinical challenges and applicationsCA. *Cancer J Clin*. 2019;**69**(2):127–157.

Boss DS, Olmos RV, Sinaasappel M, et al. Application of PET/CT in the development of novel anticancer drugs. *Oncologist*. 2008;**13**(1):25–38.

Czernin J, Ta L, Herrmann K. Does PET/MR imaging improve cancer assessments? Literature evidence from more than 900 patients. *J Nucl Med*. 2014;**55**(Supplement 2):59S–62S.

Farwell MD, Pryma DA, Mankoff DA. PET/CT imaging in cancer: current applications and future directions. *Cancer*. 2014;**120**(22):3433–3445.

Fleming IN, Manavaki R, Blower PJ, et al. Imaging tumour hypoxia with positron emission tomography. *Br J Cancer*. 2014;**112**(2):238–250.

Gerstner ER, Sorensen AG, Jain RK, Batchelor TT. Advances in neuroimaging techniques for the evaluation of tumor growth, vascular permeability, and angiogenesis in gliomas. *Curr Opin Neurol*. 2008;**21**(6):728–735.

Heron DE, Andrade RS, Beriwal S, et al. PET-CT in radiation oncology: the impact on diagnosis, treatment planning, and assessment of treatment response. *Am J Clin Oncol*. 2008;**31**(4):352–362.

Hosny A, Parmar C, Quackenbush J, et al. Artificial intelligence in radiology. *Nat Rev Cancer*. 2018;**18**(8):500–510.

Kim JH, Choi SH, Ryoo I, et al. Prognosis prediction of measurable enhancing lesion after completion of standard concomitant chemoradiotherapy and adjuvant temozolomide in glioblastoma patients: application of dynamic susceptibility contrast perfusion and diffusion-weighted imaging. *PLoS One*. 2014;**9**(11):e113587.

Iagaru A, Mittra E, Minamimoto R, et al. Simultaneous whole-body time-of-flight 18F-FDG PET/MRI: a pilot study comparing SUVmax with PET/CT and assessment of MR image quality. *Clin Nucl Med*. 2015;**40**(1):1–8.

Kuehl H, Veit P, Rosenbaum SJ, et al. Can PET/CT replace separate diagnostic CT for cancer imaging? Optimizing CT protocols for imaging cancers of the chest and abdomen. *J Nucl Med*. 2007;**48**(suppl 1):45S–57S.

Kundra V, Silverman PM, Matin SF, Choi H. Imaging in oncology from the University of Texas M. D. Anderson Cancer Center: diagnosis, staging, and surveillance of prostate cancer. *AJR Am J Roentgenol*. 2007;**189**(4):830–844.

Malviya G, Nayak TK. PET imaging to monitor cancer therapy. *Curr Pharm Biotechnol*. 2013;**14**(7):669–682.

Schaefer JF, Schlemmer HP. Total-body MR-imaging in oncology. *Eur Radiol*. 2006;**16**(9):2000–2015.

Tanvetyanon T, Eikman EA, Sommers E, et al. Response by PET scan versus CT scan to predict survival after neoadjuvant chemotherapy for resectable non-small cell lung cancer. *JCO*. 2008.

Veit P, Ruehm S, Kuehl H, et al. Lymph node staging with dual-modality PET/CT: enhancing the diagnostic accuracy in oncology. *Eur J Radiol*. 2006;**58**(3):383–389.

Wirth A, Foo M, Seymour JF, et al. Impact of [18F] fluorodeoxyglucose positron emission tomography on staging and management of early-stage follicular non-hodgkin lymphoma. *Int J Radiat Oncol Biol Phys*. 2008;**71**(1):213–219.

Wong TZ, Paulson EK, Nelson RC, et al. Practical approach to diagnostic CT combined with PET. *AJR Am J Roentgenol*. 2007;**188**(3):622–629.

Zhao B, Schwartz LH, Larson SM. Imaging surrogates of tumor response to therapy: anatomic and functional biomarkers. *J Nucl Med*. 2009;**50**(2):239–249.

40 Interventional radiology for the cancer patient

Zeyad A. Metwalli, MD ■ Judy U. Ahrar, MD ■ Michael J. Wallace, MD (deceased)

Overview

In the past decades, there has been a substantial expansion in the use of image-guided procedures for diagnosing and treating various types of cancer. There are several reasons for this increased use. Advances in cancer diagnosis and novel medical and surgical therapies have led to increased survival in this patient population. More patients now present with primary or metastatic disease confined to an organ and are consequently more likely to benefit from locoregional therapies.[1-3] Thus, a neoplasm can be defined using standard imaging modalities, and then minimally invasive percutaneous techniques can be used to establish the diagnosis and to provide locoregional or palliative therapies to treat the cancer patient. Improvements in catheter/device technology, embolic agents and chemotherapy drugs, and delivery systems are associated with improved patient outcome and have sparked renewed interest in these approaches. In this chapter, we discuss hepatic vascular interventions, genitourinary interventions, thoracic interventions, several forms of palliative therapeutic procedures, and some additional image-guided procedures.

Hepatic vascular interventions

The liver has long occupied center stage in interventional oncology, the practice of interventional radiology specific to the oncology patient. Hepatic interventions for diagnosis and treatment are popular for a number of reasons, among them that this organ is a common site of metastatic disease and can be easily accessed percutaneously. However, the key feature that makes liver tumors particularly amenable to catheter-delivered therapies stems from the unique nature of their blood supply. Hepatic tumors derive most of their blood supply from the hepatic artery, whereas normal hepatic parenchyma derives most of its supply from the portal venous system. This unique arrangement allows the interventional oncologist to direct intra-arterial therapies to hepatic lesions while relatively sparing the normal liver parenchyma.

Arterial infusion therapy

The goal of arterial infusion therapy is to achieve better tumor response by delivering chemotherapeutic agents directly into the artery that supplies the neoplasm. The rationale behind arterial infusion therapy is based on the first-pass effect, which occurs when a drug is given directly into the tissue that metabolizes it. The first-pass effect, compared with systemic administration, can lead to a several-fold increase in the drug concentration within the affected organ and, at the same time, a reduction in systemic concentration. Therefore, regional drug delivery is seen as a method of overcoming the limitations of the maximum-tolerated dose.[4]

Arterial infusion therapy has been primarily used for the treatment of metastatic colorectal cancer confined to the liver. A meta-analysis by Mocellin et al.[5] summarized the results of 10 randomized controlled trials that compared hepatic arterial infusion (HAI) with systemic chemotherapy. Although the study revealed better tumor response to fluoropyrimidine-based HAI when compared with systemic fluoropyrimidine therapy, tumor response rates for modern systemic chemotherapy regimens using a combination of fluorouracil with oxaliplatin or irinotecan were similar or superior to those for HAI. Moreover, the meta-analysis showed no survival benefit associated with fluoropyrimidine-based HAI therapy. However, a more recent meta-analysis of the literature on unresectable intrahepatic cholangiocarcinoma patients by Boehm et al.[6] showed that HAI had the longest overall survival rate amongst the trans-arterial-based hepatic therapies, including conventional chemoembolization, drug-eluting bead chemoembolization, and Yttrium-90 radioembolization. Furthermore, hepatic arterial infusion is an emerging technique for the treatment of advanced hepatocellular carcinoma primarily using fluorouracil and cisplatin-based regimens.[7] Further studies of the use of HAI for the delivery of novel anticancer agents will be instrumental in determining the role of this approach in future locoregional cancer therapy.

Arterial embolization

The aim of transcatheter hepatic arterial embolization is to completely or partially occlude the arterial supply to the tumor. The rationale is that such occlusion will cause tumor ischemia, which in turn will lead to growth arrest and necrosis. After hepatic arterial embolization, collateral hepatic circulation comes into play immediately. This collateral circulation should be identified and occluded if it supplies the neoplasm. The more central the occlusion, the more abundant is the collateral flow. Therefore, to maximize ischemia, the most effective embolization should result in distal terminal vessel occlusion. Peripheral (segmental and subsegmental) vascular embolization is best accomplished with coaxial catheters and small particles.

Many different embolic agents have been used with success for hepatic embolization. The most common agents include absorbable gelatin sponge particles and powder, polyvinyl alcohol foam granules, fibrin glue, *n*-butyl cyanoacrylate, ethiodized oil, microspheres, and absolute alcohol. Gelatin sponge segments or stainless steel coils are used for central occlusion and not often used for tumor embolotherapy.

The most common complication after hepatic arterial embolization is postembolization syndrome. This syndrome consists of fever, nausea, fatigue, and elevated white blood cell count and liver function tests. These symptoms are usually self-limited.

Holland-Frei Cancer Medicine, Tenth Edition. Edited by Robert C. Bast, John C. Byrd, Carlo M. Croce, Ernest Hawk, Fadlo R. Khuri, Raphael E. Pollock, Apostolia M. Tsimberidou, Christopher G. Willett, and Cheryl L. Willman.
© 2023 John Wiley & Sons, Inc. Published 2023 by John Wiley & Sons, Inc.

Complications resulting from nontarget embolization include cholecystitis, pancreatitis, and gastrointestinal ulcers. Hepatic embolization may also lead to liver necrosis, hepatic abscess, and liver failure. Failure to recognize intrahepatic arteriovenous shunts during embolization may cause embolic material to reach the pulmonary circulation, which can in turn lead to respiratory failure. The complications of hepatic embolization in 284 patients who underwent 410 embolizations over a 10-year period were analyzed by Hemingway and Allison.[8] Minor complications occurred in 16% of patients, serious complications in 6.6%, and death in 2%.

Arterial chemoembolization

Arterial chemoembolization consists of intra-arterial delivery of a combination of chemotherapy drugs and an embolic agent into a tumor. Although chemoembolization has been primarily utilized to treat primary and secondary liver neoplasms, preliminary investigations of its use in prostate cancer and renal cell carcinoma have been conducted.[9,10] The rationale behind chemoembolization is based on the theory that tumor ischemia caused by embolization of the dominant arterial supply has a synergistic effect with the chemotherapeutic drugs. This technique has been the mainstay of interventional radiology since it was originally introduced by Yamada in 1977 for the treatment of liver tumors.[11] The introduction of iodized oil, an iodinated ester derived from poppy-seed oil, greatly advanced this technique. Iodized oil is well suited for chemoembolization because of its preferential tumor uptake by hepatocellular carcinoma (HCC) and certain hepatic metastases; it acts simultaneously as an embolic agent and a vehicle for the chemotherapeutic agent.[12,13] These findings are partially explained by the concept of enhanced permeability and retention suggested by Maeda et al.[14] Newly formed tumor vessels are more permeable. This increased permeability coupled with a lack of lymphatics in the neoplasm, results in retention of molecules of higher molecular weight within the tumor interstitium for a more prolonged period. This retention may explain, in part, the accumulation of iodized oil or the increase in concentration of polymer conjugates of chemotherapeutic agents in neoplasms.

There are many different chemoembolization protocols. The most commonly used chemotherapeutic agent is doxorubicin. This agent may be combined with cisplatin and mitomycin C. Subsequently, the selected chemotherapeutic agents are mixed with iodized oil and slowly infused into the hepatic artery branch that supplies the tumor. Drug-eluting beads (DEBs), which are microspheres loaded with chemotherapy agents (doxorubicin or irinotecan), have more recently come into use for chemoembolization. The advantages of drug-eluting beads include delivery of higher doses of chemotherapy and prolonged tumor contact time while reducing the systemic toxic effects of chemotherapeutic agents.[15] An additional benefit of DEB chemoembolization is to standardize the dose of drug and embolic agents administered for therapy. A randomized controlled trial comparing conventional chemoembolization, using iodized oil and Epirubicin, with DEB chemoembolization for patients with HCC showed no survival benefits between the two cohorts, but patients in the DEB group had significantly less postprocedural pain.[16]

The number of chemoembolization sessions required to completely treat a patient with limited hepatic disease depends on the number and size of the lesions. For this reason, the proximal arterial supply to the tumor should be preserved to allow for repeat interventions.

Transcatheter arterial hepatic chemoembolization has been used to treat unresectable HCC, cholangiocarcinomas, and hepatic metastases and has been used in conjunction with liver resection or tumor ablation or as a bridge to liver transplant. Two randomized clinical trials showed a survival advantage when chemoembolization was performed in selected HCC patients, which helped to establish chemoembolization as part of standard therapy for patients with unresectable HCC.[17,18] A phase III clinical trial comparing chemoembolization with drug-eluting beads loaded with irinotecan and systemic therapy with irinotecan, fluorouracil, and leucovorin (FOLFIRI) in patients with metastatic colorectal cancer to the liver demonstrated significantly increased overall survival (22 vs 15 months), progression-free survival (7 vs 4 months) and improvement in the quality of life (8 vs 3 months) in the embolization group.[19] Moreover, advances in technology now allow intra-procedural acquisition of cross-sectional images using cone beam computed tomography (Figure 1). This technique enables more selective embolization as multi-planar and three-dimensional images are used to understand the arterial anatomy and assess completeness of embolization.[20] Iwazawa et al. demonstrated significantly improved technical success rate, overall survival, and local recurrence rate and progression-free survival of chemoembolization patients with the use of cone beam CT.[21] Furthermore, cone beam CT has been shown to have better diagnostic accuracy than preprocedural multidetector CT and MRI in the detection and characterization of HCC in cirrhotic patients.[22]

Hepatic radioembolization

Radioembolization or intra-arterial brachytherapy with yttrium-90 (^{90}Y) microspheres is a technique in which particles incorporating the isotope ^{90}Y are infused through a catheter directly into the hepatic arteries. Yttrium-90 is a beta emitter with a half-life of 64.1 hours. As in chemoembolization, the injected particles are selectively distributed into the tumor arterial bed. This distribution is possible because the arterial blood flow to the tumor is several times greater than the flow to the surrounding liver parenchyma. As a consequence, a much higher radiation dose can be safely achieved within the lesion than with external-beam radiation, while limiting the potential for radiation-induced hepatitis.

TheraSphere microspheres (Boston Scientific, Marlborough, Massachusetts, USA) are FDA approved for the treatment of unresectable HCC and may be used as a neoadjuvant therapy to surgical resection or as a bridge to transplantation. SIR-Spheres (Sirtex Medical, Lane Cove, Australia) are FDA approved for the treatment of metastatic colorectal cancer to the liver with concomitant use of floxuridine. Knowledge of the vascular anatomic variants in the celiac axis and superior mesenteric artery is critical to safely administering this therapy to avoid nontarget embolization of the radioactive microspheres, which can have devastating consequences such as gastrointestinal ulceration. Multiple studies have demonstrated the safety of radioembolization with yttrium-90 for the treatment of unresectable HCC and metastatic colorectal cancer.[23–25] Vouche et al. demonstrated that radioembolization is an effective treatment in patients with a solitary HCC ≤5 cm, who are not surgical or local ablation candidates due to adjacent critical structures.[26] Radioembolization has been shown to prolong progression-free survival with reduced side effects in the treatment of HCC when compared to chemoembolization.[27,28] In the first-line treatment of liver-dominant metastatic colorectal carcinoma, the addition of radioembolization to FOLFOX-based chemotherapy regimens has been shown to delay disease progression in the liver.[29] However, a mortality benefit has only been demonstrated in those patients with right-sided primary colorectal carcinoma tumors.[30]

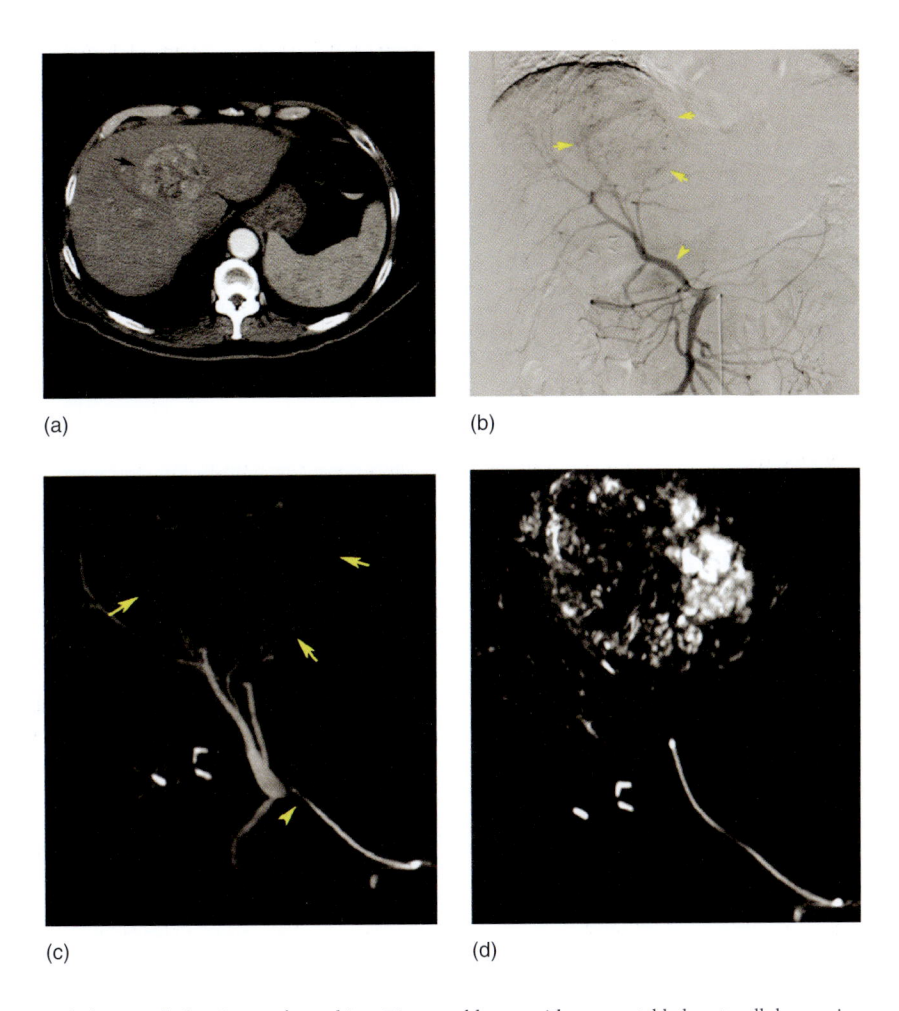

Figure 1 Transcatheter arterial chemoembolization performed in a 71-year-old man with unresectable hepatocellular carcinoma. (a) Contrast-enhanced CT scan obtained prior to chemoembolization shows a large, solitary, hypervascular mass in segment IV of the liver (arrow). (b) Anteroposterior digital subtraction angiography (DSA) of the abdomen shows a replaced right hepatic artery arising from the proximal superior mesenteric artery (arrowhead). This vessel supplies the hypervascular tumor in the left liver (arrows). (c) C-arm cone-beam CT images obtained during the procedure show tip of 3-French catheter in the distal replaced right hepatic artery (arrowhead) confirming origin of vascular supply to the hepatocellular carcinoma (arrows). (d) C-arm cone-beam CT images obtained after chemoembolization demonstrate retention of iodized oil throughout the lesion.

Local tissue ablation

Image-guided tumor ablation of focal hepatic malignancies can be accomplished using chemical agents or thermal energy. Chemical ablation options include direct intra-tumoral percutaneous ethanol injection (PEI) and ablation using hot water or saline, acetic acid, or chemotherapeutic agents that induce tumor cell death. Thermal ablation options include high-energy radiofrequency (RF), interstitial laser photocoagulation (LITT), microwave, cryotherapy, and high-intensity focused ultrasound that cause coagulation necrosis. Irreversible electroporation is an emerging ablation technique, which results in the permanent disruption of cell membranes and cell death. These procedures can be performed under imaging guidance by interventional radiologists or by surgeons in the operating suite.

Ethanol is the most commonly used agent for chemical tumor ablation worldwide.[31] Once ethanol is injected into the tumor, it causes cytoplasmic dehydration, denaturation of cellular proteins, and small-vessel thrombosis.[32] PEI is well established for the treatment of HCC, but it is much less successful in the treatment of hepatic metastases; in metastases, thermal ablation methods are more promising. This distinction appears to stem from the way in which ethanol disseminates within the different tumors. The distribution of ethanol tends to be uniform in soft lesions surrounded by hardened cirrhotic liver parenchyma, as is the case in HCC. However, when the surrounding parenchyma is softer than the tumor, as is often the case with metastases, ethanol distribution is less uniform and the treatment less effective. Ebara and colleagues[33] reported on 20 years of experience with PEI for HCC lesions ≤3 cm in a total of 270 patients. The local recurrence rate at 3 years was 10%, with overall 3- and 5-year survival rates of 81% and 60%, respectively.

Livraghi and colleagues[34] studied RF ablation versus PEI in the treatment of small HCCs (≤3 cm in diameter). Complete necrosis was achieved in 47 of 52 tumors (90%) in an average of 1.2 sessions per tumor with RF ablation and 48 of 60 tumors (80%) in an average of 4.8 sessions per tumor with PEI. One major complication (hemothorax) and four minor complications (bleeding, hemobilia, pleural effusion, and cholecystitis) occurred with RF ablation, although there was none with PEI. Lencioni and colleagues[35] reported treatment of HCC with either RF ablation or PEI in a randomized series of 102 patients with hepatic cirrhosis. Although there was no overall difference in 1- and 2-year survival, there was a significant difference in 1- and 2-year local recurrence-free survival (98% for RF ablation vs 83% for PEI at 1 year and 96% vs 62% at 2 years). The study was limited to patients with either a single HCC ≤5 cm in diameter or a maximum of three HCCs

≤3 cm in diameter. However, up to 25% of the lesions in Ebara and colleagues' study[33] of PEI could not have been treated by RF ablation because of anatomic considerations, which emphasizes that there is still a role for PEI in small tumors despite results that overall favor RF ablation. Thermal ablation for hepatic metastases from colorectal cancer has also been reported to improve survival. Median survival time after thermal ablation was increased to 39 months from 21 to 25 months in a study reported by Gillams and Lees.[36] A more recent study by Ruers and colleagues showed a longer progression-free survival in patients receiving a combination of systemic therapy and RF ablation compared to systemic therapy alone, 16.8 versus 9.9 months. Some of the limitations of RF ablation include the size of the maximum ablation zone, time for ablation, vulnerability to heat sink effect, and safety of adjacent critical structures.[37] The reported local recurrence rates are also extremely variable.

Microwave ablation overcomes some of the limitations of RF ablation by creating larger ablation zones in a shorter amount of time, without the problem of heat sink effect. However, few studies directly comparing RF and microwave ablation in the treatment of liver tumors have been performed and an improvement in overall survival or local recurrence has not been definitively demonstrated.[38] Irreversible electroporation (IRE) technology reportedly spares adjacent critical structures, such as bile ducts and vessels, from damage during an ablation procedure and thus can be used to difficult to treat lesions that would not be amenable to surgery or the more established thermal or chemical ablative therapies, but more research is needed to evaluate the safety and efficacy of the technique.

Portal vein embolization

Successful resection of the liver depends on the function of the residual hepatic parenchyma. When the portal vein is occluded, hepatocyte growth factors (hepatopoietin A, insulin, and glucagon) are shunted into the liver segments supplied by nonembolized vessels.[39] The result is atrophy of the segments supplied by the occluded vessels and hypertrophy of the other areas of the liver. Thus portal vein embolization (PVE) is used preoperatively to induce liver hypertrophy in potential surgical candidates with anticipated marginal future liver remnant (FLR) volumes (Figure 2).

PVE is performed if the FLR is estimated to be <20% of the estimated total liver volume (TLV) in patients without underlying liver disease, <30% of TLV in patients with underlying severe liver injury, and <40% of TLV in patients with cirrhosis.[40] For embolizations performed prior to extended right hepatectomy, modification of the preoperative embolization to include segment IV may optimize liver hypertrophy. The range of reported mean absolute FLR increase for PVE, in general, was 46–70% PVE results in hepatocyte apoptosis, so the postembolization syndrome associated with trans-arterial embolization and necrosis does not occur. Fibrin glue, gelatin sponge, thrombin, particles, coils, and absolute ethanol all have been used for PVE. In the United States, a combination of particles and embolization coils are the most commonly utilized embolic agents. Shindoh et al. reported on 139 patients with extensive colorectal liver metastasis who received portal vein embolization due to an inadequate FLR.[41] 62% of the patients were able to go on to curative resection after PVE with no increased major complications and similar overall survival and disease-free survival compared to a non-PVE cohort. Retrospective studies and meta-analysis suggest improved surgical outcomes after PVE.[40,42]

Recently, two-stage hepatectomy with PVE has emerged as a viable option in patients with bilobar metastases, increasing the number of potential curative resection candidates.[43] In patients with bilobar liver metastases, a first-stage surgical resection of left lobe liver metastases is followed by portal vein embolization performed concurrently or shortly after the initial surgery. Following sufficient left-lobe hypertrophy, a second-stage right hepatectomy may be performed. Mise et al. compared patients undergoing two-stage versus single-stage hepatectomy after right PVE.[44] The study showed that the first-stage resection did impair the FLR regeneration after right PVE, but that extending the PVE to segment IV of the liver resulted in similar volume gains compared to single-stage resection. Mor et al. compared patients treated with two-stage hepatectomy and PVE to a cohort of patients who underwent right hepatectomy only and found no significant difference in major complications or mortality.[45] For these reasons, PVE prior to a major hepatectomy is now considered the standard of care in many comprehensive hepatobiliary centers worldwide.

Considerations in hepatocellular carcinoma

HCC is the fifth most prevalent type of cancer and the third most common cause of cancer death in the world.[46] This disease is common worldwide because of its strong association with underlying liver cirrhosis and hepatitis. Surgical removal of the tumor is the only potentially curative treatment. However, curative resection is possible only in 20–30% of patients.[47] Recurrence rates after surgical resection are high because of dissemination of primary disease, undetected hepatic micrometastases, or metachronous lesions. Five-year survival after partial hepatic resection is approximately 50%.[48] For patients with cirrhosis and unresectable disease, liver transplantation can potentially cure both the underlying liver disease and the tumor. Intra-arterial therapies (embolization, chemoembolization, and radioembolization) and ablative techniques are viable alternatives in patients who are not candidates for partial hepatectomy or transplantation. Additionally, these liver-directed therapies may serve as a bridge to liver transplantation to achieve or maintain transplant eligibility.[49] Systemic chemotherapy for HCC has been traditionally disappointing because of the low response rates. Sorafenib, a multikinase inhibitor with antiangiogenic, pro-apoptotic, and Raf kinase-inhibitory activity, was the first agent to demonstrate a statistically significant improvement in overall survival for patients with advanced HCC.[50] More recently, additional kinase inhibitors such as regorafenib, sunitinib, and lenvatinib and checkpoint inhibitors such as nivolumab and pembrolizumab have been evaluated as the treatment landscape for HCC continues to evolve.[49,51] Combination therapy with these newer agents and liver-directed therapy is currently under investigation.[49,51]

Local etiologic factors have to be evaluated when considering locoregional therapy, because HCC in Western countries is often different from the typical HCC treated by interventional radiologists in Japan and the far east.[52] Nodular HCC is seen in fewer than 25% of Western patients but is seen in approximately 75% of patients in Japan. For patients with early to intermediate disease, ablative techniques are appealing, since the damage to the surrounding liver parenchyma is minimized, allowing for repeated treatments and serving as a bridge to transplantation. The current literature supports the use of percutaneous RF ablation in patients with HCC and either a single lesion <5 cm in diameter or up to three lesions <3 cm in diameter if partial hepatic resection or

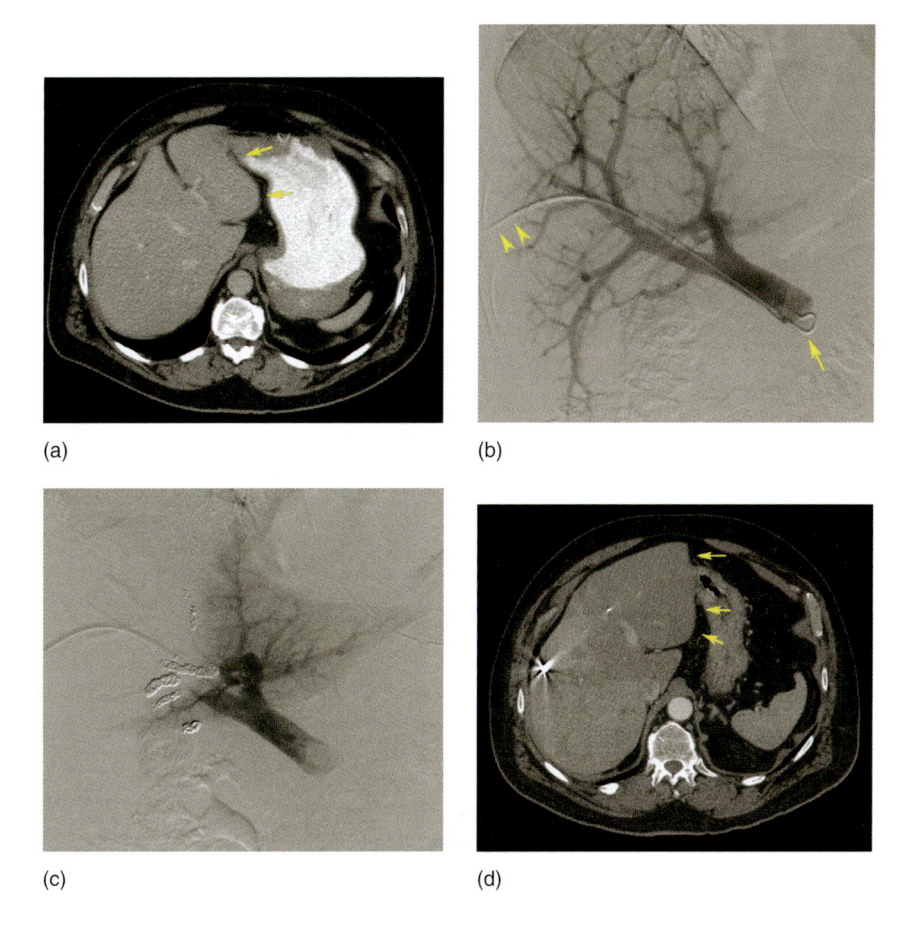

Figure 2 Transhepatic ipsilateral right portal vein embolization (PVE) extended to segment IV using tris-acryl particles and coils performed in a 52-year-old man with rectal cancer metastatic to the liver. (a) CT scan obtained prior to PVE shows marginal future liver remnant (FLR) (FLR-to-TELV (total estimated liver volume] ratio = 17%) (*arrows*). (b) Anteroposterior DSA portogram shows a 6-French vascular sheath in a right portal vein branch (*arrowheads*) and a 5-French flush catheter within the main portal vein (*arrow*). (c) Final DSA portogram shows occlusion of the portal vein branches to segments IV through VIII with continued patency of the vein supplying the left lateral liver. (d) CT scan obtained 1 month after right PVE extended to segment IV shows substantial FLR hypertrophy (FLR-to-TELV ratio = 27%) (*arrows*). The degree of hypertrophy is 10%.

transplantation is not available.[1] More recently, microwave ablation has become popularized due to ease of use, shorter ablation times, and ability to achieve large ablation zones with the use of multiple probes. Microwave ablation has been shown to be equally effective as RF ablation in the treatment of hepatocellular carcinoma with a shorter procedure time.[53] Chemoembolization is currently used for noncurative therapy for nonsurgical patients with large or multifocal HCC that has not spread to extra-hepatic sites. Two randomized studies have reported more favorable results for chemoembolization than for bland embolization, conservative therapy, or both. Llovet and colleagues[18] reported survival rates of 75% and 50% at 1 and 2 years, respectively, for 37 patients assigned to embolization alone, 82% and 63% for 40 patients assigned to chemoembolization, and 63% and 27% for 35 patients assigned to conservative treatment. The study was stopped early because of the proven survival benefit. Another study by Lo and colleagues[17] demonstrated a benefit in survival for patients with unresectable HCC treated with chemoembolization (iodized oil, cisplatin, and gelfoam) compared with a control group treated with symptomatic therapy only. Survival in the chemoembolization group was 57% at 1 year, 31% at 2 years, and 26% at 3 years, compared with 32%, 11%, and 3%, respectively, in the control group. Radioembolization with yttrium-90 is FDA-approved for neoadjuvant treatment of unresectable HCC in patients with portal vein thrombosis or as a bridge to transplantation. The study by Vouche et al.[26] demonstrated an overall survival of 53.4 or 34.5 months censored to transplantation, which is comparable to the survival rates in the literature for ablative therapies. Progression-free survival in patients treated with radioembolization for HCC has also been shown to be longer than in those treated with chemoembolization and with a more favorable side effect profile.[27,28]

Considerations in hepatic metastases

Colorectal metastases

The liver is often the first and only site of metastases from colon cancer. Many of these patients will die of their liver disease, thus local control can positively affect patient outcome. Although surgical resection is the first line of treatment for liver metastases, many patients are not surgical candidates because of extent of disease or presence of medical comorbidities. Novel systemic chemotherapy agents are now available, which have been shown to affect significant improvement in patient survival.[54] In addition, local tissue ablation can be offered to patients who are not surgical candidates because of the presence of medical comorbidities or to patients with bilobar disease that can be completely treated with a combination of ablation and surgery. Recent series of patients with up to five lesions, each measuring ≤5 cm, showed 5-year survival ranges of 24–44%.[55,56] PVE may also be employed to increase the number of patients who can be converted into surgical candidates.[33] Palliative treatment can be offered in the form of arterial infusion therapy and radioembolization. The role of novel chemotherapy agents combined with arterial infusion is currently being investigated as an alternative viable palliative therapy. Radioembolization has been shown to delay progression in hepatic colorectal cancer metastases, but a mortality benefit has only been proven in tumors originating from the right colon.[29,30]

Neuroendocrine metastases

Hepatic artery embolization or chemoembolization is indicated for patients with multiple nonresectable, hormonally active tumors. The goal of treatment is to reduce tumor bulk and hormone secretion. The 5-year postembolization survival range is 50–60%, with symptomatic and biochemical response ranges of 40–80% and 50–60%, respectively.[57] Moertel and colleagues[58] reported their 10-year experience in 111 patients with neuroendocrine hepatic metastases, usually hypervascular, who received vascular occlusion therapy by a variety of methods. As many as 71 patients received subsequent alternating chemotherapy regimens (dacarbazine combined with doxorubicin, alternating with streptozotocin combined with 5-fluorouracil) as well. Response rates of 60% with vascular occlusion alone and 80% with sequential therapy of vascular occlusion and chemotherapy were observed. Median survival times of 37 and 49 months were experienced in patients with islet cell carcinoma and carcinoid hepatic metastases, respectively. For the symptomatic treatment of hormonally active liver metastases, the use of repeated embolizations is preferred.

The best results for metastatic disease of the liver treated with hepatic artery embolization have been observed in patients with neuroendocrine tumors metastatic to the liver. Sequential and periodic embolization is required for effective palliation. Gupta and colleagues have reported on 81 patients with carcinoid syndrome who were treated with either bland embolization or chemoembolization.[59] Imaging was available for evaluation of a response in 69 patients. Partial response occurred in 67% of the patients, stable disease in 16%, and progression of tumor in 8.7%. The median response duration was 17 months in those patients with a partial response. A reduction of tumor-related symptoms occurred in 63%, with a median progression-free survival of 19 months and a median overall survival time of 31 months. In a subsequent study by Gupta and colleagues,[60] these 69 patients with carcinoid tumors were compared with 54 patients who had islet cell tumors with metastases to the liver. Patients with carcinoid tumors had a higher response rate and a longer progression-free survival than did patients with islet cell tumors (67% vs 35% and 23 months vs 16 months). Although chemoembolization, compared with bland embolization, did not prove to be beneficial for survival in patients with carcinoid tumors, it did result in improved overall survival and improved response (32 months vs 18 months and 50% vs 25) in patients treated for islet cell tumors.

RF ablation can be used to palliate symptoms associated with metastatic neuroendocrine tumors. In a series by Berber et al.,[61] RF ablation provided complete symptomatic relief in 63% of 222 patients and partial relief in 95%. Radioembolization is another minimally invasive alternative for palliating a large burden of hepatic metastases from neuroendocrine tumors. A meta-analysis by Yang et al.[62] in 2012 reviewed the data on radioembolization and found that the efficacy was similar to that of chemoembolization in patients with metastatic neuroendocrine tumors to the liver. Additionally, radioembolization may be effective in patients who have undergone unsuccessful chemoembolization or bland embolization procedures for the palliation of carcinoid syndrome.[63]

Other hepatic metastases

Other types of hepatic metastases are usually not as well suited for locoregional therapy as the tumor is likely widespread by the time of liver involvement. However, occasionally, certain types of hepatic metastases are amenable to local treatment because of the nature of the primary disease. Such hepatic metastases that can sometimes be treated by chemoembolization include ocular melanoma, leiomyosarcoma, breast carcinoma, and renal cell carcinoma. In a group of 30 patients with metastatic ocular melanoma, chemoembolization with cisplatin produced a response rate of 46% and a median survival period of 11 months.[64] The longest survival was 5 years from the initial chemoembolization. Additional studies have been reported using HAI of carboplatin-based chemotherapy and fotemustine, with response rates of 38% and 40%, respectively.[64] Hepatic artery immunoembolization has also been reported in the treatment of uveal melanoma with variable responses.[65] A group of 14 patients with metastatic leiomyosarcoma to the liver were treated with chemoembolization every 4 weeks with cisplatin and polyvinyl alcohol foam granules 150–250 μm in size, followed by vinblastine infusion.[66] The response rate was 70%, and responses lasted 4–19 months (median, 9 months). This rate compared well with the response rate of 15% obtained after systemic therapy with ifosfamide with doxorubicin. It should be noted that these are not common tumors and that most are treated on protocol studies. At MDACC, our approach to chemoembolization of hepatic metastases is similar to our approach to HCC; that is, a hypervascular tumor is more likely to benefit from the treatment than a hypovascular tumor. The goal of treatment, whether it is to provide symptomatic relief or to prolong survival, must be weighed against the risk of complications.

Genitourinary interventions

Renal arterial embolization

Renal artery embolization for renal cell carcinoma may be performed preoperatively to decrease operative blood loss in patients with extensive local disease. A study by Zielinski et al.[67] showed a survival benefit to preoperative embolization, although previous studies had not demonstrated this advantage. Embolization of renal carcinoma can also be performed for palliative relief of symptoms in patients with extensive local tumor or as a cytoreductive measure when patients are not candidates for surgery.[68] Renal artery embolization has also been used in the management of congestive heart failure caused by arteriovenous shunting through the renal carcinoma and for hypertension, hypercalcemia, polycythemia, and hemorrhage caused by the renal neoplasm. Selective segmental embolization is generally preferred, particularly in patients with impaired renal function or a solitary kidney.

Renal ablation

Thermal ablation plays an increasingly important role in the management of renal cell carcinoma. Although nephrectomy remains the gold standard for treatment of renal cell carcinoma, thermal

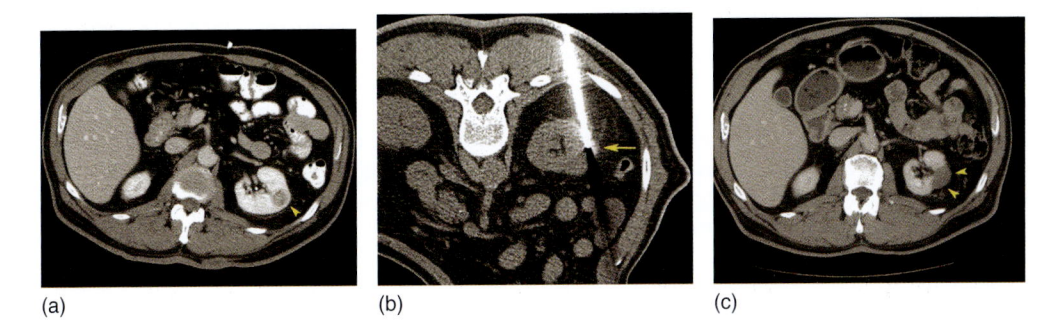

Figure 3 Percutaneous radiofrequency (RF) ablation performed in a 62-year-old man with biopsy-proven renal cell carcinoma. (a) Contrast-enhanced CT image obtained before RF ablation show an enhancing mass in the left kidney (*arrowhead*). (b) CT image obtained with patient in prone position at RF ablation shows single needle electrode in tumor (*arrow*). (c) Contrast-enhanced CT image obtained after RF ablation shows no residual enhancement in the treated kidney (*arrowheads*).

ablation, including radiofrequency ablation, microwave ablation, and cryoablation are increasingly viable alternatives (Figure 3). RF ablation for the treatment of renal tumors, first described in 1997, is minimally invasive with a low morbidity rate.[69,70] More recently, microwave ablation and cryoablation of renal tumors are techniques, which have been widely implemented with comparable efficacy and a similarly low adverse event rate.[71] Patients who are candidates for thermal ablation include those with high surgical risk secondary to medical comorbidities; patients with a solitary kidney or multifocal disease, who are not candidates for nephron-sparing surgery; and patients who do not wish to undergo surgery. Patients with hereditary syndromes, such as von Hippel-Lindau disease, are at high risk for multiple renal neoplasms over their lifetimes. These patients may be treated repeatedly with ablation, in an effort to preserve normal renal parenchyma adjacent to the tumors.

Gervais et al.[72,73] demonstrated that tumor size and location are directly related to RF ablation effectiveness. Exophytic lesions can be more effectively ablated because of surrounding fat, the presence of which makes lesions easier to target and provides heat insulation during ablation. Complete necrosis was achieved in 90% of tumors measuring less than 4.0 cm. Larger or central tumors may not be amenable to complete ablation and may require multiple ablations, or in some cases, multiple treatment sessions. This is in part owing to the proximity of medullary tumors to the renal hilar vessels resulting in an increased heat-sink effect, which affects ablation efficacy by lowering intra-lesional temperatures. A medullary tumor location also increases the risk of procedure-related complications. The most common complication of renal RF ablation is hemorrhage. This complication was observed in 5% of the patients in the series of 100 treated lesions by Gervais et al.[72,73] Hemorrhage can occur into the collecting system requiring stent placement for ureteral obstruction or it can be confined to the sub-capsular space. Aarts et al. showed a similar primary efficacy of 89% in the treatment of T1a lesions treated with microwave ablation, but a reduced primary efficacy of 52% in the ablation of T1b lesions.[74] Secondary efficacy achieved with repeated microwave ablation was similar for T1a (99%) and T1b (95%) lesions.[74]

Karam et al. at M.D. Anderson Cancer Center described their experience with 150 patients who underwent RF ablation, 130 of which were performed percutaneously.[75] The lesions had a median tumor size of 2.6 cm with a range of 0.9–7.1 cm. Mean and median follow-up intervals were 40.1 and 38.0 months, respectively. 93.7% of the patients did not show evidence of recurrence or metastasis at follow-up. Yu et al. compared propensity score-matched cohorts of 185 patients treated with microwave ablation and 1770 patients treated with laparoscopic partial nephrectomy. No significant differences in local tumor progression, cancer-specific survival, or development of metastasis were observed. Patients treated with ablation experienced smaller decreases in estimated glomerular filtration rate, smaller blood loss, shorter operative times, shorter hospitalization time, and lower cost than patients treated with partial nephrectomy.[76]

Thoracic interventions

Lung ablation

Thermal ablation can be used to treat primary and metastatic lung cancers. Lung ablation is optimal for patients with early lung cancer, where complete ablation with curative intent can be attempted. In patients with large tumor burden, ablation may provide palliation of tumor-related symptoms.[77] Lung ablation is offered primarily to patients with lung cancer who are not operative candidates as well as to patients with pulmonary metastases.

Simon et al. reported a series of 153 patients with 189 primary or metastatic inoperable lung cancers treated with percutaneous pulmonary RF ablation.[78] The overall 1-, 2-, 3-, 4-, and 5-year survival rates, respectively, for stage I non-small-cell lung cancer were 78%, 57%, 36%, 27%, and 27%; rates for colorectal pulmonary metastasis were 87%, 78%, 57%, 57%, and 57%. The incidence of pneumothorax was 28.4%. Postablation pneumothorax may be treated conservatively, if the patient remains asymptomatic. In patients with symptoms or progressively enlarging pneumothorax, placement of a chest drain is necessary. Simon et al. reported a procedure-related 30-day mortality rate of 2.6%.

Pleural effusion is also a common complication after lung ablation. In their series of 60 patients, de Baere et al.[79] reported a minor pleural effusion in 9% of patients immediately after treatment and on 60% of CT scans obtained 24–48 h after treatment. Postprocedure hemoptysis was observed in 10% of the patients. The hemoptysis started 1–9 days after the ablation and lasted 2–13 days. These complications did not require any treatment.

Lung cryoablation was first reported in 2005 and data supporting its use has been in the recent literature. Inoue et al.[80] reported on 117 patients with 396 lung tumors, primarily from metastatic disease, who were not candidates for surgery. The most common complications were pneumothorax, pleural effusion, and hemoptysis, but no CTCAE grade 4 or 5 events occurred. Only three grade 3 complications were reported, including two cases of pneumothorax requiring pleurodesis and one case of empyema requiring fenestration. Only a small number of retrospective studies, with small patient numbers, are currently available reporting survival rates but the reported ranges are similar to RF ablation.

Microwave ablation of lung metastases has become increasingly popular due to wider ablation zones and shorter ablation times when compared to RF ablation and cryoablation. Nour-Eldin et al. showed similar overall survival of 34 months for patients with noncolorectal cancer lung metastases treated with either microwave or RF ablation.[81] However, local recurrence was lower with microwave ablation (7.7% vs 20.4%) and progression-free survival was longer with microwave ablation (23.5 months vs 19.9 months). The improved efficacy of microwave ablation, which is attributed to higher intratumoral temperatures and reduced "heat sink" effect, must be weighed against a higher incidence of complications including pneumothorax (22% vs 14%) observed in patients treated with microwave ablation.

Palliative therapy

Percutaneous biliary drainage

Pancreatic carcinoma, cholangiocarcinoma, and ampullary carcinoma are the primary neoplasms that produce intrinsic biliary obstruction, whereas lymphadenopathy, HCC, and hepatic metastasis can produce extrinsic compression of the biliary system. Nonsurgical palliation of malignant biliary obstruction may be accomplished either endoscopically or percutaneously. The percutaneous methods include drainage by insertion of external or internal–external percutaneous biliary catheters as well as percutaneous biliary stent placement.

The aims of palliative therapy are to provide relief of jaundice and pruritus as well as associated cholangitis and, importantly, to prepare patients for anticancer therapy. Neither the endoscopic nor the percutaneous approach has an advantage with regard to influencing survival, and the choice of technique is often a team decision based on the available local expertise.

Internal drainage via endoscopy is preferable because of the inconvenience of an external catheter for the patient and the potential for pain at the tube entry site, bile leakage around the catheter, and sepsis from skin organisms. The percutaneous approach has the advantage of allowing prompt access to the biliary tree. Regardless of the approach, partial or complete jaundice relief can be achieved in 73–100% of treated patients.[82]

Percutaneous biliary stenting

Speer et al.[83] described 70 patients with malignant biliary obstruction who were randomized to undergo percutaneous versus endoscopic biliary stent placement. The success rate in relieving jaundice was 81% for endoscopically placed stents compared with 61% for percutaneously placed stents. The complication rate was 19% versus 67%, in favor of the endoscopic approach. In addition, the 30-day mortality rate in the two groups was 15% for endoscopic stents versus 33% for the percutaneous method. A meta-analysis performed by Duan and colleagues comparing efficacy and complications of endoscopic and percutaneous biliary drainage showed no difference in therapeutic success rate, overall complications, bile leak, 30-day mortality, sepsis, or duodenal perforation.[84] Cholangitis and pancreatitis were more common after endoscopic biliary drainage, while incidences of bleeding and tube dislodgement were greater for percutaneous biliary drains.

Cholangitis, hemorrhage, and bile leakage are the most common complications of stent placement. The incidence of cholangitis is lower in patients treated with a metallic stent than in patients treated with a plastic stent.[85] Plastic stents are also more prone to migration and remain patent on average for only 3–4 months.[85] Self-expanding metallic stents have longer patency but are more expensive. Metallic stents may be dislodged by balloon dilation immediately after deployment, but the incidence of spontaneous migration over the long term is low. Both uncovered and covered metallic biliary stents are available. Covered biliary stents were developed by placing a thin nonporous membrane on the inside of the metallic stent mesh designed to reduce tumor ingrowth and improve patency. Krokidis et al. prospectively randomized 80 patients to receive covered and uncovered stents for the treatment of biliary obstruction secondary to pancreatic cancer.[86] Primary patency rates at 3, 6, and 12 months were 77.5%, 69.8%, and 69.8% in the uncovered stent group and 97.5%, 92.2%, and 87.6% in the covered stent group. Conversely, a meta-analysis by Moole et al. showed no significant differences in survival, overall adverse event rate, or patency period of covered versus uncovered metal stents in patients with malignant biliary strictures.[87] Despite advances in stent technology, occlusion secondary to tumor ingrowth or overgrowth remains a complex issue.

Musculoskeletal ablation

The majority of patients with breast, prostate, and lung cancer show evidence of bone metastases at the time of death. These lesions are often accompanied by pain, and occasional fractures, which can dramatically decrease the quality of life of this patient population.[88] External-beam radiation therapy is the gold standard for the treatment of localized pain secondary to osseous metastases. The majority of the patients will experience symptomatic relief after radiation therapy. However, in a substantial minority of patients, radiation therapy provides suboptimal response and durability of relief.[89]

Patients are candidates for ablative therapy of painful metastases when a patient reports moderate or severe musculoskeletal pain, the patient's pain is focal in nature and correlates with abnormality evident with radiological imaging, and the painful metastatic lesion is accessible for percutaneous treatment.[90]

Lesions that are amenable to ablative therapy are typically osteolytic or mixed osteolytic and osteoblastic in nature or otherwise composed of soft tissue. RF ablation and cryoablation are safe and effective treatments for the palliation of painful metastatic lesions that are refractory to standard therapies. Importantly, the quality of life for these patients is improved with this therapy. Goetz et al.[91] reported on 43 patients with painful bone metastases treated with RF ablation. In the study, 95% of the patients experienced symptomatic relief that was considered clinically significant with a decrease in opioid usage. Prologo et al. reported on 54 painful musculoskeletal metastatic tumors treated in 50 patients using cryoablation.[92] Significant reductions in median visual analog scale score and narcotic usage were observed, and all but two patients experienced pain relief. A single ablative treatment is effective in most patients and appears to provide a long duration of pain relief.

Miscellaneous

Vena cava filter placement

Cancer patients experience an increased incidence of thrombosis and pulmonary embolism (PE). The percutaneous placement of a vena cava filter is the optimal therapeutic approach for patients with PE, who have a contraindication to anticoagulant therapy or who develop recurrent emboli despite adequate anticoagulant administration. There are numerous filters currently in use, including devices that are potentially retrievable and MRI compatible.

Wallace et al.[93] reported on the experience of vena cava filter placement in 308 patients with venous thromboembolic disease, in the setting of malignancy. Median survival times were 145 days and 207 days for 267 patients with solid tumors and 41 patients with liquid tumors, respectively. Patients with metastatic or disseminated disease were 3.7 times as likely to die as those with local disease, and patients with deep venous thrombosis and a history of hemorrhage were twice as likely to die as those with deep venous thrombosis and no history of hemorrhage. Major complications included pulmonary emboli, new caval thrombus, retroperitoneal hemorrhage, and incorrect filter deployment.

Prophylactic placement of retrievable IVC filters in the peri-operative period has also become increasingly practiced. The current indications are for patients who have a history of thromboembolic disease and must withhold anticoagulation therapy for planned surgery or for patients who will be at high risk for thrombotic events in the immediate postoperative period. McClendon et al.[94] reported significantly reduced rates of thromboembolic events, including pulmonary embolism, in patients undergoing major spinal reconstruction that had a prophylactic IVC filter placed in the peri-operative period. Once patients are eligible for systemic anticoagulation therapy, then IVC filter retrieval should be scheduled.

Stent placement for venous stenosis

Vena caval syndrome is most frequently the result of intrinsic or extrinsic malignant disease.[95] In this syndrome, neoplasms, by their local mass effect or by causing mediastinal, retroperitoneal, and pelvic lymphadenopathy, create stenosis and obstruction by extrinsic compression of the vena cava. The complications of radiation therapy and chemotherapy for this syndrome include mediastinal fibrosis and thrombophlebitis.[95]

Superior vena cava syndrome symptoms have been grouped into four classes: (1) central nervous system symptoms, including headache, blurred vision, and cognitive dysfunction; (2) laryngopharyngeal edema, producing dyspnea and hoarseness; (3) nasal or facial edema; and (4) other signs of venous congestion and dilatation.[96] In addition to stenosis or obstruction, there is frequently thrombosis complicating the mediastinal compression or intraluminal invasion by the tumor. Parish et al.[97] reported an average survival time of 7 months after the diagnosis of malignant superior vena cava obstruction. Vascular stents can effectively palliate symptoms of malignant vena cava stenosis in 68–80% of patients.[95]

Biopsy

Percutaneous biopsy has been traditionally a cost-effective modality to diagnose the patient with cancer. In the era of personalized cancer medicine, obtaining tissue for analysis is critical in aiding treatment planning. With the advent of molecular testing and genomic analysis of tissue samples, larger volumes of tissue are needed. Schneider et al.[98] reported on the adequacy of needle biopsy samples for molecular testing of lung adenocarcinomas and found that only 67% of core needle and 46% of fine needle biopsies had sufficient tissue for complete testing. Almost all tissues are accessible to percutaneous biopsy. Varied needles (11–25 gauge), as well as biopsy forceps, are efficient in obtaining representative specimens. Biopsy guns are also widely available to automate the procedure. However, a negative biopsy result does not exclude the possibility of malignancy; it may merely represent an error in sampling. Most biopsies of lesions in adults are scheduled electively on an outpatient basis.

Guidance by CT is usually adequate for biopsy of the lung or mediastinum.[99] The reported accuracy of percutaneous transthoracic needle biopsy in patients with lung cancer and pulmonary metastases is 90–98%,[100] whereas the diagnostic yield for local pulmonary infection in immunocompromised patients is 73%.[101] Serious complications of lung and mediastinal biopsies include systemic air embolization, hemorrhage, pericardial tamponade, seeding of malignant cells into the needle track, and empyema. The incidence of pneumothorax, when using CT guidance, is approximately 22–45%.[102] In a study described by Cox et al.,[103] when biopsies were done under CT guidance, smaller lesions (<2 cm) and the presence of emphysema strongly correlated with the occurrence of pneumothorax.

Abdominal biopsies guided by ultrasonography, CT, and MRI yielded adequate diagnostic material for cytologic analysis in 84–95% of patients. When a 20- to 23-gauge needle is used, biopsies of the liver, pancreas, kidney, adrenal gland, spleen, and ovary, among other organs, are performed with a sensitivity of 86%, a specificity of 98%, and an accuracy of 90%. The overall complication rate in a study of 63,180 biopsies was 0.16%. Seeding of malignant cells along the needle tract occurred in 0.05% of patients.[104,105]

The diagnostic accuracy of percutaneous skeletal biopsy is on average 80%. The overall diagnostic accuracy of 78% was reported in a series of 178 patients with primary skeletal tumors who underwent percutaneous needle biopsy.[106] The procedure was more accurate for malignant neoplasms (83%) than benign tumors (64%).

Partial splenic embolization

Thrombocytopenia is commonly encountered in the oncologic patient as a consequence of oxaliplatin-induced liver toxicity and related hypersplenism as in patients with other causes of portal hypertension.[107] Dose adjustment or suspension of chemotherapy may be required when thrombocytopenia reaches 75×10^9/L. Partial splenic embolization can be performed to reduce the degree of hematologic sequestration and increase the circulating platelet count. Luz et al. reported a 94% success rate in achieving a thrombocyte level above 130×10^9/L in 33 patients with a mean platelet count of 69×10^9/L prior to the embolization.[108] Kauffman et al. reported a 96% success rate in achieving a thrombocyte level above 150×10^9/L in 28 patients with a mean platelet count of 81×10^9/L prior to embolization.[109] Hill et al. reported a success rate of 88% in achieving a platelet count above 100×10^9/L in 98 patients with a mean platelet count of 61×10^9/L prior to embolization.[110] The most common reported adverse events after partial splenic embolization include abdominal pain, fever, and nausea.

Key references

The complete reference list can be found on Vital Source version of this title, see inside front cover.

1 Chen MS, Li JQ, Zheng Y, et al. A prospective randomized trial comparing percutaneous local ablative therapy and partial hepatectomy for small hepatocellular carcinoma. *Ann Surg.* 2006;**243**(3):321–328.

3 Tracy CR, Raman JD, Donnally C, et al. Durable oncologic outcomes after radiofrequency ablation: experience from treating 243 small renal masses over 7.5 years. *Cancer.* 2010;**116**(13):3135–3142.

6. Boehm LM, Jayakrishnan TT, Miura JT, et al. Comparative effectiveness of hepatic artery based therapies for unresectable intrahepatic cholangiocarcinoma. *J Surg Oncol*. 2015;**111**(2):213–220.
7. Obi S, Sato S, Kawai T. Current status of hepatic arterial infusion chemotherapy. *Liver Cancer*. 2015;**4**(3):188–199.
9. Pisco J, Bilhim T, Costa NV, et al. Safety and efficacy of prostatic artery chemoembolization for prostate cancer-initial experience. *J Vasc Interv Radiol*. 2018;**29**(3):298–305.
10. Gunn AJ, Patel AR, Rais-Bahrami S. Role of angio-embolization for renal cell carcinoma. *Curr Urol Rep*. 2018;**19**(10):76.
15. Namur J, Wassef M, Millot JM, et al. Drug-eluting beads for liver embolization: concentration of doxorubicin in tissue and in beads in a pig model. *J Vasc Interv Radiol*. 2010;**21**(2):259–267.
16. Golfieri R, Giampalma E, Renzulli M, et al. Randomised controlled trial of doxorubicin-eluting beads vs conventional chemoembolisation for hepatocellular carcinoma. *Br J Cancer*. 2014;**111**(2):255–264.
17. Lo CM, Ngan H, Tso WK, et al. Randomized controlled trial of transarterial lipiodol chemoembolization for unresectable hepatocellular carcinoma. *Hepatology*. 2002;**35**(5):1164–1171.
20. Wallace MJ, Murthy R, Kamat PP, et al. Impact of C-arm CT on hepatic arterial interventions for hepatic malignancies. *J Vasc Interv Radiol*. 2007;**18**(12):1500–1507.
22. Lucatelli P, De Rubeis G, et al. Intra-procedural dual phase cone beam computed tomography has a better diagnostic accuracy over pre-procedural MRI and MDCT in detection and characterization of HCC in cirrhotic patients undergoing TACE procedure. *Eur J Radiol*. 2019;**124**:108806.
27. Salem R, Gordon AC, Mouli S, et al. Y90 radioembolization significantly prolongs time to progression compared with chemoembolization in patients with hepatocellular carcinoma. *Gastroenterology*. 2016;**151**(6):1155–1163.
29. van Hazel GA, Heinemann V, Sharma NK, et al. SIRFLOX: randomized phase III trial comparing first-line mFOLFOX6 (plus or minus Bevacizumab) versus mFOLFOX6 (plus or minus Bevacizumab) plus selective internal radiation therapy in patients with metastatic colorectal cancer. *J Clin Oncol*. 2016;**34**(15):1723–1731.
30. Gibbs P, Heinemann V, Sharma NK, et al. Effect of primary tumor side on survival outcomes in untreated patients with metastatic colorectal cancer when selective internal radiation therapy is added to chemotherapy: combined analysis of two randomized controlled studies. *Clin Colorectal Cancer*. 2018;**17**(4):617–629.
35. Lencioni RA, Allgaier HP, Cioni D, et al. Small hepatocellular carcinoma in cirrhosis: randomized comparison of radio-frequency thermal ablation versus percutaneous ethanol injection. *Radiology*. 2003;**228**(1):235–240.
38. Izzo F, Granata V, Grassi R, et al. Radiofrequency ablation and microwave ablation in liver tumors: an update. *Oncologist*. 2019;**24**(10):990–1005.
41. Shindoh J, Tzeng CW, Aloia TA, et al. Portal vein embolization improves rate of resection of extensive colorectal liver metastases without worsening survival. *Br J Surg*. 2013;**100**(13):1777–1783.
44. Mise Y, Aloia TA, Conrad C, et al. Volume regeneration of segments 2 and 3 after right portal vein embolization in patients undergoing two-stage hepatectomy. *J Gastrointest Surg*. 2015;**19**(1):133–141.
45. Mor E, Al-Kurd A, Yaacov AB, et al. Surgical outcomes of two-stage hepatectomy for colorectal liver metastasis: comparison to a benchmark procedure. *Hepatobiliary Surg Nutr*. 2019;**8**(1):29–36.
47. Yamada R, Kishi K, Sato M, et al. Transcatheter arterial chemoembolization (TACE) in the treatment of unresectable liver cancer. *World J Surg*. 1995;**19**(6):795–800.
49. Viveiros P, Riaz A, Lewandowski RJ, Mahalingam D. Current state of liver-directed therapies and combinatory approaches with systemic therapy in hepatocellular carcinoma (HCC). *Cancers (Basel)*. 2019;**11**(8):E1085.
51. Cervello M, Emma MR, Augello G, et al. New landscapes and horizons in hepatocellular carcinoma therapy. *Aging (Albany NY)*. 2020;**12**:102777.
53. Chong CCN, Lee KF, Cheung SYS, et al. Prospective double-blinded randomized controlled trial of Microwave versus RadioFrequency Ablation for hepatocellular carcinoma (McRFA trial). *HPB (Oxford)*. 2020;**22**(8):P1121–P1127.
60. Gupta S, Johnson MM, Murthy R, et al. Hepatic arterial embolization and chemoembolization for the treatment of patients with metastatic neuroendocrine tumors: variables affecting response rates and survival. *Cancer*. 2005;**104**(8):1590–1602.
63. Jia Z, Wang W. Yttrium-90 radioembolization for unresectable metastatic neuroendocrine liver tumor: a systematic review. *Eur J Radiol*. 2018;**100**:23–29.
65. Sato T, Eschelman DJ, Gonsalves CF, et al. Immunoembolization of malignant liver tumors, including uveal melanoma, using granulocyte-macrophage colony-stimulating factor. *J Clin Oncol*. 2008;**26**(33):5436–5442.
71. Zhou W, Herwald SE, McCarthy C, et al. Radiofrequency ablation, cryoablation, and microwave ablation for T1a renal cell carcinoma: a comparative evaluation of therapeutic and renal function outcomes. *J Vasc Interv Radiol*. 2019;**30**(7):1035–1042.
74. Aarts BM, Prevoo W, Meier MAJ, et al. Percutaneous microwave ablation of histologically proven T1 renal cell carcinoma. *Cardiovasc Intervent Radiol*. 2020. doi: 10.1007/s00270-020-02423-7.
76. Yu J, Zhang X, Liu H, et al. Percutaneous microwave ablation versus laparoscopic partial nephrectomy for cT1a renal cell carcinoma: a propensity-matched cohort study of 1955 patients. *Radiology*. 2020;**294**(3):698–706.
81. Nour-Eldin N-EA, Exner S, Al-Subhi M, et al. Ablation therapy of non-colorectal cancer lung metastases: retrospective analysis of tumour response post-laser-induced interstitial thermotherapy (LITT), radiofrequency ablation (RFA) and microwave ablation (MWA). *Int J Hyperthermia*. 2017;**33**:820–829.
84. Duan F, Cui L, Bai Y, et al. Comparison of efficacy and complications of endoscopic and percutaneous biliary drainage in malignant obstructive jaundice: a systematic review and meta-analysis. *Cancer Imaging*. 2017;**17**(1):27.
87. Moole H, Bechtold ML, Cashman M, et al. Covered versus uncovered self-expandable metal stents for malignant biliary strictures: a meta-analysis and systematic review. *Indian J Gastroenterol*. 2016;**35**(5):323–330.
90. Callstrom MR, Charboneau JW. Image-guided palliation of painful metastases using percutaneous ablation. *Tech Vasc Interv Radiol*. 2007;**10**(2):120–131.
92. Prologo JD, Passalacqua M, Patel I, et al. Image-guided cryoablation for the treatment of painful musculoskeletal metastatic disease: a single-center experience. *Skeletal Radiol*. 2014;**43**(11):1551–1559.
93. Wallace MJ, Jean JL, Gupta S, et al. Use of inferior vena caval filters and survival in patients with malignancy. *Cancer*. 2004;**101**(8):1902–1907.
98. Schneider F, Smith MA, Lane MC, et al. Adequacy of core needle biopsy specimens and fine-needle aspirates for molecular testing of lung adenocarcinomas. *Am J Clin Pathol*. 2015;**143**(2):193–200.
107. Overman MJ, Maru DM, Charnsangavej C, et al. Oxaliplatin-mediated increase in spleen size as a biomarker for the development of hepatic sinusoidal injury. *J Clin Oncol*. 2010;**28**(15):2549–2555.
108. Luz JH, Luz PM, Marchiori E, et al. Partial splenic embolization to permit continuation of systemic chemotherapy. *Cancer Med*. 2016;**5**(10):2715–2720.
109. Kauffman CR, Mahvash A, Kopetz S, et al. Partial splenic embolization for cancer patients with thrombocytopenia requiring systemic chemotherapy. *Cancer*. 2008;**112**(10):2283–2288.
110. Hill A, Elakkad A, Kuban J, et al. Durability of partial splenic artery embolization on platelet counts for cancer patients with hypersplenism-related thrombocytopenia. *Abdom Radiol*. 2020;**45**(9):2886–2894.

41 Principles of surgical oncology

Todd W. Bauer, MD, FACS ■ Kenneth K. Tanabe, MD, FACS ■ Raphael E. Pollock, MD, PhD

> **Overview**
>
> The discipline of surgical oncology describes a surgical super specialty to which a board certification process is now attached in the United States. With specific cognitive as well as technical surgical expertise, the surgical oncologist is an oncology specialist who uses surgery as his or her mainstay therapeutic modality in treating tumors. The surgical oncologist has a thorough grounding in the natural history of solid malignancy, extensive experience in tumor biopsy and staging approaches, the knowledge needed to direct a multidisciplinary solid tumor treatment program, and the commitment required to participate in the many relevant research opportunities that will advance comprehensive care of the cancer patient.

In spite of significant advances in various systemic approaches to the care of the cancer patient, surgical therapy remains the mainstay of treatment for most solid malignancies and plays a role in various components of the cancer care continuum, from prevention to diagnosis, curative therapy, survival prolongation, and palliation. To be maximally effective, the cancer surgeon must function as a member of the oncology team and is frequently the first oncology specialist that a patient will consult. The cancer surgeon is commonly charged with the responsibility to establish a tissue diagnosis for a suspicious lesion; this may require either an operative procedure or an image-directed or other biopsy approach. The cancer surgeon will usually bear the responsibility for communicating the biopsy findings to the patient, completing the procedures needed to stage the cancer, and initiating subsequent interaction between the patient and other members of the multimodality oncology team. Because of these responsibilities, it is most often the cancer surgeon who initially explains to the patient the sequence and rationale of the various treatment components that will be used to manage the specific malignancy. To be maximally effective, the cancer surgeon must therefore be aware of the different therapeutic options, the natural history of a given malignancy, and how these factors will be integrated into a well-conceived and appropriate multimodality treatment algorithm. It is also usually the surgical oncologist's responsibility to provide initial information about prognosis and to make decisions about follow-up care and surveillance to detect tumor recurrence. In these aspects, the surgical oncologist is unlike almost any other surgical specialist in that the commitment to a given patient is for both the acute and the long-term components of the patient's disease process.

Over the years, the practice of surgical oncology has come full circle. Originally, surgeons attempted to treat cancer conservatively by removing only the gross lesion. Unfortunately, this led to extremely high rates of local recurrence and subsequent patient mortality. In the late nineteenth century, surgeons began to undertake radical en bloc resections and amputations to treat patients with malignant disease. These techniques yielded improved results, but the procedures were often mutilating. With the advent of other complementary and effective treatment modalities, notably radiation therapy in the 1920s and chemotherapy after the 1940s, the orientation of surgical resection is once again becoming conservative with a focus on organ preservation and restoring the comorbid state when possible.

Adjuvant chemotherapy, alone or in combination with radiation therapy, has improved disease-free and overall survival and prolonged quality of life for patients who have been rendered free of gross disease by surgery but who still have a high likelihood of recurrence as a consequence of microscopic residual metastases. Randomized clinical trials have demonstrated the benefit of adjuvant chemotherapy in a variety of tumors, including breast cancer, colorectal cancer, pancreatic cancer, cholangiocarcinoma, gastric cancer, osteosarcoma, testicular cancer, ovarian cancer, and certain lung cancers. In addition, adjuvant molecularly targeted therapies have improved survival for patients with high-risk gastrointestinal stromal tumors (GISTs).

Surgery is most effective in the treatment of apparently locoregionally confined primary disease. The principles of surgical resection include en bloc resection of the primary tumor that attempts to encompass gross and microscopic tumor in all contiguous and adjacent anatomic locations. For some tumor types, concomitant resection of regional lymph nodes comprises an important component of the initial surgical management. In many cases, when disease is diagnosed and removed at an early stage, resection is the single therapeutic modality, often associated with a high rate of long-term success. Intuitively, it appears logical that surgery should have little role in disease management once a neoplasm has spread from the primary location to a distant site. However, surgical therapy is being applied with increasing frequency for metastatic disease as well. Prolonged survival can be seen in selected patients following resection of various metastatic sites, including in the liver, lung, or brain. In particular, complete resection of hepatic colorectal metastases results in 5-year survival rates in excess of 50% in most contemporary series. As more active systemic cytotoxic, targeted, and immune therapies are prolonging survival in patients with various tumor types, resection or ablation of residual metastatic sites are being utilized with increasing frequency.

Surgery operates by zero-order kinetics, in which 100% of excised cells are destroyed. In contrast, chemotherapy and radiation therapy operate by first-order kinetics, where only a fraction of tumor cells are killed by each treatment. It is for this reason that these therapies can be considered complementary. Surgical resection reduces the tumor burden, which hopefully increases the efficacy of nonsurgical adjuvant therapies intended to eliminate microscopic residual disease, thereby decreasing the risk of recurrence and prolonging survival.

Holland-Frei Cancer Medicine, Tenth Edition. Edited by Robert C. Bast, John C. Byrd, Carlo M. Croce, Ernest Hawk, Fadlo R. Khuri, Raphael E. Pollock, Apostolia M. Tsimberidou, Christopher G. Willett, and Cheryl L. Willman.
© 2023 John Wiley & Sons, Inc. Published 2023 by John Wiley & Sons, Inc.

During the past several decades, a significant reduction has been seen in the morbidity and mortality associated with many complex cancer operations. These results, in part, can be attributed to improvements in surgical technique, patient selection, and regionalization to high-volume centers. For example, both perioperative risk and long-term survival after pancreaticoduodenectomy have been shown to be strongly influenced by hospital volume.[1] In addition, trends toward more limited cancer resections are being seen with comparable improvement in oncologic outcome. Specifically, breast-conserving surgery has become an alternative to mastectomy in patients with breast carcinoma, limb salvage is often possible in patients with bone and soft-tissue sarcomas, and sphincter function and sexual potency can frequently be preserved for patients with rectal cancer. Because surgery is increasingly combined with other treatment modalities, it is essential that most patients with solid neoplasms have their treatment planned by a multidisciplinary team, which includes radiation and medical oncologists as well as surgical oncologists. To retain a primary role in the management of the cancer patient, the successful surgical oncologist must be able to coordinate and integrate the efforts of the entire oncologic team while maintaining a patient-centered focus on dignity and quality of life.

The history of surgical oncology

Oncology (from the Greek words *onkos*, meaning mass or tumor, and *logos*, meaning study) is the study of neoplastic diseases. Early authors suggested that certain families, races, and working classes were predisposed to neoplastic transformations. In 1862, Edwin Smith, an American Egyptologist, discovered the apparently earliest recordings of the surgical treatment of cancer.[2] Written in Egypt circa 1600 BC, this treatise was based on teachings possibly dating back to 3000 BC. The Egyptian author advised surgeons to contend with tumors that might be cured by surgery but not to treat those lesions that might be fatal.

Hippocrates (460–375 BC) was the first to describe the clinical symptoms associated with cancer. He advised against treating terminal patients, who would enjoy a better quality of life without surgical intervention.[3] He also coined the terms carcinoma (crab legs tumor) and sarcoma (fleshy mass). In the second century AD, Galen published his classification of tumors, describing cancer as a systemic disease caused by an excess of black bile.[4] Galen cautioned that as a systemic disease, cancer was not amenable to cure by surgery, which was often promptly followed by patient death. This strong admonition against surgery for cancer persisted for more than 1500 years until eighteenth-century pathologists discovered that cancer often grew locally before spreading to other anatomic sites. Before the advent of safe general anesthetics, surgery was used primarily to manage trauma or severe infectious problems such as abscess drainage. In that era, cancer surgery consisted primarily of amputation or cauterization of surface tumors of the trunk or extremities. Patients were usually unwilling to submit to the pain of tumor surgery, when there was little likelihood of improved survival.

During the eighteenth and nineteenth centuries, advances in anatomic pathology led to an increase in autopsies, which in turn resulted in a better understanding of human anatomy and physiology. The early work of Morgagni, Le Dran, and Da Salva established that there was an initial period of local tumor growth before distant dissemination. This led to the understanding that not all tumors spread systemically and that certain malignancies cause death solely by local invasive growth. Percival Pott (1714–1788) was the first to describe a specific etiologic factor associated with cancer development. In 1775, Pott demonstrated a high incidence of cancer of the scrotum in chimney sweeps who had reached puberty and recommended wide local resection for cure. In 1829, the French Surgeon Joseph Recamier (1774–1852) first described the complicated process of tumor dissemination. The first recorded elective tumor resection was performed in 1809 by Ephraim McDowell, an American surgeon. He successfully removed a 22-pound ovarian tumor from a patient, who subsequently survived 30 years. McDowell's work, which included 12 more ovarian resections, stimulated greater interest in elective surgery for cancer patients.

Surgeons were initially hindered by the extreme discomfort that patients experienced during surgical procedures as well as the lack of agents that could reduce the incidence of infection. Crawford Long (1815–1878) was the first to use ether for general anesthesia in 1842, but it was the reported work of John Collins Warren (1778–1856) and William T.G. Morton (1819–1868) that brought the potential of anesthesia to public attention. The surgical procedure in Warren's first published account of ether anesthesia (1846) was the elective removal of a tongue carcinoma for which sub-maxillary gland resection and partial glossectomy were performed. Warren was also responsible for the first American-authored textbook of tumor surgery, *Surgical Observations on Tumors*, published in 1838. Joseph Lister (1827–1912) was the first to report the successful use of antisepsis during elective surgery. In 1867, Lister applied Pasteur's concept that bacteria caused infection, when he introduced the use of carbolic acid as an antiseptic agent in conjunction with heat sterilization of surgical instruments. Lister is also credited with the introduction of absorbable ligatures as well as the placement of drainage tubes to control secretions and dead space in surgical wounds.

Even with the advent of antisepsis and general anesthesia, surgical oncology in the second half of the nineteenth and early twentieth centuries was still associated with high mortality rates. Cancer was rarely diagnosed in the early stages; consequently, few patients were considered candidates for curative surgery. Those surgeons who did attempt surgical excision of malignant lesions were hindered by rudimentary anesthesia, which was also independently associated with high patient mortality. Antibiotics were not yet available, and surgical instruments were crude. The importance of the microscope to evaluate frozen tissues for surgical margins was not yet appreciated, and surgeons had great faith in their own unaided gross visual assessment of the tumor perimeter. However, several important developments in this era led to rapid advancements in surgical oncology. Emphasizing meticulous surgical technique, gentle tissue handling, and applications of Listerian principles, pioneers such as Albert Theodore Billroth (first gastrectomy, laryngectomy, and esophagectomy), William Stewart Halsted (en bloc resection, radical mastectomy), and many other more contemporary surgeons defined and advanced the boundaries of surgical oncology (Table 1).[3]

Ongoing innovations to advance effective surgical primary tumor control have improved surgical outcomes and quality of life. Advances in microvascular surgery now permit the free transfer of complex autologous tissues, such as free jejunal grafts to reconstitute the upper aerodigestive system or osteomyocutaneous flaps to reconstruct extremities and other mobile body parts such as the jaw. Automatic stapling devices, as well as laparoscopic/robotic instrumentation coupled with high-resolution optics, have remarkably advanced minimally invasive cancer surgery resulting in less-morbid procedures that require significantly less patient discomfort and recuperation time (Figure 1).

Table 1 Landmark advances in surgical oncology.[a]

Year	Event	Surgeon
1775	Etiologic basis of cancer	Percival Pott
1809	Elective oophorectomy	Ephraim McDowell
1829	Metastatic process	Joseph Recamier
1846	Ether as anesthesia	John Collins Warren
1867	Carbolic acid as antisepsis	Joseph Lister
1873	Laryngectomy	Albert Theodore Billroth
1878	Resection of rectal tumor	Richard von Volkman
1880	Esophagectomy	Albert Theodore Billroth
1881	Gastrectomy	Albert Theodore Billroth
1890	Radical mastectomy	William Stewart Halsted
1896	Oophorectomy for breast cancer	G.T. Beatson
1904	Radical prostatectomy	Hugh H. Young
1906	Radical hysterectomy	Ernest Wertheim
1908	Abdominoperineal resection	W. Ernest Miles
1909	Thyroid surgery (Nobel Prize)	Theodore Emil Kocher
1910	Craniotomy	Harvey Cushing
1912	Cordotomy for the treatment of pain	E. Martin
1913	Thoracic esophagectomy	Franz Torek
1927	Resection of pulmonary metastases	George Divis
1933	Pneumonectomy	Evarts Graham
1935	Pancreaticoduodenectomy	Allen O. Whipple
1945	Adrenalectomy for prostate cancer	Charles B. Huggins
1957	Isolated limb perfusion	Oliver Creech
1958	Organization of National Adjuvant Breast and Bowel Project (NSABP) to conduct prospective randomized trials	Bernard Fisher
1965	Hormonal therapy of cancer	Charles Huggins
1971	Free tissue transfer with microvascular anastomosis	Harry Buncke
1991	Lymphatic mapping and sentinel node biopsy	Donald Morton

[a]Source: Hill.[3]

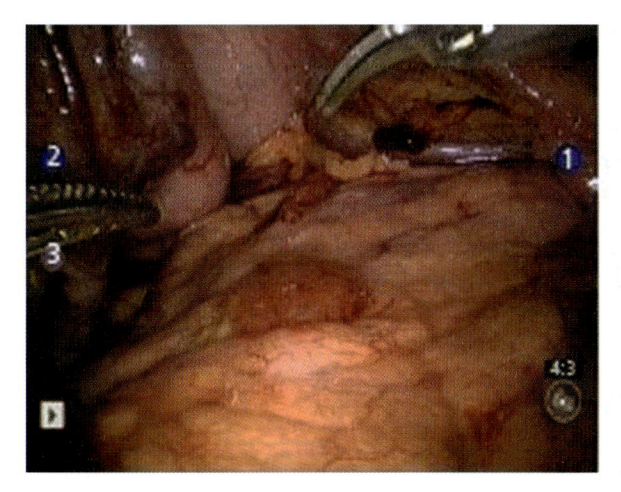

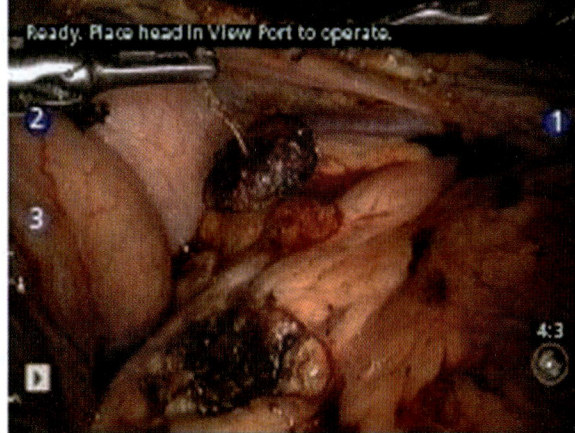

Figure 1 Robotic enucleation of insulinoma in the body of the pancreas.

The rapid deployment of robotic technologies is changing traditional surgical interventional approaches. Among the potential advantages, robotic surgery is performed as a direct extension of the operator's prehensile hand replete with multiplanar articulating robotic "wrists," thereby avoiding the crossed rigid armature impediments of laparoscopic surgical maneuvers.

Improvements in preoperative optimization of comorbid disease, advances in perioperative critical care, and enhance recovery pathways have made it possible to safely undertake increasingly complicated surgical procedures. A more sophisticated awareness of the patterns of tumor spread has also resulted in increasing opportunities for less-invasive surgical approaches. One example is the use of lymphatic mapping and sentinel node biopsy instead of formal lymphadenectomy in early-stage melanoma and breast carcinoma. In other cases, this better understanding of recurrence risk has led to more, not less, extensive surgical resections. An example of this includes the selected use of total hepatectomy and orthotopic liver transplantation for early-stage hepatocellular carcinoma.

Surgical oncology in the modern era

Surgical oncologists are surgeons who devote most of their time to the study and treatment of malignant neoplastic disease. They must possess the necessary knowledge, skills, and clinical experience to perform both the standard and extraordinary surgical procedures required for patients with cancer. Surgical oncologists must be able to diagnose tumors accurately and differentiate aggressive neoplastic lesions from benign reactive processes. In addition, surgical oncologists should have a firm understanding of radiation oncology, medical oncology, and diagnostic and interventional radiology. They must also be capable of organizing interdisciplinary studies of cancer. Surgical oncologists should also be trained in pathology because they will be called on to excise appropriate tumor samples for pathologists and make decisions about adequacy of surgical margins. Surgical oncologists should have a shared role with medical oncologists as the "primary care physicians" of cancer treatment. Almost all cancer patients will initially be managed by one of these two specialists, who will bear the ultimate responsibility for coordinating appropriate multimodality care for the individual patient.

Given the complexity of contemporary multidisciplinary approaches to the cancer patient, cancer centers have developed facilities to provide the needed planning expertise, clinical care, patient support services, and access points to clinical trials. Comprehensive cancer centers are often affiliated with academic medical institutions and offer the complete spectrum of oncology therapies, clinical trials, rehabilitation, and social services as well as basic and translational research programs to move new knowledge from the laboratory bench to the patient bedside. In this contemporary understanding of the continuum of care of the cancer patient, the role of the surgical oncologist is taking on an ever-increasing importance.

Surgical oncology is more of a cognitive than a technical surgical specialty. With the exception of a small cluster of index operations, such as pancreaticoduodenectomy, limb salvage, retroperitoneal sarcoma surgery, isolated limb perfusion, and complex liver resection, most of the surgical procedures that are performed by surgical oncologists are similar to those performed by surgeons who are not oncologically trained. What frequently differentiates these two types of surgeons is not mere knowledge about *how* to do a specific operation but an awareness of how and *when* to do that operation; that is, the cognitive knowledge of contemporary multimodality cancer care. A broad knowledge of cancer in its presenting and recurring forms as well as an awareness of the mechanisms driving tumor proliferation and dissemination is an integral part of the special cognitive database of the surgical oncologist.

As cancer management continues to march forward in the age of genomics, proteomics, and metabolomics, there is an ever-increasing need to study human tumor tissue. An unparalleled understanding of the pathophysiology of solid tumors coupled with intimate knowledge of anatomy and the workflow in the operating room and pathology department places the cancer surgeon in the central role of organizing, maintaining, optimizing, and overseeing effective tissue procurement and tumor banking; thus making the surgical oncologist a vital member of a translational science team. In addition, the cancer surgeon, working with pathologists and researchers, has the opportunity to provide meaningful clinical information, which can be used to annotate archival tissue repositories and aid in the creation of tissue microarrays. These are valuable tools whose utility can range from explorative, hypothesis-generating retrospective studies, confirmation of specific laboratory findings, and establishment of relevant preclinical animal models of cancer with patient-derived xenograft tumors.

As part of the larger surgical community, the surgical oncologist is a critical conduit for the dissemination of cancer information to colleagues in general surgery and other surgical specialties. This individual makes academic presentations at large surgical meetings, directs hospital-based tumor boards, and consults on behalf of individual cancer patients. Because of their leading role in the initial diagnosis of cancer, it is not surprising that surgical oncologists are also frequently in leadership roles in cancer prevention and screening programs. Nationally based multimodality clinical trial groups also depend on surgical oncology expertise in helping with trial design; establishing the criteria of surgical quality control; educating trial participants regarding standards of surgical care (including indications for procedures); assuring safe acquisition of research grade tumor and autologous normal tissues for correlative studies, and assisting in accurate data collection, analysis, and presentation of trial results.

Multidisciplinary management

Multidisciplinary management of solid tumors requires surgeons to play a key role in decisions concerning sequencing of treatment modalities. For example, a patient with rectal cancer and resectable liver metastases may ultimately be treated with a liver resection, rectal resection, pelvic radiation therapy, and systemic chemotherapy. Traditionally, the sequence for these treatments was preoperative chemoradiation therapy, followed by rectal resection (e.g., abdominoperineal resection or low anterior resection), subsequent liver resection, and then adjuvant chemotherapy—an aggressive approach but one that produces long-term survival in a subset of patients. However, in recognition that the greatest risk for mortality in these patients comes from systemic relapse, the current standard approach would be to start with chemotherapy, rather than leaving it to the end. Another benefit of this approach is that the nature of response to neoadjuvant treatment serves as an important prognostic marker. Moreover, tumor shrinkage may lead to a less difficult liver resection or rectal resection. While liver and bowel operations were rarely performed simultaneously, these are now more commonly performed together based on data showing safety of this approach in select patients. More often, in cases in which the two operations are performed separately, liver resection is now often performed first. The basis for this approach is that while preoperative chemotherapy rarely has any adverse impact on colon or rectal operations, accumulation of chemotherapy treatments is known to increase the risk of chemotherapy-induced liver toxicity leading to complications from liver surgery. Use of short course adjuvant radiation therapy such as 25 Gy in five fractions followed by surgery 1 week later rather than the traditional 5-week course of radiation shortens the time required for trimodality treatment and reduces the length of time off of chemotherapy. Fundamental principles that influence the sequence of multimodality treatment apply to most other solid tumors as well, and are requisite knowledge for surgical oncologists.

Unlike surgery and radiation therapy, systemic therapies, such as chemotherapy, immunotherapy, and hormonal therapy, are treatments that can kill tumor cells that have already metastasized to distant sites. These systemic modalities have a greater chance of cure in patients with minimal (or even subclinical) tumor burden as compared with those patients with clinically evident disease. Consequently, surgery and radiation therapy may be useful in decreasing a given patient's tumor burden thereby maximizing the impact of subsequent systemic approaches. Whether the goals of therapy should be cure or palliation depends on the stage of a specific cancer. If the cancer is localized without evidence of spread, it may be possible to eradicate the cancer and cure the patient. When the cancer has spread beyond the possibility of cure, the goal is to control symptoms and maintain maximum activity and quality of life for as long as possible. Patients are generally judged incurable by surgery if they have distant metastases or evidence of extensive local infiltration of critical structures adjacent to tumor. However, some patients are potentially curable even though they have distant metastases. Specifically, patients with hepatic or pulmonary metastases may still be curable by resection, and patients with melanoma or gastrointestinal stromal tumor

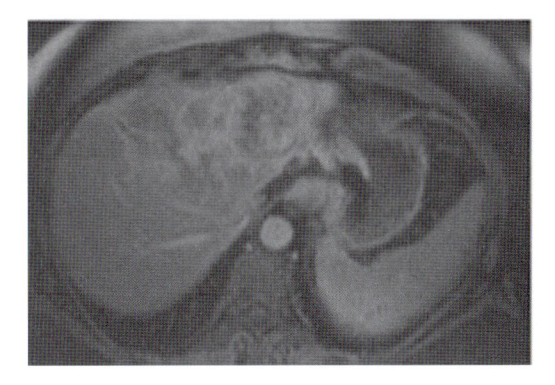

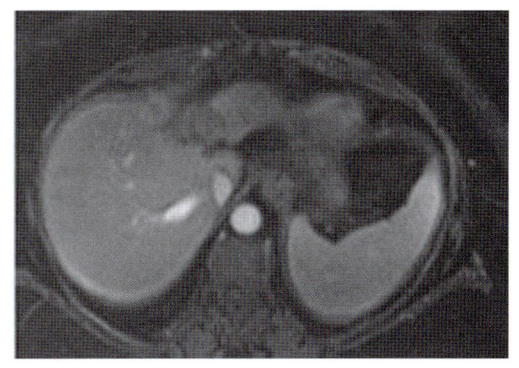

Figure 2 Previously unresectable (involvement of all three hepatic veins) intrahepatic cholangiocarcinoma downstaged using neoadjuvant gemcitabine and cisplatin.

may still be cured using systemic therapy alone. Histologic proof of distant metastases should be obtained before the patient is deemed incurable. In equivocal situations where extensive studies fail to demonstrate metastatic or incurable local extension, the patient deserves the benefit of the doubt and should be treated for cure.

The selection of therapeutic modalities depends not only on the type and extent of cancer but also on the patient's general condition and the presence of any comorbid conditions. For example, surgery may be contraindicated in a patient who has significant emphysema or liver failure. A patient with preexisting diabetes will be much more susceptible to the toxic effects of hormonal therapy with corticosteroids. Renal disease may increase the toxicity of some of the chemotherapeutic agents, such as cisplatin or ifosfamide. The presence of an autoimmune condition often precludes the use of immunotherapy. Extensive staging procedures may indicate that a tumor is localized to a primary site and/or regional lymph nodes and hence potentially curable by locoregional therapy. However, approximately 60% of localized malignant tumors ultimately recur, suggesting that many such patients must have had subclinical metastases at the time of initial diagnosis. The probability of cure may be improved if systemic approaches are coupled with local treatment. Molecularly targeted therapies and chemotherapeutic drugs may be more effective when administered at a time that the number of tumor cells is low enough to permit their destruction at doses that can be tolerated by the patient. The opportunity for cure is most likely during the early stage of disease or immediately after surgery when the tumor burden has been minimized. Adjuvant chemotherapy has remarkably improved surgical results in some malignancies, primarily because of cytocidal effects on clinically undetectable malignant cells outside the operative field. Neoadjuvant chemotherapy that is initiated before local and regional treatments also can affect micro-metastatic distant disease while significantly cytoreducing the primary tumor.

Classically, surgical extirpation has been first in the sequence of therapies for resectable solid malignancies, but increasing evidence suggests that it may be more effective when used later in the treatment plan, particularly in more advanced tumors. Molecularly targeted therapy, chemotherapy, and radiation therapy each work by first-order kinetics. However, because of tumor cell heterogeneity, it can be anticipated that resistant clones of viable neoplastic cells may persist in the primary tumor after these therapies. Such clonal heterogeneity is more likely in large tumors that are both poorly perfused by chemotherapeutic agents and are also relatively hypoxic and therefore resistant to radiation therapy. Because surgery works by zero-order kinetics, it effectively removes the local residual primary tumor cells that are resistant to these other modalities.

From a practical management standpoint, the use of chemotherapy before surgical therapy can provide useful prognostic information regarding response to therapy. Presence of response to neoadjuvant therapy can aid in the planning of additional postoperative adjuvant chemotherapy. In addition, earlier administration of systemic therapy addresses the potential occult micro-metastatic disease. In some cases, preoperative therapy (or "conversion" therapy) can be used to downsize a tumor from an unresectable to resectable status (Figure 2).

Components of surgical management in the care of the cancer patient

Surgical prevention

As the role of genetic mutations that predispose to subsequent cancer development expands, one can anticipate that prophylactic surgery will be extended to encompass some of these conditions. In such cases, it is imperative that the surgical oncologist become intimately knowledgeable about the indications, limitations, and ethical considerations regarding genetic counseling, if only because it will be the responsibility of the surgeon to alert other family members at risk and arrange for appropriate testing. The above emerging indications are being added to an already established role for prophylactic surgery in the prevention of predisposing malignancies, including ulcerative colitis with dysplasia, familial adenomatous polyposis, multiple endocrine neoplasia syndromes, and hereditary breast cancer. Assessing the risk–benefit ratio of prophylactic surgery is critical but frequently inexact. The future advent of inexpensive and reliable genetic screening technologies, coupled with emerging insights derived from the new field of molecular epidemiology, should bring more definitive understanding of prophylactic surgery benefits in populations at risk.

Biopsy and diagnosis

The diagnosis of solid tumors depends on locating and performing a biopsy of the lesion. The findings from biopsy specimens will be used to determine the histology and/or grade of a tumor, which is a prerequisite for planning definitive therapy. Significant therapeutic errors have been made when biopsy confirmation of malignancy was not obtained before treatment. Even when biopsy reports from another hospital are available, the slides of the previous biopsy must be obtained and reviewed before the initiation of therapy. This is essential because all too often an erroneous interpretation may have been made in the initial pathology assessment.

Surgeons play a key role in the initial diagnosis for many solid tumors, including the decision on whether and how to biopsy a mass. In the case of a clinically suspicious breast mass combined with an abnormal mammogram, core biopsy rather than excisional biopsy is often appropriate as a strategy to limit the number of surgical procedures and allow for multidisciplinary planning and possibly neoadjuvant therapy. Conversely, in a patient with chronic viral hepatitis, and an arterially enhancing liver mass with imaging features suggestive of a resectable hepatocellular carcinoma, needle biopsy is typically not indicated if resection represents the most appropriate treatment pathway. Proper approaches to biopsy of a cutaneous pigmented lesion for possible melanoma requires understanding of the importance of proper intraoperative tissue manipulations to avoid compromising tumor thickness measurements by leaving a positive deep margin and understanding the difficulty in clinically following an atypical nevus that has only been partially biopsied; complete excisional biopsy is appropriate in most circumstances. The strategy for biopsy of masses suspicious for soft-tissue sarcomas involves thoughtful planning to obtain sufficient tissue for histologic study, minimize disruption and potential seeding of tissue planes and allow for needle biopsy tracks to be placed within fields used for adjuvant or neoadjuvant radiation therapy. The strategy for biopsy of very small lesions causing obstruction of the common bile duct typically integrates understanding of the relatively high likelihood of false-negative results and the observation that the most curable lesions are the smallest and most difficult from which to attain a true-positive result. Resection is commonly performed in such circumstances even in the absence of a positive biopsy. And because diagnosis of distant metastases will often change overall management, surgeons commonly decide on how to achieve a tissue diagnosis at distant sites with minimal morbidity and high sensitivity. Fundamental principles that influence approaches to biopsy are requisite knowledge for surgical oncologists.

Biopsy is easiest when the tumor is near the surface or involves an orifice that can be examined with appropriate visualizing instruments, such as the bronchoscope, colonoscope, or cystoscope. Carcinomas of the breast, tongue, or rectum can be seen or palpated and a portion can be excised for definitive diagnosis. In contrast, deep-seated lesions may grow to quite a large size before causing symptoms. Ultrasonography, computed tomography (CT), and magnetic resonance imaging (MRI) are all useful techniques for localizing such lesions at the time of invasive biopsy. However, although image-directed needle biopsy may be useful in some patients, exploratory surgery is occasionally required to obtain a definitive biopsy that establishes the exact histologic diagnosis. In some cases, tissue samples larger than that which are obtained by percutaneous biopsy may be required for tumor characterization, such as lymphoma, necessitating surgical biopsy. Fortunately, such procedures can now be frequently performed on an outpatient basis using minimally invasive technology such as laparoscopic surgical approaches.

Three methods are commonly used to biopsy suspicious lesions: needle biopsy (fine needle aspiration [FNA] or core), open incisional, or excisional biopsy. Regardless of the method used, the pathologic interpretation of the tumor mass will be valid only if a representative section of tumor is obtained. The surgical oncologist must be aware that a sampling error can occur with needle and incisional biopsies where only small portions of the total tumor mass are submitted for pathologic examination. It is the surgeon's task to provide adequate tissue for diagnosis. Orientation of the specimen, as may be necessary, is also the responsibility of the surgeon.

FNA is a cytologic technique in which cells are aspirated from a tumor using a needle and syringe. The technique can be performed using image-directed guidance and is particularly helpful in the diagnosis of relatively inaccessible lesions such as deep visceral tumors. Because the aspirate consists of disaggregated cells rather than intact tissue, diagnosis of malignancy usually depends on detection of abnormal intracellular features, such as nuclear pleomorphism; thus, the margin of error is higher than with other biopsy techniques. In addition, because of the lack of intact tumor architecture, FNA cannot distinguish invasive from noninvasive malignancy. Negative results do not rule out malignancy. Depending on the clinical context, such as distinguishing carcinoma *in situ* from an infiltrating malignancy, other types of biopsy may be more appropriate.

Core biopsy is the simplest method of histologic (as opposed to cytologic) diagnosis and may be useful for biopsy of subcutaneous masses and muscular masses as well as some internal organs, such as liver, kidney, and pancreas. Needle biopsy may be less appropriate if the specimen is small, which increases the likelihood of the needle missing the lesion or the biopsy not being representative of the entire tumor. Consequently, a needle biopsy report that is negative for malignant disease should be viewed with skepticism if it is inconsistent with the clinical presentation and should be followed by incisional or excisional biopsy.

Incisional biopsy for pathologic examination involves removal of a small portion of the tumor mass. It is best performed in circumstances where the incisional wound can be totally excised in continuity with the definitive surgical resection in the event that any tumor cells are spilled at the time of biopsy. Incisional biopsy is indicated for deeper subcutaneous or intramuscular tumor masses when initial needle biopsy fails to establish a diagnosis. An incisional biopsy is also appropriate when a tumor is so large that complete local excision would violate wide tissue planes and impair a subsequent wide local resection for curative purposes. If possible, an incisional biopsy should retrieve a deep section of tumor as well as a margin of normal tissue. Incisional biopsies suffer from the same disadvantages as needle biopsies in that the removed portion may not be representative of the entire tumor. Consequently, a negative biopsy does not preclude the possibility of cancer in the residual mass.

Excisional biopsy completely removes the mass of interest. It is used for small, discrete masses that are generally <3 cm in diameter, where complete removal will not interfere with a subsequent wider excision that may be required for definitive local control. However, this method is contraindicated in large tumor masses because the biopsy procedure could scatter tumor cells throughout a large surgical field that would need to be widely and totally encompassed by the ultimate surgical resection. For this reason, excisional biopsy is usually contraindicated for skeletal and soft tissue masses when the diagnosis of sarcoma is being entertained. The excisional method is also used for polypoid lesions of the colon, for thyroid and breast nodules, lymph nodes, for small skin lesions, and when the pathologist cannot make a definitive diagnosis from tissue removed by incisional biopsy. An unbiopsied mass is also surgically removed when the suspicious character of the lesion, the need for its removal (whatever the diagnosis), and the nonmutilating nature of the operation render such an approach feasible. Examples of such procedures include subtotal thyroidectomy for thyroid nodules after an inconclusive FNA and a right hemicolectomy for a cecal mass that might be either inflammatory or neoplastic. In the latter instance, colonoscopic biopsy is informative only if positive for neoplasm.

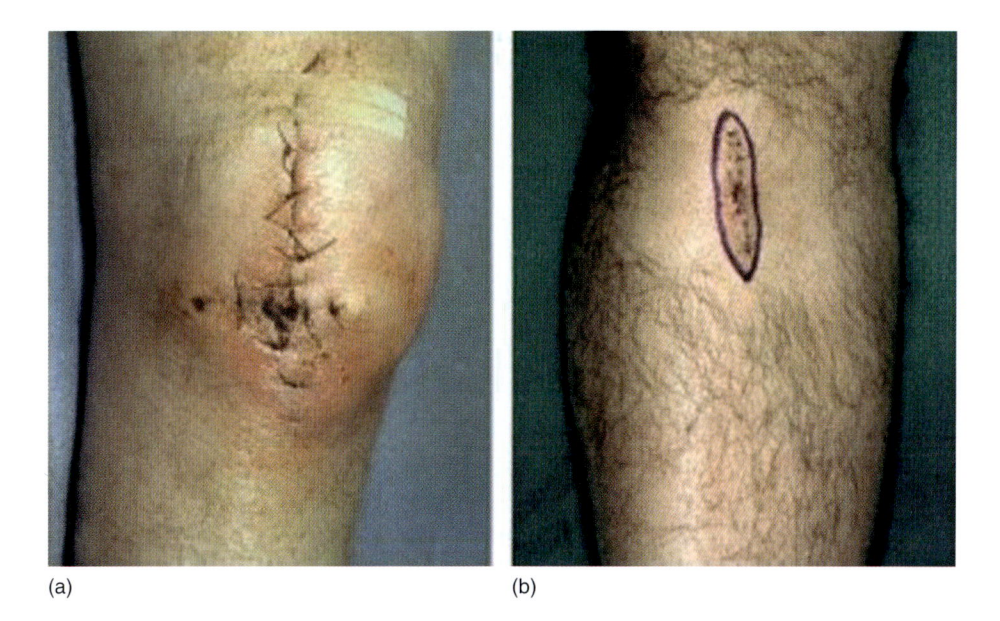

Figure 3 Appropriate and inappropriate biopsy incisions. (a) A patient with a cruciate-shaped biopsy scar overlying the patellar tendon that contained a synovial sarcoma. Note the erythema in this infected incision. This ill-conceived biopsy scar would have required a wide-field soft tissue and osseous composite resection to encompass all of the violated tissue planes. Unfortunately, tumor was *intruded* into the joint space at the time of this biopsy, and this patient ultimately required an above-knee amputation to treat this small, otherwise limb-salvageable sarcoma. (b) An appropriately oriented incisional biopsy scar in the lower extremity. Note the alignment of the scar parallel with the long axis of the extremity and the meticulous placement of small biopsy wound sutures. The entire scar could be excised at surgery (blue ellipse) with minimal concomitant normal tissue sacrifice.

Surgeons should always mark the excisional biopsy margins with sutures or metal clips so that if removal is incomplete and further excision is needed the positive margin can be accurately identified *in situ*.

Strategic orientation of biopsy incisions is also extremely important. Ill-conceived incisions can unnecessarily open up additional tissue planes, necessitating subsequent wider radiotherapy fields or more extensive ultimate surgical resections. For example, tumors of the extremities are best biopsied using incisions that run parallel to the long axis of that limb. This facilitates a definitive en bloc resection that encompasses the biopsy track (Figure 3). Biopsy incisions should be closed using meticulous hemostasis because a hematoma can lead to dissemination of tumor cells with contamination of tissue planes. Instruments, gloves, gowns, and drapes should be discarded and replaced with unused substitutes if the definitive surgical resection immediately follows the biopsy procedure.

Lymph nodes should be carefully selected for biopsy. Axillary nodes may be preferable to groin nodes if both are enlarged because of a decreased likelihood of postoperative infection. Other caveats are also noteworthy. For example, lymph node specimens preserved in formaldehyde cannot be analyzed for cytogenetics or flow cytometric immunophenotyping. The laboratory workup for lymphoma usually requires unfixed sterile tissue. Isolated cervical lymph nodes should not be biopsied until a careful search for a primary tumor has been made using nasopharyngoscopy, esophagoscopy, and bronchoscopy because enlargement of the upper cervical nodes by metastases is usually caused by laryngeal, oropharyngeal, and nasopharyngeal primary neoplasms. In contrast, supraclavicular nodes are more frequently enlarged as a result of metastases from primary tumors of the thoracic or abdominal cavities or breast.

The tumor specimen may be prepared for pathologic examination by either frozen or permanent sections. Frozen sections are made at the time of biopsy, and pathologic diagnosis can typically be obtained within 10 min. Frozen sections are used when the diagnosis is required to assess resectability at the time of major surgery, or to check tumor margins intraoperatively, or to assess adequacy of a diagnostic specimen. Frozen-section biopsy-proven carcinomatosis may mandate abandoning a procedure with a curative intent in favor of a palliative approach. Occasionally, mediastinoscopy, laparoscopy (peritoneoscopy), thoracoscopy, exploratory thoracotomy, or even laparotomy is necessary to obtain adequate representative tissue samples for microscopic examination to confirm diagnosis or tumor stage. In many instances, direct communication between the surgical oncologist and pathologist is crucial for proper tissue processing and staining.

Patterns of tumor spread

In general, a malignant tumor may spread (1) by direct extension into surrounding structures, (2) via the lymphatics, (3) by hematogenous spread, or (4) by implantation in serous cavities. However, many cancers spread by more than one route, and an orderly course of metastasis is not predictably certain. For example, patients with breast cancer or melanoma can manifest distant metastatic disease in the lungs, liver, or skeleton without ever developing evidence of lymph node metastases. Table 2 summarizes the metastatic patterns of various human tumors.

Cancer cells may also spread by direct extension through tissue spaces and planes. Some neoplasms, such as soft tissue sarcomas and adenocarcinomas of the stomach or esophagus, may extend for a considerable distance (10–15 cm) along tissue planes beyond the palpable tumor mass. Other neoplasms, such as a basal cell carcinoma of skin, rarely extend for more than a few millimeters beyond the visible margin. Even though most central nervous system (CNS) tumors infrequently metastasize, they may penetrate nearby brain tissue, and their location can cause death by interfering with vital CNS functions.

Tumor cells can readily enter the lymphatics and extend through these channels by permeation or embolization to regional lymph

Table 2 Patterns of neoplastic spread for common human malignancies.

Neoplasms	Hematogenous	Lymphatic	Local infiltration (expressed as local recurrence)
Adenocarcinoma			
Breast	++++	+++	++
Endometrium	+	++	+
Ovary	++	+++	++++
Stomach	++++	++++	+++
Pancreas	++++	++++	+++
Colon	+++	+++	+
Kidney	++	++	++
Prostate	+++	+++	+++
Liver	+	+	++++
Epidermal carcinoma			
Lung	++++	+++	++
Oropharynx	++	+++	+++
Larynx	+	+++	++
Cervix	+	++++	+++
Transitional cell carcinoma			
Bladder	++	+++	++++
Cutaneous neoplasm			
Squamous cell carcinoma	+	++	+
Melanoma	+++	+++	++
Basal cell carcinoma	0	0	+
Sarcoma			
Bone	++++	+	+
Soft tissue	++++	+	+++
Brain neoplasm	0	0	++++

Key: Does not occur; 0, <1%; +, 1–5%; ++, 15 – +++0%; 3, 30%; and ++++, 50%.

nodes. Permeation is the growth of a colony of tumor cells along the course of the lymphatic vessel. This commonly occurs in the skin lymphatics in carcinoma of the breast and in the perineural lymphatics in carcinoma of the prostate. Lymphatic involvement is extremely common in malignant epithelial neoplasms of all types, except basal cell carcinoma of the skin, which metastasizes to regional lymphatics in <0.1% of cases, or mesenchymal neoplasms, such as sarcomas, which metastasize to lymph nodes in only 2–5% of cases.

Spread along the lymphatics by embolization to regional or distant lymph nodes is of great clinical importance. Tumor cells travel within local lymphatics and can spread to proximal nodal basins via the collateral lymphatic channels. Lymph node metastases are first confined to the subcapsular space; at this stage, the node is not enlarged and may appear grossly normal. Gradually, the tumor cells permeate the sinusoids and replace the nodal parenchyma, changing the shape and texture of the node. There is little direct spread from node to node because the nodal capsule is not penetrated until a late stage. However, when an involved lymph node is more than 3 cm in diameter, tumor has usually extended beyond the capsule into the perinodal fat.

Lymph from the abdominal organs and lower extremities drains into the cisterna chyli and then into the thoracic duct, which finally opens into the left jugular vein. Using this route, tumor cells can pass freely from the lymphatic system into the bloodstream. Oncologists originally believed that solid neoplasms first involved regional lymph nodes and then spread into the bloodstream by drainage into the thoracic duct and then to other parts of the body. An alternative explanation now favored by most oncologists assumes that the presence of cancer cells in regional lymph nodes indicates an unfavorable host-tumor relationship and the concomitant higher likelihood of distant metastases.

Cancer cells may reach the bloodstream either through the thoracic duct or by direct invasion of blood vessels. Capillaries offer no resistance to tumor cell transgression. Small veins are frequently invaded, whereas thicker-walled arteries are rarely violated. Veins frequently form a plexus extending to the subendothelial regions, which provide a portal of entry through the thin vein wall. When the vascular endothelium is destroyed, a thrombus can form that is quickly invaded by tumor. This combination of thrombus and tumor may detach to form large tumor emboli. Vascular invasion is common in both carcinomas and sarcomas and is associated with a poor prognosis. GI cancers, due to their drainage by the portal venous system, have a propensity for liver metastasis after intravasated cells become trapped in the hepatic sinusoids. Some types of neoplasms have a remarkable tendency to grow as a solid column along the course of veins. For example, renal cell carcinoma can grow into the renal vein and up the inferior vena cava extending to the right atrium. In this situation, a spectacular en bloc removal requiring cardiopulmonary bypass may still result in long-term survival or even cure.

Tumor cells occasionally gain entrance to serous cavities by growing through the wall of an organ. Many tumor cells can grow in suspension without a supporting matrix and may widely spread within the peritoneal cavity or attach to serous surfaces. Thus, widespread peritoneal seeding is common with gastrointestinal and ovarian cancers. Similarly, malignant gliomas may spread widely within the CNS via the cerebrospinal fluid.

Although much is known about the routes of tumor spread, the mechanisms underlying this process remain unclear. Some cancers are metastatic at the time of clinical discovery, whereas others of the same type and in the same organ tissue may remain localized for years. Metastases may dominate the presenting clinical picture although the primary tumor remains latent and asymptomatic or even undetectable. For example, cerebral metastases from silent cancers in the bronchus or the breast are often mistaken for primary benign CNS neoplasms.

Preoperative preparation

Preparation of a patient for surgical cancer therapy is important in order to minimize perioperative complications, hasten recovery

Table 3 American Society of Anesthesiologists: Physical status classification.[a]

Class	Description
P-1	A normal healthy patient
P-2	A patient with mild systemic disease
P-3	A patient with severe systemic disease
P-4	A patient with severe systemic disease that is a constant threat to life
P-5	A moribund patient who is not expected to survive without the operation
P-6	A declared brain-dead patient whose organs are being removed for donor purposes

[a]Source: Saklad.[5]

Table 4 Eastern Cooperative Oncology Group Performance Status[6] and corresponding Karnofsky rating.[7][a]

Grade	Description
0	Fully active, able to carry on all predisease activities without restriction (Karnofsky 100)
1	Restricted in physically strenuous activity but ambulatory and able to carry out work of a light or sedentary nature, for example, light housework/office work (Karnofsky 80–90)
2	Ambulatory and capable of all self-care but unable to carry out any work activities; up and about more than 50% of waking hours (Karnofsky 60–70)
3	Capable of limited self-care; confined to bed or chair 50% or more of waking hours (Karnofsky 40–50)
4	Completely disabled; cannot carry on any self-care; totally confined to bed or chair (Karnofsky 30 or less)

[a]Source: Adapted from Oken et al.[6] and Karnofsky and Burchenal.[7]

to premorbid state of health, and avoid delay in possible initiation of postoperative adjuvant therapy. Severely deconditioned patients may benefit from a four to 6 week period of prehabilitation with a physical therapist prior to major surgery. Every effort should be made to correct nutritional deficiencies if present, restore depleted blood volume, and correct electrolyte imbalances before extensive surgical procedures. Enteral or total parenteral nutrition (TPN) can be used to prepare the extremely malnourished patient for a major operation, although reconstitution is a slow process, and TPN may chiefly serve to interrupt further deterioration by restoring positive nitrogen balance. Surgical morbidity and mortality following extensive cancer operations will predictably be problematic if critical physiologic and biochemical deficiencies are not corrected in advance.

Determining the risk inherent in a given operation is a complicated and inexact assessment based on a number of factors. The physical status of the patient, including cardiopulmonary reserve, comorbid conditions, debility inherent to a specific operation, hepatic and renal function, and the intent of surgical procedure (curative vs palliative), are all pertinent to this assessment. The technical complexity of an operation, the type of anesthetic used, and the relative experience of the involved health care personnel can all impact on the complications of a procedure. Various schema for risk assessment, such as the five-level physical status classification of the American Society of Anesthesiologists (Table 3) and the Eastern Cooperative Oncology Group Five-Step Performance Scale (Table 4), may be useful in assessing the appropriateness of a given operation for a specific patient. More recently, it has been the introduction of the American College of Surgeons surgical risk calculator (www.riskcalculator.facs.org), which takes into account 20 patient predictors that can be entered online and used to predict any of the 18 possible procedure-specific outcomes within 30 days of surgery, including death, any complication, severe complications, and surgical site infection among others. The calculator was developed based on data obtained from over 4.3 million operations at 780 hospitals participating in the ACS NSQIP project between 2013 and 2017.[8]

Operative mortality is defined as mortality that occurs within 30 days of an operative procedure. In cancer patients, the underlying disease is a major determinant of operative mortality. Although it is true that comparable operations are usually more morbid in the geriatric age group as compared with other adults, advanced age per se should not disqualify a patient from a potentially curative surgical procedure. Because of their high-risk nature, decisions about the indications for palliative surgical procedures are particularly difficult. For example, palliative surgery for extensive metastatic disease or symptomatic intestinal obstruction secondary to carcinomatosis has a 20–30% perioperative mortality. In such circumstances, the risk–benefit ratio and ultimate surgical objectives must be defined as clearly as possible and accepted by patient, family, and surgeon.

Preoperative chemotherapy and/or radiation therapy is being administered with increasing frequency in patients undergoing cancer operations. In some cases, these therapies can be associated with increased perioperative complications. For example, the antivascular endothelial growth factor antibody bevacizumab is associated with increased risk of wound healing complications when administered within several weeks before surgery.[9] As this targeted therapy has a 21-day half-life, discontinuation of bevacizumab is recommended at least 6–8 weeks before elective surgery.

Operative considerations

Once a decision has been made to proceed with surgical therapy, the operative procedure itself must be carefully planned for the specific surgical patient. It is essential to realize that the best (and often the only) opportunity for cure is with the first resection, as tumor cells may be dislodged within the operative field, potentially exposing tissue planes, lymphatics, and blood vessels to the dislodged tumor cells. A subsequent recurrence may be difficult to distinguish from the normal postsurgical inflammatory reaction and scarring.

The principle of the "no-touch technique" has maintained some traction in the surgical lore. This opinion is based on the theoretical concept that direct contact with and manipulation of the tumor during resection can lead to an increased risk in local implantation and embolization of tumor cells. Although little clinical evidence exists to support this principle, there may be some validity to this concept with respect to tumors that extend directly into the vascular system, such as hepatocellular or renal tumors with extension to the large veins or vena cava. Although not definitively proved to be detrimental, the general tenet of avoidance of forceful handling of the tumor and care to avoid any tumor disruption during surgical resection is sound technique. Similarly, every attempt should be made to extirpate a tumor with meticulous attention to detail while avoiding excessive blood loss and trauma to normal tissue. Although the need for contiguous multivisceral resection may, by its nature, result in prolonged operation with high blood loss, familiarity, and experience with such complicated operations such as major hepatectomy, pancreatectomy, and retroperitoneal tumor removal potentially minimizes operative morbidity and maximizes oncologic benefit.

Types of cancer operations

Wide local resection with removal of an adequate margin of normal peritumoral tissue may be adequate treatment of low-grade neoplasms that very rarely metastasize to regional nodes or widely infiltrate adjacent tissues. Basal cell carcinomas and mixed tumors of the parotid gland are examples of such tumors. In contrast, neoplasms that spread widely by infiltration into adjacent tissues, such as soft tissue sarcomas and esophageal and gastric carcinomas, must be excised with a wide margin of normal tissue. This wide tissue margin between the line of excision and the tumor mass may also act as a protective barrier against intraoperative tumor cell traversal into severed lymphatics and vessels. Tumor cells may have been implanted in the incision when an incisional biopsy alone had been previously performed. To encompass potentially contaminated tissues, it is extremely important to remove a wide segment of skin and underlying muscle, fat, and fascia beyond the limits of the original incision.

Malignant neoplasms are usually not truly encapsulated. The tumor is commonly encased by a pseudocapsule comprising a compression zone of normal tissue interspersed with neoplastic cells. This pseudoencapsulation offers a great temptation for simple enucleation in that the tumor may be easily dislodged from its bed. However, this approach must be resisted because microscopic extensions of tumor from the primary through the pseudocapsule will be left behind after simple enucleation, dooming the patient to a local recurrence. Ideally, the surgeon should operate through normal tissues at all times and never encounter or even directly visualize the neoplasm during its removal. Dissection should proceed with meticulous care to avoid tumor cell spillage. Many neoplasms metastasize via the lymphatics, and operations have been designed to remove the primary neoplasm and draining regional lymph nodes in continuity with all intervening tissues. Circumstances favor this type of operative approach when the lymph nodes draining the neoplasm lie adjacent to the tumor bed or when there is a single avenue of lymphatic drainage that can be removed without sacrificing vital structures. It is important to avoid cutting across involved lymphatic channels, which markedly increases the possibility of local recurrence.

At the present time, it is generally agreed that en bloc regional lymph node dissection is indicated for clinically demonstrable nodal involvement with metastatic tumor. However, in many cases, the tumor has already spread beyond regional nodes. Although the cure rates following resection in such circumstances may be quite low (20–50%), undue pessimism should not prevent such patients from receiving appropriate surgical treatment. En bloc removal of the involved lymph nodes may offer the only chance for cure and can at least provide significant palliative local control. Regional lymph node involvement should therefore not be viewed as a contraindication to surgery but as a possible indication for adjuvant therapies, such as radiation or chemotherapy. Importantly, an inadequate lymph node resection is associated with worse survival for many cancers due to either (1) locoregional recurrence in undissected positive lymph nodes, or (2) distant failure in patients who were not offered adjuvant therapy because they were presumed to be lymph node negative on the basis of a small sample of negative lymph nodes (e.g., understaging).

The routine dissection of regional nodes in close proximity to the primary malignancy is recommended for most cancer types even when these structures are not clinically involved with tumor. This recommendation is based on the high rate of locoregional recurrence following surgical resection when multiple lymph nodes are microscopically involved and the high error rate when palpation alone is used to assess possible lymph node involvement with tumor. Microscopic tumor dissemination to regional lymph nodes can be detected in 20–40% of clinically node-negative carcinomas and melanomas.

The extent of lymph node dissection has been an area of evolution. Sentinel lymphadenectomy is now a well-established technique for detection of early nodal disease in selected tumor types. First introduced by Morton et al.[10] for melanoma, it is now being applied as well for the management of breast carcinoma[11] and other neoplasms.[12] Initially, the technique relied on the injection of a vital blue dye at the tumor site and visual tracking of this dye along the lymphatics draining to the nodal basin, sentinel node mapping has been facilitated by adding a radiolabeled isotope to the dye and monitoring its path using a handheld gamma probe. Sentinel lymphadenectomy is a low-morbidity procedure that accurately stages the regional lymph nodes and identifies the 60–80% of melanoma and breast cancer patients who do not require complete lymphadenectomy.

Advances in surgical technique, anesthesia, and supportive care (blood transfusion, antibiotics, and fluid and electrolyte management) permit the more radical, extensive, and lengthy operative procedures to be done more safely. Such procedures offer a chance for a cure that cannot be achieved by other means and are justified in selected situations, if there is no evidence of distant metastases. For example, some slow-growing primary tumors may reach an enormous size and widely infiltrate locally without metastasizing to distant sites. Supra-radical operative procedures should be considered for these extensive and nearly inoperable tumors because the occasional patient is cured. However, such operations should be undertaken only by experienced surgeons who can select those patients most likely to benefit. As an example of carefully indicated radical surgery, pelvic exenteration is a well-conceived operation capable of curing patients with radiation-treated recurrent cancer of the cervix and certain well-differentiated and locally extensive adenocarcinomas of the rectum. This operation removes all pelvic organs (bladder, uterus, and rectum) and soft tissues within the pelvis. Bowel function is restored with colostomy. Urinary tract drainage is established by anastomosis of the ureters into a segment of the bowel (ileum or sigmoid colon). The 5-year relapse-free survival is 25% when pelvic exenteration is used to manage these problems. It is also imperative that the surgical oncologist be willing to accept responsibility for helping to optimize the postoperative emotional and psychological rehabilitation of the patient before embarking on extensive resections, such as hemipelvectomy, forequarter amputation, mutilating operations for head and neck carcinomas, or total pelvic exenteration.

Although logic might suggest that once a neoplasm has metastasized to a distant site, it is no longer curable by surgical resection, experience shows otherwise. The removal of metastatic deposits within the liver, lung, or other sites can occasionally result in long-term cure. In others, often with favorable biology and good response to systemic chemotherapy, metastatectomy can significantly prolong survival beyond that of chemotherapy alone, not infrequently turning advanced disease into a chronic condition. Before undertaking resection, an extensive workup should be performed to rule out metastatic spread to other body sites outside of the proposed operative field.

Some patients with liver-only metastases may benefit from surgical resection, particularly when of colorectal origin. Advances in preoperative evaluation, surgical technique, and systemic therapies have all contributed to an increasingly aggressive approach to such patients. Although in the past, resectability was defined by the number, size, and distribution of hepatic metastases, more recently, resectability is defined by the capability to resect all disease with negative margins (R0) and have a sufficient functional remnant liver, regardless of the tumor number. Even patients with limited and resectable extrahepatic disease combined with liver metastases may be candidates for surgical therapy provided all disease can be safely removed. Moreover, when not initially optimally resectable, approaches to (1) reduce tumor size with preoperative chemotherapy, (2) expand the remnant liver with preoperative portal vein embolization or staged liver resections, or (3) application of thermal ablative approaches combined with resection, all can contribute to increasing the number of patients eligible for surgical therapy of liver metastases with curative intent. Even with increasingly aggressive approaches, contemporary series are reporting 5-year survival rates following complete resection in excess of 50%.[13]

There are certain operations that are classically performed by surgical oncologists, due to the unique expertise that is commonly learned during Surgical Oncology Fellowship training. These include debulking and hyperthermic intraperitoneal chemotherapy (HIPEC) for certain disseminated intraperitoneal malignancies, hyperthermic isolated limb perfusion (ILP), or isolated limb infusion (ILI) for regional limb metastasis from melanoma, and D2 lymphadenectomy for gastric adenocarcinoma.

Surgical procedures are sometimes indicated to palliate symptoms without attempting to cure the patient, thereby prolonging a useful and comfortable life. A palliative operation may be justified to relieve pain, hemorrhage, obstruction, or infection when it can be done without untoward risk to the patient. Palliative surgery may also be applicable when there are no better nonsurgical means of palliation or when the procedure will improve the quality of life, even if it does not result in prolonged survival. In contrast, surgery that only prolongs a miserable existence is not of benefit to the patient. Examples of indicated palliative surgical procedures include (1) colostomy, enteroenterostomy, or gastrojejunostomy to relieve intestinal obstruction; (2) cordotomy or celiac block to control pain; (3) hepaticojejunostomy to relieve biliary obstruction and pruritis; (4) amputation for intractably painful tumors of the extremities; (5) simple mastectomy for carcinoma of the breast, when the tumor is infected, large, ulcerated, and locally resectable (even in the presence of distant metastases); and (6) resection of obstructing colon cancer in the presence of disseminated metastatic disease. Surgery for residual disease is a special application of palliative surgery. In some patients, extensive yet isolated local spread of malignancy precludes gross total resection of all disease. In these patients, cytoreductive surgery may be of benefit, such as biologically indolent disease or that which is producing local or hormonal symptoms such as metastatic neuroendocrine tumors.

Problems with exsanguinating hemorrhage, perforated viscus, abscess formation, or impending obstruction of a hollow viscus, such as gastrointestinal organs, critical blood vessels, or respiratory structures, are sometimes amenable to emergency surgical intervention. Emergency surgery may also be indicated to decompress tumors that are invading the CNS or that are destroying critical neurologic components by exerting pressure in closed spaces. The cancer patient being evaluated for emergency surgery may be neutropenic or thrombocytopenic as a consequence of recent myelosuppressive chemotherapy. Sometimes, a potential catastrophe can be avoided by operating on such patients expectantly just after they have gone through the nadir of their most recent myelosuppressive chemotherapy. Because of the high risks involved, each patient and the patient's family must be made aware of the dangers and benefits of the proposed surgery, as well as of other potentially effective treatments that might be available if the patient survives this emergency operation.

Reconstructive surgery after tumor resection has remarkably improved the quality of life for many cancer patients. The routine application of microvascular anastomotic techniques has enabled the free transfer of composite grafts containing skin, muscle, and/or bone to surgically created bodily defects. Breast reconstruction after mastectomy, tissue transfers as part of extremity surgery for sarcoma or mandible reconstruction, and aerodigestive reconstruction using jejunal-free grafts are examples of these dramatic improvements in the combined surgical management of complex cancer problems. In the future, applications of the new discipline of tissue engineering may remarkably extend the reconstructive armamentarium. Using these approaches in the future, it may be possible to custom-grow nerve, fat, muscle, bone cartilage, or other body components as replacements for tissues that will need to be resected as part of a composite cancer procedure.[14]

Cancer/surgical quality control

Constant and ongoing assessment of personal and institutional outcomes provides opportunity to improve systems that can result in safer operations and identify new markers or therapies that can improve oncology outcomes. Oncologists, particularly surgeons, are well positioned to develop databases that can be used to identify etiologic factors for cancer development, predictors of surgical complications, markers of cancer outcomes, and potential changes in management schemes. Such comprehensive data sets can be combined across institutions to provide insight for uncommon cancers and/or procedures. When combined to create annotated tumor banks, these become very powerful tools that can be used to identify potential targets for drug discovery in addition to process improvement. The American College of Surgeons Commission on Cancer provides a forum by which more than 1500 associated institutions monitor quality of cancer care. Through this accreditation mechanism, institutions are required to have state-of-the-art clinical cancer services, cancer committee leadership, cancer conferences for care planning and provider education, quality improvement program in part through compliance with accepted cancer treatment guidelines (e.g., NCCN), and a comprehensive cancer registry to monitor quality of care. The surgical oncologist is well suited to lead these efforts.

The future of surgical oncology

Cancer is about to replace cardiovascular disease as the leading cause of death in the United States. The aging of the population combined with increase in incidence rates for certain cancers will generate an enormous growth in demand for oncological procedures. From 2010 to 2020, the number of cancer cases in the United States increased by an estimated 19%, and from 2020 to 2030 an additional increase of 15% is expected.[15] The demand for surgical oncologists will be strained as significant increases in incidence are predicted between 2020 and 2030 for the following cancers: breast (12% increase), melanoma (36% increase), pancreas (42% increase), liver and bile duct (77% increase), and thyroid (99% increase).[15] If a shortage of surgeons performing these procedures does occur, the result will inevitably be decreased access to care. To prevent this from happening, the ability of surgeons to cope with an increased burden of work needs to be critically evaluated and improved. Given that there are a limited number of surgical oncologists produced each year (55 in the United States and 8 in Canada), it is clear that the traditional surgical oncology educational roles in academic medical centers as well as in the larger health care community will continue and perhaps come under increasing pressure to expand.

As multimodality care grows in complexity and chemotherapy/radiotherapy move more prominently into the neoadjuvant position, surgical oncologists will have to become increasingly involved in clinical trial design. To be effective in this arena, understanding the natural history of specific malignancies will require an expanded knowledge base about the mutated genes and their cognate proteins that drive solid tumor proliferation and metastasis. Surgical oncologists will have to become more knowledgeable about these factors, both during training and as a lifelong commitment to self-education.

An important effort to strengthen the position of surgical oncology in medical community has been establishing board certification in surgical oncology, beginning in 2014. The past half-century has seen the unprecedented evolution of surgical specialties into their current status as discrete disciplines, with specialized knowledge, techniques, anatomic challenges, and diseases of focus. This is especially true in surgical oncology, which has attracted many owing to its strong allure as a combination of the technical and the cognitive. There is an emerging understanding that the surgical oncologist has specialized knowledge that is not acquired in general surgical training: knowledge of the natural history of malignant disease, knowledge of the multidisciplinary care for the cancer patient, and, certainly, knowledge of how to perform some very unusual and technically demanding oncological operative procedures. These factors, coupled with an awareness of the rapidly increasing manpower need, have led to creating a board certification mechanism for surgical oncology. Entitled board certification in *complex general surgical oncology*, the assessment process includes both a written and oral examination component. Eligibility to sit for these examinations is limited to graduates of American Council of Graduate Medical Education (ACGME) accredited surgical oncology fellowship programs, meaning that graduates of such fellowship program that were not ACGME accredited at the time of an individual fellowship graduation renders such individuals ineligible for *complex general surgical oncology* board certification. This stipulation effectively limits the annual total number of board eligible candidates, yet has resulted in a significant increase of the fellowship applicant pool in the United States over the past two decades. Board certification will strengthen the position and impact of surgical oncologists practicing in the community and academic environments and might also aid in the development of comparable certification mechanisms in other countries, leading to enhanced cancer care worldwide.

References

1 Birkmeyer JD, Warshaw AL, Finlayson SR, et al. Relationship between hospital volume and late survival after pancreaticoduodenectomy. *Surgery*. 1999;**126**:178–183.
2 Breasted JH. *The Edwin Smith Surgical Papyrus*. Chicago: University of Chicago Press; 1930.
3 Hill GJII. Historic milestones in cancer surgery. *Semin Oncol*. 1979;**6**:409–427.
4 Faguet GB. A brief history of cancer: age-old milestones underlying our current knowledge database. *Int J Cancer*. 2015;**136**:2022–2036.
5 Saklad M. Grading of patients for surgical procedures. *Anesthesiology*. 1941;**2**:281.
6 Oken M, Creech R, Tormey D, et al. Toxocity and response criteria of the Eastern Cooperative Oncology Group. *Am J Clin Oncol*. 1982;**5**:649–655.
7 Karnofsky D, Burchenal J. The clinical evaluation of chemotherapeutic agents in cancer. In: MacLeod C, ed. *Evaluation of Chemotherapeutics Agents*. New York, NY: Columbia University Press; 1949:191–205.
8 Cohen ME, Liu Y, Ko CY, Hall BL. An examination of American College of Surgeons NSQIP surgical risk calculator accuracy. *J Am Coll Surg*. 2017;**224**(5):787–795.
9 Scappaticci FA, Fehrenbacher L, Cartwright T, et al. Surgical wound healing complications in metastatic colorectal cancer patients treated with bevacizumab. *J Surg Oncol*. 2005;**91**:173–180.
10 Morton DL, Wen D-R, Wong JH, et al. Technical details of intraoperative lymphatic mapping for melanoma. *Arch Surg*. 1992;**127**:392–399.
11 Giuliano AE, Kirgan DM, Guenther JM, Morton DL. Lymphatic mapping and sentinel lymphadenectomy for breast cancer. *Ann Surg*. 1994;**220**:391–398.
12 Koch WM, Choti MA, Civelek AC, et al. Gamma probe-directed biopsy of the sentinel node in oral squamous cell carcinoma. *Arch Otolaryngol Head Neck Surg*. 1998;**124**:455–459.
13 Pawlik TM, Scoggins CR, Zorzi D, et al. Effect of surgical margin status on survival and site of recurrence after hepatic resection for colorectal metastases. *Ann Surg*. 2005;**241**:715–722.
14 Sterodimas A, De Faria J, Correa WE, Pitanguy I. Tissue engineering in plastic surgery: an up-to-date review of the current literature. *Ann Plast Surg*. 2009;**62**(1):97–103.
15 Rahib L, Smith BD, Aizenberg R, et al. Projecting cancer incidence and deaths to 2030: the unexpected burden of thyroid, liver, and pancreas cancers in the United States. *Cancer Res*. 2014;**74**(11):2913–2921.

42 Principles of radiation oncology

Scott R. Floyd, MD, PhD ■ Justus Adamson, PhD ■ Philip P. Connell, MD ■ Ralph R. Weichselbaum, MD ■ Christopher G. Willett, MD

Overview

Ionizing radiation can halt the growth of cells, mainly through the induction of damage in DNA. Cancerous cells differ from normal cells in their response to this radiation-induced DNA damage, creating a therapeutic window that is exploited in the clinical practice of radiation oncology to stop cancer cells while protecting normal tissues. This article will introduce the basic concepts behind the physics of radiation interaction with tissues, radiation treatment modalities and the radiation biology of treatment responses. Current concepts from the forefront of radiation physics and biology that may shape the future of radiation oncology are also presented.

Introduction

Electromagnetic radiation of sufficient energy to ionize has cytotoxic properties. In the early twentieth century, the first users of man-made radiation sources (such as cathode ray tubes) and naturally occurring radioactive isotopes discovered this cytotoxicity as skin damage and hair loss following radiation exposure.[1] A brief summary of the cytotoxic action of radiation is that through both direct ionization and formation of highly reactive chemical species in cells, radiation damages many biomolecules. The damage sustained in DNA, however, is the most consequential, especially in rapidly dividing cells. Therefore, cytotoxic effects of ionizing radiation are manifest in highly proliferative cancer cells, as well as rapidly dividing healthy cells such as those found in continuously replenishing tissues (skin, GI tract, and bone marrow), or, in the case of children exposed to radiation, cells in many tissues that are actively growing. Over the past several decades, detection and control of ionizing radiation have greatly improved, creating new imaging and therapeutic advances. Current physics and engineering allow direction of radiation energy and fluence to precisely deposit ionizing photons and charged particles, enabling steep dose gradients to maximize radiation dose in tumors while sparing normal tissue. Many biological factors such as DNA repair capacity, intracellular signaling, and immune system state also contribute to tumor control from radiation therapy. Our growing understanding of tumor biology and the immune system's ability to control cancer now holds promise for optimal leverage of radiation therapy to improve local/regional control, and perhaps systemic cancer control, likely in combination with surgery and medical therapy. This article will summarize the basic principles behind the use of ionizing radiation for tumor therapy and give an overview of current clinical radiation therapy with some historical context.

The physics of radiation therapy

Fundamental principles

The ionization potential of a photon or charged particle is related to its energy. For photons, energy is inversely related to wavelength, while for particles, energy depends on the particle's mass and velocity. When using standard units, energies of less than 10 keV rarely ionize, while 10–100 keV photons create ionizations useful for imaging (primarily photoelectric effect) and higher energy photons (1–20 MeV) penetrate deeper in tissue before causing efficient ionizations useful for therapy (primarily Compton effect and pair production).

The fundamental unit of radiation therapy is the Gray (Gy). This unit measures the amount of energy deposited in tissue and has S.I. units of Joules/kilogram (J/kg). 1 Gy is equivalent to 1 J deposited in 1 kg and corresponds to 100 cGy (historically termed rads). Ionization events from radiation are most easily measured in air and have the unit of Roentgen (R). In tissue, 1 R = ~0.9 cGy.

Clinical radiation therapy delivery can be classified into two broad categories: teletherapy and brachytherapy. Teletherapy (also called external beam, or EBRT) constitutes the majority of current practice and involves radiation beams directed at the tumor (tele-Greek for "at a distance"). Brachytherapy involves radioactive sources placed near the tumor (brachy-Greek for "short"). High energy photons (6–20 MeV) that deposit dose deep in tissue and spare skin are most commonly used for teletherapy, while electrons can be used to treat superficial tumors. Protons and other heavy charged particles require complex specialized therapy equipment but can deposit dose at a range in tissue dependent on energy of the particle.

Beam production for external beam radiotherapy

The evolution of external beam radiation therapy begins with cathode-ray tubes, first described by Roentgen in 1895.[2] In a cathode ray tube, X-rays are produced by "Bremsstrahlung" or "braking radiation" in which electrons from a heated cathode filament are accelerated through an electrical field into a high atomic number anode (usually copper or tungsten). As the electrons collide with the anode, they change momentum, generating photons through conservation of energy. The energy of the photons corresponds to the strength of the electrical field across which the electrons are accelerated. Cathode ray tubes can generally produce electrical potentials between 50 and 360 kV and are used in diagnostic X-ray imaging equipment. Cathode ray tubes and radioactive isotopes (such as radium) were the only therapeutic source of radiation until the advent of other devices in the late 1930s, when the Van de Graf generator (~1–2 MeV), and later the betatron (2–45 MeV, 1949) and synthetic radioactive isotopes (cobalt 60, ^{60}Co, 1.1 MeV, 1951) entered use. ^{60}Co was used for much of treatment in the period between ~1950 and ~1980 and is still in use internationally as well as in the GammaKnife stereotactic treatment device.

Modern photon beams are generated from electron linear accelerators with nominal energies of 6–15 MeV. The linear accelerator uses a waveguide that maintains standing or traveling microwaves generated by a magnetron or klystron to accelerate electrons to high energies into a tungsten target, producing Bremsstrahlung photons at high dose delivery rates.

In addition to photon-based external beam radiation therapy, charged particles can also be used for radiotherapy, most commonly electrons and protons. Electrons are generated by the same linear accelerators used for photon therapy by removing the Bremsstrahlung target, substantially lowering the beam current, and incorporating specialized scattering and collimation hardware. Electron therapy is used clinically to treat to depths of 1.5–4 cm, making electron therapy especially useful for skin treatments.

Heavy charged particle therapy leverages the phenomenon of the "Bragg Peak," a concentrated deposition of energy. Particle beam energy can be modified to tune the width and depth in tissue at which this peak occurs to match the treatment volume. Thus, the Bragg Peak represents a major theoretical advantage over other radiation therapy modalities. Currently, the most comprehensive data demonstrating a benefit comes from long-term follow-up of pediatric patients treated with protons.[3,4] Because heavy charged particles such as protons and as carbon ions require highly specialized and complex equipment, fewer than 100 proton and 15 carbon ion centers are currently in use worldwide. More centers are planned and may make particle therapy available for more patients in the future.

Modern beam modulation and treatment planning

Advances in linear accelerator design involve devices that control the shape, direction, and fluence of the beam. In teletherapy machines, the photon source (the gantry) rotates around the patient, enabling avoidance of normal tissues through delivery of beams from multiple directions, or with moving "arc" therapy. The beam shape itself can also be conformed to the shape of the tumor or target region to optimize dose distribution. This is accomplished with movable "jaws" that shape the beam into rectangular fields. These fields are further conformed to nonrectangular shapes with customized blocks, historically made from lead alloy. Early radiation therapy treatment planning incorporated conventional X-ray imaging of target and normal tissue for "2D" planning, wherein idealized calculations for standardized field sizes approximated delivered dose. Computed tomography (CT)-based planning incorporates "3D" imaging and targeting of tumor tissue, and advanced forms of 3D planning incorporate tissue attenuation of the treatment beam, calculated from CT Houndsfield units, to improve accuracy of dose calculation.

Current linear accelerators contain a motorized system that allows adjustment of the field aperture based on electronic control of a series of individual tungsten "leaves" each 0.25–1.0 cm wide in a unit called a multi-leaf collimator. This greatly increases the throughput of treatment and reduces the physical labor, resource consumption, and environmental concerns of customized lead alloy blocks. The multi-leaf collimator also enables precise control over the fluence of photons throughout the treatment field. This control is coupled with CT-based treatment planning to determine optimal fluence through tissue to distribute dose in three-dimensional space. These planning techniques are now commonly used in a technique known as intensity-modulated radiation therapy, or IMRT. Combinations of IMRT with arc therapy provide some of the most advanced and precise photon treatments, yielding dose distributions that conform tightly to target tissue. Notably, the delivery of these complex treatments is critically dependent on patient immobilization and localization of the target and normal tissue during treatment.

Radiation therapy imaging and target localization

For accurate and effective radiation therapy, the locations of tumor and normal tissues in the treatment plan must be aligned to their actual position in the patient during treatment delivery. Currently, a planning session, also called a "simulation," uses CT imaging on a treatment couch designed like the treatment machine couch to create planning imaging data. Modern radiation planning is almost exclusively CT-based, as CT data provide the 3D and tissue attenuation information needed for IMRT and other advanced dosimetry calculations. However, simple 2D images can be used for rapid and emergency treatments with rectangular fields and dose estimations. Additional imaging modalities that give better anatomical information, such as MRI (brain and pelvic tumors), PET imaging (head, neck, and lung tumors), and ultrasound (prostate tumors) can also be registered with the planning CT to improve tumor and normal tissue targeting. Use of MRI as the primary data set for simulation (MRI simulation) is an ongoing recent development that offers the advantage of decreased ionizing dose from imaging for the patient. The main technical challenge for MRI simulation is that the conversion of MRI intensity to electron density for dose calculation is not straightforward.[5,6]

Currently, linear accelerators have diagnostic X-ray sources and detectors mounted at 90° to the treatment source. This diagnostic imaging equipment is used to take both static X-ray images of the treatment field and "cone-beam CT" images when the treatment gantry is rotated around the patient while X-ray images are detected.[7] These CT images allow adjustments to patient positioning to improve accuracy of radiation delivery. Other advanced techniques to improve radiation targeting and verification include X-ray equipment mounted in the treatment room with automatic feedback to correct the couch positioning and/or robotic positioning of the treatment machine.[8,9] Other imaging modalities and detection technologies can also be included to improve targeting, such as radiographic or radiofrequency fiducial marker placement in the tumor[10] or ultrasound and even MRI imaging integrated with the treatment machine.[11,12]

Brachytherapy

Brachytherapy involves placement of radioactive sources in or near the malignancy. The intrinsic physical properties of the radioactive sources are such that dose decreases dramatically with distance from the source. Therefore, by positioning the sources in direct proximity to the tumor, a conformal treatment of the tumor is achieved. Sealed sources are commonly used in brachytherapy which contain the isotope in a metal cylinder or wire so that no radioactive material is able to diffuse away from the source. Sealed sources can be implanted permanently (as in the case of ^{125}Iodine therapy for prostate cancer) or temporarily placed near tumor using an applicator (as with ^{137}Cs or ^{192}Ir for gynecological malignancies). Sealed sources (such as commonly used ^{192}Ir and ^{137}Cs) are often both beta (electron) or gamma (photon) emitters, but the energy is low such that only tissues near the source receive high dose. As mentioned above, the rate of dose deposition can be either high (HDR as with ^{192}Ir,) or low (LDR, commonly with ^{137}Cs) which dictates how the radiation is administered (i.e., in daily fractions lasting less than 1 h for HDR) or over days (36–72 h as with LDR).

Unsealed sources are often similar to natural biological compounds and are designed to enter the body and home to the disease site through the intrinsic properties of the radioactive molecule. An idealized example is radioactive iodine (usually ^{131}I) for the treatment of thyroid cancer and other thyroid conditions, as thyroid cells efficiently concentrate iodine. Other examples include radium (^{223}Ra) which is taken up by osteoblasts owing to properties similar to calcium and can be used to treat prostate cancer blastic bone metastases. MIBG (meta-iodobenzylguanidine) can be labeled with iodine isotopes and is chemically similar to norepinephrine and therefore concentrated by tumors such as neuroblastoma and pheochromocytoma. Somatostatin analogs can be labeled with the beta-emitter lutetium (^{177}Lu) and used to treat neuroendocrine tumors that overexpress the somatostatin receptor. One additional therapy that deserves mention is Yttrium microspheres, which can be thought of as intermediate between sealed sources and unsealed sources.[13,14] These 20–60 μm spheres are tiny sealed sources that are designed to flow intra-arterially and reach small capillaries that feed a tumor where they lodge and both cause tumor ischemia and deliver radiation dose from beta-emitting ^{90}Yt. This therapy can be used to treat tumors of the liver, where catheterization of the hepatic arteries is possible owing to dual circulation of the portal system.

The biology of radiation therapy

Radiation interactions with biological molecules

When tissues are exposed to high energy radiation, the resulting ionizations react with biomolecules such as DNA, RNA, lipids, and proteins in the tissue, either through "direct action" (ionization of biomolecules) or through "indirect action": ionization and hydrolysis of water, resulting in formation of highly reactive free radicals that then subsequently interact with biomolecules. Radiation-induced changes to these different biomolecules can all contribute to the cytotoxic effects of radiation therapy. Some studies have demonstrated radiation-induced membrane lipid reactions and subsequent pro-apoptotic signaling, especially in endothelial cells,[15,16] as well as intracellular signaling triggered by increased reactive oxygen species.[17,18] Radiation also alters cytokines such as TGF-beta and TNF-alpha,[19,20] which can mediate some of the toxic effects of radiation, and may be important in the context of immune therapy, as discussed in more detail below.

Radiation-induced DNA damage

While radiation-induced reactions with other biomolecules likely play a role in the tumor and normal tissue response to radiation, the damage sustained in DNA is the most consequential in terms of cytotoxicity, as unrepaired DNA damage can directly cause cell death and permanently alter the genetic code, resulting in changes in gene transcription and protein function. Ionizing radiation can cause multiple different types of DNA damage, including base damage, single strand, and double strand breaks (DSBs) of the DNA helix. Of these types of DNA damage, the most toxic is the DSB. Of note, 1 Gy of radiation typically produces about 1000 single strand breaks and ~40 double strand breaks in tissue. Cells possess a robust machinery to detect and repair DNA damage. This machinery is activated by ionizing radiation-induced DNA damage and triggers a response in cells. The DNA damage response is also important in preventing cancer initiation by enabling repair of DNA damage that occurs through natural metabolism and environmental exposures. As a consequence, many of the genes involved in the DNA damage response to ionizing radiation are also important tumor suppressor genes.

The DNA damage response

The DNA damage response can be divided into phases: (1) DNA damage sensing, (2) recruitment of signaling and repair factors, (3) propagation of the DNA damage response signal, (4) arrest of the cell cycle and repair of the damage, or signaling to cell death machinery (Figure 1). In the DNA damage detection phase of the DNA damage response, damaged DNA can cause physical changes in the structure of chromatin (which is the collection of proteins that packages DNA). Some of the earliest known events in the DNA damage detection phase involve these chromatin structure changes that are detected by the KAT5 (Tip60) acetyl-transferase enzyme, activating its enzymatic activity and causing acetylation of chromatin and the Atm kinase.[21] The ATM gene (encodes the Atm protein kinase) is named for the genetic cancer-predisposition syndrome ataxia-telangiectasia, in which mutations in the ATM gene lead to leukemia, brain tumors, and other cancers.[22] This is an important kinase, which when activated, phosphorylates many substrates to propagate the DNA damage signal throughout the cell, thereby participating in the propagation phase of DNA damage signaling. An important protein complex in the detection phase of the DNA damage response is the MRN complex, consisting of Mre11, Rad50, and Nbs1. The NBN gene (encodes the Nbs1 protein) is mutated in the Nijmegen breakage syndrome, another cancer predisposition syndrome causing defective DNA damage signaling and repair, and resulting in characteristics of microcephaly, immune dysfunction, and non-Hodgkin's lymphoma.[23] The MRN complex is recruited to sites of DNA damage (DSBs) very early in the signaling cascade and can also activate the Atm kinase.[24]

As described above, Atm is an important kinase involved in the detection and propagation phases of DNA damage signaling. The Atm kinase is a member of a family of serine-threonine protein kinases that bear sequence homology to the lipid kinase, phosphatidyl inositol-3 kinase (PI3K), and are therefore called PIK-related protein kinases (PIKKs). The other members of this kinase family are Atr (encoded by the ATR gene, named for Ataxia telangiectasia-Rad3-related), DNApkcs (encoded by the PRKDC gene), mTOR (MTOR gene, for mammalian target of rapamycin), TRAPP (transformation/transcription domain associated protein), and SMG1 (suppressor of morphogenesis of genitalia).[25] Many of these PIKK family members have important roles in DNA damage: DNApkcs is the key kinase mediator of the nonhomologous end-joining (NHEJ) pathway which is most active in the G_0 and G_1 phases of the cell cycle.[26–29] Atr mediates replication stress signaling. SMG1 regulates the splicing of many DNA damage factors.[30] MTOR is important for metabolic signaling and is an important cancer therapy target. This protein kinase family (except for TRAPP, which has sequence homology but no known kinase activity) has a similar substrate preference for serine or threonine followed by glutamine (S/T-Q, in single-letter amino acid code).[31,32] This fact enabled elegant studies to define

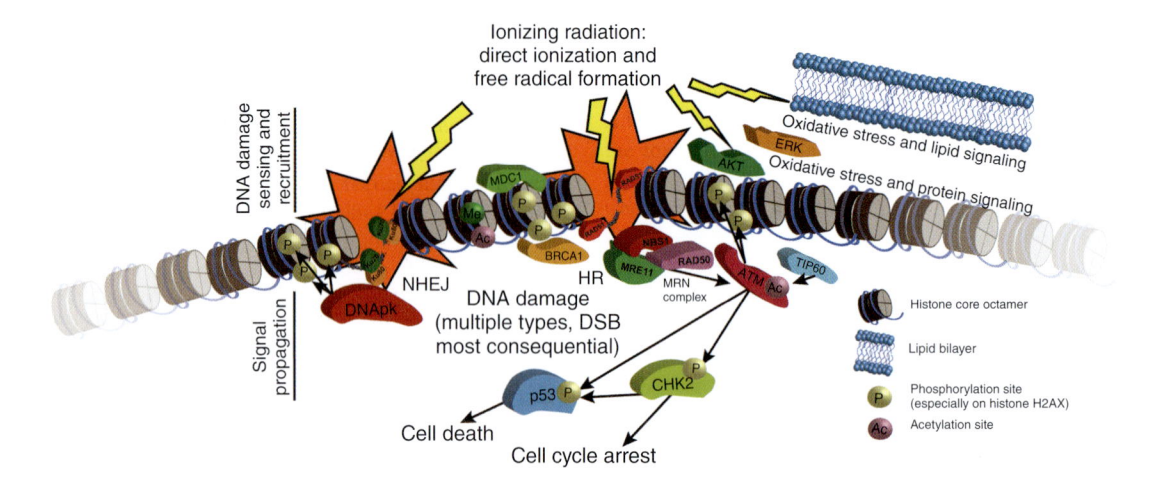

Figure 1 The cellular response to ionizing radiation. Ionizing radiation causes many cellular effects, including free radical formation, oxidative stress, and direct ionization of biological molecules. A principal consequence of ionizing radiation exposure is DNA damage. Many different types of DNA damage occur, but double strand breaks (DSB) are the most lethal to the cell. Molecular components of the major DSB repair pathways, nonhomologous end joining (NHEJ), and homologous recombination (HR) are shown.

many of the additional components of the DNA damage signaling pathway, through sequence and antibody-based screens for phosphor-serine/threonine-glutamine (pS/T-Q)-containing substrates.[31,33]

The signaling network around the recruitment phase of the DNA damage response was further elucidated by the discovery of BRCT phospho-peptide binding domains.[34,35] These protein domains are named for homology with the BRCA1 protein, another key signaling protein in the DNA damage response, and a major cancer predisposition gene. Mutations in this gene are known to cause breast, ovarian, prostate, and pancreatic cancers. The function of the BRCT domain is to interact with phosphorylated S/T-Q sites, thereby extending the signaling network. Many DNA damage response proteins contain either pS/T-Q sites or BRCT domains enabling identification of much of the signaling network. An example of how part of the signaling network functions is as follows: One important protein that contains an S-Q site is the histone H2AX. Very early in the DNA damage response, this protein is phosphorylated at the S-Q site, by either ATM, DNApkcs, or ATR, depending on the phase of the cell cycle during which the DNA damage occurs. In G_0–G_1: DNApkcs activity and NHEJ is more likely, in S-G_2-M, ATM activation and homologous recombination (HR) is more possible owing to the second copy of the DNA template made in S phase that is required for HR, while specifically in S phase, replication fork conflicts activate Atr. Regardless of which PIKK kinase is activated, the phosphorylated H2AX (at serine 139 in human cells) is an important signaling event in the DNA damage response (H2AX phosphorylation is also an important marker used in DNA damage research studies). Phosphorylated H2AX can then serve as a docking site for the BRCT domains of MDC1, an important scaffolding protein.[36] MDC1 can help assemble the MRN complex, which can further accelerate activation of Atm, and phosphorylation of other substrates, with recruitment of additional BRCT-containing signaling mediators. Alternatively, MDC1 can also recruit RNF8, a ubiquitin ligase that triggers a ubiquitin signaling cascade that recruits 53BP1.[37] 53BP1 can block the activity of MRE11, and instead trigger NHEJ.[38] In either case, the recruitment and signal propagation phases of DNA damage are promoted through a feed-forward mechanism involving kinase and ubiquitin ligase activation, with subsequent recruitment of phospho- and ubiquitin-binding proteins, further activation of kinases, and subsequent substrate phosphorylation and ubiquitylation. Other signaling cascades such as poly-ADP ribose (through poly-ADP ribose polymerase, or PARP enzymes) are also involved.[39]

Cell cycle control and checkpoints

Once activated, the DNA damage PIKK kinases can also phosphorylate other "downstream" signaling molecules to transmit the DNA damage response throughout the cell. Important downstream signaling factors include the checkpoint kinases Chk1 (phosphorylated mainly by Atr)[40] and Chk2 (phosphorylated by Atm).[41] These checkpoint kinases are activated by phosphorylation, and then trigger the halting of the cell cycle by phosphorylating key cell cycle regulators such as Cdc25a and p53. Radiation triggers a p53-dependent transcriptional program that can arrest the cell cycle and/or induce senescence or apoptotic cell death, depending on the cell type and cell state. Of note, mutations in Chk2 (breast, ovarian) and p53 (Li Fraumeni syndrome- many tumor types) also lead to cancer, again demonstrating the importance of the DNA damage response in tumor suppression. Other key regulators of cell cycle progression include Cdk4/6 and WEE1, which are now targets of clinical small-molecule inhibitors.[42,43]

DNA repair mechanisms

Repair of DNA double strand breaks is an important function of normal cells. Certain cell types, such as B and T lymphocytes, have mechanisms that introduce genomic DNA DSBs and repair them via error-prone NHEJ in order to introduce diversity in the sequences of immunoglobulins and T-cell receptors. Mutations that abrogate function of NHEJ proteins can lead to severe immune deficiency syndromes.[44,45] Of note, CRISPR (clustered regularly interspersed palindromic repeat)-Cas9 gene knockout strategies, now in common laboratory use, also utilize NHEJ to repair DSBs introduced by the Cas9 nuclease guided by RNA molecules with homology to specific genomic sites. In this way, small insertions and deletions are introduced into genes, thereby disrupting the coding sequence.[46]

A second important pathway of DNA DSB repair is HR, wherein a DNA template is copied to repair the break and preserve DNA sequence fidelity. As noted above, several important

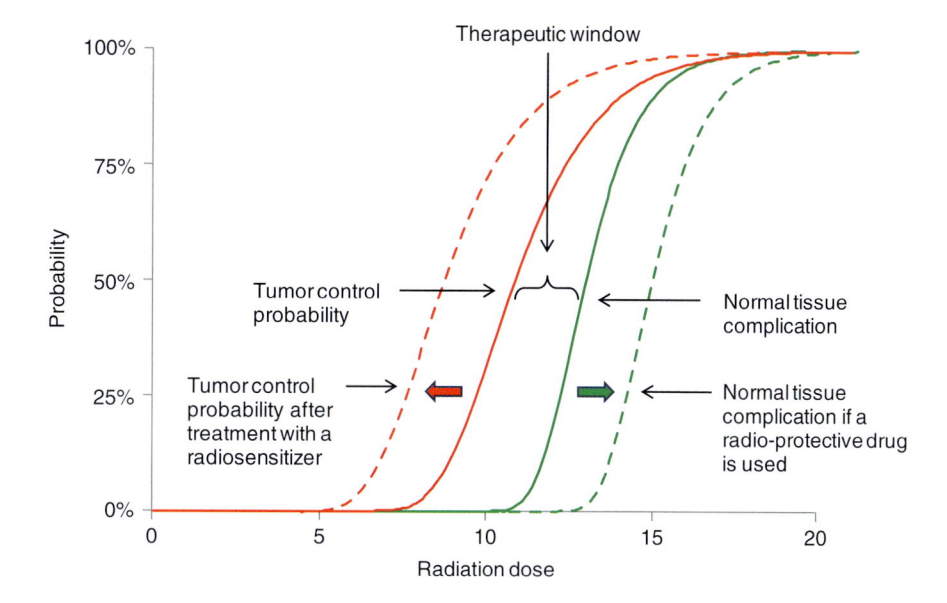

Figure 2 The therapeutic window. Efficacy of radiation therapy can be explained by a differential response of cancer cells compared to normal tissue cells. This difference in response, called "therapeutic window," is modeled by parallel curves representing the probability of cancer and normal cell lethality versus radiation dose. Factors that preferentially enhance cancer cell death (radiosensitizers), or protect normal cells (radiation protectors, dose fractionation), can widen therapeutic window.

tumor suppressor proteins are part of the HR pathway, including ATM, BRCA1, BRCA2, and Chk2. Defects in this high-fidelity DNA repair pathway can lead to cancer-causing mutations. Also, current laboratory gene editing techniques utilize HR repair of Cas9-induced DSBs and an artificially introduced template DNA to change genomic DNA sequence.[47] HR also has implications for the clinical use of PARP inhibitors. PARP inhibitors lock the PARP enzyme onto chromatin and inhibit the progression of the replication fork in dividing cells. These stalled forks are repaired and restarted by HR pathways. Normal cells can therefore tolerate PARP inhibition, as HR pathways are intact, but cancer cells that lack HR function are preferentially damaged by PARP inhibition and die. This phenomenon, known as synthetic lethality, is elegantly demonstrated for BRCA-mutant cells.[48–50]

In addition to NHEJ and HR, there are other repair pathways that have important roles in DSB repair, especially as potential therapeutic targets. DNA polymerase theta mediates microhomology-mediated repair, also called alternative-end joining (alt-EJ) or theta-mediated end joining (TMEJ), and recently, polymerase theta-specific inhibitors have been identified.[51] Other mechanisms of DSB repair include breakpoint induction replication (BIR) and microhomology-mediated template switching.

Therapeutic window

Radiation therapy can affect normal and neoplastic tissue differently. The different responses in normal neoplastic tissue form the basis of the "Therapeutic Ratio" or "Therapeutic Index" and can be represented as a dual sigmoidal curve of effect on tumors and normal tissues as a function of increasing radiation dose (Figure 2). The "therapeutic window" is the idealized area in that dual curve that indicates potent tumor kill (efficacy) with low normal tissue damage (side effects). Current clinical radiation therapy takes advantage of dose and fractionation schedules to optimize the therapeutic window for any given irradiated site. Moreover, a fundamental goal of radiation research is to widen the therapeutic window by employing strategies to radiosensitize tumor tissue, and/or radioprotect normal tissue.

Cell cycle arrest and DNA repair in normal tissues: dose fractionation

As discussed previously, many cancer cells have defects in cell cycle checkpoints and DNA damage signaling and repair pathways. It is likely that these defects are intricately tied to the development of cancer, as such circumstances facilitate the genomic instability, mutations, and other alterations in gene function that promote the unlimited cell growth, invasion, and other features that are hallmarks of cancer.[52] Therefore, one strategy to exploit this difference in DNA damage response and repair is through the delivery of a total radiation dose in multiple small doses (fractions) of radiation administered at regular times (fractionation). This is particularly useful when irradiating larger fields containing mixed tumor and normal cells. With this strategy, normal tissues usually sustain radiation doses that are not lethal (termed "sub-lethal") and can repair the DNA damage, while cancer cells with defective DNA damage response die. The DNA damage response differences between normal and neoplastic tissue are exploited by the repeated administration of small sub-lethal radiation doses to a maximum tolerated normal tissue radiation dose, which has comparatively greater lethal effect on cancer cells.

Radiosensitization

Many cytotoxic chemotherapies are used as radiation sensitizers. Examples include 5-fluorouracil (5-FU) in gastro-intestinal malignancies, and platinum compounds in squamous cell carcinomas. Combined chemo-radiation is the current standard of care for many solid tumors. While these cytotoxic chemotherapies are excellent radiosensitizers, and work by increasing DNA damage (cisplatin) and impairing DNA replication and repair (5-FU), as with radiation therapy, they rely on the same cancer cell properties of elevated replication and DNA damage response and repair inefficiencies for their therapeutic window. Therapy toxicity and side effects are therefore often elevated with these combined treatments. Optimal radiation sensitizers would exploit unique cancer cell vulnerabilities to enhance radiation effects. Some progress in this respect comes from molecularly targeted agents such as the epidermal growth factor receptor (EGFR) blocking antibody cetuximab. Combining EGFR-targeted therapy with radiation proved beneficial over radiation alone for squamous-cell head and neck cancer[53]; however, this combination has increased side effects, and later work proved inferiority to combined radiation and cisplatin chemotherapy.[54,55] Other examples include erlotinib with radiation.[56] Of note, small-molecule inhibitors of the DNA damage PIKKs (ATM, ATR, and DNAPKCs) show potent radiosensitization effects in preclinical models, and some are in clinical trials.[57,58] Careful combination with precise targeting and timing of radiation may mitigate against normal tissue toxicity, and results from these trials are anxiously awaited. Molecular biomarkers can also direct the use of cytotoxic chemotherapies as radiosensitizers, as in the case of temozolomide, where methylation of the promoter of the MGMT gene identifies a subset of glioblastoma patients who respond much better to combined temozolomide/radiation.[59]

Biomarkers, in general, can also identify tumor subtypes that are predicted to have superior response to radiation therapy. This can be especially important for treatment planning, as well as clinical trial selection, as these biomarkers can allow dose reduction and lower side effect risk. Examples include Epstein–Barr virus (EBV) positive nasopharyngeal carcinoma, and human papillomavirus (HPV) positive squamous cell carcinoma of the head and neck.[60,61] Other experimental predictive markers of radiation response show promise and are in clinical trials. Several approaches use gene expression patterns and focus on expression of DNA repair factors.[62–64]

The therapeutic window can also be widened by radioprotecting normal tissues. Successes with this approach include amifostine, which protects normal tissue mucosa and achieved FDA approval,[65] albeit with significant side effects. Other approaches include magnesium porphyrin compounds (BMX-001) that are currently in clinical trials.[66] These compounds scavenge free radicals and may also have radiosensitizing effects in cancer cells owing to abnormal tumor cell mitochondrial function. Additional approaches such as the keratinocyte growth factor palifermin promote healing and recovery of normal tissue.[67]

Current concepts in radiobiology

High dose per fraction/ablative radiation therapy

Current technologies for precise control over radiation dose and advanced, real-time imaging enable high dose radiation delivery in a single or a limited number of treatments.[68] This approach is in contrast to "conventional" fractionated radiation treatment (see above), wherein small daily doses of ~2 Gray are administered. These high-dose-per-fraction (DPF) strategies can be very effective for tumor control and rely on steep dose gradients to reduce the risk of damage to nearby normal tissue. There is evidence that high DPF radiation may achieve increased efficacy owing to enhanced biological effects on blood vessels and other tumor features.[15,16,69–72] Regardless of the biological effect, the practical consequence of more rapid delivery of radiation is that patients have reduced treatment times, and through more precise dosing to tumor and physical/anatomical protection of normal tissues, may have reduced side effects. Partly owing to the relative simplicity of immobilizing the brain and advent of neurosurgical stereotaxis techniques, this high DPF radiation approach has been used for many years in the treatment of brain tumors, especially metastatic and benign tumors, where diffuse invasion of tumor cells is less common.[73–75] More recently, as technology to immobilize and/or visualize and treat tumors has improved, this practice has gained favor for the treatment of other tumor sites, including head and neck tumors, early-stage lung cancer, spine tumors, liver, kidney, prostate and GI tumors.[76,77] These stereotactic techniques enable the routine high DPF treatment of many disease sites with the intent of ablating these tumors with low side effects. This can clearly benefit patients with early-stage disease through treatment of the primary site, as in lung[78] and prostate cancer[79]) and can effectively treat metastatic sites for symptom relief. However, the role of stereotactic ablative radiotherapy may be expanding. For many years, debate has continued over the existence of a group of cancer patients, with a limited extent of metastatic disease, who could be cured by eradication of the few metastatic sites.[80,81] With the advent of stereotactic ablative techniques, the ability to treat metastatic sites has expanded. Now, there is evidence that, for a select group of patients with limited metastatic disease, this approach may yield survival benefit.[77]

"Flash" radiation therapy

As discussed above, the concept of fractionation has relevance to repair of DNA damage, such that delivering a total dose of radiation over a longer period of time can allow normal tissues to repair radiation-generated DNA damage. A simple statement of this concept treats fractionation as a rate of dose delivery. Therefore, a slower rate of dose delivery (multiple daily fractions) allows for DNA repair, while high DPF radiation may allow less repair potential. This concept is also demonstrated with brachytherapy where low-dose-rate (LDR) and high-dose-rate (HDR) isotopes can be employed. In HDR brachytherapy, dose is delivered in daily fractions to enable some normal tissue DNA repair in the time between fractions, while LDR sources are implanted and deliver dose continually over several days, but the lower dose rate still enables normal tissue repair. A recent and surprising finding is that there appears to be an exception to this general relationship between dose rate and normal tissue radiation tolerance, such that normal tissues tolerate extremely high dose rates (usually >40 Gy/s) better than tumors.[82–85] Technological advances in linear accelerator and proton beam design enable these extremely high dose rates. The physical, chemical, and biological details of radiation effects in cells and tissues at these extremely high dose rates are under investigation, but an initial report of clinical use of this technology is encouraging.[86]

Radiation interactions with the immune system

The role of the immune system in cancer suppression has been postulated since the nineteenth century when German physicians Fehleison and Busch and later William Coley identified a relationship between *Streptococcous pyogenes* infection and sarcoma regression.[87] It was not until the late twentieth and early twenty-first century that the first successful immune therapies were harnessed to attack cancer.[88–92] Currently, biological agents that enable T-cells to attack cancer are in clinical use for many tumor types. Strong preclinical and some encouraging clinical evidence points to a synergy of immune therapy with radiation.[93–95] Immune effects are postulated as a potential mechanism for the abscopal effect, in which irradiation of a tumor results in regression of unirradiated tumors at remote sites. The abscopal effect

Table 1 Radiation therapy techniques and their clinical use.

	Fractionated XRT with photons 3D-CRT, IMRT	Ablative methods of XRT SRS, SBRT	XRT with particle beams proton or carbon ion beam therapy	Brachytherapy intracavitary or interstitial
Common indications	Many	Brain metastases Early-stage lung cancer Oligo-metastatic disease	Pediatric malignancies Uveal melanoma Chordoma	Prostate cancer Cervical cancer
Illustrations	An anal cancer was treated with different types of X-ray-based XRT	These treatments involve specialized approaches that enable delivery of ablative doses, using a single or a few[1-5] large fractions	Proton beam therapy generates specific dose distributions in tissue	Radioactive sources are positioned within or near a target volume. This limits exposure to surrounding tissue. This represent a common and effective treatment for prostate cancer, wherein permanent seeds placed from a perineal approach using real-time imaging via trans-rectal ultrasound
	The yellow shaded area denotes the target volume, which includes the anus/rectum and the draining lymph nodes. The pelvic bones and bladder represent the adjacent normal tissues in this situation	Numerous intersecting beams chosen generate very conformal plans that markedly reduce normal tissue exposure	XRT is used to treat the craniospinal axis of a child with medulloblastoma. The proton-based treatment results in less exposure to normal tissues located anterior to the spinal column	
	The IMRT-based plan conforms to the shape of the target more closely, thereby exposing less normal tissue to treatment 3D-CRT: 45 Gy at 1.8 Gy/fx IMRT: 45 Gy at 1.8 Gy/fx	SRS for brain metastasis: 18 Gy delivered in a single fraction SBRT for lung cancer: 12 Gy/fraction delivered over 5 fractions	Photons protons Craniospinal radiation: 36 Gy at 1.8 Gy/fraction	A plain film X-ray shows small seeds throughout the prostate (contrast media fills the bladder) Implant dosimetry: 145 Gy
Distinguishing features	These treatments are among the most widely used forms of radiotherapy	Advanced targeting enables steep dose gradients, which allow for tolerance of large fraction sizes. This relies heavily on precise immobilization and imaging	Requires a specialized and expensive cyclotron facility. In some clinical settings, proton-based treatment may reduce toxic risks of XRT	Results in very low exposure to adjacent normal tissue. Anatomic barriers limit brachytherapy to only a small subset of cancer types

Abbreviations: XRT, external beam radiation therapy; 3D-CRT, three-dimensional conformal radiotherapy; IMRT, intensity-modulated radiation therapy; SBRT, stereotactic body radiation therapy; SRS, stereotactic radiosurgery.

is rarely observed, however, enhanced abscopal effects have been reported in patients who receive immune therapy in combination with radiation therapy. The biological mechanisms for this synergy are under active investigation, however, high DPF radiation is implicated in the process.[96] Recent data points to a role for DNA released into the cell by high DPF radiation-induced DNA damage. This intracellular DNA triggers a potent signaling cascade through the cGAS-STING pathway to release type I interferons.[97] These type I interferons enhance immune responses and are also postulated to stimulate antitumor immunity. Preclinical work also implicates irradiation fractionation schemes in the stimulation of the cGAS-STING pathway,[98] and many clinical trials are currently underway to test these preclinical hypotheses regarding synergy between immune therapy and radiation therapy.

Conclusions

Radiation therapy is a key treatment modality in the multidisciplinary management of many malignancies. It is often combined with surgery, chemotherapy, hormonal interventions, and more recently immunotherapy. The application of radiation therapy in contemporary oncology is based on many factors including the natural history and biology of the specific malignancy, the use of other treatment modalities as well as its anatomical location and potential normal tissue toxicity that can arise from treatment. Many of the common radiation therapy techniques and uses in cancer therapy are summarized in Table 1. Detailed information as to the role of radiation therapy in the overall treatment of cancers is found in the diagnosis-specific articles in this edition. In addition to primary tumors at any given anatomic site, metastatic tumors can arise as well. Techniques for metastatic disease can range from lower-dose treatment of larger fields for palliation of symptoms such as pain, to very high dose per fraction conformal treatments with a curative goal in the case of oligo-metastatic disease.

Current radiation therapy takes advantage of our increasing ability to image the body and direct high dose ionizing radiation to tumors while protecting normal tissues from radiation dose. We still have much to learn regarding the effects of ionizing radiation on the biology of tumors and normal tissues, and how to best harness other therapies in conjunction with radiation therapy to maximize tumor response and minimize side effects. Over half of all cancer patients will receive radiation therapy at some point during treatment. Cure rates are rising, and radiation therapy plays a vital role in many cancer types. Future technological advances in the delivery of radiation and understanding and control over the biological response to radiation and interactions with the immune system hold promise for an even greater probability of cure.

Key references

The complete reference list can be found on Vital Source version of this title, see inside front cover.

1. Connell PP, Hellman S. Advances in radiotherapy and implications for the next century: a historical perspective. *Cancer Res.* 2009;**69**(2):383–392.
3. Baliga S, Yock TI. Proton beam therapy in pediatric oncology. *Curr Opin Pediatr.* 2019;**31**(1):28–34.
4. Mizumoto M, Murayama S, Akimoto T, et al. Long-term follow-up after proton beam therapy for pediatric tumors: a Japanese national survey. *Cancer Sci.* 2016;**108**(3):444–447.
13. Gates VL, Atassi B, Lewandowski RJ, et al. Radioembolization with Yttrium-90 microspheres: review of an emerging treatment for liver tumors. *Future Oncol.* 2007;**3**(1):73–81.
15. Paris F, Fuks Z, Kang A, et al. Endothelial apoptosis as the primary lesion initiating intestinal radiation damage in mice. *Science.* 2001;**293**(5528):293–297.
18. Liauw SL, Connell PP, Weichselbaum RR. New paradigms and future challenges in radiation oncology: an update of biological targets and technology. *Sci Transl Med.* 2013;**5**(173):173sr2.
22. Lavin MF. ATM: the product of the gene mutated in ataxia-telangiectasia. *Int J Biochem Cell Biol.* 1999;**31**(7):735–740.
24. Lee J-H, Paull TT. ATM activation by DNA double-strand breaks through the Mre11-Rad50-Nbs1 complex. *Science.* 2005;**308**(5721):551–554.
25. Durocher D, Jackson SP. DNA-PK, ATM and ATR as sensors of DNA damage: variations on a theme? *Curr Opin Cell Biol.* 2001;**13**(2):225–231.
27. Lees-Miller SP, Anderson CW. The DNA-activated protein kinase, DNA-PK: a potential coordinator of nuclear events. *Cancer Cells.* 1991;**3**(9):341–346.
31. O'Neill T, Dwyer AJ, Ziv Y, et al. Utilization of oriented peptide libraries to identify substrate motifs selected by ATM. *J Biol Chem.* 2000;**275**(30):22719–22727.
32. Lees-Miller SP, Sakaguchi K, Ullrich SJ, et al. Human DNA-activated protein kinase phosphorylates serines 15 and 37 in the amino-terminal transactivation domain of human p53. *Mol Cell Biol.* 1992;**12**(11):5041–5049.
33. Matsuoka S, Ballif BA, Smogorzewska A, et al. ATM and ATR substrate analysis reveals extensive protein networks responsive to DNA damage. *Science.* 2007;**316**(5828):1160–1166.
34. Manke IA, Lowery DM, Nguyen A, Yaffe MB. BRCT repeats as phosphopeptide-binding modules involved in protein targeting. *Science.* 2003;**302**(5645):636–639.
35. Yu X, Chini CCS, He M, et al. The BRCT domain is a phospho-protein binding domain. *Science.* 2003;**302**(5645):639–642.
36. Stucki M, Clapperton JA, Mohammad D, et al. MDC1 directly binds phosphorylated histone H2AX to regulate cellular responses to DNA double-strand breaks. *Cell.* 2005;**123**(7):1213–1226.
41. Matsuoka S, Huang M, Elledge SJ. Linkage of ATM to cell cycle regulation by the Chk2 protein kinase. *Science.* 1998;**282**(5395):1893–1897.
44. Woodbine L, Gennery AR, Jeggo PA. The clinical impact of deficiency in DNA non-homologous end-joining. *DNA Repair (Amst).* 2014;**16**:84–96. doi: 10.1016/j.dnarep.2014.02.011.
45. Fischer A. Human primary immunodeficiency diseases: a perspective. *Nat Immunol.* 2004;**5**:23–30. doi: 10.1038/ni1023.
46. Shalem O, Sanjana NE, Zhang F. High-throughput functional genomics using CRISPR-Cas9. *Nat Rev Genet.* 2015;**16**(5):299–311.
48. Bryant HE, Schultz N, Thomas HD, et al. Specific killing of BRCA2-deficient tumours with inhibitors of poly(ADP-ribose) polymerase. *Nature.* 2005;**434**(7035):913–917.
49. Helleday T. The underlying mechanism for the PARP and BRCA synthetic lethality: clearing up the misunderstandings. *Mol Oncol.* 2011;**5**(4):387–393.
50. Farmer H, McCabe N, Lord CJ, et al. Targeting the DNA repair defect in BRCA mutant cells as a therapeutic strategy. *Nature.* 2005;**434**(7035):917–921.
52. Hanahan D, Weinberg RA. Hallmarks of cancer: the next generation. *Cell.* 2011;**144**(5):646–674.
53. Bonner JA, Harari PM, Giralt J, et al. Radiotherapy plus cetuximab for squamous-cell carcinoma of the head and neck. *N Engl J Med.* 2006;**354**(6):567–578.
56. Wu S-X, Wang L-H, Luo H-L, et al. Randomised phase III trial of concurrent chemoradiotherapy with extended nodal irradiation and erlotinib in patients with inoperable oesophageal squamous cell cancer. *Eur J Cancer.* 2018;**93**:99–107.
61. Chen AM, Felix C, Wang P-C, et al. Reduced-dose radiotherapy for human papillomavirus-associated squamous-cell carcinoma of the oropharynx: a single-arm, phase 2 study. *Lancet Oncol.* 2017;**18**(6):803–811.
63. Weichselbaum RR, Ishwaran H, Yoon T, et al. An interferon-related gene signature for DNA damage resistance is a predictive marker for chemotherapy and radiation for breast cancer. *Proc Natl Acad Sci U S A.* 2008;**105**(47):18490–18495.
64. Pitroda SP, Pashtan IM, Logan HL, et al. DNA repair pathway gene expression score correlates with repair proficiency and tumor sensitivity to chemotherapy. *Sci Transl Med.* 2014;**6**(229):229ra42.
65. Brizel DM, Wasserman TH, Henke M, et al. Phase III randomized trial of amifostine as a radioprotector in head and neck cancer. *J Clin Oncol.* 2000;**18**(19):3339–3345.
68. Folkert MR, Timmerman RD. Stereotactic ablative body radiosurgery (SABR) or Stereotactic body radiation therapy (SBRT). *Adv Drug Deliv Rev.* 2016;**109**:3–14.
71. Shuryak I, Carlson DJ, Brown JM, Brenner DJ. High-dose and fractionation effects in stereotactic radiation therapy: analysis of tumor control data from 2965 patients. *Radiother Oncol.* 2015;**115**(3):327–334.
72. Brown JM, Carlson DJ, Brenner DJ. The tumor radiobiology of SRS and SBRT: are more than the 5 Rs involved? *Int J Radiat Oncol Biol Phys.* 2014;**88**(2):254–262.
77. Palma DA, Olson R, Harrow S, et al. Stereotactic ablative radiotherapy versus standard of care palliative treatment in patients with oligometastatic cancers (SABR-COMET): a randomised, phase 2, open-label trial. *Lancet.* 2019;**393**(10185):2051–2058.

79. Kishan AU, Dang A, Katz AJ, et al. Long-term outcomes of stereotactic body radiotherapy for low-risk and intermediate-risk prostate cancer. *JAMA Netw Open.* 2019;**2**(2):e188006.
80. Hellman S, Weichselbaum RR. Oligometastases. *J Clin Oncol.* 1995;**13**(1):8–10.
83. Hornsey S, Alper T. Unexpected dose-rate effect in the killing of mice by radiation. *Nature.* 1966;**210**:212–213.
85. Favaudon V, Caplier L, Monceau V, et al. Ultrahigh dose-rate FLASH irradiation increases the differential response between normal and tumor tissue in mice. *Sci Transl Med.* 2014;**6**(245):245ra93.
88. Rosenberg SA, Lotze MT, Muul LM, et al. A progress report on the treatment of 157 patients with advanced cancer using lymphokine-activated killer cells and interleukin-2 or high-dose interleukin-2 alone. *N Engl J Med.* 1987;**316**(15):889–897.
93. Demaria S, Ng B, Devitt ML, et al. Ionizing radiation inhibition of distant untreated tumors (abscopal effect) is immune mediated. *Int J Radiat Oncol Biol Phys.* 2004;**58**(3):862–870.
95. Postow MA, Callahan MK, Barker CA, et al. Immunologic correlates of the abscopal effect in a patient with melanoma. *N Engl J Med.* 2012;**366**(10):925–931.
96. Burnette B, Weichselbaum RR. The immunology of ablative radiation. *Semin Radiat Oncol.* 2015;**25**(1):40–45.

43 Principles of medical oncology

Apostolia M. Tsimberidou, MD, PhD ■ Robert C. Bast, Jr., MD ■ Fadlo R. Khuri, MD ■ John C. Byrd, MD

Overview

The principles of medical oncology have been established over the past seven decades and are now informed by the rules of evidence-based medicine and empirical guidelines while still focusing on the optimal care of individual patients with cancer. The medical oncologist has multiple roles that contribute to the well-being of patients diagnosed with cancer. These roles often include coordinating multidisciplinary teams; being the physician who is primarily responsible for a patient's cancer care; prescribing conventional and novel systemic therapy; modeling life-long learning; conducting translational, clinical, and practice-based research; practicing evidence-based precision medicine; and educating patients and their families in the prevention, detection, treatment, monitoring, and management of the symptoms and complications of cancer and its treatment.

The practice of medical oncology is evolving rapidly. During the past decade, improved understanding of the genetic, epigenetic, transcriptional, proteomic, and metabolomic aberrations in cancer cells and the immune response of patients to their cancers has provided exceptional opportunities to manage and ultimately to cure cancer. Technological breakthroughs in basic and translational science linked with innovative clinical trials have produced a plethora of approved drugs, targeted agents, monoclonal antibodies, and immunotherapies. After the diagnosis of cancer is confirmed, the medical oncologist must be able to describe, at appropriate times, the likely course of the disease, the benefits and risks of anticipated therapies, and opportunities to participate in clinical trials. They must also acknowledge the many unknowns and uncertainties, tailoring communication to the intellectual and emotional level and needs of the individual patient.

Effective care involves the careful choice of agents, often guided by new technologies, and the monitoring of tumor response and the effects of treatment on normal organs. The medical oncologist must be expert in supportive care and often must guide patients through advanced planning and end-of-life issues.

Recent declines in cancer mortality in the United States, Europe, and Japan reflect advances in prevention and early detection, improved multidisciplinary care and adjuvant therapy, and new drugs and immunotherapies that produce durable responses in a significant fraction of patients with cancer. Providing optimal care to cancer patients across our diverse society remains a significant challenge, and inequities have been highlighted recently by the COVID-19 crisis. Medical oncologists must champion access of all cancer patients to optimal care. In the twenty-first century, medical oncologists must overcome the challenges of keeping up with exponentially growing information, mastering new approaches to practice such as telemedicine, and maintaining resilience from burnout. In this unique moment in history, increased harmonization of discoveries, advances, policies, and practices will become increasingly important.

Introduction

Medical oncology was established as a specialty by the American Board of Internal Medicine in 1971.[1] Hematology and medical oncology focus on the diagnosis of malignant disease and its treatment using chemotherapy, hormone therapy, targeted therapy, and immunotherapy (Figure 1). Medical oncology has evolved from a specialty recognized as providing very toxic therapies to patients with modest to moderate impact to a specialty that can cure disease, extend survival, and/or improve quality of life for the majority of patients with cancer. The fields of hematology and medical oncology are rapidly expanding owing to technological breakthroughs in basic and translational research linked to innovative clinical trials.

As of August 2020, there were 12,940 practicing medical oncologists in the United States.[2,3] A global survey of the clinical oncology workforce in 2018 reported an approximate number of 66,880 clinical oncologists across 93 different countries.[4] A significant shortage of hematologists/oncologists has been projected by the American Society of Clinical Oncology (ASCO) in the United States by 2025. The aging and growing population and increasing numbers of cancer survivors would lead to a 40% growth in demand for oncologist services.

In this article, we aim to provide an overview of the principles that underlie the practice of medical oncology and how they relate to recent advances, with an emphasis on precision medicine. We will summarize the current principles of medical oncology and include components of hematology related to hematologic malignancies. These principles are informed by the rules of evidence-based medicine and empirical guidelines that are continually revised owing to frequent scientific advances. They encompass (1) cancer prevention by screening and lifestyle modification (Figure 2); (2) diagnostic approaches that include pathologic and molecular analysis; (3) anticancer therapy that includes traditional therapeutic agents novel targeted, and immunotherapeutic approaches that are approved by regulatory authorities (such as the Food and Drug Administration [FDA]), and investigational therapy; and (4) supportive/palliative care to help manage symptoms and improve patients' quality of life during treatment and at the end of the course of their disease.

Role of medical oncologists

Medical oncologists play a central role in the multidisciplinary care of patients with cancer. As accurate diagnosis, staging, and optimization of loco-regional treatment from initial diagnosis are essential for improved outcomes, medical oncologists interact with pathologists, radiologists, surgical oncologists, and radiation oncologists. Given the prevalence of co-morbid conditions and the frequency of infectious and organ system complications, medical oncologists must collaborate effectively with members of all other internal medicine subspecialties. Other collaborating physicians include geneticists, neurologists, onco-psychologists, and pain and palliative care experts.

Holland-Frei Cancer Medicine, Tenth Edition. Edited by Robert C. Bast, John C. Byrd, Carlo M. Croce, Ernest Hawk, Fadlo R. Khuri, Raphael E. Pollock, Apostolia M. Tsimberidou, Christopher G. Willett, and Cheryl L. Willman.
© 2023 John Wiley & Sons, Inc. Published 2023 by John Wiley & Sons, Inc.

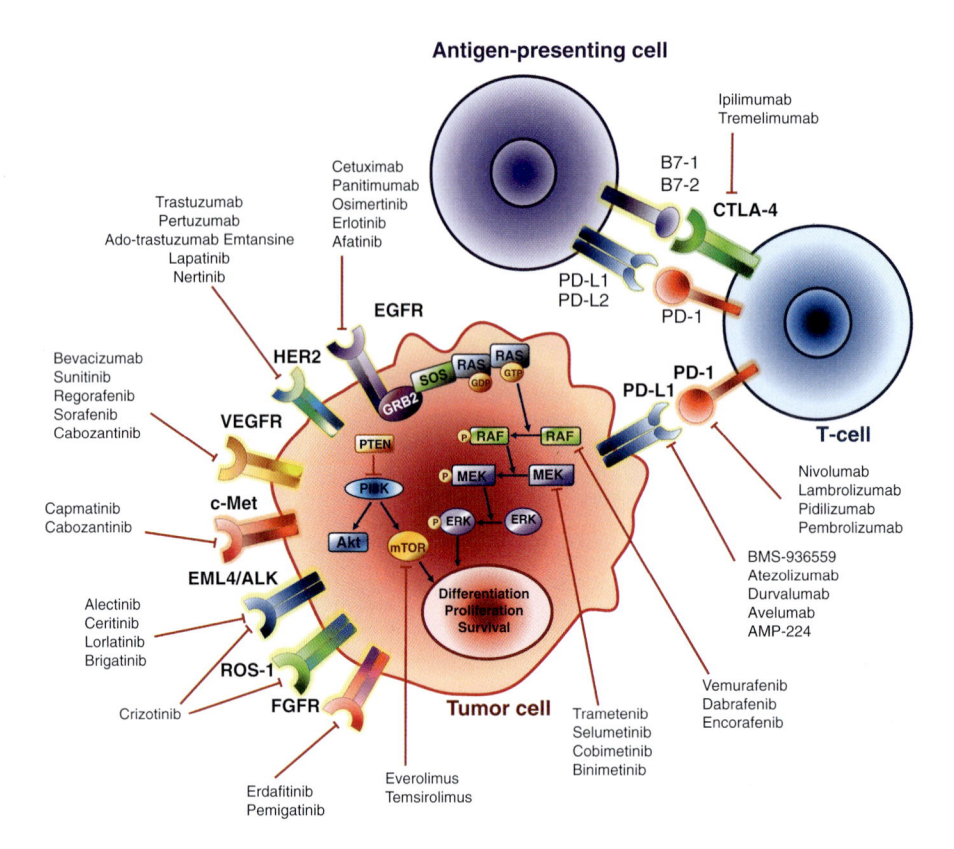

Figure 1 Targeted therapy and immunotherapy.

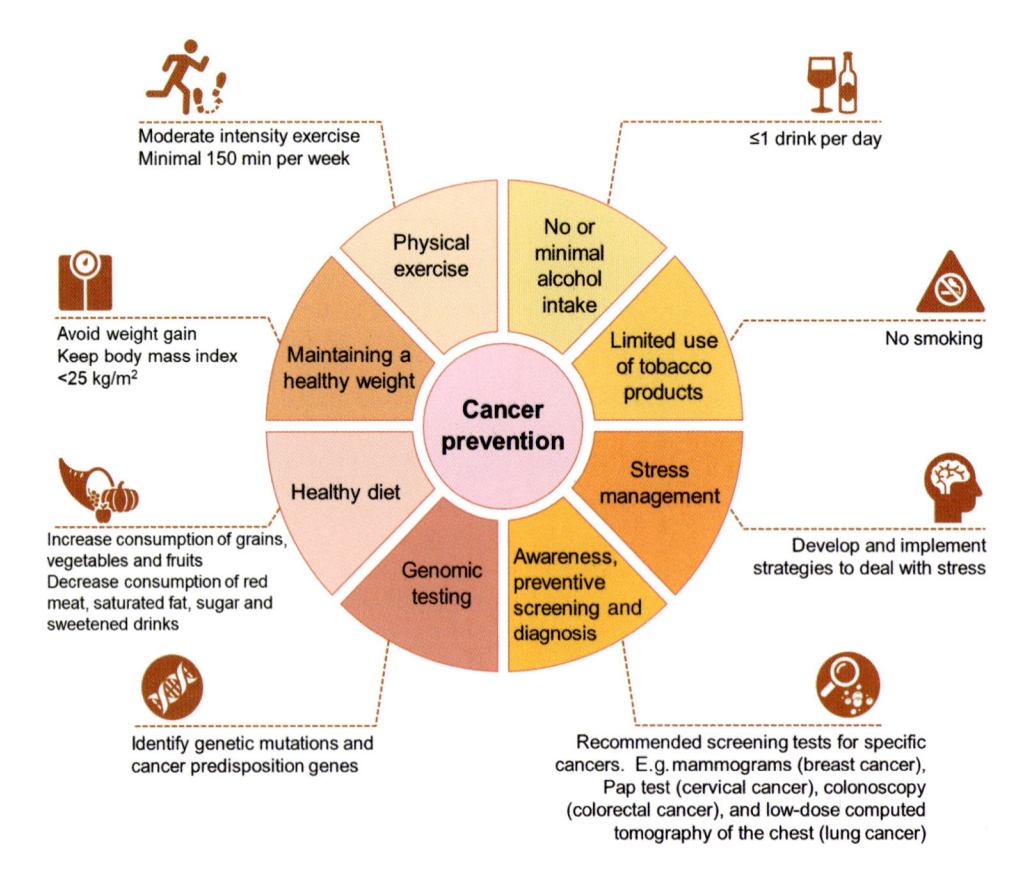

Figure 2 Cancer prevention.

The multidisciplinary approach incorporates the contributions of all specialists to reach consensus regarding the best treatment option. Novel models of multidisciplinary care are available at some institutions to expedite the assessment and treatment of patients with specific cancers. For instance, in a clinic dedicated to inflammatory breast cancer, patients can be seen the same day by multiple disciplines to optimize the treatment selection. In many cases, the medical oncologist serves as the most effective coordinator of this multidisciplinary effort.

For most cancer patients with active disease, a medical oncologist is their primary physician. This role implies responsibility for coordinating major decisions regarding treatment and supportive care, as well as continual communication with patients and their families. Medical oncologists must distinguish cancers that are curable from those that Dr. James Holland called "precurable," for which current treatment is not yet able to provide long-term disease-free survival. The choice of therapy and associated side effects may be quite different for these two groups of patients, keeping in mind that the definition of curability changes over time, given the exponential growth of new knowledge and the rapid development of new treatments.

Medical oncologists must be lifelong students. To prescribe the most effective treatment and to provide the best counsel, they must have an up-to-date understanding of not only new drugs and molecular diagnostics but also factors that predispose to cancer, the spectrum of genetic and epigenetic alterations that underlie tumor cell heterogeneity, the selection of successful clones, and the evolution of cancer and the signaling pathways on which cancers depend to become autonomous neoplasms. They must be aware of the natural history of cancers and range of virulence of cancers that arise from different sites. Some lung cancers may take >10 years for a malignant cell to undergo 30 cell divisions, producing a 1 cm mass (1 billion cells) that can be detected in time to allow for careful workup and treatment. By contrast, acute myelogenous leukemia requires immediate treatment once the diagnosis is made to prevent rapid progression to a lethal burden of 10^{12} malignant cells.

While medical oncologists must be dedicated learners, they must also be educators who provide valid and relevant information to patients and their families, raising awareness of cancer and making recommendations regarding prevention, early detection, lifestyle modification, and treatment. In addition, medical oncologists have the opportunity to educate graduate students, medical trainees, and other healthcare providers on developments in the field of oncology and on how to have quality interactions with patients and their families.

Medical oncologists are at the forefront of discovery in cancer research. While physician-scientists can be trained in any clinical discipline, medical oncologists are ideally positioned and prepared to recognize unmet medical needs that can be addressed with new technologies, agents, and ideas. Cancer clinical trials can be performed by physicians trained in any clinical discipline, but medical oncologists have been at the center of clinical investigation for more than six decades. Of great concern, the number of physician-scientists and of clinician-investigators in academic centers is continuing to decline in the United States. While translationally trained PhDs and international MDs with expertise in research can help to fill this gap, greater attention must be given to the training, support, and retention of academic medical oncologists if we are to continue to accelerate progress in cancer research. Medical oncologists in practice outside of academia must continue to participate in discovery. Most medical oncologists train at academically oriented institutions, where many participate in clinical or laboratory-based research. More opportunities are needed for participation in community-based trials, referral of appropriate patients in partnership with academic cancer centers, and sharing of data regarding best practices and outcomes in the community.

Primary, adjuvant, and neoadjuvant chemotherapy

Chemotherapy can cure a small, but significant, fraction of patients with metastatic cancer. As early as the 1950s, chemotherapy cured patients with metastatic choriocarcinoma, and this was followed by successful treatment of acute lymphoblastic leukemia and advanced non-Hodgkin lymphoma.[5] Adjuvant chemotherapy administered after complete local resection of solid tumors has improved outcomes for several different forms of cancer by eliminating micro-metastatic disease at distant sites. Early examples include Wilms tumor and osteosarcoma in children and young adults. Over the years, adjuvant chemotherapy has improved disease-free and overall survival in adults with breast, ovarian, and colon cancer. Neoadjuvant therapy, administered before surgery, can (1) produce regression of the primary lesion, (2) enhance local control with radiotherapy, and (3) make operations technically easier and possibly eliminate the need for surgery in some settings. Neoadjuvant or induction chemotherapy and the use of improved orthopedic devices has permitted limb-sparing surgery and reduced the need for amputation in the treatment of malignant bone tumors. Neoadjuvant treatment linked to postoperative radiation therapy has also facilitated segmental mastectomy for breast cancers, reducing the need for total or radical mastectomy.

Evolution of systemic cancer therapy

Cancer chemotherapy began with the observation that nitrogen mustard used in chemical warfare produced neutropenia, prompting the application of mustard derivatives such as mechlorethamine to treat patients with lymphoma. Over the next several decades, small-molecule chemotherapy has utilized other alkylating agents (cyclophosphamide, melphalan, platinum derivatives), antimetabolites (methotrexate), altered purines and pyrimidines (6-mercaptopurine, cytosine arabinoside, 5-fluorouracil), topoisomerase inhibitors (nitrosoureas and anthracyclines), and microtubule stabilizers (taxanes) and destabilizers (vinca alkaloids). These drugs are generally more effective against persistently cycling cells than against noncycling cells, providing the greatest activity against leukemias and solid tumors with a high growth fraction. Predictably, many of the toxicities encountered were related to cycling cells in marrow, hair follicles, skin, and the gastrointestinal mucosa. A principle of medical oncology that was established early was that combinations of drugs were required to overcome resistance to single agents and to produce long-lasting responses. Clinically active drugs against a cancer from a particular site and/or histotype were generally combined empirically, choosing agents, when possible, with complementary toxicities. While this approach improved outcomes for patients with acute leukemias, lymphomas, and breast, colon, and ovarian cancers, there was a limit to how many agents could be added, exemplified by the failure of the addition of three other active drugs to improve upon the benefit of carboplatin and paclitaxel for patients with ovarian cancer.[6]

Withdrawal of estrogens and androgens or blocking their receptors has contributed to the care of patients with breast and prostate cancer, respectively. Early practice utilized surgical oophorectomy, orchiectomy, and adrenalectomy, but systemic drug therapy was subsequently developed for both diseases. Endocrine-based therapy for estrogen receptor-positive breast cancer evolved with receptor blockers (tamoxifen, fulvestrant), aromatase inhibitors (anastrozole, letrozole, and exemestane), and gonadotrophin-releasing hormone (GnRH) agonists (goserelin). Assay of estrogen and progesterone receptor expression in breast cancers provided one of the first examples of personalized therapy, where the presence of biomarkers indicated the possibility of response to estrogen deprivation or receptor blockade while their absence assured a lack of response. Prostate cancer was initially managed with estrogen (diethylstilbestrol) suppression of testosterone production, but over the years, GnRH agonists (leuprolide), GnRH antagonists (degarelix, relugolix), androgen receptor inhibitors (enzalutamide, apalutamide), and CYP17 inhibitors of androgen synthesis (abiraterone) have provided more specific and effective therapy.

With increased understanding at a molecular level of the attributes and vulnerabilities of cancers at different sites, the past two decades have witnessed the development of numerous targeted drugs and antibodies that inhibit specific molecules and pathways which drive malignant growth or facilitate the survival of transformed cells. Targeted therapy includes small molecules or therapeutic antibodies directed at specific surface antigens or molecular aberrations that disrupt cancer cell proliferation and survival. Brian Druker and Charles Sawyer pioneered targeted therapy for chronic myeloid leukemia (CML), an adult leukemia where a common fusion transcript forms an oncogenic BCR-ABL fusion protein that drives myeloid proliferation. Individuals in the field of oncology were skeptical that therapies targeting BCR-ABL, such as imatinib, would work for a variety of reasons, yet they have achieved dramatic success with durable remissions and very modest toxicity.[7] The success of imatinib in CML represents the beginning of the targeted therapy era in medical oncology that is outlined extensively in **Chapter 112**. The use of targeted therapies requires tumor molecular profiling to identify genetic alterations that drive carcinogenesis in individual patients. Other landmarks include inhibition of mutant epidermal growth factor receptor (EGFR) by gefitinib and erlotinib in non-small-cell lung cancer;[8,9] targeting amplified and overexpressed HER-2 with trastuzumab in metastatic breast cancer;[10] blocking EGFR with cetuximab in colorectal cancer;[11] binding vascular endothelial growth factors (VEGFs) with bevacizumab in multiple cancer types;[12] inhibiting mutant BRAF with vemurafenib in patients with melanoma;[13] and inhibiting BTK with ibrutinib in chronic lymphocytic leukemia (CLL). In some malignancies, such as CML, the same molecular alteration is so prevalent that histologic appearance alone is sufficient to match targeted drugs to a particular type of cancer. For most targeted therapies, however, specific molecular diagnostics are required to identify target proteins or alterations in DNA that predict response. A comprehensive list of targeted agents is provided in Table 1.

One of the principles established with conventional cytotoxic chemotherapy has been found to apply to targeted therapy as well. With rare exceptions, combinations of drugs are required to eliminate subpopulations of malignant cells that resist individual agents. Considering the complexity of signaling in cancer cells, targeting more than one redundant pathway is often required to block cancer cell growth and metastasis or to trigger apoptosis or senescence. Screens for synthetic lethality[14] and collateral lethality[15] have been developed to identify effective combinations of targeted therapy. Linking molecular diagnostics to detect aberrant targets and pathways with appropriate combinations of molecularly targeted therapy will be required for effective personalized or precision therapy.

For more than a century, investigators have attempted to direct the patient's innate and adoptive immune response to eliminate cancer. Early attempts utilized a bystander effect of the immune response in rejecting intra-tumoral injection of bacterial toxins to shrink sarcomas.[16] Intra-tumoral injection of Bacillus Calmette–Guerin (BCG), an attenuated bovine tubercle bacillus, produced regression of cutaneous melanoma metastases, and intravesical administration of BCG is still used for the management of superficial bladder cancer.[17,18] Interferons,[19] interleukin-2,[20] and infusions of tumor-infiltrating lymphocytes[21] have all found application, with some success in a fraction of cases. During the past decade, however, the promise of immunotherapy has finally begun to be realized with the clinical development of immune checkpoint inhibitors (see **Chapter 63**) and CAR-T cells (see **Chapter 62**). As 2019 Nobel Laureate Dr. James Allison has suggested, immunotherapy has now been added to surgery, radiotherapy, and chemotherapy as a fourth pillar of cancer treatment. One of the challenges for medical oncology is to define how novel immunotherapies can best be combined with conventional and targeted agents to maintain and extend often transient responses.

Personalized medicine: matching drugs to the abnormalities found in individual cancers

The application of personalized medicine—with continuous refinement of technology for genomic, transcriptomic, proteomic, and other biomarker analysis and approval of novel drugs—has introduced many changes into the practice of medical oncology.

Choice of therapy based on tumor tissue analysis

The development of personalized therapy has required novel approaches to clinical investigation at many academic centers. In 2007, despite much skepticism that molecular profiling could be used to identify drugs to improve treatment for solid tumors, a personalized medicine program, called IMPACT (Initiative for Molecular Profiling and Advanced Cancer Therapy), was initiated in the Department of Investigational Cancer Therapeutics at The University of Texas MD Anderson Cancer Center. Among patients with advanced cancer who participated in Phase I clinical trials, matched targeted therapy was associated with improved rates of response, progression-free survival (PFS), and overall survival compared to patients who received nonmatched targeted therapy.[22–25] Until the initiation of IMPACT, selection of patients for Phase I studies with novel agents was not systematic, and, arguably, the impact of investigational drugs from the participating patient's perspective was suboptimal. Subsequently, additional efforts were initiated to perform comprehensive tumor testing for patients with solid tumors to support biomarker-selected, "basket" studies of targeted therapies in many institutions, such as the Memorial Sloan Kettering IMPACT study.[26]

Personalized, or precision, medicine uses traditional and emerging concepts of the genetic and environmental bases of disease to individualize prevention, diagnosis, and treatment[27,28] and integrates the tumor genetics of individual patients into medical

Table 1 FDA-approved drugs by molecular target.[a]

Target	Drug	Target	Drug
BRAF	Dabrafenib	ALK	Ceritinib
	Vemurafenib		Crizotinib
	Encorafenib		Alectinib
			Lorlatinib
			Brigatinib
FLT3	Midastaurin	IDH2	Enasidenib
	Gilteritinib		
		IDH2	Ivosidenib
BTK	Ibrutinib		
	Acalabrutinib	BCL2	Venetoclax
	Zanabrutinib		
		EZH2	Tazemetostat
MEK	Dabrafenib		
	Encorafenib	NTRK	Larotrectinib
	Trametinib		Entrectinib
	Cobimetinib		
	Selumetinib	ROS-1	Crizotinib
	Binimetinib		Entrectinib
mTOR	Everolimus	KIT, PDGFR, ABL	Imatinib
	Temsirolimus		Dasatinib
			Ponatinib
PI3K	Alpelisib		Bosutinib
	Duvelisib		Ripretinib
	Idelalisib		
	Copanlisib	KIT, PDGFRβ, RAF, RET, VEGFR1/2/3	Regorafenib
			Sorafenib
BRCA	Olaparib	VEGFR2	Ramucirumab
	Talazoparib		
	Niraparib	PDGFRα	Avapritinib
	Rucaparib		
		MET^ex14	Capmatinib
EGFR	Osimertinib		
	Erlotinib	RET	Selpercatinib
	Afatinib		Pralsetinib
	Panitumumab		
	Cetuximab	VEGF	Bevacizumab
			Sunitinib
EGFR, RET, VEGFR2	Vandetanib		
		c-MET, VEGFR2, AXL, RET	Cabozantinib
HER2	Pertuzumab		
	Trastuzumab	FGF	Erdafitinib
	Trastuzumab emtansine		Pemigatinib
	Fam-trastuzumab deruxtecan-nxki		
	Neratinib	TROP-2	Sacituzumab Govitecan-hziy
HER2, EGFR	Lapatinib	CSF1R	Pexidartinib
CDK4/6	Palbociclib	**Checkpoint Blockade**	
	Ribociclib	CTLA-4	Ipilimumab
	Abemaciclib	PD-1	Pembrolizumab
		PD-1	Nivolumab
AR	Enzalutamide	PD-L1	Avelumab
	Apalutamide	PD-1	Cemiplimab
	Abiraterone	PD-1/PD-L1	Durvalumab
		PD-L1	Atezolizumab

Abbreviations: ABL, Abelson murine leukemia virus tyrosine kinase; ALK, anaplastic lymphoma kinase; AR, androgen receptor; AXL, anexelekto; BRAF, rapidly accelerated fibrosarcoma homolog B; BRCA, breast cancer type 1; CDK4/6, cyclin-dependent kinase 4 and 6; CSFR-1, colony-stimulating factor receptor-1; CTLA-4, cytotoxic T-lymphocyte-associated protein 4; EGFR, epidermal growth factor receptor; FGF, fibroblast growth factor; HER2, human epidermal growth factor receptor 2; KIT, tyrosine-protein kinase of CD117 (cluster of differentiation 117); MEK, mitogen-activated protein kinase; MET^ex14, mesenchymal-epithelial transition exon 14 deletion; mTOR, mammalian target of rapamycin; NTRK, neurotrophin receptor kinase; PDGFR, platelets derived growth factor receptor; PD-1, programmed cell death protein 1; PD-L1, programmed death-ligand; PI3K, phosphoinositide 3-kinases; RAF, rapidly accelerated fibrosarcoma; RET, receptor tyrosine kinase; ROS-1, c-ros oncogene 1; Trop-2, trophoblast antigen 2; VEGF, vascular endothelial growth factor; VEGFR, vascular endothelial growth factor receptor.
[a]As of 6 December 2020.

practice.[29] With this approach, comprehensive tumor analysis that includes tumor DNA sequences, tumor immune markers, and transcriptomic and proteomic analyses is used to optimize treatment selection to improve clinical outcomes for patients with cancer[24,30] while taking into consideration patient comorbidities (Figure 3). Building on this concept, and addressing the genetic variability of tumors, innovative trials with adaptive design were implemented to assess drugs in patients with specific molecular characteristics, leading to expedited drug approval. To address the limitations of the initial IMPACT trial that were associated with the retrospective analysis of outcomes of patients who were prospectively profiled, the IMPACT2 trial was initiated. IMPACT2 is a randomized personalized medicine study (NCT02152254)[22,31] designed to determine whether patients treated with matched

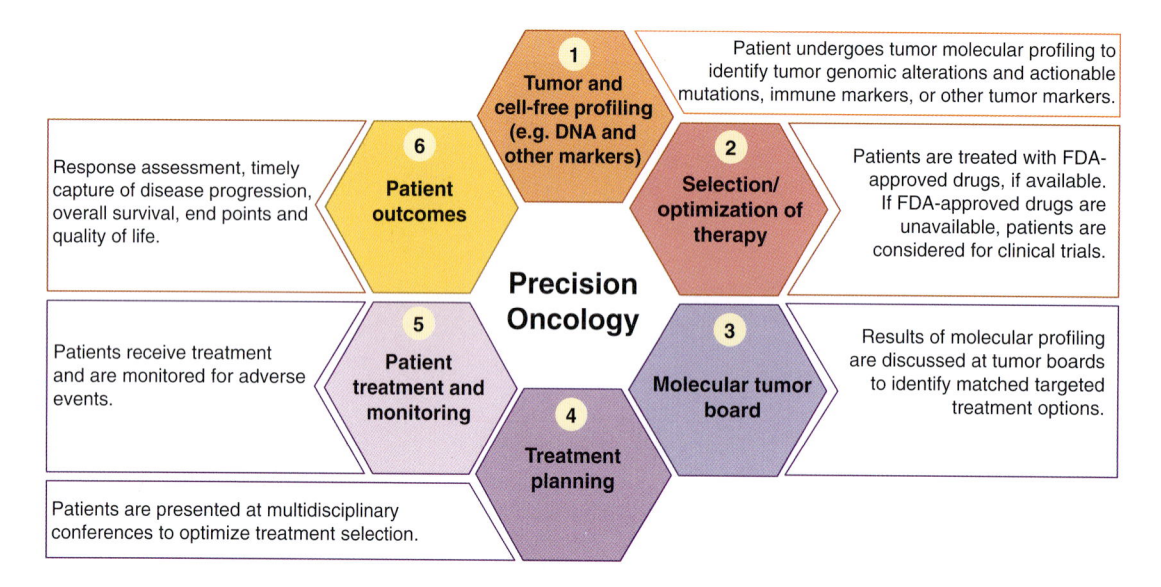

Figure 3 Precision oncology. (1) Tumor and cell-free profiling. (2) Selection and/or optimization of therapy. (3) Molecular tumor board. (4) Treatment planning. (5) Patient treatment and monitoring. (6) Patient outcomes.

targeted therapy selected on the basis of genomic alterations in their cancers have longer PFS than those whose treatment is not selected on the basis of molecular alterations. Similarly, the National Cancer Institute's MATCH (Molecular Analysis for Therapy Choice, NCT02465060) study[32] and ASCO's TAPUR (Targeted Agent and Profiling Utilization Registry, NCT02693535)[33] study are enrolling patients with advanced metastatic cancer who have exhausted standard treatments and/or have rare tumors and genetic alterations for which curative treatments do not exist. Disease-specific umbrella studies such as Beat AML, developed by the Leukemia and Lymphoma Society, have also impacted outcomes with precision medicine-directed therapy based upon a genomic target.

Multiple novel agents have been approved by the FDA or are being investigated in clinical trials (Table 1, Figure 1). Tumor-agnostic FDA approvals include larotrectinib and entrectinib, which are associated with testing of neurotrophic receptor tyrosine kinase fusion in patients with metastatic cancer and emphasize the clinical significance of comprehensive tumor analysis to select therapy.

Choice of therapy based on circulating tumor DNA (ctDNA) and liquid biopsy

Cell-free DNA analysis, or circulating tumor DNA (ctDNA) analysis, was developed as a noninvasive, cost-effective alternative to tumor biopsy when such biopsy is associated with significant risk, when tumor tissue is insufficient or inaccessible, and/or when repeated assessment of tumor molecular abnormalities is needed to optimize treatment.[34] Plasma ctDNA analysis is thought to, at least partially, overcome tissue heterogeneity, as it detects somatic abnormalities from all metastatic sites and, therefore, may be more representative of heterogeneous tumor biology compared to tissue molecular profiling from a single biopsy site. The shorter time to results and noninvasive nature of testing make ctDNA analysis an attractive approach that is indicated for the assessment of several different biomarkers and has gained significant indications associated with certain drug use. Identification of tumor genomic alterations using ctDNA analysis may also help select patients for enrollment in clinical trials.

Principles of care for the individual patient

Laws of therapeutics

Certain principles govern the use of therapy across most diseases. These principles, developed by Dr. Robert Loeb, also pertain to cancer and include (1) if what you are doing is doing good, keep doing it; (2) if what you are doing is not doing good, stop doing it; (3) if you do not know what to do, do nothing; (4) never make the treatment worse than the disease; and (5) provide reality—what is possible and what is likely.

First do no harm

The principle of Hippocrates, "ωφελέειν, ή μη βλάπτειν," i.e., "to benefit, or not to harm," is critical to the practice of medical oncology, particularly while caring for patients with "precurable" cancer. When cancer can potentially be cured, the medical oncologist must weigh the potential benefit against the toxicity of therapy in the context of each individual patient. Emphasis should be placed on providing to patients and their families information regarding disease status, prognosis, lifestyle adjustments, and potential risks and benefits of the available treatments. Broad exposure to standard treatments or investigational therapies should be provided and patients' preferences and well-being should be prioritized. Patients should be given time to understand the complexity of their disease and their treatment options so informed decisions can be made.

Prioritization of the patient's therapeutic goals

Patient-centered care is becoming a mandate of modern oncologic approaches. Continuous communication regarding descriptions of the disease, anticipated therapies, protocols in which there is randomization, and unknowns should be tailored to the intellectual and emotional levels of the individual patient. Not every patient wants to be intimately involved in the decision-making process, but where possible, shared decision-making is an important aspiration. Timely and accurate collaboration between oncologists and patients regarding goals of care is associated with care that is consistent with patients' preferences and improved quality of life, with the ultimate goals being consensus about treatment and better outcomes and experiences. The patient's decision-making preferences and goals of care should be established as early as possible. Routine reassessment of goals of care is essential. Allowing patients to process information over time and to revise goals as the situation changes enables oncologists to be better informed and increases the likelihood that patients will receive end-of-life care consistent with their preferred goals of care.

Evidence-based medicine and standards of practice

Guidelines developed by The National Comprehensive Cancer Network (NCCN), ASCO, UpToDate, and other oncologic organizations aim to support oncologists in making clinical decisions. NCCN guidelines provide details regarding sequential management decisions and interventions that apply to approximately 97% of cancers affecting patients in the United States. ASCO guidelines are intended to improve the quality of cancer care by helping oncologists make choices about treatment, prevention, supportive care, and follow-up in line with the best available evidence from oncology research. This approach sometimes appears to be antithetical to precision medicine, although the goal of these organizations is to standardize the diagnostic and treatment algorithms taking into consideration individual patient factors for the best possible treatment outcomes. Additionally, UpToDate is a clinical decision support resource that provides updated decision pathways to optimize treatment decisions tailored for specific patients. These treatment guidelines generally agree, with some exceptions.

While oncologists should respect these guidelines when making treatment decisions, no single algorithm can address the unique characteristics of each patient with cancer. Consequently, an approach different from the standard-of-care practice can be applied, when carefully justified. For instance, medical oncologists should consider molecular testing of cancers well before exhausting all conventional treatment for a patient in order to identify targets for which clinical trials with investigational agents are available. Clinical trials are often the best therapeutic approach for cancer patients. Additionally, the expansion and subspecialization that characterize the field of medical oncology have led to the development of clinics for certain tumor subtypes (e.g., triple-negative breast cancer clinics in large academic centers) that have developed algorithms which include clinical trials.

Monitoring response to therapy

While molecular markers often have a high negative predictive value and can indicate who will not respond to a given agent, most have only moderate positive predictive value. For example, less than half of breast cancers with HER-2 amplification and overexpression will respond to HER-2-targeted therapy. Consequently, medical oncologists must closely monitor their patients' disease activity during treatment to avoid unnecessary toxicity in the absence of benefit and to optimize the chance of finding effective treatment with established or experimental agents and strategies. Clinical presentation, laboratory tests, imaging studies (computed tomography, magnetic resonance imaging, positron emission tomography, etc.), and tumor markers should be assessed at baseline and longitudinally during treatment. Examples of tumor markers include serum human chorionic gonadotropin (hCG), carcinoembryonic antigen (CEA), 5-hydroxyindoleacetic acid (5-HIAA), prostate-specific antigen (PSA), cancer antigen 125 (CA125), CA15-3 (CA27.29), and CA19-9 (see **Chapter 38**).

An increase in tumor diameter by imaging studies and/or an increase in blood levels of surrogate tumor markers often indicates disease progression, requiring reevaluation of the therapeutic approach. Early recognition of inactive regimens before the development of worsening symptoms offers the opportunity for early intervention with a change in therapeutic approach, with the aim of reversing disease progression and improving clinical outcomes.

Monitoring and treatment of comorbidities

The systemic treatment of patients with cancer, with single agents or with combination regimens, can lead to end-organ damage (e.g., cardiac, renal, pulmonary, hepatic, gastrointestinal), and acute or late-onset toxicity can occur. Assessment of organ function directly or via surrogates of organ injury prior to starting therapy and sequentially following the initiation of treatment provides safety data. Examples include measurement of cardiac ejection fraction by echocardiography or radionuclotide angiography for anthracycline-based therapy, lung function by pulmonary DLCO (diffusing capacity of the lungs for carbon dioxide) for agents such as bleomycin, and renal function by serum creatinine or 24-h creatinine clearance for cisplatin. However, these diagnostic methods are limited by the lack of early detection of function loss that could result in active intervention prior to end-organ damage and long-term morbidity. Over time, the use of diagnostics such as troponin levels, β-natriuretic peptide, and cardiac MRI imaging for cardiac monitoring of early damage has emerged. These biomarkers are early surrogates of cardiotoxicity and allow for early intervention, for instance with anthracycline-based therapy. For nephrotoxic and ototoxic agents such as cisplatin, other platinum compounds (i.e., carboplatin, oxaliplatin) offer alternatives with less morbidity. Therapeutics with direct pulmonary toxicity, such as bleomycin, are less often used, even in diseases where they have curative potential, such as Hodgkin's disease.

The development of a wide range of therapeutics targeting specific signaling pathways important to cancer and overlapping with normal organ homeostasis (glucose, blood pressure, electrolytes, and enhanced immune function) has brought forth additional short-term toxicities that require a different type of monitoring. These toxicities may manifest acutely or are noted in long-term survivors, particularly those who require continued treatment with targeted agents. Examples include hypertension with vascular endothelial growth factor (VEGF) inhibitors,[35] Bruton's tyrosine kinase (BTK) inhibitors,[36] and other small-molecule kinase inhibitors used for various solid and hematologic malignancies. Prolonged use of these agents may cause cardiovascular and renal toxicity. For instance, the prolonged use of ibrutinib in patients with CLL has been associated with early- or late-onset hypertension, and untreated ibrutinib-mediated hypertension may result in long-term cardiotoxicity.

Similarly, the robust development of immune therapies with checkpoint inhibitors that target PD1 (programmed death-1), PDL1 (programmed death-ligand 1), and CTLA4 (cytotoxic T-lymphocyte-associated protein 4) for solid cancers and hematopoietic malignancies may cause immune-related adverse events (irAEs).[37] These irAEs include pneumonitis, myocarditis, hepatitis, dermatitis, endocrinopathies, including hypophysitis, and organ inflammation and require accurate reporting (Figure 4) and urgent and specialized management. Similar autoimmune complications are also observed with selective phosphoinositide 3-kinase inhibitors (duvelisib, idelalisib) that are used to treat hematologic malignancies such as CLL and non-Hodgkin lymphoma. The autoimmune complications of duvelisib and idelalisib are on-target effects on other cell types, where p110 delta isoform

Toxicity reporting

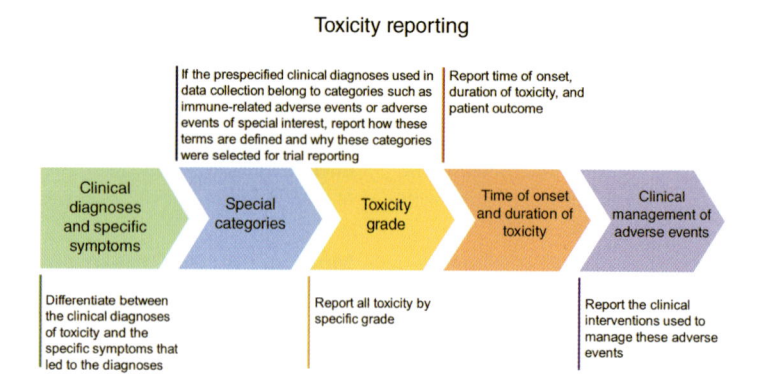

Clinical diagnoses and specific symptoms → **Special categories** → **Toxicity grade** → **Time of onset and duration of toxicity** → **Clinical management of adverse events**

- Differentiate between the clinical diagnoses of toxicity and the specific symptoms that led to the diagnoses
- If the prespecified clinical diagnoses used in data collection belong to categories such as immune-related adverse events or adverse events of special interest, report how these terms are defined and why these categories were selected for trial reporting
- Report all toxicity by specific grade
- Report time of onset, duration of toxicity, and patient outcome
- Report the clinical interventions used to manage these adverse events

Figure 4 Toxicity reporting.

inhibition in T-regulatory cells causes hepatitis, colitis, pneumonitis, and dermatitis in a small subset of patients.[38,39] Both on- and off-target effects of new and effective targeted therapies should be considered, particularly when long-term patient survival is expected. In this regard, the expansion of specific disciplines (e.g., onco-cardiology, onco-nephrology) and survivorship programs represent important resources available to medical oncologists caring for patients with cancer.[40,41]

Consideration of patient enrollment on clinical trials

Clinical trials in cancer research offer patients access to new drugs and strategies. Phase I clinical trials typically enroll 20–80 patients whose disease is incurable with standard treatments and/or who have exhausted standard treatments. The primary endpoint of Phase I studies is to determine the maximum tolerated dose (via dose escalation), select the Phase II recommended dose, and assess the safety and tolerability as well as the pharmacokinetic and pharmacodynamic parameters of the study drug. Secondary endpoints include assessment of clinical benefit, if any, and correlative parameters. Phase II studies are typically offered to 100–200 patients to further assess a drug's safety and efficacy in patients with specific characteristics, including tumor type or biologic characteristics. Drugs with efficacy in Phase I or Phase II studies are tested in randomized Phase III studies with two or more treatment arms that compare the new drug or therapeutic strategy to the standard-of-care approach in several hundred patients. Phase III clinical trials are often needed for FDA approval of a study drug. Nonrandomized studies are inherently limited in their ability to demonstrate true clinical benefit or disease control of an experimental approach owing to the absence of a comparator arm that is necessary to interpret time-to-event endpoints. However necessary, Phase III studies are cumbersome, expensive, and lengthy, and the comparator arm is often suboptimal (e.g., placebo or an approved but suboptimal available treatment). More importantly, with the large variability in patients' tumor characteristics, genomic and immune markers, microenvironment, comorbidities, and other covariates, even the best study designs cannot account for the differences in the randomized arms. Therefore, Phase II studies, including randomized Phase II studies as well as studies with adaptive design, are thought to be more efficient for drug development. As new targeted agents may potentially benefit only small populations, the performance of large trials can also be problematic owing to the rarity of the disease.

In summary, clinical trials provide early access to new treatments, offering hope for many patients, particularly to those who have exhausted standard treatments or have incurable cancer. However, access to clinical trials is limited to those patients whose insurance covers standard routine costs, that is, routine tests and physician visits. Access to clinical trials is challenging for certain minorities, women, children, and rural populations, resulting in their underrepresentation in these trials. These challenges include lack of insurance coverage for patients with life-threatening conditions (e.g., Medicaid, which covers one-fifth of the US population, is currently not federally required to cover the routine care costs for such patients).

As clinical trials have expanded, several organizations have been developed to help patients navigate the available trials for their tumor type and disease characteristics, identifying and matching patients' profiles to clinical trials (Figure 5). High-quality clinical trials include clearly defined endpoints, eligibility criteria, methodology, and treatment plans. Close monitoring of patients for adverse events, response to treatment, disease progression, and overall survival should be accompanied by documentation in real time and reporting to the appropriate regulatory authorities.

Role of supportive care and other disciplines in overall survival and quality of life

The introduction and approval of multiple novel therapeutic agents for the treatment of solid cancers and hematopoietic malignancies during the past decade has been associated with improved outcomes including overall survival. Along with these new therapeutic agents, numerous improvements have been noted in supportive care for acute toxicities such as neutropenia, anemia, thrombocytopenia, nausea, cardiotoxicity, neurotoxicity, infectious complications (bacterial, fungal, and viral), and mucositis. For instance, glucarpidase reverses methotrexate-induced toxicity in patients with delayed methotrexate clearance due to impaired renal function.[42] In addition, enhanced supportive care has led to decreased acute treatment-related mortality rates of pediatric cancers, sarcoma, acute leukemia, and autologous/allogeneic stem cell transplantation.

Cancer patient outcomes and survival are influenced by additional elements of supportive care, that include care specific to age groups (e.g., adolescents and young adults or the elderly) where specific interventions can impact compliance, toxicity, and

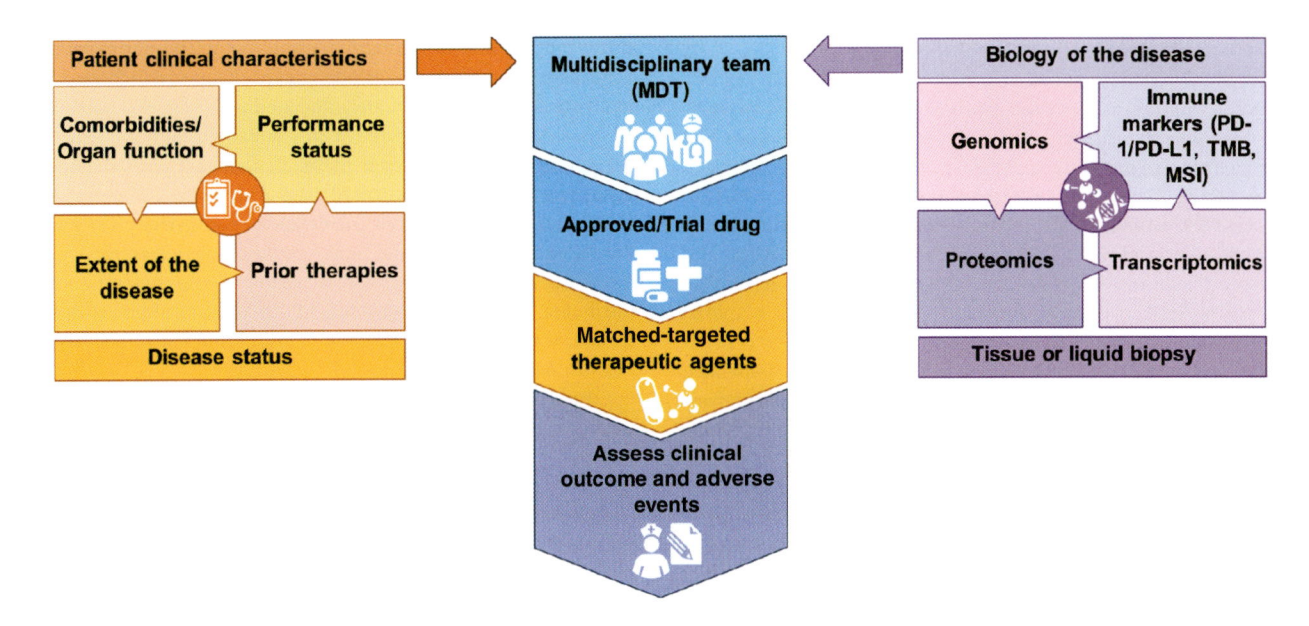

Figure 5 Oncology research. *Abbreviations*: MSI, microsatellite instability; PD-1, programmed cell death protein 1; PD-L1, programmed death-ligand 1; TMB, tumor mutational burden.

outcomes observed with therapy. Psychological support of cancer patients and their families during treatment, particularly when depression or other mental illness is present, can also contribute to better outcomes. A common intervention is alternative medicine, where agents, dietary interventions, or devices/manipulations are used by patients in combination with standard treatment. Although these interventions lack scientific proof of efficacy, as long as they do not interact with the clearance or metabolism of the cancer therapeutics administered, it is unlikely that these agents are harmful. Indeed, studies have shown that in patients participating in Phase I studies who take alternative agents, outcomes are good, and survival is not negatively impacted.[43] Clinicians caring for cancer patients receiving therapy need to inquire repeatedly, however, regarding the use of alternative therapy and interface closely with pharmacy specialists to assure that drugs used for comorbid conditions do not interact with cancer therapies.

A final component of supportive care is bringing patients to the realization that further therapeutic intervention may offer only additional morbidity, with no benefit. Options for therapy at this time often include participation in a Phase I clinical trial where the potential for benefit is uncertain or a nonconventional "standard therapy" that falls outside of traditional NCCN or other treatment guidelines for the specific cancer type.[44,45] In addition, clinical data suggest that early supportive care not only improves quality of life, but it is also associated with prolonged overall survival.[46] With the advent of targeted and immune therapies, participation in Phase I trials now offers a higher chance of patient benefit than the cytotoxic therapy of prior decades. The use of nonconventional therapy should be avoided as patients approach the end of life. Very detailed communication with the patient and their family by the primary oncology team is required in this setting to avoid unnecessary and often misunderstood interventions that do not impact long-term or short-term survival. This end-of-life communication can be effectively complemented by palliative care medicine specialists, hospital/clinic chaplains, and hospice care to achieve better quality of life.

Goals of care and advanced care planning

The relationship between medical oncologists and their patients is an intimate one, built on shared trust and treatment goals, and it should not end once therapies aimed at curing or controlling the spread of cancer are no longer effective, as feelings of abandonment may occur when a patient is abruptly released from care by their oncologist. The medical oncologist must be skilled in the principles of palliative care and collaborate with specialists in supportive care for symptom control, neurologists, psychiatrists, and hospice staff. The medical oncologist should also address end-of-life planning with the patient and their family. Advice regarding living wills, power of attorney, and resuscitation falls within the purview of the medical oncologist, and it is highlighted in states that require that "do not resuscitate" (DNR) orders be written on patient charts prior to death. In the absence of such orders, when a patient is found apparently dead, by law, emergency calls for resuscitative efforts should be initiated. Because of the legal implications involved, where religious beliefs support excessive intervention or where family members cannot accept the anticipated death of a loved one, the medical oncologist should spend considerable time planning for an eventual death. DNR forms are a technique of documentation and constitute further evidence that society has moved medicine onto a new plateau of accountability.

The medical oncologist should make known his or her intentions concerning the advisability of resuscitative efforts for individual patients in advance to forestall unnecessary trauma to the patient, family, and staff; to forestall litigation; and to settle in advance any serious disagreements with the patient or family. An impasse might occasion a medical oncologist to find a suitable substitute physician if there is irresolvable conflict concerning the plans surrounding an anticipated death.

DNR orders do not imply that there be any diminution of efforts to control or palliate the disease symptoms before death. However, if good judgment indicates that continued efforts are fruitless and can only inflict suffering, with no prospect of benefit, discontinuation of active therapy should always be accompanied by DNR orders.

Economic aspects of diagnosis and treatment

Genomic- and immune-based diagnostics are rapidly evolving as the FDA has increasingly approved new targeted therapies and companion diagnostic tests. Some payers have raised concerns about the routine use of next-generation sequencing (NGS) and associated treatments, citing lack of evidence for clinical utility and cost-effectiveness.[47,48] Two studies examining the clinical and economic value of NGS-based diagnostic testing (multi-gene panel examining ≥30 genes) for non-small-cell lung cancer compared with single-gene ALK and EGFR testing to select therapy demonstrated a moderate incremental cost-effectiveness ratio associated with the NGS testing approach and no statistical difference in overall survival.[49,50] A key practice gap was identified, as many patients with actionable mutations did not receive targeted therapies.[48] This gap was explained by limitations in NGS data availability and interpretation, access to targeted therapies, and awareness of the rapidly evolving field of personalized medicine leading to suboptimal use of targeted therapy against an actionable driver alteration. Strategies to implement personalized medicine include increasing the percentage of patients who receive testing and treating patients who are eligible for targeted therapies. These strategies will improve the cost-effectiveness of personalized medicine and will help to realize the full value of NGS testing in cancer care.[48]

Other economic challenges include the cost of highly innovative molecular tests and treatments; the lack of standardization of diagnostic, prognostic, and predictive genomic tests; and the lack of incentives for genomic medicine. Despite the current economic and associated clinical utility challenges, personalized medicine may have great potential to improve health care costs by accelerating drug discovery and potentially improving clinical outcomes. If validated, reliable tests with high negative predictive value could save billions of dollars annually and avoid toxicity in patients who would not respond to a particular targeted therapy or immunotherapy.

Oncologists in group practice are often challenged with the "step therapy" (also called "step protocol" or "fail first") requirement of patients' insurance to use the most inexpensive anticancer treatment first, depriving patients of the opportunity to have the best available treatment.[51–53] These drugs are selected on the basis of low pricing and not on efficacy, tolerability, or patient convenience. The consequences of this requirement are dismal: delayed access to optimal therapy, impaired compliance, and risk of disease progression and increased toxicity.

Ethnic diversity, genetic differences, health disparities, and impact on cancer care

Medical oncologists should be aware of differences in the incidence and clinical presentation of certain tumor types by race, as well as ethnic differences in susceptibility to the side effects of anticancer agents and response to treatment. For instance, prostate cancer is associated with younger age, higher cancer detection rate and Gleason score, and more bilateral involvement of the prostate in African American patients when compared to Caucasian patients.[54] Similarly, triple-negative breast cancer is associated with a higher incidence, earlier onset, more advanced stage at diagnosis, and more aggressive tumor phenotype in African American women when compared to European American women. These differences are attributed to lower socioeconomic status, inherent genetic risk factors, and higher rates of aberrant activation of oncogenic pathways and obesity in African American women compared to European American women.[55] Additionally, the antimetabolite 5-fluorouracil and its oral prodrug capecitabine, which are used in colon cancer treatment, are associated with poorer outcomes in African Americans compared with Caucasians and differences in the toxicity profiles between them. Leukopenia and anemia are reportedly more common in African Americans compared with Caucasians, but the overall incidence of any toxicity (including diarrhea, nausea, vomiting, and mucositis) is lower in African Americans compared with Caucasians. These differences are attributed, in part, to lower levels of dihydropyrimidine dehydrogenase, the rate-limiting enzyme of 5-fluorouracil catabolism, in African Americans compared with Caucasians.[56]

Overall, application of preventive, adjuvant, therapeutic, and palliative care across the entire field of medicine is greatly influenced by a patient's economic status, educational level, race, ethnicity, health insurance coverage, and geographic location (urban vs rural).[57] The classic measure used to access health disparities is outcome as measured by morbidity and mortality. For patients with cancer, all of these demographic characteristics have been shown to also influence outcome in terms of stage at diagnosis and toxicity associated with therapy. Patients of color and those with low socioeconomic status, rural residency, and lack of health insurance have inferior outcomes compared to others. These same features of health disparity are also often associated with increased environmental and work-related exposure to carcinogens that increase the risk of cancer. Additionally, African Americans have a significant suspicion of clinical research based upon prior injustices by unethical researchers. Efforts to diminish cancer care disparities include embedding health care navigators and educators with similar racial, ethnic, and economic backgrounds into the community involved and providing clear and distinct paths toward preventive and treatment strategies. These efforts can be augmented by strategies to provide access to care near these patients' homes to decrease their economic burden. The American Care Act (ACA) provides an excellent example of this principle within the United States, where more than 20 million otherwise uninsured patients have been provided access to cancer care. Concomitant with the introduction of the ACA, a significant reduction in cancer mortality has been observed, which is likely due to not only new, more effective therapies for specific tumor types but also improved access to these agents.[58] This improved access extended to the prevention and screening of cancer, including among minority populations.[59,60]

Opportunities and challenges facing the contemporary medical oncologist

Keeping up with new knowledge

The discipline of medical oncology represents a constantly expanding body of knowledge across many different tumor types, molecular phenotypes, multi-modality care, and supportive interventions. With the expanding amount of data related to this broad subspecialty, large practices have often become disease-subspecialized to enable focus on a given area of medical oncology. However, many oncologists practice in smaller communities where tumor type-specific specialization is challenging. In this setting, virtually continuous continuing medical education is required to provide state-of-the-art cancer care with integration of professional society and other related organization guidelines (ASCO, AACR, American Society of Hematology [ASH], NCCN,

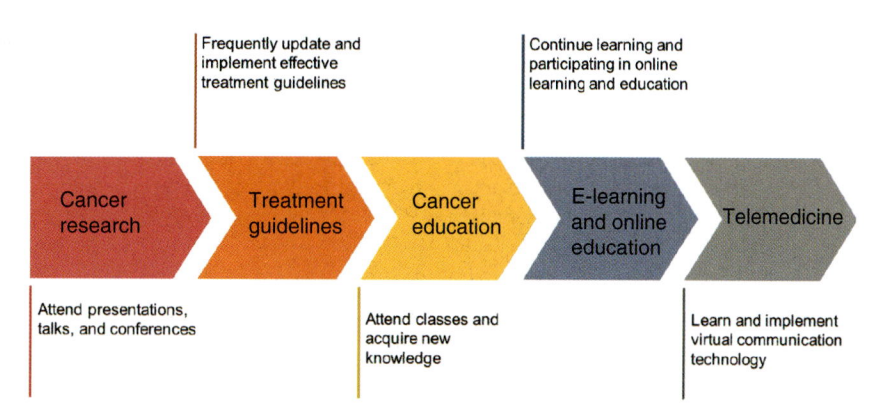

Figure 6 Continuing education for oncologists.

etc.) to assure continued quality of care (Figure 6). It is notable that oncology accrediting bodies recognize the value of continuous assessment and are modifying their re-certification processes in collaboration with other organizations (e.g., ASCO, AACR, ASH). When unusual presentations or rare diseases present to general practitioners of medical oncology, it is necessary for them to understand their knowledge limits and to consult subspecialists either by telemedicine or in person to obtain optimal recommendations for disease management. The specialty of oncology will continue to evolve rapidly with new interventions to both prevent and treat cancer. Becoming a medical oncologist commits the practitioner to continuously updating knowledge to assure optimal clinical care of patients either as a cancer subspecialist or cancer generalist.

Online education provides physicians the opportunity to update their knowledge of recent advances in clinical practice, novel therapies, and new platforms such as online consent and telemedicine services. With the rapid expansion of the field of clinical oncology toward molecular and precision medicine, online training of physicians in molecular testing and analysis helps them to optimize patient care. As clinical trials with genomic alterations have increased, molecular alterations are typically reviewed by tumor boards that include experts in genomic medicine. Optimization of treatment selection requires a multidisciplinary approach that involves consultation with experts in related subspecialties and review of treatment options.

Medical oncologists have access to websites and databases that provide up-to-date information on clinical trials that are conducted nationally and internationally.[61–63] Websites and databases also provide relevant information regarding tumor subtypes, novel biomarkers, and investigational agents, as well as summaries of clinical outcomes and adverse events associated with novel agents. The availability and sharing of databases online from clinical trials and clinical practice can enhance discovery, improve the design of clinical trials, and facilitate collaborations among medical oncologists. However, some oncologists are not in favor of making their data publicly available because of the additional interpretive, clerical, managerial, and cost burdens, as well as the risks and liabilities. Despite these concerns, the integration of these resources into patient care continues to evolve and become a valuable tool, revolutionizing many aspects of clinical oncology.

Practicing telemedicine and telehealth within and across states

Telemedicine offers patients with cancer access to care by highly specialized physicians and health professionals, minimizing the risks associated with traveling for immunocompromised patients (e.g., from the COVID-19 global pandemic). Telehealth applications have been tested in multiple clinical settings and found to produce high levels of patient and health professional satisfaction, while decreasing travel time and health care cost. Tele-oncology includes any telemedicine application used to advance cancer care and to improve patient access to treatments, including participation in clinical trials.[64] It also can provide access to relevant medical expertise that does not depend on geographic location. For instance, patients with specific genomic alterations in their cancers, such as HER-2-positive breast cancer or NTRK fusions, can be considered for clinical trials, regardless of their location. Initial patient screening and consent for clinical trials, symptom monitoring, review of laboratory tests performed in a local facility, and monitoring and management of adverse events can be supported by tele-oncology. In-person visits are still important, particularly for initiation of treatment on clinical trials, in order to fully assess patients' status and maintain the standards of high-quality research.

Telemedicine is most efficient between a patient and physician with an established relationship. However, availability of hardware and Internet access are required. Oncologists should determine whether the use of telemedicine is appropriate for a patient, whether it is secure and compliant with federal and state security and privacy regulations, and whether it can be held to the same standards of practice that would be achieved if the physician were seeing the patient in person. Despite the significantly increased use of telemedicine in oncology practice during the COVID-19 pandemic, current challenges include lack of insurance coverage from all out-of-state patients and technical difficulties. States that restrict access to telemedicine limit the optimization of anticancer therapy for patients. Providing online education and support to patients may help overcome lack of access to computer software and address technical difficulties they may experience with telemedicine. Guidelines for the appropriate use of telemedicine to improve patient outcomes should be developed.

Meeting challenges in oncology practices

Mirroring the technological and pharmaceutical developments of recent years, continued education of oncologists is essential in order to provide optimal care to patients. Understanding of tumor biology and available treatments, both standard and investigational, is required to optimize patient care. Often, utilization of combination therapies, recognition of rare adverse events, and monitoring for delayed responses, particularly with novel therapies, is needed.

Healthcare providers have been significantly impacted by the COVID-19 pandemic, particularly those who care for patients suffering from COVID-19 or for those whose COVID-19 status is unknown. The pandemic has brought new challenges to oncologists. Many clinical trials and medical research projects were disrupted during the initial phases of the COVID-19 pandemic, resulting in suspension of laboratory or clinical research and affecting the careers of young investigators. To mitigate these disruptions, baseline funding and emergency funding by the National Institutes of Health (NIH) and the National Cancer Institute should be increased to support biomedical research, catalyze cures, drive science, accelerate innovation, and develop new and better diagnostics and treatments for all patients with cancer. During the COVID-19 pandemic, oncologists have experienced shortages of personal protective equipment, reductions in support staff, limited access to office space, requirement for social distancing, missed or canceled patient visits, closed laboratories, and unavailable clinical trials.

Oncologists should work closely with other health care providers and all stakeholders to assure optimization of patient care despite the challenges posed by the COVID-19 pandemic. Harmonization in practice between health care providers, pharmaceutical companies, and regulatory agencies is needed to continue offering optimal patient care. To implement changes posed by the COVID-19 pandemic, oncologists should continue to work with other healthcare providers, particularly those with expertise in infectious diseases, the methodologies of laboratory and clinical research should be optimized, advances in technology should be incorporated into patient care, the available resources should be used more efficiently, and a greater harmonization between policy and practice is needed.

Maintaining resilience in medical oncology practice

The complexity of medical oncology practice has been amplified by an exponentially increasing number of specific interventions for different forms of cancer. Concurrent with an exponential increase in oncologic knowledge, there have been rapid changes in reimbursement for cancer care, the introduction of electronic medical records, changes in administrative requirements to practice medicine, and a reduction in daily control of patient–physician interaction time, which has placed additional emotional pressure on providers of cancer care. Patients with cancer also have emergent medical, emotional, and supportive care issues that can increase physician interaction off-hours, which disrupts emotional recovery time from work. Finally, as new medical oncologists enter the field at a younger age, issues related to gender, a desire to have a family, and work-life balance augment the stress of an ever-more-demanding specialty. Collectively, these factors have the potential to result in physician burnout, with unintended adverse effects on patients and providers.

A multitude of studies have documented the degree of physician burnout among medical oncologists at different stages of their career.[65,66] Increased attention to strategies for preventing physician burn-out in medical oncology and other specialties in medicine and in those who support them has become a focus of large hospital and health care systems through resiliency programs. Efforts to increase the resiliency of health care providers in oncology are broad in nature and include finding work-life balance along with open communication to diminish the emotional stress of continually caring for patients with life-threatening illnesses. The value of hospital chaplains, psychologists, and work coaches is essential to assure physician and staff resiliency for the entire span of a work career.

Conclusion

Medical oncology has emerged from a specialty recognized as providing very toxic therapies with modest impact in most patients to a specialty that now cures, extends survival, or improves quality of life for a majority of cancer patients. The evolution of modern molecular biology, targeted therapy, and immunologic approaches to the field of medical oncology has greatly enhanced the repertoire of impactful treatment approaches. With advances in technology and effective therapeutic interventions have also come the realization that many other aspects of cancer care require attention, including prevention, economic hardship, survivorship, and a need to develop new, more reliable models for new drug efficacy to transmit basic knowledge most rapidly to the bedside. Medical oncologists must be both empathetic and quite analytical to assure sound care of their patients. This can best be accomplished by working together with other specialists in teams focused on improving the journey of cancer patients. The horizon has never been closer to making cancer either a curable entity or a chronic disease that patients can live with for many years with an acceptable quality of life.

Key references

The complete reference list can be found on Vital Source version of this title, see inside front cover.

1 Kennedy BJ, Calabresi P, Carbone PP, et al. Training program in medical oncology. *Ann Intern Med.* 1973;**78**(1):127–130.
2 American Society of Clinical Oncology (ASCO). 2020 snapshot: state of the oncology workforce in America. *JCO Oncol Pract.* 2021;**17**(1):OP2000577.
3 American Society of Clinical Oncology (ASCO). *State of Cancer Care in America.* https://asco.org/research-guidelines/reports-studies/state-cancer-care (accessed December 2020).
4 Mathew A. Global survey of clinical oncology workforce. *J Glob Oncol.* 2018;**4**:1–12.
5 Mukherjee S. *The Emperor of All Maladies: A Biography of Cancer.* Scribner; 2010.
6 Bookman MA, Brady MF, McGuire WP, et al. Evaluation of new platinum-based treatment regimens in advanced-stage ovarian cancer: a Phase III Trial of the Gynecologic Cancer Intergroup. *J Clin Oncol.* 2009;**27**(9):1419–1425.
7 Druker BJ, Talpaz M, Resta DJ, et al. Efficacy and safety of a specific inhibitor of the BCR-ABL tyrosine kinase in chronic myeloid leukemia. *N Engl J Med.* 2001;**344**(14):1031–1037.
8 Lynch TJ, Bell DW, Sordella R, et al. Activating mutations in the epidermal growth factor receptor underlying responsiveness of non-small-cell lung cancer to gefitinib. *N Engl J Med.* 2004;**350**(21):2129–2139.
9 Shepherd FA, Rodrigues Pereira J, Ciuleanu T, et al. Erlotinib in previously treated non-small-cell lung cancer. *N Engl J Med.* 2005;**353**(2):123–132.
10 Slamon DJ, Leyland-Jones B, Shak S, et al. Use of chemotherapy plus a monoclonal antibody against HER2 for metastatic breast cancer that overexpresses HER2. *N Engl J Med.* 2001;**344**(11):783–792.
11 Cunningham D, Humblet Y, Siena S, et al. Cetuximab monotherapy and cetuximab plus irinotecan in irinotecan-refractory metastatic colorectal cancer. *N Engl J Med.* 2004;**351**(4):337–345.
12 Hurwitz H, Fehrenbacher L, Novotny W, et al. Bevacizumab plus irinotecan, fluorouracil, and leucovorin for metastatic colorectal cancer. *N Engl J Med.* 2004;**350**(23):2335–2342.
13 Flaherty KT, Puzanov I, Kim KB, et al. Inhibition of mutated, activated BRAF in metastatic melanoma. *N Engl J Med.* 2010;**363**(9):809–819.
14 Lord CJ, Ashworth A. PARP inhibitors: synthetic lethality in the clinic. *Science.* 2017;**355**(6330):1152–1158.

15 Muller FL, Colla S, Aquilanti E, et al. Passenger deletions generate therapeutic vulnerabilities in cancer. *Nature*. 2012;**488**(7411):337–342.

16 Carlson RD, Flickinger JC Jr, Snook AE. Talkin' toxins: from Coley's to modern cancer immunotherapy. *Toxins (Basel)*. 2020;**12**(4):241.

17 Bast RC Jr, Zbar B, Borsos T, et al. BCG and cancer. *N Engl J Med*. 1974;**290**(26): 1458–1469.

18 Kamat AM, Bellmunt J, Galsky MD, et al. Society for immunotherapy of cancer consensus statement on immunotherapy for the treatment of bladder carcinoma. *J Immunother Cancer*. 2017;**5**(1):68.

19 Borden EC. Interferons alpha and beta in cancer: therapeutic opportunities from new insights. *Nat Rev Drug Discov*. 2019;**18**(3):219–234.

20 Jiang T, Zhou C, Ren S. Role of IL-2 in cancer immunotherapy. *Oncoimmunology*. 2016;**5**(6):e1163462.

21 Radvanyi LG. Tumor-infiltrating lymphocyte therapy: addressing prevailing questions. *Cancer J*. 2015;**21**(6):450–464.

22 Tsimberidou AM, Iskander NG, Hong DS, et al. Personalized medicine in a phase I clinical trials program: the MD Anderson Cancer Center initiative. *Clin Cancer Res*. 2012;**18**(22):6373–6383.

23 Tsimberidou AM, Wen S, Hong DS, et al. Personalized medicine for patients with advanced cancer in the phase I program at MD Anderson: validation and landmark analyses. *Clin Cancer Res*. 2014;**20**(18):4827–4836.

24 Tsimberidou AM, Hong DS, Ye Y, et al. Initiative for molecular profiling and advanced cancer therapy (IMPACT): an MD anderson precision medicine study. *JCO Precis Oncol*. 2017;**2017**(1):1–18.

25 Tsimberidou AM, Hong DS, Wheler JJ, et al. Long-term overall survival and prognostic score predicting survival: the IMPACT study in precision medicine. *J Hematol Oncol*. 2019;**12**(1):145.

26 Hyman DM, Solit DB, Arcila ME, et al. Precision medicine at memorial sloan kettering cancer center: clinical next-generation sequencing enabling next-generation targeted therapy trials. *Drug Discov Today*. 2015;**20**(12): 1422–1428.

27 Offit K. Personalized medicine: new genomics, old lessons. *Hum Genet*. 2011;**130**(1):3–14.

28 Wheler J, Tsimberidou AM, Hong D, et al. Survival of 1,181 patients in a phase I clinic: the MD Anderson Clinical Center for targeted therapy experience. *Clin Cancer Res*. 2012;**18**(10):2922–2929.

29 Chin L, Andersen JN, Futreal PA. Cancer genomics: from discovery science to personalized medicine. *Nat Med*. 2011;**17**(3):297–303.

30 Said R, Tsimberidou AM. Basket trials and the MD anderson precision medicine clinical trials platform. *Cancer J*. 2019;**25**(4):282–286.

31 ClinicalTrials.gov. *(IMPACT II) Molecular Profiling and Targeted Therapy in Treating Patients With Metastatic Cancer* 2020. https://clinicaltrials.gov/ct2/show/NCT02152254 (accessed December 2020).

32 ClinicalTrials.gov. *Targeted Therapy Directed by Genetic Testing in Treating Patients With Advanced Refractory Solid Tumors, Lymphomas, or Multiple Myeloma (The MATCH Screening Trial)* 2020. https://ClinicalTrials.gov/show/NCT02465060 (accessed December 2020).

33 ClinicalTrials.gov. *TAPUR: Testing the Use of Food and Drug Administration (FDA) Approved Drugs That Target a Specific Abnormality in a Tumor Gene in People With Advanced Stage Cancer (TAPUR)* 2020. https://clinicaltrials.gov/ct2/show/NCT02693535 (accessed December 2020).

34 Said R, Guibert N, Oxnard GR, et al. Circulating tumor DNA analysis in the era of precision oncology. *Oncotarget*. 2020;**11**(2):188–211.

35 Dobbin SJH, Cameron AC, Petrie MC, et al. Toxicity of cancer therapy: what the cardiologist needs to know about angiogenesis inhibitors. *Heart*. 2018;**104**(24):1995–2002.

36 Dickerson T, Wiczer T, Waller A, et al. Hypertension and incident cardiovascular events following ibrutinib initiation. *Blood*. 2019;**134**(22):1919–1928.

37 Esfahani K, Elkrief A, Calabrese C, et al. Moving towards personalized treatments of immune-related adverse events. *Nat Rev Clin Oncol*. 2020;**17**(8):504–515.

38 Lampson BL, Kasar SN, Matos TR, et al. Idelalisib given front-line for treatment of chronic lymphocytic leukemia causes frequent immune-mediated hepatotoxicity. *Blood*. 2016;**128**(2):195–203.

39 Louie CY, DiMaio MA, Matsukuma KE, et al. Idelalisib-associated enterocolitis: clinicopathologic features and distinction from other enterocolitides. *Am J Surg Pathol*. 2015;**39**(12):1653–1660.

40 Alexandre J, Cautela J, Ederhy S, et al. Cardiovascular toxicity related to cancer treatment: a pragmatic approach to the American and European cardio-oncology guidelines. *J Am Heart Assoc*. 2020;**9**(18):e018403.

41 Clark RA, Marin TS, McCarthy AL, et al. Cardiotoxicity after cancer treatment: a process map of the patient treatment journey. *Cardiooncology*. 2019;**5**:14.

42 Ramsey LB, Balis FM, O'Brien MM, et al. Consensus guideline for use of glucarpidase in patients with high-dose methotrexate induced acute kidney injury and delayed methotrexate clearance. *Oncologist*. 2018;**23**(1):52–61.

43 Hlubocky FJ, Ratain MJ, Wen M, et al. Complementary and alternative medicine among advanced cancer patients enrolled on phase I trials: a study of prognosis, quality of life, and preferences for decision making. *J Clin Oncol*. 2007;**25**(5):548–554.

44 Miller VA, Cousino M, Leek AC, et al. Hope and persuasion by physicians during informed consent. *J Clin Oncol*. 2014;**32**(29):3229–3235.

45 Daugherty C, Ratain MJ, Grochowski E, et al. Perceptions of cancer patients and their physicians involved in phase I trials. *J Clin Oncol*. 1995;**13**(5):1062–1072.

46 Temel JS, Greer JA, Muzikansky A, et al. Early palliative care for patients with metastatic non-small-cell lung cancer. *N Engl J Med*. 2010;**363**(8):733–742.

47 Kris MG, Johnson BE, Berry LD, et al. Using multiplexed assays of oncogenic drivers in lung cancers to select targeted drugs. *JAMA*. 2014;**311**(19):1998–2006.

48 Tsimberidou AM, Elkin S, Dumanois R, et al. Clinical and economic value of genetic sequencing for personalized therapy in non-small-cell lung cancer. *Clin Lung Cancer*. 2020;**21**(6):477–481.

49 Hyman DM, Puzanov I, Subbiah V, et al. Vemurafenib in multiple nonmelanoma cancers with BRAF V600 mutations. *N Engl J Med*. 2015;**373**(8):726–736.

50 Schwaederle M, Zhao M, Lee JJ, et al. Impact of precision medicine in diverse cancers: a meta-analysis of phase II clinical trials. *J Clin Oncol*. 2015;**33**(32): 3817–3825.

54 Bigler SA, Pound CR, Zhou X. A retrospective study on pathologic features and racial disparities in prostate cancer. *Prostate Cancer*. 2011;**2011**:239460.

55 Siddharth S, Racial Disparity SD. Triple-negative breast cancer in African-American women: a multifaceted affair between obesity, biology, and socioeconomic determinants. *Cancers (Basel)*. 2018;**10**(12). doi: 10.3390/cancers10120514.

56 O'Donnell PH, Dolan ME. Cancer pharmacoethnicity: ethnic differences in susceptibility to the effects of chemotherapy. *Clin Cancer Res*. 2009;**15**(15): 4806–4814.

57 Patel MI, Lopez AM, Blackstock W, et al. Cancer disparities and health equity: a policy statement from the American society of clinical oncology. *J Clin Oncol*. 2020;**38**(29):3439–3448.

58 Lam MB, Phelan J, Orav EJ, et al. Medicaid expansion and mortality among patients with breast, lung, and colorectal cancer. *JAMA Netw Open*. 2020;**3**(11): e2024366.

59 Zerhouni YA, Trinh QD, Lipsitz S, et al. Effect of medicaid expansion on colorectal cancer screening rates. *Dis Colon Rectum*. 2019;**62**(1):97–103.

60 Gan T, Sinner HF, Walling SC, et al. Impact of the affordable care act on colorectal cancer screening, incidence, and survival in Kentucky. *J Am Coll Surg*. 2019;**228**(4):342–353 e1.

64 Sirintrapun SJ, Lopez AM. Telemedicine in cancer care. *Am Soc Clin Oncol Educ Book*. 2018;**38**:540–545.

65 Copur MS. Burnout in oncology. *Oncology (Williston Park)*. 2019;**33**(11):687522.

66 McFarland DC, Hlubocky F, Susaimanickam B, et al. Addressing depression, burnout, and suicide in oncology physicians. *Am Soc Clin Oncol Educ Book*. 2019;**39**:590–598.

44 Pain and palliative care

Laura Van Metre Baum, MD, MPH ■ Cardinale B. Smith, MD, PhD

Overview

Palliative care is an essential component of comprehensive cancer care. Palliative care is given concurrently with other disease-modifying, life-prolonging, and curative therapy. Palliative medicine specialists focus on helping patients and their families with a variety of care needs including symptom control, psychosocial support, physician–patient communication, addressing care goals in relation to the patient's condition, prognosis, values, and preferences, as well as with transitions in care. Cancer patients often experience significant symptom distress either from the illness itself or from the associated treatments. The beneficial effects of palliative care have been well documented. When integrated into early oncologic care, palliative care is associated with a significant improvement in quality of life, depression, and survival. As such, palliative care should be given throughout the trajectory of cancer care whether during early-stage disease in which the focus is on cure or in more advanced disease when the focus is on maximizing quality of life. Currently, national and international organizations have clinical guidelines that recommend palliative care be routinely integrated into comprehensive cancer care.

Palliative care

Palliative care is medical care focused on the relief of suffering and support for the best possible quality of life for patients and their families facing serious, life-threatening illness.[1] It aims to identify and address the physical, psychological, and practical burdens of illness and is provided as an extra layer of support for seriously ill patients. Palliative care is delivered simultaneously with all appropriate curative and life-prolonging interventions. Palliative care specialists provide assessment and treatment of pain and other symptoms; employ communication skills with patients, families, and colleagues; support complex medical decision making and goal setting based on identifying and respecting patient wishes and goals; promote medically informed care coordination, continuity, and practical support for patients, family caregivers, and professional colleagues across healthcare settings and through the trajectory of an illness. Palliative care clinicians provide support for coping and improve patient outcomes.[2] Palliative care in cancer patients should begin at the time of diagnosis. The emphasis of care will vary over the course of illness, with anticancer therapy provided concomitantly with supportive care and symptom management.

Several randomized studies have demonstrated a benefit of incorporating early palliative care into standard oncologic care.[3-5] In these studies, palliative care has been shown to improve mood, quality of life, and potentially survival among patients with advanced cancer, across different malignancies. As such, oncology guidelines now recommend the routine integration of palliative care into routine oncologic care. In 2016, the American Society for Clinical Oncology (ASCO) issued updated guidelines recommending incorporation of dedicated palliative care early in the disease course *"for any patient with advanced cancer and/or high symptom burden."*[6,7] In 2013, The Institute of Medicine's report, Delivering High-Quality Cancer Care, recommended that cancer care teams *"place primary emphasis on palliative care, psychosocial support and timely referral to hospice for end of life care."*[8] Furthermore, recent meta-analyses have shown the benefit of early, interdisciplinary outpatient palliative care integrated into the oncology practice setting.[9-12] Further attention to issues of diversity and equity is warranted, as racial and ethnic minorities are underserved and understudied in the field.[13]

There are several core components involved in providing quality palliative care for oncology patients. These include

- Whole patient assessment
- Effective communication
- Advanced care planning
- Symptom management
- Care at the end of life
- Grief and bereavement support

Whole patient assessment

The whole patient assessment is guided by the National Comprehensive Cancer Network (NCCN) guidelines and core elements of palliative care as detailed in the National Quality Forum and involves evaluating all aspects of the impact of cancer and its treatments on the patient and family.[14] In addition to routine medical history, patient assessment explores the patients' social and community support, impact of the cancer diagnosis and treatment on patients' quality of life, spiritual and social well-being, and patients' expectations of therapy and goals of care. The whole patient assessment improves patient–physician communication and assists the physician in understanding potential barriers to patient adherence with treatment plans. This assessment is optimized by utilization of the interdisciplinary team to attend to all medical and psycho-social aspects of diagnosis and treatment and to assist with patient and family distress. The whole patient assessment should also include assessment of the caregiver and other family needs, including assessing for caregiver burnout, for household coping and resiliency, and for family supportive care needs. Patients with young children have particular needs and concerns, which are often overlooked,[15,16] and may require additional support including child life expertise. Children receiving palliative care and their families are a special population outside the scope of this chapter and benefit from specialized pediatric palliative care.[17,18]

Communication

Effective communication is an important component of the oncologist–patient relationship and assists in providing the highest quality cancer care. Oncology clinicians must frequently deliver bad news to patients. Despite this, the majority of oncologists report receiving little to no formal training in delivering bad news.[19,20] Similarly, in a survey conducted at the 2004 ASCO meeting, oncology fellows reported being more likely to have observation and feedback on bone marrow biopsies than on goals of care discussions.[21] Unfortunately, this has not been improving as shown from a survey completed by hematology/oncology fellowship program directors in the United States demonstrating that only 23% of fellows receive moderate to extensive communication training.[20] This lack of training can have a negative impact on cancer patients and providers. Poor communication skills have been associated with decreased patient participation in decision making,[22] missed opportunities to respond empathically to patient concerns, ignored patient wishes to discuss health-related quality-of-life issues, and an increased likelihood of receiving chemotherapy at the end of life.[23] Alternatively, effective communication has been shown to influence desirable outcomes such as patient satisfaction, adherence with treatments, and decreased patient distress, and to reduce physician burnout.[24,25]

There are existing protocols to help deliver bad news and address goals of care (Table 1).[26,27] These protocols can be applied to most situations including a new diagnosis of cancer, cancer recurrence, progression of disease, and transition to hospice. This communication process attempts to achieve four main goals: gather information from the patient to elicit readiness to hear the news; provide information in accordance with the patient's needs and desires; reduce the emotional impact and isolation experienced by the recipient of the bad news; and develop a treatment plan that aligns with patient preferences. When communicating with patients and families it is important to use open-ended questions such as: "What are your hopes and fears?", and "What is important in your life?".[27] It is important to avoid language with unintended consequences such as "There is nothing more we can do for you," and "Do you want everything done for you?"[27] Instead, try saying "We will do everything to give you the best quality of life" or "We will manage your symptoms very aggressively." Additionally, it is important to avoid jargon or euphemisms, and instead use plain, simple language. Cultural sensitivity and cultural humility are also important components of palliative care communication. Once the goals of care are established, it becomes much easier to construct a plan of care centered on those preferences. There are currently training programs that are offered to train oncologists in these specific skills; a list if available resources can be found in Table 2.

Advance care planning

Once the patients' goals of care are established, they should be documented in the form of advance directives. Advance directives consist of two main components: the health care proxy or durable power of attorney for health care and treatment directives.[28] A commonly used comprehensive advance directive is the medical or physician orders for life-sustaining treatment (MOLST or POLST) and is currently in use or under development in over 40 states.[29] POLST is appropriate for people with cancer and a prognosis measured in 1 to 2 years. It specifically addresses medical decisions and options that are likely to arise in the near future, including cardiopulmonary resuscitation, antibiotics for infections, artificial food and fluids, and whether or not the patient would want to be re-hospitalized. Additionally, it can be transported across care settings. POLST appears to be associated with better receipt of medical care reflecting patient treatment preferences (decreased hospitalization and life-sustaining treatments) when compared to traditional practices, improved surrogate understanding of patient goals and preferences and an improved prevalence, clarity, and specificity of preferences documented.[30-32] It is important for every cancer patient to have advance directives to help avoid confusion and conflict, to prepare for future medical care, and to ensure that patients' wishes will be followed.

Table 1 Protocol for breaking bad news and addressing goals of care.[a]

Recommendation	Comments
Create the proper setting	• Prior to the meeting determine the most appropriate participants (family members and other healthcare providers) • Allow adequate time • Determine what to say prior to the meeting
Clarify what the patient and family already know	• "What have you been told about your medical situation so far?" • This allows you to correct any misinformation and tailor the conversation based on their prior knowledge
Explore hopes and expectations of patient and family	• Allows you to distinguish between attainable and unattainable goals
Suggest realistic goals	• Suggest attainable goals based on the present clinical scenario and how they can best be achieved • Review appropriateness of disease-modifying treatments • Try to explain using simple language why unrealistic goals can not be met
Use empathic responses	• Very important to allow silence and to listen • Let patient and family express emotions • Once emotions are expressed using a connector such as "I can see how upsetting this is to you"
Make a plan and follow through	• Summarize the plan to ensure that your interpretation of the conversation and decisions is in concordance with patient and family and how the plan of care will meet their goals • Make a plan for continued follow-up • Inform the patient and family how to contact you if they have further questions or concerns • Continue to review and revise the plan as needed

[a]Source: Adapted from Smith and Brawley[13] and National Consensus Project for Quality Palliative Care.[14]

Symptom management

Patients with cancer experience many physical and psychosocial symptoms either as a consequence of therapy or as a result of the disease itself. The essential components of symptom management include (1) routine and repeated formal assessment, (2) expertise in prescribing medications, including the safe use of opioid analgesics, adjuvant approaches to pain management, and management of a wide range of other common and distressing symptoms and syndromes, and (3) skillful management of treatment side effects. Currently, there is no gold standard for symptom assessment in palliative care. Although several tools

Table 2 Palliative care internet resources.

- www.capc.org: Center to Advance Palliative Care: Educational-based content to learn primary palliative care skills. Technical assistance for clinicians and hospitals seeking to establish or strengthen a palliative care program
- www.vitaltalk.org: Website to help providers learn communication skills
- www.epeconline.net: Education on Palliative and End of Life Care (EPEC): Comprehensive curriculum covering fundamentals of palliative medicine; free downloadable PowerPoint and teaching guides
- www.palliativedrugs.com: Extensive information on pharmacologic symptom management
- www.aahpm.org: American Academy of Hospice and Palliative Medicine: Physician membership organization; board review courses, publications
- www.hms.harvard.edu/cdi/pallcare: Center for Palliative Care at Harvard Medical School: Faculty development courses, other educational programs
- www.nationalconsensusproject.org: National Consensus Project for Quality Palliative Care: Clinical practice guidelines
- http://endoflife.stanford.edu/: Joint project of the US Veterans Administration and SUMMIT, Stanford University Medical School. Curriculum covering fundamentals of palliative medicine

Table 3 Guidelines for the use of analgesic drugs in cancer pain management.

Start with a specific drug for a specific type of pain

1. Clarify the patient's pain, its nature, site, duration, and intensity, and the degree of pain relief from prior nonopioid and opioid drug use
2. Complete a careful medical and neurologic history and examination. Assess the potential role of radiotherapy, surgery, and/or chemotherapy in pain control
3. Assess the psychological factors contributing to the pain complaint, and understand the meaning of the pain for the patient
4. Choose the route of administration to fit the needs of the individual patient
   (i) Choose the oral route as the simplest approach
   (ii) Consider the buccal or rectal routes for patients who cannot tolerate oral drugs and refuse parenteral routes. Start intravenous intermittent boluses or continuous infusions in patients requiring rapid escalation of opioids for pain control
   (iii) Use intermittent boluses or continuous subcutaneous infusions for patients without venous access or in patients at home
   (iv) Choose the epidural or intrathecal route in patients who develop limiting side effects from systemic opioids
   (v) Use PCA pumps for selected patients in hospital and at home
5. Know the pharmacology of the available opioid drugs. Titrate the dose to the individual needs of the patient
   (i) Start with a dose that is at least equivalent or slightly greater than the equianalgesic dose of the previous analgesic used
   (ii) Order the medication on a regular basis (oral–every 3–4 h, intravenous–every 15–60 min as needed)
   (iii) Instruct the patient to take the medication on a PRN basis if the patient is opioid naive
   (iv) Order "rescue medication" equivalent to 10% of the standing 24 h dose to begin with on a PRN basis
   (v) Inform the patient of options in taking the medication, and request that he or she report side effects of excessive sedation or confusion. Monitor the side effects closely
6. Use a combination of drugs to provide additive analgesia to reduce side effects or to control other symptoms
   (i) Know the various adjuvant drugs that provide additive analgesia, for example, anticonvulsants, corticosteroids
   (ii) Use neurostimulants to reduce sedative effects, for example, caffeine, dextroamphetamine, methylphenidate, modafinil
   (iii) Use antidepressant, anticonvulsant, and other analgesics to manage neuropathic pain
7. Anticipate and treat side effects
   (i) Watch for respiratory depression, and use naloxone if needed (in diluted doses to prevent acute withdrawal)
   (ii) Counteract sedation with neurostimulants
   (iii) Use antiemetics to suppress the emetic effect of opioids
   (iv) Define an individualized bowel regimen to prevent and manage constipation
   (v) Treat myoclonus by switching to an alternative analgesic, or suppress it with anxiolytic drugs
8. Watch for the development of tolerance
   (i) Distinguish tolerance from progression of tumor
   (ii) Recognize that there is no limit to tolerance
   (iii) Switch to an alternative opioid if the dose of the current opioid cannot be escalated
   (iv) Consider opioid rotation if one or more intractable side effects are noted

Abbreviations: PCA, patient-controlled analgesia; PRN, pro re nata (according to as circumstances may require).

exist, the most commonly used is the Edmonton Symptom Assessment System (ESAS), which consists of nine visual analog scales or numerical rating scales that evaluate a combination of the most common physical and psychological symptoms.[33] The most common symptom experienced by cancer patients is pain.[34] The most frequent nonpain symptoms are constipation, nausea and vomiting, anorexia/cachexia, dyspnea, delirium, and anxiety.[34] The management of some of these symptoms will be discussed in the following sections.

Pain

The International Association for the Study of Pain defines pain as "an unpleasant sensory and emotional experience associated with actual or potential tissue damage or described in terms of such damage."[35] Although the cause of the pain and the type of injury vary, the constellation of complex neurophysiologic phenomena of pain includes two broad categories, nociceptive pain, which include both somatic and visceral pain, and neuropathic pain.[25] Somatic pain is characterized as well localized, intermittent, or constant, and is described as aching, gnawing, throbbing, or cramping (e.g., bone metastases). Visceral pain is mediated by discrete nociceptors in the cardiovascular, respiratory, gastrointestinal, and genitourinary systems. It is usually described as deep, squeezing, or colicky, and is commonly referred to cutaneous sites, which may be tender. Neuropathic pain is clinically described as a burning, tingling, or numb sensation with paroxysms of shock-like pain. Cancer history should include description of the pain complaint, including the patient's description of pain and intensity; its quality, exacerbating, relieving factors, and its radiation if any; its exact onset and temporal pattern. Impact of pain on the activities of daily living, sleep, mood, and affect should be assessed.

The guiding principles of a therapeutic strategy for cancer pain should include: (1) detailed assessment of the patient's pain, (2) making a pain diagnosis, (3) understanding the goals of care and the patient's preferences, (4) developing and implementing the best therapeutic and diagnostic strategy, (5) continual reassessment of the degree of pain and analgesia, and (6) expertise to provide alternative therapeutic strategies. Of greatest importance, no patient should be inadequately evaluated because of patient's experiencing "too much pain." A series of algorithms have been developed for the management of cancer pain.[36,37] The World Health Organization Cancer Pain and Palliative Care Program advocates a three-step approach which advocates starting with nonopioid analgesia (e.g., nonsteroidal, anti-inflammatory drugs [NSAIDs]) and then titrating up to low- then high-potency opioids.[38] Similarly, NCCN pain management guidelines provide an algorithm of a stepwise approach to the treatment of mild, moderate, and severe pain and strategy of rapid but safe opioid titration to provide analgesia.[39] General guidelines of cancer

Table 4 Opioid analgesics commonly used for moderate to severe pain narcotic agonists.

	Parenteral (mg)	Oral (mg)	Conversion factor (IV to PO)	Comments
Morphine	10	30	1:3	Standard of comparison for opioid analgesics; lower dose for aged patients
Hydromorphone	1.5	7.5	1:5	Slightly shorter-acting
Fentanyl	25 µg = 1 mg morphine IV	–	–	Short half-life; transdermal and transmucosal preparations available
Codeine	130	200	1:1.5	Often used with nonopioid analgesics; biotransformed, in part, to morphine
Oxycodone	–	20	–	Also in combination with nonopioid analgesics, that limit dose escalation
Oxymorphone	1	10	1:10	Not available orally
Methadone[a]				

[a]Methadone has a complex pharmacokinetic and pharmacodynamic profile that makes equianalgesic dosing particularly difficult. Consult with an experienced clinician before initiating or adjusting the dose of methadone.

Table 5 Guidelines for opioids in kidney and liver disease.

	Kidney disease[a]		Liver disease	
	Renal failure	Dialysis	Stable cirrhosis	Severe disease
Morphine	Do not use	Do not use not dialyzed	Caution ↓ dose ↓ frequency[b]	Do not use
OXYcodone	Caution ↓ dose ↓ frequency[b]	Caution	Caution ↓ dose ↓ frequency[b]	Caution ↓ dose ↓ frequency[b]
HYDROmorphone	Preferred ↓ dose ↓ frequency[b]	Preferred Not dialyzed, but minimal toxicity	Caution ↓ dose ↓ frequency[b]	Caution ↓ dose ↓ frequency[b]
Fentanyl	Preferred	Preferred Not dialyzed, but minimal toxicity	Preferred	Preferred
Codeine	Do not use	Do not use	Do not use	Do not use
Methadone[c]	Preferred—with consultation only	Preferred—with consultation only. Not dialyzed, but minimal toxicity	Preferred—with consultation only	Preferred—with consultation only

[a]Avoid sustained-release oral opioids and fentanyl patches in kidney disease. Note that even the "safest" opioids are not dialyzable.
[b]↓ dose means reduce dose by 25–50%. ↓ frequency means reduce standing orders for short-acting opioids from q4h to q6h.
[c]Consult with an experienced clinician before initiating or adjusting the dose of methadone.

pain treatment are listed in Table 3. Management of cancer pain can be divided into pharmacologic approaches, interventional approaches, and psychological management.

Pharmacological approaches are the most commonly used method for managing cancer pain. The brief outline of pharmacologic approach is detailed in Table 4. The selection of the right analgesic to maximize pain relief and minimize adverse effects begins with the use of nonopioids for mild pain. In patients with moderate pain that is not controlled with nonopioids such as acetaminophen, NSAIDs, and adjuvant medications (WHO step 1), the so-called weak opioid-agonists (codeine, hydrocodone, and tramadol) alone or in combination are prescribed (step 2). In patients with severe pain, a strong opioid (morphine, hydromorphone, fentanyl, methadone, oxycodone, oxymorphone, or levorphanol) is the drug of choice (step 3). At all levels, certain NSAIDs and adjuvant drugs may be used for specific indications. A number of opioid analgesics are available for clinical use and are listed in Table 4.

Selection of the opioids should be based on patient's analgesic history, renal and hepatic function (see Table 5), side effects, and severity of pain. Short-acting opioids are usually used for opioid titration and as needed (PRN) for breakthrough pain. After an effective stable 24-h opioid requirement is established a switch to a long-acting formulation should be considered. Long-acting opioids allow patients to achieve more consistent blood levels, reduce pain recurrence, improve compliance, and reduce iatrogenic dependence. Rescue medications equivalent to 10% of the standing 24 h dose should also be made available to patients.[40,41] Overall, opioid dose, route, and titration schedule should be tailored to the patient's medical needs, treatment goals, and side-effect profile. There is no minimum or maximum dose. The opioid dose needs to be titrated to maintain the patient's desired balance between pain relief and opioid-related side effects. Though rates of misuse are low,[42,43] patients with cancer and/or receiving palliative care may still be at risk for opioid misuse and diversion;[44–46] opioid risk assessment tools and recommendations for safe storage and disposal should be integrated into care and models of universal precautions should be considered.[46,47]

Interventional approaches can be divided into six major types: (1) trigger-point injections, (2) peripheral nerve blocks, (3) autonomic nerve blocks, (4) epidural and intrathecal infusions, (5) surgical approaches, and (6) neurostimulatory approaches. The techniques for each of these procedures are outside the scope of this chapter but have been described in detail elsewhere.[48]

Psychological management of cancer pain includes the use of psychotherapeutic, cognitive-behavioral, and psychopharmacologic interventions. These techniques are most useful in three clinical situations: (1) in the management of patients with intermittent predictable pain (such as pain associated with procedures), (2) in the management of incident pain (e.g., in the patient with pain on movement), and (3) in the management of chronic cancer pain.[49,50]

Constipation

Constipation is defined as the infrequent and difficult passage of hard stool. It is a common cause of morbidity in the palliative care setting and affects more than 95% of patients who are treated with opioids for cancer-related pain.[15] The two most common etiologies are related to the side effects of opioids and the effects of progressive

Table 6 Laxatives commonly used to treat constipation.

Class of drug	Preparation	Starting dose	Mechanism of action	Comments
Oral				
Lubricant	Mineral oil	5–10 mL/d	Lubricates stool surface, allows easier passage	Adverse effects include lipoid pneumonia, leakage of oily fecal material. 255 paraffin and magnesium hydroxide considered safest
Bulk-forming agents	Methylcellulose, bran, psyllium	Bran 8 g daily Others 3–4 g daily	Increases stool bulk, stimulating peristalsis	Good for mild constipation. Caution as needs to be taken with at least 200–300 mL of water. May precipitate obstruction in a debilitated patient by forming a viscous mass. May cause flatulence and bloating
Osmotic (poorly absorbed sugars)	Lactulose	15–30 mL daily	Retention of water in the lumen via osmotic effects	Sweet taste which may not be well tolerated. Bloating, abdominal cramping, and flatulence are common
Saline	Magnesium hydroxide Sodium bisphosphonate	2.4–4.8 g daily	High osmolarity compounds cause retention of water in the lumen throughout the entire gut. Directly stimulates peristalsis	Strong cathartic. Mostly used as a bowel prep for endoscopic procedures. May alter fluid and electrolyte imbalance. Caution in patients with heart failure or renal insufficiency
Anthraquinones	Senna	Max 100 mg/d	Direct stimulation of myenteric plexus causing induction of peristalsis	Often combined with docusate. May cause abdominal cramping. Do not use if obstruction is suspected
Polyphenolic	Bisacodyl	10 mg daily	Stimulates secretion and motility of small intestine and colon	May cause abdominal cramping
Rectal				
Lubricant	Mineral oil enema	One enema	Used as retention enema to allow evacuation or manual removal of impacted stool	Efficacy is dependent on ability to retain the oil
Osmotic	Glycerin	One suppository	Softens stools via osmosis	
Saline	Sodium phosphate	One enema or suppository	Releases bound water from feces May stimulate rectal or distal colonic peristalsis	May alter fluid and electrolyte balance. Caution in patients with heart failure or renal insufficiency
Polyphenolic	Bisacodyl	10 mg suppository	Promotes colonic peristalsis	Activity depends on bisacodyl reaching the rectal wall
Subcutaneous				
Peripheral opioid receptor antagonist	Methylnaltrexone	<38 kg: 0.15 mg/kg; 38 to <62 kg: 8 mg; 62 to 114 kg: 12 mg; >114 kg: 0.15 mg/kg (round up)	Selectively blocks opioid binding at the mu receptor, in the GI tract	Only for opioid-induced constipation

disease. Severe constipation can lead to bowel and perforation and can be a cause of severe morbidity. In patients who are neutropenic, severe constipation can lead to bacterial transfer across the colon, resulting in bacteremia and potentially sepsis. The Rome criteria define constipation as the presence of two or more of the following symptoms:[51]

- Straining at least 25% of the time
- Hard stools at least 25% of the time
- Incomplete evacuation at least 25% of the time
- ≤2 bowel movements per week

Assessment of constipation should involve a history of the patient's bowel pattern, fluid intake, recent dietary changes, review of current medications, and a thorough physical examination, including a rectal exam—with caution in patients with neutropenia. In addition, abdominal radiography can be performed to look for the presence of stool if the diagnosis remains unclear.

Constipation can be managed with nonpharmacologic measures as well as pharmacologic interventions. Nonpharmacologic measures include increasing fluid intake if possible and regular toileting as colonic activity is highest early in the morning, after walking, and 30 min after meals. Pharmacologic interventions for the management of constipation may be administered orally or rectally and are summarized in Table 6. There is no single correct management approach to laxative prescribing. Initial regimens often include a stimulant, such as senna, given once or twice per day and titrated according to response. Stool-softening agents, such as docusate, are commonly prescribed but have not been shown to be efficacious in this setting.[52] Whichever bowel regimen is initiated should be individualized and titrated to response. It is important to note that the best treatment of constipation is prevention. A prophylactic bowel regimen should be initiated at the time opioids are initially prescribed and should be continued for as long as the patient remains on opioids.

Nausea and vomiting

Nausea and vomiting are reported to affect between 40% and 70% of patients with cancer.[53] Nausea and vomiting can cause substantial psychological distress for patients and families and impact overall quality of life.[54] Nausea is subjective and is defined as an

Table 7 Antiemetics commonly used to treat nausea and vomiting.

Receptor site of action	Drug name	Dosage/route	Adverse effects
Dopamine antagonists (D_2)	Chlorpromazine	10–25 mg PO every 4–6 h, 25–50 mg IM every 3–4 h	Dystonia, akathisia, sedation, and postural hypotension
	Haldol	10–20 mg PO, IV/SQ before meals and at bedtime or every 6 h	Dystonia and akathisia
	Metoclopramide	10–20 mg PO every 6 h, 5–10 mg IV every 6 h or 25 mg rectally every 6 h	Dystonia, akathisia, abdominal cramping in obstruction
	Prochlorperazine	5–10 mg PO every 6–8 h or 25 mg rectally every 12 h	Dystonia, akathisia, and sedation
	Olanzapine	5–10 mg PO once daily for up to 5–7 d, may be extended if clinical benefit	Drowsiness, akathisia, constipation
Histamine antagonists (H_1)	Cyclizine	25–50 mg PO/SQ or rectally every 8 h	Dry mouth, sedation, skin irritation at SQ sites may occur
	Diphenhydramine	25–50 mg PO/IV/SQ every 4–8 h	Sedation, dry mouth, and urinary retention
	Promethazine (also has activity on D_2 and ACH)	12.5–25 mg PO, IV/IM rectal every 4–6 h	Dry mouth, dystonia, akathisia, and sedation
Acetylcholine antagonists (ACH)	Glycopyrrolate	0.2 mg IV/SQ every 4–6 h	Dry mouth, blurred vision, confusion, urinary retention, ileus
	Hycosamine	0.125–0.25 mg PO/SL every 4 h or 0.25–0.5 mg IV/SQ every 4 h	Dry mouth, blurred vision, confusion, urinary retention, ileus
	Scopolamine	0.1–0.4 mg IV/SQ every 4 h or 1.5 mg transdermal patch every 72 h	Dry mouth, blurred vision, confusion, urinary retention, ileus
Serotonin antagonists ($5HT_3$)	Dolasetron	100 mg PO daily	Headache, diarrhea
	Granisetron	2 mg PO daily or daily	Headache, constipation, weakness
	Ondansetron	4–8 mg PO/IV or dissolvable tablet IV every 4–8 h (max 32 mg/d)	Headache, constipation, weakness
	Palonosetron	0.25 mg IV prior to start of chemotherapy[a]	Headache, constipation
Substance P antagonist	Aprepitant	125 mg PO on day 1 of chemotherapy 80 mg PO on days 2 and 3[a]	Headache
	Fosaprepitant	150 mg IV day 1 of chemotherapy	Headache, infusion site pain
Other			
Corticosteroids	Dexamethasone	10–20 mg PO/IV each treatment day	Hyperglycemia, GI Bleeding, insomnia, psychosis
Cannabinoids	Dronabinol	2–20 mg PO daily in divided doses	Dizziness, euphoria in the young and dysphoria in the elderly, paranoid reaction, somnolence
Benzodiazepines	Lorazepam[b]		
Somatostatin analogue	Octreotide	0.5–2 mg PO/IV every 4–6 h 100 mcg every 8–12 h IV/SQ or 100 mcG/h as continuous IV infusion	Sedation, respiratory depression Bradycardia, headache, malaise, hyperglycemia

[a]Have not been shown to be effective in terminating nausea or vomiting once it occurs and should not be used for this purpose.
[b]Best used for anticipatory nausea and vomiting.

unpleasant sensation of the need to vomit and can be associated with autonomic symptoms, including pallor, cold sweats, tachycardia, and diarrhea. Vomiting is the forceful discharge of gastric contents via the mouth resulting from the contraction of the abdominal musculature and diaphragm. The pathophysiology of nausea and vomiting is complex and involves four pathways (chemoreceptor trigger zone, cortex, peripheral pathways in the GI tract, and vestibular system) which when stimulated can induce nausea and vomiting.[55,56]

The etiology of nausea and vomiting is varied, but it is important to determine the exact cause in order to select targeted and effective treatment. The most common etiologies in patients with cancer are chemotherapy-induced nausea and vomiting (CINV), opioid-induced, bowel obstruction, and constipation. Once the likely etiology of nausea and vomiting is identified, directed therapy can begin. There are guidelines for the prevention and treatment of CINV in patients on antineoplastic therapy.[57] The most commonly used approach is based on identifying the etiology and administering the most potent antagonist targeted toward the implicated receptors. This strategy has been shown to be effective in up to 80–90% of patients. Some practitioners recommend starting an empirical antiemetic regimen, typically with a dopamine antagonist, regardless of the presumed etiology.[58–60]

No direct comparisons currently exist between mechanism-based and empirical therapy.

Therapy should consist of nonpharmacologic and pharmacologic measures aimed at alleviating the cause of the symptoms. Nonpharmacologic measures include avoiding strong smells or other nausea triggers, eating small, frequent meals, limiting oral intake during periods of extreme emesis,[61] relaxation techniques,[62] acupuncture, and acupressure.[63] Progressive muscle relaxation and guided mental imagery during periods of chemotherapy have also shown beneficial effects.[64] The most commonly used antiemetics worldwide are metoclopramide, dexamethasone, haloperidol, hyoscine butylbromide, and cyclizine. Olanzapine is useful for delayed and refractory nausea.[65] Antiemetics are available in the form of pills, orally dissolvable tablets, intravenous infusion, rectal suppositories, and subcutaneous infusions. Thought should be given to selection of the appropriate route of administration of the antiemetic to ensure maximum efficacy. A list of antiemetics, routes of administration and their properties can be found in Table 7.

Anorexia/cachexia syndrome (ACS)

ACS is characterized by disproportionate and excessive loss of lean body mass. ACS may occur in up to 80% of patients with advanced cancer.[66] ACS is usually a marker of disease progression. In a multicenter retrospective review of 3047 cancer patients enrolled on clinical trials from the Eastern Cooperative Oncology Group, weight loss of more than 5% of premorbid weight prior to the initiation of chemotherapy was predictive of early mortality.[67] Weight loss was independent of disease stage, tumor histology, and patient performance status in its predictive value.[67]

Management of this syndrome should first focus on trying to treat any of the contributing secondary causes. Because anorexia is a prevalent and distressing symptom suffered by most cancer patients, the basis of pharmacologic treatment has focused on alleviating this symptom. The two classes of drugs that have been shown to be effective in Phase III clinical trials are corticosteroids and progestational agents.[68,69] These drugs do not appear to improve survival but may improve quality of life. Corticosteroids, usually in the form of dexamethasone at a dose of 4 mg/day (although doses of 2–20 mg/day can be used), have been shown to alleviate cancer anorexia on a short-term basis. This finding has been replicated by other studies and both prednisolone and methylprednisolone have been shown to be effective.[70] As the duration of appetite stimulation is short lived, and the side effects increase over time, it is most useful for patients with a life expectancy of less than 6 weeks. Megestrol acetate has been shown to result in dose-dependent improvements in appetite which usually occur in about 1 week. Improvement in overall well-being has been demonstrated in more than 60% of patients starting at doses of 160 mg/day. The optimal dosing for weight gain appears to be between 480 and 800 mg per day. Effects are seen after several weeks in only 25% of patients.[71] It is important to start at a lower dose and titrate upward as adverse events are dose related. Adverse events include deep vein thrombosis, especially in those concomitantly on chemotherapy, edema, hyperglycemia, and elevated liver enzymes. Cannabinoids, in their synthetic form of dronabinol, may have some limited effects on improving appetite but do not contribute to significant weight gain. In a randomized trial comparing dronabinol to megestrol acetate significantly more patients had improvement in appetite and weight gain with megestrol acetate.[72] Combined therapy with both megestrol acetate and dronabinol had no benefit beyond that obtained with megestrol acetate alone. Adverse events with dronabinol include sedation, confusion, and perceptual disturbances.

Medical marijuana legality varies by state and is generally paid out of pocket so may be costly; reported benefits include improved pain,[73] nausea, and appetite, though data remains sparse and side effects are common.[74] Cannabidiol (CBD) formulations have lower risks of adverse effects and are more readily available than products containing tetrahydrocannabinol (THC); studies on efficacy are limited.[75]

Dyspnea

Dyspnea is the awareness of an uncomfortable or unpleasant sensation of breathing. The prevalence of dyspnea varies greatly and ranges from 21% to 79% depending on primary disease site, stage of disease, and location of metastasis.[76] The sensation of dyspnea is a subjective experience with numerous etiologies. The presence of tachypnea and hypoxia does not adequately reflect the severity of symptoms felt by the patient.[77] It is not uncommon that patients with moderate to severe tachypnea will not complain of dyspnea. In contrast, patients who are not tachypneic may report severe dyspnea. It is, therefore, of utmost importance that assessment be based on patient report. The goal of treatment is symptomatic relief of the patient's expression of dyspnea, rather than the correction of objective variables (tachypnea, low oxygen saturation).

The most common modalities used to treat dyspnea include oxygen therapy and opioids. Three randomized controlled crossover studies have evaluated the use of oxygen (4 or 5 L/min) versus air in advanced cancer patients with dyspnea. Two of these studies evaluated patients with hypoxemia on room air and found that oxygen therapy was more beneficial.[78,79] The third evaluated nonhypoxemic cancer patients and found that there was no difference between oxygen therapy and air in reducing the intensity of dyspnea.[80] Opioids are the pharmacologic treatment of choice in the management of dyspnea. Several randomized controlled trials in cancer patients with dyspnea have demonstrated their benefit. In opioid-naive patients, a starting dose of morphine sulfate 2.5–5 mg orally or its equivalent intravenously every 4 h can be effective. In those patients already on opioid therapy, an increase of 25% in the baseline dose may provide relief.[81]

The terminal phase

Death is a natural process that will occur for every patient. About 10% of people will die suddenly and unexpectedly while the other 90% die after a period of illness with gradual deterioration until an active dying phase occurs signifying the end of life.[8] There are "two roads to death,"[82] the usual road which occurs in most patients and presents as decreasing level of consciousness that leads to coma and death, and the difficult road. The difficult road is marked by terminal delirium which can manifest as restlessness, confusion, and agitation; it can be a source of great distress for patients, family, and loved ones.[82] The most common symptoms reported by families in the last week of life are fatigue, dyspnea, and dry mouth, while the most distressing are fatigue, dyspnea, and pain.[83] The Clinical Practice Guidelines for Quality Palliative Care emphasize that families should be educated regarding the signs and symptoms of approaching death in a manner that is developmentally, age, and culturally appropriate.[14] While patients and families may still be focused on glucose or blood pressure control, such preventive measures must be taken into the context of the patients' life expectancy. Discontinuation of such medications often involves a detailed discussion about the risks and adverse effects outweighing the probable lack of benefit. The least invasive rate of medication administration should be attempted initially using the most invasive route only when absolutely necessary. A variety of physiologic changes occur in the last hours to days of life and the following is a summary of the most common changes that occur[84,85]:

1. *Weakness and fatigue*. Weakness and fatigue usually increase as the patient is approaching death. Patients will begin to spend all of their time in bed and will be less interested in participating in usual activities, including visiting with others.
2. *Decreased oral intake*. Most dying patients lose their appetite and stop drinking. Many caregivers interpret this as a patient "giving up" or "starving to death." It is important to explain to patients and their family members that there is a decreased need for food and drink during this phase. There is some evidence suggesting that prolonged anorexia is not uncomfortable. One study found that 97% of dying patients who stopped eating experienced no hunger or hunger only initially.[86] It has been proposed that terminal anorexia induces a ketosis that contributes to a sense of wellbeing and diminished discomfort and may in fact be beneficial to dying patients.[84,87] Two meta-analyses of studies of both parenteral[88] and enteral[89] nutrition in patients with metastatic cancer found that neither therapy resulted in an improvement in morbidity or mortality and actually resulted in

Table 8 Pharmacologic therapy of delirium.

Drug name	Dosage/route	Comments
Haloperidol	0.5–5 mg PO/IV/IM/SC every 6–12 h	Most commonly used agent. Can prolong QT interval
Chlorpromazine	12.5–50 mg PO/IV/IM every 8–12 h	Has similar efficacy to haloperidol, but more sedating, anticholinergic, and hypotensive effects
Lorazepam	0.5–2 mg PO/SL/IV every 4–8 h and titrate as needed	Most commonly used as a second agent in combination with haloperidol. Can also be used as a continuous infusion for refractory cases where deep sedation is needed. May worsen delirium in the elderly. Caution with liver failure
Risperidone	Start at 0.5–1 mg/d PO and titrate up to 4–6 mg/d	In one study shown to have no differences in side effects when compared to haloperidol.[95] Limited use as only available in oral route
Olanzapine	5 mg PO qhs and titrated to effect (max 20 mg/d)	Risk factors for a poor response to olanzapine in cancer patients are[87] • Age >70 • History of dementia • CNS metastases • Hypoxia • Hypoactive delirium
Midazolam	1 mg/h IV and titrated to effect	Most commonly used for refractory cases where sedation is needed

an increased total complication rate. The evidence with respect to hydration in dying patients is less straightforward with many differing expert opinions.[84,90–92] Some studies suggest that parenteral hydration prevents and treats some cases of terminal delirium[90,91,93] and others correlate dehydration with adverse symptoms such as thirst.[92,94,95] Still others believe that the data does not support a correlation between dehydration and symptoms and that rehydration does not improve patient comfort.[86,93] A randomized control trial of advancer cancer patients within weeks of death demonstrated no improvement in symptoms, QOL, or survival when compared to placebo.[96] It is important that each individual patient be evaluated to determine the risk-benefit ratio. Attention should be placed on minimizing the sense of thirst and maintaining patient comfort even when dehydration is present, with oral hygiene. This can be achieved by using lollipop sponges dipped in cold fluids such as water, a lemon-flavored drink, or sorbet.

3. *Delirium.* While reversible factors may be identified in up to half of cases, terminal delirium management typically focuses on symptom control with medications.[95] Treatment should be aimed at the symptoms of delirium while simultaneously attempting to treat reversible causes. Although delirium is most often associated with the last hours to days of life, in some episodes it may be reversible with therapeutic intervention.[95,97] Neuroleptic agents are the mainstay of pharmacologic treatment as they are effective in both hypoactive and hyperactive delirium. Of these agents, haloperidol is the agent of choice as it has lower sedating properties, less anticholinergic and cardiovascular effects. The pharmacologic agents commonly used in the management of delirium can be found in Table 8.

Physician aid in dying

Physician aid in dying, or physician-assisted death (PAD), is now legal in 8 states (California, Colorado, Hawaii, Maine, New Jersey, Oregon, Vermont, and Washington) and the District of Columbia.[98] Recommendations for any patient requesting aid in dying are to provide comprehensive pain and symptom management, bolster patient's sense of control and autonomy,[99] and assess for underlying untreated depression.[100,101] The American Academy of Hospice and Palliative Medicine has revised its position on PAD from one of opposition to one of "studied neutrality" and stated that "morally conscientious individuals adhere to a broad range of positions on this issue."[102]

Grief and bereavement

Bereavement is the state of loss as a consequence of death.[103] Grief is defined as the emotional response to loss and mourning, and often refers to social expressions associated with loss.[103] Several types of grief exist including anticipatory, grief, uncomplicated grief, and complicated grief. Anticipatory grief refers to the mourning that occurs in patients and families prior to death and is a way to facilitate the adjustment to bereavement. Uncomplicated grief is the most common type of grief reaction and is socially perceived as normal. Complicated grief involves the persistence of grief reactions over a long period of time and is characterized by an inability to return to the pre-loss level of functioning.[104] Palliative care and hospice provide grief and bereavement services to patients and their caregivers before, during, and after death to help promote healthy grieving.

Both hospice and palliative care have been shown to provide effective pre-loss interventions for preventing complicated bereavement. These interventions are associated with a reduced risk of major depressive disorder in caregivers.[105] The multidisciplinary palliative care team including physicians, social workers, nurses, psychologists, and chaplains performs a psychosocial assessment of the patient and caregiver in order to identify those that may be high risk for complicated grief. The palliative care team can provide basic practical help before death such as assisting with advanced directives, assisting with financial matters, and encouraging individual medical care of the caregiver as well as providing assistance after death by offering counseling or referral to other support services.

Hospice

Hospice is a philosophy of care. The goal of hospice is to focus on maintaining the best quality of life rather than length of life in patients who have a life expectancy of 6 months or less. It is different from palliative care in that palliative care is given simultaneously with other curative and life-prolonging therapies. Hospice services have been available in the United States since 1974 and have been funded by Medicare as part of the Medicare hospice benefit since 1982.[106]

Hospice is the only Medicare benefit that includes medications, durable medical equipment, and continuous around-the-clock access to care and support. Bereavement services are also offered to family members after a patient's death. The Medicare hospice benefit covers all care related to the cancer diagnosis. The patient can still receive Medicare benefits for the treatment of other illnesses.

Most hospice care is delivered at home. It is also provided in other settings such as inpatient hospice facilities, nursing homes, assisted living facilities, and hospitals. It is estimated that approximately 45% of all people who died in the United States in 2011 were under the care of a hospice program and of all patients enrolled, 38% had a diagnosis of cancer.[107] In a study comparing survival of hospice to nonhospice patients, hospice care prolonged the lives of some terminally ill cancer patients.[108] The mean survival period was significantly longer for hospice patients with lung cancer (39 days longer) and pancreatic cancer (21 days), while marginally significant for colon cancer (33 days).[108]

Summary

Palliative care is patient and family-centered interdisciplinary care that focuses on relieving suffering and providing the best quality of life for patients undergoing curative and life-prolonging treatments as well as for patients in whom cancer-specific treatments are no longer available. It is estimated that 35% of patients with cancer will die from their disease.[109] Increasing attention has been given to improvements in quality-of-life issues in oncology, for patients undergoing chemotherapy, patients at the end of life as well as cancer survivors. Prevalence of symptoms during cancer treatment can be substantial. Palliative care is an integral part of comprehensive cancer care. Palliative care is most effective when initiated at the time of diagnosis allowing for patients to be followed through the trajectory of illness. The oncologist plays a key role in discussing treatment options, curative or palliative, from the outset of the diagnosis. Assessing the patients' goals is equally as important. Patients should be made aware that receiving anticancer treatments does not preclude them from access to palliative care services. Increasing the emphasis on palliative care in oncology should improve patient outcomes and can diminish some of the oncologist's stress of caring for patients with serious and life-threatening illness. Palliative care has had a rapid growth in the last two decades in response to the increasing number of patients living with serious, chronic conditions and as a result of a demand for high-quality symptom control, coordination of care across settings, and advanced care planning.

The number of palliative care programs within hospital settings has increased by 138% since 2000.[110] Expansion of palliative medicine education is supported by the Liaison Committee on Medical Education (LCME), which has mandated medical school education in palliative medicine and the ACGME which requires oncology fellow training in palliative medicine. There is a plethora of internet-based resources that provide physicians in practice with access to further information and education on palliative care (Table 2).

Key references

The complete reference list can be found on Vital Source version of this title, see inside front cover.

1. Morrison RS, Meier DE. Clinical practice. Palliative care. *N Engl J Med.* 2004;**350**:2582–2590.
2. Hoerger M, Greer JA, Jackson VA, et al. Defining the elements of early palliative care that are associated with patient-reported outcomes and the delivery of end-of-life care. *J Clin Oncol.* 2018;**36**:1096–1102.
3. Temel JS, Greer JA, Muzikansky A, et al. Early palliative care for patients with metastatic non-small-cell lung cancer. *N Engl J Med.* 2010;**363**:733–742.
10. Hoerger M, Wayser GR, Schwing G, et al. Impact of interdisciplinary outpatient specialty palliative care on survival and quality of life in adults with advanced cancer: a meta-analysis of randomized controlled trials. *Ann Behav Med.* 2019;**53**:674–685.
13. Smith C, Brawley OW. Disparities in access to palliative care. In: *Meeting the Needs of Older Adults with Serious Illness*. Health Affairs; 2014:19–29. doi: 10.1007/978-1-4939-0407-5_2.
14. National Consensus Project for Quality Palliative Care. Clinical practice guidelines for quality palliative care, executive summary. *J Palliat Med.* 2004;**7**:611–627.
15. Kühne F, Krattenmacher T, Beierlein V, et al. Minor children of palliative patients: a systematic review of psychosocial family interventions. *J Palliat Med.* 2012;**15**:931–945.
17. Marcus KL, Santos G, Ciapponi A, et al. Impact of specialized pediatric palliative care: a systematic review. *J Pain Symptom Manage.* 2020;**59**:339–364.e10.
20. Hebert HD, Butera JN, Castillo J, et al. Are we training our fellows adequately in delivering bad news to patients? A survey of hematology/oncology program directors. *J Palliat Med.* 2009;**12**:1119–1124.
21. Buss MK, Lessen DS, Sullivan AM, et al. A study of oncology fellows' training in end-of-life care. *J Support Oncol.* 2007;**5**:237–242.
25. Zachariae R, Pedersen CG, Jensen AB, et al. Association of perceived physician communication style with patient satisfaction, distress, cancer-related self-efficacy, and perceived control over the disease. *Br J Cancer.* 2003;**88**:658–665.
26. Baile WF, Buckman R, Lenzi R, et al. SPIKES-A six-step protocol for delivering bad news: application to the patient with cancer. *Oncologist.* 2000;**5**:302–311.
31. Hickman SE, Nelson CA, Perrin NA, et al. A comparison of methods to communicate treatment preferences in nursing facilities: traditional practices versus the physician orders for life-sustaining treatment program. *J Am Geriatr Soc.* 2010;**58**:1241–1248.
42. Jairam V, Yang DX, Verma V, et al. National patterns in prescription opioid use and misuse among cancer survivors in the United States. *JAMA Netw Open.* 2020;**3**:e2013605.
47. Broglio K, Doering A, Bassett E, et al. Universal precautions for opioid prescribing in ambulatory palliative care (FR441D). *J Pain Symptom Manag.* 2018;**55**:617–618.
52. Hawley PH, Byeon JJ. A comparison of sennosides-based bowel protocols with and without docusate in hospitalized patients with cancer. *J Palliat Med.* 2008;**11**:575–581.
53. Walsh TD. Symptom control in patients with advanced cancer. *Am J Hosp Palliat Care.* 1992;**9**:32–40.
55. Wood GJ, Shega JW, Lynch B, et al. Management of intractable nausea and vomiting in patients at the end of life: "I was feeling nauseous all of the time nothing was working". *JAMA.* 2007;**298**:1196–1207.
56. Davis MP, Walsh D. Treatment of nausea and vomiting in advanced cancer. *Support Care Cancer.* 2000;**8**:444–452.
57. NCCN. *NCCN: Antiemesis. NCCN Clinical Practice Guidelines in Oncology*, 2013; Version 1.2013.
59. Benze G, Geyer A, Alt-Epping B, et al. Treatment of nausea and vomiting with 5HT3 receptor antagonists, steroids, antihistamines, anticholinergics, somatostatinantagonists, benzodiazepines and cannabinoids in palliative care patients: a systematic review. *Schmerz.* 2012;**26**:481–499.
62. Burish TG, Tope DM. Psychological techniques for controlling the adverse side effects of cancer chemotherapy: findings from a decade of research. *J Pain Symptom Manag.* 1992;**7**:287–301.
63. Vickers AJ. Can acupuncture have specific effects on health? A systematic review of acupuncture antiemesis trials. *J R Soc Med.* 1996;**89**:303–311.
64. Cotanch PH. Use of nonpharmacological techniques to prevent chemotherapy-related nausea and vomiting. *Recent Results Cancer Res.* 1991;**121**:101–107.
65. Navari RM, Pywell CM, Le-Rademacher JG, et al. Olanzapine for the treatment of advanced cancer–related chronic nausea and/or vomiting: a randomized pilot trial. *JAMA Oncol.* 2020;**6**:895–899.
66. Del Fabbro E, Dalal S, Bruera E. Symptom control in palliative care--Part II: cachexia/anorexia and fatigue. *J Palliat Med.* 2006;**9**:409–421.
67. Dewys WD, Begg C, Lavin PT, et al. Prognostic effect of weight loss prior to chemotherapy in cancer patients. Eastern Cooperative Oncology Group. *Am J Med.* 1980;**69**:491–497.
68. Kornblith AB, Hollis DR, Zuckerman E, et al. Effect of megestrol acetate on quality of life in a dose-response trial in women with advanced breast cancer. The Cancer and Leukemia Group B. *J Clin Oncol.* 1993;**11**:2081–2089.
69. Servaes P, Verhagen C, Bleijenberg G. Fatigue in cancer patients during and after treatment: prevalence, correlates and interventions. *Eur J Cancer.* 2002;**38**:27–43.
74. MacDonald E, Farrah K. *CADTH Rapid Response Reports, Medical Cannabis Use in Palliative Care: Review of Clinical Effectiveness and Guidelines – An Update.* Ottawa (ON): Canadian Agency for Drugs and Technologies in Health Copyright © 2019 Canadian Agency for Drugs and Technologies in Health; 2019.
80. Bruera E, Sweeney C, Willey J, et al. A randomized controlled trial of supplemental oxygen versus air in cancer patients with dyspnea. *Palliat Med.* 2003;**17**:659–663.
81. Allard P, Lamontagne C, Bernard P, et al. How effective are supplementary doses of opioids for dyspnea in terminally ill cancer patients? A randomized continuous sequential clinical trial. *J Pain Symptom Manag.* 1999;**17**:256–265.

83 Hickman SE, Tilden VP, Tolle SW. Family reports of dying patients' distress: the adaptation of a research tool to assess global symptom distress in the last week of life. *J Pain Symptom Manag*. 2001;**22**:565–574.

86 McCann RM, Hall WJ, Groth-Juncker A. Comfort care for terminally ill patients. The appropriate use of nutrition and hydration. *JAMA*. 1994;**272**:1263–1266.

88 Koretz RL, Lipman TO, Klein S, et al. AGA technical review on parenteral nutrition. *Gastroenterology*. 2001;**121**:970–1001.

89 Koretz RL, Avenell A, Lipman TO, et al. Does enteral nutrition affect clinical outcome? A systematic review of the randomized trials. *Am J Gastroenterol*. 2007;**102**:412–429; quiz 468.

96 Bruera E, Hui D, Dalal S, et al. Parenteral hydration in patients with advanced cancer: a multicenter, double-blind, placebo-controlled randomized trial. *J Clin Oncol*. 2013;**31**:111–118.

97 Gagnon P, Allard P, Masse B, et al. Delirium in terminal cancer: a prospective study using daily screening, early diagnosis, and continuous monitoring. *J Pain Symptom Manag*. 2000;**19**:412–426.

105 Zhang B, El-Jawahri A, Prigerson HG. Update on bereavement research: evidence-based guidelines for the diagnosis and treatment of complicated bereavement. *J Palliat Med*. 2006;**9**:1188–1203.

108 Connor SR, Pyenson B, Fitch K, et al. Comparing hospice and nonhospice patient survival among patients who die within a three-year window. *J Pain Symptom Manag*. 2007;**33**:238–246.

45 Psycho-oncology

Diya Banerjee, MD ■ Andrew J. Roth, MD

> **Overview**
>
> Cancer increasingly is a disease of aging adults, given better diagnostic tools and improved and innovative treatments. This once uniformly deadly experience has been transformed into one that if not cured, can be lived with for longer periods of times as a chronic illness. Thus, the emotional needs of patients, family members and society has also morphed into more hope for potential and realized cures and therapies. However, dealing with a life-threatening disease and the existential reality of mortality still brings on various emotions from sadness to depression, worry to anxiety to panic, to traumatic stress. Harsh treatments can cause delirium as well as changes in cognition., and the biology of cancer itself, with an impact on hormonal axes and generation of inflammatory responses, can engender psychiatric sequelae. These emotional, medical and psychiatric sequelae of cancer and cancer treatment are important to recognize and address in order to enhance adherence with complicated cancer treatment regimens, potentially improving success of these treatments, and, if needed, coping better with adverse outcomes. This article outlines basic information oncology treatment providers need for assessment and management of the most common psychiatric complications.

This article is dedicated to the memory of Dr. Jimmie C. Holland, a pioneer in the field of Psycho-Oncology, who died December 24, 2017. She lived almost 90 years, working tirelessly to improve the quality of lives of people impacted by cancer and the oncology teams who care for them. Her endeavors to nurture the human side of cancer care engaged her heart and soul and will last for generations.

Introduction

Almost 17 million Americans who had a history of cancer were alive in 2019, and more than 1.8 million new cases were expected to be diagnosed.[1] Cancer increasingly is a disease of aging adults, given better diagnostic tools and improved and innovative treatments. This once uniformly deadly experience has been transformed into one that if not cured, can be lived with for longer periods of time as a chronic illness. Thus, the emotional needs of patients and family members and society has also changed from fighting a vicious War on Cancer 50 years ago to engaging in a Moonshot of potential and realized cures and therapies. However, dealing with a life-threatening disease and the existential reality of mortality brings on various emotions from sadness to depression, worry to anxiety to panic, to traumatic stress. Harsh treatments can cause delirium as well as changes in cognition. The biology of cancer itself, with an impact on hormonal axes and generation of inflammatory responses, can engender psychiatric sequelae. All of these emotional, medical, and psychiatric sequelae of cancer and cancer treatment are important to recognize and address.

The Institute of Medicine Report from 2008 stressed the need to focus on the emotional needs of cancer patients[2] and highlighted barriers to identifying and addressing the psychosocial problems of people with cancer. Inadequate communication between patients and prescribers, multiple demands on clinicians' time, and suboptimal coordination of care among providers due to a variety of issues in the healthcare environment may all play a role in not adequately addressing these psychosocial needs, thus limiting patients' quality of life with cancer. The stigma of suffering both a cancer diagnosis and psychological problems keep providers and patients from more fully meeting these emotional needs. Attention to emotional needs may enhance adherence with complicated cancer treatment regimens, potentially improving success of these treatments, and, if needed, coping better with adverse outcomes. This article outlines basic information oncology treatment providers need for assessment and management of the most common psychiatric complications.

Clinical management

The spectrum of psychiatric illness present in cancer patients includes mood disorders, anxiety disorders, trauma or stressor-related disorders, and delirium. One major challenge for clinicians is distinguishing what may be an understandable, common, or expected emotional response, from what constitutes a psychiatric illness, or a psychiatric presentation of a medical disorder. Situational anxiety, sadness, trouble sleeping, fatigue, and fear are frequent, and can often be well managed with reassurance and care. Psychiatric co-morbidity however can significantly impact oncologic outcomes.[3-6] This may be a question of degree of intensity and regularity of symptoms; however, a key indicator of clinical pathology includes degree of functional impairment.

Since the inception of the field of psycho-oncology in the 1970s, evidence-based studies for measurement of psychological distress and interventions to relieve that distress have been shown to make it easier for oncology teams to screen for distress and more quickly improve the quality of life of people with cancer. The National Comprehensive Cancer Network Clinical Practice Guidelines[7] provided a roadmap for state-of-the-art integration of these assessment tools and therapies into daily oncology clinical practices. The American College of Surgeons Commission on Cancer required accredited cancer centers to have programs in place to identify and refer distressed patients for appropriate care.[8]

During the arc of cancer care, from pre-diagnosis to survivorship or end of life, there are patient-specific or situational factors that contribute to increased risk of psychiatric disease. These risk factors, which include pre-existing vulnerabilities, stress related

---

Holland-Frei Cancer Medicine, Tenth Edition. Edited by Robert C. Bast, John C. Byrd, Carlo M. Croce, Ernest Hawk, Fadlo R. Khuri, Raphael E. Pollock, Apostolia M. Tsimberidou, Christopher G. Willett, and Cheryl L. Willman.
© 2023 John Wiley & Sons, Inc. Published 2023 by John Wiley & Sons, Inc.

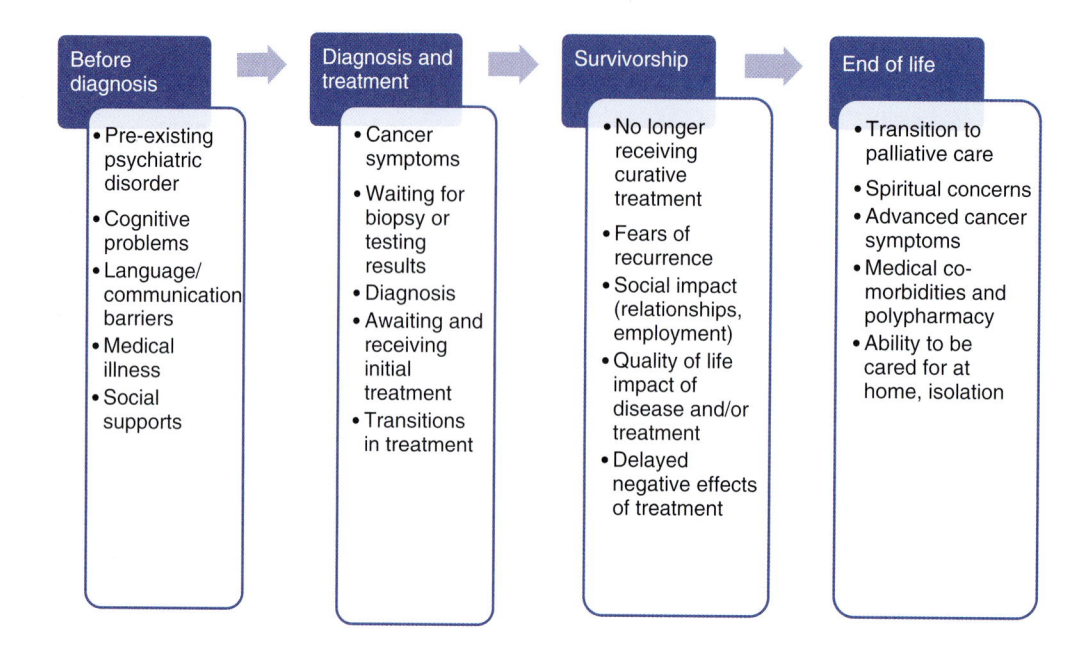

```
Before diagnosis                    Diagnosis and treatment          Survivorship                          End of life
• Pre-existing psychiatric         • Cancer symptoms                 • No longer receiving                 • Transition to palliative care
  disorder                         • Waiting for biopsy or             curative treatment                  • Spiritual concerns
• Cognitive problems                 testing results                 • Fears of recurrence                 • Advanced cancer symptoms
• Language/communication           • Diagnosis                       • Social impact (relationships,       • Medical co-morbidities and
  barriers                         • Awaiting and receiving            employment)                           polypharmacy
• Medical illness                    initial treatment               • Quality of life impact of           • Ability to be cared for at
• Social supports                  • Transitions in treatment          disease and/or treatment              home, isolation
                                                                     • Delayed negative effects
                                                                       of treatment
```

Figure 1 Risk factors for psychiatric illness at different stages of cancer care.

to diagnosis, consequences of treatment, and survivorship or transition to end of life, are identified in Figure 1 above. They are important for a primary oncologic team to be aware of and consider during cancer treatment. We will focus on the symptomatology of common psychiatric conditions as well as provide an overview of appropriate management strategies to ameliorate symptoms or unwanted psychiatric sequelae.

Depressive disorders

While sadness and distress are normal responses to cancer, depression is a distinct clinical entity with significant morbidity[9] outside of the range of normal. The incidence of depression in cancer populations is high, approximately 20%, compared to the general population, differing by type of cancer and treatment phase.[10] The common symptom cluster associated with a depressive episode includes a combination of behavioral patterns (substantial changes in sleep and/or appetite), psychomotor symptoms (apathy, slowing down or agitation), cognitive symptoms (impaired concentration), and mood (feelings of sadness and inability to experience pleasure), which are present most days, most of the day, for at least 2 weeks.

For cancer patients, in particular, disease symptoms and side effects from treatment can muddy the diagnostic picture. For example, chemotherapy is known to cause cognitive symptoms,[11] fatigue, and sleep disturbances, and advanced cancer is known to cause anorexia, fatigue, and physical weakness that lead to not being able to do usual pleasurable activities, all of which can look like signs of depression. With this in mind, there are a few cardinal symptoms that should raise concern for a primary depressive disorder. These include hopelessness; anhedonia or loss of pleasure (when there is not a physical symptom such as pain, nausea, or fatigue that might better explain avoidance of pleasurable activities); persistent low mood (for at least 2 weeks); feelings of guilt or worthlessness; and suicidal thoughts. Additionally, a careful history including a chronology of symptoms, precipitating events, correlation with onset of treatment side effects, identification of risk factors, as well as surveillance for new medical complications can provide diagnostic clarity.

Treatment of depressive disorders in people with cancer

Depression is a treatable illness, and the best evidence-based treatments suggest a multi-modal approach with pharmacotherapy, psychotherapy, and psychosocial interventions.[12] Nonpharmacologic therapy interventions include supportive psychotherapy, cognitive behavioral therapy, mindfulness-based therapy, psychodynamic psychotherapy, and group therapy.

Few clinical trials have assessed antidepressant efficacy, with mixed results in effectiveness of treatment of depression or depressive symptoms in patients with cancer.[13,14] Medications for depression fall into several different categories, including selective serotonin reuptake inhibitors (SSRIs), serotonin and norepinephrine reuptake inhibitors (SNRIs), cyclic antidepressants (TCAs), norepinephrine/dopamine-reuptake inhibitor (NDRI), and psychostimulants. Primary care physicians, advanced practice providers, and oncologists are often the prescribers of antidepressants and other psychotropic medications, because of the reluctance of patients to seek psychiatric care, inadequate insurance coverage for mental health, and the shortage of psycho-oncologists. Tables 1 and 2 feature common medications used for treating depression in cancer patients, highlighting advantages and disadvantages of different agents.

Suicide risk

Suicidality exists on a spectrum, ranging from transient passive thoughts about death (a wish to no longer be alive, or that it would be easier for the patient or others if they were to die), to active thinking, planning, enacting, and completing suicide. Suicidal thoughts are very common in cancer patients, though relatively few make suicide attempts or complete suicide. Compared to the general population, however, cancer patients are generally thought to have twice the risk of suicide, with the highest risk in cancer types that are associated with physical morbidity.[15] The risk of suicide is highest within the first year of a cancer diagnosis and can remain elevated for 5 years after diagnosis.

When assessing suicide risk, it can be helpful to identify static risk factors, modifiable risk factors, and protective factors. Static

Table 1 Pharmacology to treat depression and anxiety in cancer patients.

	Drug	Dosage	Advantages	Disadvantages
Selective Serotonin Re-update inhibitors (SSRI)	Escitalopram (Lexapro®)	Starting dose: 5 mg/d	Minimal drug interactions	Class effects: hyponatremia, nausea/diarrhea, sexual dysfunction
		Treatment dose: 10–20 mg/d	Fewer GI side effects	QT prolongation at 20 mg/d (monitor ECG)
	Citalopram (Celexa®)	Starting dose: 10 mg/d	Fewer GI side effects	Class effects: hyponatremia, nausea/diarrhea, sexual dysfunction
		Treatment dose: 10–40 mg/d	May improve quality of sleep	QT prolongation at 40 mg/d (monitor ECG)
	Fluoxetine (Prozac®)	Starting dose: 10 mg/d	Long half life (less discontinuation syndrome, better for the intermittently compliant)	Class effects: hyponatremia, nausea/diarrhea, sexual dysfunction
		Treatment dose: 20–60 mg/d		May cause agitation Strong CYP2D6 inhibitor (drug interactions)
	Sertraline (Zoloft®)	Starting dose: 25 mg/d	Few p450 interactions	Class effects: hyponatremia, nausea/diarrhea, sexual dysfunction
		Treatment dose: 50–150 mg/d		May have more GI side effects
Serotonin Neropinephrine Re-uptake inhibitors (SNRI)	Venlafaxine (Effexor XR®)	Starting dose: 37.5 mg/d	Useful for neuropathic pain	Class effects: discontinuation syndrome, sexual side effects, decreased appetite, nausea, somnolence
		Treatment dose: 75–225 mg/d	Can help with hot flashes Safe with tamoxifen	
	Desvenlafaxine (Pristiq®)	Starting dose: 50 mg/d	Fewer drug interactions than Venlafaxine	Class effects: discontinuation syndrome, sexual side effects, decreased appetite, nausea, somnolence
		Treatment dose: 50–100 mg/d		
	Duloxetine (Cymbalta®)	Starting dose: 20 mg/d	Useful for neuropathic pain and fibromyalgia	Class effects: nausea, decreased appetite, somnolence
		Treatment dose: 60 mg/d	Less likely to cause sexual side effects or discontinuation syndrome	Avoid use in liver and kidney disease

Table 2 Additional medications used to treat depression in people with cancer.

	Drug	Dosage	Advantages	Disadvantages
Tricyclic antideprasants	Antideprasant (Elavil®)	Starting dose: 25 mg/d	Useful for neuropathic pain or gastric upset	Anticholinergic side effects Sedating
		Treatment dose: 50–200 mg/d	Helpful for insomnia	Monitor EKG for arrhythmias
	Nortriptyline (Pamelor®)	Starting dose: 25 mg/d	Useful for neuropathic pain	Fewer anticholinergic side effects
		Treatment dose: 50–200 mg/d	May help sleep	Monitor EKG for arrhythmias
Other agents	Bupropion (Wellbutrin®)	Starting dose: 100 mg/d (SR) 150 mg/d (XL)	Fewer sexual side effects, less weight gain	Can worsen anxiety and insomnia
		Treatment dose: 150–300 mg/d (SR and XL)	Activating Smoking cessation	Lowers seizure threshold (do not use in patients with seizure disorder or bulimia)
	Mirtazapine (Remeron®)	Starting dose: 7.5 mg/night	Helps insomnia	Can cause daytime grogginess
		Treatment dose: 15–45 mg/night	Stimulates appetite Anti-emetic, no GI side effects Less cardiac risk	Weight gain
Stimulants	Dextroamphetamine (Dexedrine®)	Starting dose: 2.5 mg qAM and qPM	May improve fatigue and cognitive impairment from cancer treatment	Lowers seizure threshold, can cause cardiac arrhythmias
		Treatment dose: 5–30 mg total		Anxiety, insomnia, restlessness Prolonged use at high doses can cause tics and paranoia
	Methylphenidate (Ritalin®)	Starting dose: 2.5 mg qAM and qPM	May improve fatigue and cognitive impairment from cancer treatment	Lowers seizure threshold, can cause cardiac arrhythmias
		Treatment dose: 5–30 mg total		Anxiety, insomnia, restlessness Prolonged use at high doses can cause tics and paranoia
	Modafinil (Provigil®)	Starting dose: 50 mg BID	Activating, gentler than other stimulants	Medication interactions
		Treatment dose: 50–200 mg total	Usually well tolerated	Nausea, cardiac side effects

risk factors typically include demographic features (i.e., age and gender); as well as history of psychiatric illness, trauma; suicidality; substance use; or family history of suicide. Modifiable risk factors include mood symptoms, active substance use, cancer symptom burden (especially pain), access to lethal methods, and psychosocial stressors such as isolation and financial instability. Treating providers can address these risk factors by creating a safe environment, ameliorating symptoms, engaging with patient and family to modify accessible risk factors, and referring patients for additional support. Protective factors include family and community support, cultural and religious beliefs, and access to clinical interventions for mental, physical, and substance abuse disorders.

Table 3 Columbia suicide severity rating scale (applied for permissions).[a]

Columbia-suicide severity rating scale Screen with Triage Points for Primary Care (C-SSRS)	Past month	
Ask questions that are in bold and <u>underlined</u>	Yes	No
Ask questions 1 and 2		
Wish to be dead: Subject endorses thoughts about a wish to be dead or not alive anymore or wish to fall asleep and not wake up. **Have you wished you were dead or wished you could go to sleep and not wake up?**	🟨 Mild	
Non-specific active suicidal thoughts: General non-specific thoughts of wanting to end one's life/die by suicide (e.g., "I've thought about killing myself") without thoughts of ways to kill oneself/associated methods, intent, or plan during the assessment period **Have you had any actual thoughts of killing yourself?**	🟨 Mild	
If Yes to 2, ask questions 3, 4, 5, and 6. If No to 2, go directly to question 6		
Active suicidal ideation with any methods (Not Plan) without intent to act Subject endorses thoughts of suicide and has thought of at least one method during the assessment period. This is different than a specific plan with time, place or method details worked out (e.g., thought of method to kill self but not a specific plan). Includes person who would say, "I thought about taking an overdose but I never made a specific plan as to when, where or how I would actually do it… and I would never go through with it." **Have you been thinking about how you might do this?**	🟧 Moderate	🟨 Mild
Active suicidal ideation with some intent to act, without specific plan: Active suicidal thoughts of killing oneself and subject reports having some intent to act on such thoughts, as opposed to "I have the thoughts but I definitely will not do anything about them." **Have you had these thoughts and had some intention of acting on them?**	🟥 Severe	🟧 Moderate
Active suicidal ideation with specific plan and intent: Thoughts of killing oneself with details of plan fully or partially worked out and subject has some intent to carry it out. **Have you started to work out or worked out the details of how to kill yourself?** **Do you intend to carry out this plan?**	🟥 Severe	🟧 Moderate
Past 3 months		
Suicidal behavior: Have you ever done anything, started to do anything, or prepared to do anything to end your life? Examples: Collected pills, obtained a gun, gave away valuables, wrote a will or suicide note, took out pills but didn't swallow any, held a gun but changed your mind or it was grabbed from your hand, went to the roof but didn't jump: or actually took Jills, tried to shoot yourself, cut yourself, tried to hang yourself, etc.	🟥 Severe	🟧 Moderate

🟨 Mild suicide risk
🟧 Moderate suicide risk
🟥 Severe suicide risk

[a] Source: Posner et al.[18]

While static risk factors cannot change, modifiable risk factors can be mitigated, and protective factors can be reinforced.

In response to increasing suicide rates in the United States, the Joint Commission added a requirement to the National Patient Safety Goals requiring hospitals to establish assessment tools and standardize procedures to treat patients at risk of suicide.[16] The Columbia Suicide Severity Rating Scale[17] shown in Table 3 is a quick and well-established screening tool to assess suicidal thinking in patients. Acute suicidality can be a psychiatric emergency, and a patient should not be left alone until a full assessment is done.

Anxiety disorders

Across studies, over 40% of older adults with cancer report clinically significant anxiety that can persist for years following cancer treatment.[19] Yet, up to half of distressed older adults with cancer do not receive psychosocial services.[20] Anxiety is an emotional state that often impacts people's body, thoughts, and behaviors. It is a normal reaction to stress or threat, however, in anxiety disorders, these symptoms are out of proportion to the situation and hinder functioning. In cancer patients, anxiety can arise in reaction to the threat of illness or fear of recurrence after cancer treatment. The differential diagnosis for anxiety symptoms in a person with cancer must also include medication side effects, abnormal metabolic states, and delirium. Anxiety disorders can be generalized or specific; generalized presentations often result in excessive worry and avoidance of potentially distressing situations and specific presentations include particular phobias or panic attacks. There is less data assessing the incidence of anxiety compared to depression among cancer patients; however, the rate of anxiety disorders among those with cancer is approximately 10%.[21]

The treatment for anxiety tends to be similar to depression—SSRIs and SNRIs are first-line treatments for moderate to severe generalized anxiety disorder and panic disorders. However, as these medications can take weeks to have full effect, clinicians often use benzodiazepines to augment treatment or provide relief for breakthrough anxiety symptoms, especially when waiting for test results

Table 4 Pharmacology to treat anxiety in people with cancer.

Drug	Dosage frequency	Advantages	Disadvantages
Alprazolam (Xanax®)	0.25–1 mg PO q6-24 h	Fast onset, shorter half life	High addiction potential Rebound anxiety
Clonazepam (Klonipin®)	0.5–2 mg PO q6-24 h	Longer acting Less addiction potential	Slower onset of action Lower addiction potential
Diazepam (Valium®)	2–10 mg PO q6-24 h	Available as IV Long acting due to metabolite	Addiction potential
Lorazepam (Ativan®)	0.5–2 mg q4-12 h	Available as IM, IV push, IV piggyback Safer in liver impairment	Addiction potential

or undergoing medical procedures. Pharmacologic management of anxiety in older adults with cancer involves the judicious use of antidepressants, benzodiazepines, and antipsychotics.[22]

Table 4 identifies some common benzodiazepines used for treatment of anxiety. Patients and prescribers are sometimes hesitant to use these controlled substances due to concerns about addiction. Prior to prescribing, discussions about the distinction between dependence, tolerance, and addiction as well as appropriate monitoring alleviate fear of medication misuse. Buspirone is a nonbenzodiazepine that treats generalized anxiety symptoms. It needs to be taken daily and has a delayed onset, as do the antidepressants, but does not have abuse potential as do the benzodiazepines. Of note, there are some medications used off-label for anxiety that often have ameliorating effects on anxiety—these include gabapentin and pregabalin (treatments for neuropathic pain syndromes and hot flashes) and olanzapine or quetiapine (atypical antipsychotics that are also used to treat chemotherapy induced nausea and insomnia). Propranolol can treat and prevent panic attacks. As with depression, the most effective treatment usually includes medication and psychotherapy. Relaxation and meditation are useful treatments for anxiety and can equip patients with coping tools to apply to future stressful situation.

Cognitive-behavioral therapy (CBT), in particular, can be helpful for anxiety in patients with cancer.[23] CBT is a time-limited problem-focused psychological treatment, usually 2–10 sessions, that targets thoughts and behaviors that increase distress.[24] CBT has been extensively studied and shown to be effective in older adults[25,26] and cancer patients.[27] Oncologists and their team members can support patients with psychiatric symptoms in ways other than medication. Regular contact with patients and families, use of clear, empathetic and supportive communication, and involving mental health professionals in the treatment team, can all significantly ameliorate patient's suffering.

Trauma and stressor-related disorders

Trauma and stressor-related disorders are a general clinical category, encompassing acute stress reactions (such as adjustment disorders or acute stress disorder) as well as delayed and persistent symptomatology (such as posttraumatic stress disorder). Posttraumatic stress disorder (PTSD) can arise from any life-threatening traumatic event, including events associated with cancer and cancer treatment. Lifetime prevalence rates among cancer patients are approximately 12.6%,[28] higher than the general population. Symptoms of PTSD overlap with anxiety and depression but also include phenomena such as re-experiencing traumatic events (flashbacks or nightmares), hypervigilance, dissociation, and avoidance behaviors (such as missing appointments or noncompliance). Assessment of distress with the NCCN distress thermometer can help screen patients at higher risk for trauma and stressor-related disorders. Treatment for these disorders involves focusing on comorbid depression and anxiety with the interventions described above. Trauma-specific therapies such as exposure therapy and eye movement desensitization and reprocessing (EMDR) have shown some efficacy in cancer populations.[28] Not all people experience cancer as a trauma; in fact, there is a converse phenomenon of positive changes that can arise called posttraumatic growth.[29]

Personality clusters and potential impact on cancer treatment

Patients with personality disorders are often among the most difficult for clinicians to treat. They tend to exhibit atypical behavioral and communication styles in response to stressful circumstances[30] such as those in inpatient and outpatient cancer settings. Most oncology practices do not have readily available mental health workers to manage the spectrum of pervasive personality disorders typified by rigid character traits associated with impaired ability to relate to others. A quick synopsis of three general personality clusters, grouped by shared vulnerabilities and coping styles, can expedite recognition of someone with a personality disorder that can add hours to staff support requirements, frustration and unexpected anger among, and sometimes between, staff.

Cluster A personality traits

Patients with paranoid tendencies are generally distrusting and interpret other's motives as malevolent. They may make angry accusations against oncology staff and withdraw abruptly. For these patients, it is necessary to take additional time to assess understanding and provide repetition, support, and reassurance. Patients with schizoid or schizotypal tendencies have limited need for social interactions, restricted range of emotional expression, and exhibit eccentric behavior. Recognition of these character traits can help clinicians understand behaviors that might otherwise be perceived as unfriendly and avoid potentially overstimulating interpersonal contact.

Cluster B personality traits

Borderline personality characteristics are characterized by tumultuous relationships and moods, limited sense of self, impulsivity, and sensitivity to perceived threats of abandonment. These patients can present as needy and help seeking, and rapidly fluctuate between idealizing and demonizing staff, sometimes known as "splitting," because of the difficulty the patient has holding onto opposing thoughts, feelings, or beliefs.

Histrionic traits involve excessive attention seeking, with dramatic behaviors. Narcissistic personality traits arise from a need for admiration, feeling entitled to the best care and outcomes, and a tendency to view the world as hierarchical and driven by value.

Table 5 Etiologies of delirium.

CNS dysfunction	Systemic dysfunction	End organ failure	Medications
• Brain tumors (primary or metastases) • Seizures • Paraneoplastic syndromes • Encephalitis • Leptomeningeal disease • Poor cerebral perfusion	• Endocrine disorders • Hematologic processes • Rheumatologic processes • Electrolyte abnormalities	• Hepatic encephalopathy • Uremia • Cardiac failure	• Chemotherapy • Opiates • Benzodiazepines • Steroids

Table 6 Antipsychotics used to manage delirium in oncology settings.

Drugs	Route of administration	Dosages	Remarks
Haloperidol (Haldol®)	PO, IM, IV	0.5–2 mg Every 4–12 h as needed	Typical antipsychotic—risk of EPS Monitor QTc For severe agitation. Can start with 5 mg (with 2 mg of lorazepam)
Chlorpeomazine (Thorazine®)	PO, IM, IV	12.5–5 mg Every 4–12 h as needed	Typical antipsychotic—less EPS risk than haloperidol Sedating, anticholinergic Monitor QTc and blood pressure
Olanzapine (Zyprexa®)	PO, oral dissolving tablet (Zydis®), IM	2.5–5 mg Every 12 h as needed	Atypical antipsychotic—sedation (avoid combining with benzos) Helps with nausea Monitor QTc
Quetiapine (Seroquel®)	PO	25–150 mg Every 12 h as needed	Atypical antipsychotic—orthostatic hypotension during titration Monitor QTc
Risperidone (Risperdal®)	PO, oral dissolving tablet (M-tab®)	0.25–3 mg Every 12 h as needed	Atypical antipsychotic—risk of EPS
Aripiprazole (Abilify®)	PO	5–15 mg Daily	Atypical antipsychotic—risk of akathisia Activating
Ziprasidone (Geodon®)	PO, IM	20–80 mg Every 12 h as needed	Atypical antipsychotic—monitor QTc
Asenapine (Saphris®)	PO, sublingual	5 mg Daily	Sublingual form good for those who cannot swallow

Abbreviations: PO, by mouth; IM, Intramuscularly; IV, Intravenously; EPS, Extrapyramidal symptoms; QTc, cardiac conduction measure.

These patients will often have angry outbursts and when feeling especially vulnerable, can demean and humiliate others. Antisocial traits can co-occur with or without any of these other personality types and are marked by a disregard for the rights of others. For patients with cluster B traits, it is critical for staff to set appropriate boundaries and expectations without blame and to communicate frequently with each other and with staff from other services to better be aware of and manage potentially manipulative behaviors, emotional responses, and the potentially compromised clinical care these can illicit.

Cluster C personality traits

Patients with avoidant, dependent, or perfectionistic traits are more socially inhibited with feelings of inadequacy. These patients may appear fearful, uninterested, or disengaged from their medical issues. Dependent traits manifest as submissiveness, an excessive need to be taken care of, helplessness, or fears of being alone. These characteristics appear as childlike behavior and neediness, with excessive demands for care and attention. Perfectionistic patients are preoccupied with orderliness and control and can be harsh and judgmental. For these patients, clinicians should try to maintain awareness of their own reactions, and in interacting with patients provide clear options and roles in decision making as appropriate.

Delirium

Delirium refers to a pattern of alterations in attention and awareness, occurring acutely (within a span of hours to days), fluctuating over the course of a day, with possible additional disturbances in mental state, such as hallucinations, disorientation, aphasia, or amnesia. It is a response to a physiological insult and is distinct from other neurocognitive conditions, although those with neurocognitive disorders may be more susceptible to delirium. In cancer patients, rates of delirium can range from 43% in the general cancer population to 85% in patients in the terminal stages of their illness.[31] Delirium can manifest behaviorally as profound withdrawal (hypoactive), physical agitation (hyperactive), or both (mixed).

Diagnosing delirium can be challenging in the setting of cancer-related cognitive impairments, and there are several measurement scales which can be used for screening. Collateral information from family members or caretakers is often critical to making an earlier diagnosis in order to clarify time course, quality of symptoms, and possible precipitating factors. There are numerous causes of delirium that can be broadly categorized as CNS dysfunction, systemic dysfunction, end-organ failure, or medication related. Table 5 above identifies some common causes of delirium in people with cancer.

The treatment of delirium relies on ultimately addressing the underlying medical or neurological trigger. Psychotropic medications can be used to mitigate symptoms and maintain safety. These typically include antipsychotics (see Table 6); in select cases benzodiazepines may be added to an antipsychotic regimen. Routes of administration of antipsychotics may help decide which medication will be used, as intravenous medications are helpful in agitated patients who cannot take oral medications, and intramuscular agents are avoided in people with cancer who have low platelet counts and to avoid additional painful injections. Behavioral measures, such as ensuring a safe environment, encouraging appropriate sleep-wake cycles, frequent reorientation and redirection, and addressing impediments to communication such as access to and use of hearing aids, glasses, text boards, and language interpreters.

Conclusion

People treated for cancer today experience a far more psychologically supportive environment than years ago. Society is better educated about cancer which has reduced fears and stigma. The improvements in cancer diagnostics and successes of therapies have resulted in growing populations of cancer survivors. Patients today have access to a more diverse primary oncology clinical team that works more often in convenient ambulatory settings—this requires more attention to deliberate, yet nuanced communication to ensure that medical and emotional needs are addressed in an adequate and timely fashion. Psycho-oncologists, social workers, and other mental health providers, as well as dietitians, rehabilitation medicine, and complementary therapists provide important bridges to provide the finest comprehensive cancer care.

Patients with significant distress are identified earlier in their course of treatment through routine screening and are referred to counselors or to psychiatrists who can diagnose and treat the broad spectrum of depressive disorders, anxiety, or delirium, when primary oncology teams or medical teams are not able to address them sufficiently. Concern about patients' well-being during and after cancer treatment, and the development of Psycho-Oncology as a science of its own, has resulted in a range of evidence-based psychological, behavioral and pharmacologic interventions. With all of these gains over the last half-century, it is important to more seamlessly expand the integration of and access to psychosocial care into routine oncology treatment.

References

1. Society, American Cancer (2020) *Cancer Facts and Figures 2020*. https://www.cancer.org/research/cancer-facts-statistics/all-cancer-facts-figures/cancer-facts-figures-2020.html (accessed 1 July 2020).
2. Institute of Medicine (US). Committee on psychosocial services to cancer patients/families in a community setting. In: Adler NE, Page AEK, eds. *Cancer Care for the Whole Patient: Meeting Psychosocial Health Needs*. Washington (DC): National Academies Press (US); 2008.
3. Sherrill C, Smith M, Mascoe C, et al. Effect of treating depressive disorders on mortality of cancer patients. *Cureus*. 2017;9(10):e1740. doi: 10.7759/cureus.1740.
4. Pirl WF, Greer JA, Traeger L, et al. Depression and survival in metastatic non–small-cell lung cancer: effects of early palliative care. *J Clin Oncol*. 2012;30(12):1310–1315. doi: 10.1200/JCO.2011.38.3166.
5. Temel JS, Greer JA, El-Jawahri A, et al. Effects of early integrated palliative care in patients with lung and GI cancer: a randomized clinical trial. *J Clin Oncol*. 2017;35(8):834–841. doi: 10.1200/JCO.2016.70.5046.
6. Stanton AL, Wiley JF, Krull JL, et al. Depressive episodes, symptoms, and trajectories in women recently Diagnosed with breast cancer. *Breast Cancer Res Treat*. 2015;154(1):105–115. doi: 10.1007/s10549-015-3563-4.
7. Holland JC, Benedeti C, Breitbart W, et al. Update: NCCN practice Guidelines for the manament of psychosocial distress Version 1.2000. *Oncology*. 1999;11(11A):459–507. © 1999 National Comprehensive Cancer Network.
8. Jacobsen PB, Wagner L. A new quality standard: the integration of psychosocial care in to routine cancer care. *J Clin Oncol*. 2012;30:1154–1159.
9. Pinquart M, Duberstein P. Depression and cancer mortality: a meta-analysis. *Psychol Med*. 2010;40(11):1797–1810.
10. Krebber AMH, Buffart LM, Kleijn G, et al. Prevalence of depression in cancer patients: a meta-analysis of diagnostic interviews and self-report instruments. *Psycho-Oncol*. 2014;23:121–130. doi: 10.1002/pon.3409.
11. Schagen SB, Wefel JS. Chemotherapy-related changes in cognitive functioning. *EJC Suppl*. 2013;11(2):225–232.
12. Cuijpers P, Sijbrandij M, Koole SL, et al. Adding psychotherapy to antidepressant medication in depression and anxiety disorders: a meta-analysis. *World Psychiatry*. 2014;13(1):56–67. doi: 10.1002/wps.2008.
13. Laoutidis ZG, Mathiak K. Antidepressants in the treatment of depression/depressive symptoms in cancer patients: a systematic review and meta-analysis. *BMC Psychiatry*. 2013;13(1):1–21. doi: 10.1186/1471-244X-13-140.
14. Ostuzzi G, Matcham F, Dauchy S, et al. Antidepressants for the treatment of depression in people with cancer. *Cochrane Database Syst Rev*. 2018;2018(4):CD011006.
15. McFarland DC, Walsh L, Napolitano S, et al. Suicide in patients with cancer: identifying the risk factors. *Oncology (Williston Park)*. 2019;33(6):221–226.
16. The Joint Commission (2020) *Joint Commission in Accreditation of Health Care Organizations*. https://www.jointcommission.org/resources/patient-safety-topics/suicide-prevention (accessed 17 August 2020).
17. Posner K, Brown GK, Stanley B, et al. The Columbia-suicide severity rating scale: initial validity and internal consistency findings from three multisite studies with adolescents and adults. *Am J Psychiatry*. 2011;168(12):1266–1277. doi: 10-1176/appi.ajp.2011.10111704.
18. Posner K., Brent D., Lucas C, Gould M., Stanley B., Brown G., et al. Columbia-suicide severity rating scale (C-SSRS). Screener with triage for primary health settings. The Research Foundation for Mental Hygiene, Inc. 2008. http://cssrs.colum-bia.edu/the-columbia-scale-c-ssrs/cssrs-for-communities-and-heallhcare/#lilter general-use.english Free PDF download.
19. Deimling GT, Bowman KF, Sterns S, et al. Cancer-related health worries and psychological distress among older adult, long-term cancer survivors. *Psycho-Oncol*. 2006;15(4):306–320.
20. Trevino KM, Nelson CJ, Saracino RM, et al. Is screening for psychosocial risk factors associated with mental health care in older adults with cancer undergoing surgery? *Cancer*. 2020;126(3):602–610.
21. Pitman A, Suleman S, Hyde N, Hodgkiss A. Depression and anxiety in patients with cancer. *BMJ*. 2018;361:k1415.
22. Thekdi SM, Trinidad A, Roth A. Psychopharmacology in cancer. *Curr Psychiatry Rep*. 2015;17(1):529.
23. Andersen BL, DeRubeis RJ, Berman BS, et al. Screening, assessment, and care of anxiety and depressive symptoms in adults with cancer: an American Society of Clinical Oncology guideline adaptation. *J Clin Oncol*. 2014;32(15):1605–1619.
24. Moorey SG, S. *Cognitive Behaviour Therapy for People With Cancer*. New York: Oxford University Press; 2002.
25. Ayers CR, Sorrell JT, Thorp SR, Wetherell JL. Evidence-based psychological treatments for late-life anxiety. *Psychol Aging*. 2007;22(1):8–17.
26. Hall J, Kellett S, Berrios R, et al. Efficacy of cognitive behavioral therapy for generalized anxiety disorder in older adults: systematic review, meta-analysis, and meta-regression. *Am J Geriatr Psychiatry*. 2016;24(11):1063–1073.
27. Moyer A, Sohl SJ, Knapp-Oliver SK, Schneider S. Characteristics and methodological quality of 25 years of research investigating psychosocial interventions for cancer patients. *Cancer Treat Rev*. 2009;35(5):475–484.
28. Cordoba MJ, Riba MB, Spiegal D. Post-traumatic stress disorder and cancer. *Lancet Psychiatry*. 2017;4(4):330–338.
29. Heidarzadeh M, Rassouli M, Brant JM, et al. Dimensions of posttraumatic growth in patients with cancer. *Cancer Nursing*; 2018;41(6):441–449. doi: 10.1097/NCC.0000000000000537.
30. McFarland DC, Morita J, Alici Y. Personality disorders in patients with cancer. *Oncology*. 2019;33(10):4177–4422.
31. Edelstein A, Alici Y. Diagnosing and managing delirium in cancer patients. *Oncology*. 2017;31(9):686–692.

46 Principles of cancer rehabilitation medicine

Michael D. Stubblefield, MD ■ Miguel Escalon, MD, MHPE ■ Sofia A. Barchuk, DO ■ Krina Vyas, MD ■ David C. Thomas, MD, MHPE

Overview

Cancer is the abnormal and unchecked growth of cells in the body. There are many types of cancer and all of them have the potential to inflict a multitude of physical, cognitive, and psychological impairments that reduce functional capacity and quality of life. Aside from the direct physiologic impact of cancer on the human body, oncologic treatment can also have negative consequences. Cancer rehabilitation is the process of restoring function and quality of life (QOL) to cancer survivors by helping them achieve and maintain maximal physical, social, psychological, and vocational functioning within limits created by cancer and its treatments. Persons with cancer and undergoing treatment for cancer can have varied impairments including pain, weakness, sensory deficits and more, so a comprehensive team approach is crucial to ensure effective rehabilitation. Common secondary complications faced by those with cancer include fatigue, pain, neuropathy, lymphedema, and radiation fibrosis syndrome. This review aims to focus on delivering the most up to date information on cancer rehabilitation in brain, spinal cord, head and neck, as well as breast cancer with an emphasis on presenting new therapeutic techniques in the field.

Introduction

There were approximately 17 million Americans with a history of cancer in 2019 with more than 1.8 million new cases anticipated in 2020 (American Cancer Society). The number of survivors will increase to more than 22 million by the year in 2030.[1] At least half of these survivors will suffer functional impairment from their cancer and/or its treatment with potentially profound consequences for function and quality of life.[2] Common impairments include fatigue, pain, neuropathy, lymphedema, radiation fibrosis syndrome, and a variety of other sequelae.[3,4]

Cancer rehabilitation is the process of restoring function and quality of life to cancer survivors by helping them achieve and maintain the maximal possible physical, social, psychological, and vocational functioning within the limits created by cancer and its treatments.[5] Traditionally the restoration of function and quality of life was the primary value proposition of cancer rehabilitation. In an era of value-based care, the lens with which we view cancer rehabilitation services has evolved to include such benefits as reduced emergency room visits and hospitalizations, better pain control, improved compliance with oncologic treatment, return to work, reduced burden on oncology practitioners, and overall cost of care.[5]

Because impairments in cancer survivors are varied and often multiple, a comprehensive team approach is of paramount importance to ensure safe and effective rehabilitation. A well-rounded cancer rehabilitation team should include a physiatrist, physical therapist, occupational therapist, and speech–language pathologist among others (Table 1). Close collaboration with the oncology team and other medical providers is also necessary to ensure that rehabilitation efforts are coordinated with medical and oncologic treatments and restrictions. While most cancer rehabilitation is carried out in the outpatient setting, specialized inpatient cancer rehabilitation programs have also been developed to help ensure optimal outcomes for cancer patients who have required an acute care admission but are not yet functional enough to return home.

Cancer of the brain

The incidence of primary brain and central nervous system tumors in adults aged 20 years or older in the United States is estimated to be 29.9 in every 100,000 persons.[6] Nearly 700,000 Americans live with a primary brain tumor.[7] Tumors of the brain produce unique neurocognitive symptoms and a higher symptom burden compared with other cancers.[7,8] According to the 2016 Central Nervous System (CNS) World Health Organization (WHO) classification of brain tumors categorization is based on both microscopy and molecular patterns.[9] Intracranial tumors can also be divided into malignant or benign tumors with malignant tumors being primary or metastatic.[7] Refer to Table 2 for a detailed description of WHO classification, characteristics, tumor types, incidence, and prognosis.

The deficits caused by brain tumors are determined by their location, size, and mass effect.[7] Clinical presentation varies widely and often includes symptoms of increased intracranial pressure such as headache, nausea/vomiting, ocular palsies, altered mental status, loss of balance, seizures, or papilledema.[7] In one retrospective study of over 870, 135 Emergency Department visits, those diagnosed with brain tumors showed focal deficits 50% of the time.[10] Diagnosis of intracranial tumors is based on history and physical exam along with sophisticated imaging techniques including, but not limited to, computed tomography (CT or CAT scan), magnetic resonance imaging (MRI), and/or positron emission tomography scan (PET). Brain damage may result from the primary tumor itself, metastasis, or treatments. Management is best using a multidisciplinary approach including observation surveillance, surgical resection, chemotherapy, radiation therapy (RT), and social support with family meetings geared toward goals of care.[7]

Determining prognosis of brain and other CNS tumors is multifactorial. Several characteristics are taken into consideration such as patient age, neurological status, tumor location/size, histological grade, and molecular features (American Association of Neurological Surgeons). Intracranial tumors have a very high likelihood of producing long-term disabling effects.[11]

Table 1 Interdisciplinary cancer rehabilitation team.

Team member	Role
Caregiver(s)	Participates as source of support for the patient as well as developing a relationship with the team as an extension of the patient
Chaplain	Evaluates and assist with the spiritual needs of the patient and caregivers
Nutritionist	Evaluates the patient's nutritional condition, assesses the additional metabolic demands that the cancer places on the body, and recommends the optimal diet with respect to specific clinical condition, caloric intake, food ingredients of choice, optimal consistency for easy swallowing, and the individual's tastes
Occupational therapist	Evaluates and develops a plan with a focus on the upper extremities range of motion and strength as well as training in self-care activities
Patient	Participates as an active member of the team in decisions regarding all aspects of treatment
Physical therapist	Evaluates and develops a plan to improve joint range of motion, strengthen muscles, increase stamina with a focus on improving functional skills such as bed mobility, transfers, wheelchair locomotion, and ambulation with or without assistive devices
Physician (physiatrist)	Leads the rehabilitation team to establish realistic goals and prescribe an appropriate rehabilitation program including a plan for preventive, restorative, supportive, and palliative therapies
Prosthetist-orthotist	Evaluate and fabricate artificial limbs (prostheses) or special braces (orthoses) according to the patient's needs
Psychologist	Assesses the patient's cognition and behavior, including intelligence, personality, personal history, motivation, and reaction to the illness, and assists the patient and the caregivers in developing a plan for coping with the medical illness
Recreational therapist	Offers various activities to each patient to meet their individual needs such as art and/or music therapy, attending events, and other social activities important to the patient
Rehabilitation nurse	Evaluates the patient's specific nursing needs and determines a plan including education of the patient and caregivers
Speech-language pathologist	Evaluates and provides therapy for impaired oral communication and works closely with the occupational therapist and nutritionist in the assessment and care of swallowing disorders
Social worker	Evaluates and plans for the psychosocial aspects of the patients' treatment especially with respect to discharge planning, facilitating a smooth transition to the community, ensuring continuity of care, and securing appropriate follow-up services after discharge
Vocational counselor	Evaluate needs of patients who may potentially return to work and assist with planning re-entry to the workforce

Postoperative management is critical with careful neurological management and blood pressure control.[7] All patients with brain cancer and impaired function in mobility and activities of daily livings (ADLs) should be referred to rehabilitation with a goal of helping patients become independent in these areas. Evidence for effectiveness of rehabilitation is favorable and improvements are comparable to individuals with stroke or traumatic brain injury, but it is important to keep in mind reoccurrence rates and functional decline over time is seen more frequently in the brain tumor population.[11,12] When comparing these groups, they also have similar or even shorter lengths of stay with analogous discharge rates to the community.[11] Targeted inpatient rehabilitation with the help of trained therapists can address the common dysfunctions of these patient's face including strengthening of weak muscles, stretching of tight joints, reduction of spasticity through medication and botulinum toxin injections, and control of pain. Evaluation by qualified physical, occupational, and speech therapists along with detailed neuropsychological and neuro-ophthalmology assessment can help address visual deficits, speech disorders, dysphagia, memory deficits, judgment, and visual perception in this patient population. Although outcomes in the outpatient rehabilitation setting have not been systematically described, in part due to lack of standardized metrics, these resources can help to improve patient's functionality along with addressing family and caregiver needs throughout the recovery process.[11]

Spinal cord dysfunction

Primary tumors originating from the spine are relatively uncommon and account for 3% of all spinal tumors. Secondary, or metastatic, tumors originate from adjacent structures which spread hematogenously and lymphatically and account for 97% of all spinal tumors.[13] Primary neoplasms may arise from the spinal cord, surrounding leptomeninges, extradural soft tissue, or bony structures.[14] Spinal tumors are often categorized based on their location whether that be extradural, intradural–extramedullary, or intradural–intramedullary. Refer to Table 3 for a detailed description of tumor location, tumor types, incidence, and prognosis.

The most common cause of spinal cord dysfunction (SCD) resulting from a neoplasm is direct compression of the spinal cord, causing spinal cord injury (SCI), although vascular insults are possible as well. SCD can be iatrogenic resulting from radiation, chemotherapy, or surgical intervention. Nonmechanical back pain, especially in the middle or lower back, is the most frequent symptom of both benign and malignant tumors, but persons with SCI due to cancer often present in similar ways to other cancer patients. Some of these symptoms include fatigue, loss of sensation or muscle weakness in legs arms or chest, difficulty walking or standing, dysesthesias, and bowel/bladder incontinence.[7] Neurologic dysfunction of varying degrees has the potential to develop either suddenly or gradually depending on the cancer growth rate and location. Back pain related to cancer is often characterized as dull or achy; however, if a patient complains of pain that is worse at night or laying down then clinicians should have a heightened suspicion for cancer as a cause.[7]

Prompt diagnosis is crucial in treating spinal tumors. Determining whether the tumor is malignant or benign, identifying the source, and finding the total number of lesions will ultimately determine prognosis and medical management.[15] Due to advances in acute oncological treatment, patients with spinal cord tumors exhibit improved survival and those that participate in early rehabilitation programs show general improvement in function, mood, quality of life, and survival.[16] Most spinal metastasis are managed nonsurgically, but when neurological deficits occur rapidly, surgical decompression and/or radiotherapy may be indicated. Treatment of cancer can also cause SCD and in severe cases SCI. For example, RT can affect different levels of the spinal cord depending on the anatomic area irradiated. Radiation myelitis is a rare, but a dreaded complication of radiation exposure that presents in 2–4 months posttreatment.[7] Recovery can take up to 40 weeks for which early implementation of a rehabilitation program could greatly benefit the patient.

The rehabilitation of cancer patients with SCD depends on assessment of their neurologic, oncologic, medical, pain, and social support status. Refer to Figure 1 for International Standards for Neurological Classification (ISNCSCI) examination used to determine neurologic level of injury in SCI. SCD with

Table 2 World health organization (WHO) brain tumor grades.

Grade	WHO classification	Characteristics	Tumor types	Incidence	Prognosis
Low	WHO grade I	• Least malignant (benign) • Slower growing • Possibly curable via surgery alone • Noninfiltrating • Long-term survival	• Pilocytic astrocytoma • Craniopharyngioma • Gangliocytoma • Ganglioglioma • Subependymal giant cell astrocytoma • Protoplasmic astrocytoma • Xanthomatous astrocytoma • Subependymoma • Meningiomas	• Meningiomas (36.4%) • Pilocytic astrocytoma (1.4%) • Ependymal tumors (1.9%)	• Prognosis dependent on age, performance status, lower pathologic grade • 5-year survival rate all nonmalignant brain tumors is 91.5%
Low	WHO grade II	• Generally benign, may recur as higher grade • Relatively slow growing • Not cured by surgery alone • Still considered benign	• Diffuse astrocytoma • Pineocytoma • Pure oligodendroglioma • Fibrillary (gemistocytic, protoplasmic) astrocytoma • Ependymoma • Mixed oligo-astrocytoma • Optic nerve glioma	• Diffuse astrocytoma (2.3%) • Oligodendroglioma (1.1%)	• Prognosis dependent on age, performance status, lower pathologic grade • 5-year survival rate all nonmalignant brain tumors is 91.5%
High	WHO grade III	• Malignant • Infiltrative • Often reoccur as high-grade lesions • Anaplastic features	• Anaplastic astrocytoma • Anaplastic ependymoma • Anaplastic oligodendroglioma • Anaplastic mixed glioma	• Anaplastic astrocytoma (1.7%) • Anaplastic oligodendroglioma (0.5%)	• Prognosis dependent on age, performance status, lower pathologic grade • Survival rate all malignant brain tumors 35% • 5-year survival rate of anaplastic astrocytoma 30%
High	WHO grade IV	• Most malignant • Rapid growing • Widely infiltrative • Rapid recurrence • Necrosis prone • Poor prognosis	• Glioblastoma multiforme (GBM) • Pineoblastoma • Medulloblastoma • Ependymoblastoma • Gliosarcoma • Gliomatosis cerebri	• Glioblastoma (15.1%) • Malignant glioma (2.0%)	• Prognosis dependent on age, performance status, lower pathologic grade • Survival rate all malignant brain tumors 35% • 5-year survival rate of GBM 5.6%

profound paralysis and sensory loss, along with bowel and bladder dysfunction, requires specialized medical and nursing care, followed by comprehensive rehabilitation addressing each of the associated conditions. Rehabilitation interventions can provide substantial pain relief and improve stabilization of the spine with less invasiveness and risk of surgery or radiotherapy (American Association of Neurological Surgeons). Secondary issues such as urinary tract complications, pressure ulcers, deep venous thrombosis/pulmonary embolism, and joint contractures can be effectively treated using a multidisciplinary approach with a trained and qualified rehabilitation team.

Head and neck cancer

Head and neck cancer (HNC) treatment is often aggressive requiring combined modalities including surgery and RT with or without chemotherapy to maximize regional control and functional organ preservation. Surgery generally involves resection of the primary tumor as well as neck dissection. This was historically classified as radical with removal of all lymph nodes, spinal accessory nerve (SAN), sternocleidomastoid muscle (SCM), internal jugular vein (IJV); modified radical (removal of all lymph nodes but spares one or more of the SAN, SCM, IJV; or selective (preserves one or more lymph node levels normally removed in a radical neck dissection). In general, the more extensive neck dissections result in more severe dysfunction, pain, and reduced quality of life.[17]

While resection or damage to the SAN is a major cause of this morbidity, damage to other key structures including the cervical root branches and cervical plexus can play an important role.[18–20] Perturbation of scapulothoracic motion from trapezius weakness (compromised SAN) and rotator cuff (RTC) weakness (compromised root branches) can lead to musculoskeletal shoulder disorders such as RTC tendonitis and adhesive capsulitis.

Approximately 80% (range 73.9–84.4%) of all HNC patients will receive RT at least once during the course of their disease and RT is a major cause of long-term disability.[21] HNC patients who undergo RT are likely to develop radiation fibrosis syndrome which can include trigeminal neuralgia, dermal sclerosis, trismus, cervical dystonia, and migraines.[18] Late effects of radiation in HNC include radiculopathy, cervical and/or brachial plexopathy, cranial mononeuropathies (most commonly CN XII followed by CN X), dysphagia, and dysarthria.[22,23] The combination of surgery and radiation likely has additive morbidity.

The treatment of late effects in HNC survivors varies depending on the specific issues. Physical therapy is the primary modality for most disorders. In two prospective randomized trials, progressive resistance training (PRT) for HNC cancer patients with SAN neurapraxia/neurectomy and shoulder dysfunction was shown to be more effective than standard physical therapy in terms of improving shoulder pain, range of motion, and disability.[24,25]

Pharmacotherapy is typically the principal treatment modality for cancer-related pain.[26] Nociceptive pain which does not respond to physical therapy may benefit from nonsteroidal anti-inflammatory medications or opiate analgesics. Neuropathic pain and muscle spasms should initially be treated with nerve stabilizing agents (gabapentin, pregabalin, duloxetine, tricyclic antidepressants). Botulinum toxin can also be used to treat focal

Table 3 Classification of spinal tumors by location.

Location	Description	Tumor types	Incidence	Prognosis
Extradural (epidural)	• Form inside the spinal column, outside of the dura mater • Primary or secondary (metastasis) • More commonly malignant than benign • Primary tumors arise from osteoblasts, chondrocytes, fibroblasts, and hematopoietic cells • Metastases often originate from the lung breast, prostate, kidney, GI tract, and thyroid	• Hemangioma • Osteoid osteoma • Osteoblastoma • Osteochondroma • Giant cell tumor • Chordoma • Sarcomas • Lymphoma • Plasmacytoma • Multiple Myeloma • Eosinophilic granuloma	• Extradural spinal tumor incidence (50–55%)	• Prognosis depends on tumor grade, tumor location, extent of tumor involvement, duration of symptoms
Intradural-extramedullary	• Form inside the dura (may or may not involve the spinal cord) • Develop from inside the nerve roots or inside surface of dura mater • Often primary tumors can be metastases • Can cause spinal cord compression • Vast majority are benign • Often treated with minimally invasive surgery • Sometimes treated with radiation • No role of chemotherapy in treatment	• Nerve sheath tumors (Schwannoma) • Epidermoid • Teratoma • Dermoid • Lipoma • Neurenteric cyst • Meningiomas	• Intradural spinal tumor incidence (40–45%) • Majority of spinal canal tumors are intradural-extramedullary (70–80%) • Schwannoma (25%) • Meningiomas account for 37% of all primary CNS tumors	• Prognosis depends on tumor grade, tumor location, extent of tumor involvement, duration of symptoms
Intradural-intramedullary	• Grow inside the spinal cord • Often primary tumors, but can be metastases • Often treated with minimally invasive surgery • Sometimes treated with radiation • No role of chemotherapy in treatment	• Astrocytoma • Ependymoma • Oligodendrogliomas • Hemangioblastoma	• Intradural spinal tumor incidence (40–45%) • Gliomas (5%) of spinal tumors • Ependymomas (60–80%) • Anaplastic ependymoma (5%) of spinal ependymomas	• Prognosis depends on tumor grade, tumor location, extent of tumor involvement, duration of symptoms • 15-year survival rate of ependymomas is 35–75% • 10-year survival rate for myxopapillary ependymoma >90%

neuropathic pain and painful muscle spasms associated with radiation fibrosis.[27,28]

Dysphagia develops either as a direct result of the location and/or size of the primary tumor or due to RT.[29] Impaired swallowing can lead to complications, such as aspiration pneumonia and malnutrition. Dysphagia rehabilitation first involves a comprehensive evaluation, which begins with bedside swallow tests using liquids and food of different consistencies, proceeding as needed to video fluorography and endoscopy of the pharynx, larynx, and esophagus. Training to improve swallowing involves strengthening exercises for weak muscles, identification of optimal head and neck positions for swallowing, careful feeding of liquids and foods of different viscosities, providing intraoral devices and adaptive bottles, cups, plates, and utensils and sometimes by undergoing specific surgical procedures.

Cancer of the breast

According to the American Cancer Society, there is an estimated total of 3,861,520 female breast cancer survivors as of January 2019 and the numbers keep growing with a predicted value of 4,957,960 in January of 2030. Although breast cancer itself has the potential for limiting physical, social, psychological, and vocation functioning breast cancer treatments often result in impairments as well (American Association of Neurological Surgeons).[9] Cancer rehabilitation programs seek to address the physical and emotional needs of these patients as they relate to function and well-being.[7,9,10] Breast cancer treatment includes surgery, RT, chemotherapy, hormonal, and biologic therapies. There are multiple potential complications of breast cancer treatment that directly benefit from a rehabilitation program such as lymphedema, upper body dysfunction, pain, aromatase inhibitor-induced arthralgias, and neurocognitive disorders.[30]

The incidence of lymphedema varies widely due to variations in diagnostic methods and time to assessment. It is considered the most dreaded complication of surgery with diagnosis being from 6% to 28%.[31,32] Mastectomy, extent of axillary lymph node dissection, radiotherapy, and positive lymph nodes increase the risk of developing lymphedema.[83] Not only does lymphedema decrease functional mobility and ROM it also contributes to overall decreased quality of life.[83] It predisposes patients to infection and has the potential to develop into malignant lymphangiosarcoma. It takes a team of cancer rehabilitation specialists who are trained in diagnosing and treating the physical, cognitive and functional impairments of patients in an effort to restore function, reduce burden of symptoms, maximize independence, and improve quality of life in this complex population.[33–35] Comprehensive physical therapy, lower-level laser therapy, pharmacotherapy, manual lymphatic drainage, progressive exercise, low-stretch compressive bandaging, fitting of appropriate gradient compression garments, and education are some of the many tools that can be utilized to enhance the well-being of these patients.

The effects of breast cancer treatment vary widely and often include neuromuscular, musculoskeletal, mononeuropathy, and lymphovascular disorders that can lead to upper body dysfunction. More specifically, upper body dysfunction, include common diagnoses treated by rehabilitation specialists such as rotator

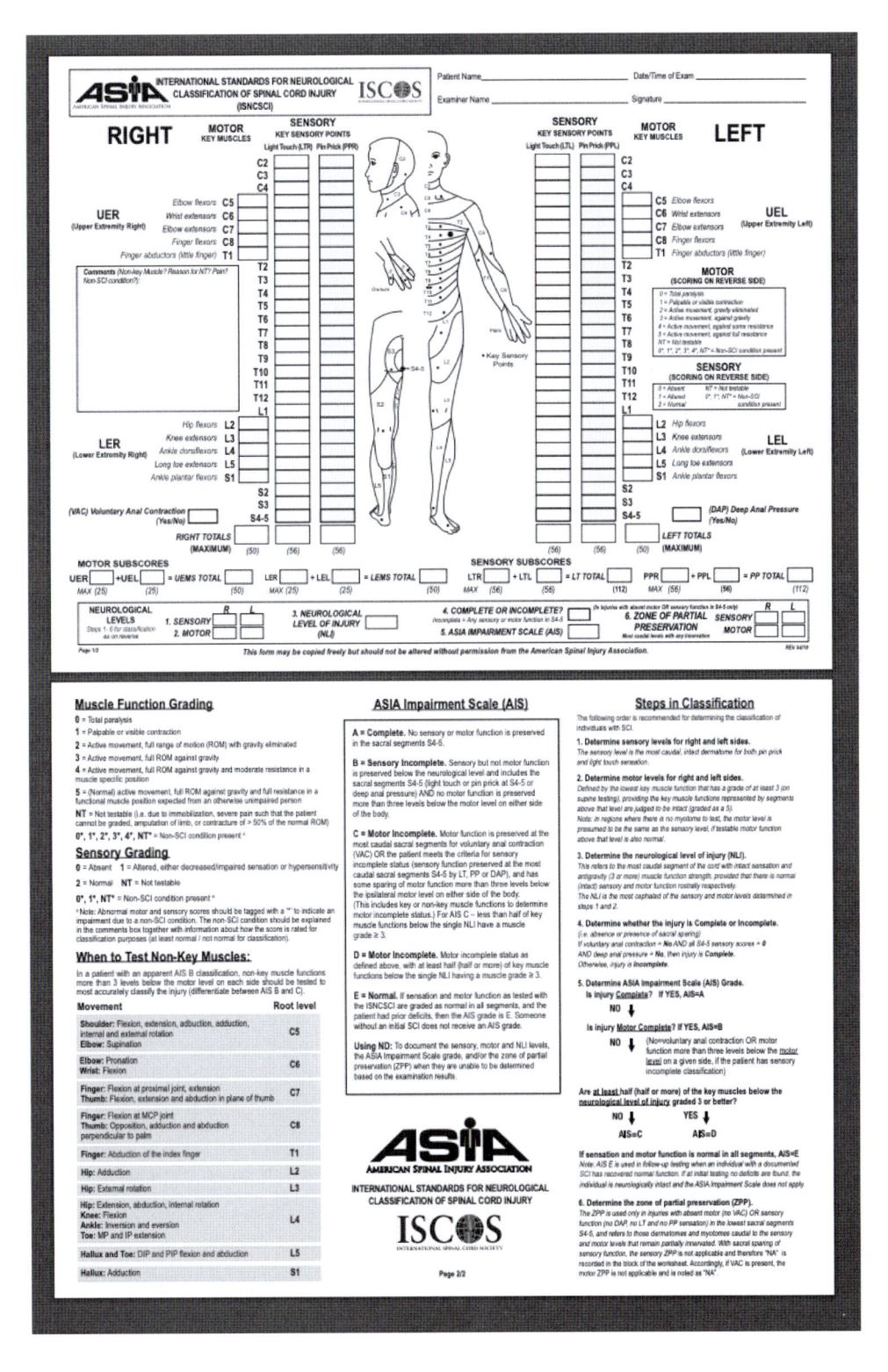

Figure 1 ISNCSCI examination.

cuff disease, bicipital tendonitis, adhesive capsulitis, epicondylitis, DeQuervain's tenosynovitis, arthralgias, arthritis, cervical radiculopathy, and brachial plexopathy.[34–36] Patients undergoing axillary lymph node dissection have the highest rate of developing impairments of the shoulder including decreased ROM, decreased strength, lymphedema, and impairment of ADLs.[30] A comprehensive review concluded that upper limb exercises, including ROM and stretching, are helpful in recovering upper limb movement following breast surgery, and initiating exercises 1–3 days postop may improve short-term gains in shoulder movement.[30] Rehabilitation has also proven to improve quality of life in a recent study in breast cancer survivors with axillary web syndrome. Despite the multitude of benefits, comprehensive rehabilitation remains an underutilized service in breast cancer treatment today.

According to the American Cancer Society, the most common side effects of breast cancer and treatment are pain, fatigue, and emotional distress (2019). Pain has been reported to affect 12–51% of women 6 months to 3 years after treatment. Cancer rehabilitation can improve pain, functioning and overall quality of life throughout every stage of the treatment process.[34,35] Common pain syndromes include radiation-induced, chemo-induced peripheral neuropathy, axillary cording, postsurgical pain, aromatase inhibitor-induced arthralgias, and postmastectomy pain syndrome.[37] In regards to chemotherapy-induced pain, taxane can cause motor and sensory neuropathies which are cumulative and dose dependent.[36] Paclitaxel induces a neuropathy that involves the sensory fibers with major manifestations including burning paresthesias of the hands and feet.[36] Vincristine can cause colicky abdominal pain which affects up to 50% of patients.[36] It often takes a multidisciplinary approach to address both the cognitive and physical difficulties affecting these patients in which qualified physiatrists, whom specialize in rehabilitation medicine, are well equipped to treat.

The long-term cognitive side effects of breast cancer treatments still remain largely unknown, but efforts have been made to identify at-risk patients.[38] In women with breast cancer receiving adjuvant chemotherapy, the estimated number of individuals who will suffer from neurocognitive effects is around 20–25% with an estimated length of deficit being 10–20 years.[38] Factors that contribute to vulnerability are increased age, cognitive reserve, and genetics.[38] In a particular subset of these individuals, brain structure and function are altered with decreased volume of the frontal lobes seen one month after chemotherapy with partial or no recovery after one year.[38] One study published in the Oxford journal also noted an increase in anxiety, depression, and suicide, along with neurocognitive and sexual dysfunction among breast cancer survivors.[34,35] Neurocognitive assessment provided by a rehabilitation specialist's with speech therapy intervention would be crucial in identifying and treating at-risk patients that exhibit neurocognitive decline.[33]

Conclusion

Cancer rehabilitation is the process of restoring function and quality of life to cancer survivors by helping them achieve and maintain the maximal possible physical, social, psychological, and vocational functioning within the limits created by cancer and its treatments. In addition to restoring function and quality of life, cancer rehabilitation services hold the promise of reducing emergency room visits and hospitalizations, improving pain control, enhancing compliance with oncologic treatment, returning patients to work, lessening the burden on oncology practitioners, and reducing overall cost of care. An integrated team approach is of paramount importance in realizing this promise.

References

1 Miller KD, Nogueira L, Mariotto AB, et al. Cancer treatment and survivorship statistics, 2019. *CA Cancer J Clin*. 2019;**69**(5):363–385. doi: 10.3322/caac.21565.
2 Ness KK, Wall MM, Oakes JM, et al. Physical performance limitations and participation restrictions among cancer survivors: a population-based study. *Ann Epidemiol*. 2006;**16**(3):197–205. doi: 10.1016/j.annepidem.2005.01.009.
3 Kline-Quiroz C, Nori P, Stubblefield MD. Cancer rehabilitation: acute and chronic issues, nerve injury, radiation sequelae, surgical and chemo-related, part 1. *Med Clin North Am*. 2020;**104**(2):239–250. doi: 10.1016/j.mcna.2019.10.004.
4 Nori P, Kline-Quiroz C, Stubblefield MD. Cancer rehabilitation: acute and chronic issues, nerve injury, radiation sequelae, surgical and chemo-related, part 2. *Med Clin North Am*. 2020;**104**(2):251–262. doi: 10.1016/j.mcna.2019.10.005.
5 Stubblefield MD, Kendig TD, Khanna A. ReVitalizing cancer survivors—making cancer rehabilitation the standard of care. *MD Advis*. 2019;**12**(2):30–33.
6 Ostrom QT, Gittleman H, Truitt G, et al. CBTRUS statistical report: primary brain and other central nervous system tumors diagnosed in the United States in 2011–2015. *Neuro-Oncology*. 2018;**20**:iv1–iv86. doi: 10.1093/neuonc/noy131.
7 Cristian A. *Central Nervous System Cancer Rehabilitation*. Elsevier; 2019.
8 Afseth J, Neubeck L, Karatzias T, Grant R. Holistic needs assessment in brain cancer patients: a systematic review of available tools. *Eur J Cancer Care*. 2019;**28**(3):e12931. doi: 10.1111/ecc.12931.
9 Louis DN, Perry A, Reifenberger G, et al. The 2016 World Health Organization classification of tumors of the central nervous system: a summary. *Acta Neuropathol*. 2016;**131**(6):803–820. doi: 10.1007/s00401-016-1545-1.
10 Comelli I, Lippi G, Campana V, et al. Clinical presentation and epidemiology of brain tumors firstly diagnosed in adults in the emergency department: a ten-year single center retrospective study. *Ann Transl Med*. 2017;**5**(13):2. doi: 10.21037/atm.2017.06.12.
11 Vargo M. Brain tumor rehabilitation. *Am J Phys Med Rehabil*. 2011;**90**(5 Suppl 1):S50–S62. doi: 10.1097/PHM.0b013e31820be31f.
12 Geler-Kulcu D, Gulsen G, Buyukbaba E, Ozkan D. Functional recovery of patients with brain tumor or acute stroke after rehabilitation: a comparative study. *J Clin Neurosci*. 2009;**16**(1):74–78. doi: 10.1016/j.jocn.2008.04.014.
13 Arnautovic K, Arnautovic A. Extramedullary intradural spinal tumors: a review of modern diagnostic and treatment options and a report of a series. *Bosn J Basic Med Sci*. 2009;**9**(Suppl 1):S40–S45; https://www.ncbi.nlm.nih.gov/pmc/articles/PMC5655171.
14 Weill Cornell Brain and Spine Center. *Spinal Tumors*, 2013; https://weillcornellbrainandspine.org/condition/spinal-tumors (accessed 3 October 2020).
15 Ciftdemir M, Kaya M, Selcuk E, Yalniz E. Tumors of the spine. *World J Orthop*. 2016;**7**(2):109–116. doi: 10.5312/wjo.v7.i2.109.
16 American Spinal Injury Association. *American Spinal Injury Association—The premier North American organization in the field of Spinal Cord Injury Care, Education, and Research*, 2020; https://asia-spinalinjury.org (accessed 10 June 2020).
17 Kuntz AL, Weymuller EA. Impact of neck dissection on quality of life. *Laryngoscope*. 1999;**109**(8):1334–1338. doi: 10.1097/00005537-199908000-00030.
18 Dilber M, Kasapoglu F, Erisen L, et al. The relationship between shoulder pain and damage to the cervical plexus following neck dissection. *Eur Arch Otorhinolaryngol*. 2007;**264**:1333–1338. doi: 10.1007/s00405-007-0357-2.
19 Roh J-L, Yoon Y-H, Kim SY, Park CI. Cervical sensory preservation during neck dissection. *Oral Oncol*. 2007;**43**(5):491–498. doi: 10.1016/j.oraloncology.2006.05.003.
20 Umeda M, Shigeta T, Takahashi H, et al. Shoulder mobility after spinal accessory nerve-sparing modified radical neck dissection in oral cancer patients. *Oral Surg Oral Med Oral Pathol Oral Radiol Endod*. 2010;**109**(6):820–824. doi: 10.1016/j.tripleo.2009.11.027.
21 Strojan P, Hutcheson KA, Eisbruch A, et al. Treatment of late sequelae after radiotherapy for head and neck cancer. *Cancer Treat Rev*. 2017;**59**:79–92. doi: 10.1016/j.ctrv.2017.07.003.
22 Dong Y, Ridge JA, Ebersole B, et al. Incidence and outcomes of radiation-induced late cranial neuropathy in 10-year survivors of head and neck cancer. *Oral Oncol*. 2019;**95**:59–64. doi: 10.1016/j.oraloncology.2019.05.014.
23 Luk YS, Shum JSF, Sze HCK, et al. Predictive factors and radiological features of radiation-induced cranial nerve palsy in patients with nasopharyngeal carcinoma following radical radiotherapy. *Oral Oncol*. 2013;**49**(1):49–54. doi: 10.1016/j.oraloncology.2012.07.011.
24 McNeely ML, Parliament MB, Seikaly H, et al. Effect of exercise on upper extremity pain and dysfunction in head and neck cancer survivors: a randomized controlled trial. *Cancer*. 2008;**113**(1):214–222. doi: 10.1002/cncr.23536.
25 McNeely ML, Parliament M, Courneya KS, et al. A pilot study of a randomized controlled trial to evaluate the effects of progressive resistance exercise training on shoulder dysfunction caused by spinal accessory neurapraxia/neurectomy in head and neck cancer survivors. *Head Neck*. 2004;**26**(6):518–530. doi: 10.1002/hed.20010.
26 Glare PA, Davies PS, Finlay E, et al. Pain in cancer survivors. *J Clin Oncol Off J Am Soc Clin Oncol*. 2014;**32**(16):1739–1747. doi: 10.1200/JCO.2013.52.4629.
27 Stubblefield MD. Cancer rehabilitation. *Semin Oncol*. 2011;**38**(3):386–393. doi: 10.1053/j.seminoncol.2011.03.008.
28 Stubblefield MD. Radiation fibrosis syndrome: neuromuscular and musculoskeletal complications in cancer survivors. *PM R*. 2011;**3**(11):1041–1054. doi: 10.1016/j.pmrj.2011.08.535.
29 Greco E, Simic T, Ringash J, et al. Dysphagia treatment for patients with head and neck cancer undergoing radiation therapy: a meta-analysis review. *Int J Radiat Oncol Biol Phys*. 2018;**101**(2):421–444. doi: 10.1016/j.ijrobp.2018.01.097.
30 Stubblefield MD. The underutilization of rehabilitation to treat physical impairments in breast cancer survivors. *PM&R*. 2017;**9**(9S2):S317–S323. doi: 10.1016/j.pmrj.2017.05.010.

31 Borman P. Lymphedema diagnosis, treatment, and follow-up from the view point of physical medicine and rehabilitation specialists. *Turk J Phys Med Rehabil.* 2018;**64**(3):179–197. doi: 10.5606/tftrd.2018.3539.

32 Tsai RJ, Dennis LK, Lynch CF, et al. The risk of developing arm lymphedema among breast cancer survivors: a meta-analysis of treatment factors. *Ann Surg Oncol.* 2009;**16**(7):1959–1972. doi: 10.1245/s10434-009-0452-2.

33 Campbell G, Reigle BS. Introduction: the case for cancer rehabilitation. *Semin Oncol Nurs.* 2020;**36**(1):150973. doi: 10.1016/j.soncn.2019.150973.

34 Fu JB, Raj VS, Guo Y. A guide to inpatient cancer rehabilitation: focusing on patient selection and evidence-based outcomes. *PM&R.* 2017a;**9**(9S2):S324–S334. doi: 10.1016/j.pmrj.2017.04.017.

35 Fu JB, Raj VS, Guo Y. A guide to inpatient cancer rehabilitation: focusing on patient selection and evidence-based outcomes. *PM&R.* 2017b;**9**(9S2):S324–S334. doi: 10.1016/j.pmrj.2017.04.017.

36 Stubblefield MD. *Cancer Rehabilitation – Principles and Practice*, 2nd ed. New York: Demos Medical; 2018.

37 Roberts K, Rickett K, Greer R, Woodward N. Management of aromatase inhibitor induced musculoskeletal symptoms in postmenopausal early breast cancer: a systematic review and meta-analysis. *Crit Rev Oncol Hematol.* 2017;**111**:66–80. doi: 10.1016/j.critrevonc.2017.01.010.

38 Ahles TA, Saykin AJ, Furstenberg CT, et al. Neuropsychologic impact of standard-dose systemic chemotherapy in long-term survivors of breast cancer and lymphoma. *J Clin Oncol Off J Am Soc Clin Oncol.* 2002;**20**(2):485–493. doi: 10.1200/JCO.2002.20.2.485.

47 Integrative oncology in cancer care

Gabriel Lopez, MD ▪ Wenli Liu, MD ▪ Santhosshi Narayanan, MD ▪ Lorenzo Cohen, PhD

> **Overview**
>
> Integrative medicine seeks to merge conventional medicine and complementary therapies in a manner that is comprehensive, personalized, evidence-based, and safe. Integrative oncology is the term used to describe the application of integrative medicine to cancer care. The field of integrative oncology is a constantly evolving set of disciplines. This article reviews the role of integrative medicine in cancer care with an emphasis on effective communication, an overview of the evidence, integrative-based resources to guide health care providers and patients, and presents a model of how to effectively incorporate integrative medicine within cancer care. Existing research suggests that the majority of cancer patients desire communication with their doctors about integrative medicine. It is the health care professional's responsibility to ask patients about their use of complementary medicines and to provide evidence-based advice to guide patients in this evolving area. Key findings in the areas of mind-body practices, massage, and acupuncture are presented. Mind-body practices help to improve mood, sleep quality, physical functioning, and overall well-being. Massage is helpful at relieving pain, anxiety, and increasing relaxation. Acupuncture has the greatest evidence to support its use in managing symptoms such as chemotherapy-induced nausea, vomiting, and pain; additional research suggests benefit in providing relief for radiation-induced xerostomia, hot flashes, arthralgias, and other symptoms. Many authoritative resources now exist to help guide patients' appropriate use of complementary therapies, allowing the medical team to follow evidence-based guidelines.

Introduction

Integrative medicine seeks to combine conventional medicine with the safest and the most effective complementary therapies. A number of comprehensive cancer centers in the United States are putting into practice the concept of integrative medicine in cancer care under the term *integrative oncology*.[1] As a result of growing interest in integrative oncology, the National Cancer Institute (NCI) formed the Office of Cancer Complementary and Alternative Medicine, the American Cancer Society (ACS) dedicated a portion of its web site to assessment of complementary therapies, the Academic Consortium for Integrative Medicine and Health formed an oncology working group, and the Society for Integrative Oncology (SIO) was formed. This article will review the role of integrative medicine in cancer care with an emphasis on effective communication, an overview of the evidence, integrative-based resources to guide health care providers and patients, and an example of how to effectively incorporate integrative medicine within cancer care.

Definitions

The National Center for Complementary and Integrative Health emphasizes the importance of distinguishing between complementary, alternative, and integrative medicine: a nonmainstream practice used together with conventional medicine is complementary; a nonmainstream practice used in place of conventional medicine is considered alternative; and integrative health brings conventional and complementary approaches together in a coordinated way.[2] Although evidence may exist for some of these modalities, it may not be sufficient to bring them into the realm of *conventional* medicine, and other complementary medicine (CM) modalities may have no support for their use. Several different types of specialty health care providers offer CM therapies and these may include physicians, nurses, physical therapists, psychologists, acupuncturists, and massage therapists who are operating within the guidelines of their licenses or accrediting organizations. Practitioners of all disciplines should be knowledgeable and aware of all treatment options and open to communication with other types of practitioners.

Integrative medicine seeks to merge conventional medicine and complementary therapies in a manner that is comprehensive, personalized, evidence-based, and safe. The Academic Consortium for Integrative Medicine and Health has defined integrative medicine as "the practice of medicine that reaffirms the importance of the relationship between practitioner and patient, focuses on the whole person, is informed by evidence, and makes use of all appropriate therapeutic and lifestyle approaches, healthcare professionals and disciplines to achieve optimal health and healing."[3] The application of integrative medicine to cancer care has come into practice under the term *integrative oncology*. An expert consensus definition for integrative oncology was proposed as part of a special *Journal of the National Cancer Institute* (JNCI) issue: "Integrative oncology is a patient-centered, evidence-informed field of cancer care that utilizes mind and body practices, natural products, and/or lifestyle modifications from different traditions alongside conventional cancer treatments. Integrative oncology aims to optimize health, quality of life (QOL), and clinical outcomes across the cancer care continuum and to empower people to prevent cancer and become active participants before, during, and beyond cancer treatment."[4] The terms "complementary and alternative medicine" (CAM) and "complementary and integrative medicine" (CIM) are often used interchangeably; however, when the term CAM is used it includes treatment that could be considered alternative and used in place of conventional care; the term CIM would not include alternative treatment approaches.

Utilization

According to the World Health Organization (WHO), although there is broad worldwide use of traditional and complementary medicine in both developing and industrialized nations, there is a need to move toward the evidence-based integration of these practices with conventional medicine.[5] Comparison of a 2012 and

2017 survey by the US Centers for Disease Control (CDC) found a significant increase in use of complementary health approaches such as yoga (9.5%–14.4%), meditation (4.1%–14.2%), and chiropractic care (9.1%–10.3%) during the comparison time period.[6]

Among patients and families touched by cancer, the use of CAM is higher than in the general population. An estimated 48% to 69% of US patients with cancer use CAM therapies and percentages increase if spiritual practices are included.[7] CAM therapies are used by up to 69% of cancer patients, with increased use in those with advanced cancers.[7,8]

In most cases, people who use CAM are not disappointed or dissatisfied with conventional medicine but want to do everything possible to regain health and to improve QOL, reduce side effects, stimulate immunity, or prevent new cancers or recurrences.[7,9] Whether or not patients use CAM therapies to treat cancer or its effects, they may use them to treat other chronic conditions such as arthritis, heart disease, diabetes, chronic pain, and other conditions.

Communication

Research indicates that neither adult nor pediatric patients receive sufficient information or discuss CAM therapies with physicians, pharmacists, nurses, or CAM practitioners.[10] It is estimated that 38%–60% of patients with cancer are taking complementary medicines without informing any member of their health care team.[8,9] Most patients do not bring up the topic of CAM because no one asks; thus, patients may believe it is unimportant. This lack of discussion is of grave concern because herbs and supplements may have direct toxicity or interact with cancer treatments. Patients are commonly unaware of the differences between the US Food and Drug Administration (FDA)-approved medications (which require evidence of efficacy, safety, and quality control manufacturing) and supplements, which are governed not by the FDA but by the Dietary Supplement Health and Education Act (DSHEA) of 1994. Supplements under this legislation are exempt from the same scrutiny the FDA imposes on medications; furthermore, these supplements are not intended to treat, prevent, or cure diseases. The common belief by patients that "natural" means safe needs to be addressed with education as some herbs and supplements have been associated with multiple drug interactions, as well as increased cancer risk and organ toxicity.[11,12]

Existing research suggests that the majority of cancer patients desire communication with their doctors about CAM.[13] There is general agreement within the oncology community that in order to provide optimal patient care, oncologists must not only be aware of CAM use but also be willing and able to discuss all therapeutic approaches with their patients. It is the health care professional's responsibility to ask patients about their use of complementary medicines, and the discussion should ideally take place before the patient starts using a complementary treatment—whether it is a nutritional supplement, mind-body therapy (e.g., massage, acupuncture, yoga, meditation), or other CAM approach.

A number of strategies can be used to increase the chance of a worthwhile dialogue. One approach is to include the topic of CAM as part of a new patient assessment. For example, when asking about medications, physicians should inquire about everything the patient ingests—including over-the-counter products, vitamins, minerals, herbs, and even the patient's diet. Physicians may consider having the patients bring in the actual bottles of herbs and supplements for evaluation. When asking about a patient's past medical history, physicians may ask about all other health care professionals involved in the patient's care to learn if the patients have visited with CAM practitioners such as naturopaths or chiropractors. If the issue of CAM arises, clinicians need to develop an empathic communication strategy that addresses the patient's needs while maintaining an understanding of the current state of the science.[14] In other words, this strategy needs to be balanced between clinical objectivity and bonding with the patient so that it can benefit both the patient and the health care provider. The physician who is receptive to patient inquiries is able to establish an environment in which a patient feels comfortable to bring up the topic of CAM therapies. Part of this strategy should be an open attitude combined with a willingness to review evidence-based references and consult with other health care professionals. Patients need reliable information on CAM from reliable resources, as well as adequate time to discuss this information with their oncologists.[15]

The evidence

The field of integrative oncology is a constantly evolving set of disciplines. There has been a dramatic increase in research in integrative oncology. Below we list some of the key findings to date in integrative oncology in the main areas of CAM where there is sufficient evidence to recommend the therapies: mind-body practices, massage, and acupuncture. Although there is ongoing research in many other areas such as healing touch, homeopathy, natural products, and special diets, there is insufficient evidence to recommend these at this point in time.

Mind-body practices

The belief that what we think and feel can influence our health and healing dates back thousands of years. The importance of the role of the mind, emotions, and behaviors in health and well-being is central to traditional Chinese, Tibetan, Greek, and Ayurvedic medicine and other medical traditions of the world.

The health-damaging effects of chronic stress are well documented in the medical literature. Research shows that chronic stress affects almost every biological system in our bodies.[16] Unmanaged chronic stress can speed the aging process through telomere shortening,[17] increasing the risk for heart disease,[18] sleeping difficulties,[19] digestive problems,[20] and depression.[21] Research has shown that stress can also decrease compliance with health screening behaviors and treatment.[22] Moreover, it can also cause patients to forego healthy eating and exercise habits that help prevent cancer and other disease.

With regard to cancer, there is little convincing evidence that chronic stress affects cancer initiation; however, there is extensive evidence that chronic stress can promote cancer growth and progression.[23] The underlying mechanisms for such effects are complex and involve chronic activation of the sympathetic nervous system (SNS) and the hypothalamic, pituitary, and adrenal axis.[24] Sustained elevations in these pathways (e.g., norepinephrine, cortisol) can result in diverse effects including stimulation of cancer invasion, angiogenesis, inflammation and immune dysregulation, reduced anoikis, and even reduced efficacy of chemotherapy drugs.[25] The underlying signaling pathways offer opportunities for designing new therapeutic approaches for disrupting the effects of stress biology on cancer biology and include both behavioral and pharmacological (e.g., β-blockers) approaches.

The clinical significance of stress-related biological changes and changes in the tumor microenvironment have not been widely studied. However, these changes may be significant enough to affect not only the immediate health of the patient, but also the course of the disease and, thus, the future health of the patient. It is, therefore, prudent to suggest that patients engage in some type of practice to reduce stress in their lives.

Mind-body practices are defined as a variety of techniques designed to enhance the mind's capacity to affect bodily function and symptoms. Mind-body techniques include relaxation, hypnosis, visual imagery, meditation, biofeedback, yoga, Tai Chi, Qigong, other movement-based therapies, cognitive-behavioral therapies (CBT), group support, autogenic training, and spirituality as well as expressive arts therapies such as visual arts, music, or dance. As research continues, the treatments that are found beneficial will hopefully become integrated into conventional medical care.

Research has shown that after being diagnosed with cancer, patients try to bring about positive changes in their lifestyles, indicating a tendency to take control of their health care.[26] Techniques of stress management that have proven helpful include progressive muscle relaxation, diaphragmatic breathing, guided imagery, and social support. Participating in stress management programs prior to treatment has enabled patients to tolerate therapy with fewer reported side effects.[25] Supportive expressive group therapy has also been found to be useful for patients with cancer. Although there is some data to support the use of expressive art therapies such as music therapy,[27] art therapy,[28] and expressive writing[29] and journaling to improve QOL, the number of trials is limited and they typically have small sample sizes and often no control groups. Psychosocial interventions have been shown to specifically reduce anxiety, depression and mood disturbance in cancer patients, and assist their coping skills.[30]

Newell and colleagues[31] reviewed psychological therapies for cancer patients, recommending hypnosis for managing nausea and vomiting, although further research is needed to examine the benefits of relaxation training and guided imagery. The beneficial effects of hypnosis, and especially self-hypnosis, are further supported by more recent research as hypnosis was found beneficial for reducing distress and discomfort during difficult medical procedures.[32] An NIH Technology Assessment Panel found strong evidence for hypnosis in alleviating cancer-related pain.[33] Hypnosis effectively treats anticipatory nausea in pediatric and adult cancer patients, reduces postoperative nausea and vomiting, improves adjustment to invasive medical procedures, and when combined with CBT, hypnosis leads to reduced fatigue in women with breast cancer at the end of radiotherapy and 1 and 6 months later.[34]

Research examining yoga, Tai Chi, and meditation, including mindfulness-based stress reduction (MBSR), incorporated into cancer care suggests that these mind-body practices help to improve aspects of QOL including improved mood, sleep quality, physical functioning, and overall well-being of cancer survivors.[35]

The meditation practice that has been researched the most is MBSR. The larger RCTs of meditation published in the past few years have used some form of MBSR for women with breast cancer. MBSR has been found to reduce self-reported levels of anxiety and depression and improve sleep quality; it has reduced the long-term emotional and physical adverse effects of medical treatments, including endocrine treatment; and resulted in a significant reduction in mood disturbance and symptoms of stress. A cancer-specific version of MBSR called Mindfulness-Based Cancer Recovery (MBCR) found that breast cancer survivors scoring 4 or greater in the distress thermometer had lower symptoms of stress and improved QOL.[36] In addition, both MBCR and a supportive-expressive therapy group resulted in more normative diurnal cortisol profiles than a control group.[36]

Yoga

The more movement-based mind-body practices such as Indian-based yoga, Tibetan yoga, and Chinese Tai Chi/Qigong typically combine physical postures or movements, breathing techniques, and meditation with the goal to enhance health and wellbeing. Indian-based Yoga ("yoga" is Sanskrit for "to yoke" or "join"), one of the most widely practiced Eastern traditions in Western cultures, focuses on the union of mind and body or the harmonic synchronization of body, breath, and mind. Yoga has increasingly gained popularity in the cancer setting. In fact, several systematic reviews and meta-analyses indicate the QOL benefits associated with practicing yoga in cancer patients and survivors.[37,38] Research demonstrates that yoga is useful for treating sleep for improving fatigue,[39,40] sleep disturbance,[41] overall health, QOL, physical function and reducing distress, anxiety, and depression.[42] Yoga has also been found to reduce inflammatory signaling and stress hormone regulation,[43] which plays a role in behavioral symptoms such as fatigue after breast cancer treatment.[44] Thus, yoga may actually impact biological pathways beyond patients' perceptions of QOL and symptoms. Although most yoga research has been conducted in women with early-stage breast cancer, efforts are underway to extend these findings to women with advanced breast cancer as well as survivors of lung cancer and to caregivers.[45]

Tai Chi and Qi Gong

Less research has examined the effects of *Tai Chi/Qigong* in oncology.[46] In our experience, patients and caregivers participating in *Tai Chi* and *Qigong* group classes experienced significant improvements in fatigue, physical distress, and global distress.[47] A randomized trial comparing *Tai Chi Chih* versus CBT for insomnia demonstrated that both could contribute to clinically meaningful improvement in insomnia.[48]

Massage

Massage has shown promise for relief of cancer and cancer treatment-related symptoms. As a manipulative touch-based therapy, massage can benefit cancer patients when performed by therapists who have an awareness of the special needs of cancer patients.[49,50] A massage therapist with special training in oncology massage is the best equipped to safely deliver the massage. Risk of bruising, bleeding, or injury can be minimized by careful application of pressure, avoiding massage into the deep tissue or bone in selected patients. Areas that have recently had surgery or radiation should be avoided. In patients with extremities subject to lymphedema, therapists will need to adjust their technique to maximize safety. Patients may benefit from formal lymphedema therapy as part of a physical therapy program.[51]

Research to date suggests that massage is helpful at relieving pain, anxiety, fatigue, distress, and increasing relaxation.[52,53] Benefit on mood and pain relief is limited to the more immediate effect of massage, with no current studies demonstrating long-term relief.[54,55] Anecdotal and case-report evidence has suggested benefit of massage for relief of chemotherapy-induced peripheral neuropathy. A massage to the feet, hands, and head can provide therapeutic benefit, as these areas are especially sensitive to tactile stimulation and can result in relaxation and increased well-being. Massage provided by caregivers may offer a unique opportunity for interaction between patient and caregiver that can help enhance the well-being of both.[56] In addition to symptomatic relief, studies have also demonstrated systemic effects of massage, with decreases in cortisol levels resulting from a massage intervention.[57] More research is needed to better understand massage mechanisms and treatment protocols (ideal massage-type, dosing) to better define the role of massage therapy in cancer symptom management.

Acupuncture

Acupuncture is a treatment modality that is part of traditional Chinese medicine (TCM). It has been practiced in China for thousands of years and is used in at least 78 countries throughout the world. According to TCM theory, placement of acupuncture needles, heat, or pressure at specific body points can help regulate the flow of Qi (vital energy) within the body. The most common form of acupuncture involves the placement of solid, sterile, stainless steel needles into various sites on the body that are believed to have reduced bioelectrical resistance and increased conductance. The needles may be stimulated manually or a mild electrical current may be applied directly to the needles after insertion. Stainless steel or gold (semi-permanent) needles, or "studs," are also sometimes placed at points on the ears and left in place for 3–5 days.

The strongest evidence supporting the use of acupuncture in cancer care is for symptom management. Studies have shown acupuncture is helpful to control nausea and vomiting from multiple causes (i.e., chemotherapy-induced nausea and vomiting (CINV), postoperative nausea and vomiting, and pregnancy),[58,59] and although there is good evidence for the use of acupuncture to control pain, there is still limited research in a cancer setting.

For the management of other treatment- or cancer-related symptoms, the evidence is not as strong as that for pain and nausea; however, initial research suggests acupuncture may help reduce the severity of radiation-induced xerostomia with a lasting benefit.[60,61] A randomized trial comparing true acupuncture versus sham for relief of aromatase inhibitor-induced arthralgia revealed a statistically significant reduction in joint pain at 6 weeks, however, with unclear clinical significance.[62] There is also some evidence to suggest acupuncture may be useful in treating or helping to manage symptoms such as constipation, loss of appetite, peripheral neuropathy, fatigue, insomnia and sleep disorders, dyspnea, anxiety/depression, and leukopenia, but the quality of research for these indications remains weak and further studies are needed.[63] When performed correctly, acupuncture has been shown to be a safe, minimally invasive procedure with very few side effects. The side effects most commonly reported are fainting, bruising, and mild discomfort. Infection is a potential risk, but very uncommon when treatment is provided by a qualified acupuncturist. Treatments should only be performed by a health care professional with an appropriate license and experience.

The mechanisms of acupuncture are not well understood, but for symptoms such as CINV and pain, there is clear evidence to support its use. Although data are still lacking for other symptom control, as a cost-effective treatment option with minimal associated risks, acupuncture may be a helpful addition to cancer care for patients suffering from uncontrolled treatment-related side effects or for those in whom conventional treatment approaches have failed, especially when offered in the context of clinical research intending to bolster the scientific evidence.

Guidelines

The **Society for Integrative Oncology** (SIO) has published clinical practice guidelines on the evidence-based use of integrative therapies during and after treatment for breast cancer.[64] The **American Society for Clinical Oncology** (ASCO) subsequently endorsed the guidelines.[65]

- Music therapy, meditation, stress management, and yoga for anxiety and stress reduction;
- Meditation, relaxation, yoga, massage, and music therapy for depression/mood disorders;
- Meditation and yoga for improvement in overall QOL;
- Acupressure and acupuncture for reducing chemotherapy-induced nausea and vomiting; and
- No strong evidence supports the use of ingested dietary supplements to manage breast cancer treatment-related side effects.

The **National Comprehensive Cancer Network** (NCCN) has updated guidelines (nccn.org) supporting the use of CM modalities alongside conventional care for symptom control:

- Acupuncture/acupressure, hypnosis, relaxation, music therapy, biofeedback, and yoga for anticipatory nausea and vomiting;
- Acupuncture and/or acupressure, massage, hypnosis, CBT, and MBSR a for pain;
- Yoga, massage, CBT, CBT-I (CBT for insomnia), and other psychoeducational interventions for cancer-related fatigue;
- Relaxation, mindfulness, meditation, creative therapies (art, dance, music), exercise for distress management.

As there is now consensus for the use of acupuncture, massage, music therapy, and multiple mind-body practices for the management of multiple symptoms in oncology, it is ideal if these modalities are offered to patients alongside conventional cancer care as part of a coordinated, evidence-based approach.

Educational resources

Comprehensive reviews can quickly become out-of-date and the ease of internet publishing has fostered the growth of comprehensive scientific review organizations that provide electronic access to their reviews. We will outline websites of organizations providing reliable information for providers and patients (Table 1).

The ACS and NCI Office of Cancer Complementary and Alternative Medicine (OCCAM) provide valuable educational resources for patients and the general public on complementary therapies. Natural Medicines Comprehensive Database provides evidence-based reviews of complementary therapies. The Cochrane Review Organization, founded in 1993 as an international nonprofit independent organization, provides systematic reviews that include complementary therapies.

The integrative medicine service at the Memorial Sloan-Kettering Cancer Center provides evidence-based reviews as part of their "About Herbs, Botanicals & Other Products" internet resource. The integrative medicine program at the University of Texas MD Anderson Cancer Center offers an internet resource with curated audio and video content for patients and providers to learn more about the evidence-based role of Integrative Medicine in cancer care.

Integrative oncology in clinical practice

Integrative oncology has the ability to enhance the care provided for cancer patients by incorporating additional treatment options that lead to improved health, symptom management, and QOL. Most major cancer centers now offer some complementary

Table 1 Recommended web sites for evidence-based CIM resources.

Organization/web site (alphabetical order)	Address/URL
American Institute for Cancer Research	www.aicr.org
American Cancer Society	www.cancer.org
Cochrane Review Organization	www.cochrane.org
Memorial Sloan-Kettering Cancer Center	www.mskcc.org/cancer-care/integrative-medicine/about-herbs
National Comprehensive Cancer Network	www.nccn.org
Natural Medicines Comprehensive Database	naturalmedicines.therapeuticresearch.com
NCI Office of Cancer Complementary and Alternative Medicine (OCCAM)	cam.cancer.gov
University of Texas MD Anderson Cancer Center Integrative Medicine Program	www.mdanderson.org/integrativemed

medicine treatment modalities alongside the conventional care.[66] In order to create comprehensive integrative cancer care, these types of therapies must be delivered in a manner that does not just avoid potential interactions but works to create synergy with ongoing treatment. To do so, the integrative oncology care plan must incorporate principles of being evidence-based, personalized, and safe. Organizations such as the American Society of Clinical Oncology and the Society for Integrative Oncology are working together to develop further evidence-based clinical practice guidelines for the use of integrative therapies during cancer care.[65]

The Integrative Medicine Center at MD Anderson Cancer Center is one example. The center utilizes a bio-psychosocial model of health care (Figure 1) as a clinical framework to guide the implementation of services to patients throughout the cancer continuum (prevention, treatment, and survivorship), and some services are also provided for caregivers. The clinical services are provided to address specific medical conditions such as pain or anxiety or the appropriate use of herbs and supplements and not available to patients as part of a spa service. The center provides patient care on an individual basis as well as in groups. Patients may receive inpatient and outpatient physician consultation, acupuncture, massage, mind-body therapy such as meditation, and music therapy. Physical therapy for exercise counseling, a dietician for nutrition counseling, and a psychologist for mood management and behavioral counseling are also available for all patients. Patients may also attend free group classes such as meditation, yoga, Tai Chi/Qigong, music therapy, exercise, and cooking classes. All staff members meet on

Physical
- Exercise
- Nutrition
- Acupuncture
- Oncology massage

  - Primary oncology team
  - Physical medicine & rehabilitation
  - Supportive care
  - Cancer pain

Mind-body
- Health psychology
- Meditation
- Music therapy
- Tai Chi/Qi Gong
- Yoga

  - Psychiatry
  - Spiritual care

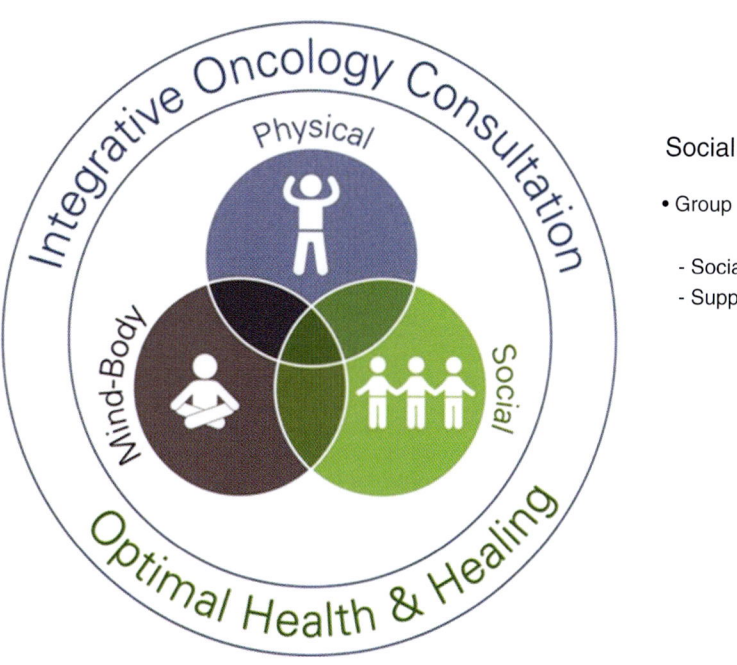

Social
- Group programs

  - Social work
  - Support groups

Figure 1 Integrative oncology model of care.

a weekly basis to discuss challenging new patients and to help coordinate care. Clinical notes are available in the electronic health record. As part of routine care, patients complete validated instruments on symptoms and QOL and are included as part of a broader clinical research initiative to understand the clinical impact of the clinical services provided. The integrative medicine center works collaboratively with supportive services such as palliative medicine, psychiatry, pain center, and rehabilitation services.

Conclusion

Integrative oncology is a rapidly expanding discipline that holds great promise for additional treatment options, expanding options for symptom control, and supporting lifestyle modification efforts for cancer prevention. For the majority of patients who are either using complementary medicines or want to know more about them, an integrative approach provides them with a more personalized system of care for meeting their needs. The clinical model for integrative care requires an evidence-informed, patient-centered approach. Enhanced communication between oncology-care teams, integrative medicine clinicians, and other providers of non-conventional therapies is critical for the successful implementation of an evidence-informed integrative oncology care plan. In this way, cancer patients will be receiving the best medical care making use of all appropriate treatment modalities.

Acknowledgment

The authors acknowledge the contributions from authors, Richard Lee, MD, Alejandro Chaoul, PhD, and M. Kay Garcia, DrPH, MSN, LAc, from the prior edition of this book.

Key references

The complete reference list can be found on Vital Source version of this title, see inside front cover.

6. Clarke TC, Barnes PM, Black LI, et al. Use of Yoga, Meditation, and Chiropractors Among U.S. Adults Aged 18 and Over. NCHS Data Brief. No. 325. Nov 2018.
7. Richardson MA, Sanders T, Palmer JL, et al. Complementary/alternative medicine use in a comprehensive cancer center and the implications for oncology. *J Clin Oncol*. 2000;**18**(13):2505–2514.
8. Navo MA, Phan J, Vaughan C, et al. An assessment of the utilization of complementary and alternative medication in women with gynecologic or breast malignancies. *J Clin Oncol*. 2004;**22**(4):671–677.
11. Ulbricht C, Chao W, Costa D, et al. Clinical evidence of herb-drug interactions: a systematic review by the natural standard research collaboration. *Curr Drug Metab*. 2008 Dec;**9**(10):1063–1120.
13. Verhoef MJ, White MA, Doll R. Cancer patients' expectations of the role of family physicians in communication about complementary therapies. *Cancer Prev Control*. 1999 Jun;**3**(3):181–187.
16. Chrousos GP, Gold PW. The concepts of stress and stress system disorders. Overview of physical and behavioral homeostasis. *JAMA*. 1992;**267**(9):1244–1252.
17. Epel ES, Blackburn EH, Lin J, et al. Accelerated telomere shortening in response to life stress. *Proc Natl Acad Sci U S A*. 2004;**101**(49):17312–17315.
21. Hammen C. Stress and depression. *Annu Rev Clin Psychol*. 2005;**1**:293–319.
22. Prasad SM, Eggener SE, Lipsitz SR, et al. Effect of depression on diagnosis, treatment, and mortality of men with clinically localized prostate cancer. *J Clin Oncol*. 2014;**32**(23):2471–2478.
23. Lutgendorf SK, Sood AK, Antoni MH. Host factors and cancer progression: biobehavioral signaling pathways and interventions. *J Clin Oncol*. 2010;**28**(26):4094–4099.
24. Lutgendorf SK, Sood AK, Anderson B, et al. Social support, psychological distress, and natural killer cell activity in ovarian cancer. *J Clin Oncol*. 2005;**23**(28):7105–7113.
25. Parker PA, Pettaway CA, Babaian RJ, et al. The effects of a presurgical stress management intervention for men with prostate cancer undergoing radical prostatectomy. *J Clin Oncol*. 2009;**27**(19):3169–3176.
26. Thaker PH, Han LY, Kamat AA, et al. Chronic stress promotes tumor growth and angiogenesis in a mouse model of ovarian carcinoma. *Nat Med*. 2006;**12**(8):939–944.
27. Archie P, Bruera E, Cohen L. Music-based interventions in palliative cancer care: a review of quantitative studies and neurobiological literature. *Support Care Cancer*. 2013;**21**(9):2609–2624.
30. Devine EC, Westlake SK. The effects of psychoeducational care provided to adults with cancer: meta-analysis of 116 studies. *Oncol Nurs Forum*. 1995;**22**(9):1369–1381.
31. Newell SA, Sanson-Fisher W, Savolainen NJ. Systematic review of psychological therapies for cancer patients: overview and recommendations for future research. *J Natl Cancer Inst*. 2002;**94**(8):558–584.
33. Integration of behavioral and relaxation approaches into the treatment of chronic pain and insomnia. NIH Technology Assessment Panel on Integration of Behavioral and Relaxation Approaches into the Treatment of Chronic Pain and Insomnia. *JAMA*. 1996;276:313–318.
34. Montgomery GH, David D, Kangas M, et al. Randomized controlled trial of a cognitive-behavioral therapy plus hypnosis intervention to control fatigue in patients undergoing radiotherapy for breast cancer. *J Clin Oncol*. 2014;**32**(6):557–563.
35. Chaoul A, Milbury K, Sood AK, et al. Mind-body practices in cancer care. *Curr Oncol Rep*. 2014;**16**:417.
36. Carlson LE, Doll R, Stephen J, et al. Randomized controlled trial of mindfulness-based cancer recovery versus supportive expressive group therapy for distressed survivors of breast cancer. *J Clin Oncol*. 2013;**31**(25):3119–3126.
37. Cramer H, Lange S, Klose P, et al. Yoga for breast cancer patients and survivors: a systematic review and meta-analysis. *BMC Cancer*. 2012;**12**:412.
38. Danhauer SC, Addington EL, Cohen L, et al. Yoga for symptom management in oncology: a review of the evidence base and future directions for research. *Cancer*. June;**125**(12):1979–1989.
39. Bower JE, Garet D, Sternlieb B, et al. Yoga for persistent fatigue in breast cancer survivors: a randomized controlled trial. *Cancer*. 2012;**118**(15):3766–3775.
40. Bower JE, Greendale G, Crosswell AD, et al. Yoga reduces inflammatory signaling in fatigued breast cancer survivors: a randomized controlled trial. *Psychoneuroendocrinology*. 2014;**43**:20–29.
41. Mustian KM, Sprod LK, Janelsins M, et al. Multicenter, randomized controlled trial of yoga for sleep quality among cancer survivors. *J Clin Oncol*. 2013;**31**(26):3233–3241.
43. Kiecolt-Glaser JK, Bennett JM, Andridge R, et al. Yoga's impact on inflammation, mood, and fatigue in breast cancer survivors: a randomized controlled trial. *J Clin Oncol*. 2014;**32**(10):1040–1049.
44. Chandwani KD, Perkins G, Nagendra HR, et al. Randomized, controlled trial of yoga in women with breast cancer undergoing radiotherapy. *J Clin Oncol*. 2014;**32**(10):1058–1065.
45. Milbury K, Chaoul A, Engle R, et al. Couple-based Tibetan yoga program for lung cancer patients and their caregivers. *Psychooncology*. 2014. doi: 10.1002/pon.3588.
51. Torres Lacomba M, Yuste Sanchez MJ, Zapico Goni A, et al. Effectiveness of early physiotherapy to prevent lymphoedma after surgery for breast cancer: randomised single blinded, clinical trial. *BMJ*. 2010;**340**:b5396.
53. Russell NC, Sumler SS, Beinhorn CM, Frenkel MA. Role of massage therapy in cancer care. *J Altern Complement Med*. 2008;**14**(2):209–214.
54. Wilkinson SM, Love SB, Westcombe AM, et al. Effectiveness of aromatherapy massage in the management of anxiety and depression in patients with cancer: a multicenter randomized controlled trial. *J Clin Oncol*. 2007 Feb 10;**25**(5):532–539.
56. Collinge W, Kahn J, Walton T, et al. Touch, caring, and cancer: randomized controlled trial of a multimedia caregiver education program. *Support Care Cancer*. 2013 May;**21**(5):1405–1414.
59. Ezzo J, Vickers A, Richardson MA, et al. Acupuncture-point stimulation for chemotherapy-induced nausea and vomiting. *J Clin Oncol*. 2005;**23**(28):7188–7198.
61. Garcia MK, Meng Z, Rosenthal DI, et al. Effect of true and sham acupuncture on radiation-induced xerostomia among patients with head and neck cancer: a randomized clinical trial. *JAMA Netw Open*. 2019;**2**(12):e1916910.
63. Garcia MK, McQuade J, Haddad R, et al. Systematic review of acupuncture in cancer care: a synthesis of the evidence. *J Clin Oncol*. 2013;**31**(7):952–960.
65. Lyman GH, Greenlee H, Bohlke K, et al. Integrative therapies during and after breast cancer treatment: ASCO endorsement of the SIO clinical practice guideline. *J Clin Oncol*. 2018;**36**(25):2647–2655.

48 Health services research

Michaela A. Dinan, PhD ∎ Devon K. Check, PhD

Overview

Health services research (HSR) describes a diverse group of research strategies and fields that seek to evaluate the impact of health care on patients and populations and has been a critical component of understanding the use, outcomes, and costs associated with oncology care since its inception over 100 years ago. In modern times, physicians and researchers often tout "bench to bedside" innovations as the goal of biomedical research. However, patients, physicians, and health care systems in the real world are subjected to a host of factors that impact patient care before, during, and after an intervention occurs at the bedside. Although HSR is a complex and evolving concept, a basic understanding of the key principles of HSR is needed to accurately assess, quantify, and optimize the real-world impact of progress in oncology today and in the future.

Introduction—what is health services research?

Health services research (HSR) comprises a diverse group of research disciplines and strategies that seek to evaluate the impact of health care on patients and populations. While the focus of the included disciplines may differ, there are similarities which allow us to group them together under the umbrella of HSR. In most cases, the same basic premise can be applied: A treatment or intervention is examined in the context of an outcome of interest in order to better understand and guide clinical practice.

According to the Institute of Medicine (IOM), HSR focuses on the investigation of three major aspects of healthcare including (1) access to care, (2) the quality of care, and (3) the cost of health care in order to inform health care consumers about their best options for medical treatment and/or prevention.[1] The IOM has also developed a list of the major issues that health services researchers are studying today (Table 1).

HSR is truly a multidisciplinary field. Health services researchers, biostatisticians, economists, and providers are all examples of critical and necessary players in the HSR arena. In oncology, the clinical expertise of medical, surgical, and radiation oncologists, as well as nurses, pathologists, and radiologists, are all needed to develop clinically relevant questions that will lead to improvements in patient care. Close collaboration between methodologists and clinical providers is essential to ensure both the scientific validity and clinical significance of HSR studies.

The goals of HSR in oncology are many. While some research focuses on the investigation of diagnostics and treatments to prolong survival, other seeks to improve quality of life (QOL), understand and inform decision making, improve access to care, ensure guideline-concordant or evidence-based care, or examine the economic impact of care for cancer patients. In addition to the wide range of these and other potential outcomes, HSR in oncology has several stakeholders with vested interests in the results including patients and their caregivers and families, physicians and other medical staff, additional providers and payers of health care, industry, advocacy organizations, and policy makers that must be considered in any effort to make advances in oncology.

The significance of health services research in cancer

HSR in oncology is the principal means by which we frame the scope of cancer care and attempt to improve cancer care delivery in the real world. Discoveries made in the controlled environments of laboratories and clinical trials may or may not translate when taken out of the context of a select group of trial participants and applied to the larger population of patients. That is to say, most clinical trials are focused on the *efficacy* of a specified intervention, or the ability of an intervention to provide benefit under tightly controlled circumstances. Such controlled settings can lead to questions as to whether a trial's findings can be considered *generalizable* to the population as a whole. In contrast, HSR focuses on the *effectiveness* of these interventions, which describes the ability of an intervention to provide benefit under real-world conditions. The goal of HSR is to improve the effectiveness of interventions as they are disseminated into broader, more diverse populations and promote the health of all members of the population.

HSR in oncology has been used to provide estimates of the scope of cancer on a national scale and as a prediction of how it will change in the future. For example, HSR using the population-based surveillance, epidemiology, and end results (SEER) registry provides the estimate that in 2020, there were an estimated 1.8 patients newly diagnosed with cancer and 606,520 people who died from their cancer. As the US population continues to age, this number is expected to increase along with the costs associated with cancer care. For example, in 2010, the total direct estimated cost of cancer care in the United States was $124.5 billion. After only accounting for demographic changes, these costs were projected to increase to $157.8 billion by 2020.[2] The most recently complete available data are from 2018 and show $150.8 billion in US cancer care costs.[3] These costs will likely continue to climb much higher due to the adoption of expensive innovative therapies, the widespread diffusion of advanced technologies without supporting evidence, inappropriate use (either over- or underuse) of existing treatments, with patient demands and unrealistic expectations being additional areas of concern. HSR provides a framework to consider how to mitigate the impact of this surge in need on current medical resources and infrastructure.

Table 1 IOM list of major health services research topics.

- Health services organization and financing
- Access to healthcare
- Behaviors of practitioners, patients, and healthcare consumers
- Quality of care
- Clinical outcomes research
- Health care decision-making and informatics
- Health professions workforce

Disciplines within health services research

In practice, HSR is often separated into multiple distinct fields of discipline—health economics, health outcomes research, epidemiology, and implementation research. The distinctions have developed over time based on the data requirements, methodologies, and expertise needed to answer questions meaningfully. Despite these potential differences, there is considerable overlap and a common goal of inferring causality and informing practice. Outcomes research revolves around the identification of a treatment or exposure of interest and a relevant outcome (i.e., the impact of a new treatment on survival). Health economists focus on health care costs and resource utilization, epidemiologists on naturally occurring exposures and patterns, and implementation researchers on strategies for improving the uptake of evidence-based practices (EBPs) in routine care.

An overview of health services research study designs

HSR can be conducted with a variety of different study designs. They may analyze primary data (collected prospectively as part of either a qualitative or quantitative study design) or secondary data (collected for some other purpose, such as for hospital billing, and are then repurposed). Clinical trial study designs are perhaps most familiar, where a specific intervention is imposed on a study group. Randomized clinical trials (RCTs) are considered the gold standard of clinical research because the intervention or exposure of interest is randomly designated across study participants. RCTs are often blinded, where the physician is not aware of a subject's assignment to a given study arm, or even double blinded, where neither the physician nor the subject is aware of the assignment. These design elements help to avoid any biases that may occur by ensuring the random distribution of interventions across subjects.

Observational analyses do not assign interventions among subjects and are most often retrospective in nature. Instead, researchers examine the relationship between exposures or events of interest that occurred and the associated effects or outcomes. The studies can be descriptive or analytic in their design. Descriptive studies include case reports or case series, ecologic studies, and cross-sectional studies, while analytic studies include longitudinal cohort and case-control studies. Descriptive analyses are used to generate hypotheses, whereas analytic analyses are used to test specific hypotheses about the association between a specific exposure and outcome.

Randomized controlled trials

RCTs have long been considered to produce the highest level of evidence among individual studies. In an RCT, patients are randomly assigned to either a control (placebo or standard of care) arm or an experimental arm. Such trials have been used in countless assessments of therapeutic benefit of medications, behavioral interventions, screening studies, and chemoprevention studies. Although such trials represent the pinnacle of evidence development and have a number of strengths, it is critical for care providers and researchers to have a thorough understanding of both the benefits and limitations of such studies so that they are able to accurately interpret and incorporate their findings in guiding clinical practice and future HSR studies.

The key strength of the RCT is its ability to ensure that a treatment was assigned at random, which serves as the single most reliable method to remove potential sources of bias. This allows the closest ability we have to study what we truly want to understand—the "counterfactual condition." Counterfactual means literally "against the facts" and describes a "what-if" situation. What we really want to know is "what if" the same patient was exposed to treatment A versus treatment B? If we could go back in time and administer a different treatment to the same patient, would it have changed their outcome? This is obviously not possible. However, through the use of RCTs, we are able to randomly assign treatment so that we can indirectly infer, on average, what would have been the impact had a patient received treatment A versus treatment B. The potential for bias introduced by confounders in observational studies is the principal weakness of observational studies and the ability to avoid confounded treatment assignment is the fundamental strength of RCTs.

Potential limitations of randomized controlled trials

RCTs are not able to address many questions in HSR. Perhaps the most significant reason is that RCTs are often impossible to conduct due to ethical concerns about a lack of equipoise, or equal validity of both proposed treatment strategies. Because of this, there is often only a limited period during which equipoise of two proposed management strategies exists. A classic example of this in oncology is the comparison of radical prostatectomy to radiation therapy in the definitive management of localized prostate cancer. In most cases, a patient's provider and the patient themselves are generally unwilling to randomly assign such substantially different treatments. Numerous RCTs attempting to compare the two strategies have resulted in limited accrual, leading to concerns about sample sizes and external validity.[4] In the United Kingdom, only 1 of 20 patients enrolled on such a study consented to randomization.[5]

Even when adequate equipoise exists to enroll meaningful numbers of patients into RCTs, there are additional limitations. Caution should always be taken whenever interpreting a "negative study" to make sure that the study was adequately powered to answer the question being asked.

Another key limitation of RCTs is that such studies are often applied to a selected group of patients that lack external validity. Patients who are eligible for clinical trials are heavily screened and reflect a group of patients whose outcomes are often superior to those seen in the community. An example of difficulties with external validity comes from a high-quality and well-known meta-analysis of multiple studies assessing the benefit of chemotherapy in localized breast cancer.[6] Despite the inclusion of 194 trials, few patients were over the age of 69, which leaves the benefit of chemotherapy unclear in women over 70.

The process of study design, enrollment, follow-up, and analysis of RCTs can take decades or longer before results are known. The studies can be outdated before they are completed, particularly in areas of cancer care where practice is changing rapidly and the natural disease history is relatively indolent or protracted such as in localized breast or prostate cancer. RCTs cannot assess how the general population is treated, examine the extent to which risks and benefits seen in controlled settings match those observed in actual practice, or characterize adoption, utilization, costs, or factors associated with the use of an intervention in real-world practice. Although RCTs remain a critical component in creating high-level evidence of the efficacy of experimental treatments, observational studies must be used as a complement in order to provide a full and balanced perspective of the true impact and effectiveness of proposed treatment strategies.

Observational studies

Observational studies do not assign or alter any factor of interest as, by definition, they cannot control which patients receive a given exposure or treatment. Prospective analyses consist of data collected with the intention of analyzing it for a given purpose. In contrast, retrospective analyses utilize data that have already been collected for a different reason, often leveraging administrative claims used to bill insurance companies or general cancer registries that include treatment data. Although a distinction is often made between prospective and retrospective analyses, the methods and approaches used to analyze the data are similar. However, prospective analyses, especially those for which a detailed analysis plan is created prior to collecting and viewing the data, are less likely to lead to extensive subgroup analyses or other approaches that may identify spurious associations due to chance and extensive data manipulation. Additional limitations of most retrospectively performed analyses include a lack of personal risk factors, detailed performance status, and other factors that might influence or more accurately characterize the exposure or outcome of interest that would have been collected had the analysis plan been known at the time of data collection. The quality of analyses performed on any data set will vary widely depending on the quality of the data. Key to the internal validity of any study is the reliability of key exposures, outcomes, and potential confounders contained within the data. In administrative claims data, for example, claim dates and procedural codes are typically heavily audited and highly reliable, since this information is used to determine payment information. However, the reliability of a diagnosis of constipation or some other minor complication that does not impact payment might be missed in a large proportion of patients. Therefore, familiarity with the data being analyzed is paramount to performing a well-conducted study.

The potential for bias or confounding is the primary limitation of observational studies, and a host of advanced statistical methods have been developed to help combat and mitigate potential biases in order to avoid invalid conclusions. Despite this fundamental weakness, observational studies continue to play an important and critical role in much of HSR that cannot be addressed by RCTs. Perhaps the single most important risk factor for developing cancer in the modern era, smoking, has never been examined within a RCT but has been firmly established by countless observational studies across numerous cancer types.

There are several principal strengths of observational studies. They examine real-world practice in the community, as opposed to that limited to major academic or cancer trial centers, and provide a representation of the actual use and outcomes associated with an intervention as it is used in practice. Compared to interventional studies, observational studies have the additional benefits of significantly reduced costs, large sample sizes, the potential to observe extended follow-up, and often the statistical power necessary to detect heterogeneous treatment effects or risks among rare patient subgroups.

Types of observational studies

Observational studies can be primarily classified as descriptive or analytic. The focus of analytic studies is similar to that of randomized trials, where the goal is to infer whether or not a causal relationship exists between an exposure or treatment and the outcome of interest. Such studies seek to test a specific hypothesis, for example, one might hypothesize that patients undergoing surgery at a high-volume center have superior outcomes compared to those treated at lower-volume centers. In contrast, descriptive studies characterize a particular set of patient characteristics or outcomes and can be used to generate hypotheses to be tested in future studies.

The two most common examples of analytic observational studies are case-control and cohort studies. *Case-control* studies are often used in cancer HSR to assess the association between environmental exposures such as smoking, genotype, geography, drugs, diet, or toxins and the likelihood of developing cancer (the outcome). Such studies identify patients with the outcome of interests (cases, i.e., cancer), and match them to patients who did not experience the outcome (controls, i.e., no cancer). Interviews or surveys are often conducted to obtain additional information from both sets of patients. The strength of such studies is that they can be used to analyze factors that might predispose people to rare cancers that would otherwise be difficult to evaluate. The primary challenge of these studies is often identifying controls that are otherwise similar to the cases except for the exposure of interest and ensuring that recall bias among cases does not over-report exposures compared to the controls.

In contrast to case-control studies, *cohort studies* select a group of patients based on their exposure and then follow them forward over time. Cohort studies are called as such because they first define the specific cohorts of interest—that is, exposure and nonexposure—before examining outcomes. There are numerous examples of cohort studies in HSR, which include analyses of clinical trials, registries, and other retrospective or prospective databases. These studies are often used to characterize the adoption and costs of emerging medical technology such as advanced imaging and positron emission tomography (PET) scans[7] or intensity-modulated radiation therapy (IMRT) in the treatment of prostate cancer.[8]

The strengths of observational cohort studies include the ability to examine rare exposures over prolonged periods of time, such as the impact of atomic bomb radiation exposure on the risk of developing leukemia and other cancers decades later. In contemporary HSR, cohort studies are perhaps the most commonly used observational study approach and are used to compare the impact of a particular treatment on patient outcomes. For example, given the difficulties of conducting large RCTs of prostatectomy versus radiation in prostate cancer, many cohort studies have compared outcomes following treatment with these two modalities.[9]

Descriptive studies include ecologic studies, cross-sectional studies, and case reports or case series. Unlike analytic studies, such studies are not designed to test hypotheses, but rather to generate hypotheses that may be tested in later studies. *Ecologic studies* describe situations where the exposure and outcomes occur at the individual level but are measured at the population level.[10] For example, ecologic studies of many cancers have been used to demonstrate changes in the risk of specific cancers such as breast or prostate between the United States and other countries, presumably due to cultural, environmental, lifestyle, or dietary differences in exposures.[11] Such studies, while hypothesis generating, suffer from the primary weakness that they cannot confirm individual-level associations between exposures and outcomes.

Table 2 Strengths and weaknesses of commonly encountered large secondary databases.

Data source	Examples	Strengths	Weaknesses
Disease registries	SEER NCDB	• High-quality short-term exposure and outcome data • Clinically rich • Collection of potential confounders • Large sample sizes across a broad population	• Lack of randomization to key exposure • Poor long-term follow-up • Lack of data for unrelated disease states
Administrative data	CMS (Medicare) VA (Veterans Affairs) Kaiser Permanente	• Broad coverage of the population • Efficiency of data collection • Long-term follow-up availability of patient-specific identifiers that can be linked to additional data sources	• Lack of randomization to key exposure(s) • Inaccurately recorded data • Limited clinical details
EMR based data research networks	Flatiron health PCORnet Cancer research network	• Access to near real-time data • Potential for interventional or adaptive studies • Potential to access test results	• Limited follow-up outside of network • Limited death data
Epidemiologic cohort studies	NHANES CCSS	• Large sample size • High-quality lifestyle/behavioral data	• Inclusion criteria of cohort may limit generalizability • Prespecified data elements at time of cohort creation
Clinical trials	Collaborative group studies Industry trials Institutional trials	• Clinically rich data • Random assignment of key exposures	• Preselected population and smaller sample sizes • Loss to follow-up

In contrast to ecologic studies, *cross-sectional* studies are used to observe individuals at a single snapshot in time and can characterize the association of exposures and outcomes among those patients. However, the primary limitation of these studies is that they cannot be used to draw causal inferences, since it is not possible to distinguish whether such an association represents the exposure causing the outcome or the outcome causing the exposure.

Lastly, *case reports or case series* describe detailed exposures and outcomes of a small number of patients. Such studies have often heralded the potential for extraordinary therapeutic efficacy of novel treatment strategies. A contemporary example of a high impact case report comes from the case of combining novel immune checkpoint inhibitors with radiation, where radiation to a single site of disease was observed to induce complete systemic resolution of all sites of disease in a patient with metastatic melanoma. The effect was attributed to a radiation-induced stimulation of a systemic immune response.[12]

Secondary data sources relevant to HSR in oncology

A common understanding among health services researchers is that the study is only as good as the data being used. There are limitations to every data source so health services researchers must consider multiple approaches to be able to address a question of interest. Primary data quality will depend largely on the instrument design and any logistic constraints involved in the collection of the data. Secondary data are often limited by the purpose for which they were originally collected. Billing data (aka claims data), collected as documentation of services provided and payments received; studies using these data must account for the inherent limitations when designing an analytic plan.

There are a few commonly encountered types of oncology databases available for secondary analyses in HSR which include clinical registries, administrative datasets, clinical trial databases, epidemiologic cohorts, and more recently an increasing body of data from aggregated electronic medical records (EMRs).

A thorough understanding of the strengths and limitations of the dataset one plans to use is critical in order to conduct a valid analysis (Table 2).

Clinical registries collect relevant data on patients with an incident cancer diagnosis within a specific population, health care system, network, or region. Strengths of clinical registries include high-quality short-term exposure and outcome data, clinically rich data specific to a disease of interest, collection of potential confounders, and the potential for large sample sizes. The principal weakness of registry data is a lack of randomization to key exposures of interest, poor intermediate and long-term follow-up and outcomes, and lack of data regarding unrelated disease states such as cardiovascular disease. Two examples of powerful cancer registries that are often leveraged in HSR studies include the SEER data and the National Cancer Data Base (NCDB).

The SEER tumor registry program collects detailed clinical and pathological information on 28% of cancer patients in the United States, aggregating it from participating registries that are representative of the national patient population. Limitations of these data include a lack of detailed information on treatments, providers, and costs. To address these needs, linkages were pursued to generate a richer set of variables. This resulted in a collaboration between the National Cancer Institute (NCI) and the Centers for Medicare and Medicaid Services (CMS) to make a SEER-Medicare dataset available that adds Medicare administrative data and health care claims. Since CMS provides health insurance to over 97% of Americans aged 65 and older, this allows a detailed assessment of health care utilization and costs among SEER patients. The SEER-Medicare data have been used to examine cancer care quality around issues of racial disparities, physician and hospital characteristics, screening, treatment choices (i.e., surgery, chemotherapy, radiation), complications, costs, and mortality.[13] While powerful, a core limitation of the SEER-Medicare dataset is that it only includes those 65 years of age and older.

Another oncology-specific dataset which is widely used is the NCDB which is a joint project of the American Cancer Society and the American College of Surgeons' Commission on Cancer (CoC). The NCDB was established in 1989 as a nationwide, hospital-based, comprehensive clinical surveillance data set. The NCDB obtains data from more than 1500 CoC-accredited facilities which captures 30 million patient records and 70% of all newly diagnosed cancer cases.[14] The key strength of the NCBD is its sheer size and its capture of the majority of cancers diagnosed within the United States. It is well poised to study nationwide patterns of care, adoption of novel surgical procedures, and the approach to rare cancers. As a surgical data set, it contains excellent data on the details of a patient's surgery and survival. However, some aspects of the data are not reliably coded; there are limited details regarding chemotherapy, radiation, or non-cancer-related health; and there is no information on relapse, recurrence, or subsequent treatments.

Administrative datasets consist of information that is routinely collected within the operations of a given health care entity, such as an insurer (i.e., Medicare), integrated health care systems (i.e., Veterans Affairs Hospitals), or large health care organizations (i.e., Kaiser Permanente). The strength of administrative data lies in its broad coverage of tens or even hundreds of millions of lives, the efficiency of data availability, and the long-term follow-up available through the use of patient identifiers. In addition, administrative data are representative of the population at large, while data collected within a clinical trial are clinically rich but limited to a carefully preselected, smaller populations due to cost and scientific considerations. The weaknesses of administrative data stem from their collection for purposes of billing and tracking health care resource utilization, often limiting the granularity of available information. Information such as dates of claims and types of procedures performed are highly accurate. However, information that is not critical to billing, such as cancer stage, is not always captured.

EMRs are foundational to a learning health system, as they provide a digital footprint of each patient's story. To the effect that data in the EMR can be codified to a common standard, then EMR data can approximate registry data. In order to solve this, information in structured data feeds (e.g., laboratory data) needs to be harmonized and normalized to a single common data model; information trapped in unstructured documents (e.g., PDFs of clinical notes, pathology reports) must be transferred to codifiable digital standards. Multiple groups are focused on solving this problem in cancer.

The contributors to these efforts are broad, spanning organizations such as traditional health organizations, government entities, and genomics companies. HSR will benefit from real-world data obtained in real time through the linking of EMRs to numerous external databases. The potential to incorporate decisions support into routine care, leveraging patient-specific data in areas such as genomics, treatment history, and predicted outcomes will require knowledge of how to manage such data from technical, medicolegal, ethical, and practical perspectives.

Electronic health record (EHR)-based Data Research Networks include data extracted directly from the EHRs and can either be data pulled into a central repository or part of a distributed research network (DRN) where each entity maintains its own data. Strengths of EHR Data Research Networks often include (1) access to near real-time data, (2) offering a potential mechanism for interventional or adaptive studies, and (3) access to test results which are not typically available in administrative datasets. Health system data networks (HSDN) are central databases that use EMR data within their health system as their primary data source, and then supplement these data by partnerships with other entities or networks. The quality, quantity, and limitations of data networks varies by the specific data network. The Flatiron Health data are an example of a HSDN. Limitations to these data include a lack of nononcologic data and imperfect death data although efforts are ongoing to improve these limitations with additional linkages and partnerships. DRNs are networks of networks in which researchers are able to generate queries that are then distributed among partnering networks. Efforts to standardize data across network partners occur through a common data model. PCORnet and the Cancer Research Network are examples of these. PCORnet is disease agnostic and is not specific to cancer, however, oncology-specific efforts are ongoing. Limitations of DRNs, in general, include that patients are limited to those within the health care network and thus a lack of generalizability.

There are also disease or population-specific caches of data collected as part of large epidemiologic or cohort studies. The National Health and Nutrition Examination Survey (NHANES) is an example of a cross-sectional data survey of about 5000 individuals per year since the 1960s. These data are rich in lifestyle data (alcohol use, smoking, BMI, etc.) but there no follow-up of patients is included, although there have been examples of researchers linking the NHANES data with mortality and cause of death data. Examples of longitudinal epidemiologic cohorts include the Women's Health Initiative (WHI) and the Childhood Cancer Survivor Study (CCSS). These cohorts have excellent follow-up and detailed information about the individual populations for which they were created but no information outside of those specific populations.

The process of linking data attempts to combine the strengths of multiple data sources into one dataset to help offset limitations of any single data set. For example, registry and clinical trial data, which often suffer from a lack of long-term follow-up and incompleteness can be supplemented with administrative claims data (such as Medicare) to augment the available follow-up and survival data.

Statistical analyses in health services research

An in-depth review of statistics is well beyond the scope of this article, so we will focus on commonly used techniques that encompass the vast majority of HSR. In HSR, statistical analyses are used to analyze data from a population of interest in order to either describe or learn something (i.e., make an inference) about the general state of affairs in that population. Descriptive statistics simply describe or summarize a set of data, by providing means, frequencies, counts, plots, or other depictions. Inferential or analytic statistics use more complex methodologies to attempt to draw generalizable inferences from a set of data, such as whether or not two groups differ from one another by more than what would reasonably be expected by chance. Generally speaking, health services researchers use quantitative methodologies to test or confirm hypotheses, quantify variation, predict causal relationships, and/or to describe characteristics of a population.

Multivariable versus univariate analyses

In HSR, one of the most common distinctions made in practice is the use of statistics to investigate single variables versus multiple variables. Single variable or "univariate" analyses are used to summarize or describe the properties of a single variable, such as what percent of a population has ever smoked. Multivariable or multivariate analyses (in practice these are used interchangeably) are more complex and seek to explain the relationship between a single variable of interest and multiple other variables at the same time.

Often univariate versus multivariable analyses are referred to as "unadjusted" and "adjusted," since the multivariable approach "adjusts" for potential confounding by uncontrolled variables. Such control variables might include clinically relevant variables associated with the outcome of interest such as age, stage, or grade and *must* include any variables that might be associated with both the exposure and outcome of interest in order to fully control for potential confounding. In a study that performs both "unadjusted" and "adjusted" analyses, the results from the adjusted (or multivariable) analyses are more likely to reflect the true relationship of interest, since these models have at least attempted to adjust for factors that might otherwise explain the observed relationship. Variables are often interrelated in HSR and a failure to account for these relationships can result in erroneous conclusions. The key question that HSR seeks to answer is often how a certain treatment, condition, or exposure impacts a specific outcome of interest after controlling for all other relevant factors.

Multivariable analyses

One of the most widely used methods in multivariable analysis in HSR is that of multivariable regression analysis. The term "regression" was originally coined in the late 1800s by Francis Galton to describe the tendency of tall or short pea plants (outliers) to produce offspring that were more similar to, or "regressed" towards the overall population height.[15] In its simplest form, this is essentially drawing a straight line through a plot of two variables that shows the mean or average of one variable as a function of the other. Significant mathematical and computational progress since has allowed for the routine use of far more complicated models that are able to predict the value of a so-called "dependent" variable whose value is predicted *depending* on the values of multiple "independent" variables. Such models come in many forms and have been refined and developed to be able to predict, model, or describe any combination of different variable types. Most often in HSR, continuous data are modeled using linear regression, dichotomous data using logistic regression (from its use of binary logic values, that is zero or one to describe the dependent variable), and survival data using cox proportional hazard models (survival variables include an event such as death or relapse versus no death or relapse combined with the time to that event). Linear regressions will predict the mean value of the dependent variable as a function of each independent variable (i.e., average weight as a function of sex and height), logistic regressions will estimate odds ratios (OR) associated with a particular exposure, and cox proportional hazards models yield hazard ratios (HR). Poisson regression is a reliable alternative to logistic regression when relative risk is the parameter of interest.[16] Other frequently used multivariable statistical analyses include variations of the χ^2 ("chi-squared") test, such as the Cochrane–Mantel–Haenszel test,[17,18] which essentially performs the χ^2 test for an association between two categorical variables while controlling for other potentially confounding variables.

One of the benefits of multivariable regression is the ability to capture "interaction effects," or an interaction between two independent or explanatory variables on the dependent variable of interest. Interaction effects can capture cases where a variable might only impact the outcome of treatment within a subset of patients. For example, a meta-analysis of three randomized controlled trials in non-small-cell lung cancer (NSCLC) found a significant interaction between squamous tumor histology, receipt of pemetrexed, and a lack of treatment response.[19] This meta-analysis confirmed that the drug pemetrexed is associated with improved outcomes, but only in patients with nonsquamous cell histology. As a result, pemetrexed is now the drug of choice in nonsquamous NSCLC.

Bias and confounders

Perhaps the single most important concept in HSR is the idea of bias or confounding. A confounder is anything that confuses, obscures, or otherwise mixes the effect of the characteristic of interest with others. The word "confound" comes from the Latin for "pour together,"[20] and so literally describes a situation where the observed association is mixed or confused by a confounder. An example of confounding can be demonstrated using a hypothetical retrospective study of patients with metastatic disease, in which patients who have less aggressive disease and receive surgery for their metastatic disease are observed to live longer. In this case, the observed association of surgery with prolonged survival is being confused with, or "confounded" by, the association of nonaggressive disease with both surgery and survival.

Bias is also used to describe confounding but can be more descriptive by additionally specifying the direction of the observed erroneous association. Bias is a related term from the old French *biais*, meaning "slant,"[20] and describes the situation where the observed association is biased, or unfairly slanted, to yield either a false positive (can bias the estimate of an association upward or downward) or false negative ("biased towards the null hypothesis") association between two variables.

One specific example of bias in the HSR oncology literature comes from analyses of survival in patients with NSCLC. Several studies had observed that receipt of PET scans are associated with improved survival, and erroneously concluded that receipt of PET *improves* survival. However, upon closer examination, we know that PET scans are generally administered to patients with early-stage disease who are candidates for curative surgery and definitive treatment. The use of PET scans is not indicated for patients with obvious advanced or metastatic disease. In this case, one would say that the association of PET with survival is confounded by selection bias, or selective administration of PET scans to patients with less advanced disease. Another way to describe this would be to say that the association of PET with survival is being confounded by selective administration of PET to lower risk patients.[21,22]

There are several commonly encountered types of bias that are important in the accurate interpretation of observational HSR studies. *Omitted variable bias* is one of the principal forms of bias in observational studies, and is nearly always present to some extent in HSR. It will occur in any situation where (1) a variable exists that is associated with both the outcome and exposure of interest and (2) is omitted as a control. For example, in the PET-NSCLC scenario, disease stage was correlated with both PET and survival but was not included in the model.

Selection bias is used to describe when a group or exposure is not randomly applied to patients, or in the example case above, where PET scans were *selectively* applied to patients with less advanced disease. *Recall bias* refers to the situation where one population is more likely to recall an event than another. For example, patients with a rare form of cancer might be more likely to recall exposure to any number of environmental stimuli that have been forgotten or would have been overlooked by patients without cancer who had the identical exposure. Bias due to *loss to follow-up* can occur if patients who remain in the study are systematically different from those who do not. *Nonresponse bias* can be seen in self-reported surveys, where survey participants are often more likely to express stronger beliefs than that held by the overall, target study population. *Misclassification bias* refers to the case where either the exposure or outcome of interest is misclassified. Lastly, *interviewer bias* can occur when the interviewer knows which exposure or treatment a patient has had, and probes more deeply than they otherwise would have in patients without that exposure.

Minimizing confounders and bias

There are several potential methods that can be used to minimize confounders. Several of these methods can only be implemented during the design phase of a study, and it is, therefore, key to involve a biostatistician or HSR methodologist early on in the design of any study, when the full set of all options are available. For example, RCTs will often stratify by key variables known to influence the outcome of interest in order to ensure that they will not wind up with an unbalanced treatment and control group in the final analysis. Multivariable regression analyses are commonly used to help adjust or control for potential confounders. However, a key limitation of such attempts is that variables that are not or cannot be observed cannot be controlled. There are nearly always such unobservable factors at play to some extent in most observational HSR studies, which is why any observed associations should not be reported as causal without further confirmation.

Commonly used methods to mitigate the impact of bias include matching, stratification, subgroup analysis, and instrumental variable analysis.

Matching is the process whereby the characteristics between two groups are matched as closely as possible, in order to create populations that are similar in all respects. The quality of the match can be indirectly assessed by checking to make sure that observable variables that were not used to match patients appear to be similar between groups.

When there are many factors that may differ between two populations, exact matching on all factors is not possible. A calculated *propensity score* may be used to predict the likelihood (or propensity) to receive the treatment or exposure of interest.[23] Patients can then either be matched directly or stratified by their propensity score to assess the exposure or treatment of interest, thereby mitigating important differences between study groups.

Related to matching approaches is the idea of *stratification or subgroup analysis*, which respectively control for, or limit analysis to, a specific subgroup of selected patients in which outcomes are predicted to be similar (i.e., stage, age, performance status).

The above approaches all have in common that they identify potential confounders and attempt to correct or adjust for them. In contrast, an approach called *instrumental variable (IV)* analysis is meant to minimize bias by avoiding confounders all together. In the IV approach, researchers attempt to identify a so-called "instrument," or proxy, that is strongly associated with the exposure of interest, but that is not associated with the outcome of interest through confounding. For example, distance to the nearest facility with PET scanners might predict the likelihood of undergoing a PET scan (the exposure of interest) but should not otherwise be directly associated with stage or survival (outcomes) except through the exposure of interest (PET). Strong "instruments" can be difficult to identify and often are unavailable.

It is important to realize that none of the above methods will completely eliminate bias in real-world HSR analyses. As such, the ability to mitigate, and test for, residual bias is paramount in conducting and accurately interpreting observational HSR.

Internal and external validity

Internal validity refers to whether or not observed findings are likely to be reflective of the examined population. In other words, internal validity describes whether the observed findings can be believed within the patients that were analyzed in the study. Any and all studies must have internal validity in order to allow for clinically meaningful interpretation. Common threats to interval validity include selection bias, differential follow-up, recall bias, confounding, misclassification, investigator or interviewer bias, or any systematic differences between control and treatment groups that are associated with the exposure of interest.

External validity (often described as "generalizability") refers to whether the associations observed within the confines of the population studied can be generalized to patients outside (external to) the study sample. Not all studies will be externally valid to the same extent. For example, many RCTs are limited to young patients with few co-morbidities. The benefit seen in RCTs may not extend to older, sicker, or heavily pretreated patients who were not included in the study.

Meta-analyses and systematic reviews

Systematic reviews are thorough, systematized reviews of the literature on a specific question in HSR and often take place as the preliminary step within a meta-analysis. Meta-analysis describes a statistical technique for combining data from multiple studies in order to try and provide a more precise estimate of the true impact of an intervention or exposure. In order for such studies to be valid, meta-analyses should first perform a quality systemic review of the existing literature, incorporate all relevant data, and check for evidence of heterogeneity in reported studies in order to assess whether or not there is evidence of a potential bias in the field to only publish positive associations. Major findings should be confirmed via the use of sensitivity analyses that ensure that observed estimates are robust to reasonable variations in the analysis. Systematic Reviews and Meta-analysis are often considered a principal component of the evidence development process and are particularly important in supporting the generalizability and understanding of clinical effectiveness.

Modeling

Modeling studies in HSR refer to the creation of algorithms to describe complex associations and relationships between exposures, outcomes, and confounders.[24] Modeling can play a particularly important role in guiding the design of policies, guidelines, treatment approaches, or reimbursement that would otherwise be too time consuming, costly, and complicated to analyze using direct interventional or conventional observational approaches. Modeling also provides a means of exploring relationships among data which cannot be directly observed or feasibly obtained in practice, such as those involving costs or long-term outcomes. Models used in HSR often examine the impact of various decision algorithms, new interventions, policies, or patient factors on associated outcomes or costs. The studies often use metrics such as quality-adjusted life-years (QUALYs) to objectively provide an indication of the balance between overall quantity and QOL for cancer patients. Cost-effectiveness analyses often report incremental cost-effectiveness ratios (ICERs), which describe the relative cost and gains of alternative management strategies or exposures.

An example in the cancer literature comes from several analyses of the impact of Oncotype DX testing in breast cancer. Use of the Oncotype DX test, which predicts the benefit associated with receipt of chemotherapy, has been previously shown to change physician recommendations to prescribe less overall chemotherapy. Modeling studies of Oncotype DX testing have been used to perform cost-effectiveness analyses and have predicted that the use of the assay has the potential to be cost-saving.[25] The advantage of modeling is that various factors and their relative impact on outcomes of interest can be dissected—for example, one could adjust estimates of cost savings from Oncotype DX testing depending on the utilization strategy, the age of the population, and the cost of chemotherapy. The obvious disadvantage of modeling is that many assumptions must be made that may impact the findings.

Comparative effectiveness research

According to the Agency for Healthcare Research and Quality (AHRQ), comparative effectiveness research (CER) is "designed to inform health-care decisions by providing evidence on the effectiveness, benefits, and harms of different treatment options."[26] The term "comparative effectiveness" was coined roughly 25 years ago and was originally used to describe research to "help patients, family, and caregivers make more informed decisions with providers."[27] In practice, the use of CER is used to describe studies (often observational) that attempt to compare the benefits of two interventions or management strategies. The 2010 Patient Protection and Affordable Care Act (PPACA) established the Patient-Centered Outcomes Research Institute (PCORI) to fund and conduct research to determine the effectiveness of various medical services. PCORI explicitly emphasized the incorporation of costs and cost-effectiveness into studies.[28] As a result, the use of CER has evolved over recent years to include a greater focus on cost and cost-effectiveness.

CER is not a specific analysis technique or approach but a re-framing of existing observational study methodologies to focus on the comparison of potential treatment strategies. Most CER studies are simply cohort-based studies, described previously in this article, with an emphasis on attempting to simulate an RCT comparing two treatment arms with the goal of performing causal inference. At the end of the day, the key challenge in CER studies, much like other observational studies, is the mitigation of potential bias and confounding.

Quality of care

The Institutes of Medicine (IOM) has defined quality of care as "the degree to which health care services for individuals and populations increase the likelihood of desired health outcomes and are consistent with current professional knowledge," and then later extended the definition to encompass "care that incorporates respect for patients' values and preferences."[29,30] It is underappreciated that, despite substantial improvements in available treatments and technology, the main determinants of patient health outcomes, quality of care, and overall costs are related to variability in clinical practice[31,32] and the failure of patients to receive basic care.[33]

One such example comes from studies of surgery at high-volume centers. For over 30 years it has been consistently observed that centers with higher volume, or total number of cases performed, are often associated with improved outcomes.[34] Twenty years after this was initially observed, this was confirmed in a meta-analysis showing that in 123 of 128 studies included, lower hospital mortality was observed in high-volume centers across 40 different procedures.[35] The risk of receiving a procedure at a low-volume center was highest for complicated procedures such as esophagectomy and pancreatectomy, where differences in 30-day mortality approach 5–10%.[36]

However, it is important to note that such studies are observational in nature, vary in their definition of "high-volume," and may be significantly biased by case selection of patients willing to travel to higher volume centers. Quality of care may also vary by geographic region due to differences in regional treatment patterns, patient populations, available oncology specialists, or other factors. For example, rates of laparoscopic colectomy[37] and end of life care[38] vary widely by geography.

The quality metrics used to describe the structure, process, and outcomes of care were proposed by Dr. Donabedian in 1950 and continue to be used to this day.[39] Structure describes the context in which care is provided and its associated financial and personnel resources. Examples might include institutional characteristics such as provider expertise, accreditation, and case volume. Processes consist of patient and provider activities in the diagnosis and treatment of an illness and are often defined in terms of guidelines issued by national organizations such as the National Comprehensive Cancer Network (NCCN) or the American Society of Clinical Oncology (ASCO). Outcomes describe the patient's health posttreatment and are defined in terms such as overall survival, disease-specific survival, objective response rates, time to progression, and toxicity. The use of outcomes in formal metrics is often debated in oncology due to variations in case-mix, disease-severity, and other potential confounders that might be outside an institution's control. Increasingly, methods are used to overcome this limitation.

Despite the potential for each of these to impact the quality of care, there are inherent challenges in using outcomes and structure-based endpoints to define quality in a way that can incentivize health care providers and systems to improve care. For example, outcomes may be significantly impacted by the case-mix seen by an institution. Efforts to "cherry-pick" or otherwise select patients may be effective at increasing profits, but not improve care. Structure-based endpoints may not be appropriate as a one size fits all solution depending on the total case volume, case mix, amount of resources, or rural versus urban location. As a result, assessments of health quality in both HSR and in practical use are dominated by procedural measures. As an example, the majority of healthcare effectiveness data and information set (HEDIS) measures currently used to assess health care performance across a wide variety of settings relies almost entirely on procedure-based definitions of quality such as the use of cancer screening, immunizations, or specific treatments for disease. Procedures can be underused, overused, or misused. In practice, under-use is often most easily studied in the setting where current guidelines recommend a specific procedure and whether or not patients received the recommended standard of care can be examined. Overuse and misuse, however, are challenging to prove, since guidelines tend to be less likely to describe situations where a specific test should not be performed under any circumstances. For example, although a PET scan may not be indicated for all patients with breast or colorectal cancer, a borderline CT scan or other equivocal study would be a reasonable indication to perform a PET. Such nuances can be difficult to describe systematically within many retrospective data sets. Lastly, misuse can be similarly difficult to confirm in the absence of detailed treatment records, which typically are not available in larger retrospective studies.

Outcomes and endpoints

Although HSR can encompass any outcome or endpoint associated with patient care, there are a number of types of outcomes and endpoints that form the bulk of current HSR, including patient-reported outcomes (PROs), QOL, cost, quality, access, patterns of care, and CER.

Patient-reported outcomes

PROs are generated by questions posed to patients regarding their symptoms and other concerns, as opposed to being documented by physicians or other members of the health care team.

Widespread internet access and advances in computational technology now provide the opportunity to engage with patients and collect longitudinal PROs, which has grown dramatically over the last few years. As a result, the collection and utilization of PROs have emerged as a distinct area of study with networks of researchers dedicated to its implementation. In support of this, researchers with expertise in the collection and utilization of PROs often collaborate with QOL researchers to efficiently achieve their research goals. For the purpose of the discussion, we will only briefly mention QOL as a subset of PRO research, noting that it in fact composes a large portion of PRO research but will be described in more detail in the next section.

The use of PROs in HSR has several strengths including efficient collection, improved accuracy as to the patient's experience when compared to physician-reported measures, and the ability to use them to predict objective clinical outcomes such as survival, patient satisfaction, and general health.[40] PRO measures can be either generic or disease-specific, each of which have their respective advantages and weaknesses.[41] Advantages of general PRO tools include wider generalizability across disease types and a larger body of literature to support both their validity and association with traditional objective endpoints.

Although a large number of PROs have been used in the literature, there are several PRO measures that have been specifically evaluated in oncology and are worth brief mention here and include the European Organization for Research and Treatment of Cancer Quality of Life Questionnaire (EORTC QLQ-C30), Functional Assessment of Cancer Therapy (FACT), MD Anderson Symptom Inventory (MDASI), patient reported outcome version of the Common Terminology Criteria for Adverse Events (PRO-CTCAE), and patient reported outcome Measurement Information System (PROMIS).[40] Efforts to validate, standardize, and compare PROs have greatly improved the quality of PRO measures, which are now used routinely in clinical trial design and the approval of new drug applications submitted to the FDA.

A recent advance in the field has been the incorporation of the patient's voice using PROs. In particular, the advantages of capturing electronic patient reported outcomes (ePROs) over conventional PROs are numerous and include reduced costs, increased efficiency in delivery and completion for both patients and providers, and the ability to use computer adaptive testing (CAT) to further economize and personalize the data gathered from these interactions. Through this cycle, these data can then be used to help inform clinical care, provide decision support, and educate patients and clinicians in real-time at the point of care.

Quality of life

Measures of QOL are numerous and complex, each containing specific domains or areas of interest (i.e., fatigue, urinary symptoms, medical events), with each domain including multiple items. Key measures of the utility of specific QOL instruments include their reliability, internal consistency, reproducibility between interviewers, and validity (content and construct). The short form—36 item (SF-36) is an example of a questionnaire that has been used in hundreds of studies and disease types with a large body of literature supporting its reliability and applicability. Alternatively, disease-specific measures provide a more targeted assessment of key factors relevant to a particular patient population. For example, for patients with prostate cancer, urologic and sexual QOL metrics should be directly assessed through disease-specific tools such as the International Index of Erectile Function (IIEF). Choosing the best measures of QOL requires a thorough understanding of the most relevant symptoms and outcomes to a specific patient population.[40] QOL research can also be used to derive utilities or quantitative measures of QOL. Such utilities can be used to adjust survival analyses to represent both quantity and QOL.

QOL measures have a number of limitations, including the fact that they often contain a large number of domains and items, with many potential permutations of measures, dysfunctions, and symptoms, impeding efforts at standardization and validation. QOL measures may also not hold the same value for all patients. For example, elderly patients may not be as concerned with sexual function and previously disabled patients may have a different baseline level of functionality that precedes their diagnosis. Lastly, as with any data, missing data or failure of patients to complete questionnaires may occur due to fatigue, apathy, decline in mental function, or overall decline in health. Such declines are notorious in palliative care settings, where nonparticipation may be strongly associated with declining patient overall performance status and can result in reporting bias.

Costs

As described previously in this article, the cost of cancer in the United States is increasing rapidly due to the aging of the population and the adoption, and increased use, of expensive emerging medical technologies. Efforts to accurately quantify current costs, understand factors driving costs, and model the impact of alternative strategies are a critical component of HSR. Such analyses may examine overall costs, cost-effectiveness, cost-utility, cost-benefits, and help provide a uniform framework and set universal thresholds to objectively and rationally inform policy, reimbursement, payer, provider, and patient decisions.

Even the most basic cost analyses are more complex and nuanced than one might initially expect. Patients undergoing the same treatment, at the same institution, for the same condition, may pay vastly different amounts for the same service (e.g., due to different insurance). Because of the nature of health care and its perception as a right (i.e., emergency care), "customers" cannot be turned away for certain services. The means by which hospitals and medical facilities balance the costs of those who can pay versus those who cannot set the stage for a widely variable, often obscure, pricing system in which the physician often is not able to know the cost of the treatment they are prescribing. This is in stark contrast to other consumer services in which charges are known in advance and discussed upfront by service providers such as is done by mechanics and veterinarians.

As a result, the method and perspective used to estimate costs of medical care must be carefully specified and can include payments made by the insurer (payer perspective), out of pocket payments by the patient (patient perspective), total payments, total charges, lost wages due to lost productivity, and the additional burden placed on family members or other caregivers (societal perspective). Many interventions may alter subsequent management strategies and outcomes, which may impact overall costs via these "indirect costs." Of all these metrics, hospital-listed charges vary the most widely, are the least reliable indicators of true cost, and are rarely used since most patients pay a lower price as negotiated by their insurance company. Marginal costs indicate the additional cost of a change in treatment strategies or additional services and are often used to examine the incremental impact of changes in treatment strategies. Because of the complexity of calculating health care costs, and the potential variation in the cost for a given service, close attention should be paid to the details and underlying assumptions of any cost estimates.

Bundled episodes of care

Many payers no longer operate using an a-la-carte, fee-for-service system where each service or good is associated with a payment. Inpatient costs are increasingly bundled and rates of reimbursements set by a Diagnosis Related Group (DRG) code which consists of a single lump sum that is paid to hospitals to cover all care administered during a hospitalization. These DRG codes are based on estimates of how much an admission should reasonably cost given the reason for the admission and potential complicating factors. Similarly, surgical procedures are often bundled, where a single reimbursement is expected to cover the surgery and all associated follow-up care, including complications within a predetermined timeframe. These systems are designed to incentivize providers and hospitals to provide efficient care and minimize complications.

Cost-effectiveness analysis

There are several types of cost analyses beyond simple summations that provide objective data with which patient, providers, payers, and policy makers can make informed decisions. Common analyses include cost-effectiveness analyses and modeling (described previously in this article). A cost-effectiveness analysis has been defined by the National Institute for Health and Clinical Excellence (NICE) as an economic study design in which consequences of different interventions are measured using a single outcome (i.e., life-years gained, deaths avoided, cases detected). Alternative interventions are then compared in terms of cost per unit of effectiveness. This key metric is referred to as the incremental cost-effectiveness ratio (ICER). Whether or not a specific intervention is considered "cost-effective" depends on the available resources and willingness to pay of the target population. A classic analysis of over 500 life-saving interventions suggested that the median cost per life year saved was approximately $42,000 per life year saved[42] (in 1995 dollars), providing a rough benchmark of the relative willingness of the American public to pay. In contrast, global health initiatives, vaccinations, and the treatment of malaria are highly cost-effective at less than $100 per life year saved. A screening colonoscopy every 10 years beginning at age 50 costs roughly $11,000 per year of life saved.[43] The World Health Organization recommends considering cost-effectiveness in terms of gross domestic product (GDP) per capita. Using this schema, interventions are considered highly cost-effective (less than GDP per capita); cost-effective (between one and three times GDP per capita); and not cost-effective (more than three times GDP per capita). For the United States (2012 GDP per capita), this would equate to <$50,000, $50,000–$150,000, and >$150,000, respectively. In the end, cost-effectiveness analyses are often phrased in terms of currently accepted ICERs. For example, if a given health system is already paying for interventions that cost $60,000 per QALY, it would make logical sense for them to cover a novel intervention with an ICER < $60,000. In current US practice interventions, ICERs of <$50,000 are generally considered cost-effective but this has changed over time and will continue to change. Such analyses provide a detailed and objective framework with which patients, providers, and policy makers can make rational tradeoffs in costs, care, and outcomes.

Qualitative methods

The previous sections discussed quantitative methodologies health services researchers use to test or confirm hypotheses, describe characteristics of a population, quantify variation, and predict causal relationships. Qualitative methodologies, on the other hand, are used to generate hypotheses and to describe variation, relationships, and individual experiences. Common qualitative data collection methods include individual interviews and focus groups. Both methods use open-ended questions organized into flexible (i.e., semi-structured or unstructured) question guides. While quantitative research studies yield numerical data, qualitative research studies yield mainly textual data, usually obtained from audio recordings and transcriptions of interviews or focus groups.

There are several categories of qualitative research. Most qualitative studies in HSR fall under the category of qualitative description, which is well suited for describing the "who, what, when, and where" of events. It involves minimal theorization or interpretive spin of data. The goal is to use everyday language that is reflective of the participant voice.[44]

In HSR, qualitative research—particularly qualitative description—is often used to understand and explore health care phenomena from the perspective of key stakeholders, including clinicians and patients. For example, cancer-related HSR studies conducted in recent years have used qualitative description to explore factors that influence patients' treatment preferences[45–47] and clinicians' adoption of EBPs and guidelines.[48–50] Qualitative description is also commonly used to inform the development, refinement, or adaptation of clinical and behavioral interventions, for example by assessing patients' or clinicians' needs and preferences with respect to intervention content and delivery. For example, in their 2019 study, Ouchi and colleagues developed an emergency department-based intervention for older adults with serious illness—including metastatic cancer—to formulate their goals of care.[51] They conducted a series of mock clinical encounters using the prototype intervention and then conducted semi-structured interviews with clinicians and patients who had participated in the mock encounters, with the goal of refining the intervention. After the authors fielded the refined intervention, they again conducted semi-structured interviews with patients to assess intervention acceptability.

Mixed methods

Mixed methods research draws upon the strengths of both quantitative and qualitative approaches to HSR. There are several advantages to integrating quantitative and qualitative methods in HSR studies. For example, qualitative data can be used to assess the validity of quantitative findings, inform the development or refinement of quantitative instruments, or generate hypotheses to be tested in the quantitative phase of a study. Quantitative data can be used to help generate the sample for the qualitative phase of a study or explain findings from qualitative data. Quantitative and qualitative results from mixed methods studies may be published together or separately.

There are three basic types of mixed methods designs: Exploratory sequential, explanatory sequential, and convergent. In sequential designs, one phase (qualitative or quantitative) of the mixed methods study builds on the other; in convergent designs, the qualitative and quantitative components of the study occur separately but in parallel.

In an *exploratory sequential* design, the research team first collects and analyzes qualitative data, and these qualitative findings inform subsequent quantitative data collection. For example, researchers might conduct semi-structured interviews with patients to understand their experiences and use those qualitative data to identify key concepts measured subsequently in a survey. Buckley and colleagues conducted qualitative interviews with patients with acute myeloid leukemia (AML) to elicit concepts for the development of an AML-specific QOL instrument.[52] They then fielded the instrument to patients with AML, collecting quantitative data on its validity and reliability.[53]

In an *explanatory sequential design*, the research team first collects and analyzes quantitative data, and the quantitative findings inform qualitative data collection and analysis. For example, the research team might use surveys followed by interviews to further explore specific concepts covered by the survey. So and colleagues conducted an explanatory sequential mixed methods study consisting of a survey of over 285 Chinese head and neck cancer survivors, to assess survivors' unmet supportive care needs. The authors then conducted semi-structured interviews with 53 survey respondents to explore several unmet needs in more detail.[54]

In a *convergent design*, the quantitative and qualitative data collection efforts occur in parallel. Often, the quantitative and qualitative data are analyzed separately and then merged in the interpretation phase of the study. For example, Roberts and colleagues conducted a quantitative analysis of a longitudinal population-based study of nearly 3000 North Carolina women diagnosed with breast cancer to examine potential racial disparities in uptake of Oncotype DX testing.[55] Concurrently, the study team collected qualitative data from oncology providers to understand factors that may impede or facilitate their use of Oncotype DX.[48]

Implementation science

Implementation science is "the scientific study of methods to promote the systematic uptake of research findings and other evidence-based practices into routine practice, and, hence, to improve the quality and effectiveness of health services."[56] An implementation research study typically begins with an EBP or evidence-based intervention (EBI) that is under-utilized, and then seeks to identify, understand, and address multi-level barriers to the uptake of that practice or intervention.

Implementation research studies focus on evaluating the process of implementation and the impact of that process on the adoption (i.e., uptake) of and/or fidelity to the EBP or EBI of interest. The process of implementation typically involves an implementation strategy or, more commonly, a collection or package of several individual implementation strategies. Implementation strategies can be thought of as interventions that implementation scientists develop and test to improve uptake of an EBP or EBI.[57] Scholars have identified 73 distinct implementation strategies[58] and organized them into 9 overarching categories: use evaluative and iterative strategies; provider interactive assistance; adapt and tailor to context; develop stakeholder relationships; train and educate stakeholders; support clinicians; engage consumers; use financial strategies; and change infrastructure.[59]

According to Bauer and colleagues,[60] implementation studies can involve one or more of three broad types of evaluation: process evaluation, formative evaluation, and summative evaluation.

Process evaluations describe use of an EBP or EBI (or lack thereof), including potential barriers to or facilitators of its use. Data are collected before, during, and/or after implementation of the EBP or EBI. Process evaluations are not intended to change the ongoing implementation process. They might be undertaken in preparation for developing an implementation strategy either as part of a purely observational study or as part of an effectiveness trial of an intervention.[60] The Oncotype DX interview study by Roberts and colleagues[48] described in the previous section provides an example of a process evaluation. The authors interviewed oncology providers in an effort to understand barriers to their use of an evidence-based practice—Oncotype DX testing.[48] To take an example from the effectiveness trial context, in their recently published study protocol, Battaglia and colleagues[61] describe a planned implementation-related process evaluation as part of their effectiveness study of a patient navigation intervention to reduce disparities in breast cancer treatment. The process evaluation will use a convergent mixed-methods design, quantitatively assessing navigator fidelity to the intervention protocol and costs associated with the intervention, and qualitatively assessing intervention acceptability, and factors that may influence intervention adoption and sustainment among navigators, clinicians, and hospital administrators.[61]

Formative evaluations are similar to process evaluations. The main distinction is that, in a formative evaluation, results are fed back to clinical and operations partners in the target implementation setting in order to adapt and improve the ongoing implementation process.[60] For example, in their study protocol published in 2018, Midboe and colleagues[62] describe a planned formative evaluation of an evidence-based collaborative care intervention for primary care patients with chronic pain. During the preimplementation phase, the study team will gather information to inform the development of an implementation strategy to support successful integration of the collaborative care intervention into primary care practice. During the implementation phase, the study team will monitor progress with respect to intervention implementation and modify the implementation strategy as needed. During the sustainment phase (i.e., after active implementation efforts have concluded), the authors plan to gather data related to implementation successes or failures and recommendation for future implementation refinements.

Summative evaluations compile data—at the conclusion of a study—on the impact of the implementation strategy or strategies evaluated as part of the study. Measures used in summative evaluations usually assess impacts on use of the EBP or EBI at the clinician or setting level.[60] For the Midboe study described above, the summative evaluation examines whether the implementation strategy leads to uptake and sustained use of the collaborative care intervention in the target primary care clinics.

Implementation science is a relatively young and continually evolving field. Traditionally, implementation research efforts start after an evidence base has been established for a given intervention. Increasingly, however, research teams are integrating an implementation science perspective into earlier stages of the intervention development and testing process. For example, "designing for dissemination and implementation" describes a recent focus on developing interventions that align with both the resources and limitations of the target setting, to increase the chances that interventions can achieve their intended goals.[63] In addition, increasing numbers of effectiveness studies—including the studies described above—use "effectiveness-implementation hybrid" designs to investigate effectiveness—and implementation-related research questions in tandem,[64] rather than sequentially. The goal of considering implementation earlier in the intervention development and evaluation process is to expedite the translation of effective interventions into practice.

Key references

The complete reference list can be found on Vital Source version of this title, see inside front cover.

1. IOM. *Committee on Health Services Research: Training and Work Force Issues. Health Services Research: Workforce and Educational Issues.* Washington, DC: National Academy Press; 1995.
9. Sun M, Karakiewicz PI, Sammon JD, et al. Disparities in selective referral for cancer surgeries: implications for the current healthcare delivery system. *BMJ Open.* 2014;**4**(3):e003921.
10. Morgenstern H. Ecologic studies in epidemiology: concepts, principles, and methods. *Annu Rev Public Health.* 1995;**16**:61–81.
14. ACS. American College of Surgeons. Inspiring Quality: Highest Standard, Better Outcomes. National Cancer Data Base, 2015; https://www.facs.org/quality%20programs/cancer/ncdb (accessed 1 July 2015).
15. Pearson K. *The Life, Letters and Labors of Francis Galton.* Cambridge University Press; 1930.
16. Zou G. A modified poisson regression approach to prospective studies with binary data. *Am J Epidemiol.* 2004;**159**(7):702–706.
17. Woolson RF, Bean JA, Rojas PB. Sample size for case-control studies using Cochran's statistic. *Biometrics.* 1986;**42**(4):927–932.
18. Mantel N, Haenszel W. Statistical aspects of the analysis of data from retrospective studies of disease. *J Natl Cancer Inst.* 1959;**22**(4):719–748.
20. Online Etymology Dictionary, 2015; http://www.etymonline.com (accessed 1 July 2015).
21. Dinan MA, Curtis LH, Carpenter WR, et al. Stage migration, selection bias, and survival associated with the adoption of positron emission tomography among medicare beneficiaries with non-small-cell lung cancer, 1998–2003. *J Clin Oncol.* 2012;**30**(22):2725–2730.
22. Chee KG, Nguyen DV, Brown M, et al. Positron emission tomography and improved survival in patients with lung cancer: the Will Rogers phenomenon revisited. *Arch Intern Med.* 2008;**168**(14):1541–1549.
23. D'Agostino RB Jr,. Propensity score methods for bias reduction in the comparison of a treatment to a non-randomized control group. *Stat Med.* 1998;**17**(19):2265–2281.
26. AHRQ. Agency for Healthcare Research and Quality. What is Comparative Effectiveness Research; http://effectivehealthcare.ahrq.gov/index.cfm/what-is-comparative-effectiveness-research1 (accessed 2015). Published 2015.
28. Kinney ED. Comparative effectiveness research under the patient protection and affordable care act: can new bottles accommodate old wine? *Am J Law Med.* 2011;**37**(4):522–566.
29. IOM and NRC (National Research Council). *Ensuring Quality Cancer Care.* Washington, DC: National Academy Press; 1999.
30. IOM. *Crossing the Quality Chasm: A New Health System for the 21st Century.* Washington, DC: National Academies Press; 2001.
37. Reames BN, Sheetz KH, Waits SA, et al. Geographic variation in use of laparoscopic colectomy for colon cancer. *J Clin Oncol.* 2014;**32**(32):3667–3672.
38. Morden NE, Chang CH, Jacobson JO, et al. End-of-life care for medicare beneficiaries with cancer is highly intensive overall and varies widely. *Health Aff (Millwood).* 2012;**31**(4):786–796.
41. Dinan MA, Compton KL, Dhillon JK, et al. Use of patient-reported outcomes in randomized, double-blind, placebo-controlled clinical trials. *Med Care.* 2011;**49**(4):415–419.

PART 7

Individualized Treatment

49 Precision medicine in oncology drug development

Apostolia M. Tsimberidou, MD, PhD ■ Elena Fountzilas, MD, PhD ■ Razelle Kurzrock, MD

Overview

In recent years, advances in technology have led to identification of complex and unique biologic mechanisms of tumorigenesis. Precision medicine uses tumor and cell-free DNA profiling, immune markers, RNA and proteomic analyses, and other biomarkers in combination with patients' unique characteristics and comorbidities to individualize anti-cancer therapy. The focus of selected clinical trials has shifted from tumor type-centered to gene-directed, and in some cases, histology-agnostic approaches. Innovative trial designs tailored to biomarker profiling aim to improve treatment outcomes. These designs enable the dynamic evolution of the studies, allow the elimination of treatment arms with inferior outcomes and modification of patient randomization, and optimize biomarker selection based on real-time study outcomes. They also accelerate regulatory approval of novel drugs by empowering seamless transition from phase I to phase II and III clinical trials. Companion diagnostic biomarkers provide essential information for the safe and effective use of the corresponding targeted or immune treatments and lead to improved clinical outcomes of patients with molecular alterations treated with matched targeted treatments. However, the complex interaction between tumors, immune cells, and the tumor microenvironment complicates the identification of robust biomarkers. To overcome biologic complexity and tumor heterogeneity, clinical trials evaluate combinations of gene-targeted therapy with immune-targeted approaches (e.g., checkpoint blockade, personalized vaccines, oncolytic viruses, and/or adoptive cell therapy), hormonal therapy, chemotherapy, and/or novel agents, customized to individuals in an N-of-1 fashion. In this article, we discuss the rapid evolution of precision medicine in oncology and the challenges and opportunities associated with its implementation into daily clinical practice.

Introduction

Precision oncology combines data from tumor genomic profiling, cell-free DNA assays, proteomic and immune profile analyses, and assessments of other markers to individualize treatment according to unique patient and tumor characteristics. Recent advances in precision oncology have altered the therapeutic landscape of cancer.

The overall survival (OS) has improved in specific tumor types with the use of treatments that target specific biomarkers. Examples of the first robust predictive biomarkers used to individualize treatment in cancer include identification of estrogen and progesterone receptors (1971)[1] and human epidermal growth factor receptor 2 (1998)[2] in patients with breast cancer and Philadelphia chromosome [t(9;22)] (2001) in patients with chronic myelogenous leukemia.[3] Later, the use of next-generation sequencing (NGS) allowed for the assessment of epidermal growth factor receptor (EGFR) activating mutations (2004) in patients with lung cancer,[4] KRAS resistance mutations (2006) in patients with colorectal cancer,[5] and BRAF activating mutations (2010) in patients with melanoma.[6] The implementation of global sequencing and multi-gene panels (2011) led to major advances in precision oncology, including the identification of multiple predictive molecular alterations simultaneously, discovery of innovative targeted treatments, and evaluation of matched therapies across tumor types.

Clinical trials across tumor types have shown improved clinical outcomes of patients with molecular alterations treated with matched targeted treatments.[7-12] For example, we have reported on the long-term OS of patients in the initiative for molecular profiling and advanced cancer therapy (IMPACT) 1 study.[13] Patients who had tumor molecular profiling received a matched therapy if they had a targetable molecular alteration and if a clinical trial was available. Among 3737 consecutive patients, 1307 (37.5%) patients had ≥1 molecular alteration and received either a matched (711, 54.4%) or a nonmatched (596, 45.6%) therapy. The rates of objective response, progression-free survival (PFS), and OS were higher in patients who received matched therapy (targeting their molecular alterations) compared to patients treated with unmatched therapy.[13] Specifically, the 10-year OS rates were 6% versus 1%, respectively for matched versus unmatched therapy (HR = 0.72; $p < 0.001$). Several other prospective precision medicine clinical trials are evaluating the role of tumor molecular profiling in treatment selection for patients with advanced solid and hematologic malignancies.[14-17] In I-PREDICT (Investigation of Profile-Related Evidence Determining Individualized Cancer Therapy), tumor genomic profiling, PD-L1 expression, tumor mutational burden (TMB), microsatellite instability (MSI) status, and circulating tumor DNA (ctDNA) analysis were used to select treatment. The disease control rate was 30% in 83 evaluable patients with refractory metastatic cancers.[18] The overview of precision oncology is depicted in Figure 1.

On the basis of the success of drug development across tumor types, the tumor agnostic approach has emerged as a new paradigm in the clinical management of patients with cancer. Consequently, clinical trials continue to evolve, shifting from tumor type-centered to gene-directed, histology-agnostic designs. Since May 2017, tumor-agnostic therapies that target molecular abnormalities regardless of primary tumor site have been approved by the US Food and Drug Administration (FDA).[19-22]

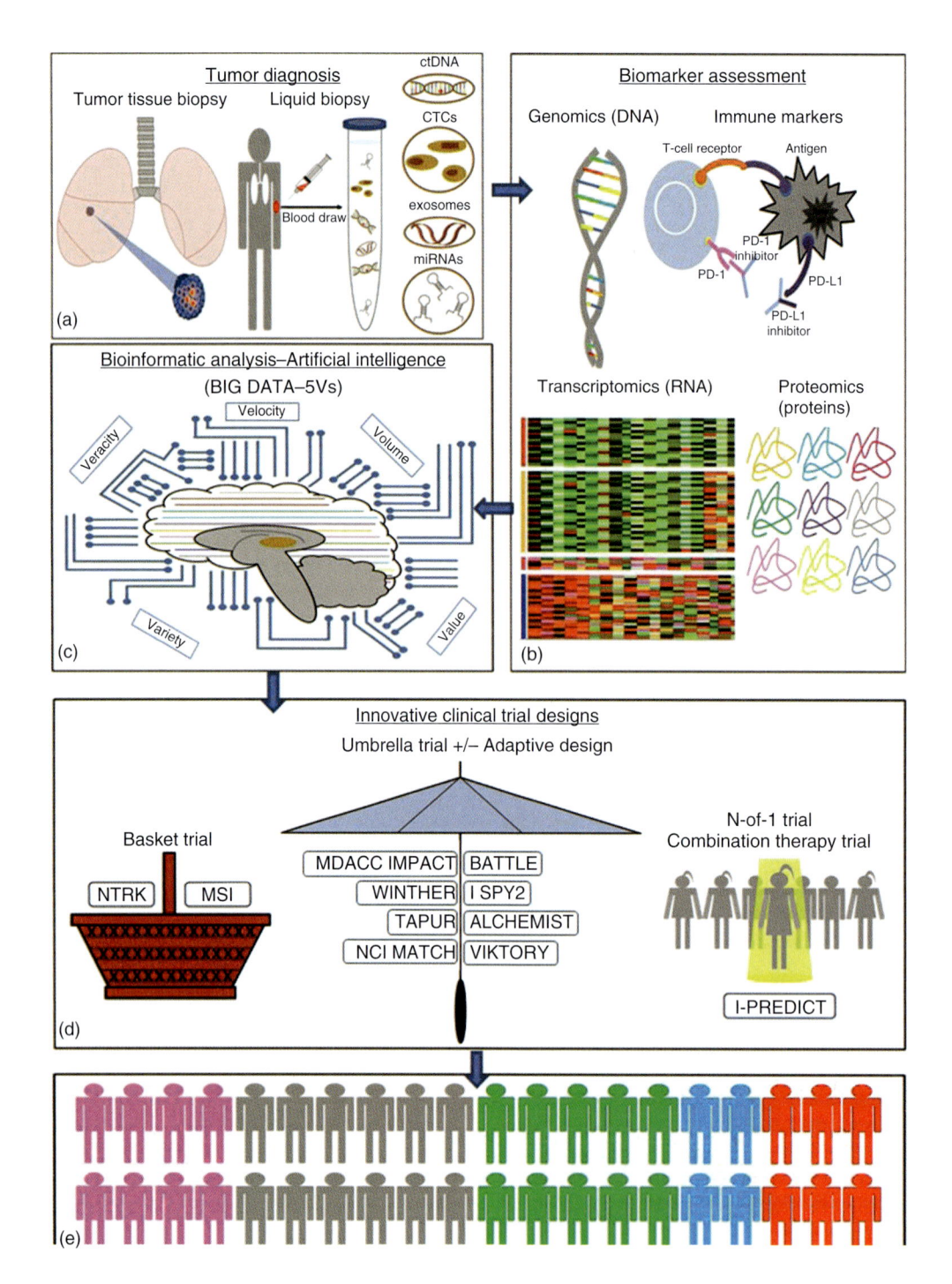

Figure 1 Precision oncology overview. (a) In addition to tumor tissue analysis, liquid biopsy is currently used for the diagnosis and management of patients with cancer. Liquid biopsy, which includes analysis of cell-free DNA, circulating tumor cells, microRNAs, and exosomes, enables noninvasive, longitudinal profiling of molecular alterations, thus overcoming challenges associated with tumor heterogeneity and evolution. (b) Complete tumor and cell-free DNA profiling using next-generation sequencing, RNA analysis, proteomics, and understanding of immune-related mechanisms are used to identify biomarkers predictive of response to innovative treatments. (c) High-throughput profiling generates massive amounts of molecular data ("big data"), characterized by five "Vs": Volume, Variety, Velocity, Value, and Veracity. Conventional methods are not adequate for data processing and, therefore, artificial intelligence and machine-learning algorithms are being incorporated into clinical practice. (d) Innovative trial designs ("N-of-1" approach, adaptive trials) hold the promise for expedited drug approval and individualization of treatment based on each patient's tumor characteristics. (e) Targeted treatments, immunotherapies, and T-cell therapy have altered the therapeutic landscape of cancer. Precision oncology trials have demonstrated that selected alterations can be successfully targeted by novel agents, with improved rates of response and progression-free survival in patients with cancer compared to standard treatments. Examples of precision oncology trials are shown in the figure. As the therapeutic management of patients with cancer shifts from tumor type-centered to a gene-directed, histology-agnostic approach, the future of precision oncology lies in the use of comprehensive tumor molecular/immune profiles to inform treatment decisions that are individualized for each patient. *Abbreviations:* CTC, circulating tumor cells; ctDNA, circulating tumor DNA; miRNA, microRNA; MSI, microsatellite instability; MDACC, MD Anderson Cancer Center; PD-1, programmed death-1; PD-L1, programmed death-ligand 1; Vs, Volume, Variety, Velocity, Value, and Veracity. Source: Based on Sicklick et al.[18]

The use of immunotherapy in the implementation of precision oncology is thought to overcome the complexity of molecular profiling by initiating an immune response against the tumor. The recent FDA approvals of immune checkpoint inhibitors in diverse tumor types highlight the clinical benefit across tumor types and the distinct mechanism of action of these agents. In 2019, more than 5000 clinical trials of immunotherapeutic agents as monotherapy or combined with other drugs were being conducted. These trials aim to enhance the host immune system against tumor cells and to overcome resistance to therapy, inducing durable responses.[23] Cutting-edge immunotherapy approaches, including adoptive cell therapy and vaccines, are being evaluated in several solid tumor types. Several meta-analyses of phase I, II, and III studies have demonstrated the benefit of personalized medicine.[24-26]

In this article, we review the rapid evolution of precision medicine in oncology and the challenges and opportunities met in anticancer drug development in daily clinical practice.

New drug approval

Clinical trials with innovative designs evaluate treatments tailored to biomarker profiling with the goal to improve treatment outcomes. On the basis of the results of these trials, since 2018 several targeted agents have been approved by the FDA for the treatment of solid tumors (Table 1).[52]

The most recent tumor-agnostic FDA approvals involved two NTRK inhibitors, larotrectinib, and entrectinib.[53,54] NTRK fusions occur rarely (0.1–3.3% of lung cancers, 0.6–1.2% of glioblastomas, 0.2–1% of sarcomas, 0.2–2.7% of colon cancers, 0.5% of head and neck cancer squamous cell carcinomas, 2.4% of thyroid cancers, 25.9% of papillary thyroid cancers, 7% of pediatric high-grade gliomas, and 50.0–96.2% of infantile fibrosarcomas).[55]

A basket trial evaluating the NTRK inhibitor larotrectinib included 55 patients with NTRK fusions across 17 different tumors.[19] The use of larotrectinib resulted in an objective response rate (ORR) of 75%, and 71% of patients who responded had sustained response for ≥12 months, leading to the FDA agnostic approval.[53] In a study of entrectinib, another NTRK inhibitor, in 54 patients with 10 tumor types and NTRK fusions the ORR was 57% and the median response duration was 10.4 months, leading to FDA tumor agnostic approval.[20] Entrectinib was also evaluated in patients with central nervous system metastases.[56] Integrating data of patients with advanced NTRK-positive tumors who participated in three-phase I/II clinical trials (ALKA-372-001, STARTRK-1, and STARTRK-2) demonstrated ORR of 57%, while the median duration of response was 10 months.[34] Given the high antitumor activity of NTRK inhibitors, NTRK fusion analysis should be performed in all patients to identify those who might gain significant benefit from the respective treatments.[19,20]

Notably, the first agent that gained tumor-agnostic FDA approval was pembrolizumab, in May 2017.[57] Pembrolizumab was approved for the treatment of adult and pediatric patients with unresectable or metastatic, microsatellite instability-high (MSI-H), or mismatch repair deficient (dMMR) solid tumors that had progressed after prior treatment and for the treatment of unresectable or metastatic MSI-H or dMMR colorectal cancer (CRC) that had progressed after treatment with a fluoropyrimidine, oxaliplatin, and irinotecan.[58] The approval was based on favorable results of five single-arm trials evaluating patients with 15 tumor types with MSI-H or dMMR tumors treated with checkpoint blockade (KEYNOTE-016, $n = 58$; KEYNOTE-164, $n = 61$; KEYNOTE-012, $n = 6$; KEYNOTE-028, $n = 5$; and KEYNOTE-158, $n = 19$). The ORR was 39.6% (complete response [CR], 7%), the response lasted ≥6 months in 78% of responders, and there was no difference in ORRs between CRC and other tumor types.[59] Additionally, a nivolumab and ipilimumab combination therapy was granted accelerated approval for the treatment of patients with MSI-H or dMMR metastatic CRC that has progressed following treatment with a fluoropyrimidine, oxaliplatin, and irinotecan.[60] The approval was based on the results of a nonrandomized, phase 2 trial in patients with advanced MSI-H/dMMR colorectal cancer who had progressed on a prior line of therapy with fluoropyrimidine and oxaliplatin or irinotecan.[61] Patients ($n = 119$) received treatment with nivolumab and ipilimumab for four doses followed by nivolumab until disease progression, serious toxicity, or study end. The rates of objective response and disease control for ≥12 weeks were 55% and 80%, respectively.[61] Nivolumab monotherapy also received accelerated approval on the basis of favorable results of a phase II trial in patients with recurrent/metastatic CRC locally assessed as dMMR/MSI-H and progressing following prior treatment (CHECKMATE 142); the ORR was 32% (24 of 74), while responses lasted ≥6 months in 67% of patients.[62,63]

Currently, there are seven FDA-approved immune checkpoint inhibitors: ipilimumab, pembrolizumab, nivolumab, avelumab, cemiplimab, durvalumab, and atezolizumab (Table 2). Novel immuno-oncology approaches, including oncolytic viruses, cell-based products, modified cytokines, CD3-bispecific antibodies, vaccine platforms, and adoptive cell therapy, are undergoing clinical investigation. The availability of multiple immuno-oncology therapies that are associated with the cure of selected patients with diverse tumor types, but also with severe toxicity, emphasizes the need to develop robust biomarkers to select appropriate patients for immuno-oncology therapy.

Tumor biology and novel biomarkers

The pathophysiology of carcinogenesis is complex. This complexity is attributed to highly variable genetic and epigenetic patterns and clonal evolution that is linked to distinct properties of cancer cells, including spatial expansion, proliferative self-renewal, migration, and invasion, that drive the tumor growth. Tumor evolution is also complicated by the dynamic, Darwinian evolutionary behavior of cancer cells, which develop sequential mechanisms to escape environmental constraints, including immune surveillance, spatial barriers, and hypoxia. This evolutionary process includes the interaction of "driver" with "passenger/hitchhiker" alterations. "Driver" alterations involve genes with known roles in carcinogenesis that provide a fundamental growth advantage to cancer cells. These alterations occur frequently in various tumor types and are associated with clonal expansion. "Passenger/hitchhiker" alterations have a neutral role, or they are not necessarily functionally relevant in driving carcinogenesis. Other factors contributing to tumor evolution include additional molecular alterations in tumor cells that increase the rate of other genomic abnormalities and changes in the microenvironment and immune machinery. The clinical significance and function of these alterations are also associated with anticancer therapy. Certain targeted therapies apply selective pressure to tumor cells leading to selection of the fittest ones for survival and proliferation and/or emergence of new subclones that may drive disease progression later in the course of the disease.

Next-generation sequencing (NGS) of tumor and ctDNA is used for the diagnosis and management of patients with cancer. Comprehensive panels, comprising hundreds of genes, in combination

Table 1 Selected new targeted therapies (with a biomarker) approved by the U.S. Food and Drug Administration for solid tumors (2015–2020), as of 5/2020.[a]

Drug	Target	Clinical outcomes[b]	Most common AEs	Month/year of FDA approval	Indication(s)	Line of therapy
Selpercatinib	RET	NSCLC: ORR: 64% (95% CI: 54%, 73%), ORR ≥ 6 m: 81%[27] Medullary thyroid cancer: ORR: 73% (95% CI: 62, 82), ORR ≥ 6 m: 61%	Dry mouth, diarrhea, hypertension, increased AST, ALP, hyperglycemia, leukopenia, decreased albumin, hypocalcemia, increased creatinine	05/2020	Advanced NSCLC with RET and advanced or radioactive iodine-refractory medullary thyroid cancer with RET mutations (adult and pediatric)	≥1
Capmatinib	MET	ORR: 39.1% (95% CI: 27.6, 51.6) in pretreated pts and 71.4% (95% CI: 51.3, 86.8) in treatment-naïve pts[28]	Peripheral edema, nausea, fatigue, vomiting, dyspnea, and decreased appetite	05/2020	Advanced NSCLC with MET exon 14 skipping	≥1
Pemigatinib	FGFR2	ORR: 36% (95% CI: 27%, 45%) Median DoR: 9.1 m, ORR ≥ 6 m: 63%[29]	Alopecia, diarrhea, nail toxicity, fatigue, dysgeusia, nausea, constipation, stomatitis, dry eye, dry mouth, decreased appetite, vomiting, hyperphosphatemia	04/2020	Advanced cholangiocarcinoma with a FGFR2 fusion or other rearrangements	≥2
Tucatinib	HER2	Median PFS: 7.8 m (95% CI: 7.5, 9.6) in tucatinib versus 5.6 m (95% CI: 4.2, 7.1) in control arm (HR: 0.54; 95% CI: 0.42, 0.71; $p < 0.00001$)[30]	Diarrhea, palmar-plantar erythrodysesthesia, nausea, fatigue, vomiting, stomatitis, hepatotoxicity	04/2020	Advanced HER2-positive breast cancer in combination with trastuzumab and capecitabine	≥3
Encorafenib/ cetuximab	BRAF	Median OS: 8.4 m (95% CI: 7.5, 11.0) in encorafenib/cetuximab versus 5.4 m (95% CI: 4.8, 6.6) in chemotherapy (HR: 0.60; 95% CI: 0.45, 0.79; $p = 0.0003$)[31]	Fatigue, nausea, diarrhea, rash	04/2020	Metastatic colorectal cancer with a BRAF V600E mutation	≥2
Avapritinib	PDGFRA exon 18, including D842V mutations	Pts with PDGFRA exon 18 mutation, ORR: 84% (95% CI: 69%, 93%), (CR: 7% and PR: 77%) ORR ≥ 6 m: 66%[32]	Edema, nausea, fatigue/asthenia, cognitive impairment, vomiting	01/2020	Unresectable/metastatic GIST with PDGFRA exon 18 mutations	≥1
Fam-trastuzumab deruxtecan-nxki	HER2	ORR: 60.3% (95% CI: 52.9%, 67.4%), (CR: 4.3%, PR: 56%). Median DoR: 14.8 m[33]	Nausea, fatigue, vomiting, alopecia, constipation, anemia	12/2019	Unresectable/metastatic HER2-positive breast cancer, after ≥2 prior anti-HER2-based regimens	≥3
Entrectinib	ROS1, NTRK	NTRK: ORR: 57% (95% CI: 43%, 71%), (CR: 7% and PR: 50%). ORR ≥ 6 m: 68%[34]	Fatigue, constipation, dysgeusia, edema, dizziness, diarrhea	8/2019	NTRK-fusion-positive solid tumors, age ≥12 years, metastatic NSCLC, ROS1-positive	≥1
Pexidartinib	CSF1R	ORR: 38% (95% CI: 27%, 50%), (CR: 15% and PR: 23%). ORR ≥ 6 m: 100%[35]	Hair color changes, neutropenia, increased LDH, AST, ALP, cholesterol	8/2019	Symptomatic tenosynovial giant cell tumors	≥1
Alpelisib	PIK3CA	PFS: 11 m (alpelisib plus fulvestrant) versus 5.7 m (placebo plus fulvestrant), HR: 0.65; 95% CI: 0.50, 0.85; $p = 0.001$[36]	Diarrhea, rash, lymphocytopenia, increased glucose, increased creatinine	5/2019	Advanced breast cancer, HR-positive, HER2-negative, PIK3CA-mutated	≥2
Erdafitinib	FGFR	ORR: 32.2% (95% CI: 22.4%, 42.0%), (CR: 2.3% and PR: 29.9%). Median DoR: 5.4 m[37]	Stomatitis, fatigue, diarrhea, increased creatinine, hypophosphatemia	4/2019	Advanced bladder cancer with susceptible FGFR3 or FGFR2 genetic alteration	≥2
Larotrectinib	NTRK	ORR: 75% (95% CI: 61%, 85%), (CR: 22% and PR: 53%). Median DoR: response had not been reached. ORR ≥ 6 m: 73%[19]	Fatigue, nausea, dizziness, vomiting, cough, increased AST and ALT	11/2018	Advanced cancer, across tumor types, NTRK-fusion-positive, any age	≥1
Lorlatinib	ALK	ORR: 48% (95% CI: 42%, 55%), (CR: 4% and PR: 44%). Median DoR: 12.5 m[38]	Edema, peripheral neuropathy, cognitive effects, dyspnea	11/2018	Advanced NSCLC, ALK-positive	≥2
Talazoparib	PARP	PFS: 8.6 m (talazoparib) versus 5.6 m (chemotherapy), HR: 0.54; 95% CI: 0.41, 0.71; $p < 0.0001$[39]	Fatigue, nausea, headache, anemia, neutropenia, thrombocytopenia	10/2018	Locally advanced/metastatic breast cancer, germline BRCA mutation	≥1

Table 1 (Continued)

Drug	Target	Clinical outcomes[b]	Most common AEs	Month/year of FDA approval	Indication(s)	Line of therapy
Dacomitinib	EGFR	PFS: 14.7 m (dacomitinib) versus 9.2 m (gefitinib), HR: 0.59; 95% CI: 0.47, 0.74; $p<0.0001$[40]	Diarrhea, rash, paronychia, stomatitis, decreased appetite, dry skin	9/2018	Metastatic NSCLC with (EGFR) exon 19 deletion or exon 21 L858R substitution mutation	First
Encorafenib/ binimetinib	BRAF/MEK	PFS: 14.9 m (binimetinib/encorafenib) versus 7.3 m (vemurafenib), HR: 0.54, 95% CI: 0.41, 0.71; $p<0.0001$[41]	Fatigue, nausea, diarrhea, vomiting, abdominal pain, arthralgia	6/2018	Unresectable/metastatic melanoma, *BRAF* mutant	≥1
Dabrafenib/ trametinib	BRAF/MEK	ORR: 61% (95% CI: 39%, 80%), (CR: 4% and PR: 57%). ORR ≥ 6 m: 64%[42]	Pyrexia, rash, chills, headache, arthralgia, cough, skin cancer	5/2018	Advanced anaplastic thyroid cancer, *BRAF* mutant, with no satisfactory locoregional treatment options.	≥1
Lutetium Lu 177 dotatate	Somatostatin receptor	Median PFS: NYR (177Lu-Dotatate group) vs 8.4m (control), HR: 0.21; 95% CI: 0.13, 0.33; $p<0.001$[43]	Vomiting, nausea, lymphopenia, hyperglycemia, increased GGT, AST, and ALT	1/2018	GEP-NETs, somatostatin receptor-positive	≥1
Vemurafenib	BRAF	ORR: 54.5% (95% CI: 32.2%, 75.6%), (CR: 4.5% and PR: 50%). Median DoR: 26.6 m[44]	Arthralgia, maculopapular rash, alopecia, fatigue, QT prolongation, skin papilloma, skin cancer	11/2017	Erdheim-Chester disease with *BRAF V600* mutation	≥1
Neratinib maleate	HER2	Median iDFS: 94.2% (neratinib) versus 91.9% (placebo), HR: 0.66; 95% CI: 0.49, 0.90; $p=0.008$[45]	Diarrhea, nausea, abdominal pain, fatigue, vomiting, rash, stomatitis	7/2017	Early-stage breast cancer, HER2-overexpressed/ amplified after adjuvant trastuzumab-based therapy	Adjuvant
Brigatinib	ALK	ORR: 48% (95% CI: 39%, 58%) in 90 mg arm and 53% (95% CI: 43%, 62%) in 180 mg arm[46]	Nausea, diarrhea, fatigue, cough, headache	4/2017	Advanced NSCLC, ALK-positive, patients who progressed/intolerant to crizotinib	≥2
Rucaparib	PARP	ORR: 54% (95% CI: 44%, 64%), Median DoR: 9.2m (95% CI: 6.6, 11.6)[47,48]	Nausea, fatigue, vomiting, abdominal pain, dysgeusia, constipation, anemia	12/2016	Advanced ovarian cancer in patients with deleterious *BRCA* mutation (germline and/or somatic)	≥3
Alectinib	ALK	12-month EFS: 68.4% (alectinib) versus 48.7% (crizotinib), HR: 0.47, 95% CI: 0.34, 0.65; $p<0.001$[49]	Fatigue, constipation, edema, myalgia, anemia	12/2015	Advanced NSCLC, ALK-positive	1
Osimertinib	EGFR	ORR: 59% (combined results from two multicenter, single-arm, open-label clinical trials)	Diarrhea, rash, dry skin, nail toxicity, eye disorders, nausea, decreased appetite, constipation	11/2015	Advanced NSCLC, EGFR-mutated. Specifically targets *EGFR* exon 20 T790M alteration	≥2
Cobimetinib	MEK	Median PFS: 12.3m (cobimetinib and vemurafenib) versus 7.2m (placebo and vemurafenib), HR: 0.58, 95% CI 0.46, 0.72; $p<0.0001$[50]	Pyrexia, dehydration	11/2015	Advanced melanoma (*BRAF* V600E or V600K mutation-positive) in combination with vemurafenib	≥1
Pembrolizumab	MSI-high	ORR: 39.6% (95% CI: 31.7%, 47.9%), ORR ≥ 6 m in 78% of responders[51]	Fatigue, pruritus, diarrhea, decreased appetite, rash, pyrexia	05/2017	Colorectal cancer, MSI-H/dMMR, having failed fluoropyrimidine, oxaliplatin, and irinotecan, and advanced solid tumors (tissue agnostic; adult and pediatric)	≥2

Abbreviations: AE, adverse events; ALP, alanine transaminase; AR, androgen receptor; AST, aspartate transaminase; CI, confidence interval; CR, complete response; DoR, depth of response; EFS, event-free survival rate; FDA, Food and Drug Administration; gBRCA, germline BRCA; GEP-NETs, gastroenteropancreatic neuroendocrine tumors; GIST, gastrointestinal stromal tumor; HER2, human epidermal growth factor receptor 2; HR, hazard ratio; HR, hormone receptor; iDFS, invasive disease-free survival; LDH, lactate dehydrogenase; m, months; MFS, metastasis free survival; MSI, microsatellite instability; NSCLC, non-small cell lung cancer; NYR, not yet reached; ORR, objective response rate; OS, overall survival; PD-1, programmed death 1; PD-L1, programmed death-ligand 1; PFS, progression-free survival; PR, partial response; pts, patients; rPFS, radiographic progression-free survival.
[a]Source: Based on Hematology/Oncology (Cancer) Approvals & Safety Notifications, U.S. Food and Drug Administration, 2021.
[b]Selected trials used for respective FDA drug approval.

Table 2 Selected indications for checkpoint inhibitors of solid tumors approved by the Food and Drug Administration in diverse tumor types, as of April 2020.

Checkpoint inhibitor	Target	Tumor type	Month, year	Indication(s)	Approved line of therapy	Sample references
Pembrolizumab	PD-1	Melanoma	September 2014	Metastatic melanoma	≥1	Ribas et al.[64]
			February 2019	Melanoma, stage III	Adjuvant	Eggermont et al.[65]
		Lung	October 2016	NSCLC, PD-L1 positive (TPS ≥ 50%)	1	Reck et al.[66]
			October 2016	NSCLC, PD-L1 positive (TPS ≥ 1%) after chemotherapy failure	≥2	Herbst et al.[67]
			August 2018	Nonsquamous NSCLC (EGFR and ALK WT), combined with chemotherapy	1	Gandhi et al.[68]
			October 2018	Squamous NSCLC, combined with chemotherapy	1	Paz-Ares et al.[69]
		Head and neck	August 2016	HNSCC, after failure of platinum-containing chemotherapy	≥2	Mehra et al.[70]
			June 2019	HNSCC, PD-L1 positive (CPS ≥ 1%), as monotherapy or in combination with chemotherapy	1	Burtness et al.[71]
		Urothelial	May 2017	Metastatic urothelial carcinoma, PD-L1+ ineligible for cisplatin-containing chemotherapy	1	Balar et al.[72]
			May 2017	Metastatic urothelial carcinoma after failure of platinum regimen	≥2	Bellmunt et al.[73]
			January 2020	Non-muscle-invasive bladder cancer, BCG-unresponsive, high-risk, who are ineligible for or have elected not to undergo cystectomy	Definitive	Balar et al.[74]
		Across tumor types	May 2017	Advanced solid tumors, MSI-H/dMMR (tissue agnostic; adult and pediatric)	≥2	Diaz et al.[51]
		Colorectal	May 2017	Colorectal cancer, MSI-H/dMMR, after failure of fluoropyrimidine, oxaliplatin, and irinotecan	≥3	Diaz et al.[51]
		Gastric	September 2017	Advanced gastric or gastroesophageal junction adenocarcinoma, PD-L1+, after failure of fluoropyrimidine- and platinum-containing chemotherapy and, if appropriate, HER2/neu-targeted therapy	≥3	Fuchs et al.[75]
		Cervical	June 2018	Cervical cancer, PD-L1+, after failure of chemotherapy	≥2	Chung et al.[76]
		HCC	July 2018	HCC after failure of sorafenib	≥2	Zhu et al.[77]
		Merkel cell	December 2018	Advanced Merkel cell carcinoma	≥1	Nghiem et al.[78]
		Renal	April 2019	Advanced renal cancer, combined with axitinib	1	Rini et al.[79]
		Esophagus	July 2019	Advanced squamous esophageal cancer, PD-L1+ (CPS ≥ 10) after failure of systemic therapy	≥2	Shah et al.[80] Kojima et al.[81]
		Endometrial	October 2019	Advanced endometrial carcinoma, combined with lenvatinib after failure of systemic therapy	≥2	Makker et al.[82]
Nivolumab	PD-1	Melanoma	December 2014	Metastatic melanoma	1	Robert et al.[83]
			December 2017	Melanoma with lymph node involvement after complete resection	Definitive	Weber et al.[84]
		Lung	March 2015	Metastatic NSCLC after failure of platinum-based chemotherapy	≥2	Borghaei et al.[85]
			August 2018	Metastatic SCLC after failure of chemotherapy	≥3	Ready et al.[86]
		Renal	November 2015	Advanced renal cell carcinoma after failure of antiangiogenic therapy	≥2	Motzer et al.[87]
		Head and neck	November 2016	Advanced HNSCC after failure of platinum-based therapy	≥2	Ferris et al.[88]
		Urothelial	February 2017	Advanced urothelial carcinoma after failed platinum-containing chemotherapy or progressed within 12 months of neoadjuvant or adjuvant treatment	≥1	Sharma et al.[89]
		Colorectal	August 2017	Colorectal cancer, MSI-H/dMMR, after failure of fluoropyrimidine, oxaliplatin, and irinotecan	≥3	Overman et al.[63]
		HCC	September 2017	HCC after failure of sorafenib	≥2	El-Khoueiry et al.[90]
Nivolumab/ ipilimumab	PD-1/CTLA-4	Melanoma	January 2016	Metastatic melanoma	1	Hodi et al.[91]
		Colorectal	July 2018	Colorectal cancer, MSI-H/dMMR, after failure of fluoropyrimidine, oxaliplatin, and irinotecan	≥3	Overman et al.[61]
		Renal	April 2018	Advanced renal cell carcinoma (intermediate or poor risk)	≥1	Motzer et al.[92]
		HCC	March 2020	HCC after failure of sorafenib	≥2	Kudo et al.[93]

Table 2 (Continued)

Checkpoint inhibitor	Target	Tumor type	Month, year	Indication(s)	Approved line of therapy	Sample references
Ipilimumab	CTLA-4	Melanoma	October 2015	Melanoma, stage III	Adjuvant	Eggermont et al.[94]
Cemiplimab	PD-1	CSCC	September 2018	Advanced CSCC, or ineligible for curative surgery or curative radiation	≥1	Migden et al.[95]
Atezolizumab	PD-L1	Urothelial	May 2016	Advanced urothelial carcinoma after failure of platinum-based therapy or progression within 12 months of neoadjuvant or adjuvant platinum-containing chemotherapy	≥2	Rosenberg et al.[96]
			April 2017	Advanced urothelial carcinoma ineligible for cisplatin chemotherapy	1	Necchi et al.[97]
		Lung	October 2016	Metastatic NSCLC after failure of platinum-based chemotherapy	≥2	Fehrenbacher et al.[98] Rittmeyer et al.[99]
			December 2018	Advanced nonsquamous NSCLC (EGFR or ALK WT), combined with bevacizumab, paclitaxel, and carboplatin	1	Socinski et al.[100]
			March 2019	Extensive-stage SCLC with etoposide and carboplatin	1	Horn et al.[101]
			December 2019	Advanced nonsquamous NSCLC (EGFR or ALK WT), combined with paclitaxel protein-bound and carboplatin	1	West et al.[102]
		Breast	March 2019	Advanced TNBC with paclitaxel protein-bound (PD-L1 +)	≥1	Schmid et al.[103]
Avelumab	PD-L1	Merkel	March 2017	Advanced Merkel cell carcinoma (adult and pediatric)	≥1	D'Angelo et al.[104]
		Urothelial	May 2017	Advanced urothelial carcinoma after failure of platinum-based therapy or progression within 12 months of neoadjuvant or adjuvant platinum-containing chemotherapy	≥2	Patel et al.[105]
Durvalumab	PD-L1	Urothelial	May 2017	Advanced urothelial carcinoma after failure of platinum-based therapy or progression within 12 months of neoadjuvant or adjuvant platinum-containing chemotherapy	≥2	Powles et al.[106]
		Lung	February 2018	NSCLC, unresectable stage III, after concurrent platinum-based chemotherapy and radiation therapy	Definitive	Antonia et al.[107]
			March 2020	Extensive-stage SCLC with etoposide and carboplatin/cisplatin	1	Paz-Ares et al.[108]

Abbreviations: BCG, Bacillus Calmette-Guerin; CSCC, cutaneous squamous cell carcinoma; CPS, combined positive score; CTLA-4, cytotoxic T lymphocyte-associated antigen 4; dMMR, deficient mismatch repair; HCC, hepatocellular cancer; HER2, human epidermal growth factor receptor 2; HNSCC, head and neck squamous cell carcinoma; MSI-H, microsatellite instability-high; NSCLC, nonsmall cell lung cancer; PD-1, programmed death 1; PD-L1, programmed death-ligand 1; SCLC, small cell lung cancer; TNBC, triple-negative breast cancer; TPS, tumor proportion score; WT, wild-type.

with immune markers and RNA profiling, are evaluated in clinical trials. Clinical trials have demonstrated that selected alterations can be successfully targeted by novel agents and improve rates of response and PFS in patients with cancer compared to standard treatments.[19,109–111] Genomic sequencing involves not only tissue, but blood-derived ctDNA, circulating tumor cells, and exosomes are increasingly used in diverse tumor types.

ctDNA analysis from peripheral blood (liquid biopsy) can be a noninvasive, cost-effective alternative to tumor biopsy used when the tumor is inaccessible or insufficient for biopsy, when biopsies are associated with significant risk, or for optimization of treatment via longitudinal profiling of molecular alterations. ctDNA analysis may overcome challenges associated with tumor heterogeneity and evolution.[112] In June 2016, the FDA approved the first "liquid biopsy test" (Cobas EGFR Mutation Test v2) for the detection of EGFR exon 19 deletions or exon 21 (L858R) substitution mutations for patients with advanced non-small cell lung cancer (NSCLC).[113,114] The approval was based on a phase 3 study (ENSURE) in patients with IIIB/IV NSCLC comparing erlotinib (EGFR inhibitor) to cisplatin/gemcitabine combination therapy. Plasma EGFR mutations were identified in 76.7% of patients whose tumor tissues had the respective mutations. This approval included the EGFR T790M mutation for the use of osimertinib (third-generation inhibitor) in NSCLC.[113] In 2020, NGS-based ctDNA testing as a companion diagnostic device was also approved by the FDA for multiple biomarkers, including BRCA1 and BRCA2 mutations in patients with ovarian cancer, EGFR mutations and ALK rearrangements in patients with NSCLC, PIK3CA mutations in patients with breast cancer, and BRCA1, BRCA2, and ATM mutations in patients with prostate cancer.[115] Identification of these alterations is currently associated with the regulatory approval of targeted agents as follows: rucaparib for BRCA1 and BRCA2 alterations in ovarian cancer,[116] erlotinib, gefitinib, and osimertinib for EGFR mutations in NSCLC,[4,117,118] alectinib for ALK rearrangements in NSCLC,[49] rucaparib and olaparib for BRCA1, BRCA2, and ATM mutations in prostate cancer[119,120] and alpelisib for PI3K mutations in breast cancer.[36] ctDNA analysis is also used for KRAS mutations in patients with colorectal cancer.[115] The clinical use of ctDNA analysis must be evaluated in prospective trials with targeted agents.[112] Limitations of this approach include discordance between ctDNA and tumor tissue genomic analysis and identification of false-positive findings.

In addition to genomic alterations, MSI-high, and PDL-1 expression, other exploratory biomarkers have been associated with tumor biology and clinical outcomes. High TMB was associated with response to immune checkpoint inhibitors in melanoma, NSCLC, and other tumor types.[121-126] The cutoff of TMB varies by tumor type and laboratory. In one study in NSCLC, high TMB was defined as >10 mutations/Mb,[122] while other investigators used the cut-off of 178 nonsynonymous mutations.[123] In melanoma, high TMB was defined as >23.1 mutations/Mb, intermediate as 3.3–23.1 mutations/Mb, and low as <3.3 mutations/Mb.[124] In patients with melanoma treated with antibodies against cytotoxic T-lymphocyte antigen 4 (CTLA-4), high TMB was defined as >100 mutations per tumor.[126] In a study of 151 patients with various tumor types treated with immunotherapeutic agents, high TMB (≥20 mutations/Mb), compared to low (1–5 mutations/Mb) or intermediate (6–19 mutations/Mb) TMB, was independently associated with higher rates of response ($p = 0.0001$), PFS ($p < 0.0001$), and OS (0.0036).[125] However, high TMB does not always correlate with response to immunotherapy, possibly owing to the complex dynamics associated with host immune response, tumor microenvironment, and immune modulation by tumor cells. Standardization of methodologies for TMB, optimization of cut-off values, and prospective validation across tumor types will further elucidate the value of TMB as a biomarker.

Other immune-related biomarkers include response markers such as PD-L1 expression, *PD-L1* amplification, and *PBRM1* molecular alterations, as well as resistance markers such as *JAK2* loss, beta-2 microglobulin mutations, *MDM2* amplification, *EGFR* alterations, *PTEN* loss, *STK11* mutations, and β-catenin pathway alterations. However, the predictive value of these biomarkers is limited in selected tumor types.[127] Selected immune-related biomarkers are summarized in Table 3. Additional studies evaluating the clinical relevance of these biomarkers in patients with various tumor types treated with immunotherapy are warranted.

Companion biomarkers provide critical information for the safe and effective use of a corresponding targeted treatment. They may identify whether a patient's tumor harbors specific molecular alterations that can be effectively targeted by drugs,[4,149] molecular alterations that denote resistance to specific treatments,[150,151] or alterations that predict serious toxicity.[152-154] Examples of FDA-approved companion diagnostic tests are gene amplifications (HER2, KIT), mutations (KRAS, EGFR, BRAF), or translocations (ALK, ROS1).[155] Targeted treatments have been approved by the FDA based on companion biomarkers used in clinical trials that have demonstrated higher rates of response, PFS, and/or OS than standard chemotherapy. In addition, the use of negative predictive biomarkers can spare patients from noneffective treatments and excessive toxicity, while saving valuable time, as well as increased costs. For instance, the EGFR inhibitor cetuximab is contraindicated in patients with colorectal cancer whose tumors harbor KRAS mutations.[150,151] MDM2 amplification has been associated with accelerated progression (hyper-progression) after the administration of immune checkpoint inhibitors.[140] Challenges associated with identification and wide implementation of companion biomarkers include tumor heterogeneity, molecular complexity, increased time, and cost. More importantly, the use of NGS testing has been extensively adopted in clinical practice as an efficacious approach requiring decreased time and cost; more importantly, it provides information for hundreds of genes rather than a single gene (as the companion diagnostic tests). Notably, in the United States, Clinical Laboratory Improvement Amendments (CLIA) certification is required to ensure standardization and quality laboratory testing.

Innovative trial designs

Although phase III randomized trials were considered the gold standard for approval of a novel agent, the majority of these trials in oncology are drug-centered, often include a suboptimal comparator arm (even placebo), and, most importantly, do not always enroll patients with characteristics associated with the mechanism of action of the study drug. Furthermore, these trials are cumbersome, expensive, time-consuming, and require a large number of patients. Innovative trial designs that take into consideration the variability in patients' characteristics, tumor molecular alterations, and immune-related markers have been developed. In recent years, clinical trials with adaptive design have been increasingly used. These designs enable the dynamic evolution of the studies, allow the elimination of treatment arms with inferior outcomes and modification of patient randomization, and optimize biomarker selection based on real-time study outcomes. These trials are also more efficient, because they allow more patients to be randomized to the treatment arm(s) that appear to be more effective and ultimately require fewer patients and shorter follow-up to evaluate the endpoints of the study.

Several innovative trial designs have been developed. **Basket trials** are tissue-agnostic trials that evaluate targeted treatments in patients with diverse tumor types who share a specific tumor molecular alteration. **Umbrella studies** enroll patients who share a specific tumor type and assign them to one of multiple study arms on the basis of potential molecular targets. Each arm represents a potentially effective treatment for the molecular marker. This design permits testing of many treatment agents simultaneously. In **"N-of-1" trials**, each patient is the sole unit of observation. Unique patient and tumor characteristics are considered separately to determine the optimal treatment for each patient; these trials can be used in cases of low-prevalence molecular aberrations, where the performance of randomized studies is challenging. **Octopus studies** have multiple arms that test different drugs or drug combinations in a single trial. **Platform studies** are based on a single analytic technique (e.g., NGS) for interrogating the presence of biomarkers across tumor types (Figure 2). These trials include multiple treatment arms and a control arm; patients are randomized, and each treatment arm is compared to the control arm. This design can be modified to be adaptive, leading to an open platform design. Following this design, treatments can be dropped or replaced by new ones with the goal of identifying effective treatments faster than with the traditional approach and of accelerating the regulatory drug approval process and improving efficiency.

Real-world data

Real-world evidence is often used to evaluate the efficacy, toxicity, and cost of a certain treatment. Since only a small fraction of patients participate in randomized clinical trials, it is critical to assess the reproducibility of toxicity and outcome data in clinical practice. Importantly, real-world efficacy and toxicity data can be valuable for certain patient populations that are often underrepresented in clinical trials, including older patients, patients with poor performance status, and patients with comorbidities. Recently, regulatory agencies have begun encouraging sponsors to provide real-world evidence to support their submissions and to use such evidence to modify indications and schedules of dose and administration. For instance, palbociclib, a cyclin-dependent kinase inhibitor, was approved by the FDA for the treatment of male breast cancer based, at least in part, on such data.[156]

Table 3 Immune-related biomarkers for checkpoint blockade agents.[a]

Biomarker	Tumor type	Role	Sample references investigator, year	Predictive value and comments
FDA approved				
PD-L1 IHC positive (≥1)	NSCLC, TNBC, bladder, gastric	PD-1/PD-L1 interaction inhibits T-lymphocyte proliferation, survival, and function	Hellmann et al. (2019)[128] Schmid et al. (2019)[103]	Predicts response However, multiple technical nuances
MSI-high (mismatch repair gene deficient)	Across tumor types	Increased mutations/neoantigens	Le et al. (2015)[21] Overman et al. (2018)[61] Marabelle et al. (2019)[129]	Predicts response FDA approved for pembrolizumab
Reported/investigational				
TMB regardless of microsatellite status	Across tumor types	Increased mutations/neoantigens	Goodman et al. (2017)[125] Hellman et al. (2018)[130] Goodman et al. (2019)[131]	Predicts response FDA priority review for pembrolizumab and high TMB
ARID1A alterations	Across tumor types	ARID1A deficiency compromises MMR proteins	Okamura et al. (2020)[132]	Predicts response Requires validation
PBRM1 molecular alterations	Renal cancer	SWI/SNF chromatin remodeling	Braun et al. (2019)[133]	Predicts response Requires validation
SMARCA4	Small cell ovarian cancer	Chromatin remodeling SWI/SNF complex	Jelinic et al. (2018)[134]	May predict response Requires validation
PDL1 amplification	Hodgkin Across solid tumors	PDL1 ligand is important in the immune checkpoint machinery	Ansell et al. (2015)[135] Goodman et al. (2018)[136]	Predicts response Requires validation in solid tumors
JAK2 loss	Melanoma, colorectal	Defects in interferon-receptor signaling pathways	Zaretsky et al. (2016)[137] Shin et al. (2017)[138]	Predicts resistance Requires validation
Beta-2 microglobulin mutations	Melanoma	Defects in antigen presentation	Zaretsky et al. (2016)[137] Sade-Feldman et al. (2017)[139]	Predicts resistance Requires validation
MDM2 amplification	Across tumor types	Unclear	Kato et al. (2017)[140] Kato et al. (2018)[141]	Predicts hyperprogression Requires validation
EGFR alterations	Across tumor types	Unclear, upregulation of PD-1 and PD-L1	Kato et al. (2017)[140]	Predicts resistance and hyperprogression Requires validation
PTEN loss	Melanoma	Upregulation of immunosuppressive cytokines, may decrease CD8+ T cell infiltration	Peng et al. (2016)[142] Trujillo et al. (2019)[143]	Predicts resistance Requires validation
STK11 mutation with *KRAS* alterations	Lung	Altered cytokines/chemokines, metabolic restriction of T cells, impaired antigenicity	Skoulidis et al. (2018)[144]	Predicts resistance Requires validation
β-catenin pathway alterations	Melanoma, Colon	Decreases T-cell infiltration	Spranger et al. (2015)[145] Abril-Rodriguez et al. (2020)[146] Grasso et al. (2018)[147]	Predicts resistance Requires validation
BAP1 alterations	Mesothelioma	Promotes immune-inflammatory environment in mesothelioma	Shrestha et al. (2019)[148]	Predicts response Requires validation

Abbreviations: FDA, Food and Drug Administration; IHC, immunohistochemistry; MMR, mismatch repair; MSI, microsatellite instability; NSCLC, nonsmall cell lung cancer; PD-1, programmed death 1; PD-L1, programmed death-ligand 1; TMB, tumor mutational burden; TNBC, triple-negative breast cancer.
[a]Source: Based on Davis and Patel.[127]

Therefore, real-world data are being collected by investigators and sponsors to accelerate the drug approval process and to increase information about already approved treatments.

Selected precision oncology trials of targeted therapy

Completed clinical trials

Historically, the vast majority of precision oncology trials used genomic biomarkers to select targeted therapy. In recent years, immune markers and transcriptomic and proteomic data have been added to the list of biomarkers that can guide therapeutic decisions. Many trials have demonstrated that therapies matched with biomarkers are associated with improved clinical outcomes compared to nonmatched therapies in diverse tumor types (Table 4).[7,11,18,159] Below, several selected precision medicine trials are detailed.

MD Anderson Cancer Center IMPACT study

The first IMPACT study was initiated in 2007.[7-9,13] This was a nonrandomized study of prospectively evaluated patients with advanced cancer who were treated in early-phase clinical trials. Of 3487 consecutive patients who had tumor molecular profiling, 1307 (37.5%) patients had ≥1 molecular alteration. Patients who received matched therapies had a higher ORR (16.4% vs 5.4%, $p < 0.0001$) and longer time-to-treatment failure (TTF) (4.0 vs 2.8 months, $p < 0.0001$) compared to patients who did not receive matched targeted therapy.[13] The median OS was 9.3 months in the matched therapy group compared to 7.3 months in the nonmatched therapy group; and the 10-year OS rates were 6% versus 1%, respectively ($p < 0.001$). Five factors, independently associated with OS (performance status >1, liver metastases, increased lactate dehydrogenase levels [>upper limit of normal], PI3K/AKT/mTOR pathway molecular alterations, and nonmatched therapy), were used to develop a prognostic score. A score was assigned to each

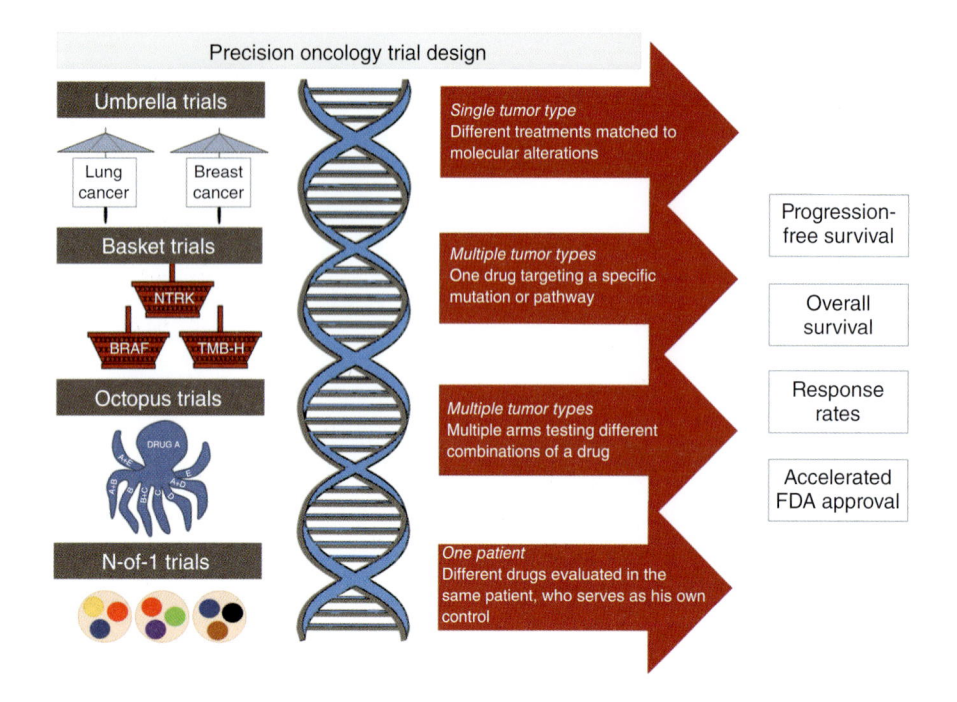

Figure 2 **Innovative trial designs.** Innovative trial designs take into consideration the variability in patients' characteristics, tumor molecular alterations, and immune-related markers. These designs include (i) umbrella studies that enroll patients with a specific tumor type who receive treatments matched to potential molecular targets in different arms, (ii) basket trials that evaluate targeted treatments in patients with diverse tumor types who share a specific tumor molecular alteration (tissue-agnostic), (iii) octopus studies with multiple arms testing different drugs or drug combinations and (iv) "N-of-1" clinical trials where unique patient and tumor characteristics are considered separately to determine the optimal treatment (optimally with customized combination of drugs) for each patient, who is the sole unit of observation.

of these factors based on its hazard ratio. The median OS differed according to the number of risk factors (0 risk factors, 18.2 months; 1 risk factor, 9.3 months; 2 risk factors, 7.3 months; 3 risk factors, 4.7 months, and 4–6 risk factors, 3.7 months).[13]

PREDICT family trials

The PREDICT trial evaluated the outcomes of 347 patients with advanced solid tumors who received "matched" versus "unmatched" therapy based on tumor molecular profiling.[159] "Matched" patients had longer PFS (4.0 vs 3.0 months, $p = 0.039$) and higher disease control rates (partial response [PR] or CR and stable disease [SD] ≥ 6 months: 34.5% vs 16.1%, $p ≤ 0.02$) compared to "unmatched" patients. Patients with a "matching core" (total number of molecular alterations matched to the drugs administered divided by the total number of identified genomic alterations) >0.2 had longer median OS (15.7 months compared with 10.6 months, $p = 0.040$).[159] Subsequently, a prospective navigation trial (I-PREDICT) included, in addition to tumor genomic profiling, other biomarkers such as PD-L1 expression, TMB, and MSI to select treatment.[18] Patients with high matching scores had increased median PFS (6.5 vs 3.1 months, $p = 0.001$) and OS (not reached vs 10.2 months, $p = 0.046$) compared to patients with low matching scores.[18]

SHIVA randomized trial

The first randomized precision oncology study was the SHIVA trial, a multicenter French trial that evaluated the use of molecular markers to select matched treatments compared to standard therapy.[158] Of 741 screened patients with advanced refractory cancer, 293 (40%) patients had ≥1 molecular alteration that was matched to 1 of 10 regimens (abiraterone, dasatinib, erlotinib, everolimus, imatinib, lapatinib plus trastuzumab, letrozole, sorafenib, tamoxifen, vemurafenib). However, the reality was that 80% of patients received monotherapy with everolimus or a hormone blocker. There was no difference in PFS between patients who received matched therapies and those who did not (HR: 0.88, 95% CI .65–1.19, $p = 0.41$).[158] The limitations of SHIVA include that patients with cancer often have multiple molecular alterations and are unlikely to respond to monotherapy; indeed, everolimus is a weak PI3K/Akt/mTOR pathway inhibitor and has been demonstrated to be ineffective as a single agent if multiple genomic alterations are present, even in the presence of a match reference.[9] Furthermore, response to hormonal monotherapy in pretreated patients with hormone receptor abnormalities is unlikely. Other issues include the fact that imatinib, an ineffective RET inhibitor, was matched to RET alterations, and patients randomly assigned to targeted therapy were treated using a predefined algorithm, in contrast with the control group, who were assigned therapy by a physician. Precision medicine is defined by the presence of biological data showing that a drug affects a targeted molecular alteration and needs to be used in the context of clinical experience—an unmet criterion for many matches in SHIVA.

These limitations highlight the importance of selecting matched therapies that effectively and consistently inhibit the function of a "driver" molecular alteration, of using drug combinations to target multiple molecular alterations when needed, and of implementing well-designed protocols that combine clinical experience with genomic data.[167]

WINTHER genomic/transcriptomic trial

The WINTHER trial was an international prospective clinical trial performed in five countries and organized by the Worldwide Innovative Network for Personalized Cancer Medicine (WIN Consortium).[11] In order to increase the number of predictive biomarkers, investigators used transcriptomic analysis in addition to genomics to match patients with advanced cancer to targeted

Table 4 Examples of key precision oncology trials across tumor types and biomarkers used.[a]

Year First/Last author	Trial name	Trial type	Biomarker used
2010[157] Von Hoff D Penny R	Bisgrove	Prospective, navigational	Protein based
2012[7] Tsimberidou A Kurzrock R	IMPACT, first cohort	Registry type, navigational	Genomic hot spot mutations
2014[8] Tsimberidou A Berry D	IMPACT, second cohort	Registry (real-world) type, navigational	PCR-based genomic analysis
2015[158] Le Tourneau Paoletti X	SHIVA	Prospective, randomized	Tissue NGS
2016[159] Schwaederle M Kurzrock R	PREDICT	Registry (real-world) type	Tissue NGS
2016[12] Wheler JJ Kurzrock R	MD Anderson Personalized Cancer Therapy Initiative	Prospective, navigational	Tissue NGS
2016[160] Park J Berry D 2020[161] Nanda R Esserman L	I-SPY 2	Prospective randomized, adaptive	IHC, Mammaprint
2017[9] Tsimberidou AM Kurzrock R	IMPACT, third cohort	Registry (real-world) type, navigational	PCR-based genomics and NGS
2018[162] Hainsworth JD Kurzrock R	MyPathway	Prospective, phase 2 multiple baskets	Tissue NGS or hot spot genomics
2019[18] Sicklick J Kurzrock R	I-PREDICT	Prospective, navigational, N-of-1 combination therapy	NGS including liquid and tissue
2019[163] Trédan O Blay JY	PROFILER	Prospective	Tissue NGS
2019[11] Rodon J Kurzrock R	WINTHER	Prospective, navigational	Tissue NGS and transcriptomics (tumor versus normal)
2019[13] Tsimberidou AM Kurzrock R	IMPACT1	Registry (real-world) type, navigational	Tissue NGS
		Ongoing or planned trials	
2014 Tsimberidou (NCT02152254)	IMPACT2	Prospective, randomized	Genomic analysis
2015[164] Flaherty KT Conley B	NCI-MATCH	Prospective, nonrandomized	Genomic analysis
2016[165] Mangat P Schilsky R	TAPUR	Prospective, nonrandomized	Genomic analysis or IHC
2020[166] Dickson D Kurzrock R	ROOT	Master observational protocol	NGS

Abbreviations: IHC, immunohistochemistry; NGS, next-generation sequencing; PCR, polymerase chain reaction.
[a]Source: Based on Tsimberidou et al.[7]; Rodon et al.[11]; Sicklick et al.[18]; Schwaederle et al.[159]

treatments. NGS of 236 genes and gene expression analysis of paired tumor and normal tissue were used for treatment selection. Of 303 patients who were enrolled on the trial, 107 (35%) were treated and evaluable for analysis, and their disease control rate was 26%.[11] The median PFS and OS were 2.01 months and 5.9 months, respectively. Other clinical trials in patients with solid and hematologic malignancies have also shown that transcriptomic analysis can increase the number of matched therapies in patients with advanced cancer and can be used successfully in guiding therapeutic decisions in selected patients.[168,169]

Collectively, these trials demonstrated that tumor molecular profiling and selection of matched targeted therapy is associated with higher rates of response, PFS and OS compared to patients not treated with matched targeted therapy. However, treatments need to be carefully selected to inhibit the function of a "driver" molecular alteration effectively and consistently. Clinical trials using novel targeted agents with preclinical antitumor activity are essential to determine whether these drugs are efficacious and well-tolerated "targeted" therapies in patients with tumors harboring specific tumor alterations. Additionally, tumor boards and clinical experience are important to optimize selection of the appropriate therapy or combinations to target molecular alterations.

Ongoing clinical trials

There are multiple ongoing precision medicine trials, many with unique designs.

MD Anderson IMPACT2 randomized trial

Following the promising results of the MD Anderson IMPACT 1 study, IMPACT 2 was initiated in 2014, providing a prospective randomized clinical trial that assessed the use of molecular profiling and matched therapy in advanced cancer (NCT02152254).[170] Patients with advanced solid malignancies who have received standard-of-care treatment and have no other efficacious treatment options or have declined standard-of-care treatment are eligible for the study. Tumor molecular profiling of fresh tissue samples is performed before study enrollment. The study's tumor board reviews molecular data, including genomic alterations, gene expression data, immune markers, TMB, and/or MSI status. Based on their suggestions, and taking into consideration the eligibility criteria of the clinical trials, patients are offered treatment with investigational drugs or with off-label FDA-approved drugs. Recently, the protocol was revised so that patients can opt to be randomized to matched therapy versus nonmatched treatment (not based on tumor profiling data). The primary endpoint of the study is PFS. The trial is still recruiting patients.

NCI-MATCH

In August 2015, the Eastern Cooperative Oncology Group–American College of Radiology Imaging Network (ECOG-ACRIN) Cancer Research Group, in collaboration with the US National Cancer Institute (NCI), launched the NCI-MATCH trial (NCT02465060). It is a phase II nonrandomized trial, which aims to evaluate the clinical benefit of targeted treatments, alone or in combination, matched to patient tumor molecular alterations, regardless of the tumor type in patients with refractory malignancies. The NCI-MATCH trial involves nearly 1100 cancer centers in the United States.[17] Targeted agents in the various arms are available through the study and are provided at no cost to patients. An interim analysis demonstrated the safety of tumor biopsies (<1% severe adverse events), time to profiling results (median, 14 days), tumor profiling success rates (87.3%), and rate of participant enrollment.[171,172] However, very few of the enrolled patients were treated (16 of 645) in this initial analysis.[171]

Results from NCI-MATCH trial subprotocols have also been reported. Of 42 evaluable patients with dMMR and advanced noncolorectal tumors (including endometrioid endometrial adenocarcinoma, prostate adenocarcinoma, and uterine carcinosarcoma) who received treatment with nivolumab, the ORR was 36% (all PRs) and the median OS was 17.3 months.[173] Of 35 patients whose tumors harbored the *AKT1* E17K mutation and who were treated with capivasertib, a pan-AKT inhibitor, the ORR was 23% (all PRs) and the PFS rate at 6 months was 52%.[174] Among 36 evaluable patients with HER2-amplified refractory tumors (excluding breast and gastric/gastroesophageal junction adenocarcinomas) who were treated with ado-trastuzumab emtansine (T-DM1), PR was observed in 2 (5.6%); the 6-month PFS rate was 23.6%.[175] Of 65 patients with activating mutations in PIK3CA (excluding patients with breast or squamous lung cancer with KRAS mutations or PTEN mutations or loss) treated with taselisib, a PI3-kinase inhibitor, no responses were noted and the PFS rate at 6 months was 27%.[176] In 31 evaluable patients with pathogenic mutations in *BRCA1/2* genes treated with a Wee1 kinase inhibitor (AZD1775), one patient had a PR and four had SD >6 months (clinical benefit rate, 3.2%); the 6-month PFS rate was 19%.[177] Finally, of 41 evaluable patients with FGFR aberrations (amplification, mutation, and fusion) who received treatment with AZD4547, a selective inhibitor of FGFR 1-3 kinases, the rate of OR was 5% (all PRs); PFS at 6 months was 17%.[178]

TAPUR

The Targeted Agent and Profiling Utilization Registry (TAPUR) study is a nonrandomized clinical trial initiated by the American Society of Clinical Oncology (ASCO) to evaluate the safety and efficacy of FDA-approved treatments in patients with advanced cancer and potentially actionable molecular alterations, collect real-world data on prescribing practices, and educate oncologists on the implementation of precision medicine.[179] Nine pharmaceutical companies provide 13 targeted agents at no cost for patients with refractory cancers based on CLIA-certified available tumor genomic profiling data. The primary end point of the study is OR at ≥8 weeks or SD documented at ≥16 weeks.[15] In the first stage, 10 participants are entered; if ≥2 patients experience OR or SD of ≥16 weeks duration, 18 more patients are enrolled in that treatment arm; otherwise, the cohort is permanently closed. After 28 patients have been evaluated for the primary outcome and ≥7 patients achieve OR or SD ≥16 weeks, the null hypothesis will be rejected, and the drug considered active in the specific cohort. Currently, seven arms have been closed, while nine have been expanded.

Results of selected TAPUR arms for specific tumor types have been published. Of 28 evaluable patients with advanced CRC whose tumors harbored BRAF V600E/D/K/R mutation and no mutation in MAP2K1/2, MEK1/2, or NRAS and who received treatment with cobimetinib and vemurafenib, the ORR was 29% (all PRs).[180] Of 28 patients with CRC with ERBB2-overexpressing/amplified tumors treated with pertuzumab and trastuzumab, the ORR was 14% (all PRs) and the median PFS was 17.2 weeks.[181] In 27 evaluable patients with advanced CRC with high TMB, defined as ≥9 mutations/Mb, after excluding patients with MSI-H tumors, the ORR was 4% (all PRs); the estimated 1-year OS rate was 45.6%.[182] In patients with refractory CRC and FLT-3 amplification treated with sunitinib, no objective response was noted among 10 enrolled patients and two patients with SD at week 16 had disease progression shortly after and, therefore, the arm was closed.[183] Of 28 evaluable women with refractory breast cancer and high TMB who received pembrolizumab, the ORR was 21% and the median PFS was 10.6 weeks.[184] In patients with breast cancer and NSCLC whose tumors did not harbor mutations in *KRAS, NRAS,* or *BRAF* treated with cetuximab, no response or disease stabilization was noted and this arm was closed.[185] Finally, PR was achieved in one of 28 patients with NSCLC with CDKN2A alterations with the use of palbociclib.[186]

NCI-MPACT

The NCI-MPACT (Molecular Profiling-Based Assignment of Cancer Therapy) is an NCI-sponsored phase II trial for patients with advanced refractory cancers.[187] Patients with tumor molecular alterations are randomized (ratio of 2:1) to receive matched treatment in one of the four predefined treatment arms targeting three molecular pathways (DNA repair, PI3K, and RAS/RAF/MEK) vs nonmatched treatment.[187] Three of the treatment arms were closed because of low enrollment rates, while an amendment employing a nonrandomized design was used to increase enrollment in the DNA repair arm.

I-SPY2

The Investigation of Serial Studies to Predict Your Therapeutic Response With Imaging And moLecular Analysis 2 (I-SPY2) is an adaptive phase II clinical trial evaluating multiple investigational arms in parallel in patients with high-risk breast cancer. Following a master protocol, the efficacy of neoadjuvant treatment with innovative drugs in combination with standard chemotherapy is evaluated in comparison to standard therapy alone. Treatments are selected based on tumor molecular characteristics. Results from selected arms have been published. In patients with HER2-positive, hormone-receptor-negative cancer, the addition of neratinib to standard treatment was associated with increased pathological complete response (pCR) rates compared to standard chemotherapy with trastuzumab (56% vs 33%).[160] In another arm, the addition of pembrolizumab to standard chemotherapy was evaluated; the combination with pembrolizumab was associated with increased pCR rates compared to standard chemotherapy in patients with hormone receptor-positive/HER2-negative and triple-negative breast cancer.[161] Patients are still being recruited in multiple experimental arms. The innovative design of the I-SPY 2 trial enables the addition of new experimental agents or combinations to its ongoing trial, by using a single control arm for all the experimental arms. The Bayesian algorithm incorporates constantly updated patient data into probability predictions about efficacy, leading to faster decisions regarding drug performance. If the efficacy of an investigational agent is greater than 85% in a molecular subtype of breast cancer, the drug graduates and phase 3 studies can be initiated. The aim of this design is seamless transition to phase 3 studies in an efficient and expedited manner, resulting in regulatory drug approval. Notably, the phase 2 part of a drug in the I-SPY 2 study can be completed as early as in 1 year.

ROOT

Recently, the Master Registry of Oncology Outcomes Associated with Testing and Treatment (ROOT) study was initiated.[166,188] It is a prospective trial that broadly accepts patients with diverse tumor types, irrespective of biomarkers, and collects comprehensive data on their demographics, tumor biomarkers, treatments, and clinical outcomes. The ROOT trial is one of the first examples of a national Master Observational Trial (MOT). It mimics on a national scale in the US trials such as PREDICT (NCT02478931) and IMPACT (NCT00851032) implemented at the University of California San Diego and at MD Anderson Cancer Center, respectively. MOTs are observational trials that prospectively combine data on real-world evidence and targeted interventions.[166] They aim to longitudinally collect data on patient clinical characteristics, tumor molecular biomarkers, and treatments (regimens, combinations of treatments, or sequenced therapies) and to use artificial intelligence and machine learning tools to associate these parameters with clinical outcomes. Interventional trials, either single-arm or randomized, can be attached to the MOT or performed externally.

Precision immunotherapy trials

Adoptive cell therapy (see Chapter 61 in addition)

Adoptive cell therapy (ACT) refers to enhancement of a patient's immune system to specifically kill tumor cells. This personalized therapeutic approach harvests a patient's blood or tissue-derived immune cells, reprograms them to recognize tumor-specific antigens, expands them *in vitro*, and then reinfuses them into the patient.[189,190] ACT includes tumor-infiltrating lymphocyte (TIL) therapy, chimeric antigen receptor (CAR) T-cell therapy, engineered T-cell receptor (TCR) therapy, and natural killer (NK) cell therapy. ACT therapy and clinical trials are more advanced in hematologic malignancies than in solid tumors.

CAR T-cells are autologous T-lymphocytes that are genetically engineered to recognize specific antigens expressed on tumor cells.[191] Adoptive CAR T-cell therapy has resulted in remarkably high rates of durable CR in patients with hematologic malignancies, even in patients with refractory disease.[192–194] In a phase 2, single-cohort, multicenter study of 75 children and young adults with relapsed or refractory CD19+ B-cell acute lymphoblastic leukemia who received tisagenlecleucel, an anti-CD19 CAR T-cell therapy, the overall remission rate was 81%, while the 12-month event-free survival and OS rates were 50% and 76%, respectively.[192] In a multicenter phase 2 trial, 101 patients with refractory large B-cell lymphoma were treated with axicabtagene ciloleucel, an autologous anti-CD19 CAR T-cell therapy; the ORR was 82% (CR, 54%) and the 18-month OS rate was 52%.[193] Patients with relapsed or refractory mantle-cell lymphoma who received prior treatment with a BTK inhibitor were treated with KTE-X19, an anti-CD19 CAR T-cell therapy; in 74 patients the ORR was 85% (59%, CR) and 12-month PFS and OS rates were 61% and 83%, respectively.[194] As a result of these studies, the FDA has approved CAR T-cell therapy for the treatment of adult patients with relapsed/refractory diffuse large B-cell lymphoma[195] and pediatric patients and young adults with relapsed/refractory B-cell precursor acute lymphoblastic leukemia.[196] Currently, CAR T-cells are being evaluated in solid tumors.[197,198] Multiple intracranial infusions of CAR T-cells targeting IL13Rα2 in a patient with recurrent multifocal glioblastoma resulted in regression of all intracranial and spinal tumors for 7.5 months.[198]

ACT of TILs is based on the expansion and activation of autologous T-cells that have infiltrated a patient's tumor. Specifically, TILS isolated from resected tumor lesions are grown *in vitro* and expanded using high-dose interleukin-2-containing culture media. Purified TILs are then harvested and administered intravenously to the patient following the administration of a lymphodepleting regimen. Promising results have been reported in metastatic melanoma,[199–202] nasopharyngeal carcinoma,[203] and cervical carcinoma.[204] One of the major advantages of TIL therapy is the long duration of response in selected patients. For instance, 19 of 20 patients with refractory melanoma who received treatment with autologous TILs and experienced a CR had ongoing complete regressions beyond 3 years.[199]

Other ACT approaches involve the use of NK cytotoxic lymphocytes that play a critical role in innate immunity and TCR engineered T-cells, where retroviruses enable integration into the genome of T-cells of new TCR transgenes targeting antigens, which are expressed at high levels on different cancers.[205] For instance, CG antigen NY-ESO-1 is expressed in several tumors, including melanomas, synovial sarcomas, and lung, breast, ovarian, and prostate cancers. Treatment of patients with NY-ESO-1+ synovial cell sarcoma and melanoma with autologous NY-ESO-1-reactive T cells resulted in ORRs of 61% and 55%, respectively.[206] The estimated 5-year survival rates were 14% for patients with synovial cell sarcoma and 33% for patients with melanoma. In another study, the administration of autologous highly reactive TCRs against MART-1 and gp100 in 36 patients with refractory melanoma resulted in an ORR of 25%.[207] Finally, in another study patients with advanced solid malignancies were treated with T cells that were retrovirally transduced with melanoma-associated antigen-A3 (MAGE-A3) TCR.[208] Of nine patients who were treated at the highest dose level, three patients had an objective response (1 patient with esophageal cancer, 1 with urothelial cancer, and 1 with osteosarcoma).

As ACT becomes more widely used, distinct adverse events, including cytokine release syndrome and a CAR T-cell-related encephalopathy syndrome, are being reported. These toxicities can result in serious complications and can be fatal, thus requiring intensive monitoring and management by specialists. Ongoing clinical trials evaluate the role and safety of TIL, CAR T-cell, TCR, and NK-cell therapies in hematologic malignancies and/or solid tumors.

Personalized vaccines (vaccinomics) (see Chapter 61 in addition)

The accumulation of somatic mutations in cancer can generate cancer-specific neo-epitopes. Autologous T-cells often identify these neo-epitopes as foreign bodies, which makes them ideal cancer vaccine targets. Every cancer has its own unique mutations, but a small number of neo-antigens are shared between cancers. Several personalized vaccines are currently being evaluated in clinical trials.[51,209]

Challenges

Biomarkers

The complex interaction between tumors, immune cells, and the tumor microenvironment complicates the identification of robust biomarkers. Therefore, complete and deep understanding of tumor biology is critical for treatment selection in individual patients. Optimization of NGS, whole-exome sequencing, immune markers, RNA profiling, proteomic analysis, and bioinformatic analysis is needed.

Drug availability and access

Despite significant progress, not every driver of carcinogenesis and tumor histology can be matched with an effective anticancer therapy (e.g., many *KRAS* alterations, *TP53*). This is particularly the case for cancers with molecular alterations in different genes. Off-label use of targeted agents is common in the United States, and collection of this real-world data is important. The efficacy and toxicities might differ in various ethnic groups, due to differences in molecular alterations and common polymorphisms associated with drug metabolism.

Due to the deregulation of multiple downstream pathways, genomic co-aberrations should be targeted simultaneously. Contrary to most precision oncology trials, which target a single gene/pathway, carefully designed clinical trials with drug combinations matched to >1 alteration are warranted. The I-PREDICT trial[18] shows that this approach can be done safely and efficaciously.

Regulatory, financial, and other challenges

Although the timeline for FDA drug approval has improved, the regulatory burden associated with the activation, implementation, and completion of clinical trials causes considerable delays and complexity, slowing drug development. Excessive eligibility criteria, complex and costly requirements, including the performance of additional biopsies, tumor molecular profiling, and frequent tests, and limited access to clinical trials rule out large numbers of patients with real-world co-morbidities. Nonstrategic initiation of multiple trials with similar agents in parallel, such as immuno-oncology trials, should be evaluated to optimize efficient drug development. However, the excessive cost of precision oncology clinical trials (molecular profiling, drugs, procedures), off-label drugs, and other logistical issues limit patient access to this approach. In many countries, precision medicine is not an option. For drugs that are effective against cancers with rare genomic defects, widespread use of comprehensive next-generation sequencing as part of the standard of care should overcome the need to screen a large number of patients to identify patients who will benefit from these drugs.

Conclusions and future perspectives

The number of patients with cancer who undergo tumor or peripheral blood DNA analysis and other biomarker assessment for the selection of therapy is continually increasing.

Improved technologies at a lower cost are needed to identify the roles of molecular, immune-related, and other biological biomarkers. In order to incorporate genomics, transcriptomics, proteomics, and epigenomics into clinical practice, profiling results should be comprehensive and available to all patients with cancer for treatment planning. Advanced bioinformatics infrastructure and artificial intelligence should be incorporated to analyze massive amounts of molecular data ("big data") efficiently.

Innovative treatments continue to evolve and are being evaluated as monotherapies or in combination with chemotherapy or other targeted treatments. New drugs demonstrate high antitumor activity and favorable toxicity profiles. Immunotherapy, in combination with cytotoxic or other effective therapeutic strategies, has changed the therapeutic landscape of cancer, improving significantly the clinical outcomes of selected patients. ACTs will continue to evolve and be assessed in patients with diverse tumor types. The FDA approval process has improved in recent years, but the process for trial activation and the restrictive eligibility criteria for clinical trials still require an overhaul. Insurance coverage remains an issue for some patients with cancer, affecting their access to cancer treatment.

Clinical trials with laboratory correlates will define the clinical relevance of specific biomarkers with antitumor activity for novel therapeutic approaches. Innovative trial design, including those that evaluate real-world data,[166] will continue to evolve to accelerate drug development and approval. The ultimate goal is to generate high-quality data and provide the resources to understand the biology of cancer in individual patients and offer them effective targeted anticancer therapy. Monitoring of evolving molecular alterations and optimization of treatment should be offered to all patients with cancer. Instituting and educating for a new and disruptive paradigm since the introduction of the field of precision oncology accelerate the implementation of this field. Large leaps in technology continue to lead us toward unprecedented progress in the cure of cancer.

Acknowledgment

The authors wish to thank Dr. Angelo Vasiliadis for his contribution to conceptualization and design of the figures.

Key references

The complete reference list can be found on Vital Source version of this title, see inside front cover.

8. Tsimberidou AM, Wen S, Hong DS, et al. Personalized medicine for patients with advanced cancer in the phase I program at MD Anderson: validation and landmark analyses. *Clin Cancer Res.* 2014;**20**(18):4827–4836.

14. Aftimos PG, Antunes De Melo e Oliveira AM, Hilbers F, et al. First report of AURORA, the breast international group (BIG) molecular screening initiative for metastatic breast cancer (MBC) patients (pts). In: *ESMO Meeting*; 2019: Abstract 30.

15. Mangat PK, Halabi S, Bruinooge SS, et al. Rationale and design of the targeted agent and profiling utilization registry study. *JCO Precis Oncol.* 2018. doi: 10.1200/po.18.00122(2):1-14.

16. Herbst RS, Gandara DR, Hirsch FR, et al. Lung master protocol (Lung-MAP)-A biomarker-driven protocol for accelerating development of therapies for squamous cell lung cancer: SWOG S1400. *Clin Cancer Res.* 2015;**21**(7):1514–1524.

19. Drilon A, Laetsch TW, Kummar S, et al. Efficacy of Larotrectinib in TRK fusion-positive cancers in adults and children. *N Engl J Med.* 2018;**378**(8): 731–739.

115. NIH. *FDA Approves Blood Tests that Can Help Guide Cancer Treatment.* https://www.cancer.gov/news-events/cancer-currents-blog/2020/fda-guardant-360-foundation-one-cancer-liquid-biopsy (accessed 10 December 2020).

132. Okamura R, Kato S, Lee S, et al. ARID1A alterations function as a biomarker for longer progression-free survival after anti-PD-1/PD-L1 immunotherapy. *J ImmunoTherapy Cancer.* 2020;**8**(1):e000438.

170. ClinicalTrials.gov. *IMPACT2.* https://clinicaltrials.gov/ct2/show/NCT02152254?term=impact2&rank=4 (accessed 10 December 2020).

201. Andersen R, Donia M, Ellebaek E, et al. Long-lasting complete responses in patients with metastatic melanoma after adoptive cell therapy with tumor-infiltrating lymphocytes and an attenuated IL2 regimen. *Clin Cancer Res.* 2016;**22**(15):3734–3745.

PART 8

Chemotherapy

50 Drug development of small molecule cancer therapeutics in an Academic Cancer Center

Christopher C. Coss, PhD ■ Jeffrey T. Patrick, PharmD ■ Damien Gerald, PhD ■ Gerard Hilinski, PhD ■ Reena Shakya, PhD ■ John C. Byrd, MD

Overview

Drug development of small molecules in the context of an academic cancer center is a challenging but imminently achievable process. The process involves stage-gated, strategic decision-making informed by the best experimental data that can be obtained. In addition to validating and comprehensively testing the drug molecule in all of the ways suggested, one of the most vital components in drug development aimed at achieving commercialization is intellectual property (IP). Most academic cancer centers are likely going to have access to an internal or external partner who establishes and maintains intellectual property. Intellectual property is in fact what a commercial partner will license with regard to a drug development program. Whether the IP is related to novelty of molecule structure, a synthesis process, an unanticipated (nonobvious) effect or a specific utility against a disease or in combination with another agent, the IP suite established for a drug development asset is the key value attribution that will garner interest from commercial entities.

A robust preclinical development data package depicting clarity of mechanism of action, a tolerable or acceptable toxicity profile along with comparative data to similar programs and finally a robust intellectual property position strongly enhances the likelihood of obtaining a commercial partner as well as enabling full clinical development and commercialization. In addition to advancing basic research to enable translation to clinical research, cancer drug development can also provide a commercial resource support mechanism that can help fuel future research at the developing center based on the financial returns to the academic center from the commercialization process. With all of the available resources, with the right team and vision in place, drug development can be a rewarding process that also aligns to the academic research goals and needs.

Introduction

Drug development in the field of cancer therapeutics represents activities across a wide spectrum of therapeutic modalities including small molecules, peptides, cellular therapies, gene therapies, and more. There are many review articles as well as textbooks dedicated to drug development processes and techniques for each of these products including more complex entities such as oncolytic viruses, monoclonal antibodies, and antibody–drug conjugates.[1-3] Attempting to cover each of these drug development entity topics thoroughly in a single text book chapter would require limiting the discussion of each so substantially that there would likely be little benefit. Instead this article will focus on our experience with preclinical and early clinical drug development of small molecule therapeutics in the setting of an academic cancer center and in the context of conventional academic budgets. Specifically, this article will attempt to provide guidance and emphasis on key elements of early stage small molecule development as well as early clinical (phase 1) development. Discussions will cover how best to develop and analyze appropriate activity assays guided by the best information obtainable on the mechanism of action (MOA). Further, it will attempt to shed light on the importance of target engagement, *in vivo* modeling, characterization of drug exposure–response relationships and therapeutic window. Thematically, we hope to convey one of the most fundamental needs in drug development, a network of collaborators. This includes both academic and commercial entities that may have expertise to advance a project to or through the critical "Go/No Go" decisions. Importantly, the notion of continually pursuing therapeutic drug development when the data do not support it is of paramount importance. Given the scarcity of funding resources available to most academic resources, a key understanding is knowing when "no" represents the best answer. A vital learning of academic drug development is to arrive at a "Go/No Go" decision without incurring excessive expenditure of scarce resources, particularly as the entity achieves the stage of investigational new drug (IND) filing.

In our opinion, drug development must be approached with the end in mind. In order for patients to receive any new cancer therapy in the United States, drug development must proceed through a rigorous process designed to demonstrate both efficacy and safety as set forth by the Food and Drug Administration (FDA). FDA requirements include characterization of many aspects of a given therapeutic. To this end, one useful process common in industrial drug development but rarely implemented by academics is the creation of a target product profile (TPP). The goal of the TPP is to establish the parameters of the final product that the development process seeks to achieve and is ultimately devised to enhance communications with FDA regarding labeling language.[4] It includes the establishment of therapeutic indication, efficacy and safety parameters, biomarkers of relevance, pharmacology and toxicology information and other key aspects of pharmaceutical products. Importantly, as a small molecule drug development project advances through the stages of hit identification, to lead identification to lead optimization, further characterization must take place in order to ensure the likely clinical candidate has the best drug like properties achievable.[5] These characterizations include features such as high oral bioavailability (if the product is to be given orally, which is preferred), a prolonged circulating half-life suitable for once daily dosing, sufficient solubility such that reliable and consistent absorption can be achieved with clinically suitable formulations, minimal impact on hepatic enzyme function or drug transport such that risk of problematic drug–drug interactions are low, and limited inhibition of well-characterized toxicological receptors associated with acute risks to patient health, to name but a few. All of these drug-like property characterizations

---

Holland-Frei Cancer Medicine, Tenth Edition. Edited by Robert C. Bast, John C. Byrd, Carlo M. Croce, Ernest Hawk, Fadlo R. Khuri, Raphael E. Pollock, Apostolia M. Tsimberidou, Christopher G. Willett, and Cheryl L. Willman.
© 2023 John Wiley & Sons, Inc. Published 2023 by John Wiley & Sons, Inc.

need to be carried out in a logical, iterative procession while concurrently optimizing the efficacy and toxicity assessments of the lead molecule in multiple repeat efficacy assessments. All of these efforts occur in concert to ensure the putative lead molecule exhibits its anticancer efficacy with defined and acceptable on- or off-target toxicity.

Considering all of the required characterization and the importance of efficacy assessments either as monotherapy and/or in concert with other medications, it is necessary to constantly assess the competitive landscape or perform competitive intelligence, as commonly defined in the pharmaceutical industry, to ensure your development program is positioned for success. Here, again we would recommend the incorporation of a collaborator. Should an academic program have a business school or a life sciences program with an entrepreneurial aim, perhaps a member of one or more of those programs could help with database access and design of analyses of similar programs in development by other academic or commercial entities. Having an understanding of competitive attributes such as improved potency, enhanced or improved pharmacokinetics (PKs), differing exposure levels to key target organs or an improved toxicity profile are all important when attempting to advance the molecule into the clinical development space and/or toward commercial partnership. Studies demonstrating direct comparisons to competitors are expected from potential industrial partners whereas they are seldom employed in the course of academic therapeutics research.

A key factor shaping every aspect of an academic drug development project is the limited budget typically available to the academician through extramural funds or internal resources. Projecting development costs is quite challenging as made clear by the wide range in reported budgets. It is not disputed that over the last couple of decades, the cost of drug development has increased dramatically.[6–8] However, estimates of this cost range from $314 million to $2.8 billion to bring a drug to the market, in part due to different analysis parameters from multiple studies. Clearly these sums exceed typical research grant support and point to the requirement of industrial, for-profit partners to bring a therapy to market. Beyond that the range of costs reported raise questions regarding the real cost of drug development, particularly in early preclinical stages, which is a primary focus of this text. Most of the available information on drug development costs focuses on clinical expenses, which should be disclosed by pharmaceutical companies to the US Securities and Exchange Commission (SEC.gov) or other governmental agencies. There are inconsistencies in how these companies report these costs, which could be explained by distinct accounting methods, indirect costs, drug acquisitions, collaboration agreements, or cost of capital.[8] However, the most critical parameter influencing the final cost is the adjustment made to offset losses incurred by failed drug programs. As this factor is typically not relevant to a company focusing on a single asset, the cost of drug development in such a setting should be significantly lower than that reported by a company with multiple assets. For example, the total cost of a pharmacologic (e.g., small molecule inhibitor) or a biologic (e.g., antibody) asset was estimated at $309 million and $391 million respectively, without adjustment for the costs of failures. Even with this consideration, these sums exceed even the most lucrative institutional research awards provided by federal agencies by at least an order of magnitude.

Another challenge for the academic drug developer or a small start-up company who is attempting to gauge drug development budget costs from reported information is determining the relative contribution of clinical and preclinical investments. Preclinical costs were previously estimated to represent 42.9% of total costs based on aggregated data and assumptions.[6,7] A more recent estimation was lower, with a median cost of 12.7%, but notably with a broad range from 0.3% to 50.7%.[8] To our knowledge, one of the only analyses describing the cost of a single new molecular entity (NME) through the distinct phases of drug discovery from target selection to drug launch was published in 2010.[9] In this study, the estimate of the total cost of the preclinical discovery phase including target-to-hit ($1 million), hit-to-lead ($2.5 million), lead optimization ($10 million), and preclinical stages ($5 million) was $18.5 million. As highlighted by the authors, their estimate did not include discovery research prior to target selection. The investments in this initial stage are challenging to estimate as they can vary highly from one target to another. Additional factors could impact the different stages of preclinical development, including the targeting modality. For example, even though the total cost of antibody versus small molecule development across preclinical and clinical stages is only slightly different, antibodies are potentially more expensive than small molecules during the late preclinical phase. One common reason is the need for scale-up production of the clinical candidate molecule for IND-enabling studies. In the case of antibodies, the cost of goods, the yield of cell culture bioreactors, and purification procedures that may still be under optimization measurably increase this cost. Other recent targeting modalities, such as cell and gene therapies, also have additional specific costs that are rapidly evolving due to the constant improvement of research tools and production methods.

In conclusion, the budgetary requirements for small molecule synthesis and testing in the preclinical setting are substantially reduced compared to the expenses associated with antibody or cell and gene therapeutics. Considering these costs, an academic researcher or a small company could choose to push a small molecule development program through the early clinical stages. However, it is quite likely that the involvement of an outsider partner will be required. These partners can be engaged through small business granting mechanisms such as SBIR/STTR or directly through coordination with an institution's technology transfer group. The specific parameters of such a partnership will be driven by the value of the therapeutic asset in the eyes of the partner and the direct result of the rigors applied to developing the preclinical data package. The remainder of this section will focus on maximizing an asset's value in the context of an academic cancer center.

Section 1: *in vitro* drug testing and development

A solid foundation of both cell-free and cell-based data that clearly demonstrates a masterful understanding of the MOA of the class of molecule in development is absolutely critical to increasing the likelihood of success in any drug development program.[10,11] At the most basic level, an understanding of MOA requires demonstration of two points:

1. The molecule interacts physically with the intended target in a known manner; and
2. The molecule elicits a biological effect that is dependent upon this physical interaction.

Regardless of the means of compound discovery (e.g. target-based screening or phenotypic screening), our experience suggests that identifying and validating or verifying the MOA is paramount to support a focused and rational therapeutic development program. In an academic drug development setting, resources are

```
Cell-free experiments                                    Cell-based assays
```

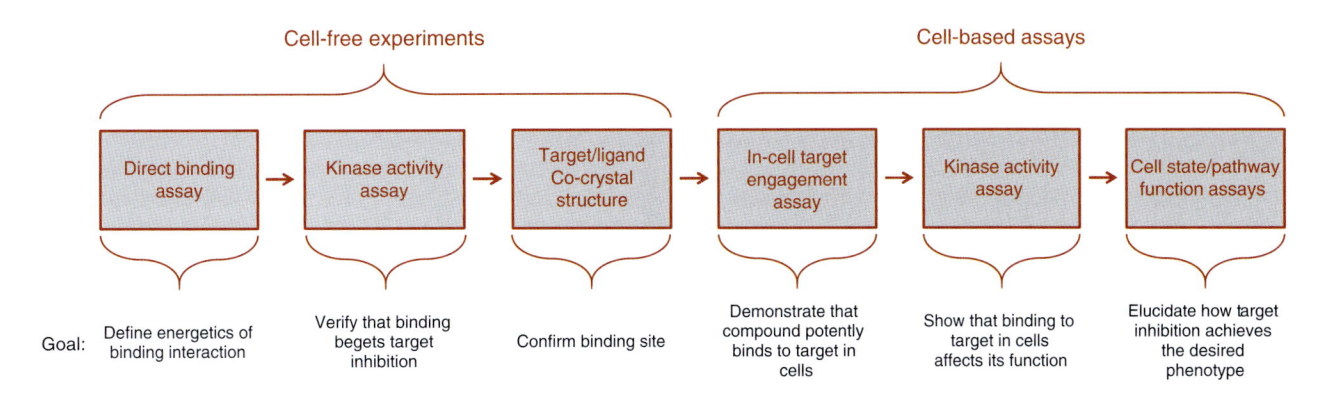

| Direct binding assay | → | Kinase activity assay | → | Target/ligand Co-crystal structure | → | In-cell target engagement assay | → | Kinase activity assay | → | Cell state/pathway function assays |

Goal: Define energetics of binding interaction | Verify that binding begets target inhibition | Confirm binding site | Demonstrate that compound potently binds to target in cells | Show that binding to target in cells affects its function | Elucidate how target inhibition achieves the desired phenotype

Figure 1 Sample *in vitro* research operating plan (ROP) for development of a kinase inhibitor for oncology.

often a precious limiting reagent, so it is important to plan a suite of in vitro experiments that complement each other to link, as clearly as possible, the molecular event of target binding to the desired phenotype of disrupted tumor cell growth.

One strategy for efficiently enabling elucidation of the MOA of a class of compounds is to follow an *in vitro* research operating plan (ROP) that comprises a progression of experiments that connects these dots (see Figure 1 for a sample *in vitro* ROP for a kinase inhibitor). As discussed previously, the FDA requires demonstration of a reasonable expectation of safety and efficacy in order to approve an IND application. In the majority of scenarios, an understanding of MOA will help identify the most relevant and meaningful experiments to facilitate demonstration that administration of the compound to humans would be safe and potentially effective. As in all scientific endeavors, one must recognize that experiments only address the specific question or set of questions that is being asked. Correspondingly, care must be taken to ensure that the interpretation of the results of any experiment is consistent with the totality of the generated data.

Even within the narrow scope of small molecule cancer therapeutics, the specific experiments comprising an optimal strategy for in vitro evaluation of a specific class of molecule can vary widely. Factors that influence the choice of experiments in an *in vitro* ROP include whether the therapeutic approach is molecularly targeted (e.g., a kinase inhibitor) or nontargeted (e.g., cytotoxic chemotherapy). Within each of these paradigms, additional factors will also influence the specifics of the optimal ROP. For example, a molecularly targeted cancer therapeutic could modulate the function of a wild type protein that is present in both malignant and normal cells, or it could selectively modulate the function of a certain oncogenic mutant protein that is only present in malignant cells. Depending on the ubiquity of the target, experiments designed to understand the possibility of undesired on-target toxicity may vary in relevance. This section aims to demonstrate how a suite of cell-free and cell-based assays can be employed to understand the details of, and validate, the putative MOA. To facilitate this pedagogical exercise within the confines of limited space, the discussion focuses on a case in which the compound in development is an adenosine triphosphate (ATP)-competitive, non-covalent small-molecule kinase inhibitor for cancer treatment. The principles underlying development of an *in vitro* ROP, however, are broadly applicable to diverse types of cancer therapeutics.

A priori, an understanding of the specific MOA of any kinase inhibitor requires a robust cell-free kinase activity assay that can reveal the intrinsic ability of a compound to inhibit the kinase activity of the target. When employing such an assay to evaluate the compounds produced during lead identification and optimization, it is important to understand how assay conditions and design can influence the stringency and translational relevance of the evaluation. One such key parameter to consider in a cell-free kinase activity assay is the concentration of ATP that is present in solution. Standard cell-free kinase activity assays often use concentrations of ATP in the 10–100 µM range, but this range is at least an order of magnitude below the typical cellular ATP levels of 1–10 mM. For an ATP-competitive inhibitor, a cell-free kinase activity assay employing micromolar ATP concentrations may vastly overestimate the potency of a compound in a cell-based or *in vivo* settings. It may be desirable, therefore, to evaluate ATP-competitive, non-covalent kinase inhibitors in two versions of a cell-free kinase activity assay: a low-stringency assay run at sub-physiologic ATP concentrations and a high-stringency assay run at physiologically relevant ATP concentrations. To supplement the interpretation of the results of kinase activity assays performed at different ATP concentrations, a cell-free binding assay that measures the energetics of the interaction between a small molecule and its target can be very illuminating. One widely employed biophysical technique for characterizing the interaction between a small molecule and a protein is surface plasmon resonance (SPR), which allows for the measurement of both the association kinetics (k_{on}, on-rate) and dissociation kinetics (k_{off}, off-rate) governing the interaction of interest.[12] An understanding of binding kinetics enables the calculation of the equilibrium dissociation constant K_D to describe the binding affinity of a molecule for a given target. Perhaps more importantly, however, the on-rate and off-rate can be used to access additional parameters such as drug-target residence time, which can help further explain the observed potency of compounds in cell-free, cell-based, and *in vivo* settings.[13] To provide a more complete understanding of the specific molecular interactions that govern the binding event and result in the observed effect on the activity of the target protein, high-resolution ligand–protein co-crystal structures that reveal the specifics of the interaction in atomic-level detail are very valuable.[14] In addition to providing confirmation of the binding site to further support the proposed MOA, such structures can accelerate the identification of a clinical candidate molecule by enabling structure-based drug design. It is important to note that, though protein crystallography and structure determination requires significant expertise and access to specialized equipment such as a synchrotron light source, many academic institutions have Principal Investigators who are highly experienced in structural biology who could serve as intra-institutional collaborators.

Armed with a thorough understanding of the manner in which a compound interacts with a target of interest and modulates its activity in a cell-free setting, it is critical to implement a cell-based assay that directly assesses how efficiently the compound accesses its intended target in a cellular environment. For such cell-based target engagement assays, there are a number of validated chemical biology techniques capable of assessing direct intracellular interaction with the target of interest.[15] Two of the most appealing techniques for cell-based target engagement assays are BRET (Bioluminescence Resonance Energy Transfer) and CETSA (Cellular Thermal Shift Assay).[16] For BRET assays directed at measuring the occupancy of a small molecule on a target such as a kinase, cells are genetically manipulated to express the target protein as a luciferase fusion protein and then treated with the inhibitor and a fluorescently labeled ligand for the target. In the case of an ATP-competitive non-covalent kinase inhibitor, this probe would typically be an ATP analog. After treatment, a substrate for luciferase is added and a plate reader is used to measure BRET between the target protein and the ligand. Compounds that interact with the target and displace the probe compound will modulate the extent of BRET that is measured. Importantly, there are BRET assay variations that enable the assessment of cellular target engagement for compounds with other mechanisms of action, such as inhibitors of intracellular protein–protein interactions. Unlike BRET assays, CETSA assays do not require any manipulation of the target protein (i.e., theoretically CETSA can be performed in any cells that feature endogenous expression of the target protein). Upon binding of a small molecule to a protein target, the three-dimensional structure of the target typically is stabilized; this stabilization manifests as an increase in the target's thermal denaturation temperature (melting temperature). To perform a standard CETSA assay, cells are treated with compound and subsequently heated to cause protein denaturation. Cellular lysates are then prepared and centrifuged to remove denatured proteins, and the soluble fraction is analyzed by Western blot or another method to assess the amount of target protein therein. A compound that is able to engage the target in cells will cause an increase in the melting temperature of the target, resulting in an increased amount of the target protein detected in the supernatant. Of particular importance for drug discovery and development in academia, BRET and CETSA assays generally require only standard laboratory equipment. For BRET, a plate reader capable of measuring fluorescence is necessary; evaluation of protein levels in a CETSA assay can be performed using standard techniques such as Western Blotting or ELISA.

Having validated that the compound can modulate the function of a target in a test tube and also engage the target inside an intact cell, cell-based functional assays are a critical step for further demonstrating that the binding event does indeed achieve the desired modulation of target activity inside the cell. It is often most informative to query the most direct readout of activity of the target protein in order to maximize the likelihood that the observed effect results from the validated target engagement event. In the case of a kinase inhibitor, a key functional assay would be to examine the effect of the inhibitor on the occurrence of a specific phosphorylation event known to be dependent on the activity of the kinase of interest.

Depending on the extent of knowledge regarding the cellular function of the drug target, there are a host of diverse assays that could be used to investigate how inhibition of the activity of the target changes the cellular phenotype.[17] One important consideration in the choice of cell-based assays to define MOA is to recognize that though generic cell proliferation or viability assays can be useful for compound triage, they often do not give much information about how the observed phenotype is achieved. Additionally, the interpretation of results from these assays must be performed with care, because the assay type (e.g., a tetrazolium reduction assay that measures mitochondrial dehydrogenase activity) may not enable unambiguous conclusions about cell number or viability.[18] Alternatively, assays probing specific processes or cell states (such as apoptosis, cell cycle arrest, or senescence) generally are much more informative in the pursuit of defining MOA than assays that generically measure cell proliferation or viability. The former type of assay typically provides a much clearer view of how cells respond to modulation of the activity of the target protein, pointing toward follow-up cell-based experiments that can help to more specifically elucidate the MOA. Experiments that monitor the effect of a compound on a specific phenotype such as phosphorylation state or the accumulation of DNA damage can also help begin to identify biomarkers to be monitored in PK–pharmacodynamic (PD) experiments that demonstrate the link between drug exposure and biological response *in vivo*.

After utilizing standard two-dimensional (2D) cell culture assays to define the MOA of a compound, more complex cell culture paradigms should be considered in order to further understand the potential to translate the compound to the clinic. Three-dimensional (3D) cell culture has gained in popularity in drug development because of the potential to better recapitulate the environment inhabited by tumor cells *in vivo*.[19,20] In addition to utilizing more physiologically relevant cell culture models to increase confidence that the effects observed in cell-based assays will reflect the effects caused by the compound *in vivo*, the rational manipulation of experimental conditions can also provide further insight into the translatability of cell-based assay results. One such way in which experimental conditions can be modified involves the supplementation of standard cell culture media (typically containing 5–10% fetal bovine serum) with physiologically relevant amounts of human serum proteins such as human serum albumin (HSA) and α1-acid glycoprotein (AAG). The kinetics and thermodynamics of the interaction of a compound with either or both of these proteins, which are significant components of human plasma, can significantly affect the amount of free (unbound) drug that is available to access the target of interest.[21]

We have found that the appropriate implementation of cell-free and cell-based assays in drug discovery and development is crucial for the demonstration that a given compound interacts physically with its intended target and that this interaction elicits a biological effect through an understood MOA. Beyond this key point, rigorous activity assay development sufficient to differentiate the activity of related compounds from each other is common place in industrial drug development whereas academic labs often focus on characterizing a single lead, giving little thought to how an activity assay might be used to refine a lead agent through a medicinal chemistry effort. Once a representative assay, or series of assays are established, we recommend careful consideration as to how this assay might scale from a single compound to potentially hundreds, and if the assays are sufficiently robust and reproducible to support structure–activity relationship (SAR)-based refinement of a chemical series. To be sure, no amount of *in vitro* data will guarantee safety and efficacy when an experimental compound is administered to patients, but a robust package of biochemical and cell-based MOA data is essential to increase the probability of achieving this goal. For a more extensive treatment of in vitro assay design for drug discovery and development, we direct you to the comprehensive Assay Guidance Manual produced and maintained by Eli Lilly & Company and the National Center for Advancing Translational Sciences.[22]

Section 2: pharmacology/toxicology in preclinical oncology research

"All substances are poisons, and it is the right dose that differentiates a poison from a remedy."
—Paracelsus (1493–1541).

In any drug development project there is a critical need to understand dose-plasma exposure–response and dose-plasma exposure–toxicity relationships. The difference between these two sets of data can be described as a drug's safety window and its range defines the design of many IND enabling safety studies per FDA guidance.[23,24] The exact moment in a development project when a refined understanding of dose level and exposure level differences between the minimum efficacious dose and the maximum tolerated or even toxic dose is largely project specific. Our opinion is that the value of this information is maximized once a lead molecule is identified. There exist multiple excellent reviews on how to integrate safety pharmacology and toxicology studies into diverse drug development programs published elsewhere.[25–27] For the purposes of this text, we will focus on oncology therapeutic development which traditionally tolerates a very narrow safety window (as low as threefold) given the severity of most malignancies and the alternative to successful therapeutic intervention is often death. Per FDA-guidance, in non-oncology settings, multi-species robust toxicology studies are needed to support first in human (FIH) dosing in healthy volunteers.[23,24] By contrast, recognizing many cancers represent a dire unmet medical need, in some cases FDA will allow single species toxicology studies for novel anti-cancer agents to support FIH dosing in actual cancer patients.[28] As we will outline in the following section, informative tolerability data are readily generated in the context of most academic oncology drug development projects but significant challenges often prevent the timely generation of IND-enabling safety data within academic institutions.

In the academic drug development setting, there is unfortunately little value placed in thorough pre-clinical pharmacological and toxicological characterization by traditional extramural funding bodies (NIH, DOD, NSF, etc.) or top tier journals. Put bluntly, this characterization is seen as non-innovative when compared to the study of novel drug targets, mechanisms of action and anti-cancer efficacy. When this "low scientific value" perception is combined with the requirement of expensive bioanalytical instrumentation (e.g., LC–MS) and specialized personnel (e.g., veterinary pathologist), an environment results whereby true IND-enabling pharmacological and toxicological characterization requires significant long-term institutional support or the recruitment of an industrial partner. To the trained drug development professional, the idea that a novel small therapeutic could be studied for years in an academic lab without the first thought given to characterizing its drug-like properties and safety is likely surprising. Likewise, to the academic researcher, the idea that potent inhibition of human cytochrome p450 3A4 would be sufficiently problematic to dissuade further development of a promising novel anti-cancer agent is similarly jarring. In our experience, academic drug development often exists within this tension between the overlapping goals of academic researchers and drug development professionals (i.e. bringing novel therapies to cancer patients) and their respective distinct goals (i.e. publishing and disseminating promising findings versus de-risking and building support for further development). Educating academic investigators on the necessary rigors of drug development and how they may differ from their own immediate project goals (grants and papers) but still serve the long term goal of translating their discoveries is absolutely essential to building a successful academic development program. To this end, even minimal consultation concerning the design of early proof-of-concept animal studies can provide considerable efficiency to the overall project as is the case when first determining test agent tolerability.

In practice, maximally tolerated doses (MTDs) in mice for many agents are determined empirically by researchers as they pursue proof-of-concept *in vivo* efficacy. Regrettably, these studies seldom mimic the immune status of disease model mice, dose route or duration of the end-product therapeutic (likely oral, for weeks) and can be misleading. At a minimum, the very first multi-dose studies in animals should involve frequent bodyweight and food consumption assessments as these are gross markers of adverse effects[29] and animal carcasses stored in formalin so that follow-up histopathology can be performed on common toxicological tissues. Even with these noted limitations, should early tolerability studies reveal potential toxicity concerns at low doses, it is worthwhile to determine if the exhibited toxicity is on-target or, in other words, related to the novel agent interacting with its intended target in normal as opposed to diseased tissue. Suspicion of unwanted on-target activity can often be confirmed using data from a comparator compound (when available) or in-depth knowledge of the drug target organism wide. If your team determines the toxicity is likely on-target then careful consideration needs to be given to the PDs of your novel agent against the human versus pre-clinical species' (likely murine) target. As nearly all development programs in oncology will include tissue of human origin in a non-human species it is imperative to understand if apparent wide safety windows are due to poor affinity for the [murine] target as compared to human. Conversely, the inability to generate preclinical antitumor efficacy absent overt toxicity may be due to increased affinity for the [murine] target as compared to human.

In any case, once proof-of-concept in vivo efficacy is established it becomes critical to understand the PKs of the test agent at the dose and route used. Very few academic labs are equipped to accurately determine drug disposition and very few academic institutions offer timely and cost-effective core facility support. As such, we recommend engaging contract research organizations who, using economies of scale, can cost effectively support academic preclinical drug development pharmacokinetic studies. With quality disposition data in hand matching efficacious doses, the development team can interpret a whole host of standard in vitro safety data including human ether-à-go-go-related gene (hERG) channel blockade and risk of cardiac arrhythmias,[30] cytochrome p450 inhibition and risk of drug-drug interactions,[31] and general toxicology receptor activity or CEREP or BioPrint screening.[32] Absent an understanding of how much of the test agent circulates following an effective dose, (C_{max}) or systemic exposure [area under the curve (AUC)], the pharmacological relevance of the concentrations at which the test agent produces a potentially problematic *in vitro* toxic signal is unknown. Once therapeutic dose–exposure–response relationships are characterized it becomes critical to determine dose–exposure–toxicity relationships.

It is increasingly seen as unethical to dose escalate in an animal until fatal toxicity is achieved.[33] As such, the combination of advanced knowledge of expected toxicities, shorter duration studies with built in recovery periods, and broad assessment of necessary physiological systems (CNS, cardiovascular, respiratory) are combined to determine nonfatal but toxic dose levels. Ideally much higher doses and exposures of a test agent are required to generate off-target toxicity, or in other words, unwanted actions of the novel agent on normal tissues that does not involve modulating the therapeutic target, relative to therapeutic doses. As broad characterization of potentially toxic effects can get very expensive, very quickly [especially in a good laboratory practice (GLP) setting], one paradigm we suggest is a one dose study where several animals are given a range of dose levels including several half-log multiples of your previously determined efficacious dose (going up to at least 10x, but as high as possible is preferred), stopping with any evidence of acute toxicity. These animals should then be closely followed for at least a week, and thoroughly examined at sacrifice to find evidence of toxicological signals to more closely evaluate in follow-up, potentially GLP studies. The most important outcome of such an acute study is to set dose levels for subsequent studies. It bears mentioning that these studies are often limited by the test agent solubility, a common issue in toxicity work discussed at length elsewhere.[34,35] Solubility challenges at high doses are non-trivial and often require formulation expertise to overcome. That said, an ideal IND enabling toxic study will include three dose of the test agent in an enabled formulation; low-no adverse effects; middle-moderate adverse but not overtly toxic; and high-overtly toxic but not fatal. These doses are given for at least 28 days, often with a 7-day recovery period at the middle and high dose levels to evaluate the reversibility of any apparent toxicity.[36] It is critical that the projected route and schedule for human studies is as closely emulated as possible in pre-clinical toxicology studies. Often, separate toxicokinetic study arms are used to understand dose-exposure relationships resulting in toxicity. More so than dose levels, the relationship between minimally efficacious exposures and toxic exposure are used to define safety window and project FIH dose levels.[23,24]

In closing, our experience is that the vast majority of academic drug development programs consider toxicity as either present or absent and generally lack the expertise to quantify the relationship between efficacious and toxic doses of a test agent. We recommend defining poorly tolerated dose levels of test agent early in characterizing *in vivo* efficacy of lead agent. Doing so will allow your drug development team to build a preclinical data set with dose levels projected to be well tolerated and best prepare your project for critical IND-enabling safety studies.

Section 3: *in vivo* tumor modeling

Preclinical efficacy studies in small animals, primarily in mice, have become the lynchpin for GO/NO GO decision for any small-molecule oncology drug development program. Readers are referred to some excellent reviews that describe in depth the pros and cons of various mouse model systems for drug discovery and development efforts.[37,38] Hence, the focus of this section will be general practical aspects of conducting these studies arising from our experience to ensure robustness and reproducibility of the data generated. To ensure that these proof-of-concept (POC) preclinical *in vivo* studies are as robust and reliable as possible, we recommend that following precautions be undertaken before starting a study: (1) tumor cell-line authentication by small tandem repeat (STR) DNA profiling to ensue cell line fidelity given the high frequency of cross-contamination among cultured cell-lines, as high as 16–35%[39]; (2) verification of mycoplasma-free status of cell-lines given high prevalence of this bacterial contaminant in research labs[40] and its negative impact on cell-biology, for example, cell growth, metabolism, gene-expression profile, antigenicity, etc.[41]; (3) creation of a large cryo-preserved stock of low-passage number cells sufficient enough to complete all preclinical studies for a particular drug-development program to ensure loss of this critical component never places a development program in jeopardy[42]; (4) proper selection of mouse strains (and sub-strains) and alleles used including consistency in vendor source, inbred versus outbred, sub-strain status, etc. since these mundane details may impact the outcome and reproducibility of therapeutic studies significantly[43–45]; (5) establishment of animal husbandry conditions and health reports, in particular the status of opportunistic pathogen prevalence (e.g., *Corynebacterium bovis*) among immune-compromised mouse strains is of great importance[46]; (6) use whenever possible of littermate controls to minimize any variation arising from control cohorts being sourced from external vendors while experimental animals are generated in house; (7) proper randomization of animals during cohort generation[47]; (8) establishment of procedure facilitating the blinding of the experimenter to cohort distribution when making relevant measurements to minimize bias; (9) inclusion of a control cohort which is un-manipulated (e.g., only tumor cells xenografted with no treatment of any kind, a disease model that is allowed to progress without any interventions) to better understand the true course of the disease model in a particular study; it is strongly advised not to rely on historical control data alone for comparison; (10) generation of a formal study report that is detailed enough to allow a third party to replicate the study independently. Lastly, another important factor to consider during study design is to include sufficiently large enough cohort sizes to provide proper statistical power to data interpretation while adhering to the principle of the "3Rs"—replace, reduce, and refine in animal studies. Proper input from a statistician both at the initial study design phase and later for data analysis is strongly encouraged. Statisticians have many statistical tools in their toolbox to help researchers to follow the "3Rs" while assisting in generating the most meaningful data that would be equally informative in designing follow-up studies.

In conclusion, in our opinion, as important as it is to understand the strengths and limitations of the animal models used to recapitulate a particular disease and/or MOA, it is equally important that these pilot preclinical efficacy studies are conducted with sufficient rigor that an independent third party can replicate the results. In most cases, external investors interested in advancing a drug development program will either sponsor independent validation of these study results, or request one before or early in their involvement before sponsoring GLP animal studies and/or toxicity studies; failure to reproduce critical *in vivo* findings are often the death knell for the program.

Section 4: early clinical development

Drug development of new therapeutics rarely initiates from academic universities due to the cost and complexity necessary to put forth a pre-clinical data package to support an investigational IND to the FDA.[48] Most often, academic laboratories identify therapeutic targets and in some cases identify lead compounds with some lead optimization accompanied by *in vitro* and *in vivo* testing using specific murine xenograft models. At this point technology transfer often occurs to for-profit companies that are much more facile at the process of commercializing therapeutics. This is essentially uniform for noncancer indications where patient survival even absent improved therapeutic intervention is expected to be prolonged. Here, extensive safety studies in animals are required before proceeding to human testing and often several large phase 3 studies are needed before approval can be sought. In contrast, cancer represents a devastating disease for which survival is short and requirements for FIH testing are reduced. Even so, the transition of new therapeutic cancer drug candidates to industrial partners most often occurs at the same juncture as non-cancer therapeutics. Why is this? As outlined earlier in this article, a great deal of additional work done using drug material acceptable for administration in patients must occur before consideration of a first in man study. Most academic institutions simply lack the capacity to move quickly and often find early public disclosures leading to competitors leap frogging over them to successful commercialization. For academic institutions with resources, expertise, and patient population to enable completion of these tasks in a rapid manner, active involvement early by the FDA staff is strongly recommended to prevent errors that can delay trial initiation. A general outline of early drug development is provided here with relevant references for the interested reader.

For many years cancer therapy was very much focused on cytotoxic DNA damaging or cell cycle specific therapies that facilitated a relatively straight forward dose escalation strategy with expected adverse event profile often manifesting as toxicity in proliferative compartments of the hematopoietic, epithelial, and gastrointestinal system. The introduction of such agents into patients with cancer often occurred using predetermined established strategies beginning dosing at 10% of the dose lethal to 10% of the most sensitive preclinical species as determined by rigid toxicology studies. Eligibility often included a broad class of solid tumor cancer patients for whom either no therapy was available or proven therapies had become ineffective. Because expected dose limiting toxicities were often relative to hematopoietic indices (neutropenia, thrombocytopenia), patients with hematologic malignancies with bone marrow disease involvement were often excluded from early studies. Dose escalation typically included incremental dosing over a defined period (dose defining period, often 4 weeks) which would proceed using a classic 3 + 3 phase 1 design. Dose limiting toxicities identified would further define a recommended phase 2 dose where expansion could occur in different diseases. Laboratory studies accompanying such phase 1 escalation included detailed pharmacokinetics to assess if dose escalation yields proportional increases in drug levels and to correlate these with selected clinical PD endpoints.[49] Accumulated experience with multiple cytotoxic therapeutics identified many limitations in this approach to development. Rodent and canine toxicity studies done for preclinical safety assessment are of short duration (4 weeks) and not predictive of central nervous system, pulmonary, or delayed cumulative toxicity observed with cancer therapies in humans. Additionally, differential interspecies metabolism of specific therapeutics can lead to either under-estimation of the starting dose which can prolong dose escalation or over-estimation in rare cases which has the potential to lead to severe early toxicity of a new agent. These limitations, along with a lack of diversity in targeted therapeutics, cumulatively resulted in cancer drug development that was: extended in duration to obtain a phase 1 dose[50]; resulted in a majority of patients receiving sub-therapeutic doses; and due to the often empiric application of phase 2 investigation, frequently resulted in the treatment of large numbers of patients across multiple cancer types before the approach was deemed ineffective. In addition, entirely separate phase 1 studies were often required in patients with hematologic malignancies which likely led to many valid treatments failing to reach this patient population. While strategies improving phase 1 dose escalation were established to accelerate dose finding,[51] ultimately, empiric phase 1 drug development in cancer patients became associated with dismal expectations of clinical response or benefit. Consistent limitations with empiric phase 1 studies resulted in broad disagreement among physicians as to the actual clinical benefit of this approach to the numerous patients enrolling in these studies such that ethical concerns have been raised and debated in the cancer field over the past decade.

The rapid advance in basic and translational science of cancer initiation and disease progression along with novel strategies to develop targeted therapies toward different biomolecules cancer cells depend upon for aberrant growth has led to a metamorphosis in drug development. For example, targeted small molecules can be effectively designed to modulate proteins resulting from specific genomic rearrangements or mutations that sub-populations of cancer cells become dependent upon for survival, specific oncogenes that are dysregulated by amplification or over-expression, and pathways of signaling for which cancer types are addicted.[52] In contrast to the empirical development of cytotoxic therapeutics, it is generally the expectation for targeted drug development that numerous aspects of clinical trial implementation will be known before the first patient with a specific agent is dosed. This includes target patient population, specific laboratory PD assay that will be utilized to confirm the small molecule is effectively influencing the expected target protein, and often down-stream measures of this inhibition. The advent of both targeted irreversible inhibitors and PROTACs (proteolysis targeting chimera) allow use of drug probes or degradation of the target protein to assess target engagement. PD assays are often done on surrogate cells (mononuclear cells, skin biopsies, etc.) unless tumor material is readily available. Depending upon the expected genotoxicity and toxicology of the targeted agent in preclinical studies, targeted molecule studies can sometimes initiate with limited dosing (1 day to 7 day) in healthy volunteers to estimate initial human pharmacology and in some cases also assess PD target engagement. In most cases, such healthy volunteer studies are enabled by a pre-clinical data package that demonstrates no/minimal toxicity in animal models with a broad therapeutic index. All of these strategies can facilitate more effective initial phase 1 dosing of targeted therapies such that doses resulting in PD target modulation are achieved more rapidly. In contrast to cytotoxic agents, targeted agents are not always dose escalated to the MTD but rather the biologically effective dose or a dose level or two above this to ensure adequate inhibition among all patients. With selection of a patient population bearing dependence upon the drug target and a validated assay to assess target engagement, phase 1 studies in this setting are more often associated with more clinical benefit than traditional phase 1 studies. For targeted agents indicated in small patient populations (i.e., rare tumor genomics), dose escalation sometimes occurs in a broader non-selected patient population and then expands to the targeted group at the projected effective phase 2 dose.[53] In contrast to cytotoxic cancer therapies previously developed, targeted therapies rarely extend beyond phase 1b testing unless some evidence of clinical activity or demonstrable target engagement is demonstrated.[54] This further emphasizes the critical importance of pre-clinical translational science prior to phase 1 initiation. Furthermore, unlike cytotoxic therapies, hematopoietic tumors are often approached initially or in parallel with solid tumors, as targeted therapies' PDs on tumor cells are readily assessed in blood or marrow cells and can be compared to effects on normal cells.[55]

Despite the success of targeted small molecules in the treatment of cancer, many notable challenges remain that can trip up even the most skilled university drug development team.[56] From the onset, this can include failure by academic institutions to adequately insure global intellectual property protection which is itself constantly in tension with academic investigators' needs to disseminate their findings. All drug development teams are subject to implicit bias toward their lead molecule making necessary the inclusion of an external board who is empowered to continually question the team on limitations to the approach taken. On the therapeutic side, targeted therapies are often overcome by redundant escape signaling pathways in the cancer cell that bypass the intended action of the therapeutic rendering the agent ineffective. Targeted therapies optimized for human drug targets can sometimes appear relatively innocuous in preclinical efficacy and toxicology models due to species differences in binding and subsequently over-estimate therapeutic window if xenograft cell line or PDX studies are the predominate source of preclinical testing. For some targets it can be difficult to develop assays that show appropriate engagement in surrogate normal tissues whereas in others, target expression or activity may be different than the tumor type. Finally, there represents a broad range of tumor types that can have specific driving mutations for which differential biology results in response rates ranging from complete to zero activity. An example of a mutation in cancer is the BRAF activating mutations where complete remissions are noted in classic hairy cell leukemia, responses among melanoma and lung cancer whereas in colon cancer it is inactive. Despite the challenges, successful development of a small molecule internally or in partnership with a for-profit company represents the ultimate goal of experimental therapeutics research and can be the most impactful and rewarding experience of an academic career.

References

1. Mould DR, Meibohm B. *Drug development of therapeutic monoclonal antibodies.* BioDrugs. 2016;**30**(4):275–293.
2. Kommineni N et al. *Antibody drug conjugates: development, characterization, and regulatory considerations.* Polym Adv Technol. 2020;**31**(6):1177–1193.
3. Engeland CE. In: Engeland CE, ed. *Oncolytic Viruses, in Methods in Molecular Biology 2058.* Humana Press; 2020.
4. FDA. (2020). *Guidance for Industry and Review Staff: The Target Product Profile – A Strategic Development Process Tool.* https://www.fda.gov/media/72566/download
5. Di L, Kerns EH. *Drug-Like Properties : Concepts, Structure Design and Methods : From ADME to Toxicity Optimization*, 2nd ed. Elsevier:560.
6. DiMasi JA, Hansen RW, Grabowski HG. The price of innovation: new estimates of drug development costs. *J Health Econ.* 2003;**22**(2):151–185.
7. DiMasi JA, Grabowski HG, Hansen RW. Innovation in the pharmaceutical industry: new estimates of R&D costs. *J Health Econ.* 2016;**47**:20–33.
8. Wouters OJ, McKee M, Luyten J. Estimated research and development investment needed to bring a new medicine to market, 2009-2018. *JAMA.* 2020;**323**(9):844–853.
9. Paul SM et al. *How to improve R&D productivity: the pharmaceutical industry's grand challenge.* Nat Rev Drug Discov. 2010;**9**(3):203–214.
10. Schenone M et al. *Target identification and mechanism of action in chemical biology and drug discovery.* Nat Chem Biol. 2013;**9**(4):232–240.
11. Kitagawa D, Gouda M, Kirii Y. Drug discoveries and molecular mechanism of action. In: Fishcer J, Rotella DP, eds. *Successful Drug Discovery.* Wiley; 2014.
12. Kitagawa D, Gouda M, Kirii Y. *Quick evaluation of kinase inhibitors by surface plasmon resonance using single-site specifically biotinylated kinases.* J Biomol Screen. 2014;**19**(3):453–461.
13. Copeland RA. *The drug-target residence time model: a 10-year retrospective.* Nat Rev Drug Discov. 2016;**15**(2):87–95.
14. Carvalho AL, Trincao J, Romao MJ. *X-ray crystallography in drug discovery.* Methods Mol Biol. 2009;**572**:31–56.
15. Schurmann M et al. *Small-molecule target engagement in cells.* Cell Chem Biol. 2016;**23**(4):435–441.
16. Stefaniak J, Huber KVM. *Importance of quantifying drug-target engagement in cells.* ACS Med Chem Lett. 2020;**11**(4):403–406.
17. Ediriweera MK, Tennekoon KH, Samarakoon SR. *In vitro assays and techniques utilized in anticancer drug discovery.* J Appl Toxicol. 2019;**39**(1):38–71.
18. Eastman A. *Improving anticancer drug development begins with cell culture: misinformation perpetrated by the misuse of cytotoxicity assays.* Oncotarget. 2017;**8**(5):8854–8866.
19. Ravi M, Ramesh A, Pattabhi A. *Contributions of 3D cell cultures for cancer research.* J Cell Physiol. 2017;**232**(10):2679–2697.
20. Langhans SA. *Three-dimensional in vitro cell culture models in drug discovery and drug repositioning.* Front Pharmacol. 2018;**9**:6.
21. Trainor GL. *The importance of plasma protein binding in drug discovery.* Expert Opin Drug Discovery. 2007;**2**(1):51–64.
22. Markossian S and Sittampalam GS. *The Assay Guidance Manual.* 2004. https://www.ncbi.nlm.nih.gov/books/NBK53196/.
23. FDA. *S7A Safety Pharmacology Studies for Human Pharmaceuticals.* 2001. https://www.fda.gov/regulatory-information/search-fda-guidance-documents/s7a-safety-pharmacology-studies-human-pharmaceuticals
24. FDA. *M3R2 Nonclinical Safety Studies for the Conduct of Human Clinical Trials and Marketing Authorization for Pharmaceuticals.* 2010. https://www.fda.gov/regulatory-information/search-fda-guidance-documents/m3r2-nonclinical-safety-studies-conduct-human-clinical-trials-and-marketing-authorization.
25. Gad SC. *Preclinical Development Handbook. Toxicology*, Vol. xiii. Hoboken, NJ: Wiley-Interscience; 2008:1059.
26. Lodola A, Stadler J. *Pharmaceutical Toxicology in Practice : A Guide for Non-clinical Development*, Vol. **vi**. Hoboken, NJ: Wiley; 2011:258.
27. Faqi AS (ed). *A Comprehensive Guide to Toxicology in Preclinical Drug Development*, Vol. xvi, 1st ed. London; Waltham, MA: Academic Press; 2013:885.
28. FDA. *S9 Nonclinical Evaluation for Anticancer.* 2010. https://www.fda.gov/regulatory-information/search-fda-guidance-documents/s9-nonclinical-evaluation-anticancer-pharmaceuticals.
29. Hoffman WP, Ness DK, van Lier RB. *Analysis of rodent growth data in toxicology studies.* Toxicol Sci. 2002;**66**(2):313–319.
30. Gintant G. *An evaluation of hERG current assay performance: Translating preclinical safety studies to clinical QT prolongation.* Pharmacol Ther. 2011;**129**(2):109–119.
31. Nettleton DO, Einolf HJ. *Assessment of cytochrome p450 enzyme inhibition and inactivation in drug discovery and development.* Curr Top Med Chem. 2011;**11**(4):382–403.
32. Bendels S et al. *Safety screening in early drug discovery: an optimized assay panel.* J Pharmacol Toxicol Methods. 2019;**99**:106609.
33. Seidle T et al. *Cross-sector review of drivers and available 3Rs approaches for acute systemic toxicity testing.* Toxicol Sci. 2010;**116**(2):382–396.
34. Li P, Zhao L. *Developing early formulations: practice and perspective.* Int J Pharm. 2007;**341**(1-2):1–19.
35. Shah SM et al. *Preclinical formulations: insight, strategies, and practical considerations.* AAPS PharmSciTech. 2014;**15**(5):1307–1323.
36. FDA, S9 Nonclinical Evaluation for Anticancer Pharmaceuticals Questions and Answers Guidance for Industry. 2010.
37. Ireson CR et al. *The role of mouse tumour models in the discovery and development of anticancer drugs.* Br J Cancer. 2019;**121**(2):101–108.
38. Guerin MV et al. *Preclinical murine tumor models: a structural and functional perspective.* elife. 2020;**9**.
39. American Type Culture Collection Standards Development Organization Workgroup, A.S.N. Cell line misidentification: the beginning of the end. *Nat Rev Cancer.* 2010;**10**(6):441–448.
40. Drexler HG, Uphoff CC. *Mycoplasma contamination of cell cultures: Incidence, sources, effects, detection, elimination, prevention.* Cytotechnology. 2002;**39**(2):75–90.
41. Miller CJ et al. *Mycoplasma infection significantly alters microarray gene expression profiles.* BioTechniques. 2003;**35**(4):812–814.
42. Hughes P et al. *The costs of using unauthenticated, over-passaged cell lines: how much more data do we need?* BioTechniques. 2007;**43**(5):575, 577-8, 581-2 passim.
43. Simpson EM et al. *Genetic variation among 129 substrains and its importance for targeted mutagenesis in mice.* Nat Genet. 1997;**16**(1):19–27.
44. Goldstein JM, Wagers AJ. *What's in a (Sub)strain?* Stem Cell Reports. 2018;**11**(2):303–305.
45. Kawashita E et al. *A comparative analysis of hepatic pathological phenotypes in C57BL/6J and C57BL/6N mouse strains in non-alcoholic steatohepatitis models.* Sci Rep. 2019;**9**(1):204.
46. Besselsen DG et al. *Lurking in the shadows: emerging rodent infectious diseases.* ILAR J. 2008;**49**(3):277–290.
47. Hirst JA et al. *The need for randomization in animal trials: an overview of systematic reviews.* PLoS One. 2014;**9**(6):e98856.
48. FDA. *Content and Format of Investigational New Drug Applications (INDs) for Phase 1 Studies of Drugs, Including Well-Characterized, Therapeutic, Biotechnology-derived Products.* 1995. https://www.fda.gov/regulatory-information/search-fda-guidance-documents/content-and-format-of-investigational-new-drug-applications-inds-phase-1-studies-drugs-including-well
49. Dancey JE et al. *Guidelines for the development and incorporation of biomarker studies in early clinical trials of novel agents.* Clin Cancer Res. 2010;**16**(6):1745–1755.
50. Penel N et al. *Justification of the starting dose as the main determinant of accrual time in dose-seeking oncology phase 1 trials.* Investig New Drugs. 2010;**28**(6):839–843.

51 Yuan Y et al. *Bayesian optimal interval design: a simple and well-performing design for phase I oncology trials.* Clin Cancer Res. 2016;**22**(17):4291–4301.

52 Mbugua SN et al. *Beyond DNA-targeting in cancer chemotherapy. emerging frontiers – a review.* Curr Top Med Chem. 2020.

53 Lemery S, Keegan P, Pazdur R. *First FDA approval agnostic of cancer site – when a biomarker defines the indication.* N Engl J Med. 2017;**377**(15):1409–1412.

54 Gormley NJ, Farrell AT, Pazdur R. *Minimal residual disease as a potential surrogate end point-lingering questions.* JAMA Oncol. 2017;**3**(1):18–20.

55 Farrell AT, Goldberg KB, Pazdur R. *Flexibility and innovation in the FDA's novel regulatory approval strategies for hematologic drugs.* Blood. 2017;**130**(11):1285–1289.

56 Silva PJ, Ramos KS. *Academic medical centers as innovation ecosystems: evolution of industry partnership models beyond the Bayh-Dole Act.* Acad Med. 2018;**93**(8):1135–1141.

51 Principles of dose, schedule, and combination therapy

Joseph P. Eder, MD ■ Navid Hafez, MD, MPH

Overview

The role of dose and schedule have always and continue to play a critical role in clinical cancer drug treatment. Dose is a significant determinant of the antitumor activity and toxicology for the established cytotoxic chemotherapeutic agents and newly developed targeted agents. The relationship for dose, or more correctly exposure, is quite consistent for the effect on normal tissues, most clearly seen in the deoxyribonucleic acid (DNA) damaging agents and mitotic tubule inhibitors. The effect of dose for biologically therapeutic agents such as the interferons, interleukins, monoclonal antibodies, hormones, and for molecularly targeted tyrosine kinase inhibitors is complicated, and there is not the same unequivocal evidence for a dose–response effect with these agents. Contemporary targeted agents have a much more specific relationship to the extent of target interaction. The schedule of drug administration may be important to the therapeutic index independent of dose. Cytokinetic studies related to drug schedule have led to the improved use of agents such as cytosine arabinoside (cytarabine, ara-C) in both experimental and clinical leukemia. Most of the molecularly targeted agents, whether small molecules or monoclonal antibodies, are dosed to provide a continuous effect, which markedly changes the clinical toxicity profile but has come for reconsideration as a general approach.

The intrinsic tumor cell sensitivity, the tumor burden, and the presence of resistance determine the outcome of therapy as much as exposure, which does correlate well with host factors and toxicity, particularly the pharmacokinetics of drug clearance and kinetics of sensitive host cell targets. Bone marrow transplantation and hematopoietic growth factors have permitted the use of increased doses of alkylating agents to improve results and increase cures in several settings.

For most chemotherapeutic agents that directly or indirectly target DNA or the mitotic spindle used alone or in combination, intermittent courses (e.g., four 5-day courses every 3–4 weeks) are generally superior to other schedules such as continuous dosing to permit normal tissue recovery and maximize dose. Cytarabine in acute myeloid leukemia (AML) and 5-fluorouracil (5-FU) in gastrointestinal (GI) cancers are notable exceptions, driven in short by the extremely rapid plasma clearance due to metabolism.

Continuous oral administration of many new targeted therapies, particularly kinase inhibitors is the current clinical schedule for reasons related to the mechanism of action. The continued suppression of proliferative growth factor signals and interruption of survival pathway signals in tumor cells or the repair of DNA appears necessary in the clinic and in preclinical models. This is the case for the poly (ADP-ribose) polymerase (PARP) inhibitor rucaparib. Monoclonal antibodies produced with contemporary means, whether alone or as a drug antibody conjugate, have predictable clearance/half-lives equivalent to native immunoglobulin G (IgG) proteins (half-life 21–23 days).

The most compelling rationale for combination chemotherapy is tumor cell heterogeneity and its implication for drug resistance, and the success of combination chemotherapy in the clinic. In practical clinical terms, the selection of specific combinations in particular types of cancer depends on the individual activity of the agents in the target cancer type and the absence of overlapping toxicities. The agents with the highest single-agent activity are preferred, particularly agents that produce complete responses (if any such agents exist), with different mechanisms of action to address the theoretical heterogeneity issue.

The vast majority of cancers are treated successfully only with combinations of agents chosen for the highest possible individual activity against a specific type of cancer. Empiricism was an essential component in the development of contemporary cancer therapy, but rational drug discovery, analog development, preclinical modeling, precise pathologic diagnosis, careful staging of disease, and clinical trial design are the foundation for the measure of success known today. The breakthroughs in molecular biology have presented the oncologist with enormous opportunities and challenges. Based on these breakthroughs, a molecular diagnosis will be able not only to determine where and how cancer originates but also the processes that are essential to its survival.

Introduction

The identification of novel, clinically active agents has been central to progress in cancer chemotherapy. Table 1 presents examples of new agents and of cellular pathways and targets being explored for new therapeutic targets. Dose is a significant determinant of the antitumor activity and toxicology for the established, "classical" cytotoxic chemotherapeutic agents.[1] These agents are deoxyribonucleic acid (DNA) damaging agents, directly or indirectly, or inhibitors of cell division and a quantitative relationship between target interaction and cell lethality is unknown. The relationship for dose, or more correctly exposure, is quite consistent for the effect on normal tissues, however. High-dose chemotherapy (4–10 times the baseline dose), made possible by hematopoietic stem cell transplantation, has proven curative for selected hematologic neoplasms. The FDA is quite explicit in the centrality of the dose–response relationship of any agent for any purpose "Exposure—response information is at the heart of any determination of the safety and effectiveness of drugs. That is, a drug can be determined to be safe and effective only when the relationship of beneficial and adverse effects to a defined exposure is known".[2]

The effect of dose for biologically therapeutic agents such as the interferons, interleukins, monoclonal antibodies, hormones, and for molecularly targeted tyrosine kinase inhibitors is complicated, and there is not the same unequivocal evidence for a dose-response effect with these agents. Contemporary targeted agents have a much more specific relationship to the extent of target interaction, such as receptor occupancy for monoclonal antibodies or extent of phosphorylation inhibition for kinase inhibitors (proof of mechanism) and a measured pharmacodynamics effect (proof of principle), such as phosphorylation inhibition expected to

Table 1 Molecular targets for cancer treatment.[a]

The cell cycle
- Cyclin-dependent kinases, cyclins, cyclin-dependent kinase inhibitors, mitotic tubule-associated proteins

Differentiation
- Retinoid and vitamin D nuclear steroid receptors

Apoptosis
- BCL2, NF-kB, TP53, TNFSF10, FAS

Angiogenesis
- KDR, the endothelial integrins, PDGFRB

Signaling cell surface receptors
- Insulin-like growth factor receptor (IGF), ERBB family of receptors, KIT

Metastasis
- Matrix metalloproteinases, chemokine receptors

Intracellular signaling elements
- BCR-ABL1, Ras, Raf, MADD, PI3 kinase, m-TOR, SRC, protein kinase C, focal adhesion kinase (PTK2: protein kinase 2), anaplastic lymphoma kinase (ALK), the STAT family of proteins, and the MAP family of protein kinases

Nuclear transcription factors
- For example, steroid hormone No. 4

Potential targets
- Telomerase
- DNA methylation [human DNA methyltransferase (MeTase)], proteasome 20S, farnesyltransferase, histone deacetylase, hsp90 (chaperone protein)

Cell surface antigens
- For example, CD20

[a]Source: Based on Frei and Canellos.[1]

Table 2 Number of agents and curative treatment for childhood acute lymphoblastic leukemia (ALL).[a]

	Number of chemotherapeutic agents							
	1	2	3	4	5	6	7	8
Year	1948	1954	1956	1960	1965	1974	1985	1988
Agent	Methotrexate	MP	Prednisone	Vincristine	Methotrexate[b]	Adriamycin	Asparaginase	Ara-C
CR (%)	20–40	40–92	80–95	>95	>95	>95	>95	>95
Cure (%)	0	0	0	15	5–35	55	75	80

[a]Source: Based on Menon-Andersen et al.[2]
[b]Intrathecal methotrexate.
Abbreviations: CR, complete response; MP, 6-mercaptopurine.

correlate with clinical efficacy in the proper molecularly selected patient segment (proof of concept) than dose alone implies, though in clinical medicine this is the surrogate used.

The schedule of drug administration may be important to the therapeutic index independent of dose. Cytokinetic studies related to drug schedule have led to the improved use of agents such as cytarabine in both experimental and clinical leukemia (see section titled "Cytokinetics of bone marrow" later in this article).[3,4] Most of the molecularly targeted agents, whether small molecules or monoclonal antibodies, are dosed to provide a continuous effect, which markedly changes the clinical toxicity profile but has come for reconsideration as a general approach.

Combination chemotherapy has been crucial in the development of curative regimens for hematologic malignancies, pediatric solid tumors, testicular cancer, and ovarian cancer, and for the adjuvant regimens for breast, lung, and bowel cancer, and for osteosarcomas.[5,6] The rationale for combination chemotherapy is discussed under the various topical headlines. The principal rationale includes (1) the empiric: almost all therapy that has proven curative in the clinic involves the use of agents in combination (Table 2); (2) the fact that genetic instability results in tumor cell heterogeneity, which manifests as drug resistance in cancer therapy[6–8]; and (3) signal transduction inhibitors molecularly targeted to specific cancer driver mutations, with the possible exception of imatinib in some patients with chronic myelogenous leukemia (CML).[9] Resistance to signal transduction inhibitors can be circumvented by either combining a second agent (dabrafenib and trametinib in melanoma)[10] or using second-generation agent with a broader spectrum of targets specific for the mutations conferring resistance [osimertinib in epidermal growth factor receptor (EGFR) mutant non-small-cell lung cancer (NSCLC)][11,12] to have significant therapeutic benefit. Although dose and combination chemotherapy are generally considered separately, they have an important and complex relationship.[13,14] There is an impressive increase in the number of putative molecular targets for cancer treatment in development (see Table 1). A major clinical research

Principles of dose, schedule, and combination therapy **643**

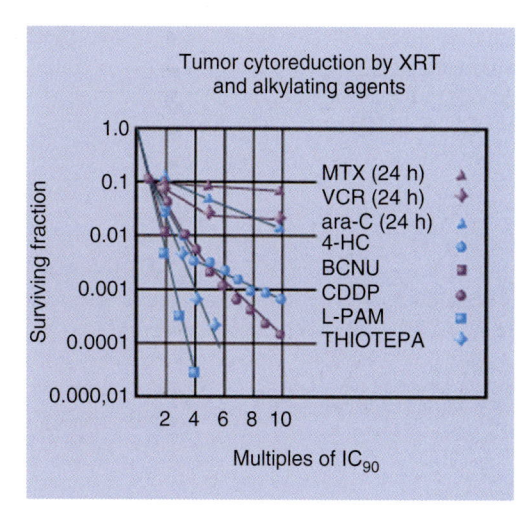

Figure 1 Log kill *in vitro*: Effect of antitumor agent concentration expressed as multiples of the IC_{90} (i.e., the dose or concentration that reduces the number of tumor cells by 90%), on the surviving fraction of human breast cancer (MCF7) cells in culture (colony assay). Abbreviation: 4-HC, 4-hydroxy-cyclophosphamide. Source: Based on Frei.[6]

challenge will be not only to maximize the effectiveness of individual agents but to integrate drugs into optimal combination strategies.

Dose

In controlled experimental systems, such as established tumor cell lines in culture, the relationship between dose and tumor cytotoxicity may be close to linear-log (i.e., exponential).[15] A linear increase in the dose of selected chemotherapeutic agents causes a log reduction of MCF7 human breast cancer cells in culture.[16] In Figure 1, dose is expressed as multiples of the IC_{90} (i.e., the dose or concentration that reduces the number of tumor cells by 90%), a very good response in terms of tumor regression in a patient. The estimated total tumor burden for patients with clinically evident cancer is $5 \times 10^{11} \pm 10^{1}$ (11 ± 1 logs). Thus, a dose that produces a good partial remission (e.g., 50–90% tumor regression) produces at most a 1-log reduction, which is less than 10% of the "exponential iceberg." Numerous factors influence the dose effect. They are presented in the subsections that follow.[17,18]

Factors influencing the dose effect

Class of antineoplastic agent
The ideal therapeutic agent would maintain a linear relationship between dose and log tumor cell reduction (log-TCR) down through multiple logs of tumor cell death (see Figure 1). Ionizing radiation comes closest to this ideal. As a group, alkylating agents maintain a dose/log-TCR in experimental models (see Figure 1). DNA damaging alkylating agents exhibit major activity during the S and M periods of the cell cycle, but unlike other chemotherapeutic agents, they maintain activity throughout the cell cycle. Although comparative studies demonstrate a dose effect in chemotherapy-sensitive tumors such as the leukemias and lymphomas, the effect of dose is less evident in solid tumors, particularly those tumors of epithelial origin.[19,20] Purine and pyrimidine-targeted antimetabolites are active mainly in proliferating cells, and therefore pharmacokinetic resistance occurs that is

overcome less by increasing dose than by increasing the duration of exposure, allowing more cells to enter the proliferative compartment. This also applies to the DNA-damaging topoisomerase I and II directed agents and microtubule-interacting agents, where the target must be encountered in the setting of DNA synthesis or mitotic spindle assembly to produce antineoplastic cytotoxicity.[21,22]

Agents directed at hormone and growth factor receptors have a different relationship since once receptor/kinase interactions are saturated, further dose increases will produce no further effect.[23] Hence these agents are analogous to antimetabolites in that dose escalation once saturation levels of drug are achieved produces no further benefit. Targeted kinase inhibitors have characteristics of the antimetabolites in schedule dependency in that continuous exposure correlates with optimal tumor cytotoxicity. Higher doses of imatinib in chronic phase or accelerated phase CML with a suboptimal response to standard dose can benefit a subgroup of patients, but the percentage is low and the duration of response brief.[24,25]

Tumor factors

Intrinsic tumor cell sensitivity
The more sensitive the tumor is to a given agent, the steeper the dose effect. Thus, if a unit dose produces a 0.5 log-TCR, then doubling that dose may produce up to a 1.0 log tumor cell kill—which clinically represents only a partial remission. In a chemotherapy-sensitive tumor, where a unit dose produces a 3 log-TCR, doubling the dose may produce up to a 6 log-TCR, depending on the degree of tumor cell heterogeneity and drug resistance (see section titled "Drug resistance" later in this subsection). A 6 log-TCR would produce a major clinical achievement in terms of complete response, duration of complete response, and, most important, an approach to tumor cure or eradication. This level of TCR can be achieved in CML by a number of BCR-ABL1-targeted therapies.[26] For patients with a metastatic common epithelial tumor, such as breast cancer, the most that can be achieved with standard single-agent chemotherapy is a partial response (<1 log-TCR) in about 30% of patients. Combinations result in higher partial response rates and a low (10–20%) complete response rate. Alternatively, combination chemotherapy regimens in patients with chemotherapy-sensitive tumors (e.g., non-Hodgkin's lymphoma, Hodgkin's disease, and germ cell tumors) may achieve multi–log-TCR as a result of combination chemotherapy.[27]

Tumor burden
Tumor burden is a consistent adverse prognostic factor for response to chemotherapy. This finding was first demonstrated for transplanted tumors in mice; in these animals, macroscopic (i.e., palpable) tumors often respond minimally to chemotherapy. The same tumor, at a microscopic tumor burden size, may be much more responsive and potentially curable.[27,28]

These observations in mice are consistent with the parallel observation that adjuvant cancer treatment can be curative for patients with breast cancer, but not for those with overt metastatic breast cancer. Postulates for the delay in growth of microscopic metastases include a balanced rate of cell loss (i.e., apoptosis) and of cell production and inability to support tumor neovascularization (angiogenesis). Resistant microscopic tumor may persist in most long-term survivors, an observation that has major implications for therapeutic strategy (see section titled "Cytokinetics of the tumor—the growth fraction" later in this subsection).

The study of microscopic metastases in patients may become increasingly possible with molecular techniques for detection and characterization of minimal residual tumor.[27] The kinetics of microscopic disease can be inferred from adjuvant chemotherapy studies (see section titled "Adjuvant chemotherapy").

Drug resistance
In the laboratory, drug resistance is usually produced by "selection pressure"—that is, by exposing target cells to progressively increasing concentrations of the selecting agent. Drug resistance is usually expressed as the concentration of drug that is required to produce 50% inhibition in a colony or growth assay (IC_{50}) for the resistant cell line, divided by the concentration required (IC_{50}) for the parent sensitive cell line. For a detailed presentation of drug resistance, see section titled "Combination chemotherapy" later in this article and *see* "Drug resistance and its clinical circumvention".

Cytokinetics of the tumor—the growth fraction
The growth fraction (GF) of the tumor and the dose of cell cycle-specific agents have a major effect on the log-TCR of tumor cells. The generation time of cycling (i.e., mitotically active) cells is much shorter than the volume doubling time.[29-33] Thus, many cells within tumors are dying or "noncycling"—that is, in G_0/G_1. The GF of a tumor is the ratio of the cycling cells to the total number of tumor cells, often measured as mitotic index or Ki67.[34]

For the common epithelial solid tumors, the GF is often less than 5%.[35,36] A solid tumor with a GF of 5% would be minimally responsive to cell cycle-specific agents and variably sensitive to other chemotherapeutic agents. Repetitive treatments, however, might "recruit" cells into cycle by allowing dormant, noncycling cells access to necessary growth conditions and thus enabling them to be more effective. Prolonged exposure to cell cycle-specific agents might be effective in low—GF tumors. In contrast, a high-GF tumor such as Burkitt's lymphoma might have a multilog response with the same treatment or even the same dose over a shorter period.[1] A recent challenge to the long-standing clonal evolution model of cancer evokes specific cancer progenitor cells (CPCs) as responsible for the continued proliferation of a tumor. By this model, self-renewing CPCs give rise to all progenitor and differentiated cells within a tumor, but remain a small proportion of all tumor cells.[37] CPCs, as with normal tissue stem cells, are extremely resistant to chemotherapy and radiotherapy.[38] The difference between curative therapeutic regimens and those that are only palliative may be attributable to the relative sensitivities of CPCs and of the progenitor and differentiated cancer cells incapable of self-renewal. Identification of therapeutic targets within the CPC population should offer significant opportunities for more effective therapies.

Tumor hypoxia
Hypoxia commonly occurs in both experimental and clinical solid tumors, a condition presumably resulting from inadequate angiogenesis and high metabolic activity (oxygen consumption). Oxygen distribution within tumors is heterogeneous and even a small fraction of hypoxic cells can profoundly affect chemotherapy responsiveness. The farther cells are from blood vessels, the lower the concentration of chemotherapeutic agents in those cells. Cellular proliferation decreases as a function of distance from blood vessels, with a significant fraction of nonproliferating cells conferring kinetic resistance to cell cycle-specific agents. Certain cancer chemotherapy agents require oxygen as an intermediate in toxicity or in metabolism.[39] Finally, hypoxia produces altered gene expression. Hypoxia-inducible factor 1 (HIF1) stops proliferation and prevents apoptosis in the hypoxic fraction of cells by increasing angiogenesis. HIF1 alpha produces an epithelial to mesenchymal transition (EMT) in cancer cells resulting in increased invasiveness, metastases, and drug resistance.[40,41] Hypoxia increases the production of hepatocytes growth factor (HGF) and its receptor MET, with a further increase in angiogenesis, and increased incidence of metastasis and drug resistance.[42,43] There may be increased expression of adenosine triphosphate-binding cassette (ABC) proteins such as p-glycoprotein (PgP) that may confer resistance to chemotherapeutic agents. Hypoxia also selects for *TP53* mutants with a reduced apoptotic response to DNA damage or cell cycle arrest targeted agents.[44] Exploiting hypoxia as a target in cancer therapy with bioreductive alkylating agents such as mitomycin C and the nitroimidazoles, which can serve as electron acceptors in lieu of oxygen, has been investigated in numerous clinical circumstances with no or minimal benefit.[45,46] Impaired chemosensitivity is not universal, and in selected cell lines (i.e., renal), some drugs appear even less effective in normoxia than hypoxia.[47] Radiotherapy, in particular, requires molecular oxygen for cytotoxicity.[48]

Oncogene addiction-growth factor signaling
The maintenance of the transformed state results in significant metabolic and genetic stress on cancer cells. Maintaining viability under these conditions requires positive antiapoptotic signaling factors and interfering with these survival pathways can result in tumor cell lethality. Mutant oncogenes such as *BCR-ABL* in CML, or mutant growth factor receptors like *EGFR (ERBB1)* in lung cancer, rapidly accelerated fibrosarcoma homolog B (*BRAF*) in melanoma and tyrosine-protein kinase KIT (*CKIT*) in gastrointestinal stromal tumors (GIST) provide essential survival signals and interruption of these pathways produces significant clinical benefit in affected patient. The emergence of diagnostic molecular testing enables identification of patients and permits selection of appropriate therapy.

Host factors

Cytokinetics of bone marrow
Because of the bone marrow's proliferative activity and relative lack of DNA repair capacity, myelosuppression is dose limiting for many chemotherapeutic agents. Exploiting the cytokinetic difference between marrow and tumor has been a basis for the construction of selected clinical strategies.[4,29]

Normal marrow recovers within 1–2 weeks after cytarabine, with little cumulative myelosuppression. For many patients, recovery of acute myeloid leukemia (AML) cells as compared with normal marrow cells between courses of cytarabine is incomplete. AML cells *in vitro* are less susceptible to growth factors such as granulocyte colony-stimulating factor (G-CSF) and granulocyte/macrophage colony-stimulating factor (GM-CSF) than are the cells of the normal marrow.[49] Thus, when marrow colony-stimulating factors (CSFs) increase in homeostatic response to cytarabine-induced myelosuppression, the interval recovery of normal marrow may be more rapid than that demonstrated by the AML cells, a factor that should, with successive dosing, result in a cumulative effect—the therapeutic advantage.

Similar changes occur in other proliferative tissues, including the gastrointestinal tract, where drugs cause mitotic arrest with loss of epithelial surface cells, including cells involved in the adsorption of fluids. This requires a recovery period just as the marrow does.[50]

Pharmacokinetics

Pharmacokinetic factors commonly affect the dose–response curve. If an inactivating enzyme for the drug becomes saturated, both toxicity and antitumor effect may increase disproportionately, an effect observed with certain dose schedules of 5-FU.[51,52]

The opposite effect may occur if a drug activation system becomes saturated. Ifosfamide, a pro-drug, is activated by the cytochrome P450, oxygen-dependent, drug-metabolizing enzymes in the liver to the biologically active 4-hydroxyl derivative. The 3-day conventional dose of ifosfamide is higher (1200–2400 mg/m^2 daily) than that for cyclophosphamide (600 mg/m^2) because the rate of P450 activation of ifosfamide is relatively slow. With increasing doses of cyclophosphamide, a constant fractional conversion to active 4-hydroxyl cyclophosphamide occurs. However, for ifosfamide, once the P450 enzyme system becomes saturated, a decreasing proportion of ifosfamide is converted to the active form, with a consequent loss of additional antitumor effect at higher doses.[39]

Clinical trials and the dose effect

Dose selection in patients

Clearance determines the total drug exposure (area under the curve [AUC] of concentration multiplied by time), and AUC in mice correlates with toxicity in that species. This relationship of AUC with drug exposure and toxicity also holds true in humans and can be predicted from mouse data.[53] The process for initial dose selection in Phase I clinical trials is detailed in **Chapter 50**. In most circumstances, the dose is determined in Phase I trials and in other situations is individualized to the body surface area (BSA), weight, or exposure (AUC) of the patient.

The Dubois BSA formula is useful in allometric scaling of drug-dose selection between species. The expectation is that similar adjustments would reduce the variability in clearance between patients and is often used in determining the initial dose in first time in human (FTIH) trials. BSA may be helpful in selecting the dose of cytotoxic agents in childhood leukemia and was subsequently incorporated into standard usage.[54,55] Recent reviews of the literature and of individual institutional experience can find no significant correlation between BSA and clearance variability with investigational or commonly used anticancer drugs except for paclitaxel, oral busulfan, and possibly temozolomide.[56,57]

BSA may correlate with glomerular filtration rate, blood volume, and basal metabolic rate.[56] However, the variability in drug clearance introduced by these factors is small (<25%) compared with that induced by hepatic metabolic enzymes, and there is no correlation between BSA and metabolic activity.[56]

Cytochrome P450 3A4 (family 3, subfamily A, polypeptide 4) is the most prevalent metabolic enzyme in humans and is responsible for more than 55% of drug metabolic clearance.[58] Recent studies utilizing noncancer drugs as indicators of *CYP3A4* metabolic activity, such as midazolam clearance,[59] suggest potential clinical utility with agents that are metabolized by this pathway—for example, docetaxel.[60] Enzymatic pathways are responsible for the clearance of 5-FU and 6-mercaptopurine (6-MP) and for glucuronidation via *UGT1A1* for clearance of SN-38, the active product of irinotecan (see **Chapter 56**). Each of these enzymes has a significant incidence of polymorphisms that affect drug disposition and correlate with toxicity. Persons with the UGT1A1*28 homozygous 7/7 genotype have a reduced capacity for glucuronidation as the major metabolic pathway of SN-38 and higher drug exposure (AUC). Several studies have confirmed a significant correlation between the SN-38 exposure, 1A1*28 genotype, and severe neutropenia and diarrhea.[61] Pharmacogenetic profiling offers the prospect of individualized dose selection in the future and is a frequent component in early clinical drug development. These DNA based tests are commercially available but as of yet do not have widespread clinical use in the United States.

Glomerular filtration rate as estimated from serum creatinine does correlate with toxicity for topotecan, etoposide, and carboplatin. Calculated AUC from serum creatinine (Calvert formula) is now used to dose carboplatin.[55] These alternatives (except for carboplatin AUC dosing) remain under investigation at present, and BSA-based dosing remains the standard of clinical practice for classical chemotherapy agents.

All the molecularly targeted kinase inhibitors approved for clinical use as well as the many more in clinical development are administered as a flat dose with no adjustment for weight or BSA. Dose selection of monoclonal antibodies used in cancer medicine also does not follow a classical dose escalation to toxicity. Receptor occupancy (RO) of a surface glycoprotein target is a quantitative measure of an appropriate dose of agents directed at surface proteins (i.e., anti PD 1 immune checkpoint agents) or depletion of a circulating protein [vascular endothelial growth factor (VEGF) and bevacizumab].

Real-time pharmacokinetics and patient safety

Pharmacokinetic studies provide important information regarding the dose effect. Such studies indicate substantial variation in serum drug levels and in the AUC per given dose. For methotrexate and 6-MP in acute leukemia and for high-dose busulfan and carmustine [bis-chloroethyl nitrosourea (BCNU)] in the transplant setting, the AUC level of drug or its active metabolites (or both) correlates with toxicity and therapeutic effect.[62-65]

Measurement of methotrexate plasma levels after high dose administration (>1 gm/m^2) used in selected settings of acute lymphocytic leukemia (ALL), or diffuse large B-cell lymphoma (DLBCL) are clinically tested and are used to determine the duration and dose of leucovorin rescue in these patients.[66] Substantial variation in the AUC per given dose of paclitaxel was also observed in patients with solid tumors. Real-time adjustment of dose on subsequent days significantly reduced mucositis requiring morphine administration and decreased the duration of hospital stay.[67]

Dose effect in sensitive tumors

Few clinical studies have included dose intensity as an independent, randomized variable. In a Cancer and Leukemia Group B (CALGB) study, 596 patients with AML were randomized to receive four 5-day courses of cytarabine at one of three dose schedules: (1) 100 mg/m^2 daily ("standard arm"); (2) 400 mg/m^2 by continuous infusion; or (3) 3 g/m^2 in a 3-h infusion every 12 h (twice daily) on days 1, 3, and 5.[3] For patients 60 years of age or younger, the probability of remaining in continuous complete remission after four years was 24% in the 100 mg/m^2 group; 29% in the 400 mg/m^2 group; and 44% in the 3 g/m^2 group ($p = 0.002$), indicating a better response with increased dose. Elderly patients were less responsive.

In all, the dose rate of maintenance chemotherapy had a major impact on the duration of response.[68] Similarly, in studies of combination chemotherapy in small-cell lung cancer, the dose effect was significant, albeit with outmoded therapy.[69] Increased doses of anthracycline combined with standard-dose cytarabine in the initial therapy of patients with AML resulted in an increased CR rate and PFS in both young and elderly patients.[70]

Dose—response effects are less well studied in the new kinase inhibitors, which tend to be dosed at the maximum-tolerated daily dose, leaving little opportunity for significant increases. Increasing doses of imatinib in patients with chronic phase or accelerated phase CML and in GIST show an increase in response rate in a subgroup of patients. In cases where resistance to imatinib is due to increased metabolic clearance, increased activity of PgP, or amplification of the *BCR-ABL* gene, this might be expected although responses were seen even in patients with mutations in the *BCR-ABL* kinase itself.[24,25,71,72]

In treating individual patients, dose is a key factor if cure is possible. Thus, for leukemias, lymphomas, testicular cancer, childhood solid tumors, and conventional-dose adjuvant treatment of breast cancer, dose should not be compromised even at the risk of significant toxicity. For more resistant tumors, where palliation is the goal, dose should be adjusted primarily on the basis of toxicity.

Peripheral blood stem cell and marrow transplantation

Allogeneic bone marrow transplantation produces a plateau in disease-free survival (i.e., cures) in patients with acute and chronic leukemias and lymphomas, but because of the effect of graft versus leukemia, the component contributed by dose cannot be independently evaluated.

The most compelling evidence regarding dose–response is in high-dose, autologous stem cell rescue studies in patients with relapsed lymphoma.[73,74] Alkylating agents and total body radiotherapy-based regimens are commonly used because their dose-limiting toxicity is myelosuppression. Depending on the agent, dose can be escalated between 3 and 20 times the baseline level, before nonmyelosuppressive toxicity becomes dose limiting. Given the considerable overlap of AUCs for serum levels of drugs at dose escalations of 2–4 times baseline, the escalations possible with stem cell support allow better comparisons of the effect of dose. High-dose therapy with autologous stem cell rescue produces high complete response rates and cures in non-Hodgkin's lymphoma and testicular cancer.[74,75] Because toxicity can be lethal, high-dose therapy should be limited to specialized centers.[76]

Adjuvant chemotherapy

Randomized studies

Cytokinetics provides an experimental basis for many therapeutic designs. A brief review of the related history follows.

Skipper and colleagues established the fundamental exponential relationship between drug treatment and surviving tumor fractions. It is the fractional tumor cell reduction that is constant for a given dose and drug.[15] Although this exponential relationship is modified by other factors, such as drug resistance and microenvironment, it remains the fundamental tenet of cytokinetics and chemotherapy. Norton and Simon applied Gompertzian theory and analysis to treatment during remission and demonstrated the potentially greater effectiveness of late intensification.[77] Goldie and Coldman introduced the mutation-to-resistance theory, relating tumor burden and inherent mutation rate to potential for cure.[78] Hryniuk and colleagues found a significant dose–response effect not only in the leukemias and lymphomas but also in the relatively less chemosensitive tumors, such as breast cancer.[79–81]

The adjuvant setting, where the tumor burden is microscopic, should be ideal for demonstrating a dose effect. Many factors that could reduce tumor cytotoxicity (tumor size, decreased and abnormal vascularity, low GF, hypoxia, and increased tumor heterogeneity) and contribute to chemotherapy resistance are less evident in the microscopic tumor (adjuvant and neoadjuvant) setting. Combination chemotherapy with cyclophosphamide, methotrexate, and 5-FU or with cyclophosphamide, doxorubicin (Adriamycin), and 5-FU, which produce only transient partial and a few complete responses in metastatic breast cancer, reduce relapse and mortality rates by 20–30% in the adjuvant breast cancer setting.[82] Similar effects are seen in colon cancer.[83]

Attempts to improve disease-free survival by increasing the adjuvant chemotherapy dose in breast cancer have produced mixed results. The first statistically robust positive study was conducted by the CALGB.[19] Patients with node-positive breast cancer were randomized to one of three cyclophosphamide, adriamycin, 5-FU (CAF) regimens. The high-dose arm involved four courses of CAF at doses of 600 cyclophosphamide, 60 doxorubicin, and 600 mg/m^2 5-fluorouracil every 3–4 weeks; in the low-dose arm, the doses were 300, 30, and 300 mg/m^2 respectively. A 10% difference in the relapse-free curve developed by 2 years and persisted through 10 years. That result represents an approximately 20% reduction in mortality. The dose effect was seen most prominently in the 20% of patients whose tumors overexpressed human epidermal growth factor receptor 2 (*ERBB2* or *HER2/neu*). For tumors without *ERBB2* overexpression, no significant dose effect was seen.[20,84,85] This subset effect would not have been identified in the absence of the molecular marker.

Two other studies conducted by the National Surgical Adjuvant Breast and Bowel Project (NSABP) failed to show that a 2- or 4-times increase in the dose of cyclophosphamide alone affected response in terms of relapse or survival in adjuvant breast cancer.[84,85] Thus, in the comparative study of CAF, the dose of doxorubicin was probably important; however, in another study of adjuvant breast cancer, patients randomized to three doses of doxorubicin[86] (60, 75, and 90 mg/m^2, all given with the standard dose of cyclophosphamide) showed no difference in disease-free or overall survival (OS). The 60 mg/m^2 is probably a threshold dose, above which no further benefit accrues.

The basis for the seemingly discordant results of dose in major clinical trials has been the subject of preclinical and mechanism-of-action studies, but it remains unexplained. It can be speculated how often in the analysis of large comparative studies an important effect has been missed within a subset not known to exist at the time. That possibility is an important limitation in the interpretation of negative studies.

Dose-dense chemotherapy

The concept behind dose-dense chemotherapy is to increase the intensity of drug administration by shortening the interval between treatments without increasing the total dose of drug administered. This increase is accomplished by compressing the number of cycles into a shorter period of time. The use of neutrophil-CSF is an essential requirement for dose-dense therapy. Over 30 such trials have been performed in breast cancer but with several variations, including additional drugs that confound the interpretation. A recent meta-analysis of every two weeks versus every three weeks administration of the same drugs (cyclophosphamide, doxorubicin followed by paclitaxel) in the same total dose in a subset of 8 trials reported a modest but significant increase in 10-year disease-free survival (DFS) (4.3%) and OS (2.2%).[87] This report supports the concept of dose-dense intensification as a means to enhance chemotherapy efficacy, albeit at a cost of increased short-term toxicity.[86]

Summary

In the clinic, the effect of dose correlates generally with the basic chemosensitivity of the tumor. Burkitt's lymphoma, ALL, and testicular cancer are all highly sensitive and highly responsive to dose intensity, including achievement of cure. On the other hand, relatively insensitive tumors such as gastrointestinal and lung cancers respond poorly to chemotherapy and are therefore not significantly affected by dose. There are clearly unknown factors at work in the human cancer patient, with the complex milieu of the inherent genetic background in the particular cell type and patient in which cancer arises, the effect of somatic and nontransformed stromal cells, the emerging role of cancer stem cells and other unappreciated factors not accounted for by the reductionist *in vitro* and *in vivo* models on which cancer researchers depend that continue to defy simple explanation.

Schedule of drug administration

Schedule effects of individual agents

Cytarabine

Skipper and colleagues performed elegant, quantitative studies of L1210 mouse leukemia using the prototype cell-cycle phase-specific agent cytarabine.[4,15] Cytarabine was shown to produce optimal therapeutic effects when given in courses of appropriate duration and with intervals that allowed for recovery of normal bone marrow. Extrapolating their work to human AML, the investigators gave patients repeated courses of a continuous infusion for 5–7 days separated by 2–3 weeks for recovery. In patients with AML, this schedule produced a 30–40% complete response rate as compared with 10% for other schedules, such as daily intravenous administration.[4,88,89] The addition of daunorubicin to cytarabine further increased the complete response rate and has become the backbone for remission induction therapy for the treatment of AML in adults for the more than five decades. (For details, see section titled "Cytokinetics of Bone Marrow," earlier in this article.)

Gemcitabine

The dose-limiting toxicity of gemcitabine, a nucleoside analog structurally related to cytarabine, is myelosuppression.[90,91] Gemcitabine, which is 2,2′difluoro-2′deoxy cytidine, resists hydrolysis and has a long intracellular half-life and unlike cytarabine, has activity in solid tumors, particularly in pancreatic, breast, and non-small-cell lung cancer. Weekly or biweekly bolus treatments are well tolerated, with toxicity largely limited to the marrow. Clinically and in experimental animals, gemcitabine given by continuous infusion necessitates a marked reduction in dose, particularly because of myelosuppression, but also because of gastrointestinal toxicity and, in some circumstances, hypotension.[91]

Methotrexate

Intermittent methotrexate (5-day bolus courses every 3–4 weeks), developed by Li and colleagues for gestational choriocarcinoma, proved to be curative.[92] Goldin and colleagues demonstrated in L1210 mouse leukemia that intermittent methotrexate was superior to continuous (daily) methotrexate.[93] In a randomized, comparative study of patients with ALL in complete remission, intermittent methotrexate was significantly superior to daily therapy.[94] This empiric observation is consistent with subsequent findings by Schimke and colleagues, indicating that continuous exposure to methotrexate *in vitro* produces drug resistance more consistently than does intermittent methotrexate.[95] Moreover, with continuous administration, resistance results from gene amplification as compared with a transport defect following intermittent methotrexate.[95,96] The kinetics of bone marrow recovery and mucosal cell replacement, important in cytarabine scheduling, may be important clinical determinants of scheduling with methotrexate as well.

Fluoropyrimidines

In clinical studies, 5-FU may be administered in daily pulse doses of 350–450 mg/m^2 for five days. Using that schedule, myelosuppression is dose limiting. Twice that dose can be delivered by continuous infusion over 2–5 days, in which case mucositis and diarrhea become dose limiting.[97]

Fluorodeoxyuridine (FUDR) is much more toxic when delivered by continuous infusion than by intermittent bolus dosing. For example, daily doses in the range 30–50 mg/m^2 produce toxicity. The biochemical basis for the schedule difference is speculative. Continuous-infusion FUDR may have a greater effect on DNA synthesis; other schedules have a relatively greater effect on host tissue ribonucleic acid (RNA) and RNA synthesis.[97] Data regarding the effect of these differences in schedule on the therapeutic index are few. (Modulation with leucovorin is discussed later in this article.) Longer durations of systemic administration currently are under study.[98]

Capecitabine is an oral prodrug of 5-FU. It has allowed protracted administration with opportunities for increased effectiveness and simplicity of administration. It has not fully supplanted intravenous 5-FU in all indications, as in the folinic acid, fluorouracil, and oxaliplatin (FOLFOX) regimen for colorectal and gastric cancer.[99]

Thus, mechanisms of action, resistance, and cross-resistance for 5-FU appear to differ depending on the analog chosen and the schedule of administration, among other factors.[100]

Alkylating agents

The alkylating agents are a heterogeneous group of compounds that have in common interaction with DNA. This interaction leads to malignant transformation of mammalian cells in culture and to carcinogenesis in patients. The cytotoxic action of these agents is produced by the addition of an alkyl (CH_3) group and/or intra- and inter-strand linkages that impair or prevent DNA replication directly or produce lethal double-stranded breaks if not fully repaired by DNA damage repair mechanisms, which are frequently defective in transformed cells. This mutagenic interaction also explains its teratogenic and carcinogenic potential.

The alkylating agents are of equal potency in terms of preclinical antitumor effect. The difference is primarily host toxicity. This variation in toxicity is particularly true for the dichloroplatinum group of compounds, which closely resemble X-radiation in terms of antitumor effect. They are substantially different in toxicity depending on the nature of the *trans*-adducts. Most experimental data regarding alkylating agents suggest that they are scheduled independent: that is, the antitumor and host effects are dose-related, independent of schedule.[101] (Please see section titled "Pharmacokinetics" and "Adjuvant chemotherapy" earlier in this article for discussions of specific aspects of cyclophosphamide and ifosfamide.)

Anthracyclines

Cardiotoxicity is an important delayed toxicity of anthracyclines. In experimental studies, peak concentrations produced more cardiotoxicity for an equivalent dose than did lower concentrations achieved by continuous infusion schedules. Weiss and Manthel first demonstrated that weekly doxorubicin administration produced less cardiotoxicity per total dose administered than did standard tri-weekly regimens.[102] Legha and colleagues demonstrated that a 4-day, continuous infusion of doxorubicin every three weeks is less cardiotoxic than bolus injections, an observation confirmed in randomized studies.[103–105] Infusion approaches allow a 30–50% increase in total cumulative dose before cardiotoxicity develops. In experimental and preliminary clinical studies, liposomal doxorubicin may be less cardiotoxic than doxorubicin.[106,107] The use of the cardioprotective agent dexrazoxane is current clinical practice in selected settings.[108]

Etoposide

An inhibitor of topoisomerase II that produces DNA double strand breaks, etoposide is selectively active against cells in cycle. Etoposide is commonly used in combination chemotherapy of solid tumors, particularly with cisplatin. Preclinical studies showed that etoposide must be present both during and immediately following cisplatin to achieve optimal effect, consistent with a possible interaction with cisplatin involving inhibition of DNA repair. In small-cell lung cancer, the optimal etoposide dose schedule of three daily doses every three weeks is consistent with the discussion earlier in this article of marrow and tumor cytokinetics and response to cell cycle-specific agents.[109]

Tubulin binders

Although the *Vinca* alkaloids vincristine and vinblastine are cell cycle-specific, no schedule appears superior to standard weekly dosing.[110] On the basis of limited data, the same is true for vinorelbine. Paclitaxel schedule considerations have been dominated by acute histamine-like toxicity, probably related to the vehicle (Cremophor EL); this toxicity is relieved by antihistamines and corticosteroids. Practical and economic considerations favoring outpatient use have resulted in 1- to 3-h intravenous infusions, although some randomized trials suggest an advantage for infusions that are even longer.[111]

Weekly infusions are superior to intermittent administration in breast and ovarian cancer.[112,113] Myelosuppression correlates with the duration of plasma concentrations of paclitaxel above the threshold of 0.1 mol/L.[111] Neutropenia appears to be related more to schedule than to dose, although neuropathy appears dose related.[114]

General use of intermittent dosing

For most chemotherapeutic agents that directly or indirectly target DNA or the mitotic spindle used alone or in combination, intermittent courses (e.g., four 5-day courses every 3–4 weeks) are generally superior to other schedules such as continuous (i.e., daily) dosing. Such is the case for cyclophosphamide and methotrexate in Burkitt's lymphoma, methotrexate, and actinomycin D in choriocarcinoma, melphalan in myeloma, cytarabine in AML, and methotrexate in ALL.[115] It is also true for combination regimens for Hodgkin's disease, ALL, and childhood solid tumors.[110,115,116] In experimental and clinical studies alike, intermittent intensive treatment for rapidly proliferating tumors is superior. The reason may be recruitment of resting G_0/G_1 cells into active cycle. Continuous treatment may be superior for more indolent, low-GF tumors, but more definitive studies are needed.[117]

Advances in supportive care now allow a novel approach to intermittent intensive chemotherapy. Neutrophil CSFs in dose-dense adjuvant breast cancer therapy[118] or leukapheresis following marrow recovery from chemotherapy and treatment with G-CSF allow the harvest of sufficient peripheral blood circulating stem cells to rescue as many as four courses of moderately intensive chemotherapy.[119]

Continuous administration

Protracted infusions (six weeks) of 5-FU combined with local radiotherapy in adjuvant rectal cancer demonstrated both a lower local recurrence rate in the irradiated field and a reduced incidence of metastatic relapse.[120] Capecitabine is an orally absorbable agent that undergoes biotransformation to 5-FU. Prolonged administration over 14 days of capecitabine as a single agent, repeated at 21-day intervals, showed a response rate that is superior to that of intravenous 5-FU and leucovorin, although no survival benefit was noted.[121,122] Capecitabine is also active in refractory breast cancer as monotherapy or in combination. The role of continuous fluoropyrimidine administration with capecitabine is being explored in combination chemotherapy and with radiation. The treatment interruption every three weeks does seem to significantly reduce dose-limiting hand-foot syndrome toxicity with capecitabine.

Targeted inhibitors

For reasons related to the mechanism of action, continuous oral administration of many new targeted therapies, particularly kinase inhibitors such as imatinib in CML and in GIST, is the current clinical schedule.[117,123] The continued suppression of proliferative growth factor signals and interruption of survival pathway signals in tumor cells or the repair of DNA appears necessary in the clinic and in preclinical models. This is the case for the poly (ADP-ribose) polymerase (PARP) inhibitor rucaparib.[124] One clinical trial of a randomized discontinuation of the multi-targeted tyrosine kinase inhibitor sorafenib in renal cell cancer patients with stable disease demonstrated a significant progression-free survival advantage at six months for patients who continued to receive sorafenib versus placebo, which supports the preclinical modeling in the clinic.[125]

This default approach has come under reconsideration. For some agents, such as sunitinib or alpelisib, intermittent schedules are used because of better tolerance, similar to the DNA damaging agents and mitotic spindle inhibitors.[126,127] EGFR targeted agents erlotinib and afatinib have been given intermittently at much higher doses to achieve efficacious concentrations in the brain to treat metastases or to target the T790M drug-resistant mutant enzyme.[128,129] In experimental models, intermittent schedules delay the emergence of resistant disease.[130,131]

Immune checkpoint inhibitors

Monoclonal antibodies targeting immune checkpoints exert their antitumor effects via host immunity as opposed to direct cytotoxic activity, and thereby require a different approach to dosing and schedule determination. These agents are described in more detail in other sections of this volume, but they are mentioned here to highlight the difference. As previously described, the dose–response and dose-toxicity relationship of immune checkpoint inhibitors (ICIs) are inconsistent at best. Traditional dose-finding studies such as maximum tolerated dose (MTD) are not appropriate. There are currently seven FDA-approved ICIs for various indications; ipilimumab, pembrolizumab, nivolumab, atezolizumab, avelumab, durvalumab, and cemiplimab. None of these agents reached an MTD in their Phase 1 evaluation.[132] Modeling of host–immune responses is an additional challenge in preclinical dose evaluation. Target occupancy considerations are paramount in dose-determination, with schedules favoring continuous dosing and target occupancy, without the need for cytotoxic recovery. Early approvals of body-weight-based dosing for nivolumab, pembrolizumab, avelumab, and durvalumab led to updates with flat-dosing approvals.[133]

Combination chemotherapy

Rationale

The most compelling rationales for combination chemotherapy are (1) tumor cell heterogeneity and its implication for drug resistance, and (2) the success of combination chemotherapy in the clinic. In practical clinical terms, the selection of specific combinations in particular types of cancer depends on the individual activity of the agents in the target cancer type and the absence of overlapping toxicities. The agents with the highest single-agent activity are preferred, particularly agents that produce complete responses (if any such agents exist), with different mechanisms of action to address the theoretical heterogeneity issue.

Combination chemotherapy in the clinic

Ample clinical precedent exists for using multiple agents. An example is the treatment of ALL in children, where multiple active agents have been identified. A direct correlation is seen between the number of agents used and the cure rate (Table 2). In fact, essentially all curative chemotherapy involves combinations of two and usually three or more agents (Table 3). Curative combinations need not incorporate each agent at each dosing encounter, as the sequential use of taxanes after doxorubicin and cyclophosphamide in breast cancer or in pediatric soft tissue cancers, but within a patient's total treatment course. Normal tissue tolerance often limits the number of agents that can be administered at one time.

Current studies have demonstrated evidence for synergy or an additive effect between established DNA/mitotic spindle targeted chemotherapeutic agents and agents representing other classes. Molecularly targeted agents, whether monoclonal antibodies or small molecules, have been combined with cytotoxic agents as well as with other targeted agents. Trastuzumab, a monoclonal antibody to *ERBB2*, is synergistic with doxorubicin and paclitaxel. *ERBB2* is present on the cancer cell surface in 25% of patients with breast cancer and benefit is restricted to only those patients with amplification of the *ERBB2* gene.[134] Toxicities may be substantial, however. Trastuzumab in combination with doxorubicin increased cardiotoxicity. A lesser risk of cardiotoxicity exists when trastuzumab is included in paclitaxel combinations. The addition of a complement-fixing monoclonal antibody, rituximab, to cyclophosphamide, doxorubicin, vincristine, and prednisone (CHOP) chemotherapy in non-Hodgkin's lymphoma increases response and OS without an increase in toxicity. The addition of the mechanistic target of rapamycin (mTOR) inhibitor everolimus to an aromatase inhibitor (AI) markedly prolongs the progression-free survival (PFS) in estrogen receptor-dependent metastatic breast cancer.[135] The addition of the CDK 4/6 inhibitor to an AI increases the OS in estrogen receptor (ER) positive breast cancer.[136] This compatibility of new and old is not to be assumed, since combinations of cytotoxic chemotherapy with both erlotinib and gefitinib fail to produce significant benefit in lung cancer.[137]

The combination of multiple targets in a single molecule can be incorporated into novel molecularly targeted agents. Certainly, multiple targets within a single small molecule, such as vascular endothelial growth factor receptor (VEGFR) and platelet-derived growth factor receptor (PDGFR), in the angiogenesis pathways produces greater clinical benefit than targeting either alone, as the success, limited as it may be, of single-agent cabozantinib or axitinib demonstrate *viz a viz* single agent, including bevacizumab and many failed compounds limited to VEGFR2 alone.[11,138]

Multiple agents can be directed at a single target protein or to sequential proteins in a single pathway essential to the neoplastic process. Combining the monoclonal antibodies trastuzumab and pertuzumab, which bind to different epitopes of the ERBB2 receptor, produces unprecedented OS in ERBB2-expressing metastatic breast cancer.[139] Sequential inhibition of BRAF and mitogen-activated protein kinase (MEK) in BRAF^{V600E} melanoma produces high rates of response, PFS and OS.[10] All-*trans*-retinoic acid and arsenic trioxide interact with the PML protein in acute pro-granulocytic leukemia cells with resultant differentiation and durable remission.[140]

Technology has reached a point where a monoclonal antibody can be conjugated to a small molecule to deliver therapy in a highly selective manner, such as the T-DMI conjugate of trastuzumab and auristatin in breast cancer or radioactive yttrium to antiCD30 in Hodgkin's lymphoma.[141,142]

Tumor cell heterogeneity and drug resistance

Tumors are clonal in origin, but the increasing DNA instability that accompanies the onset of neoplasia leads to increased variation in the daughter cells, called "clonal evolution" to tumor cell heterogeneity. This evolution is associated with selection for progeny with greater survival capacity, which is evident as higher

Table 3 Cancer chemotherapy-number of agents required for cure by tumor type.

Tumor	Number of agents required for cure	Adjuvant or neoadjuvant	Number of agents required for cure
Acute lymphoblastic leukemia (children)	4–7	Wilms tumor	2–3
Gestational choriocarcinoma[a]		Embryonal rhabdosarcoma	2–3
Early	1–3	Osteogenic sarcoma	3
Advanced	2–4	Soft tissue sarcoma	3
Acute myeloid leukemia	3+	Ovarian cancer	3–4
Testicular cancer	3	Breast cancer	2–4
Burkitt lymphoma[b]	1–4	Colorectal cancer	2
Hodgkin disease	4–5	Non-small-cell lung carcinoma, stage IIIA	2
Diffuse histiocytic lymphoma	4–5	Small-cell lung carcinoma, limited	2–4

[a]One agent is curative, but a higher cure rate results with two or more agents.
[b]One agent cures state 1 African Burkitt lymphoma, but two or more agents are better.

proliferative capacity, resistance to apoptosis, greater metastatic or invasive potential, reduced dependence on normal cellular growth factors, and angiogenesis.[143] Heterogeneity among tumor cells increases the number and diversity of potential target sites for chemotherapy and the need to combine therapeutic agents.

Initially, resistance was thought to be limited to the selecting agent (mono-drug resistance). The recognition of multidrug resistance required a reexamination of this rationale for combination chemotherapy.[144] The ABC family of transport proteins such as (ABCB1, PgP), the multidrug resistance proteins (ABCC1), and the breast cancer-related protein (ABCG2) confer multidrug resistance that relates almost exclusively to natural products. Prolonged exposure to low doses of substrate drugs such as doxorubicin may overcome resistance mediated by these transport proteins.[145] However, glutathione transferase, DNA repair capacity, and topoisomerase II alterations also may be associated with multidrug resistance.[146]

Recent studies of multicellular drug resistance indicate an altered set point for apoptosis.[147] Differences between in vitro and in vivo drug resistance are modifying the approach to combination chemotherapy.[148] Although prolonged drug exposure results in stable, resistant cell lines, acute exposure may induce short-term, reversible resistance. There is emerging evidence implicating epigenetic histone modification of protein expression as a sole or intermediate state linking short-term resistance mechanistically to the long-term, genetic, resistance.[149]

The advent of molecular profiling of patient tumors as a clinical means of treatment selection continues to emphasize the heterogeneity that exists within a single tumor at a single point in time but also the variability that occurs over time in a single tumor and the heterogeneity that exists in a single point in time in different metastases in the same patient. New treatment algorithms are being developed to address this complex problem. (Please see **Chapters 49** and **50** for a more detailed discussion.)

Cytokinetics

The discovery that solid tumors contain a large number of potentially clonogenic cells in G_1 or G_0—presumably because of tumor hypoxia and a low GF—provided a basis for combination chemotherapy.[28,29,35] Thus, cell cycle-specific agents were employed to kill mitotically active cells, and non-cell cycle-specific agents (for example, alkylating agents) were added to damage the noncycling tumor cells. The use of repeated cycles allows normal tissues to recover, so that dose need not be compromised, and G_0/G_1 tumor cells can be recruited into the proliferating fraction by increased availability of nutrients, oxygen, and vascular access.

Synchronization

Synchronization of tumor or normal cells in vitro and in vivo with drugs that inhibit DNA synthesis or that arrest cells in mitosis can be achieved. Experimentally, the most impressive synchronization has been achieved with hormonal agents that affect tumor, but not essential normal cells.

Some degree of tumor-cell synchrony follows this hormonal manipulation in experimental studies but the heterogeneity of human tumors with regard to the time course of recruitment and synchronization has limited this approach, and it remains investigational.[150,151]

Modulation

Agents that are nontoxic may still improve the therapeutic index of an established chemotherapeutic agent, either by reducing normal tissue toxicity—as leucovorin does for methotrexate, for example—or by preferentially enhancing antitumor efficacy—as 5-FU and leucovorin do in metastatic and adjuvant colon cancer studies.[152-158]

Biochemically, the product of 5-FU, fluorodeoxyuridine monophosphate (FdUMP), binds to the substrate site of thymidylate synthase (TS), thus inhibiting DNA synthesis and, therefore, cellular replication. The stability and duration of this inhibition directly relate to a third agent, 5,10-methylenetetrahydrofolate, which is a metabolic product of leucovorin that also binds to TS, producing the so-called ternary complex (FdUMP—TS—5,10-methylenetetrahydrofolate). In preclinical systems, in vitro and in vivo alike, leucovorin favorably modulated the therapeutic index of 5-FU. A number of clinical trials comparing 5-FU to 5-FU with leucovorin indicated an advantage for 5-FU/leucovorin in patients with metastatic colorectal cancer at a cost of only moderately increased mucositis and diarrhea. The combination of 5-FU with leucovorin improved survival rates in two separate studies in metastatic and adjuvant colon cancers.[157,158]

Bevacizumab (Avastin) is a monoclonal antibody that depletes serum VEGF. VEGF is an essential mitogenic and antiapoptotic factor for endothelial cells (see **Chapter 16**). Signaling through the VEGF receptor 2 kinase-insert domain-containing receptor (KDR) and platelet-derived growth factor receptor beta (PDGFRB) act to increase endothelial cell permeability, which results in increased interstitial fluid pressure (IFP) within tumors. In colon, breast, lung, head and neck, cervix, and skin carcinomas, the IFP is significantly higher than in normal tissues.[159-162] Increased tumor IFP acts as a barrier for tumor transvascular transport; reduction of tumor IFP, or modulation of microvascular pressure, increases the transvascular transport of tumor-targeting antibodies or low molecular weight tracer compounds.[163,164] Growing evidence indicates that the PDGFRB and KDR tyrosine kinases play a crucial role in increased tumor IFP. That makes them candidate targets for pharmacologic intervention for tumor interstitial hypertension[165-168] and for a novel, possibly general, combination strategy that will enhance the therapeutic effects of standard chemotherapeutics. Bevacizumab reduced the IFP in patients with advanced colorectal cancer and increases the uptake of gadolinium in the tumors. Combined with irinotecan, 5-FU, and leucovorin, bevacizumab produces a significant prolongation of survival in patients with metastatic colorectal cancer.[169] This modulation of IFP occurs only within tumors and provides a selective increase in drug levels to the tumor without increasing host toxicity, as was noted in the latter two studies. Those findings offer a general treatment strategy for solid tumors of any type.

Bevacizumab (and similar agents) combined with cytotoxic chemotherapy has shown improvements in PFS and OS in many-though not all types of cancer. Given the many mechanisms of VEGF action, it is uncertain which mechanisms mediate this effect. That VEGF—targeted therapy is more effective in combination, concurrent or sequential, than as a single agent denotes it as a modulator in most clinical circumstances.

Implications of drug resistance

Tumor cell heterogeneity in response to the potentially cytotoxic and antiproliferative effects of cancer chemotherapeutic agents has been the stimulus for a current novel approach to combination chemotherapy. Avoiding therapeutic resistance has been from the beginning a major rationale for combination chemotherapy.

Initial observations about resistance involved reduced drug levels at the site of action because of increased efflux, alteration or amplification of the target, and cellular inactivation.

Recent investigations have focused on mechanisms of drug sensitivity or resistance operative after interaction of the drug and its target receptor, including apoptosis (programmed cell death). The cell damage caused by various chemotherapeutic agents has the common property of triggering the apoptosis cascade in an active process that requires energy, enzymes, and cytostructure for completion.[170] In addition to apoptosis, under certain circumstances cells undergo necrotic cell death due to drug-induced depletion of adenosine 5′-triphosphate (ATP).[171] Finally, autophagy, a highly conserved process of cell survival under conditions of nutrient and or oxygen deprivation can lead to a previously unappreciated form of drug resistance following treatment with cytotoxic drugs, hormonal agents, and radiation.[172] Drug resistance must always be viewed in the context of therapeutic index. Resistance fundamentally means there exists no selective cancer cytotoxicity in relation to toxicity in the cancer-bearing host. This may be present at the outset or become apparent only during therapy. This narrow or lack of therapeutic index is present in most cancer therapeutic agents.

Reversal of drug resistance

Another approach to modulation involves reversal of drug resistance, the most studied of which is multidrug resistance mediated by PgP. Verapamil and several other lipid-soluble heterocyclic drugs, including cyclosporine analogs, can inhibit PgP and thus reduce the efflux of a number of natural antitumor products (doxorubicin, vincristine, taxanes, and others) from the cell, thereby increasing cytotoxicity. PgP is increased in B-cell tumors, AML, sarcoma, and tumors previously treated with drugs that led to multidrug resistance.[173] This approach has not yet produced significant clinical benefit in clinical trials or practice.

Molecular biology/targeted therapy

Implications for dose and schedule

The level of optimism among researchers has increased substantially as a result of the recent "proof of concept" regarding the clinical effectiveness of more targeted therapies. Evidence for unique molecular targets in cancer cells (e.g., fusion genes, mutations, recombinations) and on their surfaces has led to synthesis of small molecules and monoclonal antibodies with a target specificity achieved only rarely in cancer therapeutics.[174–176]

Table 1 presents a sampling of combinations of molecules and biochemical pathways that are currently being evaluated as targets for selective antitumor agents. The magnitude of such activity and the number of active agents in preclinical systems offer remarkable opportunities for the use of agents in combination. The cumulative effect of these agents on a molecular level suggests an interaction that may result from the diversity of target interaction and a sequential or simultaneous attack on critical cell behavior.

Another important area of diversity relates to anticipated toxicity. Thus, as compared with classical chemotherapy agents, where dose-delineating toxicity usually relates to proliferating tissues and is relatively uniform, the molecular biologic agents will almost certainly express toxicity that varies from agent to agent and that largely differs from the classical antitumor agents. Molecular agents are under extensive study not only for their antitumor properties but also most particularly for their interaction with each other and with other established antitumor agents.

Experimental models of combination therapy

The classical antitumor agents are limited largely to those that directly or indirectly produce DNA damage; the products of the molecular biology era markedly extend the diversity of target mechanisms. Indeed, using experimental models, a number of interesting preclinical experiments have demonstrated an additive or synergistic effect. The literature on preclinical models and computer analysis has been reviewed by Rideout and Chou.[177]

The future of combination chemotherapy will be influenced substantially by the number of these compounds and their interactions. The strategy of combining drugs whose mechanisms of action vary has been successful, even in the curative treatment of hematologic, childhood, and embryonal neoplasms.

The terms "additive" and "synergistic" are commonly used in the clinic, but they are not well defined. In considering these terms, selectivity for the tumor as compared to the host—the *therapeutic index*—is key. If two agents with additive therapeutic effect have a differing dose-limiting toxicity, so that the toxicity is nonadditive, the overall antitumor effect should be described as additive. When the effects are greater than "additive," the term "synergism" may be appropriate.

Table 4 presents the properties and comparisons of combination chemotherapy and combined modality therapy. Incorporation of many more classes of agents will force more efficient experimental designs. Such designs may include, for example, a rolling Phase II/Phase III study design. Increasingly, quantitative molecular markers and "real-time" pharmacology will be integrated operationally into clinical studies. The effectiveness of such related approaches should improve the efficiency and effectiveness of clinical trials.

Table 4 Combination chemotherapy versus holotherapy.

Combination	Chemotherapy	Holotherapy
Diversity of agents	Drawn from one class, antiproliferative	Drawn from all classes[a]
Number of agents	2–5	4–12+
Toxicity	Bone marrow and gastrointestinal (steep dose), cardiac, neuralgic, pulmonary	Major diversity, including that relative to dose and toxicity; toxicity commonly nonadditive; limited, greated selection
Experimental design of clinical trials	Rigid, establishment	Flexible, innovative, semi-Bayesian; patient participation
Endpoints	Classical; R, dR, DFS, OS	MRT
Integration with basic science	Limited	Extensive, operational; PK, PD; targets

[a]Chemotherapy, immunotherapy, endocrinology, antiangiogenesis, antimatrix, gene therapy, control of cell cycle [anticyclins (CDK family), transcriptional control, antisense].
Abbreviations: DFS, disease-free survival; dR, duration of response; MRT, microbeam radiation therapy; OS, overall survival; PD, pharmacodynamics; PK, pharmacokinetics; R, response (partial or complete).

Table 5 Therapeutic interaction between agents of different classes.

Agent	Cancer acted on
Chemotherapy + other systemic agent	
Chemo + immunotherapy	
Cisplatin + hepceptin	Breast cancer
Taxol + herceptin	Breast cancer
CHOP + rituximab	Lymphoma
Chemotherapy→MRT→recovery of immunity→vaccine	
Minitransplant chemotherapy followed by allogeneic armed lymphocyte	
Chemotherapy + hormonal therapy	
Vincristine + prednisone	Acute lymphocytic leukemia
Chemotherapy + tamoxifen	Breast cancer
Chemotherapy + differentiation agent	
Daunorubicin + ATRA	Acute progranulocytic leukemia
Chemotherapy + antiangiogenesis	
IFL + bevacizumab	Colorectal cancer

Abbreviations: ATRA, all-*trans*-retinoic acid; IFL, irinotecan/5-fluorouracil/leucovorin; MRT, microbean radiation therapy.

Oncogenes and tumor-suppressor genes may operate by modifying or exploiting abnormalities in the cell cycle, by interfering with growth factors, angiogenesis, and DNA repair. Identification of the specific genes or gene pathways driving cancer in a particular patient by tumor profiling will allow identification of the precise agents most likely to be effective in that patient, with the goal of personalizing cancer therapy.

An integrated approach to cancer chemotherapy

More than a half-century has elapsed since cancer chemotherapy began. The chemotherapy agents now in use originated as biologically targeted therapy. Hitchings and Elion developed specific inhibitors of purine synthesis such as 6-MP and 6-thioguanine (6-TG); Heidelberger targeted RNA synthesis with 5-FU; and Farber targeted the reduced folate pathway with aminopterin. These innovations not only provided the groundwork for cancer treatment, but they also became tools for discovery of the basic workings of transformed cancer cells.

Natural products such as the *Vinca* alkaloids, anthracyclines, and taxanes were selected specifically for activity against cancer proliferation. These agents were combined with other classes of agents—for example, hormones, alkylating agents, and irradiation—that are active against proliferating cells. The optimal use of the new agents requires their integration into increasingly complex combinations so that a greater therapeutic index results. The same is true for the current classical chemotherapeutic agents, which largely inhibit proliferation.

Molecular biology has expanded the classes of cancer therapeutics. Thus, hormones, immunotoxins, signal transduction inhibitors, and inhibitors of invasion and metastasis are available in addition to the classical antiproliferation and DNA damaging compounds. Receptors and kinases of unique structure and quantity, capable of targeting with specific molecular agents, continue to be discovered and the pathways activated in cancer further elucidated. Outside the scope of this article, immune checkpoint therapy has added an entire new dimension to cancer therapeutics. Decades of cancer drug development have not been erased by these new agents and combinations of immune checkpoint agents and cancer chemotherapy are superior to either modality alone.[178,179]

The vast majority of cancers will be treated successfully only with combinations of agents chosen for the highest possible individual activity against a specific type of cancer. Empiricism was an essential component in the development of contemporary cancer therapy, but rational drug discovery, analog development, preclinical modeling, precise pathologic diagnosis, careful staging of disease, and clinical trial design are the foundation for the measure of success known today.

The breakthroughs in molecular biology have presented the oncologists with enormous opportunities and challenges. Based on these breakthroughs, a molecular diagnosis will be able not only to determine where and how cancer originates but also the processes that are essential to its survival. The specific processes that initiate and propagate cancer have become the targets of unprecedented rational drug development (see Table 1). Pharmaceutical technology provides not only small molecules, but also monoclonal antibodies, immunoconjugates, ribozymes, antisense RNA, and recombinant viruses.

The therapy of cancer now has the potential to combine agents with even more mechanisms of action to confront the heterogeneity of cancer with a wider array of therapeutics. Some of these combinations are now the standard of care, as improvements in response and survival demonstrate (see Table 4). The challenges to be overcome include (1) clinical development of cytostatic agents without the expectation of significant acute toxicity; (2) combining of classes of targeted agents (see Table 5) both molecular and biologic, with regard to dose and schedule; and (3) selection of the appropriate types of cancer and individual patients for a specific therapy.

With molecular biology playing an increasing role, the clinical and laboratory sciences that address the therapy of cancer will continue to accelerate toward cancer control.

Key references

The complete reference list can be found on Vital Source version of this title, see inside front cover.

1. Frei E 3rd, Canellos GP. Dose: a critical factor in cancer chemotherapy. *Am J Med*. 1980;**69**(4):585–594.
2. Menon-Andersen D, Yu B, Madabushi R, et al. Essential pharmacokinetic information for drug dosage decisions: a concise visual presentation in the drug label. *Clin Pharmacol Ther*. 2011;**90**(3):471–474.
4. Skipper HE, Schabel FM Jr, Wilcox WS. Experimental evaluation of potential anticancer agents. XXI. Scheduling of arabinosylcytosine to take advantage of its S-phase specificity against leukemia cells. *Cancer Chemother Rep*. 1967;**51**(3):125–165.
6. Frei E 3rd., Curative cancer chemotherapy. *Cancer Res*. 1985;**45**(12 Pt 1): 6523–6537.
10. Robert C, Karaszewska B, Schachter J, et al. Improved overall survival in melanoma with combined dabrafenib and trametinib. *N Engl J Med*. 2015;**372**(1):30–39.
12. Soria J-C, Ohe Y, Vansteenkiste J, et al. Osimertinib in untreated EGFR-mutated advanced non–small-cell lung cancer. *N Engl J Med*. 2017;**378**(2):113–125.

18. Bonadonna G. Karnofsky memorial lecture. Conceptual and practical advances in the management of breast cancer. *J Clin Oncol*. 1989;**7**(10):1380–1397.
19. Wood WC, Budman DR, Korzun AH, et al. Dose and dose intensity of adjuvant chemotherapy for stage II, node-positive breast carcinoma. *N Engl J Med*. 1994;**330**(18):1253–1259.
24. Zonder JA, Pemberton P, Brandt H, et al. The effect of dose increase of imatinib mesylate in patients with chronic or accelerated phase chronic myelogenous leukemia with inadequate hematologic or cytogenetic response to initial treatment. *Clin Cancer Res*. 2003;**9**(6):2092–2097.
26. Braun TP, Eide CA, Druker BJ. Response and resistance to BCR-ABL1-targeted therapies. *Cancer Cell*. 2020;**37**(4):530–542.
43. Engelman JA, Janne PA. Mechanisms of acquired resistance to epidermal growth factor receptor tyrosine kinase inhibitors in non-small cell lung cancer. *Clin Cancer Res*. 2008;**14**(10):2895–2899.
53. Baker SD, Verweij J, Rowinsky EK, et al. Role of body surface area in dosing of investigational anticancer agents in adults, 1991–2001. *J Natl Cancer Inst*. 2002;**94**(24):1883–1888.
54. Pinkel D. The use of body surface area as a criterion of drug dosage in cancer chemotherapy. *Cancer Res*. 1958;**18**(7):853–856.
66. Green MR, Chowdhary S, Lombardi KM, et al. Clinical utility and pharmacology of high-dose methotrexate in the treatment of primary CNS lymphoma. *Expert Rev Neurother*. 2006;**6**(5):635–652.
68. Pinkel D, Hernandez K, Borella L, et al. Drug dosage and remission duration in childhood lymphocytic leukemia. *Cancer*. 1971;**27**(2):247–256.
74. Philip T, Guglielmi C, Hagenbeek A, et al. Autologous bone marrow transplantation as compared with salvage chemotherapy in relapses of chemotherapy-sensitive non-Hodgkin's lymphoma. *N Engl J Med*. 1995;**333**(23):1540–1545.
77. Norton L, Simon R. The Norton-Simon hypothesis revisited. *Cancer Treat Rep*. 1986;**70**(1):163–169.
78. Goldie JH, Coldman AJ. A mathematic model for relating the drug sensitivity of tumors to their spontaneous mutation rate. *Cancer Treat Rep*. 1979;**63**(11–12):1727–1733.
86. Citron ML, Berry DA, Cirrincione C, et al. Randomized trial of dose-dense versus conventionally scheduled and sequential versus concurrent combination chemotherapy as postoperative adjuvant treatment of node-positive primary breast cancer: first report of Intergroup Trial C9741/Cancer and Leukemia Group B Trial 9741. *J Clin Oncol*. 2003;**21**(8):1431–1439.
97. Seifert P, Baker LH, Reed ML, et al. Comparison of continuously infused 5-fluorouracil with bolus injection in treatment of patients with colorectal adenocarcinoma. *Cancer*. 1975;**36**(1):123–128.
111. ten Bokkel Huinink WW, Eisenhauer E, Swenerton K. Preliminary evaluation of a multicenter, randomized comparative study of TAXOL (paclitaxel) dose and infusion length in platinum-treated ovarian cancer. Canadian-European Taxol Cooperative Trial Group. *Cancer Treat Rev*. 1993;(19 Suppl C):79–86.
115. Wolfrom C, Hartmann R, Fengler R, et al. Randomized comparison of 36-hour intermediate-dose versus 4-hour high-dose methotrexate infusions for remission induction in relapsed childhood acute lymphoblastic leukemia. *J Clin Oncol*. 1993;**11**(5):827–833.
117. Heinrich MC, Corless CL, Demetri GD, et al. Kinase mutations and imatinib response in patients with metastatic gastrointestinal stromal tumor. *J Clin Oncol*. 2003;**21**(23):4342–4349.
121. Hoff PM, Ansari R, Batist G, et al. Comparison of oral capecitabine versus intravenous fluorouracil plus leucovorin as first-line treatment in 605 patients with metastatic colorectal cancer: results of a randomized phase III study. *J Clin Oncol*. 2001;**19**(8):2282–2292.
123. Joensuu H, Roberts PJ, Sarlomo-Rikala M, et al. Effect of the tyrosine kinase inhibitor STI571 in a patient with a metastatic gastrointestinal stromal tumor. *N Engl J Med*. 2001;**344**(14):1052–1056.
125. Ratain MJ, Eisen T, Stadler WM, et al. Phase II placebo-controlled randomized discontinuation trial of sorafenib in patients with metastatic renal cell carcinoma. *J Clin Oncol*. 2006;**24**(16):2505–2512.
129. How J, Mann J, Laczniak AN, et al. Pulsatile erlotinib in EGFR-positive non-small-cell lung cancer patients with leptomeningeal and brain metastases: review of the literature. *Clin Lung Cancer*. 2017;**18**(4):354–363.
132. Sheng J, Sanghavi K, Liang Y, et al. Abstract 4120: dose selection and dosing optimization of immune checkpoint inhibitors. *Cancer Res*. 2019;**79**(13 Supplement):4120.
135. Baselga J, Campone M, Piccart M, et al. Everolimus in postmenopausal hormone-receptor-positive advanced breast cancer. *N Engl J Med*. 2012;**366**(6):520–529.
138. Li W, Feng C, Di W, et al. Clinical use of vascular endothelial growth factor receptor inhibitors for the treatment of renal cell carcinoma. *Eur J Med Chem*. 2020;**200**:112482.
139. Swain SM, Baselga J, Kim SB, et al. Pertuzumab, trastuzumab, and docetaxel in HER2-positive metastatic breast cancer. *N Engl J Med*. 2015;**372**(8):724–734.
147. Fisher DE. Apoptosis in cancer therapy: crossing the threshold. *Cell*. 1994;**78**(4):539–542.
148. Teicher BA, Herman TS, Holden SA, et al. Tumor resistance to alkylating agents conferred by mechanisms operative only in vivo. *Science*. 1990;**247**(4949 Pt 1):1457–1461.
155. Ginsberg SJ, Anderson JR, Gottlieb AJ, et al. A randomized trial of high-dose methotrexate versus standard-dose methotrexate following cyclophosphamide, doxorubicin (adriamycin), vincristine, and prednisone with or without bleomycin in the therapy of diffuse large cell lymphoma: preliminary report of Cancer and Leukemia Group B Study 7851. *NCI Monogr*. 1987;**5**:77–80.
163. Netti PA, Hamberg LM, Babich JW, et al. Enhancement of fluid filtration across tumor vessels: implication for delivery of macromolecules. *Proc Natl Acad Sci U S A*. 1999;**96**(6):3137–3142.
167. Pietras K, Ostman A, Sjoquist M, et al. Inhibition of platelet-derived growth factor receptors reduces interstitial hypertension and increases transcapillary transport in tumors. *Cancer Res*. 2001;**61**(7):2929–2934.
171. Zong WX, Ditsworth D, Bauer DE, et al. Alkylating DNA damage stimulates a regulated form of necrotic cell death. *Genes Dev*. 2004;**18**(11):1272–1282.
173. Dalton WS, Grogan TM, Meltzer PS, et al. Drug-resistance in multiple myeloma and non-Hodgkin's lymphoma: detection of P-glycoprotein and potential circumvention by addition of verapamil to chemotherapy. *J Clin Oncol*. 1989;**7**(4):415–424.
177. Chou T-C, Rideout DC. *Synergism and Antagonism in Chemotherapy*. San Diego, CA: Academic Press; 1991.
178. Burtness B, Harrington KJ, Greil R, et al. Pembrolizumab alone or with chemotherapy versus cetuximab with chemotherapy for recurrent or metastatic squamous cell carcinoma of the head and neck (KEYNOTE-048): a randomised, open-label, phase 3 study. *Lancet*. 2019;**394**(10212):1915–1928.

52 Pharmacology of small-molecule anticancer agents

Zahra Talebi, PharmD ■ *Sharyn D. Baker, PharmD, PhD* ■ *Alex Sparreboom, PhD*

> **Overview**
>
> The biology and clinical indications relevant to systemic anticancer therapies are covered extensively in other articles in this encyclopedia. In this article, we will focus on the principles of clinical pharmacology as they apply to systemic anticancer therapies and will attempt to illustrate how an understanding of clinical pharmacokinetics and pharmacodynamics can optimize the therapeutic index of these agents.

Introduction

There have been drastic changes in our comprehension of cancer pharmacology in recent years along with an improved understanding of cancer biology and the advent of newly developed drugs that can specifically target cancer cells.[1] Depending on the stage and characteristics of tumors, pharmacotherapy can be used in three basic modalities in disease management. While almost one-third of patients with localized tumors can be managed with local treatment strategies, such as surgery or radiotherapy, in the remaining cases, early micrometastasis is a typical event, which requires a systemic approach with chemotherapy to effectively combat cancer. *Primary* chemotherapy using chemotherapy as the approach of choice in systemic diseases when no alternative treatments are available or subsequently suitable even with tumor response, such as in hematologic malignancies or advanced metastatic cancers. In advanced cancers, chemotherapy is aimed to reduce tumor burden and improve quality of life, while in some hematological cancers, such as Hodgkin's and non-Hodgkin's lymphoma, primary chemotherapy can be curative. Chemotherapy alone can be used either as *induction* therapy or in some cancers like leukemia may be administered over prolonged periods of time as *continuation* therapy after induction regimens. However, in most cases of cancers, chemotherapy is combined with radiotherapy and/or surgery. In cancers such as anal cancer, bladder cancer, breast cancer, and esophageal cancer, chemotherapy is administered as *neoadjuvant* before the surgery to ensure optimal resection of the localized tumor. In patients with breast cancer, colon cancer, gastric cancer, NCSLC, Wilms' tumor, anaplastic astrocytoma, and osteogenic sarcoma, chemotherapy is used after surgical interventions as *adjuvant* therapy to reduce the chance of recurrence and improve overall survival.[2,3]

Anticancer drugs can be categorized into three major classes: cytotoxics, biologics, and small-molecule noncytotoxics. This section is aimed to discuss pharmacologic concepts of relevance to small-molecule chemotherapeutic agents, with biologic anticancers being discussed in a different section. A summary of presumed mechanism of action and examples of cytotoxic and small-molecule noncytotoxic chemotherapeutic anticancers are presented in Table 1. It should be noted that in the case of kinase inhibitors, although several targets are identified, the exact mechanism by which the drugs exert their effects are largely unknown. For example, while regorafenib has the potential to inhibit multiple tyrosine kinases with relatively high affinity, the exact mechanism by which it prolongs survival in chemotherapy-refractory metastatic colorectal cancer remains to be fully understood.[4]

Despite the major therapeutic successes achieved by chemotherapeutic drugs and the fast-growing market of newly approved agents, they often have a narrow therapeutic index and great potential for causing harmful effects, suggesting the need for precision in administration and dosing of these drugs to ensure optimal therapeutic results.[1] The ideal dosing scheme for anticancer therapy should maximize efficacy while minimizing the potential for severe toxicities and pharmacokinetic variability between patients. With few exceptions, cytotoxic therapies are typically dosed by body surface area for historical reasons, even though height and weight are not the only variables that influence pharmacokinetic variability.[5] Biologics are typically dosed by weight, and small-molecule noncytotoxics are typically administered in a fixed dose for all patients. As the magnitude of antitumor response is assumed to be a function of the concentration of the drug, traditional phase I trials use dose–escalation designs to determine the maximum tolerated dose (MTD), which is the dose immediately below that which caused a prespecified rate of dose-limiting toxicity in an attempt to maximize efficacy.[6] However, this conventional dosing approach is considered suboptimal since for one it does not consider the sources of interpatient variability in efficacy and safety. Furthermore, the maximum efficacy for biologics and small-molecule noncytotoxics can often be achieved at doses lower than the MTD, considering the importance of receptors and transporters in their effect which can cause saturable bioavailability or a saturable effect on the targeted signaling pathway.[7,8] Thus it is necessary to understand the events that follow drug administration before deciding on the dose, frequency, and duration of the treatment. While the therapeutic efficacy requires maintaining an adequate concentration at the site of action for the duration of therapy, anticancer drugs are rarely directly administered at their sites of action. Most anticancer drugs are administered intravenously or orally when their effects are expected to be present in the brain, lungs, or elsewhere. Consequently, in order to administer drugs optimally, knowledge of the pharmacokinetic and pharmacodynamic aspects of drugs is needed.[9]

In *the pharmacokinetic* phase, the dose, dosage form, frequency, and route of administration determine drug concentration–time relationships in the body, whereas, in the *pharmacodynamic* phase, the concentration of drug at the site(s) of action determines the magnitude of the effect(s) produced. Once both of these phases have been defined, the dosage regimen can be designed to achieve the therapeutic objective. In this approach,

---

Holland-Frei Cancer Medicine, Tenth Edition. Edited by Robert C. Bast, John C. Byrd, Carlo M. Croce, Ernest Hawk, Fadlo R. Khuri, Raphael E. Pollock, Apostolia M. Tsimberidou, Christopher G. Willett, and Cheryl L. Willman.
© 2023 John Wiley & Sons, Inc. Published 2023 by John Wiley & Sons, Inc.

Table 1 Anticancer therapies and their mechanisms of action.

Class of drugs	Example drug(s)	Target/mechanism of action
A. Cytotoxics		
Alkylating agents	Cyclophosphamide	Cross-linking of DNA
Platinum agents	Cisplatin, carboplatin, oxaliplatin	Cross-linking of DNA
Antibiotics	Doxorubicin	Inhibits topoisomerase II; stabilizes topoisomerase II-DNA
Antimetabolites	Antifolates: methotrexate	Interference with the incorporation of nucleotides into DNA
	Pyrimidine analogs: 5-fluorouracil	
	Purine analogs: 6-mercaptopurine	
Tubulin-binding agents	Taxanes: paclitaxel	Enhance or inhibit tubulin polymerization
	Vinca alkaloids: vincristine eribulin, ixabepilone	
Camptothecins	Irinotecan	Stabilizes topoisomerase I-DNA to induce DNA strand breaks
B. Small-molecule noncytotoxics		
Tyrosine kinase inhibitors	Erlotinib, afatinib	EGFR inhibitor
	Lapatinib	HER2 inhibitor
	Ruxolitinib	JAK inhibitor
	Gilteritinib, midostaurin	FLT3 inhibitor
	Crizotinib, ceritinib	ALK inhibitor
	Sorafenib, sunitinib, pazopanib	VEGFR2 inhibitor
	Entrectinib, larotrectinib	NTRK inhibitor
	Vemurafenib, dabrafenib, encorafenib	BRAF inhibitor
	Trametinib, binimetinib, cobimetinib	MEK inhibitor
	Imatinib, nilotinib, bosutinib, dasatinib, ponatinib	BCR-ABL inhibitor
	Imatinib, sunitinib, regorafenib	KIT inhibitor
	Ibrutinib, acalabrutinib	Bruton's tyrosine kinase
BCL-2 inhibitor	Venetoclax	
CDK4, CDK6 inhibitor	Abemaciclib, palbociclib, ribociclib	
mTOR inhibitor	Everolimus, temsirolimus	
SMO inhibitor	Glasdegib, sonidegib, vismodegib	
Phosphatidylinositol 3-kinase inhibitor	Alpelisib, copanlisib, duvelisib, idelalisib	
PARP inhibitor	Olaparib, niraparib, rucaparib	
ER antagonist	Tamoxifen, fulvestrant	
Aromatase inhibitor	Anastrazole, letrozole, exemestane	
AR antagonist	Flutamide, bicalutamide, enzalutamide	
CYP17A1 inhibitor	Abiraterone	
Proteasome inhibitor	Bortezomib, carfilzomib	

This is intended to be an illustrative rather than a comprehensive list.

pharmacokinetic and pharmacodynamic causes of unusual drug response can be identified. As both response and toxicity are dependent on the concentration of the drug at the site(s) of action, therapeutic failure can be expected when the concentration is either too low, leading to insufficient response, or is too high, producing unacceptable toxicity. Therapeutic success is achieved between these limits of concentrations, which is commonly referred to as the *therapeutic index* or *therapeutic window*. It should be bore in mind that there are additional issues that can influence the patient's regimen independently of these factors, including cost of the treatment, convenience of regimens, and patient compliance and adherence.

Pharmacokinetic concepts

The term pharmacokinetics encompasses all processes involved in the movement of a drug in the body and is commonly described in four distinct stages: absorption, distribution, metabolism, and excretion. Some key concepts have been introduced to quantify these operations, establishing a relationship between the concentration of the drug in the body, usually plasma or blood, and time, and this relationship may help decision-making in the clinical setting. For phase I trials of anticancer agents, pharmacokinetic profiles are often assessed by sampling blood at multiple time points after the first dose of a drug and are occasionally repeated after multiple doses of a drug to establish steady-state conditions, which will be discussed later. In single-dose sampling, typical parameters that can be derived include the maximum concentration observed (Cmax), the time to the maximum concentration (Tmax), the area under the concentration–time curve (AUC), volume of distribution (Vd), clearance, and half-life. These parameters can be derived from either a noncompartmental analysis or a compartmental modeling approach. In the noncompartmental analysis, which is more readily available, cost-effective, and quick, parameters such as Cmax and AUC are estimated for each patient, and summary statistics are calculated for the population. In compartmental methods or population pharmacokinetic modeling, mathematical models are applied to concentration–time data that include one or more compartments that represent specific pharmacokinetic characteristics much like body organs. Although population pharmacokinetic modeling approaches require specialized expertise and software, such strategies can be performed with sparse (fewer time points) sampling data and are less susceptible to missing data or variability in sample collection times between individuals. Such modeling can also be utilized to identify covariates in a study population that contribute to inter-patient variability in particular parameter estimates such as clearance. It should be noted that the validity of pharmacokinetic modeling depends considerably on the quality of the data used to develop the model. Therefore, the timing of drug infusions, number, and schedule of plasma samples, and the analytic methods used should be carefully determined. In addition, any extrapolation of models outside the investigated dose, schedule, population, and conditions (e.g., single-dose vs combination regimens) must be done with great caution.[10]

Absorption is the process by which the unchanged drug moves from the site of administration to the site of measurement within the body. While many anticancer drugs are still administered intravenously, some can be administered locally to pleural or peritoneal cavities, the cerebrospinal fluid, or into the specific artery that leads to the tumor tissue.[11] The use of orally administered agents is continually growing with the development of small-molecule targeted cancer therapeutics, such as tyrosine kinase inhibitors,[12] that require chronic dosing. An orally administered agent should disintegrate and dissolve in the gastrointestinal tract and then permeate the gut membrane, where it would eventually be taken up into the portal circulation, moved through the liver, and finally reach the systemic circulation. The loss of drug due to its initial passage through the gastrointestinal membranes and the liver before entering the systemic circulation is known as the *first-pass effect*.[13]

The rate and extent of drug absorption are determined by its solubility and permeability across the mucosal lining of the gastrointestinal tract. The fraction (or percent) of the administered dose that enters the systemic circulation intact is regarded as bioavailability (F) which is the most commonly used pharmacokinetic parameter in absorption and can be estimated by dividing the AUC achieved following extravascular administration by the AUC observed after intravenous administration. By definition, bioavailability can range from 0 to 1.0 (or 0% to 100%).

Absorption as a pharmacokinetic process is a significant source of interpatient variability in AUC. In pharmacokinetic models, the rate of absorption is typically dependent on drug concentration and is estimated by a first-order rate constant, Ka. The mechanisms involved in gastro-intestinal absorption of drugs may be saturable, meaning that higher doses do not necessarily lead to proportional increase in exposure above a certain threshold dose. Examples of this phenomenon include many small-molecule tyrosine kinase inhibitors for which absorption is at least partially dependent on outward-directed efflux transport by membrane proteins such as ABCB1 (P-glycoprotein) or ABCG2 (BCRP; breast cancer resistance protein.[14] The concomitant intake of food can also alter the absorption of several orally administered anticancer agents and influence their toxicity profiles. As an example, co-administration of abiraterone with a high-fat meal can lead to a 10-fold increase in AUC compared to the exposure observed after the same dose administered following an overnight fast.[15–17] Additional examples of the effect of food on the pharmacokinetics of oral anticancer drugs are provided in Table 2. It should be noted that the drug

Table 2 Effect of food on exposure to select oral anticancer agents.

Drug	Food	Effect on drug exposure	Manufacturer's recommendations
Abiraterone	High-fat meal	↑ AUC 1000%	Without food
Afatinib	High-fat meal	↓Cmax 50%, ↓AUC 39%	Without food
Cabozantinib	High-fat meal	↑Cmax 41%, ↑AUC 57%	Without food
Capecitabine	Food not specified	↓Cmax 147%, ↓AUC 50%	With food
Cyclophosphamide	Plenty of fluids	Help flush metabolites and protect bladder	With food[a]
Dasatinib	High-fat meal	↑ AUC 14%	With or without food
Erlotinib	High-fat, high-calorie breakfast	Single dose, ↑AUC 200%	Without food[b]
Gefitinib	High-fat breakfast	Multiple dose, ↑AUC 37–66% ↓ AUC 14%, ↓ Cmax 35%	With or without food
	High-fat breakfast	↑ AUC 32%, ↑ Cmax 35%	
Imatinib	High-fat meal	No change	With food and a large glass of water[a]
Lapatinib	Low-fat meal (5% fat, 500 calories)	Variability (% CV) ↓ 37% ↑ AUC 167%, ↑ Cmax 142%	Without food[c]
	High-fat meal (50% fat, 1000 calories	↑ AUC 325%, ↑ Cmax 203%	
Lomustine			Without food[a]
Melphalan		↓AUC	Without food[d]
Mercaptopurine			
Nilotinib	High-fat meal	↑ AUC 82%	Without food
Pazopanib	High-fat meal	↑ AUC ~100%	Without food
Regorafenib	Low-fat meal containing <600 calories and <30% fat		With low-fat breakfast
Sorafenib	Moderate-fat meal (30% fat, 700 calories)	No change in bioavailability	Without food
Sunitinib	High-fat meal (50% fat, 900 calories High-fat, high-calorie meal	↓ bioavailability 29% ↑ AUC 18%	With or without food
Temozolomide	Food not specified	↓ Cmax 33%	Without food
Everolimus	High-fat meal	↓ AUC 9 % ↓ AUC 16%, ↓ Cmax 60%	With or without food
Vismodegib	High-fat meal	↑ AUC 74% for single dose; no effect at steady-state	With or without food
Vorinostat	High-fat meal	↑ AUC 37%	With food[e]

Abbreviations: AUC, area under the plasma concentration–time curve; Cmax, maximum plasma concentration.
[a]Recommended to reduce nausea.
[b]Recommended without food as the approved dose is the maximum tolerated dose.
[c]Recommended without food to achieve consistent drug exposure; was taken without food in clinical trials.
[d]Not stated in the Product information.
[e]Was taken with food in clinical trials.

label of agents for which pharmacokinetic food effects have been documented are not necessarily recommending the fast/fed condition that is associated with the strategy that provides the most desirable degree of systemic drug exposure. In addition to food, the extent of absorption of many orally-administered drugs is known to be influenced by pH-dependent solubility, and for these agents, including dasatinib, ponatinib, and vismodegib, absorption can be decreased by concomitant use of proton-pump inhibitors or other acid-reducing agents.[18]

Distribution is the process in which a drug is reversibly transferred to and from the site of measurement. Distribution processes can affect both a drug's efficacy and unwanted side effects and are determined by many factors, including physicochemical properties such as molecular structure and hydrophobicity, permeability in certain tissues, tissue-binding, binding to serum proteins, and local organ blood flow. The apparent volume into which a drug is distributed in the body after reaching equilibrium is called the Vd, and this parameter is calculated as the amount of the drug in the body divided by the plasma concentration.[9] Thus, large apparent volumes of distribution are usually indicative of high tissue binding, although they rarely represent an actual physiological compartment or tissue. Distribution of hydrophilic compounds, such as methotrexate, into fluid collections (such as pleural effusions or ascites) can significantly delay clearance of the drug from the central (plasma) compartment.[19] On the other hand, pegylated liposomal doxorubicin tends to stay in the bloodstream with a very small Vd since the liposomes cannot cross the tight junctions of endothelial cells in blood vessels and has, therefore, a Vd that is similar to the circulating volume.[20] It should be noted that distribution of certain drugs into specific body compartments might be limited by physiological protective barriers, such as the blood–brain barrier protecting the central nervous system or the blood–testes barrier, which should be considered when modeling the distribution of the drug.[21]

Elimination takes place when a drug leaves the site of measurement and does not return, and this pharmacokinetic process can involve either or both *metabolism* and *excretion*. Metabolism is the conversion of a drug into another chemical species that is often more water-soluble, whereas excretion is the irreversible loss of the parent drug (or its metabolites) from the body. Metabolism itself involves two distinct phases: direct chemical modification (phase I) and conjugation (phase II). Phase I reactions, which usually include oxidation, reduction, and hydrolysis, are typically catalyzed by cytochrome P450 (CYP) enzymes in liver microsomes. Since phase I metabolites are occasionally more pharmacologically active or potent than the parent drug, regulatory guidance documents suggest that toxicologic properties of metabolites whose exposure exceeds 10% of the parent AUC at steady-state should be evaluated in a nonclinical model. During phase II reactions, parent drugs, metabolites from phase I reactions, or both are conjugated with charged species and form more hydrophilic substances through a variety of enzymes, including the class of UDP-glucuronosyltransferases (UGT). Many of these products are then removed from liver cells in phase III reactions by members of the ATP-binding cassette (ABC) family of transporters, either by direct transport into bile (e.g., by ABCB1 or ABCG2) or transport back into the circulation (e.g., by ABCC3) for terminal excretion by the kidney into the urine. A so-called mass balance study can be performed to quantitatively establish the major routes of elimination. This method commonly applies the administration of drugs carrying a radiotracer to allow quantitative recovery of the administered dose in urine and feces that is collected over prolonged time periods and in which samples are analyzed with a technique that can distinguish between parent drug, known, and unknown metabolites.

Clearance is the most clinically relevant pharmacokinetic parameter for elimination which defines the relationship between drug dose and systemic drug exposure (AUC). In clinical practice, clearance of a drug is commonly calculated indirectly through either of the following equations:[22,23]

$$\text{Clearance} = \frac{\text{Dose}}{\text{AUC}}$$

$$\text{Clearance} = \frac{\text{Infusion rate}}{C_{ss}}$$

where C_{ss} is the concentration of the drug at steady state, which occurs when the rate of drug administration is equal to the rate of drug elimination. For many drugs, the time to reach steady state is directly dependent on the elimination half-life and is independent of the dose and dosing interval. In a clinical setting, steady state is generally assumed to be reached after 4–5 half-lives.

The plasma concentration at steady state (C_p^{ss}) can be calculated as follows:[24]

$$C_p^{ss} = F \times \frac{D}{\text{CL}} \times \tau$$

where F is the bioavailability, D is the dose, CL is clearance, and τ is the dosing interval. Nonadherence to medication as well as drug–drug interactions and prandial conditions can either increase or decrease the C_p^{ss} over time. For some anticancer therapies, C_p^{ss} tends to change over time on its own. An example is this phenomenon occurs with cyclophosphamide, where the agent can induce CYP enzymes involved in its own metabolism and cause an almost doubling of CL by the end of a 96-h infusion.[25] Similarly, for imatinib exposure was decreased by approximately 30% over the first 90 days of therapy before stabilizing in patients with gastrointestinal stromal tumors.[26]

The concept of clearance can also be presented as a function of both distribution and elimination. In the simplest pharmacokinetic model, where V is the volume of distribution, and K is the elimination constant, clearance can be calculated as follows:[4]

$$\text{Clearance} = V \cdot K$$

The half-life of the drug, or the time needed for the drug concentration in plasma to drop by half, is much more commonly considered in pharmacokinetic studies than the elimination rate constant from which it is derived. It is particularly useful in estimating the time required to reach steady state, either in a multi-dose schedule or during a continuous intravenous drug infusion. In certain circumstances, binding of drugs to serum proteins can also influence clearance. As drug–protein complexes can be considered macromolecules, only the fraction of drug that is unbound can distribute outside of the circulation, reach and interact with pharmacological target sites, and be eliminated, an increase in protein binding can potentially increase half-life and decrease clearance. One example of this phenomenon has been documented for vismodegib, which reversibly binds to alpha-1-acid glycoprotein (AAG) and albumin with high affinity.[27] For this agent, variability in AAG levels between patients accounts for almost 70% of the observed interpatient variability in pharmacokinetic parameters, and administration of concomitant drugs or disease states (e.g., hypoproteinemia) which reduce the level of these proteins can theoretically increase the fraction of unbound drug. However, the clinical significance of this is still unclear for vismodegib and many other highly protein-bound drugs.[28]

Pharmacokinetic linearity is also an important feature that should be considered for each anticancer drug. When the clearance and Vd are independent of time and dose, the AUC is not affected by changes in drug schedule and is always directly proportional to the administered dose, and this is called dose proportionality or linear pharmacokinetics. The following formula applies to drugs with a linear pharmacokinetic profile:[29]

$$\frac{dC}{dt} = -KC$$

Dose proportionality is a clinically favorable and important feature because it means that changes in dose result in cause predictable changes in exposure. However, factors such as saturable oral absorption, capacity-limited distribution, and/or saturable metabolism can lead to deviations from linearity in pharmacokinetic parameters of a given drug.[30] In nonlinear pharmacokinetics, clearance and/or Vd are either concentration or time-dependent, or both, which can reduce predictability in clinical outcomes and lead to inappropriate dose adjustments. In most instances nonlinear pharmacokinetics is the result of saturation of a critical, rate-limiting enzymatic step in metabolism or a transporter-mediated pathway. For some drugs, this may lead to decreased clearance at higher doses, and consequently a greater than proportional increase in the AUC with an increase in dose. Decreasing the duration of infusion can also lead to an increase in the AUC as clearance might be slower at the higher peak plasma concentrations. Well-documented examples of nonlinear pharmacokinetic profiles include 5-fluorouracil (5-FU) and paclitaxel. The nonlinear pharmacokinetic behavior may be one of the main factors in the notion that the side effect profile of 5-FU is highly schedule-dependent, and the AUC is higher, for a given dose, when infusion time is shorter (e.g., 3-h vs 24-h).[31] For many orally administered drugs, on the other hand, saturable absorption from the gastrointestinal tract can cause nonlinear pharmacokinetics such that an increase in dose results in a disproportional decrease in the AUC. This case is more common for drugs that structurally resemble natural compounds since their mechanism of absorption is frequently mediated by uptake transporters that display saturable kinetics. Examples of drugs with saturable absorption properties include folate analogs such as methotrexate or leucovorin and amino acid analogs such as melphalan.[32–34] Studies have also suggested that for some anticancer drugs such as cisplatin, renal tubular reabsorption can be saturable,[35,36] and this would provide an explanation of the fact that prolonged continuous infusions result in increased unbound concentrations of cisplatin in plasma compared to short i.v. infusions.[36]

Pharmacodynamic concepts

Pharmacodynamics refers to the effects that a drug exerts on patients (or tumors) and pharmacodynamic models demonstrate how clinical effects of drugs correlate with pharmacokinetic parameters that are indicative of drug exposure, such as AUC. Pharmacodynamic variability can potentiate substantial differences in clinical outcomes in oncology, even when systemic exposures are similar. Such variability can result from clinical characteristics such as age, gender, prior chemotherapy, prior radiotherapy, concomitant medications, among others.[37] In general, the specific marker of clinical effect used as the independent variable in a pharmacodynamic analysis depends on the particular characteristics of the study drug.

Pharmacodynamics models are the cornerstone of phase I clinical trials, where the goal is to assess the feasibility and safety of new therapeutic agents and determine the MTD. Ideally, the determination of pharmacodynamic effects requires repeated biopsies of the tumor. However, this approach is rather challenging depending on the location of the tumor and also it is very invasive. Therefore, surrogate normal tissues such as skin, hair follicles, and peripheral blood mononuclear cells (PBMCs) are used to indirectly obtain this information. Since surrogate tissues often lack the expression of oncogenic targets such as acquired oncogenic somatic mutations, and also the drug concentrations are different between surrogate normal tissues and tumor tissues, surrogate endpoints or biomarkers are often used as an intermediate marker of treatment effects that can be analyzed at time points earlier than the actual clinical endpoint of interest. An example of this is the use of pathological complete response and progression-free survival (PFS) as surrogate markers for overall survival in clinical trials. It should, however, be noted that surrogate markers may not always correlate well with overall survival, for instance for bevacizumab in metastatic breast cancer, PFS benefit did not translate to improved overall survival.[38]

Another surrogate endpoint is treatment-related toxicity, where the adverse effect of the drug is reflective of its therapeutic efficacy. Examples include the use of myelosuppression as a marker of efficacy for drugs that affect cell proliferation or hyperglycemia observed with phosphoinositide 3-kinase (PI3K) inhibitors, which is dependent on the therapeutic mechanism of action as the alpha subunit of PI3K is involved in insulin signaling.[38] With certain chemotherapeutic agents, the antitumor activity is particularly dependent on the dosing schedule, meaning that administrating the dose over several days can produce a different antitumor response or toxicity profile compared with giving the same dose over a shorter period. An example of this is the use of etoposide in the treatment of small-cell lung cancer, which effect is markedly increased when the same total dose is administered with a 5-day divided-dose schedule rather than a 24-h infusion.[39] Although both schedules produce very similar overall drug exposure in terms of AUC, the divided-dose schedule maintains an etoposide plasma concentration of greater than 1 μg/mL for twice the duration.

The efficacy of many traditional cytotoxic drugs relies on the tumor's high proliferation rate compared to normal tissue, rather than targeting specific tumoral pathways. In recent years, the discovery of specific biochemical alterations in signaling pathways as the driving cause in some human malignancies has led to the design and development of "targeted agents." The efficacy of these agents is often dependent on somatic mutations that create abnormal dependencies upon signaling pathways for survival ("oncogene addiction" and "network-attacking mutations"). Since this serves as a tumor-specific target not found (or needed) in healthy tissues, the therapeutic index of targeted therapy is assumed to be higher than that of cytotoxic chemotherapy. This enables targeted agents to be administrated at least theoretically at a lower "biologically effective dose" (BED), which is defined as the minimum dose that results in the level of control in the function of the molecular target required for efficacy instead of the maximum tolerated dose.[40–43] Imatinib was the first targeted therapy of this kind which received FDA approval for Philadelphia chromosome-positive chronic myelogenous leukemia in 2001 and gastrointestinal stromal tumors in 2002, based on its ability to target the tyrosine kinase activity of the Bcr-Abl fusion protein and c-Kit, respectively. Since then, many highly active small-molecule inhibitors of kinase and nonkinase targets have been developed and over 50 of these agents have been approved for human use. These new selective drugs are however mostly reserved as second-line options and for combating resistance to first-generation targeted inhibitors. For example, second-generation Bcr-Abl inhibitors such as dasatinib, nilotinib, and bosutinib are indicated in case of imatinib-resistant disease.[44–46] Although the design of these drugs is in a way that is more targeted towards specific pathways, studies conducted to optimize the dosing schedules of imatinib and dasatinib still compared dosage regimens based on rate and severity of toxicities and raised concern that lower toxicity might be indicative of inferior efficacy.[47–49] These uncertainties have been overcome to some extent with the use of receptor occupancy assays as a pharmacodynamic endpoint for certain newer agents such as ibrutinib. For this agent, a population pharmacokinetic model has been developed that included information on the occupancy of ibrutinib in the active site of its target BTK using patients' peripheral blood mononuclear cells before and after treatment as the pharmacodynamics marker. Optimal doses and systemic drug levels required to achieve maximal occupancy of BTK and consecutively, maximal inhibition of BCR signaling were thus determined.[49] Since molecular pharmacodynamic studies require accurate and applicable measurements of drug action in tumors,[50,51] the involvement of multiple medical specialties is required to define and optimize treatment regimens. Therefore, communication plays a major part in paving the path for developing clinical trial protocols that are capable of optimal pharmacodynamic evaluations and answering important questions about drug action.[52]

Sources of variability in pharmacokinetics and pharmacodynamics

Significant interindividual variability has been reported in the pharmacokinetic profile of many anticancer drugs, which will often lead to variability in the pharmacodynamic effects of the drug at a given dose.[53] As a result, the same dose of a drug may be relatively safe in one patient, induce unacceptable and possibly life-threatening toxicity in another, or achieve clinical response in one individual and cause cancer progression in another. This variability is even more pronounced with orally administered agents, especially when bioavailability is low. Some examples of pharmacokinetic variability are presented in Figure 1. Here, we discuss some of the major factors that can serve as the underlying source of these variabilities.

Body size and body composition

Traditionally anticancer drugs dosage was calculated for each individual according to their body surface area (BSA).[54] Although the usefulness of BSA as a method of normalizing the dose of anticancer drugs in adults has been questioned as there is not always a detectable relationship between BSA and clearance,[55] most attempts to replace BSA with alternate size descriptors such as lean body weight have failed for many anticancer agents.[56] Despite these findings, the routine use of BSA in drug dose calculation in oncology persists, although its use in the calculation of drug dose in pediatric patients to normalize pharmacokinetic parameters is more properly evidence based.[57] Since significant variability in the pharmacokinetic profile of drugs remains observable in patients receiving BSA-normalized dosing of the classic cytotoxic chemotherapeutics, many of the more recently developed molecularly targeted agents are currently administered using a flat-fixed dose irrespective of an individual's BSA.[56]

Age

Both the pharmacokinetic and pharmacodynamic profile of drugs can be affected by changes in body composition and organ function at the extremes of age. For example, children less than 3 years having a statistically significant lower clearance of doxorubicin than older children, after correcting for BSA.[58] As more treatment options for malignancies of infants, adolescents, and the elderly become available, it is increasingly important to understand the influence of age on the pharmacokinetics and pharmacodynamics of each individual anticancer drug.[59] While pediatric cancers are relatively rare compared with cancers in adults and the elderly, high cure rates and extended long-term survival are possible in children, and therefore it is particularly important to optimize their therapy to ensure the highest efficacy while minimizing potential long-term toxicities.

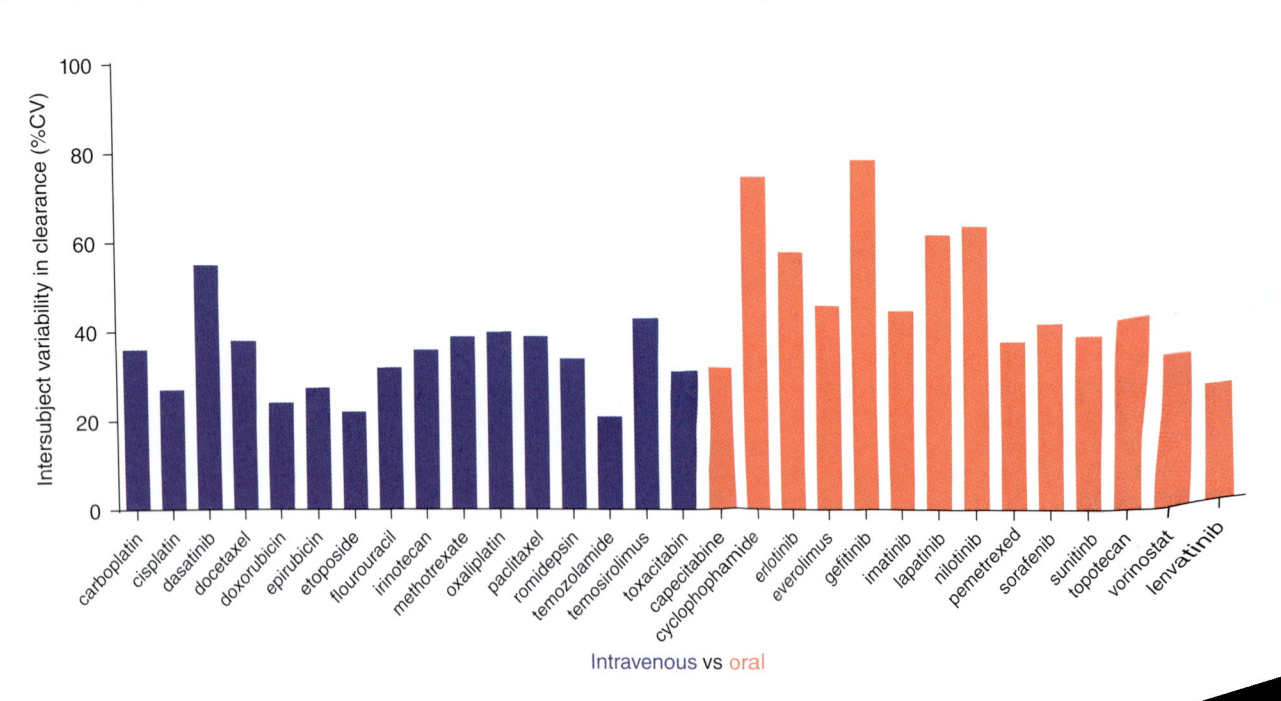

Figure 1 Inter-individual variability in pharmacokinetic of anticancer chemotherapeutics.

Pathophysiologic changes

Effects of disease
Pathophysiologic changes associated with particular malignancies can alter pharmacokinetic properties dramatically. For example, in children with acute lymphoblastic leukemia (ALL), the clearance of both antipyrine and lorazepam are increased after remission induction while the clearance of unbound teniposide is lower in relapse than during the first remission. This can be due to leukemic infiltration of the liver at the time of diagnosis, which can, in turn, reduce the clearance of drugs that undergo extensive metabolism in the liver.[9] Other disease-specific changes in pharmacokinetics have been observed with cabozantinib, where inter-individual variability in clearance is greater in patients with renal cell carcinoma compared with medullary thyroid carcinoma.[60] Furthermore, certain tumors can provoke an acute phase response which is accompanied by downregulation of CYP3A4, the main drug-metabolizing enzyme in the liver, as well as the mouse ortholog Cyp3a11,[61] and these changes have been connected to significant reduction in the metabolism of substrate drugs. These documented effects of tumor type of the pharmacokinetic properties of certain drugs support the need for a disease-specific design of early clinical trials for anticancer drugs, as has been recommended for docetaxel.[62]

Effects of renal impairment
With drugs for which urinary excretion is an important route of elimination, any decrement in renal function could lead to decreased drug clearance, and subsequent drug accumulation and toxicity.[63] Therefore, for these drugs, the administered dose should be decreased relative to the degree of impaired renal function with the aim of maintaining plasma concentrations within a target therapeutic window. Clinically important drugs for which the dose needs to be modified relative to a patient's renal function include bleomycin, lenalidomide, capecitabine, lomustine, carboplatin, melphalan, carmustine, methotrexate, cisplatin, mitomycin, cytarabine, pemetrexed, dacarbazine pentostatin, fludarabine, topotecan, and ifosfamide.[2] Although renal function differentially contributes to the elimination of these agents, assessment of renal impairment as a guide to optimize drug dose has been advocated for some agents, including carboplatin. For this drug, measures of glomerular filtration are applied as a measurement of kidney function[64] in order to derive an individualized dose of carboplatin that targets a predefined AUC. This strategy has led to a substantial reduction in pharmacokinetic variability, and carboplatin is currently one of the few drugs routinely administered to achieve a target exposure (AUC) rather than being dosed by weight or BSA.

Interestingly, renal impairment can also affect the pharmacokinetics of drugs that are predominantly eliminated by nonrenal processes such as metabolism and/or active transport. Therefore the FDA recommends that pharmacokinetic/pharmacodynamic alterations should also be evaluated in patients with renal impairment for drugs that are predominantly eliminated by nonrenal processes, as well as those that are mainly excreted unchanged by the kidneys. One example of this is imatinib, which is predominantly eliminated by hepatic metabolism but is associated with dramatically reduced drug clearance patients with reduced renal function, presumably due to a transporter-mediated process.[65]

Effects of hepatic impairment
Many cancer-related situations can inadvertently affect hepatic function, such as primary or metastatic tumor involvement of the liver, concomitant use of hepatotoxic drugs (e.g., other cytotoxics, hormones [estrogens, androgens], antimicrobials [trimethoprim–sulfamethoxazole, voriconazole]), concurrent infections (e.g., hepatic candidiasis, viral hepatitis), use of parenteral nutrition, portal vein thrombosis, and paraneoplastic syndrome.[2] Also, in contrast to the predictable decline in renal clearance of drugs when glomerular filtration is impaired, it is difficult to accurately estimate the level of hepatic impairment and predict its effect on drug concentrations. Since commonly applied criteria used to evaluate hepatic impairment are typically not good indicators of drug-metabolizing enzyme activity, alternative dynamic measures of liver function have been proposed, including the use of a hepatic dysfunction score.[66] Guidelines have been proposed for dose adjustments of several agents, including 5-FU, methotrexate, anthracyclines (daunorubicin, epirubicin), taxanes (docetaxel, paclitaxel), *Vinca* alkaloids (vinblastine, vincristine), and etoposide when administered to patients with liver dysfunction. It should be emphasized, however, that the criteria used in the conduct of these studies are not uniform and therefore determination of the hepatic activity of enzymes especially relevant to the chemotherapeutic drug(s) of interest is indicated as a more reliable way to achieve proper individualized doses, as has been done for docetaxel.[67]

Effects of serum proteins
Since only the unbound (or free) drug in plasma is available for distribution and inducing a therapeutic response, the binding of drugs to serum proteins may have significant implications for clinical outcomes. Several clinical conditions, including liver and renal disease, can cause a dramatic decrease in the extent of serum binding, and consequently pose possible risks of unexpected toxicity, while the total (free plus bound forms) plasma drug concentrations are unaltered.[68] It is worth noting that for most anticancer drugs, binding to serum proteins is independent of drug concentration after the initial dose is administrated, and so the total plasma concentration is reflective of the unbound concentration. However, for some anticancer agents, including etoposide and paclitaxel, protein binding is highly dependent on dose and schedule and therefore can be subject to variability.

Sex dependence
Several pharmacokinetic analyses have suggested higher elimination capacity for various anticancer drugs (e.g., paclitaxel) and increased clearance (e.g., imatinib) in male compared with female patients.[69] These observations add to a growing body of evidence suggesting that there is a significant sexual dimorphism in the pharmacokinetic profile of anticancer drugs. Nevertheless, these differences are rarely considered in the design of clinical trials during oncology drug development.

Drug interactions
The concurrent administration of different drugs during cancer therapy is one of the main causes for interactions that affect variability in response among individual patients. These interactions can have a pharmacokinetic or pharmacodynamics basis, and the previously mentioned factors age, disease-related changes, renal, and hepatic impairment can all potentiate drug–drug interaction and contribute more to variability.

Co-administration of other chemotherapeutic drugs
Combination chemotherapy is a common strategy to avoid or overcome resistance and improve treatment outcome as it may provide coverage against differentially resistant cells within heterogeneous

Table 3 Common substrates, inhibitors, and inducers of CYP450 subtypes in clinical drug–drug interaction studies.

CYP450 subtype	Sensitive substrate	Moderate sensitive substrate	Strong inhibitors	Moderate inhibitors	Weak inhibitors	Strong inducer	Moderate inducers	Weak inducers
CYP1A2	Caffeine, duloxetine, ramelteon, tizanidine	Theophylline	Ciprofloxacin	Methoxsalen, oral contraceptives	Acyclovir		Rifampin, smoking, teriflunomide	
CYP2B6	Bupropion	Efavirenz			Clopidogrel, voriconazole	Carbamazepine	Efavirenz, rifampin	Nevirapine, ritonavir
CYP2C8	Repaglinide	Pioglitazone,	Gemfibrozil	Clopidogrelte-riflunomide	Trimethoprim		Rifampin	
CYP2C9	Celecoxib	Warfarin		Amiodarone, fluconazole	Voriconazole	Enzalutamide rifampin	Apalutamide, aprepitant carbamazepine, ritonavir	
CYP2C19	Omeprazole	Diazepam, voriconazole	Fluconazole		Omeprazole, voriconazole	Rifampin	Apalutamide, efavirenz enzalutamide-phenytoin	Ritonavir
CYP2D6	Dextromethorphan perphenazine	Metoprolol, propafenone, propranolol, tramadol	Bupropion, terbinafine	Abiraterone	Amiodarone, celecoxib, cimetidine, clobazam, ritonavir sertraline, vemurafenib			
CYP3A	Alfentanil, everolimus, ibrutinib, midazola, simvastati, tacrolimus, budesonide, dasatinib, quetiapine, sildenafil	Alprazola, aprepitant, atorvastatin, rivaroxaban, tadalafil	Ritonavir, grapefruit juice, itraconazole, posaconazole, voriconazole, clarithromycin	Aprepitant, ciprofloxacin, crizotinib, fluconazole, imatinib, verapamil	Chlorzoxazone, fosaprepitant, ranitidine, ticagrelor	Enzalutamide, mitotane rifampin, St. John's wort	Phenobarbital, primidone	

tumor masses.[69] Several principles are used as the basis for designing a combination chemotherapy regimens, including that selected agents (1) should have demonstrable single-agent activity against the specific type of tumor; (2) should have different mechanisms of action; (3) should not cause similar or overlapping toxicities in order to reduce the severity and duration of acute and chronic toxicities; and (4) should be used in their respective optimal doses and schedule.[2] Given these principles, any unfavorable interaction will likely be a result of alteration in the pharmacokinetic profile of one drug by the other, and this type of interaction has been documented for several combinations of tyrosine kinase inhibitors with cytotoxic chemotherapeutics.[70]

Co-administration of nonchemotherapeutic drugs

Polypharmacy is particularly common in patients with cancer,[71] as these patients are often use prescription medications to minimize adverse effects of the chemotherapy (e.g., antiinfectives) or the cancer itself (e.g., pain management, anticoagulants, antidepressants). As cancer is more prevalent in the elderly, patients commonly have other comorbidities such as diabetes and hypertension, which also require pharmacotherapeutic interventions.[72] Together, this can lead to an increased risk of drug–drug interactions that usually involve changes in pharmacokinetic processes and can include absorption, metabolism, and/or excretion:

Absorption: As mentioned before, the absorption of various orally administered anticancer drugs can be affected by food and acid-suppressive agents by modulating solubility and bioavailability.[73] Similarly, administration of certain agents displaying pH-dependent solubility, including erlotinib, with an acidic beverage that can reduce stomach pH for a short period such as a cola beverages can cause potentially significant drug interactions.[74] The impact of acid suppression on drug absorption can be mitigated by providing sufficient time between administration of the chemotherapeutic drug and the acid-blocking agents like H2 antagonists.[72]

Metabolism: Many prescription drugs can influence the activity of CYP enzymes either by decreasing (inhibition) or increasing (induction) metabolism. Concomitant use of such agents with orally or intravenously administered anticancer drugs can result in significant alterations in clearance and subsequently influence safety and efficacy.[75,76] For substrates of a specific CYP isoforms such as CYP3A4, drugs with an ability to induce activity (e.g., the anticonvulsant drugs carbamazepine and phenobarbital) can potentially reduce plasma concentrations of anticancer drugs and diminish efficacy, while inhibitors (e.g., the antifungal ketoconazole) can increase drug exposure and risk of severe toxicity. Some of the most important drugs that can cause interactions through this mechanism according to regulatory agencies and are prevalent among cancer patients are listed in Table 3. Inhibition of enzymes involved in glucuronidation can also be occurred by various drugs and can lead to changes in patient outcomes, as has been demonstrated for certain tyrosine kinase inhibitors.[77]

Excretion: Certain anticancer drugs that undergo elimination primarily through transporter-mediated urinary excretion, such as methotrexate and cisplatin, are particularly sensitive to interactions with antibacterials, proton pump inhibitors, and NSAIDs that affect renal tubular secretion and can thereby modulate toxicity profiles.[78–80]

It should be noted that in all these scenarios, several pharmacokinetic parameters could be altered simultaneously. For

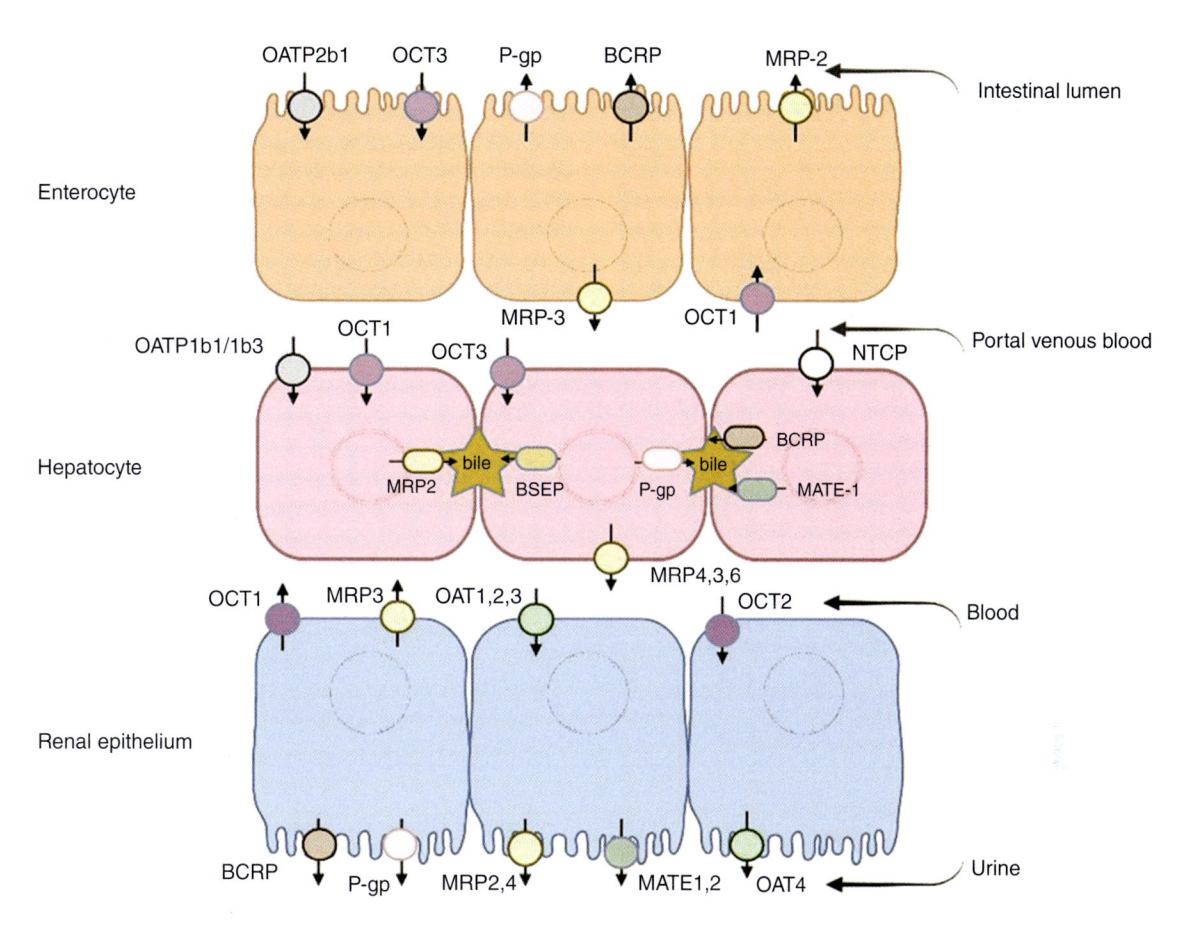

Figure 2 Major transporters involved in the intestinal absorption (enterocyte) and the hepatic (hepatocyte) and renal (renal epithelium) excretion of anticancer drugs. *Abbreviations*: OATP, members of the organic anion transporting polypeptide family; OCT, members of the organic cation transporters; OAT, members of the organic anion transporters; MRP, multidrug resistance protein; BSEP, bile salt export pump; BCRP, breast cancer resistance protein; P-gp, P-glycoprotein; MATE, members of the multidrug and toxin extrusion protein family.

example, proton pump inhibitors can alter both absorption and metabolism of some drugs. Many oral anticancer drugs are also themselves substrates or inhibitors of uptake and/or efflux transporters (Figure 2), and therefore alterations in their activity might alter multiple components of drugs pharmacokinetics. Examples of important drugs that can cause interactions through transporters are provided in Table 4.

Co-administration of complementary and alternative medicine

According to published surveys from the past decade, the prevalence of complementary and alternative medicine (CAM) use in oncology patients may be as high as 87%, and interestingly, in many cases, the treating physician is unaware of the patients' CAM use.[81] Therefore, there is an increasing need to understand possible adverse drug interactions of CAM in oncology. Most of the observed interactions of CAM with drugs involve herbs affecting several isoforms of the CYP family, either through inhibition or induction, however, the causal relationship has not always been established. St. John's wort, garlic, milk thistle, and Echinacea have been formally evaluated for their potential to cause pharmacokinetic drug–interaction in cancer patients. Nonetheless, various other herbs including ginkgo and ginseng also have the potential to significantly modulate the expression and/or activity of drug-metabolizing enzymes and drug transporters (Table 5).[81,82] Given the high prevalence of herbal medicine use, it is becoming increasingly important that the physicians include herb usage in their routine drug histories before participation in a clinical trial, to ensure that the patient is getting adequately evaluated for potential risk of interactions.

Inherited genetic factors

Pharmacogenetic is the discipline that investigates variation in genes as a predictor of responsiveness to a specific drug, in order to increase the number of responders and reduce the number of subjects affected by adverse drug reactions. Factors such as the contribution of the specific gene product to pharmacologic response, the availability of alternative pathways of elimination, and the frequency of occurrence of the variant allele determine the importance, detectability of polymorphisms for a given enzyme or transporter and the availability of the clinical data determine the importance a polymorphism in a given enzyme or transporter. Although drug-metabolizing enzymes and transporters are known to be subject to varying degrees of polymorphism and testing is available for many of them, a definitive demonstration of clinically relevant contribution of genetics to inter-individual pharmacokinetic variability has been established for only a few cancer chemotherapeutic agents and genotyping has not yet become widespread in even these cases. In most confirmed instances, elimination of certain cancer drugs was found to be critically dependent on a rate-limiting action of a polymorphic enzyme, and some examples of the use of pharmacogenetics in cancer therapy which are deemed clinically relevant[9,83] are described below.

Table 4 Examples of transporters involved in anticancer drugs' pharmacokinetics, with their most clinically important substrates and inhibitors.

Transporter	Gene	Substrate	Inhibitor
P-gp	ABCB1	Dabigatran etexilate, digoxin, fexofenadine	Amiodarone, carvedilol, clarithromycin, itraconazole, lapatinib, verapamil
BCRP	ABCG2	Rosuvastatin, sulfasalazine	Curcumin
OATP1B1 OATP1B3	SLCO1B1, SLCO1B3	Atorvastatin, docetaxel, fexofenadine, paclitaxel, pravastatin, repaglinide, rosuvastatin	Clarithromycin, gemfibrozil, rifampin (single dose)
OAT1 OAT3	SLC22A6 SLC22A8	Cefaclor, ceftizoxime, famotidine, furosemide, ganciclovir, methotrexate, oseltamivir carboxylate, penicillin G	Probenecid, teriflunomide
MATE1, MATE-2K, OCT2	SLC47A1, SLC47A2, SLC22A2	Metformin	Isavuconazole, trimethoprim, vandetanib

Table 5 Commonly used complementary medicine agents which have the potential to interact with anticancer drugs.

Botanical	Concurrent chemotherapy/condition (suspected effect)
Ginkgo	Caution with camptothecins, cyclophosphamide, TK inhibitors, epipodophyllotoxins, taxanes, and Vinca alkaloids (CYP3A4 and CYP2C19 inhibition); discourage with alkylating agents, antitumor antibiotics, and platinum analogs (free-radical scavenging)
Ginseng	Discourage in patients with estrogen-receptor-positive breast cancer and endometrial cancer (stimulation of tumor growth)
Garlic	Caution with docetaxel (CYP3A4 inhibition)
Green tea	Discourage with erlotinib and pazopanib (CYP1A2 induction)
Japanese arrowroot	Avoid with methotrexate (ABCC and OAT transporter inhibition)
St. John's wort	Avoid with all concurrent chemotherapy (CYP2B6, CYP2C9, CYP2C19, CYP2E1, CYP3A4, and ABCB1 induction)
Valerian	Caution with tamoxifen (CYP2C9 inhibition), cyclophosphamide, and teniposide (CYP2C19 inhibition)
Milk thistle	Caution with tamoxifen (CYP2C9 inhibition), irinotecan (glucuronidation), paclitaxel, docetaxel, vinorelbine, vincristine (CYP 3A4 inhibition)

Abbreviation: TK, tyrosine kinase.

Fluoropyrimidines, DPD, and TS variants
Deficiency in the metabolizing enzyme dihydropyrimidine dehydrogenase (DPD) is associated with increased toxicity in both 5-FU and its produg capecitabine and is, therefore, a contraindication for their use according to manufacturers. While testing is commercially available to detect the most common high-risk polymorphisms in DPD and at least one other enzyme associated with fluoropyrimidine toxicity, thymidylate synthase (TYMS), given the low frequency of finding a predictive allele and the fact that grade 3 or 4 fluoropyrimidine-related toxicity is still prevalent in patients who lack one of these high-risk variants preemptive genetic testing of all patients prior to receiving a fluoropyrimidine is controversial and still not widely practiced.

Irinotecan and UGT1A1 variants
The risk for neutropenia and diarrhea following treatment with the SN-38 produg irinotecan is increased in individuals who are homozygous for a variant allele in the enzymes that can inactivate SN-38 by glucuronidation, namely UGT1A1*28. The irinotecan label recommends testing to identify this allele and reduced initial irinotecan doses should be administered in those who are homozygous for UGT1A1*28. Again, routine preemptive use of this assay in all patients who are to receive irinotecan is not widely accepted, as consideration of just this single polymorphic variant appears to be account for only a modest degree of interindividual pharmacokinetic variability in exposure to SN-38 and thus may be inadequate to achieve proper individualized dosing with irinotecan.

Thoipurines and TPMT variants
Polymorphisms in thiopurine S-methyltransferase (TPMT), responsible for the metabolism of thiopurines, can result in decreased activity or inactivity of the enzyme, and an increased risk of treatment-related leukopenia in patients treated with 6-mercaptopurine. TPMT testing is not specifically recommended by the FDA but is recommended by CPIC guidelines prior to treatment with 6-mercaptopurine and dose reductions of up to 90% may be needed for patients with low or absent TPMT activity.

Tamoxifen and CYP2D6 variants
Tamoxifen biotransformation by CYP2D6 leads to the formation of the metabolites 4-hydroxytamoxifen and 4-hydroxy N-desmethyl tamoxifen (endoxifen), both of which possess greater antiestrogenic potency than the parent drug. Reduced concentrations of endoxifen and a higher risk of disease recurrence have been observed in patients with certain CYP2D6 genetic polymorphisms and in those who receive strong CYP2D6 inhibitors. Although an increase in the initial tamoxifen dose can be considered for patients in whom the function of CYP2D6 is compromised,[84] routine testing for CYP2D6 variants in subjects eligible for treatment with tamoxifen is not recommended by NCCN and ASCO and is not discussed in FDA label of tamoxifen.

In addition to drug metabolism, drug transporters can also significantly contribute to variability in a drug's pharmacokinetic properties, and inherited variations in drug transporter function or expression can influence individual responses to various commonly prescribed drugs. For example, emerging evidence indicates that the clearance and toxicity of methotrexate are dependent on the hepatic uptake transporter OATP1B1,[85] and toxicity associated with sunitinib-based therapy has been related to the polymorphic efflux transporters ABCB1 and ABCG2.[86]

Approaches to reduce variability in drug exposure and response

Therapeutic drug monitoring
Therapeutic drug monitoring (TDM) involves the measurement of drug levels in plasma or serum in order to refine individualized

drug doses. The method is particularly appealing for cancer drugs since many of these are administered intravenously and, if a link between steady-state concentration and the desired pharmacodynamic endpoint can be established, infusion rates can be modified to achieve the desired steady-state concentration for the remainder of the treatment. This method has been successfully used during continuous infusions of 5-FU and etoposide, repeated oral administrations of etoposide, mitotane and tamoxifen, and repeated intravenous administrations of cisplatin. Methotrexate plasma concentrations are also routinely monitored to identify patients at high risk of toxicity and then adjust leucovorin rescue therapy in those patients who present with delayed excretion profiles.[87]

For TKIs, even in tumors that are intrinsically very sensitive, there is a minimum threshold below which the drug is inactive, and under-dosing may then lead to ineffective treatment or acquired resistance. Therefore, TDM can be a rational step for improving the efficacy of certain TKI-based regimens. While target concentrations have been established for a number of TKIs,[88] the most compelling data in support of the use of TDM for this class of agents has been for *imatinib*, where specific trough concentrations have been proposed for patients with chronic myeloid leukemia or gastrointestinal stromal tumors.[89,90] TDM may also prove to be a promising option for optimizing treatment with antihormonal drugs, as a large number of them are administered orally and can be subject to substantial interpatient variability in pharmacokinetics.[91] Although TDM is generally considered an expensive and labor-intensive strategy, when properly and successfully implemented it may actually be cost-effective for many anticancer drugs.[92]

Feedback-controlled dosing

It remains to be determined how information on inter-individual pharmacokinetic variability can eventually be used to devise an optimal dosage regimen of a drug for the treatment of a given disease in an individual patient. Obviously, the desired objective would be most efficiently achieved if the individual's dosage requirements could be calculated prior to administering the drug. While this ideal cannot be met completely in clinical practice, with the notable exception of carboplatin (see above), some success may be achieved by adopting feedback-controlled dosing. In the adaptive dosage with feedback control, population-based predictive models are used initially, but allow the possibility of dosage alteration based on feedback revision. In this approach, patients are first treated with standard dose and, during treatment, pharmacokinetic information is estimated by a limited-sampling strategy and compared with that predicted from the population model with which treatment was initiated. On the basis of the comparison, more patient-specific pharmacokinetic parameters are calculated, and dosage is adjusted accordingly to maintain the target exposure measure producing the desired pharmacodynamic effect. Despite its mathematical complexity, this approach may be the only way to deliver the desired and precise exposure of an anticancer agent.

Population pharmacokinetic strategies

The study of population pharmacokinetics seeks to identify the measurable factors that cause changes in the dose-concentration relationship and the extent of these alterations so that, if these are associated with clinically significant shifts in the therapeutic index, dosage can be appropriately modified in the individual patient. It is obvious that a careful collection of data during the development of drugs and subsequent analyses could be helpful to collect some essential information on the drug. Unfortunately, important information is often lost by failing to analyze this data or due to the fact that the relevant samples or data were never collected. Historically, this has resulted in the notion that tools for the identification of patient population subgroups are inadequate for most of the currently approved anticancer drugs. However, the use of population pharmacokinetic models is increasingly studied in an attempt to accommodate as much of the pharmacokinetic variability as possible in terms of measurable characteristics. This type of analysis has been conducted for a number of clinically important anticancer drugs and has provided mathematical equations based on morphometric, demographic, phenotypic enzyme activity, and/or physiologic characteristics of patients, in order to predict drug clearance with an acceptable degree of precision and bias.

Conclusions

Substantial progress has been made in recent years toward optimization of cancer chemotherapy during early phases of drug development with the use of pharmacokinetics, pharmacodynamics, and pharmacogenetics, although various aspects of anticancer drug pharmacology deserve more work before they become more useful clinically. Indeed, incorporation of pharmacologic principles in drug development and clinical trials is essential to maximize the clinical potentials of new anticancer agents, as improvements in outcome can be anticipated using these principles to individualize anticancer drug administration. In addition to its importance with classical anticancer drugs, incorporation of these principles will also be essential for the rational development of new agents designed to exploit advances in molecular oncology and those acting on oncogenes, tumor suppressor genes and related signal transduction pathways, invasion, angiogenesis, and metastasis, as well as agents used for chemoprevention.

Acknowledgment

The authors would like to thank Drs. Manish Sharma and Mark Ratain for their contributions to this article in the previous edition of this encyclopedia. Some of the key concepts and content from the last edition were carried forward into the current version.

References

1. Wellstein A. General principles in the pharmacotherapy of cancer. In: Hilal-Dandan R, Brunton LL, Knollmann BC, eds. *Goodman and Gilman's: The Pharmacological Basis of Therapeutics*, 13th ed. New York: McGraw-Hill Medical; 2018:1161–1166.
2. Zeind C, Carvalho M. *Koda-Kimble and Young's Applied Therapeutics: The Clinical Use of Drugs*. Philadelphia, PA: LWW; 2018.
3. Chu E, Sartorelli AC. Cancer chemotherapy (instead of adrenocorticosteroids and adrenocortical antagonists). In: Katzung BG, Trevor AJ, eds. *Adrenocorticosteroids and Adrenocortical Antagonists*, 13th ed. New York, NY: McGraw-Hill Medical; 2015.
4. Grothey A, Van Cutsem E, Sobrero A, et al. Regorafenib monotherapy for previously treated metastatic colorectal cancer (CORRECT): an international, multicentre, randomised, placebo-controlled, phase 3 trial. *Lancet*. 2013;**381**(9863):303–312.
5. Bins S, Ratain MJ, Mathijssen RH. Conventional dosing of anticancer agents: precisely wrong or just inaccurate? *Clin Pharmacol Ther*. 2014;**95**(4):361–364.
6. Le Tourneau C, Lee JJ, Siu LL. Dose escalation methods in phase I cancer clinical trials. *J Natl Cancer Inst*. 2009;**101**(10):708–720.

7. Marshall JL. Maximum-tolerated dose, optimum biologic dose, or optimum clinical value: dosing determination of cancer therapies. *J Clin Oncol.* 2012;**30**(23):2815–2816.
8. Ratain MJ. Targeted therapies: redefining the primary objective of phase I oncology trials. *Nat Rev Clin Oncol.* 2014;**11**(9):503–504.
9. Sparreboom A, Baker SD. Pharmacokinetics and pharmacodynamics of anticancer drugs. In: DeVita VT Jr, Lawrence TS, Rosenberg SA, eds. *DeVita, Hellman, and Rosenberg's Cancer: Principles and Practice of Oncology.* United States of America: Lippincott Williams & Wilkins (LWW); 2015.
10. Mould DR, Upton RN. Basic concepts in population modeling, simulation, and model-based drug development-part 2: introduction to pharmacokinetic modeling methods. *CPT Pharmacometrics Syst Pharmacol.* 2013;**2**:e38.
11. Hasovits C, Clarke S. Pharmacokinetics and pharmacodynamics of intraperitoneal cancer chemotherapeutics. *Clin Pharmacokinet.* 2012;**51**(4):203–224.
12. Jeon JY, Sparreboom A, Baker SD. Kinase inhibitors: the reality behind the success. *Clin Pharmacol Ther.* 2017;**102**(5):726–730.
13. DeMario MD, Ratain MJ. Oral chemotherapy: rationale and future directions. *J Clin Oncol.* 1998;**16**(7):2557–2567.
14. Deng J, Shao J, Markowitz JS, An G. ABC transporters in multi-drug resistance and ADME-Tox of small molecule tyrosine kinase inhibitors. *Pharm Res.* 2014;**31**(9):2237–2255.
15. Ratain MJ. Flushing oral oncology drugs down the toilet. *J Clin Oncol.* 2011;**29**(30):3958–3959.
16. Szmulewitz RZ, Ratain MJ. Playing Russian roulette with tyrosine kinase inhibitors. *Clin Pharmacol Ther.* 2013;**93**(3):242–244.
17. Ribas A, Zhang W, Chang I, et al. The effects of a high-fat meal on single-dose vemurafenib pharmacokinetics. *J Clin Pharmacol.* 2014;**54**(4):368–374.
18. Budha NR, Frymoyer A, Smelick GS, et al. Drug absorption interactions between oral targeted anticancer agents and PPIs: is pH-dependent solubility the Achilles heel of targeted therapy? *Clin Pharmacol Ther.* 2012;**92**(2):203–213.
19. Evans WE, Pratt CB. Effect of pleural effusion on high-dose methotrexate kinetics. *Clin Pharmacol Ther.* 1978;**23**(1):68–72.
20. Tahover E, Patil YP, Gabizon AA. Emerging delivery systems to reduce doxorubicin cardiotoxicity and improve therapeutic index: focus on liposomes. *Anticancer Drugs.* 2015;**26**(3):241–258.
21. Deeken JF, Löscher W. The blood-brain barrier and cancer: transporters, treatment, and Trojan horses. *Clin Cancer Res.* 2007;**13**(6):1663–1674.
22. Wu CY, Benet LZ. Predicting drug disposition via application of BCS: transport/absorption/ elimination interplay and development of a biopharmaceutics drug disposition classification system. *Pharm Res.* 2005;**22**(1):11–23.
23. Benet LZ. The role of BCS (biopharmaceutics classification system) and BDDCS (biopharmaceutics drug disposition classification system) in drug development. *J Pharm Sci.* 2013;**102**(1):34–42.
24. Ismael G, Hegg R, Muehlbauer S, et al. Subcutaneous versus intravenous administration of (neo)adjuvant trastuzumab in patients with HER2-positive, clinical stage I-III breast cancer (HannaH study): a phase 3, open-label, multicentre, randomised trial. *Lancet Oncol.* 2012;**13**(9):869–878.
25. Hassan M, Svensson US, Ljungman P, et al. A mechanism-based pharmacokinetic-enzyme model for cyclophosphamide autoinduction in breast cancer patients. *Br J Clin Pharmacol.* 1999;**48**(5):669–677.
26. Eechoute K, Fransson MN, Reyners AK, et al. A long-term prospective population pharmacokinetic study on imatinib plasma concentrations in GIST patients. *Clin Cancer Res.* 2012;**18**(20):5780–5787.
27. Graham RA, Lum BL, Cheeti S, et al. Pharmacokinetics of hedgehog pathway inhibitor vismodegib (GDC-0449) in patients with locally advanced or metastatic solid tumors: the role of alpha-1-acid glycoprotein binding. *Clin Cancer Res.* 2011;**17**(8):2512–2520.
28. Benet LZ, Hoener BA. Changes in plasma protein binding have little clinical relevance. *Clin Pharmacol Ther.* 2002;**71**(3):115–121.
29. Stuurman FE, Nuijen B, Beijnen JH, Schellens JH. Oral anticancer drugs: mechanisms of low bioavailability and strategies for improvement. *Clin Pharmacokinet.* 2013;**52**(6):399–414.
30. Malingré MM, Terwogt JM, Beijnen JH, et al. Phase I and pharmacokinetic study of oral paclitaxel. *J Clin Oncol.* 2000;**18**(12):2468–2475.
31. Eisenhauer EA, ten Bokkel Huinink WW, Swenerton KD, et al. European-Canadian randomized trial of paclitaxel in relapsed ovarian cancer: high-dose versus low-dose and long versus short infusion. *J Clin Oncol.* 1994;**12**(12):2654–2666.
32. Alberts DS, Chang SY, Chen HS, et al. Oral melphalan kinetics. *Clin Pharmacol Ther.* 1979;**26**(6):737–745.
33. Choi KE, Ratain MJ, Williams SF, et al. Plasma pharmacokinetics of high-dose oral melphalan in patients treated with trialkylator chemotherapy and autologous bone marrow reinfusion. *Cancer Res.* 1989;**49**(5):1318–1321.
34. Straw JA, Szapary D, Wynn WT. Pharmacokinetics of the diastereoisomers of leucovorin after intravenous and oral administration to normal subjects. *Cancer Res.* 1984;**44**(7):3114–3119.
35. Reece PA, Stafford I, Russell J, Gill PG. Nonlinear renal clearance of ultrafilterable platinum in patients treated with cis-dichlorodiammineplatinum (II). *Cancer Chemother Pharmacol.* 1985;**15**(3):295–299.
36. Forastiere AA, Belliveau JF, Goren MP, et al. Pharmacokinetic and toxicity evaluation of five-day continuous infusion versus intermittent bolus cis-diamminedichloroplatinum(II) in head and neck cancer patients. *Cancer Res.* 1988;**48**(13):3869–3874.
37. Karlsson MO, Molnar V, Bergh J, et al. A general model for time-dissociated pharmacokinetic-pharmacodynamic relationship exemplified by paclitaxel myelosuppression. *Clin Pharmacol Ther.* 1998;**63**(1):11–25.
38. Pezo R, Bedard P. Definition: translational and personalised medicine, biomarkers, pharmacodynamics. In: *ESMO Handbook of Translational Research*; 2015.
39. Slevin M, Clark PI, Joel SP, et al. A randomized trial to evaluate the effect of schedule on the activity of etoposide in small-cell lung cancer. *J Clin Oncol.* 1989;**7**(9):1333–1340.
40. Fox E, Curt GA, Balis FM. Clinical trial design for target-based therapy. *Oncologist.* 2002;**7**(5):401–409.

53 Folate antagonists

Lisa Gennarini, MD ■ Peter D. Cole, MD ■ Joseph R. Bertino, MD (deceased)

Overview

Folic acid antagonists (antifols) are cytotoxic drugs used as antineoplastic, antimicrobial, anti-inflammatory, and immune-suppressive agents. While several folate antagonists have been developed, methotrexate (4-amino-4-deoxy-10-N-methyl-pteroylglutamic acid, MTX) is the antifol with the most extensive history and widest spectrum of use. MTX remains an essential drug in curative chemotherapy regimens used to treat patients with acute lymphoblastic leukemia, osteosarcoma, and choriocarcinoma, and is an important agent in the therapy of patients with lymphoma, breast cancer, bladder cancer, and head and neck cancer. In addition, it is used for patients with nonmalignant diseases such as rheumatoid arthritis, psoriasis, autoimmune diseases, and graft-versus-host disease. This article will review the clinical use of and metabolism of MTX and discuss structurally related folate antagonists that have been developed to overcome resistance or have alternate intracellular targets.

Historical overview

In the early 1940s, the combined observations that patients with acute leukemia often have serum folate deficiency and that the bone marrow megaloblasts of folate-deficient patients morphologically resemble leukemic blasts prompted some investigators to postulate that leukemia might be a result of a deficiency of this B vitamin. However, it rapidly became apparent that administration of folic acid to patients with leukemia was not only ineffective but often accelerated the course of the disease.[1] Efforts to treat these leukemias thus turned to pharmacologically mimicking folate deficiency using folate analogs with effects antagonistic to those of the vitamin. Aminopterin (AMT) (4-amino-4-deoxy pteroylglutamic acid (PGA); AMT; Figure 1) was the first of these analogs to produce temporary remissions in 5 of 16 patients with acute leukemia.[2] This report was a landmark in cancer chemotherapy, as the first successful example of the power of rational drug design leading to an effective antineoplastic agent.

Since that initial study indicating the usefulness of AMT in the treatment of acute leukemia of childhood, there has been sustained interest in folate antagonists. Although known to be less potent, MTX supplanted AMT in the clinic in the early 1950s because the toxicity caused by AMT was greater and less predictable.[3-5] Newer antifols, rationally designed analogs of folate or MTX, have been synthesized either in an effort to overcome cellular resistance to MTX or to target alternative folate-dependent processes. Two of these, pralatrexate and pemetrexed, have received FDA approval for oncologic indications.

New classes of anticancer therapies, including immunotherapeutics and small molecule inhibitors are beginning to supplant conventional chemotherapy agents like MTX in front-line regimens for some cancers.[6] Nevertheless, antifols have been in continuous use for almost three-quarters of a century and are likely to continue to play a central role in curative regimens for decades to come.

Mechanisms of action of MTX

Folate antagonists function in several ways: by competing with folates for uptake into cells, by inhibiting the formation of folate coenzymes, or by inhibiting one or more reactions that are mediated by folate coenzymes. Thus far, the clinically important antineoplastic folate analogs appear to work primarily by inhibiting dihydrofolate reductase (DHFR) or thymidylate synthase (TS). The prototypic DHFR inhibitor is a 4-amino-substituted pterin compound, such as MTX or AMT (Figure 1). Substitution of an amino group for the 4-hydroxy moiety results in a folate analog with several thousand-fold increases in affinity for DHFR. The K_i of MTX for DHFR is below 10^{-10} M, well below the micromolar K_m of the natural substrate, dihydrofolate. By stoichiometrically inhibiting DHFR at slightly acidic pH, MTX blocks the cell's ability to replenish a supply of reduced folates necessary for *de novo* thymidylate synthesis (Figure 2).[7] In rapidly dividing cells, the inhibition of thymidylate biosynthesis leads to a decrease in thymidine triphosphate pools, a decrease in DNA synthesis, and eventually cell death.[8]

Intracellular metabolism of classical antifols like MTX to polyglutamate species significantly impacts their function and mechanisms of cytotoxicity.[9] Folylpolyglutamate synthetase (FPGS) adds glutamate residues in γ-carboxyl linkage to both folate coenzymes and classical folate antagonists (those with a glutamate moiety). This addition of up to seven or eight additional glutamate molecules serves to add mass and negative charge, markedly reducing efflux and increasing total intracellular accumulation at steady-state.[10] Both quantitative differences in FPGS expression and qualitative differences in FPGS function[11] exist between neoplastic and nonneoplastic tissues, which may explain some of the selectivity of antifolates for neoplastic cells.[12] A relative lack of FPGS may explain the observation that a cell population with a large number of G_0 cells would be less affected by the same concentration and time of exposure to MTX than a population with more actively dividing cells.

MTX polyglutamates are more potent inhibitors of DHFR than the parent compound, because they bind as tightly to DHFR as MTX but dissociate less rapidly.[13] In addition, MTX polyglutamates are also potent inhibitors of other folate-requiring enzymes, including TS[14] and two of the rate-limiting steps of *de novo* purine synthesis: glycinamide ribonucleotide (GAR) and aminoimidazole carboxamide ribonucleotide (AICAR) transformylases.[15] These

Figure 1 Structure of folic acid and structurally related classical antifols, AMT and MTX. (a) Folic acid (pteroylglutamic acid; PGA). (b) Aminopterin (4-amino-PGA). (c) Methotrexate (4-amino-N-10-methyl PGA).

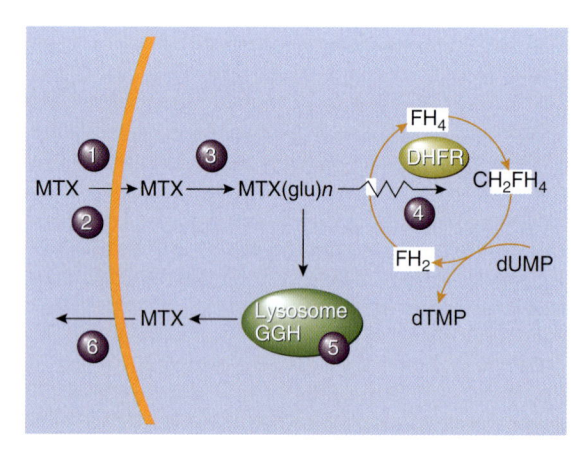

Figure 2 Primary site of action of MTX and MTX(glu)n. MTX enters cells by either the reduced folate carrier (1) or the membrane folate-binding protein (2). MTX is then metabolized by the cytosolic enzyme folylpolyglutamate synthetase (3) to MTX(glu)n, a potent inhibitor of dihydrofolate reductase (DHFR) (4). MTX(glu)n can be hydrolyzed to MTX by the lysosomal enzyme γ-glutamyl hydrolase (GGH) (5). Abbreviations: CH2FH4, N5, N10-methylene tetrahydrofolate; dTMP, deoxythymidine monophosphate; dUMP, deoxyuridine monophosphate/deoxyuridylate; FH2, dihydrofolate; FH4, tetrahydrofolate; MTX, methotrexate; MTX(glu)n, MTX polyglutamates.

two enzymes are also potently inhibited by DHF-polyglutamates and 10-formyl-DHF polyglutamates, which increase after MTX inhibits DHFR.[16] As a result, inhibition of de novo purine synthesis may be at least as relevant as DHFR inhibition to the cytotoxic effects of MTX in cancer cells[17] and for the anti-inflammatory action of MTX in patients with rheumatologic diseases.[18,19]

Other possible mechanisms by which MTX exerts antineoplastic or anti-inflammatory action are worth mentioning. First, by inhibiting folate-dependent methionine biosynthesis, MTX causes intracellular concentrations of homocysteine (Hcy) to increase, resulting in a secondary increase in S-adenosyl-homocysteine (SAH), a potent inhibitor of many folate-dependent methylation reactions. MTX exposure, therefore, can block membrane localization of Ras,[20] a member of a family of critical signal transduction proteins constitutively activated in many human cancers. Second, the anti-inflammatory effects of MTX, and some component of its antineoplastic activity may be due to its ability to inhibit endothelial cell proliferation at low concentrations.[21] Preclinical data confirm that low-dose MTX can inhibit the growth of microscopic metastatic disease through its antiangiogenic properties.[22] In addition to the mechanisms mentioned above, rapidly proliferating cancer cells overexpress enzymes of the mitochondrial and glycine-serine pathway, and this phenotype is a determinant of methotrexate sensitivity.[23]

Pharmacokinetics of MTX

MTX is one of few anticancer agents for which pharmacokinetic data are routinely used in clinical practice to modulate the balance between efficacy and toxicity.[24] Retrospective analysis of children with acute lymphocytic leukemia (ALL) shows that lower MTX clearance[25] and higher MTX concentrations[26] are associated with lower risk of relapse. Even more intriguing are data from a prospective randomized trial in patients with ALL comparing dosing by body surface area with individualized dosing based on pharmacokinetic data, which showed significantly improved complete continuous remission rates in the individualized therapy arm.[27] It is possible, however, that these results are protocol-specific, since others have found that pharmacologically guided treatment intensification led to inferior outcomes for some subpopulations.[28]

Absorption

Following oral administration, peak plasma concentrations occur 1–5 h after a dose of 15–30 mg/m^2. Absorption can be relatively poor and unpredictable,[29,30] affected by food, nonabsorbable antibiotics, bile salts, and a shortened intestine transit time. Thus, it is suggested that the drug be taken on an empty stomach with clear liquids. Nevertheless, at a dose and schedule of 25 mg/m^2, given orally every 6 h for four doses, plasma MTX concentration greater than 0.5 μM was observed in more than 85% of pediatric patients with ALL, indicating the reliability of this oral regimen.[31]

Distribution

After intravenous (IV) administration of MTX, the initial volume of distribution (V_d) is approximately 0.18 L/kg of body weight. The initial distribution phase has a $T_{1/2}$ of 30–45 min; the beta $T_{1/2}$ is 3–4 h. Steady-state V_d is between 0.4 and 0.8 L/kg.[32]

After high doses of MTX (>3 g/m^2), peak serum concentrations in the range of 10^{-4} to 10^{-3} M are achieved.[33] At these concentrations, transmembrane transport is saturated, limiting further influx of MTX to passive diffusion. Uptake of reduced folates, including leucovorin (LV), is inhibited as well. Studies of MTX metabolism in lymphoblasts in vitro have also shown that too high extracellular concentration of drug can impede metabolism of MTX to a polyglutamate.[34]

MTX binding to plasma proteins, especially to albumin, is approximately 50%.[35,36] The 7-hydroxy metabolite of MTX is 90% bound to plasma proteins, but apparently does not interfere with MTX binding to plasma proteins at clinically observed concentrations. The highest tissue-to-plasma concentrations found in humans are in the liver and kidney, followed by the gastrointestinal tract. Prolonged plasma levels after high-dose MTX infusions in humans have been attributed to decreased transit rate secondary to gastrointestinal obstruction.

Because of the blood–brain barrier and efflux mechanisms that actively remove MTX from the central nervous system (CNS),[37] cerebrospinal fluid (CSF) MTX concentrations are approximately 1% of those in the plasma. Cytocidal concentrations are, therefore, not obtained in the CSF after conventional doses but only with doses of 500 mg/m^2 and higher.[38] After high-dose systemic MTX (HDMTX) administration, lumbar CSF and ventricular CSF concentrations were similar. HDMTX may, therefore, be able to replace intrathecal drug for the treatment of patients with nonleukemic leptomeningeal disease.[39] However, a meta-analysis of CNS-directed therapy for children with acute lymphoblastic leukemia concluded that efforts to increase CSF penetration using HDMTX have not produced the desired result of lowering the rate of CNS relapse in this population.[40]

As MTX is accumulated poorly into the CSF, even small doses of LV given orally can increase CSF folates significantly. This systemic rescue, especially if given too early after MTX, may rescue leukemic cells in the CSF compartment.[41]

When injected into an indwelling ventricular catheter, MTX reaches reproducible therapeutic drug concentrations ($>10^{-6}$ M) for at least 48 h.[42] In contrast, when MTX is given by the lumbar route into the CSF, it distributes unreliably into the ventricles. An improved dose schedule utilizing the administration of multiple small doses of intrathecal MTX has been suggested.[43] Following intrathecal administration, MTX slowly exits into the systemic circulation with a $t_{1/2}$ of 8–10 h.[37] Systemic toxicity can be observed if multiple doses of intrathecal MTX are administered without LV rescue. The pharmacology of intrathecal MTX and the amount of intraventricular MTX may be altered by overt meningeal leukemia and the position of the patient at the time of lumbar puncture.[44] The clinical observation that irradiation followed by MTX treatment may predispose patients to neurotoxicity may be a consequence of the effect of radiation therapy (RT) on the blood–brain barrier.[45]

Patients with pleural or peritoneal effusions may be at increased risk for developing toxicity to HDMTX as a result of "third spacing," or MTX trapping in the infusion, and slow release leading to sustained MTX concentrations in serum.[46] In these circumstances, higher LV doses and prolonged LV rescue may be necessary until the serum level of MTX decreases to less than 0.05×10^{-6} M.

Metabolism

The major metabolite of MTX, produced by the action of hepatic aldehyde oxidase, is 7-hydroxy MTX (7-OH MTX) (Figure 3), which is only 1% as potent an inhibitor of DHFR as MTX.[47] It is also less water soluble than MTX and may contribute to renal toxicity after high doses.[48]

A second, less important pathway of metabolism of MTX occurs in the intestine. MTX is hydrolyzed by bacteria to the pteroate (4-deoxy-4-amino-N10-methyl pteroic acid; dAMPA) and glutamic acid (Figure 3).[49] dAMPA, like 7-OH MTX, is also a relatively inactive metabolite with approximately 1/200th the affinity of MTX for DHFR. dAMPA excretion in the urine accounts for <5% of the dose administered.

The third metabolic product of MTX is MTX polyglutamate. As discussed above, MTX polyglutamates are at least as potent inhibitors of DHFR as is MTX and have a slower rate of disassociation from DHFR.[13] MTX polyglutamates are not found in plasma or urine because of the abundant activity of γ-glutamyl hydrolase(s) (GGH) in plasma that convert folyl- and MTX-polyglutamates to monoglutamates. Like MTX, 7-OH MTX is also polyglutamylated intracellularly, and retention of these polyglutamate forms could contribute to MTX cytotoxicity.[50]

It has been proposed that compliance with oral MTX regimens can be monitored by measuring MTX-polyglutamate concentrations within circulating erythrocytes [red blood cells (RBCs)].[51–53]

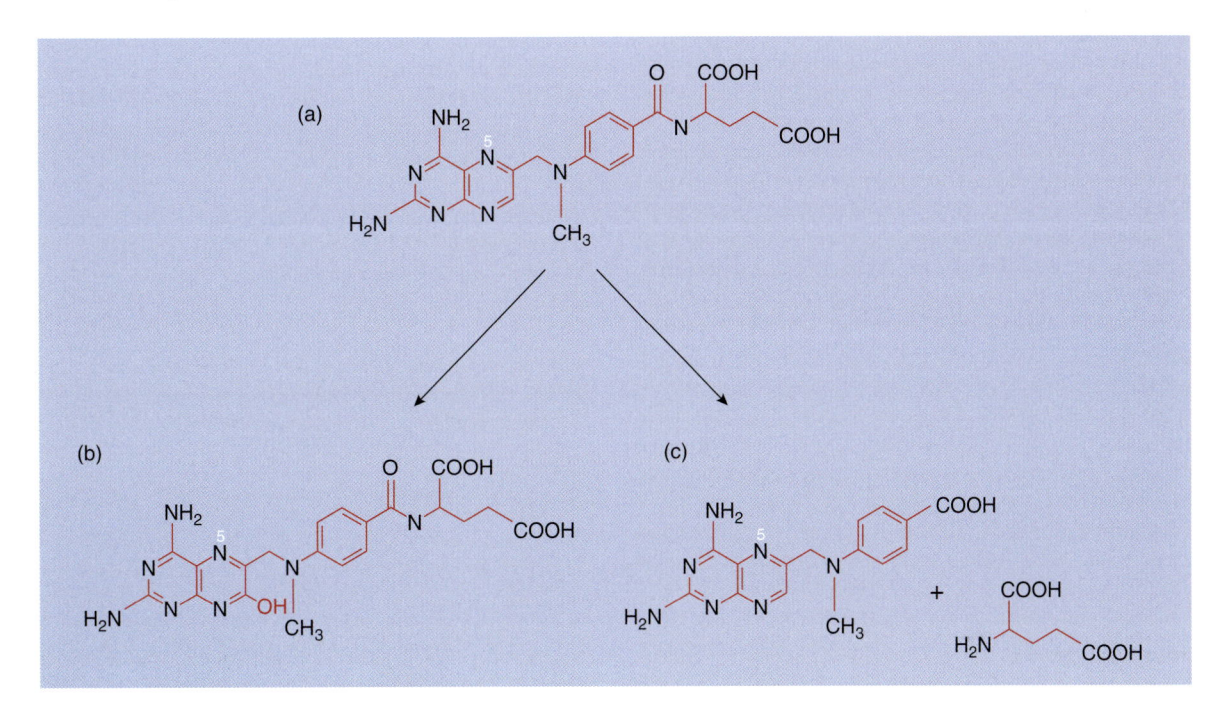

Figure 3 Catabolism of MTX. MTX (a) can be converted in the liver to 7-OH MTX (b). In addition, enteric bacteria will cleave the molecule to dAMPA plus glutamate (c).

Nucleated RBC precursors within the bone marrow will accumulate and metabolize circulating MTX. The resulting MTX polyglutamates will remain within the mature RBC throughout its lifespan,[54] while unmetabolized MTX will gradually efflux.[55]

Excretion

The majority of administered MTX (and its metabolites 7-OH MTX and DAMPA) is excreted unchanged in the urine.[56,57] Because of active secretion in the proximal tubules, renal clearance of MTX can exceed creatinine clearance.[58] There is wide inter-patient variability in MTX clearance, which does not correlate perfectly with renal function.[59] It has been reported that MTX excretion seems to be inversely related to age as plasma clearance of renal eliminated drugs is closely correlated with maturation of kidney function. Children tend to exhibit more rapid MTX clearance than adults, and a general trend toward decreasing clearance with increasing age has been observed.[60] MTX excretion through organic acid transporters can be inhibited by probenecid or competitively blocked by other weak organic acids, such as aspirin or penicillin G. MTX elimination is increased by drugs that block distal tubular reabsorption, such as folic acid, some cephalosporins, and sulfamethoxazole.

Less than 10% of MTX is typically recovered in the feces.[61] Following IV administration of doses of 30–80 mg/m^2, 0.4–20% of the administered dose is excreted through the canalicular multi-organic acid transporter (cMOAT; ABCC2; MRP2) into the bile. Using a knock-out mouse model (ABCC2$^{-/-}$; ABCG2$^{-/-}$), it was shown that both transporters play overlapping roles in the elimination of MTX and 7OH-MTX. Many polymorphisms and mutations of these transporters have been identified, leading to differences in expression and activity, affecting systemic MTX exposure. Consequently, patients with mutations or heterozygous polymorphisms in ABCC2 and/or ABCG2 might be at increased risk for MTX toxicity.[62]

Drug interactions

Several drugs used in patients with cancer, including antibiotics, may alter the renal excretion of MTX, increasing toxicity or decreasing efficacy. Deleterious and even fatal reactions have been reported between MTX and nonsteroidal anti-inflammatory drugs, in particular with naproxen and ketoprofen.[63,64] This increased toxicity may be due to decreased renal elimination, possibly as a result of competition for renal secretion.[58] Other commonly used organic drugs may also potentiate MTX toxicity, such as phenylbutazone, salicylate, and probenecid.[65,66] Probenecid increased the efficacy of MTX in tumor-bearing mice, but it has not been used clinically with this goal in mind.[67]

Increased toxicity was also reported when trimethoprim, the antibacterial agent, was used together with MTX. Presumably, this antifolate, with only weak binding affinity to mammalian DHFR, lowers folate stores, especially in patients with subclinical folate deficiency, making marrow cells more susceptible to MTX-induced toxicity.[68] Alcohol should also be avoided in patients receiving MTX because of the risk of hepatic fibrosis and cirrhosis.

Pharmacogenomics

A growing body of data implicates inherited variation in genes for enzymes responsible for folate metabolism in interpatient variability in antifolate response or toxicity. A more detailed discussion of these data is beyond the scope of this article but has been the subject of comprehensive reviews.[69–72] Briefly, functional polymorphisms have been described in either the promoter or coding regions of the genes for DHFR, methylenetetrahydrofolate reductase (MTHFR), aminoimidazole carboxamide ribonucleotide transformylase (ATIC), the reduced folate carrier (RFC), GGH, methionine synthase (MTR), methionine synthase reductase (MTRR), methylenetetrahydrofolate dehydrogenase (MTHFD), serine hydroxymethyltransferase (SHMT), TS, and solute carrier organic anion transporter gene 1B1 (SLCO1B1). Many of these polymorphisms are present at significant frequency among the population and some have been linked to higher rates of relapse or toxicity among patients with acute lymphoblastic leukemia[73–80] or rheumatoid arthritis.[81] If replicated in larger populations, these data suggest the potential for individualizing MTX therapy, based on each patient's genotype.

Gene–environment interactions may also modulate the effects of genotypic variation on toxicity. To focus on one relevant example, some of the observed variation in serum homocysteine (a marker of functional folate deficiency) is explained by two common functional polymorphisms in the MTHFR gene, C677T and A1298C, but only under conditions of decreased intake of dietary folate.[82,83] Adequate dietary folate in countries with mandated folate supplementation could, therefore, erase the effects of genetic polymorphisms.

Clinical application

Clinical dosage schedules

MTX has been administered on a variety of dosage schedules since its introduction into the clinic five decades ago (Table 1). In a trial of MTX in patients with head and neck cancer treated with either 50, 500, or 5000 mg/m^2 with LV "rescue," a trend of dose responsiveness was seen (5 of 24, 5 of 16, 9 of 18, respectively). Some responses were noted with the 5000 mg/m^2 dose regimen in patients who did not respond at lower doses.[84] The importance of dose scheduling was emphasized by an experimental study showing that resistance to high-dose pulse MTX may not extend to continuous low-dose exposure.[85] Determining the optimum dose schedule of MTX is complicated by the use of the drug in combination therapy (Table 2). Sequencing appears to be important when MTX is used with 5-fluorouracil (5-FU), with L-asparaginase, and probably with cytosine arabinoside and 6-mercaptopurine or 6-thioguanine. Table 2 summarizes the use of some common drug combinations that include MTX, along with sequence-specificity.

Table 1 Dosage schedules commonly used for methotrexate.

Schedule and dose	Use/comments
Oral	
Weekly or biweekly (15–25 mg in single or divided doses)	Mainly for nonmalignant conditions, such as psoriasis or rheumatoid arthritis
Weekly or biweekly (20–30 mg/m^2)	Maintenance therapy for ALL
Parenteral	
Pulse weekly (30–60 mg/m^2)	Choriocarcinoma, ALL
Intermediate dose (120–500 mg/m^2 weekly)	ALL, NHL; requires LV rescue, 10–15 mg/m^2 q 6 h × 6–8 doses
High dose (500–12 000 mg/m^2 weekly or every other week)	Osteosarcoma, ALL, neoplastic meningitis; requires LV rescue

Abbreviations: ALL, acute lymphoblastic leukemia; LV, leucovorin; NHL, non-Hodgkin lymphoma.

Table 2 Combination chemotherapy with methotrexate.

Used with	Schedule notes	Result	Comments
5-FU	MTX must precede 5-FU by 24 h	Synergistic	
Anthracyclines		Additive	
Bleomycin		Additive	Mucosal toxicity is increased
Corticosteroids	Used together	Synergistic	Used in ALL
Cyclophosphamide	Used together	Additive	
Cytarabine	Used together	Additive or synergistic	
L-Asparaginase	If MTX precedes l-asparaginase by 24 h	Synergistic	Used in ALL
	If used simultaneously	Aantagonistic	AML
Vinca alkaloids		Additive	

Abbreviations: ALL, acute lymphoblastic leukemia; AML, acute myelogenous leukemia; 5-FU, 5-fluorouracil.

Current uses for MTX in the treatment of neoplastic disease

Acute lymphoblastic leukemia

MTX is a component of nearly all multi-agent therapeutic regimens for patients with acute lymphoblastic leukemia postremission, and some protocols include MTX in remission induction. In addition to systemic use, MTX is administered intrathecally for the treatment of meningeal leukemia and for prophylaxis against CNS relapse.

During the intensive, early postremission phases, MTX can be administered orally or parenterally. Parenteral administration at intermediate dose (100–500 mg/m^2/dose) or high dose (≥1000 mg/m^2) has been incorporated in some protocols to increase accumulation of MTX-polyglutamates by blast cells,[86] to overcome mechanisms of resistance and to increase penetration into protected sites including the CNS and testes.[87] While the ability of HDMTX to prevent CNS relapse is not clearly proven,[40] the rate of isolated testicular relapse does appear to have decreased with the addition of intermediate or HDMTX.[88] Randomized trials comparing escalating IV doses with oral MTX showed a significant improvement in 5-year event-free survival (EFS) in those patients randomly assigned to the IV MTX-based interim maintenance compared with the oral MTX-based arm.[89-93] However, in some studies, the increase in EFS came at the expense of increased hematologic and neurologic toxicity.[94-97] Disease sensitivity to MTX differs between B-ALL and T-ALL. Two different MTX intensification strategies are commonly used in pediatric ALL trials: HDMTX with LV rescue and Capizzi-style escalating intravenous MTX without LV rescue plus pegaspargase Capizzi-style, intravenous MTX (C-MTX). Recent reports suggest that C-MTX is superior to HDMTX for those patients with T-ALL.[98]

During later maintenance phases, most current protocols rely on prolonged weekly administration of MTX at low doses (20–50 mg/m^2/dose) in combination with daily mercaptopurine. Early studies showed that twice-weekly therapy (20 mg/m^2) was superior to continuous daily oral administration for treatment during remission.[99] The effectiveness of an oral divided dose (25–30 mg/m^2 given every 6 h for 4–6 doses weekly) has also been shown.[31]

Acute myelogenous leukemia

MTX has limited value in the current treatment of patients with acute nonlymphocytic leukemia. Complete remissions can be seen in approximately one-quarter of adults with AML treated with MTX-containing regimens: prednisone, Oncovin (vincristine), methotrexate and Purinethol (mercaptopurine) (POMP)[100] or MTX with L-asparaginase (the "Capizzi Regimen").[101,102] High-dose regimens with LV rescue have a transient but rapid effect on the peripheral blood count without producing marrow remission in the large majority of these patients.[103] The lack of efficacy of MTX in this disease has been attributed to poor intracellular retention of the drug caused by a lack of polyglutamylation, and an increase of the target enzyme DHFR following treatment.[104]

Lymphoma

Based on Phase II studies that indicated that moderate to high doses of MTX (200 to 3000 mg/m^2) with LV rescue could produce transient regressions in patients with large cell lymphoma, MTX with LV rescue has been added to combination regimens for intermediate- and high-grade lymphomas. In some regimens (e.g., M-BACOD), MTX is used with LV during the leukopenic phase of drug treatment, since the MTX/LV combination has little marrow toxicity.[105] Based on experimental studies showing that MTX and cytosine arabinoside produce additive and possibly synergistic effects,[106] this combination has also been utilized in regimens to treat this disease [e.g., COMLA (cyclophosphamide, vincristine, MTX, cytosine arabinoside, and LV)]. Similarly, following documentation of responses among patients with Burkitt's lymphoma to therapy including MTX,[107,108] high-dose MTX with LV rescue has been added to cyclophosphamide, vincristine, doxorubicin, dexamethasone (CVAD), cytarabine, and intrathecal therapy as well as to other combination chemotherapy regimens for patients with Burkitt's lymphoma.[109-111]

Most treatment regimens for patients with primary central nervous system lymphoma (PCNSL) include high-dose MTX, as conventional radiation doses may lead to neurotoxicity. The optimal HDMTX-based regimen for PCNSL has not been determined, however, and there is variation in clinical practice. While single-agent MTX has significant activity, experience in other hematologic malignancies suggests that combination therapy is more effective than single-agent induction therapy.[112] In a retrospective review of 226 patients with PCNSL, those patients treated with regimens that included HDMTX followed by radiotherapy had an improved survival, with no higher risk of late neurotoxicity.[113]

Choriocarcinoma

Choriocarcinoma is unique in that single-drug treatment with either MTX or actinomycin D produces a substantial number of cures.[114,115] The basis for the unusual sensitivity of this tumor to MTX is not entirely clear, but choriocarcinoma cells may accumulate and retain this drug effectively by synthesizing long-chain polyglutamates. The JAR (human choriocarcinoma) cell line was shown to have active-receptor coupled uptake (potocytosis) of folates and antifolates.[116] Current programs for the treatment of this malignancy utilize MTX in combination with other drugs, especially for "poor risk" or relapsed patients.[117]

Breast cancer
MTX as a single agent causes regressions of breast cancer in approximately 30% of patients. When used with fluorouracil, sequential use of MTX followed by 5-FU improved response rates to 50% and it also improved disease-free survival when used as adjuvant therapy.[118] The adjuvant use of cyclophosphamide, MTX, and 5-FU (CMF), also significantly reduces the risk of relapse,[119] may allow more conservative surgery among women with localized disease when used as neoadjuvant therapy,[120] and has a role in the treatment for patients with inoperable, advanced disease.[121] The combination of MTX, 5-FU with vinorelbine (VMF) instead of cyclophosphamide has also shown activity among women with advanced breast cancer.[122] An additional advantage of this combination is the diminution of long-term toxicity (infertility, carcinogenesis) compared to regimens containing alkylating agents. Finally, it is interesting to note that low-dose oral MTX (2.5 mg BID × 2 days/week) with daily oral cyclophosphamide has shown activity among heavily pretreated women with advanced metastatic breast cancer.[123]

Gastrointestinal cancer
Antifolates have limited effectiveness in the treatment of gastrointestinal malignancies. The role of MTX in the treatment of these diseases is mainly to modulate, and possibly improve, the effectiveness of 5-FU. By inhibiting purine synthesis, MTX pretreatment increases phosphoribosyl pyrophosphate, a precursor necessary for 5FU nucleotide formation.[124] Data from trials using high-dose MTX followed by LV/5-FU in patients with colon cancer highlight the need for a 7- to 24-h interval between MTX and 5-FU administration.[125] However, a randomized Phase III study comparing 5FU plus MTX to standard, continuous infusion of 5FU demonstrated increased toxicity among those treated with MTX, and no difference in overall survival between the two arms. Based on these findings, 5FU remains the standard of care for advanced gastric cancer.[126–128]

Genitourinary cancer
MTX alone (100 mg/m^2), or in high doses ($\geq$500 mg/m^2) with LV rescue, is active in the treatment of advanced bladder cancer. The response rate reported (approximately 30%) is similar to the response rate of the other most active single drug, cisplatin. Combinations of drugs including MTX with cisplatin, vinblastine, and doxorubicin (M-VAC) have resulted in a substantial number of long-term clinical remissions.[129] A meta-analysis of randomized trials demonstrated that neoadjuvant treatment with MTX-containing regimens conferred a survival advantage.[130]

Head and neck cancer
MTX is an active agent for the treatment of patients with advanced carcinoma of the head and neck region. High-dose MTX regimens with LV rescue appear to improve response rates from 30% to 50%, but remission duration and survival rates are not improved.[131] MTX has also been used with 5-FU in this disease, with response rates as high as 60%.[132,133] The sequence and timing of drug administration have not been shown to affect the response rate, although different patterns of toxicity were observed.

Central nervous system tumors
Multiagent chemotherapy including HDMTX followed by high-dose chemotherapy with autologous hematopoietic stem cell rescue (HDCSCR) has been shown to be effective in several small studies and case series in patients with high-grade embryonal CNS tumors.[134] For those patients who are ineligible for HDCSCR, HDMTX with dose intensified chemotherapy with or without RT has proven to be a safe and efficacious treatment approach.[135]

Lung cancer
MTX as a single agent in conventional doses, or in high doses with LV rescue, has only marginal activity in non-small-cell lung cancer (NSCLC). This drug does have limited activity in small-cell lung cancer and has been used in combination regimens to treat that disease. Pralatrexate, a nonclassical antifolate later discussed in further detail, has been shown to have activity for patients with previously treated NSCLC.[136]

Osteogenic sarcoma
Osteosarcoma responds poorly to conventional dose of methotrexate. However, high-dose methotrexate has been one of the mainstays of treatment since its introduction in the 1970s.[137] Randomized trials of pre- and postdefinitive treatment demonstrated the beneficial effect of chemotherapy that includes HDMTX with LV rescue.[138] Different studies investigated whether MTX peak concentration and area under concentration–time curve (AUC) are significant prognostic factors of osteosarcoma.[139] There remains controversy as to whether there is correlation between MTX exposure and outcome.[140] Among children treated with HDMTX for osteosarcoma, there was no correlation between survival and peak concentration or AUC; however, the 48-h MTX concentration had significant correlation to survival, confirming that systemic MTX exposure was a significant prognostic factor of treatment outcome.[141]

Neoplastic meningitis
Intrathecal MTX is often a component of therapy for patients with solid-tumor neoplastic meningitis. Systemic administration of HDMTX (8 g/m^2) with LV rescue is the most widely used alternative to IT chemotherapy,[39] as therapeutic antineoplastic concentrations of MTX can be achieved more easily in the presence of neoplastic meningitis.[142]

Adverse effects

Hematologic toxicity
Expression of many folate-dependent enzymes targeted by MTX is cell-cycle specific, consistent with their role in DNA synthesis. Tissues that are self-renewing, with a higher S-phase fraction, are therefore at highest risk for damage by the folate antagonists. Bone marrow progenitor cells of all lineages are affected by MTX, but neutropenia usually predominates, with a nadir 10 days after drug administration and recovery typically between days 14 and 21. The effects on the marrow are dose related, but there is considerable variability among patients. Genetic variants,[72,143,144] subclinical folate deficiency, impaired renal function, a damaged marrow owing to previous RT, chemotherapy, or infection, and the use of trimethoprim-sulfamethoxazole for *Pneumocystis jirovecii*

Table 3 Supportive care for high-dose methotrexate treatment.

Pretreatment hydration and alkalinization
8–12 h before treatment, patients should receive 1.5 L/m² of saline or 5% glucose with 100 mEq HCO₃ and 20 mEq KCl/L. Continue hydration until urine pH is 7.0 or greater before MTX administration
Monitoring
MTX levels should be monitored at 24 h after completion of MTX infusion. Serum creatinine should be measured pretreatment, at 24, and at 48 h
Additional LV rescue
Required for an MTX level >10⁻⁶ M at 24 h. Increase LV dose to 100 mg/m² q 6 h for levels above 10⁻⁶ M and 200 mg/m² q 6 h for levels above 5 × 10⁻⁶ M. Monitor MTX levels daily and continue LV until plasma MTX concentration is <10⁻⁸ M

Abbreviations: LV, leucovorin; MTX, methotrexate.

prophylaxis may predispose patients to hematologic (and gastrointestinal) toxicity. Young patients usually tolerate MTX better than older individuals, a fact presumably related to clearance of the drug by the kidneys. The administration of LV can prevent or lessen MTX toxicity and allow larger doses of the antifolate to be administered.

Gastrointestinal toxicity

Nausea and vomiting, even with high doses of MTX, are usually mild to moderate. In contrast, mucositis is a common side effect of MTX treatment. Mucositis usually becomes manifest 3–5 days following exposure to the drug. This is an early sign of MTX toxicity, and the drug should be discontinued when it occurs. More severe gastrointestinal toxicity is manifest by diarrhea, which may progress to severe bloody diarrhea. When this occurs in association with neutropenia, patients are at high risk of typhlitis, sepsis, and death. These severe side effects generally occur in a setting of renal damage, usually a consequence of high doses of MTX ($\geq$500 mg/m²/dose) but may also occur in patients treated with conventional doses. MTX blood levels and serum creatinine levels should be followed, and appropriate doses of LV administered, along with the supportive measures instituted (see below).

Renal toxicity

Renal toxicity occurs occasionally following high-dose regimens and is rare during treatment with lower doses of MTX. When it occurs, renal toxicity leads to delayed MTX clearance and subsequently to severe marrow and gastrointestinal toxicity, which can be fatal, especially in adults.[145] This toxicity is believed to be due to precipitation of MTX and its less soluble metabolite 7-OH MTX (Figure 3) in the tubules, as well as to a possible direct effect of this drug on the renal tubule.[48] The use of vigorous hydration, often with osmotic diuresis and alkalinization of urine to increase solubility of MTX and 7-OH MTX, has markedly ameliorated this problem. Occasional patients, even with this regimen, exhibit renal impairment, and therefore it is essential to carefully monitor MTX and creatinine serum levels (Table 3). In developing and middle-income countries where resources are limited, algorithms using single determinations of serum MTX concentrations permit safe administration of HDMTX when limited resources preclude more frequent drug measurements.[146] For those patients who have markedly delayed clearance of MTX secondary to acute renal dysfunction, increasing the dose and rate of LV administration has been the routine therapeutic maneuver to counteract the consequences of prolonged exposure to high MTX levels.[147]

Methylxanthines, such as caffeine or aminophylline, may be useful in the setting of delayed MTX clearance. MTX administration has been shown to increase serum adenosine concentrations, which will decrease glomerular filtration rate.[18] Adenosine receptor competitive antagonists, like the methylxanthines, may therefore act as a specific diuretic to increase MTX elimination.[148]

Extremely high levels of MTX (>10⁻³ M) are difficult to rescue, even with high doses of LV.[149] Removal of MTX by peritoneal dialysis or hemodialysis is ineffective because the drug is extensively protein-bound. Charcoal hemoperfusion columns have been used successfully in a small number of patients, but their efficacy is limited by rebounds in MTX levels.[150] Extracorporeal methods of methotrexate removal such as high-flux hemodialysis and hemodiafiltration have had variable efficacy, but both are highly invasive procedures which have resulted in only transient and small decrease in MTX levels, necessitating their combined or repeated daily use to effectively lower MTX concentration.[151,152] Oral charcoal and cholestyramine have also been used to bind MTX in the gut, thus limiting enterohepatic recirculation and toxicity.[153] Thymidine (1–3 g/m²/d) is also capable of rescuing patients from MTX toxicity, but this metabolite is not generally available.[154] A recombinant form of bacterial carboxypeptidase, glucarpidase [carboxypeptidase-G₂ (CPDG₂)], an enzyme which hydrolytically cleaves the peptide bond in MTX resulting in glutamate and dAMPA (Figure 3), has been reported to rapidly reduce systemic MTX concentrations by >95% within 1 h of administration.[155–157] When given in combination within 96 h after the start of the MTX infusion in addition to LV, carboxypeptidase G2 is highly effective in patients at high risk for developing life-threatening MTX toxicity IV[156,158,159] or intrathecal MTX administration.[160] While most studies are reported in the adult population, a retrospective review in pediatric patients showed similar results.[161]

Hepatotoxicity

Chronic low-dose weekly MTX treatment for patients with psoriasis, rheumatoid arthritis, or ALL has been associated with portal fibrosis, and in some patients, with frank cirrhosis.[162] Among cancer patients, acute elevations of liver enzymes commonly occur within days after treatment with MTX, but rapidly return to normal, and do not appear to predict chronic liver toxicity, even when elevated to 10–20 times the upper limit of normal. Rarely, HDMTX causes a temporary elevation in serum bilirubin, which usually normalizes within a few days.[163,164] Concurrent administration of dexamethasone may increase MTX-induced hepatotoxicity.[165] Alcohol and other hepatotoxic drugs should be avoided in these patient populations.

There are at least three case reports of hepatocellular carcinoma developing in patients with MTX-induced hepatic fibrosis, all of which were in children treated for ALL. These data suggest a potential for long-term carcinogenesis following treatment with MTX, at least in the rare patient who develops hepatic fibrosis.[166–168]

Central nervous system toxicity

Intrathecal MTX and intravenous administration of high-dose MTX have been associated with acute, subacute, and long-term neurotoxicity. Neurotoxicity can be manifested as aseptic meningitis, transverse myelopathy, acute and subacute encephalopathy, and leukoencephalopathy. The manifestations of MTX neurotoxicity are largely determined by its dose and route of administration. In cases of inadvertent overdosing (>100 mg intrathecally), fatalities have been reported. Greater understanding of the pathophysiology of MTX-induced neurotoxicity is now leading to therapeutic interventions to prevent or treat this complication of therapy.

The most common immediate side effect of intrathecal MTX administration, made manifest by severe headache, fever, meningismus, vomiting, and CSF pleocytosis, is thought to be caused by a chemical arachnoiditis, or perhaps by the release of adenosine, which is a potent autocoid in the CNS.[169] This effect of adenosine has been ameliorated by systemic administration of low doses of methylxanthines, such as aminophylline and theophylline, which act as competitive antagonists at adenosine receptors.[148] Dosage adjustment or switching to cytosine arabinoside may be required if these symptoms persist. Acute toxicity occurring several days after high-dose systemic MTX treatment manifests with headache, paresis, aphasia, or seizures. It is usually transient, resolving within 2–3 days.[170]

Subacute neurotoxicity (7–14 days after administration) has been observed in 5–18% of patients receiving intrathecal MTX and/or intravenous high-dose MTX. At its most severe, it presents with motor paralysis of the extremities, cranial nerve palsies, seizures, and even coma. While the pathogenesis of subacute antifolate-induced neurotoxicity is likely multifactorial, disruption to homocysteine homeostasis may play a pivotal role. By inhibiting re-methylation to methionine, MTX leads to increased amounts of homocysteine in the plasma and CSF of patients.[171] Homocysteine may cause neurotoxicity through induction of oxidative damage to neuronal tissue and vascular endothelium.[172,173] In addition, homocysteine and its metabolites are excitotoxic amino acids (glutamate analog) that activates the N-methyl-D-aspartate (NMDA) class of glutamate receptors. Subacute neurotoxicity of MTX may, therefore, be ameliorated by an antagonist of the NMDA receptor, such as dextromethorphan or memantine.[174–176]

Delayed MTX-induced neurotoxicity may be associated with chronic demyelinating encephalopathy in as many as 80% of children with acute lymphoblastic leukemia, and the magnitude of the radiographic changes seems to correlate with both the number of individual MTX doses, as well as the level (g/m^2) of each individual MTX dose.[96,97] Computed tomography scans show cortical thinning, ventricular enlargement, and diffuse intracerebral calcifications. Although most commonly attributed to the combination of cranial radiation with intrathecal MTX, encephalopathy has been reported in patients treated only with high-dose IV MTX. The pathogenesis of delayed neurotoxicity may be a result of impairing folate-dependent methylation of components of the myelin sheath.[177]

Methotrexate exposure has also been associated with persistent cognitive deficits among survivors, including impairments of memory, attention, and executive functions. In addition, methotrexate-induced changes in neuroinflammatory markers and cellular proliferation, along with structural changes in the corpus callosum have also been observed. Further study will determine whether the observed changes are directly responsible for causing cognitive deficits or are simply biomarkers reflective of prolonged chemotherapy exposure.[178]

In patients who receive a MTX overdose intrathecally (>100 mg), immediate CSF removal with ventriculumbar perfusion is indicated.[179] Intrathecal use of carboxypeptidase G2 was shown to decrease mortality in animals given a lethal dose of MTX intrathecally and may be the preferred treatment for this complication.[180] Intrathecal or systemic LV is not indicated in these cases, since it is unlikely that this toxicity is attributable to inhibition of DHFR.

Pulmonary toxicity

Although uncommon, pulmonary toxicity due to MTX has been noted in patients treated chronically with low-dose oral MTX.[181] The clinical picture usually consists of cough, dyspnea, fever, and hypoxemia. Chest radiograph findings are nonspecific but may show patchy interstitial infiltrates. *Pneumocystis jirovecii* must be ruled out, especially in patients also receiving steroids. Histologic examinations show diffuse interstitial lymphocytic infiltrates, giant cells, and noncaseating granulomas. In some patients, peripheral eosinophilia is observed, raising the possibility that this is an allergic pneumonitis. The process may progress to fibrosis, and it is important to discontinue MTX while the pulmonary toxicity is reversible. Some patients have been retreated without recurrence of the problem.

Skin toxicity

Skin toxicity to MTX occurs in 5–10% of patients. It manifests as an erythematous rash characteristically noted on the neck and upper trunk. The rash may be pruritic and relatively insignificant and usually lasts for several days. A cutaneous vasculitis after intermediate-dose MTX has also been reported.[182] In the setting of severe systemic MTX toxicity following HDMTX or overdose, the skin manifestations may progress to severe bullous formation and desquamation.[183]

Teratogenic and mutagenic effects

Folate deficiency alters gene expression by causing hypomethylation of DNA and increases DNA strand breaks by causing misincorporation of uracil instead of thymine. Consequently, folate deficiency can directly influence carcinogenesis.[184] MTX is known to be a potent abortifacient, especially if administered during the first trimester of pregnancy. Nevertheless, there is no direct evidence that MTX has any mutagenic or carcinogenic effects.

Miscellaneous toxicity

Osteoporosis has been reported with chronic low-dose MTX administration[185] and may result from direct inhibition of osteoblastic differentiation.[186] Fever, seizures, radiation recall, phototoxicity, and anaphylactoid reactions have been reported with high-dose administration. Pleuritic and left-upper-quadrant pain, presumably attributable to splenic capsule inflammation, has been reported with a moderately high-dose regimen. An acute hemolytic anemia due to an IgG-3 antibody that reacts with erythrocytes only in the presence of MTX has been described.[187]

Resistance to antifolates

Although the development of effective chemotherapeutic regimens including MTX has significantly improved the therapy of a number of different malignancies, achieving prolonged disease-free survival is still difficult even in chemotherapy-sensitive diseases. The efficacy of MTX, as with other antineoplastic agents, is ultimately limited by either inherent resistance or resistance acquired during the course of therapy. Distinct categories of resistance mechanisms have been described: (1) decreased accumulation due to impaired transport into the cell, (2) decreased accumulation of polyglutamate forms, either due to decreased polyglutamate formation or increased removal of glutamate residues (3) an increase in DHFR and (4) altered or mutated DHFR that binds MTX less avidly than the normal enzyme. Additionally, because both DHFR and FPGS activity fluctuate with cell cycle, dysregulation of cell cycle genes may have a profound effect on antimetabolite resistance.

Intrinsic resistance to MTX

Impaired ability to transport MTX into cells through the RFC results in intrinsic resistance in many tumor types. The vast majority of mechanisms of impaired antifolate transport involve quantitative and/or qualitative alterations at the RFC level. These alterations include mutations in RFC that alter its transport activity, RFC silencing via promoter methylation and 3′-UTR alterations, RFC silencing via loss of function of transcriptional regulators and alterations in gene copy number of RFC in antifolate-resistant cells.[188] Decreased expression of RFC mRNA has been documented by quantitative RT-PCR in osteosarcoma samples at initial biopsy.[189] In other tumors, decreased expression can result from aberrant methylation in the promoter region.[190,191]

Mutations in the RFC gene corresponding to altered transport function have been documented both in resistant cell lines[192] and in leukemic blasts at diagnosis.[193] Single nucleotide polymorphisms (SNPs) in the gene for RFC can result in proteins with a decreased affinity for antifolates, while maintaining sufficient affinity for folate to allow continued cell growth. Other known polymorphisms selectively increase affinity for folates and increase the intracellular folate pool. However, in one analysis of 246 pediatric leukemia patient samples, only three were found to have potentially functional RFC polymorphisms, suggesting that RFC polymorphisms do not appear to play a major role in intrinsic MTX resistance in this population.[194]

Polyglutamylation enhances cellular retention of classical antifolates. Therefore, loss of FPGS activity can confer relative resistance. Differing ability to form long-chain MTX polyglutamates to some degree explains the relative intrinsic resistance of AML to MTX, compared with ALL.[195,196] Similarly, tumor cells from patients with soft tissue sarcomas intrinsically resistant to MTX have a low capacity to form long-chain MTX polyglutamates.[197,198] Higher MTX-polyglutamate accumulation in B-lineage ALL blasts as compared to T-lineage blasts may be explained by the finding of higher FPGS activity in B-lineage blasts.[199,200] The possibility that different isoforms (splice variants) of FPGS are expressed in different tissues is supported by the finding of differences in FPGS affinity for MTX between AML and ALL cell lines and blast samples,[201] and between resistant and sensitive sarcoma cell lines,[202] as well as by differences between FPGS isolated from L1210 cells and murine liver in degree of inhibition by long-chain folylpolyglutamates.[11]

Increased expression of the target enzyme DHFR, a well-described mechanism of acquired MTX resistance, may also confer intrinsic resistance. A polymorphism in the 3′ untranslated region that decreases binding of an inhibitory micro-RNA species (miR-24) leads to increased DHFR expression without prior MTX exposure.[203] Although this SNP was initially described as existing in 11–16% of a Japanese cohort,[204] the prevalence of this SNP may be much lower in other populations.[205]

Lack of the retinoblastoma protein, frequently deleted or altered in many tumor types, may play a role in intrinsic MTX resistance. In the absence of retinoblastoma protein, levels of the transcription factor E2F increase, resulting in an increase in transcription of several genes involved in DNA replication, including DHFR.[206]

Overexpression of p-glycoprotein does not confer resistance to MTX. However, MTX is a substrate for the related proteins, multidrug resistance proteins 1–5 (ABCC1-5),[207,208] and the breast cancer resistance protein (also called ATB Binding Cassette Subfamily G, Member 2 [ABCG2]).[209] In addition, ABCC5[208] and ABCG2[210] are able to transport both MTX and MTX-diglutamate. Overexpression of these proteins produces MTX resistance in vitro[208,211,212] and may affect the response to therapy among patients with leukemia.[213,214] It is not yet clear to what degree these proteins contribute to clinically relevant intrinsic resistance to MTX in other diseases.

Acquired resistance to MTX

Four predominant mechanisms of acquired resistance to MTX have been described in experimental tumors and clinical samples: increased DHFR activity due to amplification of this gene, altered binding of MTX to DHFR due to DHFR mutations, decreased influx of MTX through the RFC, or decreased formation of long-chain polyglutamate.

At the point of entry into the cell, either mutations or deletions in the RFC could result in decreased uptake of MTX and MTX resistance. Although polymorphisms in the gene for RFC do not seem to be a common mechanism of intrinsic resistance among patients with leukemia,[194] decreased transport of MTX through the RFC has been shown to be a common mechanism of acquired resistance to MTX in leukemic blasts from patients with relapsed ALL.[215]

Unstable or reversible resistance due to gene amplification has usually been associated with the presence of "double minute" chromosomes containing the DHFR amplicon, while high-level stable resistance has been associated with an abnormal banding region, often referred to as a homogeneously staining region.[216-220] Point mutations in DHFR in several cell lines, including human cells, have been detected that cause a change in the binding of MTX to the enzyme, and have usually involved amino acids that bind the inhibitor by hydrophobic interaction.[221]

Although defects in polyglutamylation have been described in several MTX-resistant cell lines,[222] the resistance of these cells has usually been found to be attributable to a combination of mechanisms. Increased hydrolysis of MTX polyglutamates can result from increased transport of MTX-polyglutamates into the lysosome[223] or increased levels of GGH activity.[198,224] Epigenetic regulation and SNPs in the promoter and coding region of GGH can affect GGH expression and therefore responsiveness to antifolate therapy.[225-227] However, forced overexpression of GGH in cancer cell lines does not confer resistance to short exposure to MTX.[228]

Strategies to overcome resistance to MTX using new (or older) antifols

The rational design of new folate antagonists is driven by an increasing understanding of the molecular basis of normal folate physiology, of MTX cytotoxicity, and of MTX resistance, and is guided by crystallographic data from the target enzymes.[221] Newer antifolates have been designed to have one or more of the following properties: increased transport into the cell by either increased affinity for the RFC or independence of the RFC, independence of polyglutamylation or increased polyglutamylation by virtue of increased affinity for FPGS, increased inhibition of DHFR or TS, or increased inhibition of enzymes responsible for purine synthesis.

Aminopterin (AMT), an older antifol

Preclinical and clinical data support reevaluating an antifol older than MTX, 4-amino-pteroyl-glutamic acid (AMT; Figure 1), the first antifolate to produce remissions among patients with leukemia.[2] AMT has several advantages over MTX, including 20–40 times greater clinical potency,[229] more efficient conversion (higher $V_{max}:K_m$ ratio) by FPGS to polyglutamates[230] leading to greater accumulation by patients' leukemic blasts in vitro,[231] and complete oral bioavailability.[232] Twenty-seven percent of children with refractory ALL had clinically significant responses to oral AMT in a Phase II trial,[233] and a Phase IIb trial demonstrated that AMT can be safely substituted for MTX in multiagent therapy for children with newly diagnosed children with ALL at high risk of relapse, without excessive toxicity.[143] Preclinical data suggest AMT may benefit patients with atopic dermatitis.[234]

Pralatrexate, a second-generation DHFR inhibitor

Like MTX, pralatrexate (10-propargyl-10-deazaaminopterin; PDX; Figure 4) competitively inhibits DHFR, limiting thymidine synthesis and cell division. PDX was designed to have high affinity for the RFC and FPGS, leading to enhanced and selective intracellular internalization and retention in tumor cells.[235] Consequently, PDX exhibits a 14-fold greater rate of influx[236] and more potent inhibition of tumor growth when compared to MTX.[237]

Pralatrexate is given via intravenous administration. The total systemic exposure (AUC) and maximum plasma concentration (C_{max}) increase proportionally with dose. The terminal elimination $T_{1/2}$ of PDX is 12–18 h. Approximately one-third of an intravenous dose is excreted unchanged in urine, and clearance decreases with decreasing creatinine clearance. The PK of PDX does not change significantly over multiple treatment cycles.[238]

Preclinical studies of PDX in combination with gemcitabine[239] and bortezomib[240] led to clinical trials of these combinations for patients with lymphoma. The overall response rate among those with T-cell lymphomas was significantly higher than those with B-cell lymphoma, suggesting a possible selectivity of the T-cell malignancies.[241] A prospective study looking at relapsed or refractory peripheral t-cell lymphoma (PTCL), Pralatrexate in Relapsed or Refractory Peripheral T-cell Lymphoma (PROPEL) included 115 patients, most of whom had been heavily pretreated. An overall response rate of 29% was reported, and based on these finding, the FDA approved the use of PDX for treatment of relapsed and refractory T-cell lymphoma.[242] PDX has also been shown to have high activity with acceptable toxicity in patients with NSCLC[136] and relapsed or refractory cutaneous T-cell lymphoma, and PTCL.[243,244] Both in vitro and in vivo models demonstrate the protective effect of LV on PDX toxicity.[245]

Pemetrexed, an inhibitor of multiple folate-dependent enzymes, primarily TS

Pemetrexed (N-[4-[2-(2-amino-3,4-dihydro-4-oxo-7H-pyrrolo[2,3-d]pyrimidin-5-yl)ethyl] benzoyl]-L-glutamic acid; Figure 4) inhibits TS, DHFR, and glycinamide ribonucleotide formyltransferase (GARFT). Although initially promoted as a "multitargeted" antifolate, it is primarily a TS inhibitor, as indicated by its greater affinity for this enzyme and by end-product inhibition experiments.[246,247] Pemetrexed is transported into cells via the RFC, as well as the proton-coupled folate transporter. Pemetrexed is rapidly polyglutamated by FPGS, with a K_m for the enzyme two orders of magnitude below that of MTX. Like pralatrexate, pemetrexed is administered intravenously. The AUC and C_{max} increase proportionally with dose. The elimination $T_{1/2}$ of pemetrexed is 3.5 h in patients with normal renal function. The PK of pemetrexed did not change significantly over multiple treatment cycles.[248] Clinically, pemetrexed toxicity is increased with a high concentration of plasma homocysteine, which in turn has been associated with nutritional folate deficiency or low concentrations of 5-methyl tetrahydrofolate required for methionine synthesis, secondary to mutations in methylene tetrahydrofolate reductase. Supplementation with these vitamins in all subsequent regimens reduced toxicity and allowed delivery of a greater number of courses, increasing response rates.[249]

Pemetrexed has broad-spectrum activity in multiple tumor types.[250] Based on results from a Phase III clinical trial, pemetrexed in combination with cisplatin is considered first-line therapy for advanced nonsquamous NSCLC.[251] The use of pemetrexed as maintenance therapy in NSCLC was evaluated in the PARAMOUNT Phase III (maintenance pemetrexed versus placebo immediately after induction treatment with pemetrexed plus cisplatin) study. This study proved pemetrexed to be effective with an improvement in progression-free and overall survival.[252] Pemetrexed is also used as monotherapy for relapsed or refractory NSCLC and in combination with cisplatin for the treatment of pleural mesothelioma.[249,253] There have been several preclinical and Phase I studies, investigating pemetrexed in patients with advanced solid malignancies such as breast cancer, colorectal cancer, and medulloblastoma.[254–256]

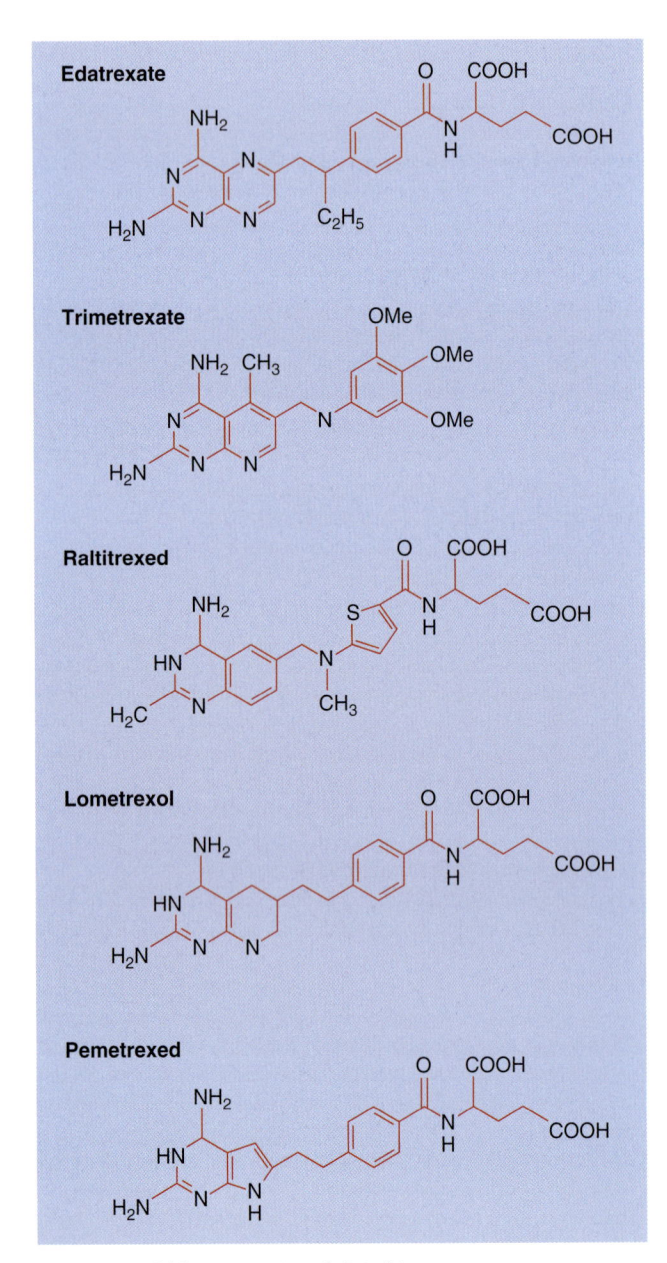

Figure 4 Novel folate antagonists of clinical interest.

Conclusion

Folic acid antagonists, epitomized by methotrexate, have been employed as anticancer agents for over 70 years, as components of curative regimens for patients with a wide array of common malignancies. As suggested by the class name, antifolates cause cytotoxicity primarily by inhibiting synthetic reactions dependent on the vitamin folic acid. Off-target toxicity leads to both acute and chronic organ dysfunction that must be monitored when antifolates are administered. Newer antifolate agents have been developed to overcome key components of the multifactorial cellular properties that contribute to antifolate resistance. Although new classes of anticancer therapies are beginning to supplant conventional chemotherapy agents like antifolates, it is likely that this class will continue to play a central role in curative regimens in the near future.

Key references

The complete reference list can be found on Vital Source version of this title, see inside front cover.

1. Farber S, Cutler EC, Hawkins JW, et al. Action of pteroylglutamic conjugates on man. *Science*. 1947;**106**:619–621.
2. Farber S, Diamond L, Mercer RD, et al. Temporary remissions in acute leukemia in children produced by folic acid antagonist, 4-aminopteroyl-glutamic acid (aminopterin). *N Engl J Med*. 1948;**238**:787.
7. Osborne MJ, Freeman MB, Huennekens FM. Inhibition of dihydrofolic reductase by aminopterin and amethopterin. *Proc Soc Exp Biol Med*. 1958;**97**:429–431.
9. Chabner BA, Allegra CJ, Curt GA, et al. Polyglutamation of methotrexate. Is methotrexate a prodrug? *J Clin Investig*. 1985;**76**(3):907–912.
14. Allegra CJ, Chabner BA, Drake JC, et al. Enhanced inhibition of thymidylate synthase by methotrexate polyglutamates. *J Biol Chem*. 1985;**260**(17):9720–9726.
17. Allegra CJ, Hoang K, Yeh GC, et al. Evidence for direct inhibition of de novo purine synthesis in human MCF-7 breast cells as a principal mode of metabolic inhibition by methotrexate. *J Biol Chem*. 1987;**262**(28):13520–13526.
18. Cronstein BN, Naime D, Ostad E. The antiinflammatory mechanism of methotrexate. Increased adenosine release at inflamed sites diminishes leukocyte accumulation in an in vivo model of inflammation. *J Clin Investig*. 1993;**92**(6):2675–2682.
20. Winter-Vann AM, Kamen BA, Bergo MO, et al. Targeting Ras signaling through inhibition of carboxyl methylation: an unexpected property of methotrexate. *Proc Natl Acad Sci U S A*. 2003;**100**(11):6529–6534.
24. Stoller RG, Hande KR, Jacobs SA, et al. Use of plasma pharmacokinetics to predict and prevent methotrexate toxicity. *N Engl J Med*. 1977;**297**(12):630–634.
25. Borsi JD, Moe PJ. A comparative study on the pharmacokinetics of methotrexate in a dose range of 0.5 g to 33.6 g/m² in children with acute lymphoblastic leukemia. *Cancer*. 1987;**60**(1):5–13.
26. Evans WE, Crom WR, Abromowitch M, et al. Clinical pharmacodynamics of high-dose methotrexate in acute lymphocytic leukemia. Identification of a relation between concentration and effect. *N Engl J Med*. 1986;**314**(8):471–477.
27. Evans WE, Relling MV, Rodman JH, et al. Conventional compared with individualized chemotherapy for childhood acute lymphoblastic leukemia. *N Engl J Med*. 1998;**338**(8):499–505.
32. Huffman DH, Wan SH, Azarnoff DL, et al. Pharmacokinetics of methotrexate. *Clin Pharmacol Ther*. 1973;**14**(4):572–579.
41. Thyss A, Milano G, Etienne MC, et al. Evidence for CSF accumulation of 5-methyltetrahydrofolate during repeated courses of methotrexate plus folinic acid rescue. *Br J Cancer*. 1989;**59**(4):627–630.
43. Bertino JR, Sawicki WL, Lindquist CA, et al. Schedule-dependent antitumor effects of methotrexate and 5-fluorouracil. *Cancer Res*. 1977;**37**(1):327–328.
44. Blaney SM, Poplack DG, Godwin K, et al. Effect of body position on ventricular CSF methotrexate concentration following intralumbar administration. *J Clin Oncol*. 1995;**13**(1):177–179.
51. Schmiegelow K, Schroder H, Pulczynska MK, et al. Maintenance chemotherapy for childhood acute lymphoblastic leukemia: relation of bone-marrow and hepatotoxicity to the concentration of methotrexate in erythrocytes. *Cancer Chemother Pharmacol*. 1989;**25**(1):65–69.
71. Robien K, Boynton A, Ulrich CM. Pharmacogenetics of folate-related drug targets in cancer treatment. *Pharmacogenomics*. 2005;**6**(7):673–689.
85. Pizzorno G, Mini E, Coronnello M, et al. Impaired polyglutamylation of methotrexate as a cause of resistance in CCRF-CEM cells after short-term, high-dose treatment with this drug. *Cancer Res*. 1988;**48**(8):2149–2155.
92. Matloub Y, Bostrom BC, Hunger SP, et al. Escalating intravenous methotrexate improves event-free survival in children with standard-risk acute lymphoblastic leukemia: a report from the Children's Oncology Group. *Blood*. 2011;**118**(2):243–251.
94. Mahoney DH Jr, Shuster JJ, Nitschke R, et al. Acute neurotoxicity in children with B-precursor acute lymphoid leukemia: an association with intermediate-dose intravenous methotrexate and intrathecal triple therapy--a Pediatric Oncology Group study. *J Clin Oncol*. 1998;**16**(5):1712–1722.
113. Blay JY, Conroy T, Chevreau C, et al. High-dose methotrexate for the treatment of primary cerebral lymphomas: analysis of survival and late neurologic toxicity in a retrospective series. *J Clin Oncol*. 1998;**16**(3):864–871.
132. Coates AS, Tattersall MH, Swanson C, et al. Combination therapy with methotrexate and 5-fluorouracil: a prospective randomized clinical trial of order of administration. *J Clin Oncol*. 1984;**2**(7):756–761.
143. Cole PD, Drachtman RA, Masterson M, et al. Phase 2B trial of aminopterin in multiagent therapy for children with newly diagnosed acute lymphoblastic leukemia. *Cancer Chemother Pharmacol*. 2008;**62**(1):65–75.
148. Bernini JC, Fort DW, Griener JC, et al. Aminophylline for methotrexate-induced neurotoxicity. *Lancet*. 1995;**345**(8949):544–547.
156. Buchen S, Ngampolo D, Melton RG, et al. Carboxypeptidase G2 rescue in patients with methotrexate intoxication and renal failure. *Br J Cancer*. 2005;**92**(3):480–487.
164. Farrow AC, Buchanan GR, Zwiener RJ, et al. Serum aminotransferase elevation during and following treatment of childhood acute lymphoblastic leukemia. *J Clin Oncol*. 1997;**15**(4):1560–1566.
171. Cole PD, Beckwith KA, Vijayanathan V, et al. CSF folate homeostasis during therapy for acute lymphoblastic leukemia. *Pediatr Neurol*. 2009;**40**(1):35–42.
174. Drachtman RA, Cole PD, Golden CB, et al. Dextromethorphan is effective in the treatment of subacute methotrexate neurotoxicity. *Pediatr Hematol Oncol*. 2002;**19**(5):319–327.
175. Cole PD, Vijayanathan V, Ali NF, et al. Memantine protects rats treated with intrathecal methotrexate from developing spatial memory deficits. *Clin Cancer Res*. 2013;**19**(16):4446–4454.
180. Adamson PC, Balis FM, McCully CL, et al. Rescue of experimental intrathecal methotrexate overdose with carboxypeptidase-G2. *J Clin Oncol*. 1991;**9**(4):670–674.
192. Zhao R, Assaraf YG, Goldman ID. A mutated murine reduced folate carrier (RFC1) with increased affinity for folic acid, decreased affinity for methotrexate, and an obligatory anion requirement for transport function. *J Biol Chem*. 1998;**273**(30):19065–19071.
196. Goker E, Lin JT, Trippett T, et al. Decreased polyglutamylation of methotrexate in acute lymphoblastic leukemia blasts in adults compared to children with this disease. *Leukemia*. 1993;**7**(7):1000–1004.
205. Mishra PJ, Longo GSA, Menon LG, et al. The 829C?T single nucleotide polymorphism in the 3' UTR of the dihydrofolate reductase gene results in methotrexate resistance and is rare among non-Japanese American patients [Abstract 1274]. *Proc Am Assoc Cancer Res*. 2006;**47**:1274.
215. Gorlick R, Goker E, Trippett T, et al. Defective transport is a common mechanism of acquired methotrexate resistance in acute lymphocytic leukemia and is associated with decreased reduced folate carrier expression. *Blood*. 1997;**89**(3):1013–1018.
222. Pizzorno G, Chang YM, McGuire JJ, et al. Inherent resistance of human squamous carcinoma cell lines to methotrexate as a result of decreased polyglutamylation of this drug. *Cancer Res*. 1989;**49**(19):5275–5280.
240. Marchi E, Paoluzzi L, Scotto L, et al. Pralatrexate is synergistic with the proteasome inhibitor bortezomib in in vitro and in vivo models of T-cell lymphoid malignancies. *Clin Cancer Res*. 2010;**16**(14):3648–3658.
242. O'Connor OA, Pro B, Pinter-Brown L, et al. Pralatrexate in patients with relapsed or refractory peripheral T-cell lymphoma: results from the pivotal PROPEL study. *J Clin Oncol*. 2011;**29**(9):1182–1189.
246. Chattopadhyay S, Moran RG, Goldman ID. Pemetrexed: biochemical and cellular pharmacology, mechanisms, and clinical applications. *Mol Cancer Ther*. 2007;**6**(2):404–417.
252. Paz-Ares LG, de Marinis F, Dediu M, et al. PARAMOUNT: final overall survival results of the phase III study of maintenance pemetrexed versus placebo immediately after induction treatment with pemetrexed plus cisplatin for advanced nonsquamous non-small-cell lung cancer. *J Clin Oncol*. 2013;**31**(23):2895–2902.

54 Pyrimidine and purine antimetabolites

Robert B. Diasio, MD ■ Steven M. Offer, PhD

Overview

Antimetabolites based on pyrimidine and purine bases are some of the most widely used anti-cancer drugs globally. Nucleotides, which consist of purine or pyrimidine bases covalently linked to five-carbon carbohydrate group and one or more phosphate groups, are the "building blocks" of DNA and RNA that underlie fundamental cellular processes such as cellular proliferation and protein synthesis. The development of pyrimidine and purine antimetabolite drugs has been based on the rationale that nucleic acids are essential for these critical functions. Purine and pyrimidine antimetabolites have been shown to be highly effective against solid tumors such as colon and breast cancers, as well in certain hematological malignancies. Effectiveness has also been shown against primary tumors and against select advanced metastatic cancers. The mechanism of action and toxicity profiles associated with each drug vary, depending on biochemical structure, predominant mechanism(s) of action, metabolism, dose, and treatment schedule. The development of prodrugs has allowed for various administration routes, including orally bio-available compounds. Combination therapies in which antimetabolites are co-administered with other drugs have generally improved the efficacy of treatments without dramatic increases in toxicity compared to monotherapy. Healthcare providers should be aware of potentially serious drug–drug interactions, particularly when co-administered drugs are metabolized by the same or linked enzymatic pathways. Furthermore, for many antimetabolites, genetic and nongenetic biomarkers have been demonstrated to be associated with varying degrees of risk for severe drug-related adverse events, which in severe cases can result in death. Genotyping and DNA sequencing are increasingly being used to identify carriers of risk genotypes. The resulting pharmacogenomic data have shown strong potential for informing optimized treatment approaches and individualized dose-adjustment to reduce the risk for developing severe drug-related toxicity. Even with pharmacogenetically guided dosing, patients receiving this class of chemotherapeutics should be monitored closely for the development of adverse events. Ongoing research in this clinical area focuses on identifying biomarkers of response and/or toxicity, optimizing bioavailability and efficacy, and evaluating combination regimens containing multiple classes of anti-cancer therapies. In this chapter, we review the various antimetabolite drugs that are analogs of uracil/thymine, cytidine/deoxycytidine, hypoxanthine/guanine, and adenosine that are used in cancer treatment. The focus is on metabolism, mechanism of action, clinical pharmacology, clinical activity, and toxicity.

The synthesis of pyrimidine and purine antimetabolite drugs has been based on the rationale that nucleic acids are critical to cell replication. The pyrimidine and purine bases, including their nucleosides and precursors, are the "building blocks" necessary to synthesize nucleic acids. These molecules are potential sites for designing drugs that could be effective in inhibiting nucleic acid synthesis, whether these be in bacteria, viruses, or tumor cells. Since neoplastic cells (e.g., leukemic cells) in contrast to their normal counterparts (e.g., lymphocytes or granulocytes) typically rapidly reproduce, it appeared logical for drug developers to design drugs similar to pyrimidine and purine bases, their nucleosides, or their precursors with the goal of disrupting nucleic acid synthesis and thereby inhibiting cell replication. The term "antimetabolite" refers to the fact that these synthetic pyrimidines and purines mimic the structures of naturally occurring pyrimidine and purine base (or nucleoside or precursor metabolites) and therefore are able to enter biochemical pathways similar to their natural counterparts, but instead of stimulating nucleic acid synthesis and cell replication, they exert an "anti" cell growth effect. Slight molecular differences in the antimetabolite analogs can result in interference with the synthesis of DNA and RNA. The resultant disruption in naturally occurring nucleic acid synthesis may occur in several ways. Thus, the pyrimidine or purine antimetabolites might compete with their naturally occurring counterparts for an enzyme that is critical in the nucleic acid synthesis pathway, thereby disturbing the pools of natural pyrimidine and purine nucleotides needed to synthesize DNA or RNA. Alternatively, the pyrimidine of purine may be incorporated directly into DNA or RNA, resulting in the formation of a dysfunctional nucleic acid or possibly resulting in nucleic acid fragmentation as the DNA or RNA repair molecular machinery seeks to correct the abnormality.[1]

Pyrimidine antimetabolites

Potential pyrimidine antimetabolite cancer chemotherapy drugs might include structural modifications of the naturally occurring pyrimidine bases uracil, cytosine, or thymine or their ribose or deoxyribose nucleosides, as well as their potential precursors (Figure 1a).

Uracil antimetabolites

Over the years, there have been several uracil antimetabolites that have shown potential activity in the treatment of various malignancies. The only uracil antimetabolites that remain actively used today in the United States are the 5-fluorouracil (5-FU) drugs (Figure 1b) including the parent drug 5-FU, its deoxyribose nucleoside 5-fluorodeoxyuridine (Floxuridine, FUdR, or FdUrd) that is used occasionally today with hepatic arterial infusion, and the prodrug of 5-FU capecitabine. In other parts of the world, particularly Asia, there has been widespread use of other 5-FU prodrugs (e.g., UFT, S-1), but in the United States capecitabine is the only one currently widely used.[2]

5-Fluorouracil (5-FU)

Background

5-FU is one of the first rationally synthesized antineoplastic agents.[3] The stimulus for developing this antimetabolite derives

Holland-Frei Cancer Medicine, Tenth Edition. Edited by Robert C. Bast, John C. Byrd, Carlo M. Croce, Ernest Hawk, Fadlo R. Khuri, Raphael E. Pollock, Apostolia M. Tsimberidou, Christopher G. Willett, and Cheryl L. Willman.
© 2023 John Wiley & Sons, Inc. Published 2023 by John Wiley & Sons, Inc.

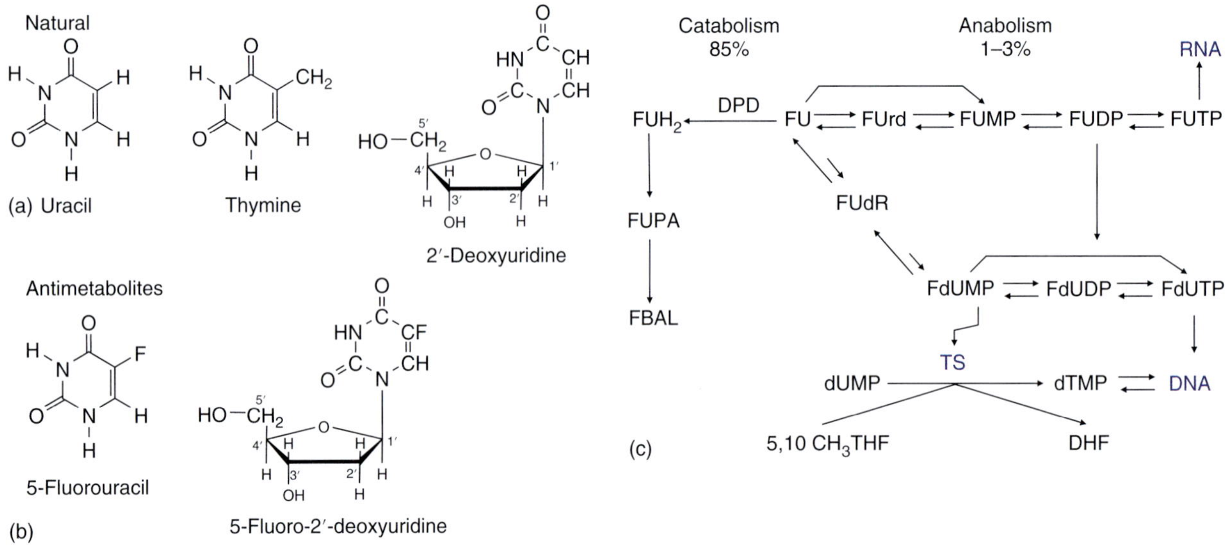

Figure 1 Uracil antimetabolites; and metabolism and sites of action of 5-Fluorouracil. (a) Natural occurring pyrimidine bases uracil and thymine together with the uracil deoxyribonucleoside (2′-deoxyuridine). (b) Antimetabolites 5-fluorouracil and 5-fluoro-2′deoxyuridine developed from structural modifications of uracil and 2′-deoxyuridine. (c) The catabolic (to left of FU) and anabolic (to right of FU) pathways that 5-FU may enter. Approximately 85% of administered 5-FU is catabolized via the rate-limiting enzymatic step (*DPD*) to dihydrofluorouracil (FUH_2) and then to fluoroureidopropionic acid (FUPA) and finally 2-fluoro-β-alanine (FBAL) with only 1–3% being anabolized (the rest being excreted into the urine). 5-FU is anabolized to nucleosides and then nucleotides as shown. These metabolites and the enzymatic steps are described in more detail in Refs. 2,3. The three primary sites of action include: (1) inhibition of thymidylate synthase (*TS*) by the 5-fluoro-2′-deoxyuridylate (FdUMP) in the presence of 5,10 methylenetetrahydrofolate (5,10 CH_3THF); (2) incorporation of 5-fluoro uridylate triphosphate (FUTP) into RNA; and (3) incorporation 5-fluoro-2′-deoxyuridylate triphosphate (FdUTP) into DNA which in turn is removed by uracil glycosylase causing DNA fragmentation.

from the observation that rapidly growing tumor cells require an exogenous source of uracil for growth (beyond what can be provided by the endogenous natural synthetic pathway forming uracil from orotic acid). Exogenously formed uracil can be converted to deoxyuridylate (dUMP), which in turn, in the presence of 5,10 methylene tetrahydrofolate, can form thymidylate required for DNA synthesis, from donation of a methyl group to the fifth position of uracil (Figure 1). 5-FU is a close analog of uracil with fluorine effectively substituting for hydrogen at the fifth position of uracil due to similar conformation, including a similar *van der Waals* radius. This allows 5-FU to enter the same biochemical pathways used naturally by uracil (Figure 1c).

Metabolism
After gaining entry into the circulation, 5-FU may undergo glomerular filtration as a small molecule and pass directly into the urine or enter the anabolic and catabolic pathways, depending on the tissues, efficiently substituting for uracil and uracil-derived metabolites as substrates for its various enzymatic steps. Approximately 85% of the 5-FU that enters the circulation is destined for catabolism with 10–15% being excreted through the urine unchanged and 1–3% being available for anabolism.[4] The reaction catalyzed by dihydropyrimidine dehydrogenase (DPD), an initial step in uracil catabolism, is the major rate-limiting step in the overall metabolism of 5-FU and is the major determinant of 5-FU available for anabolism.[4] Most 5-FU destined for anabolism will be metabolized to the ribonucleotide form by conversion through orotate phosphoribosyltransferase in the presence of PRPP or via the sequential action of uridine phosphorylase and uridine kinase. Less likely is the formation of the deoxyribonucleotide 5-fluoro-2′-deoxyuridine monophosphate (FdUMP) via the sequential action of deoxyuridine phosphorylase and deoxyuridine (or thymidine) kinase as the activity of deoxyuridine phosphorylase favors conversion to the base rather than the reverse reaction. Formation of the 5-FU nucleotides (in particular FdUMP, FUTP, and FdUTP) is critical to the activity of 5-FU (see below). More information of the individual metabolic steps is provided elsewhere.[2,3]

Resistance to 5-FU theoretically can be secondary to any barrier to formation of 5-FU nucleotides critical to the potential mechanisms of action.[5] This could include inhibition of uptake of 5-FU into the cell, or any inhibition of enzymatic conversion of 5-FU to the nucleoside and then to the nucleotide. Thus, for example, reduced uridine phosphorylase/kinase or orotate phosphoribosyltransferase could result in decreased levels of 5-FU nucleotides.

One aspect of 5-FU metabolism and pharmacology that is somewhat different from other agents is the concept of "biochemical modulation", in which the activity of 5-FU at an important enzymatic step or a critical site of action is influenced by the addition of an important chemical or precursor to a critical metabolite.[6] The best example of this is the use of leucovorin (folinic acid) that is often administered clinically with 5-FU to increase the likelihood that adequate amounts of 5,10 methylene tetrahydrofolate are available to insure combination with FdUMP and thymidylate synthase to form a ternary complex capable of inhibiting DNA synthesis.[5]

Mechanism of action
5-FU is thought to derive its anticancer activity from the effect of its nucleotide metabolites at three different sites (Figure 1c). Inhibition of the enzyme thymidylate synthase (TS) by FdUMP (which actually has a greater affinity for TS than that of the natural substrate dUMP) in the presence of 5,10-methylene tetrahydrofolate inhibits

the formation of thymidylate (TMP), which is critical for DNA synthesis. This has long been thought to be the primary mechanism by which fluoropyrimidine drugs work.[5] A second possible mechanism is the incorporation of the 5-FU ribonucleotide FUTP into RNA in place of the natural uracil ribonucleotide UTP. This form of RNA may also be important due to its effect on small RNAs.[2] The third mechanism is somewhat similar to the second with incorporation of the 5-FU deoxyribonucleotide FdUTP into DNA in place of the natural thymidylate nucleotide TTP. In this latter setting, however, it is the excision and repair of DNA containing FdUTP by uracil glycosylase resulting in DNA fragmentation that is thought to contribute to cytotoxicity.[3]

Clinical pharmacology
5-FU is typically administered either as an intravenous bolus or an intravenous infusion. Following administration as an intravenous bolus, 5-FU is rapidly cleared following first pass through the liver where it is rapidly catabolized with more than 85% of the administered dose being inactivated by initial degradation to dihydrofluorouracil (FUH_2).[3] The half-life of 5-FU in this setting is typically approximately 13 ± 7 min with the clearance being approximately 600 ± 200 mL/min/m^2.[4] Administering 5-FU by continuous infusion over 5 days or as a protracted multiday infusion by ambulatory pump, leads to a predicted, relatively constant but low level of 5-FU.[2]

Variability in the efficiency of catabolism exists with the main determinant being DPD, the rate-limiting step in 5-FU catabolism. In a small (<5%) but significant part of the population, genetic variants in the gene coding for DPD (*DPYD*) can result in decreased DPD activity that can shift more 5-FU into the anabolic pathway and in turn result in increased toxicity.[7–9]

Recently, therapeutic drug monitoring has been suggested as a method by which more pharmacokinetically rational dosing of 5-FU can be achieved.[10] Although not widely used yet in the clinic, this has potential to improve 5-FU efficacy and decrease its toxicity.

Clinical use and indications
5-FU continues to be widely used in the treatment of several common malignancies, including colorectal cancer and certain forms of skin cancer and breast cancer. It remains after more than six decades, one of the most widely used cancer chemotherapy drugs in the United States and worldwide, as the major component of both adjuvant and advanced colorectal cancer regimens, where it is typically administered in combination with other drugs.[2]

Toxicities
Toxicities from 5-FU vary depending on dose and schedule of administration. Acute toxicities associated with intravenous bolus administration include myelosuppression, mucositis, and diarrhea. Prolonged exposure to 5-FU from continuous infusion may result in palmar-plantar erythrodysesthesia (hand-foot syndrome).[2,3]

One interesting approach to countering severe, life-threatening toxicity from 5-FU or its derivative drugs (see below) has been the use of the antidote uridine triacetate. This pyrimidine analog provides increased amounts of uridine which can be easily converted to uridine monophosphate, which in turn can compete with fluorouridine monophosphate at the major sites of 5-FU in particular incorporation into the RNA thereby lessening the toxicity from 5-FU. While this has proven useful in 5-FU overdose situations and potentially with DPD deficiency, the major limitation is that it must be administered soon after the 5-FU has been administered (probably within 96 h when 5-FU nucleotide pools are high).[11]

Other 5-FU Drugs
Over the past 60 years, there have been many additional 5-fluorouracil analogs synthesized. Most of these have been prodrugs of 5-FU. Today only a few are used in the United States.

5-Fluorodeoxyuridine

Background
5-Fluorodexyuridine (FdUrd, FUDR), the deoxyuridine of 5-FU, was synthesized about the same time as 5-FU in the late 1950s. Today it has relatively limited use. Its structure is shown in Figure 1.

Metabolism
FdUrd can function as a prodrug of 5-FU, being converted by deoxyuridine or thymidine phosphorylase to 5-FU. However, because it is a very good substrate for deoxyuridine or thymidine kinase, it is more likely, rapidly, and directly converted to FdUMP, one of the primary active metabolites of 5-FU.

Mechanism of action
Formation of FdUMP can, in the presence of 5,10 methylene tetrahydrofolate, form an irreversible ternary complex with thymidylate synthase thereby blocking DNA synthesis.[4] Since most administered FdUrd will be metabolized directly to FdUMP, FdUrd is a relatively pure S-phase inhibitor.[2]

Clinical pharmacology
Today, when FdUrd is administered to cancer patients, it is mainly as a continuous hepatic arterial infusion through an implantable pump.[12]

Clinical activity
FdUrd is utilized mainly in the treatment of hepatocellular cancer and at times for colorectal cancer metastatic to the liver.

Toxicities
With prolonged hepatic arterial infusion, the most common toxicity is hepatoxicity and includes biliary sclerosis and occasional elevation of transaminases.[2,3]

Capecitabine

Background
There have been many attempts to develop an oral 5-FU drug that could provide a more convenient way to administer 5-FU, and at the same time mimic the desirable effects of a 5-FU infusion.[10] Capecitabine is the only oral 5-FU prodrug that is approved by the Food and Drug Administration (FDA) in the United States, although other oral forms of 5-FU are available in Asia and Europe.[13]

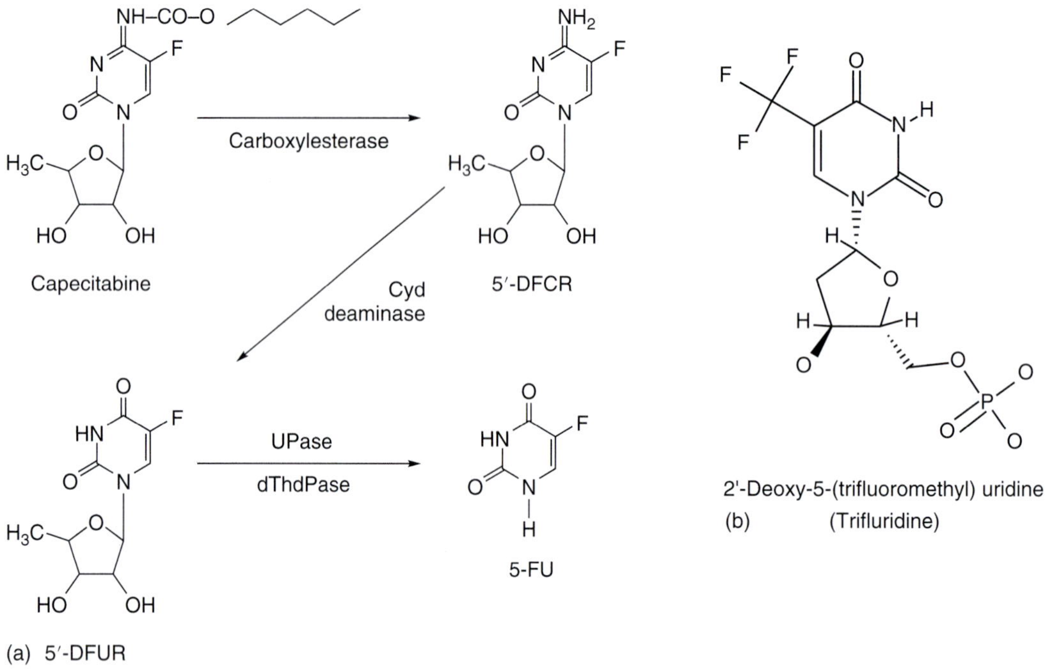

Figure 2 Structure and activation of capecitabine; and structures of thymidine antimetabolites. (a) The prodrug capecitabine is converted to 5-FU by three enzymatic steps carboxylesterase, cytidine deaminase, and uridine (or thymidine) phosphorylase. Intermediate metabolites include 5′-deoxyfluorocytidine (5′-dFCR) and 5′-deoxyfluorouridine (5′dFUR). (b) Trifluridine is the only thymidine antimetabolite that is currently used in the treatment of cancer in the United States It is used in a drug formulation combined together with the thymidine phosphorylase inhibitor tipiracil.

Metabolism

Capecitabine is converted to 5-FU by the sequential action of three enzymes: (1) hepatic carboxylesterase, which initially hydrolyzes the drug to 5′-deoxy-5-fluorocytidine; (2) cytidine deaminase, which in turn deaminates this derivative to 5′-deoxy-5-fluorouridine (5′-dFUrd) and; (3) finally thymidine phosphorylase, which converts 5′-dFUrd to 5-FU (Figure 2a). Because tumor tissue often has a higher activity of thymidine phosphorylase compared to most normal tissues, there is a potential selective benefit and in turn an improved therapeutic index.

Mechanism of action

Following conversion to 5-FU, the mechanism of action is identical with that of 5-FU (see above).

Clinical pharmacology

Capecitabine provides an alternative, more patient-friendly way of administering 5-FU to produce the effects of a 5-FU protracted infusion.

Clinical activity

Capecitabine has a similar spectrum of activity as 5-FU and is typically used in the treatment of colorectal and breast cancer.

Toxicities

The toxicities of capecitabine are similar to those of 5-FU infusion with palmar-plantar erythrodysesthesia being the major toxicity seen with continuous Capecitabine use. Capecitabine is, reportedly, tolerated differently between European and American populations. The underlying mechanism remains unclear although external factors like folate levels may contribute to this difference.[11]

Thymidine antimetabolites

There is only one thymidine antimetabolite that is currently used in the treatment of cancer in the United States. It is a combined drug formulation consisting of the thymidine-based nucleoside analog trifluridine together with the thymidine phosphorylase inhibitor tipiracil.[14]

2′-Deoxy-5-(trifluoromethyl) uridine (trifluridine) and tipiracil

Background

Trifluridine is the most recently approved pyrimidine antimetabolite drug (Figure 2b). This combined drug formulation consists of the thymidine-based nucleoside analog, trifluridine, together with the thymidine phosphorylase inhibitor, tipiracil, in a molar ratio 1:0.5 (weight ratio, 1:0.471).[14]

Metabolism

Trifluridine and tipiracil are not metabolized by cytochrome P450 (CYP) enzymes. Trifluridine is eliminated primarily by metabolism via thymidine phosphorylase to form an inactive metabolite, 5-(trifluoromethyl) uracil. Inclusion of tipiracil increases trifluridine exposure by inhibiting its metabolism by thymidine phosphorylase.

Mechanism of action

Following uptake into cancer cells, trifluridine is incorporated into DNA, where it can interfere with DNA synthesis and in turn inhibit cell proliferation.

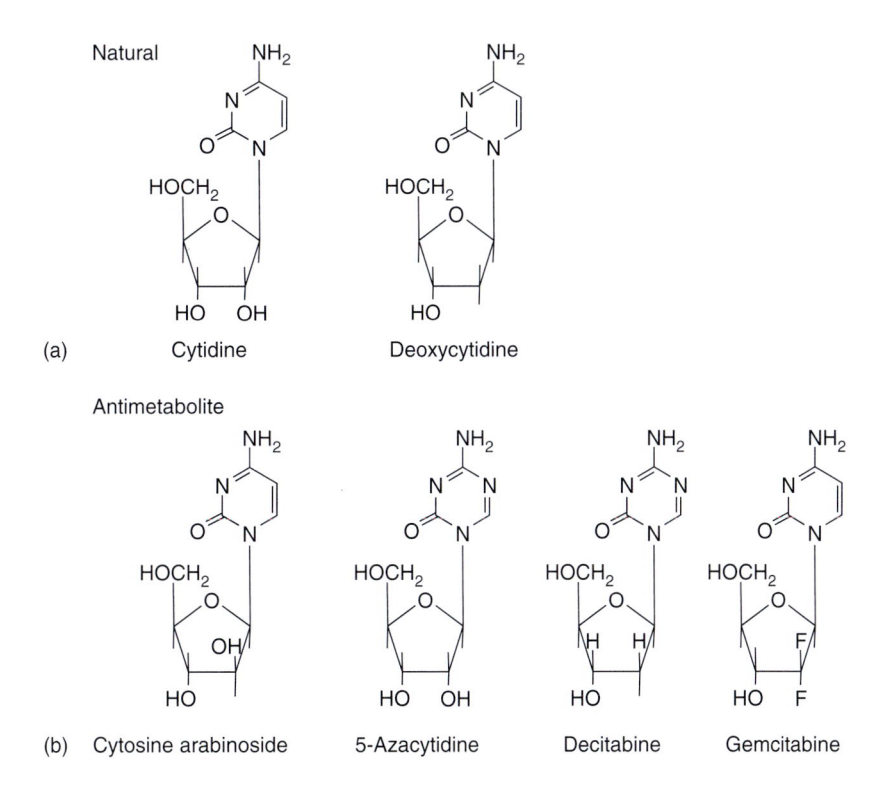

Figure 3 Structures of cytidine/deoxycytidine antimetabolites. (a) Natural occurring cytosine nucleosides cytidine and deoxycytidine. (b) Antimetabolites cytosine arabinoside, 5-azacytidine, decitabine, and gemcitabine developed from structural modifications of the sugar of the cytosine nucleosides.

Clinical pharmacology
The combined drug formulation is administered as a tablet twice daily (35 mg/m^2) with food on days 1 through 5 and days 8 through 12 of each 28-day cycle until disease progression or unacceptable toxicity. The dose is rounded to the nearest 5 mg increment. Following a single oral administration at 35 mg/m^2 in patients with cancer, the mean time to peak plasma concentration (Tmax) of trifluridine was around 2 h. The mean elimination half-life at steady state of trifluridine was 2.1 h and of tipiracil was 2.4 h.[14–17]

Clinical activity
Trifluridine and tipiracil have shown antitumor activity in both metastatic colorectal cancer and metastatic gastric cancer. For metastatic colorectal cancer, this regimen has been mainly used for patients who have been heavily pretreated with fluoropyrimidines, as well as oxaliplatin- and irinotecan-based chemotherapy, an anti-VEGF biological therapy, and if *RAS* wild type, an anti-EGFR therapy.[14] The combined trifluridine and tipiracil drug formulation has shown activity in gastric cancer and cancer of the gastroesophageal junction metastatic to other organs. It is also used for patients who have been previously treated or cannot receive indicated chemotherapy medications such as a fluoropyrimidine or a platinum compound, either a taxane or irinotecan, and if appropriate, HER2/neu-targeted therapy.[16]

Toxicities
Severe and life-threatening myelosuppression (Grade 3–4) consisting of neutropenia (38%), anemia (18%), thrombocytopenia (5%), and febrile neutropenia (3%) have been observed with this drug formulation. In addition, a few patients (0.2%) have died due to neutropenic infection. Common side effects include fatigue, weakness, nausea, decreased appetite, diarrhea, vomiting, abdominal pain, and fever.[17]

Cytosine antimetabolites
Cytosine antimetabolites with demonstrated clinical anticancer activity are mainly nucleosides, where the major structural modification is in the sugar part of the molecule and not the base. Currently, four cytosine antimetabolites are used clinically and include cytosine arabinoside, 5-azacytidine, decitabine, and gemcitabine (Figure 3).

Cytosine arabinoside

Background
Cytosine arabinoside (ara-C) was first identified as a natural product following isolation from *Cryptotethya crypta*. The arabinoside sugar differentiates this compound from the cytosine deoxyribonucleoside that is normally a component of DNA in which the 2′-OH group is in the *cis* configuration relative to the *N*-glycosyl bond between the cytosine and the sugar (Figure 3).[18] Today, ara-C is prepared synthetically for commercial use. Its effectiveness in cancer chemotherapy has led to the synthesis of other arabinoside compounds, such as the purine antimetabolites 2-fluoro-ara-adenosine monophosphate and nelarabine (see below).

Metabolism
Following uptake into cells through nucleoside transporters, ara-C must first be converted to ara-C monophosphate (ara-CMP) by the action of deoxycytidine kinase and then further phosphorylated to the diphosphate (ara-CDP) and triphosphate (ara-CTP). The latter is critical for cytostatic activity[19] (Figure 4a).

Catabolism or degradation of ara-C inactivates the anti-tumor activity and can occur either through the action of cytidine deaminase, converting ara-C to ara-U, or through the action of deoxycytidylate deaminase converting ara-CMP to ara-UMP. Increased deamination is a basis for increased resistance as is

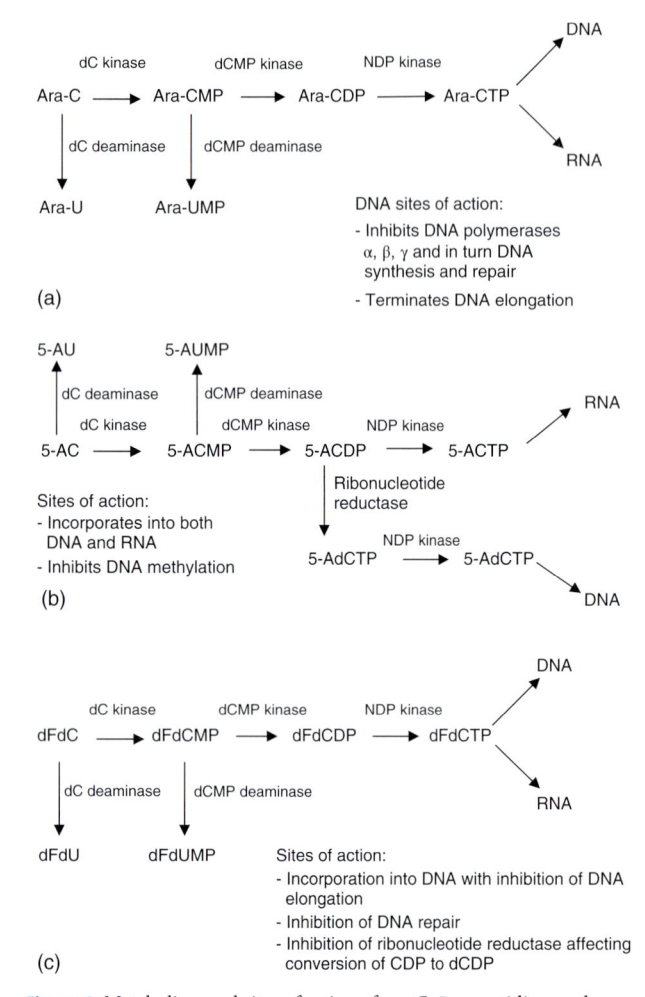

Figure 4 Metabolism and sites of action of ara-C, 5-azacytidine, and gemcitabine (dFdC). (a) The metabolic pathway used by ara-C. Ara-C is activated to ara-CTP by the sequential action of three kinases: deoxycytidine kinase (*dC Kinase*), deoxycytidine monophosphate kinase (*dCMP Kinase*), and nucleotide diphosphate kinase (*NDP Kinase*). Ara-C is inactivated by both cytidine deaminase (*CdR deaminase*) and deoxycytidine monophosphate deaminase (*dCMP deaminase*). Also listed are the sites of action of ara-C. (b) The metabolic pathway used by 5-AC. 5-AC is initially activated by the sequential action of deoxycytidine kinase (*dC Kinase*), and deoxycytidine monophosphate kinase (*dCMP Kinase*) to 5-ACDP. This can then be converted to 5-ACTP by nucleotide diphosphate kinase (*NDP Kin*) or to 5-AdCDP by the action of ribonucleotide reductase (*Rib Red*). 5-AdCDP can then be converted to 5-AdCTP by nucleotide diphosphate kinase (*NDP Kin*). 5-AC is inactivated by both cytidine deaminase (*dC deaminase*) and deoxycytidine monophosphate deaminase (*dCMP deaminase*). Also listed are the sites of action of 5-AC. (c) The metabolic pathway used by gemcitabine (dFdC). Initially, dFdC must be activated to dFdCTP by the sequential action of three kinases: deoxycytidine kinase (*dC Kinase*), deoxycytidine monophosphate kinase (*dCMP Kinase*), and nucleotide diphosphate kinase (*NDP Kinase*). Like ara-C, dFdC is inactivated by both cytidine deaminase (*dC deaminase*) and deoxycytidine monophosphate deaminase (*dCMP deaminase*). Also shown are sites of action of dFdC.

decreased transport into the cell or any other mechanism for decreased anabolism to the active metabolite ara-CTP.

Mechanism of action
The mechanism of action of ara-C is thought to occur at several potential sites. One mechanism is that ara-CTP is a potent inhibitor of DNA polymerases α, β, γ resulting in inhibition of DNA synthesis, elongation, and repair. An alternative mechanism of action occurs following incorporation of ara-CTP into DNA where it can terminate DNA elongation, acting as a DNA chain terminator.[20]

Clinical pharmacology
The bioavailability of ara-C is poor with extensive deamination occurring in the gastrointestinal tract. This has necessitated intravenous administration typically as a continuous infusion. Ara-C undergoes metabolism to ara-U within the plasma, liver, and various peripheral tissues with >80% excreted into the urine as ara-U. Ara-C can also cross the blood–brain barrier and enter the cerebrospinal fluid.

Clinical activity
Ara-C is an effective anti-leukemic agent, often used as the standard induction regimen for acute myelogenous leukemia (AML). It also has activity in acute lymphocytic leukemia (ALL) and chronic myelogenous leukemia, as well as other hematologic malignancies such as non-Hodgkin's lymphoma. Of interest, the drug has essentially no activity in solid tumors.

Toxicities
Toxicities vary depending on both dose and schedule. As expected, one of the most prominent toxicities is myelosuppression. This is seen with standard 7-day regimens with peak myelosuppression at 7–14 days, and it is particularly prominent with the use of high doses (2–3 g/m^2). Accompanying the myelosuppression are other hematologic toxicities in particular thrombocytopenia. Other toxicities include gastrointestinal manifestations such as nausea, anorexia, vomiting, diarrhea as well as, mucositis, and abdominal pain at times with pancreatitis and finally cerebellar toxicities at high doses.

5-Azacytidine or decitabine

Background
5-Azacytidine (5-AC) represents an attempt to improve on the success of cytosine arabinoside in treating leukemias. Of particular interest was identifying cytidine analogs that did not require activation by deoxycytidine kinase, the enzyme with decreased or absent activity in many cytosine arabinoside resistant tumors. A number of analogs were synthesized, in particular, ribonucleosides, where structural changes had been made in the pyrimidine ring that still allow the compound to be anabolized by uridine-cytidine kinase.[18] The most active of these was 5-azacytidine, which was also later identified occurring naturally in fungal cultures (Figure 3). 5-Azacytidine was shown to be toxic to both bacterial and mammalian cells. A related drug is decitabine (Figure 3).

Cellular uptake and metabolism
5-Azacytidine utilizes the equilabrative nucleoside transporter to enter human cells. Once within the cell, it is anabolized via the uridine-cytidine pathway to form 5-azacytidine monophosphate. This is converted to 5-azacytidine triphosphate by the sequential action of deoxycytidine monophosphate kinase and deoxycytidine diphosphate kinase (Figure 4b).[18] Decitabine's cellular uptake and metabolism are similar.

Resistance to 5-azacytidine can occur through several mechanisms. Thus, a deficient or altered nucleoside transporter on the cell surface could inhibit cellular uptake and in turn result in relative resistance. Endogenous levels of uridine and/or cytidine can compete with 5-azacytidine for phosphorylation resulting in less activity. Similarly, decreased or absent expression of uridine–cytidine kinase could confer resistance. The presence of increased activity of catabolizing enzymes (e.g., cytidine deaminase) can result in formation of 5-azauridine, which lacks cell toxicity.[18]

Mechanism of action
5-Azacytidine triphosphate is the critical metabolite. There are several suggested sites of action. 5-Azacytidine triphosphate first competes with naturally occurring CTP for incorporation into RNA. 5-Azacytidine triphosphate that is incorporated into RNA can produce several detrimental effects on RNA processing and function including inhibition of ribosomal 328S and 18S formation, alteration of acceptor function of transfer RNA, disruption of polyribosomal assembly, and resultant inhibition of protein synthesis.[21] In addition, 5-azacytidine triphosphate can be incorporated into DNA, leading to inhibition of DNA methylation following replication of DNA.[18] It is the latter effect that makes this drug particularly interesting to the study of epigenetic effects secondary to methylation.

Decitabine has a similar mechanism of action as azacytidine.[18,22] This includes demethylation or interference with the methylation of DNA. As a result, normal function to the tumor suppressor genes is restored, enabling control over cell growth. As a typical antimetabolite, decitabine can also be incorporated into nucleic acid, interacting with a number of potential targets to produce a direct cytotoxic effect that causes death of rapidly dividing cancer cells.

Clinical pharmacology
5-Azacytidine is typically administered via intravenous infusion and undergoes rapid deamination to 5-azauridine. Plasma clearance is often lower in women and the elderly, and caution should therefore be used in these groups. In 2020, the FDA approved the use of oral 5-azacytidine in AML. Also, in 2020 the FDA approved the use of the combination of decitabine with cedazuridine. Cedazuridine potentiates the effect of decitabine by inhibiting cytidine deaminase. The combination regimen is approved for use in adult patients with myelodysplastic syndrome.

Clinical activity
Both 5-azacytidine and decitabine have clinical activity in AML and myelodysplasia.[18,22] As noted above, 5-azacytidine exerts its inhibitory effect on DNA methylation by enabling a mechanism that clinically and experimentally increases expression of epigenetically suppressed genes.[23]

Toxicities
Similar to other members of this antimetabolite group, the major dose-limiting toxicity (DLT) for both 5-azacytidine and decitabine is myelosuppression, in particular neutropenia and thrombocytopenia. Nausea and vomiting occur particularly with bolus administration. Other toxicities observed mostly with high dose 5-azacytidine include hepatocellular abnormalities, hyperbilirubinemia, muscle tenderness and weakness, and central nervous system (CNS) toxicity that includes lethargy, confusion, and even coma.[18,23] Because of these latter toxicities, one should use caution in administering these drugs in patients with hepatic failure or altered mental status.

Gemcitabine

Background
Gemcitabine is a synthetic nucleoside analog in which two fluorines have been substituted for the hydrogens in deoxycytidine.[18,24] The structure of gemcitabine is shown in Figure 3.

Cellular uptake and metabolism
Similar to other antimetabolites, gemcitabine utilizes the cell's nucleoside transporter to enter human cells. Once within the cell, it must be anabolized via the cell's natural deoxycytidine pathways to form the gemcitabine triphosphate to achieve activity; it is inactive as the parent drug.[24]

There are several theoretical sites of resistance to gemcitabine. Thus, a deficient or altered nucleoside transporter can inhibit the cellular uptake of gemcitabine and result in relative resistance.[18] Metabolically, resistance can occur through either decreased activity of critical anabolizing enzymes (e.g., deoxycytidine kinase) or increased activity of catabolizing enzymes (e.g., cytidine deaminase or deoxycytidylate deaminase).

Mechanism of action
Gemcitabine triphosphate is the critical metabolite. Although there are several suggested sites of action, the most important is thought to be chain termination and inhibition of DNA synthesis and function following incorporation into DNA.[25] Gemcitabine triphosphate is also thought to directly inhibit DNA polymerases α, β, and γ, which can result in chain termination and inhibition of DNA synthesis, and also DNA repair. Lastly, gemcitabine triphosphate is capable of inhibiting ribonucleotide reductase, further contributing to inhibition of DNA synthesis by depleting critically needed deoxyribonucleotide pools.

Clinical pharmacology
Gemcitabine is typically administered via intravenous infusion, because of rapid deamination to 2′,2′-difluoro-2′-deoxyuridine (dFdU). Plasma clearance is often lower in women and the elderly, and caution should, therefore, be used in these groups.

Clinical activity
Although it has structural similarity and shares an identical site of action with cytosine arabinoside, gemcitabine has a much broader spectrum of clinical activity including several solid tumors, for example, pancreatic, lung (small cell and non-small cell), ovarian, bladder, and breast cancers as well as in hematologic malignancies, for example, both Hodgkin's and non-Hodgkin's lymphoma.

Toxicities
The major DLT is myelosuppression with both neutropenia and to a somewhat lesser extent thrombocytopenia. When infusions are increased beyond 30 min, hematologic toxicity tends to be more severe. Other frequently observed toxicities include flu-like symptoms including fever, headaches, myalgias, and arthralgias.

Purine antimetabolites

Purine antimetabolite cancer chemotherapy drugs include structural modifications of the naturally occurring purine bases, guanine, and adenine, or their ribose or deoxyribose nucleosides or potentially their precursors. As with the pyrimidine antimetabolites, the structural changes can be in either the base or the sugar.[26,27]

Guanine antimetabolites

Two guanine antimetabolites, 6-mercaptopurine (6-MP) and 6-thioguanine (6-TG), synthesized more than six decades ago, have shown anticancer activity and continue to be used today. Azathioprine, a prodrug of 6-MP that results in slow release of 6-MP, although it does not have significant antitumor activity (and therefore not discussed here), is an effective immunosuppressant that has been widely used in organ transplantation, inflammatory bowel disease (e.g., Crohn's), and rheumatologic diseases.

6-Mercaptopurine

Background
The structure of 6-MP is closely related to the naturally occurring purine base hypoxanthine (Figure 5a,b) with a thiol group substituting for the hydroxyl group at the sixth position. As is characteristic of other antimetabolites, 6-MP can enter both the anabolic and catabolic pathways used by the naturally occurring metabolites, in this case hypoxanthine.

Metabolism
Following uptake into cells, 6-MP can be immediately anabolized by hypoxanthine-guanine phosphoribosyltransferase (HGPRT) to 6-thioinosine monophosphate (TIMP). TIMP can be further anabolized to the triphosphate and then be incorporated into DNA. The metabolism of 6-MP is shown in Figure 5c.[27]

Resistance can result from decreased availability of TIMP either from decreased anabolism or increased catabolism primarily mediated by phosphatases.

Mechanism of action
TIMP is thought to be the active metabolite deriving its mechanism of action through inhibiting *de novo* purine biosynthesis in turn leading to a disturbance in the size of the natural purine nucleotide pools needed for nucleic acid synthesis (Figure 5c).

Clinical pharmacology
6-MP is administered orally (typically 90 mg/m^2), although its absorption can be erratic with variation in peak concentrations and peak times. 6-MP has minimal binding to serum proteins with the half-life of free drug being in the 20–45 min range.[28] 6-MP is metabolized by xanthine oxidase. Because other drugs used in the oncologic setting such as allopurinol also utilize this same enzyme in its metabolism, this can lead to a potentially serious drug interaction accompanied by increased toxicity (in effect more active 6-MP metabolite present). Therefore, with concomitant use, the dose of 6-MP is typically reduced 50–75%.[29] Another important clinical pharmacologic finding with 6-MP use is pharmacogenetic. Thus, because there is variability in the expression of thiopurine methyltransferase (TPMT) in the general population due to variants within the TPMT gene, the metabolism and hence the availability of active drug may vary. It is possible now to screen for these TPMT variants prior to 6-MP administration and thereby avoid toxicity.[9,30]

Clinical activity
Although introduced clinically more than 50 years ago, 6-MP continues to have a clinical role in the management of ALL, particularly in children. 6-MP lacks efficacy in solid tumors. Because of its immunosuppressive effects, it has also been used for nononcologic diseases (e.g., Crohn's disease).

Toxicities
The primary toxicity with 6-MP is myelosuppression. Other toxicities include gastrointestinal, such as anorexia, nausea, vomiting, diarrhea, and hepatotoxicity. Therefore, the concomitant use of hepatotoxic agents should be avoided. Lastly, 6-MP, like its prodrug azathioprine, can produce immunosuppression and lead to an increased risk of infections.

6-Thioguanine

Background
6-TG, like 6-MP, is one of the original purine antimetabolites, first synthesized in the 1950s. It also belongs to the family of guanine antimetabolites.[26] Its structure is shown in Figure 5b.

Metabolism
Following uptake into cells, 6-TG is anabolized by the endogenous enzymes in the guanine pathway as shown in Figure 5c. 6-TG differs from 6-MP in that it is converted directly to 6-TG nucleotide monophosphate and then subsequently to the nucleotide diphosphate and nucleotide triphosphate, which can then be incorporated into RNA and DNA.

Similar to other antimetabolites, resistance may occur from either decreased activity of anabolic enzymes or increased activity of catabolic enzymes.[26]

Mechanism of action
The mechanism of action of 6-TG is thought to be secondary to its incorporation into both RNA and DNA where it interferes with nucleic acid synthesis and function.[31]

Clinical pharmacology
6-TG is typically administered orally. Its oral bioavailability is variable with peak levels occurring 2–4 h after dosing. Its metabolism differs from that of 6-MP in that it is not metabolized by xanthine oxidase. Therefore, no drug interactions occur with concomitant administration of allopurinol, and unlike 6-MP the dose of 6-TG need not be reduced to avoid toxicity.

6-TG, however, similar to 6-MP, is a substrate for TPMT and therefore in the presence of decreased expression secondary to genetic variability in the TPMT gene expression, the dose should be adjusted in affected individuals. TPMT deficiency is found in approximately 10% of all patients and, therefore, TPMT screening is recommended prior to drug administration.[9,30]

Clinical activity
6-TG is active in AML, where it is sometimes used for remission induction and maintenance therapy; and it is also used in ALL.

Toxicities
Myelosuppression is the major toxicity. Other toxicities include stomatitis and gastrointestinal toxicities in particular anorexia, nausea/vomiting, and diarrhea. Hepatotoxicity may also be seen in a significant proportion of patients, particularly those with cholestatic jaundice and occasionally in those with transaminase elevations. For this reason, concomitant use of hepatotoxic agents should be avoided. Lastly, like 6-MP, 6-TG is also associated with immunosuppression and therefore an increased risk of infections.

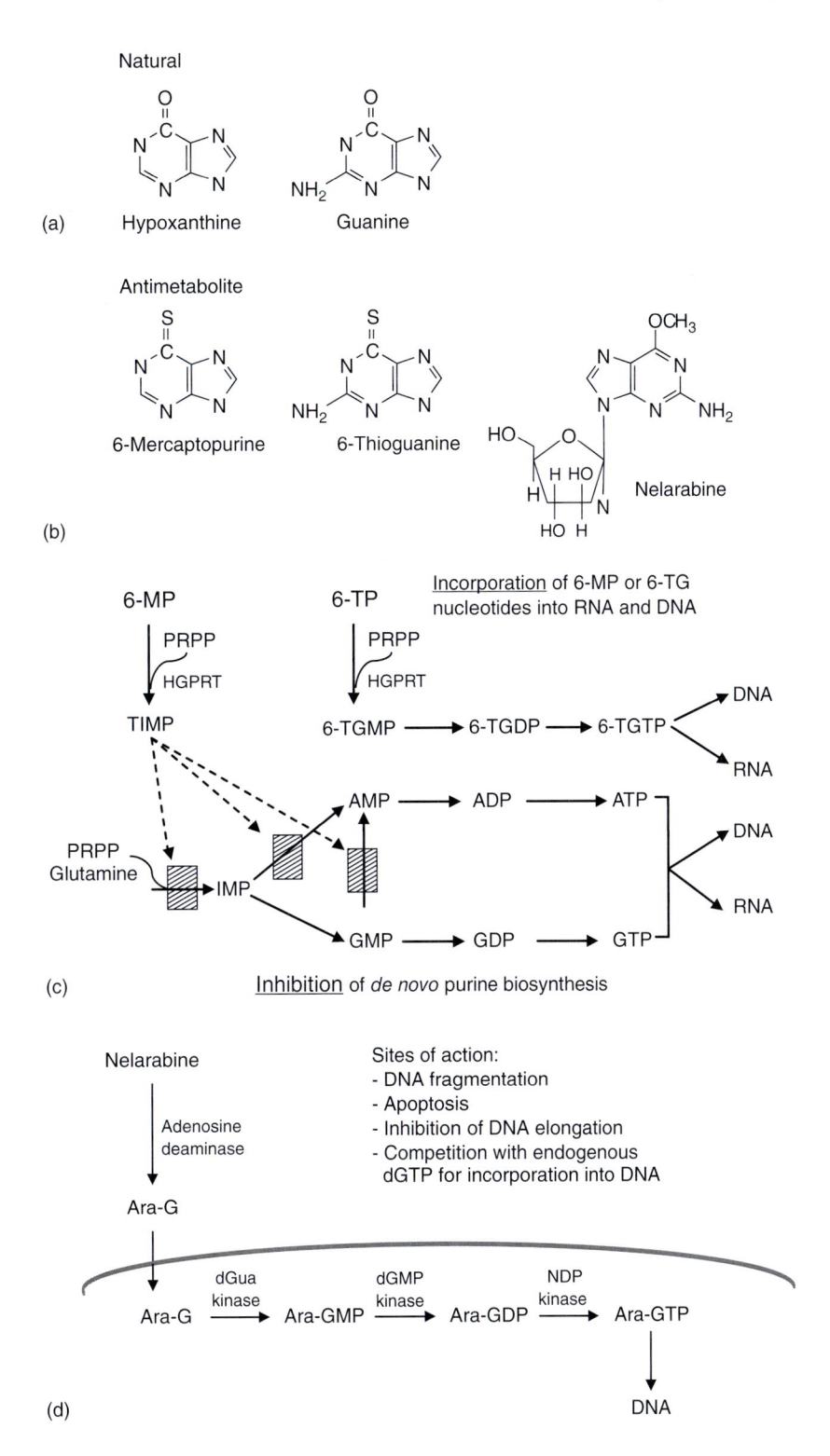

Figure 5 Structures of hypoxanthine/guanine antimetabolites; and metabolism and sites of action of 6-mercaptopurine (6-MP), 6-thioguanine (6-TG), and nelarabine. (a) Natural occurring purine bases hypoxanthine and guanine. (b) Antimetabolites 6-mercaptopurine and 6-thioguanine developed from structural modifications of hypoxanthine and guanine as well as nelarabine a prodrug of the deoxyguanosine antimetabolite 9-β-D-arabinofuranosylguanine (ara-G). (c) 6-MP is converted to 6-thioinosine monophosphate (TIMP) and 6-TG is converted to 6-thioguanine ribonucleotide monophosphate 6-TGMP) by hypoxanthine-guanine phosphoribosyltransferase (*HGPRT*) in the presence of PRPP. TIMP is active by inhibiting *de novo* purine biosynthesis at three steps: (1) inhibiting formation of inosine monophosphate (IMP) from glutamine and PRPP; (2) inhibiting conversion of IMP to AMP; and (3) inhibiting conversion of AMP to IMP. Through the sequential activation of nucleotide kinases, 6-TGMP can be eventually converted to the ribonucleotide diphosphate (6-TGDP) and then ribonucleotide triphosphate (6-TGTP). 6-TGTP is active following incorporation into both RNA and DNA, resulting in a disturbance of nucleic acid function. (d) Nelarabine is a prodrug that following intravenous administration undergoes O-demethylation in the blood by adenosine deaminase (*Ade deaminase*) to Ara-G. Ara-G is then transported into cells by nucleoside transporters where it is converted by deoxyguanosine kinases (*dGua Kinase*) to the monophosphate, ara-GMP, and then through the sequential action of nucleotide kinases, dGMP kinase, and NDP Kinase, to the active metabolite ara-GTP. Also shown are the sites of action ara-GTP.

Nelarabine

Background
Nelarabine is a prodrug of the deoxyguanosine antimetabolite 9-β-D-Arabinofuranosylguanine (ara-G), which is cytotoxic. It is one of the newer purine antimetabolites, that was developed for use in patients resistant to Fludarabine (see below).[32] Its structure is shown in Figure 5b.

Metabolism
As a prodrug, Nelarabine must first be converted to ara-G[32] by adenosine deaminase-mediated demethylation. Once transported into the tumor cells by nucleoside transporters, ara-G is anabolized to the ribonucleotide triphosphate (ara-GTP), which is the active metabolite. It utilizes the same enzymes used by naturally occurring purines in the purine anabolic pathway (Figure 5d). Like other antimetabolites, increased activity of catabolic enzymes may contribute to relative resistance.

Mechanism of action
Ara-GTP is active following incorporation into DNA where it can result in DNA fragmentation and apoptosis. Like other antimetabolites, ara-GTP competes with the naturally occurring deoxyguanosine triphosphate (dGTP) for incorporation into DNA. Following incorporation at the 3′ end of the elongating DNA, further incorporation into DNA is inhibited resulting in apoptosis and cellular death. Other mechanisms of action remain unclear.[32,33]

Clinical pharmacology
Nelarabine is a soluble prodrug typically administered by 2–3 h intravenous infusion. Neither Nelarabine nor ara-G are significantly bound by plasma proteins and are eliminated through the kidney.[33]

Clinical activity
Nelarabine was approved by the FDA in 2005 for use in patients with T-cell acute leukemia or T-cell lymphoblastic lymphoma, whose disease is unresponsive to previous chemotherapy or relapsed after at least two chemotherapy regimens.[34]

Toxicities
Common toxicities include malaise, fever, nausea, and myelosuppression. Grade 3–4 neurologic toxicities occur in 10–15% of patients and may include both CNS side effects, for example, obtundation, seizures, and encephalopathy, as well as peripheral neuropathy.[34]

Adenosine antimetabolites

The adenosine analogs represent the other major class of purine antimetabolites. In contrast to the guanine antimetabolites that depend on structural modification within the purine base, the adenosine antimetabolites rely on changes within the sugar portion of the molecule. This structural change results in decreased activity of adenosine deaminase. Halogen substitution at the two-position of the deoxyadenosine with fluorine in fludarabine and chlorine in cladribine also contributes to the desired effect. Currently, there are several adenosine antimetabolites approved for clinical use that include fludarabine, cladribine, and clofarabine (Figure 6a,b). A fourth adenosine-like analog, pentostatin (deoxycoformycin), is a naturally occurring purine analog that was first identified in fermentation broths of *Streptomyces antibioticus*. Its structure is similar to the transitional form of adenosine in the adenosine deaminase reaction. It is one of the most effective inhibitors of adenosine deaminase.[26]

Fludarabine

Background
Fludarabine, also known as 9-β-D-arabinosyl-2-fluoroadenine monophosphate or F-ara-AMP, has a structure that is shown in Figure 6b.

Metabolism
Following intravenous administration, fludarabine is rapidly dephosphorylated to F-ara A (Figure 6c). This can then cross into cells using the nucleoside transporters. Within the cells in the presence of ATP and deoxycytidine kinase, it is converted back to a nucleotide monophosphate and then sequentially converted to F-ara-ATP.[35]

Mechanism of action
F-ara-ATP is the active metabolite responsible for the mechanism of action. This results from competition with the natural metabolite deoxyadenosine triphosphate (dATP).

Clinical pharmacology
F-ara-AMP must be administered by the intravenous route. Peak concentrations are observed after 3–4 h. It is excreted into the urine with almost 25% of the administered drug being eliminated unchanged.[36]

Clinical activity
This purine antimetabolite is active in chronic lymphocytic leukemia where it was first approved. It also has activity in several other hematologic malignancies including pro-lymphocytic leukemia, indolent non-Hodgkin's lymphoma, cutaneous T-cell lymphoma, mantle cell lymphoma, and Waldenström macroglobulinemia. Fludarabine has essentially no activity in nonhematologic solid tumors.[36]

Toxicities
The two major side effects limiting F-ara-AMP in the clinic are myelosuppression and immunosuppression. The myelosuppression is often lymphocytopenia and thrombocytopenia. Fever is often seen with myelosuppression. Immunosuppression is primarily T-cell mediated with much less effect on B-cells. Lymphocyte counts, in particular CD4 cells, often decrease after F-ara-MP and may take more than a year to recover. The combined effect of myelosuppression and immunosuppression may result in an increased risk for opportunistic infections such as *Candida albicans, pneumocystis carinii*, or viral *infections with varicella-zoster*. Prophylactic antibiotic coverage for *pneumocystis carinii* is often recommended with trimethoprim-sulfamethoxazole the drug of choice to be co-administered with F-ara-AMP. Other less frequent toxicities include anorexia, nausea, vomiting, diarrhea, abdominal pain, and at times increased salivation, and parageusia (metallic taste), skin rash, and stomatitis. Laboratory abnormalities include transient elevations of hepatic enzymes as well as evidence of renal dysfunction.[36]

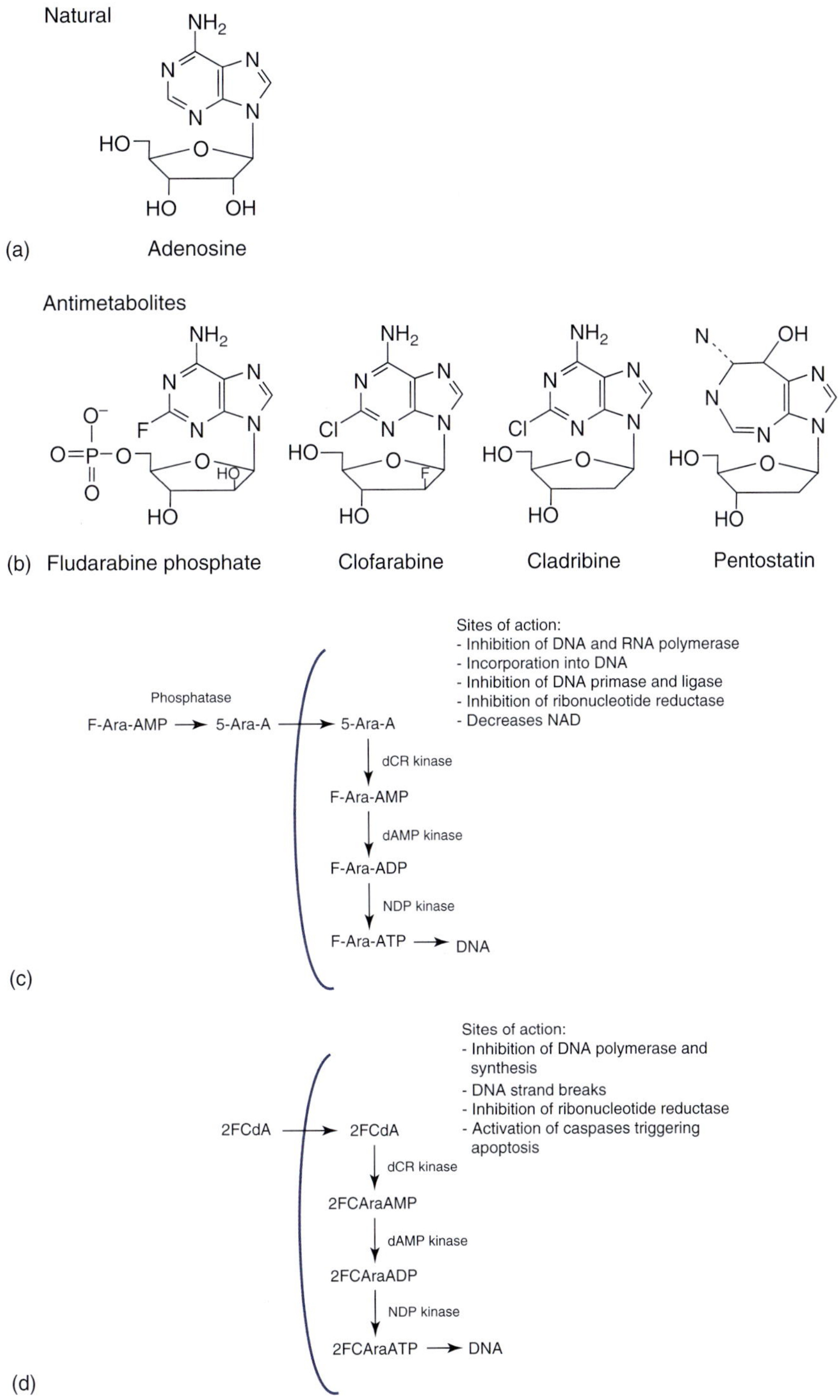

Figure 6 Structures of adenosine antimetabolites; and metabolism and sites of action of fludarabine (FAraAMP) and cladribine. (a) The naturally occurring purine base adenosine. (b) The antimetabolites fludarabine monophosphate, cladribine, and clofarabine developed from structural modifications of adenosine. In addition (although not discussed here), pentostatin, an adenosine analog first isolated from fermentation broths of *Streptomyces antibioticus*, is shown for comparison as it corresponds to the transitional form of adenosine in the adenosine deaminase reaction. (c) Following intravenous administration, FAraAMP is dephosphorylated in the blood by ubiquitous phosphatases to FAra-A. FAra-A is then transported into cells by nucleoside transporters where it is reconverted by deoxycytidine kinase (*dCR Kinase*) to the monophosphate, FAra-AMP, and then through the action of nucleotide kinases (*dAMP Kinase and NDP kinase*) converted to the active metabolite FAra-ATP. Listed are the sites of action for FAra-ATP. (d) Following intravenous administration, cladribine is transported into cells by nucleoside transporters where it is reconverted by deoxycytidine kinase (*dCR Kinase*) to the monophosphate, 2CFAra-AMP, and then through the action of nucleotide kinases (*dAMP Kinase and NDP kinase*) to the active metabolite 2CFAra-ATP. Also listed are the sites of action ara-2CFAra-ATP.

2-Chlorodeoxyadenosine (cladribine or 2FCdA)

Background
2-Chlorodeoxyadenosine is a purine deoxyadenosine analog.[37] Its structure is shown in Figure 6b.

Metabolism
Following entry into the cell using the cell's nucleoside transporters, cladribine is anabolized via deoxycytidine kinase (dCR Kinase) to 2-chlorodeoxyadenosine monophosphate eventually being converted to 2-chlorodeoxyadenosine triphosphate, the active metabolite[37,38] (Figure 6d).

Altered metabolism of 2-chlorodeoxyadenosine can contribute to resistance, specifically via decreased activity of dCR kinase, a critical step in the anabolism of this drug. Similarly, increased expression of catabolic enzymes, in particular 5′-nucleotidase, may contribute to resistance.

Mechanism of action
The active metabolite 2-chlorodeoxyadenosine triphosphate competes with naturally occurring dATP for incorporation into DNA where it can cause termination of chain elongation. There can also be inhibition of DNA synthesis and repair due to an imbalance in critical deoxyribonucleotide pools as well as inhibition of ribonucleotide reductase.[37]

Clinical pharmacology
2-Chlorodeoxyadenosine can be administered orally. The drug is primarily excreted via the kidney with approximately 50% cleared into the urine, with as much as 25% unchanged. The drug can cross the blood–brain barrier into the cerebrospinal fluid.

Clinical activity
2-Chlorodeoxyadenosine was initially approved by the FDA and remains the drug of choice for treatment of hairy cell leukemia.[39] In patients with both primary and relapsed hairy cell leukemia, the response rate is 60% or greater. The drug also has activity in low-grade lymphoproliferative diseases, and it has potential activity for patients with CLL and non-Hodgkin's lymphoma.[40,41]

Notably, 2-chlorodeoxyadenosine has also been shown to be useful in nononcologic diseases as well as having shown potential efficacy in relapsing-remitting multiple sclerosis.

Toxicities
Myelosuppression is the primary DLT at standard doses with both thrombocytopenia and neutropenia. Other toxicities include nausea, vomiting and diarrhea, and neurotoxicity. Cladribine can also cause immunosuppression with decreased lymphocyte counts particularly CD4-positive cells. These depressed counts may take years to recover after completion of therapy and the decreased CD4 counts predispose patients to developing opportunistic infections.

Clofarabine

Background
Clofarabine was synthesized to develop a potentially more effective adenine analog than fludarabine and cladribine (Figure 6b). This 2-halo-2′-halodeoxyarabinofuranosyl adenine analog has the 2-chloroadenine aglycone that conveys resistance to inactivation by adenosine deaminase (ADA). It also is thought to benefit from the fluorine in the 2′ position of the sugar in the arabinosyl configuration that potentially contributes to its DNA inhibition. The fluorine substituted at the C-2′ position is thought to inhibit the effect of PNP (phosphorolysis) in contrast to what typically occurs with fludarabine and cladribine.[42]

Metabolism
Following uptake into tumor cells, clofarabine must be anabolized to a triphosphate, which is the active metabolite. Its chemistry potentially contributes to decreased catabolism and hence increased effectiveness. Clofarabine has been reported to be a better substrate for deoxycytidine kinase than fludarabine or cladribine.[43]

Resistance can result from perturbation of metabolism either due to decreased anabolism or increased catabolism.

Mechanism of action
Several possible sites of action include inhibition of DNA synthesis due to chain termination following incorporation into DNA; inhibition of DNA synthesis by inhibiting DNA polymerases α, β, and γ, which in turn interferes with DNA chain elongation and synthesis and repair of DNA. DNA synthesis is further inhibited by depletion of intracellular deoxyribonucleotide pools through inhibition of ribonucleotide reductase.[43,44]

Clinical pharmacology
Clofarabine is typically administered as an intravenous infusion at doses between 2 and 40 mg/m^2 over 5 days. Half-life is approximately 5 h with plasma concentrations as high as 2.5 μM being achievable, although there is interpatient variability. It is estimated that 50–60% of the administered drug may be excreted unchanged into the urine. Currently, there is no data to guide use of this drug in individuals with renal or hepatic insufficiency.

Clinical activity
The FDA-approved clofarabine in 2004 for use in refractory pediatric ALL. It has also been used in adult AML and myelodysplastic syndrome.[45,46] The combination of clofarabine with ara-C is particularly interesting, because it is associated with an increased response rate and without increased toxicity compared with ara-C. This is thought to be a result of potentiation by increasing cytosine arabinoside concentrations.

Toxicities
The major toxic manifestation is myelosuppression, which results in an increased risk for infection. Hepatic transaminase elevation has also been noted in as many as 25% of patients. Other side effects include anorexia, nausea, and skin rash particularly in children.[45,46]

Conclusions

Although the first representatives of this class on cancer therapeutics were introduced several decades ago, the pyrimidine and purine antimetabolite drugs continue to be important. While there have been only a few new pyrimidine and purine antimetabolites added clinically in the last 10 years, several of these drugs are still widely used in oncology in two of the four most common malignancies. Thus, the fluoropyrimidine drugs are first-line choices particularly in colorectal cancer as both adjuvant and advanced treatments and as later line agents in the treatment of advanced breast cancer. There are also several examples of pyrimidine and purine antimetabolites that remain important therapeutic options in the treatment of both lymphocytic and myelocytic leukemias.

Understanding how to best select patients for treatment with each of the pyrimidine and purine antimetabolite drugs continues to be a major goal.

Key references

The complete reference list can be found on Vital Source version of this title, see inside front cover.

1. Wellstein A. Goodman & Gilman's the pharmacological basis of therapeutics. In: Brunton LL, Hilal-Dandan R, Knollmann BC, eds. *General Principles of Pharmacotherapy of Cancer*, 13th ed. New York: McGraw-Hill; 2018.
3. Diasio RB, Harris BE. Clinical pharmacology of 5-fluorouracil. *Clin Pharmacokinet*. 1989;**16**(4):215–237.
7. Diasio RB, Beavers TL, Carpenter JT. Familial deficiency of dihydropyrimidine dehydrogenase. Biochemical basis for familial pyrimidinemia and severe 5-fluorouracil-induced toxicity. *J Clin Invest*. 1988;**81**(1):47–51.
8. Shrestha S, Zhang C, Jerde CR, et al. Gene-specific variant classifier (DPYD-Varifier) to identify deleterious alleles of dihydropyrimidine dehydrogenase. *Clin Pharmacol Ther*. 2018;**104**(4):709–718.
9. Offer SM, Diasio RB. Pharmacogenetics and the role of genomics in cancer therapeutics. In: Chabner BA, Longo DL, eds. *Cancer Chemotherapy, Immunotherapy, and Biotherapy; Principles and Practice*, 6th ed. Walters Kluwer Lippincott Williams & Wilkins; 2018.
10. Beumer JH, Chu E, Allegra C, et al. Therapeutic drug monitoring in oncology: international association of therapeutic drug monitoring and clinical toxicology recommendations for 5-fluorouracil therapy. *Clin Pharmacol Ther*. 2019;**105**(3):598–613.
11. Saif MW, Diasio RB. Benefit of uridine triacetate (Vistogard) in rescuing severe 5-fluorouracil toxicity in patients with dihydropyrimidine dehydrogenase (DPYD) deficiency. *Cancer Chemother Pharmacol*. 2016;**78**(1):151–156.
12. Kemeny NE, Schwartz L, Gonen M, et al. Treating primary liver cancer with hepatic arterial infusion of floxuridine and dexamethasone: does the addition of systemic bevacizumab improve results? *Oncology*. 2011;**80**(3–4):153–159.
13. de Bono JS, Twelves CJ. The oral fluorinated pyrimidines. *Invest New Drugs*. 2001;**19**(1):41–59.
14. Kang C, Dhillon S, Deeks ED. Trifluridine/tipiracil: a review in metastatic gastric cancer. *Drugs*. 2019;**79**(14):1583–1590.
16. Xu J, Kim TW, Shen L, et al. Results of a randomized, double-blind, placebo-controlled, phase III trial of trifluridine/tipiracil (TAS-102) monotherapy in Asian patients with previously treated metastatic colorectal cancer: the TERRA study. *J Clin Oncol*. 2018;**36**(4):350–358.
18. Chabner BA, Nabel CS, Brunner AM. Cytidine analogues. In: Chabner BA, Longo DL, eds. *Cancer Chemotherapy, Immunotherapy, and Biotherapy; Principles and Practice*, 6th ed. Walters Kluwer Lippincott Williams & Wilkins; 2018.
19. Chou TC, Arlin Z, Clarkson BD, et al. Metabolism of 1-beta-D-arabinofuranosylcytosine in human leukemic cells. *Cancer Res*. 1977;**37**(10):3561–3570.
20. Ohno Y, Spriggs D, Matsukage A, et al. Effects of 1-beta-D-arabinofuranosylcytosine incorporation on elongation of specific DNA sequences by DNA polymerase beta. *Cancer Res*. 1988;**48**(6):1494–1498.
21. Vesely J. Mode of action and effects of 5-azacytidine and of its derivatives in eukaryotic cells. *Pharmacol Ther*. 1985;**28**(2):227–235.
22. Kantarjian H, Oki Y, Garcia-Manero G, et al. Results of a randomized study of 3 schedules of low-dose decitabine in higher-risk myelodysplastic syndrome and chronic myelomonocytic leukemia. *Blood*. 2007;**109**(1):52–57.
23. Glover AB, Leyland-Jones BR, Chun HG, et al. Azacitidine: 10 years later. *Cancer Treat Rep*. 1987;**71**(7–8):737–746.
24. Shewach DS, Hahn TM, Chang E, et al. Metabolism of 2′,2′-difluoro-2′-deoxycytidine and radiation sensitization of human colon carcinoma cells. *Cancer Res*. 1994;**54**(12):3218–3223.
25. Ruiz van Haperen VW, Veerman G, Vermorken JB, et al. 2′,2′-Difluoro-deoxycytidine (gemcitabine) incorporation into RNA and DNA of tumour cell lines. *Biochem Pharmacol*. 1993;**46**(4):762–766.
26. Hande KR, Chabner BA. Purine antimetabolites. In: Chabner BA, Longo DL, eds. *Cancer Chemotherapy, Immunotherapy, and Biotherapy; Principles and Practice*, 6th ed. Walters Kluwer Lippincott Williams & Wilkins; 2018.
27. Zimm S, Collins JM, Riccardi R, et al. Variable bioavailability of oral mercaptopurine. Is maintenance chemotherapy in acute lymphoblastic leukemia being optimally delivered? *N Engl J Med*. 1983;**308**(17):1005–1009.
28. Zimm S, Collins JM, O'Neill D, et al. Inhibition of first-pass metabolism in cancer chemotherapy: interaction of 6-mercaptopurine and allopurinol. *Clin Pharmacol Ther*. 1983;**34**(6):810–817.
29. Lennard L. Implementation of TPMT testing. *Br J Clin Pharmacol*. 2014;**77**(4):704–714.
30. Karran P, Attard N. Thiopurines in current medical practice: molecular mechanisms and contributions to therapy-related cancer. *Nat Rev Cancer*. 2008;**8**(1):24–36.
31. Nelson JA, Carpenter JW, Rose LM, et al. Mechanisms of action of 6-thioguanine, 6-mercaptopurine, and 8-azaguanine. *Cancer Res*. 1975;**35**(10):2872–2878.
32. Gandhi V, Keating MJ, Bate G, et al. Nelarabine. *Nat Rev Drug Discov*. 2006;**5**(1):17–18.
33. Sanford M, Lyseng-Williamson KA. *Nelarabine Drugs*. 2008;**68**(4):439–447.
34. Kadia TM, Gandhi V. Nelarabine in the treatment of pediatric and adult patients with T-cell acute lymphoblastic leukemia and lymphoma. *Expert Rev Hematol*. 2017;**10**(1):1–8.
35. Gandhi V, Plunkett W. Cellular and clinical pharmacology of fludarabine. *Clin Pharmacokinet*. 2002;**41**(2):93–103.
36. Montillo M, Ricci F, Tedeschi A. Role of fludarabine in hematological malignancies. *Expert Rev Anticancer Ther*. 2006;**6**(9):1141–1161.
37. Griffig J, Koob R, Blakley RL. Mechanisms of inhibition of DNA synthesis by 2-chlorodeoxyadenosine in human lymphoblastic cells. *Cancer Res*. 1989;**49**(24 Pt 1):6923–6928.
38. Fukuda Y, Schuetz JD. ABC transporters and their role in nucleoside and nucleotide drug resistance. *Biochem Pharmacol*. 2012;**83**(8):1073–1083.
39. Grever MR, Lozanski G. Modern strategies for hairy cell leukemia. *J Clin Oncol*. 2011;**29**(5):583–590.
40. Sigal DS, Miller HJ, Schram ED, et al. Beyond hairy cell: the activity of cladribine in other hematologic malignancies. *Blood*. 2010;**116**(16):2884–2896.
41. Zhou A, Han Q, Song H, et al. Efficacy and toxicity of cladribine for the treatment of refractory acute myeloid leukemia: a meta-analysis. *Drug Des Devel Ther*. 2019;**13**:1867–1878.
42. Zhenchuk A, Lotfi K, Juliusson G, et al. Mechanisms of anti-cancer action and pharmacology of clofarabine. *Biochem Pharmacol*. 2009;**78**(11):1351–1359.
43. Nagai S, Takenaka K, Nachagari D, et al. Deoxycytidine kinase modulates the impact of the ABC transporter ABCG2 on clofarabine cytotoxicity. *Cancer Res*. 2011;**71**(5):1781–1791.
44. Aye Y, Stubbe J. Clofarabine 5′-di and -triphosphates inhibit human ribonucleotide reductase by altering the quaternary structure of its large subunit. *Proc Natl Acad Sci U S A*. 2011;**108**(24):9815–9820.
45. Rubnitz JE, Lacayo NJ, Inaba H, et al. Clofarabine can replace anthracyclines and etoposide in remission induction therapy for childhood acute myeloid leukemia: the AML08 multicenter, randomized phase III trial. *J Clin Oncol*. 2019;**37**(23):2072–2081.
46. Bryan J, Kantarjian H, Prescott H, et al. Clofarabine in the treatment of myelodysplastic syndromes. *Expert Opin Investig Drugs*. 2014;**23**(2):255–263.

55 Alkylating agents and platinum antitumor compounds

Zahid H. Siddik, PhD

Overview

Alkylating agents and platinum-based compounds constitute two important classes of antitumor drugs in the war against cancer. These drugs transform spontaneously or metabolically to induce DNA monofunctional adducts and interstrand and intrastrand crosslinks. As a result, the DNA unwinds and/or bends, which are then recognized by specialized DNA damage recognition proteins to induce cell cycle arrest that allows cells time to repair the DNA and survive. If DNA damage is extensive and repair cannot be completed, then cells undergo programmed cell death to result in a positive antitumor response. Since active species in the two drug classes are not tumor-selective, they will also interact with DNA in normal cells to induce several side effects, some of which can be irreversible and cumulative and, thereby, become life threatening. Another limitation is that tumor cells can become resistance to alkylating and platinating drugs through mechanisms that are either intrinsic or acquired. Such resistance mechanisms are manifested as reduced drug accumulation, increased drug inactivation, increased DNA repair, failure of DNA damage recognition system to recognize the damage, and aberrant apoptotic signal transduction pathways. Therefore, identifications of rational personalized combination therapeutic strategies involving these two potent classes of DNA-reactive drugs are desperately needed to combat resistance mechanisms and enhance curative responses.

Introduction

Antitumor agents interacting with deoxyribonucleic acid (DNA) to inhibit cellular proliferation are critical for effectively managing cancer patients. Such therapeutics are broadly termed as DNA alkylating and platinum-based drugs. These agents form monofunctional and/or bifunctional adducts, with bifunctional adducts existing in several forms, including interstrand and intrastrand DNA crosslinks.

The foundation for modern cancer chemotherapy was laid with alkylating agents in early 1940s when the nitrogen mustard mechlorethamine, or mustine, became the first antitumor drug to enter clinical trials and demonstrate activity.[1,2] Other structural classes of alkylating agents include aziridines, hexitol epoxides, alkyl sulfonates, nitrosoureas and the triazines/hydrazines, and these, together with the platinum-containing antitumor drugs, remain of oncologic interest.

General mechanisms of cytotoxicity

Alkylating agents and platinum antitumor compounds are inert and must transform to highly reactive species, which bind covalently to DNA at electron-rich (nucleophilic) centers for their antitumor response. This covalent interaction, usually at the N7-position of guanine, can induce monofunctional or bifunctional adducts, with bifunctional interactions manifesting as cytotoxic interstrand (as with alkylating agents) or intrastrand (as with platinum drugs) crosslinks (Figure 1). Interstrand GG crosslinks with nitrogen mustards involve the 5′-GC-3′ or 5′-GXC-3′ nucleotide sequence (where X = any nucleotide) in both DNA strands.[3,4] Similarly, these crosslinks are also formed by cisplatin with guanine in the 5′-GC-3′ sequence.[5] On the other hand, N2-guanine in the 5′-CG-3′ sequence is preferred for crosslinking by mitomycin C due to its orientation in the minor groove of DNA.[6] Alkylation at O6-guanine and N3-cytosine can also occur.

Bifunctional drugs are up to 100-fold more potent than monofunctional agents in inducing cellular effects, including cell cycle arrest, DNA repair, and apoptosis.[7] These effects result from specific distortions and unwinding in DNA that induce coordinated assembly of distinct proteins at the DNA damage site to activate signal transduction pathways. A critical pathway involves the tumor suppressor p53, which is activated by a number of proteins, such as ATR, ATM, Chk1, and Chk2, to transactivate downstream target genes, such as p21 and Bax, and regulate cellular response to DNA damage (Figure 1). Indeed, a vast majority of antitumor drugs at therapeutic doses are dependent on robust p53 activation for apoptotic antitumor response.[8] Lower p53 activation from low level DNA damage by the drug instead induces cell cycle arrest, which then permits DNA repair and cell survival.[9] Interestingly, select alkylating (e.g., cyclophosphamide) and platinum (e.g., oxaliplatin) drugs induce immunogenic cell death that then prevents regrowth of the same tumor.[10] These cytotoxic events occur in both tumor and normal cells, and, therefore, side effects from therapy become inevitable.

Alkylating agents

Monofunctional alkylating agents

Drugs of interest that interact with DNA in a monofunctional manner can be classified as hydrazines, triazines and isoquinoline alkaloids, and representative drugs are shown in Figure 2. From the many hydrazines examined preclinically, only procarbazine has received clinical approval, specifically for Hodgkin's lymphoma, lung cancer, and melanoma. Its activation is poorly understood, but metabolism to azoxy-procarbazine is important. This metabolite rearranges to a reactive diazonium intermediate that forms O6- and mostly N7-methyl-guanine monoadducts, which then

---

Holland-Frei Cancer Medicine, Tenth Edition. Edited by Robert C. Bast, John C. Byrd, Carlo M. Croce, Ernest Hawk, Fadlo R. Khuri, Raphael E. Pollock, Apostolia M. Tsimberidou, Christopher G. Willett, and Cheryl L. Willman.
© 2023 John Wiley & Sons, Inc. Published 2023 by John Wiley & Sons, Inc.

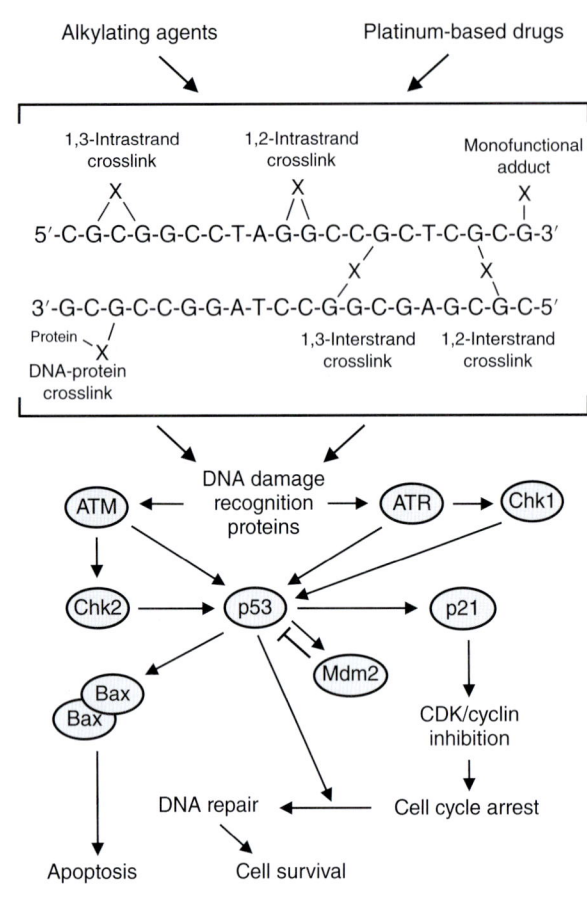

Figure 1 Monofunctional DNA adducts and bifunctional interstrand and intrastrand crosslinks induced by alkylating and platinum drugs (X = alkyl or platinum species).

Figure 2 Structures of some monofunctional alkylating agents.

Figure 3 Structures of some bifunctional alkylating agents.

induce single-strand breaks.[11–13] In the triazine family, the most significant are dacarazine (DTIC-Dome) and temozolomide (Temodar). Dacarbazine has been used against several cancers, including Hodgkin's lymphoma, sarcoma, malignant melanoma, and pancreatic islet cell carcinoma. Temozolomide, a derivative of dacarbazine, is particularly active against astrocytoma. While dacrabazine requires hepatic activation for cytotoxic alkylation at O6- and N7-guanine for DNA single strand breaks,[14,15] temozolomide generates the reactive species spontaneously.[16] Of the isoquinoline alkaloids, trabectedin (ecteinascidin-743, Yondelis) and PM00104 (Zalypsis) are the most interesting. Trabectedin, which is the first marine-derived drug to be approved,[17] initially binds non-covalently to TCG, CGG, AGC, or GGC sequence of one strand in the DNA minor groove, where it activates and then alkylates the unusual N2-site of guanine in the opposite strand.[18] The monofunctional adducts recruit the transcriptionally coupled nuclear excision repair (TC-NER) protein Rad13/ERCC5 to the DNA damage site, resulting in strand breaks and cell death. Interestingly, absence of p53 function actually increases antitumor activity threefold.[19] PM00104 is a derivative of trabectedin, but its clinical development is uncertain.[20,21]

Bifunctional alkylating agents

Some of the bifunctional alkylating drugs discussed below are shown in Figure 3.

Nitrogen mustards

Mechlorethamine, cyclophosphamide, ifosfamide, melphalan, chlorambucil, and bendamustine are examples of US Food and Drug Administration (FDA)-approved nitrogen mustards. Their reaction with DNA has been well characterized, with the structural bischloroethyl groups being essential for bifunctional alkylation to induce the favored interstrand 1,3-crosslinks.[22] This crosslink to form requires drug activation, either spontaneous, as with mechlorethamine, or metabolic, as with cyclophosphamide.[23] The most significant metabolite of cyclophosphamide is 4-hydroxy-cyclophosphamide, which can also be formed directly from the prodrug 4-hydroperoxycyclophosphamide for use in purging tumor cells in bone marrow aspirates from bone marrow transplant patients.[24] Ifosfamide, an isomer of cyclophosphamide, is important in managing testicular cancer and sarcomas. It also requires metabolic activation in the liver,[25] but its poor activation decreases potency approximately fourfold.[26,27] Melphalan, chlorambucil, and bendamustine have the aromatic ring, instead of the oxazaphosphorine in cyclophosphamide and ifosfamide (see Figure 3), that moderates spontaneous activation of the bischloroethyl group to minimize side effects. An advantage of melphalan is that its phenylalanine-based structure facilitates its active transport into cells and across the blood–brain barrier.[28] Bendamustine, however, is better tolerated and, therefore, is clinically more cost-effective.[29] These nitrogen mustards are active against several cancers, including multiple myeloma, chronic lymphocytic leukemia (CLL), Hodgkin's and non-Hodgkin's lymphoma, and breast and ovarian cancers.

Nitrosoureas

The nitrosourea group in the chemical structure is the basis for activity of these alkylating agents, which are also known as 2-chloroethyl-nitrosourea (CENU) due to the presence of at least one chloroethyl alkylating moiety (Figure 3). The second moiety may be identical [bis-chloroethyl-nitorosourea (BCNU) or Carmustine], a cyclohexane (CCNU or Lomustine) or a phosphonate (fotemustine or Muphoran). Streptozotocin (Zanosar) is unique in not having the chloroethyl group, but the glucosamine group in its structure imparts activity against pancreatic islet tumors by facilitating substantial drug uptake via the overexpressed glucose transport protein GLUT2 in this cancer.[30] With the ability to cross the blood–brain barrier, BCNU and CCNU are effective against brain cancers, but also against gastrointestinal (GI) and breast cancers and multiple myeloma. Fotemustine has received approval in several countries, but not USA, for its activity in brain cancer and metastatic melanoma.[31,32]

CENUs in general are activated rapidly, as exemplified by a short half-life of about 50 min for BCNU.[33] Interestingly, CENUs alkylate at both O6-guanine[34] and N7-guanine.[35] These DNA monoadducts form rapidly (within an hour), but then rearrange to N7-GG interstrand crosslink within 8 h.[33] From steric considerations, a conflicting report proposes that the cytotoxic GG crosslink is intrastrand.[34]

Aziridines

The aziridine class includes thio-tepa (N,N′,N″-triethylenethiophosphoramide), mitomycin C, and triethylenemelamine. Of these, thio-tepa and mitomycin C (Figure 3) are of clinical interest for the treatment of several cancers, including refractory osteosarcoma and bladder cancer, respectively.[36] High-dose thio-tepa has also been used in drug combination regimens with[37] or without[38] autologous stem cell support for breast cancer.

Although less reactive, the three-membered heterocyclic aziridine ring in thio-tepa still spontaneously alkylates all four nucleotides, with N7-guanine being preferred.[39] The interstrand 1,2-crosslinks may also form via metabolism of thio-tepa to tepa.[40] Cytotoxic DNA monoadducts are also formed that induce DNA single strand breaks.[41,42] Unlike thio-tepa, interaction of mitomycin C with DNA requires metabolic reduction to form the initial monofunctional adduct,[43] with glutathione as the reducing agent.[44] Spontaneous intramolecular rearrangement then induces the cytotoxic 1,2-GG interstrand crosslinks. In contrast, alkylation at N2-guanine of DNA is preferred by mitomycin C.[6] Triethylenemelamine also has the aziridine ring, and its alkylation of DNA likely follows the same path as thio-tepa.

Alkyl sulfonates

Busulfan is the best known alkyl sulfonate, and is structurally composed of two sulfonates separated by a linear alkyl chain (Figure 3). It was approved in 1999 for chronic myelogenous leukemia (CML), but is used today in the allogeneic stem cell or bone marrow transplantation setting.[45,46] Cytotoxicity is mediated through alkylation by the sulfonate group of N7-guanine to form GG interstrand crosslinks.[47,48]

Hexitol epoxides

Like the aziridines, the hexitol epoxide 1,2 : 5,6-dianhydrogalactitol (DAG) (Figure 3) also alkylates DNA at N7-guanine via a strained tricyclic ring to form interstrand crosslinks,[49] but monofunctional DNA adducts are also formed in significant amounts.[49–52] DAG, however, may be mechanistically distinct since it demonstrates activity against tumor cells resistant to alkylating BCNU.[53] Based on its clinical activity in brain cancer,[54] DAG has received orphan drug designation in United States, but its future is uncertain. In China, however, it is approved for the treatment of CML and lung cancer.

Decomposition and metabolism

For DNA-damage, the neutral alkylating agent must first be activated to mediate antitumor response, but the activated species also interact with nucleophiles in cells, such as glutathione and metallothionein, to become inactivated. Consequently, depletion of glutathione by inhibiting its synthesis can enhance antitumor activity of alkylating agents.[55] Their metabolic activation and/or inactivation in the liver and extrahepatic tissues also play a major role in drug disposition. Specific unique reactions may also occur, as exemplified with dechlorination and denitrosation of nitrosoureas.[56] Moreover, metabolism can be influenced by other agents, such as phenobarbital,[57,58] which can increase microsomal enzymatic activity and modulate both activation and inactivation of the drug.

Resistance to alkylating agents

A major clinical limitation of alkylating agents is resistance of tumor cells. Reduced intracellular drug uptake from downregulation of the L-type amino acid transporter is a specific resistance mechanism with melphalan.[59,60] Increased cellular inactivation as another mechanism can result from elevated levels of thiols, such as glutathione and metallothionein, or thiol-related biosynthetic (γ-glutamylcysteine synthase) or drug neutralizing (glutathione-S-transferase) enzymes.[61–65] Increased inactivation of cyclophosphamide and related alkylating agents can also occur by elevated levels of aldehyde dehydrogenase.[66,67]

Since DNA adducts are cytotoxic, repair of O6-guanine adducts by upregulated O6-alkylguanine–alkyltransferase induces BCNU resistance,[68] which can be prevented by O6-benzylguanine to inhibit the enzyme.[34,69,70] Repair of crosslinks by nucleotide excision repair (NER) and non-homologous end-joining (NHEJ) also induce resistance to cyclophosphamide, melphalan, and chlorambucil.[71–74] Conversely, since cytotoxicity of O6-alkylguanine adducts are facilitated by mismatch repair (MMR) recognition proteins,[75] resistance to temozolomide arises when MMR becomes dysfunctional.[76]

Interstrand crosslinks of alkylating agents kill cells by apoptosis.[77,78] A number of proteins are involved, such as ATR, Chk1, Chk2, p53, and Bax, and defect in any one entity may lead to resistance. As an example, loss of p53 function through mutation or by overexpression of its negative regulator Mdm2 leads to temozolomide resistance.[79–81] Similarly, Bax downregulation[82,83] or overexpression of its negative regulator Bcl-2[77] also inhibits apoptosis. Resistance from poor tumor perfusion or changes in the tumor microenvironment may occur *in vivo*,[84–86] and this has been implicated for a EMT-6 mammary tumor model that demonstrates resistance to cyclophosphamide only in mice.[87]

Co-existence of multiple mechanisms in tumor cells is common, as has been reported for melphalan[59] and temozolomide.[80] Thus, treatment of refractory cancers may require multi-targeted therapy. However, a single target may be exploitable with a synthetic lethality strategy.[88] Alternatively, functional restoration of a dominant trigger of apoptosis, such as p53, could alone provide therapeutic benefits.

Clinical pharmacology

The pharmacokinetics (PK) of a drug dictates its pharmacodynamics (PD), and this PK–PD relationship is integral to designing regimens that maximize antitumor activity and minimize side effects. The essential knowledge on the clinical pharmacology of alkylating agents of interest is summarized below.

Monofunctional alkylators

Temozolomide and trabectedin are the two monofunctional alkylators investigated in detail. Temozolomide given iv or orally at 150 mg/m^2 results in peak plasma levels of 38–40 µmol/L and an AUC of 116–127 µmol h/L, and this indicated that the oral dose is fully bioavailable.[89,90] Elimination from the plasma was rapid ($T\frac{1}{2}$, 1.8 h), and food intake reduced peak concentration by 32% and AUC by 9%. About 38% of temozolomide dose was excreted in the urine, mostly (~95%) as transformed products. Trabectedin has high potency and, therefore, was studied at 0.6 mg/m^2 as a 1- or 3-h iv infusion.[91] At this dose, the peak concentration of 8–15 nmol/L, mean AUC of 31–43 nmol h/L, and terminal phase plasma $T\frac{1}{2}$ of about 2–4 days were observed. Several metabolites of trabectedin have also been noted in the urine and feces of patients.[92]

Bifunctional alkylators

All bifunctional alkylators are eliminated from the plasma rapidly, with a $T\frac{1}{2}$ of 0.5–3 h. With cyclophosphamide, a systemic dose of 50–75 mg/kg results in peak plasma levels of up to 400 µmol/L as intact drug, with 50–100 µmol/L as the phosphoramide mustard metabolite.[93–95] Interestingly, the AUC of this metabolite and the 4-hydroxy-cyclophosphamide product after intravenous and oral administration were similar, which indicated that both routes are beneficial. However, PK varies considerably among patients, but this does not alter its toxicity or therapeutic effects.[96] Urinary excretion of cyclophosphamide, predominantly as inactive metabolites, accounts for about 60–70% of the dose.[97,98] The relatively limited PK data on ifosfamide, including oral bioavailability, resembles that of cyclophosphamide.[95,99] However, the greater inter-patient variation in ifosfamide metabolism may, therefore, favor cyclophosphamide as the drug of choice.[100–102]

Like cyclophosphamide and ifosfamide, chlorambucil is also subject to auto-induction of its metabolism and excretion. This conclusion stems from progressive decline in plasma AUC with each treatment cycle[103] that may contribute to inter- and intra-individual variation of up to fourfold in the PK of oral drug.[104] Interestingly, AUC of chlorambucil or its metabolite phenylacetic acid mustard was unaffected by food intake.[105] The variation in oral bioavailability (range 25–94%) is also observed with bendamustine. Total excretion of this drug in urine and feces of patients accounts for 76% of the iv dose, with hepato-generated metabolites as the major species (~95% of excreted dose).[106] Melphalan also has good oral bioavailability, and conventional oral doses of 0.15–0.25 mg/kg result in peak plasma levels of up to 0.2–0.6 µmol/L by 1–2 h.[107] However, food can reduce drug absorption. An iv dose of 0.6 mg/kg results in peak melphalan plasma levels of 4–13 µmol/L and urinary excretion of parent drug over 24 h of about 13% of the dose, which indicates significant drug transformation.[108,109]

Administration iv of the aziridine thio-tepa at 12 mg/m^2 resulted in peak plasma levels of about 5 µmol/L for the parent drug, with an AUC of about 9 µmol h/L.[110] The metabolite tepa reached peak levels of about 1 µmol/L at 2 h after drug administration. Urinary excretion accounted for about 30% of the dose in 24 h, mostly (>98%) as transformed products. Thio-tepa given intraperitoneally resulted in rapid absorption, with plasma levels comparable to iv administration.[111] However, its persistence in the peritoneum justifies the intraperitoneal route. PK of high-dose BCNU iv (300–750 mg/m^2) demonstrated only 23% of the total plasma BCNU as bioavailable for activity.[112] The PK study of CCNU given orally at 130 mg/m^2 failed to detect unchanged drug in the plasma, likely due to rapid conversion to *cis*- and *trans*-4-hydroxy CCNU.[113] Busulfan is distinct among bifunctional alkylators in that its insolubility in aqueous solutions makes oral PK highly variable.[114] However, since 2002, busulfan has been available as iv-formulated Busulfex, which has reduced this variability.[115]

Adverse effects

Given that alkylating agents target DNA, these drugs also impact normal tissues, particularly those having a high proliferation rate. Thus, hematopoietic toxicity is common, but reversible, as with temozolomide.[90] Interestingly, cyclophosphamide and ifosfamide are associated with less myelosuppressive and GI toxicity than other alkylating agents, with aldehyde dehydrogenase facilitating the protection of the GI tract by inactivating the toxic aldophosphamide metabolite. GI toxicity, however, is serious with melphalan and thio-tepa, particularly in high doses. Moreover, with DNA as a target, alkylating agents are highly teratogenic[116] and induce secondary leukemia.[117]

Busulfan, and to a limited extent melphalan, cyclophosphamide, and chlorambucil, also induce pulmonary damage.[118] This toxicity occurs within a few weeks, impacting 3–43% of the patients. Hepatotoxicity and fatal veno-occlusive disease syndrome have been observed in up to 26% of patients receiving cyclophosphamide, BCNU or busulfan.[119,120] Gonadal damage is a serious complication with these drugs, but is mostly reversible.[121] Procarbazine, on the other hand, may render permanent infertility in men and ovarian failure in women.[122]

Hemorrhagic cystitis of the bladder is serious with cyclophosphamide and ifosfamide,[123] but use of mesna to inactivate the acrolein by-product[124] and adequate hydration have provided some protection. In a study using six courses of BCNU or methyl-CCNU, renal impairment was common.[125] The nitrosourea streptozotocin, on the other hand, induces toxicity to pancreatic beta cells due to its absorption via the GLUT2 transporter.[126] Cardiotoxicity with cyclophosphamide, ifosfamide, and busulfan is known, but is fatal with high-dose cyclophosphamide due to electrolyte imbalance from renal impairment.[127–129] Severe alopecia has also been observed with these three agents, but is usually reversible.[130] This toxicity has been attributed to lipophilic metabolites penetrating into the hair follicles.[131] Likewise, neurotoxicity with busulfan or BCNU is a serious complication with intracarotid delivery or at high iv doses.[132–134]

Platinum antitumor compounds

The most recognizable platinum compound is cisplatin (*cis*-diammine-dichloro-platinum(II)), which structurally has two labile chloro and two stable ammine ligands in a square planar cis-configuration (Figure 4). This configuration is critical, since the analogous transplatin with trans-geometry is 20-fold less active. The antitumor activity of cisplatin was discovered serendipitously in 1969, and clinical development followed, with eventual approval by the FDA in 1978.[135] The analogs carboplatin and oxaliplatin have since been approved also by the FDA and have also become indispensable in the clinic.[136] Like cisplatin, the two analogs have the cis-configuration, with platinum in a divalent state (Figure 4).

The analogs also first require activation by aquation to form cytotoxic intrastrand crosslinks as the major lesion. However, each analog is unique in its spectrum of activity, side effects and/or molecular characteristics.

Cisplatin

About 85–90% of DNA adducts formed by cisplatin are 1,2-AG and -GG intrastrand crosslinks, with 1,3-intrastrand GXG crosslinks (where X = any nucleotide), interstrand GG-crosslinks and monofunctional adducts each representing 2–6%. Only a few intrastrand crosslinks are sufficient to inhibit DNA replication, and this conveys the high potency of the drug.[137] Cisplatin is effective against several neoplasms, including testicular, ovarian, head and neck, bladder, and cervical cancers.[138] The cure rate for testicular cancer is about 85%, but the actual rate may depend on the cisplatin schedule.[139] Since crosslinks are repaired in part by homologous recombination, dysregulation of this repair from mutated *BRCA1* gene in ovarian and breast cancers increases their response rates with cisplatin.[140,141] Responses are further enhanced by inclusion

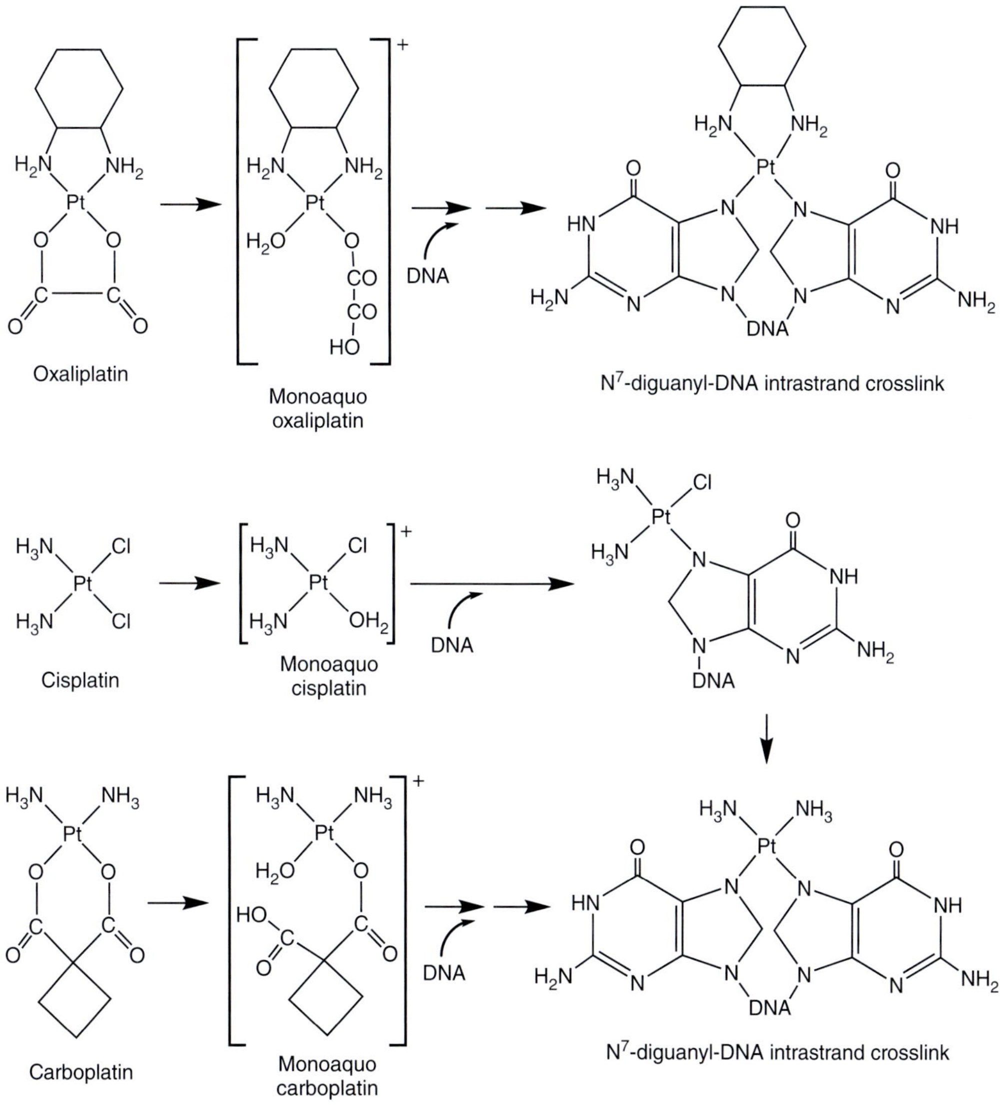

Figure 4 Structures of oxaliplatin, cisplatin, and carboplatin and their interactions with DNA to form crosslinks. Although cisplatin and carboplatin form identical crosslinks, that of oxaliplatin is structurally distinct by virtue of the diaminocyclohexane ligand tethered to the platinum atom.

of PARP inhibitors, such as olaparib, to inhibit the salvage base excision repair (BER) pathway.[142]

Carboplatin

Carboplatin was selected from preclinical studies for its lack of nephrotoxicity, and this was confirmed clinically.[136] The explanation may be due to the presence in carboplatin of the bidentate cyclobutanedicarboxylate (CBDCA) ligand, which, unlike the chloro-ligands in cisplatin, prevents rapid activation of the analog.[143] However, renal clearance of carboplatin by glomerular filtration compared to active tubular secretion of cisplatin may also explain the differential nephrotoxicity of the two agents at the tubular level.[144] The greater stability of carboplatin, on the other hand, increases the clinical dose by fourfold compared to cisplatin for a similar level and spectrum of clinical activity.[143] Thus, cancers refractory to cisplatin demonstrate full cross-resistance to carboplatin.[145,146] This similarity in antitumor profiles is ascribed to DNA adducts of cisplatin and carboplatin being identical (Figure 4). Therefore, slight differences in response or relapse rates (as in testicular cancer) and the patient's renal function before or during therapy may dictate preference of one drug over the other.[147]

Oxaliplatin

The interest in identifying an analog that has activity in cisplatin-resistant tumor cells resulted in the development of oxaliplatin, in which the bidentate oxalate group is sufficiently labile to make the clinical dose requirements similar to cisplatin.[148] Oxaliplatin is structurally distinct in having the non-labile bidentate 1,2-diaminocyclohexane (DACH) moiety in place of the two ammine ligands in cisplatin and carboplatin (Figure 4). The DACH ligand in oxaliplatin appears to be critical for activity in refractory cancers. Indeed, oxaliplatin is active against colorectal cancers, including those that are refractory to 5-fluorouracil (5FU).[136,148] Interestingly, oxaliplatin also synergizes with 5FU, and provides the rationale for the FOLFOX regimen (oxaliplatin, 5FU, and leucovorin) as frontline therapy for refractory advanced metastatic colorectal cancer, with an exceptional response rate of about 50%.[148]

New analogs in development

The search for effective platinum drugs against refractory cancers has led to clinical development and approval of nedaplatin and miriplatin in Japan, haptaplatin in Korea, and lobaplatin in China.[149] This effort continues using innovative strategies. In one strategy, the cisplatin-prodrug BTP-114 has been designed as a parent platinum(IV) drug, with an axial maleimide group that interacts covalently with plasma albumin once it enters the circulation.[149] It is then transported intracellularly into tumor cells, where the albumin-bound prodrug releases cisplatin following reduction to platinum(II). The resultant elevated concentration of cisplatin can then circumvent resistant tumor cells. The drug is currently in clinical trials.[150] In an analogous strategy, the tumor-homing texaphyrin has been linked via the axial ligand to a DACH-platinum(IV)-oxalate core to form the oxaliplatin prodrug oxaliTEX, which reduces to form the platinum(II) oxaliplatin. This drug, therefore, has all the characteristics of oxaliplatin, but accumulates in cells to a greater extent to circumvent not only cisplatin resistance, but also oxaliplatin resistance induced by reduced drug uptake.[151] It is currently in development for clinical trials. A third platinum drug to highlight is phosphaplatin (PT-112), which, like oxaliplatin, also induces immunogenic cell death and is in clinical trials.[152] It is a platinum(II) drug, with DACH as the stable ligand and a bifunctional phosphate moiety as the leaving ligand. However, its activity is claimed to be independent of DNA interaction,[153] as has also been speculated for oxaliplatin.[154,155]

Resistance to cisplatin, carboplatin, and oxaliplatin

As with alkylating agents, resistance to platinum drugs may be intrinsic or acquired, but mechanisms are invariably multifactorial.[156] Moreover, mechanisms for these two classes of drugs may overlap. Indeed, biochemical mechanisms of resistance to all platinum drugs occur from reduced drug accumulation, increased thiol levels, and/or increased DNA adduct repair in tumor cells.[157,158] Reduced accumulation has been linked to reduced influx and/or increased efflux transporter proteins.[156,159,160] Resistance due to high thiol levels that inactivate the platinum drug has been observed in cancer patients[156,161] as has enhanced DNA repair of adducts.[162] Molecular mechanisms of resistance are associated with dysfunctional DNA adduct recognition, cell cycle checkpoint activation, and apoptosis. Downregulation of MMR proteins (hMLH1, hMSH2, and hMSH6) involved in DNA damage recognition have been well examined.[156] An example in defective checkpoint activation is provided by mutation or silencing of Chk2 in cancer patients that also impedes stabilization and activation of p53 and, thereby, cell cycle and apoptosis.[163] The p53 itself can become inactivated through mutation.[164,165]

Based on these resistance mechanisms, an important question to address is how oxaliplatin circumvents cisplatin resistance mechanisms. This ability relates to specific, but not all, mechanisms. For instance, oxaliplatin is also dependent on p53, mutation of which in tumor cells results in resistance to both agents.[164,166] On the other hand, dysfunction of wild-type p53 through loss of Chk2 can be circumvented by oxaliplatin, which upregulates Chk2-independent pathways to activate p53.[155,166] Similarly, oxaliplatin does not rely on MMR proteins for recognition of DNA adducts, even though intrastrand GG-adducts are formed, as with cisplatin.[167] The differential recognition, however, may be ascribed to distinct conformational changes in DNA by virtue of ammine ligands in cisplatin adducts and DACH ligand in oxaliplatin adducts (see Figure 4).[168–171]

Clinical pharmacology

The plasma PK of cisplatin or oxaliplatin as the intact molecule is complicated by their rapid and spontaneous transformation to active species, which are then inactivated through irreversible binding to plasma proteins. Thus, analysis involves estimating "total" platinum in the plasma and "free" (active) platinum in plasma ultrafiltrates, usually by flameless atomic absorption spectrophotometry (FAAS).[172,173] However, the more stable carboplatin in plasma ultrafiltrates produces similar PK profiles whether analyzed by high performance liquid chromatography (HPLC) or FAAS.[174,175]

Cisplatin

The plasma PK has been investigated at 100 mg/m² cisplatin using a bolus (4–15 min infusion) or a 3- and 24-h infusion schedule, which gave similar AUC of 25–28 μmol h/L and explains why clinical activity is independent of schedule.[176] However, toxicity is usually lower with longer infusions, which, therefore, may be preferred. After bolus administration, free platinum levels decline rapidly in a biphasic manner, with $T\frac{1}{2}$ of less than an hour.[173,177] Total plasma platinum, in contrast, declines with a long terminal $T\frac{1}{2}$ of about

5 days,[172] which is consistent with platinum becoming covalently bound to plasma proteins. Thus, urinary excretion is low, accounting for only 28–33% of the dose in 24 h.[173,178]

Carboplatin

The greater stability and, therefore, low reactivity of carboplatin results in high urinary excretion of about 77% of the dose in 24 h, mostly (41%) as intact carboplatin.[173,175] Peak total plasma platinum concentration of 251 μmol/L was observed after a dose of 550 mg/m^2, and this represents predominantly intact drug.[172,173] As with the other platinum drugs, free platinum from carboplatin has a short $T\frac{1}{2}$ of ≤2 h, with total platinum displaying a prolonged terminal $T\frac{1}{2}$ of 5.8 days. The AUC for free platinum and intact carboplatin were similar (506 vs 456 μmol h/L), and this confirms intact carboplatin is the major free drug component.

Oxaliplatin

As with cisplatin, oxaliplatin is cleared rapidly through covalent interaction with plasma proteins that results in urinary excretion of 37% in 24 h of a standard 130 mg/m^2 dose.[173] Peak plasma concentration of free and total platinum are lower than with cisplatin, but the AUC values are comparable to those with cisplatin.[172,173] The free plasma platinum with oxaliplatin has a typical short initial $T\frac{1}{2}$ of 17 min and a prolonged terminal $T\frac{1}{2}$ of about 270 h.

Adverse effects

The dose-limiting complication with cisplatin is the cumulative and irreversible nephrotoxicity from tubular damage,[179,180] likely due to active uptake of cisplatin by tubular cells.[181] However, prior hydration reduces the severity and/or incidence of kidney damage. Nephrotoxicity is rare with oxaliplatin and carboplatin, which are cleared exclusively by glomerular filtration.[173,182] Based on this, the Calvert formula was devised and is used routinely to individualize carboplatin dose based on renal glomerular function.[182] Cumulative ototoxicity is also significant with cisplatin,[183] particularly with cumulative doses >400 mg/m^2.[184] This may be due to high cochlear cisplatin uptake, particularly since lower uptakes of carboplatin and oxaliplatin correlates with absence of this side effect.[185–187]

Peripheral neuropathy is associated with all three platinum drugs.[186] It is cumulative and irreversible with cisplatin at total doses exceeding 300 mg/m^2. Tingling paresthesia, weakness, tremors, and loss of taste are also described, and these can be severe following intra-arterial administration of cisplatin in head and neck patients. Peripheral neuropathy with oxaliplatin, however, is dose-limiting, but symptoms improve slowly after treatment stops in 40% of the patients. Chemoprotective strategies with thiol compounds and vitamin E may reduce the severity of this side effect.[186] Carboplatin is the least neurotoxic, affecting only 4–6% of the patients. Cisplatin is considered one of the most emetic antitumor agents at doses >50 mg/m^2, but is managed with antiemetics.[188] This side effect is moderate with carboplatin and oxaliplatin.

Severe, but reversible, myelosuppression is associated with the platinum drugs.[189] With cisplatin, this is manifested as leucopenia, whereas carboplatin induces thrombocytopenia as its dose-limiting toxicity. Neutropenia and thrombocytopenia, on the other hand, have been reported with oxaliplatin. Other side effects, such as pulmonary toxicity, hepatotoxicity, alopecia, and/or allergic reactions may also be observed in some patients with these platinum drugs.[189]

Acknowledgments

The research support from the U.S. Public Health Service grants CA211975 to Zahid H. Siddik and Support Grant CA16672 to MD Anderson Cancer Center awarded by the National Cancer Institute, and in part from the Megan McBride Franz Endowed Research Fund, is gratefully acknowledged.

Key references

The complete reference list can be found on Vital Source version of this title, see inside front cover.

2. Gilman A. The initial clinical trial of nitrogen mustard. *Am J Surg*. 1963;**105**:574–578.
6. Borowy-Borowski H, Lipman R, Tomasz M. Recognition between mitomycin C and specific DNA sequences for cross-link formation. *Biochemistry*. 1990;**29**:2999–3006.
8. Jiang H, Pritchard JR, Williams RT, et al. A mammalian functional-genetic approach to characterizing cancer therapeutics. *Nat Chem Biol*. 2011;**7**:92–100.
9. el Deiry WS. The role of p53 in chemosensitivity and radiosensitivity. *Oncogene*. 2003;**22**:7486–7495.
10. Bezu L, Gomes-de-Silva LC, Dewitte H, et al. Combinatorial strategies for the induction of immunogenic cell death. *Front Immunol*. 2015;**6**:187.
17. D'Incalci M, Badri N, Galmarini CM, Allavena P. Trabectedin, a drug acting on both cancer cells and the tumour microenvironment. *Br J Cancer*. 2014;**111**:646–650.
22. Colvin ME, Sasaki JC, Tran NL. Chemical factors in the action of phosphoramidic mustard alkylating anticancer drugs: roles for computational chemistry. *Curr Pharm Des*. 1999;**5**:645–663.
29. Woods B, Hawkins N, Dunlop W, et al. Bendamustine versus chlorambucil for the first-line treatment of chronic lymphocytic leukemia in England and Wales: a cost-utility analysis. *Value Health*. 2012;**15**:759–770.
33. Gnewuch CT, Sosnovsky G. A critical appraisal of the evolution of N-Nitrosoureas as anticancer drugs. *Chem Rev*. 1997;**97**:829–1014.
46. Hassan M. The role of busulfan in bone marrow transplantation. *Med Oncol*. 1999;**16**:166–176.
53. Institoris E, Szikla K, Otvos L, Gal F. Absence of cross-resistance between two alkylating agents: BCNU vs bifunctional galactitol. *Cancer Chemother Pharmacol*. 1989;**24**:311–313.
55. Hamilton TC, Winker MA, Louie KG, et al. Augmentation of adriamycin, melphalan, and cisplatin cytotoxicity in drug-resistant and -sensitive human ovarian carcinoma cell lines by buthionine sulfoximine mediated glutathione depletion. *Biochem Pharmacol*. 1985;**34**:2583–2586.
59. Hazlehurst LA, Enkemann SA, Beam CA, et al. Genotypic and phenotypic comparisons of de novo and acquired melphalan resistance in an isogenic multiple myeloma cell line model. *Cancer Res*. 2003;**63**:7900–7906.
67. Rekha GK, Sreerama L, Sladek NE. Intrinsic cellular resistance to oxazaphosphorines exhibited by a human colon carcinoma cell line expressing relatively large amounts of a class-3 aldehyde dehydrogenase. *Biochem Pharmacol*. 1994;**48**:1943–1952.
73. Spanswick VJ, Craddock C, Sekhar M, et al. Repair of DNA interstrand crosslinks as a mechanism of clinical resistance to melphalan in multiple myeloma. *Blood*. 2002;**100**:224–229.
78. Roos WP, Batista LF, Naumann SC, et al. Apoptosis in malignant glioma cells triggered by the temozolomide-induced DNA lesion O6-methylguanine. *Oncogene*. 2007;**26**:186–197.
83. Shi L, Chen J, Yang J, et al. MiR-21 protected human glioblastoma U87MG cells from chemotherapeutic drug temozolomide induced apoptosis by decreasing Bax/Bcl-2 ratio and caspase-3 activity. *Brain Res*. 2010;**1352**:255–264.
88. Reinhardt HC, Jiang H, Hemann MT, Yaffe MB. Exploiting synthetic lethal interactions for targeted cancer therapy. *Cell Cycle*. 2009;**8**:3112–3119.
89. Hammond LA, Eckardt JR, Baker SD, et al. Phase I and pharmacokinetic study of temozolomide on a daily-for-5-days schedule in patients with advanced solid malignancies. *J Clin Oncol*. 1999;**17**:2604–2613.
93. Egorin MJ, Forrest A, Belani CP, et al. A limited sampling strategy for cyclophosphamide pharmacokinetics. *Cancer Res*. 1989;**49**:3129–3133.
99. Boddy AV, Cole M, Pearson AD, Idle JR. The kinetics of the auto-induction of ifosfamide metabolism during continuous infusion. *Cancer Chemother Pharmacol*. 1995;**36**:53–60.
103. Silvennoinen R, Malminiemi K, Malminiemi O, et al. Pharmacokinetics of chlorambucil in patients with chronic lymphocytic leukaemia: comparison of different days, cycles and doses. *Pharmacol Toxicol*. 2000;**87**:223–228.

115. Madden T, de Lima M, Thapar N, et al. Pharmacokinetics of once-daily IV busulfan as part of pretransplantation preparative regimens: a comparison with an every 6-hour dosing schedule. *Biol Blood Marrow Transplant*. 2007;**13**:56–64.
123. Manikandan R, Kumar S, Dorairajan LN. Hemorrhagic cystitis: a challenge to the urologist. *Indian J Urol*. 2010;**26**:159–166.
127. Pai VB, Nahata MC. Cardiotoxicity of chemotherapeutic agents: incidence, treatment and prevention. *Drug Saf*. 2000;**22**:263–302.
134. Vassal G, Deroussent A, Hartmann O, et al. Dose-dependent neurotoxicity of high-dose busulfan in children: a clinical and pharmacological study. *Cancer Res*. 1990;**50**:6203–6207.
136. Kelland LR, Sharp SY, O'Neill CF, et al. Mini-review: discovery and development of platinum complexes designed to circumvent cisplatin resistance. *J Inorg Biochem*. 1999;**77**:111–115.
144. Siddik ZH, Newell DR, Boxall FE, Harrap KR. The comparative pharmacokinetics of carboplatin and cisplatin in mice and rats. *Biochem Pharmacol*. 1987;**36**:1925–1932.
145. Gore M, Fryatt I, Wiltshaw E, et al. Cisplatin/carboplatin cross-resistance in ovarian cancer. *Br J Cancer*. 1989;**60**:767–769.
148. Alcindor T, Beauger N. Oxaliplatin: a review in the era of molecularly targeted therapy. *Curr Oncol*. 2011;**18**:18–25.
151. Thiabaud G, He G, Sen S, et al. Oxaliplatin Pt(IV) prodrugs conjugated to gadolinium-texaphyrin as potential antitumor agents. *Proc Natl Acad Sci U S A*. 2020;**117**:7021–7029.
154. Bruno PM, Liu Y, Park GY, et al. A subset of platinum-containing chemotherapeutic agents kills cells by inducing ribosome biogenesis stress. *Nat Med*. 2017;**23**:461–471.
155. He G, Xie X, Siddik ZH. Protein expression profiling identifies differential modulation of homologous recombination by platinum-based antitumor agents. *Cancer Chemother Pharmacol*. 2020;**85**:1129–1140.
156. Siddik ZH. Cisplatin: mode of cytotoxic action and molecular basis of resistance. *Oncogene*. 2003;**22**:7265–7279.
164. Martinez-Rivera M, Siddik ZH. Resistance and gain-of-resistance phenotypes in cancers harboring wild-type p53. *Biochem Pharmacol*. 2012;**83**:1049–1062.
165. Siddik ZH, Mims B, Lozano G, Thai G. Independent pathways of p53 induction by cisplatin and X-rays in a cisplatin-resistant ovarian tumor cell line. *Cancer Res*. 1998;**58**:698–703.
172. van Hennik MB, van der Vijgh WJ, Klein I, et al. Comparative pharmacokinetics of cisplatin and three analogues in mice and humans. *Cancer Res*. 1987;**47**:6297–6301.
182. Calvert AH, Newell DR, Gumbrell LA, et al. Carboplatin dosage: prospective evaluation of a simple formula based on renal function. *J Clin Oncol*. 1989;**7**:1748–1756.
183. Rybak LP, Mukherjea D, Jajoo S, Ramkumar V. Cisplatin ototoxicity and protection: clinical and experimental studies. *Tohoku J Exp Med*. 2009;**219**:177–186.
189. Oun R, Moussa YE, Wheate NJ. The side effects of platinum-based chemotherapy drugs: a review for chemists. *Dalton Trans*. 2018;**47**:6645–6653.

56 DNA topoisomerase targeting drugs

Anish Thomas, MD ■ Susan Bates, MD ■ William D. Figg, Sr, PharmD ■ Yves Pommier, MD, PhD

Overview

Topoisomerases are an important class of enzymes that are ubiquitously expressed across all organisms, and function to resolve deoxyribonucleic acid (DNA) supercoiling and prevent and resolve ribonucleic acid (RNA) entanglements. These biochemically distinct enzymes play a critical role in DNA replication, transcription, and cellular division. Inhibitors that target specific topoisomerases, therefore, represent a major component of the anticancer chemotherapeutic armamentarium. In this chapter, we provide an overview of topoisomerase biology and topoisomerase inhibitors. We review the common and specific mechanisms of action and the molecular pharmacology of the drugs that target the topoisomerase cleavage complexes by interfacial inhibition. Molecular pathways for cancer cell death and DNA repair associated with each specific topoisomerase inhibitor are discussed. Other mechanisms of anticancer activity of selected topoisomerase inhibitors that include DNA intercalation and/or generation of oxygen radicals destabilizing and damaging chromatin structure are described. We summarize the clinical use, toxicity profile, and the molecular basis of sensitivity and resistance to topoisomerase inhibitors. We also discuss the pharmacogenomics focusing on genetic variants in drug-metabolizing enzymes, transporters, and other proteins associated with topoisomerase inhibitors. Evolving data demonstrate the important role of molecular profiling and analysis of genetic variants in individuals that enable personalized dosing and enhance therapeutic efficacy, minimizing toxicity. Ongoing efforts focus on optimization of treatment selection, identification of novel combination therapies, elucidation of the molecular basis of response and resistance, and development of strategies for tumor-targeted delivery based on tumor molecular signatures.

Introduction

The human genome consists of long double-stranded and helical deoxyribonucleic acid (DNA) polymers (46 chromosomes) densely packaged in the cell nucleus (approximately 1.8 meter of DNA squeezed in a nucleus almost 1 million times smaller in diameter). Relaxing DNA supercoiling by topoisomerases is obligatory when the two genomic strands separate for transcription and replication, because the nucleosomal structure of chromatin constrains and generates DNA supercoiling. Type II topoisomerases are required at mitosis for the even distribution of the genome between daughter cells following replication. Thus, topoisomerases are ubiquitous and essential for all organisms as they prevent and resolve DNA and ribonucleic acid (RNA) entanglements and resolve DNA supercoiling during transcription and replication.

Topoisomerases were named historically with the first topoisomerase being Topo I in *Escherichia coli*[1] and TOP1 in mouse.[2] Notably, most of the anticancer and antibacterial agents, which are highly specific for their topoisomerase targets are integral to the anticancer chemotherapeutic armamentarium and were discovered independently and before the term topoisomerase was even coined.

Topoisomerase biology

The human genome contains six topoisomerase genes, with three of the encoded enzymes targeted by anticancer drugs: TOP1, TOP2α, and TOP2β (Table 1).[3-6]

The type of topoisomerase-mediated DNA break is specific to each topoisomerase (Figure 1 and Table 1). These catalytic intermediates are referred to as cleavage complexes (Figure 1, middle panels b, e). The reverse rejoining reaction is carried out by the attack of the ribose hydroxyl ends toward the tyrosyl-DNA bond.

TOP1 (and TOP1mt) covalently attaches to the 3′-end of the break, whereas the other topoisomerases (TOP2α and β) act by cutting and resealing the DNA backbone without assistance of nucleases and ligases. TOP1 and TOP1mt cleave and religate one strand of DNA duplex, whereas TOP2α and β cleave and reseal both strands with a 4-base pair staggered cut (Figure 1). The DNA cutting-rejoining mechanism is common to all topoisomerases and utilizes an enzymatic tyrosine residue acting as nucleophile and becoming covalently attached to the end of the broken DNA. The polarity of the attachment to the 3′- versus the 5′-ends of the DNA (TOP3α and β) have the opposite polarity with covalent attachment to the 5′-end of the breaks (Table 1; Figure 1b, e).

Topoisomerases are biochemically distinct.[6] TOP1 and TOP1mt act as monomers in the absence of nucleotide or metal cofactor, whereas TOP2α and β act as dimers, requiring adenosine triphosphate (ATP) and Mg^{2+} for catalysis. TOP3 α and β also require Mg^{2+} but function as monomers without ATP. Notably, the DNA substrates differ for TOP3 enzymes. Whereas both TOP1 and TOP2 process double-stranded DNA, the TOP3 substrates need to be single-stranded nucleic acids (DNA for TOP3α and DNA or RNA for TOP3β).

Mechanisms of action

Common mechanism of action and molecular pharmacology of topoisomerase inhibitors: trapping the topoisomerase cleavage complexes by interfacial inhibition

Topoisomerase cleavage complexes (TOPccs) are normally highly reversible and therefore transient and hardly detectable in the absence of topoisomerase inhibitor. This occurs because the rejoining of the cleavage complexes is driven by the realignment of the broken ends, which is determined by two basic structural

Table 1 Characteristics of topoisomerases.[a]

Genes	Chromosome	Proteins	Drugs	Mechanism	Polarity[b]	Main functions
TOP1	20q12-q13.1	Top1 100 kDa monomer	Camptothecins Indenos	Swiveling rotation	3'-Y	Nuclear supercoiling relaxation
TOP1MT	8q24.3	Top1mt 100 kDa monomer	None			Mitochondrial supercoiling relaxation
TOP2A	17q21-q22	Top2α 170 kDa dimer	Anthracyclines, Anthracediones Epipodophyllotoxins	Strand passage ATPase	5'-PY	Decatenation/replication
TOP2B	3p24	Top2β 180 kDa dimer				Transcription
TOP3A	17p12-p11.2	Top3α 100 kDa monomer	None	Strand passage	5'-PY	DNA replication with BLM[c]
TOP3B	22q11.22	Top3β 100 kDa monomer				RNA topoisomerase

[a]Source: Adapted from Pommier[3,4]; Gheeya et al.[5]; Pommier et al.[6]
[b]Covalent linkage between the catalytic tyrosine and the end of the broken DNA.
[c]Bloom syndrome, RecQ helicase.

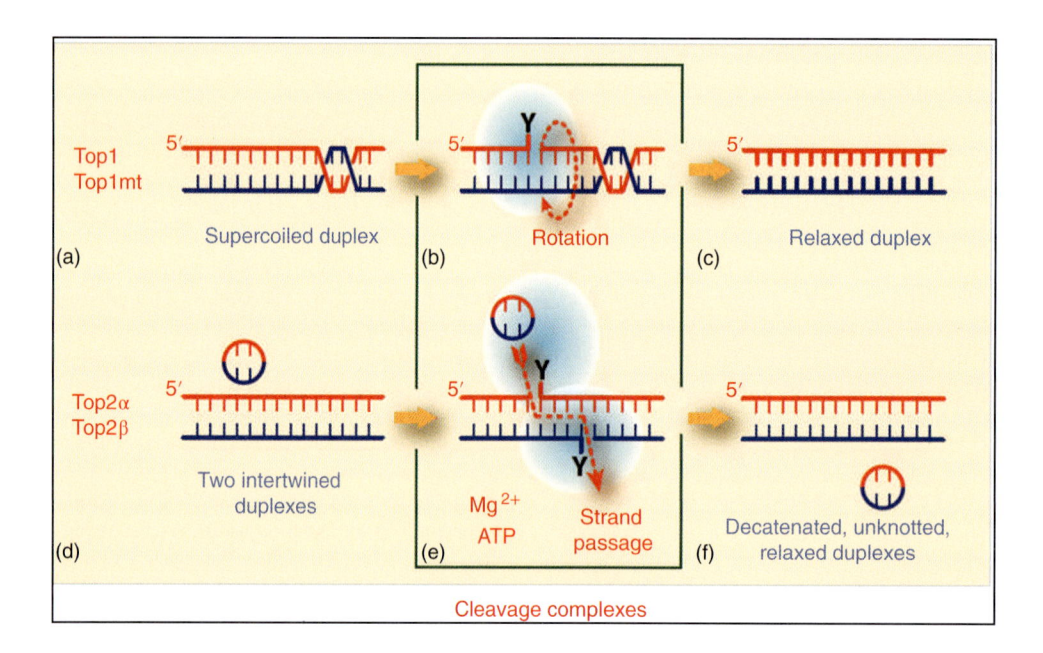

Figure 1 Topoisomerase molecular mechanisms. (a–c) Topoisomerases I (TOP1 for nuclear DNA and TOP1mt for mitochondrial DNA) relax supercoiled DNA (a) by reversibly cleaving one DNA strand, forming a covalent bond between the enzyme catalytic tyrosine and the 3'-end of the nicked DNA (the TOP1 cleavage complex: TOP1cc; (b) This reaction allows the swiveling of the broken strand around the intact strand. Rapid rejoining allows the dissociation of TOP1 (c). (d–f) Topoisomerases II acts on two DNA duplexes. They act as homodimers, cleaving both strand by forming a covalent bond between their catalytic tyrosine and the 5'-end of the DNA break (TOP2cc; e). This reaction allows the passage of the intact duplex through the TOP2 homodimer (red dotted arrow; e). TOP2 inhibitors trap the TOP2cc and prevent the normal rejoining (f). Topoisomerase cleavage complexes (b and d) are the targets of topoisomerase inhibitors.

features of double-stranded DNA: (1) the stacking of adjacent base by π–π interactions within each strand, and (2) the pairing of bases across the opposite strands by hydrogen bond interactions (duplex DNA can be viewed as a "powerful molecular zipper").

The clinical topoisomerase inhibitors act by generating topoisomerase-linked DNA breaks as they block the rejoining of the cleavage complexes when a single drug molecule tightly binds at the interface of the topoisomerase–DNA cleavage complex. The selectivity and strength of the drug binding are established by (1) the stacking of the drug with the bases flanking the cleavage site, and (2) a network of hydrogen bonds with the topoisomerase (Figure 2). As the drug is bound within the cleavage site, it prevents DNA rejoining by misaligning the DNA end, which is normally required to attack the phosphotyrosyl bond. This mode of binding led to the concept of "interfacial inhibition", which applies not only to protein–DNA interfaces but also to protein–protein interfaces, as in the case of tubulin and mTOR inhibitors.[7] Crystal structures of drug-bound cleavage complexes have firmly established this mechanism for both TOP1- and TOP2-targeted drugs.[7] The structural characteristics of each drug (differences in chemical scaffold and arrangement of hydrogen-bond donors and

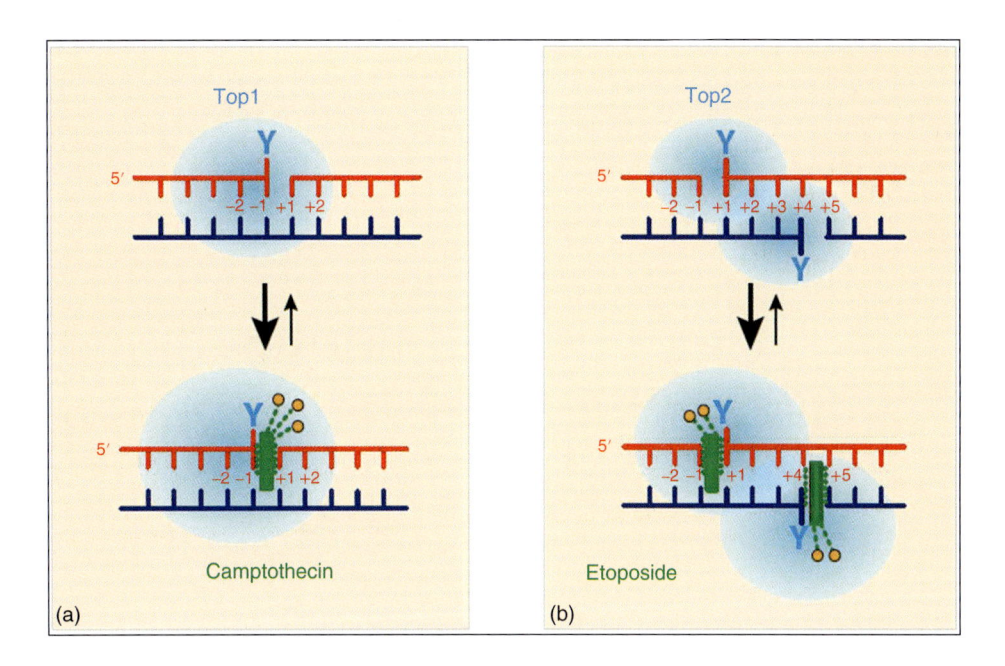

Figure 2 Trapping of topoisomerase cleavage complexes by interfacial inhibition. (a) Binding of camptothecin and noncamptothecin TOP1 inhibitors (green rectangle) at the cleavage site generated by the TOP1. A single drug molecule binds reversibly to the TOP1cc by stacking against the bases flanking the cleavage site (intercalation) and by a network of hydrogen bonds with TOP1 (orange circles and dashed green lines). (b) Same for etoposide with a single drug molecule (green) intercalated in the cleavage site formed by each TOP2 monomer. Hydrogen bonds with TOP2 are shown as orange circles and dashed green lines.

acceptors) (Figure 3) accounts for the selectivity of each drug for TOP1 versus TOP2 cleavage complexes (TOP2ccs), and for the differential DNA sequence selectivity and genomic targeting for different topoisomerase inhibitors within each class.[5,8]

It is important to understand that the cytotoxicity of topoisomerase inhibitors is due to the trapping of TOPccs as separate from the associated topoisomerase catalytic inhibition. Except in molecularly defined settings, it is the TOPccs (the DNA breaks and associated topoisomerase–DNA covalent complexes) that kill cancer cells. This distinguishes topoisomerase inhibitors from classical enzyme inhibitors such as antifolates. Indeed, knocking out TOP1 renders yeast cells totally immune to camptothecin[9] and reduction of enzyme levels renders cancer cells drug resistant.[3,5] Additionally, mutations of TOP1 and TOP2 that render cells insensitive to the trapping of TOPccs confer high resistance to TOP1 or TOP2 inhibitors. Conversely, amplification of TOP2A, which is on the same locus as HER2 on human chromosome 17, contributes to the selectivity and activity of doxorubicin in breast cancer with amplification at this locus.

The outcome of topoisomerase trapping is determined by the ability of the cell to repair the cleavage complexes, and by two common pathways: the apoptotic and the cell cycle checkpoint pathways. Topoisomerase repair pathways are specific to TOP1 or TOP2. Defects in pro-apoptotic molecules and excess of antiapoptotic molecules, which are commonly associated with cancer, confer global resistance to topoisomerase inhibitors and to other anticancer agents. Systematic analyses of cell lines with specific DNA repair alterations revealed that cells deficient in DNA double-strand break (DSB) repair may be selectively sensitive to topoisomerase inhibitors.[10] Genomic analyses recently uncovered a previously unsuspected common pathway that determines cellular sensitivity to both TOP1 and TOP2 inhibitors (and also other DNA damaging agents, including cisplatin and carboplatin). This novel pathway is centered on the gene SLFN11 (Schlafen 11)[11–13] and represents a paradigm for discovering genomic determinants and signatures to predict response to topoisomerase inhibitors and staging of patients who are most likely to respond to topoisomerase inhibitors.

Molecular pathways specific for cancer cell killing and DNA repair by TOP1 inhibitors

TOP1 cleavage complex (TOP1cc)-targeted drugs (topotecan, irinotecan, belotecan, exatecan, and indenoisoquinoline derivatives) kill cancer cells primarily by replication collisions. TOP1ccs by themselves are not cytotoxic as they remain reversible even in the presence of drugs that increase their persistence.[14] TOP1ccs damage DNA by replication and transcription fork collisions. This explains why cytotoxicity is directly related to drug exposure and why arresting DNA replication protects cells from camptothecin.[4] Collisions arise from the fact that the drugs, by slowing down the nicking-closing activity of TOP1, uncouple the TOP1 from the polymerases and helicases, leading polymerases to collide into TOP1cc. Such collisions have two consequences. They generate DSBs (replication and transcription run-off) and irreversible TOP1–DNA adducts, which are an integral part of the cleavage complexes. The replication DSBs are repaired by homologous recombination, which explains the hypersensitivity of BRCA-deficient cancer cells to TOP1cc-targeted drugs.[10,15,16] The TOP1-covalent complexes can be removed by two pathways, the excision pathway involving tyrosyl-deoxyribonucleic acid-phosphodiesterase 1 (TDP1) and the endonuclease pathway involving 3′-flap endonucleases such as XPF-ERCC1.[17,18] It is also possible that drug-trapped TOP1cc directly generate DNA DSBs when they are within 10 base pairs on opposite strands of the DNA duplex or when they occur next to a preexisting

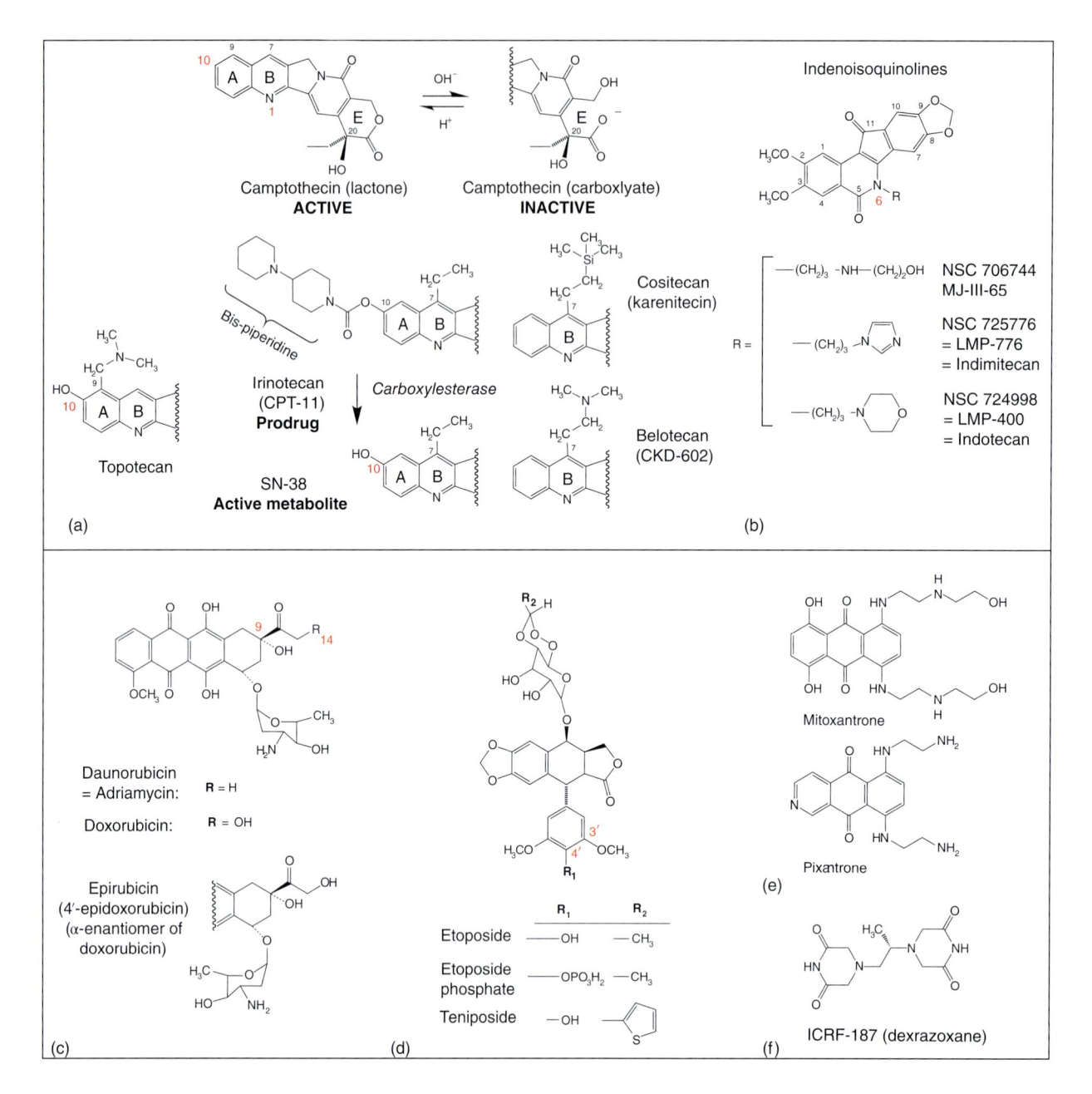

Figure 3 Clinical topoisomerase inhibitors. (a) Camptothecin derivatives are instable at physiological pH with formation of a carboxylate derivative within minutes. Irinotecan is a prodrug, which needs to be converted to SN-38 to trap TOP1cc. (b) Noncamptothecin indenoisoquinoline derivatives in clinical trials. (c) Anthracycline derivatives. (d) Demethylepipodophyllotoxin derivatives. (e) Mitoxantrone. (f) Dexrazoxane, which acts as a catalytic inhibitor of TOP2.

single-strand break on the opposite strand.[6,19] Finally, it is not excluded that topological defects contribute to the cytotoxicity of TOP1cc-targeted drugs (accumulation of supercoils[20]) and formation of alternative structures such as R-loops[21] and reversed replication forks.[22]

Molecular pathways specific for cancer cell killing and DNA repair by TOP2 inhibitors

Contrary to TOP1 inhibitors, TOP2 inhibitors can kill cancer cells independently of DNA replication fork collisions. The collision mechanism in the case of TOP2cc-targeted drugs involves transcription and proteolysis of both TOP2 and RNA polymerase II, leading to DNA DSBs by disruption of the TOP2 dimer.[18,23] Alternatively, the TOP2 homodimer interface could be disjoined by mechanical tension. Notably, 90% of TOP2cc trapped by etoposide are not concerted (i.e., only one of the two subunits of the TOP2 homodimer is trapped by etoposide) and therefore consist in single-strand breaks, which is different from doxorubicin, which produces a majority of TOP2-mediated DNA DSBs.[4,5] Finally, it is not excluded that topological defects resulting from TOP2 sequestration by the drug-induced cleavage complexes could contribute to the cytotoxicity of TOP2cc-targeted drugs. Such topological defects would include persistent DNA knots and catenanes, potentially leading to chromosome breaks during mitosis. TOP2 covalent complexes are removed by TDP2 (tyrosyl-deoxyribonucleic acid-phosphodiesterase 2)[17] in conjunction with the end-joining pathway [Ku, deoxyribonucleic acid-dependent protein kinase (DNA-PK), ligase IV, and XRCC4].[10,24]

The anticancer activity of intercalating TOP2 inhibitors (anthracyclines and anthracenediones) extends beyond the trapping of TOP2 cleavage complexes

Some TOP2 inhibitors, such as anthracyclines (Figure 3c) and mitoxantrone (Figure 3e) are also potent DNA intercalating agents. Consequently, anthracyclines and mitoxantrone affect TOP2cc in two mechanisms: at low drug concentrations, they trap TOP2cc, whereas at higher concentrations (>5 μM), high levels of intercalation outside of the TOP2cc suppress the binding of TOP2 to DNA and thereby inhibit the formation of TOP2cc. As a result, the concentration-response curve of doxorubicin is "bell-shaped."[4,25] Intercalation of anthracylines also destabilizes chromatin structure with nucleosome eviction.[26,27] Another property of the anthracyclines is the generation of oxygen radicals due to their quinone structure.[28]

Topoisomerase I inhibitors

Topotecan

Camptothecin and its derivatives demonstrated a high degree of *in vitro* antitumor activity in the 1960s, which was then confirmed in early clinical trials.[29-31] Clinical development was limited by unpredictable toxicities, including severe myelosuppression and diarrhea, and incomplete understanding of the mechanism of antitumor activity. Topotecan has since been shown to be a specific inhibitor of the nuclear enzyme TOP1.[32] Consequently, topotecan has been developed for several clinical indications (Table 2).

Clinical pharmacology
Topotecan (9-dimethylaminomethyl-10-hydroxycamptothecin) (Figure 3a) is a semisynthetic analogue of camptothecin, an alkaloid derived from the oriental tree *Camptotheca acuminata*. The side chain at the 9-position of the A-ring (Figure 3a), provides water solubility. Lactone topotecan, the active form of the drug is unstable as it is rapidly and reversibly converted to the open-ring carboxylate in a pH-dependent reaction[14] (Figure 3a). At neutral pH, the open-ring form predominates.[33]

Topotecan pharmacokinetics fit a two-compartment model with a terminal half-life of 2–3 h. The plasma concentrations increase linearly with increasing doses but do not show evidence of accumulation on the 30-min infusion, 5-day schedule.[34] Binding of topotecan to plasma proteins is approximately 35%.[34]

Topotecan lactone is widely distributed, with a steady-state mean volume of distribution of 75 L/m^2. Topotecan is predominantly eliminated in the urine after its conversion to the carboxylate species. Although large inter-individual variability exists, about 30% of the administered dose is excreted unchanged in urine.[34]

Renal dysfunction decreases topotecan plasma clearance, such that mild (creatinine clearance 40–60 mL/min) and moderate dysfunction (creatinine clearance 20–39 mL/min), lead to reductions to 67% and 34% of normal values, respectively.[35] Dose adjustments are therefore recommended for renal impairment. Liver impairment does not influence topotecan clearance and doses do not need to be adjusted for patients with hepatic dysfunction.[36]

Although the typical route of administration is intravenous (IV), an oral formulation is available. The oral formulation of topotecan was aimed at maintaining sufficiently prolonged drug exposures, which produce high in *in vitro* and *in vivo* antitumor efficacy,[14] without the need for infusion pumps.[37] The approved oral dose is 2.3 mg/m^2 once daily for 5 consecutive days repeated every 21 days. The oral bioavailability of topotecan is approximately 35%.[34] The low bioavailability may be caused by hydrolysis of topotecan lactone in the gut, yielding the poorly absorbed open-ring form. Oral topotecan has shown clinical activity comparable to the IV dose in small-cell lung cancer (SCLC).[38]

Clinical use
Topotecan monotherapy is approved in the United States and Europe for patients with metastatic ovarian cancer after failure of initial or subsequent chemotherapy, and in patients with relapsed SCLC. It is also approved in combination with cisplatin for recurrent or resistant (stage IVB) cervical cancer.[39]

Topotecan has shown clinical activity in other tumor types, including pediatric medulloblastoma,[40] non-small-cell lung cancer (NSCLC),[41] myelodysplastic syndrome, chronic myelomonocytic leukemia,[42] Ewing's sarcoma,[43] rhabdomyosarcoma,[44] and multiple myeloma.[45] In addition to the combination with cisplatin approved in cervical cancer, combinations of TOP1 inhibitors with other antitumor agents have been pursued. Synergistic and additive combinations have been observed in preclinical models, including with histone deacetylase inhibitors and poly (ADP-ribose) polymerase (PARP) inhibitors, and a number of drug combination strategies have been investigated in patients.[46,47] Topotecan diffuses into the spinal fluid and can be considered for treating brain metastases.[48]

Table 2 DNA topoisomerase targeting drugs.[a]

Drug class	Drugs	Year of FDA approval	Approved indication
Camptothecin	Irinotecan	1996	Colorectal cancer
	Topotecan	1996	Cervical cancer, ovarian cancer, small-cell lung cancer
Anthracycline	Doxorubicin	1974	Breast cancer, acute lymphoblastic leukemia, acute myeloid leukemia, Wilms tumor, neuroblastoma, soft tissue and bone sarcomas, ovarian cancer, transitional cell bladder carcinoma, thyroid carcinoma, gastric carcinoma, Hodgkin lymphoma, non-Hodgkin lymphoma, bronchogenic carcinoma
	Pegylated liposomal doxorubicin	1999	AIDS-related Kaposi sarcoma, multiple myeloma, ovarian cancer
	Daunorubicin	1979	Acute lymphocytic leukemia, acute myeloid leukemia
	Idarubicin	1990	Acute myeloid leukemia
Anthraquinone	Mitoxantrone	1987	Acute nonlymphocytic leukemias, advanced hormone-refractory prostate cancer
Podophyllotoxin	Etoposide	1984	Small-cell lung cancer, testicular cancer
	Teniposide	1992	Acute lymphoblastic leukemia

[a]Source: Based on Hsiang and Liu.[32]

Schedule of administration

Various schedules of topotecan have been evaluated in Phase I studies. The Food and Drug Administration (FDA)-recommended dose of topotecan in recurrent ovarian cancer and SCLC is 1.5 mg/m^2 by IV infusion over 30 min on days 1–5 of a 21-day cycle.

Despite its high incidence of grade 3–4 myelosuppression, this dose and schedule of topotecan remain the standard of care. To mitigate this toxicity, multiple-dose and schedule variations have been evaluated in Phase I and II trials.[49,50] In ovarian cancer, weekly topotecan (4 mg/m^2/week administered on days 1, 8, and 15) has been reported to have efficacy comparable to the standard schedule, but with less toxicity.[50] The weekly schedule has not been directly compared with the 5-day schedule in SCLC.[38] In cervical cancer, topotecan is approved in combination with cisplatin; the recommended dose of topotecan is 0.75 mg/m^2 IV over 30 min on days 1, 2, and 3 and of cisplatin is 50 mg/m^2 IV on day 1 repeated every 21 days.[51]

Toxicity

The dose-limiting toxicity (DLT) of topotecan is bone marrow (BM) suppression, primarily neutropenia, but thrombocytopenia and anemia may also occur. At 1.5 mg/m^2/day for five days, topotecan produces an 80–90% decrease in white blood cell count at nadir after the first cycle of therapy. The degree of neutropenia has been correlated with the area under the curve (AUC) of the intact lactone or total drug concentrations.[52] Topotecan should not be administered to patients with baseline neutrophils <1500/mm^3 or platelets <100,000/mm^3.

Renal dysfunction decreases topotecan clearance and increases toxicity. Additional factors associated with greater hematologic toxicity include advanced age and prior therapy, including platinum administration (especially carboplatin) and radiation therapy.[53] In high-risk patients receiving topotecan for five consecutive days, the incidence of severe myelosuppression may be mitigated by reducing the topotecan dose to 1.0 or 1.25 mg/m^2/day. Hematopoietic growth factors, transfusions, and schedule adjustments may also help manage myelosuppression. Alternative schedules of 3-day, weekly dosing or oral administration are associated with less myelosuppression.[54]

Less common toxicities of topotecan include rash, fever, fatigue, nausea and vomiting, mucositis, and elevated serum transaminases.[55] Most nonhematological toxicities are generally manageable. Diarrhea is uncommon with IV administration, but it has been reported with oral topotecan. Rare, but life-threatening nonhematologic toxicities include interstitial lung disease (ILD) and neutropenic colitis.

Irinotecan

Irinotecan is a potent water-soluble camptothecin-derivative.

Clinical pharmacology

Irinotecan (CPT-11) is the prodrug of the potent 7-ethyl-10-hydroxy analogue of camptothecin (SN-38) (Figure 3a).[52] It contains a bispiperidine substituent at C-10, to confer water-solubility for parenteral administration. Irinotecan undergoes extensive metabolic conversion by esterases to its active metabolite SN-38 (Figure 3a). Irinotecan prodrug is activated by carboxylesterases to SN-38, the biologically active compound. This explains why in *in vitro* cytotoxicity assays, irinotecan is orders of magnitude less active than SN-38.[56,57]

Irinotecan peak plasma concentration and AUC increase proportionally with the administered dose suggestive of linear pharmacokinetics. The plasma AUC of SN-38 is only 2–8% of irinotecan indicating that only a small fraction of irinotecan is converted to SN-38, its active form. Both irinotecan and SN-38 exist in the active lactone form and the inactive carboxylate form. Similar to topotecan, both forms are in a pH-dependent equilibrium.[14]

Irinotecan plasma concentrations decline in a multi-exponential manner after IV infusion. The mean terminal elimination half-life of irinotecan is 6–12 h and that of SN-38 10–20 h, both much longer than that of topotecan. The relatively large percentage of the lactone form of both irinotecan and SN-38 that persists in plasma after drug administration is attributable to the preferential binding of the lactone forms to albumin.[33] SN-38 is 95% bound to plasma proteins compared to approximately 50% for irinotecan.[52]

Unlike topotecan, irinotecan elimination occurs predominantly by biliary excretion.[56] Renal excretion of SN-38 and irinotecan represents only a fraction of the administered dose. The 1A1 isoform of UDP-glucuronosyl transferase (UGT1A1; encoded by the *UGT1A1* gene) mediates glucuronidation of SN-38 to the inactive metabolite SN-38G (see section titled "Pharmacogenomics"). There is wide inter-patient variability in UGT1A1 enzyme activity related to UGT1A1 gene polymorphisms.[58,59] Additionally, polymorphisms of this enzyme are associated with conditions causing familial hyperbilirubinemia such as Crigler–Najjar syndromes and Gilbert's disease.[60] UGT1A1 polymorphisms can significantly alter the metabolism of irinotecan and thereby impact its toxicity in individual patients, and dose reduction is recommended for patients bearing particular variants of UGT1A1. Irinotecan is also inactivated by CYP3A4-mediated oxidative metabolism.[61]

Clinical use

Irinotecan is approved in the United States and Europe for first-line therapy in combination with 5-fluorouracil and leucovorin for metastatic colorectal cancers. It is also approved for metastatic colorectal cancer in patients whose disease has recurred or progressed following fluorouracil-based therapy.[56,62]

Irinotecan monotherapy or combined with other agents have shown clinical activity in diverse tumor types, including extensive-stage SCLC,[63] squamous cell carcinoma of the cervix,[64] recurrent glioblastoma,[65] gastric cancer, esophageal cancer,[66] NSCLC,[67] pancreatic cancer,[68] rhabdomyosarcoma,[69] and ovarian cancer.[70]

Schedule of administration

Monotherapy with irinotecan is usually administered at 125 mg/m^2 IV infusion over 90 min on days 1, 8, 15, and 22 followed by two weeks rest (6-week treatment cycles). An alternative dosing regimen is 350 mg/m^2 given as a 90-min IV infusion once every three weeks. In patients with 5-fluorouracil-refractory, metastatic colorectal cancer, the weekly and once every three weeks schedule demonstrated similar efficacy and quality of life. The regimen of once every three weeks was associated with a significantly lower incidence of severe diarrhea.[71]

In combination with 5-fluorouracil and leucovorin, irinotecan is used at 125 mg/m^2 IV infusion over 90 min on days 1, 8, 15, and 22 (6-week treatment cycles). An alternative dosing regimen is 180 mg/m^2 over 90 min on days 1, 15, and 29 (6-week treatment cycles).

Toxicity

Diarrhea and myelosuppression are the most concerning toxicities of irinotecan. Late-onset diarrhea occurs more than 24 h after

Table 3 Investigational TOP1 inhibitors in clinical development.

	Drugs/drug class	Comments
Camptothecin analogs	Belotecan	Water-soluble camptothecin analogue
	Cositecan	Lipophilic, semisynthetic camptothecin
	Lipotecan	Lactone ring modified to increase antitumor potency
	Simmitecan	Ester prodrug of the TOP1 inhibitor chimmitecan
Targeted camptothecin delivery	*Liposomal/nanoparticle/PEGylated formulations*	
	MM-398	Nanoliposomal formulation of irinotecan
	CPX-1	Liposome-encapsulated formulation of irinotecan and floxuridine
	Firtecan pegol	Pegylated formulation of SN-38
	CRLX101	Cyclodextrin-based polymer conjugate of camptothecin
	Antibody–drug conjugates	
	Sacituzumab govitecan	Antibody drug conjugate [antibody that binds to trophoblast cell-surface antigen (TROP-2) and SN-38]
	Camptothecin conjugates	
	HA–irinotecan	Irinotecan complexed with hyaluronic acid
	Etirinotecan pegol	Irinotecan bound to polyethylene glycol core by a biodegradable linker
Noncamptothecin TOP1 inhibitors	Indenoisoquinoline derivatives	Better chemical stability, produces stable DNA–TOP1 cleavage complexes

irinotecan. When prolonged, it can lead to life-threatening dehydration and electrolyte imbalance.[72] Grade 3–4 late-onset diarrhea occurs in approximately a third of patients receiving weekly dosing. The median time to the onset of late diarrhea was 5 days with 3-week dosing and 11 days with weekly dosing.[56,62] Free intestinal luminal SN-38, either from bile or SN-38G deconjugation is responsible for late-onset diarrhea. SN-38 induces direct mucosal damage with resultant water and electrolyte malabsorption and mucous hypersecretion.[73] Late diarrhea should be treated without delay with loperamide, and fluid and electrolytes as needed. Antibiotic therapy is warranted if the patient develops ileus, fever, or severe neutropenia. Predisposing factors for late-onset diarrhea include increasing age, poor performance status, and prior abdominopelvic radiotherapy.[74] A reduced starting dose should be considered in patients with risk factors. Treatment-related diarrhea should have fully resolved before initiating the next course of treatment. Dose reductions are recommended for grade 3–4 diarrhea. Various measures to reduce its severity have been studied, but none have an established role in practice.[75] In 2005, the FDA approved a diagnostic test for the UGT1A1 variant allele *28, which has been associated with reduced expression leading to impaired clearance and increased toxicity.[76] However, other variant alleles that impair expression of the enzyme are also identified and impact clearance of drugs requiring glucuronidation in *in vitro* cytotoxicity assays.

Less commonly irinotecan can also cause early-onset diarrhea during or within 24 h of the infusion. It is usually transient and only infrequently severe. It is attributed to a cholinergic syndrome mediated by anticholinesterase activity of irinotecan.[77] This cholinergic syndrome tends to occur at higher irinotecan dose levels at peak irinotecan plasma levels. Other cholinergic symptoms including abdominal cramping, rhinitis, tearing, and increased salivation may occur. The mean duration of symptoms is 30 min and usually responds rapidly to atropine.

Other common toxicities observed with irinotecan are nausea, vomiting, abdominal pain, constipation, anorexia, asthenia, fever, weight loss, and alopecia. Rare, but life-threatening nonhematological toxicities include ILD and hypersensitivity reactions.

Risk factors for pulmonary toxicity include preexisting lung disease, use of pulmonary toxic medications, radiation, and use of colony-stimulating factors. Patients with risk factors should be monitored for respiratory symptoms during irinotecan and for several weeks after treatment.[78]

Camptothecin analogs and noncamptothecin TOP1 inhibitors

As discussed above, camptothecin derivatives have several well-established limitations. They are inactivated within minutes at physiological pH by lactone E-ring opening (Figure 3a). This results in a loss of antitumor activity since the lactone form is essential for antitumor activity. Other limitations include fast reversal of the trapped DNA–TOP1cc following drug removal, drug resistance mediated by ATP-binding cassette (ABC) transporters.[14]

Several newer derivatives of camptothecin currently in clinical development aim to mitigate some of the shortcomings of camptothecins and their derivatives (Table 3). Camptothecin analogs, derived from modifications to the parent drug, have been an area of active research.[79] Belotecan hydrochloride, a water-soluble camptothecin analogue is approved in Korea for SCLC and ovarian cancer.[80]

Several approaches have been taken to stabilize the lactone ring of camptothecins without interfering with their antitumor activity.[25] Indenoisoquinolines are noncamptothecin inhibitors of TOP1, but with better chemical stability, producing stable DNA-TOP1ccs. They also have a preference for unique DNA cleavage sites, compared with their camptothecin counterparts, and have demonstrated activity against camptothecin-resistant cell lines and produce DNA protein cross-links, which are resistant to reversal. They also show less or no resistance to cells overexpressing the ABC transporters, ATP-binding cassette subfamily G member 2 (ABCG2), and multidrug resistance (MDR)-1.[81] Like the camptothecins, they are selectively active in homologous recombination-deficient (HRD) and BRCA1/2-deficient (BRCAness) cancer cells, as well as cancer cells overexpressing SLFN11 and RB1-deficient.[15,16] Other approaches to address E-ring instability include the conversion of the E-ring to a five-membered ring that completely stabilizes the drug.[82]

Targeted delivery of TOP1 inhibitors

Several approaches are being explored to improve the targeted delivery, and tumor localization of camptothecins.[83] Broadly, they involve (1) liposomal or nanoparticle formulation to increase plasma half-life and tumor localization, (2) antibody conjugation for targeted delivery, and (3) conjugation to agents to improve pharmacokinetic properties and exposure.

Liposomal/nanoparticle formulations

Liposomes are microscopic phospholipid spheres with an aqueous core.[84] Due to their biphasic character, they can act as carriers for both lipophilic and hydrophilic drugs; hydrophilic drugs tend to be entrapped in the core whereas the hydrophobic agents are entrapped within the lipid bilayers. Stable liposomal encapsulation of camptothecin minimizes its conversion to inactive carboxylate form by reducing the direct exposure of the drug to physiologic pH and prolonging the residence time of the lactone active drug. PEGylation increases the size and molecular weight of conjugated biomolecules.[85] PEGylated molecules show increased half-life, decreased plasma clearance, and different biodistribution compared with non-PEGylated counterparts. PEGylation of liposomes further improves the stability and circulation time. Polymeric nanoparticles are drug carriers that are designed to have defined size and surface properties to favor drug deposition and retention in tumors.[86] These formulations are thought to improve the "passive" targeting of tumors, through a process known as the enhanced permeation retention effect, wherein macromolecules penetrate and are trapped in tumor tissue due to the abnormally leaky vasculature of tumors.[87]

Liposomal irinotecan

Clinical Pharmacology

Liposomal irinotecan (MM-398, nal-IRI) comprises irinotecan-free base encapsulated in liposome nanoparticles. The liposome is designed to keep irinotecan in the circulation—sheltered from conversion to its active metabolite SN-38—longer than free (unencapsulated) irinotecan, which would increase and prolong intratumoral levels of both irinotecan and SN-38 compared with free irinotecan.[88]

Clinical use

Liposomal irinotecan is approved for use in combination with fluorouracil and leucovorin, for the treatment of patients with metastatic pancreatic adenocarcinoma after disease progression following gemcitabine-based therapy.[89]

Schedule of administration

Patients should receive premedication with a corticosteroid and an antiemetic. The recommended dose of liposomal irinotecan is 70 mg/m^2 intravenous infusion every two weeks. Patients homozygous for UGT1A1*28 should receive a lower starting dose of 50 mg/m^2 every two weeks.

Toxicity

The most common adverse events in patients treated with liposomal irinotecan include diarrhea, nausea, and vomiting.

Antibody–drug conjugates

Two antibody–drug conjugates (ADCs) generated by conjugating the most potent camptothecins to monoclonal antibodies are approved for clinical indications: Fam-trastuzumab deruxtecan-nxki and sacituzumab govitecan-hziy.

Fam-trastuzumab deruxtecan-nxki

Clinical Pharmacology

Trastuzumab deruxtecan (DS-8201) is an ADC composed of antihuman epidermal growth factor receptor 2 (HER2) antibody, a cleavable tetrapeptide-based linker, and TOP1 inhibitor deruxtecan (DXd), with approximately eight molecules of DXd per antibody.[90] Dxd is an exatecan derivative and is 10 times more potent than SN-38. The linker is stable in plasma and is selectively cleaved by lysosomal cathepsins that are upregulated in cancer cells. DXd is cell membrane permeable allowing for bystander cytotoxic effect, whereby the released TOP1 inhibitor diffuses across the target-cell membrane, affecting nearby cells regardless of their HER2-expression.[91]

Clinical use

Trastuzumab deruxtecan has remarkable antitumor activity in patients who previously received other HER2-targeted treatments such as pertuzumab, trastuzumab, and trastuzumab emtansine. It received accelerated approval (based on surrogate endpoints such as response rate and duration of response rather than clinical endpoints such as overall survival (OS) improvement, often from small uncontrolled trials, in order to bring a promising drug to market sooner) for unresectable or metastatic HER2-positive breast cancer who have received ≥2 prior anti-HER2-based regimens in the metastatic setting.[92,93]

Schedule of administration

The recommended dose of trastuzumab deruxtecan is 5.4 mg/kg given as an intravenous infusion once every three weeks (21-day cycle).

Toxicity

Two common classes of adverse events during trastuzumab deruxtecan treatment are gastrointestinal and hematological.[90] Nausea and vomiting occur in about 50–80% of patients, while they are severe in only <5% of cases. Approximately 30% of patients develop anemia and neutropenia; neutropenia can be severe in 20% of patients. Patients treated with trastuzumab deruxtecan are at increased risk of developing left ventricular dysfunction, a known class effect of anti-HER2 therapies. While these events are rare (<3%), left ventricular ejection fraction (LVEF) assessment is recommended prior to initiation of treatment and at regular intervals during treatment. LVEF decrease is generally managed through treatment interruption, but permanent discontinuation is warranted for LVEF <40%, absolute LVEF decrease from baseline of >20%, or symptomatic congestive heart failure.

Trastuzumab deruxtecan is associated with a substantial risk of ILD and/or pneumonitis, occurring in 9% of patients with unresectable or metastatic HER2-positive breast cancer, including fatal events in 2.6% of patients.[92,93] In clinical trials, the median time to onset of these symptoms was 4.1 months. Patients should be advised to report cough, dyspnea, fever, and/or any new or worsening respiratory symptoms, and such symptoms should be promptly investigated. Management of ILD generally consists of corticosteroids and treatment interruption for asymptomatic ILD, and discontinuation of trastuzumab deruxtecan for symptomatic disease.

Sacituzumab govitecan-hziy

Clinical pharmacology
Sacituzumab govitecan (IMMU-132) is a humanized antibody against trophoblast cell-surface antigen (TROP-2) conjugated by a pH-sensitive linker (CL2A) to SN-38, with an average 7–8 molecules of SN-38 per antibody molecule.[94,95] TROP-2 is a type I transmembrane, calcium-transducing, protein expressed by many epithelial cancers, but with limited normal tissue expression. The antibody internalizes selectively into cancer cells following binding to TROP-2 to deliver SN-38 into the tumor cell.[96] In addition, because of the cleavable linker, SN-38 is released in tumors both intracellularly and in the tumor microenvironment, thereby allowing for the delivery of the drug in bystander cells to which the conjugate has not bound. Sacituzumab-bound tumor cells are killed by intracellular uptake of SN-38, and adjacent tumor cells are killed by the extracellular release of SN-38.[97] Sacituzumab govitecan provides substantially longer plasma half-life of SN-38 (mean half-life of sacituzumab govitecan is 16 h and free SN-38 18 h) compared with irinotecan and results in increased intra-tumoral accumulation of SN-38 in animal models.

Clinical use
Sacituzumab govitecan received accelerated approval for the treatment of patients with metastatic triple-negative breast cancer who have received at least two prior therapies for metastatic disease.[98] It is also being investigated as monotherapy and in combination with PARP inhibitors in multiple solid tumors.

Schedule of administration
Premedications should include two or three antiemetics following established guidelines to prevent chemotherapy-induced nausea and vomiting, and medications (e.g., antipyretics, H1 and H2 antagonists, and corticosteroids) to prevent hypersensitivity reactions. The recommended dose of sacituzumab govitecan is 10 mg/kg once weekly on Days 1 and 8 of continuous 21-day treatment cycles.

Toxicity
Major toxicities include nausea, vomiting, neutropenia, and diarrhea.[98] Nausea and diarrhea are frequent adverse events, occurring more than 60% of patients, with severe events in 6–8% of patients. Febrile neutropenia occurs in approximately 8% of patients who receive sacituzumab govitecan after ≥2 prior therapies. Individuals who are homozygous for the UGT1A1 variant allele *28 are at increased risk for neutropenia. In a retrospective analysis of patients who received sacituzumab govitecan and had UGT1A1 genotype results available, the incidence of grade 4 neutropenia was 26% and 13% in patients homozygous and heterozygous for the UGT1A1*28 allele, and 11% in patients homozygous for the wild-type allele. Hypersensitivity reactions within 24 h of dosing occur in approximately 40% of patients, including severe or life-threatening events in 1%.

Camptothecin conjugates
Etirinotecan pegol is a long-acting TOP1 inhibitor consisting of irinotecan conjugated to a polyethylene glycol core by a biodegradable linker. The linker slowly hydrolyses *in vivo* to form SN38, the active moiety. The drug is designed to provide prolonged continuous exposure to SN38 while reducing the toxicities associated with excessively high irinotecan and SN38 plasma concentrations. Etirinotecan pegol is being studied in a Phase III trial in women with advanced breast cancer.[99] Hyaluronic acid-irinotecan is an IV formulation of irinotecan conjugated with hyaluronic acid.[100] Hyaluronic acid selectively binds cancer cells via CD44, thereby enhancing membrane fluidity and potentially reducing side effects.

PEN-866 is an esterase-cleavable conjugate which links a HSP90 binding small molecule to SN-38.[101–103] PEN-866 selectively binds activated HSP90—which is highly expressed in advanced malignancies—and releases its cytotoxic payload resulting in selective drug accumulation tumors cells.

TOP2 inhibitors

TOP2 targeting drugs used in the clinic can be divided into intercalating and nonintercalating "poisons." The intercalators are chemically diverse, and include doxorubicin and other anthracyclines, and anthracenediones (Figure 3c,e). Nonintercalating TOP2 poisons include the epipodophyllotoxins, etoposide, and teniposide (Figure 3d) (Table 2).

Anthracyclines

Anthracycline antibiotics, originally isolated from fermentation products of *Streptomyces peucetius*, were shown to have antineoplastic activity decades ago, before topoisomerase enzymes were identified. It was not until 1984 that the anthracyclines were found to inhibit TOP2.[104] Doxorubicin represents first generation anthracyclines; epirubicin and idarubicin are second-generation compounds aimed at reducing cardiotoxicity and drug efflux by ABC transporters. Anthracyclines have wide-ranging activity against human cancers and are used extensively in the curative, adjuvant, and palliative settings, both as single agents and in combination regimens.

Doxorubicin is the most commonly used anthracycline (Figure 3c). The anthracycline ring is lipophilic, but the presence of abundant hydroxyl groups adjacent to the amino sugar produces an amphoteric molecule. Doxorubicin binds to the cell membranes and membrane-associated molecules including cardiolipin as well as plasma proteins. Daunomycin differs from doxorubicin by a single hydroxyl group on carbon-14 (Figure 3c) and has a distinct spectrum of antitumor activity. Idarubicin is a semisynthetic derivative of daunomycin (4-demethoxy daunorubicin) without the 4-methoxy group (Figure 3c). Epirubicin is an epimer of doxorubicin: the C4′ hydroxyl group on the amino sugar is in the equatorial rather than in the axial position which increases its lipophilicity. None of these analogs have stronger antitumor efficacy than the original two anthracyclines, but they tend to limit the toxicity of doxorubicin and daunorubicin.[105]

Clinical pharmacology
Doxorubicin displays linear pharmacokinetics and exhibits a triphasic disposition after IV injection. The initial half-life is very short, approximately 5 min, suggesting rapid tissue uptake. The second phase of approximately 10 h represents its metabolism and the slow final phase of 24–48 h, the gradual release of doxorubicin from multiple sites of binding including the DNA.[106] Doxorubicin and its major metabolite, doxorubicinol, are substantially bound to plasma proteins, approximately 50–90%.[107] Doxorubicin does not cross the blood–brain barrier.

Plasma clearance of doxorubicin is predominantly accomplished by metabolism and biliary excretion. The drug is extensively metabolized in the liver by aldo-keto reductase to yield the dihydrodiol derivative doxorubicinol, which retains antitumor activity, and by the nicotinamide adenine dinucleotide phosphate (NADPH)-dependent cytochrome P450 reductase to cleave the glycosidic bond and release aglycone metabolites.[108] The clearance of doxorubicin and doxorubicinol are reduced in patients with impaired hepatic function.[109] Renal clearance is quantitatively unimportant, and dose modification is not required in renal failure.

Liposome encapsulation of doxorubicin has been successfully used as a strategy to reduce toxicity without losing efficacy.[110] Pegylated liposomal doxorubicin is a liposomal formulation of doxorubicin, which compared with unencapsulated doxorubicin has a long half-life and delayed uptake by the reticuloendothelial system due to the attachment of polyethylene glycol polymers to a lipid anchor and stable retention of the drug as a result of liposomal entrapment via an ammonium sulfate chemical gradient.[111] The pharmacokinetic profile of this drug is characterized by an extended circulation time and a reduced volume of distribution, which promotes tumor uptake.

Clinical use

Doxorubicin is utilized in many human cancers. It is also FDA approved for adjuvant chemotherapy following resection of primary breast cancer for patients with axillary lymph node invasion. Doxorubicin is also used for the treatment of acute lymphoblastic and myeloblastic leukemias and in combination regimens for non-Hodgkin's and Hodgkin's lymphoma. Doxorubicin has activity in many solid tumors including breast, ovarian, bladder, thyroid, gastric and lung cancers, soft tissue and bone sarcomas. Pegylated liposomal doxorubicin is used in treatment of acquired immunodeficiency syndrome (AIDS)-related Kaposi sarcoma after failure of or intolerance to prior systemic therapy and in multiple myeloma as a component of combination therapy.[112,113] It is also used in the treatment of progressive or recurrent ovarian cancer after platinum-based treatment.[114]

Epirubicin has a spectrum of activity very similar to doxorubicin, but with lower toxicity.[115] Epirubicin is used as a component of adjuvant therapy for primary breast cancer and for esophageal and gastric cancers, soft tissue, and uterine sarcomas.[116]

Daunomycin (Figure 3c) is used mostly as part of an induction regimen in acute lymphocytic leukemia (ALL) and acute myeloid leukemia (AML). It is also active in pediatric solid tumors, but it has little activity against adult solid tumors. Idarubicin is used predominantly in the treatment of AML and ALL.[117]

Schedule of administration

Single-agent doxorubicin is administered IV at 60–75 mg/m^2 every 21 days. In combination therapy, it is administered at 40–75 mg/m^2 every 21–28 days. Daunorubicin is given IV at 30–60 mg/m^2 daily for 3 days. Idarubicin is given IV at 12 mg/m^2 daily for 3 days. Epirubicin is given IV at 100–120 mg/m^2 by bolus injection every 3 weeks. Pegylated liposomal doxorubicin is given IV at 20 mg/m^2 every 21 days for AIDS-related Kaposi sarcoma and 50 mg/m^2 once every 28 days in ovarian cancer.

Toxicity

All anthracyclines produce cardiac damage that can result in serious and even life-threatening complications.[118,119] It is the major DLT of prolonged treatment with doxorubicin. Cardiotoxicity is more common with doxorubicin and daunorubicin than with epirubicin or idarubicin.[115] Cardiotoxicity manifests acutely with electrocardiographic abnormalities, including ST-T elevation and arrhythmias and can occur at any time from initiation of treatment to several weeks afterward. Cardiomyopathy, a manifestation of chronic cardiotoxicity, may also occur early, within one year after termination of the treatment, or it may be delayed beyond one year after treatment.

Doxorubicin-associated cardiomyopathy and congestive heart failure are dose-dependent. Risk increases proportionally to the total accumulated dose in a nonlinear fashion (1–5% up to 550 mg/m^2, 30% at 600 mg/m^2, and 50% at 1 g/m^2 or higher) with marked inter-individual variation.[120] The frequency of these complications is unacceptably high when the cumulative dose of the drug exceeds 550 mg/m^2 of body-surface area.[121] The mode of administration plays an important role in cumulative cardiotoxicity and bolus administration appears to be involved.[122] Continuous infusion regimens have been studied in an effort to reduce cardiotoxicity. Infusion over 48 or 96 h has been shown to shift the toxicity profile, resulting in lower incidence of nausea, vomiting, and cardiotoxicity and increased incidence of mucositis,[123] but allowing dosing above conventional limits. Despite evident advantages, the difficulty of administering a continuous infusion schedule suggested that this approach has not had significant uptake in the community.

The cardiotoxicity of doxorubicin had been attributed to redox cycling and reactive oxygen species (ROS) generation; however, ROS scavengers have failed to prevent this toxicity.[121,124] More recent data implicate TOP2β.[125] TOP2α is overexpressed in tumors and represents the molecular basis of doxorubicin antitumor activity, whereas TOP2β is expressed by cardiomyocytes and nonreplicating cells.[17,126] Multiple lines of evidence indicate the role of TOP2β in contributing to the development of doxorubicin-induced cardiomyopathy. TOP2β-doxorubicin-DNA ternary cleavage complex can induce DNA DSBs leading to cell death in cardiomyocytes. TOP2β-deleted mouse embryonic fibroblasts have been shown to be resistant to doxorubicin-induced cell death.[127] Recent studies also indicate that the mitochondrial topoisomerase, TOP1mt counteracts the cytotoxicity of doxorubicin by enabling mitochondrial DNA replication and maintaining functional oxidative phosphorylation.[126]

Several factors increase the risk for anthracycline cardiotoxicity. The strongest predictor is cumulative drug dose.[128] Age at the time of drug exposure, concomitant administration of other cardiotoxic drugs, radiation to the chest, and preexisting cardiovascular disease are other risk factors. Several approaches have been taken to decrease the risk of cardiotoxicity while maintaining efficacy. These include alternate schedules of drug administration, modifications of the anthracycline molecule, and adjunctive treatment with beta-adrenergic blockers or dexrazoxane.[127] Recent evidence implicates mitochondrial *TOP1* (*TOP1mt*) mutations, which exist as normal single nucleotide polymorphisms (SNPs), as potential determinants of doxorubicin-induced cardiotoxicity.[126]

Dexrazoxane (Figure 3f) is an ethylenediaminetetraacetic acid (EDTA)-like chelator that prevents anthracycline damage by binding to iron released from intracellular storage secondary to lipid peroxidation.[129] Patients with breast cancer treated with dexrazoxane experienced fewer cardiac events compared with those treated with anthracycline alone.[130] Dexrazoxane is approved in the United States and Europe for patients with advanced or metastatic breast cancer who have already received 300 mg/m^2 of doxorubicin or 540 mg/m^2 of epirubicin. However, concerns exist regarding the possibility of lower response to chemotherapy and more myelosuppression with dexrazoxane use.[131] Dexrazoxane is therefore not recommended for routine use in breast cancer with doxorubicin-based chemotherapy. Continued cardiac monitoring is recommended in patients receiving doxorubicin.[132]

Other toxicities of anthracyclines include myelosuppression, mucositis, and alopecia, nausea, vomiting, diarrhea, and increased skin pigmentation. Myelosuppression is the acute DLT. After a bolus dose, the leukocyte count begins to fall in 7 days, reaches a nadir at 10–14 days, and recovers 1–2 weeks later. Thrombocytopenia and anemia are less severe. Erythema at the injection site ("flare reaction") is benign, in contrast to extravasation, which can lead to serious local complications, such as severe necrosis of surrounding tissues. Inflammation at sites of previous radiation ("radiation recall") can lead to unanticipated complications, including pericarditis, pleural effusion, and skin rash. The incidence of nausea, vomiting, and alopecia is lower with epirubicin compared with doxorubicin.[115]

The toxicity profile of pegylated liposomal doxorubicin is characterized by mucosal and cutaneous toxicities, mild myelosuppression, decreased cardiotoxicity compared with doxorubicin and minimal alopecia. Palmar-plantar erythrodysesthesia is the most common grade 3–4 toxicity, frequently at the second or third cycle, and occurs at a higher frequency than with patients receiving conventional doxorubicin.[133] The mucocutaneous toxicities are dose-limiting. The pathophysiology of palmar-plantar erythrodysesthesia is not well understood. It has been hypothesized that following the local trauma, pegylated liposomal doxorubicin may extravasate via the eccrine glands from the deeper microcapillaries in the hands and feet where its accumulation is facilitated by the hydrophilic coating of the liposomes.[134] Reduced cardiotoxicity of pegylated liposomal doxorubicin allows a larger cumulative dose than that of doxorubicin. Acute hypersensitivity reaction may occur usually with the first infusion.[135]

Newer anthracyclines
Although anthracyclines have a wide spectrum of activity, structural, pharmacokinetic, and pharmacodynamic characteristics somewhat limit their efficacy and safety. To circumvent these limitations and to further exploit its activity, newer anthracyclines and anthracycline conjugates have been developed.

Amrubicin is a completely synthetic anthracycline with a structure similar to doxorubicin and potent TOP2 inhibitory activity that is available only in Japan where it is approved for use in NSCLC and SCLC.[136] Amrubicin itself has weak antitumor effects and needs to be converted to its active form, amrubicinol, to be effective.[137] In preclinical studies amrubicin caused almost no cardiotoxicity. The lower cardiotoxicity of amrubicin has been attributed to lower levels of accumulation and metabolic advantages over doxorubicin.[138] In second-line treatment of SCLC, although it was associated with better response rates, amrubicin did not improve survival compared with topotecan.[139] As first-line treatment for SCLC, amrubicin plus cisplatin was inferior to irinotecan plus amrubicin.[140]

Anthracenediones

Mitoxantrone (Figure 3e) is a potent inhibitor of TOP2 derived in part from an early hypothesis that the cardiotoxicity of the anthracyclines might depend on the presence of an amino sugar.[141] Since the aglycones of the cardiac glycosides have less cardiotoxic potency than the parent compounds, it was thought that a polycyclic aromatic molecule that intercalates with DNA but does not have an amino sugar, might be an effective antitumor agent without cardiotoxicity. The antitumor spectrum of mitoxantrone is limited compared to that of doxorubicin. Mitoxantrone is used in the initial treatment of acute nonlymphocytic leukemias and is active in advanced castrate-resistant prostate cancer and breast cancer. The DLT of mitoxantrone is leukopenia in patients with solid tumors, whereas stomatitis may be dose limiting in patients with leukemia. Other adverse effects are usually mild or moderate. Cardiotoxicity, particularly congestive heart failure, may be of concern, especially in patients previously treated with anthracyclines, mediastinal irradiation, or patients with cardiovascular disease.

Pixantrone (Figure 3e) is an aza-anthracenedione with structural similarity to mitoxantrone. In preclinical models, compared with doxorubicin, pixantrone showed enhanced activity and decreased cardiotoxicity with decreased free radical formation.[142] Salvage therapy with pixantrone monotherapy has received conditional marketing authorization in the European Union for the treatment of patients with multiply relapsed or refractory aggressive non-Hodgkin's B-cell lymphoma.[143] The recommended dose of pixantrone is 50 mg/m^2 administered on days 1, 8, and 15 of each 28-day cycle for up to six cycles. The most common side effects with pixantrone are myelosuppression (particularly neutropenia) nausea, vomiting, and asthenia. It is not approved for use in the United States.

Epipodophyllotoxins

Podophyllotoxin is a natural product isolated from *Podophyllum peltatum* and *Podophyllum emodi*.[144] Although the anticancer activity of podophyllotoxin and selected derivatives were known in the 1940s, the prohibitive toxicity of podophyllin precluded further development. Demethylepipodophyllotoxin TOP2 inhibitors are podophyllotoxin derivatives, that resulted from efforts to identify agents that retained antineoplastic activity but had less toxicity.

Etoposide

Etoposide (VP-16) (Figure 3d) was the first agent to be identified as a TOP2 inhibiting anticancer drug.[145] As with several other topoisomerase inhibitors, the appreciation of its clinical activity and approval preceded the understanding of its mechanism of action and pharmacology.

Clinical pharmacology
Etoposide is not water-soluble, which presents difficulties for rapid administration and drug hypersensitivity reactions related to the vehicles utilized as solubilizers. Etoposide phosphate, an ester of etoposide that is soluble at concentrations up to 20 mg/mL, is a result of efforts to overcome this issue and is FDA-approved for IV use.[146] The water solubility of etoposide phosphate also alleviates the risk of drug precipitation during IV administration. *In vivo* etoposide phosphate is rapidly converted to the active moiety, etoposide, by dephosphorylation. The pharmacokinetic profile, toxicity, and clinical activity of etoposide phosphate are similar to that of etoposide.

Etoposide exhibits biphasic pharmacokinetics with a distribution half-life of approximately 1.5 h and terminal elimination half-life ranging from 4–11 h. There is a linear relationship between the AUC and peak plasma concentrations achieved following IV administration.[147] CSF concentrations of etoposide, albeit lower than in extracerebral tumors and in plasma, may exceed minimum cytotoxic levels and may be useful in CNS-directed therapy.[148]

Etoposide is highly bound to plasma proteins with an average free plasma fraction of 6%. Since free drug is biologically active, conditions that decrease protein binding increase the pharmacological effect of the drug.[149] Etoposide clearance is modestly decreased in patients with renal failure, and dose modification is recommended in patients with moderate renal impairment. Biliary excretion represents a minor route of elimination and clearance is not affected in hepatic obstruction.[150]

Although the typical route of administration is IV, an oral formulation of etoposide is available.[151] Bioavailability of oral etoposide is widely variable both within and between patients as compared to the IV route and ranges from 40% to 75%. Oral bioavailability also varies with drug dose and is better at lower doses.[152] Despite its limitations, oral etoposide allows long-term drug administration and is FDA-approved.

Clinical use

Etoposide is approved for use in combination with other agents in refractory testicular tumors and in first-line treatment of SCLC. Etoposide has also shown clinical activity in other tumor types, including non-Hodgkin's lymphomas, leukemias, Kaposi's sarcoma, neuroblastoma, and soft-tissue sarcomas. It is also an important component of preparatory regimens given prior to BM and peripheral stem-cell rescue.

Schedule of administration

Etoposide is administered combined with other agents at 35–50 mg/m^2 IV for 4–5 days every 21–28 days in SCLC. The typical doses for testicular cancer are 50–100 mg/m^2/day for days 1–5 or 100 mg/m^2/day on days 1, 3, and 5 repeated every 21–28 days.

The duration of exposure to etoposide is an important determinant of activity with many studies indicating that prolonged administration maximizes activity.[153,154] In SCLC, the 3- to 5-day schedule has greater efficacy than single-day administration.[154,155] To determine whether administration schedules longer than a standard 3- to 5-day treatment might further improve the therapeutic index of etoposide, prolonged oral dose-regimens were developed. However, in Phase III trials, patients with SCLC who were treated with oral etoposide for 21 days did not have any improvement in response rates or survival compared with those receiving the drug for 3–5 days.[156]

Toxicity

Myelosuppression is the major DLT of etoposide, IV or orally. Granulocyte and platelet nadirs occur 7–14 days and 9–16 days, respectively, after drug administration. BM recovery is usually complete by day 20. Other possible toxicities include allergic or other infusion reactions, which manifest as fever, bronchospasm, and hypotension. Toxicities associated with oral etoposide include nausea, vomiting, and mucositis.

Teniposide

Teniposide (VM-16) (Figure 3d), an etoposide analogue, is a semisynthetic derivative of podophyllotoxin. Teniposide differs from etoposide by its sugar ring. Although it was isolated and evaluated in patients before etoposide, early concerns about hypersensitivity reactions and use at low doses led to slower development of this drug.[151] *In vitro*, teniposide is more potent than etoposide in killing cancer cells possibly related to its better cellular uptake.[157–159] A greater fraction of teniposide is protein-bound relative to etoposide,[160] and renal function is less relevant to teniposide clearance.[161] Myelosuppression is the DLT for teniposide. It can also produce hypersensitivity reactions. Teniposide is approved for the treatment of refractory childhood ALL. Few studies have directly compared the activity of these two agents.

Therapy-related secondary AML (t-AML)

One of the major complications of TOP2 inhibitors, especially etoposide and mitoxantrone, is acute secondary leukemia, occurring in approximately 5% of patients. Therapy-related acute myelocytic leukemias (t-AMLs) are characterized by their relatively rapid onset (they can occur only a few months after therapy) and the presence of recurrent balanced translocations involving the mixed lineage leukemia (MLL) locus on 11q23 and over 50 partner genes.[162] The proposed molecular mechanism is by the disjoining of two drug-trapped TOP2ccs on different chromosomes in relationship with transcription collisions and illegitimate rejoining.[163] TOP2β has been implicated in the generation of these disjoined cleavage complexes.[163,164]

Pharmacogenomics

Genetic variants in drug-metabolizing enzymes, transporters, and other proteins have been shown to influence the pharmacology of topoisomerase inhibitors including irinotecan and doxorubicin. An understanding of these genetic variants will allow for individualized dosing of each drug, with the aim of increasing therapeutic efficacy and minimizing toxicity.

Irinotecan

UDP-glucuronosyl transferase 1A

Several enzymes and drug transporters are involved in the elimination of irinotecan. Variations in irinotecan dosing are affected by genetic polymorphisms in the *UGT1A*, *CYP3A*, and *ABC* gene families. Several allelic variants of these genes alter functional activity, thereby contributing to inter-individual differences in irinotecan metabolism and predisposing patients to variable toxicity.

SNPs have been described in the promoter and coding regions of the *UGT1A1* gene, which significantly impact irinotecan metabolism and toxicity.[165,166] The variants are described as alleles denoted by the * symbol followed by a number. While there are over 113 gene variants, only several variants have been described to influence irinotecan pharmacodynamics (*6, *27, *28, *36, *37, *60, *93). Clinically relevant variants are *28 and *6. Clearance of SN-38 via this pathway contributes to inter-individual variability in irinotecan-induced toxicity that is associated with a variant allele in the proximal promoter region of *UGT1A1* (*UGT1A1*28*). The *UGT1A1*28* (rs8175347, also referred to as the UGT1A1 7/7 genotype) allele has a seventh dinucleotide repeat in the TATA box of the promoter region, while the wildtype *UGT1A1*1* allele has six repeats, resulting in reduced rates of transcription, protein expression, and enzyme activity. The frequency of *UGT1A1*28* in the Caucasian and African American populations is 0.26–0.31 and 0.42–0.56, respectively.[167,168] Patients with the UGT1A1*28 homozygous variant have significantly higher systemic exposure to SN-38 and lower plasma SN-38G/SN-38 ratio than *1/*1 patients and commonly develop dose-limiting severe diarrhea or neutropenia.[59,169–172] The *UGT1A1*6* polymorphism is characterized by a single-nucleotide substitution in exon 1 of *UGT1A1* resulting in decreased expression and increased toxicity similar to *UGT1A1*28*. The *UGT1A1*6* (rs4148323) variant occurs at a higher frequency (0.13–0.25) in Asians[173] and has been associated with irinotecan-related diarrhea and neutropenia in Asians.[169,174,175]

The concept of *UGT1A1* genotype-directed dosing of irinotecan has been evaluated in patients receiving irinotecan monotherapy in an every-2-week regimen[176] or an every-3-week regimen[177] or in combination therapy involving irinotecan with fluorouracil,[178,179] capecitabine,[180] or capecitabine and oxaliplatin.[181] Despite differences in patient population and regimens, the general consensus with these studies is that patients with the *28/*28 genotype are at the highest risk of irinotecan-related toxicity and require a dose reduction of up to 40%. Since 2005, the US FDA has recommended a reduction of the initial irinotecan dose (by at least one level) for individuals who are UGT1A1*28 homozygous variant because they are at increased risk for neutropenia.

Numerous meta-analyses have evaluated the association of *28/*28 genotype to the risk of toxicity as a function of irinotecan dose. Hoskins et al. ($n = 821$) showed that severe hematotoxicity was significantly higher in *28/*28 patients for both high/intermediate doses.[58] Hu et al. ($n = 1998$) demonstrated that the risk of grade 3–4 neutropenia is significantly increased in *28/*28 patients, and is higher for high doses compared to intermediate or low doses.[182] A recent meta-analysis of 16 colorectal cancer studies ($n = 2328$), revealed that regardless of irinotecan dose, grade 3–4 neutropenia occurred more frequently in patients with *28/*28 as compared to *1/*1 (OR = 4.79, 95% CI = 3.28–7.01, $p < 0.000,01$) or *1/*28 (OR = 3.44, 95% CI = 2.45–4.82, $p < 0.000,01$).[183]

Studies of irinotecan pharmacogenetics have mainly focused on the association of UGT1A1*28 allele to irinotecan-related toxicity. The clinical utility of UGT1A1*28 genotyping for preemptive dose reductions depends on whether UGT1A1*28 also affects treatment efficacy and studies to date have been contradictory. A recent meta-analysis found no difference between the UGT1A1*28 genotypes (homozygous, heterozygous, or wild-type) and patient survival related to irinotecan therapy and included data for OS ($n = 1524$ patients) and progression-free survival (PFS) ($n = 1494$ patients).[184] Therefore, while genotyping for *28 was shown to be cost-effective, clinical utility was classified as unclear.[185,186] Clinical implementation remains to be determined since studies to date on whether *28 affects treatment efficacy have been contradictory and since most episodes of severe toxicity (neutropenia or diarrhea) are managed by dose reduction in subsequent cycles.

In addition to UGT1A1, variants in the UGT1A7 and UGT1A9 genes are also involved in inter-patient irinotecan-related toxicity differences. UGT1A7 is primarily involved in extra-hepatic metabolism (located in the intestine) and is responsible for detoxifying SN-38, whereas UGT1A9 is necessary for conjugation of SN-38 to SN-38G in the liver.[187] UGT1A7*2, UGT1A7*3, or UGT1A7*4, polymorphisms may result in altered irinotecan metabolism and related toxicity.[188–191] Patients homozygous for UGT1A9*1 have been reported to have more severe diarrhea than UGT1A9*9 or UGT1A9*22 carriers.[191,192]

Collectively, these studies suggest that clinical outcomes are likely the result of complex combined signature of the haplotypes involving key genomic variations in UGT metabolic detoxification (UGT1A1, UGT1A7, and UGT1A9) pathways.[187,190]

CYP3A and drug transporters

The CYP3A4 and CYP3A5 genes are crucial for oxidative metabolism of irinotecan to inactive metabolites 7-ethyl-10-[4-N-(5-aminopentanoic acid)-1-piperidino]-carbonyloxycamptothecin (APC) and 7-ethyl-10-(4-amino-1-piperidino)-carbonyloxycamptothecin], (NPC). In vitro studies have shown variants (CYP3A4*16 or CYP3A4*18 or CYP3A5*3) with decreased activity, resulting in reduced rates of oxidative metabolism and hence less APC and NPC metabolite production.[192,193] However, correlations between these genetic variants and irinotecan treatment outcomes remain to be elucidated.

Elimination of irinotecan is also dependent on the ABC drug transporters, present on the bile canalicular membrane that facilitates the secretion of irinotecan and its metabolites.[194] Specific polymorphisms of ABCB1 and ABCC2 can influence irinotecan drug disposition and tumor response.[195] While the ABCC2*2 haplotype is associated with lower rates of irinotecan-induced diarrhea,[196] patients with ABCC2 (rs3740066) and ABCG2 (rs2231137) variants experience higher rates of grade 3 diarrhea.[192,197,198] A pharmacogenomic profile of irinotecan-induced gastrointestinal toxicity using the novel drug-metabolizing enzyme and transporter (DMET) microarray genotyping platform identified three additional SNPs mapping to the ABCG1, ABCC5, and OATP1B1/SLCO1B1 transporter genes in patients with colorectal cancer.[199] Another study demonstrated that OATP1B1 and tumor OATP1B3 modulated exposure, toxicity, and survival after irinotecan-based chemotherapy.[200]

Doxorubicin

Genetic polymorphisms exist in genes that mediate the metabolism, transport, and pharmacological actions of doxorubicin, but the clinical significance of these variants and their impact on doxorubicin efficacy and toxicity has only been evaluated in recent years. Doxorubicin is characterized by substantial interindividual variations in pharmacokinetic parameters[201] and the cumulative dose is the most significant risk factor for doxorubicin-induced cardiotoxicity.

The major metabolite of doxorubicin is 13-C alcohol, doxorubicinol; metabolized by enzymes carbonyl reductase 1 (CBR1), carbonyl reductase 3 (CBR3), and aldo-keto reductase 1C3 (AKR1C3). Functional SNPs have been characterized in CBR1, CBR3, and AKR1C3. Two SNPs (rs1143663 and rs9024) have been described in CBR1 that have a functional impact on CBR1 activity[202] or expression.[203] To date, there are limited studies investigating the influence of genetic polymorphisms in the CBR1 gene and no association was seen in a population of patients with breast cancer.[204] However, patients who were heterozygous for rs9024 and another CBR1 variant with which it is in linkage disequilibrium (LD) had a lower clearance of doxorubicin.[205]

Two common SNPs in CBR3 G730A (rs1056892) and G11A (rs8133052) in LD were shown in vitro to have reduced catalytic efficiency compared with wildtype.[206] It has been suggested that the wild-type CBR3 G730A allele, which exhibits higher activity and increased expression, is associated with the risk of anthracycline-related congestive heart failure among childhood cancer survivors.[207] Higher CBR3 expression was found in tumor tissues from Asian patients with breast cancer with the variant being associated with higher doxorubicinol AUC.[204] In the same cohort, the G11A minor allele was associated with greater hematologic toxicity and efficacy in addition to an influence on doxorubicin pharmacokinetics and CBR expression.[204] Voon et al. also showed that the G11A minor allele correlated with lower doxorubicinol AUC and longer OS.[208] However, other studies in patients with breast cancer showed no effect of these variants on doxorubicin pharmacokinetics[205] or survival.[209]

An in vitro study has demonstrated that two nonsynonymous SNPs in exon 5 of the aldo-keto reductase 1C3 (AKR1C3) gene 508 C>T (rs35575889) and 538 C>T (rs34186955) encode enzymes that significantly reduced doxorubicin metabolism compared with wild type.[210] In Asian patients with breast cancer, the above two SNPs were not identified; however, two intronic variants IVS4−212 C>G (rs1937840) and IVS4+218 G>A (rs1937841) were detected. The *AKR1C3* IVS4−212 GG allele was associated with greater hematologic toxicity and longer OS and PFS after doxorubicin-based therapy.[208]

Several transporters have been shown to be involved transporting doxorubicin including ABCB1, ABCC1, ABCC2, ABCG2, RALBP1, and SLC22A16. Doxorubicin is a substrate for ABCB1, and doxorubicin efflux mediated by ABCB1 can lead to decreased efficacy in laboratory and animal models. Inhibition of ABCB1 may lead to increased doxorubicin-induced toxicity. Three high frequency *ABCB1* polymorphisms, 1236C>T (rs1128503), 2677G>A/T (rs2032582), and 3435C>T (rs1045642) have been proposed to alter pharmacokinetics of substrate drugs, but there has been some controversy in the literature, with both positive and negative studies. This is likely due to different patient populations, other co-variants, and individual substrate drug. One small study in Asian patients noted impaired doxorubicin pharmacokinetics, resulting in significantly increased exposure levels and reduced clearance; however, the study involved only a small number of patients.[211] Moreover, while the 2677A allele was associated with a shorter OS and PFS in patients with breast cancer treated with adjuvant doxorubicin and cyclophosphamide, the C1236T, G2677T, and C3435T SNPs had no effect on survival.[212] In Asian patients with breast cancer on a doxorubicin-based regimen, *ABCB1* G2677T/A was associated with drug clearance and platelet toxicity, and *ABCB1* IVS26+59 T>G was associated with OS.[208] The 3435T allele was significantly correlated with a prolonged PFS in patients with multiple myeloma treated with doxorubicin and bortezomib, consistent with the hypothesized loss of function or expression.[213] Other studies have found no impact of ABCB1 genotypes in response to doxorubicin.[214] An additional *ABCB1* G1199T/A (rs2229109) variant found in European populations, not in LD with the other three, is less well studied clinically but has been shown to have a functional impact on doxorubicin efflux and toxicity.[215] Given the inconsistencies in studies across populations, the functional significance of *ABCB1* SNPs on the disposition of doxorubicin remains controversial.

ABCG2-mediated resistance to doxorubicin is dependent on an acquired mutation (R482T/G).[216] In patients with breast cancer, no significant influences on doxorubicin pharmacokinetic parameters were observed in relation to the *ABCG2* 421C>A polymorphism,[211] which has been previously demonstrated to have less ATPase activity than wild type.[217] Expression of other ABC family members, including ABCB5, ABCB8, ABCC5, and RALBP1, also confers resistance to doxorubicin; however, the clinical implications remain unknown.

The organic cation exporter SLC22A16 transports doxorubicin into the cell. Homozygotes of the *SLC22A16* A146G (rs714368) may have a higher AUC for doxorubicin[218] and carriers of the same minor allele, and other SLC22A16 SNPs (T312C and T755C variants) in LD, are less likely to have a dose delay during adjuvant doxorubicin and cyclophosphamide therapy for breast cancer.[212] A higher incidence of dose delay, indicative of increased toxicity, was seen in SLC22A16 T1226C (rs12210538) carriers.[212]

In a study of pharmacogenomic predictors of anthracycline-induced cardiotoxicity involving SNPs of 82 genes from 1697 patients, 3.2% of whom developed the toxicity acutely or chronically, five significant associations were identified and the polymorphisms were located in genes of the NAD(P)H oxidase complex (CYBA rs4673, NCF4 rs1883112, and RAC2 rs13058338), and doxorubicin transporters (*ABCC1* rs45511401, *ABCC2* rs8187694, and rs8187710).[219] Rossi et al. also showed *CYBA* rs4673 and *NCF4* rs1883112 being associated with toxicity in patients with lymphoma treated with doxorubicin-containing chemotherapy.[220] Polymorphisms in genes that reduce ROS may result in increased efficacy or toxicity following doxorubicin treatment and may include variants of superoxide dismutase II (*SOD2*), glutathione S-transferases (GSTs), or NAD(P)H:quinone oxidoreductase 1 (*NQO1*). Furthermore, pharmacogenetic studies have evaluated gene copy number of *ERBB2* and *TOP2A* as predictors of response to doxorubicin with contradictory results.[221–223]

Daunorubicin, epirubicin, and etoposide

Limited data are available on pharmacogenomics of daunorubicin, epirubicin, or etoposide. In pediatric patients, the use of the DMET platform showed associations between *FMO3* and *GSTP1* haplotypes with daunorubicin PK that could potentially affect efficacy and toxicity.[224] The major inactivation pathway for epirubicin and epirubicinol is glucuronidation catalyzed by uridine diphosphate–glucuronosyltransferase 2B7 (UGT2B7). Patients with breast cancer with the *UGT2B7* 802 C>T homozygous minor allele may benefit most from adjuvant epirubicin-based chemotherapy.[225] In a adjuvant breast cancer treatment with cyclophosphamide, epirubicin, and 5-fluorouracil, an NQO2 exonic SNP was associated with a higher exposure to epirubicinol relative to epirubicin. Other polymorphic variants of NQO1, carbonyl reductase, UGT enzymes, and transporters had no influence on epirubicin or its metabolite.[226] Finally, 63 genetic variants that contribute to etoposide-induced cytotoxicity were identified through a whole-genome association study using data generated on the HapMap cell lines.[227]

Perspectives

Topoisomerase inhibitors represent a basic component of the anticancer armamentarium. Four points are relevant to their future use: (1) novel formulations and targeted delivery approaches (exemplified by liposomes and antibody conjugates) may enable the selective targeting of tumors while limiting DLTs; (2) detailed understanding of the chemical limitation of the drugs (chemical instability of the camptothecins and redox reactions of the anthracyclines) and molecular mechanisms of toxicities should enable the design of novel topoisomerase inhibitors, such as the noncamptothecin TOP1 inhibitors (indenoisoquinoline LMP derivatives) and TOP2α-specific inhibitors that would avoid serious toxicities related to TOP2β inhibition (cardiotoxicity of the anthracyclines and secondary leukemia induced by the epipodophyllotoxins); (3) better understanding of the molecular basis of sensitivity will optimize combinations of anticancer agents[11,12] including PARP, ATR, and CHK1 inhibitors for TOP1 inhibitors.[83] To date, combinations have been developed empirically, but going forward a better understanding of genomics and epigenomics will allow development of rational combination therapies. (4) Finally, it remains critically important to predict the activity of topoisomerase inhibitors and precisely select patients based on modern technology such as tumor genomic signatures[11,12,228] including BRCAness and SLFN11.[13] These agents, while identified before the era of personalized medicine, do have specific cellular targets, and it is important to understand them as such. It is also important to identify the molecular basis of sensitivity and resistance, so that future strategies of optimal tumor-targeted therapy can be developed with predicted sensitivity based on tumor molecular signatures.

Key references

The complete reference list can be found on Vital Source version of this title, see inside front cover.

25. Pommier Y, Leo E, Zhang H, et al. DNA topoisomerases and their poisoning by anticancer and antibacterial drugs. *Chem Biol.* 2010;**17**(5):421–433.
34. Herben VMM, Huinink WWTB, Beijnen JH. Clinical pharmacokinetics of topotecan. *Clin Pharmacokinet.* 1996;**31**(2):85–102.
35. OReilly S, Rowinsky EK, Slichenmyer W, et al. Phase I and pharmacologic study of topotecan in patients with impaired renal function. *J Clin Oncol.* 1996;**14**(12):3062–3073.
47. Kummar S, Chen A, Ji JP, et al. Phase I study of PARP inhibitor ABT-888 in combination with topotecan in adults with refractory solid tumors and lymphomas. *Cancer Res.* 2011;**71**(17):5626–5634.
50. Sehouli J, Stengel D, Harter P, et al. Topotecan weekly versus conventional 5-day schedule in patients with platinum-resistant ovarian cancer: a randomized multicenter phase II trial of the North-Eastern German society of gynecological oncology ovarian cancer study group. *J Clin Oncol.* 2011;**29**(2):242–248.
57. Tanizawa A, Fujimori A, Fujimori Y, et al. Comparison of topoisomerase I inhibition, DNA damage, and cytotoxicity of camptothecin derivatives presently in clinical trials. *J Natl Cancer Inst.* 1994;**86**:836–842.
59. Iyer L, Das S, Janisch L, et al. UGT1A1*28 polymorphism as a determinant of irinotecan disposition and toxicity. *Pharmacogenom J.* 2002;**2**(1):43–47.
71. Fuchs CS, Moore MR, Harker G, et al. Phase III comparison of two irinotecan dosing regimens in second-line therapy of metastatic colorectal cancer. *J Clin Oncol.* 2003;**21**(5):807–814.
73. Takasuna K, Hagiwara T, Hirohashi M, et al. Involvement of beta-glucuronidase in intestinal microflora in the intestinal toxicity of the antitumor camptothecin derivative irinotecan hydrochloride (CPT-11) in rats. *Cancer Res.* 1996;**56**(16):3752–3757.
77. Stein A, Voigt W, Jordan K. Chemotherapy-induced diarrhea: pathophysiology, frequency and guideline-based management. *Ther Adv Med Oncol.* 2010;**2**(1):51–63.
81. Pommier Y, Cushman M. The indenoisoquinoline noncamptothecin topoisomerase I inhibitors: update and perspectives. *Mol Cancer Ther.* 2009;**8**(5):1008–1014.
82. Takagi K, Dexheimer TS, Redon C, et al. Novel E-ring camptothecin keto analogues (S38809 and S39625) are stable, potent, and selective topoisomerase I inhibitors without being substrates of drug efflux transporters. *Mol Cancer Ther.* 2007;**6**(12 Pt 1):3229–3238.
89. Wang-Gillam A, Li CP, Bodoky G, et al. Nanoliposomal irinotecan with fluorouracil and folinic acid in metastatic pancreatic cancer after previous gemcitabine-based therapy (NAPOLI-1): a global, randomised, open-label, phase 3 trial. *Lancet.* 2016;**387**(10018):545–557.
92. Modi S, Saura C, Yamashita T, et al. Trastuzumab deruxtecan in previously treated HER2-positive breast cancer. *N Engl J Med.* 2020;**382**(7):610–621.
98. Bardia A, Mayer IA, Vahdat LT, et al. Sacituzumab govitecan-hziy in refractory metastatic triple-negative breast cancer. *N Engl J Med.* 2019;**380**(8):741–751.
101. Bobrov V, Skobeleva N, Restifo D, et al. Targeted delivery of chemotherapy using HSP90 inhibitor drug conjugates is highly active against pancreatic cancer models. *Oncotarget.* 2017;**8**(3):4399–4409.
102. Gaponova AV, Nikonova AS, Deneka A, et al. A novel HSP90 inhibitor-drug conjugate to SN38 is highly effective in small cell lung cancer. *Clin Cancer Res.* 2016;**22**(20):5120–5129.
104. Tewey KM, Rowe TC, Yang L, et al. Adriamycin-induced DNA damage mediated by mammalian DNA topoisomerase II. *Science.* 1984;**226**(4673):466–468.
113. Orlowski RZ, Nagler A, Sonneveld P, et al. Randomized phase III study of pegylated liposomal doxorubicin plus bortezomib compared with bortezomib alone in relapsed or refractory multiple myeloma: combination therapy improves time to progression. *J Clin Oncol.* 2007;**25**(25):3892–3901.
121. Singal PK, Iliskovic N. Doxorubicin-induced cardiomyopathy. *N Engl J Med.* 1998;**339**(13):900–905.
125. Zhang S, Liu X, Bawa-Khalfe T, et al. Identification of the molecular basis of doxorubicin-induced cardiotoxicity. *Nat Med.* 2012;**18**(11):1639–1642.
126. Khiati S, Seol Y, Agama K, et al. Poisoning of mitochondrial topoisomerase I by lamellarin D. *Mol Pharmacol.* 2014;**86**(2):193–199.
131. Swain SM, Whaley FS, Gerber MC, et al. Cardioprotection with dexrazoxane for doxorubicin-containing therapy in advanced breast cancer. *J Clin Oncol.* 1997;**15**(4):1318–1332.
132. Hensley ML, Hagerty KL, Kewalramani T, et al. American society of clinical oncology 2008 clinical practice guideline update: use of chemotherapy and radiation therapy protectants. *J Clin Oncol.* 2009;**27**(1):127–145.
135. Uziely B, Jeffers S, Isacson R, et al. Liposomal doxorubicin: antitumor activity and unique toxicities during two complementary phase I studies. *J Clin Oncol.* 1995;**13**(7):1777–1785.
140. Satouchi M, Kotani Y, Shibata T, et al. Phase III study comparing amrubicin plus cisplatin with irinotecan plus cisplatin in the treatment of extensive-disease small-cell lung cancer: JCOG 0509. *J Clin Oncol.* 2014;**32**(12):1262–1268.
143. Pettengell R, Coiffier B, Narayanan G, et al. Pixantrone dimaleate versus other chemotherapeutic agents as a single-agent salvage treatment in patients with relapsed or refractory aggressive non-Hodgkin lymphoma: a phase 3, multicentre, open-label, randomised trial. *Lancet Oncol.* 2012;**13**(7):696–706.
148. Relling MV, Mahmoud HH, Pui CH, et al. Etoposide achieves potentially cytotoxic concentrations in CSF of children with acute lymphoblastic leukemia. *J Clin Oncol.* 1996;**14**(2):399–404.
154. Slevin ML, Clark PI, Joel SP, et al. A randomized trial to evaluate the effect of schedule on the activity of etoposide in small-cell lung cancer. *J Clin Oncol.* 1989;**7**(9):1333–1340.
156. Miller AA, Herndon JE 2nd, Hollis DR, et al. Schedule dependency of 21-day oral versus 3-day intravenous etoposide in combination with intravenous cisplatin in extensive-stage small-cell lung cancer: a randomized phase III study of the cancer and leukemia group B. *J Clin Oncol.* 1995;**13**(8):1871–1879.
158. Long BH, Musial ST, Brattain MG. Single- and double-strand DNA breakage and repair in human lung adenocarcinoma cells exposed to etoposide and teniposide. *Cancer Res.* 1985;**45**(7):3106–3112.
163. Cowell IG, Sondka Z, Smith K, et al. Model for MLL translocations in therapy-related leukemia involving topoisomerase IIbeta-mediated DNA strand breaks and gene proximity. *Proc Natl Acad Sci U S A.* 2012;**109**(23):8989–8994.
164. Azarova AM, Lyu YL, Lin CP, et al. From the cover: roles of DNA topoisomerase II isozymes in chemotherapy and secondary malignancies. *Proc Natl Acad Sci U S A.* 2007;**104**(26):11014–11019.
168. Beutler E, Gelbart T, Demina A. Racial variability in the UDP-glucuronosyltransferase 1 (UGT1A1) promoter: a balanced polymorphism for regulation of bilirubin metabolism? *Proc Natl Acad Sci U S A.* 1998;**95**(14):8170–8174.
171. Innocenti F, Undevia SD, Iyer L, et al. Genetic variants in the UDP-glucuronosyltransferase 1A1 gene predict the risk of severe neutropenia of irinotecan. *J Clin Oncol.* 2004;**22**(8):1382–1388.
182. Hu ZY, Yu Q, Pei Q, et al. Dose-dependent association between UGT1A1*28 genotype and irinotecan-induced neutropenia: low doses also increase risk. *Clin Cancer Res.* 2010;**16**(15):3832–3842.
190. Cecchin E, Innocenti F, D'Andrea M, et al. Predictive role of the UGT1A1, UGT1A7, and UGT1A9 genetic variants and their haplotypes on the outcome of metastatic colorectal cancer patients treated with fluorouracil, leucovorin, and irinotecan. *J Clin Oncol.* 2009;**27**(15):2457–2465.
195. Han JY, Lim HS, Yoo YK, et al. Associations of ABCB1, ABCC2, and ABCG2 polymorphisms with irinotecan-pharmacokinetics and clinical outcome in patients with advanced non-small cell lung cancer. *Cancer.* 2007;**110**(1):138–147.
198. Michael M, Thompson M, Hicks RJ, et al. Relationship of hepatic functional imaging to irinotecan pharmacokinetics and genetic parameters of drug elimination. *J Clin Oncol.* 2006;**24**(26):4228–4235.
200. Teft WA, Welch S, Lenehan J, et al. OATP1B1 and tumour OATP1B3 modulate exposure, toxicity, and survival after irinotecan-based chemotherapy. *Br J Cancer.* 2015;**112**(5):857–865.

57 Microtubule inhibitors

Giuseppe Galletti, MD, PhD ∎ *Paraskevi Giannakakou, PhD*

> **Overview**
>
> Central to the ever-growing list of anticancer therapies is the microtubule inhibitors (MTIs), a class of naturally derived compounds that bind tubulin or microtubules and disrupt the function of the cell's cytoskeleton. The vinca alkaloids were among the first drugs to receive FDA approval for the treatment of cancer, even before the α/β-tubulin dimer was identified as their target. Today, 60 years from their entry to the clinic, these microtubule-destabilizing drugs continue to be central in current and widely used chemotherapy regimens. Paclitaxel was the first natural product identified to bind microtubule polymers instead of soluble tubulin dimers, and the prototype of the new class of microtubule-stabilizing drugs. Together, both destabilizing and stabilizing drugs form the family of MTIs, which continues to expand with the clinical approval of several other plant-, marine sponge- and bacteria-derived compounds, such as epothilones, haliconrin B, maytansinoids, and auristatins. Even in the current era of targeted therapies and immune checkpoint inhibitors, MTIs are among the most effective drugs for the treatment of solid tumors and hematologic malignancies. For decades, these drugs were thought to exert their antitumor activity solely by inhibiting cancer cell division. Current evidence demonstrates that MTIs can effectively kill not only dividing but also nondividing interphase cells, which represent the most abundant cell population in patient tumors. In this chapter, we will discuss MTI mechanism of action or "inaction," all the way from molecular interactions to cancer cell effects to patient treatment. Fundamental to this chapter is the thesis that MTIs are "targeted therapies," which is a big departure from the established view that these drugs are nonspecific, generally cytotoxic chemotherapy drugs. Once accepted, this thesis provides previously unrecognized opportunities for precision oncology, taking advantage of the distinct functions and alterations of the MT cytoskeleton in different tumor types and individual patients.

Tubulin and microtubules as drug targets in oncology

Microtubules (MTs) are the backbone of all eukaryotic cells cytoskeleton. They are cylindrical protein polymers composed of α/β-tubulin heterodimers, which are the building block of MTs. These tubulin dimers assemble in a head-to-tail fashion longitudinally to form linear protofilaments, which then associate laterally to form the MT.[1] MTs are highly dynamic structures, as their ends undergo rapid lengthening (polymerization) or shortening (depolymerization), by the addition or removal of tubulin heterodimers, respectively; and their rapid switch between these two states, using energy provided by GTP hydrolysis, is called "dynamic instability."[2–4]

MTs exist in a dynamic chemo-mechanical equilibrium between the soluble pool of tubulin dimers and MT polymers (Figure 1) and their dynamic behavior is a highly regulated process that constitutes the basis for many biological functions such as cell motility, intracellular transport, and cell division.[5] In addition, MTs have inherent polarity characterized by a fast-growing plus-end oriented toward the cell periphery and a less dynamic minus-end embedded in the centrosome, where MTs are nucleated from during interphase, forming a fine and intricate array that fills the entire cytoplasm. Interphase MTs are critically important in cell signaling and intracellular transport as their polarity is recognized by motor proteins that move cargos (organelles, RNA, and proteins) toward the MT minus (dyneins) or plus (kinesins) ends.[6]

During mitosis, the interphase MT array quickly dissolves and reorganizes to form the bipolar mitotic spindle to enable cell division. Mitotic MTs are highly dynamic, continuously surveying the three-dimensional space to capture and align chromosomes at the metaphase plate so that effective separation of sister chromosomes to the opposite poles can proceed.[7] Any interference with MT dynamics or mass will affect the proper chromosome alignment and separation causing mitotic arrest and programmed cell death (apoptosis).[8]

Thus, drugs that bind tubulin or MTs will interfere with all MT functions both during interphase and mitosis.[9]

The basic premise that cancer cells divide much faster than their normal counterparts, together with the profound interruption of mitotic progression induced by microtubule inhibitors (MTIs) observed at the initial preclinical studies,[10] prompted the classification of these drugs as purely "antimitotics."

However, cancer cells spend the majority of their time in interphase, as mitosis occupies less than 2% of cell cycle; which, together with the extremely low mitotic index of tumors in patients (<1%), suggests that the antimitotic effects of MTIs cannot solely account for their overall antitumor activity.[11] Moreover, there is increasing evidence from preclinical and clinical studies that MTI antitumor activity is likely attributed to both the disruption of interphase and mitotic MTs.[12,13] Therefore, we posit that the old classification of this class of drugs as "Anti-Mitotics" is obsolete and does not accurately capture their mechanism of action. Therefore, we propose their reclassification as MTIs, a term that more precisely describes their mechanism of action as functional inhibitors of the microtubule cytoskeleton.

Microtubule inhibitors (MTIs)

MTIs represent one of the most successful classes of cancer chemotherapy drugs. MTIs have the broadest range of clinical indications in oncology as compared to all other classes of cancer chemotherapeutics (Table 1). MTIs are classified based on their effect on the MT polymer mass, into MT-stabilizing and MT-destabilizing drugs. The class of *MT-stabilizing drugs* includes agents that stimulate MT polymerization such as the taxanes (paclitaxel, nab-paclitaxel, docetaxel, and cabazitaxel) and epothilones (ixabepilone). The second group is known as

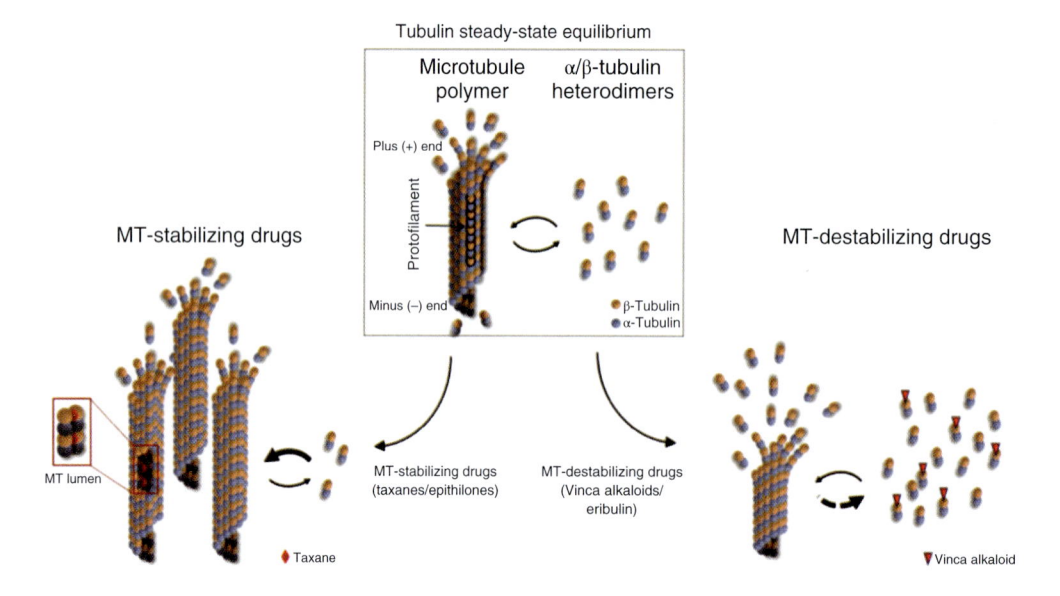

Figure 1 Tubulin dynamic equilibrium and the effect of MTIs. Tubulin exists in a dynamic equilibrium between microtubule (MT) polymers and the pool of soluble tubulin dimers (top panel). This complex and tightly regulated equilibrium is characterized by alternating periods of MT elongation (polymerization) and MT shortening (depolymerization). MT elongation occurs when α/β-tubulin heterodimers are added to the growing end of an existing MT (plus-end) promoting polymerization. When MTs shorten, α/β-tubulin heterodimers are released from the polymer shifting the dynamic equilibrium toward the soluble pool of tubulin and decreasing the MT polymer mass. **The effect of MTIs on tubulin steady-state equilibrium** (bottom panel). MT-stabilizing drugs (e.g., taxanes, epothilones) bind β-tubulin in the MT lumen which "locks" MTs in the polymerized form preventing release, while promoting addition, of α/β-tubulin dimers to the plus-ends of MTs, thereby inducing an increase in the MT polymer mass (thick arrow) (bottom left panel). MT-destabilizing drugs (e.g., vinca alkaloids) bind β-tubulin in the soluble tubulin dimers preventing their incorporation into MT polymers, thereby causing MT depolymerization with a net increase of the soluble tubulin compartment (thick dashed arrow) (bottom right panel).

MT-destabilizing drugs and includes drugs that inhibit MT polymerization, such as the vinca alkaloids (vincristine, vinblastine, vinorelbine, vinflunine, vindesine) and eribulin. In addition, MT-destabilizing drugs make excellent payloads in antibody–drug conjugates (ADCs), such as maytansine conjugated to anti-HER2 antibody (T-DM1) and auristatin conjugated to anti-CD30 antibody (brentuximab vedotin).

Microtubule-stabilizing drugs

Taxanes

Originally isolated from the bark of the yew tree *Taxus Brevifolia*, paclitaxel was the first compound to be identified as MT-stabilizing.[58] Paclitaxel (Taxol®) was approved by the Food and Drug Administration (FDA) for the treatment of ovarian cancer in 1992, and since then it became the prototype of the taxane family of MT-stabilizing drugs (Table 1 and Figure 2a). Subsequently, docetaxel (Taxotere®), a paclitaxel semisynthetic analogue, was FDA approved for the treatment of breast cancer in 1996. More recently, cabazitaxel (Jevtana®), another paclitaxel analog, received FDA approval for the treatment of prostate cancer. As taxanes are large lipophilic drugs with complex chemical structures and poor water solubility, efforts to improve on taxane pharmacology and intratumoral drug delivery resulted in the development and approval of the albumin-bound paclitaxel (nab-paclitaxel, Abraxane®). Currently, taxanes are FDA approved for most of the major solid tumor types including breast, lung, pancreatic, gastric, and prostate cancers (Table 1); while several novel taxane formulations are currently being clinically developed in the USA and other countries (Table 2).

Mechanism of action
All taxanes bind to the β-subunit of the α/β-tubulin dimer in a pocket that faces the inner lumen of MTs.[90,91] The MT polymer is the preferred binding substrate for taxanes, as *in vitro* studies identified early on that taxanes bind MTs with far greater affinity than dimers.[92,93] Taxane binding promotes MT polymerization by favoring addition of new α/β-tubulin dimers to MT plus-ends in the polymer, stabilizing the lateral interactions of protofilaments in the polymer, thereby increasing MT polymer mass[94] (Figure 1).

In cells, taxane binding stabilizes MTs, suppressing MT dynamics and inducing a profound rearrangement of the MT network into thick bundles that cannot execute any of their biological functions in interphase and in mitosis.[13]

This extensive reorganization and stabilization of interphase MTs disables MT-based trafficking, inhibiting the nuclear translocation of several oncogenic transcription factors and DNA repair proteins, causing their inactivation which considerably contributes to the overall taxane antitumor activity.[95-99]

In addition, the taxane-induced suppression of MT dynamics has a deleterious effect in mitotic progression, as MTs are no longer able to properly assemble a functional bipolar spindle that segregates chromosomes into the two daughter cells; instead, they form multipolar spindles with uncongressed chromosomes causing aberrant mitotic arrest and subsequent cell death.[100]

Both MT bundling and aberrant mitotic arrest indicate effective drug-target engagement and are considered hallmarks of taxane cellular activity. The presence of drug-target engagement in patient tumors and patient-derived circulating tumor cells has been clinically associated with response to taxane-based chemotherapy, in prostate and gastric cancers.[101,102]

Table 1 MTIs in clinical oncology.

MTIs	Origin/chemical structure	FDA approved indications (year of approval)	Toxicities	Registration trials (References)
MT-stabilizing drugs				
Paclitaxel (Taxol®; Bristol-Myers Squibb)	Natural product, (originally isolated from the bark of the pacific yew tree *Taxus Brevifolia*), first-in-class MT stabilizing drug	Ovarian Cancer (1992), Breast Cancer (1994), AIDS-related Kaposi's sarcoma (1997), NSCLC (1998)	Myelosuppression (neutropenia), neurotoxicity (peripheral neuropathy), hypersensitivity, nausea, vomit, alopecia	*Ovarian*: Eisenhauer EA et al. J Clin Oncol 1994; 12(12): 2654.[14] *Breast*: Nabholtz JM et al. J Clin Oncol 1996; 14(6): 1858.[15] *Kaposi sarcoma*: Welles L et al. J Clin Oncol 1998; 16:1112.[16] *NSCLC*: Giaccone G et al. J Clin Oncol 1998; 16: 2133.[17]
Docetaxel (Taxotere®; Sanofi-Aventis)	Semisynthetic analog of paclitaxel	Breast Cancer (1996), NSCLC (1999), Prostate Cancer (2004), Gastric Cancer (2006), HNSCC (2006)	Myelosuppression (neutropenia), neurotoxicity (peripheral neuropathy), hypersensitivity, nausea, vomit, alopecia, fluid retention, cardiotoxicity, nail alterations	*Breast*: Nabholtz JM et al. J Clin Oncol 1999; 17(5): 1413.[18] *NSCLC*: Shepherd FA et al. J Clin Oncol 2000; 18(10): 2095.[19] *Prostate*: Tannock IF et al. NEJM 2004; 351(15): 1502.[20] *Gastric*: Van Cutsem E et al. J Clin Oncol 2006; 24(31): 4991.[21] *HNSCC*: Vermorken JB et al NEJM 2007; 357:1695.[22]
Cabazitazel (Jevtana®; Sanofi-Aventis)	Semisynthetic analog of paclitaxel	Prostate Cancer (2010)	Myelosuppression (neutropenia- lower than with paclitaxel or docetaxel), neurotoxicity (peripheral neuropathy, lower than paclitaxel or docetaxel), hypersensitivity, nausea, vomit, alopecia	*CRPC*: de Bono JS et al. Lancet 2010; 376: 1147.[23]
Nab-paclitaxel (Abraxane®; Bristol-Myers Squibb)	Nanoparticle albumin-bound formulation of paclitaxel	Breast Cancer (2005), NSCLC (2012), Pancreatic Cancer (2013)	Myelosuppression (neutropenia), neurotoxicity (peripheral neuropathy), alopecia, nausea, vomit	*Breast*: Gradishar WJ et al. J Clin Oncol 2005; 23(31): 7794.[24] *NSCLC*: Socinski MA et al. J Clin Oncol 2012; 30(17): 2055.[25] *Pancreatic*: von Hoff DD et al. NEJM 2013; 369(18): 1691.[26]
Ixabepilone (Ixempra®; Bristol-Myers Squibb)	Semisynthetic analog of Epothilone B (natural product isolated from the soil bacterium *Sorangium cellulosum*)-binds MTs at the taxane-binding site	Breast Cancer (2007)	Myelosuppression (neutropenia), neurotoxicity (peripheral neuropathy), alopecia	*Breast*: Thomas ES et al. J Clin Oncol 2007; 25(33): 5210.[27]
MT-destabilizing drugs				
Vinblastine (Velban®; Eli Lilly)	Natural product (originally isolated from the Madagascar periwinkle, *Catharanthus roseus*)	Hodgkin's and Non-Hodgkin's Lymphomas (1961), Testicular Cancer, Mycosis Fungoides, Kaposi's Sarcoma, Breast Cancer, Choriocarcinoma, Histiocytosis X	Myelosuppression (neutropenia), injection site reactions, neurotoxicity (peripheral neuropathy), constipation or diarrhea, alopecia, nausea, vomit	*Testicular*: Warwick OH et al. Canada Med Ass J 1961; 85:579.[28] *Hodgkin Lymphoma*: Stutzman L et al. JAMA 1966; 195(3): 173.[29] *Non-Hodgkin Lymphoma*: Mihich E et al. Single agents in cancer chemotherapy; 1971.[30] *Mycosis fungoides*: Scheulen ME et al. J Cancer Res Clin Oncol 1986; 111: S40.[31] *Choriocarcinoma*: Schlaerth JB et al. Am J Obstet Gynecol 1980; 136: 983.[32] *Breast*: Yau JC et al. Cancer 1985; 55(2): 337.[33] *Histiocytosis X*: Gadner H et al. J Pediatr 2001; 138: 728.[34] *Kaposi sarcoma*: Volberding PA et al. Ann Intern Med 1985; 103: 335.[35]

(continued overleaf)

Table 1 (Continued)

MTIs	Origin/chemical structure	FDA approved indications (year of approval)	Toxicities	Registration trials (References)
Vincristine (Oncovin®; Eli Lilly)	Natural product (originally isolated from the Madagascar periwinkle, Catharanthus roseus)	Acute leukemia (1963), Hodgkin's and Non-Hodgkin's Lymphoma, Neuroblastoma, Rhabdomyosarcoma, Wilms' Tumor	Myelosuppression (neutropenia), injection site reactions, neurotoxicity (peripheral neuropathy), constipation or diarrhea, alopecia, nausea, vomit	Acute leukemia: Karon M et al. Pediatrics 1962; 30:791.[36] Neuroblastoma: Windmiller JW et al. Am J Dis Child 1966; 111(1): 75.[37] Wilm's tumor: Sullivan MP et al. JAMA 1967; 202(5): 381.[38] Hodgkin lymphoma: DeVita VT et al. Ann Intern Med 1970; 73:881.[39] Non-Hodgkin lymphoma: Schein PS et al. Ann Intern Med 1976; 85:417.[40] Rhabdomyosarcoma: Maurer HM et al. Cancer 1977; 40(5): 2015.[41]
Vincristine sulfate liposomal injection (Marqibo®; Talon Therapeutics)	Liposomal formulation of vincristine	Philadelphia chromosome-neg acute Lymphoblastic Leukemia (2012)	Myelosuppression (neutropenia); neurotoxicity (peripheral neuropathy), constipation or diarrhea, nausea, vomit	Ph- ALL: O'Brien S et al. J Clin Oncol 2013; 31:676.[42]
Vinorelbine (Navelbine®; Pierre Fabre Group)	Semisynthetic analogue of vinblastine	NSCLC (1994)	Myelosuppression (neutropenia), injection site reactions, neurotoxicity (peripheral neuropathy), constipation or diarrhea, alopecia, nausea, vomit	NSCLC: Le Chevalier T et al. J Clin Oncol 1994; 12: 360.[43]
Vindesine (Eldisine®; Eli Lilly)[a]	Semisynthetic analogue of vinblastine	Acute Lymphocytic Leukemia (1981)[a], Chronic Myelocytic Leukemia (1981)[a], Melanoma (1982)[a], Breast Cancer (1985)[a]	Myelosuppression (neutropenia), injection site reactions, neurotoxicity (peripheral neuropathy), constipation, alopecia, nausea, vomit	ALL: Anderson J et al. Cancer Treat Rep 1981; 65:1015.[44] CML: Mathe G et al. Cancer Treat Rep 1978; 62:805.[45] Melanoma: Carmicheal J et al. Eur J Cancer Clin Oncol 1982; 18(12): 1293.[46] Breast: Paridaens R et al. Eur J Cancer Clin Oncol 1985; 21(5): 595.[47]
Vinflunine (Javlor®; Pierre Fabre Group)[b]	Semisynthetic analogue of vinorelbine	Metastatic Transitional Cell Carcinoma of the Urothelium (2009)[b]	Myelosuppression (neutropenia), injection site reactions, neurotoxicity, constipation or diarrhea, alopecia, nausea, vomit	mTCCU: Bellmund J et al. J Clin Oncol 2009; 27:4454.[48]
Eribulin (Halaven®; Eisai)	Synthetic analogue of halicondrin B (natural compound isolated from the marine sponge Halicondria okadai); binds tubulin near at or the vinca-alkaloid binding site	Breast Cancer (2010), Liposarcoma (2016)	Myelosuppression (neutropenia), injection site reactions, neurotoxicity (peripheral neuropathy), constipation or diarrhea, alopecia, nausea, vomit	Breast: Cortes J et al. Lancet 2011; 377; 914.[49] Liposarcoma: Schoffski P et al. Lancet 2016; 387:1629.[50]

MT-destabilizing drugs as payload in antibody–drug conjugates

MTIs	Origin/chemical structure	FDA approved indications (year of approval)	Toxicities	Registration trials (References)
T-DM1 or ado-trastuzumab emtansine (Kadcyla®; Genentech)	Anti-HER2 antibody conjugated to emtansine–a drug maytansinoid (DM) that binds tubulin at the vinca-alkaloid binding site. Maytansinse was originally isolated from the bark of the African shrub Maytenus ovatus	HER2+ Metastatic (2013) and Early-stage (2019) Breast Cancer	Myelosuppression (thrombocytopenia), neurotoxicity (peripheral neuropathy), cardiotoxicity (left ventricular disfunction), hepatotoxocity.	Metastatic breast: Verma S et al. NEJM 2012; 367:1783.[51] Early-stage breast: von Minckwitz G et al. NEJM 2019; 380: 617.[52]
Brentuximab vedotin (Adcetris®; Seattle Genetics)	Anti-CD30 antibody conjugated to monomethyl auristatin E (MMAE)–a synthetic analog of the natural product Dolastatin 10, originally isolated from the sea hare Dolabella auricularia; binds tubulin near or at the vinca-alkaloid binding site	Relapsed and Refractory Hodgkin Lymphoma and Systemic Anaplastic Large Cell Lymphoma (2011)	Myelosuppression (neutropenia), neurotoxicity (peripheral neuropathy), hypersensitivity reactions, diarrhea, progressive multifocal leukoencephalopathy	Hodgkin lymphoma: Younes A et al. J Clin Oncol 2012; 30(18): 2183.[53] ALCL: Pro B et al. J Clin Oncol 2012: 30(18): 2190.[54]

Table 1 (Continued)

MTIs	Origin/chemical structure	FDA approved indications (year of approval)	Toxicities	Registration trials (References)
Enfortumab vedotin (Padcev®; Astellas)	Antinectin 4 monoclonal antibody conjugated to monomethyl auristatin E (MMAE)	Locally advanced or Metastatic Urothelial Cancer (2019)	Neurotoxicity (peripheral neuropathy), dysgeusia, diarrhea, dry eyes, skin rash, alopecia, pruritus, nausea	*Urothelial cancer*: Rosenberg JE et al. J Clin Oncol 2019; 37(29): 2592.[55]
Polatuzumab vedotin (Polivy®; Genentech)	Anti-CD79b monoclonal antibody conjugated to monomethyl auristatin E (MMAE)	Relapsed or refractory diffuse large B-cell lymphoma (2019)	Myelosuppression (neutropenia, thrombocytopenia, anemia), peripheral neuropathy, hypersensitivity reactions, progressive multifocal leukoencephalopathy, fatigue, diarrhea, decreased appetite, pneumonia	*DLBCL*: Sehn LH et al. J Clin Oncol 2020; 38(2): 155.[56]
Belantamab mafodotin (Blenrep®; GlaxoSmithKline)	Anti-BCMA monoclonal antibody conjugated to monomethyl Auristatin F (MMAF)	Relapsed and Refractory Multiple Myeloma (2020)	Myelosuppression (thrombocytopenia), keratopathy, decreased visual acuity, infusion-related reactions, nausea	*Multiple Myeloma*: Lonial S et al Lancet Oncol 2020; 21(2): 207.[57]

[a] Approved in UK and South Africa.
[b] Approved in Europe and Australia.

Clinical pharmacology and indications

Taxanes are generally insoluble in water and this chemical characteristic critically affects taxane pharmacology and their clinical administration. Taxanes are generally delivered as an intravenous infusion that could span from less than one hour to several hours, depending on the drug and the selected schedule. With the exception of nab-paclitaxel, all taxane require prophylactic premedication with corticosteroids (dexamethasone 20 mg, given 14- and 7-h prior infusion) and H2 receptor antagonists (given 30 min before) to reduce the incidence of mild and severe allergic reactions.[103] Paclitaxel is conventionally formulated in 50% alcohol and 50% polyoxyethylated castor oil (Cremophor EL) vehicle, which improves water solubility followed by *i.v.* infusion.[104] Despite its extensive clinical utilization, serious toxic effects such as hypersensitivity reactions are associated to castor oil.[105] To circumvent the requirements of solvent vehicles and to increase paclitaxel solubility in water, a solvent-free formulation of paclitaxel bound to albumin nanoparticles (nab-paclitaxel) was developed and it's now standard treatment in solid tumors.[106]

Docetaxel is formulated in the nonionic surfactant polysorbate 80 (Tween-80) to compensate its poor solubility in water. Similar to Cremophor, polysorbate 80 has been associated with the occurrence of acute hypersensitivity reactions, which can be ameliorated via prophylactic medications.[107] No different than the other two taxanes, cabazitaxel has a lipophilic structure that makes it water-insoluble; thus, the drug is formulated in polysorbate 80, which still necessitates the prophylactic medications required for the other taxoids.

The major pathway of elimination for taxanes is hepatic metabolism through cytochrome P (CYP450) 3A4 and 2C8, followed by biliary excretion.[103,108,109]

Today, taxanes are among the most widely used chemotherapeutics worldwide due to their high antitumor activity and clinical benefit in patients with cancer and are currently used for the treatment of several solid tumors, as monotherapy or as part of multidrug chemotherapy regimens (Table 1). *Paclitaxel* was the first taxane to receive FDA approval for the treatment of ovarian cancer in 1992; since then, it was successfully tested for many cancer types and it is now routinely used for the treatment of early-stage and metastatic breast cancer, non-small-cell lung cancer, and gastric cancer, among the most clinically relevant.[110–113] Based on the observation of severe hypersensitivity reactions during early studies, original Phase I and II clinical trials adopted long infusions (24–96 h infusion) of paclitaxel with doses ranging from 135 to 250 mg/m^2.[114] Subsequently, more convenient shorter infusion schedules (1–3 h), coupled with the administration of proper premedication, were adopted without affecting patient safety.[114] Now the recommended doses of paclitaxel as single agent or in combination range from 135 to 250 mg/m^2 generally as a 3-h infusion repeated every 3 weeks. Weekly schedules of paclitaxel at lower doses (80–100 mg/m^2) have been studied in solid tumors, with good tolerability and reasonable activity, and are now part of the NCCN guidelines for the treatment of breast cancer.[115]

Following the clinical success of paclitaxel, *docetaxel* was extensively tested and it is currently a therapeutic option for several solid tumors, such as breast cancer, non-small-cell lung cancer, prostate cancer, gastric cancer, and head and neck cancer.[20,111,116,117] Docetaxel is routinely administered according to a wide range of schedules (weekly or once every 3 weeks) and dosages (from 80 to 115 mg/m^2)[118] with the most frequently recommended dose being 60–100 mg/m^2 administered as a 1-h *i.v.* infusion every 3 weeks.

Cabazitaxel entered the clinical scene later as a novel potent taxane that showed promising clinical objective response rates in patients who had progressed following docetaxel treatment. Today, cabazitaxel is approved for the treatment of castration-resistant prostate cancer[23,119] at recommended doses ranging from 20 to 25 mg/m^2 as a 1-h infusion every 3 weeks.

Nab-paclitaxel, due to its chemical formulation and the drastically different pharmacokinetics, is delivered as a short (30–40 minutes) *i.v.* infusion without the need of prophylactic medications. It is usually administered as single agent at a dose of 260 mg/m^2 on day 1 of a 21-day cycle; schedules and doses of administration vary when the drug is part of a combination regimen (days 1, 8, and 15 of a 21-day cycle at 100 mg/m^2 or day 1 of a 3–4 week cycle at 125 mg/m^2). Nab-paclitaxel is now routinely used as first-line treatment of advanced/metastatic breast cancer, regardless of prior exposure to other taxanes, and it is also approved for the treatment of pancreatic cancer, in combination with gemcitabine, and for NSCLC, in combination with carboplatin.[24,26,120]

Table 2 MTIs in clinical development.

MTIs	Characteristics	Stage and indication	Clinical trial ID
MT-stabilizing Agents			
Tesetaxel (Odonate Therapeutics™)	Oral taxane (semisynthetic taxane with the addition of two nitrogen-containing functional groups to the taxane core)[59]	Phase III (Breast Cancer)	NCT03326674
Oraxol (Athenex)	Oral formulation of paclitaxel combined with HM30181 P-gp inhibitor[60]	Phase III (Breast Cancer); Phase II (solid tumors)	NCT02594371
			NCT04180384
Liporaxel® (Daehwa Pharmaceutical Co)[a]	Oral paclitaxel[61]	Phase III (Breast Cancer)	NCT03315364
ANG1005/paclitaxel trevatide (Angiochem)	Paclitaxel conjugated to Angiopep-2, a synthetic peptide that binds to LRP1 protein expressed on endothelial cells, to enable BBB crossing[62]	Phase III (Leptomeningeal disease from Breast Cancer)	NCT03613181
ModraDoc006/r (Modra Pharmaceuticals)	Docetaxel combined with ritonavir (P450 and P-gp inhibitor)[63]	Phase II (Prostate Cancer; Breast Cancer)	NCT03890744
			NCT04028388
CPC634 (Cristal Therapeutics)	CriPec® Docetaxel (nanoparticle entrapping docetaxel)[64]	Phase II (Ovarian Cancer)	NCT03742713
Nanoxel®M (Samyang Biopharm)	Docetaxel PM: nanoparticle-based formulation consisting of polymeric micelles (PMs), made with poly(N-vinylpyrrolidone)-block-poly(D,L-lactide) (PVP-b-PDLLA) block polymers, encapsulating the taxane molecule[65]	Phase II (HNSCC; Esophageal Squamous Carcinoma)	NCT02639858
			NCT03585673
NanoDoce® (NanOlogy)	Submicron particle suspension of docetaxel that allows extended drug release (depot) when injected intratumorally[66]	Phase II (Urothelial Cancer)	NCT03636256
NanoPac® (NanOlogy)	Submicron particle suspension of paclitaxel that allows extended drug release (depot) when injected intratumorally[67]	Phase II (NSCLC, Prostate Cancer, Pancreatic Cancer)	NCT04314895
			NCT04221828
			NCT03077685
Genexol® PM (Samyang Biopharm)	Polymeric micelle formulated paclitaxel free of Cremophor EL[68]	Phase II (Hepatocellular Carcinoma)	NCT03008512
SOR007 (NanOlogy)	Nanoparticle paclitaxel ointment[69]	Phase II (Cutaneous metastases)	NCT03101358
TSD-001 (Lipac Oncology)	Proliposomal paclitaxel formulation for intravesical instillation[70]	Phase II (Bladder Cancer)	NCT03081858
Iso-Fludelone (Bristol-Myers Squibb)	Synthetic epothilone B analogue (non-Cremophor EL formulation)[71]	Phase I (advanced solid tumors)	NCT01379287
Oradoxel (Athenex)	Oral formulation of docetaxel combined with HM30181 P-gp inhibitor	Phase I (advanced solid tumors)	NCT02963168
FID-007	Polyethylozaxoline (PEOX) polymer encapsulated paclitaxel[72]	Phase I (advanced solid tumors)	NCT03537690
AR160 (Mayo Clinic)	Nab-paclitaxel noncovalently bound to anti-CD20 monoclonal antibody (rituximab)[73]	Phase I (B-cell Non-Hodgkin Lymphoma)	NCT03003546
Lipusu® (Nanjing Luye Sike Pharma)[b]	Lyophilized liposome-based paclitaxel[74]	Phase IV (squamous NSCLC)	NCT02996214
MT-destabilizing Agents			
Plinabulin (BeyonSpring)	Synthetic analog of the natural product phenylahistin, originally isolated from *Aspergillus ustus*[75,76]; colchicine-binding site MTI with profound vascular disrupting activity (VDA)[77]. Originally developed for the reduction of chemotherapy-induced neutropenia (CIN)[78] [b]	Phase III (NSCLC as anti-CIN); Phase I/II (NSCLC as VDA)	NCT02504489
			NCT02812667
RC48-ADC (RemeGen)	Anti-HER2 monoclonal antibody conjugated to monomethyl auristatin E (MMAE)[79]	Phase III (Breast Cancer)	NCT04400695
SAR408701 (Sanofi)	Anti-CECAM5 monoclonal antibody conjugated to the drug maytansinoid DM4[80]	Phase III (NSCLC)	NCT04154956
Mirvetuximab Soravtansine (ImmunoGen)	Anti-Folate Receptor-α monoclonal antibody conjugated to the drug maytansinoid DM4[81]	Phase III (Ovarian Cancer)	NCT04296890
Depatuximab Mafodotin (Abbvie)	Anti-EGFR monoclonal antibody conjugated to the drug monomethyl auristatin F (MMAF)[82]	Phase III (EGFR-amplified Glioblastoma)	NCT02573324
Lorvotuzumab Mertansine (ImmunoGen)	Anti CD56 (neural cell adhesion molecule) monoclonal antibody conjugated to the drug maytansinoid DM1[83]	Phase II (Neuroblastoma, Rhabdomyosarcoma)	NCT02452554
Anetumab ravtansine	Antimesothelin antibody conjugated to the drug maytansinoid DM4[84]	Phase II (Ovarian Cancer, Mesothelioma, Pancreatic Cancer)	NCT03587311
			NCT03126630
			NCT03816358
Eribulin ORA (Athenex)	Oral formulation of eribulin combined with HM30181 P-gp inhibitor[85]	Phase I (solid tumors)	NCT04013217
BNC105P	Synthetic analog of combretastatin A4 (CA4),[86] a colchicine-binding site MT inhibitor with potent vascular disrupting activity, originally isolated from African tree *Combretum caffrum*[87]	Phase I (CML)	NCT03454165
BAT8001 (Bio Thera Solutions)	Anti-HER2 monoclonal antibody conjugated to a maytansine derivative via an uncleavable linker to reduce toxicity[88]	Phase I (Breast Cancer)	NCT04189211
OXi4503 (Mateon Therapeutics)	Combretastatin A1 di-phosphate (CA1P), a colchicine-binding site MT inhibitor with potent vascular disrupting activity, originally isolated from African tree *Combretum caffrum*[89]	Phase I/II (AML)	NCT02576301

[a] Approved in South Korea in 2016 for the treatment of gastric cancer.
[b] Approved in China for clinical use in cancer patients in 2006.

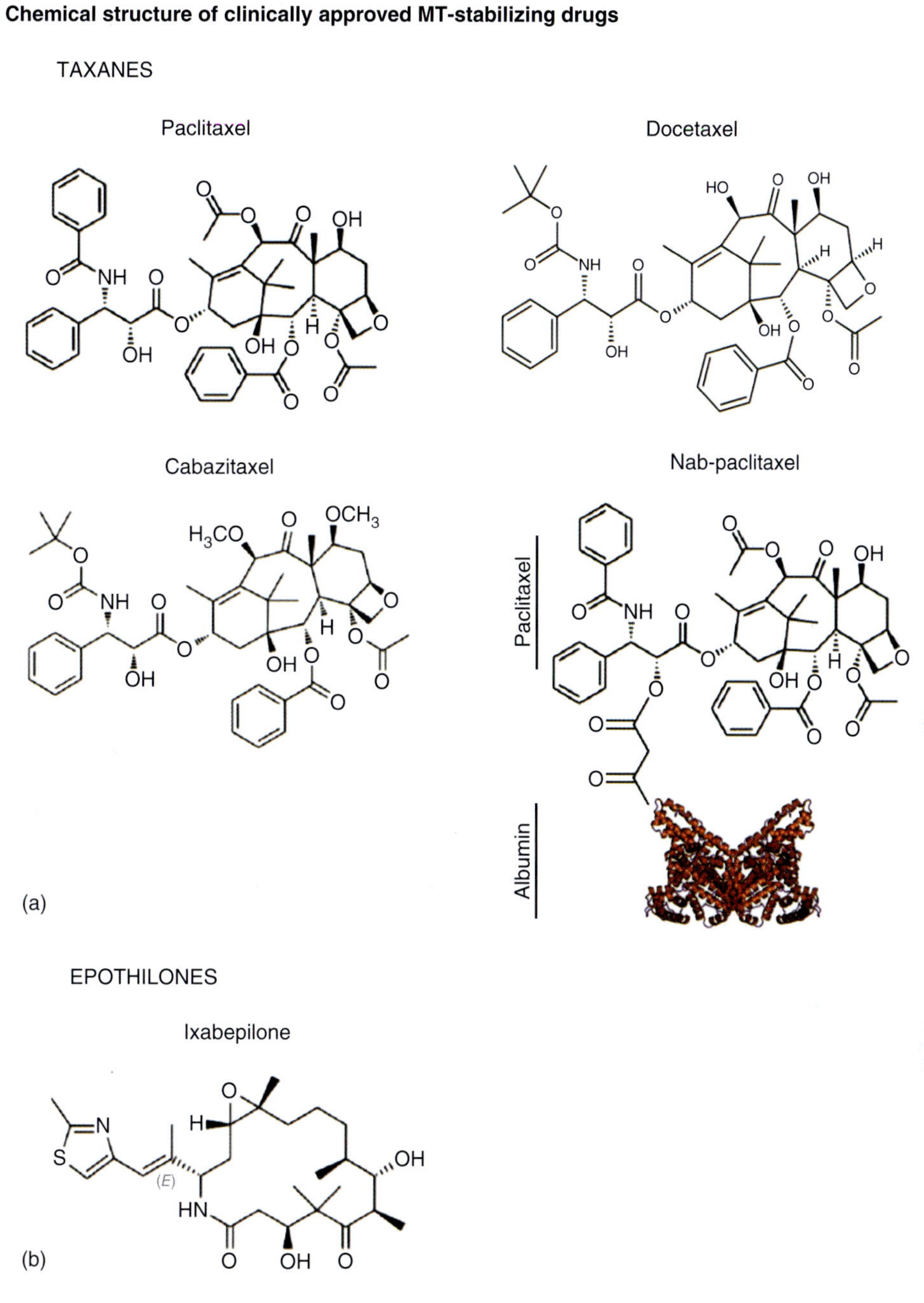

Chemical structure of clinically approved MT-stabilizing drugs

TAXANES

Paclitaxel

Docetaxel

Cabazitaxel

Nab-paclitaxel

(a)

EPOTHILONES

Ixabepilone

(b)

Figure 2 Chemical structures of clinically approved MT-stabilizing drugs: taxanes (a) and epothilones (b).

In addition to these FDA-approved taxanes, there is a large number of novel formulations of paclitaxel and docetaxel currently being tested in clinical trials (Phase I–III) (Table 2). Finally, tesetaxel is an oral formulation of a novel semisynthetic taxane, which has demonstrated promising activity in a Phase III clinical study of patients with metastatic breast cancer previously treated with a taxane, and which is currently undergoing further clinical testing.[121]

Drug interactions

As taxane metabolism is catalyzed by CYP450, caution should be exercised when taxanes are co-administered with known inducers (i.e., rifampicin, carbamazepine, Hypericum perforatum–St John's wort) or inhibitors (erythromycin, azole antifungal drugs such as itraconazole and ketoconazole, and grapefruit juice) of CYP450 activity. It has been shown that docetaxel plasma levels increased twofold in patients receiving ketoconazole, increasing the risk of severe adverse events.[122]

Interestingly, a Phase 1 trial showed that myelosuppression was more pronounced when paclitaxel was given following cisplatin compared to the alternate sequence, likely due to paclitaxel's decreased clearance by 25% after cisplatin, indicating that paclitaxel should always precede cisplatin when these drugs are administered in combination.[123]

Adverse events

Most of the clinical adverse events and dose-limiting toxicities are commonly shared among the clinically approved taxanes (paclitaxel, docetaxel, cabazitaxel, and nab-paclitaxel), and drug-specific toxic effects are rare. Nevertheless, the frequency and the grade of these adverse events vary significantly based on the schedule of administration, the performance status of the patient, and co-administration with other chemotherapy drugs.

All taxanes are associated with the development of significant myelosuppression, principally neutropenia, with a nadir at the second week from the administration followed by a rapid recovery due to bone marrow turnover. While only high-grade neutropenia (G3/G4) requires medical intervention such as co-administration of growth factors (e.g., G-CSF) and modulation of the schedule of drug administration, it is a common adverse effect that requires close monitoring. The long 24 h infusion of paclitaxel as single agent was traditionally associated with high-grade neutropenia (G3/4 in 71% of patients); this effect is mitigated with shorter drug infusion (1 or 3 h) schedules without compromising the drug's efficacy (G3/4 in 18% of patients).[14] However, high-grade neutropenia can still occur with short infusion schedules when paclitaxel is part of multidrug regimens. Neutropenia has been a dose-limiting adverse event for docetaxel (all grades in up to 97% of patients), with the risk of febrile neutropenia ranging from 14% with single-agent docetaxel to 38% when the drug was part of multidrug regimens.[124–126] Both of the next-generation taxanes, nab-paclitaxel, and cabazitaxel, have a better hematologic toxicity profile with high-grade neutropenia observed in about 9% of patients, likely due to their improved clinical pharmacology.[24,119,127]

Other hematologic toxicities such as anemia and thrombocytopenia are also frequently noted but usually at lower grade.

Mild *hypersensitivity reactions* (skin rash, dyspnea, hypotension) are commonly observed with all taxanes in as many as 20–30% of the patients and can be attributed primarily to the allergenic properties of the formulation solvent (i.e., Cremophor) and to a lesser extent to the taxanes themselves.

Neurotoxicity represents the Achilles' heel of taxane treatment, presenting either as an acute transient neuropathy (acute pain syndrome), or as a subacute but long-lasting *peripheral sensory neuropathy* (i.e., hand and feet tingling, numbness, and cold sensitivity) also referred to as a "glove-and-stocking" distribution with the most distal portions of the limb exhibiting the greatest deficits.[128]

Peripheral sensory neuropathy, which interferes with basic daily functions affecting the quality of life, typically resolves in half of the patients within the first year after treatment discontinuation and is by far the most debilitating adverse effect of taxane treatment and the key reason for treatment discontinuation in more than 17% of the patients.[129]

Paclitaxel is associated with peripheral sensory neuropathy in 57–83% of patients, and docetaxel in 11–64% of patients.[130,131] Interestingly, cabazitaxel is associated with less neurotoxicity than the other taxanes, with only 14% of patients reporting peripheral sensory neuropathy, which is rarely of grade 3 or higher and whose onset is delayed compared with docetaxel.[23] The high-grade peripheral neuropathy associated with nab-paclitaxel is the lowest reported, ranging from 3% to 10% of patients.[24,25]

Mechanistically, the peripheral sensory neuropathy is attributed to the effect of taxane treatment on the highly polarized dorsal root ganglion sensory neurons, where proper MT dynamics are required for axonal transport. Taxane treatment compromises the integrity and dynamics of these neuronal MTs, leading to loss of axonal integrity and decreased synaptic signaling which result in the degeneration of peripheral nerve fibers.[128,132]

Other frequently reported but severe not adverse events associated with taxane treatment are mostly *gastrointestinal* (diarrhea, nausea, vomit, and constipation), *fatigue, asthenia, fluid retention, and alopecia*.

Epothilones

Epothilones are natural compounds that were isolated from myxobacterium *Sorangium Cellulosum* at the beginning of the 1990s and showed a remarkable antineoplastic activity in preclinical models.[133] Epothilones are the only nontaxane MT-stabilizing class of compounds, sharing with the taxanes the same binding site on β-tubulin inside the MT polymer.[134–136] Similar to taxanes, they promote MT polymerization and stability and suppress MT dynamics causing cell death due to their effects on both interphase and mitotic MTs.[137]

Of the many epothilones than have been tested clinically, only *ixabepilone* (Ixempra®, Figure 2b) received FDA approval for the treatment of taxane-resistant advanced/metastatic breast cancer as single agent or in combination with capecitabine.[138] Ixabepilone is administered as a 1 h intravenous infusion at 40–50 mg/m^2 on day 1 of a 3-week cycle. It also showed clinical activity in prostate, lung, and pancreatic cancers.[139–141] Ixabepilone is also dissolved in Cremophor-EL and is mostly metabolized in the liver by CYP450 3A4.[142] Similar to taxanes, a concomitant prophylactic medication protocol is adopted for ixabepilone to prevent the onset of hypersensitivity reactions.[143–146] Due to ixabepilone's hepatic metabolism via cytochrome CYP450, co-administration with either CYP450 inhibitors or inducers, can increase ixabepilone's plasma concentration leading to excess toxicity; or decrease it to subtherapeutic levels, respectively. Thus, ixabepilone co-administration with such drugs should be avoided. Interestingly, when ixabepilone is co-administered with capecitabine (prodrug of the antimetabolite 5FU) both drugs' plasma concentrations are reduced, however, the enhanced clinical efficacy of this regimen for the treatment of patients with breast cancer, overrides the concern about their decreased pharmacokinetics.

The adverse reactions to ixabepilone are similar to those observed with taxanes with the most clinically relevant being the dose-limiting peripheral sensory neuropathy (seen in up to 45% of patients) (Table 1).

Microtubule-destabilizing drugs

Microtubule-destabilizing agents fall into two main categories, the ones that bind tubulin at the vinca alkaloid-binding site and the ones that bind tubulin at the colchicine-binding site. They are all-natural products known for their medicinal (often poisonous) properties since antiquity. Colchicine was the first compound ever found to bind tubulin, which led to the discovery of tubulin itself, as the "cellular protein that binds colchicine."[147]

Both classes of MT-destabilizing drugs bind to the tubulin heterodimer, at distinct sites, and promote MT destabilization. Currently, only drugs that bind tubulin at the vinca site are clinically approved in oncology (Table 1). Colchicine-site binding agents, also known for their vascular-disrupting properties, are in clinical development for oncology indications (Table 2), while they are approved for other medical conditions such as gout and other inflammatory diseases.

Vinca alkaloids

Vinca alkaloids were among the first anticancer agents to be introduced into the clinic during the 1960s. The prototype of this class is vinblastine (Velban®), a natural alkaloid isolated from the Madagascar periwinkle *vinca rosea*. Since the FDA approval of vinblastine in 1961 for the treatment of testicular cancer, four additional compounds from the vinca alkaloid family (vincristine, Oncovin®;

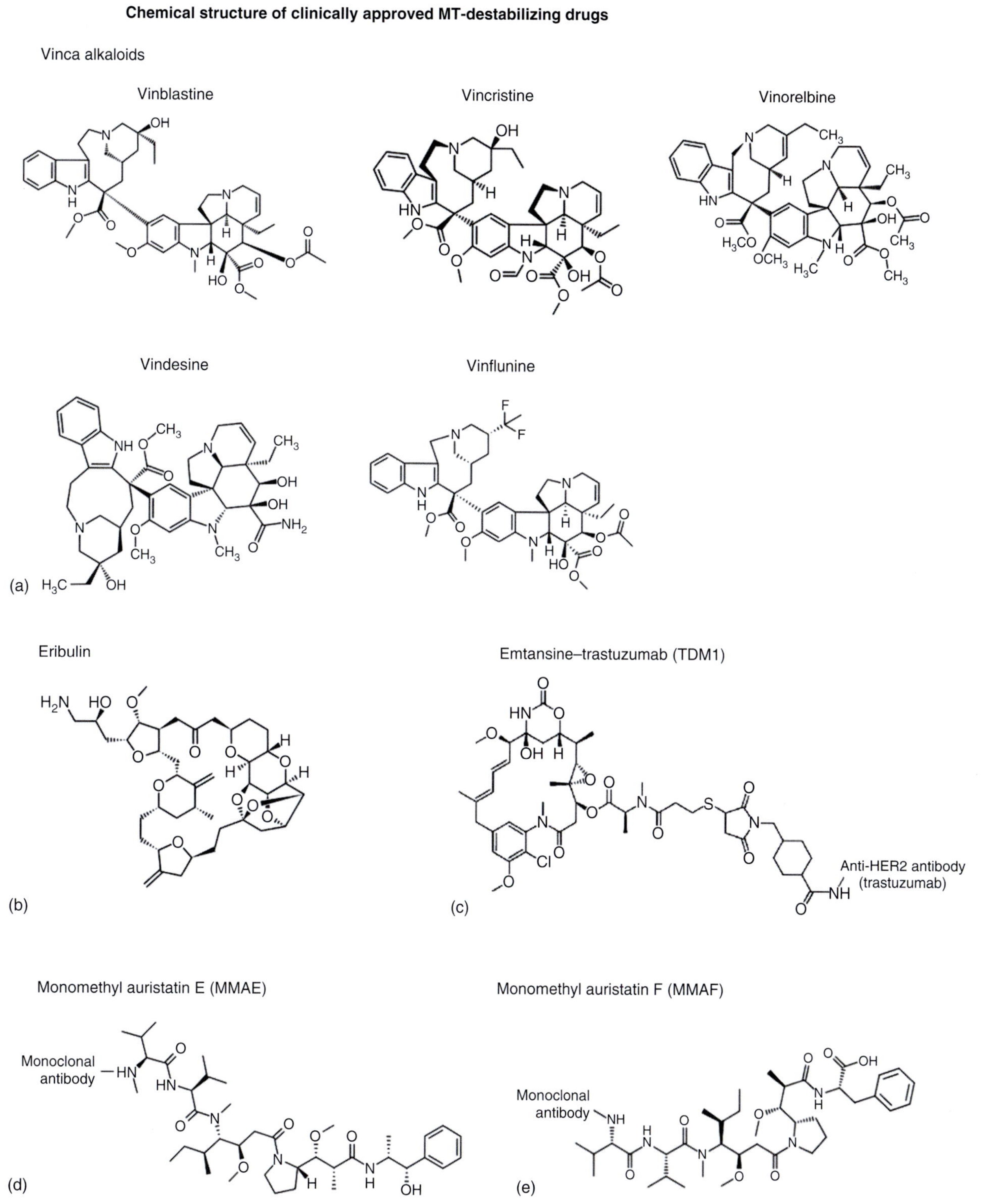

Microtubule inhibitors

Chemical structure of clinically approved MT-destabilizing drugs

Vinca alkaloids

Vinblastine Vincristine Vinorelbine

Vindesine Vinflunine

(a)

Eribulin

Emtansine–trastuzumab (TDM1)

Anti-HER2 antibody (trastuzumab)

(b) (c)

Monomethyl auristatin E (MMAE) Monomethyl auristatin F (MMAF)

Monoclonal antibody Monoclonal antibody

(d) (e)

Figure 3 Chemical structures of clinically approved MT-destabilizing drugs: vinca alkaloids (a), eribulin (b), emtansine–trastuzumab (TDM1, c), monomethyl auristatin E and F (d and e, respectively).

vinorelbine, Navelbine®; vindesine, Eldisine®; and vinflunine, Javlor®) (Figure 3a) have been approved and are currently utilized as either monotherapy or as part of multi-drug regimens for the treatment of hematologic malignancies and solid tumors (Table 1). The broad spectrum of clinical indications associated with the use of vinca alkaloids has led to ongoing clinical development of novel MT-destabilizing compounds, which are currently being clinically developed in the United States and other countries (Table 2).

Mechanism of action

The vinca alkaloids bind to the β-subunit of the α/β-tubulin heterodimer and prevent its incorporation into the MT polymer, thereby destabilizing MTs. Although the vinca-binding site was broadly identified decades ago, only recently a high-resolution X-ray structure of vinblastine bound to tubulin was obtained.[148] This study identified that vinblastine binds the tubulin dimer in solution near the α/β-tubulin interface introducing a "wedge" between two tubulin molecules and interfering with MT assembly while also causing self-assembly of tubulin aggregates. These new insights readily explain the clinical findings of a report published more than 50 years ago, when vincristine was administered intrathecally to one of the first pediatric patients with ALL[149]; the patient died shortly after drug administration and the autopsy identified irregular rhombohedral crystals in the patient's cerebrospinal fluid, indicative of what would be identified today as drug-induced tubulin aggregates or tubulin paracrystals.[148]

Interestingly, vinca alkaloids affect microtubule behavior in a concentration-dependent fashion.[150] At high concentrations (10–100 nmol/L), vinca alkaloids depolymerize microtubules, leading to the dissolution of the microtubule cytoskeleton. At lower concentrations (<10 mmol/L), vinca alkaloids do not affect microtubule polymer mass but act by suppressing microtubule dynamics, by binding to the microtubule plus-ends, reducing rate, and extent of MT growth (treadmilling) and shortening (dynamic instability).

In cells, treatment with vinca alkaloids dissolves the fine and intricate MT network, shifting the equilibrium toward the soluble pool of tubulin dimers (Figure 1), inhibiting all interphase MT functions such as intracellular protein and organelle shuttling, cell shape preservation, and regulation of signaling pathways (i.e., JNK).[151–156]

In addition, and similar to taxanes, the vinca-induced suppression of MT dynamics inhibits the formation of the mitotic spindle causing aberrant mitotic arrest and subsequent apoptotic cell death.[10]

Clinical pharmacology and indications

Vinca alkaloids are typically given by *i.v.* administration (bolus), followed by rigorous venous flushing to reduce the risk of phlebitis and local reactions at the injection site. However, longer infusions to maintain high drug concentrations can be also adopted; in addition, vinorelbine is also available as oral formulation, with similar pharmacokinetics as the *i.v.* injection. The major pathway for vinca alkaloid elimination is their hepatic metabolism through CYP450, followed by biliary excretion.[157,158]

Vinca alkaloids are clinically used for the treatment of various and diverse tumor types, ranging from solid tumors to hematologic malignancies (Table 1), as single agent or as part of multidrug regimens.

Vinblastine was the first vinca alkaloid to receive FDA approval in 1961 for the treatment of germ cell tumors, and the third approved chemotherapy drug. Since then, vinblastine's indications have exponentially expanded as monotherapy or as part of multi-drug combination regimens for the treatment of several types of solid tumors, including breast, bladder, and central nervous system malignancies. Even though it is now often replaced by other drugs, vinblastine is still widely used for the treatment of newly diagnosed Hodgkin lymphoma as part of the ABVD (adriamycin, bleomycin, vinblastine, and dacarbazine) multidrug regimen, in which it is administered at the dose of 6 mg/m^2 at day 1 and 15 of a 4-week cycle.[159]

Vincristine was the second vinca alkaloid to be approved by the FDA in 1963, for the treatment of acute childhood lymphoblastic leukemia and in 1967 for the treatment of lymphomas (Burkitt lymphoma, Hodgkin lymphoma).[39] Vincristine is currently routinely used for the treatment of several pediatric tumors, such as neuroblastoma and Wilms tumor, and it is an integral part of the CHOP (cyclophosphamide, doxorubicin, vincristine, and prednisone) multidrug regimen as first-line treatment of non-Hodgkin lymphomas.[160,161] Vincristine is usually administered at a dose range of 1.4–2 mg/m^2, usually weekly as single agent or every three weeks as part of multi-drug regimens. More recently, a liposomal formulation of vincristine (Marqibo®) has been approved for the treatment of acute lymphoblastic leukemia, based on its enhanced safety profile and improved drug delivery to the target tissue due to the drug's encapsulation in a sphingomyelinic/cholesterol envelope.[42]

Vinorelbine is the most recent FDA-approved vinca alkaloid, and it is widely used for the treatment of non-small-cell lung cancer, either as monotherapy or in combination with cisplatin, where vinorelbine is administered every four weeks at a dose of 25 mg/m^2.[162] Vinorelbine also demonstrated clinical benefit for the management of lung malignancies in elderly and frail patients and for other solid tumors such as breast cancer, for which it is currently approved in Europe as monotherapy at a dose of 30 mg/m^2.[163,164]

Vinflunine and vindesine are synthetic analogs of vinorelbine and vinblastine, respectively, and are not yet approved for cancer treatment in the United States. Vinflunine is currently approved as monotherapy (320 mg/m^2 every 3 weeks) for the treatment of advanced transitional cell carcinoma of the urothelial tract in Europe and Australia.[48] Similarly, vindesine is currently used only outside the United States as a therapeutic option for several tumor types such as melanoma, leukemia, and breast cancer, for which this drug is usually administered weekly at a dose of 3 mg/m^2.[165,166]

Drug interactions

Due to the hepatic CYP450 metabolism of the vinca alkaloids, any drug that affects cytochrome metabolic processes should be avoided during vinca alkaloid-based chemotherapy. In particular, drugs that induce the metabolic activity of CYP450, such as rifampicin, carbamazepine, and Hypericum perforatum (St John's worth) might accelerate the clearance of vinca alkaloids, thus potentially reducing drug exposure and clinical activity.[167] On the contrary, drugs that inhibit CYP450, such as erythromycin, azole antifungal drugs (i.e., itraconazole, ketoconazole), and grapefruit juice might decrease vinca alkaloids metabolism, thus increasing drug plasma concentrations and leading to increased severity of adverse reactions.

Vinca alkaloid can also affect the pharmacokinetics of other drugs, for example, causing reduction of blood levels of the anticonvulsant phenytoin, with the increased risk of seizures.[168]

Adverse events

Vinca alkaloid drugs have each a distinct toxicity profile despite their structural and pharmacological similarities. Neurotoxicity and myelosuppression are the two most clinically relevant side effects to consider for this class of drugs.

All vinca alkaloids induce *neurotoxicity* characterized primarily by peripheral, symmetric sensory-motor, and autonomic polyneuropathy, which is more clinically complex than the peripheral neuropathy induced by MT-stabilizing drugs. Mechanistically, neurotoxicity, which is more severe with vincristine and less frequent with vinorelbine,[169] is attributed to the inhibition of fast axonal transport, secondary to perturbation of neuronal microtubules. In agreement, preclinical studies demonstrated that vincristine was the most potent MTI to inhibit anterograde axonal transport, recapitulating the clinical findings.[170]

Toxic manifestations of the autonomic toxicity include constipation, abdominal cramps, paralytic ileus, and urinary retention. These side effects generally depend on the cumulative dose of the drug and generally resolve after treatment suspension; dose reduction or treatment discontinuation are the only effective interventions for vinca alkaloid-induced neurologic side effects.

Myelosuppression is the principal dose-limiting adverse event of vinca alkaloids, particularly applicable for vinblastine and vinorelbine. Myelosuppression is not cumulative, and it mostly consists of neutropenia (G3/4 in about 10% of the patients), which occurs between day 7 and 11 from the onset of treatment and resolves by day 21.[171] Thrombocytopenia and anemia can also be present, but to a lesser extent.

Gastrointestinal adverse events (i.e., mucositis, stomatitis, nausea, vomit, diarrhea) are also associated with vinca alkaloid administration and can be due to either the vinca-induced autonomic dysfunction (abdominal pain and diarrhea), or to direct drug effect on the gastrointestinal tract. *Cardiovascular complications* (i.e., chest pain with or without cardiac ischemia, edema, hyper/hypotension), *respiratory adverse events*, and changes in hepatic function can also be observed, together with the onset of dermatologic toxicity (i.e., alopecia, hand-and-foot syndrome).[172]

It is important to note that vinca alkaloids are effective vesicants that can cause extensive tissue damage at the site of venous injection in case of extravasation.

Eribulin

Eribulin mesylate (Halaven®) is a synthetic analogue of the natural product Halicondrin B and acts as a potent inhibitor of tubulin polymerization[173] (Figure 3b). Biochemical studies with purified tubulin have shown that eribulin is a noncompetitive inhibitor of vinblastine and of GTP-hydrolysis, placing its binding site near the exchangeable GTP-site on β-tubulin, largely overlapping with the vinca alkaloid-binding site.[174] More recently, X-ray crystallography studies further confirmed eribulin's binding at the vinca domain while also showing that eribulin, unlike the vinca alkaloids, also binds on β-tubulin at the plus-ends of MTs, terminating protofilament elongation and inducing MT disassembly.[175] In cells, similarly to the other MTIs, eribulin exerts its antitumor activity by inhibiting the function of both interphase and mitotic MTs, ultimately inducing cell death.

Eribulin was first approved by the FDA in the United States in 2010 for the treatment of patients with heavily pretreated advanced/metastatic breast cancer who had previously received anthracyclines and taxanes, and it is now also used as first-line treatment for patients with HER2-negative and triple-negative breast cancer.[49,176–178] In addition, eribulin is used for the treatment of liposarcoma that has progressed on anthracycline therapy.[50] Similar to vinca alkaloids, eribulin is administered as rapid *i.v.* injection, at a dose of 1.4 mg/m^2 on day 1 and day 8 of a 21-day cycle and has a similar clinical toxicity profile. However, peripheral neuropathy is observed at significantly lower frequency and severity as compared with the vinca alkaloids or with the microtubule-stabilizing MTIs both in preclinical models and in patients.[179–181] It is important to note that CYP450 does not play a role in eribulin metabolism and that the drug is primarily eliminated in feces unchanged. Due to the negligible cytochrome metabolism, no drug–drug interactions are expected with CYP450 inducers or inhibitors, neither eribulin is known to affect CYP450 enzymatic activity.

Microtubule-destabilizing drugs as payload for antibody–drug conjugate therapies

The clinical success of recently developed ADCs has re-ignited interest in MT-destabilizing drugs, as they represent the most common payload for ADCs in oncology (Table 1). Currently, there are four FDA approved ADCs carrying as a payload either a maytansinoid (ado-trastuzumab emtansine, T-DM1) or auristatin (brentuximab vedotin, enfortumab vedotin, belantamab mafodotin) (Table 1), with seven additional ADCs carrying the abovementioned payloads conjugated to different therapeutic antibodies, in clinical development (Table 2).

Emtansine

Emtansine (DM1), a derivative of maytansine, is a potent inhibitor of tubulin polymerization (Figure 3c). Originally thought to bind at the vinca domain on β-tubulin, recent X-ray studies identified that maytansine binds on β-tubulin at a unique site, and works by inhibiting longitudinal dimer interactions in the MT thereby inhibiting polymerization.[182,183] Treatment with maytansine results in mitotic arrest in dividing cells, and in impaired interphase MT functions in nondividing cancer cells.[184] Previously tested as anticancer single agent, it showed limited clinical efficacy likely due to its significant toxicity profile. Upon conjugation with the anti-HER2 antibody trastuzumab (T-DM1), emtansine showed extensive antitumor activity as cytotoxic payload of an ADC compound in patients with HER2$^+$ breast cancer, leading to its approval in 2013 for the treatment of patients with HER2$^+$ advanced/metastatic breast cancer whose disease progressed following treatment with anti-HER2 monoclonal antibodies (trastuzumab, pertuzumab).[51,185] More recently, in 2019, T-DM1 was approved as adjuvant therapy in patients with resected HER2$^+$ breast cancer who have residual disease after anti-HER2 neoadjuvant treatment.[52] In addition to HER2-based ADCs in breast cancer, maytansine analogs have been conjugated with different tumor-targeting antibodies, which are currently in clinical trials in NSCLC (anti-CECAM 5), ovarian (antifolate receptor α), and pancreatic (antimesothelin) cancers among others (Table 2).

Monomethyl auristatin E (MMAE, vedotin) and auristatin F (MMAF, mafodotin)

Auristatin is a synthetic analog of the natural product dolastatin 10, an ultrapotent cytotoxic microtubule inhibitor, which binds tubulin at the vinca alkaloid site and induces extensive and rapid MT depolymerization.[186,187] Although its toxicity profile prevented its clinical development as a stand-alone treatment, auristatin demonstrated profound antitumor activity at clinically tolerated doses as payload for several ADCs (Table 1).

Today, monomethyl auristatin E (MMAE, vedotin; Figure 3d) has been successfully used as payload of the anti-CD30 monoclonal antibody brentuximab, which received FDA approval in 2011 for the treatment of relapsed/refractory Hodgkin lymphoma after autologous stem cell transplantation, as well as for the treatment of systemic anaplastic large-cell lymphoma.[53] In 2019, MMAE conjugated with antinectin 4 or with anti-CD79b antibodies received FDA approval for the treatment of urothelial cancer[55] and relapsed/refractory diffuse large B-cell lymphoma, respectively.[56] Auristatin F (MMAF, mafodotin, Figure 3e) has been successfully conjugated with the anti-BCMA (B-cell maturation antigen) monoclonal antibody and was granted accelerated approval by the FDA in 2020 for the treatment of relapsed or refractory multiple myeloma.[57] Currently, auristatin analogs conjugated with anti-HER2 or anti-EGFR monoclonal antibodies are clinically tested in breast cancer and glioblastoma, respectively (Table 2).

Mechanisms of resistance to MTIs

Despite their clinical success and broad spectrum of indications, the therapeutic benefit from treatment with MTIs is limited owing to drug resistance. Drug resistance can be either preexistent in cancer cells (intrinsic) or treatment-induced (acquired). Key mechanisms of drug resistance to MTIs can be grouped into three main categories: (1) mechanisms upstream of drug-target engagement (e.g., altered cellular drug uptake or retention), (2) mechanisms affecting drug-target engagement (e.g., molecular alterations of the target itself, such as tubulin mutations, or altered expression of proteins/pathways that affect MT stability), (3) mechanisms downstream of drug-target engagement (e.g., alterations of downstream apoptotic signaling or MT-based trafficking of oncogenic transcription factors). As MTI resistance, coupled with limited alternative therapeutic options, is the main cause of cancer mortality, there is an urgent need to identify and clinically validate actionable genes/pathways that underlie MTI resistance.

Mechanisms upstream of drug-target engagement largely involve expression of the plasma membrane ATP-binding cassette (ABC) family of transporters. Both taxanes and vinca alkaloids have large lipophilic chemical structures, which make them ideal substrates for these cellular pumps, with the multidrug resistance protein 1 (MDR1), also known as P-glycoprotein or P-gp, being the first discovered and most investigated.[188,189] Extensive in vitro studies have established the structure and function of P-gp as an MTI transporter, which confers drug resistance by binding to and "pumping out" MTIs from the cells, lowering their effective intracellular concentration to sub-therapeutic levels.[190] Functional inhibition of P-gp with the use of pharmacologic inhibitors such as verapamil and cyclosporin A has demonstrated complete reversal of multidrug resistance in preclinical models, which generated considerable excitement for the development and clinical testing of next-generation inhibitors of P-gp and related family members.[191] Nevertheless, clinical trials using several of these inhibitors in combination with MTIs did not show any clinical benefit while they were also associated with increased toxicity.[192,193] As P-gp is a natural detoxification mechanism expressed in many normal tissues, including the GI tract, an interesting new application of these inhibitors involves their addition to the oral taxane formulation to increase the drug's absorption by the small intestine and enhance its bioavailability (Table 2).

Mechanisms that affect MTI interaction with its target (drug-target engagement) involve primarily point mutations in β-tubulin, altered expression of tubulin isotypes, and posttranslational modifications in tubulin and MT-associated proteins. The first point mutation at the taxane-binding site was identified in 1997 in a human ovarian cancer cell line with acquired paclitaxel resistance. The β270$^{Phe \rightarrow Val}$ mutation inhibited the aromatic interaction between paclitaxel's C13 phenyl ring and phenylalanine's phenyl group, lowering paclitaxel's binding affinity for tubulin.[194] Since then, several reports identified point mutations in tubulin that differentially affected the binding of both MT-stabilizing and MT-destabilizing drugs conferring MTI resistance in preclinical models.[134,195,196] These data generated a lot of excitement as they could provide a mechanistic explanation for the clinical MTI resistance and could also serve as the basis for patient selection. Although an initial clinical study in patients with NSCLC identified tubulin mutations in about 33% of patient tumors, which were significantly associated with clinical taxane resistance,[197] it soon became evident that the high mutation rate was due to co-amplification of tubulin pseudogenes that do not give rise to a protein product,[198,199] while the actual tubulin mutation rate was very low and unlikely to contribute to MTI resistance in patients.

In addition to point mutations, differential expression of tubulin isotypes has been reported as a mechanism of MTI resistance. Mammalian tubulin is encoded by a multigene family with 7 α- and 8 β-tubulin isotypes, encoded by different genes whose protein products have high sequence homology and some tissue specificity[200] and are interchangeably incorporated into the MTs.[201]

As all MTIs bind β-tubulin, the role of β-tubulin isotype expression has been extensively studied in MTI resistance.[202] Interestingly, in vitro studies demonstrated that β-tubulin isotypes display different polymerization properties and that MTs enriched in the neuronal-specific β-III isotype (encoded by TUBB3 gene) are more dynamic[203,204] and less susceptible to the suppressive effects of taxanes,[205,206] thus suggesting that β-III tubulin could play a crucial role in clinical resistance to MT-stabilizing MTIs. Even though early clinical studies in ovarian and lung cancers supported this notion,[207–209] additional clinical studies including large meta-analyses[210] identified that high expression of β-III tubulin in tumors is associated with poor clinical outcomes,[211] but not with clinical response to MTI treatment.[212] Taken together, these data suggest that β-III tubulin expression is not a predictive biomarker of MTI resistance but rather a prognostic marker of poor outcomes, while its exact role in tumor biology and progression is still under investigation.

Tubulin, MTs, and a large number of proteins that associate with them, known as MT-associated proteins (MAPs), are subject to a large number of posttranslational modifications (PTMs) such as acetylation and phosphorylation that regulate their function. These PTMs can affect MT stability and shift the steady-state equilibrium between tubulin dimers and MTs, thus ultimately affecting their susceptibility to MTIs.[213,214] For example, β-tubulin phosphorylation at Ser^{172}, precludes the incorporation of tubulin dimers into MT polymers, thus affecting MT steady-state equilibrium shifting the balance toward the pool of soluble tubulin, which is the preferred substrate of MT-destabilizing drugs.[215]

Another example of the effect of PTMs on the steady-state equilibrium of cellular tubulin is the phosphorylation status of several MAPs. MAP4, a ubiquitously expressed non-neuronal MAP, in its unphosphorylated state binds to the MT wall and stabilizes MTs against depolymerization; and stathmin, a phosphoprotein that regulates cell cycle, binds tubulin dimers and sequesters them away from MTs, thus promoting microtubule depolymerization.[216–220] Although several studies have demonstrated that altered expression levels and/or phosphorylation status of these proteins is associated with altered sensitivity to both MT-stabilizing and destabilizing MTIs, they have yet to impact clinical care.

As phosphorylation is a key PTM that affects both tubulin and MAPs, several studies have implicated kinases having tubulin or MAPs as substrates in MTI resistance. For example, both tubulin and MAPs were identified as phosphorylation substrates for the spleen tyrosine kinase (SYK), whose pharmacological inhibition was reported to revert taxane resistance, by enhancing MT stability shifting the equilibrium toward MTs which are the preferred substrate for taxane binding.[221] Similarly, pharmacologic inhibition of the FER tyrosine kinase that phosphorylates CRMP2, a MT-associated protein known to stabilize MTs, greatly enhanced taxane antitumor activity by increasing MT stability and expanding drug-target engagement by paclitaxel.[222] Finally, ERG protein, a transcriptional factor that is found overexpressed in 40–50% of patients with prostate cancer, has been shown to bind to tubulin heterodimers altering microtubule dynamics and reducing microtubule polymerization, and it has been repeatedly associated with lower rates of response to taxane-based chemotherapy in patients with prostate cancer.[223,224]

It should be noted that regardless of which specific protein and PTM affects MT stability, the end effect is that they all impair effective drug-target engagement (DTE) resulting in MTI resistance. DTE can be readily visualized in cells and tumor biopsies by tubulin immunofluorescence and its hallmarks include aberrant mitotic figures or in interphase changes in the MT array in response to MTI treatment. However, it was only recently that DTE was clinically tested as a biomarker of response to taxane treatment in patients with prostate or gastric cancer. DTE quantification in patient-derived tumor biopsies or circulating tumor cells, collected before and during taxane treatment identified that DTE was significantly associated with clinical response to treatment with docetaxel, cabazitaxel, or a nanoparticle formulation of docetaxel.[101,102,225,226] Future prospective clinical studies are currently being planned to validate DTE as an early predictive and actionable biomarker of clinical response.

Finally, MTI resistance can arise by alteration in pathways downstream of drug-target engagement, including altered trafficking of oncogenic transcription factors or activation of prosurvival pathways. These include activation of Notch and Hedgehog signaling, shown to induce taxane resistance in prostate cancer by inducing PI3K/AKT prosurvival signaling pathways[227]; and overexpression of the antiapoptotic BCL2 family of proteins.[228] In addition, expression of microtubule-independent androgen receptor (AR) splice variants, whose nuclear accumulation and oncogenic activity is not affected by taxane treatment, have been associated with taxane resistance in preclinical models of prostate cancer and with lower tumor response in patients with prostate cancer receiving taxane-based therapies.[229,230]

Key references

The complete reference list can be found on Vital Source version of this title, see inside front cover.

1. Desai A, Mitchison TJ. Microtubule polymerization dynamics. *Annu Rev Cell Dev Biol.* 1997;**13**(1):83–117. doi: 10.1146/annurev.cellbio.13.1.83.
2. Mitchison T, Kirschner M. Dynamic instability of microtubule growth. *Nature.* 1984;**312**(5991):237–242. doi: 10.1038/312237a0.
5. Avila J. Microtubule functions. *Life Sci.* 1992;**50**(5):327–334. doi: 10.1016/0024-3205(92)90433-p.
9. Gascoigne KE, Taylor SS. Cancer cells display profound intra- and inter-line variation following prolonged exposure to antimitotic drugs. *Cancer Cell.* 2008;**14**(2):111–122. doi: 10.1016/j.ccr.2008.07.002.
10. Jordan MA, Wilson L. Microtubules as a target for anticancer drugs. *Nat Rev Cancer.* 2004;**4**(4):253–265. doi: 10.1038/nrc1317.
11. Komlodi-Pasztor E, Sackett D, Wilkerson J, Fojo T. Mitosis is not a key target of microtubule agents in patient tumors. *Nat Rev Clin Oncol.* 2011;**8**(4):244–250. doi: 10.1038/nrclinonc.2010.228.
13. Field JJ, Kanakkanthara A, Miller JH. Microtubule-targeting agents are clinically successful due to both mitotic and interphase impairment of microtubule function. *Bioorg Med Chem.* 2014;**22**(18):5050–5059. doi: 10.1016/j.bmc.2014.02.035.
20. Tannock IF, de Wit R, Berry WR, et al. Docetaxel plus prednisone or mitoxantrone plus prednisone for advanced prostate cancer. *N Engl J Med.* 2004;**351**(15):1502–1512. doi: 10.1056/NEJMoa040720.
26. Von Hoff DD, Ervin T, Arena FP, et al. Increased survival in pancreatic cancer with nab-paclitaxel plus gemcitabine. *N Engl J Med.* 2013;**369**(18):1691–1703. doi: 10.1056/NEJMoa1304369.
49. Cortes J, O'Shaughnessy J, Loesch D, et al. Eribulin monotherapy versus treatment of physician's choice in patients with metastatic breast cancer (EMBRACE): a phase 3 open-label randomised study. *Lancet.* 2011;**377**(9769):914–923. doi: 10.1016/S0140-6736(11)60070-6.
51. Verma S, Miles D, Gianni L, et al. Trastuzumab emtansine for HER2-positive advanced breast cancer. *N Engl J Med.* 2012;**367**(19):1783–1791. doi: 10.1056/NEJMoa1209124.
53. Younes A, Bartlett NL, Leonard JP, et al. Brentuximab vedotin (SGN-35) for relapsed CD30-positive lymphomas. *N Engl J Med.* 2010;**363**(19):1812–1821. doi: 10.1056/NEJMoa1002965.
57. Lonial S, Lee HC, Badros A, et al. Belantamab mafodotin for relapsed or refractory multiple myeloma (DREAMM-2): a two-arm, randomised, open-label, phase 2 study. *Lancet Oncol.* 2020;**21**(2):207–221. doi: 10.1016/S1470-2045(19)30788-0.
58. Schiff PB, Fant J, Horwitz SB. Promotion of microtubule assembly in vitro by taxol. *Nature.* 1979;**277**(5698):665–667. doi: 10.1038/277665a0.
90. Nogales E, Wolf SG, Khan IA, et al. Structure of tubulin at 6.5 A and location of the taxol-binding site. *Nature.* 1995;**375**(6530):424–427. doi: 10.1038/375424a0.
95. Mabjeesh NJ, Escuin D, LaVallee TM, et al. 2ME2 inhibits tumor growth and angiogenesis by disrupting microtubules and dysregulating HIF. *Cancer Cell.* 2003;**3**(4):363–375. doi: 10.1016/s1535-6108(03)00077-1.
96. Giannakakou P, Sackett DL, Ward Y, et al. p53 is associated with cellular microtubules and is transported to the nucleus by dynein. *Nat Cell Biol.* 2000;**2**(10):709–717. doi: 10.1038/35036335.
97. Darshan MS, Loftus MS, Thadani-Mulero M, et al. Taxane-induced blockade to nuclear accumulation of the androgen receptor predicts clinical responses in metastatic prostate cancer. *Cancer Res.* 2011;**71**(18):6019–6029. doi: 10.1158/0008-5472.CAN-11-1417.
101. Gjyrezi A, Xie F, Voznesensky O, et al. Taxane resistance in prostate cancer is mediated by decreased drug-target engagement. *J Clin Investig.* 2020;**130**(6):3287–3298. doi: 10.1172/JCI132184.
105. Szebeni J, Muggia FM, Alving CR. Complement activation by Cremophor EL as a possible contributor to hypersensitivity to paclitaxel: an in vitro study. *J Natl Cancer Inst.* 1998;**90**(4):300–306. doi: 10.1093/jnci/90.4.300.
111. Schiller JH, Harrington D, Belani CP, et al. Comparison of four chemotherapy regimens for advanced non-small-cell lung cancer. *N Engl J Med.* 2002;**346**(2):92–98. doi: 10.1056/NEJMoa011954.
129. Shimozuma K, Ohashi Y, Takeuchi A, et al. Taxane-induced peripheral neuropathy and health-related quality of life in postoperative breast cancer patients undergoing adjuvant chemotherapy: N-SAS BC 02, a randomized clinical trial. *Support Care Cancer.* 2012;**20**(12):3355–3364. doi: 10.1007/s00520-012-1492-x.
134. Giannakakou P, Gussio R, Nogales E, et al. A common pharmacophore for epothilone and taxanes: molecular basis for drug resistance conferred by tubulin mutations in human cancer cells. *Proc Natl Acad Sci U S A.* 2000;**97**(6):2904–2909. doi: 10.1073/pnas.040546297.
135. Nettles JH, Li H, Cornett B, et al. The binding mode of epothilone A on alpha,beta-tubulin by electron crystallography. *Science.* 2004;**305**(5685):866–869. doi: 10.1126/science.1099190.
138. Sparano JA, Vrdoljak E, Rixe O, et al. Randomized phase III trial of ixabepilone plus capecitabine versus capecitabine in patients with metastatic breast cancer previously treated with an anthracycline and a taxane. *J Clin Oncol.* 2010;**28**(20):3256–3263. doi: 10.1200/JCO.2009.24.4244.
147. Borisy GG, Taylor EW. The mechanism of action of colchicine: binding of colchicine-3H to cellular protein. *J Cell Biol.* 1967;**34**(2):525–533. doi: 10.1083/jcb.34.2.525.
148. Gigant B, Wang C, Ravelli RB, et al. Structural basis for the regulation of tubulin by vinblastine. *Nature.* 2005;**435**(7041):519–522. doi: 10.1038/nature03566.
150. Jordan MA, Thrower D, Wilson L. Mechanism of inhibition of cell proliferation by Vinca alkaloids. *Cancer Res.* 1991;**51**(8):2212–2222.
152. Giannakakou P, Nakano M, Nicolaou KC, et al. Enhanced microtubule-dependent trafficking and p53 nuclear accumulation by suppression of microtubule dynamics. *Proc Natl Acad Sci U S A.* 2002;**99**(16):10855–10860. doi: 10.1073/pnas.132275599.
155. Mabjeesh NJ, Escuin D, LaVallee TM, et al. 2ME2 inhibits tumor growth and angiogenesis by disrupting microtubules and dysregulating HIF. *Cancer Cell.* 2003;**3**(4):363–375. doi: 10.1016/S1535-6108(03)00077-1.
159. Santoro A, Bonadonna G, Valagussa P, et al. Long-term results of combined chemotherapy-radiotherapy approach in Hodgkin's disease: superiority of ABVD plus radiotherapy versus MOPP plus radiotherapy. *J Clin Oncol.* 1987;**5**(1):27–37. doi: 10.1200/JCO.1987.5.1.27.
160. Johnson IS, Armstrong JG, Gorman M, Burnett JP. The vinca alkaloids: a new class of oncolytic agents. *Cancer Res.* 1963;**23**:1390–1427.
161. Coiffier B, Lepage E, Briere J, et al. CHOP chemotherapy plus rituximab compared with CHOP alone in elderly patients with diffuse large-B-cell lymphoma. *N Engl J Med.* 2002;**346**(4):235–242. doi: 10.1056/NEJMoa011795.
194. Giannakakou P, Sackett DL, Kang YK, et al. Paclitaxel-resistant human ovarian cancer cells have mutant beta-tubulins that exhibit impaired paclitaxel-driven polymerization. *J Biol Chem.* 1997;**272**(27):17118–17125. doi: 10.1074/jbc.272.27.17118.
203. Panda D, Miller HP, Banerjee A, et al. Microtubule dynamics in vitro are regulated by the tubulin isotype composition. *Proc Natl Acad Sci.* 1994;**91**(24):11358. doi: 10.1073/pnas.91.24.11358.
214. Janke C, Magiera MM. The tubulin code and its role in controlling microtubule properties and functions. *Nat Rev Mol Cell Biol.* 2020;**21**(6):307–326. doi: 10.1038/s41580-020-0214-3.

223 Galletti G, Matov A, Beltran H, et al. ERG induces taxane resistance in castration-resistant prostate cancer. *Nat Commun.* 2014;5:5548. doi: 10.1038/ncomms6548.

225 Antonarakis ES, Tagawa ST, Galletti G, et al. Randomized, noncomparative, phase II trial of early switch from docetaxel to cabazitaxel or vice versa, with integrated biomarker analysis, in men with chemotherapy-naïve, metastatic, castration-resistant prostate cancer. *J Clin Oncol.* 2017;35(28):3181–3188. doi: 10.1200/JCO.2017.72.4138.

229 Thadani-Mulero M, Portella L, Sun S, et al. Androgen receptor splice variants determine taxane sensitivity in prostate cancer. *Cancer Res.* 2014;74(8):2270–2282. doi: 10.1158/0008-5472.CAN-13-2876.

230 Tagawa ST, Antonarakis ES, Gjyrezi A, et al. Expression of AR-V7 and ARv^{567es} in circulating tumor cells correlates with outcomes to taxane therapy in men with metastatic prostate cancer treated in TAXYNERGY. *Clin Cancer Res.* 2019;25(6):1880. doi: 10.1158/1078-0432.CCR-18-0320.

58 Drug resistance and its clinical circumvention

Jeffrey A. Moscow, MD ■ *Shannon K. Hughes, PhD* ■ *Kenneth H. Cowan, MD, PhD* ■ *Branimir I. Sikic, MD*

> **Overview**
>
> Tumors initially sensitive to chemotherapeutic agents frequently develop resistance to them, resulting in the familiar clinical pattern of initial response followed by a recurrence that no longer responds to therapy. Laboratory and clinical investigation have identified a plethora of drug resistance mechanisms, some that are particular to an individual agent and others that are applicable across classes of agents. These mechanisms include altered cellular accumulation and detoxification of drugs, mutation of the drug target, change in expression of the drug target, and activation of alternative signaling pathways. The identification of drug resistance mechanisms has led to strategies to overcome resistance and improved clinical outcomes.

Introduction

Systemic therapy with cytotoxic drugs or targeted agents is the basis for most of the effective treatments of disseminated cancers. Additionally, adjuvant chemotherapy can offer a significant survival advantage to selected patients, following the treatment of localized disease with surgery or radiotherapy, presumably by eliminating undetected, minimal, or microscopic residual tumor. However, the responses of tumors to therapeutic regimens vary, and failures are frequent owing to the emergence of drug resistance.

The phenomenon of clinical drug resistance has prompted studies to clarify mechanisms of drug action and to identify mechanisms of antineoplastic resistance. It is expected that through such information, drug resistance may be circumvented by rational design of new non-cross-resistant agents, by novel delivery or combinations of known drugs, and by the development of other treatments that might augment the activity of or reverse resistance to known antineoplastics. While earlier mechanisms of drug resistance were identified experimentally by generation of resistant cell lines, recent advances in bulk and single-cell genomic and epigenomic technologies and in experimental models, such as patient-derived xenografts and *ex vivo* organoid cultures, have allowed the direct determination of resistance mechanisms present in clinically resistant tumors.

General mechanisms of resistance to single agents

Experimental selection of drug resistance by repeated exposure to single antineoplastic agents will generally result in cross-resistance to some related agents of the same drug class, especially when employed at a maximum tolerated dose. This phenomenon may best be explained by a combination of multiple mechanisms, including shared drug transport carriers, drug-metabolizing pathways, and intracellular cytotoxic targets of structurally and biochemically similar compounds.

Generally, the resistant cells retain sensitivity to drugs of different classes with alternative mechanisms of cytotoxic action. Thus, cells selected for resistance to alkylating agents or antifolates will usually remain sensitive to unrelated drugs, such as anthracyclines. Exceptions include emergence of cross-resistance to multiple, apparently structurally and functionally unrelated drugs, to which the patient or cancer cells were never exposed during the initial drug treatment and may be driven by tumor heterogeneity. Despite apparent differences in their presumed sites of action within cells, the drugs associated with multidrug resistance (MDR) phenotypes frequently share common metabolic pathways or efflux transport systems.

Although there are exceptions, in general resistance to cytotoxic chemotherapy has been ascribed to metabolic mechanisms of resistance while resistance to targeted agents has been ascribed to genetic mechanisms. In this section, several processes related to drug resistance will be described. A more comprehensive discussion of selected mechanisms of resistance to specific classes of drugs will be discussed in subsequent sections.

Metabolic mechanisms

Decreased drug accumulation

Decreased intracellular levels of cytotoxic agents are one of the most common mechanisms of drug resistance. Since polar, water-soluble drugs cannot penetrate the lipid bilayer of the cell membrane and require specific mechanisms of cell entry, resistance to these drugs is readily mediated by downregulation of drug uptake mechanisms in tumor cells. For example, antifolates such as methotrexate require specific transporters to gain intracellular access, including high-affinity folate receptors, the reduced folate carrier (SLC19A1), and the proton-coupled folate transporter (SLC46A1), and downregulation of these mechanisms of uptake has been described as contributors to methotrexate resistance.[1] For hydrophobic, nonpolar drugs that can easily diffuse across the cell membrane, decreased intracellular drug concentrations can be achieved by increasing the activities of drug efflux pumps. For example, overexpression of the P-glycoprotein (*MDR1/ABCB1*) drug efflux pump is an important example of this mechanism of resistance, especially in MDR phenotypes.[2]

Although preclinical studies in murine models showed efficacy of P-glycoprotein inhibitors, most clinical studies involving the use of MDR-reversing agents in the treatment of solid human tumors have been disappointing, and despite the plethora of MDR reversing agents identified in hundreds of preclinical studies, none have evolved into clinically useful agents. Clinical trials of MDR reversing agents encountered significant obstacles, including (1) increased toxicity of the chemotherapy agents caused profound effects on the pharmacokinetics and pharmacodynamics of MDR1 reversing agents on the cytotoxic drugs associated with MDR, (2) the toxicity of some of the early MDR1 reversing agents themselves, such as verapamil, prevented adequate exposure to them; (3) lack of screening of patients for *MDR1/ABCB1* expression in tumors; (4) involvement of other transporters and other mechanisms of resistance at the time of recurrence; and (5) lack of understanding of how polymorphisms affect susceptibility to MDR1 inhibition.[3] While P-glycoprotein and other ATP-binding cassette (ABC) transporters may play important roles in tumor biology and drug resistance, no pharmacologic strategy has emerged that can improve clinical outcomes by inhibiting the activity of these transporters once clinical drug resistance has been established.

Altered drug metabolism

The three phases of drug metabolism—activation, inactivation, and elimination—may all play a role in drug resistance. Drug activation may involve phase 1 drug metabolism mediated by cytochrome P-450 mixed-function oxidase, where the drug or xenobiotic is rendered into a more electrophilic, reactive intermediate—a process that may enhance toxicity. These metabolites may then be converted to a less reactive, presumably less toxic form in phase 2 reactions, which include the formation of drug/xenobiotic conjugations with glutathione (GSH), glucuronic acid, or sulfate—reactions that are catalyzed by multiple isozymes each of glutathione *S*-transferases (GSTs), uridine diphosphate (UDP)-glucuronosyl transferases, and sulfatases, respectively. Phase 3 detoxification consists of export of the parent drug/xenobiotic or its metabolites by energy-dependent transmembrane efflux pumps, including multidrug resistance-associated protein (MRP/ABCC) family members. For example, decreased conversion of nucleobase analogs to their active cytotoxic nucleoside and nucleotide derivatives by alterations in specific kinases and phosphoribosyl transferase salvage enzymes can lead to resistance to these anticancer drugs.[4,5] Another example of decreased activation associated with resistance is decreased levels of carboxyesterase—an activity necessary to convert the topoisomerase I inhibitor irinotecan, CPT-11, to its active metabolite, SN-38.[6,7] On the other hand, enhanced inactivation of pyrimidine and purine analogs by increased expression of deaminases is linked to resistance toward these agents.[5,8] Also, alterations in cofactor levels can also modify drug toxicity. For example, optimal formation of inhibitory complexes between 5-fluorodeoxyuridine monophosphate (FdUMP) and its target enzyme, thymidylate synthase, require the cofactor 5,10-methylene tetrahydrofolate.[9] Alterations in the intracellular levels of this cofactor can lead to resistance to fluoropyrimidines.

Increased repair or tolerance to drug-induced DNA damage

Cells contain multiple complex systems involved in the repair of damage to deoxyribonucleic acid (DNA), and changes in the balance of these repair processes can influence drug sensitivity. For example, the cytotoxic action of cisplatin relies upon the inability of cells to resolve intrastrand DNA cross-links. One mechanism of cisplatin resistance is the DNA damage tolerance process of translesion synthesis (TLS). Small molecular inhibitors of TLS were effective in overcoming TLS-mediated resistance in preclinical models.[10] Defects in mismatch repair (MMR) may also be associated with tolerance to cisplatin-induced DNA damage. In this form of platinum resistance, the MMR machinery is unable to recognize platinum–DNA adducts thus allowing the more efficient nucleotide excision repair pathway to recognize and repair the lesion.[11]

Genetic mechanisms

Mutation of drug targets

Qualitative changes in the enzyme targets of antineoplastic drugs can compromise drug efficacy and have been associated with resistance to targeted agents, especially tyrosine kinase inhibitors (TKIs). The mutations that arise through selective pressure during treatment often occur in locations that alter the binding site of the TKI. These so-called "gatekeeper" mutations have been found to be near-universal mechanisms of resistance to therapeutic TKI's, and have prompted the development of second, third, and even fourth-generation inhibitors that overcome these resistance mutations and may even be more potent against cells with both the activating and resistance mutation. Similarly, mutations in the direct targets of multiple enzyme inhibitors promote resistance to cytotoxic chemotherapy agents, including dihydrofolate reductase (DHFR) resistance to methotrexate, thymidylate synthase resistance to fluoropyrimidines, and topoisomerases I and II resistance to camptothecins.

Altered gene and protein expression

Increased or decreased expression of target enzymes can also lead to drug resistance. These alterations may result from changes that occur at any point along the pathways of gene expression and regulation, including DNA deletion or amplification, altered transcriptional or posttranscriptional control of ribonucleic acid (RNA) levels, and altered posttranslational modifications, trafficking, and degradation of proteins. For example, increased expression of DHFR is a mechanism of resistance to methotrexate, while decreased expression of topoisomerase I is a mechanism of resistance to camptothecins.

Activation of alternative signaling pathways

Resistance to targeted agents can be mediated by activation of alternative signaling pathways that provide continued growth signaling despite successful inhibition of a primary oncogenic event. Activation of several bypass signaling pathways has been found in lung cancer patients treated with inhibitors of mutant EGFR and ALK.[12] These alternative pathways include amplification of *MET*, increased hepatocyte growth factor (HGF) expression, *PIK3CA* mutation, *BRAF* mutation, and *HER2* amplification. In melanomas treated with inhibitors of mutant BRAFV600, mechanisms of resistance include *BRAF* amplification, increased activity of A-RAF and C-RAF, mutations of *NRAS* and *MEK1*, and loss of *NF1*.[13] Nongenetic mechanisms also exist, including sporadic fluctuations in ERK signaling that allow a small number of cells to survive and persist during treatment with BRAF inhibitor[14] or paradoxical decreases in protease activity that lead to upregulation of alternative receptors that drive proliferation and cell survival.[15] One strategy for overcoming drug resistance to BRAF inhibitors is concurrent inhibition of more than one kinase in the RAF–MEK–ERK pathway. This strategy was successfully tested in a randomized clinical trial of the BRAF inhibitor vemurafenib alone versus vemurafenib plus the MEK inhibitor cobimetinib in metastatic melanoma.[16] The combination resulted in a median progression-free survival of 9.9 months and remission rate of 68%, compared to 6.2 months and 45% for vemurafenib alone, respectively.

General mechanisms of resistance to multiple agents

Transport-mediated multiple drug resistance (MDR)

De novo and acquired cross-resistance to multiple antineoplastic agents can result from increased expression of a host of promiscuous drug efflux pumps known as ABC proteins. ABC proteins constitute a large family of 48 transport proteins organized into seven subfamilies, ABCA–ABCG.[2] Of these, at least three have been directly shown to cause MDR, namely MDR1/P-glycoprotein (ABCB1), MRP1, (ABCC1), and BCRP/MXR/ABC-P (ABCG2). Classic MDR associated with resistance to drugs is mediated by P-glycoprotein (MDR1 or ABCB1). A similar but distinct MDR phenotype was attributed to the energy-dependent drug efflux activities of multidrug resistance protein (MRP) family members, including MRP1 or ABCC1.[17]

The genetic basis of acquired MDR has been studied by longitudinal whole genome sequencing of tumor samples from high-grade serous ovarian and breast cancers. Multiple fusions of *ABCB1* were found to be associated with increased expression of the *ABCB1* multidrug transporter gene in approximately 60% of patients with recurrent disease after chemotherapy.[18] Fusion-positive patients had all been treated with chemotherapies that are substrates for the P-glycoprotein transporter. At least 16 different fusions were located with fusion frequency increasing with lines of chemotherapy.

Inhibition of P-glycoprotein during exposure of cancer cells to taxanes such as cabazitaxel has revealed other, alternative mechanisms of resistance to taxanes.[19] These alternate mechanisms of resistance include induction of an epithelial to mesenchymal transition (EMT) and increased dynamic instability of microtubules by overexpression of the TUBB3 isoform of β-tubulin.

Multidrug resistance related to suppression of cell death pathways

Although chemotherapeutic drugs initiate cytotoxicity through their interactions with a variety of molecular targets, cancer drugs affect cell death, at least partially, via downstream events that converge upon regulated cell death (RCD) pathways.[20] In addition to the well-studied pathways of apoptosis and autophagy, several additional forms of RCD are recognized by the Nomenclature Committee on Cell Death, including necroptosis, ferroptosis, pyroptosis, NETotic cell death, entotic cell death, and others.[21] Apoptosis refers to an orderly cellular death program with predictable molecular and morphologic changes, including nuclear pyknosis and fragmentation, internucleosomal endonucleolytic DNA fragmentation, formation of cytoplasmic apoptotic bodies, and plasma membrane changes, such as transposition of phosphatidylserine to the extracellular surface.[22,23] Autophagy is a pathway for bulk degradation of subcellular constituents that occurs in response to stresses such as nutrient deprivation.[24] It involves the creation of autophagosomes/autolysozymes and can be inhibited by PI3 kinase inhibitors such as 3-methyladenosine and wortmannin.

Although their mechanisms of action are incompletely known, the balance of expressed antiapoptotic family members (Bcl-2, Bcl-XL) and proapoptotic family members (Bax, Bak, Bad, and Bid) can influence the relative sensitivity of cells to toxic stressors.[25] Indeed, increased Bcl-2 family members are associated with increased resistance of lymphoid cells to the cytotoxic effects of corticosteroids, radiation, and DNA damage from chemotherapeutic drugs.[26,27] It has been proposed that increased levels of antiapoptotic proteins Bcl-2 or Bcl-XL may result in reduced sensitivity to DNA-damaging cancer drugs—a resistance phenotype characterized by cell survival and increased tolerance to DNA damage and genomic instability. This genomic instability may lead to further mutations activating additional resistance mechanisms and conferring more aggressive tumor behavior.[25]

Another paradigm for the role of apoptosis resistance in the development of clinical drug resistance is the concept that there is an intermediate state between sensitivity and resistance that has been termed "persistence." The clinical experience of patients who develop prolonged partial responses to targeted therapies, only to ultimately relapse with frank progression, is mirrored by the observation that cells can exist in culture under selective pressure for months without dying or growing, only to ultimately develop familiar mechanisms of agent-specific resistance. During the persister stage, these cells show increase resistance to apoptosis and increase sensitivity to Bcl-xL inhibition.[28]

Other members of the BCL2 family also play important roles in resistance to targeted therapies.[28] BIM and PUMA are both pro-apoptotic BCL2 family members whose expression is induced by targeted kinase inhibitors of oncogenes such as mutated EGFR and BRAF, the BCR-ABL fusion protein, and amplified HER2. Loss of BIM expression has been shown to inhibit apoptosis and results in resistance to inhibitors of these oncogenes. Thus, the expression of mutant and wild-type TP53, Bcl-2 family members, MAPK family members, and other proteins associated with the control of apoptosis and/or autophagy may contribute significantly to the clinical sensitivity of tumor cells. Each of these proteins is the targets of investigational agents.[25,29]

Exploiting alternative RCD pathways that induce apoptosis or autophagy in resistant cells is an emerging area of interest. Ferroptosis, a form of regulated necrosis, occurs through excessive peroxidation of polyunsaturated fatty acids in an iron-dependent manner and can be induced using one of four classes of ferroptosis inducers.[30,31] Cancer cells that are resistant to targeted and chemotherapies are generally susceptible to ferroptosis inducers. Examples include carcinoma cells with increased expression of mesenchymal gene programs[32] and also of persister cells as described above that are characteristic of minimal residual disease across a wide range of tumors.[33] Although promising in preclinical models, bioavailability, and drug transport have been roadblocks to moving effective ferroptosis inducers to the clinic,[30] but recent discoveries promise to increase the battery of potential compounds[34] and employment of nanomedicines with improved targetability are promising steps forward.[31]

Resistance factors due to host–tumor interactions and the tumor microenvironment

The failure of chemotherapy to eradicate a tumor *in vivo* despite exquisite sensitivity to drug *in vitro* might be a result of pharmacologic sanctuaries, suboptimal environmental niches, or tumor cell interactions with nontumor cells of the microenvironment. For example, failure to deliver adequate amounts of many drugs across blood–brain and blood–testicular barriers probably accounts for the relatively high frequency of acute lymphoblastic leukemia relapse at these sites prior to addition of central nervous system (CNS)-directed therapy to the treatment plans.[35] In large solid tumors, chemotherapeutic failures are frequently attributed to decreased drug delivery to a tumor that has overgrown its vascular supply and the development of acidosis and hypoxia may interfere with the cytotoxicity of some drugs.[36] Additionally, altered prodrug activation within specific anatomic sanctuaries, such as the liver may profoundly influence the efficacy of drugs such as cyclophosphamide.

Therapeutic resistance is not always tumor cell autonomous or driven by a tumor-specific gene mutation but can instead be promoted by interactions between tumor and nontumor cells within the microenvironment. For example, when exposed to therapy, cancer-associated fibroblasts remodel the extracellular matrix and release paracrine signaling factors, both of which can contribute to drug resistance in estrogen receptor positive (ER+) breast cancer,[37] prostate cancer,[38] melanoma,[39] and other tumor types.[40] Cancer drugs also directly impact cells of the immune system and can induce unexpected and paradoxical interactions that facilitate resistance.[41] The advent of single-cell sequencing and imaging technologies is allowing for more careful dissection of the subtypes of stromal and immune cells within the tumor microenvironment and will likely provide significant insight into the specific cellular populations and receptor–ligand interactions that promote therapy resistance.[42–44]

Cancer stem cells, lineage plasticity, and drug resistance

The concept of cancer stem cells (CSCs) developed from observations that individual malignant cells within a cancer differ in their capacity to form tumors. These CSCs, or "tumor-initiating cells" form a few to less than 1% of the population, have the property of plasticity or ability to change between tumorigenic and nontumorigenic states, and are a significant factor in the drug resistance of cancers.[45] Relapsed cancers are enriched in CSCs, and this subpopulation is known to express high levels of multidrug transporters as well other drug resistance genes. At the same time, CSCs offer new targets for cancer therapy, including inhibition of the Notch, Wnt, Hedgehog, and Hippo pathways.[46]

Cellular transitions during development and disease, such as the well-known EMT, facilitate acquisition of cell phenotypes not achievable in well-differentiated cells and contribute to increased therapy resistance. While EMT and other transitions may share characteristics of CSC plasticity, they are not strictly limited to the tumor-initiating cell population. Lineage plasticity is a characteristic of acquired treatment resistance across some solid tumors. Up to 5% of non-small-cell lung cancers harboring EGFR mutations and up to 20% of castrate-resistant prostate cancers exhibit histological transformation from adenocarcinoma to neuroendocrine tumor upon treatment with EGFR and antiandrogen targeted therapies, respectively.[47] A common molecular characteristic is the loss of Rb1 and p53 activity,[48–51] although deficiencies in these tumor suppressors is not sufficient to drive neuroendocrine transition, and microenvironmental context is likely important.[52,53] Lung and prostate neuroendocrine tumors can be treated with chemotherapy regimens for primary small-cell lung cancer, including the chemotherapy doublet platinum-etoposide and/or taxanes.[54,55] Adaptive therapy regimens that draw on principles of evolutionary biology may also be effective in reducing the frequency of transformation and have recently been tested in androgen resistant prostate cancer.[56]

Genetic basis of acquired drug resistance and tumor heterogeneity

Whole-genome, exome, and targeted DNA sequencing can disclose "actionable mutations" such as BRAFV600E or HER2 amplification that can guide selection of specific targeted drugs, a concept that is being tested in several clinical trials, such as NCI-MATCH (NCT02465060), DARWIN (NCT02183883), and BATTLE-2 (NCT01248247). U.S. Food and Drug Administration (FDA)-approved sequencing tests, such as Memorial Sloan Kettering integrated mutation profiling of actional cancer targets (MSK-IMPACT™) and FoundationOne CDx, are facilitating precision medicine approaches and providing publicly available knowledge bases (https://www.oncokb.org) for matching genetic alterations to possible therapies.

In addition to suggesting individual precision therapy, high resolution, deep sequencing of individual cancer genomes, and single tumor cells has revealed intratumoral heterogeneity of many cancers.[57] These data support a branched evolutionary model of tumor growth, with competing subclones differing in growth rate, metastatic potential, and sensitivity to therapy. The oncogenic truncal mutations that cause a cancer and are likely to exist in all subsequent subclones can contribute to drug sensitivity, by driving cell replication and increasing cancers' vulnerability to chemotherapy drugs that kill proliferating cells, but all true truncal mutations may be difficult to detect due to sensitivity of the sequencing assay. One mechanism of acquired resistance to an anticancer therapy is the development of resistant subclones, some of which were present before treatment and some that develop as a result of genomic instability or mutagenesis due to therapy. Evolutionary biology and population genetics have offered insight to the dynamics of positive subclonal selection in tumors exposed to therapy, as well as the challenges associated with detecting and quantifying tumor evolution.[58] In general, the emergence of drug resistance is reflected in the disappearance of drug-sensitive clones and overgrowth of resistant clones, an example of Darwinian "survival of the fittest" within cancer populations.[58] The challenge of dynamic tumor heterogeneity, as evidenced by changing subclonal structures, is evident from comparisons of DNA sequences of sequential specimens from individual patients, as well as the evolution of resistance among different patients.[59] The availability of longitudinal sampling provides the opportunity to identify new druggable vulnerabilities[60] and could facilitate strategies that exploit evolutionary principles, such as adaptive therapy.[61] More recent, large-scale efforts, including TRACERx (NCT01888601) in lung cancer, are providing new evolution-guided principles for treatment plans[62] and clinical trials such as the serial measurements of molecular and architectural response to therapy (SMMART) PRIME trial (NCT03878524) utilize multi-omic analysis to nominate combination therapy regimens based upon truncal mutations and subclone heterogeneity arising from treatment history.[63]

Deep sequencing is also revealing differences in genomic instability and apparent rates of mutation among cancers. Differences in genomic instability are generally not well understood but are correlated with mutations in genes associated with DNA damage repair pathways.[64] For example, MMR deficiency, which can underlie cisplatin resistance, is associated with a high rate of point mutations, and this may actually lead to more favorable outcomes for immunotherapies that enhance antitumor immunity via immune checkpoint controls (e.g., CTLA4, PD-1, and PDL-1).[65] Additionally, mutations in other DNA repair pathway genes can create opportunities for synthetic lethal approaches to cancer therapy.[66]

In summary, the concept that tumor masses and their metastases are composed of genetically identical clones has given way to a model that pictures each tumor as a tree-like structure with cells of origin at the center and multiple evolving subclones branching out from the trunk. Therefore, evolution of the growing tumor contributes to a heterogeneous collection of related but not identical cells in the primary mass and in distant metastases. Selection pressures such as prior therapy and the tumor microenvironment can shape the characteristics of the overall tumor cell population in a patient, and spatially separated subclones can develop different mechanisms of resistance. This appearance of a tumor with its own organism-like qualities has emerged from studies that have performed deep sequencing on multiple biopsies from primary tumor masses and their metastases. The heterogeneity of a tumor extends to genetic, epigenetic, and phenotypic diversity. Thus, strategies to overcome drug resistance must take into account diverse mechanisms of resistance to any agent because distinct populations of cells within a patient may harbor different resistance mechanisms.

Potential clinical application of strategies to avert or overcome drug resistance

Approaches to overcome chemotherapeutic failures include efforts to prevent the emergence of drug resistance. An appreciation of factors that induce resistance mechanisms may lead to the choice of more efficacious treatment regimens. Classically, aggressive combination chemotherapy with non-cross-reacting drugs was developed to eliminate tumor cells rapidly enough to prevent the selection of tumor cell clones with multiple resistance. These multi-agent chemotherapy regimen development strategies were based on the accepted concept that cells were unlikely to simultaneously develop cross-resistance to agents with different mechanisms of action. Drug combinations chosen to overcome resistance were therefore developed empirically on the basis of mechanisms of action and nonoverlapping toxicities, so that the combinations would be clinically tolerable, but without reference to, or understanding of, the molecular mechanisms of resistance to the agents.

The identification of specific mechanisms of resistance to chemotherapeutic agents, such as those conferred by the *MDR1* gene, started investigation into the possibility that drug resistance mechanisms could be identified and overcome. However, clinical strategies to circumvent mechanisms related to xenobiotic protection overall have not resulted in enhanced clinical efficacy. More recently, the clinical approach to drug resistance has been based on knowledge of how cancer cells develop resistance to each agent, and the drug combinations tested in the clinic are ones that are tailored to specific oncogenic pathways and to the observed cellular responses when those pathways are inhibited.

One strategy for preventing resistance is to use eligibility screening to select tumors that have inactivated a potential resistance mechanism. This strategy is an adaptation of the concept of "synthetic lethality" where inactivation of two genes in different pathways results in lethality, but inactivation of only one of the two genes does not. Synthetic lethality partners are often the very rescue pathways that result in resistance. By identifying synthetic lethality pairs of genes, where one is inactivated as a genetic driver mutation, tumors can be selected for treatment that will target the synthetic lethal partner of an inactivated gene, and thus avoid toxicity in normal cells while preventing the development of resistance. One of the most common approaches to the successful application of the synthetic lethality concept is the use of PARP inhibitors, which inhibit DNA repair, in tumors with inactivation of other DNA repair pathways, such as those with mutations of BRCA1 and BRCA2. Synthetic lethal combinations may involve one or more pathways, so understanding of the biology of the tumor mutations and the pathways that adapt to those mutations is essential for development of these approaches.[67]

Although some insight into these mechanisms of resistance has been gained using laboratory models of drug resistance, much of the current insight into how tumors respond to inhibition of cancer-causing signaling pathways has been hard-fought knowledge derived from biopsies of tumors of patients whose disease progressed on targeted therapies coupled to reverse translation approaches at the bench. The molecular study of these biopsies and their subsequent validation in other experimental models have led to combinations of targeted agents that directly address the mechanisms described above, including combinations where the second drug inhibits an alternative signaling of the first; a pro-apoptotic agent is added to a cytotoxic regimen; a synthetic lethal strategy might be possible; or where dual inhibition of an oncogenic target can be achieved.

In fact, the concept of overcoming drug resistance as a specialized goal of a clinical trial has evolved to the point where almost all drug combination studies can be viewed through the lens of a strategy to overcome at least one mechanism of resistance. Clinical studies of these strategies in relapsed populations, if promising, are advanced into the frontline setting, so there has become little distinction between strategies to overcome and strategies to prevent drug resistance.

Conclusion and future directions

The diversity of mechanisms of antineoplastic drug resistance combined with the biologic heterogeneity of tumors presents a formidable therapeutic challenge. Nevertheless, the identification of the drug resistance mechanisms has led to useful approaches to overcoming clinical drug resistance and improving therapeutic outcomes. These approaches include the design of novel drugs that are less likely to share resistance mechanisms and the development of combination therapies that target resistance pathways. Despite these efforts, many tumors will remain refractory to conventional and targeted chemotherapeutic agents.

Key references

The complete reference list can be found on Vital Source version of this title, see inside front cover.

1. Matherly LH, Wilson MR, Hou Z. The major facilitative folate transporters solute carrier 19A1 and solute carrier 46A1: biology and role in antifolate chemotherapy of cancer. *Drug Metab Dispos*. 2014;**42**(4):632–649.
2. Robey RW, Pluchino KM, Hall MD, et al. Revisiting the role of ABC transporters in multidrug-resistant cancer. *Nat Rev Cancer*. 2018;**18**(7):452–464.
3. Amiri-Kordestani L, Basseville A, Kurdziel K, et al. Targeting MDR in breast and lung cancer: discriminating its potential importance from the failure of drug resistance reversal studies. *Drug Resist Updat*. 2012;**15**(1–2):50–61.
5. Tsesmetzis N, Paulin CBJ, Rudd SG, et al. Nucleobase and nucleoside analogues: resistance and re-sensitisation at the level of pharmacokinetics, pharmacodynamics and metabolism. *Cancers (Basel)*. 2018;**10**(7):240.

7. Capello M, Lee M, Wang H, et al. Carboxylesterase 2 as a determinant of response to irinotecan and neoadjuvant FOLFIRINOX therapy in pancreatic ductal adenocarcinoma. *J Natl Cancer Inst.* 2015;**107**(8):djv132.
8. Hunt SW 3rd, Hoffee PA. Amplification of adenosine deaminase gene sequences in deoxycoformycin-resistant rat hepatoma cells. *J Biol Chem.* 1983;**258**(21):13185–13192.
9. Houghton JA, Maroda SJ Jr, Phillips JO, et al. Biochemical determinants of responsiveness to 5-fluorouracil and its derivatives in xenografts of human colorectal adenocarcinomas in mice. *Cancer Res.* 1981;**41**(1):144–149.
10. Wojtaszek JL, Chatterjee N, Najeeb J, et al. A small molecule targeting mutagenic translesion synthesis improves chemotherapy. *Cell.* 2019;**178**(1):152–159 e11.
11. Galluzzi L, Vitale I, Michels J, et al. Systems biology of cisplatin resistance: past, present and future. *Cell Death Dis.* 2014;**5**(5):e1257.
12. Camidge DR, Pao W, Sequist LV. Acquired resistance to TKIs in solid tumours: learning from lung cancer. *Nat Rev Clin Oncol.* 2014;**11**(8):473–481.
13. Van Allen EM, Wagle N, Sucker A, et al. The genetic landscape of clinical resistance to RAF inhibition in metastatic melanoma. *Cancer Discov.* 2014;**4**(1):94–109.
14. Gerosa L, Chidley C, Fröhlich F, et al. Receptor-driven ERK pulses reconfigure MAPK signaling and enable persistence of drug-adapted BRAF-mutant melanoma cells. *Cell Syst.* 2020;**11**(5):478–494 e9.
15. Miller MA, Sullivan RJ, Lauffenburger DA. Molecular pathways: receptor ectodomain shedding in treatment, resistance, and monitoring of cancer. *Clin Cancer Res.* 2017;**23**(3):623–629.
16. Larkin J, Ascierto PA, Dreno B, et al. Combined vemurafenib and cobimetinib in BRAF-mutated melanoma. *N Engl J Med.* 2014;**371**(20):1867–1876.
17. Cole SP. Multidrug resistance protein 1 (MRP1, ABCC1), a "multitasking" ATP-binding cassette (ABC) transporter. *J Biol Chem.* 2014;**289**(45):30880–30888.
18. Christie EL, Pattnaik S, Beach J, et al. Multiple ABCB1 transcriptional fusions in drug resistant high-grade serous ovarian and breast cancer. *Nat Commun.* 2019;**10**(1):1295.
19. Duran GE, Wang YC, Francisco EB, et al. Mechanisms of resistance to cabazitaxel. *Mol Cancer Ther.* 2015;**14**(1):193–201.
20. Tang D, Kang R, Berghe TV, et al. The molecular machinery of regulated cell death. *Cell Res.* 2019;**29**(5):347–364.
21. Galluzzi L, Vitale I, Aaronson SA, et al. Molecular mechanisms of cell death: recommendations of the Nomenclature Committee on Cell Death 2018. *Cell Death Differ.* 2018;**25**(3):486–541.
23. Hanahan D, Weinberg RA. Hallmarks of cancer: the next generation. *Cell.* 2011;**144**(5):646–674.
24. Levine B, Kroemer G. Autophagy in the pathogenesis of disease. *Cell.* 2008;**132**(1):27–42.
25. Thomas S, Quinn BA, Das SK, et al. Targeting the Bcl-2 family for cancer therapy. *Expert Opin Ther Targets.* 2013;**17**(1):61–75.
27. Stahnke K, Fulda S, Friesen C, et al. Activation of apoptosis pathways in peripheral blood lymphocytes by *in vivo* chemotherapy. *Blood.* 2001;**98**(10):3066–3073.
28. Hata AN, Engelman JA, Faber AC. The BCL2 family: key mediators of the apoptotic response to targeted anticancer therapeutics. *Cancer Discov.* 2015;**5**(5):475–487.
31. Liang C, Zhang X, Yang M, et al. Recent progress in ferroptosis inducers for cancer therapy. *Adv Mater.* 2019;**31**(51):e1904197.
32. Viswanathan VS, Ryan MJ, Dhruv HD, et al. Dependency of a therapy-resistant state of cancer cells on a lipid peroxidase pathway. *Nature.* 2017;**547**(7664):453–457.
33. Hangauer MJ, Viswanathan VS, Ryan MJ, et al. Drug-tolerant persister cancer cells are vulnerable to GPX4 inhibition. *Nature.* 2017;**551**(7679):247–250.
34. Eaton JK, Furst L, Ruberto RA, et al. Selective covalent targeting of GPX4 using masked nitrile-oxide electrophiles. *Nat Chem Biol.* 2020;**16**(5):497–506.
35. Poplack DG, Reaman G. Acute lymphoblastic leukemia in childhood. *Pediatr Clin N Am.* 1988;**35**(4):903–932.
36. Pillai SR, Damaghi M, Marunaka Y, et al. Causes, consequences, and therapy of tumors acidosis. *Cancer Metastasis Rev.* 2019;**38**(1–2):205–222.
37. Shee K, Yang W, Hinds JW, et al. Therapeutically targeting tumor microenvironment-mediated drug resistance in estrogen receptor-positive breast cancer. *J Exp Med.* 2018;**215**(3):895–910.
38. Sun Y, Zhu D, Chen F, et al. SFRP2 augments WNT16B signaling to promote therapeutic resistance in the damaged tumor microenvironment. *Oncogene.* 2016;**35**(33):4321–4334.
39. Hirata E, Girotti MR, Viros A, et al. Intravital imaging reveals how BRAF inhibition generates drug-tolerant microenvironments with high integrin β1/FAK signaling. *Cancer Cell.* 2015;**27**(4):574–588.
40. Leask A. A centralized communication network: recent insights into the role of the cancer associated fibroblast in the development of drug resistance in tumors. *Semin Cell Dev Biol.* 2020;**101**:111–114.
41. Wang SJ, Li R, Ng TSC, et al. Efficient blockade of locally reciprocated tumor-macrophage signaling using a TAM-avid nanotherapy. *Sci Adv.* 2020;**6**(21):eaaz8521.
42. Tirosh I, Izar B, Prakadan SM, et al. Dissecting the multicellular ecosystem of metastatic melanoma by single-cell RNA-seq. *Science.* 2016;**352**(6282):189–196.
43. Elyada E, Bolisetty M, Laise P, et al. Cross-species single-cell analysis of pancreatic ductal adenocarcinoma reveals antigen-presenting cancer-associated fibroblasts. *Cancer Discov.* 2019;**9**(8):1102–1123.
44. Azizi E, Carr AJ, Plitas G, et al. Single-cell map of diverse immune phenotypes in the breast tumor microenvironment. *Cell.* 2018;**174**(5):1293–1308 e36.
45. Mertins SD. Cancer stem cells: a systems biology view of their role in prognosis and therapy. *Anti-Cancer Drugs.* 2014;**25**(4):353–367.
46. Clara JA, Monge C, Yang Y, et al. Targeting signalling pathways and the immune microenvironment of cancer stem cells - a clinical update. *Nat Rev Clin Oncol.* 2020;**17**(4):204–232.
47. Quintanal-Villalonga Á, Chan JM, Yu HA, et al. Lineage plasticity in cancer: a shared pathway of therapeutic resistance. *Nat Rev Clin Oncol.* 2020;**17**(6):360–371.
48. Ku SY, Rosario S, Wang Y, et al. Rb1 and Trp53 cooperate to suppress prostate cancer lineage plasticity, metastasis, and antiandrogen resistance. *Science.* 2017;**355**(6320):78–83.
49. Lee JK, Lee J, Kim S, et al. Clonal history and genetic predictors of transformation into small-cell carcinomas from lung adenocarcinomas. *J Clin Oncol.* 2017;**35**(26):3065–3074.
51. Offin M, Chan JM, Tenet M, et al. Concurrent RB1 and TP53 alterations define a subset of EGFR-mutant lung cancers at risk for histologic transformation and inferior clinical outcomes. *J Thorac Oncol.* 2019;**14**(10):1784–1793.
52. Nyquist MD, Corella A, Coleman I, et al. Combined TP53 and RB1 loss promotes prostate cancer resistance to a spectrum of therapeutics and confers vulnerability to replication stress. *Cell Rep.* 2020;**31**(8):107669.
53. Patel GK, Chugh N, Tripathi M. Neuroendocrine differentiation of prostate cancer-an intriguing example of tumor evolution at play. *Cancers (Basel).* 2019;**11**(10):1405.
55. Marcoux N, Gettinger SN, O'Kane G, et al. EGFR-mutant adenocarcinomas that transform to small-cell lung cancer and other neuroendocrine carcinomas: clinical outcomes. *J Clin Oncol.* 2019;**37**(4):278–285.
56. Zhang J, Cunningham JJ, Brown JS, et al. Integrating evolutionary dynamics into treatment of metastatic castrate-resistant prostate cancer. *Nat Commun.* 2017;**8**(1):1816.
57. Swanton C. Intratumor heterogeneity: evolution through space and time. *Cancer Res.* 2012;**72**(19):4875–4882.
58. Turajlic S, Sottoriva A, Graham T, et al. Resolving genetic heterogeneity in cancer. *Nat Rev Genet.* 2019;**20**(7):404–416.
59. Patch AM, Christie EL, Etemadmoghadam D, et al. Whole-genome characterization of chemoresistant ovarian cancer. *Nature.* 2015;**521**(7553):489–494.
60. Brady SW, McQuerry JA, Qiao Y, et al. Combating subclonal evolution of resistant cancer phenotypes. *Nat Commun.* 2017;**8**(1):1231.
61. West J, You L, Zhang J, et al. Towards multidrug adaptive therapy. *Cancer Res.* 2020;**80**(7):1578–1589.
62. Swanton C. Take lessons from cancer evolution to the clinic. *Nature.* 2020;**581**(7809):382–383.
63. Mitri ZI, Parmar S, Johnson B, et al. Implementing a comprehensive translational oncology platform: from molecular testing to actionability. *J Transl Med.* 2018;**16**(1):358.
64. Knijnenburg TA, Wang L, Zimmermann MT, et al. Genomic and molecular landscape of DNA damage repair deficiency across the cancer genome atlas. *Cell Rep.* 2018;**23**(1):239–254 e6.
65. Zhao P, Li L, Jiang X, et al. Mismatch repair deficiency/microsatellite instability-high as a predictor for anti-PD-1/PD-L1 immunotherapy efficacy. *J Hematol Oncol.* 2019;**12**(1):54.
66. Srivas R, Shen JP, Yang CC, et al. A network of conserved synthetic lethal interactions for exploration of precision cancer therapy. *Mol Cell.* 2016;**63**(3):514–525.
67. Li S, Topatana W, Juengpanich S, et al. Development of synthetic lethality in cancer: molecular and cellular classification. *Signal Transduct Target Ther.* 2020;**5**(1):241.

PART 9

Biological and Gene Therapy

59 Cytokines, interferons, and hematopoietic growth factors

Narendranath Epperla, MD, MS ■ Walter Hanel, MD, PhD ■ Moshe Talpaz, MD

Overview

Cytokines are a diverse family of signaling molecules encompassing interleukins, interferons, and hematopoietic growth factors. As important mediators of immune responses, cytokines play critical roles and have clinical relevance in cancer. Interleukins have numerous diverse effects in cancer, including influencing the growth, differentiation, or survival of endothelial cells; attracting inflammatory cell types or induce secondary cytokines to regulate angiogenesis; influencing the tumor environment and infiltrating hematopoietic effector cells; inhibiting or stimulating tumor growth; and regulating immune responses. Various immunostimulatory cytokines, including ILs, are administered to patients in an attempt to initiate or augment antitumor immune responses. Interferons are a large family of multifunctional secreted proteins involved in antiviral defense, cell growth regulation, and immune activation. The three types of IFNs, types I, II, and III, signal via specific cell surface receptors and the JAK-STAT pathway to transcriptionally activate IFN-regulated genes (IRGs). Alterations in IRG expression result in modulation of receptors for other cytokines, concentration of regulatory proteins on the surface of immune effector cells, and activation of enzymes that control cellular growth and function. Both natural and recombinant IFNs have shown antitumor activity as single agents in more than a dozen malignancies. Hematopoietic growth factors, most notably epoetin, thrombopoietin, and granulocyte colony-stimulating factor (G-CSF), are used in the clinic to stimulate the growth and differentiation of red blood cells, platelets, or neutrophils in clinical settings including after chemotherapy or bone marrow transplantation in a restorative role.

Cytokines, a diverse family of signaling molecules, are important mediators of immune responses and are produced by almost every cell in the body including various cancer cells. Some cytokines are growth stimulatory and others are inhibitory. Cytokines with clinical relevance in cancer can be subclassified as interleukins (ILs), monokines, chemokines, interferons (IFNs), and hematopoietic growth factors. ILs designate any soluble protein or glycoprotein product of leukocytes that regulates the responses of other leukocytes. ILs produce their effects primarily through paracrine interactions. In cancer, certain cytokines act directly on the growth, differentiation, or survival of endothelial cells. Others act by attracting inflammatory cell types affecting angiogenesis or by inducing secondary cytokines or other mediators regulating angiogenesis. Proinflammatory and chemotactic cytokines influence the tumor environment and control the quantity and nature of infiltrating hematopoietic effector cells and can inhibit or stimulate tumor growth. They may also regulate immune responses and can either stimulate a more robust antitumor immune response or dampen immune responses by suppressing the function of antigen-presenting cells (APC). Various immunostimulatory cytokines, including ILs, are now administered to patients in an attempt to initiate or augment antitumor immune responses. In addition to immune response stimulation, some cytokines, most notably epoetin, thrombopoietin (TPO), and granulocyte colony-stimulating factor (G-CSF), are frequently used in the clinic to stimulate the growth and differentiation of red blood cells, platelets, or neutrophils in several clinical settings including after chemotherapy or bone marrow transplantation (BMT) in a restorative role. It is now clear that the pleiotropic nature of many cytokines allows them to influence virtually all organ systems (Figure 1). Cytokines may have their own private receptor but may also share a "public" receptor with other cytokines (Tables 1 and 2).

In this article, we will discuss the biologic characterization of selected ILs, IFNs and growth factors, the rationale for their use in therapy for patients with cancer, and the most current clinical data of each. Although anticytokine therapies, including anticytokine antibodies and decoy receptors, have revolutionized the treatment of many diseases, most notably autoimmune diseases, this article will mainly focus on therapy with cytokines rather than anticytokine therapy.

Interleukins

Interleukin-1

IL-1 (IL-1α and IL-1β) is the prototypic pleiotropic cytokine and influences nearly every cell type.[1,2] IL-1 is a highly inflammatory cytokine and has been found to play a central role in many autoimmune disorders. IL-1 can increase its own expression as well as the expression of other cytokines (including IL-1RA), cytokine receptors, inflammatory mediators (such as cyclooxygenase and inducible nitric oxide synthase), hepatic acute phase reactants, growth factors, clotting factors, neuropeptides, lipid-related genes, extracellular matrix molecules, and oncogenes (e.g., *c-jun, cabl, c-fms, c-myc, c-fos*).[1]

The IL-1 family has been implicated in the function and dysfunction of virtually every human organ system. Indeed, increased IL-1 production has been reported in patients with infections (viral, bacterial, fungal, and parasitic), intravascular coagulation, cancer (both solid tumors and hematologic malignancies), Alzheimer's disease, autoimmune disorders, trauma, ischemic diseases, pancreatitis, graft-versus-host disease (GvHD), transplant rejection, and in healthy subjects after exercise.[1] The IL-1 axis plays a pivotal role in cancer-associated inflammation, as further discussed in the following paragraph.[3] In addition, IL-1 is a proangiogenic stimulus of both physiological and pathological angiogenesis.

Holland-Frei Cancer Medicine, Tenth Edition. Edited by Robert C. Bast, John C. Byrd, Carlo M. Croce, Ernest Hawk, Fadlo R. Khuri, Raphael E. Pollock, Apostolia M. Tsimberidou, Christopher G. Willett, and Cheryl L. Willman.
© 2023 John Wiley & Sons, Inc. Published 2023 by John Wiley & Sons, Inc.

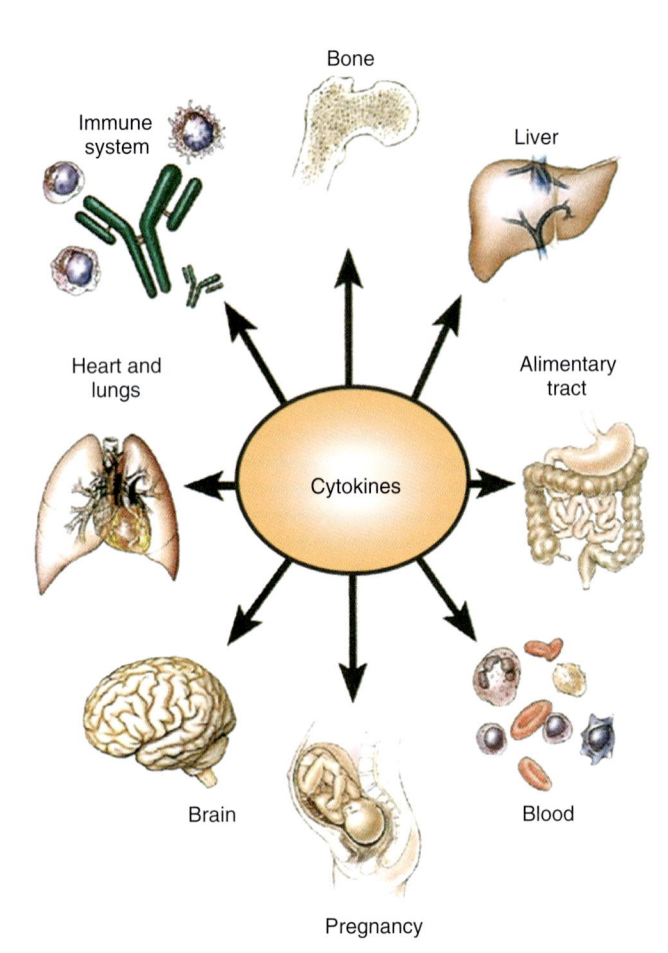

Figure 1 In addition to their effects on hematopoiesis and immunocompetence, "hematopoietic" growth factors influence multiple organ systems, including (but not limited to) bone remodeling, cardiorespiratory function, hepatic function, and the gastrointestinal tract.

IL-1 and its naturally occurring antagonists must each be considered because it is the balance between these various cytokines, and not just one individual member, which is most relevant to illness.[4] This balance may be altered in different ways, depending on the disease. In acute myelogenous leukemia (AML), IL-10 is spontaneously expressed, but IL-1RA gene expression is suppressed even when stimulated with granulocyte-macrophage colony-stimulating factor (GM-CSF).[5,6] Chronic myeloid leukemia (CML) patients with advanced disease and poor survival have suppressed IL-1RA accompanied by high IL-1β.[7] In AML and CML patients, IL-1β acts as an autocrine growth factor; exposure to molecules that decrease the activity of IL-1 suppresses leukemic proliferation.[8,9] Constitutive production of IL-1α, IL-1β, and/or IL-1RA in solid tumors (melanomas, hepatoblastoma, sarcomas, squamous cell carcinomas, transitional cell cancers, and ovarian carcinomas) has been described and may, at least in some cases, contribute to metastatic potential. However, the relationship between IL-1 and tumor growth is complex.

IL-1 in the clinic

IL-1α and IL-1β have both been administered in clinical cancer trials, to induce bone marrow recovery or cancer treatment.[1] In general, the acute toxicities of both isoforms were greater after intravenous than subcutaneous injection. Subcutaneous injection was associated with significant local pain, erythema, and swelling. Dose-related chills and fever were observed in nearly all patients, and even a 1 ng/kg dose was pyrogenic. Nearly all patients receiving intravenous IL-1 at doses of 100 ng/kg or greater experienced significant hypotension, probably because of the induction of nitric oxide.

IL-1 infusion into humans significantly increased circulating IL-6 levels and resulted in a rise in leukocyte counts, even at doses as low as 1 or 2 ng/kg. Increases in platelets, peripheral monocyte count, and phorbol-induced superoxide production were also observed in patients with normal marrow reserves. In contrast, patients with aplastic anemia treated with five daily doses of IL-1α (30–100 ng/kg) had no increases in peripheral blood counts or bone marrow cellularity.[10] However, after chemotherapy, two doses of IL-1α significantly shortened the duration of neutropenia,[11] and IL-1α (5 days) significantly reduced thrombocytopenia.[12] IL-1 therapy has proved to be exceedingly difficult due to the toxicity involved. With the advent of more targeted and less toxic agents to induce count recovery, such as G-CSF and TPO agonists, IL-1 therapy for this purpose is no longer appropriate. Overall, in cancer-related studies, including therapies for hematological malignancies, GvHD, and chemotherapy-induced mucositis, the focus has shifted to blocking the IL-1 axis, such as with anakinra (recombinant IL-1RA) rather than augmenting it for therapy.[13]

Interleukin-2

Originally discovered as a T-cell growth factor, the function of IL-2 has since extended beyond lymphocyte activation and population expansion to B-cells, natural killer (NK) cells, and lymphokine-activated killer (LAK) cells.[14] The IL-2R consists of

Table 1 Types of hematopoietic growth factor receptors.

Type	Characteristics	Receptor examples
Type I cytokine receptor	Does not possess intrinsic kinase activity. Receptor acts as docking site for adaptor molecules, which leads to phosphorylation of cellular substrates	IL-1, IL-2, IL-3, IL-4, IL-5, IL-6, IL-7, IL-9, IL-13, IL-18, IL-21, GM-CSF, G-CSF, EPO, TPO, leukemia inhibitory factor
Type II cytokine receptor	Contains extracellular fibronectin III type domain	Interferon and IL-10
Receptors with tyrosine kinase domains (type III)	Large extracellular immunoglobulin-like domain, single transmembrane spinning region, and a cytoplasmic tyrosine kinase domain(s)	fms (M-CSF receptor), FLT-3, c-kit (SCF receptor), PDGFR
Chemokine receptor	Seven transmembrane spanning G protein-linked regions	IL-8
Tumor necrosis factor family	Cysteine-rich repeats in the extracellular domain, and cytoplasmic 80 amino acid "death domain"	Tumor necrosis factor and Fas

Abbreviations: EPO, erythropoietin; G-CSF, granulocyte colony-stimulating factor; GM-CSF, granulocyte macrophage colony-stimulating factor; IL, interleukin; M-CSF, macrophage colony-stimulating factor; SCF, stem cell factor; TPO, thrombopoietin.

Table 2 Interleukins.

	Chromosomal location	Receptors	Selected biologic activities
IL-1	2q13	IL-1RI and IL-1RII	Promotes acute phase response IL-1 acts on nearly every organ system. Induces production of multiple cytokines Up-regulates cell-surface cytokine expression Synergizes with other cytokines to stimulate hematopoietic progenitor proliferation Influences immune regulation Modulates endocrine function Affects bone formation IL-1R acts as a cofactor in neural transmission
IL-2	4q26-q27	$\alpha\beta\gamma$ heterotrimeric complex	Induces proliferation and activation of T cells, B cells, and NK cells
IL-3	5q31	IL-3 receptor (heterodimer of IL-3 specific asubunit and β subunit)	Stimulation of multilineage hematopoietic progenitors, especially when used in combination with other cytokines (SCF, IL-1, IL-6, G-CSF, GM-CSF, EPO, TPO)
IL-4 and IL-13	5q31	Type I IL-4 receptor (IL-4Rα and IL-2 receptor γc chain subunits) transduces IL-4 Type II IL-4 receptor (IL-4Rα and the IL-13 Rα1 subunits) transduces IL-4 and IL-13 IL-4Rα and IL-13 Rα2 complex or two IL-13 Rα transduce IL-13	IL-4 and IL-13 are involved in allergic reaction (induce switch to IgE)
IL-5	5q31	Consists of IL-5Rα (IL-5-specific) and a β subunit β subunit is common to IL-3 and GM-CSF complexes	Regulates production, function, survival, and migration of eosinophils Enhances basophil number and function
IL-6	7p21	IL-6Rα together with gp130	B- and T-cell development and function Thrombopoiesis Acute-phase protein synthesis Inhibition of hepatic albumin excretion Osteoclastic bone resorption Neural differentiation
IL-7	8q12-q13	Composed of IL-7Rα (CD127) and the common γc chain subunits	Critical for T- and B-cell development
IL-8	4q12-q13	IL-8Rα and IL-8Rβ exist	Potent chemoattractant agent for a variety of leukocytes, especially neutrophils Suppresses colony formation of immature myeloid progenitors Increases keratinocyte and endothelial cell proliferation
IL-9	5q31.1	IL-9 receptor	Supports clonogenic maturation of erythroid progenitors Acts as a mast cell differentiation factor Protects lymphomas from apoptosis Cooperates with IL-4 in B-cell responses Enhances neuronal differentiation
IL-10	1q31-q32	IL-10 receptor interferon receptors	Inhibits cytokine synthesis by Th1 cells and monocytes/macrophages Stimulates B cell proliferation Involved in transformation of B cells by Epstein–Barr virus and tumor necrosis factor (TNF) receptors
IL-11	19q13.3-q13.4	IL-11Rα and gp 130 subunits gp 130 = CD130 on 5q11 IL-6, oncostatin M, and leukemia inhibitory factor also use gp130 subunit	Best known as a thrombopoietic factor Stimulates multilineage progenitors, erythropoiesis, myelopoiesis, and lymphopoiesis Decreases mucositis in animal models Stimulates osteoclast development Inhibits adipogenesis Stimulates proliferation of neuronal cells
IL-12	IL-12A:3p12-q13.2 IL-12B:5q31.1-q33.1	IL-12Rβ1 and IL-12Rβ2 chains are related to gp 130	Proinflammatory cytokine important in resistance to infections Th1 development Stimulatory and inhibitory effects on hematopoiesis
IL-15	4q31	High affinity receptor requires IL-2Rβ and γ chains and IL-15 Rα chain	Triggers proliferation and immunoglobulin production in preactivated B cells Number of CD8+ memory T cells may be controlled by balance of IL-15 (stimulatory) and IL-12 (inhibitory) Stimulates proliferation of NK cells and activated CD4+ or CD8+ T cells Facilitates the induction of LAK cells and CTLs Stimulates mast cell proliferation Promotes proliferation of hairy-cell leukemia and chronic lymphocytic leukemia cells

(continued overleaf)

Table 2 (Continued)

	Chromosomal location	Receptors	Selected biologic activities
IL-16	15q26.1	Requires CD4 for biologic activities Tetraspanin CD9	Chemoattractant for CD4+ cells (T cells, monocytes, eosinophils) May be involved in asthma and in granulomatous inflammation Has antiviral effects on HIV-1
IL-17	2q31	IL-17 receptor	May mediate, in part, T-cell contribution to inflammation Stimulates epithelial, endothelial, fibroblastic, and macrophage cells to express a variety of inflammatory cytokines Promotes the capacity of fibroblasts to sustain hematopoietic progenitor growth Promotes differentiation of dendritic cell progenitors May be involved in the pathogenesis of rheumatoid arthritis and graft rejection
IL-18	11q22.2-q22.3	IL-18 receptor	Promotes production of IFN-γ, TNF Targets are T cells, NK cells, and macrophages Promotes Th1 responses to virus
IL-19	1q32	IL-20Rl and IL-20R2	Induces IL-6 and TNF-α
IL-20	1q32	IL-20R1 and IL-20R2	Induction of genes involved in inflammation such as TNF-α, MRP14 and MCP-1
IL-21	4q26–27	IL-21 receptor	Mainly, regulates T-cell proliferation and differentiation Regulates cell-mediated immunity and the clearance of tumors
IL-22	12q14	IL-22R1 and IL-10R2	Up-regulates the production of acute-phase reactants Induces the production of ROS in resting B cells
IL-23	12q13	IL-12Rb1 and IL-23R	A unique function of IL-23 is the preferential induction of proliferation of the memory subset of T cells
IL-24	1q32	IL-20R1 and IL-20R2	Induces IL-6, TNF-a, IL-1b, IL-12 and GM-CSF
		IL-22R1 and IL-20R2	Functionally it has opposite effects with IL-10 Infection with Ad-IL24 results in down-regulation of Bcl-2 and Bcl-XL (anti-apoptotic proteins) and up-regulation of Bax and Bak (pro-apoptotic proteins) in cancer cells
IL-25	14q11	IL-17BR	IL-25 induces IL-4, IL-5, and IL-13 gene expression and protein production
IL-26	12q14	IL-20R1 and IL-10R2	Immune-protective role against viral infection
IL-27	12q13	TCCR/WSX-1 and GP130	Early Th1 initiation Synergizes with IL-12 in inducing IFN-γ production by T cells and NK cells
IL-28A, 28B, and 29	19q13	IL-28R1 and IL-10R2	Antiviral activities
IL-31	12q24	IL-31 receptor A and oncostatin M receptor	Responsible for promoting the dermatitis and epithelial responses that characterize allergic and nonallergic diseases
IL-32	16p13.3	Proteinase 3	Induces other proinflammatory cytokines and chemokines such as TNF-α, IL-1β, IL-6, and IL-8 Induces ικβ degradation Phosphorylates p38 MAPK signaling pathway
IL-33	9p24.1	ST2	Activates NF-κβ and MAP kinases Drives production of Th2-associated cytokines from in vitro polarized Th2 cells Induces the expression of IL-4, IL-5, and IL-13 Leads to severe pathologic changes in mucosal organs
IL-35	19p13.3	IL-12Rβ2 and gp130	Contributes Treg suppressor activity Induces IL-10 and IFN-g serum levels Reduces induction of IL-17
IL-36	IL36A;2q12-q14.1 IL36G:2q12-q21 IL36RN:2q14	IL-1Rrp2 and IL-1RAcP	Activates NF-κβ and MAP kinases Play important role in skin biology Involved in the initiation and regulation of immune responses
IL-37	2q12-q14.1	IL-18R	Regulates inflammatory responses
IL-38	2q13	IL36R	Reduces IL-36g induced IL-8 production

three distinct proteins, α, β, and the common γ chain (γc), which together form a high affinity receptor for IL-2. The β and γc chains can form an intermediate affinity IL-2R while the α chain by itself is a low-affinity IL-2R. Binding of IL-2 results in internalization and cell-cycle progression induced by the expression of a defined series of genes.[15] A second functional response occurs through the dimeric β/γc receptor and involves the differentiation of several subclasses of lymphocytes into LAK cells.[16] This response occurs in patients with cancer who receive IL-2[17,18] and was originally considered to be a critical part of the anticancer effect of IL-2.

IL-2 in the clinic

IL-2 has had a profound impact on the development of cancer immunotherapy. The administration of IL-2, as well as the adoptive transfer of antitumor T cells grown in IL-2, represented the first effective immunotherapies for cancer in humans.[19] Since 1992, numerous clinical trials using high dose IL-2 (HD IL-2) have delivered a remarkably consistent 7% complete response rate in two advanced cancer types, renal cell carcinoma (RCC) and malignant melanoma.[20–24] Many of these complete responses have been durable beyond 10 years. HD IL-2's anticancer activity is strongly related to its ability to act as a growth factor for T lymphocytes, its capacity to stimulate antigen-independent NK cells and LAK cells, and its ability to increase lymphocytes at the site of malignancy. The significant and sometimes fatal adverse effects of HD IL-2 are largely the result of severe vasodilation and capillary leak syndrome and include hypotension, arrhythmias, and liver and renal toxicities. Expert guidelines exist for the safe administration of IL-2,[25] and require staff who are trained in its administration and the recognition of severe side effects so supportive care can be provided promptly. The 1–2% risk of mortality with IL-2 highlights the importance of choosing a well-suited patient for this treatment modality.[26]

Historically, HD IL-2 was first used in a combinational biochemotherapy (BCT) setting, usually involving cisplatin, vinblastine, and dacarbazine (CVD) or cisplatin, vinblastine, and temozolomide (CVT), plus the biologic agents interferon α (IFN-α) and IL-2. However, a modest increase in survival came with a substantial increase in toxicity.[27] More recently, as the immune checkpoint inhibitors (ICIs), such as nivolumab and ipilimumab, have revolutionized the treatment of melanoma after demonstrating durable responses with a safer profile without the need for inpatient administration, HD IL-2 has become less frequently used. Combining ICIs with HD IL-2 has been the subject of multiple past and ongoing clinical trials, but their role together as a combination therapy still needs to be more clearly defined. No data are currently available regarding the correct sequencing of immunotherapies. Some melanoma experts believe that IL-2 is best used very early on in therapy when subjects have more limited disease (M1a disease) and good performance status. A small study has indicated that there may be a higher response rate (47%) in patients with NRAS-mutant melanoma, but further validation of this finding is needed.[28] A 2005 study in 36 patients with advanced melanoma who received a combination of ipilimumab (0.1–3 mg/kg every 3 weeks) and IL-2 demonstrated an overall response rate of 22%.[29] Studies evaluating the role of ipilimumab with adoptive cell therapy are ongoing. Another approach to extend or enhance the efficacy of HD IL-2 is to combine immunotherapy with BRAF inhibitors for the treatment of patients with BRAFV600-mutant advanced melanoma.[30] Preclinical studies showed an increase in melanoma antigen expression and the number of tumor-infiltrating lymphocytes in tumor biopsies after BRAF inhibitor therapy, which correlated with a reduction in tumor size and an increase in necrosis.[31,32] However, a recent small Phase II study combining vemurafenib with IL-2 showed progression of all six patients enrolled, with an increase in Tregs potentially abrogating the efficacy of the combination.[33]

Interleukin-3

IL-3 was first described as a T-cell product involved in the pathogenesis of Moloney leukemia virus-induced T-cell lymphomas.[34] This molecule is of interest because of its ability to stimulate multilineage hematopoietic progenitors both *in vitro* and *in vivo*.[34–41] *In vitro*, IL-3, in combination with other cytokines, such as stem cell factor (SCF), IL-6, IL-1, G-CSF, GM-CSF, erythropoietin (EPO), or TPO, induces the proliferation of colony-forming unit (CFU)-GM, CFU-Eo, CFU-Baso, BFU-E, and CFU-granulocyte, erythrocyte, monocyte, megakaryocyte (GEMM) in semisolid medium, and stimulates the proliferation of purified CD34+ cells in suspension culture.[35] Indeed, IL-3 is combined with other cytokines, in particular SCF, IL-6, IL-1, FL, G-CSF, and/or EPO, in almost all protocols to expand hematopoietic stem and progenitor cells *in vitro*.

IL-3 in the clinic

IL-3 has been used in a variety of clinical trials; peripheral blood stem cell mobilization, postchemotherapy and transplantation, and bone marrow failure states. The majority of studies show only modest effects of IL-3 by itself, but significant salutary effects in conjunction with other growth factors. For instance, in mobilization studies, treatment with IL-3 did not mobilize by itself but significantly potentiated G-CSF-induced yield of all progenitor cell types used to restore hematopoiesis after high-dose chemotherapy. After transplantation, the combination of IL-3 and GM-CSF proved more efficient to support bone marrow engraftment than IL-3 or GM-CSF alone. The combination of IL-3 and GM-CSF was more efficient than G-CSF for supporting platelet recovery but was of similar benefit for the reconstitution of myelopoiesis. Following chemotherapy, IL-3 was found to attenuate neutropenia and/or thrombocytopenia in some but not all clinical studies. However, given the success of G-CSF and TPO agonists in the induction of myelopoiesis and thrombopoiesis in various settings, the role of IL-3 therapy in the clinic has not been defined.

Interleukin-4 and interleukin-13

IL-4 and IL-13 are closely related.[42–44] They share biologic and immunoregulatory functions on B cells, monocytes, dendritic cells, and fibroblasts. They can stimulate the growth of T and B-cells, differentiate B-cells to plasma cells, and allow B-cell IgE class switching. In addition, IL-4/IL-13 can polarize macrophages into the anti-inflammatory M2 phenotype. Both IL-4 and IL-13 genes are located in the same vicinity on chromosome 5. The major regulatory sequences in the IL-4 and IL-13 promoters are identical, thus explaining their restricted expression pattern in activated T cells and mast cells. Furthermore, the IL-4 and IL-13 receptors are multimeric and share at least one common chain—IL-4RA. This, together with similarities in IL-4 and IL-13 signal transduction, explains the striking overlap of biologic properties between these two cytokines as IL-13 elicits many, but not all, of the biologic actions of IL-4. IL-4 is, however, distinguished from IL-13 by its T-cell growth factor activity and its ability to drive differentiation of Th0 precursors toward the Th2 lineage. Th2 cells secrete IL-4 and IL-5 and lead to a preferential stimulation of humoral immunity. In contrast, Th1 cells, which produce IL-2 and IFN-γ, lead to a preferential stimulation of cellular immunity. The inability of IL-13 to regulate T-cell differentiation is due to a lack of IL-13 receptors on T lymphocytes. Therefore, despite the redundancy of these two molecules, regulatory mechanisms are in place to guarantee their distinct functions.

IL-4 and IL-13 possess potent antitumor activity *in vivo* in mice.[45] They can inhibit the proliferation of some human cancer cell lines *in vitro* and *in vivo* in nude mice. A similar antiproliferative effect of IL-13 on human breast cancer cells has been described. Moreover, a chimeric protein composed of IL-13 and a truncated form of *Pseudomonas* exotoxin A exhibits specific cytotoxic activity toward human RCC but not against normal hemopoietic cells.[46]

IL-4 in the clinic
Despite the preclinical promise of IL-4, clinical trials in humans demonstrated that although the molecule is safe and nontoxic, only sporadic antitumor activity is observed in a variety of cancers, including melanoma, lung cancer, and AIDS-related Kaposi's sarcoma.[47–49] It is likely that at least part of the reason for the limited antitumor activity is its immune-suppressive activity, especially given the now established importance of the immune antitumor responses in these malignancies.

Interleukin-6
IL-6 was first cloned in 1986.[50] It is a typical cytokine, exhibiting functional pleiotropy and redundancy. IL-6 is involved in immune response, inflammation, and hematopoiesis. IL-6 is a 21- to 30-kDa glycoprotein of 212 amino acids that binds to a specific receptor that requires the same 130-kDa membrane glycoprotein (CD130) for several other cytokines, including leukemia inhibitor factor (LIF) and IL-11.[51,52] IL-6 affects the hypothalamic–pituitary axis, bone resorption, and both humoral and cellular arms of the immune system[53–57] and is a potent and essential factor for the normal development and function of both B and T lymphocytes.[58] IL-6 is also involved in megakaryocyte maturation, neural differentiation, and osteoclast development. As a major inducer of acute-phase protein synthesis in hepatocytes,[59] IL-6 plays an important role in the pathogenesis of sepsis.

IL-6 acts as a growth factor for myeloma cells, keratinocytes, mesangial cells, RCC, and Kaposi sarcoma and promotes the growth of hematopoietic stem cells. On the other hand, IL-6 inhibits the growth of myeloid leukemic cell lines and certain carcinoma cell lines. IL-6 has been implicated as a mediator of B symptoms in lymphoma.[60] Elevated serum IL-6 levels have also been associated with an adverse prognosis in both Hodgkin and non-Hodgkin lymphoma (NHL).[61–64] In diffuse large-cell lymphoma, IL-6 levels were found to be the single most important independent prognostic factor selected in multivariate analysis for predicting complete remission rate and relapse-free survival.[62] IL-6 level is a prognostic factor in RCC, pancreatic cancer, and multiple myeloma (MM) and high levels are observed in prostate and ovarian cancers. IL-6 also plays a key etiologic role in the systemic manifestations of the lymphoproliferative disorder Castleman's disease.[65]

IL-6 in the clinic
Clinical studies have shown that the toxicities of IL-6 therapy include fever and anemia.[66–68] IL-6 has also been tested as an antitumor agent in melanoma and RCC with low overall response rates (<15%).[59] This is not surprising given the fact that high levels of IL-6 correlate with an adverse outcome in many cancers. Thus, studies have focused on the utility of anti-IL6 therapy in the treatment of cancer. Given the striking responses seen in multicentric Castleman's disease (MCD), the anti-IL-6 monoclonal antibody siltuximab is currently food and drug administration (FDA) approved for the treatment of idiopathic MCD.[69] Anti-IL-6 therapies siltuximab or tocilizumab have been previously studied or are currently involved in ongoing investigations in various malignancies including MM, prostate cancer, myelodysplastic syndromes (MDS), and breast cancer, and remain investigational at this time.

Interleukin-7
IL-7 was identified and cloned based on its ability to induce proliferation of B-cell progenitors in the absence of stromal cells.[70–78] It is now known that this cytokine is secreted by stromal cells in the bone marrow and thymus and is irreplaceable in the development of both B and T cells.[71–73] Indeed, while most single cytokine knockout mice show relatively normal B- and T-cell compartments, indicating that many cytokine functions are redundant, IL-7-deficient mice present with striking lymphocyte depletion in both the thymus and bone marrow. Collectively, these genetic experiments identify clearly distinct *in vivo* roles for various lymphoid factors. IL-2 and IL-4 function by influencing mature lymphocyte populations during immune responses, whereas IL-7 plays a singularly dominant role for the production and expansion of both CD4+ and CD8+ lymphocytes. The upregulation of IL-7R occurs at the stage of the clonogenic common lymphoid progenitor that can give rise to all lymphoid lineages at a single-cell level.[76] There are at least three principal means by which IL-7R-mediated signals act in lymphocyte development: enhancement of proliferation, triggering of lineage-specific developmental programs, and maintenance of viability of appropriately selected cells, in part due to its upregulation of BCL2 thereby preventing apoptosis.

High IL-7 levels are found in states of T-cell depletion and may, therefore, play a role in promoting T-cell expansion.[77] High levels of IL-7 are also found in CLL and Burkitt lymphoma, and transgenic mice overexpressing the IL-7 gene show dramatic changes in lymphocyte development, which, in some instances, can result in the formation of lymphoid tumors.[78] Recombinant IL-7 (CYT107) has been studied in a variety of lymphopenic conditions, including HIV, hepatitis C, septic shock, and bone marrow reconstitution after stem cell transplant with a favorable safety profile and several-fold expansion in lymphocytes in most cases.[79–81] To date, IL-7 therapy has not been approved for clinical use.

Interleukin-8
IL-8 was first identified in 1987 as a potent, proinflammatory chemokine that induces trafficking of neutrophils across the vascular wall (chemotaxis).[82] This molecule belongs to a chemokine superfamily whose members include neutrophil-activating peptide-2, platelet factor-4, growth-related cytokine (GRO), and IFN-inducible protein-10, all of which are responsible for the directional migration of various cells.[83] IL-8 receptor demonstrates strong homology to a gene encoded by human herpesvirus-8 (HHV-8).[84,85] Among the neutrophil-affecting chemokines, IL-8 is one of the most potent.[86] On exposure to a chemokine, neutrophils are activated, and within seconds, their shapes change by perturbations of cellular integrins and the actin cytoskeleton. The activation and upregulation of integrins also permit the adherence of neutrophils to the endothelial cells of the vessel wall, to allow for subsequent migration into the tissues. Leukocytes follow the IL-8 concentration gradient and accumulate at the location of elevated concentration. These processes play a fundamental role in the host

defense since activated leukocytes act to kill and engulf invading bacteria at the site of injury.

IL-8 can induce tumor growth, an effect attributed to its angiogenic activity. On the one hand, the administration of anti-IL-8 to severe combined immunodeficiency (SCID) mice bearing xenografts of IL-8-expressing human lung cancer has been shown to have beneficial effects.[87] On the other hand, antitumor effects of IL-8 have also been reported. Increased levels of IL-8 have been found in lung carcinomas and melanomas. IL-8 may be a growth factor for pancreatic cancer and melanoma.[83] In melanomas, IL-8 levels correlate with the growth and metastatic potential of tumor cells, and exposure of the cells to IFN, which has known antitumor activity in melanoma, decreases IL-8 levels and cancer cell proliferation.[88] Thus, blocking IL-8 or IL-8R has been suggested as a therapeutic strategy.[83] In a recent Phase I study, Hu-Max-IL8, a fully human monoclonal antibody that inhibits IL-8 in patients with metastatic or unresectable tumors, was found to be safe and well tolerated.[89]

Interleukin-9

Human IL-9 was initially identified and cloned as a mitogenic factor for a human megakaryoblastic leukemia. Subsequently, IL-9 was found to target a wide range of cells, including erythroid progenitors, human T cells, B cells, fetal thymocytes, thymic lymphomas, and immature neuronal cell lines.[90,91] IL-9 can support the clonogenic maturation of erythroid progenitors in the presence of EPO. In contrast, granulocyte or macrophage colony formation (CFU-GM, CFU-G, or CFU-M) is usually not influenced by IL-9. IL-9 is more effective on fetal than adult progenitors, and in cells that are activated. In addition to its proliferative activity, IL-9 also seems to be a potent regulator of mast cell effector molecules. A distinct CD4+ T-helper subset produced in the presence of TGF-beta and IL-4 has been identified that secretes IL-9 (Th9).[92]

There is an interesting paradox between the unresponsiveness of normal T cells to IL-9 and the potent activity of this molecule on lymphoma cells. This is illustrated by the observation that murine T cells acquire the ability to respond to IL-9 after a long period of *in vitro* culture, while they simultaneously acquire characteristics of tumor cell lines. Observations made with transgenic mice also demonstrate the oncogenic potential of dysregulated IL-9 production since 5–10% of mice that overexpress this cytokine develop lymphoblastic lymphomas.[91] In line with these data, constitutive IL-9 production by human Hodgkin lymphomas and large-cell anaplastic lymphomas has been clearly documented.[90] IL-9 is an important mediator of asthma. An anti-IL-9 antibody (MEDI-528) has been developed and studied in the treatment of asthma but did not show evidence of clinical benefit.[93]

Interleukin-10

IL-10 is a pleiotropic cytokine discovered in 1989 as an activity produced by murine type 2 helper T cells (Th2).[94,95] It was initially designated as cytokine synthesis inhibitory factor because of its ability to inhibit the production of certain cytokines.[96] IL-10 inhibits the synthesis of Th1-derived cytokines, including IL-2, IFN-γ, GM-CSF, and lymphotoxin, and of monocyte-derived IL-1α and β, IL-6, IL-8, tumor necrosis factor (TNF)-α, GM-CSF, and G-CSF. Exogenous IL-10 can also suppress expression of IL-10.[95] At the same time, IL-10 induces synthesis of the IL-1 receptor antagonist by macrophages. IL-10 also suppresses the CD28 costimulatory pathway, and hence, acts as a decisive mechanism in determining if a T cell will contribute to an immune response or become anergic.

From the molecular standpoint, IL-10 suppresses cytokine expression at a transcriptional and posttranscriptional level.[97] Both these mechanisms appear to require new protein synthesis. At a cellular level, Th1 cytokine synthesis inhibition is mediated indirectly through the effect of IL-10 on APC, since suppression occurs when macrophages, but not B cells, are used as APCs.[98] In the presence of monocytes/macrophages, IL-10 inhibits the proliferation of resting T cells, including Th0, Th1, and Th2 CD4+ T-cell clones. This inhibition can only be partially reversed by high concentrations of IL-2, suggesting that the reduced proliferation is only partially a reflection of reduced IL-2 production. IL-10 can also enhance the cytotoxic activity of CD8+ T cells. These effects support an important role of IL-10 in regulating inflammatory responses. In contrast to the inhibitory effects on other lineages, IL-10 has a stimulatory effect on B cells and mast cells.[99] For instance, IL-10 strongly stimulates the proliferation and differentiation of activated B cells.

The role of IL-10 in cancer should be considered within the frame of a highly complex biological puzzle. It is known that IL-10 can have pleiotropic effects on adaptive and innate immune cell mediators. Although several studies show that IL-10 can actively mediate immune suppression, IL-10 has also been shown to mediate T-cell immune surveillance and suppression of metastasis.[100–102] In addition, IL-10 can increase the cytolytic activity of NK cells, particularly in combination with IL-18.[103]

Interleukin-11

Originally characterized as a thrombopoietic factor, IL-11 is now known to be expressed and have activity in a multitude of organ systems, including the gut, testes, and the central nervous system.[104,105] IL-11 was originally isolated from cells derived from the hematopoietic microenvironment and may act as a paracrine or autocrine growth factor in this environment. IL-11 acts synergistically with other early- and late-acting growth factors, including IL-3, IL-4, IL-7, IL-12, IL-13, SCF, FLT-3 ligand, and GM-CSF, to stimulate various stages and lineages of hematopoiesis.[104] IL-11 acts synergistically with IL-3, TPO, or SCF to stimulate various stages of megakaryocytopoiesis and thrombopoiesis[106,107] and in combination with other IL-3, SCF, or EPO to stimulate multiple stages of erythropoiesis. IL-11 also modulates the differentiation and maturation of myeloid progenitor cells. IL-11 in combination with SCF stimulates myeloid colony formation. The combination of IL-11 with IL-13 or IL-14 can reduce the proportion of granulocytes and blasts in myeloid colonies, with a concomitant increase in macrophages. IL-11 in combination with SCF or IL-4 effectively supports the generation of B cells in primary cultures. IL-11 and IL-4 can also reverse the inhibitory effect of IL-3 on early B-lymphocyte development. The promotion of B-cell differentiation may be mediated by T cells.

IL-11 acts not only on normal cells but also on leukemic cells. It acts synergistically with IL-3, GM-CSF, and SCF to stimulate the proliferation of human primary leukemia cells, myeloid leukemia cell lines, megakaryoblastic cell lines, and erythroleukemic cell lines and to stimulate leukemic blast colony formation. IL-11 mRNA expression in leukemic cells and inhibition of leukemic cell growth by IL-11 antisense oligonucleotides suggest that IL-11 may function as an autocrine growth factor in leukemic cell lines.[108] Although IL-11 stimulates the proliferation of murine plasmacytoma cells and murine hybridoma cells, the effect of IL-11 on the growth of human myeloma/plasmacytoma cells is controversial.[104] IL-11 has also been found to enhance the survival and metastasis of solid tumor cells.[109]

Clinical use of IL-11
IL-11 was the second IL to receive FDA approval and was approved for the secondary prevention of chemotherapy-induced thrombocytopenia and the reduction of the need for platelet transfusion in patients with nonmyeloid malignancies. However, it has since been discontinued in the United States and has largely been replaced by the TPO agonists romiplostim and eltrombopag.

Interleukin-12

IL-12 was first identified as an NK-cell stimulatory factor.[110] Subsequently, it was demonstrated that IL-12 is crucial to the development of Th1 cells.[111] Indeed, there appears to be a common pathway leading from the innate immune response to adaptive immunity; intracellular pathogens stimulate macrophages to produce IL-12, which then promotes the development of Th1 cells from a naïve cell population. Thus, IL-12 is essential for resistance to bacterial, fungal, and parasitic infections. It is produced within a few hours of infection, activates NK cells, and, through its ability to induce IFN-γ production, enhances the phagocytic and bactericidal activity of phagocytic cells. IL-12 also leads to the release of proinflammatory cytokines, including IL-12 itself. IL-12 does not induce proliferation of resting peripheral blood T cells or NK cells. However, it can potentiate the proliferation of T cells induced by various mitogens and has a direct proliferative effect on preactivated T and NK cells.

IL-12 synergizes with other hematopoietic factors to promote survival and proliferation of early multipotent hematopoietic progenitor cells and lineage-committed precursor cells.[112] Although *in vitro* IL-12 has mostly stimulatory effects on hematopoiesis, *in vivo* IL-12 treatment results in decreased bone marrow hematopoiesis and both transient anemia and neutropenia, an effect mediated by IFN-γ.

IL-12 in the clinic
IL-12 has the potential for allergy treatment via its Th2 suppression and as an adjuvant for infectious disease therapy.[113] Additionally, the ability of IL-12 to revert existing states of tolerance and stimulate both innate and adaptive immunity made it an ideal candidate for use in vaccines for infectious agents and cancer therapy. However, IL-12 was found to have only modest antitumor effects with significant adverse events with hematopoietic, hepatic, and gastrointestinal (GI) toxicities. The severe toxicities seen in early studies could be reduced by giving a single priming dose of IL-12 before starting consecutive dosing 1–2 weeks later. However, even with improved safety profile with this dosing strategy, antitumor effects were modest, which may be due to the inability to overcome immune-suppressive microenvironment milieu.[114] Tumor-targeted IL-12, in conjunction with other immune therapies, such as ICIs, are currently being investigated which can reduce the toxicity associated with systemic administration while potentially overcoming intratumoral immune resistance.[115]

Interleukin-15

IL-15 shares biologic activities with IL-2,[116] including triggering both proliferation of and immunoglobulin production by normal B lymphocytes. These biologic functions may be acquired, however, only when B cells are preactivated *in vitro* with polyclonal mitogens or cultured in association with other stimuli. IL-15 also stimulates the proliferation of NK cells and activated CD4+ and CD8+ T cells, and facilitates the induction of cytolytic effector cells (such as LAK cells). Finally, the numbers of CD8+ memory T cells are maintained in animals by a balance between the stimulatory effect of IL-15 and the suppressive effects of IL-12.[117]

IL-15 responsiveness distinguishes malignant B cells from normal B lymphocytes. In contrast to normal B lymphocytes, which require preactivation to proliferate in response to IL-15, leukemic cells from patients with chronic B-cell malignancies proliferate in response to IL-15 regardless of *in vitro* preactivation, which is mainly related to the presence of the β and γ chains of the IL-2R system on the malignant B lymphocytes.[116] Even so, IL-15 cannot be considered an autocrine factor in these leukemias, since it is not produced by the leukemic cells themselves. Rather, the major reservoir of IL-15 in these patients is from cells belonging to the monocyte/macrophage lineage.[116] IL-15 plays an important role in the pathogenesis and progression of cutaneous T-cell lymphoma (CTCL) and overexpression of IL-15 can produce the manifestations of CTCL in mice, suggesting targeting IL-15 in this disease may provide therapeutic benefit.[118]

IL-15 has been studied as an immune-stimulatory cytokine with antitumor activity, with continuous IV infusion having a more acceptable toxicity profile than bolus dosing.[119] The combination of IL-15 with IL-15Rα (termed IL-15 superagonist) produces a much greater effect than IL-15 alone and can selectively expand NK and memory CD8+ lymphocytes.[120] This complex (ALT-803) has been studied in treating patients who relapsed after hematopoietic stem cell transplant (HSCT), demonstrating safety and expansion of NK and CD8+ in human patients.[121] IL-15 is now being combined with various immunotherapies in multiple ongoing clinical trials.[122]

Interleukin-17

Human IL-17 has 72% overall amino acid sequence identity with open reading frame 13 of herpesvirus Saimiri (HVS).[123] IL-17 is produced by a dedicated T-helper cell population (Th-17 cells) and induces inflammation by its synergistic action with other inflammatory cytokines, such as TNF-α.[124,125] IL-17 can stimulate epithelial, endothelial, and fibroblastic cells, and macrophages to express a variety of cytokines,[112] which appear to be cell-specific. For instance, fibroblast cells produce IL-1, G-CSF, IFN-γ, IL-6, and IL-8 in response to IL-17, while macrophages produce TNF-α, IL-lβ, IL-1Rα, IL-6, IL-10, and IL-12.[126]

IL-17 exhibits indirect hematopoietic activity by enhancing the capacity of fibroblasts to sustain the proliferation of CD34+ hematopoietic progenitors and their differentiation into neutrophils.[124,127] IL-17 can also promote the maturation of dendritic cell progenitors, and thus has been implicated in host T-cell allostimulation and graft rejection.[128] IL-17 has been implicated in a large number of autoimmune disorders, including rheumatoid arthritis, psoriasis, multiple sclerosis, Crohn's disease, systemic lupus erythematosus, and asthma.[129] Several anti-IL17 antibodies, including secukinumab, ixekizumab, and broadalumab, are approved for the treatment of moderate-to-severe plaque psoriasis.[130]

Interleukin-18

IL-18 (IFN-inducing factor) was first described as a serum activity that induced IFN-γ production in mouse spleen cells.[131] IL-18 has a molecular weight of 18–19 kDa and has homology to IL-1.[132,133] Like IL-1β, IL-18 is initially synthesized as an inactive precursor molecule (pro-IL-18) lacking a signal peptide and is cleaved by interleukin-1 beta converting enzyme (ICE) to yield an active molecule.[134,135] T lymphocytes, NK cells, and macrophages are primary targets for IL-18. For example, IL-18 directly stimulates the production of TNF in human blood CD4+ T lymphocytes and NK cells and plays an important role in promoting a long-lasting

Th1 lymphocyte response to viral antigens. IL-18 does not appear to be an endogenous pyrogen but may nevertheless contribute to inflammation and fever because it is a potent inducer of TNF, chemokines, and IFN.[136] In the case of IFN-γ induction, IL-18 acts as a costimulant with mitogens or IL-2. Indeed, mice deficient in ICE, the molecule that cleaves pro-IL-18 to its mature form, fail to produce IFN-γ in response to endotoxin.

IL-18 has had moderate toxicity upon administration in humans. It is currently being studied in combination with rituximab for the treatment of B-cell lymphomas.[137] On the converse side, IL-18 binding protein (BP), an inhibitor of IL-18, is currently in clinical trials for macrophage activation syndrome (MAS) and adult-onset Still's disease.[138]

Interleukin-21

IL-21, a cytokine most closely related to IL-2 and IL-15, is involved in the proliferation and maturation of NK-cell populations from bone marrow, as well as in the proliferation of mature B-cell and T-cell populations.[139] IL-21 has been implicated in the activation of innate immune responses and the Th1 response. IL-21 also plays a critical role in B-cell differentiation to plasma cells, the development of T-follicular helper cells, and promotes the antiviral and antitumor activity of CD8+ T-cells.[140,141] Phase I and II studies have shown IL-21 to have an acceptable safety profile but with antitumor activity in only a small number of patients, thus IL-21 would likely need to be combined with other immune therapies to have clinical utility.[142]

Interleukin-24

IL-24 was originally named melanoma differentiation-associated gene-7 (*mda-7*) when it was identified in 1995 by subtractive hybridization after treatment of melanoma cells with IFN-β and mezerein, which caused their terminal differentiation and growth arrest.[143] In 2001, *mda-7* was shown to encode a secreted protein with significant homology to IL-10, which was officially designated IL-24.[144] Human IL-24 is secreted by activated peripheral blood mononuclear cells and is the ligand for two heterodimeric receptors, IL-22R1/IL-20R2 and IL-20R1/IL-20R2.[145] IL-24 also acts as a tumor-suppressor gene and the protein product was found to be constitutively expressed by melanocytes, nevus cells, and some primary melanomas, but not metastatic lesions of melanoma.[146,147] This is possibly the first example of a tumor-suppressor gene exhibiting immune-stimulatory properties.[148] IL-24 has several interesting and unique properties, including direct cancer-killing activity via diverse signaling pathways, potent bystander antitumor activity, immune-modulating activity, and antiangiogenic properties.

IL-24 in the clinic
Based on its remarkable attributes and effective antitumor therapy in animal models, this cytokine has entered clinical trials. In Phase 1 clinical trial, intratumoral injection of adenovirus-administered *mda-7*/IL-24 (INGN 241) was safe, elicited tumor-regulatory and immune-activating processes, and provided clinically significant activity.[149,150] Improved vector delivery methods of *mda-7*/IL-24 are being developed to improve further on these responses.[151]

Interleukin-26

Subtraction hybridization coupled with representational differential analysis identified IL-26/AK155 as a gene upregulated in human T cells following infection with vesicular stomatitis virus (VSV), human cytomegalovirus (HCMV), and herpes simplex virus type 1 (HSV-1).[152] IL-26 has the capacity to transform these cells in culture. The IL-26 protein is part of the IL-10 family of cytokines and has 24.7% amino acid identity and 47% amino acid similarity with IL-10. Structural analysis revealed that IL-26 contains six helices with four highly conserved cysteine residues, which are assumed to be relevant for dimer formation as is the case with IL-10. IL-26 is produced by Th17 cells, plays a role in neutrophil mobilization, and has many antiviral and antimicrobial activities. It is present at high levels in multiple auto-immune disorders.[153]

Interleukin-27

In 2002, Pflanz and colleagues[154] described a new heterodimeric cytokine related to IL-12, designated IL-27. It acts together with IL-12 to trigger IFN-γ production by naïve CD4+ T cells. They also identified IL-27 as the ligand for TCCR/WSX-1, a novel member of the class I cytokine receptor family shown to be important for Th1 development.[155] IL-27 has also been found to play a role in infectious disease and autoimmunity.[156] Interestingly, in mouse models of inflammatory bowel disease (IBD), administration of IL-27 has been found to improve colitis, and mice deficient in IL-27 have more severe colitis, suggesting IL-27 cytokine therapy may provide benefit to humans with IBD.[157,158] IL-27 is elevated in the serum and intestinal mucosa of patients with IBD, which is thought to more likely represent an inadequate anti-inflammatory response than a pro-inflammatory response.[159]

Studies revealed that IL-27 can induce tumor-specific antitumor activity and protective immunity and that the antitumor activity is mediated mainly through CD8+ T cells, and IFN-γ.[160] Conversely, IL-27 may also induce Treg activity in the tumor microenvironment and increase expression of PD-L1 on multiple tumor types.[161] However, a more recent study demonstrated that adenovirus-based IL-27 gene therapy-induced depletion of Tregs thus enhancing tumor immunotherapy in a mouse model of melanoma as well as enhancing the efficacy of anti-PD1 therapy.[162] As of yet, clinical trials of IL-27 therapy in humans have not been conducted.

Interleukin-28 and interleukin-29

The IL-28 family was identified from searching the human genome for homologous cytokine sequences and designating IL-28A, IL-28B, and IL-29. These molecules were originally described as distantly related to type I IFNs and the IL-10 family. IL-28 and IL-29 are induced by viral infection and show antiviral activity. Moreover, IL-28 and IL-29 interact with a heterodimeric class II cytokine receptor that consists of IL-10Rβ and an orphan class II receptor chain, designated IL-28Rα. Now, they are subclassified as Type III IFNs and seem to be promising candidates for the development of alternatives to type I IFNs, as suggested by their potent antiviral and antitumor properties. Given the fact that IL-28/29 primarily influences epithelial cells, melanocytes, and tumor cells derived from melanocytes, as well as hepatocytes, there are several potential therapeutic fields in which these cytokines could be applied, including as antitumor therapy for carcinoma and melanoma.[163] Anti-IL28 therapy may have a role in preventing mortality in sepsis, as been shown recently in mouse cecal ligation and puncture model of sepsis.[164] A pegylated form of IL-29 (PEG-rIL-29 or PEG-IFN Lambda) has been previously studied in the treatment of chronic hepatitis C infection as an alternative to IFN-α, but since the advent of highly active antivirals for hepatitis C treatment, IFN treatment for this disease has generally fallen out of favor.[165]

Table 3 Interferons (IFN).

Type		Stimuli	Receptors	Signaling molecules
Type I IFNs	IFN α IFN β	• Viruses • Other microorganisms	IFNAR: IFNAR1–IFNAR2	• JAK1 and TYK2 • STAT1–STAT2–IRF9 complexes • STAT1–STAT1 complexes
Type II IFN	IFN γ	• Antigen–MHC complexes • Activating NK-cell ligands • IL-12 plus IL-18 • TLRs	IFNGR: IFNGR1–IFNGR2	• JAK1 and JAK2 • STAT1–STAT1 complexes
Type III IFN	IFNλ	• Viruses • Other microorganisms	IL10R2 and IFNLR1	• JAK1 and TYK2 • STAT1–STAT2–IRF9 complexes • STAT2–STAT2 complexes

Interleukin-31

IL-31 has been identified as a four-helix bundle cytokine that is preferentially produced by T helper type 2 cells.[166] IL-31 signals through a receptor composed of IL-31 receptor A and oncostatin M receptor. Expression of IL-31 RA and oncostatin M receptor mRNA is induced in activated monocytes, whereas epithelial cells expressed both mRNAs constitutively. The IL-31 RA/oncostatin M complex signals through the Jak/STAT, phosphatidylinositol-3-kinase (PI3K), and extracellular signal-regulated kinase (ERK) pathways.

IL-31 is a pro-inflammatory cytokine that plays an important role in cell-mediated immunity and has been identified in several inflammatory disorders. More specifically, data indicate that IL-31 may be involved in promoting dermatitis and epithelial responses that characterize allergic and nonallergic diseases.[167] IL-31 plays an important role in the induction of the sensation of pruritis, as the IL-31 RA/oncostatin M complex is expressed on sensory neurons.[168] Lokivetmab is an anti-IL31 antibody approved for the treatment of atopic dermatitis in dogs. Nemolizumab is an anti-IL-31RA humanized monoclonal antibody that showed improvement in the clinical symptoms and pruritis in patients with atopic dermatitis in a randomized, double-blind Phase II study.[169] Nemolizumab was granted a Breakthrough Therapy Designation by the FDA recently and a Phase III pivotal study is planned.

Interleukin-35

IL-35 represents a new member of the heterodimeric IL-12 cytokine family. IL-35 is a novel anti-inflammatory cytokine that is produced by Treg cells and contributes to their suppressive activity. Ectopic expression of IL-35 confers regulatory activity on naive T cells, whereas recombinant IL-35 suppresses T-cell proliferation. IL-35 was found to suppress inflammatory mediators such as TNF-α in a collagen-induced arthritis mouse model.[170] Because IL-35 may be secreted exclusively by Treg cells and other cell populations with regulatory potential, it represents a novel potential target for the therapeutic manipulation of Treg activity to treat cancer and autoimmune diseases.[171] However, anti-IL-35 therapy still remains at the preclinical stage despite its potential for antitumor therapy.[172]

Interleukin-37

Since the discovery of IL-1 in 1977, the list of IL-1 cytokine family members is continually evolving.[173] IL-37 was originally defined as IL-1 family member 7 (IL-1F7) and transcripts are detected in lymph nodes, thymus, bone marrow, lung, testis, uterus, and placenta.[174] TGF-β and several Toll-like receptor (TLR) ligands induce production of high levels of IL-37 by PBMCs; proinflammatory cytokines such as IL-18, IFN-γ, IL-1β, and TNF moderately increase IL-37 levels.[175] In addition, expression of IL-37 in monocytic cells has been shown to reduce several intracellular kinases important for transducing proinflammatory signals, such as focal adhesion kinase (FAK), STAT1, p38 mitogen-activated protein kinase (MAPK), and c-jun, and thus it is considered one of many key anti-inflammatory cytokines, inhibiting both innate and adaptive immune responses. IL-37 is expressed in a variety of cancers, chronic inflammatory, and autoimmune disorders.[176] Further studies are needed to fully clarify the role in human disease to realize its therapeutic potential.

Interferons

The IFNs are a large family of multifunctional secreted proteins involved in antiviral defense, cell growth regulation, and immune activation. There are three types of IFNs: types I (IFNα1-13, β, ε, κ, ω), II (IFNγ), and III (IFNλ1-4). Each IFN type has sequence similarity, signals via specific cell surface receptor complexes (Table 3) and mediates its effect generally through the Janus kinase-signal transducer and activator of transcription (JAK-STAT) pathway. Canonical signaling through JAK-STAT leads to the activation of STAT1 and STAT2, which bind to interferon-stimulated response element (ISRE), gamma-activated sequence (GAS), and STAT-binding sites in promoters of interferon-regulated genes (IRGs), resulting in the transcriptional activation of those IRGs.[177] IFNs have also been shown to signal through alternative pathways, including other STATs, p38, Erk1/2, Pyk2, and CrkL.[178]

Almost all cell types can produce type I IFNs in response to a variety of stimuli.[179] NK and T cells are the primary sources of type II IFN, mainly in response to mitogens or cytokines such as IL-12 and IL-18. The source of type III IFNs is broad; however, they primarily act on epithelial surfaces. Cellular action follows binding to a small number of high-affinity receptors. IFNs regulate gene expression, modulate expression of proteins on the cell surface, and induce synthesis of new enzymes. Thousands of IRGs have been identified; however, IFN signaling only induces a subset of IRGs, depending on context and cell type.[179] The products of these IRGs underlie the pleiotropic biologic effects: virus inhibition, immunomodulation, inhibition of cell proliferation, alterations in differentiation, increased apoptosis, and angiogenesis inhibition. However, which of the specific IRG products control various biologic and therapeutic effects remains undefined, as do the specific cellular mechanism(s) underlying their antitumor action. Because IFN signaling controls many important cellular functions, it is tightly regulated by positive and negative feedback loops, including the suppressor of cytokine signaling (SOCS) proteins, which limit the IFN response.[179] Alterations in IRG expression result in modulation of receptors for other cytokines, concentration of regulatory proteins on the surface of immune effector cells, and activation of enzymes that control cellular growth and function. On a cellular basis, these effects translate into alterations of the state of differentiation, rate of proliferation and death, and functional activity of many cell types. Induced proteins and their products can be identified on cells and in serum of patients treated with IFN. Their measurement or the quantitation of immune effector cell function can be used to define biologically active molecules, doses, schedules, and routes of administration of IFN.

Antitumor effects in humans

Both natural and recombinant IFNs have shown antitumor activity as a single agent in more than a dozen malignancies. The unique molecular and cellular effects of IFNs also complement the mechanisms of actions of other therapies. Type II and III IFNs still have limited clinical application, whereas IFN-α2 has been used to treat a variety of diseases, including malignancies, multiple sclerosis, and chronic viral hepatitis.[180] Most gene and biologic modulatory effects of IFN-α2 peak at 24–48 h, which contrasts with maximal serum levels of minutes to hours after intravenous or subcutaneous administration.[181–183] After intravenous bolus administration, the t½α of IFN-α2 is short (<60 min); mean terminal half-life is 4–5 h with no serum levels measurable at 12 h. After intramuscular or subcutaneous administration, peak levels are 3–8 h.[181] The pharmacologic hallmark of IFN-β is virtual absence of serum levels with subcutaneous or intramuscular administration, yet pharmacodynamic and therapeutic effects occur.[183] Pegylated IFNs have markedly different kinetics than do unmodified IFNs.[184–186] Once-weekly administration has resulted in measurable serum levels of IFN-α2 at 7 days in excess of that required for gene induction and cellular effects *in vitro*. Pegylated IFN-α2 (PegIFNα) has resulted in tumor responses in metastatic RCC, CML, and melanoma.[186,187] Ropeginterferon alfa-2b (ropeg; Besremi®; PharmaEssentia) is a novel monopegylated IFN with a longer half-life, requiring a shorter dose interval than PegIFNα. The European Medicine Agency in February 2019 approved ropeg for the treatment of polycythemia vera (PV) without symptomatic splenomegaly, and the US FDA granted approval for ropeg use in PV in November 2021.[188]

Hematologic malignancies

In CML, IFN-α2 resulted in sustained therapeutic response in a majority (>75%) of newly diagnosed patients in early clinical studies.[189,190] Complete cytogenetic remissions were noted in a minority of patients and the rate was higher in younger patients. However, due to the considerable side effects from IFN-α2, many clinicians chose to stop therapy if cytogenetic improvement was not seen after approximately one year of treatment. Prior to the development of the tyrosine kinase inhibitors (TKIs), IFNs were the treatment of choice for most patients with CML. With the development of imatinib mesylate and the increased toxicity of IFN-α2 compared with TKIs, IFN has been used much less commonly for the treatment of CML. However, up to one-third of CML patients on imatinib will become resistant or intolerant to therapy.[191] Furthermore, each drug targets different molecules and their different mechanisms of action (e.g., TKIs cause disease debulking while IFN-α2 activates antitumor immunity) offer opportunities for therapeutic synergism. Thus, IFN-α2 has been incorporated into various treatment schedules with TKIs in clinical trials. The Phase III French SPIRIT trial demonstrated higher rates of molecular response using the combination of imatinib and PegIFNα compared with IFN alone,[192] but another study failed to demonstrate an improvement in progression-free survival (PFS).[193] Studies investigating the combination of IFN-α2 with second-generation TKIs are ongoing and show that IFN-α2 may deepen molecular responses over time.[194–200] The German TIGER study (CML V; NCT01657604) is investigating whether IFN-α2 should be administered with nilotinib or as maintenance therapy once major molecular response (MMR) has been achieved in CML patients.[197] At 18 months, the rates of MR[4] and MR[4.5] on this trial were superior for nilotinib plus PegIFNα versus nilotinib alone. In addition, several reports have cited long-term cytogenetic remission after IFN-α2 therapy was discontinued in CML patients.[201–206] However, even patients in long-term remission show evidence of molecular disease.[207,208] Therefore, IFN-α2, like TKIs, is not curative in CML but offers an opportunity to improve responses to TKIs and eventually even discontinue therapy in some cases.

IFN-α2 has demonstrated responses in other myeloproliferative neoplasms (MPNs), particularly PV and essential thrombocythemia (ET). Phase II trials with IFN-α2 reported complete hematologic responses in 75–95% of PV or ET patients, and 15–20% complete molecular responses, as defined by an inability to detect *JAK2V617F* mutation.[209–213] These responses are encouraging considering conventional therapies hydroxyurea (HU) and anagrelide have had minimal impact on molecular disease. A Phase III randomized trial PROUD-PV and its extension CONTINUATION-PV compared monopegylated IFN-α2 ropeg to HU. Hematological and molecular responses were superior with ropeg,[214] and tolerability was comparable between treatments. Another Phase III study did not find a difference between responses with PegIFNα-2a and HU.[215] Encouragingly, similar to CML, long-term treatment with IFN-α2 has allowed some patients with PV to discontinue therapy.[213,216–219] In myelofibrosis (MF), IFN-α2 has shown less therapeutic activity.[220–224] Moving forward, the use of IFN-α2 in MPNs will likely focus on combinations with conventional (HU or anagrelide) or targeted (TKI, JAK1-2 inhibitors, HDACi, and chromatin-modifying) agents.[225]

Solid tumors

Numerous tumor models suggest type I IFN signaling has antitumor effects, and loss of IFN signaling in preclinical models and patients with solid tumors is associated with tumor development and metastasis.[179] In melanoma, type I IFN has direct pro-apoptotic and antiproliferative effects on tumors, and indirect immunomodulatory effects by activating various immune cells and inhibiting immunosuppressive elements.[180] Approximately 15% of patients with metastatic melanoma respond to IFN-α2 as a single agent, comparable to cytotoxic agents used alone.[226–229] When combined with chemotherapy and IL-2, response rates can exceed 45%, but with increased toxicity and no marked prolongation in PFS or overall survival (OS).[27,229–233] However, some trials have shown prolonged disease-free survival with use of IFN-α2 as an adjuvant to surgery for patients with melanoma at high risk for disease recurrence (stage IIb or stage III).[187,234–237] Analysis of quality-of-life-adjusted survival in the adjuvant setting has also identified an advantage for use of IFN-α2.[238] Thus, IFN-α2 became a standard of care for patients with high-risk melanoma in the US, until 2015.[238,239] Responses in metastatic melanoma patients led to an innovative trial design of long-duration IFN-α2 treatment with dose adjustments for fatigue and anorexia, which led to improvements in disease-free survival,[187,240,241] More recent meta-analyses demonstrated IFN-α2 adjuvant therapy has a modest impact on OS compared with observation alone, with ulceration of the primary tumor predicting sensitivity to IFN.[241–243] The recent E1609 trial update showed that adjuvant therapy with ipilimumab at 3 mg/kg had a survival benefit over high-dose IFN-α2 in melanoma adjuvant therapy, disputing the role of IFN as an initial adjuvant for advanced melanoma.[242,244] In addition, anti-PD-1 antibodies and BRAF plus MAPK/extracellular signal–regulated kinase kinase (MEK) inhibitors have shown higher efficacy and lower toxicity than either ipilimumab or IFN-α2 in advanced melanoma, and the FDA has approved these newer agents for adjuvant therapy of melanoma.[245,246] Nonetheless, several lines of evidence suggest IFN-α2 can synergize with conventional, targeted, and immunotherapy approaches, including ICIs and BRAF-targeted therapies. Thus, combination studies of IFN-α2 with BRAF inhibitor vemurafenib and antiprogrammed cell death protein 1 (PD-1) pembrolizumab in melanoma are ongoing and tentatively show promising results.[247,248]

IFN has been extensively used in the treatment of RCC. Response rates from 4% to 26% have been reported in trials of IFN-α2 in metastatic RCC, with a mean response of 15% in a cumulative summary of several trials.[249] IFN-α2 has been combined with other biological response modifiers including IL-2 and chemotherapeutic agents, in particular, 5-fluorouracil (5-FU) with limited benefit to survival for patients with RCC.[250] Combining IFN-α with bevacizumab, a VEGF inhibitor, significantly improved PFS, but not OS, compared with IFN-α alone.[251] More recently, the success of anticytotoxic T-lymphocyte-associated protein 4 (CTLA-4) and anti-PD-1/PD-L1 checkpoint inhibitors in treating melanoma led to their application in RCC. Due to their significant impact on response rates and survival, first-line agents recommended for RCC now include pazopanib, ipilimumab plus nivolumab, axitinib plus pembrolizumab, and axitinib plus avelumab, whereas bevacizumab–IFN-α2 combination is considered an alternative treatment.[252,253] In summary, as several targeted therapies have improved outcomes for metastatic RCC, combination cytokine therapy is no longer recommended as standard treatment. Other solid tumors, such as ovarian, bladder, and basal cell carcinomas, have responded to IFN-α administered regionally, particularly in patients with lesser tumor bulk.[254–256]

The shared gene induction profile of types I and III IFN has led to investigations of the potential role of type III IFN in cancer therapy. The hope is that type III IFN will be effective against responsive cancer cells while showing fewer side effects than type I IFN due to the restricted distribution of its receptor, primarily on epithelial cells.[257] The favorable side effect profile of type III over type I IFN was demonstrated in a Phase I study of the effect of type III IFN against hepatitis C virus (HCV). While some patients treated with type I IFN developed neutropenia or anemia, patients treated with type III IFN remained symptom free.[258] However, new evidence indicates that type III IFN can also promote tumor cell migration and invasiveness in experimental tumor models and can block release of reactive oxygen species, which may impede immune killing of tumor cells.[259] Overall, type III IFN may play a positive role in cancer therapy with few or no side effects, yet more studies of its dual effects in different cancer models are needed before advancing its clinical development. Likewise, type II IFN has demonstrated antitumor and protumor effects, the latter through suppressing antitumor immune responses and increasing proliferation and survival of tumor cells in experimental tumor models. Thus, its future place in cancer therapy is not clear.[260]

Hematopoiesis and the role of growth factors

Through a series of well-orchestrated divisions, hematopoietic stem cells give rise to all blood cells. Functionally, these early progenitors are capable of self-renewal as well as proliferation and differentiation. The development, homeostasis, trafficking, and response capacity of the hematopoietic system are tightly regulated by a complex communications network that is mediated by intercellular signals. These signals are triggered by direct cell-to-cell or cell-to-matrix contact or by the release of soluble cytokine mediators.

The identification and cloning of hematopoietic growth factors have revolutionized hematology practice. Raising white blood cell counts in neutropenic patients was unimaginable until the advent of G-CSF and GM-CSF. Today, growth factors are routinely used to alleviate neutropenia and, to a lesser extent, thrombocytopenia and anemia after chemotherapy. They can also help mobilize stem cells for transplantation, reverse cytopenias in a variety of nonmalignant illnesses, and may have the potential to mobilize the immune system against infection or cancer.

Erythropoietin

EPO is the major hormone regulator of erythropoiesis. It has an established role in the treatment of anemia associated with a variety of illnesses (Table 4).

Biologic activities of EPO

EPO provides a proliferative signal to early erythroid progenitors [burst-forming unit erythroid (BFU-E)] and a differentiation signal to a later erythroid precursor [colony-forming unit erythroid (CFU-E)]. EPO can also promote megakaryocyte differentiation, B-cell proliferation, and endothelial cell chemotaxis.

EPO in malignancy

High levels of endogenous EPO are often found in patients with anemia due to cancer, especially hematologic malignancies. In contrast, in many patients with anemia, even anemia due to cancer, there is a relative deficiency in endogenous EPO. In other words, though the levels of this molecule are elevated, they are not as high as they should be for the degree of anemia. Certain cases of familial erythrocytosis have been attributed to the presence of EPO-hypersensitive cells. This heightened EPO response results from the formation of a truncated EPO receptor, which is missing a negative regulatory domain.[261]

EPO in the clinic

EPO is most useful in those anemias where there is an absolute or a relative deficiency in endogenous EPO levels. First used successfully as replacement therapy to correct the anemia associated with chronic renal failure, EPO is also effective in increasing hemoglobin in some patients with both solid tumors and hematologic malignancies as well as in those with a variety of other conditions.[262]

EPO has generally been used for patients with significant anemia, that is, hemoglobin <10 g/dL. The US FDA suggests that EPO should be used conservatively to avoid transfusion, but not to normalize hemoglobin levels. In the case of cancer, however, not all patients respond, and those with the highest levels of endogenous EPO are probably less likely to benefit.

Table 4 Hematopoietic growth factors.

	Chromosomal location	Receptors	Selected biologic activities
EPO	7q21	EPO receptor	• Promotes the proliferation, differentiation, and survival of erythroid precursors
GM-CSF	5q31.1	Type I receptor with α (CD116) and β (CDw131) subunits	• Stimulates growth of multilineage progenitors, BFU-E, granulocyte, macrophage, and eosinophil colonies • Induces migration and proliferation of vascular endothelial cells • Activates mature phagocytes (neutrophils, macrophages, eosinophils)
G-CSF	17q11.2-q12	G-CSF receptor (CD114)	• Regulates production and function of neutrophils
M-CSF	1p21-p13	Fms (CD115)	• Influences most aspects of monocyte/macrophage development and function • Stimulates hematopoiesis • Induces osteoclast production • Helps maintain pregnancies • Lowers cholesterol levels • Affects microglial function
SCF	12q22-12q24	c-kit (CD117)	• Promotes hematopoiesis at multiple levels • Influences primordial germ cell and melanocyte migration during embryonic life • Affects immunoregulatory cells (B and T cells, mast cells, NK cells, dendritic cells) • Influences hematopoietic cell adhesive properties
TPO	3q27-q28	Mpl (CD110)	• Major regulator of platelet production • Acts in synergy with EPO to stimulate growth of erythroid progenitors • Acts in synergy with IL-3 and SCF to stimulate proliferation and prolong survival of hematopoietic stem cells

Granulocyte-macrophage colony-stimulating factor

GM-CSF was the first CSF to enter clinical trials. It has now been approved in many countries for treatment of neutropenia after chemotherapy or transplantation, for treatment of graft failure, and for peripheral blood stem cell mobilization.

Major biologic activities of GM-CSF
GM-CSF stimulates proliferation of multilineage progenitors and the growth of BFU-E, granulocyte, macrophage, and eosinophil colonies. GM-CSF also enhances the functional activity of most phagocytes, including neutrophils, macrophages, and eosinophils.

GM-CSF in malignancy
Autocrine expression of GM-CSF in myeloid leukemia cells and cell lines has been proposed to play a role in neoplasia.[263] Autonomous production of GM-CSF (or G-CSF) by the tumor has also been implicated as one possible pathophysiologic mechanism underlying leukemoid reactions in cancer patients.[264] In addition, the presence of GM-CSF biologic activity in synovial fluid from patients with rheumatoid arthritis suggests that it may enhance the tissue destruction associated with this disorder.

GM-CSF has been shown to be safe and effective in the treatment of patients with AML who are undergoing induction therapy. This molecule shortens the neutropenic period and decreases the rate of serious infections in older individuals. GM-CSF is also indicated for accelerating myeloid reconstitution after allogeneic BMTs. It also enhances survival in patients who experience engraftment failure or delay after allogeneic or autologous transplantation. Finally, peripheral blood stem cells mobilized in the presence of GM-CSF yield significantly higher colony counts than those mobilized without this molecule and, after transplantation, recipients of GM-CSF-mobilized progenitors have quicker neutrophil, platelet, and red blood cell recovery and shorter hospital stays.

Granulocyte colony-stimulating factor

G-CSF has revolutionized the treatment of neutropenia and its sequelae (infection). It has been used worldwide and has been found to be remarkably effective and virtually devoid of side effects.[265,266]

Biologic activities of G-CSF
G-CSF is a relatively specific stimulator of the growth and differentiation of hematopoietic progenitor cells committed to the neutrophil lineage. It also protects neutrophils from apoptosis and enhances their function. Finally, G-CSF moves mature neutrophils from the marrow into the circulation.

G-CSF in human disease
In healthy persons, mean ± SD G-CSF levels are 25 ± 19.7 pg/mL. G-CSF levels increase by 30-fold in infection and by 10 000-fold in septic shock.[267] Some patients with solid tumors present with significantly increased leukocyte counts. In several of these individuals, elevated serum levels of G-CSF (or GM-CSF) have been demonstrated and probably account for the rise in white blood cell count.[264] Presumably, G-CSF (or GM-CSF) is produced by the tumor itself.

Point mutations in the gene for the G-CSF receptor have been described in patients with AML, which evolved from severe congenital neutropenia. These mutations truncate the C-terminal cytoplasmic region of the G-CSF receptor and hence are presumed to disrupt the maturation signal of the receptor.[268]

Studies of G-CSF as an adjunct to standard-dose cytotoxic chemotherapy for solid tumors and lymphomas demonstrate that the duration of neutropenia, the number of days of hospitalization, and the number of days of antibiotic treatment are reduced significantly during G-CSF cycles. Placebo-controlled studies in patients with small-cell lung cancer showed a clinically significant protective effect of G-CSF against febrile neutropenia.[269] After high-dose chemotherapy, recovery from neutropenia and its associated complications is more rapid when patients receive G-CSF. These studies suggest that the dose intensity of nonmyeloablative chemotherapy can be increased with G-CSF support. In the transplantation setting, the administration of G-CSF results in reductions in neutropenia and infection.[270] G-CSF also mobilizes autologous peripheral blood progenitor cells; these cells are used to accelerate hematopoietic recovery in patients who have received myeloablative or myelosuppressive chemotherapy.[271]

A new form of G-CSF has been developed; a conjugate of G-CSF and monomethoxypolyethylene glycol. PEGylated G-CSF has a prolonged half-life because of its reduced renal clearance. Serum clearance is directly related to neutrophil number. As a result, only a single SC dose of PEGylated G-CSF (Neulasta) is required after chemotherapy. Based on the results of randomized, blinded trials, this molecule is indicated to decrease the incidence of infection in patients with nonmyeloid malignancies receiving myelosuppressive chemotherapy with a significant incidence of febrile neutropenia.[272]

Macrophage colony-stimulating factor

Although macrophage colony-stimulating factor (M-CSF) is known to affect a variety of organ systems, its cardinal effect remains its ability to influence most aspects of monocyte/macrophage development and function.

Biologic activities of M-CSF

M-CSF stimulates differentiation of progenitor cells to mature monocytes and prolongs the survival of monocytes. It enhances cytotoxicity, superoxide production, phagocytosis, chemotaxis, and secondary cytokine production (G-CSF, IL-6, and IL-8) in monocytes and macrophages. In addition to stimulation of hematopoiesis, M-CSF also promotes differentiation and proliferation of osteoclast progenitor cells and has profound effects on lipid metabolism.

M-CSF in malignancy

M-CSF is intricately involved in atherosclerosis, but information about its role remains contradictory. For instance, M-CSF administration lowers cholesterol levels. Paradoxically, it appears that an absence of M-CSF protects against atherosclerosis even in the presence of hyperlipidemia.[273] M-CSF and Fms are expressed in the brain. This cytokine induces microglial proliferation, activation, and survival.

In malignancy, mutations in Fms (the M-CSF receptor) have been reported at codon 969 in about 10% of cases of human myeloid malignancies (including myelodysplasia and AML).

M-CSF in the clinic

In a large-scale study, it has been shown that the administration of M-CSF to AML patients after consolidation chemotherapies shortens the periods of neutropenia and thrombocytopenia after chemotherapy and reduces the incidence and shortens the duration of febrile neutropenia.[274] Similar benefits have been reported after chemotherapy or BMT. M-CSF can elevate neutrophil counts in children with chronic neutropenia. Finally, preliminary results in uncontrolled trials suggest that this molecule may improve outcome after fungal infections.[275]

Stem cell factor

SCF is also known as kit ligand, mast cell growth factor, or steel factor. It functions as a hematopoietic cytokine that triggers its biologic effect by binding to c-kit (the SCF receptor).[276]

Biologic activities of SCF

SCF is constitutively produced by marrow stromal elements. It is now well established that SCF acts on hematopoietic stem cells and, in some lineages, mature cells.

SCF synergizes with other cytokines (including EPO and IL-3) to support the direct colony growth of BFU-E, CFU-GM, and CFU-granulocyte/erythroid/macrophage/megakaryocyte in semisolid media, and current data suggest that SCF can act on a more primitive cell (pre-CFU-C) capable of generating the direct colony-forming cells. SCF can also promote progenitor cell survival, accelerate stem cell entry into cell cycle, and function as a chemotactic and chemokinetic factor for these cells. Synergistic proliferative effects on megakaryocytic progenitor cells are observed when SCF is combined with TPO or IL-3.[277] SCF is also involved in processes of cell adhesion and trafficking. SCF induces progenitor cell adhesion to fibronectin, a process that may involve alteration of integrin avidity through an inside-out signal initiated in response to c-kit receptor kinase activation after ligand binding. Alternatively, it is possible that the transmembrane form of SCF displayed on fibroblasts binds directly to the c-kit receptor on the surface of hematopoietic cells and, thus, helps to anchor the hematopoietic cells in the microenvironment.[277]

The effects of SCF when combined with G-CSF are even more pronounced.[278] Phase 1 clinical studies show that treatment with SCF increases the numbers of progenitor cells of many types (including BFU-E, CFU-GM, CFUM, e.g., and CFU-GEMM) in the marrow.[279]

SCF and c-kit in malignancy

The concentration of SCF in normal human serum is, on average, 3.3 ng/mL. Serum SCF levels are not elevated in patients with aplastic anemia, myelodysplasia, chronic anemia, or after marrow ablative therapy.[277] Thus, the level of SCF in the circulation, unlike the level of EPO, is not inversely related to the hematocrit.

Alterations in the local distribution of SCF within the skin have been implicated in the pathogenesis of cutaneous mastocytosis.[277] Point mutations in the c-kit receptor cytoplasmic domain have been identified in murine and human mast cell lines and in hematopoietic cells from patients with mast cell disorders.[277] Activating mutations in kit characterize a type of leiomyosarcoma known as gastrointestinal stromal tumors.

Neoplastic human hematopoietic cells can also display the c-kit receptor. Receptor density is highest in erythroleukemia cell lines, which may express up to 50 000–100 000 c-kit receptors per cell. Solid tumor cell lines as well as a variety of fresh human tumor tissues also express c-kit receptor protein.[277]

SCF in the clinic

Clinical trials of SCF in a number of situations have been undertaken. SCF factor seems to be reasonably well tolerated, with the predominant side effects being transient local erythema and long-lasting hyperpigmentation at injection sites. The most worrisome toxicity is a mast cell effect resulting in allergic-like reactions characterized by urticaria, with or without respiratory symptoms.[277] The side effects of SCF, including the allergic phenomenon, appear to be dose-dependent.

Of special interest is the role of mutations in the SCF receptor (kit) in gastrointestinal stromal tumors. These mutations activate the kinase enzymatic activity of kit. A kinase inhibitor targeted against kit (STI571 or imatinib mesylate) has been found to be dramatically effective in these notoriously chemotherapy-resistant tumors.[280]

Thrombopoietin

The humoral basis of megakaryocyte and platelet production has been more enigmatic than that of other lineages. Factors that have now been implicated in at least some aspects of thrombocyte development include IL-3, IL-6, IL-9, IL-11, G-CSF, GM-CSF, SCF, leukemia-inhibiting factor, and TPO. The latter molecule is believed to be of paramount importance in the physiologic regulation of platelet production. Unfortunately, however, compared with the striking effects of the granulopoietic factors in neutropenic patients, use of the thrombopoietic molecules in the clinic setting has met with less success.

Biologic properties of TPO
TPO participates in hematopoiesis in general, in addition to thrombopoiesis, as supported by experiments demonstrating that genetic elimination of TPO or its receptor causes a 65–95% reduction in the numbers of transplantable stem cells. The survival of TPO in the circulation is longer than that of other hematopoietic growth factors (half-life = 30 h).

TPO in malignancy
High serum levels of TPO have been found in patients with autosomal dominant hereditary thrombocythemia.[281] Overproduction has been attributed to a splice donor mutation in the gene for TPO, which leads to a shortened 5′-untranslated region that is more efficiently translated than its normal counterpart.[281] Because platelets themselves regulate the level of circulating TPO, high levels of TPO are also found in patients with bone marrow failure states. Homozygous elimination of *c-mpl* (TPO receptor) results in congenital amegakaryocytic thrombocytopenia.

TPO in the clinic
Two forms of TPO have entered clinical trials: TPO (the full-length polypeptide) and PEG-conjugated recombinant human megakaryocyte growth and development factor (PEG-rHuMGDF).[282,283]

Because its biologic action is prolonged, parenteral administration of TPO for 7–10 days results in increased platelet production 6–16 days later.[284] Results of clinical trials of PEG-rHuMGDF or recombinant human TPO in patients with cancer who were receiving chemotherapy, albeit with regimens that produce only moderate thrombocytopenia, suggest that platelet counts return to baseline significantly faster and the nadir platelet counts are higher.[285,286] However, the effectiveness of these molecules in accelerating platelet recovery after myeloablative therapy has not been impressive.[287] Furthermore, in patients with delayed platelet recovery after peripheral blood stem cell or BMT, recombinant human TPO did not significantly raise platelet counts in most patients.[288]

Future perspectives

The inchoate understanding of cytokines of some decades ago has now emerged as a complex picture of interacting stimulatory and inhibitory factors. Many of the molecules that govern this process have been cloned and have entered clinical trials. It is now clear that regulatory cytokines are characteristically pleiotropic and, at the same time, exhibit significant functional redundancy.

The history of medicine is replete with examples that show how innovative technologies improve clinical outcomes. The genetic engineering techniques that permitted the rapid cloning of newly identified cytokines and their translation into clinical therapies in hematology and oncology are an exciting example of this phenomenon.[289] However, it should be remembered that many, if not most, cytokines and their respective natural inhibitors are ubiquitously expressed and have myriad biologic properties that influence virtually every organ system (see Figure 1). It is already apparent that these molecules may also be effective in allergic and inflammatory conditions. Furthermore, the emerging understanding of their role and the availability of recombinant molecules for therapeutics suggests that the clinical role of these agents will continue to grow and may ultimately impact most fields of medicine.

Acknowledgments

This article combined and updated from the earlier articles, called "Interferons" and "Cytokines and Hematopoietic Growth Factors," in the prior edition of Cancer Medicine. In this earlier edition, these articles were written by the authors, Dr. Ernest C. Borden (Interferons) and in collaboration with Dr. Razelle Kurzrock (Cytokines and Hematopoietic Growth Factors), whose prior contributions provided an important basis for this update.

Key references

The complete reference list can be found on Vital Source version of this title, see inside front cover.

41 Kurzrock R, Talpaz M, Estrov Z, et al. Phase I study of recombinant human interleukin-3 in patients with bone marrow failure. *J Clin Oncol*. 1991;**9**(7):1241–1250.

100 Fujii S, Shimizu K, Shimizu T, Lotze MT. Interleukin-10 promotes the maintenance of antitumor CD8(+) T-cell effector function in situ. *Blood*. 2001;**98**(7):2143–2151.

101 Mumm JB, Emmerich J, Zhang X, et al. IL-10 elicits IFNgamma-dependent tumor immune surveillance. *Cancer Cell*. 2011;**20**(6):781–796.

108 Kobayashi S, Teramura M, Sugawara I, et al. Interleukin-11 acts as an autocrine growth factor for human megakaryoblastic cell lines. *Blood*. 1993;**81**(4):889–893.

109 Putoczki TL, Ernst M. IL-11 signaling as a therapeutic target for cancer. *Immunotherapy*. 2015;**7**(4):441–453.

110 Kobayashi M, Fitz L, Ryan M, et al. Identification and purification of natural killer cell stimulatory factor (NKSF), a cytokine with multiple biologic effects on human lymphocytes. *J Exp Med*. 1989;**170**(3):827–845.

111 Hsieh CS, Macatonia SE, Tripp CS, et al. Development of TH1 CD4+ T cells through IL-12 produced by Listeria-induced macrophages. *Science*. 1993;**260**(5107):547–549.

113 Trinchieri G. Interleukin-12: a cytokine at the interface of inflammation and immunity. *Adv Immunol*. 1998;**70**:83–243.

117 Ku CC, Murakami M, Sakamoto A, et al. Control of homeostasis of CD8+ memory T cells by opposing cytokines. *Science*. 2000;**288**(5466):675–678.

122 Waldmann TA, Dubois S, Miljkovic MD, Conlon KC. IL-15 in the Combination Immunotherapy of Cancer. *Front Immunol*. 2020;**11**:868.

129 McGeachy MJ, Cua DJ, Gaffen SL. The IL-17 Family of Cytokines in Health and Disease. *Immunity*. 2019;**50**(4):892–906.

130 Ly K, Smith MP, Thibodeaux Q, et al. Anti IL-17 in psoriasis. *Expert Rev Clin Immunol*. 2019;**15**(11):1185–1194.

137 Robertson MJ, Kline J, Struemper H, et al. A dose-escalation study of recombinant human interleukin-18 in combination with rituximab in patients with non-Hodgkin lymphoma. *J Immunother.* 2013;**36**(6):331–341.

139 Parrish-Novak J, Dillon SR, Nelson A, et al. Interleukin 21 and its receptor are involved in NK cell expansion and regulation of lymphocyte function. *Nature.* 2000;**408**(6808):57–63.

140 Ozaki K, Spolski R, Feng CG, et al. A critical role for IL-21 in regulating immunoglobulin production. *Science.* 2002;**298**(5598):1630–1634.

152 Braum O, Klages M, Fickenscher H. The cationic cytokine IL-26 differentially modulates virus infection in culture. *PLoS One.* 2013;**8**(7):e70281.

154 Pflanz S, Timans JC, Cheung J, et al. IL-27, a heterodimeric cytokine composed of EBI3 and p28 protein, induces proliferation of naive CD4(+) T cells. *Immunity.* 2002;**16**(6):779–790.

163 Witte K, Witte E, Sabat R, Wolk K. IL-28A, IL-28B, and IL-29: promising cytokines with type I interferon-like properties. *Cytokine Growth Factor Rev.* 2010;**21**(4):237–251.

169 Ruzicka T, Hanifin JM, Furue M, et al. Anti-interleukin-31 receptor a antibody for atopic dermatitis. *N Engl J Med.* 2017;**376**(9):826–835.

176 Wang L, Quan Y, Yue Y, et al. Interleukin-37: a crucial cytokine with multiple roles in disease and potentially clinical therapy. *Oncol Lett.* 2018;**15**(4):4711–4719.

179 Parker BS, Rautela J, Hertzog PJ. Antitumour actions of interferons: implications for cancer therapy. *Nat Rev Cancer.* 2016;**16**(3):131–144.

180 Sanlorenzo M, Vujic I, Carnevale-Schianca F, et al. Role of interferon in melanoma: old hopes and new perspectives. *Expert Opin Biol Ther.* 2017;**17**(4):475–483.

185 Talpaz M, O'Brien S, Rose E, et al. Phase 1 study of polyethylene glycol formulation of interferon alpha-2B (Schering 54031) in Philadelphia chromosome-positive chronic myelogenous leukemia. *Blood.* 2001;**98**(6):1708–1713.

192 Preudhomme C, Guilhot J, Nicolini FE, et al. Imatinib plus peginterferon alfa-2a in chronic myeloid leukemia. *N Engl J Med.* 2010;**363**(26):2511–2521.

194 Nicolini FE, Etienne G, Dubruille V, et al. Nilotinib and peginterferon alfa-2a for newly diagnosed chronic-phase chronic myeloid leukaemia (NiloPeg): a multicentre, non-randomised, open-label phase 2 study. *Lancet Haematol.* 2015;**2**(1):e37-46.

196 Hjorth-Hansen H, Stentoft J, Richter J, et al. Safety and efficacy of the combination of pegylated interferon-alpha2b and dasatinib in newly diagnosed chronic-phase chronic myeloid leukemia patients. *Leukemia.* 2016;**30**(9):1853–1860.

197 Hochhaus A, Burchert A, Saussele S, et al. Nilotinib vs nilotinib plus pegylated interferon α (Peg-IFN) induction and nilotinib or Peg-IFN maintenance therapy for newly diagnosed BCR-ABL1 positive chronic myeloid leukemia patients in chronic phase (TIGER Study): the addition of Peg-IFN is associated with higher rates of deep molecular response. *Blood.* 2019;**134**(Supplement_1):495.

214 Gisslinger H, Klade C, Georgiev P, et al. Ropeginterferon alfa-2b versus standard therapy for polycythaemia vera (PROUD-PV and CONTINUATION-PV): a randomised, non-inferiority, phase 3 trial and its extension study. *Lancet Haematol.* 2020;**7**(3):e196–e208.

225 Hasselbalch HC. A new era for IFN-alpha in the treatment of Philadelphia-negative chronic myeloproliferative neoplasms. *Expert Rev Hematol.* 2011;**4**(6):637–655.

235 Kirkwood JM, Manola J, Ibrahim J, et al. A pooled analysis of eastern cooperative oncology group and intergroup trials of adjuvant high-dose interferon for melanoma. *Clin Cancer Res.* 2004;**10**(5):1670–1677.

248 Atkins MB, Hodi FS, Thompson JA, et al. Pembrolizumab plus pegylated interferon alfa-2b or ipilimumab for advanced melanoma or renal cell carcinoma: dose-finding results from the phase Ib KEYNOTE-029 study. *Clin Cancer Res.* 2018;**24**(8):1805–1815.

250 Dizman N, Adashek JJ, Hsu J, et al. Adjuvant treatment in renal cell carcinoma. *Clin Adv Hematol Oncol.* 2018;**16**(8):555–563.

251 Rini BI, Halabi S, Rosenberg JE, et al. Phase III trial of bevacizumab plus interferon alfa versus interferon alfa monotherapy in patients with metastatic renal cell carcinoma: final results of CALGB 90206. *J Clin Oncol.* 2010;**28**(13):2137–2143.

260 Zaidi MR. The interferon-gamma paradox in cancer. *J Interf Cytokine Res.* 2019;**39**(1):30–38.

262 Adamson JW. Epoetin alfa: into the new millennium. *Semin Oncol.* 1998;**25**(3 Suppl 7):76–79.

265 Bonilla MA, Dale D, Zeidler C, et al. Long-term safety of treatment with recombinant human granulocyte colony-stimulating factor (r-metHuG-CSF) in patients with severe congenital neutropenias. *Br J Haematol.* 1994;**88**(4):723–730.

266 Root RK, Dale DC. Granulocyte colony-stimulating factor and granulocyte-macrophage colony-stimulating factor: comparisons and potential for use in the treatment of infections in nonneutropenic patients. *J Infect Dis.* 1999;**179**(Suppl 2):S342–S352.

276 Williams DE, Eisenman J, Baird A, et al. Identification of a ligand for the c-kit proto-oncogene. *Cell.* 1990;**63**(1):167–174.

280 Demetri GD, von Mehren M, Blanke CD, et al. Efficacy and safety of imatinib mesylate in advanced gastrointestinal stromal tumors. *N Engl J Med.* 2002;**347**(7):472–480.

285 Fanucchi M, Glaspy J, Crawford J, et al. Effects of polyethylene glycol-conjugated recombinant human megakaryocyte growth and development factor on platelet counts after chemotherapy for lung cancer. *N Engl J Med.* 1997;**336**(6):404–409.

60 Monoclonal antibody and targeted toxin therapy

Robert C. Bast, Jr., MD ■ Michael R. Zalutsky, PhD, MA

Overview

Monoclonal antibodies have impacted significantly on the care of patients with cancer. Overall, the US FDA has approved 100 different monoclonal antibodies for the treatment of human diseases. More than 40 monoclonal antibodies, cytotoxic drug conjugates, radionuclide conjugates, and targeted toxins have been approved for the treatment of more than two dozen different malignancies. Useful monoclonal antibodies have most frequently targeted structural proteins and receptors on the cancer cell surface (CD20 by rituximab, HER2 by trastuzumab, and pertuzumab), inhibiting growth, inducing apoptosis, and enhancing chemotherapy, but some have targeted cytokines (IL-6 by siltuximab), growth factors (vascular endothelial growth factor (VEGF) by bevacizumab), and growth factor receptors (VEGFR2 by ramucirumab) that affect both cancer cells and normal stromal cells including endothelial cells and lymphocytes. Monoclonal antibodies have disrupted checkpoint inhibition of effector T lymphocytes by blocking CTLA4 (ipilimumab), PD1 (pembrolizumab, nivolumab, and cemiplimab), and PD-L1 (atezolizumab, durvalumab, and avelumab). In the case of trastuzumab and pertuzumab, binding of the two antibodies to different sites on the HER2 cell surface receptor has produced greater antitumor activity than either alone. Enhanced cancer cell killing has also been achieved by conjugation of antibodies with cytotoxic drugs (emtansine to anti-HER2 trastuzumab and vedotin to anti-CD30 brentuximab) or radionuclide conjugates (^{90}Y to anti-CD20 ibritumomab tiuxetan) permitting effective treatment of patients who had failed therapy with unconjugated antibodies. There are several barriers to effective therapy with monoclonal antibodies including antigen specificity, antigenic modulation, heterogeneity of antigen expression, effective delivery of antibodies to cancer cells, potency of effector mechanisms, and response to immunologically foreign globulin. The latter problem has been circumvented with the use of chimeric constructs, humanization of murine antibodies, and developing genetically engineered mice with the ability to develop fully human antibodies. Use of unconjugated antibodies is likely to improve as our knowledge of tumor biology and immunology grows, identifying targets such as OX-40 ligand. Use of smaller molecularly engineered binding constructs may improve pharmacokinetics and pharmacodynamics of monoclonal antibody and conjugate therapy. Combinations of antibodies may be required to compensate for antigenic heterogeneity. Development of more effective antibody–drug conjugates will require the identification of monoclonal reagents that target tumor-initiating stem cells. Use of antibody fragments, pretargeting, and the use of alpha-emitters are promising approaches to improving antibody–radionuclide conjugates. Development of targeted toxins must be further explored.

Introduction

Following the initial report of Kohler and Milstein,[1] monoclonal antibody technology exerted a prompt and substantial impact on laboratory investigation. Over the last four decades, the availability of monoclonal reagents has permitted the development of novel markers for *in vitro* applications, including monitoring response to treatment, detecting malignant cells histochemically, identifying subsets of patients with particularly favorable or unfavorable prognoses, and distinguishing some tumors of unknown origin. Application of monoclonal antibodies for the *in vivo* treatment of human cancer has been more gradual, but serotherapy with monoclonal antibodies and their conjugates now has an established role in the management of more than two dozen hematopoietic and solid cancers.[2-5]

In 2021, the United States Food and Drug Administration (FDA) approved the 100th monoclonal antibody or antibody conjugate for therapeutic indications, including transplant rejection, coronary thrombosis, respiratory syncytial virus, COVID-19 and anthrax infections, rheumatoid arthritis, systemic lupus erythematosus, paroxysmal nocturnal hemoglobinuria, macular degeneration, inflammatory bowel disease, psoriasis, asthma, and cancer.[6,7] Forty-one of the first 100 antibodies and conjugates were approved for the treatment of different cancers, as were three targeted toxins (Table 1).[8] Unmodified monoclonal antibodies contribute to the care of patients with acute lymphoblastic and chronic lymphocytic leukemias (CLLs), acute myelogenous leukemia, Hodgkin and non-Hodgkin lymphomas (NHLs), multiple myeloma (MM), Castleman disease, neuroblastoma, HER2-amplified breast cancer, non-small-cell, and small-cell lung cancer, head and neck cancer, renal cell cancer (RCC), colorectal cancer, gastro-esophageal junction (GEJ), and gastric cancer. With the general availability of these agents, it appears that monoclonal serotherapy has a well-established role in clinical oncology.

In an attempt to exert greater antitumor activity *in vivo*, monoclonal antibodies have been linked to cytotoxic drugs, radionuclides, and immunotoxins. Extensive preclinical and clinical studies have now been performed with each type of immunoconjugate, with several approved by the FDA for the treatment of different cancers.[9] This article considers the current use as well as some of the challenges and additional opportunities for the further clinical application of monoclonal reagents, drug conjugates, radionuclide conjugates, and targeted toxins for the treatment of patients with cancer.

Serotherapy for leukemia and lymphoma with unmodified monoclonal antibodies

With rare exceptions, murine monoclonal antibodies raised against human neoplasms recognize tumor-associated antigens, which are also expressed by normal adult or fetal tissues. Some antigens are expressed by only a small number of normal cells that may not be essential to a patient's well-being, exemplified by idiotypes on immunoglobulins associated with lymphoma cells. Others

---

Holland-Frei Cancer Medicine, Tenth Edition. Edited by Robert C. Bast, John C. Byrd, Carlo M. Croce, Ernest Hawk, Fadlo R. Khuri, Raphael E. Pollock, Apostolia M. Tsimberidou, Christopher G. Willett, and Cheryl L. Willman.
© 2023 John Wiley & Sons, Inc. Published 2023 by John Wiley & Sons, Inc.

Table 1 Monoclonal antibodies, radionuclide conjugates, and targeted toxins approved in the United States for Treatment of Cancer.[7]

Antibody	Product name	FDA approved	Type	Antigenic target	Indication
Rituximab	Rituxan	1997	Chimeric	CD20	Relapsed or refractory follicular and low-grade non-Hodgkin lymphoma
Trastuzumab	Herceptin	1998	Humanized	HER2	Metastatic breast cancers that overexpress HER-2 (HER-2+)
Denileukin diftitox	Ontak	1999	Targeted toxin	CD25	Cutaneous T-cell leukemia
Gemtuzumab ozogamicin	Mylotarg	2000	Humanized ADC	CD33	Relapsed acute myelogenous leukemia (AML) in elderly patients
		2017			Newly diagnosed AML
		2020			Newly diagnosed AML
Alemtuzumab	Campath	2001	Humanized	CD52	B-cell chronic lymphocytic leukemia
⁰Y-ibritumomab tiuxetan	Zevalin	2002	Murine ARC	CD20	Relapsed or refractory follicular and low-grade non-Hodgkin lymphomas in elderly patients and rituximab-resistant disease
¹³¹I-tostuzumab	Bexxar	2003	Murine ARC	CD20	Relapsed or refractory follicular and low-grade non-Hodgkin lymphomas in elderly patients and rituximab-resistant disease
Cetuximab	Erbitux	2004	Chimeric	EGFR	Metastatic colorectal cancer with irinotecan
		2006			Head and neck cancers with radiotherapy
		2020			CRC with BRAF V600E mutation
Bevacizumab	Avastin	2004	Humanized	VEGF	Metastatic colorectal cancer
		2006			Non-small-cell lung cancer
		2008			Breast cancer (withdrawn)
		2009			Renal cell
		2009			Glioblastoma
		2014			Ovarian
Panitumumab	Vectabix	2006	Human	EGFR	Colorectal cancer
Ofatumumab	Azerra	2009	Human	CD20	Chronic lymphocytic leukemia
Ipilimumab	Yervoy	2011	Human	CTLA4	Metastatic melanoma
Brentuximab vedotin	Adcetris	2011	Chimeric ADC	CD30	Hodgkin lymphoma; anaplastic large-cell lymphoma
		2017			Primary cutaneous large-cell lymphoma
		2018			Hodgkin disease, T-cell lymphoma
Pertuzumab	Perjeta	2012	Humanized	HER2	HER2+ breast cancer
		2018			Adjuvant HER2+ breast cancer with trastuzumab
Ado-trastuzumab emtansine (TDM-1)	Kadcyla	2013	Humanized ADC	HER2	HER2+ breast cancer
		2019			Adjuvant HER2+ breast cancer
Obinutuzumab	Gazyva	2013	Humanized	CD20	Chronic lymphocytic leukemia
		2017			Bulky follicular lymphoma
Siltuximab	Sylvant	2014	Chimeric Human	IL-6	Castleman disease
Ramucirumab	Cyramza	2014	Humanized	VEGFR2	Gastric cancer
		2018			Cervical cancer
		2019			Esophageal cancer, SCC lung, HNSCC
		2020			HNSCC with erlotinib
Pembrolizumab	Keytruda	2014	Humanized	PD1	Melanoma
		2018			Cervical cancer, Large B-cell lymphoma
Blinatumomab	Blincyto	2014	Bi-specific tandem ScFv	CD19, CD3	Acute lymphoblastic leukemia
Nivolumab	Opdivo	2015	Human IgG4	PD1	Melanoma, non-small-cell lung cancer, renal cell carcinoma, Hodgkin disease
Dinutuximab	Unituxin	2015	Chimeric	GD2	Neuroblastoma
Necitumumab	Portrazza	2015	Human IgG1	EGFR	Non-small-cell lung cancer
Elotuzumab	Emplicti	2015	Human IgG1	SLAMF7	Multiple myeloma
Daratumumab	Darzalex	2015	Human IgG1	CD38	Multiple myeloma
Atezolizumab	Tecentriq	2016	Human IgG1	PD-L1	Metastatic non-small cell lung cancer, triple negative breast cancer
Olartumab	Lartruvo	2016	Human IgG1	PDGFRα	Sarcoma
Durvalumab	Imfinzi	2017	Human IgG1	PD-L1	Urothelial cancer
		2018			NSCLC
Avelumab	Bavencio	2017	Human IgG1	PD-L1	Merkel cell carcinoma
Mogamulizomab kpkc	Potelgio	2018	Humanized IgG4kIgG4	CCR4	T-cell leukemia, mycosis fungoides
Cemiplimab	Libtayo	2018	IgG1	PD-1	Advanced cutaneous squamous cell cancer
		2021			NSCLC, basal cell cancer, cervical
Fam trastuzumab deruxtecan	Enhertu	2019	IgG1K	HER-2	HER-2 positive breast cancer, gastric, GEJ
Polatuzumab vedotin	Polivy	2019	Human IgG1 Fc altered	CD79b	Diffuse B-cell lymphoma
Tafasituzumab vedotin	Monjuvi	2020	Human IgG1	CD19	Multiple myeloma
Isatuximab	Sarclisa	2020	Humanized IgG1	CD38	Multiple myeloma
Naxitamab	Danielza	2020	Humanized IgG1	GD2	Neuroblastoma
Sacituzumab govitican Hzik	Trodelvy	2020	IgG1K and topotecan inhibitor	Trop-2	TNBC, gastric, Bladder Cancer
Belantamab mafodotin	Blenreb	2020	IgG1 altered FC ADC	BCM	Multiple myeloma
Amivantamab-vmjw	Rybrevant	2021	IgG4 human Low fucose Bi-specific	mEGFR MET	NSCLC with exon 21 mutation
Dostarlimab	Jemperli	2021	Humanized IgG4	PD1	Endometrial cancer, defective mismatch repair

differentiation antigens such as CD20 are more widely distributed on normal B cells, but antibody binding produces manageable toxicity. Unconjugated monoclonal antibodies against idiotypes and differentiation antigens have contributed significantly to the care of patients with lymphoma[3] and leukemia.[10,11]

Anti-idiotypic antibodies

In the early 1980s, Levy and colleagues prepared tumor-specific murine monoclonal antibodies against the unique idiotypes associated with cell surface membrane immunoglobulin present on human B-cell lymphomas but expressed by a very small subset of normal B cells.[12,13] Treatment of 18 lymphoma patients with anti-idiotypic antibodies alone produced an objective response rate of 67% with little toxicity, and one patient remained in complete remission for 72 months and survived for >17 years.[6] In subsequent trials, anti-idiotypic antibodies were combined with interferon (IFN)-α, chlorambucil, or interleukin (IL)-2. Most of the antibodies that produced responses *in vivo* were of the murine immunoglobulin G1 (IgG1) isotype, which is generally least efficient in fixing complement or participating in antibody-dependent cell-mediated cytotoxicity (ADCC). Anti-idiotypic antibodies that bind to the B-cell receptor complex appear to induce apoptosis (programmed cell death) by delivering a death signal. In a fraction of patients treated with anti-idiotypic antibodies, recurrence of lymphoma is associated with loss of the relevant antigen from the cancer cells. Genes encoding the cell surface membrane immunoglobulin continue to undergo point mutations, resulting in the loss of idiotypic determinants.[14] Use of anti-idiotypic antibodies provided critical proof of concept, but widespread application was hindered by the logistic challenge of developing reagents for each patient.

Anti-CD20 antibodies

Rituximab (Rituxan®)

Monoclonal antibodies against B-cell differentiation antigens expressed by malignant cells from different patients have been used to treat NHL, as well as acute and chronic leukemias. One useful target is CD20, a 35-kDa phosphoprotein calcium channel expressed on the surface of all normal B cells and on 80% of NHLs, but not on other normal tissues. Antibodies specific for different epitopes on CD20 are classified as Type I antibodies that translocate CD20 into detergent-insoluble lipid rafts in the cell membrane, facilitating complement-dependent cytotoxicity (CDC); or Type II antibodies that do not induce lipid rafts and facilitate ADCC by Fcγ receptor-bearing natural killer (NK) cells and macrophages.[3] Repeated weekly administration of the Type I chimeric mouse/human IgG1 anti-CD20 antibody rituximab produced a 48–50% response rate in patients with relapsed low-grade follicular NHL, with a median time to progression of 10.2–13.2 months.[15,16] In 37 newly diagnosed patients, treatment with rituximab produced an overall response rate of 72%, with 36% complete responses and median time to disease progression of 2.2 years.[17] Consequently, rituximab was used initially to treat patients with relapsed or refractory indolent follicular NHL. Use was extended to treat newly diagnosed low-grade NHL patients with rituximab alone or in combination with chemotherapy as well as for maintenance therapy.[18] Rituximab has also contributed to the care of patients with diffuse large B-cell NHL, CLL, and autoimmune diseases.

Follicular and indolent NHL. Since regulatory approval by the US FDA in 1997 for the treatment of patients with recurrent or refractory follicular or indolent NHL, indications have been extended to provide 8 rather than 4 weekly courses and to retreat patients who had previously responded.[19] After relapse, retreatment with a similar course of rituximab produced an overall response rate of 38% in 60 patients, with 10% complete remissions. Median time to progression exceeded 15 months.[20] Combination of rituximab with cyclophosphamide, doxorubicin, vincristine, and prednisone (CHOP) chemotherapy (R-CHOP) in 40 patients with low-grade follicular lymphoma, some of whom had been previously treated, resulted in an overall response of 100%, with 58% complete remissions and 42% partial remissions. Median time to progression exceeded 40.5 months.[21] In a meta-analysis of seven trials with 1943 patients with follicular lymphoma, other indolent lymphomas, and the more aggressive mantle cell lymphoma, the addition of rituximab to chemotherapy improved overall survival (OS), although the statistical significance was higher with indolent lymphomas than with the mantle cell histotype.[22] The addition of rituximab to cyclophosphamide, vincristine, and prednisone (CVP) chemotherapy prolonged time to progression in patients with newly diagnosed follicular NHL, resulting in FDA approval in 2006 for use of rituximab in first-line therapy.[23] Maintenance therapy with rituximab has prolonged progression-free survival (PFS) in four randomized trials, while OS has been extended in some but not all studies.[24] In 2011, the US FDA approved rituximab for maintenance therapy based on a randomized comparison of rituximab (up to 12 8-week cycles) to no maintenance therapy in 1018 patients with high tumor burden follicular NHL who had complete or partial response to rituximab plus one of three chemotherapy regimens. Maintenance rituximab reduced the risk of a PFS event by 46% ($p < 0.0001$). At 3 years, PFS in the rituximab maintenance group was 74.9% versus 57.6% in the observation group ($p < 0.0001$).[25]

Diffuse large B-cell NHL. More aggressive diffuse large B-cell lymphoma (DLBCL) has been less responsive to rituximab alone. Among 54 patients with disease in relapse, the overall response rate to eight cycles of rituximab was 31%, including 9% complete remissions with a median time to progression in responders of 8 or more months.[26] Subsequently, 399 elderly patients with more aggressive DLBCL were randomized to receive R-CHOP or CHOP alone. A complete response rate of 76% was observed with the combination, compared with 60% with CHOP alone.[27] Event-free survival (EFS) ($p < 0.005$) and OS ($p < 0.01$) were significantly prolonged by the addition of rituximab. Similar results were obtained in two confirmatory trials,[28,29] both in young and elderly individuals, resulting in FDA approval in 2006 for the use of R-CHOP in DLBCL, and providing the first improvement in the systemic treatment of DLBCL in some two decades. In a meta-analysis of seven trials involving 1,470 patients with relapsed or refractory DLBCL, maintenance therapy with rituximab provided numerically improved PFS and OS, but the differences were not statistically significant, whereas incorporation of rituximab in salvage therapy led to statistically significantly better OS ($p = 0.02$) and PFS ($p < 0.05$) than rituximab-free regimens.[30] However, the rate of infection-related adverse events was higher with rituximab treatment (RR = 1.37; $p = 0.001$).

CLL and Waldenstrom macroglobulinemia. Treatment with rituximab, alone or in combination with fludarabine, has been extended to CLL.[31] In early studies, only a very modest response rate (15%) was observed with low standard doses of rituximab, possibly related to the lower concentration of CD20 on the CLL cell surface (8–15,000 vs 90,000 sites/cell) and to the shedding of soluble CD20, creating an "antigenic sink."[32,33] Treatment with higher doses of rituximab or thrice weekly administration achieved an overall response rate of 46% in CLL, with an even higher response rate in previously untreated patients.[32] A cancer and leukemia group B (CALGB) trial of fludarabine and rituximab in 42 patients with CLL yielded a 100% response rate, with 48% of patients achieving complete remission.[34] Based on two randomized phase III studies where the addition of rituximab to fludarabine and cyclophosphamide extended PFS by 10–19 months in previously treated and untreated patients with CLL,[35,36] the US FDA approved rituximab in combination with fludarabine and cyclophosphamide in 2010. Rituximab has also been used with alkylating agents to treat Waldenstrom macroglobulinemia. One study reported a 74% response rate and 67% 2-year PFS with a combination of rituximab, dexamethasone, and cyclophosphamide.[37]

Autoimmune disease. Depletion of B lymphocytes has contributed to the management of autoimmune diseases. Rituximab has been approved in combination with methotrexate for the treatment of rheumatoid arthritis that has failed antitumor necrosis factor (TNF) therapy, as well as for treatment of granulomatosis polyangiitis (Wegener's Granulomatosis) and microscopic polyangiitis (MPA) with glucocorticoids.[38]

Toxicity. Rituximab therapy is generally well tolerated. Most side effects are infusion related and occur within the first few hours of treatment. Adverse events generally last minutes to hours and include chills, fever, nausea, vomiting, fatigue, headache, pruritus, and the sensation of throat swelling.[39] Although side effects are experienced by up to 77% of patients, they are severe in only 10%.[40] Normal B-lymphocyte counts can decrease to zero after initial infusion; recovery begins by 6 months and is generally complete by 9–12 months. As CD20 is not expressed on mature plasma cells, immunoglobulin levels are maintained, and intercurrent infections requiring hospitalization occurred in only 2% of patients during 1-year follow-up. Following FDA approval in 1997 and prior to 2002, >125,000 patients were treated with rituximab in the United States. Among these individuals, only eight deaths were associated with treatment and were related to the development of infusion reactions, paraneoplastic pemphigus, Stevens–Johnson syndrome, and toxic epidermal necrolysis.[41] More than 120 cases of interstitial lung disease have been reported, generally when rituximab has been given with chemotherapy but associated with monotherapy in 25%.[42] In recent years, rituximab treatment has been linked to reactivation of hepatitis B virus (HBV) in HBsAg-negative/HBcAb-positive patients. In one meta-analysis of 578 patients across 15 studies, the risk of reactivation was estimated at 6.3%,[43] suggesting that patients should be tested and antiviral prophylaxis given to those with evidence of previous HBV infection who are receiving rituximab.

Mechanism of action and resistance. The mechanism(s) by which rituximab kills leukemia and lymphoma cells is not completely understood, but probably involves ADCC, CDC, and the direct effect of CD20 ligation.[44] In cancer cells, cross-linking CD20 can induce cell cycle arrest, inhibit DNA synthesis, activate caspases, and induce apoptosis.[34] Sensitization to chemotherapy may relate to inhibiting the constitutive activation of AKT, thus downregulating the antiapoptotic protein Bcl-XL.[45] NK cells, macrophages, and polymorphonuclear leukocytes can be important effectors for ADCC,[34] and a correlation has been observed in some studies, but not all, between clinical response to rituximab and the presence of specific allelic polymorphisms in the FcγRIIIa and FcγRIIa receptors for IgG that are required to mediate ADCC.[46] Individual NK cells are capable of "serial killing" of multiple lymphoma cells, particularly in the presence of rituximab which creates a "cap" at one pole of the cancer cell containing CD20, ICAM-1, and the microtubule-organizing center, which enhances sensitivity to NK-killing.[3,47] The response to rituximab is impaired in mice genetically deficient in C1q that lack the first component of the CDC pathway but that have intact ADCC.[48] Clinical resistance to rituximab treatment rarely involves loss of CD20 expression but can be associated with upregulation of complement resistance proteins CD55 and CD59.[49] Interestingly, different patterns of gene expression have been observed in lymphoma cells obtained prior to treatment from responders and nonresponders to rituximab.[50] Gene expression in tumors that failed to respond resembled that in normal lymphoid tissues and exhibited higher expression of genes encoding certain complement components and genes involved in cytokine, T-cell, and TNF signaling.

Ofatumumab

Ofatumumab (Arzerra^R) is a Type I human anti-CD20 IgG1 that binds to an epitope distinct from that recognized by rituximab, and with greater avidity and slower off-rates, facilitating both CDC and ADCC. Ofatumumab was approved by the US FDA in 2009 for treatment of CLL based on a multicenter, randomized, open-label trial comparing ofatumumab in combination with chlorambucil to single agent chlorambucil.[51] The trial enrolled 447 patients for whom fludarabine-based therapy was considered inappropriate by the investigator for reasons that included advanced age (median 69 years) or presence of comorbidities (72% with two or more comorbidities). Median PFS was 22.4 months for patients receiving ofatumumab in combination with chlorambucil compared to 13.1 months for patients receiving single-agent chlorambucil ($p < 0.001$).

Toxicity. The most common (>5%) adverse reactions with ofatumumab in combination with chlorambucil were infusion reactions, neutropenia, asthenia, headache, leukopenia, herpes simplex, lower respiratory tract infection, arthralgia, and upper abdominal pain. Overall, 67% of patients who received ofatumumab experienced one or more symptoms of infusion reaction and 10% experienced a grade 3 or greater infusion reaction.

Obinutuzumab

Obinutuzumab (Gazyva^R) is a Type II humanized anti-CD20 IgG1 that acts predominantly through ADCC and has been glycoengineered to enhance binding to FcγR on effector cells.[3] Binding of obinutuzumab to CD20 can initiate intracellular signaling, reorganizing actin fibers, increasing lysosomal membrane permeability, and producing nonapoptotic cell death.[52] When compared to rituximab and ofatumumab, obinutuzumab exerted greater direct toxicity for B cells.[53] Obinutuzumab was approved by the US FDA in 2013 for treatment of CLL based on a randomized open-label multicenter trial comparing chlorambucil alone and in combination with obinutuzumab in 781 previously untreated participants who were elderly or had comorbidities.[54] Patients receiving obinutuzumab in combination with chlorambucil demonstrated a significant improvement in average PFS—26.7 months compared to 11.1 months with chlorambucil alone.

Activity has been observed in in patients with previously treated indolent and aggressive NHL[55,56] and in patients with rituximab-refractory indolent NHL.[57] When treatment with obinutuzumab-based chemotherapy was compared to rituximab-based chemotherapy in 1202 patients with newly diagnosed bulky follicular lymphoma, similar response rates were observed (88.5% vs 86.9%), but 3-year PFS was greater using induction and 2 years of maintenance with obinutuzumab than with rituximab (80.0% vs 73.3%; $p = 0.001$).[58] However, high-grade adverse events, generally infusion-related, were more frequent with obinutuzumab.

Toxicity. The most common side effects in participants receiving obinutuzumab in combination with chlorambucil or multidrug regimens are infusion-related reactions, neutropenia, thrombocytopenia, anemia, musculoskeletal pain, and fever. Obinutuzumab was approved with a boxed warning regarding HBV reactivation observed with other anti-CD20 antibodies and rare cases of progressive multifocal leukoencephalopathy identified in participants on other trials of obinutuzumab. So, chlorambucil with obinutuzumab or ofatumumab now provides alternatives for elderly CLL patients with comorbidities who are unlikely to tolerate fludarabine-based therapy.[11]

Antibodies against other B lymphocyte-associated cell surface proteins

Over the last three decades, clinical trials have been conducted to evaluate antibodies against CD19, CD22, CD23, CD40, CD74, and CD80 in patients with different B-cell-derived cancers.[24] In early studies of CD10-positive acute lymphoblastic leukemia (ALL), anti-CD10 antibody-induced prompt modulation of the common ALL antigen, preventing effective therapy.[59] Intravenous infusion of anti-CD5 also produced antigenic modulation and only transient, partial regression in a fraction of patients with T-cell leukemia/lymphoma and CLL.[60] In one of the first studies of serotherapy with monoclonal reagents, a serum-blocking factor was demonstrated that prevented binding of the monoclonal antibody to circulating lymphosarcoma cells, consistent with the presence of shed tumor antigen.[61]

CD19 is a 95 kDa transmembrane cell surface protein that is expressed by normal and neoplastic B cells, and that is required for effective B-cell signaling.[62] The molecule appears to play a role in maintaining the balance between antigen-induced stimulation of the humoral immune response and tolerance induction. CD19 on diffuse large B-cell lymphoma (DLBCL) has been targeted effectively in approximately half of the cases of recurrent, refractory disease by CAR T cells, resulting in the FDA approval of axicabtagene ciloleucel and tisagenlecleucel (see **Chapter 62**).

Tafasitamab
CD19 has been targeted with monoclonal antibodies as well. Tafasitamab (Monjuvi®) is a humanized IgG1 monoclonal with two amino acids altered in its Fc region to enhance affinity for the Fcγ Receptor. Lenalidomide has direct activity against lymphomas and can also enhance NK and antibody-dependent cell-mediated cytotoxicity (ADCC). Patients with relapsed and refractory DLBCL who were not eligible for autologous stem cell transplantation were given a combination of tafasitamab and lenalidomide for up to 12 months followed by tafasitamab monotherapy, resulting in 43% CR and 18% PR with severe neutropenia (48%) and thrombocytopenia (17%).[63] Accelerated approval was given by the FDA in 2020.

Antibodies against T lymphocyte-associated cell surface proteins

Mogamulizumab-kpkc
Cytokine receptors have been targeted on T-cell malignancies. Mogamulizumab-kpkc (Poteligio®) is a defucosylated, humanized IgG4K that binds to C–C chemokine receptor 4 (CCR4) that is expressed by both malignant and normal T cells, triggering ADCC. Responses have been observed in 31–50% of patients with CCR4+ T-cell leukemias and lymphomas[64] and mogamulizumab was approved by the FDA in 2018 for treatment of relapsed or refractory mycosis fungoides (MF) and Sezary syndrome (SS). When treatment with mogamulizumab was compared to treatment with vorinostat in 372 patients with MF and SS, median PFS was improved from 3.1 to 7.7 months.[65] Grade 3–4 toxicities were observed in 41% of both groups with pyrexia in 4% and cellulitis in 3% of antibody-treated patients. An erythematous plaque-like cutaneous granulomatous drug eruption can occur during treatment with mogamulizumab that can mimic progression of MF but that has been associated with prolonged PFS in small numbers of patients.[66] Skin biopsy and flow cytometric analysis of peripheral blood mononuclear cells is required to differentiate progression from pseudo-progression.

Antibodies that recognize multiple myeloma
Three monoclonal antibodies have been FDA approved for the treatment of relapsed/refractory MM. Elotuzumab is directed against signaling lymphocyte activation molecule F7 (SLAMF7), whereas darmatumumab and isatuximab recognize different epitopes on CD38, an antigen that is overexpressed on the surface of MM cells.

Elotuzumab
Elotuzumab (Emplicti®) is a humanized IgG1 that activates NK cells that express SLAMF7 (CD319) as well as targeting SLAMFZ on MM cells that are killed by NK-mediated ADCC.[67] In a study of refractory MM, 646 patients were randomized to elotuzumab, lenalidomide, and dexamethasone or to lenalidomide and dexamethasone alone. After a median of 24 months follow-up, relative risk of disease progression or death was reduced by 30% by the addition of elotuzumab[68] and a reduction of 29% was maintained at 4 years.[69] Lymphocytopenia, neutropenia, fatigue, and pneumonia were observed in both groups. The immunostimulatory agent pomalidomide has shown activity in MM that has become resistant to lenalidomide and proteasome inhibitors. The addition of elotuzumab to pomalidomide and dexamethasone in this group of patients extended progression-free survival from 4.7 to 10.3 months, reduced the hazard ratio for disease progression or death to 0.54 ($p = 0.008$), and increased the response rate from 26% to 53%.[70] Infections occurred in 65% of patients in both groups and infusion reactions were observed in only 5% of patients receiving elotuzumab.

Daratumumab
Daratumumab (Darzlex®) is a human IgG1 that targets CD38 that is overexpressed on MM cells, mediating ADCC, complement-mediated cytotoxicity, and cellular phagocytosis.[71] As NK cells also express CD38, daratumumab can deplete NK cells, which may contribute to increased susceptibility to acute viral infections and to reactivation of herpes simplex, varicella-zoster, and cytomegalovirus.[72] Daratumumab can bind to CD38

on human erythrocytes, interfering with blood compatibility testing and phenotyping for Rh and Kell before initiating therapy as has been recommended.[73] Increased PFS and increased rates of response were observed in patients with relapsed and/or refractory MM when daratumumab was added to lenalidomide and dexamethasone,[74,75] bortezomib and dexamethasone,[76–79] carfilzomib and dexamethasone,[80] or pomalidomide and dexamethasone.[81,82] In newly diagnosed patients, addition of daratumumab to bortezomib, thalidomide, and dexamethasone, before and after autologous stem cell transplant improved the depth of response and PFS.[83] Maintenance therapy with daratumumab also improved PFS with acceptable toxicity.[84] Infusion reactions were observed in 54.5% of daratumumab-naive patients but in only 2.2% of patients previously treated with the antibody. Subcutaneous injection of daratumumab with recombinant human hyaluronidase has been shown noninferior to conventional intravenous infusion of daratumumab,[85] permitting more convenient administration.

Isatuximab

Isatuximab (Sarclisa®) is a human IgG1 antibody that recognizes an epitope on CD38 that is distinct from that recognized by daratumumab. Mechanisms of action are similar to those of daratumumab.[86] Interference with Coombs testing for matching of blood is also observed. In patients with recurrent or refractory MM, addition of isatuximab increases PFS and depth of response achieved with pomalidomide and dexamethasone,[87] or carfilzomib and dexamethasone.[88] With isatuximab, pomalidomide, and dexamethasone, the benefit was seen in renal response[89] and in myeloma with high-risk genetics.[90] Initial infusion reactions have occurred in 38–46% of patients.[86] Respiratory infections and diarrhea were slightly more prevalent in patients receiving isatuximab in addition to pomalidomide and dexamethasone.

Antibodies against IL-6

Castleman disease is a lymphoproliferative disorder caused by release of IL-6 or other cytokines that can be localized to a single lymph node group or can be multicentric. Cytokine release can be stimulated by HHV-8 infection, but a fraction of Castleman disease cases are HHV-8 negative and the source of IL-6 has not been well defined.

Siltuximab

Siltuximab (Sylvant®) was approved by the US FDA and the European Union in 2014 for the treatment of HIV-negative, HHV-8-negative multicentric Castleman disease. Approval was based on an international, multicenter, randomized (2 : 1), phase 2 study comparing intravenous infusions of siltuximab and best supportive care (BSC) in 53 patients to placebo and BSC in 26 patients.[91] Siltuximab produced a greater fraction of durable (18 weeks) tumor and symptomatic responses (34% vs 0%; $p = 0.0012$), tumor responses (38% vs 4%; $p < 0.05$), median time-to-treatment failure (>422 days vs 134 days; $p < 0.05$), and increased hemoglobin (36% vs 0%; $p < 0.05$) relative to the placebo controls. Despite success in the management of Castleman disease, siltuximab has failed to demonstrate clinical activity against other malignancies where IL-6 signaling is thought to be important, including MM, RCC, and prostate cancer.[92] Common adverse reactions (>10% compared to placebo) during treatment with siltuximab include pruritus, increased weight, rash, hyperuricemia, and upper respiratory tract infections. Consequently, siltuximab provides an excellent example of a targeted therapy directed against a cytokine that drives a rare but debilitating lymphoproliferative disease.

Serotherapy for solid tumors with unmodified monoclonal antibodies

The HER family of transmembrane tyrosine kinase growth factor receptors has provided useful targets for serotherapy in solid tumors. As outlined in **Chapter 10**, interaction of peptide growth factor ligands with HER family receptors triggers signaling through the Ras-mitogen-activated protein kinase (MAPK) pathway and the phosphatidylinositol 3-kinase (PI3K) pathways, enhancing cell cycle progression, proliferation, and survival in normal cells and cancer cells. Of the four HER family receptors, most attention has been given to HER-1 (epidermal growth factor receptor or EGFR) and to HER-2.

Anti-EGFR antibodies

Several monoclonal antibodies have been prepared against the extracellular domain of the 170-kDa EGFR that is overexpressed in several carcinomas, including non-small-cell lung cancer (NSCLC), head and neck cancer, pancreatic cancer, and colorectal cancer.

Cetuximab

Cetuximab (Erbitux®) is a chimeric IgG1 monoclonal antibody that blocks the ligand-binding site of EGFR, preventing receptor activation, inducing internalization, and downregulating receptor levels. In experimental systems, treatment of human cancer cells with cetuximab produces cell cycle arrest in G0–G1, induces p21, directs hypophosphorylation of Rb, inhibits proliferation, and blocks the production of angiogenic factors such as vascular endothelial growth factor (VEGF).[93] In addition, treatment with cetuximab potentiates the activity of doxorubicin, paclitaxel, topotecan, and irinotecan as well as radiation therapy in nude mouse heterografts of human cancer. Potentiation of cytotoxic chemotherapy and radiation therapy may relate to inhibition of MAPK and PI3K with induction of BAX, activation of caspase 8, and downregulation of BCL-2 and NFκB, rendering cancer cells more sensitive to apoptotic stimuli.[94] In addition, cetuximab can induce ADCC in the presence of peripheral blood mononuclear cells. Very little EGFR expression is required to mediate cancer cell death from ADCC.[95] As in the case of rituximab, FcγR polymorphisms correlated with PFS after treatment with cetuximab, consistent with the importance of ADCC as a mechanism of cancer cell killing.[96]

Colorectal cancer. Weekly treatment with cetuximab alone produced partial remissions in 9% of 57 patients with chemotherapy-refractory colorectal cancer.[97] In two larger trials, a combination of irinotecan and cetuximab was used to treat a total of 450 patients with documented metastases from EGFR-positive colorectal cancer that had previously been treated with irinotecan.[98] A combination of cetuximab and irinotecan produced a partial response in 17–23% compared with 11% of patients retreated with irinotecan alone. In one study, PFS, but not OS, was significantly prolonged from 1.1 to 4.1 months with the combination. In a subsequent phase III study, 1289 patients with recurrent EGFR expressing colorectal cancer who had been previously treated with first-line fluorouracil and oxaliplatin containing regimens were randomized to cetuximab plus irinotecan or irinotecan alone. Cetuximab significantly improved disease-free survival (DFS), but not OS, possibly related to cross-over in 47% of patients.[99] Interestingly, the level of EGFR expression has not correlated with response to cetuximab-based therapy. Consistent with this observation, 4 of 16 previously treated patients (25%) with EGFR immunohistologically negative cancers responded to a combination of cetuximab and irinotecan.[95] Consequently, patients should not be excluded from treatment based on immunohistochemical evaluation of EGFR. In 2004, the US FDA provided accelerated approval for cetuximab in combination with irinotecan to treat patients with irinotecan-resistant colorectal cancer. In 2007, regular approval was given, based on a trial where 572 patients with advanced EGFR-positive colorectal cancers that had failed oxaliplatin- and irinotecan-based regimens were randomized to BSC with or without cetuximab until progression. Cetuximab improved OS from 4.6 to 6.1 months ($p = 0.0048$).[100] Approval also was given for use of cetuximab as a single agent to treat colorectal cancer that had failed oxaliplatin- and irinotecan-based regimens. Similar to clinical results with small molecule inhibitors and other monoclonal antibodies reactive with EGFR, responses to cetuximab are rare in cancers with *KRAS* mutations.[101] Exclusion of patients with *KRAS* mutations substantially affected the outcome, in retrospect, of the CRYSTAL trial. Here, 1217 previously untreated patients with metastatic colorectal cancer were randomized to FOLFIRI alone or in combination with cetuximab, irrespective of *KRAS* mutation status.[102,103] Addition of cetuximab prolonged median PFS from 8.1 to 8.9 months ($p = 0.036$) and did not affect OS. When cancers were tested for KRAS mutations, the addition of cetuximab to FOLFIRI increased OS (19.5–23.5 months), PFS (8.1–9.5 months), and ORR (39% vs 57%) in patients with *KRAS* wild-type tumors. In patients with *K-RAS* mutant cancers, no improvement in OS, PFS, or ORR was associated with the addition of cetuximab to FOLFIRI. Supportive data were found in two other randomized trials where only patients with KRAS wild-type cancers benefitted,[104,105] resulting in approval in 2012 for cetuximab in combination with FOLFIRI for previously untreated patients with colorectal cancer. Patients with metastatic colorectal cancer with a BRAF V600E mutation survive 4–6 months after failure of initial therapy. A phase 3 trial was conducted where 665 patients whose cancer had this mutation were randomized to a combination of encorafenib, cetuximab, and binimetinib (triplet therapy), encorafinib and cetuximab (doublet therapy), or the investigators' choice of either cetuximab and irinotecan or cetuximab and FOLFIRI (control group).[106] Median OS was 5.4 months in the control, 8.4 months in the doublet group ($p < 0.001$), and 9.0 months in the triplet group ($p < 0.001$). Based on these results, the combination of cetuximab and encorafinib was approved by the FDA for this group of patients.

Head and neck cancer. Cetuximab has also been approved for use in squamous cell carcinoma of the head and neck (SCCHN). In a pivotal multinational, phase III study, 424 patients with locally advanced head and neck cancers were randomized to high-dose radiotherapy or to a combination of radiotherapy with cetuximab.[107] The addition of cetuximab increased the duration of locoregional control from 15 to 24 months and increased OS from 29 to 49 months. When cetuximab was administered to patients with recurrent SCCHN who had progressed on platinum-based therapy, response rates of 10–13% were observed over three prospective trials ($n = 103$) with disease control rates of 46–56%.[108] The median time to disease progression ranged between 2.2 and 2.8 months, and the median OS ranged between 5.2 and 6.1 months. Cetuximab has also improved the efficacy of platinum-based chemotherapy for SCCHN. Approval by the US FDA in 2011 was based on a multicenter trial in 442 patients with locoregionally recurrent or metastatic head and neck cancer who were randomly assigned to receive cisplatin (or carboplatin) with 5-FU with or without cetuximab.[109] Significant improvements were seen in OS (10.1 vs 7.4 months; $p = 0.34$), PFS (5.5 vs 3.3 months; $p < 0.0001$) and objective response rates (35.6% vs 19.5%; $p = 0.0001$) in patients receiving cetuximab plus chemotherapy.

Toxicity. Side effects in a majority of patients included an acneiform rash, predominantly on the face and upper torso, and a composite syndrome of asthenia, fatigue, and malaise or lethargy. Treatment with minocycline can reduce the severity of the acneiform rash.[111] Meta-analysis found that the intensity of the rash correlates with OS, PFS, and ORR.[112] Hypomagnesemia results from the direct effect of cetuximab on EGFR in distal renal tubules, producing magnesium wasting.[113] A small minority of patients have experienced severe anaphylactic reactions, often on the initial infusion of cetuximab, related to a preexisting IgE antibody against galactose–α-1,3-galactose oligosaccharide, which is present on the Fab portion of the cetuximab heavy chain.[114]

Panitumumab

Panitumumab (Vectibix®) is a fully humanized IgG2 anti-EGFR antibody that was given accelerated approval by the US FDA in 2006 based on a trial in 463 patients with EGFR-positive colorectal cancer resistant to standard drugs who were randomized to single-agent antibody therapy or best supportive care (BSC). Treatment with panitumumab produced an objective response of 10% compared to 0% in the BSC control group and extended mean PFS from 60 to 96 days.[115] As with cetuximab, responses were limited to patients with wild-type nonmutated *KRAS*.[116] Interestingly, in a recent meta-analysis, neither panitumumab nor cetuximab improved OS, PFS, or ORR in patients with *HRAS* wild type but *BRAF* mutant colorectal cancer, suggesting that sequencing *BRAF* might also identify patients who would not benefit from anti-EGFR treatment.[117] Approval of the antibody by the European Union for use in colorectal cancer occurred in 2007. In previously untreated recurrent colorectal cancer, attempts to add panitumumab to bevacizumab plus FOLFOX-4 or FOLFIRI were discontinued when interim analysis of >1000 patients showed a statistically significant advantage in the control arm without panitumumab.[118]

Toxicity. A similar spectrum of side effects has been observed with panitumumab and cetuximab. Acneiform rash and hypomagnesemia have been most notable.[118] To date, fewer allergic reactions have been observed with panitumumab than with cetuximab.

Necitumumab

Necitumumab (Portrazza®) is a recombinant human IgG1 that binds to EGFR with high affinity, blocking binding of ligands. An international trial was conducted in 26 countries randomizing 1093 patients with stage IV NSCLC to gemcitabine and cisplatin with or without necitumumab.[119] Addition of necitumumab prolonged survival from 9.9 to 11.5 months ($p = 0.01$). Acneiform rash and hypomagnesemia were more prevalent in the necitumumab group.

Anti-HER-2 antibodies

Approximately 20–30% of breast cancers overexpress the 185-kDa tyrosine kinase growth factor receptor c-erbB2 (HER-2).[120] While HER-2 lacks a functioning ligand-binding domain, it is the preferred dimerization partner for the other HER family members including EGFR, HER-3, and HER-4.[121] Overexpression of HER-2 by breast cancer cells is associated with poor prognosis, particularly in node-positive disease, as well as with resistance to paclitaxel, CMF, and tamoxifen, but with an improved response to doxorubicin.[122,123] Resistance to systemic therapy, increased risk of recurrence, and shortened survival all reflect the biological consequences of HER-2 overexpression, which include increased proliferation, increased cell survival, increased invasion and metastasis, and increased angiogenesis. Monoclonal antibodies directed against the extracellular domain of this receptor can inhibit growth of cancer cells that overexpress HER-2.[124,125] In addition, treatment with anti-HER-2 antibodies can increase the susceptibility of cancer cells to platinum compounds, taxanes, doxorubicin, and 4-hydroperoxy-cyclophosphamide.[126,127] Interestingly, binding of anti-HER-2 antibodies to HER-2 in the juxtamembrane region[128] can activate the tyrosine kinase[125] but may prevent ligand-driven interaction of HER-2 with HER-3 to activate the PI3 kinase pathway, decreasing the antiapoptotic activity of phospho-AKT.[125,129,130] Antibodies have been developed that bind to different sites on the HER-2 molecule.

Trastuzumab

Trastuzumab (Herceptin®) is a humanized IgG1 antibody that binds to subdomain 4 of the extracellular domain of the HER-2 receptor, preventing homodimerization to other HER-2 receptors and downregulation of HER-2 levels. *In vivo*, inhibition of proangiogenic factors and mediation of ADCC may also play a role. Trastuzumab has received FDA approval for treatment of metastatic breast cancer, early breast cancer, gastric cancer, and GEJ cancer.

Breast cancer. In early clinical studies, trastuzumab produced objective regression of recurrent breast carcinoma in 12–15% of 269 heavily pretreated women.[131,132] Although cisplatin had demonstrated marginal activity against breast cancer in previous studies, a combination of cisplatin and trastuzumab produced an objective clinical response in 24% of 37 patients, with median duration of 8.4 months.[133] A critical international multi-institutional study was performed in 469 women with recurrent breast cancer.[134] Patients who had not previously received adjuvant therapy with doxorubicin were randomized to doxorubicin (or epirubicin) and cyclophosphamide, with or without trastuzumab. Women who had received adjuvant doxorubicin were randomized to paclitaxel with or without trastuzumab. The addition of trastuzumab to chemotherapy was associated with longer time to disease progression (median 7.4 vs 4.6 months; $p < 0.001$), higher objective response rate (50% vs 32%; $p < 0.001$), longer duration of response (median 9.1 vs 6.1 months; $p < 0.001$), and longer survival (median 25.1 vs 20.3 months; $p = 0.01$). This study resulted in the approval of trastuzumab by the US FDA in 1998 and the European Union in 2000 for the treatment of recurrent HER-2-overexpressing breast cancers. Subsequently, six large, multicenter adjuvant trials were undertaken (reviewed in **Chapter 105**) to test whether the addition of trastuzumab improved the ability of chemotherapy to prevent recurrence of primary HER-2-positive breast cancer. Interim analysis in five of the six trials demonstrated sufficiently dramatic improvement in DFS to terminate the clinical studies and to recommend the use of trastuzumab in this setting.[135–137] Addition of trastuzumab produced a 46–58% reduction in risk of recurrence, associated with an absolute reduction of 8–12% at 3 years in the five positive trials. Similarly, mortality was reduced 33–59%, producing an absolute decrease of 2–6% at 3 years. Based on the results of two of these trials (NSABP B31 and NCCTGN9831) including 3752 women, the FDA granted approval in 2006 for the addition of trastuzumab to cyclophosphamide, doxorubicin, and paclitaxel for adjuvant therapy of women with HER-2-overexpressed cancer.

Trastuzumab enhances the response rate to several other cytotoxic agents used to treat breast cancer, including vinorelbine, gemcitabine, and platinum compounds.[138–142] A randomized trial in 81 patients with metastatic HER-2-positive breast cancer who had not received chemotherapy for recurrent disease demonstrated a 51% response rate to vinorelbine and trastuzumab compared to a 40% response rate with paclitaxel and trastuzumab.[143] In most studies, only those breast cancers with strong expression of HER-2, driven by gene amplification, responded to the antibody alone or to a combination of antibody with chemotherapy. Immunohistochemistry can provide an initial screen for HER-2 overexpression, but 2+ and 3+ reactions should be confirmed with the more reliable fluorescence in situ hybridization assay.[144] HER-2 gene amplification can be acquired as breast cancers progress, arguing for repeated testing for HER-2 overexpression.[145] Because only a fraction of patients respond, overexpression of HER-2 is necessary but not a sufficient reason to ensure response to trastuzumab. Lack of response to trastuzumab correlated with lack of expression of the PTEN phosphatase, the enzyme that removes phosphate groups from PI3 and interrupts signaling through AKT.[146] Treatment with trastuzumab increased PTEN membrane localization and phosphatase activity by reducing PTEN tyrosine phosphorylation through inhibition of Src that could no longer dock on the HER-2 receptor.

Gastric and GEJ cancers. In 2010, the FDA granted approval for trastuzumab in combination with cisplatin and a fluoropyrimidine (either capecitabine or 5-fluorouracil) for the treatment of patients with HER-2-overexpressing metastatic gastric or GEJ carcinomas that had not received prior treatment for metastatic disease. The approval was based on results of a single international multicenter open-label randomized clinical trial, BO18255 (ToGA trial), which enrolled 594 patients with locally advanced or metastatic HER2-overexpressing adenocarcinoma of the stomach or GEJ.[147] Patients were randomly assigned to receive trastuzumab plus chemotherapy or chemotherapy alone. The trial was closed after the second interim analysis, when the addition of trastuzumab was associated with improved median survival (13.5 vs 11.0 months; $p = 0.0038$). An updated survival analysis demonstrated a persistent advantage for trastuzumab (13.1 vs 11.7 months) with the greatest benefit seen in HER-2 overexpressing cancers.

Toxicity. Treatment with trastuzumab is well tolerated and is associated with low-grade fever, chills, and fatigue that are generally observed with the first administration. In many studies, trastuzumab has been administered weekly, but it has been administered every 3 weeks at higher dosage with acceptable toxicity and trough levels.[148] When trastuzumab has been combined with doxorubicin or paclitaxel, increased cardiotoxicity has been observed. In the pivotal trial that demonstrated the efficacy of trastuzumab in recurrent breast cancer, American Heart Association class III and IV cardiac dysfunction occurred in 27% of the group given trastuzumab with anthracycline and cyclophosphamide compared to 8% of the group given anthracycline and cyclophosphamide alone.[149] A similar degree of cardiac dysfunction was observed in 13% of patients who received paclitaxel and trastuzumab compared with 1% who received paclitaxel alone. Long-term treatment of 218 breast cancer patients with trastuzumab-based therapy for at least 1 year was associated with an 11% incidence of class III cardiac dysfunction.[150] In the six adjuvant trials where trastuzumab was given sequentially or concurrently with paclitaxel or carboplatin, but not doxorubicin, class III/IV cardiac dysfunction was observed in 0.5–4.1%.[136,137] Cardiac dysfunction generally responds to discontinuing trastuzumab and providing medical management. Thus, the benefits of trastuzumab for recurrent disease or adjuvant treatment generally outweigh the risks in patients with normal baseline cardiac function. The mechanism for trastuzumab-induced cardiac dysfunction remains obscure. Only low levels of HER-2 are found on cardiac myocytes, but trastuzumab can localize to the myocardium, and the ligand heregulin that binds to HER-2–HER-3 and HER2–HER-4 dimers appears critical to the fetal development and survival of cardiac tissue under apoptotic stress.[151]

Pertuzumab

Pertuzumab (Perjeta®) is an IgG1 humanized monoclonal antibody that binds to the dimerization domain of HER-2 at a site distinct from trastuzumab, preventing ligand-driven dimerization of HER-2 with multiple HER family members.[152,153] Use of pertuzumab in combination with trastuzumab synergistically inhibited survival of a breast cancer cell line that overexpressed HER-2 associated with increased apoptosis and blockade of signaling through AKT, but not through MAPK.[154]

Metastatic HER-2 positive breast cancer. Pertuzumab was approved by the US FDA in 2012 and by the European Union in 2013 for treatment of HER-2 amplified breast cancer based on a single clinical trial, Cleopatra, involving 808 patients with HER2-positive metastatic breast cancer who were randomly assigned to receive pertuzumab, trastuzumab, and docetaxel, or trastuzumab and docetaxel with a placebo.[155] Patients receiving pertuzumab had a median PFS of 18.7 months, versus 12.4 months in the placebo group. With further follow-up, the addition of pertuzumab to trastuzumab and docetaxel increased OS by 15.7 months from 40.8 to 56.5 months ($p < 0.001$) and improved PFS by 6.3 months.[156]

Early-stage HER-2 positive breast cancer. In 2013, pertuzumab became the first FDA-approved drug for the neoadjuvant treatment of breast cancer in patients with HER-2-positive, locally advanced, inflammatory, or early-stage breast cancer (>2 cm in diameter or with positive lymph nodes) who are at high risk for recurrence and death. Pertuzumab was approved for use in combination with trastuzumab and other chemotherapy prior to surgery and, depending upon the treatment regimen used, can be followed by chemotherapy after surgery. Following surgery, patients should continue to receive trastuzumab to complete one year of treatment. Pertuzumab's accelerated approval for neoadjuvant treatment was based on a study designed to measure pathological complete response (pCR) in accordance with a new FDA advisory that this could be used as a surrogate endpoint. In the NeoSphere study, 417 participants were randomly assigned to receive one of four neoadjuvant treatment regimens: trastuzumab plus docetaxel, pertuzumab plus trastuzumab and docetaxel, pertuzumab plus trastuzumab, or pertuzumab plus docetaxel.[157] About 39% of participants who received pertuzumab plus trastuzumab and docetaxel achieved pCR, compared to 21% who received trastuzumab plus docetaxel. The confirmatory trial for this accelerated approval randomized 4805 women with HER2 positive breast cancer with positive nodes or absence of hormone receptors to postoperative trastuzumab and chemotherapy with or without the addition of pertuzumab. The addition of pertuzumab significantly improved 3-year invasive DFS ($p = 0.02$).

Toxicity. The most common side effects reported in participants receiving pertuzumab plus trastuzumab and paclitaxel or docetaxel were hair loss, diarrhea, nausea, and neutropenia. Diarrhea is much less frequently observed with trastuzumab than pertuzumab. Other significant side effects included decreased cardiac function, infusion-related reactions, hypersensitivity reactions, and anaphylaxis.

Margetuximab-cmkb

Margetuximab-cmkb (Margenza®) is a chimeric Fc-engineered IgG1k that binds to HER-2. Five amino acids are altered from normal human IgG to increase Fc affinity for activating FcγR IIIA CD16a and to decrease affinity for inhibitory FcγR IIB CD32B, enhancing the ability of effector cells to mediate ADCC.

Metastatic HER-2 positive breast cancer. Patients with HER2 positive breast cancer who had progressed on previous treatment with trastuzumab, pertuzumab, and/or ado-trastuzumab emtansine were randomized to treatment with one of four cytotoxic drugs (capecitabine, eribulin, gemcitabine, or vinorelbine) with or without margetuximab.[158] The addition of margetuximab increased PFS from 4.4 to 5.7 months ($p < 0.001$), OS from 19.8 to 21.6 months ($p = 0.33$), and the objective response rate from 14% to 25% ($p < 0.001$).

Toxicity. The incidence of infusion reactions was higher with margetuximab (13.3% vs 3.3%), but other toxicity was comparable with and without monoclonal antibody therapy.

Antiganglioside antibodies

Ganglioside D2 (GD2) is a disialoganglioside expressed on neuroblastomas and melanomas as well as on normal neurons, melanocytes, and pain fibers. Expression on cancer cells is relatively uniform and GD2 is not lost from the cell surface after treatment with monoclonal antibodies.[159]

Dinutuximab

Dinutuximab (Unituxin®) is a chimeric anti-GD2 IgG1 antibody that was approved by the US FDA in 2015 for treatment of newly diagnosed pediatric patients with high-risk neuroblastoma who have achieved at least a partial response to first-line multiagent, multimodality therapy. Addition of dinutuximab improved outcomes for patients who received maintenance therapy with granulocyte-macrophage colony-stimulating factor (GM-CSF), IL-2, and 13-cis-retinoic acid (RA).[160] The pivotal COG trial randomized 226 patients to either dinutuximab/RA or RA alone for six cycles of treatment. An improvement in EFS (HR 0.57; $p = 0.01$, log-rank test) was demonstrated during follow-up and the trial terminated. At that time, the median EFS was not reached (3.4 years, NR, in the dinutuximab/RA arm and 1.9 years (1.3, NR) in the RA arm). An analysis of OS conducted 3 years later documented an improvement in OS in the dinutuximab/RA arm compared to the RA arm (HR 0.58), although median OS had not yet been reached in either arm.

Toxicity. The most common (>25%) adverse drug reactions in the dinutuximab/RA group were pain, pyrexia, thrombocytopenia, infusion reactions, hypotension, hyponatremia, increased alanine aminotransferase, anemia, vomiting, diarrhea, hypokalemia, capillary leak syndrome, neutropenia, urticaria, hypoalbuminemia, increased aspartate aminotransferase, and hypocalcemia. The most common (>5%) serious adverse reactions in the dinutuximab/RA group were infections, infusion reactions, hypokalemia, hypotension, pain, fever, and capillary leak syndrome.

Naxitamab

Naxitamab (Danyelza®) is a humanized IgG1 that recognizes GD2 on the surface of neuroblastoma, osteosarcoma, and other GD2-positive cancers. The antibody can mediate direct and antibody-mediated neuroblastoma cell killing but can also drive differentiation of cancer.[161] FDA approval for neuroblastoma resulted from two single-arm studies in patients with relapsed and/or refractory disease.[162,163] In a phase II study of 22 patients, objective responses were observed in 45% and complete responses in 36% to treatment with naxitamab and GM-CSF. In a phase I–II study with an expansion phase, substantial activity was observed, among 38 patients with refractory disease, with an ORR of 34% and a CR of 26%.

Toxicity. Adverse reactions included pain and infusion reactions in all patients of some grade and grade 3–4 in 72% and 68%, respectively. The spectrum of toxicities was similar to other ant-GD2 antibodies with serious adverse events in 32% and discontinuation of treatment in 12%.

Antivascular therapy

Angiogenesis is critical for normal fetal growth and wound healing but is also required for tumor growth and metastasis.[164] Novel approaches to inhibiting angiogenesis have exploited the presence of antigens displayed on tumor-associated endothelium or on the proangiogenic factors produced by tumor cells.

Bevacizumab

Bevacizumab (Avastin®) is a humanized IgG1 that binds to the proangiogenic VEGF-A that has also been characterized as vascular permeability factor (VPF). Blockade of VEGF/VPF can inhibit tumor-driven angiogenesis in xenografts.[165] Expression of VEGF/VPF has correlated with the formation of ascites in mice with ovarian cancer xenograft.[166] Treatment with bevacizumab can completely inhibit ascites formation.[167] In addition, cancer cells themselves can express VEGF receptors. Autocrine stimulation with VEGF can enhance proliferation and resistance to chemotherapy. Bevacizumab has received FDA approval for treatment of colorectal cancer (2004, 2006, and 2013), NSCLC (2006), breast cancer (2008; withdrawn 2011), RCC (2009), glioblastoma (2009), cervical cancer (2014), and ovarian cancer (2014), but its place in oncologic practice is still being defined.[168]

Colorectal cancer. In patients with previously untreated metastatic colorectal carcinoma, the addition of bevacizumab to irinotecan, fluorouracil, and leucovorin increased the overall response rate (34.8 vs 44.89 months) and significantly prolonged median PFS (7.4 vs 10.4 months) and median OS (15.6 vs 20.3 months).[169] This trial led to the initial FDA approval in 2004 of bevacizumab for use with chemotherapy for first-line therapy of colorectal cancer. Two subsequent randomized phase 2 trials demonstrated improved response rate, PFS, and OS when bevacizumab was added to 5-FU and leucovorin.[170–172] In phase 3 studies where bevacizumab was added to more effective first-line regimens including FOLFOX-4 and XELOX, response rate and OS were not significantly improved.[173,174] A number of combinations of bevacizumab and multiple drug combinations have provided similar results in noninferiority studies.[175] In second-line therapy, however, addition of a higher dose of bevacizumab to FOLFOX-4 significantly increased response rate (9 vs 23%), PFS (4.7 vs 7.3 months), and OS (10.8 vs 12.9 months) in bevacizumab-naive patients, leading to the approval of bevacizumab for second-line therapy in 2006.[176] In patients with metastatic colorectal cancer who had progressed on bevacizumab in combination with irinotecan-based chemotherapy or oxaliplatin-based regimens, continued use of bevacizumab in combination with the complementary chemotherapy regimen improved OS (11.2 vs 9.8 months; $p = 0.0062$) and PFS (5.7 vs 4.0 months; $p < 0.0001$), leading to approval for continued use of bevacizumab in second-line therapy.[177]

Non-small-cell lung cancer. In previously untreated metastatic NSCLC, three-phase III trials have studied the addition of bevacizumab to carboplatin/paclitaxel,[178,179] or to gemcitabine/cisplatin.[180] Significant increases have been observed in response rates (range 14 vs 28%) with a more modest increase in PFS (0.6 vs 2.7 months) or OS (0.5 vs 2.0 months).[176]

Breast cancer. Addition of bevacizumab to paclitaxel in first-line treatment of patients with recurrent metastatic breast cancer significantly increased response rate (21 vs 37%) and PFS (5.9 vs 11.8 months).[181] A modest, but significant, increase in PFS (8.0 vs 8.8 months) was observed when bevacizumab was added to docetaxel.[182] In second-line therapy, the addition of bevacizumab to capecitabine significantly increased the response rate (9 vs 20%), but not PFS (4.2 vs 4.9 months) or OS (14.5 vs 15.1 months).[183] Given the limited effect of bevacizumab in confirmatory trials, approval of the drug was withdrawn for breast cancer.

Renal cell cancers. A majority of sporadic RCCs exhibit inactivation of the von Hippel Lindau (VHL) gene with consequent overexpression of VEGF.[184] In a randomized phase II trial that compared two doses of bevacizumab (3 or 10 mg/kg every 2 weeks) with placebo in previously treated patients with RCC, a significant prolongation of PFS was observed when high-dose bevacizumab was compared with placebo (2.4 vs 4.8 months; $p < 0.01$).[185] IFN-α was a standard initial therapy for RCC with a modest response rate and a survival advantage demonstrated in randomized trials. Two-phase III trials compared treatment with IFN-α and bevacizumab to IFN-α alone in previously untreated patients with RCC.[186,187] PFS was increased significantly from 5.2 vs. 5.4 to 8.5 vs. 10.2 months.

Glioblastoma multiforme (GBM). Bevacizumab demonstrated activity against GBM in two single-armed trials, AVF3708g and NCI 06-C-0064E, where monotherapy produced a 20 vs 25% response rate lasting a median of 3.9 vs 4.2 months in a total of 141 patients who had relapsed after surgery, radiotherapy, and temozolomide.[188] This prompted accelerated FDA approval for use in this setting. A double-blinded, randomized trial evaluated whether the addition of bevacizumab to radiotherapy and temozolomide would improve outcomes in 637 patients with newly diagnosed GBM.[189] Addition of bevacizumab increased PFS from 7.3 to 10.7 months ($p = 0.007$) but did not affect OS.

Ovarian cancer. In heavily pretreated patients with recurrent ovarian cancer, administration of bevacizumab, alone[190,191] or in combination with daily oral low-dose cyclophosphamide to provide "metronomic" therapy,[192] produced response rates of 16–24% with PFS of 4.4–7.2 months. Stabilization of disease for 6 months has been observed in approximately 40% of ovarian cancer patients. Four randomized studies have been performed evaluating the addition of bevacizumab to standard chemotherapy for front-line treatment (GOG 218[193] and ICON7[194]) and for recurrent "platinum-sensitive" (OCEANS[195]) and "platinum-resistant"

(AURELIA[196]) disease.[197] PFS was improved in these studies by 3.8 months ($p < 0.001$), 1.7 months ($p = 0.001$), 3.3 months ($p = 0.001$), and 4.0 months ($p < 0.0001$), respectively. OS was not improved in any of the studies, but subsets of patients in GOG 218 and ICON7 with poor prognosis appeared to benefit. Lack of impact on OS overall and similar enhancement of PFS in first-line and recurrent disease has raised the question of whether treatment with bevacizumab should be delayed until disease recurrence. Approval for use of bevacizumab in combination with chemotherapy for recurrent disease was granted based on the AURELIA trial.

Cervical cancer. Addition of bevacizumab to a combination of carboplatin with paclitaxel or topotecan increased OS by 3.7 months (from 13.3 to 17.0 months; $p = 0.004$) and increased the rate of response from 36% to 88% ($p = 0.008$) in a randomized trial including 452 women with recurrent, persistent, or metastatic cervical cancer.[198]

Toxicity. In patients with NSCLC, RCC, colorectal, breast, cervical, and ovarian cancer, bevacizumab administration has been well tolerated by the majority. Grade 3 hypertension has been observed in approximately 20% of patients. While hypertension has been readily managed in most cases, malignant hypertension and fatal hemorrhagic stroke have been observed, arguing for aggressive monitoring and management of blood pressure. Significant proteinuria occurs in less than 5% of cases. Nasal bleeding has been observed. Greater risk for delayed wound healing and bleeding has been observed when bevacizumab was administered within 60 days of surgery.[199] In patients with NSCLC, major hemoptysis was associated with 4 deaths among 35 patients in one early trial. Life-threatening hemoptysis occurred most frequently in elderly males with squamous cell histology, tumor necrosis, and cavitation, as well as disease close to major vessels. Patients with these characteristics have been excluded from many trials. Thromboembolic events have been observed in 5–7.4% of participants on randomized trials in ovarian cancer.[198] Arterial thromboembolism has been observed in 2% of patients in large phase 3 trials across disease sites. In heavily pretreated patients with ovarian cancer, perforation of the bowel has been observed in 5–7% of cases, generally in the setting of partial small bowel obstruction and of treatment response in lesions that involve the bowel wall. Bowel perforation has occurred in 2.6–3% of ovarian cancer patients on front-line adjuvant trials[198] compared with only 1% of colorectal cancer patients when bevacizumab was administered with FOLFOX.[177]

Ramucirumab

Ramucirumab (Cyramza®) is a fully human IgG1 monoclonal antibody that binds to the human VEGFR2 and prevents interaction with VEGF ligands. Ramucirumab has been approved by the US FDA for the treatment of gastric and GEJ cancers (2014), NSCLC (2014, 2020), colon cancer (2015), and hepatocellular cancer (2019).

Gastric and GEJ cancers. Ramucirumab can be used for the treatment of fluoropyrimidine-resistant or platinum-resistant gastric or GEJ cancer as a single agent or with paclitaxel. Approval of ramucirumab as a single agent was based on a multinational, randomized double-blinded trial in 655 patients with previously treated advanced or metastatic disease who were randomized (2:1) to ramucirumab or placebo plus BSC. Addition of ramucirumab to paclitaxel significantly improved OS (9.6 vs 7.4 months; $p = 0.017$) and PFS (4.4 vs 2.9 months; $p < 0.001$).[200]

Lung cancer. Ramucirumab in combination with docetaxel was approved for the treatment of metastatic NSCLC that had progressed on platinum-containing regimens or anti-EGFR or anti-ALK targeted therapy. Approval of ramucirumab in combination with docetaxel was based on a double-blinded, placebo-controlled clinical trial that enrolled 1253 patients with previously treated metastatic NSCLC.[201] Addition of ramucirumab to docetaxel significantly increased OS (9.1 vs 10.5 months; $p = 0.024$) and PFS ($p < 0.001$). In 2020, approval was given for first-line treatment of NSCLC in combination with erlotinib, for the first-line treatment of people with metastatic NSCLC with EGFR exon 19 deletions or exon 21 (L858R) mutations, based on the improvement of PFS from 12.4 to 19.4 months ($p < 0.0001$).[202]

Colorectal cancer. Ramucirumab was combined with FOLFIRI for the treatment of patients with metastatic colorectal cancer whose disease had progressed on a first-line bevacizumab-, oxaliplatin-, and fluoropyrimidine-containing regimen. Approval by the US FDA was based on the results of a randomized, double-blind, multinational trial enrolling 1072 patients who were randomly allocated to receive FOLFIRI plus placebo or FOLFIRI plus ramucirumab.[203] Addition of ramucirumab to FOLFIRI improved OS (11.7 vs 13.3 months; $p = 0.023$) and PFS (4.5 vs 5.7 months; $p < 0.001$).

Hepatocellular cancer. Treatment with ramucirumab was evaluated in a randomized, double-blinded trial in 292 patients with hepatocellular cancer with serum alpha-fetoprotein of 400 ng/mL who had already been treated with sorafenib.[204] Ramucirumab increased OS from 7.3 to 8.5 months ($p = 0.0199$) and PFS from 1.6 to 2.8 months ($p < 0.0001$).

Toxicity. Ramucirumab treatment can be associated with fatigue, weakness, hypertension, hyponatremia, diarrhea, and nose bleeds. When combined with paclitaxel or docetaxel, neutropenia, febrile neutropenia, and anemia have been observed. Other rare, but important risks described in product labeling include hemorrhage, arterial thromboembolic events, infusion-related reactions, gastrointestinal obstruction, gastrointestinal perforation, impaired wound healing, clinical deterioration in patients with cirrhosis, and reversible posterior leukoencephalopathy. Hypothyroidism has been observed in patients with colorectal cancer.

Immune checkpoint inhibitors

The principles that mediate therapy with immune checkpoint inhibitors are discussed in depth in **Chapter 63**. Here, we will focus on FDA-approved clinical indications and toxicities of these agents. Monoclonal antibodies approved to date have targeted cytotoxic T-lymphocyte antigen 4 (CTLA4), programmed cell death protein 1 (PD-1), and its ligand PD-L1. These include anti-CTLA4 (ipilimumab), anti-PD-1 (pembrolizumab, nivolumab, and cemiplimab), and anti-PD-L1 (atezolizumab, durvalumab, and avelumab).

Anti-CTLA4

Anti-CTLA4 monoclonal antibodies have been used to intervene in immunoregulation. CD4+CD25+ T regulatory (Treg) cells constitutively express CTLA4. The presence of Treg cells in tumor tissue has been associated with a poor prognosis in human cancers from several sites and their elimination can potentiate antitumor responses in preclinical models. In addition, CTLA4 is upregulated by immune stimulation of T cells and effective activation of tumor immunity can be blocked by the interaction of CD80/86 on antigen-presenting cells with CTLA4 (CD152) on T lymphocytes. Inhibiting this interaction with anti-CTLA4 antibody can enhance tumor-specific immunity.[205]

Ipilimumab

Ipilimumab (Yervoy®) is a fully human IgG1 monoclonal antibody that reacts with CTLA4.

Melanoma. Ipilimumab was approved for use against metastatic melanoma by the US FDA and the European Union in 2011 based on a single international study of 676 patients with melanoma who had stopped responding to other FDA-approved or commonly used treatments and were randomized to ipilimumab, ipilimumab plus a gp100 vaccine, or vaccine alone. Those who received the combination of ipilimumab plus vaccine or ipilimumab alone lived an average of about 10 months, while those who received only the experimental vaccine lived an average of 6.5 months. Administration of ipilimumab as a single agent has produced a 7–15% objective response rate in human melanomas and RCC.[206,207] Greater activity might be anticipated using these reagents to augment the effects of specific tumor vaccines. Among 1861 patients, median OS was 11.4 months which included 254 patients with at least 3 years of survival follow-up. The survival curve began to plateau around year 3. Three-year survival rates were 22%, 26%, and 20% for all patients, treatment naïve patients and previously treated patients, respectively.[208] In a study that led to FDA approval of adjuvant monotherapy in 2015, 951 patients with completely resected stage III melanoma were randomized to ipilimumab or placebo. Median recurrence-free survival (RFS) was prolonged by ipilimumab (17.1 vs 26.1 months; $p = 0.0013$). Five (1%) patients died of drug-related events in the ipilimumab group.[209] Response to CTLA4 blockade correlated with mutational load, neo-antigens, and expression of cytolytic markers.[210,211]

Toxicity. Common side effects that can result from autoimmune reactions associated with ipilimumab use include fatigue, diarrhea, skin rash, uveitis, hypophysitis, endocrine deficiencies, inflammation of the intestines (colitis), and hepatitis.[208] Severe to fatal autoimmune reactions were seen in 12.9% of patients treated with ipilimumab. When severe side effects occurred, ipilimumab was stopped and corticosteroid treatment was started. Not all patients responded to this treatment. Patients who did respond in some cases did not see any improvement for several weeks.

Anti-PD1

Anti-PD1 antibodies target PD1, a second regulator of T cell immunity preventing interaction with the PD-L1 and PD-L2 ligands, releasing inhibition of immune responses, including those to tumor-associated antigens.[212]

Nivolumab

Nivolumab (Opdivo®) is a human IgG4 anti-PD1 antibody.

Nivolumab was approved by the USDA in 2014 for the treatment of previously treated unresectable or metastatic melanoma that had failed ipilimumab and BRAF inhibitors.[213] Approval was based on a trial including 120 participants with a 32% ORR where approximately one-third of responders remained in remission for 6 months or more. When nivolumab was compared to dacarbazine in 418 previously untreated patients with BRAF wild-type melanoma, nivolumab produced greater 1 year OS (42% vs 72.9%; $p < 0.001$), PFS (2.2 vs 5.1 months; $p < 0.001$), and objective response rate (13.9% vs 40%; $p < 0.001$).[214] In patients who had progressed on anti-CTLA4, nivolumab improved ORR compared to the investigator's choice of chemotherapy (10.6% vs 37.7%).[215] Nivolumab was compared to ipilimumab in 906 patients with stage IIIB/C or IV melanoma that had been completely resected. Nivolumab was associated with an increase of 9.7% in 12-month rate of RFS (HR, 0.65; $p < 0.001$). Treatment was discontinued because of any adverse event in 9.7% of the nivolumab and 42.6% of ipilimumab group.[216]

Non-small-cell lung cancer. US FDA approval was obtained in 2013 for nivolumab to treat patients with NSCLC who had failed platinum-based therapy based on a randomized trial where patients with metastatic squamous NSCLC who had experienced disease progression during or after one prior platinum-based chemotherapy regimen were assigned to nivolumab ($n = 135$) or docetaxel ($n = 137$).[217] Nivolumab provided a statistically significant improvement in OS as compared with docetaxel (6 vs 9.2 months; $p = 0.00025$). Approval was supported by a single-arm, multinational, multicenter trial in patients with metastatic squamous NSCLC who had progressed after receiving a platinum-based therapy and at least one additional systemic regimen. Patients ($n = 117$) who received nivolumab, exhibited an ORR of 15%. A similar trial was performed in nonsquamous NSCLC with patients who had failed one prior platinum doublet or targeted therapy directed toward EGFR or ALK who were randomized to nivolumab ($n = 292$) or docetaxel ($n = 290$). Nivolumab prolonged OS by 2.6 months ($p = 0.0015$) and improved overall response rate by 7% ($p = 0.02$).

Small-cell lung cancer. Nivolumab was tested in 109 patients with small-cell lung cancer (SCLC) that had progressed on platinum-based therapy, producing an ORR of 12% with 62% of responses lasting 12 or more months.

Squamous cell carcinoma of the head and neck. Patients with SCCHN who had progressed on platinum-based therapy were randomized to nivolumab or the investigator's choice of therapy with cetuximab, methotrexate, or docetaxel. The check point inhibitor increased survival by 2.4 months ($p = 0.0101$) compared to chemotherapy. When only PD-L1 positive cancers were considered, OS was improved by 4.1 months.

Renal cell cancer. A combination of nivolumab and cabozantinib provided 8.3 months greater PFS ($p < 0.0001$), improved OS (HR 0.60; $p < 0.001$) and increased ORR by 28.6% compared to sunitinib as front-line therapy in advanced or recurrent RCC. In previously treated patients, nivolumab improved OS by 6.1 months ($p = 0.0018$), improved the ORR by 19% ($p < 0.001$), and median duration of response by 9.3 months when compared to everolimus.[218]

Urothelial cancer. In advanced urothelial cancers that had recurred on platinum-containing regimens or progressed within 12 months on adjuvant studies, nivolumab produced a 20% response rate with a median duration of 10.3 months.

Esophageal squamous cell cancer. Patients with unresectable advanced, recurrent or metastatic squamous cell esophageal cancer that was resistant to at least one platinum- and fluoropyrimidine-based regimen were randomized to nivolumab or the investigator's choice of paclitaxel or docetaxel. The immune check point inhibitor improved OS by 2.5 months ($p = 0.0189$), without affecting PFS or ORR.

Gastric, G-E junction, or esophageal adenocarcinoma. Addition of nivolumab to each of two chemotherapeutic regimens (FOL-FOX6 or CapeOX) for adenocarcinomas of the stomach, GE junction and esophagus increased OS by 2.2 months ($p = 0.0002$) and ORR by 10%

Hepatocellular carcinoma. In patients who had progressed on or were intolerant to sorafenib, nivolumab produced a 14% response rate with 55% lasting 12 or more months.

Hodgkin lymphoma. In classical Hodgkin disease patients ($n = 80$) who had failed autologous stem cell transplantation and posttransplant brentuximab vedotin, single-agent nivolumab produced a 66% ORR lasting a median of 13.1 months.[219]

Toxicity. The most common (>30%) adverse reactions among patients receiving nivolumab in the above single-arm trial were fatigue, dyspnea, musculoskeletal pain, decreased appetite, and cough. The most frequent grade 3 and 4 adverse drug reactions observed in at least 5% of patients treated with nivolumab were dyspnea, fatigue, and musculoskeletal pain. Clinically significant immune-mediated adverse reactions included pneumonitis, colitis, hepatitis, nephritis/renal dysfunction, hypothyroidism, and hyperthyroidism.

Nivolumab plus Ipilimumab

The combination of Nivolumab plus Ipilimumab, targeting PD-1 and CTLA4, respectively, has been evaluated in several forms of cancer.[220]

Melanoma. A combination of nivolumab and ipilimumab improved objective response rate when compared to ipilimumab alone (61% vs 11%; $p < 0.001$) in 142 previously untreated patients with BRAF wild type melanoma. Complete responses were observed in 22% of patients receiving the combination and 0% in patients receiving ipilimumab alone. PFS was prolonged in the combination arm ($p < 0.001$). Similar results were observed in patients with BRAF mutant melanomas.[221] A second randomized phase III study compared nivolumab plus ipilimumab to nivolumab or ipilimumab monotherapy in previously untreated stage III or stage IV melanoma. ORR was 50% with the combination, 40% with nivolumab, and 14% with ipilimumab. PFS was 11.7, 6.9, and 2.9 months, respectively ($p < 0.001$ for the combination or nivolumab alone vs ipilimumab). OS was improved with the combination (HR 0.44; $p < 0.001$) or with nivolumab alone (HR 0.50; $p < 0.001$) compared to ipilimumab alone. Grade 3–4 treatment-related adverse events occurred in 55% of patients in the combination arm compared to 27.3% in the ipilimumab arm.[222] With 6.5 years follow-up, OS was 72.1, 36.9, and 19.9 months in the combination, nivolumab, and ipilimumab groups, respectively, with plateau's on the survival curves.[223] In patients with Stage IV melanoma without evidence of disease after surgery or radiotherapy, a combination of nivolumab plus ipilimumab produced recurrence-free survival of 75% at 1 year and 70% at 2 years compared to 52% and 42% for nivolumab alone and 32% and 14% for placebo.[224] Treatment-related adverse events required discontinuation in 62% of the combination group compared to 13% in the nivolumab alone group.

Non-small-cell lung cancer. A combination of nivolumab and ipilimumab improved OS by 2.2 months (HR 0.79; $p = 0.0066$) compared to platinum doublet chemotherapy in previously untreated patients with squamous and nonsquamous NSCLC. ORR was improved by 6% and the duration of response from a median of 6.2 vs 23.2 months. When nivolumab and ipilimumab in combination with platinum doublets were compared to platinum doublets alone, addition of the immune checkpoint inhibitors improved OS by 3.4 months ($p = 0.0006$), PFS by 1.8 months ($p = 0.0001$), ORR by 13% ($p = 0.0003$), and median duration by 4.9 months.

Malignant pleural mesothelioma. Combined treatment with nivolumab and ipilimumab extended OS by 2 months ($p = 0.002$), but not PFS or ORR, when compared to pemetrexed and cisplatin or pemetrexed and carboplatin in previously untreated patients with malignant pleural mesothelioma.

Renal cell cancer. When compared to sunitinib, treatment with a combination of nivolumab and ipilimumab improved OS (HR 0.63; $p < 0.0001$) and ORR by 15.1% ($p < 0.0001$), but not PFS, in previously untreated advanced RCC patients.

Colorectal cancer. Addition of ipilimumab to nivolumab increased ORR in patients with advanced MSI-Hi or dMMR colorectal cancer that had progressed on standard chemotherapy from 28% to 46%.

Hepatocellular cancer. A combination of nivolumab and ipilimumab was compared to nivolumab alone in patients with hepatocellular cancer who had progressed on or were intolerant to sorafenib. Addition of ipilimumab increased ORR by 19%.

Pembrolizumab

Pembrolizumab (Keytruda®), a humanized IgG4 that targets PD1 and prevents interaction with PD-L1 and PD-L2. Clinically useful activity has been demonstrated against 17 different forms of cancer.[225]

Melanoma. Ipilimumab was approved by the US FDA in 2014 for the treatment of melanomas that had progressed on ipilimumab, but that had not yet been treated with BRAF inhibitors. Approval was based on the results of a multicenter, open-label, randomized, dose-comparative, activity-estimating cohort including 173 patients with unresectable or metastatic melanoma who were randomized to receive 2 mg/kg ($n = 89$) or 10 mg/kg ($n = 84$) of pembrolizumab intravenously once every 3 weeks until disease progression or unacceptable toxicity. The ORR was 24% in the 2 mg/kg arm, consisting of one complete response and 20 partial responses. Among the 21 patients with an objective response, 3 (14%) had disease progression at 2.8, 2.9, and 8.2 months after initial response. The remaining 18 patients (86%) had ongoing responses, ranging from 1.4+ to 8.5+ months; eight patients had ongoing responses of 6 months or longer. Similar ORR results were observed in the 10 mg/kg arm. In an extended randomized phase II trial, 6-month PFS was 34% in the 2 mg/kg arm, 38% in the 10 mg/kg arm, and 16% in a group receiving chemotherapy of the investigator's choice.[226] Pembrolizumab every 2 or 5 weeks has been compared to ipilimumab in a randomized trial with 834 patients. Six-month PFS was 47.3% for pembrolizumab every 2 weeks, 46.4% for pembrolizumab every 3 weeks, and 26.5% for ipilimumab ($p < 0.001$).[227] Pembrolizumab has also been approved for use as an adjuvant, based on a randomized, double blind placebo controlled trial (EORTC1435/KEYNOTE-054) in 1019 patients with completely resected Stage III A, B, and C melanoma where treatment every 3 weeks increased one year RFS from 61% to 75% ($p < 0.001$).[228] At the time of initial analysis, median RFS was 20.4 months in the placebo arm and had not been reached in the pembrolizumab arm. An update with 42.3 months median follow-up indicted that 3.5-year RFS was increased from 49% to 65%.[229]

Non-small-cell lung cancer. Addition of pembrolizumab to four cycles of pemetrexed and cisplatin or carboplatin followed by four cycles of pemetrexed in patients with previously untreated metastatic nonsquamous NSCLC increased OS (HR 0.49; $p < 0.0001$), increased PFS by 3.9 months ($p < 0.0001$), and increased ORR by 29% ($p < 0.0001$), increasing duration of response from 7.8 to 11.2 months. Similarly, the addition of pembrolizumab to carboplatin and protein-bound paclitaxel or paclitaxel in previously untreated metastatic squamous NSCLC increased OS by 4.6 months ($p = 0.0017$), PFS by 1.6 months ($p < 0.0001$), ORR by 23%, and duration of median response by 2.3 months. When pembrolizumab was used as a single agent and compared to pemetrexed-carboplatin or paclitaxel-carboplatin in unresectable or metastatic NSCLC, the immune check point inhibitor was superior to chemotherapy in OS and the effect was more marked in cancers with 50% or greater PD-L1 positivity. When single-agent pembrolizumab was compared to one of several chemotherapy regimens in a second trial in NSCLC that required high expression (50% or greater) of PD-L1, PFS was extended by 4.3 months ($p < 0.001$), OS by 15.8 months ($p = 0.005$), and ORR increased by 17% ($p = 0.001$). In previously treated metastatic NSCLC, pembrolizumab was superior to docetaxel in OS ($p < 0.001$) and ORR ($p < 0.001$).

Small-cell lung cancer. In single-arm studies, 83 SCLC patients who had progressed through at least two lines of therapy exhibited a 19% ORR lasting 6 months or more in 96%, 12 months or more in 63%, and 18 months or more in 56% of patients.

Head and neck squamous cell cancer. Pembrolizumab in combination with 5-fluorouracil and carboplatin or cisplatin was compared to cetuximab in combination with the same drugs for frontline treatment of metastatic SCCHN. While there was no significant difference in ORR or PFS, pembrolizumab increased overall median survival by 2.3 months ($p = 0.0067$). Treatment of platinum-resistant SCCHN in a single-arm study produced a 16% ORR, with 82% lasting 6 months or more.

Urothelial carcinoma. Pembrolizumab monotherapy produced a 29% ORR lasting >7.8 months in patients with locally advanced or metastatic urothelial cancer who were ineligible for platinum-based therapy. When treatment with pembrolizumab was compared to treatment with paclitaxel, docetaxel, or vinflunine in previously treated urothelial cancers, the immune check point inhibitor did not prolong PFS but did increase ORR by 9.7% ($p = 0.001$) and OS by 2.9 months ($p = 0.005$).[230] Fewer adverse events and fewer severe adverse events were observed with antibody therapy. Pembrolizumab has also been evaluated in BCG-unresponsive urothelial cancers in patients who could not or did not want to undergo cystectomy. A 41% CR rate was achieved that lasted a median of 16.2 months.

Renal cell cancer. Pembrolizumab is approved as first-line treatment for advanced RCC in combination with axitinib. When a combination of pembrolizumab and axitinib was compared to sunitinib, the two-agent combination improved OS (HR 0.53; $p < 0.0001$), PFS by 4.1 months ($p < 0.0001$), and ORR by 23% ($p < 0.0001$). In a randomized, placebo-controlled study, adjuvant pembrolizumab prolonged 2-year DFS by 9.2% ($p = 0.001$),[231] but failed to prolong OS.

Esophageal cancer. When pembrolizumab was compared to chemotherapy (paclitaxel, docetaxel, or irinotecan) in previously treated recurrent or metastatic esophageal cancer with a PD-L1 CPS of 10 or more, pembrolizumab improved OS by 3.6 months and ORR by 15%.

Gastric cancer. Among microsatellite stable gastric cancers with a PD-L1-CPS of 1 or more and two or more previous systemic regimens, pembrolizumab produced an ORR of 13% with 58% lasting 6 months or more and 26% 12 months or more.

Colorectal cancer. When pembrolizumab was compared to two standard regimens of front-line chemotherapy, previously untreated metastatic colorectal cancer that was MSI-H or mismatch repair deficient, pembrolizumab improved PFS by 8.3 months ($p = 0.0004$) and ORR by 11% with 75% lasting 12 months or more and 43% 24 months or more.

Hepatocellular cancer. In patients whose hepatocellular cancer had progressed on sorafenib or who were intolerant of the drug, pembrolizumab produced a 17% ORR with 89% lasting 6 and 12 months or more in 89% and 56% of patients, respectively.

Cervical cancer. Pembrolizumab produced an ORR of 17% with 91% lasting more than 6 months in recurrent or metastatic cervical cancer with a composite positivity score (CPS) of 1 or more.

Endometrial cancer. Pembrolizumab in combination with lenvatinib produced a 38.3% ORR with 69% lasting 6 months or more in endometrial cancers.

Triple-negative breast cancer. Addition of pembrolizumab to chemotherapy with protein-bound paclitaxel, paclitaxel or gemcitabine, and carboplatin for front-line recurrent unresectable or metastatic triple-negative breast cancer increased median PFS by 4.1 months ($p = 0.0012$), ORR by 13%, and duration of response by 12 months. Neoadjuvant therapy with pembrolizumab in addition to doxorubicin, cyclophosphamide, and paclitaxel improved pathologic complete response by 7% and reduced EFS (HR 0.63; $p = 0.00031$) in triple-negative breast cancer that was >1 cm with nodal involvement or >2 cm without nodal involvement.

Cutaneous squamous cell cancer. Monotherapy with pembrolizumab produced a 34% ORR for a median of >9.4 months in recurrent or metastatic cutaneous squamous cell cancer.

Merkel cell cancer. Pembrolizumab was evaluated as front-line monotherapy in 50 patients with locally advanced or metastatic Merkel cell cancer, producing an ORR of 56% with 96% of responses lasting 6 months or more and 54% 12 months or more.

Classical Hodgkin disease. Administration of pembrolizumab to 210 patients with relapsed or refractory classical Hodgkin disease was associated with a 69% ORR lasting a median of 11.1 months. Subsequently, when similar patients were randomized to pembrolizumab or brentuximab vedotin, pembrolizumab provided 4.9 months longer PFS and 12% higher ORR lasting a median of 6.9 months longer.

Primary mediastinal large B-cell lymphoma. In a single-arm trial of monotherapy in 53 patients with relapsed or refractory primary mediastinal large B-cell lymphoma, pembrolizumab achieved a response rate of 45% with a median duration >9.7 months.

Basket indications. In addition, FDA approval has been granted for use in unresectable or metastatic cancers that have high Microsatellite Instability (MSI-Hi), Mismatch Repair Deficiency, or high Mutational Burden (10 or more mutations per mega base DNA). Pembrolizumab is generally recommended for use against cancers with PD-L1 positivity of 1% or more. In several cancer types, a greater response was observed with pembrolizumab when >50% of cancer cells are PD-L1 positive.

Toxicity. The most common (>20%) adverse reactions among patients receiving pembrolizumab 2 mg/kg every 3 weeks are fatigue, cough, nausea, pruritus, rash, decreased appetite, constipation, arthralgia, and diarrhea. The most frequent (greater than or equal to 2%) serious adverse drug reactions observed with pembrolizumab were renal failure, dyspnea, pneumonia, and cellulitis. Additional clinically significant immune-mediated adverse reactions included pneumonitis, colitis, hypophysitis, hyperthyroidism, hypothyroidism, nephritis, and hepatitis.

Cemiplimab
Cemiplimab (Libtayo®) is an IgG4 anti-PD1 monoclonal antibody that blocks PD-L1 and PD-L2 ligands from binding to PD1 on T lymphocytes and has been approved for three indications in cancers that express PD-L1.[232]

Cutaneous squamous cell cancers. Treatment with cemiplimab in two trials that included patients with locally advanced or metastatic cutaneous squamous cell cancers achieved ORRs of 46% and 41% with responses lasting six months or more in 79% and 85%, respectively.

Basal cell carcinoma. Monotherapy with cemiplimab produced an ORR of 21% in metastatic cutaneous basal cell cancer and an ORR of 29% in locally advanced disease with 100% and 79% lasting 6 months or more.

Non-small-cell lung cancer. In a randomized trial with 710 patients with locally advanced or metastatic NSCLC with high (50% or greater) PD-L1 expression, cemiplimab treatment prolonged OS by 7.8 months ($p = 0.0022$), PFS by 0.6 months ($p < 0.0001$), ORR by 16% and duration of response by 15 months when compared to chemotherapy.

Toxicity. Musculoskeletal pain, fatigue, rash, and diarrhea were the most common adverse reactions (≥15%) encountered. Severe laboratory abnormalities (≥2%) included lymphopenia, hyponatremia, hypophosphatemia, increased aspartate aminotransferase, anemia, and hyperkalemia. As with other anti-PD1 antibodies, autoimmune reactions can cause colitis, pneumonitis, hepatitis, endocrinopathies, nephritis, exfoliative dermatitis, myocarditis, and neurologic toxicities.

Anti-PD-L1
Anti-PD-L1 monoclonal antibodies target the ligand for the PD-1 receptor that is expressed on many cancers.

Atezolizumab
Atezolizumab (Tecentric®) is a humanized IgG1 kappa immunoglobulin directed against PD-L1 that prevents its interaction with PD-1 and B7.1 receptors found on T lymphocytes and antigen-presenting cells.[233]

Non-small-cell lung cancer. Treatment with atezolizumab improved OSS by 7.1 months ($p = 0.01$) when compared to platinum-based chemotherapy in previously untreated stage IV NSCLC having >1% PD-LI positive tumor cells or immune cells.[234] Addition of atezolizumab to bevacizumab, carboplatin, and paclitaxel improved OSS by 4.5 months ($p = 0.016$), PFS by 1.5 months ($p = 0.0002$) and ORR by 13%, and median duration by 4.3 months in previously untreated metastatic nonsquamous NSCLC. With similar patients, addition of atezolizumab to protein-bound paclitaxel and carboplatin increased OSS by 4.7 months ($p = 0.0384$), PFS by 0.7 months ($p = 0.0024$), and ORR by 12% with an improved median duration of response of 3 months. In NSCLC patients who had failed a platinum-containing regimen, atezolizumab improved OS by 4.2 months ($p = 0.0004$), but not PFS; ORR was improved by only 1%, but the duration of response was extended by 10 months when compared to docetaxel chemotherapy.

Small-cell lung cancer. In previously untreated patients with extensive SCLC, addition of atezolizumab to carboplatin and etoposide improved OSS by 2 months ($p = 0.0069$) and PFS by 0.9 months ($p = 0.0170$).[235]

Urothelial cancer. Monotherapy in 119 patients with urothelial cancers who were ineligible for platinum-based therapy or had progressed within 12 months on adjuvant therapy exhibited an ORR of 23.5%. ORR in 310 patients with metastatic urothelial cancer that had progressed on platinum chemotherapy was 14.8% with a median duration of 27.7 months. ORR in the subset of 100 patients with >5% PD-LI immune cells in their cancers was 26% with median duration of 29.7 months.

Melanoma. Addition of atezolizumab to cobimetinib and vemurafenib in unresectable or metastatic melanoma with a BRAF V600 mutation improved PFS by 4.5 months ($p = 0.0249$) and the ORR by only 1%, but with an improved median duration of response of 7.9 months.

Hepatocellular cancer. A combination of atezolizumab and bevacizumab improved OSS (HR 0.58; $p = 0.001$), PFS by 2.5 months ($p < 0.001$), and ORR by 25% ($p = 0.001$) compared to sorafenib.[236]

Toxicity. Side effects (≥20%) as a single agent include fatigue, nausea, cough dyspnea, and decreased appetite.[237] Additional toxicities in combination with antineoplastic drugs for NSCLC and SCLC include alopecia, constipation, and diarrhea. As with other immune checkpoint inhibitors, immune-mediated pneumonitis, hepatitis, colitis, endocrinopathies, and uveitis were observed in some patients.

Durvalumab
Durvalumab (Imfinzi®) is a human IgG1 monoclonal antibody that binds PD-L1.

Non-small-cell lung cancer. Durvalumab delayed progression of Stage III lung cancer following primary chemoradiotherapy by 11.3 months.[238]

Small-cell lung cancer. Addition of durvalumab to etoposide and either cisplatin or carboplatin in patients with previously untreated SCLC increased median OS by 2.7 months (HR 0.73; $p = 0.0047$) and increased the ORR by 10% compared to chemotherapy alone.[239,240]

Toxicity. Side effects include cough, fatigue, upper respiratory infections including pneumonitis, dyspnea, and rash. Autoimmune pneumonitis, hepatitis, colitis, endocrinopathies, and nephritis occur. Infusion reactions have also been observed.

Avelumab

Avelumab (Bavencio®) is a human IgG1 lambda immunoglobulin reactive with PD-L1 that prevents binding to PD-1 and to B7.1 inhibitory receptors on T cells.

Merkel cell cancer

Monotherapy with avelumab in 88 patients with metastatic Merkel cell cancer produced an ORR of 33% with 86% lasting 6 months or more and 45% lasting 12 months or more.[241]

Urothelial cancer. In 161 patients with metastatic urothelial cancer that had progressed within 12 months of neoadjuvant or adjuvant platinum-based therapy, avelumab produced a response rate of 16%. Addition of maintenance avelumab to BSC significantly prolonged OS by 7.1 months ($p = 0.001$). Avelumab also significantly prolonged overall 1-year survival in the PD-L1–positive population by 18.3% (HR, 0.56; 95% CI, 0.40–0.79; $p < 0.001$).[242]

Renal cell cancer. A combination of avelumab and axitinib extended PFS by 5.4 months ($p = 0.0002$) and improved the ORR by 25.7% when compared to sunitinib in a randomized trial of previously untreated patients with metastatic RCC.

Toxicity. Adverse reactions (≥20%) in treating Merkel cell carcinoma included fatigue, musculoskeletal pain, diarrhea, nausea, infusion reaction, rash, decreased appetite, and peripheral edema.[243] Additional side effects in treating urothelial cancers included urinary tract infections. Use of avelumab in combination with axitinib to treat RCC was associated with additional side effects of hypertension, mucositis, palmar-plantar erythrodysesthesia, dysphonia, hypothyroidism, hepatotoxicity, cough, dyspnea, abdominal pain, and headache. Autoimmune pneumonitis, hepatitis, colitis, endocrinopathies, and nephritis occur, as with other immune checkpoint inhibitors.

Bispecific antibodies

Immunoglobulins can be engineered to contain binding sites with two different specificities. The same can be done with smaller single-chain variable fragments (scFv) that contain the relevant binding sites and have better tissue penetration. Bispecific constructs with one scFv fragment that recognizes a determinant found only on B cells with a second scFv fragment that binds to a determinant found only on T cells can enhance contact between cytotoxic T cells and malignant B cells, encouraging immunologic cancer cell killing.

Blinatumomab

Blinatumomab (Blincyto®) is a bispecific antibody with scFv fragments that bind to the CD3 T cell determinant and the CD19 B-cell determinant that is expressed on ALL cells.

Acute lymphoblastic leukemia. Blinatumomab was approved by the US FDA in 2014 for the treatment of ALL refractory to conventional therapy based on a study involving 185 adults with Philadelphia chromosome-negative relapsed or refractory precursor B-cell ALL. All participants were treated with blinatumomab for at least 4 weeks via infusion producing CR in 32% for 6.7 months.[244] When heavily pretreated patients with ALL were randomized to blinatumomab or best available chemotherapy, blinatumomab improved the OS rate by 3.3 months (HR 0.71; $p = 0.01$). CR with full hematologic recovery was increased by 18% ($p < 0.001$) with 2.7 months longer duration of remission.[245]

Toxicity. Blinatumomab carries a boxed warning that some clinical trial participants had experienced cytokine release syndrome at the start of the first treatment and experienced a short period of encephalopathy. The most common side effects seen in blinatumomab-treated participants were fever, headache, peripheral edema, febrile neutropenia, nausea, hypokalemia, fatigue, constipation, diarrhea, and tremor.

Barriers to treatment with unmodified monoclonal antibodies

Antigen specificity

Few, if any, monoclonal antibodies react only with tumor cells and fail to react with any normal tissues. The remarkable efficacy and modest toxicity of anti-idiotypic antibodies reflect, at least in part, their limited reactivity with the vast majority of human B cells. The toxicity of Campath-1 reflects reactivity with normal lymphocytes and monocytes. To treat cancers in some organs, such as ovary or thyroid, tissue-specific antibodies rather than tumor-specific antibodies may suffice because all normal tissue is removed during primary therapy.

Antigenic modulation

Antigens that modulate and are shed into the circulation, such as CD10 in ALL, have generally proven to be poor targets for serotherapy. An exception to this generalization has been observed with trastuzumab treatment of breast cancers that overexpress HER-2. A part of the extracellular domain of HER-2 can be cleaved and has been used as a marker for receptor overexpression.

Heterogeneity of antigen expression

Heterogeneity has been observed in antigen expression within and among cancers from different individuals. Cells that lack antigen expression cannot be effectively targeted. With unconjugated antibodies that lack "bystander" activity, a combination of several reagents may be required to target all cells. In the case of different breast cancers, a combination of five monoclonal reagents can target >90% of cells in >90% of cancers from different individuals.[246]

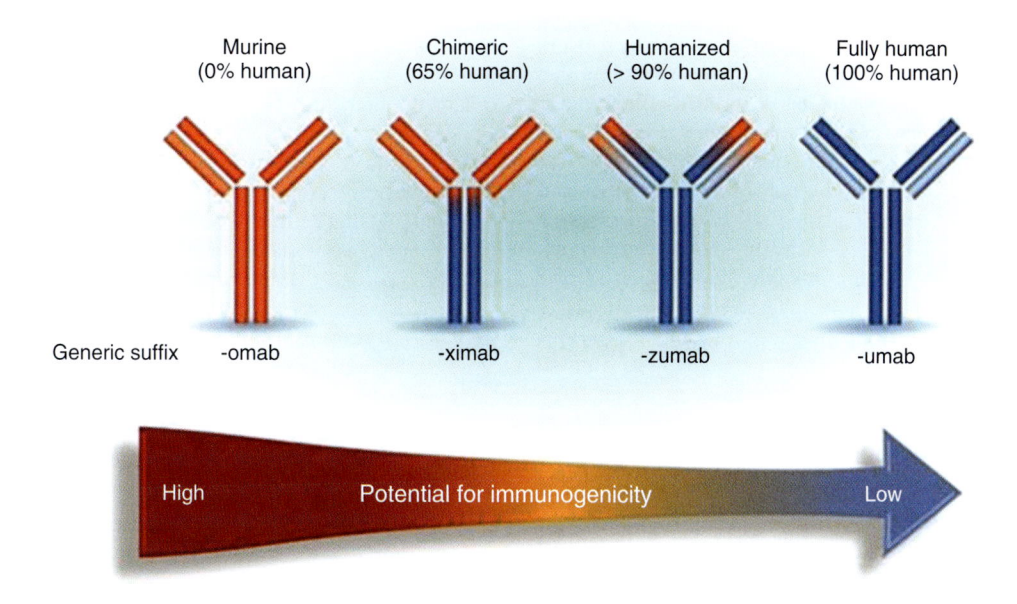

Figure 1 Immunogenicity decreases with humanization of murine monoclonal antibodies. Source: Foltz et al.[110]

Effective delivery of antibody to tumor cells

Most attempts to develop effective serotherapy have utilized IgG antibodies with an Mr of 150 kDa. In contrast, most conventional cytotoxic drugs have a mass of <1 kDa. Consequently, monoclonal antibodies have slower kinetics of distribution and less tissue penetration than conventional drugs.[247] For example, intravenous injection of an IgG2a murine monoclonal antibody against a 250-kDa melanoma-associated chondroitin sulfate proteoglycan core protein resulted in selective localization of antibody in metastatic nodules of malignant melanoma.[248] The greater the amount of antibody administered, the greater was the accumulation of murine immunoglobulin that could be demonstrated immunohistochemically in biopsied material. Even after the infusion of 500 mg of antibody, complete saturation of antigenic sites was not achieved in all patients, consistent with limited access of antibody to tumor cells outside the vascular compartment. Successful tumor localization of an antibody depends on several factors. The ability of monoclonal antibodies to reach tumor cells can be limited by abnormal vascularity, elevated interstitial pressure, and relatively large distances for the transport of immunoglobulins through the interstitium.[249,250] Disordered tumor vessels permit greater leakage of albumin and other plasma proteins into the interstitial space around cancer cells. Blockage of lymphatic outflow by tumor cells prevents clearance of interstitial protein, increasing oncotic pressure, and fluid accumulation. Increased interstitial pressure impedes the effective translocation of antibodies. Biodistribution studies indicate that distance from blood vessels is an important factor affecting antigen recognition and binding. The central areas of bulky disease not only have increased fluid pressure but are also poorly perfused, making these regions less accessible to antibodies.[251] In addition, large tumor masses can act as antigenic sinks, decreasing drug delivery to other tumor sites.[252] Modeling studies led Juweid and colleagues to formulate the hypothesis of the binding-site barrier, which postulated that antibody molecules could be prevented from penetrating tumors by the very fact of their successful binding to peritumoral antigen.[253] Subsequent experimental studies have supported this hypothesis. Intracavitary therapy has been used in an attempt to improve access of the antibody to tumor cells, but the antibody generally penetrates only a few millimeters beneath the serosal surface.

Immune response to foreign immunoglobulin

Substantial effort has been expended on the development of human monoclonal antibodies that should be less immunogenic.[254-256] Because a large number of antibodies used clinically are derived from mice, they can induce the development of human antimouse antibodies (HAMAs). The presence of HAMAs can prevent the effective delivery of murine monoclonal antibodies to tumor cells, particularly when multiple doses must be administered to obtain optimal antitumor activity. Genetic manipulation of murine monoclonal antibodies has been used to generate less immunogenic reagents (Figure 1). Chimeric (60% human) and humanized (95% human) antibodies have been engineered to retain the murine antigen-binding complementarity regions in association with human framework regions.[255] Although the immunogenicity of such antibodies can be substantially reduced and HAMA responses can be limited, their injection can still evoke an anti-idiotypic response. The availability of antibodies derived entirely from humans, isolated from combinatorial libraries using the process of phage display, has revolutionized therapeutic strategies.[257] Transgenic genetically engineered mice have also been created with human immunoglobulin genes that can produce fully human antibodies. Unlike murine antibodies, human or humanized antibodies that contain the human Fc antibody portion trigger ADCC and CDC. The Fc fragment can also be modified to increase interaction with Fc receptors on effectors for ADCC. An array of novel affinity maturation techniques such as bacterial cell surface scFv display and cell-free ribosome display is emerging to isolate rare high-affinity clones.[257] Genetic engineering has also been used to produce single-chain antigen-binding proteins that may have more favorable pharmacokinetic properties than intact immunoglobulin or Fab fragments.[258]

Potency of effector mechanisms

To the extent that unmodified monoclonal antibodies inhibit tumor growth, several mechanisms may be important for antitumor activity, including direct growth inhibition, induction of apoptosis, inhibition of angiogenesis, CDC, and ADCC, in addition to possible intervention in the specific immunoregulatory network of the host with immune checkpoint inhibition. Antibodies that react with EGFR or HER-2 can inhibit the growth of tumor cells ex vivo in the absence of complement components or host effector cells.[259,260] Antibodies that block EGF binding to the EGFR such as cetuximab affect growth more readily than do antibodies that bind to other sites on the receptor. Inhibition of ligand binding appears important for the inhibition of anchorage-dependent, but not anchorage-independent, growth. Antibodies have been described that produce apoptosis in some lymphoid cell lines, activated T cells, and certain carcinoma cell lines.[261] Murine antibodies of the IgM, IgG2a, and IgG3 isotypes can fix human complement, but often rather poorly. The rat monoclonal antibody, Campath-1G, is an important exception to this generalization in that the antibody can mediate lysis of human cells that bear the appropriate antigen in the presence of human complement components.[262] ADCC can be mediated by large granular lymphocytes (LGLs), monocytes, macrophages, or polymorphonuclear leukocytes bound to tumor cells through Fc receptors after the antibody has bound to specific antigenic determinants on the tumor cell surface. Defucosylation of IgG1 humanized antibodies has enhanced their ability to mediate ADCC.[263] Antibodies that react against GD3 on melanoma cells can also bind to GD3 on the surface of T cells, enhancing their cytotoxic and proliferative responses.[264] Hybrid antibodies have been generated with one binding site for T-cell-associated antigens and one binding site for tumor-associated antigens.[265] Such hybrid antibodies enhance tumor cell killing by IL-2-activated T cells, possibly by encouraging contact between effector cells and tumor targets.[266]

Serotherapy with monoclonal antibody–drug conjugates (ADCs)

Murine monoclonal antibodies have been coupled to a variety of conventional cytotoxic agents, including antifolates, anthracyclines, vinca alkyloids, and alkylating agents (Figure 2). Prepolymerization of some drugs such as doxorubicin prior to conjugation can achieve higher ratios of drug to antibody. Drugs can be bound to the amino side chains of lysine residues, provided that the most reactive residues are not found in the antigen-binding site. Linkage of drugs to antibody through the carbohydrate moieties of the murine immunoglobulin has provided site-specific conjugation that generally does not impair antibody binding.[267,268]

One concern raised by some investigators is based on the observation that many cell surface antigens have fewer than 10^5 copies per cell. Release of $1–3 \times 10^6$ drug molecules at the cell surface might or might not be sufficient to eliminate tumor. Another concern relates to the ability of large immunoglobulin carrier complexes to translocate across tumor capillaries. In preclinical studies, however, drug-monoclonal antibody conjugates proved substantially more effective than did the free drug. Only some of these conjugates are more potent, but many are less toxic, providing an improved therapeutic index. Therapeutic advantage may relate to different rates or patterns of drug uptake when linked with monoclonal reagents. In some instances, novel linkages have been devised that would release drug at low pH or only in the presence of lysosomal proteases.

Gemtuzumab Ozogamicin

Gemtuzumab Ozogamicin (Mylotarg®) conjugates calicheamicin with an anti-CD33 antibody.[269]

Acute myelogenous leukemia (AML). CD33 is a 67-kDa glycoprotein expressed on the surface of >90% of acute myelogenous leukemias (AMLs) and on early myeloid progenitor cells but not on normal pluripotent stem cells. Gemtuzumab ozogamicin, a conjugate of humanized anti-CD33 antibody and the cytotoxic antibiotic calicheamicin, is rapidly internalized by myeloblasts and induces apoptosis.[270] Three multicenter trials evaluated gemtuzumab ozogamicin in 142 patients with CD33 + AML in first relapse, administering two doses of 9 mg/m^2 on days 1 and 15 by 2-h intravenous infusion.[271] Complete remission, with or without full platelet recovery, was observed in 30% of patients. In newly diagnosed AML patients, the addition of gemtuzumab ozogamicin to a standard induction regimen of daunorubicin and cytarabine extended EFS by 7.8 months (HR 0.56; $p < 0.001$), but did not change OS.[272] Monotherapy was evaluated in newly diagnosed AML patients aged >75 or 61–75 years with poor performance status who did not want conventional induction therapy. Gemtuzumab ozogamicin improved OS by 1.3 months when compared to BSC.

Toxicity. Because CD33 is expressed on hematopoietic precursors, grade 3 or 4 neutropenia and thrombocytopenia were observed in 99% of 101 patients aged 60 years or above. Infections (27%) and mucositis (4%) were less frequently observed.[273] Veno-occlusive disease occurred in 14 of 119 patients (12%) who received

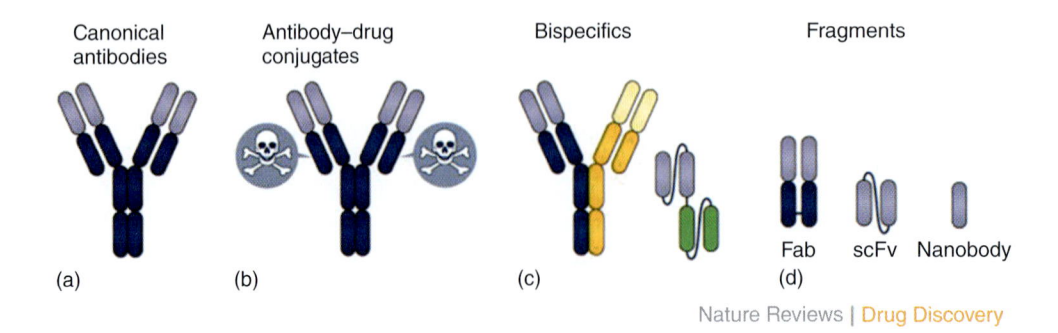

Figure 2 Antibody formats include (a) canonical, (b) antibody–drug conjugates, (c) bispecifics, and (d) fragments. Fragments include antigen-binding fragments (Fabs), single-chain variable region (scFv) constructs and domain antibodies. Radiolabeled antibodies and antibody–immunotoxins are not shown. Source: Modified from Mullard[8].

gemtuzumab ozogamicin-based regimens, including five patients who had not previously undergone stem cell transplantation.274 Despite these toxicities, gemtuzumab ozogamyycin was given accelerated approval by the FDA in 2000. The confirmatory trial was stopped in 2004 due to lack of benefit at interim analysis and the conjugate was voluntarily withdrawn from the market in 2010. Once antigenic sites are saturated with antibody drug conjugates, higher doses only increase toxicity without improving efficacy. Based on a new dose and schedule, the conjugate was approved once again by the FDA in 2017 for newly diagnosed or relapsed CD33+ AML with the judgment that benefit was greater than toxicity.275

Brentuximab vedotin

Brentuximab vedotin (Adcetris®), a conjugate of an anti-CD30 chimeric IgG1 antibody and three to five units of vedotin (monomethyl auristatin E), a small molecule microtubule disrupting agent and inhibitor of mitosis, was granted accelerated approval by the US FDA in 2011 and by the European Union in 2012.

Classic Hodgkin lymphoma (cHL). The effectiveness of brentuximab vedotin in patients with relapsed cHL was initially evaluated in a single-arm clinical trial involving 102 patients where 73% achieved either a complete or partial response to the treatment for an average of 6.7 months. In newly diagnosed stage III and stage IV cHL patients, brentuximab vedotin in combination with doxorubicin, vinblastine, and dacarbazine (AVD) improved PFS (HR 0.77; $p = 0.035$) when compared to doxorubicin, bleomycin, vinblastine, and dacarbazine (ABVD).276,277 Monotherapy with brentuximab vedotin after autologous stem cell transplantation for cHL prolonged PFS by 18.8 months ($p = 0.0001$).278

Anaplastic large-cell lymphoma (ALCL). The effectiveness of brentuximab vedotin in relapsed anaplastic large-cell lymphoma (ALCL) was evaluated in a single-arm clinical trial in 58 patients where 86% experienced either a complete or partial response on average for 12.6 months.279 In patients with previously untreated ALCL and CD30-positive peripheral T-cell lymphoma, brentuximab vedotin in combination with cyclophosphamide, doxorubicin, and prednisone increased the ORR by 11% ($p = 0.003$), extended PFS by 27.4 months ($p = 0.011$), and improved OS (HR 0.66; $p = 0.024$) when compared to conventional treatment with cyclophosphamide, doxorubicin, vincristine, and prednisone (CHOP).

Primary cutaneous large-cell lymphoma and mycosis fungoides. Monotherapy of CD30+ primary cutaneous large cell lymphoma and MF increased ORR lasting at least 4 months by 43.8% ($p < 0.001$) and PFS by 13.2 months ($p < 0.001$) when compared to the physician's choice between methotrexate or bexarotene.

Toxicity. The most common adverse reactions (>20%) in patients treated with brentuximab vedotin are neutropenia, peripheral sensory and motor neuropathy, thrombocytopenia, anemia, upper respiratory tract infection, fatigue, nausea, and diarrhea.280 Twenty-five percent of patients reported serious adverse reactions. The most common serious adverse reactions were pneumonia, pyrexia, vomiting, nausea, hepatotoxicity, and peripheral sensory neuropathy. In the registration trial, adverse reactions led to discontinuation of treatment in 32%. Cases of JC virus infection resulting in Progressive Multifocal Leukoencephalopathy have been observed in patients receiving brentuximab vedotin. Other serious and potentially fatal complications include interstitial lung disease, acute respiratory distress syndrome, Stevens–Johnson syndrome, toxic epidermal necrolysis, pancreatitis, and intestinal perforation.

Polatuzumab-vedotin-piiq

Polatuzumab-vedotin-piiq (POLIVY®) is an antibody–drug conjugate that combines a humanized IgG1K antibody directed against CD79b with vedotin.

Diffuse large B-cell lymphoma (DLBCL). Evidence for efficacy was obtained in patients with diffuse large B-cell lymphoma (DLCBL) who had failed one prior regimen of therapy. Addition of polatuzumab-vedotin to bendamustine and rituximab (BR) improved complete response rate by 22% ($p = 0.026$), the PFS by 5.8 months ($p = 0.0001$), and OS by 7.7 months ($p = 0.0002$) when compared with BR alone.281

Toxicity. Side effects in ≥30% of recipients included nausea, diarrhea, neutropenia, peripheral neuropathy, fatigue, thrombocytopenia, and pyrexia, while ≥20% experienced decreased appetite, anemia, constipation, vomiting, and abdominal pain.282 Infections occurred in >10% of patients including upper respiratory tract infection, pneumonia, febrile neutropenia, and herpesvirus infection.

Belantamab-mafodotin-cxu

Belantamab-mafodotin-cxu (Blenrep®) is an antibody–drug conjugate that combines an afucosylated IgG1 monoclonal antibody against B-cell maturation antigen (BCMA) conjugated with MMAF, a microtubule inhibitor.

Multiple myeloma. Belantamab-mafodotin-cxu was US FDA approved in 2020 for treatment of relapsed or refractory MM in patients who have received at least four prior therapies. Among 87 heavily pretreated MM patients, an ORR of 31% was observed.283

Toxicity. The most frequent toxicities (≥20%) include corneal keratopathy, decreased visual acuity, blurred vision, nausea, fever, infusion-related reactions, and fatigue. The most common grade 3 or 4 laboratory abnormalities are decreases in platelets, lymphocytes, hemoglobin, and neutrophils and increases in creatinine.

Ado-Trastuzumab-emtansine

Ado-Trastuzumab-emtansine (TDM-1; Kadcyla®) is a conjugate of the anti-HER-2 humanized IgG1 antibody trastuzumab and a 148 Da cytotoxic drug emtansine (DM1) that binds to tubulin.

HER-2-positive breast cancer. The conjugate was approved by the US FDA and the European Union in 2013 for treatment of recurrent HER-2-positive breast cancer based on a randomized, multicenter, open-label trial enrolling 991 patients who had failed prior taxane and trastuzumab-based therapy prior to enrollment. Patients were randomly allocated to receive intravenous ado-trastuzumab emtansine or oral lapatinib and capecitabine. Ado-trastuzumab emtansine produced greater PFS (6.4 vs 9.4 months; $p < 0.0001$) and OS (25.1 vs 30.9 months; $p = 0.0006$) compared to lapatinib and capecitabine.284 Ado-trastuzumab-emtansine has also been tested in the adjuvant setting in patients with HER-2-positive breast cancer that had persisted in the tumor or nodes despite trastuzumab-based neoadjuvant therapy. Completing adjuvant therapy with trastuzumab emtansine improved invasive DFS (HR 0.5; $p < 0.0001$) with an 11.3% increase in 3-year invasive DFS when compared to completion of adjuvant therapy with trastuzumab.[285,286]

Toxicity. The most common adverse reactions observed in patients receiving ado-trastuzumab emtansine are fatigue, nausea, musculoskeletal pain, thrombocytopenia, headache, increased transaminases, anemia, and constipation. The most common (>2%) grade 3–4 adverse reactions were thrombocytopenia, increased transaminases, anemia, hypokalemia, peripheral neuropathy, and fatigue. The most common adverse events leading to discontinuing ado-trastuzumab emtansine were thrombocytopenia and increased transaminases. Serious hepatobiliary disorders, including fatal cases of severe drug-induced liver injury and associated hepatic encephalopathy, have been reported in clinical trials with ado-trastuzumab emtansine. Other significant adverse reactions include left ventricular dysfunction, interstitial lung disease, and infusion-associated reactions.

Fam-trastuzumab-deruxtecan-nxki

Fam-trastuzumab-deruxtecan-nxki (Enhertu®) is an antibody–drug conjugate that contains a humanized IgG1 monoclonal directed against the HER-2 receptor, a topoisomerase I inhibitor, DXd, and a tetrapeptide-based cleavable linker.

HER-2-positive breast cancer. Fam-trastuzumab-deruxtecan-nxki has been approved by the US FDA for the treatment of HER-2-positive unresectable or metastatic breast cancer in patients who have received two or more anti-HER-2 therapies. Accelerated approval was based on a single-armed trial of monotherapy in 184 patients with these characteristics who experienced a 60.3% ORR with a median duration of 14.8 months.[287,288]

HER-2-positive gastric and gastroesophageal junction adenocarcinoma. The antibody–drug conjugate is approved for adults with locally advanced or metastatic HER-2-positive gastric or gastroesophageal junction adenocarcinomas who have received at least one previous anti-HER-2 therapy. In a randomized trial with 188 patients in Japan and South Korea with these characteristics, fam-trastuzumab-deruxtecan-nixki increased ORR by 29.2% ($p < 0.0001$), increased duration of response by 7.4 months, increased PFS by 2.1 months, and improved OS by 4.1 months ($p = 0.0097$) when compared to treatment with irinotecan or paclitaxel.[289,290]

Toxicity. Side effects include decreased neutrophils, hemoglobin, and platelets; fatigue; decreased apatite, nausea, vomiting, constipation, and diarrhea; alopecia; increased aspartate aminotransferase and alanine aminotransferase; hypokalemia, and cough.[291] Less common but serious complications include interstitial lung disease, pneumonitis, and left ventricular dysfunction.

Sacituzumab-govitecan-hziy

Sacituzumab-govitecan-hziy (Trodelvy®) is an antibody–drug conjugate that includes a monoclonal IgG1k immunoglobulin directed against trophoblast cell surface antigen (Trop-2), a topoisomerase inhibitor SN-38, and a hydrolyzable linker, CL2A.

Triple-negative breast cancer. Sacituzumab-govitecan has received US FDA approval for the treatment of metastatic triple-negative breast cancer in patients who have received at least two courses of systemic therapy, with at least one of them for metastatic disease.[292] In a randomized trial with 468 patients with locally advanced or metastatic triple-negative breast cancer, monotherapy with sacituzumab-govitecan increased median PFS by 3.9 months ($p < 0.0001$) and OS by 5.4 months ($p < 0.001$) compared to the physician's choice of eribulin, capecitabine, gemcitabine, or vinorelbine.[293] In a single-arm study of 108 patients, sacituzumab-govitecan produced a 33.3% response rate lasting a median of 7.7 months.[294]

Urothelial cancer. The antibody–drug conjugate has also been granted accelerated approval for treatment of locally advanced or metastatic urothelial cancers, in patients who have received platinum-based therapy and an anti-PD-1 or an anti-PD-L1 immune checkpoint inhibitor. In a single-arm trial with 112 patients, monotherapy produced an ORR of 27.7% with a duration of 7.2 months.[295]

Toxicity. Side effects (>25%) include neutropenia, nausea, diarrhea, fatigue, alopecia, anemia, vomiting, constipation, decreased appetite, rash, and abdominal pain.

Enfortumab vedotin-ejfv

Enfortumab vedotin-ejfv (PADCEV®) is an antibody–drug conjugate that contains an immunoglobulin directed against Nectin-4, the small molecule microtubule disrupting agent monomethyl auristatin E (MMAE), and protease-cleavable maleimidocaproyl valine.

Urothelial cancer. In 2019, the US FDA approved enfortumab vedotin for the treatment of advanced or metastatic urothelial cancer in patients who have previously received a PD-1 or PD-L1 inhibitor and platinum-containing chemotherapy or are ineligible for cisplatin-containing chemotherapy and have previously received one or more prior lines of therapy.[296] In a randomized trial that involved 608 patients, monotherapy increased ORR by 22.7% ($p = 0.0001$), enhanced PFS by 1.8 months ($p < 0.001$), and improved OS by 3.9 months ($p = 0.001$) compared to the investigator's choice of chemotherapy.[297] In a single-arm study, treatment with enfortumab vedotin produced a 44% ORR with a median duration of 7.6 months.

Toxicity. Common side effects (≥20%) include rash, dry skin, pruritus, fatigue, peripheral neuropathy, alopecia, decreased appetite, weight loss, nausea, diarrhea, and dysgeusia. Laboratory abnormalities include decreased hemoglobin, neutrophils, lymphocytes, platelets, albumin, and sodium; and increased alanine aminotransferase, urate, lipase, aspartate aminotransferase, glucose, and creatinine. Changes in vision and symptoms of peripheral neuropathy can occur. Extravasation can cause inflammation and necrosis. Uncommon, but potentially life-threatening, side effects include Sevens–Johnson syndrome, toxic epidermal necrolysis, pneumonitis, and diabetic ketoacidosis.

Radioimmunotherapy of cancer

Radioimmunotherapy (RIT) is a method of cancer treatment that involves the selective delivery of a radionuclide emitting cytotoxic radiation to tumor cells via an antibody or an antibody fragment. While the concept of antibody-based targeting of radionuclides to cancer cells has long been appreciated, this approach did not become practical until the development of monoclonal reagents, which permitted more specific targeting and large-scale production of conjugates for clinical trials. With external beam therapy, only a limited area of the body is irradiated, with the dimensions defined to match the known limits of tumor location. While conventional radiotherapy can be effective for localized disease, diffuse cancers generally are difficult to treat because of normal tissue toxicity concerns and metastatic disease beyond the margins of the radiation field escaping treatment. With RIT, if the targeted antigen or receptor is also present on metastases, sites of occult disease can also be treated even if their presence and location are unknown at the time of treatment.

RIT offers several important advantages compared with other antibody-based strategies discussed in this article. First, one can employ a theragnostic strategy—the antibody can be labeled with a small dose of either the therapeutic radionuclide (or an analogous one) and then pharmacokinetics and targeting in individual patients can be determined by nuclear medicine imaging before performing RIT. The imaging results can then be used to select patients most likely to benefit from RIT and determine patient-specific administered radioactivity levels required to deliver the desired radiation dose to tumor.[298] Second, unlike ADCs and immunotoxins that kill only the targeted cell, the cytotoxic effects of radionuclides, summarized in a review,[123] can extend beyond the targeted cell and include self-irradiation, crossfire irradiation, and a biological bystander effect. Crossfire occurs due to the fact that the range of most therapeutic radiation is multicellular, while the biological bystander effect can kill neighboring cells not directly traversed by radiation by a mechanism not fully understood.[299,300] Both can result in the destruction of adjacent cells not taking up the labeled antibody, helping to compensate for heterogeneities among cancer cells in antibody delivery, target molecule expression, or both. Perhaps the largest impediment to the acceptance of RIT is fear of radioactive materials among physicians and patients, which can be ameliorated by better education as well as clinical success.

Role of the radionuclide

An advantage of RIT is the potential to match the range of action of the radionuclide to the need, for a given clinical application, to balance normal toxicity constraints with the desire to maximize homogeneity of tumor dose deposition. Other factors that must be considered in the selection of radionuclides for RIT include (1) compatibility of its physical half-life with antibody pharmacokinetics, (2) existence of labeling chemistry that provides acceptable stability, and (3) commercial availability of the radionuclide in a form suitable for clinical use. The characteristics of the radionuclides that have been most widely investigated for RIT and other targeted radiotherapy approaches have been discussed in a review.[301] The vast majority of RIT studies utilized radionuclides decaying by the emission of beta particles or alpha particles, which have tissue ranges of 1–10 mm and 50–90 μm, respectively. Recently, radionuclides that emit subcellular range (<1 keV) Auger electrons, originally thought to only be cytotoxic when localized in close proximity to the cell nucleus, have been evaluated.[302] However, at least one study suggests that Auger electron emitters also can be effective when delivered by noninternalizing antibodies.[303]

Beta emitters

The only two FDA-approved RIT products involve radionuclides that emit beta particles. The cytotoxic effects of radiation agents depend largely on their linear energy transfer (LET), which is the amount of energy they deposit over a given distance. Beta particles have an LET of approximately 0.2 keV/μm similar to conventional external beam radiotherapy, are considered sparsely ionizing radiation, and produce mostly single strand DNA lesions that are readily repairable.[299] Given their tissue path length, beta emitters are most appropriate for treating tumors >0.5 cm in diameter as under these circumstances, most of their decay energy will be absorbed by the tumor and not by neighboring normal tissues. Shorter-range beta emitters such as ^{131}I, ^{177}Lu, and ^{67}Cu are the focus of current work and might be better in minimum residual disease settings while longer-range beta emitters such as Y and ^{186}Re are better suited to larger tumors and compensating for heterogeneities in receptor expression or poor vascularity.

Alpha emitters

Alpha particles have higher energies than beta particles and exhibit very short path lengths (<100 μm) in tissue. Alpha particles have an LET of about 100 keV/μm, are densely ionizing, and produce clusters of DNA damage, including double strand DNA breaks that are difficult to repair.[299] Moreover, the cytotoxic effectiveness of alpha particles is largely independent of dose rate and oxygenation, offering the possibility of treating hypoxic tumor regions. Because of their short range, alpha emitters were initially investigated for the treatment of blood-borne tumor cells, micrometastatic disease, and cancer cells on the surface of cavities, such as ovarian carcinoma and neoplastic meningitis. The alpha emitters that have been most widely investigated in RIT include 61-min ^{212}Bi, 46-min ^{213}Bi, 7.2-h ^{211}At, 10-day ^{225}Ac, and 18.7-day ^{227}Th.[304,305] The half-lives of ^{212}Bi and ^{213}Bi are so short that they are difficult to use and to achieve effective tumor targeting before they decay. The much longer half-lives of ^{225}Ac and ^{227}Th, while advantageous in terms of convenience and commercialization potential, are challenging from a radiochemistry perspective because of the need to maintain a stable link between the radionuclide and the antibody over a multiweek time course. This is further complicated by the need to trap their multiple alpha-emitting daughters in the tumor and avoid dose-limiting toxicities to normal tissues, particularly the kidney in the case of ^{225}Ac. For these reasons, ^{211}At has been considered the most promising alpha emitter for labeling antibodies and their fragments.[306]

Radioimmunotherapy of lymphoma

Hematological malignancies, particularly lymphomas, are attractive targets for RIT because of their inherent radiosensitivity. The only two RIT agents that have FDA approval are indicated for relapsed or refractory low-grade B-cell NHL (Table 2). These are ^{90}Y-ibritumomab tiuxetan and ^{131}I-tositumomab, which received clearance in 2002 and 2003, respectively. Both target the CD20 cell surface antigen that is expressed on about 95% of B-cell lymphoma but also on normal B cells. For this reason, an essential part of the treatment protocol is the administration of a relatively large dose of unlabeled antibody in order to saturate normal B-cell–binding sites before administration of the radiolabeled antibody. Standard protocols and other practical aspects for the use of these RIT agents have been described.[307,308]

Table 2 Approved radioimmunotherapy treatments for non-Hodgkin lymphoma.

Property	^{90}Y-Ibritumomab Tiuxetan	^{131}I-Tositumomab
Product name	Zevalin	Bexxar
Antibody for labeling	Ibritumomab	Tositumomab
Form	Murine IgG1	Murine IgG2a
Antibody for blocking	Chimeric rituximab	Murine tositumomab
Dose	250 mg/m^2	450 mg
Therapy radionuclide	Yttrium-90 (^{90}Y)	Iodine-131 (^{131}I)
Half-life	2.7 days	8.1 days
Maximum beta energy	2.28 MeV	0.61 MeV
Maximum tissue range	11.3 mm	2.3 mm
Gamma ray emission	No	Yes
Labeling method	Bifunctional chelate (tiuxetan)	Electrophilic radiohalogenation
Imaging radionuclide	Indium-111 (^{111}In)	Iodine-131 (^{131}I)
Role of imaging	Demonstrate acceptable biodistribution	Determine whole-body clearance kinetics
Patient-specific dosimetry	No	Yes
Administered activity	20–30 mCi	50–200 mCi
Parameter for dosing	mCi per kg body weight	Calculated whole-body dosimetry
Benchmark if platelets >150,000/mm^3	0.4 mCi/kg	75 cGy
Benchmark if platelets 100,000–149,000/mm^3	0.3 mCi/kg	65 cGy

^{90}Y-ibritumomab tiuxetan

^{90}Y-ibritumomab tiuxetan (Zevalin®) consists of the anti-CD20 murine monoclonal antibody parent of the chimeric antibody rituximab covalently linked to ^{90}Y via the MX-DTPA (tiuxetan) bifunctional chelator. Initially, imaging the patient with ibritumomab labeled with another radiometal,^{112}In, was performed to document acceptable antibody biodistribution prior to treatment with ^{90}Y.[309] A number of early studies demonstrated significantly enhanced therapeutic effectiveness for ^{90}Y-ibritumomab tiuxetan RIT compared with rituximab immunotherapy in patients with recurrent follicular lymphoma. In a randomized trial comparing ^{90}Y-ibritumomab tiuxetan and rituximab treatment in 143 patients with relapsed lymphoma, ^{90}Y-ibritumomab tiuxetan produced an 80% response rate compared with 56% with rituximab ($p = 0.002$).[310] Treatment of 54 patients with rituximab-refractory follicular NHL with ^{90}Y-ibritumomab tiuxetan resulted in an overall response rate of 74%, with 15% achieving complete remission.[311] Extended follow-up of 211 patients documented long-term responses of >12 months in 37% of patients with a median time to progression in the long-term responder group of 29.3 months.[312] The therapeutic potential of ^{90}Y-ibritumomab tiuxetan has been evaluated in combination with high-dose chemotherapy protocols,[313] as consolidation after induction therapy, including in other forms of B-cell lymphoma,[314–317] and as a front line monotherapy in patients with follicular lymphoma[318,319] with significant improvements in PFS and OS observed in most studies. However, FDA approval includes only treatment of relapsed and refractory low grade or follicular B-cell NHL and consolidation of treatment in patients with low grade or follicular B-cell NHL who have had a PR or CR to primary therapy.[320]

^{131}I-tositumomab

^{131}I-tositumomab (Bexxar®). Clinical procedures with ^{131}I-tositumomab are similar to those for ^{90}Y-ibritumomab tiuxetan except that in order to minimize thyroid radiation dose from dehalogenation of the radio-iodinated antibody, a thyroid protective dose of potassium iodide (or Lugols solution) is administered before treatment.[321] Also, injection of a 5 mCi dosimetry dose of ^{131}I-tositumomab is performed to determine the whole-body clearance rate in order to calculate total body dose—the antibody is then labeled with the ^{131}I activity estimated to yield a total body dose of 65 or 75 cGy, depending upon whether the platelet count is above or below 150,000/mm^3. Objective response rates of 47–68% and complete response rates of 20–38% following ^{131}I-tositumomab treatment were reported in a long-term analysis of 250 heavily pretreated patients with indolent lymphoma.[322] For complete responders, the median duration of response after the last qualifying chemotherapy was 6.1 months, whereas after RIT the median duration of response was >47 months. These results were similar to those obtained with the chimeric anti-CD20 antibody rituximab when labeled with ^{131}I.[323] On long-term follow-up, 6 of 12 patients with relapsed indolent lymphoma treated with ^{131}I-tositumomab remained disease free for a mean of 9.8 years after RIT.[324] RIT with ^{131}I-tositumomab at myeloablative doses followed by autologous stem cell infusion in relapsed/refractory NHL patients resulted in an overall response rate of 87%, and median PFS of 47.5 months and OS of 101.5 months.[325] Two phase III studies have shown similarly encouraging responses for single doses of ^{131}I-tositumomab and multiple doses of rituximab when combined with BEAM and CHOP chemotherapy for the treatment of relapsed DLBCL[326] and previously untreated follicular NHL,[327] respectively.

Despite the positive response data obtained with Zevalin and Bexxar, neither agent has become the standard first-line treatment for patients with lymphoma. Moreover, more than 60 RIT clinical trials have been reported in nonsolid tumors, largely CD20-positive, without additional FDA approvals.[328] Because of poor sales, GlaxoSmithKline stopped selling Bexxar in 2014, and there is speculation that Zevalin (Spectrum Pharmaceuticals) could suffer a similar fate. This situation can be attributed to several factors, some related to these drugs and others of a more general nature. Current regulations require radioactive drugs to be administered by nuclear medicine or radiation oncology staff, not by the oncologists who are responsible for the care of NHL patients. This results in a financial disincentive for oncologists who are paid to administer chemotherapy and rituximab but not RIT agents. Moreover, RIT is performed in the hospital setting, not in an outpatient facility, and performance of the companion imaging study to determine patient-specific dosing complicates scheduling of other procedures including the RIT. Finally, with these RIT treatments, there is a risk of developing secondary malignancies including acute myeloid leukemia (AML) and myelodysplasia (MDS).[329] However, a meta-analysis of 29 studies indicated that 3% of patients treated with RIT developed MDS/AML, comparable to 3% with CHOP alone and 5% with other NHL regimens.[330]

Radioimmunotherapy of solid tumors

The successful treatment of solid tumors with RIT has been much more difficult to achieve. Over the last decade, there have been more than 10 clinical trials reported that evaluate RIT in solid tumors with two in phase III and with no US FDA approvals.[331] Clinical trials activity in patients with solid tumors has fallen considerably during the past 20 years.[305,332] Despite a substantial amount of promising preclinical research, the lack of success in the clinic can be related to several factors, not the least of which is the lower sensitivity of solid tumors to radiation. With external beam radiation, doses as low as 4 Gy can be effective in lymphoma while with solid tumors including breast, lung, prostate, colorectal, and pancreatic carcinoma as well as glioblastoma, clinical responses generally require doses ranging from 50 to 80 Gy.[333] The fact that apoptosis is the predominant mechanism in cell killing in NHL but not solid tumors plays a role in their differential response to radiation.[299] Other barriers to effective treatment of solid tumors by RIT include accessibility of large intact antibodies to tumor cells in the face of tumor interstitial pressure and heterogeneous blood flow, and tumor hypoxia. The results of trials in patients with solid tumors have been summarized in several reviews[305,334,335] and in general, variable tumor responses were observed that were less impressive than those seen in hematological malignancies. Some of the most encouraging results have been obtained in minimum residual disease settings, which can minimize the deleterious effects of heterogeneous dose deposition and are difficult to treat by conventional approaches. Examples of promising work evaluating this strategy are the treatment of colorectal cancer, prostate cancer, and brain tumors after surgical debulking.

Strategies for improved radioimmunotherapy

Particularly for the treatment of patients with solid tumors, improving RIT therapeutic outcomes will require the development of more sophisticated strategies both in terms of the antibody-derived delivery vehicle and the nature of the radionuclide. Full-length immunoglobulins are approximately 150 kDa and are not readily cleared by the kidney, which excludes proteins of >70 kDa. Long half-lives of intact immunoglobulins result in greater exposure of normal tissues including bone marrow and liver to radiation from radionuclide conjugates. A variety of enzymatically and genetically derived antibody fragments of varying size have been evaluated[336,337] with the goal of seeking the best balance between better tumor penetration and more rapid normal tissue clearance, achievable with smaller constructs, and longer tumor residence time, generally better with intact IgG antibodies. Enzymatic preparation of F(ab)$_2$ (~110 kDa) and F(ab) (50–55 kDa) fragments can be labor intensive and inefficient and these fragments are often unstable in vivo. Smaller genetically engineered constructs include minibodies (75 kDa), diabodies (55 kDa), scFvs (26 kDa), nanobodies (12 kDa), and affibodies (6 kDa).[338] Radionuclide-fragment conjugates have shown promise in preclinical and early phase clinical studies with studies using HER2-targeted affibodies and nanobodies rapidly advancing to the clinic.[339]

Tumor vasculature plays an important role in that it provides an impediment to homogeneous antibody delivery, which might be overcome through the use of vascular disruptive agents such as combretastatin.[340] On the other hand, tumor vasculature provides an intriguing target for RIT, because damaging tumor blood vessels could increase the efficiency and homogeneity of treatment.[341] Approaches for improving RIT that have received particular attention including pretargeting and alpha-particle emitting radionuclides.

In pretargeting, the antibody is administered first, and after a delay period to achieve sufficient uptake in the tumor and normal tissue clearance, a radiolabeled lower-molecular-weight compound is injected. By shifting the label from the antibody to a smaller molecule, enhanced tumor-to-normal tissue ratios and tumor radiation dose can be achieved.[342] Initial approaches used antibody–streptavidin conjugates followed by radiolabeled biotin, with or without an intermediate clearing agent;[343] however, immunogenicity and interference by endogenous biotin were confounding factors. A second pretargeting tactic that has also entered the stage of clinical investigation involves the use of bispecific antibodies that bind to a tumor-associated molecular target as well as to a small molecule or peptide containing a radiometal-chelate complex.[344] The feasibility of this approach has been evaluated in patients with recurrent medullary thyroid carcinoma.[345] Patients first received a bispecific anti-CEA antibody and then after 4 days, ^{131}I-labeled peptide bearing two hapten groups. Median OS was 110 months, significantly longer than that observed in untreated patients (61 months). The technology for pretargeting continues to improve[346] raising hope that this strategy may have meaningful impact on the treatment of patients with solid tumors in the not too distant future.

The most attractive feature of alpha-particle–emitting radionuclides for RIT is their markedly increased potency compared with other types of radiation, given the high rate of LET. Studies in cell culture have demonstrated that human tumor cells can be killed after only a few alpha particles traverse a cell.[347] Furthermore, the cytotoxicity of alpha particles is nearly independent of dose rate, oxygen concentration, and cell cycle stage.[299] While the conceptual advantages of alpha particles for RIT were known for a long time, practical investigation in patients required developments in radionuclide production, protein-labeling chemistry, and radiation dosimetry. Alpha-emitting isotopes including ^{213}Bi, ^{225}Ac, ^{227}Th, and ^{211}At have been conjugated with monoclonal antibodies and their fragments to treat patients with brain tumors, melanoma, bladder cancer, neuroendocrine tumors, and prostate cancer, as well as leukemias and lymphomas.[348,349]

Therapy with targeted toxins

Targeted toxins are recombinantly derived fusion proteins that link cytokines or monoclonal antibody fragments with toxic moieties, generally derived from bacteria. For the three US FDA approved targeted toxins, fragments of bacterial toxins (diphtheria or pseudomonas) have been genetically engineered to eliminate binding to normal tissues and then fused with cytokines (IL-2 or IL-3) or antibody fragments (anti-CD22 Fv) that direct their binding to the surface of cancer cells, rather than to normal tissues. After internalization, the bacterial toxin domain catalytically inactivates cytosolic protein synthesis and triggers cancer cell death. This approach has produced useful clinical activity against three rare neoplasms: cutaneous T-cell leukemia, blastic plasmacytoid dendritic cell neoplasm, and hairy cell leukemia (HCL).

Targeted toxins for leukemia and lymphoma

Denileukin diftitox

Denileukin diftitox (Ontak®) is a recombinantly derived cytokine-toxin fusion protein that replaces the C-terminal cell-binding domain of diphtheria toxin with human interleukin-2 (IL-2) to kill cancer cells that express the CD25 component of the IL-2 receptor. Once bound to IL-2 expressing cancer cells, the central domain of the toxin facilitates transfer of the protein to the cytosol where the N-terminal domain of the toxin catalyzes ADP-ribosylation of elongation factor-2 (EF-2) that inactivates cellular protein synthesis leading to cell death.

Cutaneous T-cell lymphoma. Denileukin diftitox was approved by the US FDA in 1999 for treatment of persistent or recurrent cutaneous T-cell lymphoma (CTCL) based on two trials.[350] The first was a 3-arm randomized trial of 144 patients with stage Ia to III CTCL, comparing two dose levels of the agent versus placebo. The two dose levels enhanced ORR by 31% and 22% ($p = 0.002$ and $p = 0.03$) with median durations of 220 and 270 days. PFS was also prolonged (HR 0.27 and 0.42; $p = 0.0002$ and $p = 0.02$). The second was in 71 patients with previously treated persistent or recurrent CTCL, comparing two dose levels without a placebo control.[351] Clinical responses were seen in 30% of patients receiving denileukin diftitox lasting a median of 6.9 months. In later follow-up, there were a number of patients with maintained responses over 2 years.[352] The IL-2 cytokine-toxin also yields responses in other T- and B-cell neoplasms with Il-2 receptors.[353–360] Denileukin diftitox was, however, removed from the market in 2014.

Toxicity. Adverse events included flu-like symptoms (fever/chills, nausea/vomiting, and myalgias/arthralgias), acute infusion-related events (hypotension, dyspnea, chest pain, and back pain), and a vascular leak syndrome (hypotension, hypoalbuminemia, and edema), transient elevations of hepatic transaminase levels, and hypoalbuminemia. Most patients developed antibodies to the agent, but this did not correlate with toxicity or inversely with response. Further, rare toxicities of thyrotoxicosis and vision loss were reported.[361,362]

Tagraxofusp-erzs

Tagraxofusp-erzs (Elzonris®) utilized the same principle to generate a recombinant cytokine-toxin fusion protein where the catalytic and translocation domains of diphtheria toxin are linked to human interleukin-3 (IL-3) that targets CD123, the Interleukin-3 receptor A. US FDA approval was granted in 2018 for treatment of blastic plasmacytoid dendritic cell neoplasm (BPDCL), based on a single-arm trial with 13 previously untreated patients where 7 (53.8%) had CRs.[363] In 15 patients with relapsed or refractory BPDCL, one CR was observed lasting 111 days and 1 complete clinical response lasted 424 days. The median duration of response was 5 months, but 2 patients remained in remission for greater than 2 years.[364]

Toxicity. The most common side effects (>30%) include capillary leak syndrome, nausea, fatigue, peripheral edema, fever, chills, and increased weight. Frequently occurring laboratory abnormalities (>50%) include anemia, thrombocytopenia, hypoalbuminemia, hyponatremia, and increases in transaminases and glucose. Antidiphtheria antibodies were present in 96% of patients prior to treatment related to routine diphtheria immunization. Some 99% of patients evaluable for treatment-emergent antidiphtheria antibodies tested positive, with most having an increase in titer by the end of the second cycle of Tagraxofusp-erzs.

Moxetumomab pasudotox.tdfk

Moxetumomab pasudotox.tdfk (Lumoxiti®) is a recombinantly derived 63 kDa fusion protein that links an anti-CD22 Fv immunoglobulin fragment with a modified pseudomonas exotoxin fragment of 38 kDa that had been molecularly engineered to eliminate normal tissue binding through deletions in its N- and C-terminal domains while retaining its ability to translocate from the cell surface to the cytosol and to ADP ribosylate elongation factor 2, inhibiting protein synthesis and inducing apoptosis. The immunotoxin was approved by the US FDA in 2018 for treatment of refractory HCL in patients who have received at least two prior systemic therapies including treatment with a purine nucleoside analog.[365] Approval was based on a single-arm study in 80 patients with HCL who had an ORR of 75% with a 41% CR. With long term follow-up, 34% of all patients were minimal residual disease (MRD) negative and 61% of CRs lasted ≥60 months.[366]

Toxicity. Side effects (≥20%) included infusion-related reactions, edema, nausea, fatigue, headache, pyrexia, constipation, anemia, and diarrhea. Laboratory abnormalities (≥50%) included elevated creatinine, ALT, AST and decreased albumin, calcium, and phosphorus. Hemolytic uremic and capillary leak syndromes were each reported in ≤10% of patients, and ≤5% had grade 3–4 events. Adverse events were generally reversible and no treatment-related deaths were reported. Only 5% of patients developed neutralizing antibodies beyond cycle 1 of treatment.

Conclusions

Toxicities associated with targeted toxins can relate to the presence of targets on normal tissue—IL-2, IL-3, and CD22—or to nonspecific uptake by hepatocytes, vascular epithelia, or macrophage protein receptors, producing elevation of hepatic enzymes, vascular leak syndrome, and acute infusion reactions. Prophylactic corticosteroids can ameliorate some of these toxicities.

Most of the targeted toxins have short circulating half-lives with rapid clearance in the kidney and liver. Given their large size and rapid clearance, penetration of these drugs into solid tumors has been limited and the greatest activity has been seen against leukemias and lymphomas. As diphtheria and pseudomonas toxins are foreign proteins, an immune response is either present prior to treatment or develops soon after treatment is initiated, potentially neutralizing the targeted toxin and hastening its clearance. Retreatment can prove problematic. Despite these limitations, long-term remissions have been induced with a particularly impressive effect of moxetumomab pasudotox on heavily pretreated HCL. This may relate in some cases to the immunosuppression observed with these malignancies, decreasing the humoral response to the bacterial protein fragments.

Acknowledgment

The authors gratefully acknowledge Arthur E. Frankel, MD, a previous contributor to this chapter in earlier editions.

Key references

The complete reference list can be found on Vital Source version of this title, see inside front cover.

1. Kohler G, Milstein C. Continuous cultures of fused cells secreting antibody of predefined specificity. *Nature*. 1975;**256**:495–497.
3. Teo EC, Chew Y, Phipps C. A review of monoclonal antibody therapies in lymphoma. *Crit Rev Oncol Hematol*. 2016;**97**:72–84.
6. Levy R. Karnofsky lecture: Immunotherapy of lymphoma. *J Clin Oncol*. 1999;**17**:7–12.
7. Reichart, J.M. http://www.antibodysociety.org/news/approved_mabs.php
12. Miller RA, Maloney DG, Warnke R, et al. Treatment of B-cell lymphoma with monoclonal anti-idiotype antibody. *N Engl J Med*. 1982;**306**:517–522.

24 Cheson BD, Leonard JP. Monoclonal antibody therapy for B-cell non-Hodgkin's lymphoma. *N Engl J Med.* 2008;**359**:613–626.

27 Coiffier B, Lepage E, Briere E, et al. CHOP chemotherapy plus rituximab compared with CHOP alone in elderly patients with diffuse large B-cell lymphoma. *New Engl J Med.* 2002;**346**:235–242.

43 Mozessohn L, Chan KKW, Feld JJ, et al. Hepatitis B reactivation in HBsAg-negative/HBcAb-positive patients receiving rituximab for lymphoma: a meta-analysis. *J Viral Hepat.* 2015;**22**:842–849.

51 Hillmen P, Robak T, Janssens A, et al. Ofatumumab + chlorambucil versus chlorambucil alone in patients with untreated chronic lymphocytic leukemia (CLL): results of the phase III study complement 1 (OMB110911). *Blood.* 2013;**122**:528a.

54 GoedeV FK, Busch R, et al. Obinutuzumab plus chlorambucil in patients with CLL and coexisting conditions. *N Engl J Med.* 2014;**370**:1101–1110.

57 Sehn LH, Chua N, Mayer J, et al. A randomized controlled trial of obinutuzumab plus bendamustine versus bendamustine alone in patients with rituximab-refractory indolent non-Hodgkin lymphoma: primary results of the GADOLIN study. *Lancet Oncol.* 2016;**17**:1081–1093.

63 Salles G, Duell J, González Barca E, et al. Tafasitamab plus lenalidomide in relapsed or refractory diffuse large B-cell lymphoma (L-MIND): a multicentre,prospective, single-arm, phase 2 study. *Lancet Oncol.* 2020;**21**:978–988.

65 Kim YH, Bagot M, Pinter-Brown L, et al. Mogamulizumab versus vorinostat in previously treated cutaneous T-cell lymphoma (MAVORIC): an international, open-label, randomised, controlled phase 3 trial. *Lancet Oncol.* 2018;**19**:1192–1204.

70 Dimopoulos MA, Dytfeld D, Grosicki S, et al. Elotuzumab plus pomalidomide and dexamethasone for multiple myeloma. *N Engl J Med.* 2018;**379**:1811–1822.

74 Dimopoulos MA, Oriol A, Nahi H, et al. Daratumumab, lenalidomide, and dexamethasone for multiple myeloma. *N Engl J Med.* 2016;**375**:1319–1331.

88 Moreau P, Dimopoulos MA, Mikhael J, et al. Isatuximab, carfilzomib, and examethasone in relapsed multiple myeloma (IKEMA): a multicentre, open-label, randomised phase 3 trial. *Lancet.* 2021;**397**:2361–2371.

91 Van Rhee F, Wong R, Nikhil M, et al. Siltuximab for multi-centric Castleman's disease: a randomised, double-blind, placebo-controlled trial. *Lancet Oncol.* 2014;**15**:966–974.

100 Jonker DJ, O'Callaghan CJ, Carpetis CS, et al. Cetuximab for treatment of colorectal cancer. *New Engl J Med.* 2007;**357**:2040–2048.

106 Kopetz S, Grothey A, Yaeger R, et al. Encorafenib, binimetinib, and cetuximab in BRAF V600E–mutated colorectal cancer. *N Engl J Med.* 2019;**381**:1632–1643.

109 Vermorken JB, Mesia R, Rivera F. Platinum-based chemotherapy and cetuximab in head and neck cancer. *New Engl J Med.* 2008;**359**:1116–1127.

123 Pouget JP, Navarro-Teulon I, Bardies M, et al. Clinical radioimmunotherapy – the role of radiobiology. *Nat Rev Clin Oncol.* 2011;**8**:720–734.

134 Slamon DJ, Leyland-Jones B, Shak S, et al. Use of chemotherapy plus a monoclonal antibody against HER2 for metastatic breast cancer that overexpresses HER2. *N Engl J Med.* 2001;**344**:783–792.

147 Bang YJ, Van Cutsem E, Feyereislova A. Trastuzumab in combination with chemotherapy versus chemotherapy alone for treatment of HER-2 positive advanced gastric or gastro-esophageal junction cancer (ToGA): a phase 3, open label, randomized controlled trial. *Lancet.* 2010;**376**:687–697.

156 Swain SM, Baselga J, Kim S-B, et al. Pertuzumab, trastuzumab and docetaxel in HER-2 positive metastatic breast cancer. *New Engl J Med.* 2015;**372**:724–734.

160 Yu AL, Gilman L, Oskaynak MF, et al. Anti-GD2 antibody with GM-CSF, interleukin-2, and isotretinoin for neuroblastoma. *N Engl J Med.* 2010;**363**:1324–1334.

169 Hurwitz H, Fehrenbacher L, Novotny W, et al. Bevacizumab plus irinotecan, fluorouracil, and leucovorin for metastatic colorectal cancer. *N Engl J Med.* 2004;**350**:2335–2342.

185 Yang JC, Haworth L, Sherry RM, et al. A randomized trial of bevacizumab, an anti-vascular endothelial growth factor antibody, for metastatic renal cancer. *N Engl J Med.* 2003;**349**:427–434.

189 Gilbert MR, Dignam JJ, Armstrong TS, et al. A randomized trial of bevacizumab for newly diagnosed glioblastoma. *New Engl J Med.* 2014;**370**:699–708.

193 Burger RA, Brady MF, Bookman MA, et al. Gynecologic Oncology Group. Incorporation of bevacizumab in the primary treatment of ovarian cancer. *N Engl J Med.* 2011;**365**:2473–2483.

201 Garon EB, Ciuleanu TE, Arrieta O, et al. Ramucirumab plus docetaxel versus placebo plus docetaxel for second-line treatment of stage IV non-small-cell lung cancer after disease progression on platinum-based therapy (REVEL): a multicentre, double-blind, randomised phase 3 trial. *Lancet.* 2014;**382**:665–673.

213 https://www.accessdata.fda.gov/drugsatfda_docs/label/2021/125554s091lbl.pdf

214 Robert C, Long GV, Brady B, et al. Nivolumab in previously untreated melanoma without BRAF mutation. *N Engl J Med.* 2015;**372**:320.30.

216 Weber J, Mandala M, Del Vecchio M, et al. Adjuvant Nivolumab versus Ipilimumab in Resected Stage III or IV Melanoma. *N Engl J Med.* 2017;**377**:1824–1835.

221 Postow MA, Chesney J, Pavlick A, et al. Nivolumab and ipilimumab in untreated melanoma. *New Engl J Med.* 2015;**372**:2006–2017.

222 Larkin J, Chiarion-Sileni V, Gonzalez R, et al. Combined nivolumab and ipilimumab in untreated melanoma. *New Engl J Med.* 2015;**373**:23–34.

223 Wolchok JD, Charion-Silenti V, Gonzales R, et al. Long-term outcomes with nivolumab plus ipilimumab or nivolumab alone versus ipilimumab in patients with advanced melanoma. *Clin Cancer Res.* 2021;**40**:127–137.

228 Eggermont AMM, Blank CU, Mandala M, et al. Adjuvant pembrolizumab versus placebo in resected stage III melanoma. *N Engl J Med.* 2018;**378**:1789–1801.

229 Eggermont AMM, Blank CU, Mandalà M, et al. Adjuvant pembrolizumab versus placebo in resected stage III melanoma (EORTC 1325-MG/KEYNOTE-054): distant metastasis-free survival results from a double-blind, randomised controlled phase 3 trial. *Lancet Oncol.* 2021;**22**:643–654.

231 Choueiri TK, Tomczak P, Park SH, et al. Adjuvant pembrolizumab after nephrectomy in renal cell carcinoma. *New Engl J Med.* 2021;**385**:683–694.

234 Herbst RS, Giaccone G, de Marinis F, et al. Atezolizumab for first-line treatment of PD-L1–selected patients with NSCLC. *N Engl J Med.* 2020;**383**:1328–1339.

236 Finn RS, Qin S, Ikeda M, et al. Atezolizumab plus bevacizumab in unresectable hepatocellular carcinoma. *N Engl J Med.* 2020;**382**:1894–1905.

242 Powles T, Park SH, Voog E, et al. Avelumab maintenance therapy for advanced or metastatic urothelial carcinoma. *N Engl J Med.* 2020;**383**:1218–1230.

245 Kantarjian H, Stein A, Gökbuget N, et al. Blinatumomab versus chemotherapy for advanced acute lymphoblastic leukemia. *N Engl J Med.* 2017;**376**:836–847.

271 Sievers EL, Larson RA, Stadtmauer EA, et al. Efficacy and safety of gemtuzumab ozogamicin in patients with CD33-positive acute myeloid leukemia in first relapse. *J Clin Oncol.* 2001;**19**:3244–3254.

277 Connors JM, Jurczak W, Straus DJ, et al. Brentuximab Vedotin with chemotherapy for stage III or IV Hodgkin's lymphoma. *N Engl J Med.* 2018;**378**:331–344.

281 Sehn LH, Herrera AF, Flowers CR, et al. Polatuzumab vedotin in relapsed or refractory diffuse large B-cell lymphoma. *J Clin Oncol.* 2019;**38**:155–165.

284 Amiri-Kordestani L, Blumenthal GM, Xu QC, et al. FDA approval: ado-trastuzumab emtansine for the treatment of patients with HER2-positive metastatic breast cancer. *Clin Cancer Res.* 2014;**20**:4436–4441.

286 von Minckwitz G, Huang CS, Mano MS, et al. Trastuzumab emtansine for residual invasive HER2-positive breast xancer. *N Engl J Med.* 2019;**380**:617–628.

288 Modi S, Saura C, Yamashita T, et al. Trastuzumab deruxtecan in previously treated HER2-positive breast cancer. *N Engl J Med.* 2020;**382**:610–621.

294 Bardia A, Mayer IA, Vahdat LT, et al. Sacituzumab govitecan-hziy in refractory metastatic triple-negative breast cancer. *N Engl J Med.* 2019;**380**:741–751.

297 Powles T, Rosenberg JE, Sonpavde GP, et al. Enfortumab vedotin in previously treated advanced urothelial carcinoma. *N Engl J Med.* 2021;**384**:1125–1135.

298 Sgorous G, Hobbs RF. Dosimetry for radiopharmaceutical therapy. *Semin Nucl Med.* 2014;**44**:172–178.

300 Prise KM, O'Sullivan JM. Radiation-induced bystander signaling in cancer therapy. *Nat Rev Cancer.* 2009;**9**:351–360.

304 Huclier-Markai S, Alliot C, Varenot N, et al. Alpha-emitters for immunotherapy: a review of recent developments from chemistry to clinics. *Curr Top Med Chem.* 2012;**12**:2642–2654.

307 Macklis RM, Pohlman B. Radioimmunotherapy for non-Hodgkin's lymphoma: a review for radiation oncologists. *Int J Radiat Oncol Biol Phys.* 2006;**66**:833–841.

328 Rondon A, Rouanet J, Degoul F. Radioimmunotherapy in oncology: overview of the last decade clinical trials. *Cancer.* 2021;**13**:5570.

348 Zalutsky MR, Reardon DA, Akabani G, et al. Clinical experience with alpha-particle emitting 211At: treatment of recurrent brain tumor patients with 211At-labeled chimeric antitenascin monoclonal antibody 81C6. *J Nucl Med.* 2008;**49**:30–38.

351 Olsen E, Duvic M, Frankel A, et al. Pivotal phase III trial of two dose levels of denileukin diftitox for the treatment of cutaneous T-cell lymphoma. *J Clin Oncol.* 2001;**19**:376–388.

364 Frankel AE, Woo JH, Ahn C, et al. Activity of SL-401, a targeted therapy directed to interleukin-3 receptor, in blastic plasmacytoid dendritic cell neoplasm patients. *Blood.* 2014;**124**:385–392.

366 Kreitman RJ, Deardon C, Zinzani PL, et al. Moxetumomab pasudotox in heavily pre-treated patients with relapsed/refractory hairy cell leukemia (HCL): long-term follow-up from the pivotal trial. *J Hematol Oncol.* 2021;**14**:35.

61 Vaccines and immunomodulators

Jeffrey Schlom, PhD ■ Sofia R. Gameiro, PhD ■ Claudia Palena, PhD ■ James L. Gulley, MD, PhD, FACP

> **Overview**
>
> This article provides an overview of vaccine trials for a range of human cancers. It is not meant to be a compendium of all completed and ongoing trials. The vast majority of ongoing trials involve combination therapies with checkpoint inhibitor monoclonal antibodies and/or other immunomodulators. This article also deals with two concepts that are emerging as important to consider in cancer vaccine trials: tumor cell plasticity and epigenetic modulation of tumor cells and immune cells.

Introduction

Therapeutic cancer vaccines are designed to elicit a T-cell-based antitumor immune response by immunizing the patient against one or more antigens expressed by the cancer cells. Although the development of vaccines to treat established tumors has so far been challenging, recent advances in our understanding of the complexity of the tumor, its microenvironment, and the immune system are providing insights on how to best utilize cancer vaccines in the context of other therapeutics. Here, we discuss advances on the use of cancer vaccines in the context of standard-of-care therapies, targeted therapies, and other immunotherapeutics, including checkpoint inhibitors and immunomodulatory agents. This article summarizes clinical studies conducted with cancer vaccines both as monotherapy and in combination studies and emphasizes novel directions of the cancer vaccine field.

Targets for vaccine therapy

Many potential tumor-associated antigen (TAA) targets for cancer immunotherapy have been identified. Targets of vaccine therapy need not be cell-surface proteins. When a molecule is a target for vaccine therapy, the activated T cells induced by vaccination recognize complexes of tumor antigen peptide and major histocompatibility complex (MHC) molecules on the cell surface. TAA vaccine targets can be grouped into several major categories (Table 1).

Tumor-specific antigens

Tumor-specific antigens comprise gene products that are uniquely expressed in tumors, such as point-mutated *ras* oncogenes, p53 mutations, and products of ribonucleic acid (RNA) splice variants and gene translocations. Three mutations at codon 12 represent the vast majority of *ras* mutations, which are found in approximately 20–30% of some human tumors.[2] Although the *ras* protein is not found on the cell surface, one can envision vaccine therapy directed against peptide–MHC complexes on the cell surface. Indeed, there have been clinical trials in pancreatic carcinoma that target *ras*.[3,4] B-cell lymphomas overexpress a single immunoglobulin variant on their cell surface; therefore, each B-cell lymphoma displays a unique target for immunotherapy.[5–7] Mutation-associated neoantigens have also been targeted with personalized vaccine strategies. The gene products of RNA splice variants and deoxyribonucleic acid (DNA) translocations also represent unique fusion proteins that can be specific targets for immunotherapy, including c-erb-B2 RNA splice variants and the bcr/abl product of DNA translocation of chronic myelogenous leukemia.

Several viruses are associated with the etiology of some cancers. An excellent example of this is the connection between the human papillomavirus (HPV) and cervical cancer. This has led to approval by the US Food and Drug Administration (FDA) of the HPV vaccine for prevention of cervical cancer.[8]

Tumor-associated antigens

TAAs can be categorized into three major groups: oncofetal antigens, oncogene products, and tissue-lineage antigens (Table 1). Oncofetal antigens, normally found during fetal development, are greatly downregulated after birth. This class of antigens, which includes prostate-specific membrane antigen (PSMA), carcinoembryonic antigen (CEA), and the cancer mucin MUC-1, are often overexpressed in tumors compared with normal tissues. The MUC-1 TAA is overexpressed in the majority of human carcinomas and several hematologic malignancies. Much attention has been paid to the hypoglycosylated variable number of tandem repeats (VNTR) region of the N-terminus of MUC-1 as a vaccine target. While previous studies have described MUC-1 as a tumor-associated tissue differentiation antigen, studies have now determined that the C-terminus of MUC1 is an oncoprotein, and its expression is an indication of poor prognosis in numerous tumor types.[9]

Oncogene and suppressor gene products, such as nonmutated HER2/neu and p53, are analogous to oncofetal antigens in that they can be overexpressed in tumors and may be expressed in some fetal and normal tissues. Similarly, telomerase, an enzyme important in cellular replication and chromosomal stability, is overexpressed in malignant cells as compared with most normal cells. Epitopes derived from human telomerase have been reported and presumably may be overexpressed by neoplastic cells.[10]

Tissue-lineage antigens such as prostate-specific antigen (PSA) and the melanocyte antigens MART-1/Melan A, tyrosinase, gp100, and TRP-1/gp75 are usually expressed in a tumor of a given type and the normal tissue from which it is derived. Tissue-lineage antigens are potentially useful targets for immunotherapy if the normal organ/tissue in which they are expressed is not essential, such as the prostate, breast, or melanocyte.

Table 1 Spectrum of current and potential therapeutic cancer vaccine targets.[a]

Tumor-specific antigens	
Neoantigen	Undefined unique tumor mutations, frame shift mutations
Oncogene	Point mutated: ras, B-raf
Viral	HPV, HCV
B-cell lymphoma	Anti-id
Tumor-associated antigens	
Oncofetal antigen	CEA, MUC-1
Stem cell/EMT	Brachyury, SOX-2, OCT-4, TERT, CD133
Oncogene	MUC-1 C terminus, p53, EGFR, HER2/neu, WT1
Cancer—testis	MAGE-A3, BAGE, SEREX-defined, NY-ESO, survivin
Tissue lineage	PAP, PSA, gp100, tyrosinase, glioma antigen
Glycopeptides	STn-KLH
Anti-angiogenic	VEGF-R

Abbreviations: BAGE, B melanoma antigen; CEA, carcinoembryonic antigen; EMT, epithelial–mesenchymal transition; gp100, glycoprotein 100; HCV, hepatitis C virus; HPV, human papillomavirus; MAGE-A3, melanoma-associated antigen-A3; MUC-1, mucin 1; NY-ESO, New York esophageal carcinoma antigen 1; OCT-4, octamer-binding transcription factor 4; PAP, prostatic acid phosphatase; PSA, prostate-specific antigen; SOX-2, (sex-determining region Y)-box-2; STn-KLH, sialyl-Tn–keyhole limpet hemocyanin; TERT, telomerase reverse transcriptase; VEGF-R, vascular endothelial growth factor receptor; WT-1, wild-type 1.
[a]Source: Adapted from Schlom et al.[1]

Types of vaccines

Numerous vaccine-delivery platforms have been analyzed in experimental models and many of these are now being evaluated in the clinic (Table 2). Each of these platforms has advantages and disadvantages. Some of these modalities may eventually prove to be most beneficial when used in combination or in tandem.

Table 2 Spectrum of current vaccine platforms in Phase 2/3 clinical studies.[a]

Vaccine platform	Example	Cancer type
Peptides/proteins		
Peptide	gp100, MUC-1, HER2/neu	Melanoma, lung
Protein	MAGE-A3, NY-ESO	Melanoma
Antibody	Anti-idiotype	Lymphoma
Glycoproteins	sTn-KLH	Melanoma
Recombinant vectors		
Adenoviruses	Adeno-CEA-MUC1-brachyury	Carcinoma
Poxvirus	rMVA, rFP-brachyury-TRICOM	Carcinoma
	CV301 (rMVA,rFP-CEA-MUC1)	
	rV, rF-PSA-TRICOM	Prostate
Saccharomyces cerevisiae-yeast	Yeast-CEA	Pancreatic
Listeria	Listeria–mesothelin	Pancreatic
Tumor cells		
Allogeneic	GVAX (+ GM-CSF)	Pancreatic
DC/autologous tumor cell fusions		Myeloma
Autologous	Adeno-CD40L, colon (BCG)	CLL, colon, melanoma
Dendritic cells/APCs		
DC–peptide	Glioma peptides	Glioma, melanoma
DC–vector infected	rV, rF-CEA-MUC1-TRICOM (Panvac-DC)	Colorectal
APC–protein	Sipuleucel-T (PAP-GM-CSF)	Prostate

Abbreviations: APC, antigen-presenting cell; BCG, Bacillus Calmette–Guerin adjuvant; CD40L, CD40 ligand; CEA, carcinoembryonic antigen; CLL, chronic lymphocytic leukemia; gp100, glycoprotein 100; GM-CSF, granulocyte-macrophage colony-stimulating factor; MAGE-A3, melanoma-associated antigen 3; MUC-1, mucin 1; NY-ESO, New York esophageal carcinoma antigen 1; PAP, prostatic acid phosphatase; PSA, prostate-specific antigen; rF, recombinant fowlpox; rV, recombinant vaccinia; STn-KLH, sialyl-Tn–keyhole limpet hemocyanin.
[a]Source: Adapted from Schlom et al.[1]

Vaccine clinical trials

HPV-associated malignancies

Human papillomavirus vaccines protect against infection with human papillomaviruses. About a dozen HPV types can cause certain types of cancer–cervical, anal, oropharyngeal, penile, vulvar, and vaginal.[11,12] Three vaccines that prevent infection with disease-causing HPV types are now licensed for use in the United States. All three vaccines prevent infection with HPV types 16 and 18.[13] Trials that led to the approval of Gardasil®9 found it to be nearly 100% effective in preventing cervical, vulvar, and vaginal disease caused by the five additional HPV types that it targets.[14]

While HPV preventive vaccines that induce antibodies to HPV have been extremely effective, T-cell-directed vaccines will be necessary for the treatment of HPV-induced cancers. Numerous clinical studies have previously been carried out employing vaccines targeting HPV-induced cancers. Employing HPV16 E6/E7 long peptides (25-mers) and adjuvants in trials in patients with vulvar intraepithelial neoplasia (VIN) showed clinical activity, an acceptable safety profile, and the generation of HPV-specific T cells.[15] The same vaccine was employed in patients with gynecological carcinoma with a similar safety profile (no adverse events greater than grade 2).[16,17] Recently, this HPV long peptide vaccine was employed in patients with advanced HPV-associated cancers in combination with the anti-programmed cell death 1 (PD-1) nivolumab. There were no toxicities above those seen with nivolumab alone. The response rate of 33% and median overall survival (mOS) were greater than that previously seen with vaccine alone or nivolumab alone.[18] While this trial was not randomized, it does support the concept of initiating trials of HPV vaccines in combination with checkpoint monoclonal antibodies (MAbs), and/or the bifunctional agent anti-programmed cell death protein-1 ligand (PD-L1)/TGFβ-RII (bintrafusp alfa).[19] Other vaccines directed against HPV have also been evaluated in clinical studies with good safety profiles. For example, two different plasmid DNA-based vaccines showed evidence of clinical responses in patients ($n = 152$) with cervical intraepithelial neoplasia, along with the generation of HPV-specific T cells and no serious adverse events.[20–22] In support of an HPV therapeutic vaccine, several reports in the literature demonstrate that the existence of human T-cell responses in patients with HPV-associated malignancies may predict survival or may be associated with a better clinical outcome.[23–27]

Melanoma

The vast majority of clinical studies involving therapeutic vaccines and, for that matter, immunotherapeutics have been carried out in patients with melanoma. This is attributable to two main factors: (1) melanoma lesions are accessible and thus studies of the effects of a given agent on the tumor microenvironment (TME) can be monitored both clinically and mechanistically, and (2) melanoma was shown to be an immunogenic or "hot" tumor type due to its response to type 1 cytokines such as IL-2 and interferons (IFN). Prior studies have shown that most melanoma lesions contain relatively high levels of T cells compared to other solid tumor types; this is due, in part, to their high mutational burden.[28] Clinical studies of melanoma vaccines have been undertaken targeting a range of TAAs and employing multiple vaccine platforms, including peptide-pulsed dendritic cells (DCs), peptide in adjuvant, and recombinant vectors. For the most part, many of these trials showed that vaccines generated T-cell responses to melanoma

TAAs, but little clinical improvement.[1,29,30] In a randomized, placebo-controlled, Phase 3 trial[31] using granulocyte-macrophage colony-stimulating factor (GM-CSF), versus peptide vaccine versus GM-CSF plus vaccine versus placebo in patients with no evidence of disease after complete surgical resection of locally advanced and/or stage IV melanoma, neither adjuvant GM-CSF nor vaccine significantly improved relapse-free survival or overall survival in patients with high-risk resected melanoma. On the other hand, some trials showed promise. A randomized Phase 3 trial was conducted involving patients expressing human leukocyte antigen HLA-A0201 ($n = 185$) with stage 4 or locally advanced stage 3 melanoma who met the criteria to receive high-dose IL-2 therapy. Patients were randomly assigned to receive IL-2 alone or vaccine containing gp100 peptide plus incomplete Freund's adjuvant, followed by IL-2. The vaccine–IL-2 group, as compared with the IL-2-only group, had a significant improvement in overall clinical response (16% vs 6%, $P = 0.03$) and mOS (17.8 months vs 11.1 months; $P = 0.06$).[32] In another trial, using three melanoma peptides, multiple groups were evaluated: peptide vaccine alone, or peptide vaccine combined with either GM-CSF, IFN-α2b, or both. At 25 months' follow-up, the mOS of patients with vaccine immune response was significantly longer than that of patients with no immune response (21.3 vs 13.4 months; $P = 0.046$).[33]

A Phase 2 study of autologous monocyte-derived mRNA electroporated DCs plus ipilimumab in patients ($n = 39$) with pretreated advanced melanoma showed promising results.[34] The overall tumor response rate was 38%, including seven complete responses with a median follow-up of 36 months. More recently, several studies are employing neoantigen vaccines with evidence of neoantigen T-cell responses and some clinical benefit.[35–37] At this time, however, no reports exist of a multicenter randomized trial employing a neoantigen vaccine.

Intratumoral injection of vectors is, in essence, a form of vaccination to induce the host to reject tumor cells expressing TAAs, following the initial lysis of a subpopulation of tumor cells. Talimogene laherparepvec (TVEC) has been approved by the FDA for the treatment of melanoma. In a Phase 3 trial, 29.5% of patients treated with TVEC had a complete response versus 0% treated with GM-CSF. The probability of maintaining a response to TVEC after 12 months was 73%.[38] A subsequent study showed that if PD-1 inhibition was combined with TVEC, the objective response rate in melanoma was 62%, with 33% of patients having a complete response.[39] This is a better response rate than that seen with PD-1 inhibition alone and suggests that vaccines can successfully create an inflammatory gradient needed to sustain a more effective immune-mediated killing.

Prostate cancer

Multiple vaccine trials in patients with prostate cancer have been carried out.[1] It should be noted that prostate cancer has been characterized as a "cold tumor," which does not respond to checkpoint antibody therapy. For example, in a randomized, double-blind, Phase 3 trial of ipilimumab versus placebo in asymptomatic or minimally symptomatic patients with metastatic chemotherapy-naive castration-resistant prostate cancer (mCRPC), there was no increase in OS in patients receiving ipilimumab versus control.[40] In prior studies, prostatic acid phosphatase (PAP), which is expressed on over 95% of prostate cancer cells, has been used as a target of the vaccine sipuleucel-T, also called Provenge® (PAP–GM-CSF-pulsed antigen-presenting cells). After early clinical trials of the sipuleucel-T vaccine demonstrated safety, larger trials were conducted in a symptomatic or minimally symptomatic mCRPC population. A Phase 3 trial[41] was conducted with OS as the endpoint, enrolling more than 500 patients. No change in time to progression was seen, but OS was improved in the vaccine arm (25.8 months vs 21.7 months; $P = 0.032$). In April 2010, the FDA approved sipuleucel-T for the treatment of minimal or nonsymptomatic mCRPC. GVAX, a GM-CSF-secreting vaccine, is an admixture of two prostate cancer cell lines that have been transduced with a replication-defective retrovirus for GM-CSF expression. In two separate multicenter Phase 2 trials, patients with asymptomatic CRPC given GVAX had a median survival of 26.2–35.0 months.[42,43] By estimating predicted survival based on a commonly used nomogram,[44] patients exceeded anticipated survival by >6 months.[45] A Phase 3 study of GVAX in the prechemotherapy setting compared GVAX to docetaxel with similar OS seen (HR 1.03) and about 20% of the serious adverse events in the vaccine arm (8.8% vs 43%).[46,47] A Phase 2 adenovirus/PSA vaccine trial was conducted in patients with recurrent or hormone-refractory prostate cancer. The majority of patients demonstrated anti-PSA T-cell responses above preinjection levels. Sixty-four percent of the patients demonstrated an increase in PSA doubling time.[48] PROSTVAC is a vector-based therapeutic cancer vaccine comprising a series of poxviral vectors (vaccinia during the initial priming vaccine and fowlpox for all boosts) engineered to express PSA and a triad of human T-cell costimulatory molecules.[49] In a Phase 2 study of PROSTVAC there was prolonged mOS by 8.5 months versus placebo in mCRPC.[49] In a Phase 3 trial, patients were randomly assigned to PROSTVAC, PROSTVAC plus GM-CSF, or placebo, and stratified by PSA.[50] Whereas PROSTVAC was safe and well tolerated, there was no effect on OS in mCRPC. This and other vaccine monotherapy trials were designed and initiated prior to the era of checkpoint inhibitor MAbs. Studies are ongoing combining PROSTVAC with checkpoint inhibitor MAbs and other immune-modulating agents. Recently, a pilot trial evaluated a DNA encoding PAP plus pembrolizumab. Eight of 13 (62%) patients treated concurrently and one of 12 (8%, $P = 0.01$) treated sequentially achieved PSA declines from baseline. Of these, two were over 50% and one was a complete PSA response, and some patients treated concurrently had decreases in tumor volume. PSA declines were associated with the development of PAP-specific T-cell immunity and CD8⁺ T-cell infiltration in metastatic tumor biopsy specimens. The results of this clinical trial showed for the first time that the efficacy of an antitumor vaccine can be improved by using concurrent PD-1 blockade.[51]

Breast cancer

In studies employing HER2/neu peptides with or without GM-CSF, patients with breast cancer were able to generate HER2-specific immune responses.[52–54] In a Phase 1/2 clinical trial in which breast cancer patients were vaccinated with E75, an HLA-A2/A3-restricted HER2/neu peptide and GM-CSF, based on a 24-month analysis, disease-free survival (DFS) was 94.3% in the vaccinated group and 86.8% in the control group ($P = 0.08$). In subset analyses, patients who benefited most from vaccination had lymph node-positive, HER2 IHC 1 to 2+, or grade 1 or 2 tumors and were optimally dosed.[55] The results of early phase clinical trials conducted to evaluate HER2-derived peptide vaccines administered to HER2⁺ breast cancer patients in the adjuvant setting suggest synergy between those vaccines and trastuzumab, the MAb targeting the HER2 protein.[56] In a related trial, a group of patients whose tumors have low HER2 expression was identified as benefiting from E75 vaccination with a much more robust immunologic response after vaccination than patients whose tumors overexpress HER2.[55] Fusion-cell (dendritic cells and tumor cells) vaccination of patients with metastatic breast cancer was shown to induce both immunological and clinical responses.[57] In a Phase 1/2 study, patients (n = 22) with stage IV HER2/neu+ breast cancer receiving trastuzumab therapy were vaccinated with an HER2/neu T-helper peptide-based vaccine.[58] Concurrent trastuzumab and HER2/neu vaccinations were well tolerated. Many patients had preexisting immunity specific for HER2/neu while being treated only with trastuzumab; that immunity was significantly boosted with vaccination. Epitope spreading within HER2/neu and to additional tumor-related antigens was stimulated by immunization. The magnitude of the T-cell response was significantly inversely correlated with serum TGF-β levels. In a randomized trial, 54 patients with biopsy-proven HER2+ ductal carcinoma in situ (DCIS) were vaccinated via intralesional or intranodal, or a combination of both before surgery.[59,60] The majority of patients had an increased immune response following vaccination.[59] The pathological complete response rate in patients with DCIS without invasive cancer was 28.6%.[59] Compared to historical responses of invasive cancers to DC vaccine, this provides evidence suggesting that vaccines may be more effective in patients with preinvasive or early disease with low tumor burden. Several clinical trials have also been carried out using the cancer mucin MUC-1 as a target, including the use of MUC-1 peptides,[61–63] recombinant vaccinia virus encoding MUC-1 and IL-2,[64] a modified vaccinia virus Ankara (MVA) expressing human MUC-1[65] and a mannan–MUC-1 fusion protein.[66,67]

Lung cancer
In a randomized Phase 3 trial employing a peptide-based MAGE-A3 vaccine in patients with resected MAGE-A3 tumors, there was no improvement in disease-free survival versus placebo.[68] An MVA encoding the MUC-1 and IL-2 genes was assessed in combination with first-line chemotherapy in patients (n = 74) with advanced non-small-cell lung cancer (NSCLC). Six-month progression-free survival (PFS) was 43.2% in the vaccine plus chemotherapy group versus 31.5% in the chemotherapy alone group.[69] Recent results employing this vaccine have shown a relationship between specific T-cell responses and improved survival.[70] Epitope spreading postvaccination was also observed.[70] Several other vaccine trials in patients with NSCLC have been previously described.[1]

Pancreatic cancer
Allogeneic whole tumor cell vaccines modified to secrete GM-CSF have been employed in patients with pancreatic cancer. Evidence of vaccine-induced immune responses was observed as measured by delayed-type hypersensitivity.[71,72] A 60-patient Phase 2 study of the same vaccine in the adjuvant setting showed that postchemotherapy induction of mesothelin-specific CD8 cells correlated with PFS.[73] The mOS was about 26 months compared with 21 months for chemotherapy alone in this same patient population at the same institution.[74]

GVAX and CRS-207 are cancer vaccines that have been evaluated in pancreatic ductal adenocarcinoma. In a Phase 2b, randomized, multicenter study, patients with previously treated metastatic pancreatic adenocarcinoma were randomized 1 : 1 : 1 to receive cyclophosphamide/GVAX + CRS-207 (live, attenuated Listeria monocytogenes expressing mesothelin) (arm A), CRS-207 (arm B), or physician's choice of single-agent chemotherapy (arm C). The study did not meet its primary efficacy endpoint.[75]

T-cell immunity has been associated with some long-term pancreatic cancer survivors. Using whole-exome sequencing and in silico neoantigen prediction, investigators found that tumors with both the highest neoantigen number and the most CD8+ T-cell infiltrates, but neither alone, stratified patients with the longest survival. Lasting circulating T-cell reactivity to neoantigens in long-term survivors of pancreatic cancer was also observed, including clones with specificity to high-quality neoantigens.[76]

Bladder and renal cell carcinoma
Intravesical bacillus Calmette-Guerin adjuvant (BCG) has been used successfully in the treatment of bladder cancer, implicating immune mechanisms.[77] Intravesical administration of wild-type vaccinia virus was shown to be safe in a small trial with three of four treated patients disease free at 4-year follow-up.[78] Recently, clinical studies have shown that an IL-15 superagonist[79] has antitumor activity when given intravesically, further indicating the potential immunogenicity of bladder carcinoma cells.

The response of renal carcinoma to high-dose IL-2 and IFNα also implicates immune mechanisms in therapeutic responses.[80] An autologous renal cell carcinoma (RCC) tumor-cell vaccine that was genetically modified to overexpress B7-1 to provide co-stimulation to tumor-reactive T cells was employed.[81] In this single-arm Phase 2 study, patients received vaccine and low-dose IL-2. Best responses were complete response (3%), partial response (5%), and stable disease (64%). A post hoc analysis suggested that lymphocytic infiltration of the vaccine site determined by biopsy directly correlated with survival (28.4 vs 17.8 months, $P = 0.045$).

In a Phase 2 study in patients with metastatic renal cell carcinoma (mRCC), OS was associated with T-cell responses against a vaccine (IMA901) comprising 10 tumor-associated peptides. A subsequent Phase 3 trial added IMA901 to sunitinib, first-line treatment in mRCC; study findings indicated that IMA901 did not improve OS when added to sunitinib.[82] AGS-003 is an autologous immunotherapy prepared from fully matured and optimized monocyte-derived DCs, which are co-electroporated with amplified tumor RNA plus synthetic CD40L RNA. In a Phase 2 trial in intermediate and poor risk, treatment-naive patients with metastatic clear cell RCC, patients were treated with AGS-003 in combination with sunitinib. Thirteen of 21 patients (62%) experienced clinical benefit (nine partial responses, four with stable disease). Seven (33%) patients survived for at least 4.5 years, while five (24%) survived for more than 5 years. Data from this trial indicated that AGS-003 in combination with sunitinib were well tolerated and generated immunologic responses and extension of median and long-term survival in intermediate and poor risk mRCC patients.[83]

Mesothelioma
CRS-207 is a live-attenuated Listeria monocytogenes engineered to express mesothelin, a TAA highly expressed in malignant pleural mesothelioma (MPM). In a multicenter, open-label Phase 1b study, patients with unresectable MPM received two priming infusions of CRS-207, followed by pemetrexed/cisplatin chemotherapy, and CRS-207 booster infusions. Of evaluable patients, 89% (31/35) had disease control with one complete response (3%), 19 partial responses (54%), and 10 stable disease (29%). The combination of CRS-207 and chemotherapy induced significant changes in the local TME and objective tumor responses in the majority of treated patients.[84]

Glioblastoma

A recent Phase 3 trial was conducted to evaluate the addition of DCVax®-L, an autologous tumor lysate-pulsed DC vaccine to standard therapy for newly diagnosed glioblastoma patients. After surgery and chemoradiotherapy, patients were randomized (2:1) to receive temozolomide plus DCVax-L or temozolomide and placebo. Following recurrence, all 331 patients were allowed to receive DCVax-L. Median OS was 23.1 months from surgery. Because of the cross-over trial design, nearly 90% of the intention-to-treat patients received vaccine. Two hundred twenty-three patients were ≥30 months past their surgery date. A population of extended survivors ($n=100$) achieved mOS of 40.5 months. The addition of DCVax-L to standard therapy is not only feasible in glioblastoma patients but also may extend survival.[85]

Leukemia

In four clinical trials,[86–90] patients with acute myeloid leukemia (AML) or myelodysplastic syndrome (MDS) were treated with Wilms Tumor Gene 1 (WT1) peptide vaccine. Vaccination was found to be well tolerated and resulted in the induction of WT1-specific T cells. Evidence of clinical activity was seen in a subset of patients, as demonstrated by prolonged remission and resolution of bone marrow blasts. In a recent Phase 1/2 trial, 66 patients with AML ($n=42$), chronic myelogenous leukemia ($n=13$), or MDS ($n=11$) were treated with a PR1 peptide vaccine consisting of an HLA-A2-restricted peptide derived from both proteinase 3 and neutrophil elastase; immune response was observed in 53% of these patients.[91] Clinical response was observed in 23% of patients with active disease, predominantly in patients with low disease burden, and correlated with immune response.[91] In patients with lymphoma, antigen-based vaccine approaches targeting idiotype demonstrated immune response, with promising clinical outcomes seen in several Phase 2 clinical trials.[92–94] However, results from three large randomized Phase 3 clinical trials did not demonstrate a survival advantage in vaccinated patients.[95,96] In chronic lymphocytic leukemia, vaccination with GVAX following reduced-intensity transplant was safe, induced immune response, and demonstrated a 2-year PFS of 82%.[97] A personalized cancer vaccine was developed in which patient-derived AML cells were fused with autologous DCs.[98] Vaccination of patients who were in remission postchemotherapy was well tolerated and associated with a significant increase in circulating T cells recognizing whole AML cells and leukemia-specific antigens, which persisted for more than 6 months. Twelve of 17 vaccinated patients (71%) remained alive without recurrence at a median follow-up of 57 months. The results demonstrated that a personalized vaccine for patients with AML who are in remission induces the expansion of leukemia-specific T cells and may be protective against disease relapse.[98]

Targeting of cancer plasticity

Cancer plasticity in tumor progression

Carcinoma cells are highly plastic and able to undergo remarkable phenotypic changes during progression toward metastasis or in response to therapies.[99] One of the phenomena driving these phenotypic changes is the epithelial–mesenchymal transition (EMT), a process that normally occurs along embryonic development, wound healing, and tissue regeneration, which can be co-opted by tumor cells.[100] The process of EMT can be driven by signals originating in one or more soluble factors in the TME, including TGF-β, IL-8, IL-6, or via the oncogenic activation of "EMT transcription factors," including brachyury, snail, slug, twist1, zeb1, and others, which ultimately control the expression of the genes involved in the phenotype switch. During this process, tumor cells lose epithelial features, including apical-basal cell polarity and intercellular junctions, while simultaneously acquiring mesenchymal qualities such as the expression of vimentin, enhanced cell motility, and increased invasiveness.[101,102] More importantly, the acquisition of mesenchymal phenotypic traits by carcinoma cells also leads to the acquisition of resistance to a variety of cell death-inducing signals, including chemotherapy, radiation, epidermal growth factor receptor (EGFR) kinase inhibitors,[103–105] and HER-2 directed therapy,[106] among others (Figure 1a). The relevant role of tumor phenotypic plasticity *in vivo* has now been recognized in multiple studies where tumor gene signatures indicative of an EMT have been associated with poor prognosis or therapy failure. In colorectal cancer, for example, tumors characterized by the expression of TGF-β and enriched in EMT features have been associated with the worst survival among all other molecular subtypes.[108] Similarly, an EMT-related gene signature in urothelial cancer has been correlated with worse OS and resistance to PD-1 blockade.[109] In light of these data, preventing or reverting the occurrence of tumor plasticity is being proposed as a novel approach to improve the outcome of antitumor therapies, including immunotherapies.

Brachyury as a driver of plasticity

One of the proteins relevant to tumor plasticity is brachyury, a transcription factor of the T-box family that plays an essential role during normal embryonic development by promoting the formation of the mesoderm,[110] a process that requires the generation of mesenchymal cells from primitive epithelial cell layers via an EMT. During this process, brachyury is temporarily expressed in the primitive streak,[111] where it promotes cell motility and migration.[112] In most adult normal tissues, expression of brachyury is undetectable, with the exception of very low levels found in normal testis, thyroid, and B cells.[113,114] These negligible levels of brachyury seen in normal tissues contrast with the expression in some human tumors, including in chordoma, lung adenocarcinoma, small cell lung cancer, embryonal carcinoma, triple-negative breast cancer, prostate, and colorectal carcinomas, which have been shown to express variable levels of brachyury in at least a fraction of the tumor cells.[115–121] More importantly, in several cancer types, the expression of brachyury in the primary tumor has been associated with poor prognosis, as it has been shown for breast, prostate, lung, colon, testicular cancer, and gastrointestinal stromal tumors (GIST).[118,119,122,123] Studies conducted with various preclinical cancer models have now shown that brachyury drives carcinoma cells into a mesenchymal-like, invasive phenotype, and cells with very high levels of brachyury have been shown to be more resistant to cell death[124–126] (Figure 1a).

Several studies have now shown the ability of brachyury to activate an immune response both *in vitro* and *in vivo* in preclinical studies and, more recently, in patients vaccinated with brachyury-targeting vaccines. In initial preclinical studies,[114] an HLA-A2-restricted epitope of brachyury, identified by an HLA-binding prediction algorithm, was used *in vitro* to expand brachyury-specific CD8+ T cells that were cytotoxic against brachyury-positive carcinoma cells.[118] In a later study, this peptide was modified by substitution of an amino acid at the MHC anchor

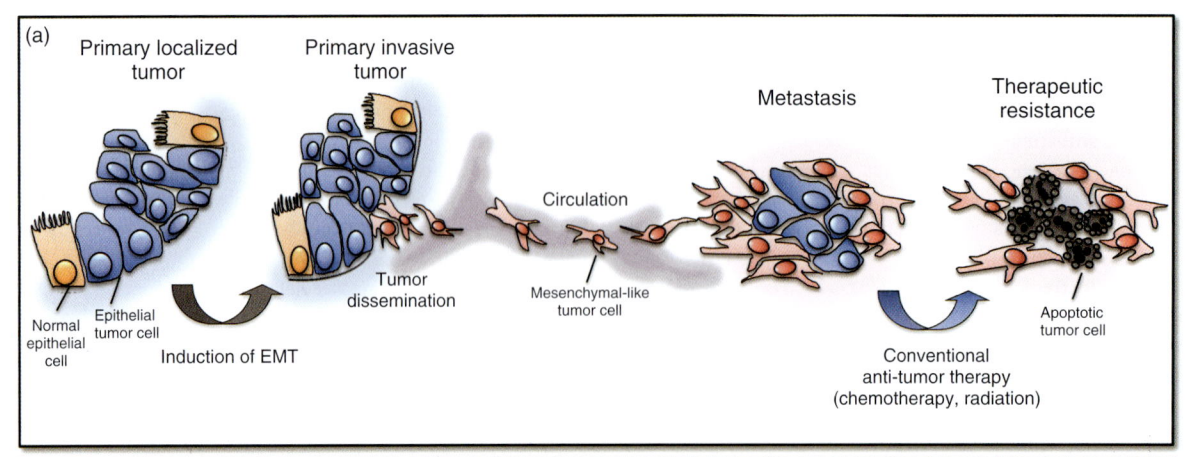

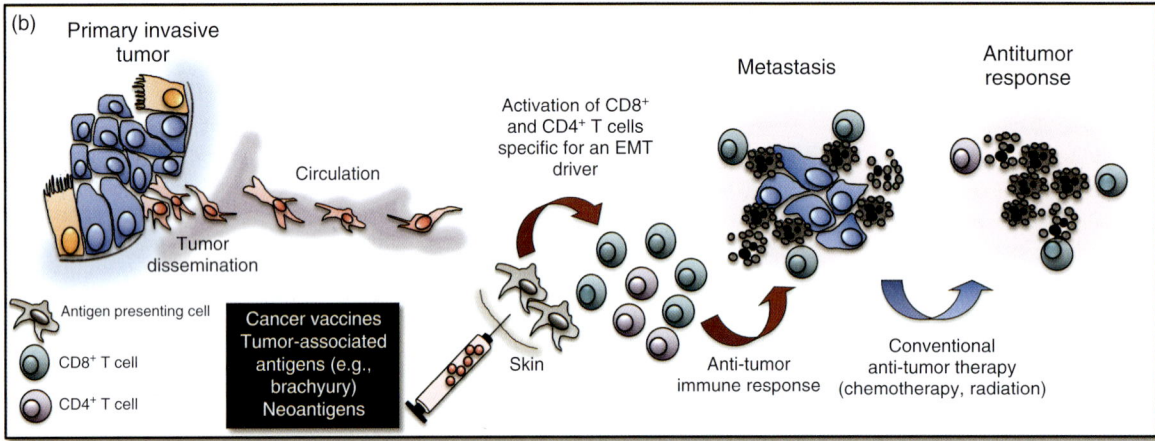

Figure 1 Targeting the epithelial–mesenchymal transition (EMT) to block metastatic dissemination and alleviate resistance to therapy. (a) EMT promotes the invasive potential of cancer cells, their propensity to generate distant metastases, and their resistance to chemo- and radiotherapy. (b) A vaccine directed against a driver of EMT could elicit an immune response that effectively targets malignant cells undergoing EMT. Combining this immunotherapeutic approach with conventional treatments targeting epithelial cancer cells might result in effective tumor eradication. Source: Adapted from Palena et al.[107]

position 9, resulting in an enhanced agonist able to better stimulate brachyury-specific T cells *in vitro* and *in vivo* in HLA-A2 transgenic mice.[127] The immunogenicity of brachyury was also shown with blood of cancer patients immunized against other tumor antigens, including CEA and PSA, whereby brachyury-specific T cells were observed posttreatment, thus indicating cross-presentation of tumor-associated brachyury to the immune system following vaccination.[128]

There are currently three vaccine platforms targeting the transcription factor brachyury. A recombinant *Saccharomyces cerevisiae* (yeast)–brachyury vaccine (GI-6301), consisting of heat-killed yeast that expresses the full-length human brachyury protein,[129] was first evaluated in a Phase 1 clinical trial in patients with chordoma or advanced carcinomas.[130] The vaccine was well tolerated and elicited brachyury-specific CD8+ and/or CD4+ T-cell responses in approximately 60% of patients postvaccination with some evidence of clinical activity in two of the chordoma patients enrolled in the study.[130] Based on these results, a Phase 2 clinical trial of the yeast-brachyury vaccine was also conducted in patients with chordoma randomized to receive radiation plus or minus vaccine.[131] Poxvirus-based brachyury vaccines encoding a triad of costimulatory molecules (TRICOM: B7-1, ICAM-1, LFA-3) have also been developed, including an MVA-brachyury-TRICOM for priming and a fowlpox-brachyury-TRICOM vaccine for boosting. These vaccines have been tested in Phase 1 clinical trials in patients with advanced carcinomas,[132,133] showing safety and the ability to elicit CD4+ and/or CD8+ T-cell responses in patients postvaccination. A third platform is composed of an adenoviral-based vaccine consisting of a mix of three recombinant adenoviral (Ad5) vectors encoding for brachyury, MUC-1, and CEA (termed TriAd5).[134] This vaccine has recently been evaluated in a Phase 1 clinical study in patients with advanced cancer demonstrating safety and the ability to induce CD4+ and/or CD8+ T-cell responses after vaccination to at least one TAA encoded by the vaccine, with approximately 83% of patients developing T-cell responses to MUC-1, 67% to CEA, and 50% to brachyury.[135] Altogether, these results demonstrated for the first time in humans that a transcription factor involved in the process of cancer plasticity could be immunologically targeted via vaccination. Multiple ongoing and planned Phase 2 clinical studies are incorporating brachyury-targeting vaccines in combination with other standard-of-care agents or immunotherapeutics, including checkpoint inhibitors and other immune modulators (Figure 1b).

Epigenetic therapies

Vaccine plus epigenetic modulators

Mounting preclinical evidence suggests that epigenetic therapies may synergize with therapeutic cancer vaccines and other immunotherapies by epigenetically modulating cancer cells as well as immune cells, resulting in increased tumor control.[136–140] Extensive alterations in the epigenome of human cancers, including dysregulated DNA methylation and/or histone deacetylation, and global changes to the chromatin landscape, contribute to tumor initiation and development, including by promoting immune evasion. Aberrant DNA methylation of tumor suppressor genes and others implicated in malignant transformation and progression can be reversed with DNA methyltransferase inhibitors (DNMTi). Mounting evidence suggests that DNMTi can increase tumor visibility to the immune system by inducing the expression of neoantigens[141–143] and eliciting immune responses characterized by production of types I and III interferons, and increased infiltration of cytotoxic T lymphocytes (CTLs) into the TME.[136,144] Similar immune-modulatory effects have been demonstrated with other epigenetic modulators, including inhibitors of histone deacetylases (HDACi) and of the enhancer of zeste homologue 2 (EZH2i).[145,146] Epigenetic modulation of tumor by HDACi upregulates natural killer (NK) ligands and multiple components of the antigen-processing machinery, including MHC class I, resulting in increased tumor recognition by antigen-specific CD8$^+$ T cells and NK cells.[147,148]

Epigenetic modulation can also reprogram the epigenome of tumor-infiltrating immune cells, including CTLs, which can become exhausted due to chronic stimulation in the TME.[149–152] This exhaustion signature is characterized by abnormal DNA methylation of genes associated with T cell effector function, including IFNγ.[149] DNMTi can alleviate the onset of CTL exhaustion and epigenetically re-establish effector functions, which is not always achieved by current immune checkpoint blockade therapies.[149–152] In preclinical carcinoma models, the class I HDAC inhibitor entinostat has been shown to promote synergistic antitumor activity in combination with a therapeutic cancer vaccine and an IL-15 superagonist.[139] This synergy was shown to be mediated by tumor MHC Class I upregulation, increased infiltration of granzyme B$^+$ CD8$^+$ T cells, and deletion of both regulatory T cells and myeloid-derived suppressor cells in the TME.

Clinical trials

Currently, there are several clinical trials examining combinations of cancer vaccines with either HDACi or DNMTi. In an ongoing Phase 1b study, 20 patients with smoldering multiple myeloma are receiving a multi-peptide cancer vaccine (PVX-410) targeting the highly expressed tumor antigens XBP1, CD138, and CS1, in combination with the HDAC6 inhibitor citarinostat. An ongoing Phase 1b trial is examining the sequential combination of a vaccine targeting brachyury with the HDACi entinostat, ado-trastuzumab emtansine (T-DM1), and bintrafusp alfa (M7824) in advanced-stage breast cancer.

Recent Phase 1 clinical studies examined the DNMTi decitabine in combination with cancer vaccines, including an antigen autologous dendritic cell vaccine in patients with neuroblastoma or sarcoma, and NY-ESO-1 peptide vaccine plus liposomal doxorubicin in patients with recurrent ovarian, fallopian, or peritoneal cancers. In a Phase 1 study, six out of seven patients with MDS who received an HLA-unrestricted NY-ESO-1 vaccine (CDX-1401 + poly-ICLC) in combination with decitabine mounted NY-ESO-1-specific CD4$^+$ and/or CD8$^+$ T-cell responses.[153] An ongoing clinical study is now examining this therapy in combination with nivolumab in MDS and AML patients. In another Phase 1 study also in patients with MDS and AML, azacytidine is being combined with a peptide vaccine against NY-ESO-1, PRAME, MAGE-A3, and WT-1. The combination of guadecitabine (SGI-110) with an allogeneic colon cancer cell

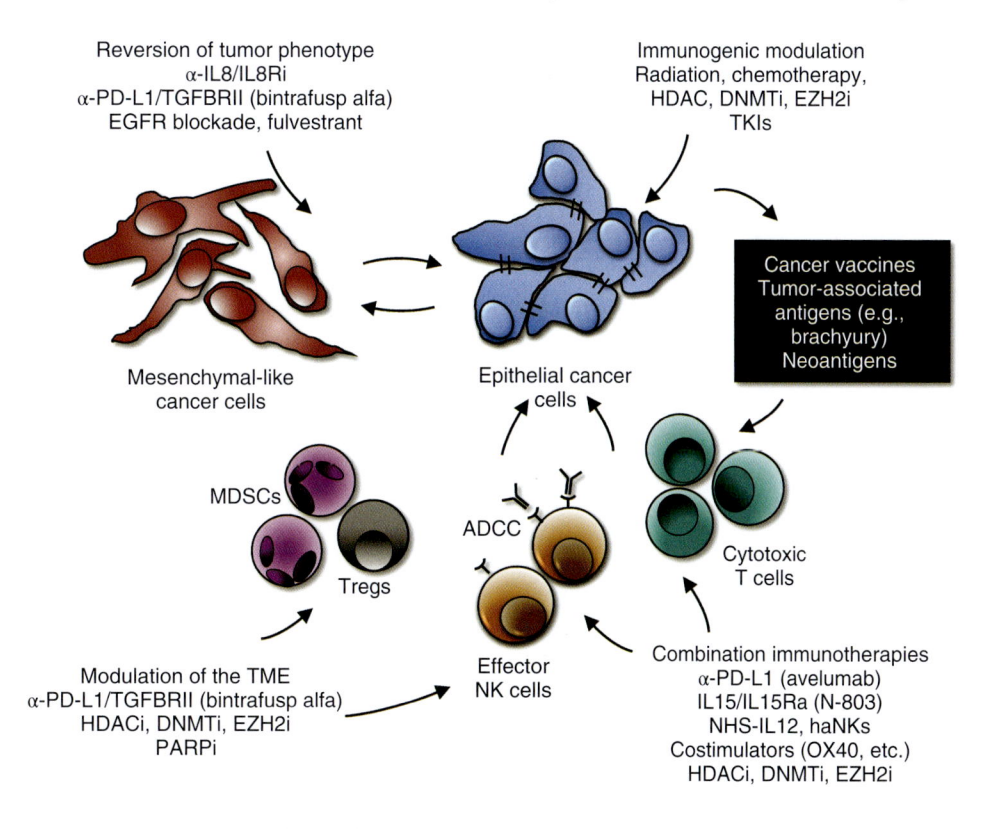

Figure 2 Schematic representation demonstrating the use of cancer vaccines as a component of a multifaceted anticancer approach. Source: Adapted from Schlom and Gulley[163].

vaccine expressing GM-CSF (GVAX), and cyclophosphamide is being examined in metastatic colorectal cancer patients.

Vaccine plus other immunomodulators

Multiple preclinical studies have shown that the antitumor efficacy of therapeutic cancer vaccines can potentially be increased in combination with other immune-modulatory agents, such as IL-8 inhibitors,[154,155] anti-PD-L1/TGFβRII (bintrafusp alfa),[156–158] IL-15 superagonists,[79,139,159] and NHS-IL12,[160–162] among others, establishing the foundation for clinical studies combining cancer vaccines with these agents (Figure 2). For example, bintrafusp alfa, a first-in-class anti-PD-L1/TGFβRII bifunctional agent that simultaneously inhibits PD-L1 and TGFβ, has significant antitumor efficacy in preclinical models of solid tumors, including those refractory to anti-PD-L1 antibodies, either as a monotherapy or in combination with a cancer vaccine targeting CEA.[157] NHS-IL12 is an immunocytokine targeted to the necrotic regions of the tumor.[161,162,164] Combination therapy with NHS-IL12 plus a MUC-1-targeted cancer vaccine resulted in greater antitumor efficacy than each individual therapy alone.[160]

Summary

The success of checkpoint inhibitor MAbs (CIM) in the treatment of many cancer types has transformed immunotherapy into the center of cancer management. For most cancer types, only a subset of patients, however, responds to CIM therapy. This is believed to be due to the fact that many so-called "cold" tumors lack mutations and thus lack expression of neoantigens and subsequent T-cell infiltration and/or many suppressive elements in the tumor microenvironment or the periphery dampen or eliminate antitumor immune responses. The last decade has revealed a renaissance in our understanding of the complexity and plasticity of the human immune system. Over 100 immune cell phenotypes have now been identified[165,166] along with the immunostimulatory or immunosuppressive function of many of these phenotypes. Figure 2 illustrates these complexities and interactions of agents that can (1) induce antitumor responses, (2) potentiate those responses, (3) reduce or eliminate immunosuppressive entities, and/or (4) alter the phenotype of the tumor to render tumor cells more susceptible to immune attack induced by vaccine and/or other immune-mediating entities.

Acknowledgments

The authors gratefully acknowledge the assistance of Debra Weingarten in the preparation of this article.

Key references

The complete reference list can be found on Vital Source version of this title, see inside front cover.

13 Koutsky LA, Ault KA, Wheeler CM, et al. A controlled trial of a human papillomavirus type 16 vaccine. *N Engl J Med*. 2002;**347**:1645–1651.

18 Massarelli E, William W, Johnson F, et al. Combining immune checkpoint blockade and tumor-specific vaccine for patients with incurable human papillomavirus 16-related cancer: a phase 2 clinical trial. *JAMA Oncol*. 2019;**5**:67–73.

32 Schwartzentruber DJ. Gp100 peptide vaccine and interleukin-2 in patients with advanced melanoma. *N Engl J Med*. 2011;**364**:2119–2127.

38 Andtbacka RH, Agarwala SS, Ollila DW, et al. Cutaneous head and neck melanoma in OPTiM, a randomized phase 3 trial of talimogene laherparepvec versus granulocyte-macrophage colony-stimulating factor for the treatment of unresected stage IIIB/IIIC/IV melanoma. *Head Neck*. 2016;**38**:1752–1758.

41 Kantoff PW, Higano CS, Shore ND, et al. Sipuleucel-T immunotherapy for castration-resistant prostate cancer. *New Eng J Med*. 2010;**363**:411–422.

51 McNeel DG, Eickhoff JC, Wargowski E, et al. Concurrent, but not sequential, PD-1 blockade with a DNA vaccine elicits anti-tumor responses in patients with metastatic, castration-resistant prostate cancer. *Oncotarget*. 2018;**9**:25586–25596.

58 Disis ML, Wallace DR, Gooley TA, et al. Concurrent trastuzumab and HER2/neu-specific vaccination in patients with metastatic breast cancer. *J Clin Oncol*. 2009;**27**:4685–4692.

69 Quoix E, Ramlau R, Westeel V, et al. Therapeutic vaccination with TG4010 and first-line chemotherapy in advanced non-small-cell lung cancer: a controlled phase 2B trial. *Lancet Oncol*. 2011;**12**:1125–1133.

76 Balachandran VP, Luksza M, Zhao JN, et al. Identification of unique neoantigen qualities in long-term survivors of pancreatic cancer. *Nature*. 2017;**551**:512–516.

84 Hassan R, Alley E, Kindler H, et al. Clinical response of live-attenuated, Listeria monocytogenes expressing mesothelin (CRS-207) with chemotherapy in patients with malignant pleural mesothelioma. *Clin Cancer Res*. 2019;**25**:5787–5798.

85 Liau LM, Ashkan K, Tran DD, et al. First results on survival from a large Phase 3 clinical trial of an autologous dendritic cell vaccine in newly diagnosed glioblastoma. *J Transl Med*. 2018;**16**:142.

91 Qazilbash MH, Wieder E, Thall PF, et al. PR1 peptide vaccine induces specific immunity with clinical responses in myeloid malignancies. *Leukemia*. 2017;**31**:697–704.

97 Burkhardt UE, Hainz U, Stevenson K, et al. Autologous CLL cell vaccination early after transplant induces leukemia-specific T cells. *J Clin Invest*. 2013;**123**:3756–3765.

98 Rosenblatt J, Stone RM, Uhl L, et al. Individualized vaccination of AML patients in remission is associated with induction of antileukemia immunity and prolonged remissions. *Sci Transl Med*. 2016;**8**:368ra171.

99 da Silva-Diz V, Lorenzo-Sanz L, Bernat-Peguera A, et al. Cancer cell plasticity: impact on tumor progression and therapy response. *Semin Cancer Biol*. 2018;**53**:48–58.

126 Huang B, Cohen JR, Fernando RI, et al. The embryonic transcription factor Brachyury blocks cell cycle progression and mediates tumor resistance to conventional antitumor therapies. *Cell Death Dis*. 2013;**4**:e682.

130 Heery CR, Singh BH, Rauckhorst M, et al. Phase I trial of a yeast-based therapeutic cancer vaccine (GI-6301) targeting the transcription factor brachyury. *Cancer Immunol Res*. 2015;**3**:1248–1256.

139 Hicks KC, Knudson KM, Lee KL, et al. Cooperative immune-mediated mechanisms of the HDAC inhibitor entinostat, an IL15 superagonist, and a cancer vaccine effectively synergize as a novel cancer therapy. *Clin Cancer Res*. 2020;**26**:704–716.

62 T cell immunotherapy of cancer

M. Lia Palomba, MD ■ Jae H. Park, MD ■ Renier Brentjens, MD, PhD

> **Overview**
>
> Bone marrow transplantation (BMT) represents the first known example of using the anti-tumor potential of T cells; a phenomenon later known as the graft versus tumor effect. Since the recognition in BMT that T cells are a significant source for therapeutic anti-cancer potential, investigators have sought for the next 6–7 decades to better harness the potential of T cells as an anti- cancer therapeutic. This road to discovery early on included utilizing virus specific T cells to target virus induced malignancies which express viral proteins. Recognition that T cells infiltrating tumors also mediate anti-tumor efficacy, investigators next harnessed these tumor infiltrating T cells (TILs), expanded in the laboratory, to demonstrate therapeutic benefit primarily in the setting of melanomas. With the advent of viral vector mediated gene engineering, the field of adoptive T cell therapies made a remarkable step forward in the setting of T cells engineered to specifically recognize tumor antigens through the introduction of genes encoding tumor targeted T cells receptors (TCRs) as well as the more novel chimeric antigen receptors (CARs). These TCR and CAR engineered T cells have to date demonstrated anti-tumor efficacies with the potential to markedly change cancer therapy in the foreseeable future. More significantly, with further understanding of the tumor immunology and consequent innovation, the ceiling on adoptive therapy using genetically engineered T cells is extremely high.

Introduction

T cell therapy of cancer has its origins in the 1950s with the advent of bone marrow transplantation (BMT). Investigators soon realized that donor immune cells contained in the bone marrow graft infused into the patient mediated a wasting disease, subsequently termed graft-versus-host disease (GvHD). These immune cells, identified as T cells, recognized, and attacked host tissues as nonself, through the recognition of recipient's histocompatibility antigens by the T cell receptor (TCR). While toxicity induced by these alloreactive donor T cells was appreciated early on, investigators further realized that the mechanisms mediating GvHD could concurrently mediate a graft-versus-leukemia (GvL) effect, wherein donor T cells could recognize tumor cells as nonself and subsequently eradicate residual disease. These early findings demonstrated for the first time that properly targeted T cells have the capacity to eradicate tumor cells. Over the subsequent 60 or so years, investigators have exhaustively explored how to convert the tumoricidal potential of cytotoxic T cells into an effective antitumor therapy. With each passing decade, slow incremental progress has advanced T cell cancer therapies from crude and highly toxic modalities to more targeted and refined approaches. Most recently, this progress has led to the commercialization of T cells genetically engineered to express tumor-targeted chimeric antigen receptors (CARs). While the current status of T cell therapies for cancer shows ever more promise to become a frontline therapy for both hematological and solid tumor malignancies, much work remains to be done in order to achieve higher and more sustained efficacy, while avoiding the potential for increased toxicity.

Bone marrow transplantation and the GvL effect

Allogeneic BMT and hematopoietic stem-cell transplants (HSCT) eradicate tumor through dual mechanisms. The first mechanism is via the cytotoxic effect of high-dose chemotherapy and/or radiation, which eradicate most diseases and limits the ability of graft rejection. A second mechanism is mediated by cytotoxic donor T cells, which recognize eradicate residual tumor (Figure 1a). Two major pathways of tumor eradication have been described, one involving release of perforin and granzyme at the site of the immunologic synapse,[1] and the second involving fas–fas ligand interaction, resulting in direct target cell apoptosis.[2] Evidence for T cell-mediated GvL is largely indirect, as it has been observed retrospectively that those patients who experience GvHD, especially chronic GvHD, are less likely to relapse. Patients with chronic myeloid leukemia (CML) receiving a T cell-depleted transplant to minimize GvHD are more likely to relapse. Likewise, those patients who receive a transplant from an identical twin donor are most likely to relapse.[3,4] More direct evidence for T cell-mediated GvL is demonstrated in patients who relapse after allogeneic HSCT, receive donor leukocyte infusions (DLI) and experience a second remission. DLI therapy is particularly efficacious in the setting of patients with relapsed CML but far less so in other leukemias and in lymphoma.[3,5–7] Evidence of GvL in the setting of leukemias prompted further investigation as to whether a similar graft versus tumor (GvT) could be appreciated in the setting of solid tumor malignancies in the context of allogeneic transplant and initial highly publicized anecdotal data suggested potential for this approach most notably in the setting of renal cell carcinoma and metastatic breast cancer.[8–10] However, lack of reproducibility and significant toxicity has largely relegated this approach in solid tumor malignancies to a footnote in T cell cancer therapy.[9,10]

Cancer treatment with virus-specific T cells

One in 10 of all cancers are associated with viral infections.[11] Most prominent of these oncogenic viruses are Epstein–Barr virus (EBV), Hepatitis B and C virus, and Human Papilloma virus (HPV). Virally encoded proteins drive signaling pathways that directly stimulate uncontrolled cell proliferation. The expression of these immunogenic viral proteins may be recognized by cytotoxic T cells.[11] Isolation and expansion of T cells targeted to immunogenic viral antigens provides a therapeutic option for the treatment of these virally induced malignancies, an option that is particularly appealing due to the ability of virus-specific T cells to specifically target virus-infected cells but not uninfected, healthy cells (Figure 1b). Most notably in

---

Holland-Frei Cancer Medicine, Tenth Edition. Edited by Robert C. Bast, John C. Byrd, Carlo M. Croce, Ernest Hawk, Fadlo R. Khuri, Raphael E. Pollock, Apostolia M. Tsimberidou, Christopher G. Willett, and Cheryl L. Willman.
© 2023 John Wiley & Sons, Inc. Published 2023 by John Wiley & Sons, Inc.

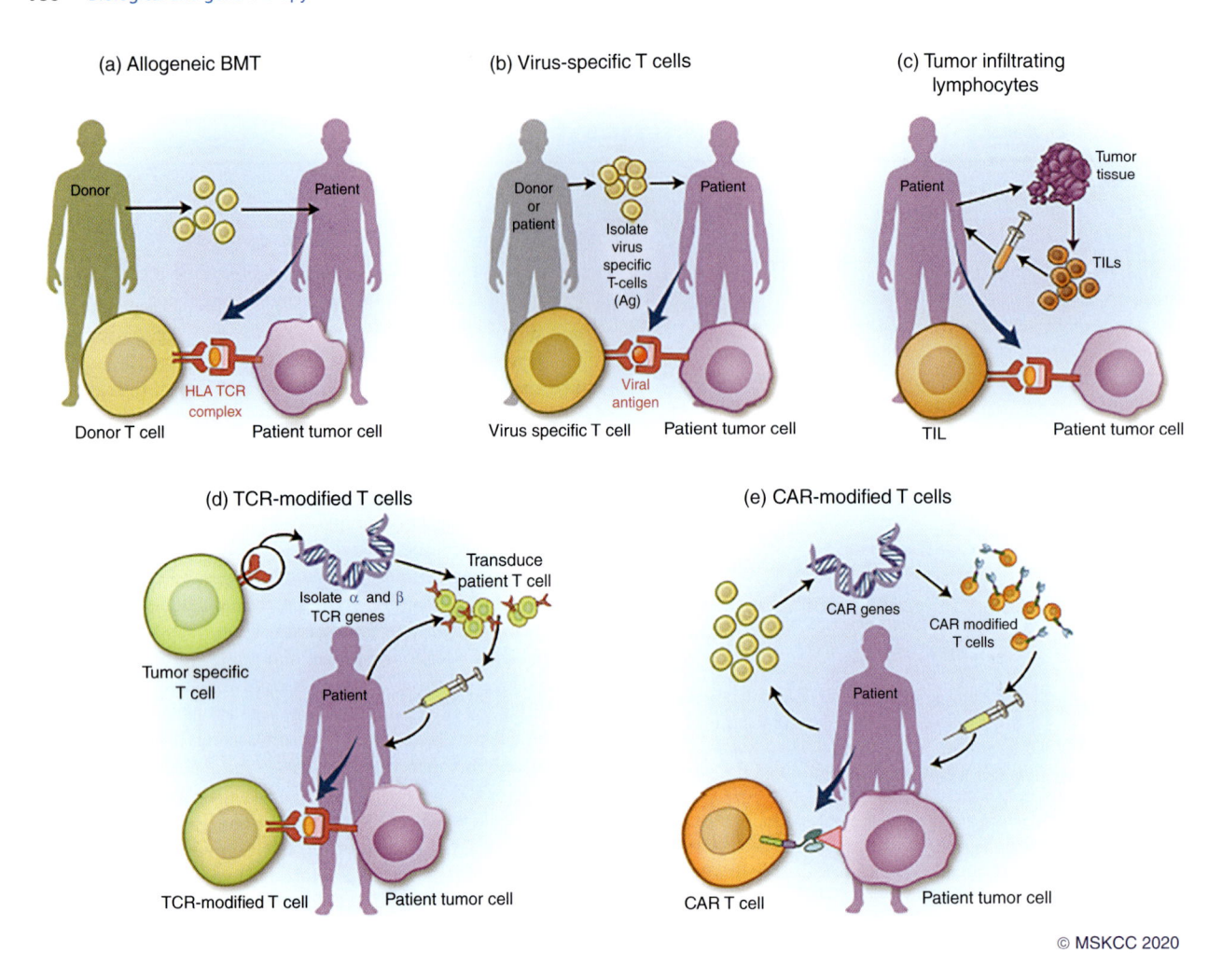

Figure 1 *The evolution of cancer T-cell therapy.* Initial T cell-mediated anti-cancer therapy was conducted through BMT wherein GvL or GvT T cells from the donor recognized antigen on residual tumor cells either through T cells contained in the bone marrow graft or through post-BMT infusion of DLI (a). Identification of donor or patient T cells specific to viral oncogenes expressed on virally induced tumors has allowed for isolation and expansion of T cells specific to target viral antigens expressed on the surface of tumor cells and infused into the patient generating a potent anti-tumor T cell response (b). Alternatively, anergic presumptive tumor specific T cells (TILs) may be harvested from tumor tissues and expanded *ex vivo* and infused back into patients to mediate a more potent anti-tumor T cell effect (c). The TCR coding domains from a TIL or tumor specific T cell may be cloned and subsequently transduced into a patient's own T cells generating TCR-modified tumor targeted T cells, expanded *ex vivo* and reinfused back into the patient generating a T cell-mediated anti-tumor response (d). Finally, a patient's own T cells may be genetically engineered to express a chimeric antigen receptor (CAR) specific to a tumor associated antigen and expanded *ex vivo*. The resulting tumor specific CAR T cells are reinfused back into the patient and mediate an anti-tumor effect (e).

hematologic malignancies, EBV infection of B cells can lead to the development of B cell lymphoma, termed Epstein–Barr virus-associated lymphoproliferative disorders (EBV-LPD). In immunocompetent individuals, latently EBV-infected B cells (for instance those that have escaped immune surveillance after a full-blown EBV infection resulting in mononucleosis) are held in check by an intact immune system, specifically by EBV-specific T cells. Conversely, in the immune-suppressed settings, such as in the context of solid organ transplantation or HSCT (especially T cell-depleted transplantations), patients may experience uncontrolled proliferation of EBV-infected B cells.[12] Initial attempts at utilizing EBV specific T cells to treat EBV-LPD was carried out in the context of HSCT, wherein unselected T cells from EBV+ donors were infused as a DLI.[12,13] Five of 5 of the first reported HSCT patients with EBV-LPD achieved complete remissions with bulk donor T cell DLI.[13] Subsequent attempts to specifically isolate and expand donor EBV-reactive T cells *ex vivo* enhanced the safety and efficacy of this approach and demonstrated marked efficacy as a prophylaxis of EBV-PLD in the setting of T cell-depleted HSCT in patients at high risk for the disease. In the initial report of 39 treated patients, none developed lymphoma.[14] Long-term efficacy and safety of this approach was recently reported both as prophylaxis as well as treatment of established EVB-LPD.[15] Given the fact that EBV-specific donor T cells carry little risk of inducing GvHD, partially HLA-matched donor T cells may be safely used to treat patients in this setting. This led to the establishment of EBV-specific T cell banks allowing for third party, or "off the shelf," source of T cells to treat these disorders.[16–18] Outside the setting of EVB-LPD, which develops in the context of immune suppression, a significant number of lymphomas which occur spontaneously express the EBV latent antigens, named latent membrane protein 1 (LMP1) and LMP2. LMP1- and LMP2-specific T cells may be isolated and expanded *ex vivo*. Isolated and expanded LMP1 and LMP2-targeted autologous T cells were found to be well-tolerated and demonstrated significant clinical activity both as an adjuvant in high-risk patients and in patients with relapsed disease.[19]

Similarly, as an adjuvant treatment, LMP-specific donor-derived T cells infused into high-risk patients in the post allogeneic HSCT setting demonstrated good safety profile as well as marked durability of disease remissions.[20] In the case of solid malignancies, nasopharyngeal carcinoma (NPC) is similarly associated with EBV infection, and tumor cells express EBV viral oncoproteins. In a series of clinical studies, investigators were able to successfully isolate and expand autologous EBV-specific T cells. Infusion of these T cells in patients with remissions or with active disease demonstrated either prolonged remissions or, in a subset of patients, durable antitumor responses, most prominently in patients with loco-regional disease when compared to patients with metastatic NPC.[21–23] Less developed are studies investigating T cell therapies for HPV-associated epithelial cancers, including cervical cancer. While HPV-specific T cells can be successfully isolated from these patients,[24] to date only anecdotal clinical data has been published with overall modest outcomes.[25,26]

Cancer treatment with tumor-infiltrating lymphocytes

Tumor-infiltrating lymphocytes (TILs) are T cells found within the tumor microenvironment. These T cells are presumably specific to tumor antigens, however, they have become exhausted or anergic within the tumor. These presumed endogenous tumor-targeted T cells may be isolated from biopsied tumor tissue and expanded *ex vivo*[27] (Figure 1c). Investigators at the National Cancer Institute were the first to clinically apply this approach to patients with metastatic melanoma, infusing 20 melanoma patients with TILs isolated from their own resected tumor metastasis in combination with IL-2. Adoptive transfer of TILs led to objective tumor regressions in 11 of 20 treated patients.[28] Limited responses using this approach were thought to be related in part to a lack of TIL persistence after infusion. Subsequent studies utilized ever-increasing chemotherapeutic conditioning regimens to deplete endogenous lymphocytes providing physical space for TILs as well as create cytokine "sinks" to enhance expansion and persistence. Resulting studies demonstrated enhanced antitumor efficacy in the setting of melanoma[29–32] and have established lymphodepleting conditioning chemotherapy as a standard for most future adoptive T cell therapies. Efficacy of TILs was further demonstrated in the setting of metastatic uveal melanomas as well as melanomas with brain metastases.[33,34] Clinical outcomes are largely focused in the setting of melanoma while smaller early-stage published clinical trials have demonstrated potential of TIL therapy in other malignancies including for example multiple myeloma (MM) and NPC where in the latter setting not surprisingly many TILs were found to be specific to EBV antigens.[35,36]

Early on, TIL specificity was largely unknown. Work at the NCI led to the identification of immunogenic un-mutated antigens such as tumor differentiation and cancer germline antigens targeted by TILs in the context of melanoma (MART-1, gp100, NY-ESO-1).[27] More recently investigators appreciated that tumor somatic mutational burden leads the tumor cells to present neo-antigens which result from these mutations.[37] Neoantigens have since been found to be expressed on multiple solid tumor malignancies and more significantly found to be immunogenic, leading to the induction of endogenous T cells.[37–39] More efficient approaches to identify and isolate these neoantigen-targeted T cells are being developed.[40–43] Early-stage clinical trials in a variety of solid tumor malignancies have demonstrated anecdotal evidence of clinical antitumor efficacy following adoptive T cell therapy with neoantigen-reactive T cells.[44–47] The ability to identify highly immunogenic tumor neoantigens and subsequently isolate T cells targeted to these neoantigens allows for the isolation of the epitope-specific T-cell receptor coding regions, which in turn can be utilized to generate TCR-modified T cells.[41]

Cancer treatment with TCR-modified T cells

TCRs are antigen-specific receptors expressed on the surface of all T cells that recognize small peptides (epitopes) presented on the surface of antigen-presenting cells (APCs). They are heterodimers composed of two disulfide-linked transmembrane proteins, in most cases an alpha and beta chain, less frequently a gamma and delta chain, which contain an antigen-binding region, an extracellular constant region, and a transmembrane domain. Their short cytoplasmic tail does not contain any signaling activity per se, and the function of signal transduction relies on their interaction with the adaptor protein CD3, which, through its immunoreceptor tyrosine-based activation motifs (ITAMs), initiate a signaling cascade upon binding of the TCR to its cognate antigen. Cellular proteins are constantly degraded by the proteasome into small fragments, which are released into the cytosol and then transported to the endoplasmic reticulum, where they form a complex with major histocompatibility complex (MHC) molecules. The peptide–MHC complex is then transported to the cell surface via the Golgi apparatus. The interaction between TCRs and cells expressing the target antigen results in the downstream activation of the TCR signaling cascade and the release of cytotoxic molecules such as perforin and granzymes.[48] Through the process of negative selection, T cells that recognize self-antigens are clonally deleted in the thymus, protecting the body from autoimmune responses. Cancer cells, despite originating from autologous tissues and therefore for the most part expressing self-antigens, can elicit an immune response, as evidenced by the presence of TILs in the tumor microenvironment, as detailed above. TILs can recognize with variable affinity a wide spectrum of tumor antigens, including tissue differentiation antigens, cancer germline antigens, viral oncoproteins, and neoantigens resulting from the transcription of mutated genes. However, clinically meaningful immune responses are usually insufficient or self-limited due to a process of immune evasion.[49,50]

The ability to clone cancer-specific TCRs from *in vitro* expanded TILs, insert them into viral vectors and transduce them into autologous T cells[51] has allowed for the development of a number of TCR-mediated immunotherapy strategies (Figure 1d). The advantage of TCR-mediated antigen recognition over antibody recognition is that peptides loaded on MHC molecules of APCs are the product of intracellular and membrane proteins degradation, circumventing the need for the tumor antigen to be membrane-bound. This is important because it is predicted that 27% of the human proteome contains transmembrane proteins, leaving almost 70% of other potential targets not amenable to antibody-mediated immunotherapy.[52] Moreover, T cells can become activated even if only a small number of TCR-MHC complexes are formed, therefore low antigen density is not as essential as in antibody-mediated immunity.[53,54] To manufacture TCR-mediated T cells, double-stranded DNA encoding the tumor-specific TCRs identified via high-throughput screening of TILs or circulating T cells are inserted into gammaretroviral or lentiviral vectors. Patients' own T cells expanded *in vitro* are then infected with the TCR-containing viral DNA, which integrates randomly into the T cells genome, where it is transcribed and expressed on the cell surface. The endogenous TRCs in the patient's T cells remain intact and continues to be expressed. Newer technologies such as CRIPR-Cas9 have allowed targeting of the exogenous TCR to a specific genomic locus (the T cell receptor alpha chain locus, TRAC), while simultaneously allowing the disruption of the endogenous TCR.[55] This allows a more homogeneous and stable expression of the transduced TCR.

Initial clinical experience with TCR-T cells therapy was reported against tumor differentiation antigens that are commonly expressed by melanoma cells and melanocytes, including MART-1 and gp100, and the colorectal antigen CEA.[56,57] These studies showed that effective antitumor immunity could be achieved, but at the expense of severe autoimmune activity against normal tissues such as melanocytes in the skin, eye and inner ear, and colonic mucosa in several of the treated patients, underlying that antigens that are shared between cancer and normal cells are not ideal targets.

A second class of potentially targetable tumor antigens are the cancer germline antigen (CGAs). The advantage of targeting CGAs is that their expression is confined to germ cells and cancer cells, but not to normal tissues.[58] Over one hundred such antigens have been identified. Of those, NY-ESO-1 and MAGE-3 have been most commonly tested in TCR-mediated T cell trials.[59,60] In a study of 38 patients with NY-ESO-1 positive synovial cells sarcoma or melanoma, 61% of patients with sarcoma and 55 patients with melanoma treated with T cells transduced with a TCR against HLA-A*0201 restricted NY-ESO-1 epitope exhibited objective responses, in some cases persisting up to 5 years.[61] In another study of 12 patients with metastatic synovial sarcoma, half had confirmed antitumor responses that lasted several months. Importantly, while most of the infused NY-ESO-1 T cells were of the effector memory phenotype, the persisting T cells pool had mostly central memory and stem-cell memory phenotype and showed no evidence of T cell exhaustion over time.[62] MAGE-A3 was the target of a small clinical trial of TCR T cells. Of the nine patients treated, five experienced a clinical response, and two developed severe neurotoxicity, unfortunately including one patient who succumbed to necrotizing leukoencephalopathy.[63] In a separate study, patients with solid tumors including melanoma, cervical, and breast cancer treated with autologous CD4-selected T cells transduced with MAGE-A3 TCR, in combination with IL-2, exhibited a modest and often transient clinical response, though a few patients had responses approaching or exceeding 2 years. The treatment was complicated by severe transaminitis in two patients and fever and hematologic toxicity in most patients, but no treatment-related deaths were reported.[60] A number of CGAs-targeting TCR-mediated T cell trials are ongoing at this time, alone or in combination with checkpoint inhibitors.

Viral oncoproteins are expressed by some solid tumors and constitute one more category of targetable antigens. Clinical trials are ongoing of TCR-engineered T cells directed against the E6 and E7 human papillomavirus proteins[64,65] as well as the EBV-associated oncoprotein LMP1 for patients with nasopharyngeal cancer as detailed in the section on virus-specific T cells above.[22]

Finally, immunogenic neoantigens created by somatic point mutations, insertions, or gene fusions are restricted to cancer cells and potentially capable to elicit T cell-mediated immunity by high affinity TCRs. When these neoantigens are restricted to a certain HLA, they are known as public neoantigens. Public neoantigens associated with oncoproteins such as KRAS, BRAF, and beta-catenin, as well as tumor suppressor genes such as TP53 have been recently identified. Treatment with public neoantigens-specific T cells has offered the proof-of-concept that this strategy is feasible and able to induce durable responses in some patients.[46,66–68]

Cancer treatment with CAR-modified T cells

Membrane-bound antigens can be targeted by antibodies that recognize extracellular epitopes with high specificity. The use of monoclonal antibodies therapy has revolutionized the concept of passive immunotherapy of cancer since it was introduced in the 1990s. Combining the high affinity of antibodies for their target antigen and the cytotoxic effect of activated T cells, chimeric antigen receptor (CAR)-modified T cells represent one of the most successful example of personalized cellular cancer therapy (Figure 1e).

Prototypical CARs are designed to include four major components: the extracellular single-chain variable fragment (scFv) of a monoclonal antibody, a hinge domain, a transmembrane (TM) domain, and an intracellular signaling domain (Figure 2).

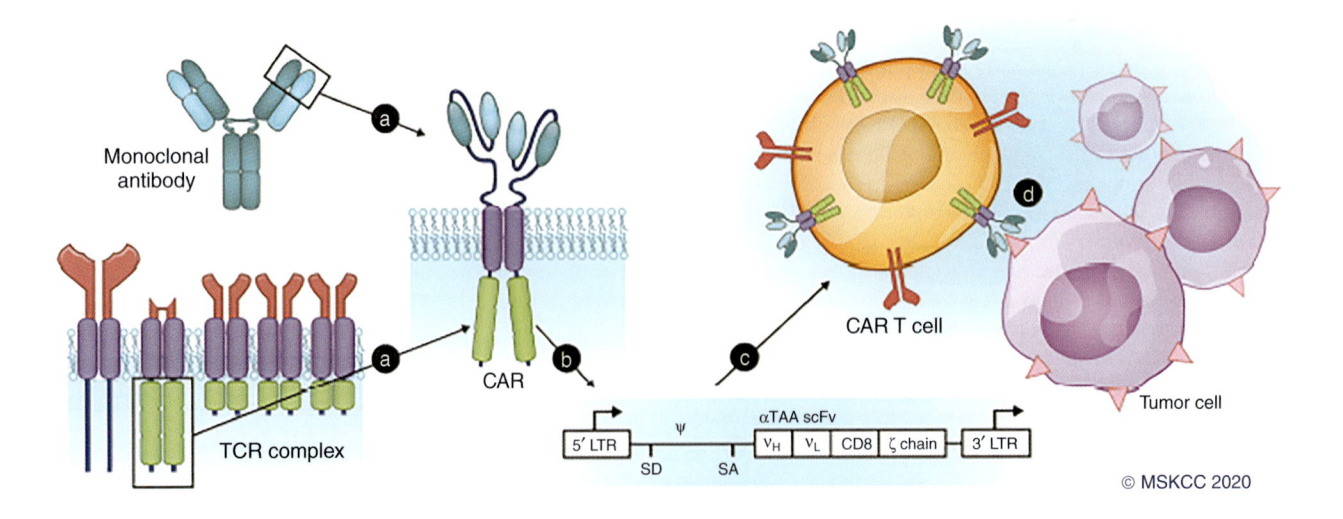

Figure 2 *Generation of a tumor targeted CAR T cell.* T cells can be genetically modified to express a chimeric antigen receptor (CAR) which typically involves the fusion of the binding domain of a monoclonal antibody, termed an scFv, fused to the signaling domain of the T cell receptor (the CD3η chain) (a). The gene encoding this CAR is cloned into a replication incompetent retro or lentiviral vector (b) and viral supernatant is used to transduce replicating T cells (c). Transduced CAR T cells which now express the CAR can recognize and lyse tumor cells which express the tumor associated antigen (d).

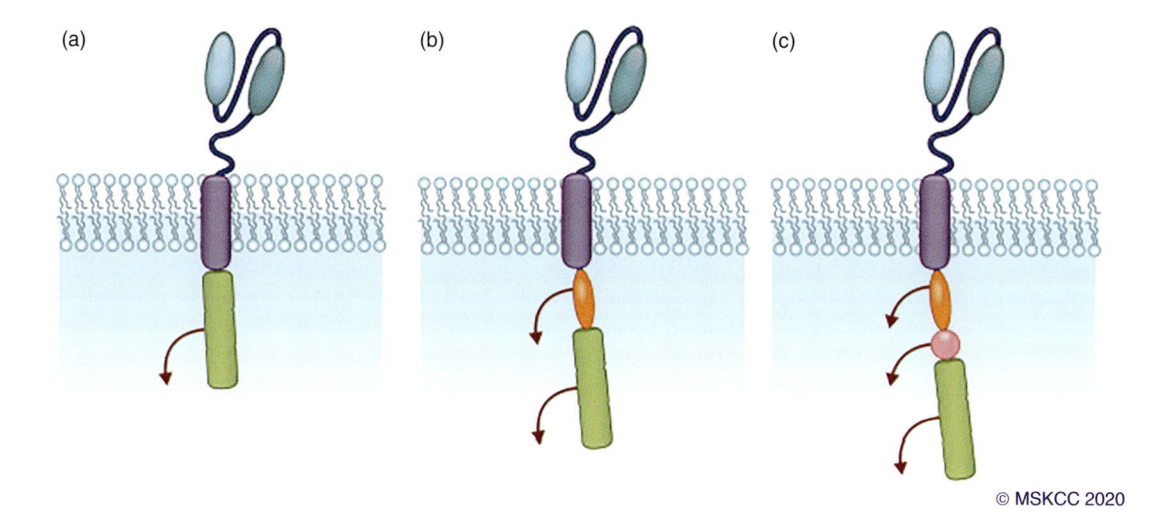

Figure 3 *Evolution of CAR design.* Initial CARs contained the target binding domain (an scFv from a MAb) fused to a transmembrane domain (typically derived from CD8 or CD28), fused to the TCR CD3η signaling domain (green rectangle) (a). Second generation CARs are designed to contain 2 cytoplasmic signaling domains wherein the membrane proximal domain is derived from a T cell costimulatory receptor (typically derived from CD28 or 4-1BB) (orange oval) fused to the CD3η chain (b) resulting in both primary and co-stimulatory T cell signaling (red arrows). Third generation CARs utilize 2 costimulatory cytoplasmic signaling domains (i.e. CD28, OX40, and/or 4-1BB) fused to the CD3η TCR signaling domain mediating dual co-stimulatory signals (c).

The scFv is composed of the variable heavy (V_H) and variable light chains (V_L) of monoclonal antibodies, connected by a flexible linker to form a single-chain variable fragment. The scFv sequence is typically derived from murine antibodies, though humanized versions of CARs exist that utilize human antibody sequences. The function of the hinge domain is to allow flexibility to the epitope-binding scFv, while the TM domain anchors the chimeric protein to the cell surface. The intracellular domain typically utilizes the signaling motifs from the CD3-ζ chain.[69,70] Since the scFv domain binds directly to target cell surface epitopes, CARs can bypass the need for MHC-restricted antigen presentation and therefore are immune to tumor escape mechanisms related to HLA downregulation. CARs can overcome T-cell triggering limitations related to epitope density, since the scFv can have a high affinity for the tumor-associated antigen (TAA). Multi-generation CARs have been developed, which possess a combination of signaling domains attached to the cytosolic activation domain.

For optimal activation and proliferation, T cells require both TCR engagement and signaling (termed "signal 1"), as well as co-stimulatory signaling through co-stimulatory receptors on T cells binding to cognate ligands expressed either by the target tumor cell or APCs (termed "signal 2"). Initial first-generation CARs were constructed through the fusion of a scFv-based TAA binding domain to an inert TM domain (e.g. the CD8 transmembrane domain), fused to a cytoplasmic signaling domain typically derived from the CD3-ζ or Fc receptor γ chains (Figure 3a).

The resulting CAR, when expressed by a T cell, engages the targeted antigen and delivers a signal 1 to the T cells, rendering tumor-targeted T cells susceptible to anergy or apoptosis[71,72] resulting in truncated *in vivo* persistence due to the lack of T cell co-stimulation (i.e. "signal 2").[73] To overcome the lack of T cell co-stimulation, first-generation CARs have been further modified by incorporating the cytoplasmic signaling domains of T cell co-stimulatory receptors such as CD28, 4-1BB (CD137), or OX40 (CD134) (Figure 2b). These second-generation CARs, when expressed in T cells, upon activation with targeted antigen, resulted in enhanced IL-2 production, superior *in vitro* antigen-dependent proliferation, and T cell upregulation of the antiapoptotic proteins (e.g. Bcl-X_L).[74–76] Third generation CARs have also been created that incorporate tandem cytoplasmic signaling domains from two co-stimulatory receptors (i.e. CD28-4-1BB or CD28-OX40) demonstrating a potential enhanced T cell signaling capacity when compared to second-generation CARs.[77–79] (Figure 3c).

Most of the clinical experience to date with CAR T cell therapies is derived from second-generation CARs. Autologous CD19 CAR T cells with either CD28 or 41BB costimulatory domains have revolutionized the treatment and outcome of patients with relapsed or refractory (R/R) B-cell hematologic malignancies. The initial data that demonstrated efficacy of CD19 CAR T cells in B-cell lymphoma came from several academic institutions in the United States including the National Cancer Institute, University of Pennsylvania, and Memorial Sloan Kettering Cancer Center, all of whom reported sustained complete response (CR) in patients with heavily treated R/R indolent B-cell lymphomas, for example, follicular lymphoma, marginal zone lymphoma, and chronic lymphocytic leukemia.[80–86]

Subsequently, two pivotal clinical trials, ZUMA-1 and JULIET, demonstrated high CR rates and durable responses in R/R aggressive large B cell lymphoma, leading to approval of axicabtagene ciloleucel and tisagenlecleucel by the FDA, respectively, for treatment of large cell lymphoma relapsed after two or more lines of therapy.[87,88] The ZUMA-1 was a phase 1/2 study that investigated the safety and efficacy of axicabtagene, a CD19 CAR with CD28 co-stimulation, in 119 patients with R/R aggressive B-cell lymphoma [77 *de novo* diffuse large B cell lymphoma (DLBCL), 24 transformed DLBCL, or primary mediastinal B-cell lymphoma].[87] Of 101 evaluable patients, 84 attained objective response including CR in 58 patients. With the median follow-up of 27 months, the 2-year overall survival (OS) was 50.5%. The JULIET trial explored the safety and efficacy of tisagenlecleucel, a CD19 CAR T containing the 4-1BB costimulatory domain, in aggressive B-cell lymphoma.[88] A total of 111 patients was treated, including 88 *de novo* DLBCL, 21 transformed follicular lymphoma (FL), and 2 other high-grade B-cell lymphoma. The best overall response and CR rate were 52% and 40%, respectively. The long-term follow-up data of both ZUMA-1 and JULIET-1 confirmed the durability of remission and sustained progression-free survival (PFS) without any subsequent therapy, especially in those who have achieved

CR.[89,90] Both studies demonstrated that the efficacy of CD19 CAR T cells was consistent across all patient subgroups irrespective of baseline patient or disease characteristics, and suggested that patients with lower tumor burden attained more durable remissions and lower incidences of toxicities.[91-93]

Recently, another CD19 CAR T cells with 41BB costimulatory domain and 1 : 1 mixture of CD4:CD8 CAR+ T cells, called lisocabtagene malaleucel, has demonstrated similar response rates in R/R DLBCL in a multi-centered phase 1/2 TRANSCEND-NHL-001 trial.[94] Of 268 treated patients, the overall response rate was 73% with 53% CR rate. Median PFS and OS were 6.8 months and 19.9 months, respectively. Based on this encouraging result, this product is currently under FDA review for approval.

Given the encouraging results of CD19 CAR T cells in R/R large cell lymphoma after two or more prior lines of chemotherapy, one of the current research endeavors is exploring the early use of the CD19 CAR T cells, specifically comparing against the efficacy of autologous stem cell transplant (ASCT).[41,42,87-94] To that end, several randomized clinical trials are ongoing with each of the three respective CD19 CARs (axicabtagene, tisagenlecleucel, and lisocabtagene) versus ASCT in first relapse of DLBCL.[95] Until these data are published, it is not clear if CAR T cells therapy can obviate for ASCT as the first salvage option.

In addition to the studies in DLBCL, CD19 CAR T cells have demonstrated clinical activities in other B-cell non-Hodgkin Lymphoma (B-NHL) subtypes. In follicular lymphoma, CD19/4-1BB CAR T cells elicited a very high CR rate and durable remission, including 88% and 46% CR rates in nontransformed and transformed FL in a phase 1/2 study.[96] Importantly, all patients with FL who achieved a CR remained in remission at a median follow-up of 24 months. The interim analysis of a study of follicular and marginal zone lymphoma patients treated with axicabtagene, the Zuma 5 trial, was recently presented: at a median follow up of 11.5 months, in 87 patients evaluable for efficacy, overall response rate was 94%, of which 79% were CRs.[97] In mantle cell lymphoma, the phase 2 ZUMA-2 study of KTE-X19 (brexucabtagene autoleucel) demonstrated a very high overall response rate of 93% and CR rate of 67% with 1-year PFS and OS of 61% and 83%, respectively,[98] leading to the FDA approval of the product in July 2020.

Beyond B-cell lymphomas, CD19 CAR T cells have demonstrated exceptional antitumor activities in R/R B-cell acute lymphoblastic leukemia (ALL). In children and adults with R/R B-ALL, CD19 CAR T cells have yielded CR rates of 60–90% with measurable residual disease (MRD) negativity of 50–90%.[99-105] The phase 2 ELIANA study of tisagenlecleucel demonstrated a very high CR rate of 81% at 3 months with the 12-month EFS and OS of 50% and 76%.[101] The result of this study led to the FDA approval of tisagenlecleucel for treatment of patients up to age 25 with R/R B-ALL. Similarly, the single-center phase I studies from MSKCC and Fred Hutch Cancer Center reported CR rates of 80% in adult patients with R/R B-ALL.[99,103] Several multi-center trials are currently investigating the efficacy of different CD19 CAR T cells in adult patients with R/R B-ALL, and preliminary results from such studies have demonstrated very similar high CR rates,[106] raising hopes for anticipated approval of one or more CD19 CAR T cells for adult patients with R/R B-ALL.

Successful CAR T cells strategies have also been employed against other antigens, specifically B-cell maturation antigen (BCMA) for patients with R/R MM. BCMA is an ideal target because it is consistently expressed in MM cells and not in critical healthy tissues. Several BCMA-specific CAR T constructs are being evaluated. The NCI and the BB2121 products both utilize a murine scFv.[107,108] Newer BCMA constructs utilize human-derived scFv sequences, including the MCARH171, JCARH125, and FCARH143.[109,110] The overall response rate in nine of the currently enrolling BCMA trials varies between 20% at low dose level to 100% at optimal dose level, and includes, CRs and stringent CRs and very good partial responses (VGPRs). Response duration is variable among the studies, but in some cases quite durable.[111] Given the very significant results in a patient population that is generally heavily treated, often including a prior ASCT, there is now a strong desire to utilize BCMA-directed CAR T cells in the early disease setting, including in first line for high-risk patients. Approval of one or more BCMA-directed CAR T cell product is expected to be granted soon.

These early phase clinical trials have also highlighted the potential toxicities for CAR T cell therapies. On-target, but off-tumor, toxicities are a consequence of varying levels of expression of the targeted tumor-associated antigen in normal tissues. Redirected T cells can be highly potent and toxic to normal tissues that express low levels of the targeted antigen. This can be extremely detrimental as described in 2006 by the Erasmus University in Rotterdam.[112] Here, patients infused with T cells modified with a CAR specific for carbonic anhydrase 9, which is physiologically expressed on bile duct epithelial cells had significant levels of cholestasis. The severity of on-target, but off-tumor toxicities is dependent on whether the tissues expressing the targeted antigen are essential for survival, and if the injuries are manageable by other means. For example, in clinical trials investigating T cells modified with a CD19-specific CAR, the resulting profound B cell aplasia posttherapy has been successfully managed by gamma-globulin replacement.[113] Conversely, low-level ERBB2 expression on lung epithelia may have led to fatal lung toxicity in a patient with colon cancer who received a high dose of third-generation CAR-modified T cells after intensive lymphodepletion, as reported by the NCI.[114]

The most severe toxicity observed in patients treated with CAR-modified T cells has been the cytokine-release syndrome (CRS) and neurotoxicity. CRS reflects a systemic inflammatory response syndrome in the hours to days following CAR T cell infusion, characterized by elevation of proinflammatory cytokines, T cell activation, and expansion, with clinical features including fevers, myalgias, malaise, tachycardia, hypoxia, and hypotension.[115] Neurological symptoms range from confusion, disorientation, dysarthria, aphasia, seizure, and global encephalopathy. A range of precautions have been proposed for mitigating the risk of life-threatening CRS including splitting the initial dose of CAR-modified T cells, early detection of clinical and laboratory signs heralding the syndrome such as C reactive protein (CRP),[116] and early therapeutic interventions, including IL-6 receptor inhibitor, tocilizumab, and/or high-dose corticosteroids.[115] Due to these measures, CRS has become much more manageable side effects of CAR T cell therapy. On the other hand, mechanisms of neurotoxicity remain largely unknown, although activation of myeloid cells or macrophages have been implicated, and therefore neurotoxicity is typically managed with corticosteroids and remain the most concerning side effect of CAR T cell therapy.

Other CAR-modified immune effector cell strategies

Currently approved and most experimental immune effector cells place the focus on autologous CAR T cells. Nonetheless, there are several different approaches to expand the adoptive immune effector cell therapy field with different cell sources. Allogeneic CAR T cells have been an area of active research to bypass the manufacturing time encountered in autologous CAR T cells by providing the "Off-the-shelf" product. Furthermore, T cells acquired from healthy donors may hold a better "fitness" advantage over the T cells collected from patients with active disease.[117] The potential concerns of allogeneic CAR T cell products may involve the possibility of graft-versus-host disease and the CAR T cell rejection. Various strategies involving novel engineering techniques and immunosuppressants are applied to mitigate such unopposed effects, and have demonstrated encouraging early clinical data with comparable response rates to autologous CAR T cells in patients with ALL and large cell lymphoma.[97,118–126]

In addition to T cell-derived immunotherapy, the natural killer cell is another component being investigated as a therapeutic platform of adoptive cellular therapy. The advantage of NK cells includes its direct HLA-independent antigen recognition through the KIR mismatch effect. This unique mechanism could potentially enhance the efficacy of CAR in recognizing and killing cancer cells. In addition, NK cells could solve the concern of GVHD, thus provide the flexible use of both autologous and allogeneic derived NK cells. Similar to CAR T cells, most ongoing studies and available data on CAR NK cells have been focused on B-cell hematologic malignancies.[127–130] Recently, Liu et al. reported the result of first-in-human phase 1/2 clinical trials of umbilical cord blood-derived CAR NK cells in CD19 expressing lymphoid malignancy (NCT03056339).[131] The study enrolled a total of 11 patients with R/R CD19+ hematologic malignancy (6 NHL, 4 CLL, and 1 Richter's transformation), and reported overall response rate of 73% (8/11; all 8 achieved CR on the aggressive component with residual CLL in 1 patient). This study provided a proof of concept that CAR NK cell therapy is a safe and effective off-the-shelf cellular immunotherapy option for patients with hematologic malignancies, and several other studies of CAR NK-cell-based therapies are ongoing internationally.

Next-generation tumor-targeted T cells

Despite clinical success achieved to date with T cell therapies of cancer, to date success treating solid tumor malignancies other than melanomas remains largely elusive. Even in the setting of CD19-targeted CAR T cells for the treatment of B cell malignancies, patients may fail therapy or experience relapsed disease after achieving initial responses. The mechanisms of treatment failure are multifold. First and foremost, many patients treated with CD19-targeted CAR T cells relapse with CD19 negative disease termed immune escape.[132,133] Lack of persistence of adoptively transferred tumor-targeted T cells has been linked to treatment failures.[134] Further, it has been well understood that tumors, especially solid tumors, scaffold themselves with immune-suppressive cells, ligands, and cytokines which may markedly suppress T cell function. This "hostile" tumor microenvironment (TME) mediates immune suppression through infiltrating regulatory CD4+ T cells, suppressive tumor-associated macrophages (TAMs), and myeloid-derived suppressor cells (MDSCs); secretion by tumor and associated immune cells of immune suppressive cytokines including IL-10 and TGF-β, and expression of inhibitory ligands including PD-L1 and PD-L2.[135] Unfortunately, this list is far from exhaustive. However, mechanistic insights into treatment failures in the context of adoptive T cell therapies have led to novel approaches designed to overcome the currently known limitations. While most of the current next-generation approaches have been studied and developed predominantly in the context of CAR T cells, these genetic modifications clearly have application to other T cell therapies including TILs and TCR-modified T cells.

CD19 targeted CAR T cell therapies have highlighted antigen escape as a primary source of treatment failure given the fact that the T cells are targeted to a single antigen. Investigators have looked into several approaches to generate multiply targeted CAR T cells including the introduction of multiple CAR genes targeted to more than tumor antigen[136] or alternatively targeting two antigens with a single bispecific CAR containing tandem scFv.[137,138] (Figure 4). Best studied in the latter setting is a single CAR specific to both the CD19 and CD20 or CD22 B cell antigens.[137,138] T cells may be genetically engineered to secrete pro-inflammatory cytokines (Figure 4b). IL-12 is a proinflammatory cytokine shown to enhance T cell cytotoxicity and proliferation as well as modulate the tumor microenvironment including modulation of TAMs changing from a suppressive M2 to a proinflammatory M1 phenotype.[139,140] In addition IL-12 may activate endogenous anergic tumor-infiltrating T cells while inhibiting regulatory CD4+ T cells.[139,141,142] This approach has been clinically studied in the setting of TILs in melanoma where these cells were found to be prohibitively toxic[143] as well as in CAR T cells in the setting of ovarian cancer.[144] IL-18 is a similarly proinflammatory cytokine and while not yet tested in the clinical setting has been shown by multiple groups in preclinical models to enhance the persistence of CAR T cells modified to secrete the cytokine, demonstrate bystander activation of endogenous tumor-infiltrating T cells leading to recruitment of endogenous T cells targeted to other tumor antigens which in turn may minimize the risk of antigen escape.[145–147] IL-18 similarly has been shown to modulate the suppressive TME.[145,146] TCR-modified T cells also demonstrate enhanced antitumor efficacy in murine models when modified to secrete IL-18.[148] CAR T cells have been modified to constitutively express otherwise transiently expressed co-stimulatory ligands. CAR T cells modified to express 4-1BBL mediate co-stimulatory activating signaling to the CAR T cell itself and well as providing co-stimulatory activation of bystander endogenous T cells and has demonstrated the ability to activate dendritic cells which in turn secrete proinflammatory cytokines and enhance tumor antigen presentation to endogenous T cells[149] (Figure 4c). CAR T cells modified to constitutively express the CD40L T cell activation marker has been found to enhance the efficacy of CAR T cells in preclinical models of disease[150,151] (Figure 4c). CD40L constitutively expressed on CAR T cells mediate maturation of antigen-presenting cells including dendritic cells and macrophages which in turn leads to secretion of IL-12 which in turn enhances tumor antigen presentation, recruitment of endogenous tumor-targeted T cells, and cytokine activation of these tumor-targeted T cells.[150,151] In addition, interaction with CD40L on the CAR T cell with CD40 on certain tumor cells may inhibit tumor cell growth or induce tumor cell death directly.[151] Expression of PD-L1 by tumor and the tumor stroma markedly limit the efficacy of adoptively transferred tumor-targeted T cells. To this end, multiple groups are testing the combination of T cell therapies in combination with systemic infusion of commercially available blocking antibodies to PD-1 or PD-L1. However, systemic immune checkpoint blockade is associated with significant toxicities. CAR T cells may be further engineered to overcome immune checkpoint through the introduction of a PD-1 dominant negative receptor (DNR) containing the PD-1 extracellular domain but either lacking a cytoplasmic PD-1 signaling domain[152] or alternatively fused to the CD28 co-stimulatory signaling domain[153] (Figure 4d). This approach specifically protects the CAR T cell from PD-L1-mediated inhibition. An alternative approach is to engineer the tumor-targeted T cell to secrete an antagonistic single fragment length variable (scFv) domain antibody binding domain specific to PD-1.[154,155] This approach allows for PD-1

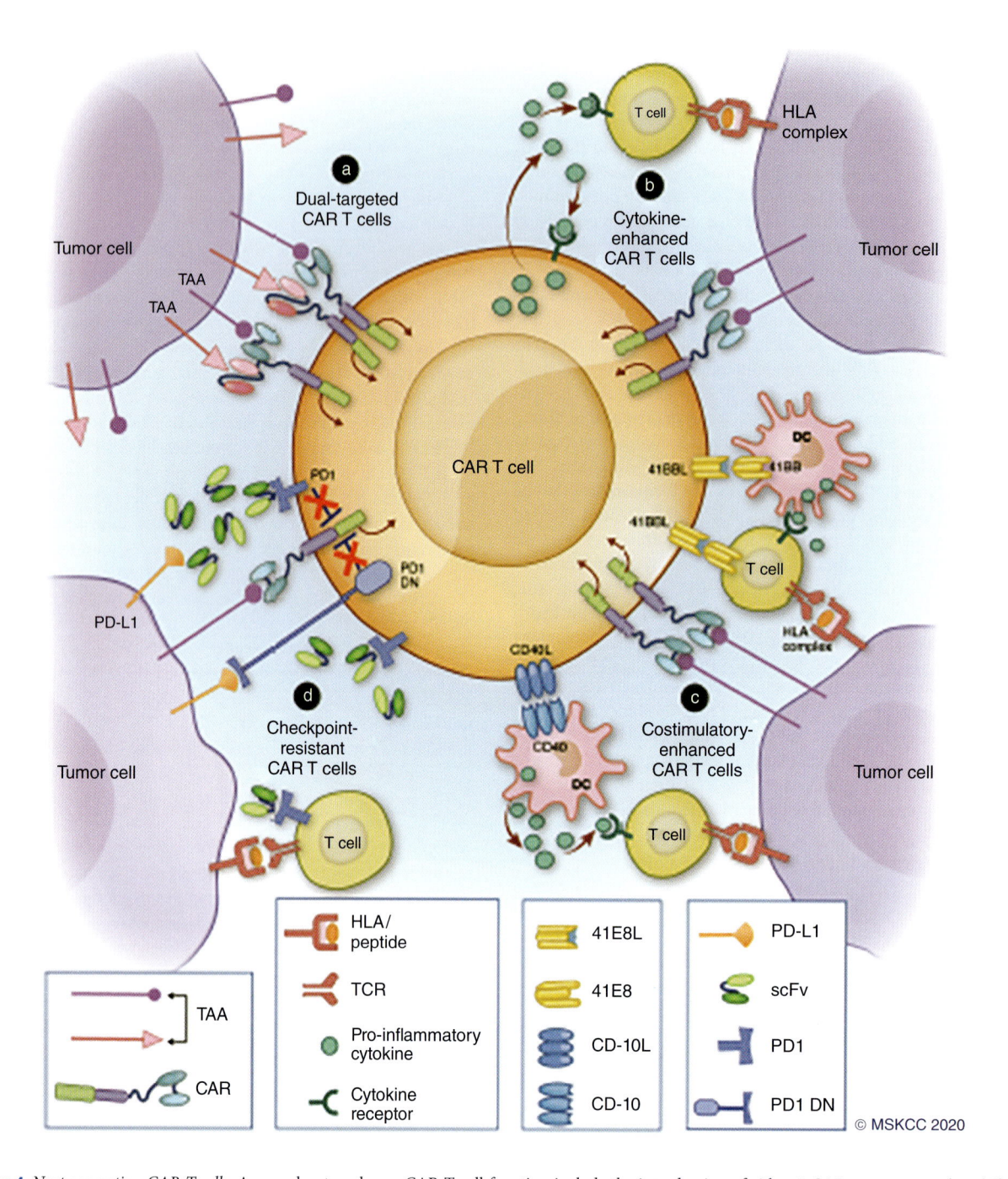

Figure 4 *Next generation CAR T cells.* Approaches to enhance CAR T cell function include the introduction of either 2 CAR genes targeted to different antigens or introduction of a single CAR gene specific to 2 tumor associated antigens (a). Additionally, CAR T cells and tumor specific T cells in general may be further genetically enhanced to secrete Pro-inflammatory cytokines such as IL-12 and IL-18 to enhance CAR T cell function as well as modulate the TME to recruit endogenous tumor-targeted T cells (b). CAR T cells may be additionally genetically modified to augment costimulation and modulate the TME through constitutive expression of costimulatory ligands including 4-1BBL and CD40L (c). Finally, CAR T cells resistant to immune checkpoint inhibition may be generated through the introduction of PD-1 dominant negative (DN) receptors of activating receptors or through the engineering of CAR T cells to secrete scFvs which block PD-1/PD-L1 interaction which protect the CAR T cells as well as potentially rescue inhibited endogenous anti-tumor T cells (d).

blockade on the CAR T cell and additionally protects endogenous tumor-targeted T cells from checkpoint inhibition (Figure 4d).

A mechanistic understanding of cancer T cell therapy treatment failures has allowed for the development of next generation of T cells designed to enhance clinical efficacy. The examples of next-generation tumor-targeted T cells discussed above are likely to those approaches to be clinically tested in the foreseeable future but these are simply examples and are by no means a comprehensive list of novel approaches.[156] However, as more becomes understood about how these T cells interact with both hematological and solid tumors, this knowledge will no doubt give rise to ever more innovative next-generation tumor-targeted T cells. Furthermore, one must appreciate that these technologies are not "one size fits all" given the fact that each tumor presents unique obstacles to the tumor-targeted T cells and one could foresee a future wherein the next generation design of the tumor-targeted T cell is specifically modified to personally address each patient's tumor and TME.

Conclusion

Over the last five to six decades, with the advent of allogeneic BMTs in the context of acute leukemias, cancer investigators have been aware of the potential of tumor-targeted T cells as a highly potent anticancer therapeutic. For many of the subsequent years, the ability of these investigators to utilize the potential of T cell therapies was limited due to the ability to isolate these tumor-targeted T cells for adoptive therapy. With the recognition of virus-induced malignancies and the fact that these foreign and immunogenic viral proteins are expressed by the tumor cells, investigators have focused on the isolation and expansion of virus-specific T cells demonstrating the potential of this adoptive T cell infusion approach in both the setting of hematologic and solid tumor malignancies. Further, the recognition that TILs have the capacity to induce tumor recognition and could be isolated and expanded *ex vivo* further promoted the concept that endogenous tumor-targeted T cells mediate significant antitumor responses and has led to the use of these TILs as a therapeutic approach. The more recent advent of T cell genetic engineering in combination with a better understanding of tumor immunology has led to the next generation of T cell adoptive immunotherapy of cancer wherein patient and/or donor T cells may be genetically manipulated to recognize tumor antigens through the introduction of CARs and tumor-targeted TCRs. Initial Food and Drug Administration (FDA) approval of CD19-targeted T cells for the treatment of relapsed and refractory B cell malignancies is just the first step in the optimization of targeted T cells for the treatment of cancer, however, multiple limitations to the CAR T cell approach have been recognized. These limitations have led to preclinical studies of genetically engineered tumor-targeted T cells designed to overcome these perceived limitations and in both the context of TCR and CAR-modified T cells demonstrate enhanced antitumor efficacy in the preclinical setting. The ceiling for genetically tumor-targeted T cells remains very high and the currently proposed approaches to enhance these engineered T cells remain to be investigated in the clinical setting. Adoptive therapy with tumor-targeted T cells remains at the forefront of novel cancer therapies and as a rapidly progressing technology will likely influence clinical therapy of cancer moving forward.

Key references

The complete reference list can be found on Vital Source version of this title, see inside front cover.

15. Heslop HE, Slobod KS, Pule MA, et al. Long-term outcome of EBV-specific T-cell infusions to prevent or treat EBV-related lymphoproliferative disease in transplant recipients. *Blood*. 2010;**115**(5):925–935. doi: 10.1182/blood-2009-08-239186; Epub 2009/11/03. PubMed PMID: 19880495; PMCID: PMC2817637.

19. Bollard CM, Gottschalk S, Torrano V, et al. Sustained complete responses in patients with lymphoma receiving autologous cytotoxic T lymphocytes targeting Epstein-Barr virus latent membrane proteins. *J Clin Oncol*. 2014;**32**(8):798–808. doi: 10.1200/jco.2013.51.5304; Epub 2013/12/18. PubMed PMID: 24344220; PMCID: PMC3940538 found at the end of this article.

28. Rosenberg SA, Packard BS, Aebersold PM, et al. Use of tumor-infiltrating lymphocytes and interleukin-2 in the immunotherapy of patients with metastatic melanoma. A preliminary report. *N Engl J Med*. 1988;**319**(25):1676–1680. doi: 10.1056/nejm198812223192527; Epub 1988/12/22. PubMed PMID: 3264384.

29. Rosenberg SA, Yannelli JR, Yang JC, et al. Treatment of patients with metastatic melanoma with autologous tumor-infiltrating lymphocytes and interleukin 2. *J Natl Cancer Inst*. 1994;**86**(15):1159–1166. doi: 10.1093/jnci/86.15.1159; Epub 1994/08/03. PubMed PMID: 8028037.

31. Rosenberg SA, Yang JC, Sherry RM, et al. Durable complete responses in heavily pretreated patients with metastatic melanoma using T-cell transfer immunotherapy. *Clin Cancer Res*. 2011;**17**(13):4550–4557. doi: 10.1158/1078-0432.Ccr-11-0116; Epub 2011/04/19. PubMed PMID: 21498393; PMCID: PMC3131487.

73. Brentjens RJ, Latouche JB, Santos E, et al. Eradication of systemic B-cell tumors by genetically targeted human T lymphocytes co-stimulated by CD80 and interleukin-15. *Nat Med*. 2003;**9**(3):279–286. doi: 10.1038/nm827; Epub 2003/02/13. PubMed PMID: 12579196.

77. Kochenderfer JN, Feldman SA, Zhao Y, et al. Construction and preclinical evaluation of an anti-CD19 chimeric antigen receptor. *J Immunother*. 2009;**32**(7):689–702. doi: 10.1097/CJI.0b013e3181ac6138; Epub 2009/06/30. PubMed PMID: 19561539; PMCID: PMC2747302.

79. Wang J, Jensen M, Lin Y, et al. Optimizing adoptive polyclonal T cell immunotherapy of lymphomas, using a chimeric T cell receptor possessing CD28 and CD137 costimulatory domains. *Hum Gene Ther*. 2007;**18**(8):712–25. doi: 10.1089/hum.2007.028.

80. Kochenderfer JN, Wilson WH, Janik JE, et al. Eradication of B-lineage cells and regression of lymphoma in a patient treated with autologous T cells genetically engineered to recognize CD19. *Blood*. 2010;**116**(20):4099–4102. doi: 10.1182/blood-2010-04-281931; Epub 2010/07/30. PubMed PMID: 20668228; PMCID: PMC2993617.

81. Kochenderfer JN, Dudley ME, Feldman SA, et al. B-cell depletion and remissions of malignancy along with cytokine-associated toxicity in a clinical trial of anti-CD19 chimeric-antigen-receptor-transduced T cells. *Blood*. 2012;**119**(12):2709–2720. doi: 10.1182/blood-2011-10-384388; Epub 2011/12/14. PubMed PMID: 22160384; PMCID: PMC3327450.

82. Kochenderfer JN, Dudley ME, Kassim SH, et al. Chemotherapy-refractory diffuse large B-cell lymphoma and indolent B-cell malignancies can be effectively treated with autologous T cells expressing an anti-CD19 chimeric antigen receptor. *J Clin Oncol*. 2015;**33**(6):540–549. doi: 10.1200/JCO.2014.56.2025; Epub 2014/08/27. PubMed PMID: 25154820; PMCID: PMC4322257.

83. Turtle CJ, Hanafi LA, Berger C, et al. Immunotherapy of non-Hodgkin's lymphoma with a defined ratio of CD8+ and CD4+ CD19-specific chimeric antigen receptor-modified T cells. *Sci Transl Med*. 2016;**8**(355):355ra116. doi: 10.1126/scitranslmed.aaf8621; PubMed PMID: 27605551; PMCID: PMC5045301.

84. Kochenderfer JN, Somerville RPT, Lu T, et al. Lymphoma remissions caused by anti-CD19 chimeric antigen receptor T cells are associated with high serum interleukin-15 levels. *J Clin Oncol*. 2017;**35**(16):1803–1813. doi: 10.1200/JCO.2016.71.3024; Epub 2017/03/14. PubMed PMID: 28291388; PMCID: PMC5455597.

86. Ramos CA, Savoldo B, Torrano V, et al. Clinical responses with T lymphocytes targeting malignancy-associated kappa light chains. *J Clin Invest*. 2016;**126**(7):2588–2596. doi: 10.1172/JCI86000; Epub 2016/06/09. PubMed PMID: 27270177; PMCID: PMC4922690.

87. Neelapu SS, Locke FL, Bartlett NL, et al. Axicabtagene ciloleucel CAR T-cell therapy in refractory large B-cell lymphoma. *N Engl J Med*. 2017;**377**(26):2531–2544. doi: 10.1056/NEJMoa1707447; Epub 2017/12/10. PubMed PMID: 29226797; PMCID: PMC5882485.

88. Schuster SJ, Bishop MR, Tam CS, et al. Tisagenlecleucel in adult relapsed or refractory diffuse large B-cell lymphoma. *N Engl J Med*. 2019;**380**(1):45–56. doi: 10.1056/NEJMoa1804980; Epub 2018/12/07. PubMed PMID: 30501490.

89. Schuster SJ, Bishop MR, Tam CS, et al. Long-term follow-up of tisagenlecleucel in adult patients with relapsed or refractory diffuse large B-cell lymphoma: updated analysis of juliet study. *Biol Blood Marrow Transplant*. 2019;**25**(3, Supplement):S20–S21. doi: 10.1016/j.bbmt.2018.12.089.

90. Locke FL, Ghobadi A, Jacobson CA, et al. Long-term safety and activity of axicabtagene ciloleucel in refractory large B-cell lymphoma (ZUMA-1): a single-arm, multicentre, phase 1-2 trial. *Lancet Oncol*. 2019;**20**(1):31–42. doi: 10.1016/S1470-2045(18)30864-7; Epub 2018/12/02. PubMed PMID: 30518502; PMCID: PMC6733402.

91. Neelapu SS, Jacobson CA, Oluwole OO, et al. Outcomes of older patients in ZUMA-1, a pivotal study of axicabtagene ciloleucel in refractory large B-cell lymphoma. *Blood*. 2020. doi: 10.1182/blood.2019004162; Epub 2020/03/18. PubMed PMID: 32181801.

94. Abramson JS, Palomba ML, Gordon LI, et al. Pivotal safety and efficacy results from transcend NHL 001, a multicenter phase 1 study of lisocabtagene maraleucel (liso-cel) in relapsed/refractory (R/R) large B cell lymphomas. *Blood*. 2019;**134**(Supplement_1):241. doi: 10.1182/blood-2019-127508 %J Blood.

99. Park JH, Rivière I, Gonen M, et al. Long-term follow-up of CD19 CAR therapy in acute lymphoblastic leukemia. *N Engl J Med*. 2018;**378**(5):449–459. doi: 10.1056/NEJMoa1709919; PubMed PMID: 29385376; PMCID: PMC6637939.

101. Maude SL, Laetsch TW, Buechner J, et al. Tisagenlecleucel in children and young adults with b-cell lymphoblastic leukemia. *N Engl J Med*. 2018;**378**(5):439–448. doi: 10.1056/NEJMoa1709866; PubMed PMID: 29385370; PMCID: PMC5996391.

103. Turtle CJ, Hanafi LA, Berger C, et al. CD19 CAR-T cells of defined CD4+:CD8+ composition in adult B cell all patients. *J Clin Invest*. 2016;**126**(6):2123–2138. doi: 10.1172/JCI85309; Epub 2016/04/25. PubMed PMID: 27111235; PMCID: PMC4887159.

104. Maude SL, Frey N, Shaw PA, et al. Chimeric antigen receptor T cells for sustained remissions in leukemia. *N Engl J Med*. 2014;**371**(16):1507–1517. doi: 10.1056/NEJMoa1407222; Epub 2014/10/16. PubMed PMID: 25317870; PMCID: PMC4267531.
105. Curran KJ, Margossian SP, Kernan NA, et al. Toxicity and response after CD19-specific CAR T-cell therapy in pediatric/young adult relapsed/refractory B-ALL. *Blood*. 2019;**134**(26):2361–2368. doi: 10.1182/blood.2019001641; PubMed PMID: 31650176.
109. Smith EL, Staehr M, Masakayan R, et al. Development and evaluation of an optimal human single-chain variable fragment-derived BCMA-targeted CAR T cell vector. *Mol Ther*. 2018;**26**(6):1447–1456. doi: 10.1016/j.ymthe.2018.03.016; Epub 2018/04/22. PubMed PMID: 29678657; PMCID: PMC5986730.
110. Mailankody S, Htut M, Lee KP, et al. JCARH125, anti-BCMA CAR T-cell therapy for relapsed/refractory multiple myeloma: initial proof of concept results from a phase 1/2 multicenter study (EVOLVE). *Blood*. 2018;**132**(Supplement_1): 957. doi: 10.1182/blood-2018-99-113548.
113. Grupp SA, Kalos M, Barrett D, et al. Chimeric antigen receptor-modified T cells for acute lymphoid leukemia. *N Engl J Med*. 2013;**368**(16):1509–1518. doi: 10.1056/NEJMoa1215134; PubMed PMID: 23527958; PMCID: 4058440.
115. Maude SL, Barrett D, Teachey DT, Grupp SA. Managing cytokine release syndrome associated with novel T cell-engaging therapies. *Cancer J*. 2014;**20**(2): 119–122. doi: 10.1097/PPO.0000000000000035; PubMed PMID: 24667956; PMCID: 4119809.
133. Rafiq S, Brentjens RJ. Tumors evading CARs-the chase is on. *Nat Med*. 2018;**24**(10):1492–1493. doi: 10.1038/s41591-018-0212-6; Epub 2018/10/10. PubMed PMID: 30297897.
134. Sadelain M, Rivière I, Riddell S. Therapeutic T cell engineering. *Nature*. 2017;**545**(7655):423–431. doi: 10.1038/nature22395; Epub 2017/05/26. PubMed PMID: 28541315; PMCID: PMC5632949.
139. Yeku OO, Purdon TJ, Koneru M, et al. Armored CAR T cells enhance antitumor efficacy and overcome the tumor microenvironment. *Sci Rep*. 2017;**7**(1):10541. doi: 10.1038/s41598-017-10940-8; Epub 2017/09/07. PubMed PMID: 28874817; PMCID: PMC5585170 Therapeutics Inc.
142. Pegram HJ, Lee JC, Hayman EG, et al. Tumor-targeted T cells modified to secrete IL-12 eradicate systemic tumors without need for prior conditioning. *Blood*. 2012;**119**(18):4133–4141. doi: 10.1182/blood-2011-12-400044; Epub 2012/02/23. PubMed PMID: 22354001; PMCID: PMC3359735.
144. Koneru M, O'Cearbhaill R, Pendharkar S, et al. A phase I clinical trial of adoptive T cell therapy using IL-12 secreting MUC-16(ecto) directed chimeric antigen receptors for recurrent ovarian cancer. *J Transl Med*. 2015;**13**:102. doi: 10.1186/s12967-015-0460-x; Epub 2015/04/19. PubMed PMID: 25890361; PMCID: PMC4438636.
145. Avanzi MP, Yeku O, Li X, et al. Engineered tumor-targeted T cells mediate enhanced anti-tumor efficacy both directly and through activation of the endogenous immune system. *Cell Rep*. 2018;**23**(7):2130–2141. doi: 10.1016/j.celrep.2018.04.051; Epub 2018/05/17. PubMed PMID: 29768210; PMCID: PMC5986286.
148. Drakes DJ, Rafiq S, Purdon TJ, et al. Optimization of T-cell receptor-modified T cells for cancer therapy. *Cancer Immunol Res*. 2020;**8**(6):743–755. doi: 10.1158/2326-6066.Cir-19-0910; Epub 2020/03/27. PubMed PMID: 32209638; PMCID: PMC7269835.
150. Curran KJ, Seinstra BA, Nikhamin Y, et al. Enhancing antitumor efficacy of chimeric antigen receptor T cells through constitutive CD40L expression. *Mol Ther*. 2015;**23**(4):769–778. doi: 10.1038/mt.2015.4; Epub 2015/01/15. PubMed PMID: 25582824; PMCID: PMC4395796.
152. Cherkassky L, Morello A, Villena-Vargas J, et al. Human CAR T cells with cell-intrinsic PD-1 checkpoint blockade resist tumor-mediated inhibition. *J Clin Invest*. 2016;**126**(8):3130–3144. doi: 10.1172/jci83092; Epub 2016/07/28. PubMed PMID: 27454297; PMCID: PMC4966328.
154. Rafiq S, Yeku OO, Jackson HJ, et al. Targeted delivery of a PD-1-blocking scFv by CAR-T cells enhances anti-tumor efficacy in vivo. *Nat Biotechnol*. 2018;**36**(9):847–856. doi: 10.1038/nbt.4195; Epub 2018/08/14. PubMed PMID: 30102295; PMCID: PMC6126939.
156. Rafiq S, Hackett CS, Brentjens RJ. Engineering strategies to overcome the current roadblocks in CAR T cell therapy. *Nat Rev Clin Oncol*. 2020;**17**(3):147–167. doi: 10.1038/s41571-019-0297-y; Epub 2019/12/19. PubMed PMID: 31848460; PMCID: PMC7223338 consultant for JUNO Therapeutics/Celgene. The other authors declare no competing interests.

63 Cancer immunotherapy

Padmanee Sharma, MD, PhD ■ Swetha Anandhan MSc ■ Bilal A. Siddiqui, MD ■ Sangeeta Goswami, MD, PhD ■ Sumit K. Subudhi, MD, PhD ■ Jianjun Gao, MD, PhD ■ Karl Peggs, MB, BCh ■ Sergio Quezada, PhD ■ James P. Allison, PhD

Overview

The basic principles that guide cancer immunology are immune surveillance, immune editing, and immune tolerance. Rapid increase in the knowledge of mechanistic details of these basic principles has led to clinical success in the treatment of cancer. In this article, we discuss the basic principles and recent advances in the field of basic and clinical immunotherapy that has given credence to the long-held belief that the immune system can be used to treat cancer. Further, we also focus on the challenges associated with immunotherapies in the clinic, the role of combining different types of immunotherapies and other therapeutic modalities in the treatment of cancer.

Introduction

Harnessing the immune system to target malignant cells in the body was first postulated by William Coley in the early 1900s, who developed a mixture of heat-killed *Streptococcus pyogenes* and *Serratia marcescens* (Coley's toxins) to treat patients with sarcoma, resulting in complete tumor regression in some patients.[1] These early studies with Coley's toxins prompted clinical trials aimed at stimulating the immune system to eradicate cancer. However, incomplete understanding of the mechanistic details of immune responses led to the failure of many early clinical trials.

In 1909, Paul Ehrlich speculated that the incidence of cancer would be much higher if the immune system failed to identify and eliminate nascent tumor cells in the body, a concept that later came to be known as the **immune surveillance**.[2] However, the proof of the theory remained elusive in murine models. Whereas chemically induced tumors were highly immunogenic, naturally occurring tumors were not similarly rejected in murine model systems.[3] Though it was shown that tumor-specific antigens in spontaneously arising tumors could be recognized by the immune system,[4] realization grew that antigenicity was necessary but insufficient to enhance immunogenicity. In the early 2000s, the theory of **immune editing** described how tumor cells become less immunogenic by different mechanisms to eventually escape immune recognition. Over many years, the concept of immune evasion has evolved to encompass three phases, occurring either independently or sequentially[5–8]: (1) the *"elimination phase,"* where immunity functions as an extrinsic tumor suppressor (equivalent to the original concept of immune surveillance); (2) the *"equilibrium phase,"* where the cancer cells survive but are held in check by the immune system; and (3) the *"escape phase,"* where the tumor cell clones grow into clinically apparent cancers. From a therapeutic standpoint, immune editing suggested that efficacy of immunotherapy for established tumors could be enhanced if the tumors were made more visible to the immune system by increasing their antigen expression. As the field progressed to understand the mechanism of immune editing, the final principle of cancer immunotherapy of **immune tolerance** was developed that suggested tumors could evade immune detection not just by becoming less immunogenic but also by inducing tolerance.[9] The idea posited that cancer progression may not solely depend on intrinsic adaptations of the tumor cells but rather on changes in host immunity to induce a state of functional inertia. Therefore, the concepts of immune surveillance, immune evasion, and immune tolerance have become the basic principles that guide the development of cancer immunotherapy.

In addition to our improved knowledge of the host immune system–tumor interaction, we have also gained further insights into the mechanisms that regulate T cell functions. T cell activation requires two major signals. The first signal involves the interaction of the T cell receptor (TCR) on naïve T cells with cognate peptide antigen-major histocompatibility complex (MHC) molecules on antigen-presenting cells (APCs). The second, costimulatory signal, is generated by the binding of CD28 on T cells and B7 (CD80/86) molecules on APCs.[10] Upon activation, T cells undergo rapid and extensive proliferation to help clear foreign agents and infections. In addition to the activation receptor signaling, the surrounding cytokine milieu and other regulatory molecules present on the APCs and T cells also influence the T cell activation process. An effective T cell-mediated anti-tumor response occurs broadly in three stages[11]: (1) detection of tumor-specific and tumor-associated antigens presented by the cancer cells and other APCs in the tumor microenvironment (TME), (2) priming and activation of the T cells by APCs in the tumor-draining lymph nodes, and (3) T cell trafficking to tumor site and T-cell mediated killing, which can occur either directly by release of cytotoxic granules such as granzyme B and perforin that kill the target cells or indirectly by producing cytokines such as interferon γ (IFNγ) and tumor necrosis factor (TNF). This process eventually leads to T cell exhaustion and T cell memory production.

The advances in our scientific understanding have given rise to novel cancer-targeting strategies such as immune checkpoint therapy (ICT) and adoptive T cell therapy. In fact, cancer immunotherapy is now established as an important pillar and a paradigm shift in the treatment of cancer. Ongoing research and clinical studies are driving novel treatment options and combination therapies that are likely to revolutionize the treatment of cancer to benefit a larger patient population. The current options of clinical immunotherapies are discussed in this article and are illustrated in Figure 1.

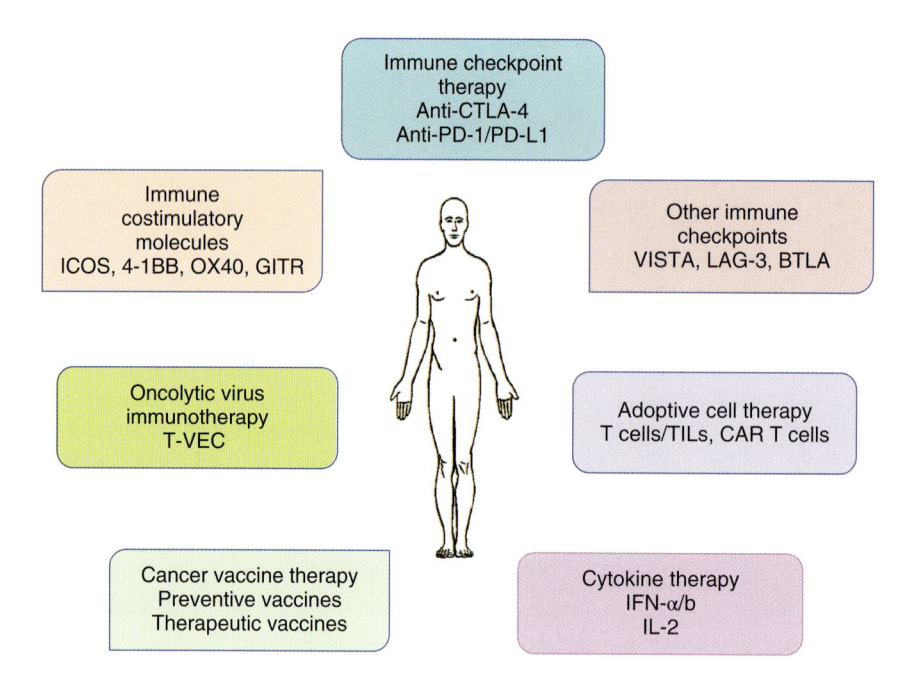

Figure 1 Clinically effective immunotherapeutic strategies.

Immune checkpoint therapy

As discussed above, T cell activation is a complex event, and a balance between co-activating and co-inhibitory signals is essential for proper homeostasis and effective immune response generation. The signaling events involved in such processes are called immune checkpoints. Several inhibitory immune checkpoints on the T cells ensure their regulation to prevent tissue damage and autoimmunity. One such inhibitory receptor is cytotoxic T lymphocyte antigen-4 (CTLA-4) which is expressed as a feedback inhibitory mechanism in activated T cells at the T cell priming phase. Seminal work by James P. Allison's group showed that anti-tumor immunity of tumor-infiltrating T cells can be enhanced by transiently blocking the inhibitory interaction of CTLA-4.[12] This strategy, known as ICT or immune checkpoint blockade, revolutionized the field of cancer immunotherapy. Soon after, another receptor programmed cell death-1 (PD-1) was identified, which is expressed on TCR-activated T cells and induces T cell dysfunction and exhaustion,[13] and its inhibition caused increased in T cell activation and proliferation.[14] Figure 2 depicts a basic overview of the mechanism of ICT. Since then, many other receptor/ligands such as **programmed cell death-ligand 1** (PD-L1), V-domain Ig suppressor of T cell activation (VISTA), and lymphocyte activation gene-3 (LAG-3) have been identified to have similar effects. An alternative strategy to blocking inhibitory immune checkpoints is to enhance costimulatory checkpoints. Other important co-stimulatory molecules such as inducible T cell costimulator (ICOS), 4-1BB, OX-40, glucocorticoid-induced TNFR (GITR), and CD27 are discussed in the subsequent section.

Many immune checkpoint molecules have been identified in the past two decades and these have now been categorized into superfamilies. The most extensively studied is the **B7-CD28 superfamily**, which consists of molecules delivering signals through the CD28 family of receptors on lymphocytes from the B7 family of ligands. CTLA-4, PD-L1/PD-L2, PD-1, ICOS, TIM-3, and VISTA are all members of this superfamily. The **tumor necrosis factor receptor superfamily (TNFRSF)** consists of members known to have necrosis-inducing and anti-tumor cytokine-producing ability. These molecules are involved in regulation of various biological processes such as cell proliferation, differentiation, apoptosis, and survival. Some examples are HVEM, OX-40, CD27, GITR, and 4-1BB. The **immunoglobulin superfamily (IgSF)** consists of immune checkpoint receptors resembling the immunoglobulin molecules. T cell immunoreceptor with Ig and ITIM domains (TIGIT) and LAG-3 are molecules that belong to this group. A schematic overview of various co-inhibitory and stimulatory ligand–receptor interactions is illustrated in Figure 3. Clinical trials of monoclonal antibodies (mAbs) targeting several of these immune checkpoints have shown considerable efficacy, specifically CTLA-4, PD-1, and PD-L1, leading to their Food and Drug Administration (FDA) approval (as shown in Table 1). Selected immune checkpoint pathways are discussed below with an emphasis on FDA-approved therapies. Additionally, novel and potentially targetable immune checkpoint molecules are discussed briefly.

Targeting inhibitory immune checkpoint molecules

Cytotoxic lymphocyte antigen-4 (CTLA-4)

CTLA-4 is expressed upon activation of naïve CD4+ and CD8+ T cells,[15] as well as in natural and inducible Foxp3+ regulatory T cells (Tregs).[16] CTLA-4 has homology to CD28 and binds with much higher affinity to the B7 molecules than CD28. It mediates its inhibitory function in two ways: (1) by outcompeting CD28 for B7 ligand binding thereby reducing T cell activation signaling, and (2) by recruiting phosphatases to its cytoplasmic domain leading to dampening of TCR signaling.[17] Furthermore, CTLA-4 ligation induces decreased production of cytokines (particularly interleukin [IL]-2 and its receptor) and cell cycle arrest in G_1 suggesting that both ligation-dependent and ligation-independent mechanisms contribute to its negative regulatory function. The function of CTLA-4 as a negative regulator of CD28-dependent T cell responses is most strikingly demonstrated by the phenotype of

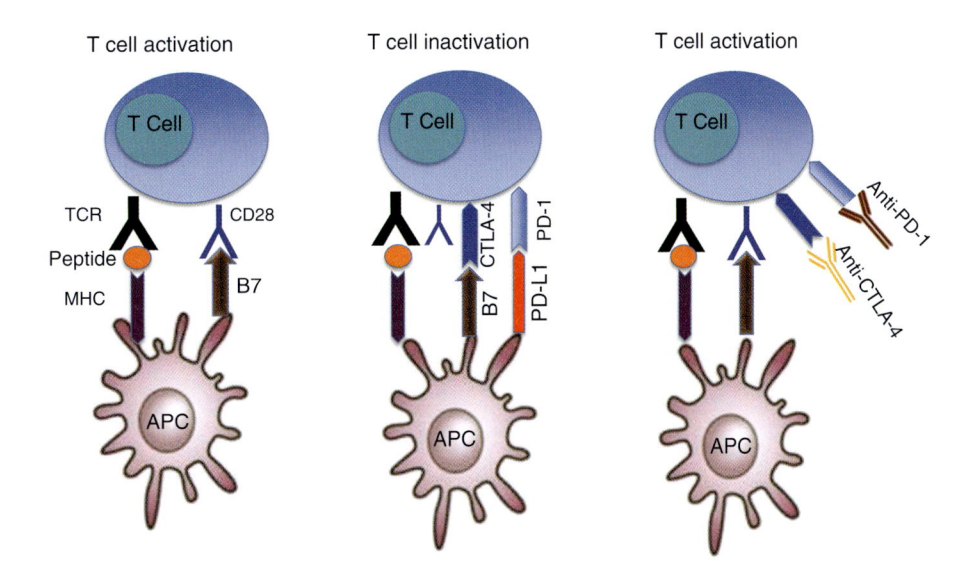

Figure 2 Regulation of T cell response. Signal 1 occurs when the T cell receptor (TCR) on a T cell recognizes the MHC–peptide complex on an APC or a target cell. Signal 2, occurs following interaction of the co-stimulatory receptor B7 (CD80/ 86) on the APC with the co-stimulatory receptor CD28 on the T cell. The activated T cells perform various effector functions. Following T cell activation, CTLA-4 an inhibitory receptor is expressed on the T cells. It binds to the co-stimulatory receptor B7 with higher affinity than CD28, leading to inhibitory signaling and suppression of activated T cell. Similarly, the ligation of another inhibitory T-cell molecule PD-1 by PD-L1 on the APC leads to the formation of PD-1/PD-L1 complex and the recruitment of phosphatases, which dephosphorylate multiple members of the TCR signaling pathway and thereby downregulate T cell responses. Targeting CTLA-4 with anti-CTLA-4 antibodies frees CD28 to interact with the B7 molecules and similarly blocking PD-1 with anti-PD-1 antibodies blocks these inhibitory interactions, further amplifying T cell responses against the tumor.

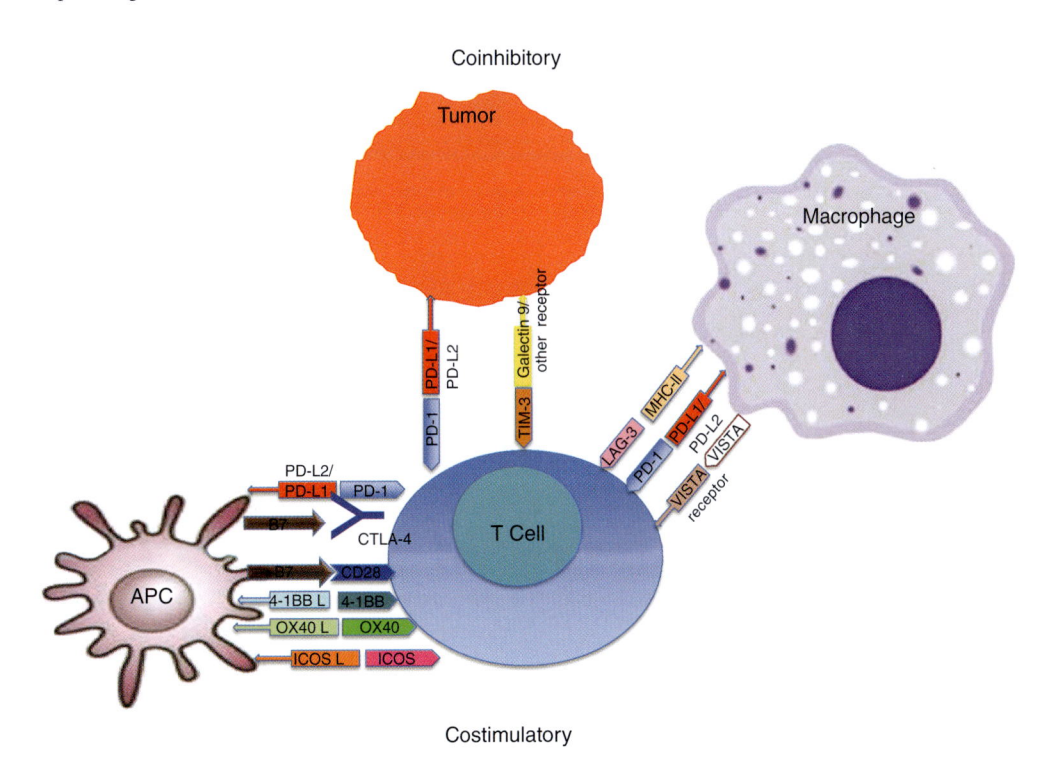

Figure 3 Costimulatory and coinhibitory ligand–receptor interactions. An overview of costimulatory and coinhibitory ligand–receptor interactions in the tumor microenvironment between T cell and APC; T cell and macrophage; T cell and tumor cell.

CTLA-4 knock-out (KO) mice, which succumb to a rapidly lethal polyclonal CD4-dependent lymphoproliferative disease within 3–4 weeks of birth. Antibody-mediated blockade of CTLA-4 enhanced secondary immune responses, more markedly in CD4+ T cells, and led to durable regression of established tumors in syngeneic mice.[12,17] These promising preclinical results of CTLA-4 inhibitors led to the clinical development of humanized mAbs that block the functions of CTLA-4.

Ipilimumab is a fully human IgG1 mAb against CTLA-4. Ipilimumab monotherapy has been FDA-approved in unresectable

Table 1 FDA approved checkpoint immunotherapy.

Agent/target	Indication	Year of approval
1. Ipilimumab/anti-CTLA-4	1. Unresectable or metastatic melanoma	2011
	2. High risk stage III melanoma after complete resection (adjuvant)	2015
	3. Pediatric patients 12 years and older with unresectable or metastatic melanoma	2017
2. Nivolumab/anti-PD-1	1. Unresectable or metastatic melanoma	2014
	2. Metastatic squamous non-small cell lung cancer (NSCLC) with progression on or after platinum-based chemotherapy	2015
	3. Metastatic nonsquamous NSCLC with progression on or after platinum-based chemotherapy	2015
	4. Metastatic renal cell carcinoma (RCC) who have received prior therapy	2015
	5. Classical Hodgkin lymphoma (cHL) that has relapsed or progressed after autologous hematopoietic stem cell transplantation and post-transplantation brentuximab vedotin or after ≥3 lines of therapy	2016
	6. Recurrent or metastatic squamous cell carcinoma of the head and neck (HNSCC) with disease progression on or after platinum-based therapy	2016
	7. Locally advanced or metastatic urothelial carcinoma (UC) with disease progression during or following platinum-based chemotherapy	2017
	8. Adult and pediatric patients with microsatellite instability-high (MSI-H) or mismatch repair deficient (dMMR) metastatic colorectal cancer that has progressed following chemotherapy	2017
	9. Hepatocellular carcinoma (HCC) previously treated with sorafenib	2017
	10. Melanoma with lymph node involvement (adjuvant) or metastatic disease following complete resection	2017
	11. Metastatic RCC, first-line (intermediate/poor risk)	2018
	12. Metastatic SCLC, with progression after platinum-based chemotherapy and at least one other line of therapy	2018
	13. Unresectable advanced, recurrent or metastatic esophageal squamous cell carcinoma after prior fluoropyrimidine- and platinum-based chemotherapy	2020
3. Pembrolizumab/anti-PD-1	1. Advanced or unresectable melanoma that no longer responds to other drugs	2014
	2. Metastatic NSCLC with PD-L1 positive tumors and disease progression after other treatments	2015
	3. First-line treatment of unresectable or metastatic melanoma	2015
	4. Recurrent or metastatic HNSCC with disease progression on or after platinum-based chemotherapy	2016
	5. First-line treatment of metastatic NSCLC, with high PD-L1 expression and no EGFR or ALK genomic tumor	2016
	6. Adult and pediatric refractory cHL or disease relapse after three or more prior lines of therapy	2017
	7. First-line treatment of metastatic nonsquamous NSCLC, irrespective of PD-L1 expression (in combination with carboplatin/pemetrexed)	2017
	8. Locally advanced or metastatic UC with disease progression on or after platinum-based chemotherapy	2017
	9. Adult and pediatric unresectable or metastatic solid tumors that are MSI-H or dMMR	2017
	10. Recurrent locally advanced or metastatic gastric or gastroesophageal junction adenocarcinoma, with PD-L1 positive tumors and disease progression on or after two or more prior lines of therapy	2017
	11. Recurrent or metastatic cervical cancer, with tumor PD-L1 CPS ≥1 and disease progression on or after prior chemotherapy	2018
	12. Primary mediastinal B cell lymphoma, refractory disease or relapse after two or more lines of therapy	2018
	13. Metastatic, non-squamous NSCLC (in combination with pemetrexed and cisplatin/carboplatin)	2018
	14. Metastatic, squamous NSCLC (in combination with carboplatin and paclitaxel or nab-paclitaxel)	2018
	15. HCC, following treatment with sorafenib	2018
	16. Merkel cell carcinoma, recurrent locally advanced or metastatic	2018
	17. Melanoma with lymph node involvement following complete resection	2019
	18. Locally advanced or metastatic NSCLC with PD-L1 TPS ≥1%	2019
	19. Advanced RCC, first line (in combination with axitinib)	2019
	20. HNSCC, first line treatment for metastatic or unresectable recurrent disease with tumor PD-L1 CPS ≥1	2019
	21. HNSCC, first line treatment for metastatic or unresectable recurrent disease (in combination with platinum and fluorouracil)	2019
	22. SCLC, metastatic, with disease progression on or after platinum based chemotherapy and at least 1 other prior line of therapy	2019
	23. Esophageal cancer, recurrent locally advanced or metastatic squamous cell, with tumor PD-L1 CPS ≥10 and disease progression after one or more prior lines of systemic therapy	2019
	24. Endometrial carcinoma, advanced, non-MSI-H/dMMR with disease progression after prior systemic therapy and not candidate for curative surgery or radiation (in combination with lenvatinib)	2019
	25. UC, high-risk, BCG-unresponsive, non-muscle invasive with carcinoma in situ with or without papillary tumors, ineligible for or declined cystectomy	2020
	26. Recurrent or metastatic cutaneous squamous cell carcinoma not curable by surgery or radiation	2020
	27. Unresectable or metastatic tumor mutational burden-high (TMB-H, ≥10 mut/Mb) solid tumors that have progressed on prior treatment with no satisfactory alternative treatment options.	2020
	28. Unresectable or metastatic MSI-H or dMMR colorectal cancer, first-line	2020
	29. Locally recurrent unresectable or metastatic triple negative breast cancer with tumor PD-L1 CPS ≥10	2020
4. Ipilimumab +Nivolumab/ anti-CTLA-4 + anti-PD-1	1. BRAF V600 wild-type unresectable or metastatic melanoma	2015
	2. BRAF V600 wild-type and BRAF V600 mutation-positive unresectable or metastatic melanoma	2016
	3. Poor/Intermediate risk or previously untreated advanced renal cell carcinoma	2018
	4. Previously treated MSI-H/dMMR colorectal cancer	2018
	5. HCC following treatment with sorafenib	2020
	6. Metastatic NSCLC with PD-L1 ≥1%	2020
	7. Unresectable malignant pleural mesothelioma	2020

Table 1 (Continued)

Agent/target	Indication	Year of approval
5. Durvalumab/anti-PD-L1	1. Locally advanced or metastatic UC	2017
	2. Unresectable stage III NSCLC with non-progressive disease following concurrent platinum-based chemotherapy and radiation therapy (adjuvant)	2018
	3. SCLC, extensive stage, first line (in combination with etoposide and carboplatin/cisplatin)	2020
6. Atezolizumab/anti-PD-L1	1. Locally advanced or metastatic UC, with disease progression during or following platinum-based chemotherapy, either before or after surgery	2016
	2. Metastatic NSCLC with disease progression during or following platinum-based chemotherapy, and progression on an FDA-approved targeted therapy if the tumor has EGFR or ALK gene abnormalities	2016
	3. Locally advanced or metastatic UC not eligible for cisplatin chemotherapy	2017
	4. First line, metastatic, non-squamous SCLC without *EGFR* or *ALK* genomic alterations (in combination with bevacizumab, paclitaxel, and carboplatin)	2018
	5. SCLC, extensive stage, first line (in combination with etoposide and carboplatin)	2019
	6. Unresectable locally advanced or metastatic triple negative breast cancer with PD-L1 ≥1%	2019
	7. Metastatic NSCLC without *EGFR* or *ALK* genomic alterations (in combination with carboplatin/nab-paclitaxel)	2019
	8. Metastatic NSCLC, first line, PD-L1 high (tumor cells ≥50% or immune cells ≥10%) without *EGFR* or *ALK* genomic alterations	2020
	9. Metastatic or unresectable HCC, first line (in combination with bevacizumab)	2020
	10. BRAF V600 mutation-positive unresectable or metastatic melanoma in combination with cobimetinib and vemurafenib	2020
7. Avelumab/anti-PD-L1	1. Adult and pediatric patients with metastatic Merkel cell carcinoma, including those who have not received prior chemotherapy	2017
	2. Locally advanced or metastatic UC with disease progression during or following platinum-based chemotherapy	2017
	3. Advanced RCC, first line (in combination with axitinib)	2019
	4. Maintenance treatment for locally advanced for metastatic UC that has not progressed with first-line platinum-containing chemotherapy	2020
8. Cemiplimab/ anti-PD-1	1. Metastatic or locally advanced cutaneous squamous cell carcinoma	2018

Updated as of January 1, 2021.

or metastatic melanoma and as adjuvant treatment for high risk, stage III melanoma. In a randomized Phase III trial in patients with metastatic melanoma who received either ipilimumab with or without a peptide (gp100) vaccine, or vaccine treatment alone, ipilimumab monotherapy improved median overall survival (OS). Importantly, approximately 20% of patients who received ipilimumab had long-term survival of greater than 3 years. These data led to the FDA approval of ipilimumab for metastatic melanoma in 2011.[18] Another Phase III trial in patients with previously untreated metastatic melanoma demonstrated that median OS was significantly longer for patients who received ipilimumab plus dacarbazine chemotherapy as compared to patients who received dacarbazine alone.[19] Additionally, ipilimumab versus placebo was investigated in patients with high-risk stage III melanoma after complete resection. Recurrence-free survival at 3 years was 46.5% in patients treated with ipilimumab versus 34.8% for patients who received placebo, which led to the FDA approval of ipilimumab in the adjuvant setting.[20] A pooled analysis of 10 prospective and 2 retrospective studies, including the above-mentioned Phase III trials showed ipilimumab increased long-term survival of approximately 20% of patients, with survival of 10 years noted for some patients. The results were independent of ipilimumab dosing or prior therapy.[21] Thus, currently, three FDA approvals of ipilimumab monotherapy are available for melanoma (Table 1).

Another humanized mAb (IgG2) targeting CTLA-4, tremelimumab, demonstrated durable responses in early clinical studies;[22–24] however, in a Phase III randomized clinical trial, it failed to demonstrate an OS benefit when compared with chemotherapy (dacarbazine or temozolomide) in patients with advanced melanoma.[25] The failure to demonstrate a survival advantage by tremelimumab may have been due to trial design, dosing, and schedule (e.g., dosing of tremelimumab 15 mg/kg every 90 days), rather than lack of biological activity of the agent.

Programmed cell death-1 (PD-1)

PD-1 is another inhibitory immune checkpoint that belongs to the CD28/CTLA-4 family. It can be detected on activated $CD4^+$ and $CD8^+$ T cells, B cells, monocytes, and at lower levels on natural killer-T (NKT) cells. PD-1 mediates its inhibitory function by the SHP-2 tyrosine phosphatase domain that de-phosphorylates signaling molecules downstream of the TCR.[26] It binds to two separate ligands, PD-L1 and **programmed cell death-ligand 2** (PD-L2), which exhibit distinct expression profiles (reviewed in Ref. 27). PD-L1 is a broadly expressed molecule and can be detected on resting and activated T cells (including $CD4^+CD25^+Foxp3^+$ Tregs), B cells, macrophages, dendritic cells (DCs), and mast cells. In addition, its expression on nonhematopoietic cells (including cornea, lung, pancreatic islets, placental syncytiotrophoblast, keratinocytes, and vascular endothelium) suggests that PD-L1 perhaps also plays a role in preventing immune-mediated tissue damage directly at the tissue interface. By comparison, PD-L2 has a much more limited expression profile, restricted to activated macrophages, myeloid DCs, and mast cells, suggesting that it fulfills a role that differs from that of PD-L1. PD-L1 is expressed on several human carcinomas (breast, cervical, lung, ovarian, colonic, renal), as well as melanoma, glioblastoma, and some hematopoietic malignancies.[28–33] Its expression has been directly correlated with poor prognosis in bladder, breast, kidney, gastric, and pancreatic cancers.[31,34,35] mAbs targeting PD-1 and PD-L1 have shown clinical benefit in various tumor types. To date, there have been three mAbs against PD-1 (nivolumab, pembrolizumab, cemiplimab) and three against PD-L1 (durvalumab, atezolizumab, avelumab) that were FDA-approved in a diverse array of cancers, including skin, genitourinary, lung, head and neck, lymphoma, gynecologic, gastrointestinal, and select tumor-agnostic indications. These are listed in Table 1.

The anti-PD-1 mAb pembrolizumab was the first immunotherapy to garner a cancer-agnostic approval in biomarker-selected patients. A study in the treatment of unresectable or metastatic microsatellite instability/deficient mismatch repair (MSI-H/dMMR) solid tumors demonstrated a better response to pembrolizumab than mismatch proficient tumors.[36] This observation led to the Phase II trial across 12 different cancer types, all with mismatch repair defects. Objective responses were noted in 53% of patients with 21% achieving complete response. This study led to the accelerated FDA approval of pembrolizumab in 2017 for unresectable and metastatic solid tumors with dMMR, the first tumor-agnostic approval of a cancer treatment based on a common biomarker. Building on this success, pembrolizumab has also been approved by the FDA to treat adult and pediatric patients with advanced solid tumors that harbor tumor mutational burden (TMB) of ≥10 mutations/megabase and have progressed through prior therapy without alternative treatment options.

CTLA-4 and PD-1/PD-L1 inhibitory interactions represent only a fraction of the potential targets that inhibit antitumor immune responses. A selection of additional inhibitory pathways that are currently being studied to improve antitumor immune responses are discussed below.

Lymphocyte activation gene-3 (LAG-3)

LAG-3 is an immune checkpoint expressed on a subset of activated T cells, B cells, DCs, and natural killer (NK) cells. Due to its homology to CD4, it was identified to interact with MHC class II as its canonical ligand to regulate T cell responses. Studies indicate that LAG-3 negatively regulates activation, proliferation, and cytokine secretion of Th1 cells.[37] LAG-3 and PD-1 are co-expressed on activated T cells.[38] Preliminary data in ovarian cancer patients showed that blockade of LAG-3 and PD-1 increased proliferation and cytokine production from tumor-infiltrating LAG-3$^+$PD-1$^+$CD8$^+$ T cells.[39] Based on preclinical data, anti-LAG-3 mAbs are showing promising results in the clinic.[40] IMP321 (eftilagimod alpha), an anti-LAG-3 mAb, showed encouraging results in Phase I studies in metastatic breast and advanced pancreatic cancer and is being explored in combination with anti-PD1 or with a cancer vaccine as an adjuvant.[41,42] Another anti-LAG-3 mAb, BMS-986016, in combination with anti-PD-1 (nivolumab) in melanoma patients showed an objective response rate (ORR) of 13% in patients who had relapsed on anti-PD-1 monotherapy.[43] LAG525 is a humanized anti-LAG-3 mAb which is currently under investigation in Phase I/II trials in combination with anti-PD-1 for advanced cancers.[44]

V-domain Ig suppressor of T cell activation (VISTA)

VISTA is another immune checkpoint molecule highly expressed on myeloid cells such as macrophages, conventional DCs, monocytes, and circulating neutrophils and moderately expressed on T cells, mostly Tregs.[45] It is known to suppress T cell activation and cytokine production. It was recently shown that VISTA is an acidic selective ligand for PSGL1.[46] Preclinical studies with VISTA blockade have demonstrated improved antitumor immunity.[47,48] Our group recently reported that anti-CTLA-4 immunotherapy can induce increased expression of VISTA on macrophages, which manifest an M2 phenotype as a resistance mechanism in prostate and pancreatic cancer.[49,50] Clinical trials with anti-VISTA mAbs are currently ongoing.[51,52]

T-cell Ig and mucin-domain-containing-3 (TIM-3)

TIM-3, also called hepatitis A virus cellular receptor 2 (HAVCR2), is an inhibitory receptor expressed on T cell subsets, DCs, NK cells, monocytes, and macrophages. It is known to bind to soluble ligands galectin-9 and HMGB1 and surface ligands CEACAM-1 and PtdSer. TIM-3 interaction with its ligands induces T cell apoptosis and dampened antitumor responses.[40,53] Both clinical and preclinical studies have shown that TIM-3$^+$ T cells display an exhausted phenotype and contribute to immunosuppressive TME[54,55] and concomitantly, addition of anti-TIM-3 mAb can restore the activated phenotype and T cell function.[56] mAbs targeting TIM-3 are under development in early phase clinical trials alone and in combination with anti-PD-1 and anti-PD-L1 therapy in solid tumor malignancies (NCT02817633, NCT03099109, NCT03446040, and NCT02608268).

Other inhibitory members of the Ig superfamily offer further possible targets for coinhibitory blockade; although the impact such interventions would have on antitumor activity remains speculative at present.

T cell immunoreceptor with Ig and ITIM domains (TIGIT)

TIGIT, a transmembrane glycoprotein, is an inhibitory receptor expressed on activated, memory, and regulatory T cells and NK cells. TIGIT is weakly expressed on naïve T cells and its expression increases following T cell activation. Preclinical studies showed promising results in restoring T cell function following TIGIT blockade. Currently, multiple clinical trials are testing anti-TIGIT monoclonal antibody in combination with other immune checkpoint therapies (NCT04047862, NCT04354246, NCT04256421, NCT04294810, and NCT03628677).

Combined targeting of inhibitory checkpoints

Combinatorial blockade of CTLA-4 and PD-1 concomitantly eliminates cell-intrinsic negative signaling through CTLA-4, B7-1, PD-L1, and PD-1 while favoring positive signaling through CD28. Inhibitory signaling of both CTLA-4 and PD-1 are largely distinct; as CTLA-4 plays a more essential role in the control of CD8$^+$ T cell priming responses,[57] whereas PD-1/PD-L1 interactions may be important in the regulation of CD8$^+$ effector T cell responses within the tumor.[58] Further, mechanistic studies in murine models of cancer indicate that anti-CTLA-4 and anti-PD-1 blockade result in expansion of distinct phenotypic T cell subsets.[59] Also, studies from our lab and others have shown that expression of PD-1/PD-L1 increases post anti-CTLA-4 treatment in human and murine bladder cancers and murine melanoma tumors.[54,60,61] Thus, combination strategies targeting both these molecules could prove to be a more effective approach than monotherapy. The combination of ipilimumab and nivolumab has demonstrated clinical efficacy in multiple tumor types.

A Phase III trial compared ipilimumab, nivolumab, and the combination in patients with untreated, unresectable, or metastatic melanoma with co-primary endpoints of progression-free survival (PFS) and OS. Treatment with combination therapy was statistically superior to either drug alone, with a median PFS of 11.5 months versus 6.9 months for nivolumab alone versus 2.8 months for ipilimumab alone. Based on these findings, the FDA-approved combination therapy with ipilimumab plus nivolumab as first-line treatment for patients with previously untreated, unresectable, or metastatic melanoma, regardless of PD-L1 expression status on tumor cells.[62] In the long-term follow-up of this trial, the estimated five-year OS was 52% for the combination versus 44% for nivolumab and 26% for ipilimumab.[63]

In a Phase III randomized trial in patients with advanced or metastatic clear cell renal cell carcinoma (RCC), a total of 1096 patients were assigned to receive nivolumab plus ipilimumab (550 patients) or sunitinib (546 patients). At a median follow-up of 25.2 months in intermediate- and poor-risk patients, the 18-month OS rate was 75% with nivolumab plus ipilimumab and 60% with sunitinib; the median OS was not reached with nivolumab plus ipilimumab versus 26.0 months with sunitinib. The ORR was 42% versus 27%, the complete response rate was 9% versus 1%, and the median PFS was 11.6 and 8.4 months, respectively.[64] This led to FDA approval of ipilimumab plus nivolumab in the metastatic RCC in the first-line setting. The combination has also been approved in advanced hepatocellular carcinoma (HCC) as second-line treatment,[65] metastatic or recurrent non-small cell lung cancer (NSCLC),[66] as well as in patients with previously treated metastatic colorectal cancer with MSI-H or dMMR.[67]

Targeting stimulatory immune receptors

Whereas inhibitory checkpoints have been targeted with *antagonist* mAbs, *agonist* mAbs targeting stimulatory immune receptors similarly seek to augment preexisting T cell responses and enhance immunological memory. A schematic overview of various costimulatory ligand–receptor interactions is illustrated in Figure 3. A brief description of selected stimulatory checkpoints is provided below.

Inducible T cell costimulator (ICOS)

ICOS is a member of the CD28/CTLA-4 family. The interaction of ICOS with its ligand (ICOSL), expressed on APCs, provides a key costimulatory signal to T cells for proliferation and survival. The expression of ICOS is increased upon T cell activation.[68] Studies indicate that ICOS signaling is necessary and essential for optimal antitumor responses mediated by anti-CTLA-4 therapy.[55] Sustained ICOS expression on CD4$^+$ T cells has also been observed to correlate with survival of melanoma patients treated with anti-CTLA-4 therapy.[69,70] Consistent with these observations, increased frequency of ICOS$^+$ CD4$^+$ T cells can also serve as a pharmacodynamic biomarker for anti-CTLA-4 therapy.[71]

4-1BB (CD137)

4-1BB, a member of the TNFR family, is expressed on early activated T cells (including Tregs and NKT cells), activated NK cells and DCs, and endothelial cells in some metastatic tumors.[72–75] Its ligand, 4-1BBL, is expressed on activated DCs, B cells, and macrophages. Engagement of 4-1BB on T cells results in upregulation of antiapoptotic genes and protection from activation-induced cell death (AICD)[76] and enhancement of durable memory cytotoxic T lymphocytes (CTLs).[77] 4-1BBL may also promote production of inflammatory mediators or enhanced cell adhesion; facilitating egress of immune effectors into sites of inflammation.[78,79] Clinical studies with utomilumab (PF-05082566, Pfizer) in combination with rituximab in B cell lymphoma and pembrolizumab (MK-3475, anti-PD-1) in solid tumors has completed Phase I.[80] Phase I clinical studies to assess the safety and immuno-regulatory activity of urelumab (BMS-663513) in patients with advanced and/or metastatic tumors and relapsed/refractory B-cell non-Hodgkin's lymphoma have also been completed.[81] Urelumab was associated with significant transaminitis, whereas utomilumab, though well-tolerated, demonstrated an overall ORR of 3.8% across solid tumors.

OX-40

OX-40 is expressed transiently on activated CD4$^+$ and CD8$^+$ T cells, functioning as a late co-stimulatory receptor.[72,82] It is also expressed by NKT cells, where triggering may be required for optimal activation by a-GalCer[83] and Tregs. Its ligand, OX-40L, is expressed on activated DCs, B cells, and macrophages, as well as on activated T cells and endothelial cells.[72] OX-40 ligation regulates CD4$^+$ and CD8$^+$ T cell survival and memory generation, preventing T cell tolerance and impairing the suppressor functions of Tregs. 4-1BB and OX-40 act independently to facilitate robust CD8 and CD4 recall responses, overlapping in their intracellular signaling pathways. A Phase I clinical trial using one course of the agonistic mouse anti-OX-40 mAb (9B12) in patients with advanced cancer showed that the treatment had an acceptable toxicity profile and regression of at least one metastatic lesion in 12 of 30 patients.[84] Currently, there are different clinical trials in metastatic colorectal cancer, RCC, lymphoma, and others where anti-OX-40 mAb and OX-40 agonists are being evaluated for efficacy.[85]

Glucocorticoid-induced TNFR (GITR)

GITR is transiently expressed on activated T cells with delayed upregulation at 24–72 h.[86,87] It is also constitutively expressed at high levels on Tregs with further induction following activation.[88,89] Its ligand, GITRL, is expressed at low levels on B cells, macrophages, and some DCs, transiently increasing following activation. GITR ligation stimulates both proliferation and function of CD4$^+$ and CD8$^+$ T cells. Injection of adenovirus expressing recombinant GITRL into B16 melanoma promoted T cell infiltration and reduced tumor volumes,[90] whereas agonistic anti-GITR mAbs have been shown to enhance both rejection of established fibrosarcomas and enhancement of systemic antitumor responses following B16 melanoma challenge.[91,92] A Phase I clinical trial with the anti-GITR mAb, TRX-518, showed Treg reductions and increased Teff:Treg ratios, though substantial clinical responses were observed.[93] This agent is now being studied in combination with PD-1 blockade (NCT02628574).

CD40

CD40 is a member of the TNFR superfamily. CD40 is constitutively expressed by B cells and DCs and is also expressed by macrophages, T cells, and nonhematopoietic cells, such as vascular endothelium.[94] Its ligand, CD40L, is principally expressed by activated CD4$^+$ T helper cells. CD40 ligation is critical for licensing of DCs and its expression on number of lymphoma and carcinoma tumor cells suggests that mAbs to CD40 could elicit complement- or antibody-dependent cellular cytotoxicity (CDC or ADCC). CD40 signaling has been reported to directly induce apoptosis in some tumor cells, notably in high-grade B cell non-Hodgkin lymphomas and epithelial carcinomas.[95–97] Clinical trials with recombinant CD40L trimer or anti-CD40 mAbs induced response in a small cohort of B cell lymphomas or melanoma patients; although toxicities including systemic inflammatory syndromes and venous thromboses have been documented.[98–100] A novel approach utilized electroporation to introduce mRNA encoding CD40L, constitutively active TLR4, CD70, and multiple melanoma tumor antigens into autologous DCs (TriMix-DC), and tumor regressions were observed in 6 of 17 patients who had received interferon-α-2b in combination with TriMix-DC.[101] Furthermore, combination of anti-CD40 mAb and a chemotherapy, gemcitabine, showed tumor regression in both human and mice.[102]

CD27

CD27, also known as TNFRSF7, is a member of TNFR family.[103] It is expressed on T cells, B cells, and NK cells. Constitutive expression of CD27 on T cells suggests a role in T cell priming. The known ligand for CD27 is CD70. The antitumor effect of CD27 has been demonstrated in multiple mouse tumor models. Varlilumab (CDX-1127) is a fully humanized mAb that targets and stimulates CD27. A Phase I study demonstrated safety and antitumor effect of varlilumab in patients with solid as well hematological malignancies.[104] Currently, there are multiple ongoing clinical trials testing CD27 in advanced cancers.

Clinical challenges with immune checkpoint therapy

Despite subsets of patients achieving durable responses with immune checkpoint therapies, challenges abound. Many patients do not respond to initial therapy (primary resistance) or relapse with disease after initially responding to treatment (acquired resistance).[105] There is a critical need to improve response rates to allow more patients with incurable cancers to benefit. The number of candidates for potential combination strategies to overcome resistance is ever growing. Proof-of-principle studies that test biologically based hypotheses are required to efficiently prioritize the development of these combinations. Multiple factors influence resistance and response to immune checkpoint therapies. In this section, we will briefly discuss the current state of knowledge on selected aspects that play a role in resistance and response to immune checkpoint therapies and future areas of research. Several factors determine the response to checkpoint therapy.

Activation of immunosuppressive oncogenic pathways

Recent studies have identified an intricate interplay between oncogenic pathways and antitumor immunity. In one such study, whole-exome sequencing and gene expression profiling of melanoma biopsies revealed that tumor-cell intrinsic activation of the WNT/β-catenin pathway correlates with the absence of T cells in the TME.[106] Further investigation in a genetically engineered autochthonous mouse melanoma model confirmed that increased oncogenic β-catenin signaling results in a failure to recruit CD8α$^+$ and CD103$^+$ DC populations in the tumor due to repressed expression of the chemokine CCL4. Consequently, mice with tumors expressing active β-catenin responded poorly to anti-CTLA-4 and anti-PD-L1 therapy, when compared to mice with tumors lacking β-catenin expression.[106]

Apart from the activation of active β-catenin, the loss of phosphatase and tensin homolog (PTEN) expression is a frequent event in melanoma, especially in tumors with v-raf murine sarcoma viral oncogene homolog B1 (BRAF) mutations. PTEN is a negative regulator of the PI3K-AKT pathway and the complete loss of PTEN is associated with increased signaling through this pathway, correlating with shorter OS in patients with advanced melanoma.[107] Another study in a murine model of melanoma demonstrated that the loss of PTEN expression can reduce the therapeutic activity of ICT. The study additionally demonstrated that a selective PI3K-β-isoform inhibitor could induce synergy with ICT in the preclinical model.[108] Similarly, findings in human melanoma specimens confirmed that the loss of PTEN correlates with exclusion of CD8$^+$ T cell in the tumor and increased PI3K activation. Importantly, patients with tumors lacking PTEN expression demonstrated poor clinical responses to anti-PD-1 therapy compared to patients with retained PTEN expression.[108]

Loss of interferon-gamma signaling

It is well established that IFNγ is a critical cytokine produced by T cells and other immune cells, which plays a key role in promoting innate and adaptive immune responses and in inhibiting tumor cell proliferation. IFNγ functions by binding to the IFNγ-receptor, which initiates signaling through the Janus kinase/signal transducer and activator of transcription proteins (JAK/STAT) pathway to regulate gene expression.[109] Data from many independent studies have established that the loss of genes involved in IFNγ signaling pathway may lead to both primary and adaptive resistance to ICT.[110–112]

Previously published data from a study in patients with bladder cancer demonstrated increased frequency of a CD4$^+$ ICOS^{hi} T cell subset that produced IFNγ, following anti-CTLA-4 therapy.[69] Evaluation of genomic alterations of IFNγ pathway genes in melanoma patients treated with ipilimumab demonstrated that the tumors of the non-responders had loss of IFNγ pathway genes at significantly higher frequencies when compared to the responders. Furthermore, mice bearing melanoma tumors with knockdown of IFNγ receptor resulted in impaired tumor rejection when treated with anti-CTLA-4 therapy. Similarly, another study compared paired tumor biopsies, which were collected from four melanoma patients prior to treatment with anti-PD-1 (pembrolizumab) and at the time of disease relapse.[110] In two out of the four patients whose disease relapsed after initial responses to pembrolizumab therapy, mutations were detected in the genes encoding interferon-receptor-associated Janus kinase 1 (*JAK1*) or Janus kinase 2 (*JAK2*), two critical components of IFNγ signaling pathway. Taken together, these findings indicate that the loss of IFNγ signaling limits the effectiveness of the immune system to eliminate tumor cells and induces resistance to ICT.

Tumor microenvironment

The TME includes cancer cells, stromal components which include fibroblasts, platelets, extracellular matrix, and recruited immune cells. As the tumor develops, ongoing communication occurs among the cellular components of the TME. These signals modulate the functions of the infiltrating lymphoid and myeloid cells and can lead to the formation of dysfunctional immune cells that are incapable of generating effective responses against ICT. The past decade has provided deeper insight into understanding of these cell phenotypes using technology such as single-cell RNA sequencing (scRNAseq) to study the transcriptomes and mass cytometry using time-of-flight (CyTOF) to study the protein expression. We briefly discuss the important lymphoid and myeloid subsets present in the TME below:

T cells

Optimal and efficient T-cell activation is the most important determinant of treatment outcome. However, recent studies indicate that CD8$^+$ T cells present in the TME are both functionally and phenotypically very heterogeneous, and only specific subsets of CD8$^+$ T cells in the TME are responsible for effective response to ICT.[58,59,113] Several groups have shown that epigenetic regulation by transcription factors such as T cell factor (TCF) and thymocyte selection-associated high mobility group box (TOX) dictate the state of exhaustion in CD8$^+$ T cells present in the TME which further determines response to therapy. Self-renewing T cells are TCF$^+$ and possess memory-like and progenitor-exhausted characteristics. These cells undergo proliferation in the presence of an appropriate stimulus.[114,115] Clinically, the presence of this specific T cell is associated with higher PFS in melanoma patients.[116]

TOX has been shown to play a key role in promoting survival of TCF1+CD8+ T cells.[117,118] However, terminally differentiated T cells express high PD-1, lose their TCF expression and thereby lose their proliferative ability. Thus, the phenotype of the T cells within the TME both at baseline and after ICT may serve as an important indicator of treatment response. Furthermore, the cytokine milieu in TME also determines effective T cell response. TGFβ present in the TME causes exclusion of T cells, thereby attenuating the response to ICT.[119] Thus, both T cell-intrinsic and extrinsic factors play a vital role in determining treatment outcome.

Myeloid cell subsets
Myeloid cells are a group of heterogeneous innate immune cells which are highly plastic and diverse in phenotype. High abundance of immune-suppressive myeloid cells in the TME is correlated with poor prognosis in most cancer types and associated with resistance to ICT.[120–123] The cumulative cues from their microenvironment, including tumor-secreted cytokines (IL-10, IL-35, TGF-β) and chemokines (CCL2, CXCL2, CXCL8) favor the recruitment and/or induce polarization of tumor-associated immune suppressive M2 macrophages, myeloid-derived suppressor cells (MDSCs), and neutrophils. These immunosuppressive cells secrete various inducible mediators such as enzymes (iNOS, Arginase1 and indoleamine-2,3-deoxygenase [IDO]), cytokines (IL-10, IL-4, and TGF-β) and express multiple inhibitory receptors such as PD-L1, VISTA, CD73, CSF1R, CCR2.[123,124] Currently, there are multiple ongoing clinical trials evaluating strategies to target immune-suppressive myeloid cells by targeting the inhibitory receptors, enzymes, and cytokines molecules.

Gut microbiome
There is increasing evidence of the importance of the gut microbiome and its influence on the clinical impact of ICT. Two independent preclinical studies showed that modulating the gut microbiome can have dramatic effects on the response to ICT. Mice harboring the commensal *Bifidobacterium* species had enhanced spontaneous antitumor immunity compared to mice with a different gut microbiota composition. Importantly, the direct administration of the *Bifidobacterium* species into mice with established melanoma tumors improved tumor-specific immunity and response to anti-PD-L1 therapy.[125]

Similarly, another study demonstrated that the efficacy of anti-CTLA-4 therapy is associated with T cell responses specific for the microbiota species, *Bacteroides fragilis*. Additionally, the study reported that ipilimumab-responsive patients with metastatic melanoma tend to have *B. fragilis* as a significant component of their microbiome.[126] These observations were further corroborated with recent clinical studies in advanced melanoma patients that show that anti-PD-1 therapy responders had higher gut microbiome diversity and a larger population of *Clostridiales* as compared to nonresponders.[127] In a different study, it was observed that patients who were treated with antibiotics prior to or during immunotherapy, showed poorer responses to the treatment.[128] These studies need further validation with larger cohorts and across different tumor types, but nonetheless, the effect of the microbiome on antitumor immunity seems to be an important factor to be considered when designing therapeutic strategies.

Epigenetic regulation
Epigenetic regulation encompasses a broad range of reversible changes in DNA and the histone proteins. These events regulate gene expression without affecting the DNA sequence. Disruption of epigenetic regulation can lead to alterations in gene expression and malignant transformation. Recent advances in the field of epigenetics have shown that epigenetic reprogramming of tumor cells, as well as immune cells, can modulate the efficacy of ICT.[129–131] Ipilimumab can induce the expression of the enhancer of zeste homolog 2 (EZH2) in T cells. EZH2 is a key epigenetic enzyme that interacts with FoxP3 and maintains a repressive chromatin structure in regulatory T cells. Inhibition of EZH2 can change the phenotype of regulatory T cells to effector-like T cells and increase the effector function of T cells resulting in enhanced efficacy of anti-CTLA-4 therapy in preclinical models.[132] Further, EZH2 inhibition increased the antigenicity of tumor and infiltration of cytotoxic CD8+ T cells.[133,134] Another study showed that DNA methyltransferase (DNMT) and histone deacetylase (HDAC) regulate PD-1 and PD-1 ligand expression. Inhibition of DNMT and HDAC upregulate PD-1 ligand in tumor cells and increase PD-1 expression in T cells.[135] Given that epigenetic agents can affect multiple immuno-modulatory pathways in both tumor cells and immune cells, it provides a strong rationale for combination of drugs that modulate epigenetic regulation with ICT. Currently, early-stage clinical trials of the epigenetic modulator with ICT are ongoing in multiple tumor types. However, epigenetic modulators have broad effects on transcription. Therefore, it will be essential to understand the tumor-specific regulation of the epigenetic agents to design rational combination therapy.

Metabolism
In recent years, the field of immunometabolism has expanded as critical metabolic pathways and checkpoints have been implicated in the activation, function, and migration of immune cells.[136] These processes are vital for T cell-mediated antitumor responses and therefore understanding immunometabolic determinants may help improve immunotherapy outcomes.[137] Further, factors in the TME and tumor cell metabolism itself induce potent and direct suppressive effects on T cell function due to competition for nutrients in limited supply.[138,139] Decreased oxidative stress activates memory T cell precursors which show enhanced antitumor immunity,[140] however, high oxygen tension in the TME induces differentiation of regulatory T cells which suppress the tumor response.[141] Hypoxic conditions further support inhibitory myeloid cells which release arginase-1 and IDO in the TME that inhibit T cell activity and suppress APC function.[142–144]

Since tumor-infiltrating lymphocyte (TIL) function is affected by metabolic checkpoints, multiple targets have the potential to be exploited clinically to improve ICT outcomes. Interestingly, it has been shown that ICT not only inhibits negative signaling in T cells but also increases glucose concentration in the TME probably due to tumor killing. Consequently, strategic use of metabolic inhibitors in combination with ICT might be beneficial. To date, however, IDO inhibition in combination with PD-1 blockade has not yet improved clinical outcomes, although this limited efficacy may be due to study design rather than to a failure of the concept.[145] Currently, multiple early-stage clinical trials are ongoing in different cancer types, combining immune checkpoint inhibition with adenosine pathway inhibitors, modulators of glucose metabolism, and cyclooxygenase (COX) enzyme inhibitors.[146]

Availability of biomarkers that predict response
Since immune checkpoint therapies benefit a subset of patients, there is an unmet need to identify predictive biomarkers to optimize patient selection for therapy. These biomarkers may

broadly be categorized under four headings: (1) target expression (e.g., surface expression of PD-L1); (2) tumor-specific features (e.g., TMB); (3) TME; and (4) host features (e.g., the gut microbiome).

In the first category, immunochemical detection of PD-L1 expression on tumor and/or immune cells is the most commonly used biomarker. Expression of PD-L1 in the tumor correlates with poor disease prognosis. Though several studies have demonstrated that PD-L1 expression on tumor cells correlates with clinical response in certain tumors such as urothelial cancer and NSCLC, these findings are not uniform. Indeed, significant responses can be observed in certain patients with PD-L1 negative tumors.[147] Additionally, PD-L1 expression is not static and can change over time and depend on the area sampled. Dynamic biomarkers, such as the finding that sustained ICOS expression on CD4+ T cells correlates with survival of melanoma patients treated with anti-CTLA-4 therapy (as described above) represent a possible avenue. Differences in the antibodies employed, tissue handling protocols, and thresholds for positivity remain challenges in the use of PD-L1 expression as a predictive biomarker.

Tumor-intrinsic biomarkers include TMB and neoantigen load, DNA damage repair (DDR) pathways, viral infection, MHC expression, and transcriptional signatures. High TMB has been associated with response to ICT in several cancer types, potentially related to neoantigen formation and compensatory upregulation of inhibitory immune checkpoints by the tumor. TMB is an imperfect biomarker, however, as certain tumor types with a low TMB also have high response rates to ICT, such as clear cell RCC. Further research is necessary into immunogenicity of different mutations, assay development, and validation of TMB thresholds. Nevertheless, the FDA has approved pembrolizumab for the treatment of patients with high TMB solid tumors (defined as ≥10 mutations/mega base) that are unresectable or metastatic and have no satisfactory alternative treatment option, based on a retrospective analysis of 102 patients with various solid tumors with high TMB and ORR of 29% (NCT02628067). Additionally, DDR pathways may play a key role in ICT (as described above with pembrolizumab in dMMR/MSI-H patients). Defects in homologous recombination DNA repair such as BRCA 1/2, leading to generation of double-stranded breaks, and release of cytosolic DNA with concomitant upregulation of cGAS-STING and promotion of type I interferon signaling has also been postulated as a possible response mechanism.

Third, the TME is essential for biomarker development. Increased TILs have been associated with response to ICT in melanoma and in breast cancer,[148] with a spectrum of tumor-infiltrating T cell populations that have been identified.[59] Anti-PD-1 therapy induces exhausted-like CD8+ T cell subsets, while anti-CTLA-4 therapy induces expansion of ICOS+ Th1-like CD4 effector cells and engages subsets of exhausted-like CD8+ T cells.[59] B cells and tertiary lymphoid structures have also been found to be associated with response to ICT in patients with melanoma and RCC.[149] Transcriptional signatures such as markers of interferon-γ signaling have been associated with response to ICT.[150]

Finally, as described above, host factors independent of the primary tumor, such as a gut microbiome have been shown to be key in predicting response to ICT. Overall, there is growing recognition that a single biomarker will be insufficient to properly integrate the dynamic interactions of tumor cells, immune cells, and the host in order to enable improved patient selection. Recent studies highlighted combinatorial biomarkers integrating genomic attributes of the tumor cells and immune microenvironment could improve predictive outcome compared to single biomarkers.[151,152]

Pseudoprogression

In the initial trials of ICT, patients were observed to develop classical findings of tumor growth (i.e., tumor flare), which subsequently regressed into deep and durable responses; this phenomenon was deemed pseudoprogression.[153] Since that time, several modified criteria for response assessment have emerged, details of which are beyond the scope of this article. Newer imaging techniques such as volumetric imaging and quantitative imaging biomarkers that may identify T cell infiltration in tumors have exciting potential to better characterize tumor dynamics.

Immune-related adverse events (irAEs)

Whereas ICT can induce T cell-mediated antitumor responses, it can also trigger inflammation of normal tissue through breach of immune self-tolerance mechanisms, deemed immune-related adverse events (irAEs).[154] These toxicities are distinct from that of conventional anticancer agents.[155] The spectrum of irAEs related to anti-CTLA-4 and anti-PD-1/PD-L1 immunotherapy includes common reactions involving the gastrointestinal tract (diarrhea, colitis), skin (rash, dermatitis), liver (transaminitis), or endocrine axis (hypophysitis, thyroiditis, and/or adrenal insufficiency). Less commonly, these irAEs can be severe and fatal, including involvement of the heart (myocarditis), muscles (myositis), and neuromuscular junction (myasthenia gravis). These toxicities can occur in different patterns depending on the ICT employed; for example, colitis is generally more associated with CTLA-4 blockade as compared to PD-(L)1 therapy.[156] It is important to recognize and manage the irAEs in the growing patient population treated with ICT, with close multidisciplinary collaboration. Active areas of investigation include development of more sophisticated treatment strategies, options for ICT re-challenge, biomarkers of toxicity, and determining immunological mechanisms of toxicity.

Current treatment guidelines for irAEs recommend withholding ICT and administration of corticosteroids, generally adapted from their spontaneous autoimmune counterparts. However, there is growing recognition of the diversity of immunopathogenic mechanisms involved in the development of irAEs including not only breach of self-tolerance with development of autoreactive T cells and autoantibody formation, but also cross-antigen reactivity between tumor and normal tissue, cytokine and chemokine production, and effects of the host microbiome.[157] Moreover, corticosteroids carry their own side effects (including risk of severe infection, myopathy, and hyperglycemia), as well as limiting resumption of antitumor therapy.[158] Accordingly, targeted immunosuppressive strategies for irAEs that have been explored include the anti-IL-6 monoclonal antibody tocilizumab, the anti-TNFα monoclonal antibody infliximab, anti-$\alpha_4\beta_7$ integrin mAb vedolizumab,[159] CTLA-4 fusion Ig abatacept and the anti-CD52 monoclonal antibody alemtuzumab.[160–162] Additionally, fecal microbiota transplantation is an emerging therapy that may be beneficial in refractory immune-mediated colitis.[163]

Finally, there is substantial interest in identifying predictive biomarkers of toxicity that can help influence patient selection for ICT. A retrospective study involving two clinical trials in patients with prostate cancer treated with ipilimumab identified CD8+ T-cell clonal expansion within the systemic circulation as a potential correlative biomarker of irAEs.[164] In addition, autoimmune antibodies have also been identified in patients with irAEs including pneumonitis and hypophysitis.[165] Overall, active research is underway in better predicting irAEs and understanding mechanisms to minimize toxicity and to improve efficacy.

Combinatorial strategies with immunotherapy

Combination treatment approaches may boost the efficacy of immunotherapy. Complementary advantages of combining immunotherapy with other targeted therapies can increase durable responses as well as reduce toxicities by targeting different pathways and molecules. Further, neoadjuvant therapy can help enhance antigen release and modulate the TME thereby making the tumors more responsive to ICT, which may also be achieved by surgical "debulking" of tumors.[166]

Recent attention has also focused on the potential for immunotherapies to augment conventional chemotherapy or radiotherapy,[167] and on trying to optimize the immunogenicity of cell death. A combination of radiotherapy and immunotherapy is currently being tested clinically.[168] Increasing evidence demonstrates that radiotherapy mediates tumor-specific immune responses by recruiting immune mediators and by increasing the vulnerability of tumor cells to T cell-mediated attack.[169–171] A Phase I trial of hypofractionated radiotherapy in combination with MEDI4736 (an anti-PD-L1 antibody) and tremelimumab (anti-CTLA-4 antibody) is being tested in patients with solid tumors (NCT02639026). Several Phases I and II trials combining ICT, cytokines, or targeted therapies plus radiotherapy in solid tumors and hematologic malignancies are currently underway to determine the safety and efficacy of these combinations.[172]

Chemotherapy in combination with immunotherapy

Combinations with chemotherapy have also provided promising results. Cytotoxic chemotherapies appear capable of inducing an appropriate milieu for presentation of tumor antigens.[173] Further beneficial effects likely include increased antigen cross-presentation,[174] partial activation of DCs,[175] and partial sensitization of tumor cells for cytotoxic T cell-mediated lysis.[176]

The combination of ICT with chemotherapy has now been approved in four tumor types: NSCLC, small cell lung cancer (SCLC), head and neck squamous cell carcinoma (HNSCC), and triple-negative breast cancer (TNBC). A Phase III clinical trial of PD-L1-unselected nonsquamous NSCLC randomized to chemotherapy (cisplatin or carboplatin with pemetrexed) with or without pembrolizumab, demonstrated improvement in OS and PFS with the combination, with the greatest benefit in PD-L1-expressing tumors.[177] In squamous cell lung carcinoma, a Phase III study in PD-L1-unselected patients, chemotherapy (carboplatin with either paclitaxel or nab-paclitaxel) with pembrolizumab or placebo improved the co-primary endpoints of OS (15.9 vs 11.3 months; hazard ratio (HR) for death 0.64, 95% CI 0.49–0.85) and PFS (median, 6.4 vs 4.8 months; HR for disease progression or death 0.56, 95% CI 0.45–0.70), leading to approval in this patient population.[178]

The combination of atezolizumab with carboplatin and etoposide has been approved for extensive-stage SCLC based on a Phase III trial comparing atezolizumab with or without carboplatin/etoposide (induction phase), followed by a maintenance phase of atezolizumab or placebo. At a median follow-up of 13.9 months, the median OS was 12.3 months for atezolizumab and 10.3 months for placebo (HR for progression or death 0.77, 95% CI: 0.62–0.96, $p = 0.02$).[179] Similarly, durvalumab plus platinum-etoposide exhibited an OS benefit in SCLC compared to chemotherapy alone.[180]

A combination of atezolizumab and nab-paclitaxel was approved by the FDA for advanced TNBC with PD-L1 tumor-infiltrating immune cell staining ≥1% on the basis of a Phase III trial of nab-paclitaxel with or without atezolizumab demonstrating a statistically significant improvement with the combination in PFS (7.2 vs 5.5 months, HR 0.62, 95% CI: 0.49–0.78, $p<0.001$), with an OS benefit in PD-L1 positive patients (25.0 vs 15.5 months, HR for death 0.62, 95% CI: 0.45–0.86).[181] Finally, in HNSCC, the combination of pembrolizumab with fluoropyrimidine and platinum-based chemotherapy has been approved based on a Phase III study comparing pembrolizumab alone to pembrolizumab plus chemotherapy (platinum and 5-fluorouracil) to cetuximab plus chemotherapy, with primary endpoints of OS and radiographic PFS.[182] Pembrolizumab with chemotherapy improved OS versus cetaximab with chemotherapy in the overall population (13.0 vs 10.7 months, HR 0.77 [95% CI: 0.63–0.93, $p = 0.0004$]). Currently, there are more than 170 studies that are investigating combination of anti-PD-1/PD-L1 inhibition with chemotherapy in multiple cancer types.[183]

Targeted therapy combinations with immunotherapy

The combination of targeted therapy with ICT is best established in RCC. For patients with advanced RCC without prior systemic therapy, a Phase III trial compared pembrolizumab plus the tyrosine kinase inhibitor axitinib versus sunitinib and demonstrated an improved OS in the entire study population (18-month OS 82% vs 72% with the combination), with the effect most pronounced in intermediate or poor-risk disease.[184] The combination of avelumab with axitinib was compared to sunitinib in a Phase III trial of 886 treatment-naïve patients, which demonstrated an improvement in PFS for the entire study population with the combination (13.8 vs 8.4 months), but did not demonstrate an improvement in OS for the overall population nor for the subgroups.[185] Finally, a Phase III trial investigated the combination of atezolizumab plus the vascular endothelial growth factor (VEGF)-targeted monoclonal antibody bevacizumab versus sunitinib, demonstrating a median PFS of 11.2 months with the combination versus 7.7 months with sunitinib in the PD-L1 positive patients.[186] In first-line HCC, a Phase III trial of atezolizumab plus bevacizumab prolonged OS compared to sorafenib, leading to its approval (HR for death 0.58, $p < 0.001$).[187] The combination of pembrolizumab with lenvatinib in endometrial cancer was approved based on a single-arm trial of non-dMMR or MSI-H patients demonstrating an ORR of 38% with a complete remission (CR) rate of 11%.[188]

Cellular immunotherapies

Another breakthrough in the field of immunotherapy has been cellular immunotherapy or **adoptive cell therapy (ACT)** which engineers a patients' own T cells to attack tumors. Initial preclinical and clinical studies have established that the reinfusion of autologous lymphocytes in cancer patients, isolated from their own tumor or peripheral blood, could inhibit tumor growth, improve survival by increasing reactive T cell numbers and provide long-term immunity and antigen specificity.[189,190] These observations formed the primary basis for ACT (Figure 4). The failure of active immunization to affect major clinical responses does not always necessarily reflect a lack of systemic antitumor immunity but also a stimulation

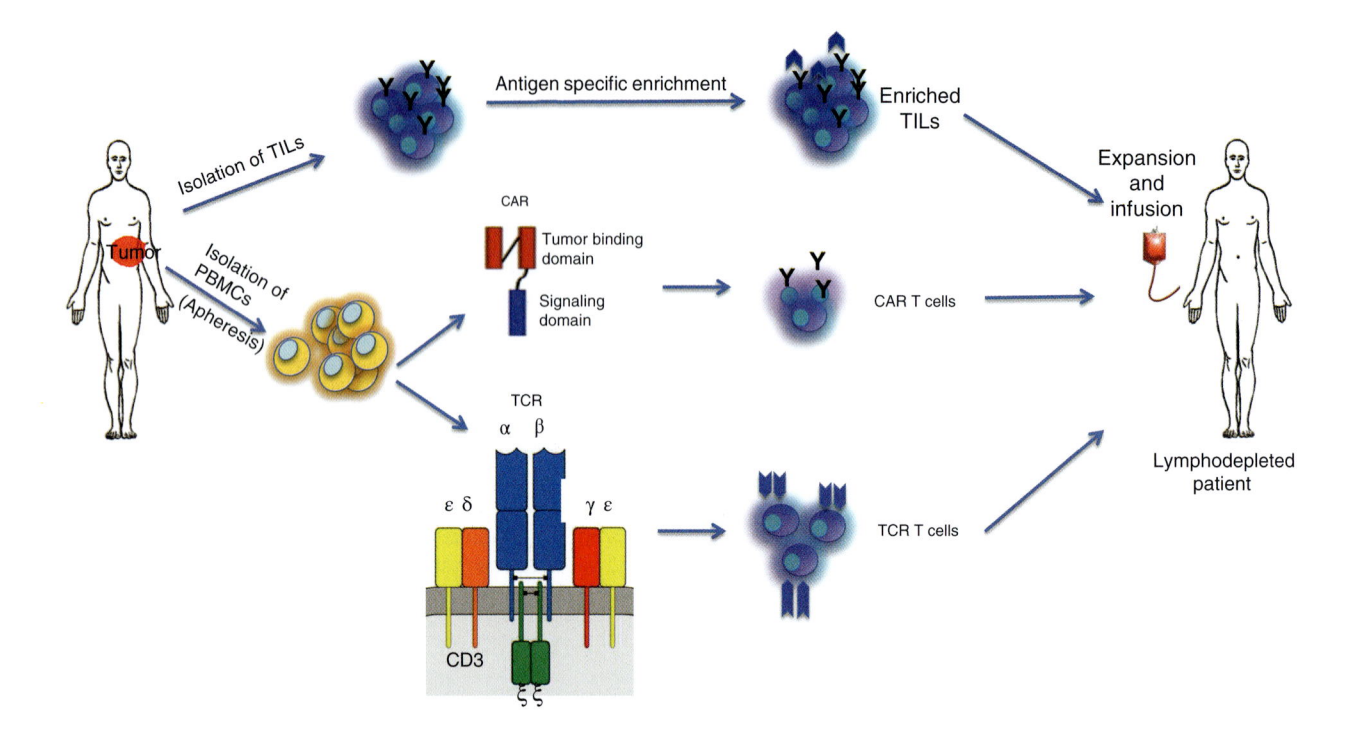

Figure 4 Adoptive cell therapy. Three approaches of adoptive cellular therapy using T cells includes: (1) Isolation, enrichment and expansion of TILs, (2) the genetic transfer of CAR-recognizing surface tumor protein, or (3) genetic transfer of TCR-recognizing tumor antigen-derived peptide–MHC target.

of low avidity effector T cells in the TME. ACT allows the identification of rare cells with a relatively high affinity for tumor antigen that can be selected *in vitro* and expanded before transfer to the host. These cells can be activated *ex vivo* and directly administered to the patient.

Much of the pioneering work that laid the foundations for subsequent investigation of anticancer immunotherapy through ACT was performed in the early 1950s.[191,192] Following this, the concept of "chemoimmunotherapy" gained popularity in the late 1960s when it was shown that an established lymphoma could be eradicated after therapeutic combination of high doses of the alkylating agent cyclophosphamide and the transfer of immune cells from a mouse previously sensitized (or challenged) with the same tumor.[193] Later studies showed that antitumor activity was enhanced in cells that had been re-sensitized and expanded with irradiated tumor *in vitro*,[194–200] or even with cells that had been only primarily sensitized *in vitro*.[197] An important advance during this work was the introduction of IL-2 in the *in vitro* system which is known to play a role in not just activation but also maintenance of the T cells. IL-2 thus allowed further expansion of tumor-reactive T cells,[197] and this observation was further corroborated with similar results with *in vivo* administration of IL-2.[198–200] Importantly, human lymphocytes grown in IL-2 were shown capable of killing autologous tumor cells *in vitro*.[201] This initial observation led to a series of publications documenting the role of IL-2 in the "lymphokine-activated killer (LAK)" cell phenomena.[202] In early 1984, the first Phase I study on the use of LAK cells in humans provided evidence of the expanded lymphocytes migrating to different organs including tumors.[203]

Following this, a much larger study combining LAK and IL-2 administration was performed[204,205] in which more than 100 patients were treated with several courses of IL-2 and very high numbers of autologous LAK cells (up to 18.4×10^{10} cells). Complete or partial responses were seen in 21% of patients.[205] However, data from murine models suggested a better approach of isolation and *in vitro* expansion of TILs with IL-2,[206] which were 50–100 times more efficient than LAK cells in the treatment of various types of tumors. Furthermore, their potency was significantly enhanced when their transfer was combined with *in vivo* administration of cyclophosphamide and IL-2.[207] Clinical trials using this strategy of combining cyclophosphamide, TILs, and IL-2 have yielded complete and partial responses in up to 31% of patients with metastatic melanoma.[208] These studies have helped to inform the evolution of ACT as a form of personalized immunotherapy.[209–211]

Adoptive transfer of tumor-specific cytotoxic T cells

In the early 1990s, it was observed that patients with relapsed chronic myeloid leukemia (CML) after allogeneic bone marrow transplantation (BMT) demonstrated complete and durable remission by the infusion of donor mononuclear cells from the original human leukocyte antigen (HLA)-identical sibling marrow donor, indicating the first evidence of efficacy in humans. Likewise, other studies also reported that transfer of autologous TILs could mediate objective regression in patients with metastatic melanoma and other cancers.[212–215] Strategies to isolate, activate, and expand T cells are being developed to target a broader population of patients.[216]

One major limitation in about 60–70% of cases has been the difficulty in accessing tumor samples containing sufficient numbers of viable TILs for successful isolation and expansion.[213] Alternative approaches for isolation of tumor-reactive lymphocytes (TRLs) include the use of T cells from peripheral blood or lymph node biopsies,[217–220] and stimulation and *ex vivo* expansion with mAbs directed against CD3 and the co-stimulatory receptor, CD28 and/or 4-1BB expressed on T cells.[220–224] The identification and cloning of T cells with specificity to antigens that are either more abundant on or, less commonly, specific to tumor cells (NY-ESO-1, MART-1, tyrosinase, gp100, p53) have also contributed greatly to the development of alternatives to isolation of TILs.

Recent studies show that IL-2 may not be the optimal cytokine to use to enhance activity *in vivo* since it also expands Tregs and is associated with significant toxicity. However, co-transfer of CD4$^+$ T cells can supply IL-2 and sustain TRLs for long periods of time and therefore, increase the antitumor effect of ACT.[225–227] Numerous studies have demonstrated the requirement for CD4$^+$ T cell help in the generation and/or maintenance of CD8$^+$ T cell memory. In addition to provision of cytokine support, they have roles in DC conditioning, and in recruitment and activation of macrophages and eosinophils, which can mediate antitumor effects.[228–230]

An alternate and perhaps complementary approach is to engineer cells in ways to enhance survival, for example, by transducing cells with chimeric GM-CSF-IL-2 receptors (designed to deliver an IL-2 signal when binding GM-CSF in an autocrine loop),[241] CD28,[242] or the catalytic subunit of telomerase.[243] The ability to further modify these lymphocytes could potentially further enhance their activity by making them less subject to the suppressive influences present in the TME, such as the introduction of genes encoding dominant-negative TGF-β, or inhibitory RNAs to prevent the expression of inhibitory molecules (e.g., CTLA-4 and PD-1).[244] Alternatively, overexpression of selected costimulatory ligands may induce auto- and trans-costimulation, resulting in potent antitumor activity.[245]

Adoptive immunotherapy with genetically modified lymphocytes

More recent efforts have focused on genetic modification of T cells to engineer improved antitumor effects through expansion of a tumor-associated antigen-specific T cell population and engineering of specific costimulatory domains. Such approaches include the transfer of chimeric antigen receptors (CARs) that have antibody-based external receptor structures and cytosolic domains that encode signal transduction modules of the TCR.[231] These allow redirection of T cell specificity in an MHC unrestricted manner, whilst delivering the equivalent intracellular signaling of TCR ligation. Furthermore, this impact can be enhanced by engineering the cytosolic domain for additional provision of counterfeit co-stimulatory signaling following ligation (mimicking CD28, 4-1BB, or OX40 ligation).

A number of early trials have suggested that persistence of transgene-expressing cells may be limited to periods of days to weeks following transfer.[232–236] This may relate in part to the potential immunogenicity of the CARs. An alternative strategy to redirect T cell specificity relies on transduction of TCR genes from tumor-reactive clones; although this has the relative disadvantage of conferring MHC-restricted targeting.[237–239] In the first clinical trial using this approach, a MART-1-reactive TCR was transduced into human lymphocytes, inducing the capacity to secrete effector cytokines and display lytic activity when coincubated with MART-1$^+$ tumor cells. Following lymphocyte depletion in the recipient, these cells were infused into patients with melanoma who subsequently received infusions of IL-2 with the suggestion that the T cells may have affected clinical responses in 2 of 17 patients.[190] Potential factors limiting efficacy in this study include variable persistence of gene-modified cells and relatively low levels of surface expression of the introduced TCR. Indeed, gene optimization that elicits only modest increases in TCR expression may result in marked enhancement of antitumor activity.[240]

Effect of ACT in the clinical setting

Significant progress has been made in the field of adoptive T cell therapy, and the recent successes hold promise and tremendous potential to harness the immune system to fight against cancer. This section provides a very brief overview of ACT in the clinical setting, which is reviewed in greater detail elsewhere[246] and in **Chapter 62**. Experience with ACT has been generally encouraging, but it is important to recognize that use of TILs may favor inclusion of those with an immune system inherently more capable of mediating antitumor activity. Tisagenlecleucel, a second-generation CAR T cell, comprising of a CD19 extracellular scFv and CD3-ζ and 4-1BB intracellular signaling domains, is FDA-approved for the treatment of patients up to 25 years of age with relapsed or refractory B-cell precursor acute lymphoblastic leukemia (ALL). The efficacy of tisagenlecleucel was evaluated in a multicenter single-arm trial (*ELIANA*) of 63 patients with relapsed or refractory pediatric precursor B-cell acute lymphoblastic leukemia (B-cell ALL), including 35 patients who had prior hematopoietic stem cell transplantation. In this study, 83% of the patients achieved CR, of which 63% of patients achieved CR and 19% achieved CR with incomplete hematological recovery.[247]

Similarly, axicabtagene ciloleucel was the second CAR T cell therapy to be approved by the FDA for the treatment of adult patients with certain types of large B-cell lymphoma who have relapsed or whose cancer has progressed after receiving at least two prior treatment regimens. The approval of axicabtagene ciloleucel CAR T cell therapy was established from the ZUMA-1 pivotal trial in patients with refractory or relapsed large B-cell lymphoma. In this study, 72% of patients treated with a single infusion responded to therapy, and the CR rate was 51%.[248,249] Table 2 shows the FDA-approved CAR T cell therapies.

Since the frequency of TILs has been shown to correlate with outcome in several therapeutic studies of human malignancies, the ability to generate a therapeutic product from TILs could be

Table 2 FDA approved adoptive T cell therapy.

Agent	Target/mechanism	Indication	Year of approval
1. Tisagenlecleucel	CAR T-cell therapy	Relapsed or refractory B-cell acute lymphoblastic leukemia (ALL) in patients up to 25 years of age in the second or later relapse	2017
		Relapsed or refractory large B-cell lymphoma in adjust after 2 or more lines of systemic therapy	2018
2. Axicabtagene ciloleucel	CAR T-cell therapy	Relapsed or refractory large B-cell lymphoma, with disease progression after receiving at least two prior treatment regimens	2017
3. Brexucabtagene autoleucel	CAR T-cell therapy	Relapsed or refractory mantle cell lymphoma	2020

Updated as of 1 January 2021.

a predictive biomarker for outcome. The achievement of higher response rates in the significantly less selected groups receiving CAR- or TCR-transduced ACT will be an important step forward in this regard, but current results have demonstrated results more typical of other single-agent immunotherapeutic approaches. Generation of appropriate cellular products is labor-intensive and requires significant laboratory expertise. Furthermore, each patient essentially requires the generation of new reagent limiting the opportunities for easy commercialization and suggesting that delivery may be considered more service-oriented rather than product-related (as in the case of most drugs). This aspect, combined with increasing awareness that minimizing *ex vivo* T cell manipulation may be advantageous in terms of clinical outcomes, is driving the current evolution of clinical strategies. The issue is also informed by topical debate concerning the nature of the best targets for immunotherapy in terms of public versus private antigens. While we have historically focused on "public" or shared tumor antigens such as MART-1 and gp100, accepting that antitumor efficacy may then be inextricably linked to tissue-specific toxicity, "private" or patient-specific antigens generated as a consequence of the evolution of the malignant phenotype and inherent genetic instability within these lesions have a number of attractive advantages.[250–252] The acceptance of tissue-specific toxicity leads to the concept of "dispensable tissues",[253] which may be acceptable in the case of vitiligo with therapies targeting melanoma or B cell deficiency following anti-CD20 therapy but will be more of an issue if the target is shared by a vital organ.[234] The parallel development of "off the shelf" reagents for enhancing immunity offers several interesting approaches to further enhance the efficacy of ACT. Indeed, a Phase I/II study of HLA-mismatched anti-CD19 CAR-NK cells derived from cord blood was administered to 11 patients with relapsed or refractory CD19-positive cancers (non-Hodgkin's lymphoma or chronic lymphocytic leukemia), and found a 73% response rate, without development of cytokine release syndrome (CRS), neurotoxicity, or graft-versus-host disease.[254] The recently reported clinical successes with genetically modified T cell therapies,[255] and renewed interest by pharmaceutical companies to develop these strategies for eventual approval of ACT for the treatment of patients holds great promise for the future.

Clinical challenges in adoptive T cell immunotherapy

The transition of ACT into the clinical setting has not been without difficulties; those primarily being related to generation of appropriate products for adoptive transfer and host or tumor resistance to transferred populations. The adoptive transfer of T cells is generally well tolerated but may be associated with the occurrence of life-threatening toxicities. Serious toxicities following adoptive T cell therapy may occur when T cells targeting differentiation antigens in the tumor also recognize these antigens on normal cells. For example, patients with melanoma who receive adoptive T cell therapy with T cells that target differentiation antigens such as MART-1 and gp100 may develop vitiligo and uveitis as toxicities since these antigens are also expressed on normal cells.[209,256] Additionally, patients with metastatic RCC who were treated with carbonic anhydrase-IX (CAIX)-specific CAR T cells developed liver toxicity.[234] In addition, fatal toxicities were reported in cancer patients who received anti-MAGE-A3 TCR-transduced T cells.[257] Another possible issue with ACT could be that the tumors can downregulate the expression of the tumor-specific antigens making the therapy less effective.

Adoptive T-cell therapy with CAR T cells may also be associated with another potentially life-threatening toxicity termed as *cytokine release syndrome* (CRS). The hallmark of CRS is elevated circulating levels of cytokines including IL-6, TNF-α, and IFN-γ; resulting in fever, rigors, hypotension, and hypoxia.[258,259] Treatment of irAEs associated with adoptive T cell therapy, such as uveitis and colitis can often be managed with topical or systemic corticosteroids. CAR T-cell therapy-related CRS is generally managed with either high-dose corticosteroids or agents such as tocilizumab or siltuximab (IL-6 receptor-blocking antibody).[260] CAR T-cell therapy is also associated with neurotoxicity which is managed similarly.[261]

Unlike ICT, ACT is not generally available "off-the-shelf" and hence can be a more expensive and labor-intensive process. However, extensive research is underway to make this possible with CAR-T cell therapy.[262]

Other strategies for immunotherapy

Apart from ICT and adoptive cell immunotherapies, several other approaches that boost the immune system for better cancer therapy show promising results. These are briefly discussed below and are reviewed in greater detail elsewhere in this text.

Bispecific antibodies (see Chapter 60 as well)

Bispecific antibodies represent a promising technology to promote specific T cell killing of tumor cells. The only FDA-approved bispecific antibody is blinatumomab, which binds to CD19 expressed on B cells and CD3 expressed on T cells, thereby forming a cytolytic synapse and activating the T cell in a non-MHC-dependent fashion.[263] Blinatumomab was studied in heavily pretreated patients with relapsed or refractory Philadelphia chromosome-positive B-cell ALL compared to chemotherapy and demonstrated an OS benefit of 7.7 versus 4.0 months as well as CR with full hematologic recovery of 34% versus 12%.[264] Bispecific antibodies are now being explored in solid tumors as well as other hematologic malignancies and are reviewed in detail elsewhere.[265]

Cytokine-based therapies (see Chapter 59 as well)

Cytokine-based therapies have long been part of the armamentarium of cancer immunotherapy, with high dose IL-2 approved for use in metastatic RCC in 1992. However, cytokines exert pleiotropic effects and adverse side effect profiles at high doses (e.g., IL-2 and type I IFN). For example, high dose IL-2 is associated with capillary leak syndrome and hypotension, limiting this therapy to highly selected situations in specialized centers. However, a novel prodrug of IL-2 conjugated with polyethylene glycol (PEG-IL-2) has been developed that masks the IL2 alpha receptor binding region preventing Treg activation, and thereby promoting only CD8$^+$ cytotoxic T cell activity.[266] This drug has shown promising results as monotherapy and in combination with anti-CTLA-4 in preclinical models and in phase 1/2 clinical trials in patients with locally advanced and metastatic tumors.[267,268]

IL-21, a member of the common γ-chain group, has attracted recent attention. IL-21 is produced by NKT and CD4$^+$ T cells and enhances the proliferation and function of CD8$^+$ T cells, NK, and NKT cells, as well as influences B cell differentiation.[269]

Table 3 FDA approved cancer vaccines.

Agent	Target/mechanism	Indication	Year of approval
1. Sipuleucel-T	Stimulates an immune response to prostatic acid phosphatase	Metastatic hormone-refractory prostate cancer	2010
2. Talimogene-laherparepvec (T-VEC)	Oncolytic virus immunotherapy	Metastatic melanoma that cannot be surgically removed	2015

Furthermore, it appears to reduce the suppressive capacity of Tregs.[270] It has been demonstrated to enhance antitumor activity in a number of preclinical murine models either as monotherapy or in combinatorial approaches with other cytokines (e.g., IL-15, IL-2), apoptosis-inducing mAbs (anti-DR5), CD1d reactive glycolipids (aGalCer), or costimulatory agonists.[271–274] Early phase clinical studies of recombinant human IL-21 suggest that it is relatively well-tolerated and mediates biological activity in terms of activation of NK and $CD8^+$ T cells; although it is too early to assess possible antitumor efficacy.[275,276] Recent studies with combination of IL-21 primed cytotoxic $CD8^+$ T cells and anti-CTLA-4 (ipilimumab) showed long-term $CD8^+$ memory T cell persistence and tumor regression in stage IV melanoma patients.[277,278] IL-15 is another such cytokine produced by monocytes, macrophages, DCs and is known to activate NK cells and is critical for the maintenance of durable high avidity $CD8^+$ memory T cells.[279] IL-15 based superagonist, ALT803, promotes the antigen-independent conversion of $CD8^+$ memory T cells into innate effector cells in murine models of cancer and is currently under Phase I trials for hematological and solid malignancies. Pegylated IL-10 (pegilodecakin) demonstrated objective tumor responses in patients with RCC and uveal melanoma and was found in combination with anti-PD-1 to increase responses in RCC and lung cancer.[280] Pegilodecakin was found to induce hallmarks of $CD8^+$ T cell immunity, including interferon-γ and GranzymeB induction, expansion and activation of intratumoral $CD8^+$ T cells, and proliferation and expansion of $LAG-3^+PD-1^+CD8^+$ T cells.[281]

Not all cytokines are immunostimulatory. Tumor cells can produce immunosuppressive cytokines or induce their production by regulatory infiltrates or stromal cells. Immune suppressive cytokines such as TGF-β are a putative target for therapeutic intervention. Targeting TGF-β has shown efficacy in murine tumor models[282,283] and is currently being tested in the clinical setting.

Cancer vaccines (see Chapter 61 as well)

Cancer vaccines aim to boost the body's natural defenses to fight against cancer. These can be either preventive or therapeutic. Preventive cancer vaccines target infectious agents including certain strains of human papillomavirus (HPV), which are known to cause head and neck, anal, and cervical cancers. The goal of therapeutic cancer vaccines is to increase the immunogenicity of tumor antigens that are poorly presented by the tumor to generate a high frequency of tumor-specific T cells.

The FDA has approved three preventive cancer vaccines to date, including Cervavix HPV (against HPV-16,-18,-31,-33,-45), Gardasil (against HPV-6,-11,-16,-18), and Gardasil 9 (against HPV-6,-11,-16,-18,-31,-33,-45,-52,-58).[284] Sipuleucel-T was the first therapeutic vaccine to be FDA approved for the treatment of asymptomatic or minimally symptomatic metastatic castrate-resistant prostate cancer (CRPC). The cell-based vaccine requires the collection of autologous peripheral blood mononuclear cells (PBMCs). This is followed by ex vivo activation of DCs with PA2024, a recombinant fusion protein consisting of a tumor-associated antigen (prostatic acid phosphatase, PAP) and granulocyte-macrophage colony-stimulating factor (GM-CSF), and re-infusion into the patient. This approval was based on results from a randomized double-blind placebo-controlled multicenter trial demonstrating a significant improvement in median OS following treatment with sipuleucel-T versus placebo in men with metastatic CRPC.[285] Presented in Table 3 is the published literature for FDA-approved cancer vaccines to date.

Oncolytic virus immunotherapy

Oncolytic viruses function by selective tumor cell killing (viral oncolysis) and induction of systemic antitumor immunity (Figure 5 and Table 3).[286] Native and genetically modified viruses have been extensively studied as oncolytic vectors. Talimogene iaherparepvec (T-VEC), a genetically modified herpes simplex virus type, was the first FDA-approved oncolytic viral immunotherapy for the treatment of advanced melanoma. T-VEC improved survival in a Phase III study (OPTiM) in patients with advanced melanoma.[287] T-VEC is currently being clinically investigated for use as neoadjuvant or combination therapy (anti-PD-L1) in malignant melanoma and other tumor types.

TLR agonists

DCs are uniquely specialized to present processed antigens to stimulate antigen-specific effector responses and thus DC-induced immunogenicity has informed the development of clinical therapeutics. Toll-like receptor (TLR) agonists are showing some early promise in clinical studies, particularly in combination with other therapeutic modalities. Unmethylated CpG oligodeoxynucleotides (ODNs) bind TLR9 on pDCs and B cells, inducing Th1 polarized immune responses and regression of established tumors in mice, as well as activity in Phase I and II clinical trials.[288–295] TLR9-activated APCs activate NK cells, enhance expression of Fc receptors on polymorphonuclear leukocytes, and promote CTL activation. TLR9 agonists are under active study in clinical trials (NCT03410901, NCT03410901, NCT04270864, NCT04050085, and NCT03618641). The imidazoquinolone and imiquimod ligate TLR7 (and to a lesser degree TLR8) and stimulates recruitment of pDCs and myeloid-derived DCs into tumors, both of which are implicated in subsequent antitumor activity.[296] However, it is important to remain aware that in some settings TLR ligands provoke immunosuppressive or tolerogenic responses.[297,298]

Future perspectives

Cancer immunotherapy has brought about a paradigm shift in cancer treatment and has resulted in durable clinical responses

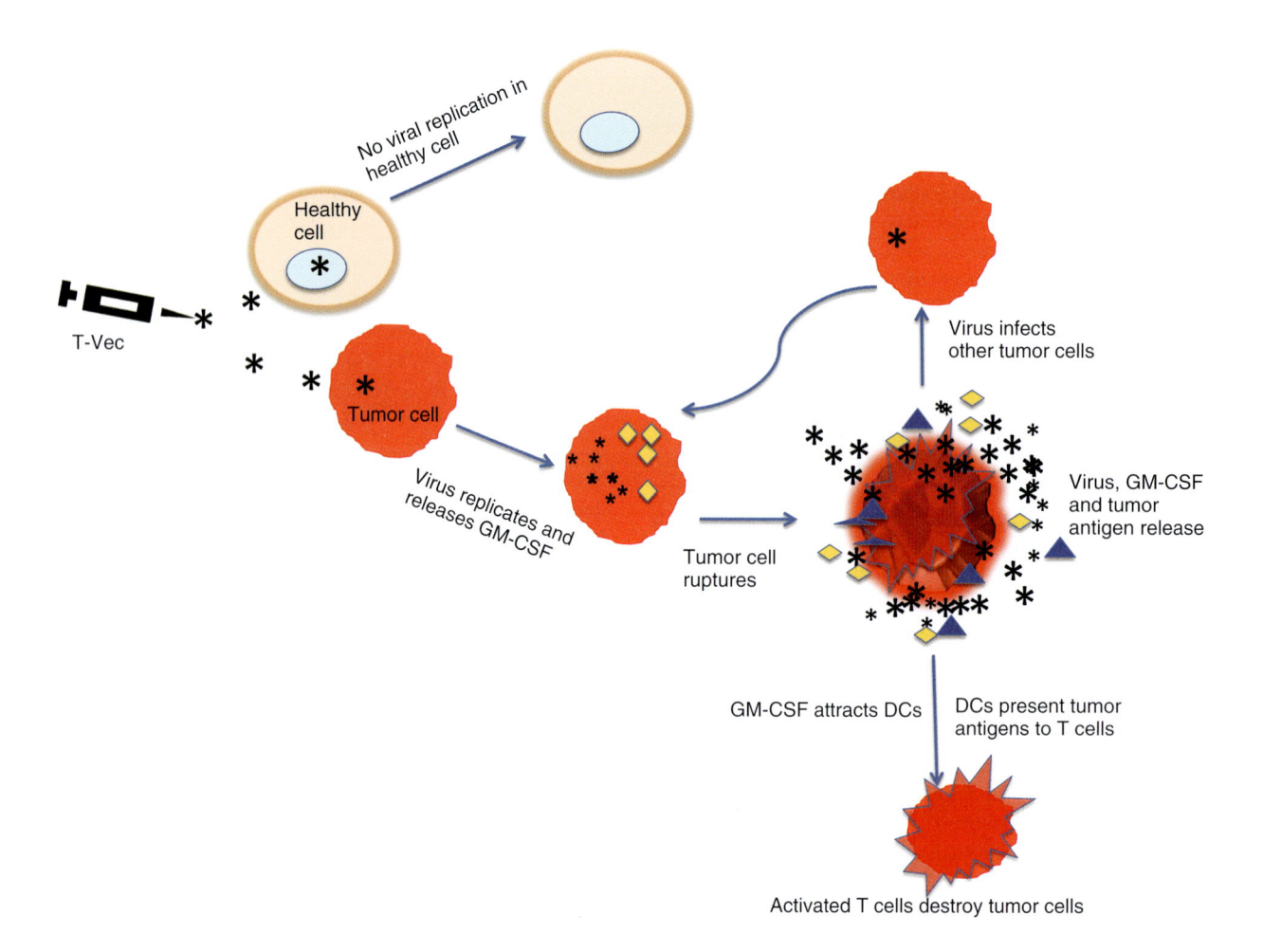

Figure 5 Oncolytic virus immunotherapy. Upon T-Vec injection, the oncolytic virus invades both healthy cells and tumor cells. Since T-vec is an attenuated virus it does not replicate in the healthy cells. On invading the tumor cell, the oncolytic virus replicates in the tumor cells and secretes GM-CSF inside the tumors cells. The tumor cell undergoes oncolysis, thus releasing the virus, which further invades and infects the residual tumor cells. The ruptured tumor cell also releases GM-CSF and tumor antigens into the tumor microenvironment. GM-CSF attracts DCs, which present the tumor antigens to the T cells, which in turn destroy other tumor cells including those that are not infected by the virus.

in patients resistant to other conventional therapies. However, effective responses are seen only in a subset of patients and in specific tumor types. Therefore, several active areas of investigation remain to improve cancer immunotherapy for patients. These include (among others), discovery and validation of additional immune checkpoints for targeting, refinement of CAR cellular therapies and the emergence of allogeneic cellular therapies, testing of immunotherapy earlier in the disease state (e.g., moving from the metastatic into the neoadjuvant or adjuvant setting), continuing exploration of combination treatments (including not only chemotherapy and radiation therapy, but also targeted therapy, epigenetic modulators and other immunotherapies, such as vaccines), improved understanding of irAEs, and development of predictive biomarkers for toxicities and response.

Thus, understanding the resistance mechanisms and factors influencing response rates would help to identify better and more robust targeting approaches. As the field of cancer immunotherapy continues to develop in the coming years, the goal will remain to improve patient selection to minimize toxicities and maximize efficacy.

Key references

The complete reference list can be found on Vital Source version of this title, see inside front cover.

11 Chen DS, Mellman I. Oncology meets immunology: the cancer-immunity cycle. *Immunity*. 2013;**39**(1):1–10.
12 Leach DR, Krummel MF, Allison JP. Enhancement of antitumor immunity by CTLA-4 blockade. *Science*. 1996;**271**(5256):1734–1736.
13 Francisco LM, Sage PT, Sharpe AH. The PD-1 pathway in tolerance and autoimmunity. *Immunol Rev*. 2010;**236**:219–242.
18 Hodi FS, O'Day SJ, McDermott DF, et al. Improved survival with ipilimumab in patients with metastatic melanoma. *N Engl J Med*. 2010;**363**(8):711–723.
20 Eggermont AM, Chiarion-Sileni V, Grob JJ, et al. Adjuvant ipilimumab versus placebo after complete resection of high-risk stage III melanoma (EORTC 18071): a randomised, double-blind, phase 3 trial. *Lancet Oncol*. 2015;**16**(5):522–530.
27 Keir ME, Butte MJ, Freeman GJ, et al. PD-1 and its ligands in tolerance and immunity. *Annu Rev Immunol*. 2008;**26**:677–704.
36 Overman MJ, McDermott R, Leach JL, et al. Nivolumab in patients with metastatic DNA mismatch repair-deficient or microsatellite instability-high colorectal cancer (CheckMate 142): an open-label, multicentre, phase 2 study. *Lancet Oncol*. 2017;**18**(9):1182–1191.
40 Anderson AC, Joller N, Kuchroo VK. Lag-3, Tim-3, and TIGIT: co-inhibitory receptors with specialized functions in immune regulation. *Immunity*. 2016;**44**(5):989–1004.

49 Gao J, Ward JF, Pettaway CA, et al. VISTA is an inhibitory immune checkpoint that is increased after ipilimumab therapy in patients with prostate cancer. *Nat Med*. 2017;**23**(5):551–555.

50 Blando J, Sharma A, Higa MG, et al. Comparison of immune infiltrates in melanoma and pancreatic cancer highlights VISTA as a potential target in pancreatic cancer. *Proc Natl Acad Sci U S A*. 2019;**116**(5):1692–1697.

55 Fu T, He Q, Sharma P. The ICOS/ICOSL pathway is required for optimal antitumor responses mediated by anti-CTLA-4 therapy. *Cancer Res*. 2011;**71**(16):5445–5454.

56 Sakuishi K, Apetoh L, Sullivan JM, et al. Targeting Tim-3 and PD-1 pathways to reverse T cell exhaustion and restore anti-tumor immunity. *J Exp Med*. 2010;**207**(10):2187–2194.

58 Wei SC, Sharma R, Anang NAS, et al. Negative co-stimulation constrains T cell differentiation by imposing boundaries on possible cell states. *Immunity*. 2019;**50**(4):1084–1098 e10.

59 Wei SC, Levine JH, Cogdill AP, et al. Distinct cellular mechanisms underlie anti-CTLA-4 and anti-PD-1 checkpoint blockade. *Cell*. 2017;**170**(6):1120–1133 e17.

61 Wei SC, Anang NAS, Sharma R, et al. Combination anti-CTLA-4 plus anti-PD-1 checkpoint blockade utilizes cellular mechanisms partially distinct from monotherapies. *Proc Natl Acad Sci U S A*. 2019;**116**(45):22699–22709.

62 Larkin J, Chiarion-Sileni V, Gonzalez R, et al. Combined nivolumab and ipilimumab or monotherapy in untreated melanoma. *N Engl J Med*. 2015;**373**(1):23–34.

71 Tang DN, Shen Y, Sun J, et al. Increased frequency of ICOS+ CD4 T cells as a pharmacodynamic biomarker for anti-CTLA-4 therapy. *Cancer Immunol Res*. 2013;**1**(4):229–234.

72 Watts TH. TNF/TNFR family members in costimulation of T cell responses. *Annu Rev Immunol*. 2005;**23**:23–68.

85 Deng J, Zhao S, Zhang X, et al. OX40 (CD134) and OX40 ligand, important immune checkpoints in cancer. *Onco Targets Ther*. 2019;**12**:7347–7353.

93 Zappasodi R, Sirard C, Li Y, et al. Rational design of anti-GITR-based combination immunotherapy. *Nat Med*. 2019;**25**(5):759–766.

102 Beatty GL, Chiorean EG, Fishman MP, et al. CD40 agonists alter tumor stroma and show efficacy against pancreatic carcinoma in mice and humans. *Science*. 2011;**331**(6024):1612–1616.

104 Burris HA, Infante JR, Ansell SM, et al. Safety and activity of varlilumab, a novel and first-in-class agonist anti-CD27 antibody, in patients with advanced solid tumors. *J Clin Oncol*. 2017;**35**(18):2028–2036.

105 Sharma P, Hu-Lieskovan S, Wargo JA, et al. Primary, adaptive, and acquired resistance to cancer immunotherapy. *Cell*. 2017;**168**(4):707–723.

106 Spranger S, Bao R, Gajewski TF. Melanoma-intrinsic beta-catenin signalling prevents anti-tumour immunity. *Nature*. 2015;**523**(7559):231–235.

108 Peng W, Chen JQ, Liu C, et al. Loss of PTEN promotes resistance to T cell-mediated immunotherapy. *Cancer Discov*. 2016;**6**(2):202–216.

114 Im SJ, Hashimoto M, Gerner MY, et al. Defining CD8+ T cells that provide the proliferative burst after PD-1 therapy. *Nature*. 2016;**537**(7620):417–421.

115 Jadhav RR, Im SJ, Hu B, et al. Epigenetic signature of PD-1+ TCF1+ CD8 T cells that act as resource cells during chronic viral infection and respond to PD-1 blockade. *Proc Natl Acad Sci U S A*. 2019;**116**(28):14113–14118.

117 Khan O, Giles JR, McDonald S, et al. TOX transcriptionally and epigenetically programs CD8(+) T cell exhaustion. *Nature*. 2019;**571**(7764):211–218.

118 Alfei F, Kanev K, Hofmann M, et al. TOX reinforces the phenotype and longevity of exhausted T cells in chronic viral infection. *Nature*. 2019;**571**(7764):265–269.

123 DeNardo DG, Ruffell B. Macrophages as regulators of tumour immunity and immunotherapy. *Nat Rev Immunol*. 2019;**19**(6):369–382.

124 Goswami S, Walle T, Cornish AE, et al. Immune profiling of human tumors identifies CD73 as a combinatorial target in glioblastoma. *Nat Med*. 2020;**26**(1):39–46.

125 Sivan A, Corrales L, Hubert N, et al. Commensal *Bifidobacterium* promotes antitumor immunity and facilitates anti-PD-L1 efficacy. *Science*. 2015;**350**(6264):1084–1089.

127 Gopalakrishnan V, Spencer CN, Nezi L, et al. Gut microbiome modulates response to anti-PD-1 immunotherapy in melanoma patients. *Science*. 2018;**359**(6371):97–103.

130 Dunn J, Rao S. Epigenetics and immunotherapy: the current state of play. *Mol Immunol*. 2017;**87**:227–239.

132 Goswami S, Apostolou I, Zhang J, et al. Modulation of EZH2 expression in T cells improves efficacy of anti-CTLA-4 therapy. *J Clin Invest*. 2018;**128**(9):3813–3818.

137 Chang CH, Pearce EL. Emerging concepts of T cell metabolism as a target of immunotherapy. *Nat Immunol*. 2016;**17**(4):364–368.

146 Li X, Wenes M, Romero P, et al. Navigating metabolic pathways to enhance antitumour immunity and immunotherapy. *Nat Rev Clin Oncol*. 2019;**16**(7):425–441.

147 Taube JM, Klein A, Brahmer JR, et al. Association of PD-1, PD-1 ligands, and other features of the tumor immune microenvironment with response to anti-PD-1 therapy. *Clin Cancer Res*. 2014;**20**(19):5064–5074.

149 Helmink BA, Reddy SM, Gao J, et al. B cells and tertiary lymphoid structures promote immunotherapy response. *Nature*. 2020;**577**(7791):549–555.

151 Goswami S, Chen Y, Anandhan S, et al. ARID1A mutation plus CXCL13 expression act as combinatorial biomarkers to predict responses to immune checkpoint therapy in mUCC. *Sci Transl Med*. 2020;**12**:548, eabc4220.

152 Cristescu R, Mogg R, Ayers M, et al. Pan-tumor genomic biomarkers for PD-1 checkpoint blockade-based immunotherapy. *Science*. 2018;**362**(6411):eaar3593.

162 Michot JM, Bigenwald C, Champiat S, et al. Immune-related adverse events with immune checkpoint blockade: a comprehensive review. *Eur J Cancer*. 2016;**54**:139–148.

164 Subudhi SK, Aparicio A, Gao J, et al. Clonal expansion of CD8 T cells in the systemic circulation precedes development of ipilimumab-induced toxicities. *Proc Natl Acad Sci U S A*. 2016;**113**(42):11919–11924.

165 Tahir SA, Gao J, Miura Y, et al. Autoimmune antibodies correlate with immune checkpoint therapy-induced toxicities. *Proc Natl Acad Sci U S A*. 2019;**116**(44):22246–22251.

168 Sharabi AB, Lim M, DeWeese TL, et al. Radiation and checkpoint blockade immunotherapy: radiosensitisation and potential mechanisms of synergy. *Lancet Oncol*. 2015;**16**(13):e498–e509.

183 Tang J, Shalabi A, Hubbard-Lucey VM. Comprehensive analysis of the clinical immuno-oncology landscape. *Ann Oncol*. 2018;**29**(1):84–91.

190 Morgan RA, Dudley ME, Wunderlich JR, et al. Cancer regression in patients after transfer of genetically engineered lymphocytes. *Science*. 2006;**314**(5796):126–129.

198 Cheever MA, Greenberg PD, Fefer A, et al. Augmentation of the anti-tumor therapeutic efficacy of long-term cultured T lymphocytes by in vivo administration of purified interleukin 2. *J Exp Med*. 1982;**155**(4):968–980.

215 Rosenberg SA, Restifo NP. Adoptive cell transfer as personalized immunotherapy for human cancer. *Science*. 2015;**348**(6230):62–68.

217 June CH. Adoptive T cell therapy for cancer in the clinic. *J Clin Invest*. 2007;**117**(6):1466–1476.

227 Wilson EB, Livingstone AM. Cutting edge: CD4+ T cell-derived IL-2 is essential for help-dependent primary CD8+ T cell responses. *J Immunol*. 2008;**181**(11):7445–7448.

246 June CH, O'Connor RS, Kawalekar OU, et al. CAR T cell immunotherapy for human cancer. *Science*. 2018;**359**(6382):1361–1365.

255 Maude SL, Frey N, Shaw PA, et al. Chimeric antigen receptor T cells for sustained remissions in leukemia. *N Engl J Med*. 2014;**371**(16):1507–1517.

262 Depil S, Duchateau P, Grupp SA, et al. 'Off-the-shelf' allogeneic CAR T cells: development and challenges. *Nat Rev Drug Discov*. 2020;**19**(3):185–199.

265 Labrijn AF, Janmaat ML, Reichert JM, et al. Bispecific antibodies: a mechanistic review of the pipeline. *Nat Rev Drug Discov*. 2019;**18**(8):585–608.

266 Charych DH, Hoch U, Langowski JL, et al. NKTR-214, an engineered cytokine with biased IL2 receptor binding, increased tumor exposure, and marked efficacy in mouse tumor models. *Clin Cancer Res*. 2016;**22**(3):680–690.

267 Caudana P, Nunez NG, De La Rochere P, et al. IL2/anti-IL2 complex combined with CTLA-4, but not PD-L1, blockade rescues antitumor NK cell function by regulatory T-cell modulation. *Cancer Immunol Res*. 2019;**7**(3):443–457.

284 Petrosky E, Bocchini JA, Hariri S, et al. Use of 9-valent human papillomavirus (HPV) vaccine: updated HPV vaccination recommendations of the advisory committee on immunization practices. *MMWR*. 2015;**64**(11):300–304.

286 Kaufman HL, Kohlhapp FJ, Zloza A. Oncolytic viruses: a new class of immunotherapy drugs. *Nat Rev Drug Discov*. 2015;**14**(9):642–662.

292 Krieg AM. Development of TLR9 agonists for cancer therapy. *J Clin Invest*. 2007;**117**(5):1184–1194.

64 Cancer gene therapy

Haruko Tashiro, MD, PhD ■ Lauren Scherer, MD ■ Malcolm Brenner, MA, MB, BChir, PhD

Overview

The encouraging results of cancer gene therapies have increased their entry into mainstream oncological practice. Gene transfer or gene editing can modify the cellular phenotype and behavior of malignant cells or of host cells, thereby modulating tumor responses. In this article, we discuss both of the above approaches and describe the vector systems that are able to produce the intended genetic modifications. We describe current clinical successes of gene therapy and outline the challenges it has yet to overcome. The success of any gene therapy for cancer requires efficient, safe gene transfer with vectors that can either integrate into the human genome (e.g., retroviral, lentiviral, adeno-associated viral, or nonviral transposons) or remain largely or completely episomal (e.g., adenoviral, herpesviral, or nonviral plasmids). To date, genetic "correction" of consequential numbers of cancer cells has not proven feasible, but infectious cytolytic viral therapy, used with accompanying immunomodulatory genes within the oncolytic virus, is beginning to demonstrate an impact in the clinic. Enhancement of active cancer immunotherapy with forced expression of antigens and cytokines or the enhancement of adoptive immunotherapy by engineering T lymphocytes with specific T-cell receptors and/or chimeric antigen receptors shows greatest immediate promise, although ultimately a combination of multiple approaches will prove optimal.

Introduction

A range of tumor-targeted and immunomodulatory antibodies have recently been added to the conventional therapeutic tools of cancer, which until recently consisted of surgery, chemotherapy, and radiotherapy. In this article, we describe gene modification, another treatment approach that is now showing remarkable clinical results, though currently only in a limited range of disorders. The intent of gene transfer in normal cells or cancer cells is to modify the cellular phenotype and behavior of these cells and thereby control or eradicate the tumor. The new genetic material may be transferred to cells *ex vivo* followed by cell infusion, or directly to the cells *in vivo*; the modification may be intended to be permanent or temporary.

Gene transfer

The ideal gene delivery system (vector) is safe, efficient, and suitable for use in a wide range of applications; such a vector does not yet exist. Instead, gene delivery vectors, which may be of viral or nonviral origin, each have their own strengths and limitations (Table 1) and should be chosen for any given application based on balancing their desirable properties with their limitations.

Viral vectors

Viruses reproduce by efficiently inserting their genetic information into target cells. Investigators have exploited this property by modifying viruses in such a way that they retain their ability to insert therapeutic genetic material but no longer cause disease in the host. Several different vectors have been used for this purpose.

Integrating vectors

Retrovirus vectors

Retroviruses are enveloped, single-stranded RNA viruses, and vectors have been derived from several different retroviral family members, including γ-retroviruses (e.g., murine leukemia virus or MLV—one of the first and still most widely used retroviral vectors)[1] and human immunodeficiency virus (HIV-1, also now widely used[2,3]). Other retroviruses including simian immunodeficiency virus (SIV), bovine immunodeficiency virus, feline immunodeficiency virus, equine infectious anemia virus (EIAV), foamy virus, bovine leukemia virus, Rous sarcoma virus (RSV), spleen necrosis virus, and mouse mammary tumor virus have also been developed as potential vectors. These vectors integrate in the host cell DNA and therefore can provide stable expression even in a dividing cell population.

γ-Retroviral vectors (e.g., MLV) Wild-type MLV retrovirus contains 5′ and 3′ long-terminal repeats (LTRs) that are responsible for integration and act as promoters. Between the LTRs are three sequences necessary for viral replication and packaging: *gag*, which encodes three proteins that contribute to the virion structure; *pol*, which encodes reverse transcriptase, integrase, and ribonuclease H (RNase H) necessary for replication; and *env*, which encodes the envelope glycoprotein. Recombinant retroviral vectors are made replication-defective by removing the *gag*, *pol*, and *env* gene sequences from the viral nucleic acid backbone and replacing them with a cargo consisting of the therapeutic sequences of interest. These "gutted" vectors are manufactured in a producer cell line, in which the missing viral genes have been stably integrated in trans and are therefore able to produce infectious but nonreplicative particles containing enough reverse transcriptase to initiate the formation of a double-stranded DNA molecule that is then integrated into the DNA of the cell targeted for gene transfer.

As mentioned above, stable integration of retroviral sequences into the host cell genome[4] means that any modification is stable and will be passed to all daughter cells. Although this property is a critical advantage when stable alteration is required in a rapidly dividing population, γ-retroviral vectors have several limitations. As stable transduction and integration occur in S-phase cells and the preintegration complex is unstable, γ-retroviruses only integrate efficiently in actively dividing cells and not in

---

Holland-Frei Cancer Medicine, Tenth Edition. Edited by Robert C. Bast, John C. Byrd, Carlo M. Croce, Ernest Hawk, Fadlo R. Khuri, Raphael E. Pollock, Apostolia M. Tsimberidou, Christopher G. Willett, and Cheryl L. Willman.
© 2023 John Wiley & Sons, Inc. Published 2023 by John Wiley & Sons, Inc.

Table 1 Advantages and disadvantages of cancer gene therapy vectors.

	Advantages	Disadvantages
Viral vectors		
Integration of vector sequence into the genome		
Retrovirus	Stable genome integration	Integration only in dividing cells
	Long-term gene expression	Insertional mutagenesis
	Low immunogenicity	Inefficient *in vivo* gene delivery
	Relatively larger insert size: 7–8 kb	
Lentivirus	Transduces nondividing cells	Potential insertional mutagenesis
	Long-term gene expression	Inefficient *in vivo* gene delivery
	Low immunogenicity	
Adeno-associated virus	Long-term gene expression	Potential insertional mutagenesis
	Transduces nondividing cells	Limited insert size 4 kb
Nonintegration of vector sequence into the genome		
Adenovirus	High titer	Transient expression
	High transduction efficacy	Immune-related toxicity with repeated administration
	Transduces nondividing cells	Limited insert size: 7–8 kb (first generation)
	Limited immunogenicity	
Herpes virus	Large insert size: 30 kb	Cytotoxic
	Neuronal tropism	Transient expression
Nonviral DNA delivery		
	Large insert size	Transient gene expression
	Low immunogenicity	Inefficient *in vivo* delivery
	Can be used repeatedly	
Transposons	Long-term gene expression	Insertional mutagenesis
	Large insert size (10 kb SB, 100 kb PB)	Inefficient *in vivo* delivery

slowly dividing or quiescent cells. Moreover, retroviral vector integration is by definition a mutational event, and as integration may favor the control regions of active genes, insertional mutagenesis can result—and has resulted—in transformation of the transduced target cell.[5–7] In addition, insert size is limited. Replication-incompetent γ-retroviral vectors made by a producer cell contain only the retroviral LTRs and the packaging signal. In principle, therefore, these vectors should have room for 7–8 kb of sequences of interest. Unfortunately, packaging constraints of the substituted "alien" sequences substantially reduce this limit.[8] Finally, retroviruses are unstable in primate complement and cannot be used readily for *in vivo* transduction. Owing to these limitations, generally, retroviruses have been used for *in vitro* transduction of specific target cells before their transfer to the patient.

Lentiviral vectors Lentivirus vectors were first developed from HIV and have been widely used both experimentally and clinically. Lentiviral vectors are usually engineered from the HIV-1 genome that contains the *gag-pro-pol* and *env* genes and two regulatory genes, *rev* and *tat* that are required for viral replication. The HIV-1 genome also has four accessory genes, *vif*, *vrp*, *vpu*, and *nef* that encode critical virulence factors. These genes are flanked by two LTRs. Recombinant lentiviral vectors are engineered by removing the majority of the HIV genes leaving the LTRs, packaging signal, and other regulatory elements.[9] First-generation packaging plasmids provide all *gag* and *pol* sequences, the viral regulatory genes, and the accessory genes. In second-generation lentiviral vectors, the four accessory genes are removed. To further reduce the risk of recombination and production of genetically modified infectious lentiviruses, third-generation vectors consist of a split-genome packaging system in which the *rev* gene is expressed from a separate plasmid and the 5′ LTR from the transfer construct;[10,11] and more recent designs further improve safety by providing *rev* and *tat* genes by a fourth plasmid[12] or by entirely excluding packaging sequences.[13] As opposed to the stable packaging cell lines used for γ-retroviruses, the requirement for a multiple plasmid system to produce lentiviral vectors for human use has made it difficult to scale up production or reduce costs of manufacture for larger clinical trials. Efforts continue to be made to generate a stable producer line that is safe and produces high-titer vector. Despite difficulties in production, lentiviruses have several advantages over γ-retroviruses. They can more readily infect nondividing and dividing cells,[14] although integration of the stable preintegration complex occurs at a high rate only when the cell enters cycle. Substitution of different viral envelopes modifies and broadens the viral tropism for target cells.[15] Initial clinical studies with lentiviral vectors evaluated the safety of an antisense gene against the HIV envelope in patients with HIV, but more recent attention has focused on the increasingly wide use of lentiviral vectors to transduce T cells to express tumor-directed receptors.[16]

Adeno-associated virus vectors
Adeno-associated viruses (AAV) are small, nonenveloped, single-stranded DNA viruses that are not known to cause disease in human or other animals[17] and require a helper virus (adenovirus, herpes simplex, or vaccinia virus) for the replication and production of new viral particles.[18] The AAV genome is composed of *rep*, which is required for virus replication, and *cap*, which encodes the viral capsid. There are at least 11 naturally occurring serotypes of AAV that differ primarily in their external capsid proteins and that bind to different cellular receptors and hence infect different targets. Recombinant AAV (rAAV) vectors are engineered by the removal of *rep* and *cap* genes but retain the AAV inverted terminal repeats (ITRs) flanking a gene of interest. rAAV has limited cargo capacity, and although widely and successfully used clinically for the treatment of monogenic disorders, production is difficult to scale. Because of the limitations of naturally occurring variants of AAV, research has focused on engineering hybrid viral-capsids to selectively bind to unique proteins or other molecules on malignant cells. This approach has demonstrated success in preclinical *in vivo* models and affords the possibility of tissue-selective gene expression. Although multiple phase I studies have demonstrated the safety of AAV-vector-based therapy in patients with malignant disease, effective clinical cancer gene therapy with these agents has yet to be established.[19]

Nonintegrating viral vectors

Adenovirus vectors

Adenoviruses are nonenveloped, linear double-stranded large DNA viruses. A set of early genes (*E1A*, *E1B*, *E2A*, *E2B*, *E3*, and *E4*) encode regulatory proteins that serve to initiate cell proliferation, DNA replication, and down-modulation of host immune defenses. The late genes (*L1–L5*) encode structural proteins. Importantly, adenoviruses are assigned to a species (A–F) and serotype according to the composition of their capsid, the knob/fiber of which attaches to one or more cellular receptors; cellular receptor usage is influenced by both species and serotype.[20] These molecular interactions lead to receptor-mediated endocytosis,[21] internalization, and uncoating of the virus. Adenoviruses can infect many normal and malignant cell types, irrespective of whether they are dividing or nondividing, but they do not integrate in host cell DNA and so the genetic modification is gradually lost in succeeding generations of dividing cells.

Recombinant adenovirus vectors are engineered from adenoviruses by the removal of one or more early genes including *E1*, which regulates replication, and *E3*, which diminishes immune recognition. The missing *E1* genes are provided in trans by a packaging (or helper) cell line to produce replication-incompetent adenoviruses with room for up to 7–8 kb of new genetic material.[22] Second-generation adenoviruses have been developed in which *E2* and *E4* along with *E1* and *E3* are deleted, providing up to a 14 kb insert.[21] They are, however, usually produced at a lower titer.[23] As adenovirus vectors do not integrate into the host cell genome, insertional mutagenesis does not occur but gene expression is only transient in dividing cells. Adenoviral vectors are also highly proinflammatory and favor an immune response against transduced cells and the transgenes they express.[24,25] While both of these characteristics make adenoviral vectors unsuited for long-term treatment of monogenic disorders, they may be beneficial for applications in cancer therapies, such as tumor vaccines, in which transient, high-level expression of an immunogenic transgene may be highly desirable.

Two major variants of adenoviral vectors are currently in clinical development.[26–28] Removal of all viral genes, except those that are required for packaging and replication, produces helper-dependent ("gutted" or "gutless") adenoviral vectors (HD-Ad) that have lower immunogenicity and greater cargo capacity. Conversely, limitation or modification of the gene deletions can produce conditionally replication-competent adenoviral vectors (CRAD), capable of replicating in—and hence destroying—malignant cells, while sparing normal tissues. These oncolytic CRADs are made selective for tumor cells either because of their requirement for transcriptional regulators present at higher level in malignant than in normal cells or because investigators substitute tumor-specific promoters for viral promoters of critical replicative genes,[29–31] which can be "armed" to increase potency by inserting a therapeutic transgene.[32,33]

Other nonintegrating virus vectors

Herpes viruses (HSV) are large (~186 nm), enveloped, double-stranded DNA viruses. Their linear double-stranded DNA genome is composed of unique long (UL) and unique short (US) coding regions, both flanked by terminal repeat sequence.[34] Although HSV encodes ~90 genes, many of these genes can be removed without inhibiting genome replication or the packaging of the virus.[35] Therefore, HSV vectors are able to carry large DNA sequences (up to 30 kb). Replication-competent HSV have also been developed and are being studied as oncolytic viruses (OV) in several different tumor types.[36–40] Vaccinia viruses are large DNA viruses that replicate cytoplasmically. Modified vaccinia virus Ankara (MVA) has had 31 kb deleted from the parental vaccinia genome, including the *K1L*, *N1L*, and *A52R* genes that regulate innate immune responses,[41,42] while MVA and Copenhagen-derived vaccine strains are being investigated currently as OV in cancer.[43] High immunogenicity that terminates the oncolytic response is one of the problems for clinical use.[44]

Nonviral vectors including transposons

Although viral vectors deliver genes with reasonably high efficiency, they have several drawbacks including cost and complexity of manufacture and the scalability of the production of some of the agents (e.g., lentiviruses and rAAV). Moreover, recognition of viral proteins by antibodies or cell-mediated immunity may limit systemic and/or repeated delivery of the vector, or the durability of transgene expression. Other limitations of viral vectors include insertional mutagenesis produced by some viral vectors and the limited size of the encoded transgenes.

Therefore, much effort has been devoted to increasing the efficiency of nonviral delivery of plasmid DNA in a way that efficiently allows the DNA to escape nuclease-mediated degradation.[45,46] Plasmid delivery can be affected by physical methods that disrupt the cell membrane (e.g., by electroporation, ultrasound, and hydrodynamic injection) or by chemicals that induce endocytosis,[47] such as cationic polymers or lipids.[48] Nonviral gene delivery methods are generally less immunogenic and toxic and often cost-effective, but efficiency of these vectors *in vivo* remains lower than viral vectors and transgene expression is modest, with up to three-fold less expression compared to viral vectors.[49–52]

Overcoming these limitations of nonviral vectors has required improvements in vector efficacy and the substantial further development of transposon-based plasmids using Sleeping Beauty or PiggyBac.[53–59] Unlike other nonviral vectors, transposons integrate into the target cell genome, thereby enabling persistent expression of the inserted gene. For example, a two-plasmid system, one containing the transposase enzyme and the other containing the expression cassette flanked by ITRs can readily be co-transfected into a T cell. By this means, *ex vivo* transfer of T-cell receptor (*TCR*) or chimeric antigen receptor (*CAR*) genes has generated tumor-directed T lymphocytes,[60,61] that are now in clinical trial for treatment of hematologic malignancies[62–64] and several early phase clinical reports of feasibility using transposon-based CAR-T cells are emerging.[65,66] Preclinical models directed against solid tumors[67–69] are also being explored, and there are efforts to optimize *in vivo* delivery of these products.[70–72]

Gene editing

A wide range of nuclease-based editing technologies are available that produce highly targeted sequence excision and/or incorporation in defined sites in the genome. These include zinc-finger-nucleases and transcription activator-like effector nucleases (TALENs).[73,74] The specificity of these techniques, however, is offset by the time and complexity of their design, manufacture, and validation. As a consequence, the less specific but speedier technique of *CRISPR/Cas9* gene editing is increasingly used for applications in human gene therapy. Cas proteins are endonucleases that combine with a single guide RNA to form complementary base pairs with target DNA and then cleave the DNA at specific sites.[75,76] The CRISPR/Cas9 system has been exploited to correct gene mutations that drive development and progression of cancers, create OV,[77] and to replace specific genome sequences of human T cells with modified sequences[78] that show promise in preclinical models.[79–81] Delivery of CRISPR/Cas9 can be accomplished by either viral[82–85] or nonviral vector[86,87] delivery, and three strategies currently dominate the field:[88] (1) use of a plasmid-based CRISPR/Cas9 system encoding Cas9 and single guide RNA from the same vector,[89] (2) combination of Cas9 mRNA and single-guide RNA,[90] or (3) combination of Cas9 protein and guide RNA,[91] the most widely used. Despite the therapeutic promise of gene-editing in cancer treatment, the major obstacle remains safe and effective delivery of CRISPR/Cas9 systems to target cells in patients. In particular, translation of this therapy to patients has been slower than anticipated[92] owing to off-target effects (although these are diminishing with newer systems), lack of safe and efficient delivery systems, and ethical considerations surrounding targeted gene therapy,[93] but several clinical trials are evaluating this further (NCT04426669). Ex vivo use of CRISPR/Cas9 to edit surface antigen expression on normal[94,95] and therapeutic[96] T cells has been demonstrated to be effective for the application of CAR T-cells in preclinical and early clinical models, allowing nonmalignant cells to evade CAR T cell targeting (NCT03690011).

Targets of gene therapy

As cancer is an acquired genetic disorder, in principle, gene therapy could be used to correct the disorder by, for example, replacing an inactive gene with an active one or neutralizing hyperfunctional genes. Interest in this option has been revived with the expansion of gene editing technologies described in the preceding section. Although gene transfer to tumor cells has shown some benefit for the treatment of p53-deficient tumors,[97] engineering gene therapies that directly target cancer cells remains highly problematic, irrespective of the strategy used. Unlikely monogenic hereditary diseases, gene therapies targeting cancer cells require modification of the complete population of tumor cells, which is usually extremely large. As described above, highly efficient gene delivery systems have not yet been established. Even if they were available, correction of a single abnormality may be insufficient to repair the transformed phenotype. Therefore, alternative strategies have been explored that target normal host tissue and enhance their capacity to eradicate cancer.

Gene therapy strategies that directly attack tumors

Prodrug-metabolizing enzymes
Transfer of genes encoding prodrug-metabolizing enzymes may partially overcome inefficient gene transfer, as these genes encode enzymes that convert harmless small-molecule prodrugs into lethal cytotoxins that are then released into the general area of the tumor. A well-studied example is that of the herpes simplex virus-derived thymidine kinase (*HSV-tk*) gene, which has been widely investigated for this purpose. The HSV-tk, which is encoded by the transferred gene, phosphorylates nontoxic prodrugs, such as acyclovir, valacyclovir, and ganciclovir, into toxic metabolites that inhibit cellular DNA synthesis and replication. Aside from the direct cytotoxic effect on the transduced cancer cells, this approach also has an indirect bystander cytotoxic effect,[98] as the metabolites can be transported from the transgene-expressing cells to adjacent nontransduced cells through gap junction intercellular communication.[99,100] Cytosine deaminase (CD) derived from *Escherichia coli* represents another prodrug-metabolizing enzyme and has been studied both independently and in conjunction with HSV-Tk.[101] One randomized Phase 3 clinical trial of *HSV-tk* gene therapy for patients with glioma employed this concept by injecting adenoviral vectors peri-lesionally.[102] As perilesional injections are not always feasible, tumor cells can be targeted through other means, such as vectors that can only transduce dividing cells, the use of enzyme-prodrug systems whose products are pharmacologically active only in dividing cells, or the use of a vector that is targeted to a receptor of tumor-restricted distribution.[103]

Virotherapy or viral oncolysis
Several case reports have documented spontaneous tumor regressions after viral infections.[104,105] As more detailed knowledge of the molecular biology of viruses and cancers has developed, OV that enter or replicate only in tumor cells have been engineered. Several of these OV are natural viral species that selectively infect and kill cancer cells. For example, H1 autonomously replicating parvovirus, reovirus, Newcastle disease virus, Mumps virus, and Moloney leukemia virus are all cancer specific. Other viruses such as measles, adenovirus, vesicular stomatitis virus, vaccinia, and herpes simplex virus require genetic modification to become cancer specific.[106] For example, in ONYX-015, there is deletion of the E1B region that normally binds to and inactivates the *p53* gene to allow viral replication. As a result, ONYX-015 is unable to block *p53* function and can replicate only in malignant cells, most of which are functionally *p53* defective.[107]

Oncolytic virus can kill tumor cells not only by direct lysis (their cytopathic effect) but also by indirect mechanisms such as the destruction of tumor blood vessels or amplification of specific anticancer immune responses. Thus, OV can be further modified to deliver therapeutic genes that induce T-cell chemotaxis (e.g., Rantes) or immunomodulation (e.g., GM-CSF [granulocyte-macrophage colony-stimulating factor], IL-2, IL-12, or IL-15)[108–115] or to deliver a prodrug-converting enzyme that turns an otherwise inert agent into a cytotoxic drug at high concentration in the tumor (see section titled "Prodrug-metabolizing enzymes").[116] Talimogene laherparepvec is GM-CSF-encoding second-generation oncolytic HSV and it is the first approved oncolytic immunotherapy in Europe, US, and Australia.[117]

Despite the licensing of talimogene and the apparent safety and efficacy of several other oncolytic virus clinical trials,[118,119] broader clinical application has not yet met investigators' expectations. A number of obstacles hamper the spread of OV into human tumors. When viruses are injected systemically, they can be cleared from the bloodstream before they reach the tumor cells by neutralizing antibodies, complement proteins, the reticuloendothelial system, or tumor microenvironment.[120–124] In addition, the initial tumor transduction rate may not be high enough for efficient subsequent viral replication. To overcome these obstacles, several strategies have been investigated, such as delivering OV using mesenchymal stem cells to shield them from the immune response,[125,126] prior administration of immunosuppressive drugs,[127] use of vasoactive or vaso-normalizing treatments,[128] and combination therapy with other gene or immunotherapy strategies.[129]

Induce host immunity by cancer vaccines
Unlike vaccines against infectious agents, cancer vaccines are not used for the prevention of disease, but for its treatment, by augmenting the patients' own immune systems to recognize and attack

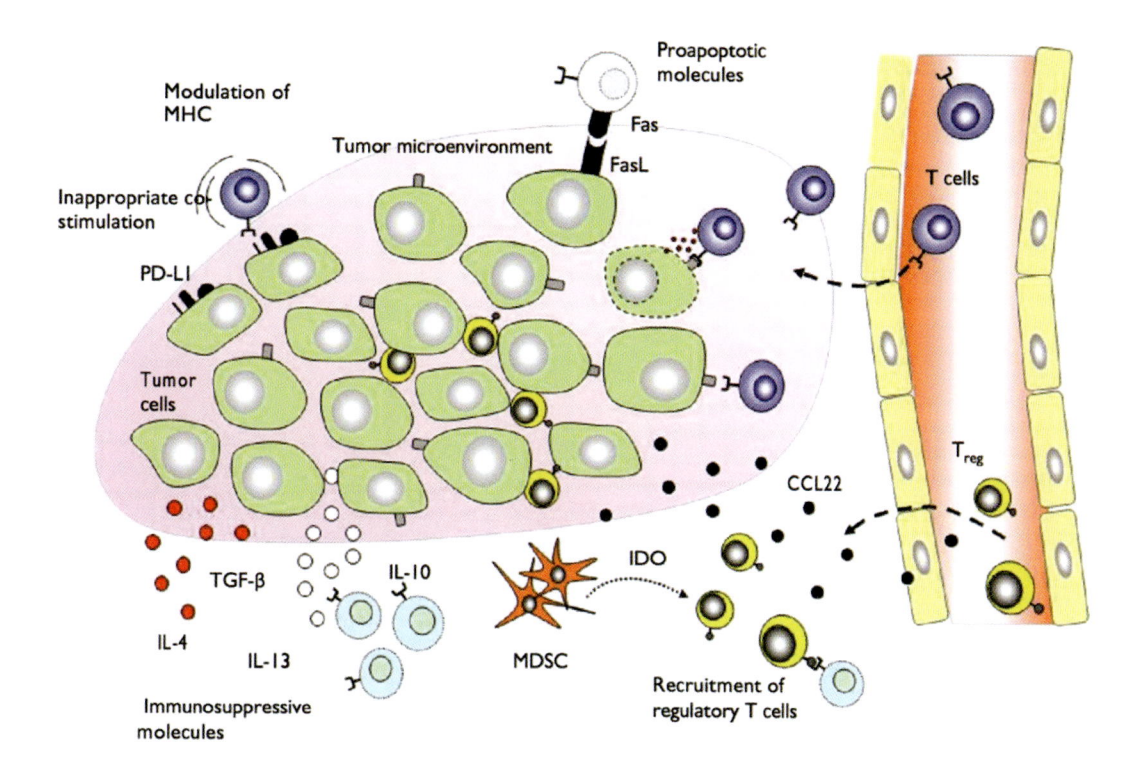

Figure 1 Tumor evasion mechanism. The tumor microenvironment consists of tumor cells and several kinds of immunosuppressive cells, such as T_{reg} and MDSCs. Tumor cells themselves express FasL to induce cytotoxic T lymphocytes (CTLs) apoptosis and PD-L1 to inhibit CTL functions. In addition, they secrete immunosuppressive molecules TGF-β, IL-10, IL4, and IL-13. Source: Based on Han et al.[130]

the cancer cells. Although vaccines against human tumors have been investigated for more than 100 years, effective agents have yet to be fully established, and less than 10% of cancer vaccine recipients benefit from the treatment.[103] There is nonetheless a strong rationale for the continued exploration of these agents. Many cancer cells express tumor-associated antigens (TAAs), but effective immunity against TAAs may be lacking because cancer cells escape from host immune surveillance (Figure 1). Tumor escape mechanisms include the downregulation of costimulatory molecules, expression of immune-inhibitory receptors/ligands such as PDL-1, secretion of a multiplicity of soluble immune-inhibitory factors, such as transforming growth factor-β (TGF-β), IL-10 and enzyme inhibitory ligands such as FasL or TRAIL, and the induction of regulatory T cells (T_{reg}) or myeloid-derived suppressor cells.[131] Vaccination is intended to elicit host immunity against tolerized TAAs by coadministering the antigen with potent immunostimulatory signals. Target antigens have included oncoproteins, oncofetal antigens, differentiation-associated proteins, and viral proteins. Efforts have also been made to capture immune responses against an individual's unique tumor-associated neoantigens (antigens arising from mutations specific to each tumor).[132] Thus, TAAs have been given as (1) injections of peptides or proteins in immune adjuvants,[133] (2) components of recombinant viruses or other recombinant microorganisms to capitalize on the proinflammatory innate and adaptive immune responses induced by these organisms,[134] (3) protein, peptide-activated dendritic cells (DCs),[135] or (4) mRNA from tumor cells or tumor cells themselves modified to express immunostimulatory genes, both of which are intended to capture immune responses against neoantigens.[136] For this last application, investigators often use combinations of immunomodulatory genes to elicit robust T-cell responses including IL-2[136] and GM-CSF[137] with costimulatory molecules such as CD40L.[136,138]

Despite many years of effort, only one cancer vaccine (Provenge) has been licensed by the U.S. Food and Drug Administration (FDA). This vaccine is used to treat advanced prostate cancer and expresses a fusion protein of prostatic acid phosphatase with GM-CSF.[135] Provenge is produced following the *ex vivo* transduction of the patients' own antigen-presenting cell population in peripheral blood. Unfortunately, the complexities of manufacturing and distribution limited the uptake of this agent. While vaccine therapy alone has rarely been powerful enough to elicit curative immune responses, the combination of vaccines and checkpoint antibodies for T cells, such as CTLA4 mAb or PD-1 mAb, may augment the efficacy of this therapy and reanimate the field.

Modifying host immune effector cells

One of the limitations of cancer vaccines is that the immune responses they are supposed to induce *in vivo* may be blocked or subverted by the immune evasion strategies of malignant cells and the tumor microenvironment these cells produce (Figure 1). An alternative approach is to prepare effector cells *ex vivo* that are engineered to be specific for the tumor and are also engineered to counteract whatever immune evasion strategies the tumor uses. These modified effector cells can then be returned to the patient.

Generating tumor specificity

T cells can be engineered to be tumor specific by transferring sequences encoding standardized TAA-specific receptors into bulk T-cell populations. Two types of receptors have been used: "natural" α and β TCRs or artificial CARs, so-called because

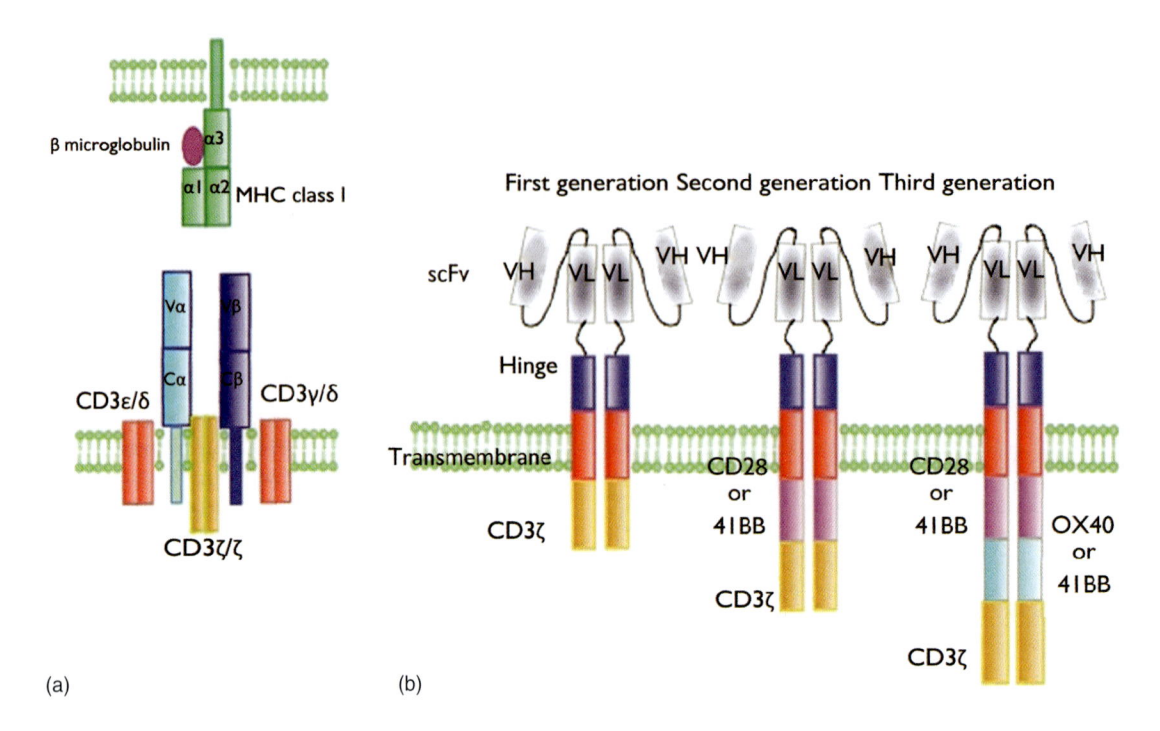

Figure 2 Transgenic T-cell receptors. (a) Transgenic α and β T-cell receptors, which need HLA to recognize the targeted antigen, and (b) chimeric antigen receptors, which recognize the antigen in HLA unrestricted manner. For endodomains, first-generation CAR has only CD3ζ and second- and third-generation CARs also have costimulatory molecules. scFV, single-chain variable fragment.

they are chimeras of a tumor–antigen-binding domain and a TCR-signaling domain. The TCR α and β chains are encoded by *TRA* and *TRB* genes and have been cloned for several different TAA epitopes.[139] These synthetic TCR can be modified to be of high affinity in an attempt to increase their effectiveness once transferred into T cells,[140] but sometimes at the cost of generating unwanted cross-reactivities.[141–143] Several clinical trials have been performed,[144–148] some of which have shown significant efficacy such as in melanoma, colorectal cancer, and myeloma, although off-target or "on-target antigen but off-tumor" toxicities remain a concern.

The major limitations of TCR-gene therapy are that each TCR recognizes only a small portion of a total tumor antigen (an epitope), which may be lost ("edited") by the tumor and that the recognition of this epitope is moreover limited to a particular major histocompatibility complex (MHC) polymorphism, restricting activity to those individuals who share that human leukocyte antigen (HLA) type. CAR-transduced T cells may allow engagement of a larger antigenic component than the 9–14 peptides recognized by the TCR. CAR T cells can also overcome the limitation of HLA restriction and recognize carbohydrate and other nonprotein antigens. CARs are composed of an extracellular domain that binds to the intended antigen, a transmembrane domain, and one or more intracellular signaling domains (Figure 2). Most commonly, the extracellular domain is derived from the antigen-binding portion of a monoclonal antibody targeting the intended antigen and the intracellular signaling domain (endodomain) comes from the CD3ζ component of the TCR.[103] Initial CAR T-cell efficacies were modest because CAR stimulation alone was insufficient to fully activate CAR T cells, producing limited expansion and persistence *in vivo*. Second-generation CARs were created that added one or more of the costimulatory signals that T cells need to pass through sequential activation barriers, such as the signaling domains from CD27, CD28, 41BB, OX40, or ICOS. When these second-generation CARs are coupled with an exodomain that binds CD19, an antigen present on most normal and many B-cell malignancies, CAR T cells produce striking results in the treatment of B cell malignancies. For example, CD19 CAR T cells have a 90% CR rate for relapsed/resistant B cell-acute lymphoblastic leukemia (B-ALL).[16,149] Thus far three CO19 CAR T cells products, Kymriah®, Yescarta®, and Breyanzi® have been approved by regulatory agencies in the US, Europe, and Japan for the treatment, of refractory patients wirh CD19+ B cell leukemia or diffuse large B cell lymphoma. Also one BCMA CAR T cells product, and one BCMA CAR T cells product, Abecma® has been approved in the US for the treatment of relapsed or refractory multiple myeloma patients. This approach has led to development of CAR T cells now in clinical trials for other hematologic malignancies including T-cell malignancies[150,151] acute myeloid leukemia,[152] and Hodgkin Disease[153] although none have yet established consistently high and sustained tumor control in multi-center studies comparable to CD19 in B cell malignancies.

Extending CAR T cell successes from B cell malignancies to solid tumors has proved challenging. One of the unwanted effects of CD19 CAR T cells is the destruction of normal B cells, which also express CD19, but this effect may be compensated for by infusion of immunoglobulin preparations. Solid tumors also share antigens with other organs, and few other normal cell types are as dispensable as B cells. There are a limited number of truly unique TAAs that can be recognized by antibodies or other antigen-recognition domains suitable for inclusion in CARs. Human epidermal growth factor receptor 2 (HER2)-CAR T cells directed against sarcomas[154] and disiaIoganglIoside (GD2)-CAR T cells directed to neuroblastoma have shown antitumor activity and in a minority of patients have been associated with sustained complete remissions, but overall activity remains well below that needed for these approaches to be widely used.[155] Several other antigen targeting CARs clinical trials have been started (carcinoembryonic antigen (CEA), Mesothelin, IL13Ra2, epidermal growth factor receptor (EGFR), epidermal growth factor receptor variant III (EGFRvIII), alpha-folate receptor, CD171, carboxy-anhydrase-IX (CAIX), prostate specific membrane antigen (PSMA), mucin 1, cell surface associated (MUC1), tumor-associated glycoprotein 72 (TAG-72), mesenchymal–epithelial transition factor (c-MET)).[156]

Engineering immune cells to combat the immunosuppressive tumor microenvironment
T cells traffic poorly to many tumor sites and once there, they encounter an immunosuppressive tumor microenvironment[130] (Figure 1) mediated by the recruitment of inhibitory cells (e.g., myeloid suppressor cells and regulatory T cells), the expression of inhibitory molecules (e.g., PDL1 and FasL), and the production of soluble inhibitory molecules/Th2-polarizing cytokines (e.g., adenosine, tumor indoleamine 2,3-dioxygenase (IDO), TGF-β, IL-6, IL-10, and prostaglandin E2 (PGE-2)). Therefore, investigators are engineering T cells to improve the tumor migration of adoptively transferred T cells and their proliferation and survival *in vivo*. For example, to resist TGFβ, a dominant-negative TGF-β receptor type II has been expressed in tumor-directed T cells. TGF-β receptor type II expression induces resistance to tumor-secreted TGF-β and is showing promising clinical benefits.[157,158]

Adding signal 3 to improve the persistence of immune cells
Once therapeutic T cells have been trafficked to the site of the tumor, they must be able to persist, expand, and eliminate tumor cells. Immunostimulatory cytokines provide signal 3, which is absent in the design of second-generation CAR T cells.[159] Preclinical studies have demonstrated improved T cell persistence and enhanced cytotoxicity with the addition of immunostimulatory cytokines including IL-7, IL-15, IL-12, and IL-21 independently and in combination.[160–165] Translation of these findings into clinical trials has been more difficult owing to systemic side effects of increased circulating cytokines.[166–169] More recently, genetic modification of T cells to secrete cytokines or express tethered cytokines (or receptors) to enhance their antitumor activity and maintain higher levels of cytokines preferentially at the tumor site have shown promise, with enhanced T cell cytotoxicity that can be achieved at lower T cell numbers.[170–172] Further studies have utilized the inhibitory molecules in the tumor microenvironment, such as IL-4, to engage extracellular receptors that in turn provide immunostimulatory cytokines such as IL-7 on adoptively transferred T cells.[173] A summary of engineering countermeasures to tumor immune evasion currently under investigation is detailed in Table 2.[174–180]

Table 2 Countermeasures to tumor immune evasion and inhibition.[a]

Targets	Gene modification	References
TGF-β	Dominant-negative TGF-β receptor	157, 158
Fas L	Downregulation of Fas	174
IDO, arginase	GCN2 knockdown	175
IL-10	IL-10 receptor 1/IgG1-Fc fusion proteins	176
IL-4	IL-4/IL-7 chimeric receptor	173, 177
IL-7 or IL-7Ra	Expression of IL-7 or IL-7Ra	171, 178, 179
IL-12	Expression of IL-12	164, 180
IL-15	Expression of IL-15	160, 162, 165
IL-21	Expression of IL-21	163, 165

[a]Source: Based on Tschumi et al.[174]; Munn et al.[175]; Sato et al.[176]; Mohammed et al.[177]; Yang et al.[178]; Perna et al.[179]; Mirzaei and Hadjati.[180]

Genetic modification of other immune system cells

The success of gene-modified T cells in cancer treatment has increased interest in genetic modification of other cells of the immune system. These include gamma–delta T cells and mucosal-associated invariant chain T cells (MAIT).[181,182] The most advanced of these alternative approaches, however, explore natural killer (NK) cells and invariant chain natural killer T cells (iNKT). These cells form part of the bridge between the innate and adaptive immune responses. They can be expanded and activated *ex vivo*, and once retargeted, may have significant antitumor activity. All of the studies described for T cells are in the process of being replicated for NK and NKT cell populations. Recently, these platforms have garnered additional interest for their potential advantages over T lymphocyte-based therapy, specifically with the expression of CARs.[183] Unlike CAR T-cells, which target tumor through their CAR alone, NK and NKT cells have multiple mechanisms of antitumor cytotoxicity that can be antigen-independent.[184–188] One mechanism of tumor evasion of CAR therapy is antigen downregulation, which poses a major limitation of CAR T cell therapy, but NK and NKT cells would retain the ability to target tumor even with antigen downregulation.[186,187] This has led to evaluation in multiple preclinical models and some early clinical trials[189] evaluating their potency and safety in diseases such as B cell lymphoma,[190,191] T cell malignancies,[192,193] and neuroblastoma.[194,195] As NK and NKT cells are more difficult to isolate and expand, with relatively short half-life there are some disadvantages, and continued work over the next few years will reveal the durability of any antitumor activity.

Safety

Although immunotherapy with adoptively transferred T cells has produced striking results, like any potent therapy, the risk is considerable. Apart from fatal cross-reactivities with normal tissues, induction of cytokine release syndrome (or systemic inflammatory response syndrome) has been reported after the administration of some T-cell therapies, particularly CD19 CAR T cells. As these events may be lethal, investigators are developing and testing several safety or suicide systems that may allow rapid control of the treatment. They include cytotoxic antibodies, prodrug-metabolizing enzymes, and inducible apoptosis genes.[196–200]

Conclusion: how will cancer gene therapy enter clinical practice?

Now that the role of gene therapy for cancer is becoming clearer, the pharmaceutical industry and healthcare providers will have to begin to assess the high cost of developing, manufacturing, and delivering these individualized therapies. As optimal results may be obtained only when multiple biological therapies are combined (e.g., engineered T cells, OV, and checkpoint antibodies), the pharmacoeconomics will need to be carefully addressed by healthcare services experts and an adequate case made for their widespread substitution for conventional therapy. Although we believe that such a case will indeed be made, this remains one more in the long list of the challenges that cancer gene therapy will face before it truly becomes frontline treatment of cancer.

Key references

The complete reference list can be found on Vital Source version of this title, see inside front cover.

8. Mann R, Mulligan RC, Baltimore D. Construction of a retrovirus packaging mutant and its use to produce helper-free defective retrovirus. *Cell*. 1983;**33**(1):153–159.
14. Durand S, Cimarelli A. The inside out of lentiviral vectors. *Viruses*. 2011;**3**(2):132–159.
16. Porter D, Levine BL, Kalos M, et al. Chimeric antigen receptor-modified T cells in chronic lymphoid leukemia. *N Engl J Med*. 2011;**365**(8):725–733.
19. Nathwani A, Tuddenham EG, Rangarajan S, et al. Adenovirus-associated virus vector-mediated gene transfer in hemophilia B. *N Engl J Med*. 2011;**365**(25):2357–2365.
20. Wold W, Ison MG. Adenoviruses. In: Knipe DM, Howley PM, eds. *Fields Virology*. Philadelphia, PA: Lippincott Williams & Wilkins; 2013:1732–1767.
21. Berk A. Adenoviridae. In: Knipe DM, Howley PM, eds. *Fields Virology*. Philadelphia, PA: Lippincott Williams & Wilkins; 2013:1704–1173.
24. Sumida S, Truitt DM, Lemckert AA, et al. Neutralizing antibodies to adenovirus serotype 5 vaccine vectors are directed primarily against the adenovirus hexon protein. *J Immunol*. 2005;**174**:7179–7185.
26. Gomez J, Curiel DT. Conditionally replicative adenoviral vectors for cancer gene therapy. *Lancet Oncol*. 2000;**1**(3):148–158.
28. Rosewell A, Vetrini F, Ng P. Helper-dependent adenoviral vectors. *J Genet Syndr Gene Ther*. 2011:001. doi: 10.4172/2157-7412.s5-001.
33. Rosewell-Shaw A, Suzuki M. Immunology of adenoviral vectors in cancer therapy. *Mol Ther Methods Clin Dev*. 2019;**15**:418–429.
37. Coffin R. T-Vec: the first oncolytic immunotherapy approved for the treatment of cancer. *Immunotherapy*. 2016;**8**(2):103.
47. Niidome T, Huang L. Gene therapy progress and prospects: nonviral vectors. *Gene Ther*. 2002;**9**(24):1647–1652.
48. Wang W, Li W, Ma N, Steinhoff G. Non-viral gene delivery methods. *Curr Pharm Biotechnol*. 2013;**14**:46–60.
57. Galvan D, Nakazawa Y, Kaja A, et al. Genome-wide mapping of PiggyBac transposon integrations in primary human T cells. *J Immunother*. 2009;**32**:837–844.
61. Lim W, June CH. The principles of engineering immune cells to treat cancer. *Cell*. 2017;**168**:724–740.
62. Nakazawa Y, Matsuda K, Kurata T, et al. Anti-proliferative effects of T cells expressing a ligand-based chimeric antigen receptor against CD116 on CD34(+) cells of juvenile myelomonocytic leukemia. *J Hematol Oncol*. 2016;**9**:27.
74. Qasim W, Zhan H, Samarasinghe S, et al. Molecular remission of infant B-ALL after infusion of universal TALEN gene-edited CAR T cells. *Sci Transl Med*. 2017;**9**(374):eaaj2013.
78. Schumann K, Lin S, Boyer E, et al. Generation of knock-in primary human T cells using Cas9 ribonucleoproteins. *Proc Natl Acad Sci U S A*. 2015;**112**:10437–10442.
79. Yin H, Xue W, Chen S, et al. Genome editing with Cas9 in adult mice corrects a disease mutation and phenotype. *Nat Biotechnol*. 2014;**32**:551–553.
85. Shalem O, Sanjana NE, Hartenian E, et al. Genome-scale CRISPR-Cas9 knockout screening in human cells. *Science*. 2014;**343**:84–87.
86. Mali P, Aach J, Stranges PB, et al. CAS9 transcriptional activators for target specificity screening and paired nickases for cooperative genome engineering. *Nat Biotechnol*. 2013;**31**:833–838.
88. Liu C, Zhang L, Liu H, Cheng K. Delivery strategies of the CRISPR-Cas9 gene-editing system for therapeutic applications. *J Control Release*. 2017;**266**:17–26.
89. Ran F, Hsu PD, Wright J, et al. Genome engineering using the CRISPR-Cas9 system. *Nat Protoc*. 2013;**8**(11):2281–2308.
90. Niu Y, Shen B, Cui Y, et al. Generation of gene-modified cynomolgus monkey via Cas9/RNA-mediated gene targeting in one-cell embryos. *Cell*. 2014;**156**(4):836–843.
92. Cyranoski D. CRISPR gene-editing tested in a person for the first time. *Nature*. 2016;**539**:479.
103. Brenner M, Gottschalk S, Leen AM, Vera JF. Is cancer gene therapy an empty suit? *Lancet Oncol*. 2013;**14**(11):e447–e456.
112. Atherton M, Lichty BD. Evolution of oncolytic viruses: novel strategies for cancer treatment. *Immunotherapy*. 2013;**5**:1191–1206.
121. Bessis N, GarciaCozar FJ, Boissier MC. Immune responses to gene therapy vectors: influence on vector function and effector mechanisms. *Gene Ther*. 2004;**11**:S10–S17.
167. Rosenberg S. IL-2: the first effective immunotherapy for human cancer. *J Immunol*. 2014;**192**:5451–5458.
170. Leen A, Sukumaran S, Watanabe N, et al. Reversal of tumor immune inhibition using a chimeric cytokine receptor. *Mol Ther*. 2014;**22**:1211–1220.
171. Shum T, Omer B, Tashiro H, et al. Constitutive signaling from an engineered IL7 receptor promotes durable tumor elimination by tumor-redirected T cells. *Cancer Discov*. 2017;**7**(11):1238–1247.
172. Shum T, Kruse RL, Rooney CM. Strategies for enhancing adoptive T-cell immunotherapy against solid tumors using engineered cytokine signaling and other modalities. *Expert Opin Biol Ther*. 2018;**18**(6):653–664.
200. Straathof K, Pule MA, Yotnda P, et al. An inducible caspase 9 safety switch for T-cell therapy. *Blood*. 2005;**105**:4247–4254.

65 Cancer nanotechnology

Xingya Jiang, PhD ■ Yanlan Liu, PhD ■ Danny Liu, BS ■ Jinjun Shi, PhD ■ Robert Langer, ScD

Overview

The advances in state-of-the-art nanotechnologies have offered enormous opportunities to overcome many obstacles in cancer therapy, such as suboptimal pharmacokinetics and therapeutic efficacy of anticancer drugs, their severe adverse effects, and the development of drug resistance. Here, we highlight clinical-stage nanoparticle technologies applied in conventional cancer therapies and the development of novel classes of anticancer therapeutics. We also discuss recent cutting-edge research efforts in this exciting field, which could lead to the development of novel and more effective cancer nanomedicines.

Introduction

Despite the exciting progress in cancer biology, diagnosis, and therapy, the global burden of cancer—one of the most devastating diseases worldwide—continues to grow at an alarming pace. According to the *World Cancer Report 2014*, it is expected that new cancer cases will rise from an estimated 14 million annually in 2012 to 22 million within the next 20 years, and cancer deaths from 8.2 million to 13 million per year over the same period.[1] Limitations in conventional cancer therapeutics, such as unfavorable pharmacokinetics, adverse effects, and the development of drug resistance are obstacles in current cancer therapy,[2] and new strategies are essential in improving patient outcomes and addressing the rising cancer burden.

Since the FDA approval of the first anticancer therapeutic nanoparticle Doxil (Liposomal Doxorubicin) in 1995, nanotechnology has demonstrated tremendous potential in enhancing cancer treatment.[3-5] For example, nanoparticles can favorably modulate pharmacokinetic and biodistribution profiles of drug molecules to improve their therapeutic efficacy and/or reduce unintended adverse effects.[6] With unique physicochemical features, some nanomaterials themselves possess therapeutic action, such as iron oxide nanoparticles for hyperthermia cancer treatment.[7] To date, over 10 cancer nanotherapeutics have been approved for clinical use, and many are currently in clinical trials (Table 1).[8] This article overviews the clinical-stage nanotechnologies in cancer treatment and discusses recent cutting-edge research in the cancer nanotechnology field.

Clinical stage cancer nanotechnologies

What makes nanotechnology particularly impactful in cancer therapy is that it possesses a variety of distinctive features for drug delivery. With nanotechnology, it may be possible to (1) improve the delivery of therapeutic molecules (e.g., hydrophobic drugs) and protect them from premature degradation, clearance, or interaction with biological environments[9,10]; (2) deliver drugs more selectively to tumor cells by modifying the nanoparticles with targeting ligands[11,12]; (3) package both imaging and therapeutic agents together for real-time feedback on drug delivery and for patient selection[13]; (4) cross tight endothelial and epithelial barriers[14,15]; (5) co-deliver multiple drugs to improve therapeutic efficacy through synergistic effects and/or to overcome drug resistance[16,17]; (6) control sustained drug release to reduce administration frequency; (7) protect nucleic acids from enzymatic degradation and facilitate their intracellular uptake and endosomal escape[18]; among others. Furthermore, some nanoparticles have inherent thermotherapy capabilities activated upon local stimulation, which make them invaluable in overcoming resistance to chemotherapeutic drugs and avoiding systemic adverse effect. Given these merits, nanotechnology has extraordinary potential to address obstacles existing in conventional cancer therapies and to develop novel classes of anticancer therapeutics. Here, we discuss the clinical-stage nanotechnologies used in different cancer treatment modalities, such as image-guided surgery, chemotherapy, radiotherapy, hyperthermia therapy, gene therapy, and immunotherapy (Table 1).

Image-guided surgery

Surgical resection remains the cornerstone and first-line treatment for many solid tumors. However, incomplete resection of cancerous tissues often leads to recurrence of cancer and poor prognosis as it is difficult to distinguish tumor from normal tissues solely based on visual and haptic cues, especially at their borders and/or in the presence of small nodules. Intraoperative imaging techniques that can clearly mark the boundaries between cancerous and noncancerous tissues are therefore desired. Fluorescence-guided surgery (FGS) is the one that attracts the most attention because of the high sensitivity, low cost, and safety of fluorescence imaging as well as a number of FDA-approved fluorescence imaging systems.[19] Central to FGS are fluorescent probes that illuminate the target of interest (e.g., tumor) with high sensitivity and selectivity. Currently, several nanoparticle-based fluorescent probes are in clinical trials. ONM-100, an intravenously administered fluorescence imaging agent developed by OncoNano Medicine, is under Phase II clinical trial for patients with solid tumors undergoing routine surgery. ONM-100 is an ultra pH-sensitive polymeric nanoparticle loaded with indocyanine green (ICG) (an FDA-approved near-infrared dye), which dissociates and lights up tumors with ICG fluorescence in response to the acidic tumor microenvironment (TME), while remaining intact and nonfluorescent in normal tissues.[20] In multiple murine tumor models, this pH-activatable fluorescence nanoprobe outperformed various commercial probes in terms of sensitivity and selectivity and could detect occult nodules of less than 1 mm^3.[21] cRGDY-PEG-Cy5.5-C dot, a fluorescent silica nanoparticle conjugated with targeting ligands, is another intraoperative fluorescence imaging probe

Table 1 Representative clinical-stage nanotechnologies in cancer therapies.[a]

Category		Product	Description	Indications	Clinical stage
Image-guided surgery		ONM-100	pH-sensitive fluorescent polymeric nanoparticle	Solid tumors undergoing routine surgery	Phase 2
		cRGDY-PEG-Cy5.5-C dot	Dye-labeled silica nanoparticle conjugated with tumor-targeting ligand	Mapping of nodal metastases in breast cancer, colorectal cancer, and melanoma	Phase 2
		^{64}Cu-NOTA-PSMAi-PEG-Cy5.5-C′ dot	Radioisotope- and dye-labeled silica nanoparticle conjugated with prostate cancer targeting ligand	Prostate cancer	Phase 1
Chemotherapy	Passive targeting	Doxil	PEGylated liposomal doxorubicin	Ovarian cancer, Kaposi sarcoma, multiple myeloma	FDA approval in 1995
		DaunoXome	Daunorubicin-loaded lipid vesicles	Advanced HIV-related Kaposi sarcoma	FDA approval in 1996
		Mepact	Liposomal muramyl tripeptide phosphatidyl-ethanolamine	Nonmetastatic, resectable osteosarcoma	Approved in Europe, Phase III in the United States
		Myocet	Liposomal doxorubicin	Metastatic breast cancer	Approved in Europe and Canada
		Abraxane	Nanoparticle albumin-bond (Nab)-paclitaxel	Metastatic pancreatic cancer, non-small-cell lung cancer, breast cancer	FDA approval in 2005
		Genexol-PM	Paclitaxel-loaded polymeric micelles	Breast cancer	Approved in South Korea, Phase IV in the United States
		Marqibo	Vincristine sulfate liposome	Acute lymphoblastic leukemia	FDA approval in 2012
		Onivyde	Irinotecan liposome	Metastatic pancreatic cancer	FDA approval in 2015
		Vyxeos	Daunorubicin and cytarabine co-loaded liposome	Acute myeloid leukemia	FDA approval in 2017
	Active targeting	BIND-014	Docetaxel-loaded polymer nanoparticle coated with a small molecule for targeting PSMA	Non-small-cell lung cancer, metastatic castration-resistant prostate cancer	Phase II(completed)
		MM-302	Doxorubicin-loaded liposome modified with antibody fragment for targeting tumor antigen	HER2 positive breast cancer	Phase III (terminated)
		MBP-426	Oxaliplatin-loaded liposome coated with transferrin for targeting transferrin receptor	Gastric, esophageal, gastroesophageal adenocarcinoma	Phase Ib/II
		2B3-101	PEGylated liposomal doxorubicin with glutathione ligand for targeting brain	Solid tumor brain metastases, malignant glioma	Phase I/II
		Anti-EGFR-IL-dox	Anti-EGFR-immunoliposomes loaded with doxorubicin	Advanced triple-negative EGFR positive breast cancer	Phase II
	Stimuli-responsive targeting	MTC-DOX	Doxorubicin is bound to microscopic beads of activated carbon and iron as a magnetic-targeted carrier (MTC)	Adult primary hepatocellular carcinoma liver cancer	Phase III (terminated)
		ThermoDox	Doxorubicin is encapsulated in thermally sensitive liposomes.	Hepatocellular carcinoma	Phase III
Radiotherapy		NBTXR3	Hafnium oxide nanoparticles	Soft tissue sarcoma, locally advanced squamous cell carcinoma of the oral cavity or oropharynx	Approved in Europe, Phase II in the United States
Hyperthermia therapy		NanoTherm	Aminosilane-coated iron oxide nanoparticles	Glioblastoma	Approved in Europe
		AuroLase	Silica core with a gold nanoshell	Refractory head and neck cancer, and primary and/or metastatic lung tumors	Pilot study
Gene therapy		CALAA-01	Transferrin-decorated cyclodextrin polymer nanoparticle-containing siRNA against the M2 subunit of ribonucleotide reductase	Solid tumors	Phase I (terminated)
		ALN-VSP02	A lipid nanoparticle-containing siRNAs against kinesin spindle protein and VEGF	Solid tumors	Phase I

(continued overleaf)

Table 1 (Continued)

Category	Product	Description	Indications	Clinical stage
	Atu027	Liposome containing a modified siRNA against protein kinase N3	Advanced or metastatic pancreatic cancer	Phase I/II
	SGT53	p53 gene-loaded liposome coated with antibody fragment for targeting transferrin receptor	Solid tumors, metastatic pancreatic cancer	Phase II
	PNT2258	Liposomal DNA oligonucleotide against BCL-2	Relapsed or refractory non-Hodgkin lymphoma and diffuse large B-cell lymphoma	Phase II
	SNS01-T	Polyethylenimine nanoparticle incorporating siRNA against eIF5A and plasmid expressing eIF5A-K50R	Relapsed or refractory B cell malignancies	Phase I/II
	TKM-080301	Lipid nanoparticle-containing anti-PLK1 siRNA	Neuroendocrine tumors, adrenocortical carcinoma, and advanced hepatocellular carcinoma	Phase I/II
	ALN-VSP02	Lipid nanoparticle-containing anti-KSP and -VEGFA siRNA	Solid tumors	Phase I
	siRNA-EPHA2-DOPC	Liposomal siRNA against EPHA2	Advanced cancers	Phase I
	pbi-shRNA STMN1 LP	Lipid nanoparticle-containing anti-stathmin 1 shRNA	Advanced and/or metastatic cancer	Phase I
Immunotherapy	Lipovaxin-MM	Liposome-based vaccine loaded with melanoma antigens	Melanoma	Phase I
	dHER2 + AS15	Liposomal vaccine consisting of a HER2/neu peptide (dHER2) combined with the immunoadjuvant AS15	Metastatic breast cancer	Phase I/II
	DPX-0907	Multi-tumor associated antigens-loaded liposome	HLA-A2 positive advanced stage ovarian, breast, and prostate cancer	Phase I
	Tecemotide	Liposome-encapsulated MUC1 antigen	Non-small-cell lung cancer	Phase III
	mRNA-2146	lipid nanoparticle-encapsulated mRNA	Solid tumor malignancies or lymphoma, ovarian cancer	Phase I/II
	mRNA-4157	lipid nanoparticle-encapsulated mRNA	Solid tumors, melanoma	Phase I/II
	JVRS-100	Liposomal plasmid DNA	Relapsed or refractory leukemia	Phase I
	CYT-6091	Colloidal gold nanoparticle bound with tumor necrosis factor	Advanced solid tumors	Phase I
	Lipo-MERIT	Liposome-encapsulated mRNA	Melanoma	Phase I

[a]Source: Based on Shi et al.[8]

currently under Phase II clinical trial. It is peritumorally injected for nodal metastasis detection and sentinel lymph node mapping in patients undergoing head and neck cancer surgery.[22] A similar structured radioactive and fluorescent silica nanoparticle targeting the prostate-specific membrane antigen (PSMA), ^{64}Cu-NOTA-PSMAi-PEG-Cy5.5-C′ dot, is also under Phase I clinical trial for use as an intravenously injected probe to guide prostate cancer surgery.

Chemotherapy

One major advantage of chemotherapy lies in its ability to systemically attack cancers. Unfortunately, due to suboptimal pharmacokinetic profiles, only a small fraction of the administered drugs can be delivered to tumor. Their nonspecific delivery to healthy cells also makes severe side effects inevitable. Nanoparticle technologies have thereby emerged as a promising way for efficient delivery of drugs to tumor tissue while reducing their side effects.[23,24] For solid tumors, it has been recognized that the tumor surroundings are dense with leaky blood vessels. Together with the lack of functional lymphatic drainage, nanoparticles can extravasate out of circulation and accumulate in tumor tissue (Figure 1a), which is denoted as the Enhanced Permeability and Retention (EPR) effect.[25] Various nanoparticle platforms have been developed and approximately ten were introduced into the market for cancer treatment, such as Doxil, Abraxane, Genexol-PM, and more recently Onivyde.[8,26]

To further improve specificity of nanoparticle delivery, active targeting has been proposed and has advanced into clinical investigation. By surface modification with targeting ligands, such as antibodies, aptamers, peptides, and carbohydrates, the

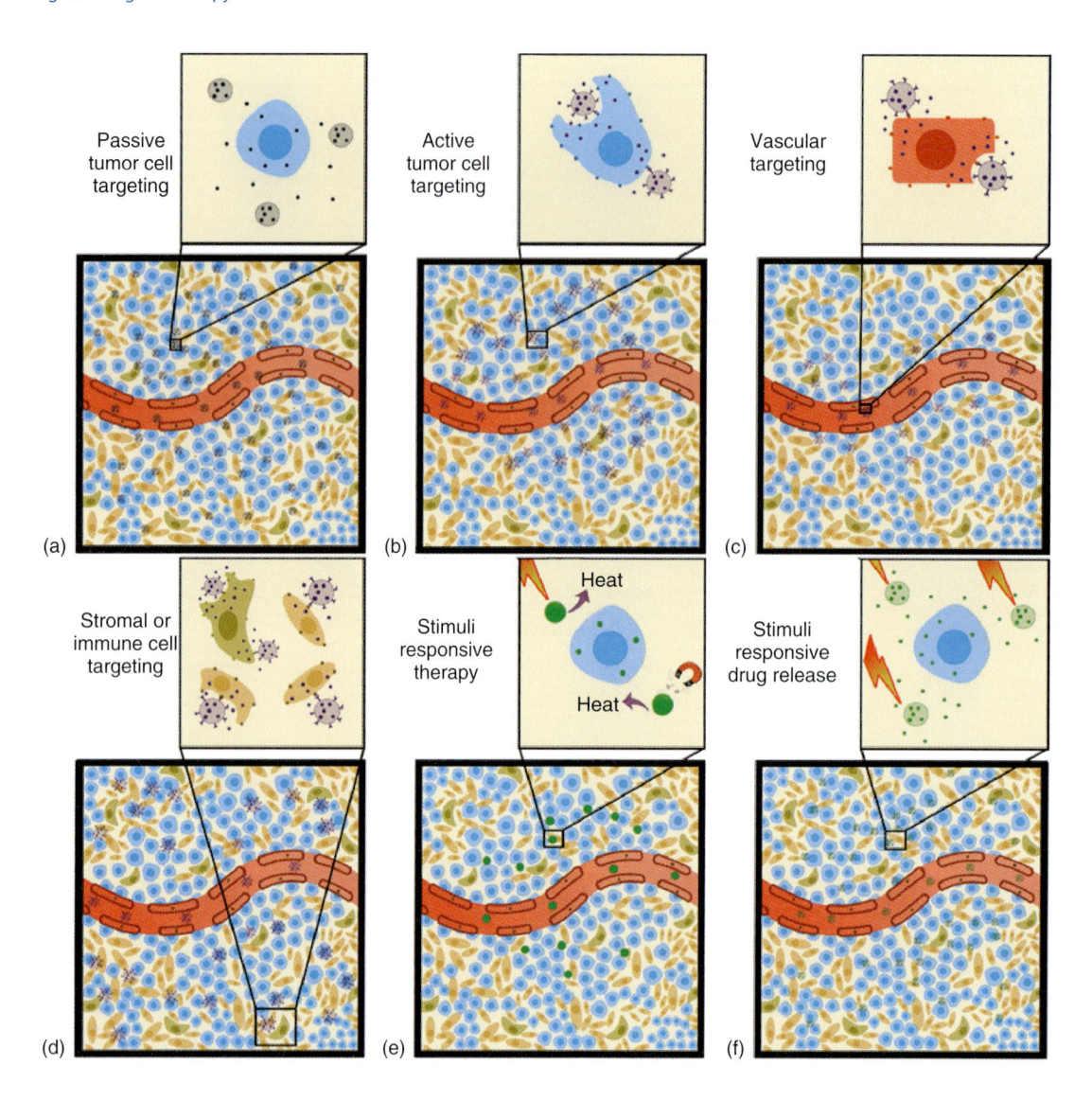

Figure 1 Schematic illustration of different nanotherapy strategies in treatment of solid tumors. (a) Nontargeted nanoparticles passively extravasate out of the leaky vasculature for tumor accumulation through the EPR effect. The drug molecules may be released from the nanoparticles and diffuse throughout the tissue for bioactivity. (b) For active tumor cell targeting, the nanoparticles are modified with targeting ligands which recognize receptors present on tumor cell surface. The receptor-mediated endocytosis leads to enhanced accumulation and cell uptake of nanoparticles. (c, d) By incorporating ligands that bind to the receptors on the surface of endothelial cells (c) or stromal/immune cells (d), nanoparticles can actively target tumor microenvironment for cancer therapy. (e) Some nanoparticles can generate heat under an alternating magnetic field or laser irradiation for cancer hyperthermia therapy. (f) Some nanoparticles become therapeutically active by releasing the payloads under either endogenous stimuli (e.g., pH, enzyme, and redox) or exogenous stimuli (e.g., light, heat, magnetic field, or ultrasound).

targeted nanoparticles can selectively recognize tumor cell-specific receptors.[27] Through receptor-mediated endocytosis, targeted delivery can increase nanoparticle retention and cellular uptake, thus significantly enhancing therapeutic efficacy (Figure 1b).[28] A representative example is BIND-014, a docetaxel-loaded polymeric nanoparticle decorated with small molecules against PSMA, which was previously developed by BIND Therapeutics. In xenograft animals treated with BIND-014, the docetaxel concentration in tumor was sevenfold higher than that treated with conventional docetaxel (Taxotere) 12 h after intravenous injection. Clinical data in a patient with metastatic cholangiocarcinoma showed that tumor shrinkage was achieved at a dose of docetaxel that corresponds to only 20% of the typical dose for docetaxel.[29]

In addition to increasing specificity, avoiding the premature release of drugs before they reach the tumor may be equally important for maximizing therapeutic efficacy and minimizing adverse effects. Stimuli-responsive nanoparticles have shown promising potential for this purpose, as they only become active in the TME (Figure 1).[30] Generally, these nanoparticles are designed to recognize subtle environmental changes associated with tumor pathological situations (e.g., pH, redox, and enzyme) or to be activated by external stimuli (e.g., heat, light, magnetic field, and ultrasound).[31] To some extent, external stimulation allows for tailored drug release profiles with excellent temporal, spatial, and dosage control.[32] In particular, noninvasive magnetic field- and ultrasound-responsive nanoparticle delivery systems have gained a lot of attention as there are nominal limits in tissue penetration for these modalities.[30,31] At present, doxorubicin-loaded thermo-responsive liposomes (ThermoDox) are being investigated in Phase II trials for the treatment of breast cancer and in Phase III trials for hepatocellular carcinoma therapy.[31]

Radiotherapy

In conventional radiotherapy, high-energy ionizing radiations such as gamma and X-rays are generally used to ionize cellular components and/or water to generate free radicals for DNA damage in tumor cells. However, the effectiveness of radiotherapy is limited by the tolerance of normal tissue to ionizing radiation dose and the development of radiation resistance of cancer cells.[33] Several approaches have been proposed to address these issues. Introducing nanoscale radiosensitizers (e.g., gold, gadolinium, and iron oxide nanoparticles) into the X-ray pathway is considered an effective way to eradicate tumors at a lower dose of radiation.[34] These materials have higher electron density than water in tissues, enabling strong interaction with X-rays and allowing for more localized and consolidated damage to tumor. Currently, a new radioenhancer (NBTXR3, developed by Nanobiotix) based on hafnium oxide nanoparticles has been approved in Europe for patients with different soft tissue sarcoma and is also under Phase II evaluation for other types of cancer in the United States.

An alternative way to enhance radiotherapeutic efficacy is to protect surrounding healthy tissues from damage or make them less radiation sensitive. Nanoparticles containing small molecules with radioprotective effects (e.g., cysteine, citicoline, and amifostine) have been investigated. Oral administration of these particles has shown radioprotective effects in both mammalian cells and rats during radiation exposure.[35–37] Furthermore, nanoparticles loaded with therapeutics against radiation-resistant biological pathways (e.g., survivin and epidermal growth factor receptor) have shown the ability to overcome the resistance of tumor to radiation therapy.[38,39] All these nanoparticle strategies could lead to further improvement in clinical radiotherapy.

Hyperthermia therapy

Owing to low host toxicity, ease of control, and absent/low resistance, hyperthermia treatment methods such as photothermal therapy (PTT) and magnetothermal therapy may be considered for cancer therapy, especially for drug-resistant cancers. Distinct from traditional therapies, PTT relies on photosensitizers to absorb light and convert it into heat to kill cells in its vicinity.[40] Its key advantage over traditional chemotherapy is that photosensitizers are minimally toxic without light exposure and thus damage to healthy tissues is minimal even with photosensitizer accumulation. Unlike radiotherapy, the light used in PTT is nonionizing (usually near-infrared (NIR) light), hence its effect on tissues is much less invasive. Considering hypoxia in most tumors, PTT is more attractive for cancer treatment than photodynamic therapy (PDT) currently used in the clinic because PTT does not require oxygen, while PDT utilizes UV or visible light to activate photosensitizers to generate toxic reactive oxygen in the presence of oxygen.[41] Moreover, NIR light involved in PTT has much deeper penetration than UV or visible light typically used in PDT.[42] Nevertheless, low molecular weight PTT agents tend to aggregate in aqueous solution, nonspecifically bind to proteins, and lack target specificity. A large number of nanoparticles have been investigated as PTT agents including carbon-based nanomaterials, semiconductor nanocrystals, metallic nanoparticles, rare earth ion-doped nanocrystals, and organic nanoparticles. *In vivo* preclinical results of these PTT nanoparticle agents demonstrated that tumor shrinking was achieved with minimal damage to surrounding healthy tissues.[43] Currently, AuroLase (a gold nanoshell-encapsulated silica nanoparticle developed by Nanospectra) is under pilot study for PTT of refractory head and neck cancer, primary and/or metastatic lung tumors, and neoplasms of the prostate. In addition to PTT, magnetothermal therapy also shows significant potential for cancer treatment. One successful example is NanoTherm (iron oxide nanoparticles) which received EU regulatory approval as a medical device for glioblastoma treatment. Interestingly, these nanoparticles could also be used for X-ray CT or MRI imaging, thus enabling diagnosis, patient selection, and/or response tracking.

Gene therapy

Advances in cancer genetics and tumor-specific signaling pathways that are critical for tumor development/metastasis have given rise to the application of gene therapy in cancer treatment. The advantage of gene therapy over other anticancer strategies is that, in principle, we can rationally design nucleic acids (e.g., DNA, siRNA, antisense, and mRNA) to specifically regulate the expression of virtually any gene of interest. RNA interference (RNAi) technology, which can specifically silence the expression of target genes, represents a revolution in gene therapy and holds great promise for cancer research and therapy.[44–46] For instance, it provides a rapid approach to study the genetic alterations in human cancers, many of which are considered as "undruggable" targets and/or require complex and time-consuming development of effective inhibitors.[47,48] However, the ubiquitous application of RNAi in cancer treatment is hindered by the challenge of safe and effective delivery of RNAi agents such as small interfering RNA (siRNA) to tumors. As siRNA molecules are susceptible to degradation by endogenous enzymes and cannot readily cross cellular membrane due to their polyanionic and macromolecular characteristics, a variety of nanoparticle vehicles have been extensively explored to protect siRNA and facilitate its delivery into the tumor cell cytosol where the RNAi machinery resides.[18,49] RNAi nanotechnology has also shown potential in reversing drug resistance. By down-regulating overexpressed antiapoptotic regulators (e.g., Bcl-2) and transporters (e.g., P-glycoprotein), or by suppressing of DNA repair pathways, drug-resistant tumor cells can be re-sensitized.[50–52] Several cationic lipid- or polymer-based siRNA nanoparticles, including CALAA-01, ALN-VSP02, Atu027, and others, entered Phase I or II clinical trials to treat different types of cancer,[18] but the clinical outcomes of these siRNA nanoparticles thus far have not been highly promising. Nevertheless, it is worth noting that the first siRNA product using lipid nanoparticles as the delivery vehicle was approved by the FDA in August 2018 for the rare hereditary disease transthyretin-mediated amyloidosis, which may encourage the continuous development of siRNA-based cancer nanomedicines.

Contrary to gene silencing by siRNA or antisense, DNA-mediated gene therapy aims to replace a mutated gene in tumor cells with a functional, therapeutic gene. But similar to siRNA delivery, the main obstacle restricting the *in vivo* applications of DNA gene therapy is the difficulty of delivering the fragile, large, and negatively charged DNA molecules into the nucleus of tumor cells. Over the past few decades, an astounding amount of positively charged materials have been designed for enhancing the safety and efficacy of DNA delivery.[53] Today, SGT53-01, a p53 gene-loaded liposome coated with transferrin, has advanced to Phase II clinical trials for treatment of metastatic pancreatic cancer.[54] In addition to DNA, mRNA is also emerging as a promising therapeutic nucleic acid in recent years. Its therapeutic mechanism is similar to that of DNA-mediated gene therapy, but to some extent, mRNA would be more efficient as it does not require nuclear localization/transcription. Furthermore, mRNA can avoid interacting with the host genome, thus excluding potentially detrimental genomic integration.[55] A growing number of studies have shown that mRNA formulated in nanoparticles exhibited enhanced translation owing to improved intracellular uptake/endosomal escape.[56] It has recently been demonstrated in animal models that systemically delivered nanoparticles incorporating tumor suppressor PTEN or p53 mRNAs were able to restore tumor growth suppression and improve drug sensitivity.[57,58]

Taken together, the idea of using nucleic acids as therapeutics for cancer therapy is straightforward, but successful application of gene therapy faces the major challenge of safe and effective delivery in vivo. While remaining elusive, development of nanoparticle delivery vehicles with long blood circulation time, high tumor accumulation, uniform tissue penetration, and efficient cellular uptake and endosomal escape, represents a great opportunity in the gene therapy field.

Immunotherapy

In contrast to the therapy modalities mentioned above, immunotherapy provides a unique strategy for cancer treatment by provoking the host's immune system to fight tumor cells. Since immune systems are robust, have the capacity for memory, and possess exquisite specificity, active immunotherapy (or therapeutic cancer vaccine) might achieve complete and long-lasting cancer cures with minimal detriment to health.[59] However, only a few vaccines have demonstrated sufficient efficacy for clinical use. Major factors that may contribute to the limited clinical response include the physical barriers imposed by the TME, host-derived immunosuppressive effects, and mechanisms in immune evasion.[60] Nanotechnology is gaining momentum in this field and becoming increasingly attractive as potent carriers for effective delivery of vaccine antigens and adjuvants. First, nanoparticles can be engineered for rapid phagocytosis by immune cells and can protect antigens (e.g., peptides, proteins, and nucleic acids) from premature enzymatic and proteolytic degradation.[61] In particular, they allow for more effective antigen-uptake in some immune cells such as dendritic cells (DCs), as compared to free antigens.[62] By surface coating with a proprietary DC-specific antibody fragment, a targeted liposomal vaccine, lipovaxin-MM (currently in Phase I study) can deliver multiple antigens to DCs effectively due to the ligand–receptor interactions. Second, nanoparticles can package antigen and adjuvant for transport to the targeted site simultaneously, which could be crucial for ideal immunotherapy. For instance, by co-loading tumor-associated antigen HER2/neu and adjuvant AS15 with potential immune stimulatory and antineoplastic activities into the liposome, this vaccine can stimulate the host immune response to mount a cytotoxic T-lymphocyte response, leading to tumor cell lysis, and is now in Phase II clinical studies for metastatic breast cancer. Compared to liposomes, biodegradable polymer nanoparticles can not only regulate the pharmacokinetic and distribution profile of antigens/adjuvants but also exhibit additional unique features such as sustained release of antigens/adjuvants at the target site and eliminating the need for repeated doses.[63] For example, a report by Selecta Biosciences further shows that adjuvant-carrying polymeric nanoparticles can augment the immune response to encapsulated antigen and exhibit strong local immune activation without inducing systemic cytokine release.[64] Besides conventional antigen-based vaccines, mRNA cancer vaccines are also in active development due to the aforementioned merits. Multiple naked and protamine-protected mRNA vaccines are in clinical trials for cancer treatment.[65,66] To overcome the premature degradation of mRNAs and enhance their delivery efficiency, mRNAs were encapsulated in nanoparticles for a more robust generation of immune response. Currently, several lipid nanoparticle-based mRNA vaccine formulations (e.g., mRNA-4157 and mRNA-2416 by Moderna), either acting alone or in combination with immune checkpoint inhibitors, are in clinical trials for cancer treatment.[67]

In addition to cancer vaccine, adoptive cell therapy [e.g., chimeric antigen receptor (CAR) T-cell therapy] and checkpoint inhibitor therapy (e.g., anti-PD1/PD-L1 therapy) have also emerged as powerful tools for cancer immunotherapy. Adoptive cell therapy often requires ex vivo activation and expansion of immune cells such as T cells with artificial antigen-presenting cells (aAPCs), of which the antibody-conjugated superparamagnetic microspheres (Dynabeads™) are the most popular currently. Nanoparticle- and nanostructure-based aAPCs have also been developed with various activation strategies to further improve the yield and function of cultured immune cells, and some have already shown superiority over Dynabeads.[68] To maximize the potential of adoptive cell therapy, nanoparticles loaded with immune modulators can be coupled to the engineered immune cells to boost their proliferation and function after transplantation.[69] Moreover, reprogramming T cells directly in vivo by T cell-targeting nanoparticles carrying CAR-encoding genes is also under investigation to bypass the elaborate and costly cell-manufacturing process ex vivo.[68] Immune checkpoint inhibitors could block the immune evasion of cancer cells and have demonstrated substantial potential either as a monotherapy or in combination with other therapies in the clinics. However, systemic administration of free immune checkpoint inhibitors often leads to autoimmune adverse effects, which severely limit the applicable dose. Nanoparticles that deliver and release checkpoint inhibitors specifically to tumors while maintaining the immune homeostasis of normal tissues are in active pursuit.[70,71]

Although with great promise, the status quo of cancer immunotherapy is still far from satisfying. Clinical challenges such as low patient response rates and immune-related side effects remain unsolved. Nanotechnology may play an important role in addressing those challenges and unleash the full potential of cancer immunotherapy.

Recent advances in cancer nanotechnologies

Despite the fascinating achievements mentioned above, the potential of cancer nanotechnologies may be far from being fully realized. Below we briefly discuss some recent exciting advances in this field, which from our perspective may enable the development of more effective cancer nanotherapeutics.

One major challenge for effective systemic drug delivery to tumor tissues is to avoid the recognition of nanoparticles by mononuclear phagocyte system (MPS) in liver and spleen for long blood circulation. This can therefore facilitate time-dependent extravasation of nanoparticles through the leaky tumor microvasculature, and lead to effective tumor accumulation. Nanoparticle physicochemical properties, such as size, shape, surface charge, and surface modification (e.g., PEGylation), were previously shown to impact the circulation and tumor accumulation.[72–76] Recently, a unique concept for effectively evading the MPS system by incorporating cellular membranes on NP surface has moved into the spotlight. By using natural erythrocyte membranes as coating shells, it was observed that the circulation half-life of cell membrane-coated nanoparticles in blood was 2.5-fold higher than PEG-coated nanoparticles.[77] Furthermore, the cellular membrane can also retain its inherent functions, leading to the active delivery of nanotherapeutics to tumor. For example, by coating with leukocyte membranes, a new generation of nanotherapeutics has demonstrated the ability to avoid opsonization, delay liver clearance, and recognize and bind tumor endothelium in an active manner.[78] Another thought-provoking concept to inhibit phagocytic clearance is to decorate nanoparticles with a "marker of self" ligand such as CD47 or its peptide variant.[79] Such ligands can impede phagocytosis of "self" cells or nanoparticles by signaling through the phagocyte receptor CD172a, thus delaying macrophage-mediated clearance of nanoparticles and promoting blood circulation for more effective drug delivery to tumors. The adsorption of proteins on nanoparticle surface (protein corona) is a key factor governing the bio-nano interactions *in vivo*, including the pharmacokinetics, biodistribution, clearance, and tumor targeting of nanoparticles. Numerous studies have been devoted to understanding the composition, arrangement, kinetics, and biological outcome of the protein corona.[80–82] For example, it is now known that surface PEG density is critical for effective prolonging of circulation and low-density-lipoprotein receptor plays an important role in the blood clearance of nanoparticles.[83] The knowledge derived from these studies could offer guidance for the design of optimal nanoparticles and may also predict the *in vivo* behavior of nanoparticles based on the fingerprints of their protein corona.[84]

The EPR effect has long been considered as the foundation to cancer nanomedicines for solid tumors, which was generally explained by the leaky tumor vasculature and poor lymphatic drainage in the tumor tissue. However, recent studies have complemented our traditional and somehow oversimplified perceptions of the EPR effect and how nanoparticles enter the tumor. Contrary to the impression that endothelium gaps in tumor are static, it was found that tumor endothelium leakage could be dynamic and characterized by many transient endothelium openings in addition to the static pores.[85] These transient endothelium vents could enhance the permeability of tumor blood vessels and improve the extravasation of nanoparticles, especially for larger ones. The entry of nanoparticles to tumor interstitium also does not solely depend on inter-endothelial gaps. A very recent study revealed that nanoparticles could be extravasated into the tumor predominately through active trans-endothelial transport.[86] This discovery may offer new insights into the design of future nanomedicines, as the vasculature of human cancer is known to be less leaky than that in animal models.[87] Moreover, the engineered nanoparticles themselves may impact the integrity and permeability of tumor vasculatures, which deserves more investigations to further assess the associated risks and opportunities.[88] With a more thorough understanding of the EPR effect and tumor-targeting of nanoparticles, it is expected that new strategies will be developed to further improve the tumor accumulation and targeting of nanomedicines.

The TME has been gradually recognized as a key contributor to tumor growth, progression, and metastasis, and can therefore be considered as a potential target for effective cancer therapy.[89] Vascular endothelium performs critical functions such as transporting oxygen and nutrients from the bloodstream to tissues, controlling blood flow, and trafficking blood cells. Its abnormalities are always implicated in the pathogenesis of tumor progression and metastasis.[90] Nanoparticles carrying drugs or siRNAs targeting dysfunctional tumor vascular endothelium have thus been a growing interest in cancer treatment (Figure 1c).[91] A specific polymeric nanoparticle platform has recently been developed for selective siRNA delivery to lung endothelial cells, leading to effective silencing of five endothelial genes (Tie1, Tie2, VEcad, VEGFR-2, and ICAM-2) without significant reduction of gene expression in pulmonary immune cells, hepatocytes or peritoneal immune cells.[92] Another strategy is to target tumor-associated inflammation, such as inhibiting the infiltration of or reprogramming tumor-associated macrophages (Figure 1d).[93,94] Attention has also been given to targeting the communication between cancer cells and the TME. One recent example is the active delivery of Bortezomib using biodegradable PLGA-PEG polymer to increase osteogenic differentiating and bond strength, which in turn significantly inhibited tumor growth in bone, the most common metastatic site for many cancers.[95] In addition, some highly cytotoxic chemotherapeutic drugs can be administrated as "prodrugs" and then activated by the TME (e.g., pH, enzyme and hypoxia) into cytotoxic products.[96]

Although in an early stage, the development of nanotherapeutics for noninvasive administration through oral, nasal, or ocular routes is constantly growing and showing many merits over systematic injection. Drug delivery through a nasal route is advantageous for treatment of lung cancer because it allows nanotherapeutics to bypass high liver uptake and avoid repeated administration. In a recent *in vivo* study using inhalable doxorubicin-encapsulated nanoparticles to treat lung cancer, highly significant improvement in survival was observed compared to intravenous injection groups.[97] On the other hand, cancer patients who require frequent administration of drugs would benefit from oral delivery because of the convenience and compliance, but this approach is limited by insufficient intestinal absorption of drugs due to intestinal mucosal barrier. One strategy to improve transportation across intestinal epithelium after oral administration is through receptor-mediated transcytosis. For example, IgG Fc fragments have been conjugated to polymer nanoparticles, which can effectively target neonatal Fc (FcRn) receptors, cross the epithelial barrier, and then reach systemic circulation with mean absorption efficiency ten times higher than nontargeted nanoparticles.[15] Such targeted nanoparticles offer new hope for developing oral delivery nanotherapeutics for cancer treatment.

Summary

Clinical success in cancer nanomedicine has become a driving force behind the development of new nanoparticle technologies for safer and more effective treatment, and the pursuit of personalized nanotherapeutics. Meanwhile, we have also realized how challenging the cancer nanotechnology field is due to the complexity and heterogeneity of cancer and the encumbrances in clinical translation. The convergence of nanotechnology with tumor biology and other biological/biomedical sciences will therefore be crucial for realizing the full potential of cancer nanotechnology. We expect that this article can encourage physicians, scientists, engineers, and others from different areas of expertise to become involved in this exciting field and promote the widespread application of nanotechnologies for cancer management.

Acknowledgments

This work was supported by NIH grants R00CA160350 (J.S.), R01CA200900 (J.S.), and U54-CA151884 (R.L.); David Koch—Prostate Cancer Foundation Program in Nanotherapeutics (R.L.); Movember-PCF Challenge Award (J.S.); and PCF Young Investigator Award (J.S.).

Competing interests

For a list of entities with which R.L. is involved, compensated or uncompensated, see https://www.dropbox.com/s/yc3xqb5s8s94v7x/Rev%20Langer%20COI.pdf?dl=0.

Key references

The complete reference list can be found on Vital Source version of this title, see inside front cover.

1. Bernard WS, Christopher PW. *World Cancer Report 2014*. World Health Organization; 2014.
3. Barenholz YC. Doxil®—the first FDA-approved nano-drug: lessons learned. *J Control Release*. 2012;**160**:117–134.
4. Hubbell JA, Langer R. Translating materials design to the clinic. *Nat Mater*. 2013;**12**:963–966.
5. Davis ME, Chen Z, Shin DM. Nanoparticle therapeutics: an emerging treatment modality for cancer. *Nat Rev Drug Discov*. 2008;**7**:771–782.
8. Shi J, Kantoff PW, Wooster R, Farokhzad OC. Cancer nanomedicine: progress, challenges and opportunities. *Nat Rev Cancer*. 2017;**17**:20.
9. Farokhzad OC, Langer R. Impact of nanotechnology on drug delivery. *ACS Nano*. 2009;**3**:16–20.
11. Langer R. Drug delivery and targeting. *Nature*. 1998;**392**:5–10.
12. Kamaly N, Xiao Z, Valencia PM, et al. Targeted polymeric therapeutic nanoparticles: design, development and clinical translation. *Chem Soc Rev*. 2012;**41**:2971–3010.
15. Pridgen EM, Alexis F, Kuo TT, et al. Transepithelial transport of Fc-targeted nanoparticles by the neonatal fc receptor for oral delivery. *Sci Transl Med*. 2013;**5**:213ra167.
18. Kanasty R, Dorkin JR, Vegas A, Anderson D. Delivery materials for siRNA therapeutics. *Nat Mater*. 2013;**12**:967–977.
21. Zhao T, Huang G, Li Y, et al. A transistor-like pH nanoprobe for tumour detection and image-guided surgery. *Nat Biomed Eng*. 2016;**1**:1–8.
25. Matsumura Y, Maeda H. A new concept for macromolecular therapeutics in cancer chemotherapy: mechanism of tumoritropic accumulation of proteins and the antitumor agent smancs. *Cancer Res*. 1986;**46**:6387–6392.
26. Zhang H. Onivyde for the therapy of multiple solid tumors. *Onco Targets Ther*. 2016;**9**:3001.
27. Peer D, Karp JM, Hong S, et al. Nanocarriers as an emerging platform for cancer therapy. *Nat Nanotechnol*. 2007;**2**:751.
28. Xu S, Olenyuk BZ, Okamoto CT, Hamm-Alvarez SF. Targeting receptor-mediated endocytotic pathways with nanoparticles: rationale and advances. *Adv Drug Deliv Rev*. 2013;**65**:121–138.
29. Hrkach J, Von Hoff D, Ali MM, et al. Preclinical development and clinical translation of a PSMA-targeted docetaxel nanoparticle with a differentiated pharmacological profile. *Sci Transl Med*. 2012;**4**:128ra139.
31. Mura S, Nicolas J, Couvreur P. Stimuli-responsive nanocarriers for drug delivery. *Nat Mater*. 2013;**12**:991–1003.
34. Kwatra D, Venugopal A, Anant S. Nanoparticles in radiation therapy: a summary of various approaches to enhance radiosensitization in cancer. *Transl Cancer Res*. 2013;**2**:330–342.
36. Capizzi RL, Oster W. Chemoprotective and radioprotective effects of amifostine: an update of clinical trials. *Int J Hematol*. 2000;**72**:425–435.
40. Cheng L, Wang C, Feng L, et al. Functional nanomaterials for photothermal therapies of cancer. *Chem Rev*. 2014;**114**:10869–10939.
42. Liu Y, Ai K, Liu J, et al. Dopamine-melanin colloidal nanospheres: an efficient near-infrared photothermal therapeutic agent for in vivo cancer therapy. *Adv Mater*. 2013;**25**:1353–1359.
43. Jaque D, Maestro LM, del Rosal B, et al. Nanoparticles for photothermal therapies. *Nanoscale*. 2014;**6**:9494–9530.
46. Whitehead KA, Langer R, Anderson DG. Knocking down barriers: advances in siRNA delivery. *Nat Rev Drug Discov*. 2009;**8**:129–138.
57. Islam MA, Xu Y, Tao W, et al. Restoration of tumour-growth suppression in vivo via systemic nanoparticle-mediated delivery of PTEN mRNA. *Nat Biomed Eng*. 2018;**2**:850–864.
59. Vanneman M, Dranoff G. Combining immunotherapy and targeted therapies in cancer treatment. *Nat Rev Cancer*. 2012;**12**:237–251.
61. Smith DM, Simon JK, Baker JR Jr. Applications of nanotechnology for immunology. *Nat Rev Immunol*. 2013;**13**:592–605.
65. Weide B, Pascolo S, Scheel B, et al. Direct injection of protamine-protected mRNA: results of a phase 1/2 vaccination trial in metastatic melanoma patients. *J Immunother*. 2009;**32**:498–507.
68. Goldberg MS. Improving cancer immunotherapy through nanotechnology. *Nat Rev Cancer*. 2019;**19**:587–602.
69. Tang L, Zheng Y, Melo MB, et al. Enhancing T cell therapy through TCR-signaling-responsive nanoparticle drug delivery. *Nat Biotechnol*. 2018;**36**:707–716.
70. Riley RS, June CH, Langer R, Mitchell MJ. Delivery technologies for cancer immunotherapy. *Nat Rev Drug Discov*. 2019;**18**:175–196.
71. Hu Q, Sun W, Wang J, et al. Conjugation of haematopoietic stem cells and platelets decorated with anti-PD-1 antibodies augments anti-leukaemia efficacy. *Nat Biomed Eng*. 2018;**2**:831–840.
77. Hu C-MJ, Zhang L, Aryal S, et al. Erythrocyte membrane-camouflaged polymeric nanoparticles as a biomimetic delivery platform. *Proc Natl Acad Sci U S A*. 2011;**108**:10980–10985.
79. Rodriguez PL, Harada T, Christian DA, et al. Minimal" Self" peptides that inhibit phagocytic clearance and enhance delivery of nanoparticles. *Science*. 2013;**339**:971–975.
80. Kelly PM, Åberg C, Polo E, et al. Mapping protein binding sites on the biomolecular corona of nanoparticles. *Nat Nanotechnol*. 2015;**10**:472.
82. Chen F, Wang G, Griffin JI, et al. Complement proteins bind to nanoparticle protein corona and undergo dynamic exchange in vivo. *Nat Nanotechnol*. 2017;**12**:387.
83. Bertrand N, Grenier P, Mahmoudi M, et al. Mechanistic understanding of in vivo protein corona formation on polymeric nanoparticles and impact on pharmacokinetics. *Nat Commun*. 2017;**8**:1–8.
85. Matsumoto Y, Nichols JW, Toh K, et al. Vascular bursts enhance permeability of tumour blood vessels and improve nanoparticle delivery. *Nat Nanotechnol*. 2016;**11**:533.
86. Sindhwani S, Syed AM, Ngai J, et al. The entry of nanoparticles into solid tumours. *Nat Mater*. 2020:1–10.
88. Peng F, Setyawati MI, Tee JK, et al. Nanoparticles promote in vivo breast cancer cell intravasation and extravasation by inducing endothelial leakiness. *Nat Nanotechnol*. 2019;**14**:279–286.
89. Albini A, Sporn MB. The tumour microenvironment as a target for chemoprevention. *Nat Rev Cancer*. 2007;**7**:139–147.
92. Dahlman JE, Barnes C, Khan O, et al. In vivo endothelial siRNA delivery using polymeric nanoparticles with low molecular weight. *Nat Nanotechnol*. 2014;**9**:648.
96. Wilson WR, Hay MP. Targeting hypoxia in cancer therapy. *Nat Rev Cancer*. 2011;**11**:393–410.

66 Hematopoietic cell transplantation

Qaiser Bashir, MD ■ *Elizabeth J. Shpall, MD* ■ *Richard E. Champlin, MD*

> **Overview**
>
> Hematopoietic cell transplantation (HCT) is an essential component of therapy for various malignant and nonmalignant conditions and provides the only curative modality for several high-risk disorders. While HCT can be associated with significant morbidity, meaningful progress has been made to reduce treatment-related toxicities and improve patient outcomes following HCT. Together with the development of international donor registries and the feasibility of alternative donor transplants, these advances have broadened the indications of HCT in recent years.

Introduction

Hematopoietic cell transplantation (HCT) involves engraftment of hematopoietic progenitor cells (HPCs) from a donor to the recipient. The HPCs can be derived from another individual (*allogeneic*), umbilical cord blood, a genetically identical twin (*syngeneic*), or patient's own (*autologous*).

The advancements in histocompatibility, the establishment of international registries and cord blood banks, and the clinical feasibility of alternative donor transplants have made it possible to have a donor for practically all patients needing a transplant. Furthermore, the refinements in conditioning regimens, graft-versus-host disease (GVHD) management, and supportive care have reduced treatment-related toxicity and improved outcomes. For these reasons, the indications of HCT have expanded since its inception, and it is now considered a well-established treatment for a variety of malignant, immune, metabolic, and hematologic conditions (Table 1).

Autologous transplantation

Autologous HCT exploits the dose-dependent response to chemotherapy or radiation by different malignancies. Myelosuppressive therapy is given to elicit antitumor response followed by infusion of the autologous hematopoietic cells to restore hematopoiesis and immunity. The patient's HPCs are used; therefore, human-leukocyte antigen (HLA) matching is not needed. Contamination of the autograft by the tumor cells may contribute towards relapse after autologous HCT. However, studies evaluating *ex vivo* or *in vivo* purging of the autografts have not shown to improve outcomes.[1,2]

Among other mechanisms, the binding of stromal-derived factor-1 (SDF-1) to its receptor (CXCR4) on HPCs is responsible for HPC retention within the bone marrow. The administration of growth factors with or without preceding chemotherapy promotes granulocyte expansion and disruption of the SDF-1/CXCR4 axis. This leads to enrichment of the pool of circulating HPCs. The HPCs are identified by the expression of CD34+ on the cell surface and collected by leukapheresis. The dose of CD34+ cells infused predicts neutrophil and platelet engraftment. For autologous HCT, the minimum accepted dose is 2×10^6 CD34+ cells/kg, which results in consistent multilineage engraftment.[3]

Allogeneic transplantation

Allogeneic HCT transplants combine cytotoxic treatments with the immune-mediated graft-versus malignancy (GVM) effect. Donor-derived lymphoid cells may react against and eradicate malignant cells that survive high-dose cytotoxic therapy. The appropriately HLA-matched HPCs can be obtained from bone marrow, peripheral blood, or UCB. A CD34+ cell dose $\geq 4.0 \times 10^6$/kg is desirable. Doses exceeding 8×10^6 cells/kg increase the risk of GVHD.[3]

Several studies have compared peripheral blood versus bone marrow grafts. A meta-analysis including randomized trials of HLA-identical sibling transplants showed that compared to bone marrow, peripheral blood graft was associated with a higher risk of chronic (c) GVHD and a reduced relapse rate, resulting in improved survival in patients with late-stage hematological malignancies.[4] In the unrelated donor setting, a large randomized trial showed a higher risk of graft failure and lower risk of cGVHD with bone marrow grafts. There was no significant survival difference.[5] The long-term follow-up of patient-reported outcomes showed that recipients of bone marrow grafts had less symptom burden and were more likely to return to work than recipients of peripheral blood graft five years after transplantation.[6] In the context of reduced-intensity conditioning (RIC), an extensive registry analysis did not show any difference in survival or cGVHD incidence between peripheral blood or bone marrow grafts.[7]

Histocompatibility

The major histocompatibility complex (MHC) region, also called the HLA complex, is the most polymorphic gene locus in the human genome. Polymorphism, derived from Greek word *Poly*, meaning many, and *morphe*, meaning shape, is a place in the DNA sequence where there is variation, and the less common variant is present in at least one percent of the people tested.[8] The IMGT/HLA database currently contains 26,214 HLA alleles, and hundreds of new alleles are reported every month.[9] The HLA complex is located within the 6p21.3 region on the short arm of human chromosome 6 and contains more than 220 genes of diverse function. The most relevant to allogeneic HCT are class I (HLA-A, -B, -C) and class II (HLA-DRB1, -DQB1, DPB1) molecules. These are glycoproteins that bind and present self, abnormal self, and foreign peptide antigens on the surface of nucleated cells.[10] T lymphocytes recognize the antigens presented by HLA molecules, leading to an immune response.

The HLA molecules were initially detected by serological typing. However, DNA-based HLA typing techniques can identify single

Table 1 Diseases treated with hematopoietic cell transplantation.

Malignant conditions
- Acute myeloid leukemia
- Myelodysplastic syndromes
- Acute lymphoblastic leukemia
- Chronic myelogenous leukemia and myeloproliferative disorders
- Chronic lymphocytic leukemia
- Non-Hodgkin lymphoma
- Hodgkin lymphoma
- Multiple myeloma and other plasma cell disorders
- Solid tumors: breast, testicular, ovarian, and small-cell lung cancer
- Pediatric solid tumors: neuroblastoma, Ewing sarcoma
- Medulloblastoma, renal cell cancer, melanoma

Nonmalignant
- Aplastic anemia and related bone marrow failure states
- Hemoglobinopathies: thalassemia, sickle cell anemia
- Congenital disorders of hematopoiesis
- Fanconi anemia and related syndromes
- Congenital immune deficiencies: severe combined immune deficiency, Wiskott–Aldrich syndrome, chronic granulomatous disease, and related syndromes
- Inborn errors of metabolism
- Autoimmune disorders
- Histiocytic disorders: Hemophagocytic lymphohistiocytosis

alleles as defined in the World Health Organization (WHO) HLA nomenclature (http://hla.alleles.org/nomenclature/index.html). A high-resolution typing result identifies alleles that encode the same protein sequence for the region of the HLA molecule called the antigen-binding site.[11] It excludes alleles that are not expressed as cell-surface proteins. Low-resolution typing can be DNA-based or a serological result at the first field (allele group) level in the DNA-based nomenclature.

Probability of finding an allogeneic donor

HLA alleles are inherited as haplotypes from each parent. This gives a 25% possibility of a full HLA match for each sibling and a chance of 50% for a single common haplotype (haploidentical).[12] For patients who do not have a full match sibling donor, an unrelated donor search is conducted. There are >37 million unrelated donors and cord blood units listed in the World Marrow Donor Association database (www.bmdw.org/accessed April 2020). The probability of finding a suitable unrelated donor varies according to ethnic and racial factors, ranging from 16% for blacks of South or Central American descent to 75% for whites of European descent.[13] The matching requirements for cord-blood are less stringent, and regardless of racial or ethnic background, more than 80% of patients age 20 or older will have a cord-blood unit mismatched at one or two HLA loci available.[13]

Impact of HLA matching and donor selection

HLA-identical siblings are typically considered the most suitable donors. The acquisition is fast, the impact of donor-specific antibodies low, resulting in an extremely low incidence of graft failure, and engraftment is usually rapid. The incidence of GVHD is also low compared to unrelated donors, and survival is usually the best.

In unrelated donor HCT, the best outcomes are achieved with high-resolution matching for HLA-A, -B, -C, and -DRB1 alleles (8/8 match).[14] A single mismatch detected at low- or high-resolution typing is associated with higher mortality and shorter survival compared to 8/8 matched pairs. Mismatching at two or more loci compounds the risk. An important feature of MHC is linkage disequilibrium, where certain alleles are inherited together more frequently than would occur by chance. HLA-DPB1, however, is usually not in linkage disequilibrium with the rest of the HLA haplotype, which reduces the probability of finding an allele level HLA-DPB1 match to <20% in 8/8 matched-unrelated donors (MUDs). The T-cell epitope grouping can classify HLA-DPB1 into nonpermissive (associated with high T-cell reactivity and increased risk of GVHD) and permissive (comparably better tolerated) mismatches. Large registry studies have shown that nonpermissive HLA-DPB1 allele mismatches are associated with higher treatment-related mortality (TRM) and overall mortality compared with permissive HLA-DPB1 mismatch in 8/8 matched UD transplants.[15] Nevertheless, in the case of 8/8 MUD transplants, the studies report survival comparable to HLA-identical sibling donors.[16]

The cord blood has the benefit of the fast acquisition. The histocompatibility is less restrictive, and a higher degree of HLA mismatching is tolerated.[17] This increases the applicability of allografting to ethnic minorities, usually underrepresented in donor registries. The main drawbacks include a low cell dose for adult patients, slower engraftment and immune reconstitution, and unavailability for donor-lymphocyte infusions (DLIs) and subsequent infusions. Strategies to overcome the issue of low cell dose include double cord-blood transplants and various techniques to expand the stem cells in the cord blood unit.[18,19]

Haploidentical HCT is another suitable option for allografting. The benefits include nearly universal availability, fast procurement, and the donor's availability for DLI and subsequent infusions. Like cord blood transplants, donor-specific antibodies, when detected, increase the risk of graft failure.[20] The speed of engraftment is slower, and graft failure is relatively more common compared to HLA-matched sibling or MUD transplants. Traditionally, the risk of severe GVHD was higher with the haploidentical transplants, but with the posttransplant cyclophosphamide platform, this risk is equivalent to that of unrelated donor transplants.[21]

Patients should undergo high-resolution typing at HLA-A, -B, -C, and -DRB1 (8/8 match). Also, HLA-DQB1, -DPB1, and -DRB3/4/5 may be added with the idea of maximizing matching and avoiding nonpermissive mismatches. In general, if an HLA-matched sibling donor is not available, an 8/8 MUD is preferred followed by alternative donors such as haploidentical, cord-blood, or mismatched unrelated donors. The clinical data suggest similar survival outcomes between cord blood and haploidentical donor transplants.[22] An ongoing national study by the Bone Marrow Transplant Clinical Trials Network (BMT-CTN 1101) comparing cord blood versus haploidentical marrow grafts hopes to answer this question.

In addition to HLA-matching, non-HLA immunogenetic factors such as killer immunoglobulin-like receptor (*KIR*), minor histocompatibility antigens, MHC class I-chain related (MIC) A gene, and immune response gene polymorphisms are increasingly being recognized as having important clinical implications for transplant outcomes.[23]

Conditioning

Conditioning involves the administration of chemotherapeutic agents, with or without total body irradiation (TBI) before infusion of the hematopoietic cells. The primary aim of conditioning is to eradicate the malignancy and provide sufficient suppression of the host immune system, which allows the engraftment of the donor hematopoietic cells. A less well-defined objective of conditioning is to provide a stem cell niche in the host marrow for the donor hematopoietic cells. The conditioning regimens are categorized based on the intensity of the treatment (Table 2).[24] *Myeloablative*

Table 2 Conditioning regimens.[24,25]

	Myeloablative conditioning (MAC)	Reduced-intensity conditioning (RIC)	Non-myeloablative conditioning (NMA)
Definition	Induce irreversible cytopenia, which is fatal in most cases without hematopoietic cell support	Does not fit MAC or NMA definitions. RIC can cause prolonged cytopenia, requiring hematopoietic cell support	Induce minimal cytopenia that may not require hematopoietic cell support Provides sufficient immunosuppression to allow engraftment (*immunoablative*)
Goal	Eradicate disease		Eradicate disease (more reliance on graft-versus-malignancy effect)
	Ensure rapid engraftment of donor hematopoietic cells		Minimize TRM
Advantages	Lower risk of relapse More rapid engraftment compared to NMA		Less inflammatory cytokine release Lower rate of GVHD Lower TRM More tolerable in elderly and patients with comorbidities
Risks	Higher rate of GVHD Higher TRM Limited role in elderly and frail		Higher risk of relapse
Examples	TBI ≥ 5 Gy (single dose), or ≥8 Gy (fractionated)	TBI > 2 Gy and <5 Gy (single dose)	TBI ≤ 2 Gy ± purine analog
	Busulfan >8 mg/kg orally or IV equivalent	TBI < 8 Gy (fractionated ± another agent)	Flu + Cy ± ATG
	Melphalan > 140 mg/m² ± another agent	Bu ≤ 9 mg/kg (oral) or IV equivalent ± another agent	Flu + AraC + Ida
	Thiotepa ≥ 10 mg/kg	Melphalan ≤ 140 mg/m² ± another agent Thiotepa < 10 mg/kg	Cladribine + AraC TLI + ATG

Abbreviations: TRM, treatment-related mortality; GVHD, graft-versus-host disease; TBI, total body irradiation; Bu, busulfan; IV, intravenous; Flu, fludarabine; Cy, cyclophosphamide; ATG, antithymocyte globulin; AraC, cytarabine; Ida, idarubicin; TLI, total lymphocyte irradiation.

conditioning (MAC) regimens induce irreversible cytopenia, which in the absence of hematopoietic cell support, is fatal in most cases. These regimens can result in significant toxicity, which limits their use in the elderly and frail. MAC regimens often involve a combination of TBI (5–15 Gy, single dose or fractionated) and cyclophosphamide (Cy 60 mg/kg × 2 days). In some regimens, TBI is substituted with busulfan (Bu 12.8 mg/Kg over 4 days, or pharmacokinetically guided dosing). Several other combinations are also commonly used. Studies have shown a similar survival rate between TBI and non-TBI-containing MAC regimens in patients with myeloid malignancies.[26] *Nonmyeloablative conditioning (NMA)* and *RIC* were developed to reduce the organ toxicity and expand the applicability of hematopoietic cell transplantation to elderly or frail patients who are not fit for MAC. Compared to MAC, a lower dose of cytotoxic agents is used in NMA and RIC regimens. Cytopenia is less severe, but sufficient immunosuppression is achieved to allow engraftment of donor hematopoietic cells.

Generally, the higher intensity of conditioning is associated with a lower risk of relapse but also higher TRM. The usual result of these opposing effects is comparable leukemia-free survival (LFS) and overall survival (OS) between MAC and RIC regimens. Prospective data comparing MAC with RIC is limited. The BMT CTN 0901 study compared RIC; fludarabine plus busulfan (Bu/Flu) or fludarabine plus melphalan (FM) with MAC; busulfan plus cyclophosphamide (Bu/Cy), busulfan plus fludarabine (Bu/Flu), or cyclophosphamide plus TBI (Cy/TBI)[27] in patients with acute myeloid leukemia (AML) or myelodysplastic syndrome (MDS). Compared to MAC, the TRM was lower, and relapse incidence was higher with RIC. A statistically significant advantage in relapse-free survival (RFS) and a trend towards longer OS was observed with MAC. Another randomized phase 3 study conducted within the European Society of Blood and Marrow Transplantation (EBMT) demonstrated similar 2-year RFS and OS between busulfan based RIC versus MAC in patients with MDS or secondary AML.[8] Specifically, in the setting of allogeneic HCT from alternative donors, cord blood and haploidentical, comparisons of RIC and MAC have shown comparable LFS and OS.[28,29] Recent trends in the United States show increasing use of RIC regimens for haploidentical transplants.[30]

The intensity of conditioning is more relevant in the setting of autologous HCT since there is no GVM effect. The primary indications for autologous HCT are multiple myeloma (MM) and lymphoma.[30] The most commonly used conditioning regimen for MM is high-dose melphalan. For malignant lymphomas, BEAM (BCNU, etoposide, cytarabine, melphalan) remains the most popular conditioning; however, several other variations also exist.

Risk assessment in allogeneic HCT

Allogeneic HCT can be associated with considerable toxicity. The risks of complications and relapse should be carefully weighed against benefits when selecting the appropriate patient. Significant variables to consider are listed in Table 3. These should not be viewed in isolation, rather facilitate a comprehensive patient assessment.

Several models are utilized to gauge the risk-benefit ratio for patients undergoing allogeneic HCT. Hematopoietic cell transplantation comorbidity index (HCT-CI) was originally developed in 2005 as a modification of the Charlson Comorbidity Index (CCI).[32] It identifies 17 comorbidities, which are assigned a score of 0, 1, 2, or 3 depending on the adjusted hazard ratios of nonrelapse mortality (NRM) for each comorbidity. The adjusted hazard ratios are converted to integer weights, and the HCT-CI score is a sum of these integer weights. The 2-year NRM for patients with HCT-CI score of 0, 1–2, and ≥ 3 were 14%, 21%, and 41%, respectively. In order to increase the predictive capacity, the model was modified in 2014 to a composite comorbidity/age index, where age ≥ 40 years was assigned a weight of 1, equivalent of a single co-morbidity in HCT-CI.[33] Another useful model was developed by the EBMT and validated in a large cohort of 56,505 patients.[34,35] The EBMT score combines five patient and donor characteristics to give a reasonable estimate of risk with allogeneic

Table 3 Important variables when selecting patients for allogeneic HCT.

Variable	Comments
Age	Higher risk of complications in elderly
	Consider when selecting conditioning intensity, that is, RIC in patients >60 year
Performance status	Generally, Karnofsky performance status ≥ 70% is considered eligible
Organ function	*Pulmonary:* Corrected diffusion capacity of the lung for carbon monoxide (DLCo) of <60% is associated with a higher risk of complications. However, this is not an absolute contraindication
	Cardiac: Generally, a left ventricular ejection fraction of ≥40% is required
	Hepatic: Lower liver reserve increases the risk of complications, for example, sinusoidal obstruction syndrome (SOS). A thorough baseline assessment of liver function and any abnormalities is critical
	Renal: Lower glomerular filtration rate is associated with higher risk of complications. Allogeneic HCT is usually not offered to patients with serum creatinine > 2 mg/dL
Psychosocial factors	Adequate caregiver support throughout the transplant process and beyond is necessary
	Underlying psychological issues should be addressed
Economic factors	Time off from work is significant
	Continued access to specialized care is needed after transplant
Disease-related factors[a]	Outcomes are worse for patients not in remission
Availability of a suitable donor[a]	Disease risk index (DRI)[31][b]
Comorbidities[a]	Commonly used predictive models include:
	Hematopoietic cell transplantation comorbidity index (HCT-CI)[32,33]
	EBMT score[34,35]
	Pretransplantation assessment of mortality (PAM) score[36,37]

Abbreviations: RIC, reduced-intensity conditioning; EBMT, European Society for Blood and Marrow Transplantation.
[a]Discussed elsewhere in the chapter.
[b]Prognostic index to estimate the impact of disease and disease status in patients undergoing allogeneic HCT.

HCT. Like HCT-CI, EBMT risk score has also been validated in multiple studies. A composite model for EBMT and HCT-CI showed that in patients with HCT-CI of ≥3, a higher EBMT score was associated with worse outcome.[38]

Complications associated with allogeneic hematopoietic cell transplantation

Intensive chemoradiotherapy and hematopoietic transplantations may be associated with several serious complications, as listed in Table 4. These include immune-mediated processes such as graft rejection and GVHD, toxicities resulting from the pretransplant conditioning regimen, infections owing to neutropenia, and posttransplant immune deficiency.

Graft failure

Engraftment is defined as the first of three consecutive days with an absolute neutrophil count higher than 0.5×10^9/L (platelets $>20 \times 10^9$/L and hemoglobin >8 g/dL, without transfusion support). Graft failure is a life-threatening complication after allogeneic HCT with an incidence ranging between 4% in matched unrelated transplantations and up to 20% after alternate donor transplantations.[39]

Graft failure can manifest in several forms. Graft rejection is when the anti-HLA antibodies[39] or remaining T-cells in the recipient eliminate donor stem cells. Primary graft failure is a failure to achieve initial donor cell engraftment. Secondary graft failure is the loss of donor graft after successful initial engraftment. Poor graft function is characterized by pancytopenia in the presence of donor chimerism >5%.[40] Several factors contribute to affecting the kinetics of engraftment (Table 5).

The outcomes after graft failure are invariably poor. It is essential to remove any modifiable factor before transplant. Once graft failure sets in, the most crucial strategy is to identify and treat the underlying cause, such as stopping the offending drugs, treating the viral illness, growth factor support, and optimizing immunosuppression. In the setting of mixed chimerism, donor lymphocyte infusion (DLI) can help restore donor chimera. Sometimes, a boost of CD34+ selected cells is given to improve poor graft function. A second allogeneic HCT after lymphodepleting conditioning can salvage a subset of patients. In this case, the donor can be the same as the first transplant or a different donor. However, if the graft rejection was immune-mediated, a different donor is preferred.

Graft-versus-host-disease

GVHD is a significant cause of morbidity and mortality after allogeneic HCT. It is a multiorgan disease caused when the immune cells from the donor (graft) react against the disparate major or minor HLA of the recipient (host).

Acute (a)GVHD is traditionally distinguished from cGVHD based on its presentation within the first 100 days after allogeneic HCT. However, this definition is not entirely explicit, as aGVHD can also present after 100 days. Increasing HLA disparity between the donor and the patient increases the risk of aGVHD. Allogeneic HCT from MUD or HLA-mismatched donors has a higher incidence of aGVHD compared to matched sibling donors. Some additional risk factors are; older age of the donor or the patient, gender mismatch (female to male), CMV seropositivity (donor or recipient), peripheral blood versus bone marrow, choice of GVHD prophylaxis regimen, and use of MAC compared to RIC regimens.

The skin, hepatobiliary system, and gastrointestinal (GI) tract are the most commonly affected organs. The symptoms depend on the organ involved. Skin manifestations generally include a maculopapular rash, which is typically pruritic and confluent. In severe forms, generalized erythroderma, desquamation, or epidermal necrolysis can occur. The diagnosis can be challenging to distinguish from viral or drug exanthems and often necessitates a biopsy. Liver involvement can occur with or without concomitant skin involvement. The patients can present with jaundice. Laboratory tests reveal marked elevation of bilirubin and alkaline phosphatase. Elevation in transaminases is seen, but the picture is usually more cholestatic. Liver GVHD should be differentiated from drug injury, sinusoidal obstruction syndrome, and viral infections; a tissue diagnosis helps establish the diagnosis. Acute GVHD of the GI tract usually presents with secretory diarrhea, abdominal pain,

Table 4 Complications after hematopoietic cell transplantation.[a]

Immune complications
- Graft failure
- Graft-versus-host disease

Organ specific
- Oral
  - Mucositis
  - Xerostomia
- Gastrointestinal (GI)
  - Esophagitis
  - Gastritis
  - Nausea and vomiting
  - Gastroenteritis
  - GI bleeding
  - Typhlitis
- Hepatic
  - Sinusoidal obstruction syndrome
- Pulmonary complications
  - Diffuse alveolar hemorrhage
  - Idiopathic pneumonia syndrome
  - Cryptogenic organizing pneumonia
  - Bronchiolitis obliterans syndrome
- Genitourinary system
  - Acute kidney injury
  - Hemorrhagic cystitis
- Cardiac
  - Congestive heart failure
  - Pericarditis
  - Arrhythmia
- Neurological
  - Posterior reversible encephalopathy syndrome (PRES)[b]
  - Encephalopathy
  - Hemorrhage or ischemic stroke

Infections and immunodeficiency
- Posttransplant lymphoproliferative disorders
- Progressive multifocal leukoencephalopathy
- Other infections

Hematologic
- Hemolytic anemia
- Transplant associated thrombotic microangiopathy

Late complications
- Metabolic syndrome[c]
- Hypothyroidism
- Diabetes mellitus
- Osteoporosis
- Gonadal dysfunction
- Infertility
- Cataract
- Avascular necrosis
- Psychological complications
- Secondary malignancies

[a]Source: Based on IDF Consensus Worldwide Definition of the Metabolic Syndrome, 2006, International Diabetes Federation.
[b]Usually in association with the use of calcineurin inhibitors use.
[c]The metabolic syndrome is a cluster of risk factors that increase the risk of a heart attack: diabetes and prediabetes, abdominal obesity, high cholesterol, and high blood pressure. https://www.idf.org/e-library/consensus-statements/60-idfconsensus-worldwide-definitionof-the-metabolic-syndrome.html (accessed 10 July, 2020).

and on rare occasions, ileus. Isolated upper GI GVHD produces nausea, vomiting, anorexia, and generalized food intolerance. The symptoms of GI GVHD should be differentiated from gut infections and conditioning regimen-related toxicity. Peripheral cytopenias and ocular manifestations such as conjunctivitis and photophobia are also frequently encountered.

Acute GVHD is graded based on signs and symptoms. Histologic grades are reported with the pathology results, but they do not correlate with clinical presentation. Glucksberg et al.[47] and International Blood and Marrow Transplant Registry (IBMTR)[48] grading systems are commonly used scales (Tables 6–8). The interpretation of these scales has the limitation of being observer-dependent, but studies have shown that high grades of aGVHD with either score are predictive of survival.

Strategies to prevent GVHD are directed towards modulating the immune response. Pharmacologic immunosuppression using a combination of a calcineurin inhibitor (tacrolimus or cyclosporine) with a short course of methotrexate is commonly used. The randomized phase 3 trials showed a lower incidence of aGVHD with tacrolimus plus methotrexate than cyclosporine plus methotrexate, but the overall survival was not different.[49,50] Newer agents, including mycophenolate mofetil (MMF) and sirolimus in varying combinations, are also being investigated. Another strategy is the use of posttransplant cyclophosphamide, which leads to selective elimination of host and donor alloreactive T cells, while sparing the hematopoietic progenitor cells and regulatory T cells.[51] In the haploidentical HCT setting, the use of posttransplant cyclophosphamide on day +3 and day +4 after allogeneic HCT in combination with tacrolimus and MMF has been successful in significantly reducing the incidence of severe aGVHD.[52] Since donor T cells play a pivotal role in GVHD cascade, several studies investigated *ex vivo* T-cell depletion. The studies showed a marked decrease in the incidence of aGVHD; however, the results were marred by a higher risk of infection and leukemia relapse.[53]

Grade 1 aGVHD involving skin can usually be treated with topical steroids alone. Most patients, however, require systemic treatment. Corticosteroids remain the mainstay of first-line systemic therapy for aGVHD. Responses are seen in approximately 50% of cases but are durable in approximately 35% of patients. A combination of other agents with corticosteroids for upfront treatment of aGVHD has not shown to provide better outcomes.[54] For patients who are refractory to corticosteroids therapy, defined as progression after 3 days, no change after 5–7 days, or incomplete response after 14 days; the survival is poor with 1-year mortality approaching 80–90%. There are several options for second-line therapy, but currently, there is no standard of care in these patients.

Chronic GVHD is the leading of long-term morbidity and mortality after allogeneic HCT. The underlying pathophysiology is poorly understood. There is a loss of recognition of self and the development of autoimmune manifestations. The risk factors of cGVHD are similar to aGVHD. Also, having a history of aGVHD is a strong predisposing factor for cGVHD. While the occurrence of cGVHD may lower the disease relapse rate, the nonrelapse mortality can range from 35% for *de novo* to 89% in cases where cGVHD occurs before the resolution of prior aGVHD and completion of its therapy.[55] The clinical manifestations mimic autoimmune disorders and vary depending on the organs involved. Oral mucosa is commonly involved, and findings can include erythema, ulcerations, and xerostomia resembling Sjögren syndrome. Skin may show lichenoid or sclerodermatous cutaneous changes. Chronic liver GVHD frequently presents a picture of cholestasis and can resemble primary biliary cirrhosis. GI involvement may present in the form of esophageal strictures, anorexia, dysphagia, malabsorption, and wasting. The involvement of lungs resulting in progressive, irreversible obstruction (bronchiolitis obliterans)

Table 5 The significant risk factors for graft failure.

Factor	Comments
HLA-mismatch	MUD have a higher risk compared to HLA identical siblings[41]
	HLA-mismatched grafts have a higher risk of GF compared to MUD or HLA identical siblings
ABO incompatibility	Major ABO incompatibility[a] between the donor and recipient increases the risk of GF[42]
Conditioning regimen	Higher rate of GF with RIC compared to MAC regimens[40]
Graft source	Bone marrow associated with a higher incidence of GF in the setting of UD transplants[5]
Graft composition	Total nucleated cell and CD34+ cells dose are essential determinants of engraftment[43][b]
Donor specific anti-HLA antibodies	Presence of DSA increases the risk of GF in the setting of UD, haploidentical, and CBT[44–46]
Viral infections	Cytomegalovirus, parvovirus B19, HHV-6, adenovirus, Epstein-Barr virus, and BK virus, etc. can impact the graft function
Miscellaneous	Several other factors, such as the donor's gender, underlying disease, graft manipulation, etc. can impact engraftment

Abbreviations: MUD, matched unrelated donor; GF, graft-failure; RIC, reduced-intensity conditioning; DSA, donor-specific anti-HLA antibodies; CBT, cord-blood transplantation.
[a]Major ABO incompatibility in the transplant setting is defined by the presence of isohem-agglutinins in the recipient plasma against the donor red blood cells.
[b]The optimum recommended number of progenitor cells in the graft is a matter of debate. Suggested guidelines have been published.[40]

Table 6 Acute GVHD organ staging.

Organ	Skin	Liver	Gastrointestinal
Stage	Body surface area	Bilirubin (mg/dL)	Diarrhea (mL/day)
1	Rash < 25%	2–3	>500
2	Rash 25–50%	3.1–6	>1000
3	Rash > 50%	6.1–15	>1500
4	Bullae formation	>15	>2000, or severe abdominal pain ± ileus

Table 7 Glucksberg grading system.

Grade	Skin	Liver[a]	Gastrointestinal[a]	Performance status (ECOG)
1	Stage 1–2	None	None	0
2	Stage 1–3	Stage 1	Stage 1	1
3	Stage 2–3	2–3	2–3	2
4	Stage 2–4	2–4	2–4	3

Abbreviation: ECOG, Eastern Cooperative Oncology Group.
[a]Liver and/or gastrointestinal involvement.

Table 8 International bone marrow transplant registry grading system.

Grade	Skin	Liver[a]	Gastrointestinal[a]
A	Stage 1	None	None
B	Stage 2	Stage 1 or 2	Stage 1 or 2
C	Stage 3	Stage 3	Stage 3
D	Stage 4	Stage 4	Stage 4

[a]Liver and/or gastrointestinal involvement.

is a dreaded complication. There is profound immune deficiency associated with cGVHD that can result in a myriad of serious infections.

The National Institute of Health consensus criteria is used to diagnose and grade cGVHD.[56] These criteria have been validated in prospective studies. The first-line treatment for cGVHD is steroids, followed by a slow taper. It is not uncommon for patients to require extended therapy. There is no standard of care therapy for patients with steroid-refractory cGVHD. A calcineurin inhibitor (cyclosporine or tacrolimus) is usually added to corticosteroids. The choice of agent depends on the side effect profile and the individual patient's tolerance. In some patients, photopheresis can provide objective responses and facilitate steroids dose reduction. Particular care should be given towards preserving the quality of life and preventing infections. Participation in clinical trials should be strongly encouraged.

Immunodeficiency and infections

Recipients of hematopoietic transplants have a severe immunodeficiency following high-dose conditioning. The innate immune system consisting of cell populations such as neutrophils, monocytes, natural killer cells (NK-cells), and dendritic cells (DCs) recovers faster. In comparison, recovery of adaptive immunity, comprised of B-cells and T-cells, can take years.[57] HLA-mismatched or unrelated and cord blood transplants have a more severe and prolonged immunodeficiency and risk for opportunistic infections. Recipients of autologous and syngeneic transplants also have a period of immunodeficiency, but recovery is more rapid.

Infections after transplant are frequent and account for up to 29% of deaths after autologous HCT and up to 27% of deaths after MUD allogeneic HCT within the first 100 days.[58] Prophylactic strategies against an array of potential infections and rapid recognition and treatment of infections are essential for the successful management of transplant recipients. Detailed international guidelines for preventing infectious complications in HCT recipients have been published.[59] Immunoglobulin replacement therapy should be considered in patients with documented immunoglobulin deficiency. Revaccinations should be performed upon immune recovery and are typically carried out 6 months posttransplant.

Posttransplant lymphoproliferative disorders (PTLDs) are a life-threatening complication of allogeneic transplantation.[60] PTLDs in hematopoietic transplant recipients arise from Epstein–

Barr virus (EBV) induced transformation of donor-derived B-lymphocytes in the presence of impaired cellular immunity. The cumulative incidence of PTLD at 10-year is 1% and most cases occur within the first year after transplantation.[61] It is more prevalent in recipients of mismatched or cord blood grafts, and especially in those treated with T-cell targeting therapies such as higher doses of ATG, alemtuzumab, or recipients of T-cell depleted allografts. Patients usually present with fever and lymphadenopathy. Diagnosis is established on histopathology. The increase in EBV DNA level precedes clinical symptoms development and should be monitored in patients at higher risk. These patients are candidates for preemptive immunotherapy with rituximab. Treatment includes the withdrawal of immunosuppression and administration of rituximab.[62] Cellular therapy with donor or EBV-sensitized lymphocyte infusions can have dramatic results in controlling PTLD.[63] Other approaches, usually employed in the second line, include donor lymphocyte infusions or chemotherapy with or without rituximab.[62]

Miscellaneous noninfectious complications

Myeloablative preparative regimens used to cytoreduce the malignancy approach the limit of tolerance for several tissues. The GI tract, kidneys, lungs, and liver are the most susceptible to toxic damage, but severe toxicity may also involve the heart, bladder, nervous system, and other tissues. The actual risk for toxicity varies among regimens and their relative dose intensity. Specific determinants include the toxicity profiles of the involved agents and their interactions affected by coexisting organ dysfunction, the effects of the diseases and prior therapy, and infections. Most toxicities are experienced during the first 30 days posttransplant, but regimen-related hepatic injury [sinusoidal obstruction syndrome (SOS)], pulmonary toxicity, and neurologic effects may be delayed for several months.

SOS, also called veno-occlusive disease of the liver, is characterized by painful hepatomegaly, jaundice, fluid retention, and weight gain, usually during the first three weeks following the conditioning regimen. Several risk factors that increase the risk of SOS have been identified. Generally, preexisting liver damage, higher intensity of conditioning regimen, and alloreactivity (allogeneic vs autologous) increase the risk of SOS.[64] Supportive care is the standard treatment. The use of ursodeoxycholic acid (Ursodiol) lessens the liver toxicity but does not have efficacy in the treatment of existing SOS.[64] Defibrotide, a potent thrombolytic agent, reduced SOS incidence in a randomized trial involving 356 children undergoing allogeneic HCT.[65] Retrospective studies have shown that defibrotide is also useful in the treatment of established SOS.[66]

Pulmonary toxicity can manifest in various forms. Diffuse alveolar hemorrhage (DAH) is a catastrophic condition that can present with nonspecific symptoms of chest pain, cough, and dyspnea. Bronchoalveolar lavage yields progressively bloody secretions. Patients often require mechanical ventilation. Correction of underlying coagulopathy and high-dose corticosteroids are the mainstay of treatment. Idiopathic pneumonia syndrome (IPS) consists of widespread alveolar injury in the absence of active lower respiratory tract infection, cardiac dysfunction, acute renal failure, or iatrogenic fluid overload as etiology for pulmonary dysfunction.[67] There is no specific treatment for IPS. Patients are treated with supportive measures, broad-spectrum antibiotics, and corticosteroids. Bronchiolitis obliterans syndrome (BOS) is a late-onset complication, typically presenting 3–36 months after transplant.[68] It has an insidious onset followed by progressive decline. Mortality is high, and patients often succumb to worsening respiratory failure. Inhaled fluticasone, azithromycin, and montelukast (FAM) with a brief steroid pulse could halt the pulmonary decline in new-onset BOS.[69] Some patients can benefit from lung transplantation.[70] Peri-engraftment respiratory distress syndrome (PERDS) is suspected in patients undergoing autologous HCT who develop fever, hypoxemia, noncardiogenic pulmonary edema, or maculopapular rash within 5–7 days of neutrophil engraftment.[71,72] Chest imaging may show diffuse opacities.[71] Mild cases may not require therapy. For severe cases, corticosteroids result in a prompt resolution of symptoms.

Cardiac toxicity usually manifests as temporary myocardial injury and a decline in cardiac ejection fraction and is produced by a variety of alkylating agent regimens. Patients with prior radiotherapy are at risk of pericarditis.[73] Cardiac arrhythmias are commonly encountered, particularly in patients receiving anthracycline and etoposide-based conditioning. The presence of prior cardiovascular risks increases the incidence of cardiac toxicity.[73]

Late effects

Late complications of hematopoietic transplantation include delayed effects of high-dose therapy, indolent infections, transfusion-related complications, and cGVHD. Late toxicity of high-dose therapy can produce cataracts, pulmonary fibrosis, dental abnormalities, hypothyroidism, hypogonadism, growth retardation, osteoporosis, and avascular necrosis of the hip or other bones. Permanent sterility occurs in most patients. There is an increased risk of solid and hematologic secondary tumors after hematopoietic transplantation. Solid tumors such as head and neck cancers, squamous cell carcinomas, melanomas, and brain, breast, and thyroid cancers may be more common in recipients of TBI-containing regimens, and the cumulative incidence is up to 7–10% at 15 years.[74] Myelodysplasia and secondary leukemia occur more commonly after autologous transplant, occurring in 4–18% of patients within 2.5–8.5 years of transplant.[73,75]

Indications for hematopoietic cell transplantation

Acute myeloid leukemia

Hematopoietic cell transplantation has been extensively evaluated for the treatment of patients with AML. The goal is to reduce the long-term risk of disease relapse while keeping the treatment-related toxicity minimum. The registry data from the Center for International Blood and Marrow Transplantation Research (CIBMTR) for 13,163 patients receiving an HLA-matched sibling allogeneic HCT for AML between 2007 and 2017 showed 3-year probabilities of survival of 59% ± 1%, 53% ± 1%, and 29% ± 1% for patients with early, intermediate, and advanced disease, respectively.[58] Significant determinants of outcome after transplant are disease status at the time of transplant (remission *versus* refractory disease), genetic abnormalities, patient age, and histocompatibility between donor and recipient. The European LeukemiaNET (ELN) panel segregates AML into three prognostic groups (Table 9).[76] Typically, allogeneic HCT is not considered in favorable-risk patients in first complete remission (CR1).[77] Adverse risk patients have a high risk of relapse and are offered allogeneic HCT in CR1. The decision to proceed with allografting in patients in the intermediate-risk category is less clear and should be made on a case-by-case basis after carefully weighing the risks of allografting against the benefit. For

Table 9 2017 European leukemiaNET risk stratification[a],[76]

Risk category	Genetic abnormality
Favorable	t(8;21)(q22;q22.1); *RUNX1-RUNX1T1*
	inv(16)(p13.1q22) or t(16;16)(p13.1;q22); *CBFB-MYH11*
	Mutated *NPM1* without *FLT3*-ITD or with *FLT3*-ITD^{low}
	Biallelic mutated *CEBPA*
Intermediate	Mutated *NPM1* and *FLT3*-ITD^{high}
	Wild-type *NPM1* without *FLT3*-ITD or with *FLT3*-ITD^{low} (without adverse-risk genetic lesions)
	t(9;11)(p21.3;q23.3); *MLLT3-KMT2A*
	Cytogenetic abnormalities not classified as favorable or adverse
Adverse	t(6;9)(p23;q34.1); *DEK-NUP214*
	t(v;11q23.3); *KMT2A* rearranged
	t(9;22)(q34.1;q11.2); *BCR-ABL1*
	inv(3)(q21.3q26.2) or t(3;3)(q21.3;q26.2); *GATA2,MECOM(EVI1)*
	−5 or del(5q); −7; −17/abn(17p)
	Complex karyotype[b], monosomal karyotype[c]
	Wild-type *NPM1* and *FLT3*-ITD^{high}
	Mutated *RUNX1*[d]
	Mutated *ASXL1*[d]
	Mutated *TP53*

[a] Source: Adapted from Dohner et al.[76]
[b] Three or more unrelated chromosome abnormalities in the absence of 1 of the WHO-designated recurring translocations or inversions, that is, t(8;21), inv(16) or t(16;16), t(9;11), t(v;11)(v;q23.3), t(6;9), inv(3) or t(3;3); AML with *BCR-ABL1*.
[c] Defined by the presence of 1 single monosomy (excluding loss of X or Y) in association with at least 1 additional monosomy or structural chromosome abnormality (excluding core-binding factor AML).
[d] These markers should not be used as an adverse prognostic marker if they co-occur with favorable-risk AML subtypes.

instance, allogeneic HCT is considered in patients with *FLT3-ITD* but deferred in patients with mutated NPM1 in the absence of *FLT3-ITD* or homozygous mutated *CEBPA*.[78] Other high-risk situations where allografting is considered for eligible patients include; primary induction failure, second CR, therapy-related AML,[79] secondary AML arising from antecedent MDS,[80] and minimal residual disease (MRD) positivity.[81]

Myeloablative transplant is preferred in younger patients. A prospective randomized trial for MAC versus RIC allografting by the Bone Marrow Transplant Clinical Trials Network (BMT-CTN) was concluded early when the data showed significantly longer disease-free survival with MAC in patients with AML or MDS.[27] However, RIC regimens remain a viable alternative, especially in older patients and those with comorbidities.[82]

Despite a high percentage of patients achieving durable remission, disease relapse after allogeneic HCT remains a significant cause of treatment failure. Posttransplant maintenance therapies show promise in this context. Different strategies to prevent relapse include targeted maintenance therapy using small molecule inhibitors against driver mutations (e.g., FLT3 inhibitors), epigenetic modulation (e.g., azacitidine, decitabine, vorinostat, panobinostat), use of prophylactic donor lymphocyte infusions, and the institution of preemptive treatment based on MRD monitoring.[83]

Myelodysplastic syndromes

Allogeneic HCT remains the only curative option for patients with MDS.[84,85] Besides the patient eligibility for allogeneic HCT, the risk of transformation to AML and survival of MDS patients are key elements considered when deciding to proceed with allografting. Several prognostic scoring systems have been established; the International Prognostic Scoring System (IPSS)[86] and revised IPSS (IPSS-R)[87] are most widely used. An international expert panel within the EBMT, ELN, BMT CTN, and the International MDSs Foundation developed recommendations for allogeneic HCT in patients with MDS based on IPSS-R and HCT-CI.[88] Eligible patients with higher-risk IPSS-R should be referred for immediate allografting. Patients with very low/low IPSS-R can have extended survival with conservative therapy and transplant can be safely postponed. However, patients with lower-risk IPSS-R are also candidates for allogeneic HCT in case of initial treatment failure, development of additional cytogenetic abnormalities, refractory cytopenias, or increasing bone marrow blasts.[88,89] The conditioning regimens used are similar to those used for AML, and prospect for long-term remission is equal to or perhaps slightly better than that for AML. Relapse is the leading cause of treatment failure. Although not standard of care, strategies to mitigate the risk of relapse after allogeneic HCT, such as preemptive DLI or maintenance therapy with hypomethylating agents, have shown promising early results.[90,91]

Acute lymphoblastic leukemia

Allogeneic HCT in the first remission is recommended for patients with Philadelphia chromosome (Ph)-positive ALL.[92–94] The incorporation of tyrosine kinase inhibitors (TKIs) into chemotherapy regimens has increased the response rate and depth of response; it has allowed more patients to undergo allogeneic HCT in a deeper level of remission. Posttransplant use of TKIs given prophylactically can further reduce the incidence of molecular relapse after allografting.[95] An expert panel from the Acute Leukemia Working Party of EBMT has issued a consensus paper regarding the use of TKIs after allogeneic HCT.[96] The panel suggested that for patients undergoing transplantation during CR1, TKI treatment should be given for 12 months of continuous MRD negativity. For patients undergoing allogeneic HCT during CR2 or a later remission, indefinite treatment was recommended.

The suitable timing for allogeneic HCT in Ph-negative ALL is less well defined. A donor versus no-donor analysis of the large prospective study by the Medical Research Council/Eastern Cooperative Oncology Group (MRC/ECOG, E2993) showed that Ph-negative patients with a donor had an improved 5-year OS, 53% versus 45% ($P = 0.01$), and a significantly lower relapse rate ($P \leq 0.001$) in standard-risk patients.[97] The American Society for Blood and Marrow Transplantation (ASBMT) Evidence-Based Review Steering Committee, in a policy statement, suggested that allogeneic HCT is appropriate for adult (<35 years) patients in CR1 in all risk groups. Allogeneic HCT is also recommended over chemotherapy for ALL in second complete remission or greater. The outcomes with related and unrelated donors are similar, and in the absence of an HLA-matched donor, cord blood transplantation can be considered.[98]

The prognosis of patients with chemotherapy-resistant relapse is poor. The most common preparative regimen used for transplants in ALL includes high-dose cyclophosphamide and TBI with or without other chemotherapeutic agents. TBI-containing regimens may be associated with improved disease-free survival, in comparison to non-TBI-containing regimens.[98] Chemotherapy-only regimens are being actively explored.[99]

Chronic myelogenous leukemia

The use of transplantation to treat CML has declined markedly due to the success of the BCR-ABL TKIs, such as imatinib, to treat this condition. These oral medications produce multiyear remissions for most patients. As a result, transplant is reserved for a minority of patients in the first chronic phase who have the disease, resistant or intolerant to multiple TKIs, and for patients with an inadequate recovery of normal hematopoiesis.[100] Patients who progress to accelerated phase during therapy or those who present with accelerated phase but have a suboptimal response to TKIs are also appropriate candidates for allografting.[100] Patients presenting in or progressing to the blast phase should immediately proceed to allogeneic HCT after gaining control of the disease.[100] Allogeneic HCT may also be a more cost-effective option in resource-constrained countries where the costs of ongoing TKI therapy are prohibitive.[100]

Transplant regimens are those commonly used for AML and produce similar and often slightly superior outcomes. Early transplant failures can often be returned to complete remission through the administration of DLI. While these infusions risk GVHD, CML is very sensitive to their use.

Chronic lymphocytic leukemia

Allogeneic HCT can provide durable remissions in selected patients with advanced CLL. The ASBMT clinical practice guidelines recommend allogeneic HCT for standard risk CLL in the absence of response or disease progression after therapy with B cell receptor (BCR) inhibitors. For high-risk patients, defined as the presence of Del17p and/or TP53 mutations and the presence of complex cytogenetics, allogeneic HCT is recommended for patients showing response to BCR inhibitors, BCL-2 inhibitors, or clinical trials. Patients who do not respond or progress after BCL-2 inhibitors are also candidates for allogeneic HCT.[101] Patients with Richter syndrome have dismal outcomes with the currently available therapies.[102] Such patients should be offered allogeneic HCT after achieving an objective response to therapy.[101] There is no particular conditioning regimen that is considered standard; however, RIC regimens are favored due to low nonrelapse mortality and slightly improved survival compared to MAC allogeneic HCT.[103] Autologous HCT has been studied for CLL treatment; however, it has not shown to improve survival.[104] It is not offered outside of a clinical trial.

Diffuse large B-cell lymphoma

Diffuse large B-cell lymphoma (DLBCL) is the most common form of non-Hodgkin lymphoma (NHL).[105] Most patients achieve durable remission with first-line therapy; however, a third of them have a refractory or relapsed disease.[106] Autologous HCT is indicated for patients with relapsed or refractory disease who are sensitive to salvage therapy.[107] Studies have shown no survival benefit for autologous HCT in CR1 for high-risk patients.[108] BEAM conditioning, with or without rituximab remains the conditioning regimen of choice; however, newer regimens such as GBM (gemcitabine, busulfan, melphalan) have shown promise in high-risk patients.[109] Allogeneic HCT is usually reserved for patients who are unable to undergo autologous HCT due to mobilization failure or who relapse after autologous HCT.[107]

Follicular lymphoma

Follicular lymphoma (FL) is an indolent lymphoma, which does not always require treatment. The role of transplant is less well defined than in DLBCL, and patients with a relapsed disease can often be successfully salvaged with available novel therapies. An evidence-based review by ASBMT noted insufficient data to make a recommendation on the use of autologous HCT after rituximab-based salvage therapy.[110] In the current era, autologous HCT can be considered in patients with early relapse (<12 months) after initial therapy or those with transformed disease.[111,112] Posttransplant maintenance therapy with rituximab can prolong PFS without significantly prolonging the OS in rituximab-naïve patients.[113] Allogeneic HCT is reserved for select high-risk patients, such as those relapsing after autologous HCT. RIC are considered acceptable alternatives to MAC regimens.[110]

Mantle cell lymphoma

Mantle cell lymphoma (MCL) has a diverse clinical spectrum. A minority of patients can remain on observation for an extended period, but the disease follows a more aggressive course in the majority. Autologous HCT as an adjunct to initial therapy is recommended, particularly if less intense induction therapy, such as R-CHOP (rituximab, cyclophosphamide, hydroxydaunorubicin, vincristine, prednisone) is used.[114,115] Maintenance rituximab every two months for a maximum of 3-year after autologous HCT is recommended regardless of the type of induction regimen used.[113] Despite encouraging results with autologous HCT, most patients with MCL experience disease relapse. Allogeneic HCT has curative potential and is used for patients who have a chemosensitive relapse after autologous HCT or have a primary chemoresistant disease.[116]

T-cell and NK/T-cell lymphoma

T-cell lymphomas consist of a multitude of histologic subtypes, comprising approximately 10–15% of lymphoid malignancies.[117] In general, autologous HCT is recommended in front-line consolidation and chemosensitive relapse. Autologous HCT is not recommended in refractory disease. Allogeneic HCT is considered part of front-line consolidation in NK/T cell (disseminated), adult T cell leukemia/lymphoma, and hepatosplenic lymphomas. Specific subtypes with chemosensitive relapse and those with refractory disease are also candidates for allogeneic HCT.[118]

Hodgkin lymphoma

Patients failing to achieve a complete remission with initial chemotherapy can be salvaged with autologous transplantation in approximately one-third of cases. For patients with recurrent Hodgkin's lymphoma, particularly with shorter relapse-free intervals, autologous HCT results in a complete remission rate of 50–80% and a 40–60% disease-free survival at 3–5 years posttransplant.[119,120] The BEAM conditioning is most frequently used.[121,122] A Cochrane systematic review and meta-analysis of randomized controlled trials showed that high-dose therapy followed by autologous HCT significantly prolongs PFS with a trend for improved OS compared to conventional chemotherapy in patients with relapsed or refractory HL after first-line treatment.[123]

Allogeneic transplants using nonmyeloablative techniques have been primarily reserved for patients who are progressing after autotransplantation or patients with inadequate marrow reserves.[124]

Multiple myeloma

Multiple myeloma is the most common indication for autologous HCT in the United States.[58] Several randomized trials have shown that autologous HCT performed as part of first-line therapy is associated with significantly higher complete remission rate, MRD-negativity, and improved PFS than nontransplant options.[125,126] Even elderly patients, including those above age 75, can be safely transplanted at experienced centers.[127] Although early transplant is favored, autologous HCT can be safely delayed until relapse in some patients, without compromising the OS. In these patients, peripheral blood progenitor cells should be collected and cryopreserved early in therapy to prevent mobilization failure due to chemotherapy's cumulative effects. Melphalan 200 mg/m^2 has remained the standard conditioning therapy for decades; however, a recent randomized trial showed that a combination of busulfan plus melphalan conditioning provides superior PFS compared to melphalan alone.[128] Maintenance therapy after autologous HCT prolongs PFS and OS and is offered to all patients.[129] Some studies have shown that a tandem approach, involving a second autologous HCT, performed 2–3 months after the first transplant prolongs PFS (and OS in one study)[126] compared to one autologous HCT.[130] However, this approach needs further investigation.

Allogeneic HCT can induce long-lasting remissions in selected patients, but randomized trials have failed to show a consistent survival benefit in patients with newly diagnosed myeloma. RIC and exploitation of GVM effects have increased the effectiveness of allotransplant, but its use after failure of autotransplant also remains investigational. In the current era, allogeneic HCT is best offered in the setting of a clinical trial.[131,132]

Solid tumors

High-dose chemotherapy with autologous HCT has been studied in both breast and ovarian cancer, but results are conflicting, and this technique is not currently a part of routine treatment of these diseases.

Germ cell tumors are chemotherapy-responsive, and single or sequential high-dose chemotherapy followed by autologous HCT provides a 2-year event-free survival of approximately 45–50% in patients with recurrent or refractory disease.[133]

Autologous transplants have been studied in a range of pediatric solid tumors such as neuroblastoma and Ewing sarcoma; tumors that are highly sensitive to chemotherapy and irradiation yet have a poor prognosis in patients with advanced disease.[134]

Concluding remarks

Hematopoietic cell transplantation is an integral part of therapy for a multitude of malignant and nonmalignant conditions. The epitome of immunotherapies, allografting continues to hold the mantle of being the only curative modality for many otherwise fatal disorders. Further development of international unrelated donor registries and the feasibility of alternative donor transplants have enhanced this approach's availability. Considerable progress in supportive care has made allogeneic transplants increasingly safe by preventing infections and transplant-related complications. As a result, procedural mortality continues to decrease.

Going forward, we are likely to see additional refinements in conditioning regimens and peri-transplant care. The availability of newer agents will increase the proportion of patients with better disease control before transplant. Posttransplant maintenance strategies aim to reduce the relapse rate. Cellular therapies will further complement transplantation in several ways, including better infection control (virus-specific T-lymphocytes), refinement of GVHD management (regulatory T-cells, mesenchymal stem cells), and enhancement of antitumor effects in the form of DLI, adoptive transfer of tumor-specific cytotoxic T-lymphocytes, or chimeric antigen receptor (CAR)-transduced T and NK-cells.

Key references

The complete reference list can be found on Vital Source version of this title, see inside front cover.

2. Schouten HC, Qian W, Kvaloy S, et al. High-dose therapy improves progression-free survival and survival in relapsed follicular non-Hodgkin's lymphoma: results from the randomized European CUP trial. *J Clin Oncol.* 2003;**21**(21):3918–3927.
5. Anasetti C, Logan BR, Lee SJ, et al. Peripheral-blood stem cells versus bone marrow from unrelated donors. *N Engl J Med.* 2012;**367**(16):1487–1496.
6. Lee SJ, Logan B, Westervelt P, et al. Comparison of patient-reported outcomes in 5-year survivors who received bone marrow vs peripheral blood unrelated donor transplantation: long-term follow-up of a randomized clinical trial. *JAMA Oncol.* 2016;**2**(12):1583–1589.
8. Kroger N, Iacobelli S, Franke GN, et al. Dose-reduced versus standard conditioning followed by allogeneic stem-cell transplantation for patients with myelodysplastic syndrome: a prospective randomized phase III study of the EBMT (RICMAC trial). *J Clin Oncol.* 2017;**35**(19):2157–2164.
11. Nunes E, Heslop H, Fernandez-Vina M, et al. Definitions of histocompatibility typing terms. *Blood.* 2011;**118**(23):e180–e183.
13. Gragert L, Eapen M, Williams E, et al. HLA match likelihoods for hematopoietic stem-cell grafts in the U.S. registry. *N Engl J Med.* 2014;**371**(4):339–348.
14. Lee SJ, Klein J, Haagenson M, et al. High-resolution donor-recipient HLA matching contributes to the success of unrelated donor marrow transplantation. *Blood.* 2007;**110**(13):4576–4583.
16. Saber W, Opie S, Rizzo JD, et al. Outcomes after matched unrelated donor versus identical sibling hematopoietic cell transplantation in adults with acute myelogenous leukemia. *Blood.* 2012;**119**(17):3908–3916.
17. Rocha V, Gluckman E. Eurocord-netcord r, European B, marrow transplant g. Improving outcomes of cord blood transplantation: HLA matching, cell dose and other graft- and transplantation-related factors. *Br J Haematol.* 2009;**147**(2):262–274.
21. Santoro N, Labopin M, Giannotti F, et al. Unmanipulated haploidentical in comparison with matched unrelated donor stem cell transplantation in patients 60 years and older with acute myeloid leukemia: a comparative study on behalf of the ALWP of the EBMT. *J Hematol Oncol.* 2018;**11**(1):55.
22. Brunstein CG, Fuchs EJ, Carter SL, et al. Alternative donor transplantation after reduced intensity conditioning: results of parallel phase 2 trials using partially HLA-mismatched related bone marrow or unrelated double umbilical cord blood grafts. *Blood.* 2011;**118**(2):282–288.
24. Bacigalupo A, Ballen K, Rizzo D, et al. Defining the intensity of conditioning regimens: working definitions. *Biol Blood Marrow Transplant.* 2009;**15**(12):1628–1633.
25. Lily Yan BAG. In: Bashir Q, Hamadani M, eds. BCOP. Hematopoietic Cell Transplantation for Malignant Conditions. Elsevier; 2019.
27. Scott BL, Pasquini MC, Logan BR, et al. Myeloablative versus reduced-intensity hematopoietic cell transplantation for acute myeloid leukemia and myelodysplastic syndromes. *J Clin Oncol.* 2017;**35**(11):1154–1161.
31. Armand P, Kim HT, Logan BR, et al. Validation and refinement of the Disease Risk Index for allogeneic stem cell transplantation. *Blood.* 2014;**123**(23):3664–3671.
38. Barba P, Martino R, Perez-Simon JA, et al. Combination of the hematopoietic cell transplantation comorbidity index and the european group for blood and marrow transplantation score allows a better stratification of high-risk patients undergoing reduced-toxicity allogeneic hematopoietic cell transplantation. *Biol Blood Marrow Transplant.* 2014;**20**(1):66–72.
47. Glucksberg H, Storb R, Fefer A, et al. Clinical manifestations of graft-versus-host disease in human recipients of marrow from HL-A-matched sibling donors. *Transplantation.* 1974;**18**(4):295–304.
48. Rowlings PA, Przepiorka D, Klein JP, et al. IBMTR Severity Index for grading acute graft-versus-host disease: retrospective comparison with Glucksberg grade. *Br J Haematol.* 1997;**97**(4):855–864.
49. Ratanatharathorn V, Nash RA, Przepiorka D, et al. Phase III study comparing methotrexate and tacrolimus (prograf, FK506) with methotrexate and cyclosporine for graft-versus-host disease prophylaxis after HLA-identical sibling bone marrow transplantation. *Blood.* 1998;**92**(7):2303–2314.
51. Ciurea SO, Al Malki MM, Kongtim P, et al. The European Society for Blood and Marrow Transplantation (EBMT) consensus recommendations for donor selection in haploidentical hematopoietic cell transplantation. *Bone Marrow Transplant.* 2020;**55**(1):12–24.
54. Rashidi A, DiPersio JF, Sandmaier BM, et al. Steroids versus steroids plus additional agent in frontline treatment of acute graft-versus-host disease: a systematic review and meta-analysis of randomized trials. *Biol Blood Marrow Transplant.* 2016;**22**(6):1133–1137.
56. Jagasia MH, Greinix HT, Arora M, et al. National Institutes of Health Consensus Development Project on Criteria for Clinical Trials in Chronic

Graft-versus-Host Disease: I. The 2014 Diagnosis and Staging Working Group report. *Biol Blood Marrow Transplant*. 2015;**21**(3):389–401 e1.
58. D'Souza A, Fretham C, Lee SJ, et al. Current use of and trends in hematopoietic cell transplantation in the United States. *Biol Blood Marrow Transplant*. 2020;**11**:S1083-8791(20)30225-1.
59. Tomblyn M, Chiller T, Einsele H, et al. Guidelines for preventing infectious complications among hematopoietic cell transplantation recipients: a global perspective. *Biol Blood Marrow Transplant*. 2009;**15**(10):1143–1238.
60. Dierickx D, Habermann TM. Post-transplantation lymphoproliferative disorders in adults. *N Engl J Med*. 2018;**378**(6):549–562.
66. Richardson PG, Riches ML, Kernan NA, et al. Phase 3 trial of defibrotide for the treatment of severe veno-occlusive disease and multi-organ failure. *Blood*. 2016;**127**(13):1656–1665.
73. Muhammad A, Saif FLD. Miscellaneous complications related to hematopoietic cell transplantation. In: Qaiser Bashir MH, ed. *Hematopoietic Cell Transplantation for Malignant Conditions*. Elsevier; 2019:341.
76. Dohner H, Estey E, Grimwade D, et al. Diagnosis and management of AML in adults: 2017 ELN recommendations from an international expert panel. *Blood*. 2017;**129**(4):424–447.
77. Koreth J, Schlenk R, Kopecky KJ, et al. Allogeneic stem cell transplantation for acute myeloid leukemia in first complete remission: systematic review and meta-analysis of prospective clinical trials. *JAMA*. 2009;**301**(22):2349–2361.
87. Greenberg PL, Tuechler H, Schanz J, et al. Revised international prognostic scoring system for myelodysplastic syndromes. *Blood*. 2012;**120**(12):2454–2465.
88. de Witte T, Bowen D, Robin M, et al. Allogeneic hematopoietic stem cell transplantation for MDS and CMML: recommendations from an international expert panel. *Blood*. 2017;**129**(13):1753–1762.
92. Fielding AK, Rowe JM, Buck G, et al. UKALLXII/ECOG2993: addition of imatinib to a standard treatment regimen enhances long-term outcomes in Philadelphia positive acute lymphoblastic leukemia. *Blood*. 2014;**123**(6):843–850.
96. Giebel S, Czyz A, Ottmann O, et al. Use of tyrosine kinase inhibitors to prevent relapse after allogeneic hematopoietic stem cell transplantation for patients with Philadelphia chromosome-positive acute lymphoblastic leukemia: a position statement of the acute leukemia working party of the european society for blood and marrow transplantation. *Cancer*. 2016;**122**(19):2941–2951.
98. Oliansky DM, Larson RA, Weisdorf D, et al. The role of cytotoxic therapy with hematopoietic stem cell transplantation in the treatment of adult acute lymphoblastic leukemia: update of the 2006 evidence-based review. *Biol Blood Marrow Transplant*. 2012;**18**(1):16–17.
108. Stiff PJ, Unger JM, Cook JR, et al. Autologous transplantation as consolidation for aggressive non-Hodgkin's lymphoma. *N Engl J Med*. 2013;**369**(18):1681–1690.
119. Schmitz N, Pfistner B, Sextro M, et al. Aggressive conventional chemotherapy compared with high-dose chemotherapy with autologous haemopoietic stem-cell transplantation for relapsed chemosensitive Hodgkin's disease: a randomised trial. *Lancet*. 2002;**359**(9323):2065–2071.
120. Smith EP, Li H, Friedberg JW, et al. Tandem autologous hematopoietic cell transplantation for patients with primary progressive or recurrent Hodgkin lymphoma: a SWOG and blood and marrow transplant clinical trials network phase II trial (SWOG S0410/BMT CTN 0703). *Biol Blood Marrow Transplant*. 2018;**24**(4):700–707.
123. Rancea M, Monsef I, von Tresckow B, et al. High-dose chemotherapy followed by autologous stem cell transplantation for patients with relapsed/refractory Hodgkin lymphoma. *Cochrane Database Syst Rev*. 2013;**6**:CD009411.
128. Bashir Q, Thall PF, Milton DR, et al. Conditioning with busulfan plus melphalan versus melphalan alone before autologous haemopoietic cell transplantation for multiple myeloma: an open-label, randomised, phase 3 trial. *Lancet Haematol*. 2019;**6**(5):e266–e275.
129. McCarthy PL, Holstein SA, Petrucci MT, et al. Lenalidomide maintenance after autologous stem-cell transplantation in newly diagnosed multiple myeloma: a meta-analysis. *J Clin Oncol*. 2017;**35**(29):3279–3289.

PART 10

Special Populations

67 Principles of pediatric oncology

Theodore P. Nicolaides, MD ■ *Elizabeth Raetz, MD* ■ *William L. Carroll, MD*

> **Overview**
>
> Pediatric malignancies differ from those that occur in adults in their relative incidence, pathological type, clinical presentation, and prognosis. The last several decades of the twentieth century have been a period of enormous accomplishment in the field of pediatric cancer research and outcomes have steadily improved largely due to results from large well-controlled clinical trials conducted by various cooperative groups at the national and international level. This article seeks to provide a broad overview of pediatric oncology, outlining the several common cancer types that are unique to the pediatric age group.

Introduction and epidemiology

Cancer is a relatively rare disease in childhood yet cancer remains the second leading cause of death in children after accidents. The spectrum of cancer types in children is distinctly different compared to adults. While epithelial tumors (carcinomas) dominate the adult cancer spectrum, childhood cancers tend to be of hematopoietic (e.g., leukemias, lymphomas), mesenchymal (sarcomas), and neuroectodermal (e.g., neuroblastomas (NBs), gliomas, medulloblastomas) origin. Acute lymphoblastic leukemia (ALL) and brain tumors are the most common childhood cancers accounting for 25% and 20%, respectively of all cases. The incidence of the most common childhood tumors is illustrated in Figure 1 and Table 1, but it should be noted that incidence can vary according to ethnic and geographic factors. For example, Burkitt Lymphoma accounts for 50% of all childhood cancer in equatorial Africa.

There is a suggestion that the incidence of cancer is rising particularly among certain subtypes of childhood tumors as detailed in Table 1 but better reporting of cases and improved diagnostic imaging may account for some of this trend.[2,3] The etiologies of most childhood cancers remain uncertain. Environmental influences are less likely to play a role in children with radiation being the most well-established risk factor. Breakthroughs in next-generation sequencing technologies also indicate that childhood tumors have a much lower mutational burden compared to malignancies of adults and this would suggest also that the environment plays a less important role in tumor initiation.[4]

Genetic predisposition causes about 5% of all cancers in the pediatric age group although this figure may increase with recent results from next-generation sequencing revealing unrecognized mutations in cancer predisposition genes. About a third of all cases of retinoblastoma (RB) are caused by a germline mutation in *RB1* and children with Down syndrome (DS) are at a 20-fold increased incidence of leukemia (lymphoid and myeloid). Other hereditary syndromes such as Neurofibromatosis 1 (brain tumors), Beckwith–Widemann (Wilms tumor [WT], hepatoblastoma [HB], rhabdomyosarcoma [RMS]), Li–Fraumeni (sarcomas, carcinomas), Gorlin (medulloblastoma, skin cancer), and Ataxia-telangiectasia (leukemia, lymphoma) account for a small, but important fraction of childhood cancers. Often these familial syndromes paved the way for identification of genes that play a role in the much more common sporadic forms of the disease.

In addition more subtle "host" genetic variation (compared to the syndromes described above) has been suggested by the identification of genetic variations (single-nucleotide polymorphisms or "SNPs") that account for an increased risk of cancer and may impact outcomes and side effects of therapy. For example, germline SNPs in *ARID5B, IKZF1, CEBPE, PIP4K2A, and CDKN2A-CDKN2B* influence susceptibility to ALL and *GATA3* variants are associated with a particular subtype of ALL called "Ph-like" ALL (see below).[5]

The dramatic improvement in outcome for childhood cancer represents one of the greatest success stories in the history of the "War on Cancer" that began in earnest in 1971. At that time, roughly 60% of all children under 20 years of age survived 5 years from diagnosis whereas today the figure is more than 80% (Table 2). There are many reasons for these advances including the commitment to multidisciplinary care and highly disciplined clinical trials directed by national and worldwide consortiums such as the Children's Oncology Group. Interestingly many of the same chemotherapeutic agents developed decades ago are still used today but augmentation of doses and schedules have been realized through advances in supportive care and treatment intensification has improved outcome for almost all tumors. Lastly, risk-adapted therapy, tailoring treatment based on prognostically relevant clinical and laboratory variables, has allowed intensification of treatment for those patients most likely to benefit while avoiding more toxic therapy for those patients predicted to have an excellent outcome with standard treatment. Survival rates have been most dramatic for ALL (10% in the 1960s to greater than 90% today) the most common malignancy but survival rates remain low for patients with certain brain tumors, metastatic solid tumors, and relapsed disease. Moreover, while mortality has decreased by approximately 50%, close to 2000 children die each year in the United States,[6] demonstrating that more effective treatments are urgently needed. The cost of cure is substantial with significant short and long-term side effects so more targeted, less toxic treatments are also a priority. Finally, 175,000 children less than 15 years of age are diagnosed annually worldwide and it is estimated than less than 40% receive adequate care.[3] The implementation of treatment protocols customized to the availability of local resources are underway to improve outcome.

Acute lymphoblastic leukemia (ALL)

ALL is the most common malignancy in children in the United States. The peak incidence is between 2 and 3 years of age and

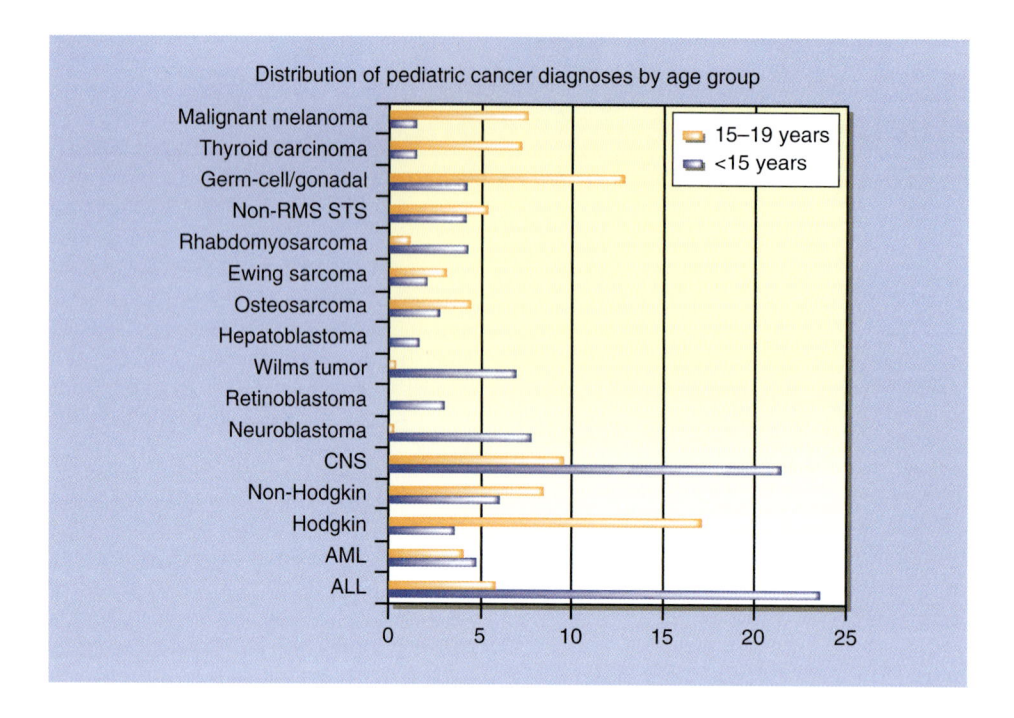

Figure 1 Distribution of pediatric cancer diagnoses by age group. *Abbreviations*: ALL, acute lymphoblastic leukemia; AML, acute myelogenous leukemia; CNS, central nervous system; RMS, rhabdomyosarcoma; STS, soft-tissue sarcoma.

Table 1 Age-adjusted SEER cancer incidence rates[a] by primary site and year of diagnosis (ages 0–19). https://seer.cancer.gov/csr/1975_2017/.[b]

Site	1975	2005	2017
All sites/races	13.0	17.9	18.1
All sites/white	13.4	19.2	18.5
All sites/black	10.8	13.3	14.6
Bone and joint	0.7	0.9	0.9
Brain and other CNS	2.1	3.0	3.1
Hodgkin lymphoma	1.5	0.9	1.1
Kidney and renal pelvis	0.5	0.8	0.7
Leukemia	3.0	4.7	4.8
NHL[c]	1.0	1.3	1.4
Soft tissue	0.8	1.5	1.1

[a]Per 100,000.
[b]Source: Data from Howlader et al.[1]
[c]Non-Hodgkin Lymphoma.

there is a slight male predominance. The incidence is higher in white than in black children and highest in children of Hispanic descent. Stepwise gains in outcome in childhood ALL equal or surpass those in other childhood cancers and have resulted from cooperative group clinical trials conducted worldwide. Refined risk-adapted approaches for therapy allocation with selective treatment intensification has led to 5-year overall survival rates of >90%.[7]

While the exact etiology of childhood ALL is unclear, genetic factors play a role in selected cases. Various constitutional genetic conditions have been associated with pediatric ALL, such as DS, Bloom syndrome, Fanconi anemia, neurofibromatosis (NF1), Li–Fraumeni syndrome, and ataxia-telangiectasia. Of these, DS-ALL deserves special attention. Children with DS have 10- to 20-fold higher risk of developing leukemia compared to children without DS. These children have unique clinical and biological characteristics that affect their treatment and outcome. Notably, T-cell and mature B-cell immunophenotype, and favorable cytogenetic features such as hyperdiploidy and the *ETV6-RUNX1* translocation are not as common in DS-ALL. Novel somatic alterations such as *JAK2* activating mutations are found in about 20% of DS-ALL, while *CRLF2* alterations (most commonly the *P2RY8-CRLF2* fusion) have been observed in about 50% of DS ALL cases.[8,9] Children with DS-ALL are more prone to methotrexate-related toxicities, with more frequent mucositis and infectious complications. In general, prognosis of DS-ALL is worse than non-DS ALL, however, enhanced supportive measures have improved recent outcomes.[10,11]

In recent years, there has also been growing evidence for inherited genetic susceptibility to ALL.[12] Several genome-wide association studies (GWAS) have identified germline genetic polymorphisms associated with the development of ALL.[13] For example, inherited genetic variation at the *GATA3* locus is associated with ALL in adolescents and young adults (AYA) population,[14] variants at the *ERG* locus have been associated with ALL in Hispanics[15] and a risk allele in the *USP7* gene have been associated with the development of T-ALL.[16]

Children with ALL usually present with signs and symptoms suggestive of bone marrow infiltration, manifesting as fever (60%), bleeding symptoms (50%), and bone pain (30%). A child may present with a limp or refusal to walk due to leukemic infiltration of the bone marrow. Lymphadenopathy and hepatosplenomegaly are present in about half to two-thirds of cases and usually asymptomatic. Rarely, patients may present with symptoms of extramedullary spread, such as neurological changes due to central nervous system (CNS) involvement, testicular enlargement, or ocular changes. Children may also present with respiratory compromise due to an anterior mediastinal mass, which is more common in patients with T-cell ALL (T-ALL). The diagnosis is typically made by bone marrow aspiration and/or biopsy. Multiple cell-surface antigen markers and cytogenetic alterations in the leukemic cells are used to establish ALL subtype and determine treatment.[17] About 85% of cases of childhood ALL are of B-precursor lineage whereas 15% are T-lineage. Rarely, children

Table 2 Five years relative survival (percent) (SEER.cancer.gov/csr/1975_2015).[a]

	Ages 0–14			Ages 0–19		
	1974–1977	1993–1995	2008–2014	1974–1977	1993–1995	2008–2014
All sites	58.0	77.4	83.8	61.5	77.3	84.0
Bone and joint	49.9	74.2	80.7	50.4	69.0	73.4
Brain and CNS	57.2	70.7	75.0	59.1	71.5	75.5
Hodgkin lymphoma	80.9	94.6	97.9	86.2	93.9	98.3
ALL[b]	57.2	83.9	90.6	53.8	81.5	89.2
AML[c]	18.8	40.6	68.8	18.7	38.6	67.1
Neuroblastoma	52.5	66.5	74.8	53.1	66.5	75.2
NHL[d]	43.2	80.7	88.5	44.6	78.0	84.3
Soft tissue	61.3	76.7	80.9	64.8	73.8	80.1
Wilms tumor	73.1	91.7	91.0	72.6	91.8	90.4

[a] Source: Data from Howlader et al.[1]
[b] Acute lymphoblastic leukemia.
[c] Acute myelogenous leukemia.
[d] Non-Hodgkin lymphoma.

develop mature B-cell leukemia, which are a form of Burkitt lymphoma requiring different treatment or acute leukemias that have characteristics of both ALL and acute myeloid leukemia (AML).

The biological heterogeneity of childhood ALL is reflected in recent genomic and epigenomic studies.[18,19] DNA copy number abnormalities were identified in genes that encode regulators of B cell development, as *CDKN2A/B, PAX5, IKZF1,* and *EBF1*.[20] In addition, somatic mutations in *JAK2*, alterations in RAS pathway genes (*NRAS, KRAS, PTPN11,* and *NF1*), and *CRLF2* genomic alterations have been identified with increased frequency in high-risk patients.[21,22] *JAK1* and *JAK2* mutations have previously been shown to be mutated in DS-ALL and T-cell ALL as well.[9] New biological subtypes continue to be discovered. For example, gene expression profiling has identified a subset of patients whose blasts share a gene expression profile observed in patients with Ph-positive ALL but who lack the BCR-ABL1 fusion protein.[23] Such patients have "BCR-ABL1-like" or "Ph-like" ALL. Ph-like ALL occurs in 10–20% of children with ALL and the frequency increases with age peaking in young adults.[24] It is characterized by a number of genetic alterations that activate kinase signaling and deletions or mutations of *IKZF1* are a characteristic feature of both Ph-positive and Ph-like ALL.[24,25] *CRLF2* genomic alterations are present in 50% of the cases of Ph-like ALL with half of those harboring *JAK* mutations. Tyrosine kinase fusions other than BCR-ABL1, including *ABL1, ABL2, CSF1R,* and *PDGFRB* fusions are present in another subset of Ph-like ALL.[26] Outcomes for Ph-like ALL are poor with chemotherapy alone and treatment regimens including the addition of JAK or ABL-class tyrosine kinase inhibitors, similar to the approach taken in Ph+ ALL,[17] are currently under evaluation in high-risk pediatric and AYA ALL.[27–29]

While age and initial WBC count at the time of disease presentation remain important predictors of outcome in B-ALL, other factors such as blast immunophenotype and cytogenetics, CNS involvement, and early response to chemotherapy are currently being utilized for risk stratification. Cytological confirmation of leukemic cells in CSF is required for the diagnosis of CNS leukemia. Standard or average-risk patients are defined as age between 1 and 9 years with an initial WBC count of less than 50,000/mm^4 while patients with age >10 years or a presenting WBC of more than 50,000/mm,^{4} regardless of age, are classified as high risk. Risk assessment is further refined by presence or absence of favorable (e.g., hyperdioloidy with trisomies of chromosomes 4 and 10 or *EVT6/RUNX1* fusion)[30,31] and unfavorable cytogenetic features (e.g., hypodiploidy (<44 chromosomes), *KMT2A* rearrangements or iAMP21),[32–35] overt CNS and testicular disease at diagnosis and minimal residual disease (MRD) at the end of induction chemotherapy, which is the most significant prognostic factor.[36]

Contemporary therapies include several components, namely, induction, presymptomatic or prophylactic CNS therapy, postinduction intensification, and maintenance therapy. This design of current treatments will cure more than 80–90% of patients.[7] In recent years, several promising new immunotherapeutic agents, including monoclonal antibodies, bi-specific T-cell engagers (BiTEs) and CAR T-cells have been studied in children with relapsed/refractory B-ALL.[37,38] Given the favorable response rates and toxicity profiles, efforts are currently underway to investigate these agents in children with newly diagnosed leukemia.

Additional recent advances in therapy include

- Current frontline therapy regimens are tailored to risk category as assessed by clinical features and biologic profile.[17]
- The substitution of dexamethasone for prednisone has improved the survival for standard-risk patients, while no EFS advantage has been noted for patients >10 years of age. In addition, there was significantly increased rate of osteonecrosis in patients >10 years of age.[39]
- Initial response to therapy determined by day 8 peripheral blood and/or bone marrow assessment of MRD at end induction (day 29) is an important predictor of outcome and is now utilized in risk-adapted treatment approaches.[36]
- Postinduction intensification (or delayed intensification) improves outcome for both high and standard risk (SR), B-precursor and T-lineage patients particularly when augmented regimens were utilized.[40] However, there is no additional benefit of second delayed intensification.[40]
- Improved outcome is associated with specific cytogenetic aberrations including hyperdiploidy, trisomy 4, 10, and t(12;21)(*ETV6-RUNX1*) and these patients are now classified as having low-risk disease and receive less intensive chemotherapy if MRD is negative at day 8 and at day 29.[41]
- High-dose methotrexate given during interim maintenance improves outcome in high-risk B-ALL.[42]
- Outcomes for children with T-ALL treated on a recent COG trial now parallel those in B-ALL with superiority of escalating Capizzi-based methotrexate and peg-asparaginase during interim maintenance and the addition of nelarabine.[43,44]

- Current systemic therapy allows elimination of cranial irradiation for almost all patients except those who have overt CNS disease at diagnosis.[45]
- Review of comparative outcome results of AYA treated with pediatric or adult protocol-based therapy has shown improved outcomes for those treated utilizing the pediatric approach.[46–48]
- Ph+ pediatric ALL can be treated with aggressive chemotherapy and concomitant targeted therapy with tyrosine kinase inhibitor-imatinib or dasatinib leading to remarkable improvement in event-free survival (EFS) without the need for stem cell transplantation.[49]
- Hematopoietic stem cell transplantation (HSCT) has a limited role in newly diagnosed ALL, except in refractory settings and possibly those patients with persistently high MRD at later time points. Early relapsed ALL (bone marrow relapse within 36 months from initial diagnosis or while in therapy) generally undergo HSCT, while late relapsed cases are treated with chemotherapy, and HSCT is considered based on treatment response.
- Immunotherapeutic approaches offer promise for children with relapsed/refractory B-ALL.[37,38,50]

In addition to the disease and treatment-related prognostic variables, recent studies have highlighted the importance of host factors in governing the disease outcome as well. Host factors refer to differences among patients with regard to drug absorption, metabolism, and sensitivity. Considerable heterogeneity has been described with respect to host pharmacology of thiopurines[51] and vincristine.[52] Furthermore, SNPs have been associated with unfavorable pharmacokinetics of various antileukemic chemotherapeutics, suggesting that drug disposition influences the risk of relapse.[53]

While significant advances have been made in the outcomes of newly diagnosed ALL over the past four decades, infant ALL and early relapsed ALL are the two subgroups whose outcome remains dismal and there is an urgent need for innovative strategies to improve outcomes for these patients.

Acute myeloid leukemia (AML)

AML comprises about 20% of pediatric leukemia and chronic myeloid leukemia is detected in about 1–2%. Similar to ALL, the development of AML has also been associated with various inherited and acquired predisposition syndromes, such as DS, bone marrow failure syndromes such as Fanconi anemia, dyskeratosis congenital, severe congenital neutropenia (Kostman syndrome), Diamond Blackfan anemia as well as acquired aplastic anemia. Patients treated with chemotherapy (particularly alkylating agents and topoisomerase inhibitors) and radiation therapy are at risk of developing therapy-related acute myeloid leukemia (t-AML). The presentation of AML is similar to that of ALL. Occasionally, a child may present with violaceous, raised, plaque-like lesions on the skin or gums, called chloromas, which are an extramedullary manifestation of AML. Patients with acute promyelocytic leukemia (APL), a distinct AML subtype, characterized by t(15;17), or PML-RARA fusion, often present with severe coagulopathy.

Compared with ALL, pediatric AML is less responsive to available chemotherapy. AML survival has recently improved with cure rates approaching up to 60–70% in the pediatric population.[54] This has been achieved by dose intensification, improved supportive measures, results from large clinical trials, and better understanding of the biology and heterogeneity of this disease. Unlike ALL, age and WBC are not considered as independent prognostic variables for stratification. In fact, cytogenetic and molecular characteristics and response to induction chemotherapy are utilized in current treatment schema for risk-adapted therapy.[55,56] Presence of inversion 16, t (8;21) and t(15;17), biallelic CEBPA mutations and NPM1 mutations are considered as favorable, while monosomy 7, monosomy 5/del(5q), KMT2A rearrangements, and FLT3-ITD with high allelic ratio are considered unfavorable characteristics. Additional poor prognosis rearrangements, many of which occur in young children, may not be picked up by conventional genotyping assays and therefore require next-generation sequencing to detect.[57]

AML therapy consists of remission-induction, prophylactic CNS-directed therapy, and postremission therapy. Chemotherapy regimens (for the most part composed of an anthracycline and cytarabine) are intensive requiring prolonged hospitalizations and aggressive supportive measures. After initial 1–2 induction courses and upon achieving morphological remission (less than 5% blasts in marrow) postremission therapy is administered, which may comprise additional intensive chemotherapy (four to five cycles total depending on risk group) or HSCT depending on the cytogenetic risk factors and the depth of response (MRD status) to induction chemotherapy. Prolonged maintenance chemotherapy courses have been shown to be inferior and are not incorporated in current regimens except in APL.

Since the more intensive induction regimens have been maximally intensified, new active agents and strategies are needed. Many promising new approaches are now available. Gemtuzumab ozogamicin is an anti-CD33 immunotoxin with proven efficacy and is now incorporated into standard induction.[58] FLT3/ITD and other FLT3 mutations provide an opportunity for targeted therapy and many tyrosine kinase inhibitors have been tested including sorafenib which improved outcome for children with a high FLT3/ITD allelic ratio when given with chemotherapy and during maintenance.[59] The impact of newer TKIs including gilteritinib is being explored. Likewise, CPX-351, a liposomal formulation of daunorubicin and cytarabine, has shown promise in relapsed/refractory patients and is now being tested in patients at initial diagnosis.[60] In addition, epigenetic modifiers such as vorinostat and 5-azacytidine, as well as BCL-2 inhibitors (e.g., venetoclax) are under evaluation. Immunotherapeutic approaches such as monoclonal antibodies, BiTEs, and CAR-T cell against myeloid cell surface antigens offer great promise, but these targets may be shared by normal hematopoietic stem cells thereby resulting in collateral myelosuppression.

APL is the most curable of all AML subtypes. Based on the unique biology of the PML-RARA fusion protein therapy has migrated from chemotherapy (cytarabine and daunorubicin) along with maintenance therapy to reduced-intensity chemotherapy with the differentiating agent all-trans retinoic acid (ATRA) to pure biologic therapy with ATRA and arsenic trioxide (ATO).[61] Patients are stratified by the initial WBC with those less than 10,000 cells/μL being classified as SR. Early deaths can occur due to bleeding and/or differentiation syndrome (fever, respiratory distress, edema, and pulmonary infiltrates) secondary to maturing myeloid cells can be seen. Outcomes are excellent with an EFS of 92% for SR and 83% for high-risk (HR) patients.[62]

Non-Hodgkin lymphoma (NHL)

Approximately 15% of all childhood cancers diagnosed in the United States are lymphomas. Sixty percent of all childhood lymphomas are classified as NHLs, representing 3% of all childhood malignancies for children younger than 5 years, and 8–9% for children and adolescents 5–19 years of age. Both primary and secondary immunodeficiency increases the risk for NHL.

In contrast to adults where most NHLs are low or intermediate grade, almost all NHL in children are high grade. There are three major subtypes of childhood NHL: (1) mature B cell lymphoma predominantly Burkitt lymphoma (classic and atypical) or diffuse large B-cell lymphoma (DL-BCL), (2) precursor T-cell lymphoma or lymphoblastic lymphoma, and (3) mature T-cell or null cell lymphomas, anaplastic large-cell lymphoma (ALCL). The WHO classifies ALCL as a peripheral T-cell lymphoma. The distribution of these histologic subtypes includes approximately 40% Burkitt lymphoma, 30% lymphoblastic lymphoma, 20% diffuse large B-cell, and 10% ALCL. Burkitt lymphoma tumor cells are characterized by a chromosomal translocation juxtaposing the *c-myc* oncogene and immunoglobulin locus regulatory elements t(8;14), rarely t(8;22), or t(2;8). Similarly, >90% of pediatric ALCL have a characteristic chromosomal rearrangement involving the *ALK* gene t(2;5).

Presence of bulky disease poses two potentially life-threatening situations that are often the presenting feature in children with NHL. First is the tumor lysis syndrome resulting in major electrolyte imbalances, most notably, hyperuricemia, hyperkalemia, and hyperphosphatemia. Aggressive hydration, allopurinol, or rasburicase (urate oxidase) are used in such situations along with other supportive measures. Second is the presence of large mediastinal masses especially seen in lymphoblastic lymphoma, posing a risk of superior vena cava syndrome and cardiac or respiratory arrest.

The primary modality of treatment of all histologic types and stages of childhood NHL is multiagent chemotherapy. The exact regimen of chemotherapy with or without intrathecal therapy and the intensity and length of treatment are usually dictated by the extent of disease and the histologic subtype. While Burkitt lymphoma, DL-BCL, and ALCL are treated with short intensive courses of chemotherapy, lymphoblastic lymphoma is generally treated with ALL-based regimens with a prolonged maintenance phase. The role of surgery is critically important in the diagnosis and staging process but has a limited role in the overall treatment of childhood NHL. There is minimal to no role of radiation therapy in the overall treatment of childhood NHL.

The prognosis for children and adolescents with NHL, both with limited-stage and advanced-stage disease, has improved significantly over the past two decades with overall survival rates exceeding 80%.[63] Except for rare subtypes, the chance of being alive and disease free at 5 years for limited-stage and advanced-stage disease B-NHL is 95% and 80%, respectively.[64] An exception, however, is primary mediastinal large B-cell lymphoma, that is distinguished from other DLBCL and has a lower EFS of approximately 70%. The prognosis for advanced lymphoblastic NHL in children and adolescents has improved with 85% 4-year EFS on a recently completed COG study.[65] The prognosis for the most advanced childhood and adolescent ALCL still lags behind the other histologies with EFS rates of approximately 75%.[63,66] There is evidence that the immune system plays a significant role in the pathogenesis of ALCL and antibodies against ALK have been inversely correlated with the risk of relapse.[67]

Recently, therapeutic strategies for childhood NHL are incorporating surface, intracellular, and molecular targets in order to not only improve the overall cure rates of advanced-stage disease but to minimize the collateral damage from the chemotherapy agents. Rituximab is a monoclonal antibody targeting the CD20 antigen, expressed by Burkitt lymphoma and DLBCL in children. The COG demonstrated the safety and tolerability of adding rituximab to a standard French-American-British (FAB)/Lymphome Malins de Burkitt (LMB)96 chemotherapy backbone in children and adolescents, with a 3-year EFS of 90% in patients with advanced Burkitt lymphoma (with bone marrow and/or CNS involvement).[68] The benefits of rituximab in combination with LMB chemotherapy were further validated in an international, randomized phase 3 trial in children with advanced-stage mature B-NHL.[69] EFS at 3 years was 93.9% with the addition of rituximab compared to 82.3% with chemotherapy alone and combination therapy was well tolerated.[69] Likewise, the promising activity of crizotinib (targeting *ALK*)[70] and brentuximab vedotin (monoclonal anti CD30 antibody),[12,71,72] in relapsed ALCL has prompted investigation of these agents in combination with chemotherapy in newly diagnosed ALCL.

Hodgkin lymphoma (HL)

Hodgkin lymphoma (HL) accounts for approximately 5% of pediatric malignancies in developed countries and is divided into two pathologic categories. Classic HL (cHL) accounts for 90% of cases and has four subtypes: nodular sclerosis, mixed cellularity, lymphocyte depleted, and lymphocyte rich. Reed-Sternberg (RS) cells (multinucleated giant cells) are the hallmark of cHD, which are present in a background of inflammatory cells consisting of eosinophils, small lymphocytes, plasma cells, neutrophils, histiocytes, and fibroblasts. RS cells nearly always express CD30, while CD15 is expressed in approximately 70% of cases. Nodular lymphocyte-predominant Hodgkin lymphoma (NLPHL) occurs only in 5–10% cases. Like cHD NLPHL is composed of rare large atypical cells ("popcorn cells") in an inflammatory background, but these cells express CD20 and lack CD30.

The cure rate for pediatric patients with HL is greater than 90%. Major prognostic factors include stage, the presence of bulky disease, and the presence or absence of "B" symptoms. More recently, prognostic scoring systems have been validated similar to those used in the treatment of adult HL.[73] Patients are classified into low-, intermediate-, and high-risk categories. Historically standard therapy for pediatric patients with HL includes combination chemotherapy based on the classic ABVD (adriamycin, bleomycin, vinblastine, dacarbazine) regimen and low-dose involved-field radiotherapy (RT). Clinical research in pediatric HL aims to delineate minimal treatment necessary for cure and eliminate or minimize late sequelae of treatment. Thus, a variety of approaches have been employed and the number of cycles of chemotherapy usually ranges from two to six cycles depending on risk group and whether consolidative RT is used. PET scans have been demonstrated to be useful in response-based therapy approaches to determine which patients would be eligible for treatment with chemotherapy alone or those that require intensification of therapy. Low-stage HL patients may be treated with three cycles of ABVD reserving RT only for those with residual PET activity.[74] Likewise the COG demonstrated successful omission of involved-field RT without comprising outcome in intermediate-risk patients who show rapid response (PET-CT negative disease), to two cycles of ABVE-PC (doxorubicin, bleomycin, vincristine, etoposide, prednisone, cyclophosphamide) and a complete response after four cycles.[75] Brentuximab vedotin, a CD30 directed antibody–drug conjugate, has shown promise in relapsed/refractory HL and is now integrated into front-line therapy for high-risk HL. Given the dense inflammatory network observed in HL, it is not surprising that immune checkpoint inhibitors have been shown to be efficacious in relapsed HL and are now also being moved into patients with newly diagnosed disease.

Patients with NLPHL usually presented with localized disease and those with a single node that is completely resected may be observed without chemotherapy and those with unresected low

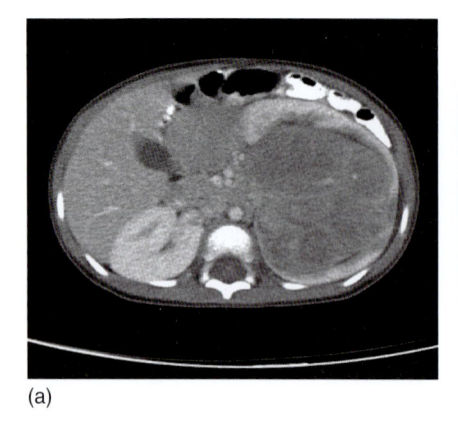

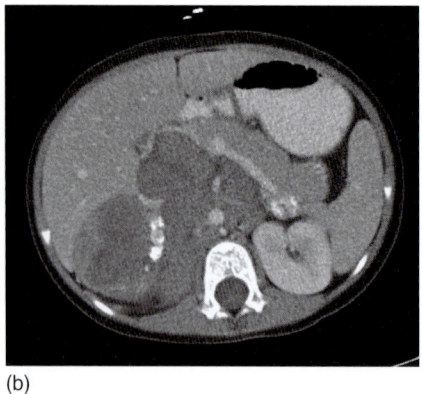

Figure 2 Computed tomographic (CT) imaging characteristics of common childhood abdominal tumors (a) Wilm's tumor: Axial contrast-enhanced CT images of the abdomen showing a large well-circumscribed heterogeneous left renal mass that does not cross the midline. (b) Neuroblastoma: Axial contrast-enhanced CT images of the abdomen demonstrating a large lobulated heterogeneous mass in the right upper quadrant that crosses the midline with characteristic encasement of aorta and displacement of superior mesenteric vein, splenic vein and pancreas anteriorly. Dense calcifications are present within the mass.

stage may be managed with three cycles of AV-PC (Adriamycin, vincristine, prednisone, cyclophosphamide) again reserving RT only for those patients with PET avid disease after chemotherapy.[76] Management of relapsed/refractory HL remains challenging, and currently, high-dose chemotherapy followed by autologous HSCT is considered standard of care for most patients especially those relapsing early following treatment.

Renal tumors

Wilms tumor

WT accounts for over 90% of renal tumors in children and 6% of childhood cancers in general. Today, survival rates for all patients exceed 90% and even patients presenting with metastatic disease have an EFS rate of 80% at 2 years.[77] The typical clinical presentation is that of a well-appearing child who has an abdominal mass noted as an incidental finding. Over 90% of patients have a unilateral tumor with multicentric or bilateral tumors accounting for the remainder of cases. Patients with unilateral tumors present on average at 36.5 months (males) to 42.5 months (girls) while those with bilateral disease present earlier in life (33–35 months) reflecting a genetic predisposition.[78]

Many congenital syndromes are associated with WT and analyses of such cases led to the discovery of tumor suppressor genes involved in the pathogenesis of both inherited as well as sporadic cases. Children with the WAGR (WT, aniridia, genitourinary abnormalities, and mental retardation) syndrome have a greatly increased risk of WT and this syndrome is associated with constitutional (germline) deletions at 11p13. Within the deleted region lies the WT1 gene responsible for the risk of WT (as well as PAX5 responsible for aniridia). Disease pathogenesis follows a classic two-hit model with the tumor having lost both WT1 alleles. Likewise, the Denys–Drash syndrome (pseudo-hermaphroditism, degenerative renal disease) is associated with constitutional mutations of *WT1* and tumors contain mutations in both alleles. Somatic mutations of *WT1* are seen in 10–20% of sporadic WT.[79]

A second tumor suppressor gene, *WT2*, has been mapped to 11p15.5. Abnormalities of this region are associated with another syndrome where the risk of WT is particularly high, the Beckwith–Wiedemann syndrome (macroglossia, omphalocele, visceromegaly, and hemihypertrophy). This region encodes a large number of imprinted genes including insulin-like growth factor II (*IGF2*) and *H19* which encodes a noncoding RNA that acts as a tumor suppressor gene.[80] Somatic loss of heterozygosity (LOH) of WT2 is the most common defect in sporadic WT occurring in up to 80% of cases.[79]

WT presents typically as a well-circumscribed heterogeneously enhancing mass originating from kidney (Figure 2a). Pathologically, WT typically shows a triphasic pattern composed of blastemal, epithelial, and stromal cell types although in some cases only one or two of these cell types may be visualized. Anaplasia is characterized by markedly enlarged nuclei, pleomorphism, and polyploidy mitotic features, and these are associated with a poor prognosis. Anaplasia may be focal or diffuse and is seen in 5% of tumors.[81] In the absence of anaplasia, WTs are classified as having "favorable histology." Nephrogenic rests are precursor lesions and represent persistent nephroblastic tissue that has not undergone full differentiation.[82] Patients with nephrogenic rests (30% sporadic and 100% bilateral WTs) may be at risk for the development of a subsequent WT.

Therapy for WT involves surgical resection and chemotherapy with radiation reserved for more advanced stages. Worldwide, there are two general approaches that lead to equivalent outcomes. In North America (based on practices established by the National Wilms Tumor Study Group (NWTSG) and now COG), most cases are treated by initial surgery (nephrectomy and lymph node sampling) followed by chemotherapy.[77] In Europe (Societe Internationale d'Oncologie Pediatrique or SIOP), neoadjuvant therapy is advocated with delayed surgery. The advantage of the North American approach is that it allows for full, unaltered evaluation of all tumor tissue and accurate staging while the SIOP approach allows for preoperative tumor shrinkage thereby making resection easier and decreasing the risk of spillage.[83,84]

The usual definitive surgical approach to WT is a radical nephrectomy through a wide abdominal incision. The adrenal gland is removed and regional lymph nodes are sampled.[85] Given the risk of second WTs, a partial nephrectomy or "nephron-sparing" surgery is used for patients with bilateral tumors but also this is increasingly being considered for unilateral favorable histology tumors, especially in the neoadjuvant setting where there is assurance of negative margins due to an excellent response to chemotherapy.

Treatment of WT includes nephrectomy and stage-dependent chemotherapy with or without radiation to the abdomen and/or lungs. There are subtle differences in staging between the COG and SIOP approaches, but in general, complete resection of tumor with an intact capsule and no extension to the renal sinus is stage I. Stage II tumors are those completely resected but the tumor extends beyond the capsule or into the renal sinus while incompletely resected tumors or those with lymph node involvement, tumor spillage, and/or positive surgical margins are declared stage III. Stage IV indicates metastatic hematogenous spread (usually lung but also liver, brain, or bone). Preoperative evaluation includes a CT of the abdomen and pelvis and doppler ultrasound if there is concern about tumor thrombus in the inferior vena cava. Magnetic resonance imaging (MRI) may be useful for following nephrogenic rests and aid in surgical planning for patients with bilateral tumors.

Once removed the tumors are evaluated pathologically to validate the diagnosis and examine sections for the presence of anaplasia. In addition, certain molecular markers may portend for a worse prognosis such as LOH at 1p and 16q and these genetic lesions have been uniformly assessed on recent protocols.[77]

Patients under 2 years of with stage I favorable histology tumors weighing less than 550 g may be treated with nephrectomy only since the small minority who relapse can be salvaged with chemotherapy and RT. Patients with stages I and II tumors (without LOH at 1p and 16q) are treated with vincristine and dactinomycin (18 weeks) while stage III patients receive vincristine, dactinomycin, and doxorubicin with abdominal irradiation (24 weeks). Patients with LOH at 1p and 16q are upstaged and require additional therapy. Many different drug combinations have been assessed for favorable histology stage IV patients but none have seemed to improve outcome over the three-drug combination given with abdominal and chest irradiation. Those patients whose metastatic lesions regress early in therapy may not require chest XRT whereas those patients whose lesions do not regress early require chest irradiation and may benefit from additional chemotherapy. The presence of anaplasia is associated with an inferior prognosis and therapy is modified based on whether the anaplasia is diffuse or focal as well as stage. For example, patients with stages II–IV tumors showing diffuse anaplasia are treated with combination therapy including vincristine, doxorubicin, cyclophosphamide, carboplatin, etoposide although the optimal regimen has yet to be established.

Patients with bilateral tumors and those with unilateral tumors and a congenital predisposition syndrome pose a special challenge since these patients are at risk for subsequent tumors. These patients can be treated with preoperative chemotherapy (vincristine, dactinomycin (unilateral tumors with predisposition syndrome) +/−doxorubicin (bilateral tumors) and undergo nephron-sparing surgery at weeks 6 or 12 depending on optimal response. Such patients usually do not require an initial biopsy given the typical clinical and radiographic presentation. Therapy after resection is guided by stage and histology of the resected specimen.

The outcomes for all stages of favorable histology WT is excellent with 10-year relapse-free survival rates of 91% (stage I), 85% (stage II), 84% (stage III), and 75% (stage IV) while historically patients with anaplastic tumors have a worse outcome (10-year relapse-free survival of 43% (stages I–III), and 18% (stage IV)). Patients with bilateral tumors have an intermediate 10-year relapse-free outcome of approximately 65% (overall survival 78%).[77]

Other renal tumors

Renal cell carcinomas, clear cell sarcomas of the kidney, and malignant rhabdoid tumors constitute 5.9%, 3.5%, and 1.6% of all renal tumors in children. Children with renal cell carcinoma present with abdominal pain, hematuria, and an abdominal mass on examination. Many conditions are associated with renal cell carcinoma including von Hippel–Lindau disease, familial renal cell carcinoma, and previous therapy for malignancy.[86,87] Most tumors in childhood are characterized by translocations between the *transcription factor E3* gene (*TFE3*) located on Xp11.2 with a variety of fusion partners. Children tend to present at a more advanced stage compared to adults. Radical nephrectomy with lymph node dissection remains the primary treatment. Survival rates at 4 years are 92%, 85%, and 73% for stages I, II, and III, respectively while outcome for stage IV disease remains dismal (14%).[77,88] Optimal therapy for patients with unresectable or metastatic disease has not been defined but there is great interest in using tyrosine kinase inhibitors (sunitinib and others) in translocation positive renal cell carcinoma.[77]

Clear cell sarcomas are a distinct group of tumors with the histological appearance of nests of cells separated by organized fibrovascular septa. The molecular pathogenesis is unknown for most tumors although a t(10;17)(q22,p13) is noted in a small subgroup of these cases. Clear cell sarcomas can metastasize to bone and the brain in addition to lung and liver but most patients present with localized disease. Historically, these patients have been classified as unfavorable but incremental improvements have been achieved over successive NWTS trials. Patients treated on a regimen of vincristine, doxorubicin, cyclophosphamide, and etoposide with radiation therapy to the tumor bed had a 5-year EFS of 79%.[77,89]

Malignant rhabdoid tumors present at a younger age compared to WT and symptoms include fever and gross hematuria.[90] The majority of patients have advanced disease and up to 15% have associated CNS lesions. Histologically the tumor is composed of large cells, prominent nucleoli, and eosinophilic cytoplasmic granules. These tumors are due to biallelic inactivation (mutation and/or deletion) of the *SMARCB1* gene on 22q (also known as *INI1*) which encodes a member of a chromatin remodeling complex.[91] About a third of patients harbor a germline mutation in *SMARCB1* and these children present at an earlier age (median 5 months compared to 18 months). Most patients are treated with surgery, radiation, and multiagent chemotherapy but optimal drug combinations have yet to be identified. Young age, advanced stage, and the presence of CNS disease are adverse prognostic factor. Four-year relapse-free survival is 50%, 33%, 33%, and 21% for stages I, II, III, and IV, respectively.[77]

Congenital mesoblastic nephroma typically occurs in infancy and presents as a unilateral abdominal tumor. Two patterns exist, classic and cellular. The cellular form of mesoblastic nephroma is characterized by the *ETV6/NTRK3* fusion transcript (t(12;15)(p13;q25) identical to infantile fibrosarcoma.[92] These tumors are treated by complete resection without the need for adjuvant therapy since metastasis is quite rare. Overall survival rates are approximately 95%.[93]

Neuroblastoma

NB is the most common extracranial solid tumor of children and accounts for 8–10% of all childhood cancers. This tumor represents transformation of precursor neural crest cells that were destined to form sympathetic ganglia and the adrenal medulla. It is the most common tumor of infancy and the median age at presentation is 19 months with 90% younger than 5 years at diagnosis.[94] Curiously, the disease has a wide clinical and biological spectrum ranging from spontaneous regression of widespread disease in infants to unrelenting, aggressive disease usually in older children. About 2% of cases are familial in nature and approximately 75% of familial cases carry germline mutations in the anaplastic lymphoma kinase gene, *ALK,* while a much smaller number of familial cases are due to mutations in *PHOX2B* in association with other neurocristopathies like Hirschsprung's disease.[95–97] It is likely that additional steps are required for full transformation since only 50% of germline carriers of *ALK* mutations develop NB.[98] Indeed GWAS have identified a number of predisposition loci, yet their contribution to most sporadic cases is likely to be quite modest.[99] *ALK* mutations and amplifications are seen in 8–12% and 2–3%, respectively of sporadic cases and *PHOX2B* mutations have been detected in 2% of sporadic tumors.[100]

The clinical presentation of NB is dependent on the location of the primary tumor, but the majority of patients have symptoms and signs due to widespread disease at initial diagnosis such as fever, weight loss, irritability, bone pain, and cytopenias. Two-thirds of cases are associated with an abdominal primary and the great majority of NBs are located in the adrenal gland (Figure 2b). Children may present with abdominal pain, constipation, and distention. A large abdominal mass that typically crosses the midline is detected on physical examination. Cervical and thoracic tumors (posterior mediastinum) can be associated with Horner syndrome. Distinctive clinical presentations also include metastatic skin nodules and proptosis with "raccoon eyes" due to orbital involvement. Presacral and paraspinal tumors may present with cord compression with urinary retention, motor weakness, and clonus. Finally, NB may present with an unusual paraneoplastic syndrome characterized by opsoclonus/myoclonus syndrome (OMS) where children typically manifest darting eye movements and myoclonic jerks with or without ataxia.[101] Interestingly, OMS is often associated with favorable prognosis tumors but unfortunately, neurological symptoms persist after effective treatment of the NB.

Initial evaluation of NB includes cross-sectional imaging with CT or MRI of the chest, abdomen, and pelvis to determine local, regional (including extradural extension), and distant sites of disease. Metastatic disease at diagnosis is present in about 70% of patients. Meta-iodo-benzyl-guanidine (MIBG) is a norepinephrine analogue selectively taken up by sympathetic nervous tissue and is used to assess disease location not detected by CT or MRI. Approximately 90% of tumors are MIBG avid, but for those that are not avid, FDG-PET may be used. Bilateral bone marrow aspirates and biopsies are required to detect bone marrow involvement. The diagnosis is confirmed by biopsy of the primary or distant site involvement, or characteristic tumor cell in the bone marrow with elevated levels of vanillylmandelic acid (VMA) and homo-vanillic acid (HVA) in the urine.

Histologically, tumors can display a range of cellular differentiation from ganglioneuroma (differentiated) to ganglioneuroblastoma to typical NB. Typically, the tumor is composed of small round blue cells with rosettes. Tumors can be classified as favorable or unfavorable based on age, the degree of differentiation (differentiated associated with better prognosis), Schwannian stromal content, and the mitosis-karyorrhexis index (MKI, the number of mitoses and karyorrhexis (fragmented nuclei) per 5000 cells). An MKI less than 100 or 200, depending on stroma, age, and degree of differentiation, is associated with a better prognosis.[102]

Table 3 International neuroblastoma risk group staging system (INRGSS).[a]

L1	Localized tumor not involving vital structures as defined by the list of image-defined risk factors and confined to one body compartment
L2	Locoregional tumor with presence of one or more image-defined risk factors.
M	Distant metastatic disease (except stage MS)
MS	Metastatic disease in children younger than 18 months with metastases confined to skin, liver, and/or bone marrow

[a]Source: Monclair et al.[104]

An International Neuroblastoma Staging System (INSS) was initially developed to harmonize approaches and analyses of outcome worldwide.[103] It is noteworthy that children with 4S disease had a high degree of spontaneous regression in spite of widespread disease. More recently, this has been replaced by the International Neuroblastoma Risk Group) Staging System (INRGSS) based on radiographic features that indicate resectability and the presence of widespread metastatic disease (Table 3): L1 (localized tumors confined to one body compartment), L2 locoregional tumor with involvement of adjacent structures), M (distant metastasis), and MS (metastatic disease in children<18 months confined to skin, liver and/or bone marrow).[104]

Treatment stratification is based on a number of clinical and biological variables that allow classification into low-, intermediate- and high-risk categories. Two of the most important risk factors are age and stage with children <18 months of age having a distinctly better prognosis than older children stage for stage. The overall survival of children with INSS stages 1, 2, 3, and 4s was 91 +/− 1% compared to 42 +/− 1% for stage 4 disease.[105] NB was one of the first human tumors where genetic stratification has had a significant impact. *MYCN* amplification (>10 copies) is observed in 20% of cases and portends aggressive disease. Ploidy is also predictive of survival especially in infants and patients with localized disease where hyperdiploidy (i.e., whole chromosome gains) is associated with a good prognosis. The COG uses age, stage, histology, *MYCN* status and ploidy to classify patients into low- (40% tumors, EFS >95%), intermediate- (20%, EFS 80–95%), and high-risk (40%, EFS 40–50%) categories.[100] Additional genetic risk factors impact prognosis including allelic gains at 17q and LOH at 1p36 and 11q deletion, which are associated with a poor prognosis. In addition to the variables used for the COG risk classification 11q aberrations are used in the INRG classification system.[105] Newer classification approaches include the integration of segmental chromosome gains or losses. While gains of whole chromosomes have been associated with a good prognosis, segmental gains or losses are associated with a poor prognosis, particularly segmental loss at 1p, 3p, 4p, 11q or gains at 1q, 2p, or 17q.[106] Future studies will factor these variables into classification of lower-risk disease.[107,108]

Treatment for patients with low-risk disease (INSS 1, biologically favorable INSS 2A, 2B, 4S; INRGSS L1, MS without *MYCN* amplification) is surgery alone with chemotherapy reserved for patients with life-threatening symptoms or for the minority of patients whose disease progresses or recurs.[107] Notably, complete resection is not mandatory. Outcomes are excellent for low-risk patients with survival rates exceeding 95%. There is a subset of patients less than 6 months of age with small adrenal primaries whose tumors may regress without surgery.[109] Most INSS stage 4S/INRG stage MS patients undergo spontaneous regression but some infants present with massive hepatomegaly and associated respiratory distress necessitating immediate management with low dose chemotherapy and/or irradiation.

Intermediate-risk patients (e.g., INSS stage 3 and most stage 4 < 18 months, INRGSS L2 and M < 18 months if diploid and without *MYCN* amplification) are treated with surgery and moderately intensive chemotherapy that includes carboplatin or cisplatin, etoposide, cyclophosphamide, and doxorubicin for two to eight cycles depending on initial tumor response and other prognostic markers such as segmental chromosome abnormalities. In some cases, surgery may be avoided altogether as well as chemotherapy (L2 < 18 months). A study conducted by the COG demonstrated outstanding outcomes for intermediate-risk patients with 3-year overall survival exceeding 95% with risk-based reduced-intensity chemotherapy.[110]

Treatment of high-risk disease (*MYCN* amplification, INSS stage 4, INRGSS M and age ≥ 18 months or 12–18 months with unfavorable histology or genetics) remains a challenge, but stepwise improvements have occurred through the use of myeloablative regimens, differentiation therapy, and most recently immunotherapy.[111,112] Initial therapy consists of six cycles of dose-intensive chemotherapy with cyclophosphamide, topotecan, cisplatin, etoposide, doxorubicin, and vincristine or similar agents. Surgery (before consolidation with myeloablative chemotherapy) and irradiation therapy (after consolidation) to minimize tumor burden are routinely used in the high-risk setting. Studies have demonstrated that consolidation with myeloablative chemotherapy followed by autologous peripheral blood stem cell re-infusion improves outcome.[113] No benefit to purging the stem cell source and stem cells are usually harvested after two cycles of chemotherapy has been demonstrated.[114] Data exist to indicate that myeloablation with busulfan-melphalan is superior to other regimens[115] and that "tandem" courses of high-dose chemotherapy with stem cell rescue may be beneficial over a single course.[116,117] An ongoing COG study is assessing the benefit of targeted[118] I-MIBG prior to consolidation in the newly diagnosed setting.[107]

The use of biological approaches has also improved outcome for patients with high-risk disease. Isotretinoin has long been noted to differentiate tumor cells in culture but early use in the treatment of relapsed or refractory disease was disappointing. However, a randomized trial examining its impact when delivered after cytotoxic therapy in the setting of MRD for high-risk patients showed a substantial benefit and its use is currently being evaluated in patients with lower-risk disease[119] The additional use of the anti-GD2 monoclonal antibody (mab) dinutuximab in conjunction with granulocyte monocyte colony-stimulating factor (GMCSF) and interleukin-2 (IL-2) increased the 2-year survival significantly (66 +/− 5% with mab vs. 46% +/− 5% without mab).[112] More recently, IL-2 has not been shown to improve outcomes and it has been eliminated from contemporary postconsolidative regimens.[120]

Pediatric bone tumors

Malignant primary bone tumors that occur in both younger and older patients have important differences in pathogenesis, presentation, and treatment, and these differences will be highlighted. Although primary bone tumors are rare, they are the sixth most common malignant neoplasm in children and the third most frequent neoplasm in AYA. Malignant bone tumors occur in the United States at an annual rate of approximately 8.7 cases per million children and adolescents younger than 20 years. Only half the bone tumors in childhood are malignant, and of these, osteosarcoma (OS) is the most frequent, accounting for approximately 35% of all primary sarcomas of bone. Ewing sarcoma (EWS), the second most frequent primary bone cancer, is more common than OS in children younger than 10 years.

Osteosarcoma

OS, the most common primary malignant bone tumor, is composed of spindle cells producing osteoid. It is a highly aggressive neoplasm for which dramatic progress has been made in treatment and outcome during the past several decades. OS is primarily a disease of AYA; although it can also occur in older patients. OS has a bimodal age distribution, with the first peak in the second decade of life during the adolescent growth spurt, and the second among older adults. It is estimated that approximately 400 children and adolescents less than 20 years of age are diagnosed each year in the United States. It is extremely rare before the age of 5 years. The most common clinical presentation is pain, with or without an associated soft tissue mass in the involved region of bone. Among young patients, the most common location is the metaphysis of a long bone. Approximately half of all OSs originate around the knee joint.

The peak age coincides with a period of rapid bone growth in young people, suggesting a correlation between rapid bone growth and the evolution of OS. Radiation exposure is another well-documented etiologic factor. The incidence of OS is dramatically increased among survivors of RB. In the hereditary form of this disorder, germ-line mutations of the RB gene are common. This is the likely basis for the increased frequency of secondary cancers in this population, since the rate in survivors of unilateral sporadic RB is much less.[121] Germ-line mutations in the *TP53* gene can lead to a high risk of developing malignancies, including OS, which has been described as the Li–Fraumeni syndrome. Most OSs, including those in children and adolescents, are of the osteoblastic subtype. The current WHO classification recognizes two additional subtypes of conventional OS: chondroblastic (Figure 4) and fibroblastic based on the predominant pattern of differentiation. Telangiectatic OS is a rare subtype, which appears as a purely lytic lesion on plain radiographs and thus, may be confused with aneurysmal bone cyst or giant cell tumor.

Similar to other sarcomas in young patients (typically high-grade), OS metastasizes very early in its evolution. Approximately 20% of patients present with radiographically detectable metastases, most frequently to the lung, while almost all newly diagnosed patients with OS have at least micro-metastatic disease as evidenced by the fact that if treated by surgical resection alone, 80% will relapse in the lung within 2 years.[122] Death from OS is almost always the result of progressive pulmonary metastasis with respiratory failure, pulmonary hemorrhage, pneumothorax, or superior vena cava obstruction. The diagnosis of OS is typically suspected by the radiographic appearance of the affected lesion. OS can present as a lytic, sclerotic, or a mixed lytic-sclerotic lesion. The diagnosis of OS is dependent on a biopsy for histologic examination providing a pathological diagnosis. OS is a pleomorphic, spindle cell tumor that forms an extracellular matrix consisting mostly of osteoid. Immunohistochemistry and cytogenetics are not helpful in diagnosing OS. Patients with OS should undergo a staging work-up to determine the extent of disease at presentation, which includes plain radiographs and MRI of the involved bone and should capture the adjoining joints, noncontrast chest CT, a bone scan, and/or a PET scan.

Multiagent systemic chemotherapy, along with local and metastatic disease control with surgery is the standard of care.[122] The standard chemotherapy of patients with nonmetastatic OS, although variable, includes the use of cisplatin and doxorubicin with the addition of high-dose methotrexate. Advances made in surgical techniques have significantly improved the clinical practice and functional limb salvage options available for patients. Rosen et al. introduced the concept of chemotherapy prior to surgical resection.[123] While no differences in outcome are reported with the incorporation of neoadjuvant chemotherapy versus upfront surgery followed by adjuvant chemotherapy, neoadjuvant chemotherapy does provide several potential advantages, including better resectability if tumor shrinks, improved surgical planning and endoprosthetic customization, treatment of micro-metastatic disease, and above all, the ability to assess the response to chemotherapy. A strong correlation between the degree of necrosis and the probability of subsequent DFS was observed,[124] which has subsequently been confirmed in multiple clinical trials. Soon after the identification of the prognostic value of the degree of necrosis following induction chemotherapy, it was suggested that chemotherapy be modified for the patients with less necrosis. Despite an early report of benefit, intensified regimens including ifosfamide and etoposide have not improved outcome for poor responders.[125] Because complete surgical resection is imperative for the cure of OS, surgical resectability is an important prognostic factor, therefore, patients presenting with axial skeleton tumors fare worse than those having tumors in appendicular skeleton.

The standard management for patients with metastatic disease at the time of initial diagnosis follows the same general principles as those who present with localized disease. The outcome of OS patients depends on several factors. The most consistent prognostic factor at diagnosis is the presence of clinically detectable metastases, which confers an unfavorable prognosis. In patients with metastatic disease at diagnosis, the number of pulmonary nodules, as well as whether they are unilateral or bilateral is also of prognostic significance. With currently available regimens, approximately 60–70% of patients with nonmetastatic OS of the extremity will survive without evidence of recurrence. In most large reported studies, only 10–20% of patients who present with clinically detectable metastatic disease survive. OS is resistant to radiation therapy, thus it is not a part of standard OS treatment and is reserved for pain/symptoms relief in palliative care settings only.

The survival of patients with OS appears to have reached a plateau. At present, none of the agents in early phase clinical trials have shown promise to move them in the frontline therapy. Research is ongoing to elucidate novel molecular targets in OS, of which anti-GD2 antibody and RANKL antibody are of particular interest.[126]

Ewing sarcoma

EWS is the second most common primary malignant bone tumor in children and adolescents. EWS is a part of peripheral primitive neuroectodermal tumors (PPNET). In the early 1980s, EWS and PPNET were both found to contain the same reciprocal translocation between chromosomes 11 and 22, t(11;22) (q24;q12).[127,128] Later that decade, similar patterns of oncogene expression (c-myc, N-myc, c-myb, and c-mil/raf-1) were seen among these tumors. The combination of the shared translocation, cellular physiology, and clinical response has led to categorizing these tumors into the Ewing sarcoma family of tumors (EWSFT). The EWSFT includes EWS, PPNET, neuroepithelioma, atypical EWS, and Askin tumor (an EWSFT of the chest wall).

Most cases are thought to be sporadic, but family members of EWSFT patients have an increased incidence of neuroectodermal and stomach malignancies.[129] EWSFT are thought to derive from cells of neuroectodermal origin, possibly postganglionic cholinergic neurons, although the exact cell of origin has yet to be identified. The immunohistochemical hallmark of EWSFT is diffuse membranous staining for CD99 (MIC2), which is present in greater than 90% of EWSFT. Undifferentiated tumors are negative for other markers except vimentin and FLI-1, whereas more differentiated tumors variably express additional markers, including neuron-specific enolase, S-100, neurofilaments, CD57, and synaptophysin. Muscle and lymphoid markers are negative. The translocation t(11;22)(q24;q12), or another related translocation, occurs in greater than 95% of EWSFT. Some argue that such a translocation is pathognomonic and is both necessary and sufficient for a diagnosis of EWSFT. The classic t(11;22)(q24;q12) translocation joins the EWS gene located on chromosome 22 to an ets-family gene, *FLI1* (Friend Leukemia Insertion), located on chromosome 11. Other ETS family partners are *ERG* t(21;22), *ETV1* t(7;22), and *E1AF* t(17;22). Standard cytogenetics and fluorescence in situ hybridization (FISH) can reveal this anomaly and additional karyotypic abnormalities, including trisomies 8 and 12, and chromosomes 1 and 16 abnormalities. Some of the t(21;22) translocations remain cryptic by standard cytogenetic techniques and require reverse transcription-polymerase chain reaction (RT-PCR) or FISH.

The incidence of EWSFT peaks in the latter half of the second decade of life. An enigma in EWSFT is its racial distribution. The incidence in whites is at least nine-fold higher than in blacks. EWS arises most commonly in the bone but can also originate in extraosseous soft tissues. Frequent primary sites include the pelvis (25%), femur (16%), ribs (12%), and spine (8%). Approximately 25% of patients present with metastatic disease. Of these, 37% (or 9% of all patients) have metastases confined to the lung or pleura. The remaining patients have bone and/or bone marrow metastases, either alone or in addition to pulmonary/pleural disease. Rarely, patients with bone marrow metastases have extensive infiltration and present with systemic symptoms. Diagnosis is typically done by tumor biopsy. Staging work-up typically includes MRI/CT of the primary site, CT scan of the chest to evaluate for lung metastasis, bone scan, and bone marrow aspiration and biopsy. Recently, FDG-PET/CT is replacing bone scan for EWS metastatic work-up. The most consistent prognostic factor is the presence of metastatic disease at diagnosis. The presence of an axial tumor, older age at diagnosis, larger size of primary tumor, and poor histologic response after induction chemotherapy are other adverse prognostic indicators in EWS.

The successful management of patients with ESFT requires the use of both local and systemic therapy. Both surgery and radiation therapy are utilized for local control while systemic control is achieved by chemotherapy. EWS, unlike OS, is quite radio-responsive, and RT is considered a standard option for definitive local control. RT can be used as an alternative to disfiguring surgery such as amputation. Alkylating agents (cyclophosphamide, ifosfamide, melphalan, and busulfan) and doxorubicin are the most active single agents in EWS, while addition of ifosfamide plus etoposide has led to significant increase in EFS and OS, particularly for localized disease.[130] Recently, the COG has shown superior efficacy of dose-intensive therapy administered every 2 weeks with filgrastim support compared to the conventional every-3-week therapy for patients with initially localized disease.[131] Altogether, these measures have increased 5-year EFS of localized EWS to approximately 75%.

EWS patients with disease metastatic at initial diagnosis have a poor outcome. Patients with multiple sites of metastases have the lowest survival rates. Patients with metastases confined to the lungs may represent a group of patients with better prognosis than patients with bone or bone marrow metastases. Overall cure rates for metastatic EWS remain 20%, utilizing the standard interval compressed chemotherapy including ifosfamide and etoposide as described above for localized disease along with local control of primary and metastatic sites utilizing surgery and radiation therapy. Myeloablative chemotherapy followed by autologous stem cell rescue has not shown significant improvement in overall survival.[132]

Moving forward, based on feasibility of adding topotecan/cyclophosphamide in a pilot study, COG is running a phase 3 randomized trial for patients with localized EWS. The insulin-like growth factor type I receptor (IGF-1R) is critical for transformation and growth of ESFT[118] and incorporation of antibody against IGF-1R with intensified chemotherapy backbone is being investigated through the COG for newly diagnosed metastatic EWS patients. In addition, mTOR inhibitors are being tested in relapse and refractory EWS.[126]

Soft tissue sarcomas

Soft tissue sarcomas represent a widely heterogeneous group of malignancies that in aggregate account for 7.4% of cancers in children and adolescents up to 19 years of age. Approximately 800–900 cases are diagnosed per year in the United States.[2] The most common soft tissue sarcoma is RMS that is derived in large part from striated muscle while others originate from fibrous connective tissue (fibrosarcoma), smooth muscle (leiomyosarcoma), and fat (liposarcoma). Synovial cell sarcoma is now thought to originate in precursor cells distinct from those that lead to synovium.

Rhabdomyosarcoma

RMS accounts for 50% of soft tissue tumors in children under 14 years of age. By far most cases of RMS are sporadic although cases have been described in association with NF-1, Costello syndrome, Beckwith–Wiedemann syndrome, and Li–Fraumeni syndrome. The histologic hallmark of RMS, a small round blue cell tumor, is evidence of skeletal muscle differentiation most often validated by immunohistochemistry (MyoD, myogenin, muscle-specific actin, myoglobin, and desmin). RMS is composed of two histologic subtypes. Embryonal RMS (ERMS, 60–75% of cases) is characterized by spindle cells with myxoid areas whereas alveolar RMS typically shows oval cells forming alveolar spaces surrounded by fibrous septae.[133] The majority of alveolar cases are characterized by translocations between the DNA-binding domains of PAX3 (55% of ARMS) or PAX7 (20%) and FOXO1. About 15% of ARMS are fusion negative. The outcome for ERMS is superior to that of ARMS and patients with fusion negative ARMS have a better outcome compared to fusion-positive cases.[134] Interestingly, ERMS is associated with a higher mutational burden and frequent alterations of RAS pathway genes.[135]

The clinical presentation of RMS depends on location. Forty percent of RMS occur in the head, neck, and orbit. Symptoms can include a painless mass (superficial head and neck primary tumors), proptosis and esotropia (orbital tumors), snoring, recurrent unilateral epistaxis, sinusitis, and cranial nerve palsies (nasopharyngeal and paranasal lesions). Genitourinary RMS accounts for 20% of cases and bladder/prostate lesions can lead to urinary obstruction. Approximately 20% occur in the extremities and usually present as a painless mass. Extremity tumors tend to be of the alveolar subtype whereas the majority of tumors located in the head, neck, and GU sites are ERMS. The botryoid variant of ERMS arises under mucosal surfaces (e.g., vagina, nasopharynx) and can present as a protruding grape-like mass.

The clinical evaluation of patients includes cross-sectional imaging CT or MRI) of the primary with evaluation of possible metastatic disease (chest CT, bilateral bone marrow aspirates and biopsies, and bone scan). Approximately 15% of patients will have metastatic disease at diagnosis, most commonly lung followed by bone marrow, lymph node, and bone. RMS is classified according to well-documented determinants of prognosis such as age, location of the primary tumor, extent of disease (group), histologic subtype, and stage. The stage incorporates the site of the primary (favorable site vs. unfavorable site) and a pretreatment assessment of tumor size (confined to organ, T1 vs. extension, T2; size ≤ 5 cm or >5 cm), nodal status (N_0 uninvolved, N_1, involved, N_X unknown) and metastasis (M_0 or M_1). Favorable sites include the orbit, nonparameningeal head and neck, biliary, and non-bladder/prostate genitourinary sites. The group is dependent on the surgical resectability (Group 1—completely resected, Group II—gross total resection with evidence of regional spread, Group III—gross residual disease, Group IV—distant metastasis at diagnosis). Regional lymph nodes should be sampled in cases of RMS located in the extremities and retroperitoneal LN sampling is recommended in patients with paratesticular primaries who are over 10 years of age. Of note, initial response to chemotherapy has not been proven to be prognostic in COG studies. These variables have been used to develop a risk stratification used in COG trials (Table 4).[136]

Table 4 COG risk stratification for rhabdomyosarcoma[a].

Risk group	Stage	Group	Histology	Percent of cases (%)	EFS (%)
Low, subset 1	1	I–II	ERMS	27	85–95
	1	III (orbit)	ERMS		
	2	I–II	ERMS		
Low, subset 2	1	III (nonorbit)	ERMS	5	70–85
	3	I–II	ERMS		
Intermediate	2–3	III	ERMS	27	73
	1–3	I–III	ARMS	25	65
High	4	IV	ERMS	8	35
	4	IV	ARMS	8	15

[a]Source: Hawkins et al.[136]

Treatment for RMS requires a multidisciplinary approach. The chemotherapeutic agents most beneficial are vincristine, dactinomycin, and cyclophosphamide (VAC). Patients with low-risk disease, subset 1, can be effectively managed with a short course of VAC treatment where the dose of cyclophosphamide is minimized to avoid infertility whereas a higher dose of the drug is required for subset 2 patients.[137] Patients with Group II and III tumors receive irradiation. There have been many attempts to improve outcome for intermediate-risk patients with the addition of agents such as etoposide, carboplatin, ifosfamide, and topotecan to VAC, but to date such efforts have been disappointing. A COG study looked at the addition of vincristine/irinotecan (V/I) to VAC and while EFS was not improved there was less hematologic toxicity and the total dose of cyclophosphamide was lower. Thus, moving forward VAC/VI is likely the standard of care for intermediate-risk RMS.[138] A major breakthrough in treatment for patients with intermediate-risk RMS is the recent observation that a 6-month maintenance course of vinorelbine and cyclophosphamide is associated with significantly improved outcome and is now the standard of care.[139] In contrast, there has been little improvement in outcome for high-risk disease but the use of interval compressed Ifosfamide/etoposide and vincristine/doxorubicin/cyclophosphamide may be associated with a substantial gain for a subset of patients with limited additional risk factors based on age, primary site, bone/bone

Table 5 Nonrhabdomyosarcoma prognostic groups.[a]

Risk group	Gross resection	Grade	Size	Distant metastasis	Percent of NRSTS (%)	Five-year survival (%)
Low	Yes	Low	Any	No	60	90
	Yes	High	<5 cm	No		
Intermediate	Yes	High	>5 cm	No	30	50
	No	Any	Any	No		
High	Any	Any	Any	Yes	10	15

[a]Source: Adapted from Toretsky et al.[136]; Spunt and Anderson[142].

marrow disease and the number of metastatic sites.[140] A number of drugs are being considered or are under investigation including some of which are aimed at molecular targets such as tyrosine kinase signaling, IGF-1R (autocrine activation), ALK (amplified), C- Met (overexpressed), and RAS (mutated in ERMS).[136,141] Finally, while immune checkpoint inhibition, in general, has not yielded promising results, other immunotherapeutic approaches are being developed including CAR T cells.

Nonrhabdomyosarcoma soft tissue sarcomas

Nonrhabdomyosarcoma soft tissue sarcomas (NRSTS) represent a wide variety of tumors with distinct genetic, pathologic, and clinical profiles. They tend to occur in older patients and most are located in the extremities. Many are associated with distinct genetic lesions that are diagnostic such as synovial sarcoma (t(X;18)p11;q11) (*SYT-SS1* and *SYT-SSX2*). The mainstay of treatment is surgery and irradiation is used for patients with high-grade lesions and positive margins. The impact of chemotherapy is less certain but neoadjuvant therapy may be indicated to improve chances of surgical excision. The use of adjuvant chemotherapy in addition to irradiation for larger grossly resected tumors is more controversial but was recommended in the recent COG protocol for these tumors.[142] Table 5 summarizes risk groups and outcomes.[136,143] Note some subtypes including infantile fibrosarcoma contain chromosomal fusions involving neurotrophic receptor tyrosine kinase genes (*TRK*) and these may be targeted by NTRK inhibitors such as larotrectinib.[144]

Central nervous system tumors

Significant differences in epidemiology, molecular genetics, and biology distinguish CNS tumors of the infant and child from those arising in adulthood. Because of these differences, important aspects of clinical presentation, treatment, and outcome are uniquely related to childhood CNS tumors.

CNS tumors are the most common solid tumor of childhood, with 5000 new cases per year in the United States.[145] Pediatric brain tumors vary considerably in their histological, topographical, and gender distribution throughout childhood and adolescence. Boys are more commonly affected than girls in all age groups, but this increase is accounted for mostly by medulloblastoma, embryonal tumors, and ependymoma. Over 90% of CNS tumors in children are primary brain tumors, in contrast to adults where up to 90% are metastases from other organs. Survival has improved from 60% in 1975 to 1984 to 65% in 1985–1994 to 73.3% in 1995–2011 and survival is noted to improve with increasing age: 45% in those aged less than 1 year, 59% in those aged 1–4 years, 64% in 5- to 9-year-old, 70% in 10- to 14-year-old, and 77% in 15- to 19-year-old. The main histological entities in children are pilocytic astrocytomas (PAs) (15%), followed by malignant gliomas (14%), benign tumors of the pituitary (13%), embryonal tumors (10%), and craniopharyngiomas (3.4%),[145,146] while high-grade glial tumors, anaplastic astrocytoma, and glioblastoma accounts for majority of adult brain tumors, followed by meningiomas and other mesenchymal tumors.

In the United States, CNS tumors are the most common cause of death due to cancer in childhood, accounting for 24% of cancer-related deaths. Morbidity as a result of increasingly successful treatment approaches remains high and includes cognitive, memory and learning impairment, neuroendocrine deficiencies, hearing deficits, sterility, and secondary cancers.

The etiology of CNS tumors remains mostly unknown. The known risk factors include (1) gender (male), (2) therapeutic doses of ionizing radiation to the head (e.g., for leukemia or prior brain tumor), and (3) genetic syndromes such as neurofibromatosis, tuberous sclerosis, nevoid basal cell carcinoma syndrome (Gorlin syndrome), Turcot's syndrome, and Li–Fraumeni syndrome.

Embryonal tumors of the CNS comprise a group of tumors that share a histologically similar, undifferentiated morphology, and represent the second most common malignant brain tumor group in children (10%). The incidence is constant from infancy to 3 years of age and then a steady decline is observed thereafter. This group includes the CNS-PNETs (primitive neuroectodermal tumors), pineoblastomas, and atypical teratoid rhabdoid tumor (AT/RT). CNS-PNETs are a group of highly malignant tumors composed of small round blue cells of neuroectodermal origin. Controversy has existed regarding the class division between CNS-PNET, pineoblastoma, and medulloblastoma but the preponderance of molecular genetic, biologic, and clinical evidence validates this division.[147,148]

Medulloblastoma is the most common malignant brain tumor in children, with a bimodal peak age distribution first being between 3 and 4 years and again between 8 and 10 years of age. It has a typical radiographic presentation of a solid midline posterior fossa mass that arises from cerebellum and occupies the fourth ventricle (Figure 3a). Surgery (preferred gross total resection) and craniospinal irradiation have been essential elements of successful therapy for medulloblastoma. However, to reduce late effects, especially in very young children, the incorporation of chemotherapy has permitted a reduction in radiation dose. Recently, tandem high-dose chemotherapy with stem cell rescue has demonstrated even further benefit without compromising survival in high-risk medulloblastomas.

More recently, medulloblastomas have been categorized into 4 groups by transcriptional profiling: WNT, Sonic Hedgehog (SHH), group 3, and group 4.[149] Tumors displaying WNT pathway activation, comprise 10% of tumors while approximately 30% exhibit activation of SHH pathway as a result of mutations in genes including *PTCH1* and *SMO*, both associated with favorable prognosis. Group 3 constitutes tumors with a poor prognosis, irrespective of their metastatic status. Ongoing research is examining treatment stratification by subgroup and potentially new targets for more effective and less toxic therapies.

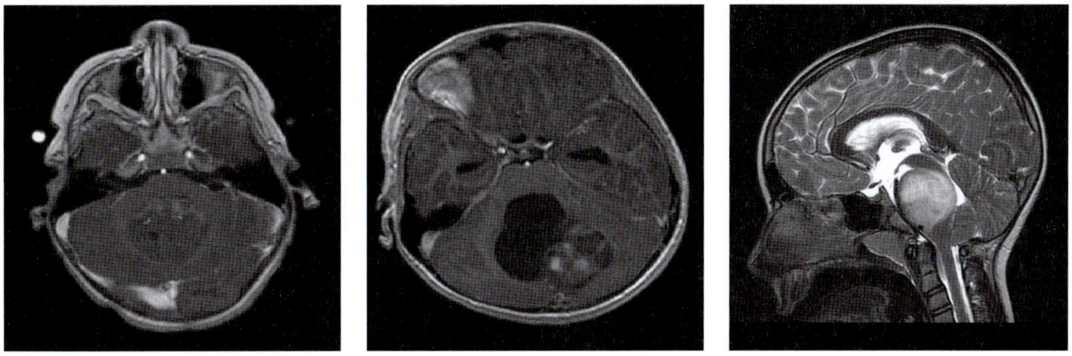

Figure 3 MRI imaging findings of common pediatric brain tumors: (a) Axial T1 image with contrast showing a midline tumor in the cerebellum, and pathology consistent with medulloblastoma. (b) T1 weighted axial MRI image with contrast of typical pilocytic astrocytoma in the cerebellum of a 5-year-old child showing heterogeneously enhancing mural nodule and intratumoral cysts, dilated temporal horns bilaterally suggestive of hydrocephalus. (c) T2 weighted sagittal view showing diffuse enlargement of pons in a patient with Diffuse Intrinsic Pontine Glioma.

AT/RT is an aggressively malignant, primitive tumor most often arising in children younger than 2 years of age. Approximately half of AT/RTs arise in the infratentorial compartment with a propensity to invade the cerebellopontine angle. Because of its association with chromosome 22 deletion and mutation of *SMARCB1/INI1* (tumor suppressor gene), analysis of these markers in infants and children with presumed medulloblastoma/CNS-PNET is being used as a molecular diagnostic tool for this tumor. Germline mutations of SMARCB1 are found in approximately 50% of infants with AT/RT and put the child at risk for rhabdoid tumors throughout the body. Once thought of as an incurable disease, treatment regimens including radiation and/or high-dose chemotherapy with stem cell rescue have recently demonstrated long-term survival approaching 50%.

Ependymoma makes up approximately 5% of childhood CNS tumors with approximately two-thirds occurring infratentorially. Greater than half of these tumors occur in children less than 5 years of age with a peak during the second year of life. The addition of chemotherapy to surgery and RT for childhood ependymoma has not been proven to impact overall survival, although studies are ongoing to investigate this further.

Glial neoplasms range from benign low-grade gliomas which can be resected and/or observed to aggressive high-grade gliomas which have extremely poor outcome. Low-grade gliomas broadly encompass both PAs (WHO grade 1) and diffuse fibrillary astrocytomas (WHO grade 2), while high-grade gliomas comprise of anaplastic astrocytoma (WHO grade 3), glioblastomas, and diffuse midline gliomas with H3K27M mutation (both WHO grade 4). The incidence of cortical astrocytomas increases with age, having a first peak at age 5 and again at age 13. In children, brain stem and cerebellar astrocytomas are as common as cortical tumors. Cerebellar astrocytoma is found almost exclusively in children, occurring most frequently between ages 4 and 9. PA is the most common subtype, accounting for 85% of cerebellar astrocytomas (Figure 3b). Diffuse astrocytoma is the next most common, whereas malignant astrocytoma is rare in this location. Total surgical resection is curative in 95–100%. PAs may stabilize for long periods of time or even spontaneously regress; however, the behavior of cerebellar astrocytomas in children with neurofibromatosis type I (NF-1) may be more aggressive. Gliomas of the visual pathway, hypothalamus, and thalamus comprise a relatively common form of childhood astrocytoma. Tumors of the optic chiasm and hypothalamus are usually low-grade, whereas thalamic tumors tend to be more variable. Twenty percent of children with NF-1 will develop visual pathway tumors, predominantly PA, during childhood. These tumors present most frequently between 5 and 10 years of age. Recent studies have highlighted the role of MAPK/ERK pathway in the oncogenesis of these tumors. While IDH1 mutations characterize the vast majority of low-grade and secondary high-grade gliomas in adults,[150] the majority of pediatric low-grade gliomas harbor BRAF alterations in the form of *BRAF* gene rearrangement or point mutation.[151,152] Tumors with these driver molecular alterations have shown sensitivity at recurrence to either BRAF inhibitors (for the BRAF V600E point mutant tumors) or MEK inhibitors (for the BRAF gene rearranged tumors) but these approaches have only recently started phase 3 randomized trials comparing them to standard cytotoxic chemotherapy, and so the optimal upfront therapy is still unclear.

Brain stem gliomas (BSG) comprise 10–15% of all pediatric CNS tumors and are generally uncommon in the adult population. Peak incidence is between the ages of 5 and 9 years of age but may occur anytime during childhood. BSGs most commonly arise in the pons (diffuse intrinsic), in which location they typically behave like adult glioblastomas multiforme (GBM) and have an almost uniformly dismal prognosis (Figure 3c). In contrast, those arising from midbrain or medulla are likely to be low-grade lesions that have a more indolent course and better outcome. Surgery and postoperative radiation therapy is the mainstay of therapy in children with high-grade gliomas. Recently, sequencing studies have shown recurrent but mutually exclusive mutations in histone H3F3A and HIST1H3B in about 30–40% of pediatric glioblastomas,[153] suggesting disrupted epigenetic regulatory mechanisms, which can be further exploited for therapeutic targeting.

Intracranial germ-cell tumors (IGCTs) account for less than 5% of pediatric CNS tumors but are primarily seen in children and adolescents, with 90% occurring in those less than 20 years. Incidence peaks at age 10–12 years. They account for nearly 50% of all pineal region tumors of childhood. Germinomas account for approximately two-thirds of IGCTs, while the remaining third are nongerminomatous germ-cell tumors (GCTs), including yolk sac tumor, choriocarcinoma, mixed GCTs, and mature and immature teratomas. Elevation of serum and CSF tumor markers as AFP and β-hHCG along with radiologic findings can be used as surrogate diagnostic markers, but when the results of tumor markers are equivocal, tumor biopsy is performed for definitive diagnosis.

Germinomas are highly radiosensitive and 5-year overall survival is >90% with radiation alone. COG is currently investigating the effect of chemotherapy followed by response-based radiation therapy, in order to minimize the radiation dose and subsequent long-term side effects.

Less-frequently encountered tumors

Individually, RB, GCTs, liver tumors, and carcinomas are less frequently encountered tumors in pediatric but collectively, however, these neoplasms account for up to 18% of all cancers seen in children and adolescents. Moreover, the incidence of some of these tumors, such as GCT malignancies and certain carcinomas, is significantly higher in older patients, those aged between 15 and 19 years, a population that has been under-represented in prospective cooperative national trials.

Retinoblastoma

RB is the most frequent neoplasm of the eye in childhood and represents 3% of all pediatric cancers. An estimated 200–300 children develop RB each year. Most patients present in infancy during the first 2 years of life (two-thirds of cases, 95% <5 years), and the tumor originates in the retina with usual extension into the vitreous cavity.[154] Common symptoms are leukocoria and strabismus. RB presents in two distinct clinical forms: (1) bilateral or multifocal, hereditary (25% of cases), characterized by the presence of germline mutations of the RB1 gene either inherited from an affected parent (25%) or as a result of a new germline mutation, and (2) unilateral (75% of cases). Ninety percent of unilateral cases are nonhereditary. Patients with bilateral RB present at an earlier age (<1 year) compared to children with unilateral nonhereditary disease (2–3 years).

Based on clinical forms of the disease, Knudsen proposed the classic "two-hit" hypothesis in 1971 where two mutational events were needed in a retinal cell for transformation.[155] Further analyses indicated that the two events were in fact disruption of both alleles of a single gene, a tumor suppressor gene. The RB1 gene, located in chromosome 13q14, was identified and cloned in 1986.[156] The product of RB1 (pRb) is a 110 kD nuclear phosphoprotein that acts by influencing the transcription of several genes involved in cell cycle progression. The level of pRb phosphorylation varies throughout the cell cycle and inactivation removes the pRb constraint on cell-cycle control, with the consequence of deregulated cell proliferation.

Patients with hereditary RB are born with a germline defect in RB1 and inactivation of the other RB1 allele is a somatic event whereas unilateral or nonhereditary tumors have somatic inactivation of both alleles. The RB1 gene is large containing 27 exons over about 200 kb of DNA, and mutations have been described in almost every exon. Nonsense and frameshift mutations are the most common germ-line and somatic events (>80%), although deletions are seen (10–20%).[157] While loss of RB1 is the critical step in tumor pathogenesis it is clear additional events are required for tumor development. All patients with RB require genetic counseling and genetic testing. While there are no mutational hotspots, technology has advanced so that almost all cases of germline predisposition can be identified. A recent study reported testing of the aqueous humor of the affected eye(s) for cell-free DNA as a method of rapid diagnosis of tumor RB1 status, as well as the presence of poor prognostic tumor alterations such as gain of 6p, and this approach may soon become part of prospective clinical trials.[158]

Suspected cases of RB are diagnosed by an experienced ophthalmologist by an exam under anesthesia with a dilated pupil. Imaging studies such as MRI, CT, and ultrasound are helpful in distinguishing RB from other causes of leucocoria (retrolental fibrodysplasia, Coats disease, toxocariasis, and toxoplasmosis) and to assess extraocular extension. CT may be used with caution given the increased risk of secondary tumors associated with radiation in patients with hereditary forms of the disease. Many staging systems are currently in use to predict outcome and guide therapy.[159]

The goals of therapy are to: eradicate the tumor optimizing cure, preserve vision, and avoid long-term complications particularly second malignancies. Typically, patients with unilateral tumors present with large tumors where there is little chance for preserving vision. Enucleation is curative in >90% of cases of unilateral tumors. Careful pathological examination of the resected specimen by an experienced ocular pathologist is needed to determine if any features associated with metastatic disease are present: vitreous seeding, massive choroidal involvement, tumor beyond lamina cribrosa, and scleral/extra-scleral extension. These features would dictate the use of chemotherapy, usually with combinations of the effective drugs including vincristine, doxorubicin, cyclophosphamide, carboplatin, and etoposide. For small tumors where vision preservation is possible, chemotherapy and local control with photocoagulation, cryotherapy and thermotherapy may be considered.[160] Direct ocular delivery of chemotherapy via the ophthalmic artery has been used with increasing frequency.[161] RB is particularly radiation sensitive but given concerns about second malignancies it is usually reserved for salvage. Chemotherapy (systemic +/− periocular or subtenon administration) is given to patients with bilateral tumors to lower tumor burden followed by local control measures.[154,162,163] This has resulted in higher eye salvage rates and decreased and delayed use of radiation therapy.

The risk of secondary tumors is strikingly higher for patients with the hereditary form of RB and risk is further increased by irradiation therapy.[121] Bone (OS) and soft tissue sarcomas, tumors of the nasal cavity, and melanoma are the most common secondary cancers. Given the association with radiation many tumors originate on the head and neck area but since germline mutations predispose to subsequent cancers independent of irradiation (and chemotherapy) many tumors are outside of the original radiation field.

Germ cell tumors

GCTs account for about 3.5% of tumors in children and adolescents and 60% originate in extragonadal sites. This distribution is related in part to the aberrant migration of primordial germ cells in the developing embryo and persistence at sites outside their normal destination into the ovary or testes. GCTs display a wide spectrum of clinical presentations depending on primary site and pathological features that range from benign to malignant. A single tumor may show a variety of tissue types and both benign and malignant elements. The age distribution follows a bimodal pattern, with a peak during the first 3 years of life and a second peak in late adolescence. In general, females have a higher overall incidence of GCT, although males are more at risk of malignant GCT. Cryptorchidism is a risk factor for the subsequent development of testicular GCT and interestingly this increased risk extends to the normally descended contralateral testis.[164] Surgical or hormonal correction ameliorates but does not eliminate the risk. Klinefelter syndrome (47 XXY) is also associated with an increased risk of GCT and all males with mediastinal GCT should

Table 6 Malignant germ cell tumors.

Tumor	Frequency	Clinical Features	Histology	Common locations	Tumor markers
Unipotential variants					
Germinoma seminoma (testes)	12%	Older age	Large cells with clear cytoplasm	Ovary, anterior mediastinum, brain, testes (much older pts.)	Negative (*mildly* elevated HCG may be seen in selected cases)
Dysgerminoma (ovary)					
Germinoma (extragonadal)					
Totipotential variants					
Embryonal Carcinoma	8%		Similar to yolk sac tumors but cells are larger, with a major epithelial pattern	Testes, many locations	Negative or mildly elevated
Yolk sac (endodermal sinus tumor)	55%		Pseudopapillary (Schiller–Duval bodies), reticular, polyvessicular, and solid patterns	Ovary, testicle sacrococcygeal location	Elevated AFP, normal HCG
Choriocarcinoma	1% (nongestational)	High likelihood of dessiminated disease	Cytotrophoblasts and syncytiotrophoblasts	Ovary, testicle, extragonadal	Elevated HCG
Malignant germ cell tumors of mixed histology	24%		Composed of immature and mature teratoma but also composed of one or more types of malignant GCT	Ovary, testicle, extragonadal	Elevated AFB and/or HCG

be screened for this condition.[165] Likewise, children with 46 XY gonadal dysgenesis (Swyer syndrome) are predisposed to GCTs.

The pathological classification of GCTs is partly predicated on their histopathological origin (germinoma vs. nongerminoma) and whether they are benign or malignant (mature teratomas, immature teratomas, and malignant GCTs).[166] Teratomas contain tissues from multiple embryonic germ layers (endoderm, mesoderm, and ectoderm) with varying degrees of differentiation. They are classified into three categories: benign, immature, and malignant teratomas [malignant GCT of mixed histologies (discussed below)]. Benign teratomas contain well-differentiated tissues such as cartilage, squamous epithelium, smooth muscle and some may contain more complex structures like teeth, salivary glands, etc. Mature teratomas are commonly observed in the sacrococcygeal region and ovary. Immature teratomas contain immature elements usually neuroepithelium but can also be immature mesenchyma or renal blastema. Immature teratomas usually occur in the ovaries, and rarely in extraovarian sites. They are graded into four categories according to the degree of maturation. Grades 0–2 usually have a benign behavior. Another benign GCT is gonadoblastoma that occurs exclusively in dysgenetic gonads.

Malignant GCTs include a spectrum of tumors that are summarized in Table 6. Symptoms are related to the site of the primary tumor. Cytogenetic and molecular studies have confirmed that childhood GCTs constitute a group of distinct entities. A distinct chromosomal aberration, i(12p), is often seen in adult GCT. In children, however, the i(12p) is found almost exclusively in gonadal and extragonadal (usually mediastinal) tumors of adolescent males.[167] Gains in chromosomes 1q, 2, 3, 7, 8, 12, and 14 have been described in tumors originating in prepubertal females, whereas tumors in prepubertal males have been found to have gains in chromosomes 1q, 7, and 21, and losses in chromosome 1p.[167] Finally, del 1p36 is a common finding in extragonadal and testicular tumors in young children with YST.[168] Recently, LIN28 a key regulator of BLIMP1 which is essential for the development of embryonic germ cells has been shown to be overexpressed in GCTs.[169] The sacrococcyx is the most common location of GCTs in children.[170] Most occur in the first 2 years of life. Two-thirds of these tumors are mature or immature teratomas and symptoms include a visible mass, urinary retention, constipation, and weakness of the lower extremities due to compression. The ovary is the second most common site and abdominal pain is the most common symptom. Torsion of the ovary may precipitate acute pain. Almost 70% of ovarian GCTs are benign teratomas. Dysgerminoma and malignant tumors of mixed histology account for 80% of malignant ovarian GCTs with most of the remainder being yolk sac tumors. Ten percent occur in the testes and these cases present as slowly growing masses. Two-thirds of these cases are yolk sac tumors. Mediastinal GCTs account for 4% of bases and patients present with wheezing, cough, and shortness of breath. There is a strong male bias and most cases occur in children over ten. About 3% of GCTs occur in the CNS.

The diagnostic evaluation includes cross-sectional imaging to assess the extent of primary disease and potential dissemination (lymph nodes, intracavitary seeding, lungs, liver, and possibly the CNS) and tumor markers. Many staging systems exist for GCTs and there are current efforts to decide on a consensus staging system to be shared by pediatric, adult, and gynecologic oncologists.[171] Most of the current systems rely on age, extent of disease including resectability, lymph node involvement, and presence of metastasis.[171] Therapy is based on the biology of individual tumor subtypes and stage.[172] Mature teratomas are treated with surgery alone as are immature teratomas. The use of chemotherapy in incompletely resected immature teratomas is controversial. Stage I completely resected testicular and ovarian (dysgerminoma) tumors can be treated with surgery alone and observation (including regression of tumor markers) since most patients (>80%) are cured and salvage with chemotherapy is quite high for the minority who recur. In general, retroperitoneal lymph node dissections are not performed in children with testicular GCT. Note stage I nongerminoma ovarian tumors may also be treated with surgery followed by observation. The relapse rate is significantly higher than for ovarian dysgerminoma but salvage is also high.[173] Surgery and chemotherapy are recommended for stages II–IV ovarian and testicular tumors. The standard chemotherapy used includes *cis*-platinum, etoposide, and bleomycin (PEB) for four to six cycles depending on stage and response to chemotherapy (including assessment after second-look surgery). The cure rate for these tumors is > 90%. Likewise, all patients with extragonadal GCT benefit from surgery and chemotherapy (four cycles stages I–II, six cycles stages III–IV) with overall survival of 90% and 70% (metastatic mediastinal)—80%, respectively for stages I–II and II–IV disease.[174]

Liver tumors
Malignant tumors of the liver account for 1% of all childhood cancers with HB accounting for 43% of all hepatic tumors (benign and malignant) followed by hepatocellular carcinoma (HCC). HB is a disease of young infants with cases infrequently observed after 4 years of age. The incidence of HB has been rising possibly due to its association with prematurity and low birth weight.[175] HB has been associated with constitutional syndromes including familial adenomatous polyposis and Beckwith–Wiedemann syndrome. Patients usually present with an asymptomatic abdominal mass noted by parents or pediatrician. HB is an embryonal tumor that histologically recapitulates liver development and there are four recognized subtypes: epithelial (embryonal and fetal patterns, 67%), mesenchymal (epithelial and mesenchymal, 21%), pure well-differentiated fetal (7%), and small cell undifferentiated (5%).[176] The fetal histology is associated with a particularly favorable outcome. The most prevalent somatic lesion in HB is deletion or mutation of exon 3 of *CTNNB1* (beta-catenin) that leads to activation of the Wnt pathway.[177,178]

The outcome for children with HB has improved due to enhanced surgical techniques and the introduction of platinum-based chemotherapy. Currently, the 5-year overall survival rate is approximately 70%. A pretreatment extent of disease (PRETEXT) is now used to stratify therapy for HB and therefore a detailed assessment of the primary hepatic lesion is mandatory to determine resectability.[179] Since 20–30% of patients may present with lung metastasis, cross-sectional imaging of the lung is also part of staging. AFP is a very sensitive diagnostic marker and is essential for assessing response to therapy. PRETEXT is based on involvement of the four major liver sections and the presence of venous, portal, and extrahepatic involvement as well as metastatic disease. Surgical resection with clear margins is the primary goal of treatment. While PRETEXT I and II tumors may be candidates for upfront resection many centers favor neoadjuvant therapy for all PRETEXT stages. Tumors are usually sensitive to therapy (usually cisplatin, 5-fluorouracil, and vincristine +/− doxorubicin). The use of dose-dense treatment and integration of new agents including irinotecan and temsirolimus are currently being evaluated for children with high-risk disease.[172] Patients with PRETEXT IV disease or venous and/or portal involvement following chemotherapy are referred for liver transplantation although complete regression (by chemotherapy +/− surgery) of all metastatic lesions is required before proceeding with organ transplantation.

HCC is a disease of older adolescents and adults. While HCC in adults is associated with preexisting liver disease (hepatitis B and C, inflammatory liver disease, cirrhosis [tyrosinemia, biliary]) less than a third of patients diagnosed in Western countries have a history of liver disease.[180] In contrast to patients with HB, patients with HCC usually have constitutional symptoms like weight loss, anorexia, and vomiting. Microscopically HCC differs from HB in that tumor cells are larger, have defined borders, distinct nucleoli and tumors have a high degree of vascular invasion. Transitional liver tumors display pathologic and genetic features of both HB and HCC. HCCs show an increased overall mutational burden than HB but far fewer mutations in *CTNNB1* and have multiple copy number variations.[181] Mutations in *TP53* and epigenetic modifiers are frequent. Outcomes for HCC have been disappointing with no improvement over the past two decades in sharp contrast to advances made for other childhood tumors.[182] Complete surgical excision is the most important prognostic variable but most patients present with advanced disease. For early-stage tumors, complete resection followed by adjuvant chemotherapy is recommended while neoadjuvant chemotherapy (with the hope of improving resection) is recommended for more advanced stages (e.g., PRETEXT III). Patients who present with metastatic disease have a dismal outcome.

Carcinomas and melanoma
Carcinomas and melanoma account for approximately 9% of all cases of cancer in children. In the SEER database, the distribution of these malignancies is as follows: thyroid carcinoma, 35%; melanomas, 31%; adrenocortical carcinomas, 1.3%; nasopharyngeal carcinoma, 4.5%; and other skin carcinomas, 0.5%. Most carcinomas (75%) occur in the 15- to 19-year-old age group. In patients aged 15–19 years, thyroid cancer and melanoma account for more than 14% of the malignancies seen in this age group.

Ninety percent of thyroid carcinomas are papillary carcinomas and the *BRAFV600E* mutation seen in adults is rare in children.[183] These tumors are treated by surgical resection and radioactive iodine ablation with 10-year survival rates exceeding 90%.[184] Patients require lifelong thyroid hormone replacement. Medullary carcinoma is usually familial (Multiple Endocrine Neoplasia II) and is particularly aggressive.[185] Patients may be candidates for inhibitors of RET kinase. Most patients (90%) with melanoma have localized disease at initial evaluation, the most common site being the trunk, although patients younger than 20 years are more likely than adults to have disease primarily in the head and neck.[186] Like their adult counterpart, the majority of pediatric melanomas contain the *BRAFV600E* mutation. Survival rates are similar for patients younger than 20 and older than 20 years of age, and the prognosis appears to be stage dependent.[187] In the 15- to 19-year-old age group, the incidence of cutaneous melanoma increased at a rate of 2% per year between 1973 and 2006, but more recent reports show a decreasing trend among children.[2]

Late effects and quality of survivorship
With the use of multimodal and risk-based treatment, the overall 5-year survival rate of the more than 12,500 children and adolescents (age 0–19) diagnosed with cancer each year in the United States is approaching 80% (SEER). The improvement in survival has resulted in about 1 in 810 individuals under the age of 20 and 1 in 640 individuals between the ages 20 and 39 years representing childhood cancer survivors.

The late sequelae of cancer treatment can cause chronic medical problems and involve all organ systems. Overall mortality among childhood cancer survivors has been described to be 10-fold that of the general population. The Childhood Cancer Survivor Study (CCSS) assessed overall and cause-specific mortality in a retrospective cohort of 20,227 5-year survivors and demonstrated a 10.8-fold excess in overall mortality.[188] Risk of death was statistically significantly higher in females, individuals diagnosed with cancer before the age of 5 years, and those with an initial diagnosis of leukemia or brain tumor. The excess mortality was due to death from primary cancer, second cancer, cardiotoxicity and noncancer death, and existing up to 25 years after the initial cancer diagnosis.

The more commonly reported second primary cancers are breast, bone, and thyroid cancers, therapy-related myelodysplasia, and AML. Female survivors who were treated with chest or mantle radiation for a pediatric malignancy face a significantly increased risk of breast cancer.

Genetic predisposition was first noted to have a substantial impact on the risk of secondary sarcomas among patients with the genetic form of RB. This risk is further increased by radiation treatment and increases with the total dose of radiation delivered. Patients with a family history of early-onset cancers have also been shown to be at an increased risk of developing a second cancer. Members of families with Li–Fraumeni syndrome have been reported to be at increased risk of multiple subsequent cancers, with the highest risk observed among survivors of childhood cancer.[189] The subsequent cancers reported in this population were characteristic of Li–Fraumeni syndrome. It, therefore, appears that germ-line mutations in tumor-suppressor genes, as occurring in Li–Fraumeni syndrome, might interact with therapeutic exposures to result in an increased risk of second cancers.

Several genetic polymorphisms of enzymes capable of metabolic activation or detoxification of anticancer drugs, such as NAD(P)H: quinone oxidoreductase (NQO1), glutathione-S-transferase (GST)-M1 and -T1, and CYP3A4, have been examined for their role in the development of therapy-related leukemia or myelodysplasia. These studies indicate that NQO1 polymorphism is significantly associated with the genetic risk of therapy-related acute leukemia and myelodysplasia. In addition, individuals with CYP3A4-W genotype may be at increased risk of treatment-related leukemia, presumably by increasing the production of reactive intermediates that damage DNA.[190,191]

Because subsequent malignancies remain a significant threat to the health of survivors treated for cancer during childhood, vigilant screening is important for those at risk. Risk of secondary AML is associated with exposure to topoisomerase II inhibitors (i.e., epipodophyllotoxins and anthracyclines) for up to 10 years and with alkylating agents for up to 15 years. In addition, there is a significant risk of breast cancer (females) and other solid tumors for survivors of Hodgkin disease who were treated with radiation therapy.

Neurocognitive sequelae of treatment of childhood cancer occur because of radiation to the whole brain, systemic therapy with high-dose methotrexate or cytarabine, or with intrathecal methotrexate and other agents. Children with a history of brain tumors, ALL, or NHL are most likely to be affected. Risk factors include increasing radiation dose, young age at the time of treatment, treatment with both cranial radiation and systemic or intrathecal chemotherapy, and female gender.[192–194] Severe deficits are most frequently noted in children with brain tumors treated with radiation therapy, and in children who were less than 5 years of age at the time of treatment.

Chronic cardiotoxicity usually manifests itself as cardiomyopathy, pericarditis, and congestive heart failure. Childhood cancer survivors in the CCSS who were treated with chest or spinal radiation had a more than two-fold increased risk of death related to cardiac disease in comparison with the standard US population.[195] The anthracyclines doxorubicin and daunomycin are well-known causes of cardiomyopathy.[196,197] The incidence of cardiomyopathy is dose-dependent and may exceed 30% among patients who received cumulative doses of anthracyclines in excess of 300 mg/m^3. A cumulative dose of anthracyclines greater than 300 mg/m^3 was associated with an increased risk of clinical heart failure (relative risk 11.8) compared with a cumulative dose lower than 300 mg/m^3. The estimated risk of clinical heart failure increased with time and approached 5% after 15 years. These studies and others emphasize that cardiomyopathy can occur many years after completion of therapy (15–20 years) and that the onset may be spontaneous or coincide with exertion or pregnancy.

Pulmonary fibrosis and pneumonitis can result from pulmonary radiation. Thus, these problems are seen most often in patients with thoracic malignancies, notably Hodgkin disease. In addition to radiation therapy, a growing list of chemotherapeutic agents appears to be responsible for pulmonary disease in long-term survivors. Bleomycin toxicity is the prototype for chemotherapy-related lung injury. Although interstitial pneumonitis and pulmonary fibrosis have been reported in children, clinically apparent bleomycin pneumonopathy is most frequent in older adults. The chronic lung toxicity usually follows persistence or progression of abnormalities developing within 3 months of therapy. Alkylating agents also are believed to cause chronic lung injury. Following HSCT, both restrictive and obstructive lung disease, including bronchiolitis obliterans are well described.[198]

Chronic fibrosis of the liver is associated with radiation. Chemotherapy, even in the absence of radiation therapy, may be a cause of chronic hepatopathy. Viral hepatitis, most often related to transfusion of blood products prior to 1992, is another cause of chronic liver disease in long-term survivors.[199]

Damage to the proximal renal tubule from chemotherapy can cause Fanconi renal syndrome (hypokalemia, hypophosphatemia, glucosuria, proteinuria, renal tubular acidosis, and rickets). Children at particular risk include those who received treatment with more than one nephrotoxic agent and those with concomitant renal damage related to surgery or radiation.[200] Electrolyte wasting associated with ifosfamide therapy and hypomagnesemia associated with cisplatin therapy appear to persist in some children. Cyclophosphamide and ifosfamide are both capable of inducing hemorrhagic cystitis as a result of accumulation of acrolein in the bladder. Radiation to the pelvis or bladder can result in fibrosis and scarring, with resultant decreased bladder capacity and predisposition to urinary tract infections. Bladder cancer has developed in some patients who received bladder-toxic agents during treatment of childhood cancer. Yearly urinalysis should be done in these patients to evaluate for the presence of microscopic hematuria.

Decreased linear growth is a common problem during therapy in children with cancer. Although catch-up growth may occur, such that the premorbid growth status is regained, in some instances short stature is permanent or even progressive. Severe growth retardation, defined as a standing height below the fifth percentile, has been observed in as many as 30–35% of survivors of childhood brain tumors[201] and in 10–15% of patients treated with some antileukemia regimens.[202] Whole-brain irradiation is a major risk factor for short stature, especially in doses exceeding 18 Gy.

Observational studies indicate that obesity as measured by weight or body mass index (BMI) has been reported in children with ALL and brain tumors treated with conventional therapy or BMT.[203] This problem has its onset either during therapy or within the first year after discontinuation of therapy and may either progress or stabilize. In addition, hypothyroidism is a common late effect and usually is due to radiation to the neck for a nonthyroid malignancy, which contributes to obesity.

All therapeutic modalities (radiation, surgery, or chemotherapy) cause both germ-cell depletion and abnormalities of gonadal endocrine function among male cancer survivors.[204] Radiation to the testes is known to result in germinal loss with decrease in testicular volume and sperm production, and increases in follicle-stimulating hormone (FSH). Effects are dose-dependent, following fractionated exposures of 0.1–6 Gy. All males treated with inverted-Y radiation for HD at a cumulative testicular dose of 1.4–3.0 Gy become azoospermic without recovery after 2–40 months of follow-up, despite lead shielding of the scrotum. At doses of 4–6 Gy, azoospermia may persist for at least 3–5 years, and at doses above 6 Gy, usually appears to be irreversible. Alkylating agents decrease spermatogenesis in long-term survivors of cancer, and the effects are dose-dependent. Gonadal damage following cumulative doses lower than 7.5 mg/m^3 of mechlorethamine or 200 mg/kg of cyclophosphamide as used in HSCT has been shown to be reversible in up to 70% of patients after therapy-free intervals of several years.

The gonadal toxicities are of serious concern to patients and their families. This concern has popularized pretreatment sperm banking. Unlike the males, germ-cell failure and loss of ovarian endocrine function usually occur concomitantly in females. Following radiation therapy, manifestations are both age-dependent and dose-dependent. Prepubertal ovaries are relatively radioresistant because of the higher number of primordial follicles. Ovarian failure has also been associated with chemotherapy, such as single alkylating agents (cyclophosphamide, busulfan, nitrogen mustard) or as combination therapy. A report from the CCSS of 4029 pregnancies in 1915 female 5-year survivors of childhood cancer did not identify excess adverse outcomes for chemotherapeutic agents.[205] A companion study of 2323 pregnancies in partners of 1427 male survivors reported 69% live births, 1% stillbirths, 13% miscarriages, and 13% abortions (5% of outcomes were not accounted for).[206] The probability of a pregnancy ending in a live birth was significantly less than that for partners of male sibling controls (RR 0.8, $p = 0007$).

Patients who desire to have children after completion of therapy may require care in high-risk obstetrical clinics, especially those who have a discussion of sperm banking storage received abdominal or pelvic irradiation. Because much remains unknown about the problems of children born to survivors of childhood cancer, long-term general follow-up should be emphasized.

Several potentially ototoxic agents are commonly used in the treatment of children with malignancies, including platinum-based chemotherapy, aminoglycoside antibiotics, loop diuretics, and RT. These agents are all capable of causing sensorineural hearing loss. Very young children who received ototoxic agents during their cancer treatment and whose speech has not yet developed should undergo audiologic evaluations to determine whether they require intervention. Interventions to assist children experiencing hearing loss because of cancer treatment include the use of hearing aids and other assistive devices, along with preferential seating in the front of the classroom. Musculoskeletal problems after childhood cancer involve bony abnormalities, such as scoliosis, atrophy, or hypoplasia; avascular necrosis (AVN); and osteoporosis (bone density ≥2.5 SD below mean)/osteopenia (bone density 1–2.5 SD below mean), especially with the use of steroids in ALL treatment.

Providing appropriate health care for survivors of cancer is emerging as one of the major challenges in medicine. Childhood cancer survivors, an especially high-risk population, seek and receive care from a wide variety of health care professionals, including oncologists, medical and pediatric specialists, surgeons, primary care physicians, gynecologists, nurses, psychologists, and social workers. The challenge arises from the heterogeneity of this patient population treated with numerous therapeutic modalities in an era of rapidly advancing understanding of late effects. The COG has recently updated risk-based, exposure-related guidelines (Long-Term Follow-Up Guidelines for Survivors of Childhood, Adolescent, and Young-adult Cancers, version 5.0, 2018) specifically designed to direct follow-up care for patients who were diagnosed and treated for pediatric malignancies. These guidelines represent a set of comprehensive screening recommendations that are clinically relevant and can be used to standardize and direct the follow-up care for this group of cancer survivors with specialized health care needs (www.survivorshipguidelines.org).

Acknowledgments

The authors acknowledge the previous contributors to this chapter since their work enabled the summary present here and the bibliography. They are Maura O'Leary, MD; Gregory H. Reaman, MD; Les Robison, PhD; Smita Bhatia, MD, MPH; Paul Gaynon, MD; Anne Angiolillo, MD; Janet Franklin, MD; Richard Aplenc, MD, MSCE; Beverly Lange, MD; Tobey McDonald, MD; Brian Rood, MD; James Nachman, MD; Mitchell Cairo, MD; Sherrie Perkins, MD; Carlos Rodriguez-Galindo, MD; Alberto Pappo, MD; Paul Grundy, MD; Jeffrey Dome, MD; John Kalapurakal, MD; Elizabeth Perlman, MD; Michael Ritchey, MD; John Maris, MD Suzanne Shustermann, MD; William Meyer, MD; Kadria Sayed, MD; David Parham, MD; Richard Gorlick, MD, FAAP; Mark Bernstein, MD, FRCP(C); Jeffrey Toretsky, MD; R. Lor Randall, MD, FACS; Mark Gebhardt, MD; Lisa Teot, MD; Suzzane Wolden, MD; Neyssa Marina, MD; Teena Bhatla, MD.

Key references

The complete reference list can be found on Vital Source version of this title, see inside front cover.

2 Siegel DA, King J, Tai E, et al. Cancer incidence rates and trends among children and adolescents in the United States, 2001-2009. *Pediatrics*. 2014;**134**:e945–e955.

4 Vogelstein B, Papadopoulos N, Velculescu VE, et al. Cancer genome landscapes. *Science*. 2013;**339**:1546–1558.

7 Hunger SP, Lu X, Devidas M, et al. Improved survival for children and adolescents with acute lymphoblastic leukemia between 1990 and 2005: a report from the children's oncology group. *J Clin Oncol*. 2012;**30**:1663–1669.

17 Schultz KR, Pullen DJ, Sather HN, et al. Risk- and response-based classification of childhood B-precursor acute lymphoblastic leukemia: a combined analysis of prognostic markers from the Pediatric Oncology Group (POG) and Children's Cancer Group (CCG). *Blood*. 2007;**109**:926–935.

30 Harris MB, Shuster JJ, Carroll A, et al. Trisomy of leukemic cell chromosomes 4 and 10 identifies children with B-progenitor cell acute lymphoblastic leukemia with a very low risk of treatment failure: a Pediatric Oncology Group study. *Blood*. 1992;**79**:3316–3324.

36 Borowitz MJ, Devidas M, Hunger SP, et al. Clinical significance of minimal residual disease in childhood acute lymphoblastic leukemia and its relationship to other prognostic factors: a Children's Oncology Group study. *Blood*. 2008;**111**:5477–5485.

64 Cairo MS, Gerrard M, Sposto R, et al. Results of a randomized international study of high-risk central nervous system B non-Hodgkin lymphoma and B acute lymphoblastic leukemia in children and adolescents. *Blood*. 2007;**109**:2736–2743.

72 Locatelli F, Mauz-Koerholz C, Neville K, et al. Brentuximab vedotin for paediatric relapsed or refractory Hodgkin's lymphoma and anaplastic large-cell lymphoma: a multicentre, open-label, phase 1/2 study. *Lancet Haematol*. 2018;**5**:e450–e461.

75 Friedman DL, Chen L, Wolden S, et al. Dose-intensive response-based chemotherapy and radiation therapy for children and adolescents with newly diagnosed intermediate-risk hodgkin lymphoma: a report from the Children's Oncology Group Study AHOD0031. *J Clin Oncol*. 2014;**32**:3651–3658.

94 London WB, Castleberry RP, Matthay KK, et al. Evidence for an age cutoff greater than 365 days for neuroblastoma risk group stratification in the Children's Oncology Group. *J Clin Oncol*. 2005;**23**:6459–6465.

96 Mosse YP, Laudenslager M, Longo L, et al. Identification of ALK as a major familial neuroblastoma predisposition gene. *Nature*. 2008;**455**:930–935.

111 Matthay KK, Villablanca JG, Seeger RC, et al. Treatment of high-risk neuroblastoma with intensive chemotherapy, radiotherapy, autologous bone marrow transplantation, and 13-cis-retinoic acid. Children's Cancer Group. *N Engl J Med*. 1999;**341**:1165–1173.

129 Novakovic B, Goldstein AM, Wexler LH, et al. Increased risk of neuroectodermal tumors and stomach cancer in relatives of patients with Ewing's sarcoma family of tumors. *J Natl Cancer Inst*. 1994;**86**:1702–1706.

143 Spunt SL, Poquette CA, Hurt YS, et al. Prognostic factors for children and adolescents with surgically resected nonrhabdomyosarcoma soft tissue sarcoma: an analysis of 121 patients treated at St Jude Children's Research Hospital. *J Clin Oncol*. 1999;**17**:3697–3705.

144 Drilon A, Laetsch TW, Kummar S, et al. Efficacy of larotrectinib in TRK fusion-positive cancers in adults and children. *N Engl J Med*. 2018;**378**:731–739.

149 Northcott PA, Korshunov A, Witt H, et al. Medulloblastoma comprises four distinct molecular variants. *J Clin Oncol*. 2011;**29**:1408–1414.

155 Knudson AG Jr,. Mutation and cancer: statistical study of retinoblastoma. *Proc Natl Acad Sci U S A*. 1971;**68**:820–823.

201 Mulder RL, Kremer LC, van Santen HM, et al. Prevalence and risk factors of radiation-induced growth hormone deficiency in childhood cancer survivors: a systematic review. *Cancer Treat Rev*. 2009;**35**:616–632.

68 Cancer and pregnancy

Jennifer K. Litton, MD

Overview

The diagnosis of cancer during pregnancy is a clinical and emotional challenge for both the patient and the caregivers. A multidisciplinary approach including medical oncologists, surgeons, radiation oncologists, and obstetrics is vital to coordinate the treatment of the mother and the monitoring of the fetus. The available data regarding the treatment of cancer during pregnancy, including staging, surgery, radiation, and systemic therapy as well as outcomes for the patients and the children exposed to chemotherapy *in utero* is reviewed.

Table 1 Issues related to cancer and pregnancy.

Impact of cancer on pregnancy
Impact of pregnancy on cancer
Termination of pregnancy/fetal death with cancer treatment
Diagnostic procedures and staging during pregnancy
Cancer treatment, maternal effects
Cancer treatment, fetal effects
Placental metastasis
Transplacental malignancy
Long-term outcome for children
Ethical, moral, legal concerns
The UNKNOWN

The diagnosis of cancer during pregnancy presents a complex set of challenges for the patient, family members, and physicians. The welfare of the mother may be perceived to be threatened by the pregnancy due to concerns regarding the disease, diagnostic and therapeutic procedures required for treatment, and a desire to avoid harm to the fetus during treatment for the mother's malignancy. Many have perceived that treatment may require compromise of the wellbeing of either the mother or the fetus. Although, in some circumstances, fetal death may be an unavoidable consequence of cancer treatment. Frequently, however, judicious decision making not only can provide appropriate cancer care for the pregnant woman but also will preserve the pregnancy through successful labor and delivery.

Many issues arise in the realm of concurrent cancer and pregnancy (Table 1). The data for specific tumor types, diagnostic procedures, therapeutic interventions, and long-term cancer outcomes have been derived primarily from case reports, small case series, and retrospective reviews. Controlled studies and prospective data are rare. Data on labor and delivery outcomes for patients completing pregnancy continues to have a small number of cohort reports, long-term data on growth and development of children exposed to cancer treatment *in utero* also remains scarce, although reports on new cohorts are emerging. Over the past several decades, the treatment for cancer during pregnancy has evolved and is now within guidelines of care for several tumor types as cohort descriptions and prospective case series have been reported.[1–3] With that there is emerging data on outcomes of patients as well as small, but emerging data on the children exposed to chemotherapy *in utero*.

Cancer and pregnancy epidemiology

Tracking the true diagnosis of cancer during pregnancy appears to be increasing, but tracking the true incidence remains challenging. Much of the data includes pregnancy-associated breast cancers (PABCs), defined as those cancers diagnosed both during pregnancy and within the 1-year period after delivery. With emerging data that biology and outcomes may be influenced by the timing of diagnosis, evaluating and reporting these incidences separately may be important. Smith et al. used the California Cancer Registry, evaluating 4,846,505 women of whom 4539 had an identified invasive malignancy either during pregnancy or within 12 months after delivery.[4] In this analysis, cancer occurred in approximately 1 in 1000 deliveries from 1991 through 1999. However, 64% of these cases occurred within the 12 months after delivery. Per 1000 live singleton births, the most common tumor types were breast (0.19), thyroid (0.14), cervix (0.12), melanoma (0.09), Hodgkin disease (0.05), ovarian (0.05), acute, and leukemia (0.04). In an Australian linkage study between 1994 and 2008, 1798 pregnancy-associated cancers, encompassing diagnoses both during and within 1 year from delivery, were identified in 1,309,501 deliveries.[5] Four hundred ninety-five of these cancers were identified during pregnancy. During pregnancy, the most common cancer identified in this cohort was melanoma (15.1/100,000), breast (7.3/100,000), thyroid (3.2/100,000), and gynecological (3.9/100,000). However, cancer from nearly any anatomic location can occur with pregnancy.

Interestingly, in this study from Australia, and others, the incidence of PABC has been increasing. This may be secondary to increasing maternal age as well as other changes in epidemiological risk factors. In the Australian cohort, from 1994 to 2007, the incidence of PABC increased from 112.3 to 191.5/100,000 deliveries. A Swedish registry also showed a trend to increasing incidence that may be partially explained by advancing maternal age, with an increase of 16.0–37.4 cases per 100,000 deliveries from the beginning to the end of cohorts collected from 1963 to 2002.[6] This may also be influenced as further advances in reproductive technologies are making pregnancies more accessible to older women.

Diagnosis and staging

A biopsy, with review of cytologic and histologic material, is required for the diagnosis of any malignancy during pregnancy.

Holland-Frei Cancer Medicine, Tenth Edition. Edited by Robert C. Bast, John C. Byrd, Carlo M. Croce, Ernest Hawk, Fadlo R. Khuri, Raphael E. Pollock, Apostolia M. Tsimberidou, Christopher G. Willett, and Cheryl L. Willman.
© 2023 John Wiley & Sons, Inc. Published 2023 by John Wiley & Sons, Inc.

The type of biopsy is determined by the accessibility of the disease site and the quantity of material required.

If a surgical biopsy if required, the anatomic location of the biopsy and the gestational age of the fetus are factors to be considered prior to proceeding. A surgical biopsy can be performed safely.[1,7,8] It is imperative that adequate material for pathologic diagnosis and required studies be obtained; for example, hormone receptors and HER-2/neu status are necessary for the proper evaluation of breast cancer, and morphologic and immuno-phenotyping of lymphomas and leukemias are essential to their optimal assessment and treatment.

Staging provides guidance for discussions regarding cancer prognosis, recommended loco-regional and/or systemic therapies, and potential risks of treatment in relation to benefit and outcome for the patient. Frequently, staging assessment in the nonpregnant patient involves exposure to ionizing radiation, which is to be avoided whenever possible during pregnancy. The impact of radiation upon the fetus varies with respect to fetal gestational age. Preimplantation and fetal organogenesis are most sensitive to the negative effects of radiation exposure.[9] Fetal exposures of <5 cGy are not thought to be harmful.[10] With abdominal computerized tomography, exposure may be as high as 30 mSv. As a consequence of known fetal toxicity associated with exposure to ionizing radiation during pregnancy, abdominal shielding, and nonionizing techniques should be used whenever possible during these imaging procedures.[10] Ultrasonography (US) for breast, liver, and other abdominal organ imaging can also contribute to the staging evaluation without ionizing radiation. Magnetic resonance imaging (MRI) can be used to assess for bone and liver disease, as well as fetal abnormalities, if required.[11,12] The use of gadolinium as a contrast agent for MRI during pregnancy remains controversial. Although multiple case reports have not demonstrated an increase in adverse effects to the fetus, gadolinium is often avoided if possible due to lack of toxicity information.[13–15] Accurate determination of disease stage is essential in ensuring accurate cancer treatment decisions, and findings during the staging process also may influence the woman's decision regarding the maintenance of her pregnancy.

The use of PET/CT scanning has become standard in the treatment and evaluation of lymphomas and has had an increase in use in evaluation of metastatic disease in solid tumors as well. There is very limited data regarding the use of PET/CT in the pregnant breast cancer patient. Evidence that FDG crosses the placenta and can accumulate in fetal brain, bladder, and cardiac tissue has been demonstrated in animal studies.[16] Zanotti-Fregonara et al. estimated the FDG uptake by embryo tissues in early pregnancy is at least 3.3E-2mGy/MBq in a patient found to be pregnant at the time of scanning.[17] Few other case reports exist. Hove et al. describe an 18-year-old woman with Hodgkin disease who underwent PET/CT. There was significant uptake in the fetal myocardium. The patient developed hemolysis, elevated liver enzymes levels and low platelets (HELLP) syndrome and the child was delivered at 31 weeks by caesarian section.[18] Therefore, there is insufficient safety data to support the use of PET/CT scanning during pregnancy and should be delayed until if it does not affect the safety and management of the patient and modifying the imaging protocol should be considered.[19,20]

Cancer treatment during pregnancy

The optimal treatment of cancer during pregnancy requires a meticulously coordinated multidisciplinary approach. Careful and repeated consultations with the obstetrician and/or maternal-fetal medicine specialist are essential during the course of the pregnancy. Accurate assessment of fetal age, maturation, and the expected delivery date must be performed prior to treatment planning. The therapeutic options for the pregnant patient do not differ from those of the nonpregnant patient with cancer, but the application of treatment may be more complex. When evaluating multiple tumor types during pregnancy, Stensheim et al. described 516 women from Norwegian health registries with no difference identified in cause-specific death.[21] However, it is interesting to note that when diagnosed instead during lactation, there was an increase in both breast and ovarian death rates. Outcomes in large cohorts are otherwise described with cancer-specific sites and the timing and treatment are important in relation to the outcomes of the patient.

Surgery

Surgery remains the mainstay for treatment of solid tumors, and pregnancy is not a contraindication for cancer surgery. Mazze and Kallen have reported on a registry series of 5405 pregnant patients on whom emergency surgery was performed.[8] They did not observe an increased incidence of congenital malformations or stillbirths in women who had surgical procedures while pregnant. An increased frequency of low- and very low birth-weight infants was noted and attributed to prematurity and intrauterine growth retardation (IUGR) and may have been influenced by the underlying reason behind the necessary surgery. No specific type of surgical procedure or anesthesia was associated with an increase in adverse reproductive outcomes. In a case-control study, Duncan and colleagues did not observe an increase in congenital anomalies in 2565 pregnant women who had surgery while pregnant, when compared to control patients who did not have surgery.[22] If warranted by tumor type and disease stage, surgery should proceed and should be coordinated with the obstetrician, anesthesiologist, and neonatal specialist.

Radiation

Pregnancy has been considered an absolute contraindication to radiation therapy for cancer. Radiation therapy for cervical cancer during pregnancy usually leads to fetal death and spontaneous abortion.[23] The fetus is most sensitive to malformation from radiation exposure 2–8 weeks after conception, whereas exposure from 8 to 25 weeks of gestation may have a greater risk of mental retardation.[9] Nevertheless, successful radiation therapy of pregnant women with Hodgkin's disease has been reported.[24] If radiation is warranted, appropriate fetal shielding, careful dosimetry calculations, and estimates of fetal dose exposure are necessary. However, due to the very limited safety data should be considered only in very select cases.[25–29] Radiation therapy for breast cancer, following mastectomy or breast conservation surgery, can usually be delayed until the postpartum period, especially if chemotherapy is administered.

Systemic therapy

Many different agents have been reported to have been used in pregnancy. Systemic therapy is of concern because of the potential deleterious effects on the fetus. Physiologic changes associated with pregnancy (elevated blood volume, increased cardiac output, amplified glomerular filtration rate, and changes in circulating protein levels) make predictions about drug pharmacokinetics uncertain at best.[30] In addition, systemic agents are designed to be antiproliferative compounds, and their administration during pregnancy poses genuine risk to the developing fetus. Potential concerns include stillbirth, spontaneous abortion, fetal malformations/teratogenesis, organ-specific toxicities, IUGR with low birth weight, and premature delivery.[31]

In addition to cytotoxic therapy, there are also reports regarding supportive medications. Erythropoietin use during pregnancy was reported by Scott and colleagues as well as others. No maternal or fetal toxicities have been noted.[32] FDA Black Box warnings about the use of erythropoietin in breast cancer patients would apply to the pregnant patient as well, even in the absence of specific risk data in these patients. There have been increasing case reports of the safe use of pegfilgrastim during pregnancy after dose-dense chemotherapy for breast cancer.[33] Dexamethasone and lorazepam have also been reported as premedications without significant toxicity.[11]

Outcomes in the children exposed to chemotherapy *in utero*

The fetal risks related to chemotherapy appear to be greatest during the first trimester of pregnancy. Doll and colleagues reviewed antineoplastic agents and fetal malformations in relation to the trimester of pregnancy.[31] They reported *in utero* exposure to systemic agents was associated with fetal malformation risks of 14% and 19% for alkylating agents and antimetabolites, respectively. A similar review of second- and third-trimester exposure demonstrated a 1.3% incidence of fetal malformation and a voluntary registry reported a 3.8% risk of congenital malformation in a subset of breast cancer patients.[33] Similarly, in a review of cytotoxic agents used during pregnancy, Ebert and colleagues collected 217 cases from the literature published between 1983 and 1995.[30] They classified the use of the agents by disease category and analyzed outcome of pregnancy in relation to agent, dose, and gestational age at exposure. There were 94 cases of leukemia, 57 cases of lymphoma, 26 cases of breast or ovarian cancer, 16 cases of cytotoxic therapy used for rheumatic diseases, and the remainder of the malignancies. Eighteen newborns were reported to have congenital developmental abnormalities. Of these 18 newborns, 15 neonates had been exposed to cytotoxic drugs during the first trimester. Chromosomal abnormalities were noted in two neonates who had experienced exposure to cytotoxic agents during the first trimester.[30] Antimetabolite use was found in 50% of the neonates with congenital abnormalities following first-trimester exposure to chemotherapy. Of the reviewed cases, 82% of leukemia patients, 75% of lymphoma patients, and 75% of breast or ovary cancer patients with associated pregnancies were reported to have live births with normally developed neonates. Germann et al. collected data involving 160 patients who received anthracyclines during pregnancy.[34] In this group, five cases of fetal malformations (3%) were found, with three cases occurring with the use of chemotherapy in the first trimester. The remaining two cases of fetal malformation occurred after chemotherapy administration in the second trimester; one involved Down's syndrome unrelated to chemotherapy, and the other involved a congenital adherence of the iris to the cornea that demonstrated no clinical consequence. The combination chemotherapy regimens associated with fetal malformations included cytosine arabinoside or cyclophosphamide. Since these initial reports, there have been multiple case studies showing safety of systemic therapy with anthracyclines and taxanes as well as limited information regarding platinum compounds when treated in the second and third trimester.[35–37] Systemic treatment, especially with antimetabolites such as methotrexate, should be avoided during the first trimester of pregnancy except in circumstances in which delay in cancer treatment would jeopardize the life of the patient, such as acute leukemia.

A long-term report on children exposed to chemotherapy *in utero* during treatment of mothers for a variety of hematologic malignancies has been presented by Aviles and Neri.[38] They described 84 children followed a median of 18.7 years. Thirty-eight had been exposed to chemotherapy *in utero* during the first trimester of pregnancy. Fertility was reported to be preserved, some of the chemotherapy-exposed children having become parents. No learning, neurologic, or psychological problems were reported for any of the *in utero* chemotherapy-exposed subjects. Van Calsteren et al. reported on 10 children from 9 pregnancies exposed to chemotherapy *in utero* for differing primary cancers. The children who were born prematurely had multiple abnormalities ranging from speech delay to mental and motor retardation. These were children born at less than 33 weeks gestation. Echocardiograms were also obtained demonstrating a tendency towards a thinner ventricular wall.[39] Abdel-Hady et al. describe 118 children born to mothers who received chemotherapy during pregnancy with no significant difference when compared to a control group of children.[40] Given these findings, there have been consensus guidelines recommending chemotherapy in the second and third trimester.[2]

Much of the data in the children exposed to chemotherapy has come from studies of breast cancer diagnosed and treated during pregnancy. Murthy et al. have updated on the outcomes of the children exposed to chemotherapy *in utero*.[41] Complications for the neonate included: prematurity, neutropenia, tachypnea of the newborn, and respiratory distress syndrome. One case of spontaneous cryptogenic intracranial hemorrhage occurred which all resolved. There were 3 congenital abnormalities reported which included Down syndrome (1), congenital ureteral reflux (1), and clubfoot (1).[41] Cardonick et al. also described a voluntary registry of outcomes in children exposed to chemotherapy demonstrating a 3.8% rate of congenital malformations which is similar to the national average of pregnant patients without cancer.[42] Loibl et al. reviewed a registry of patients diagnosed with breast cancer during pregnancy from multiple different European sites. Of the 447 patients followed, 197 received chemotherapy during pregnancy from 2003 to 2011.[43] Of these, 22 babies had reported complications and were delivered before the 37th week with 4 congenital malformations (trisomy 18, rectal atresia, polydactyly, and craniosynostosis). Nine of these babies were delivered after the 37th week with 3 malformations (asymmetric head, polydactyly, and Mobius syndrome). When evaluating for longer-term outcomes in children exposed to chemotherapy in utero, Amant et al. described 129 children and evaluated for neurocognitive and cardiac outcomes as well as general health there was no significant finding except for those children who were born prematurely.[44] Both of these studies highlight the need for to avoid iatrogenic preterm delivery whenever possible, with holding treatment past the 35th week of pregnancy in order to avoid blood nadirs and allowing the children to proceed full term.

Specific cancers

Breast cancer

The diagnosis of breast cancer during pregnancy is often delayed, presumably due to the anatomical and physiologic changes in the pregnant breast.[45] However, women with breast cancer during pregnancy have demonstrated the same survival rates, stage for stage, as nonpregnant patients with breast cancer.[37,46–48] Imaging, local, and systemic therapy have been well described in the successful treatment of breast cancer diagnosed during pregnancy.

Imaging of the breast in women with a palpable mass or thickening is warranted, especially if it persists for 2 weeks or longer. Mammography and US may confirm the presence of a malignant mass. Breast US has been well used with minimizing risks to the fetus. Liberman reported positive findings in six of six patients, and Samuels found positive findings in two of four patients.[49,50] Yang et al. diagnosed 100% of the masses as well as axillary metastases in 18 of 20 women.[51] US was also shown to be effective for restaging to evaluate response to preoperative chemotherapy in the pregnant breast.[51] US may be useful for guiding either fine-needle aspiration (FNA) or core biopsy in order to confirm a diagnosis of malignancy.[52–54] Chest radiography, liver US, and MRI of the thoracic/lumbar spine can be used to assess for extant organ metastasis.[1,11]

Lymph node evaluations can be tailored to clinical findings. If clinically suspicious regional nodes are identified on physical examination or by imaging techniques, an FNA that is guided by palpation or US can be utilized to confirm metastases. The theoretical dosage of radiation that would be absorbed by the fetus following sentinel lymph node (SLN) biopsy has been calculated to be less than 5 cGy.[55,56] There were multiple early reports of safety.[12,57,58] Han et al. reported on 145 women who underwent SLN biopsy during pregnancy and had comparable recurrence rates and no adverse events noted in the children exposed in utero.[59]

Breast-conserving surgery is possible with postpartum breast irradiation. Pre- or postoperative chemotherapy is used with the same criteria for selection of therapy as in the nonpregnant patient. However, breast-conserving therapy should be considered when radiation can be given in a timely fashion after delivery. Often, given the timing of chemotherapy, this will allow for postpartum radiation. Dominici et al. have described a single institution experience of mastectomy versus breast-conserving surgery as well as biopsy procedures with no significant difference in wound complications or complications from FNA or core biopsies.[52]

Other agents have been described in the literature to treat breast cancer and include vinorelbine, paclitaxel, docetaxel, and cisplatin.[60,61] The use of taxanes, both paclitaxel and docetaxel have been described also in the second and third trimesters.[60,62–69] with all available follow-up data reported healthy children.[60] Vinorelbine has been reported to be used in both adjuvant and metastatic settings, with 5 of the 6 children reported healthy at 6–35 months of follow-up. Information on one of the children was not available in the literature. Neonatal complications included one episode of grade 4 neutropenia and transient cytopenia at day 6 of life.[67,70–72] Multiple case reports of trastuzumab administered during pregnancy have been identified. This has been associated with oligo- and anhydramnios with its use was described in case reports.[66,70,73–77] One case was of reversible heart failure in the mother with no anhydramnios in the fetus was reported.[75] One of the children born developed respiratory failure, capillary leak syndrome, infections, and necrotizing enterocolitis, dying from multiple organ failure 21 weeks after delivery.[77] Additionally, Bader et al. described a case of reversible renal failure in the fetus.[66] One report of the use of lapatinib was recently described in a patient who conceived while on lapatinib. Despite approximately 11 weeks of exposure, the pregnancy was otherwise uncomplicated with the delivery of a healthy baby.[78] Routine administration of biologic agents is not recommended during pregnancy and trastuzumab now has an FDA Category D rating.

Tamoxifen is a standard treatment for hormone receptor-positive tumors in premenopausal women. Although some case reports of tamoxifen fetal exposure demonstrated no effect on the newborn, there are other reports including Goldenhar syndrome (microtia, preauricular skin tags, and hemifacial microsomia),[79] ambiguous genitalia, and other birth defects. Additionally, vaginal bleeding and spontaneous abortion have also been reported.[79–83] Braems et al. described 11 babies with congenital malformations out of 44 live births and 3 stillbirths.[84] Aromatase inhibitors with ovarian suppression also should be delayed until after delivery.

Outcomes of pregnant breast cancer patients appear to be similar to nonpregnant cancer patients when treated with appropriate therapies in the second and third trimesters. Litton et al. have described the outcomes of a single institution cohort treated at The University of Texas MD Anderson Cancer Center since 1989 where all women presented for early-stage breast cancer and received chemotherapy with 5-fluorouracil, doxorubicin, and cyclophosphamide (FAC) in the second and third trimesters of pregnancy. There were all live births.[85] Rouzier et al. reviewed 48 patients with PABC and have concluded that chemosensitivity and pathological response rates were modeled to be similar in pregnant and nonpregnant breast cancer patients.[86] Amant et al. compared 311 women to 865 nonpregnant breast cancer patients with no statistically significant difference in OS.[46]

Azim et al. performed a meta-analysis of 30 studies of PABC which did show a higher risk of relapse and death.[36] However, this did not hold true for the diagnosis during pregnancy which may further emphasize the importance of separating the situations of being diagnosed during versus after pregnancy. This analysis also included multiple older studies that either delayed or gave substandard therapy to pregnant patients that may also have affected survival outcomes.

Thyroid cancer

In pregnant women, thyroid cancer presents most often as an asymptomatic nodule in the neck. Ultrasound evaluation can confirm the size and solid character of the nodule. FNA biopsy is the most reliable diagnostic test and is safe and accurate during pregnancy.[87–90] Most often, pregnancy-associated thyroid cancers are differentiated thyroid cancers (DTC). Radioiodine scans and therapeutic radioiodine should not be given during pregnancy and can be safely delayed until after delivery.[91] Thyroid surgery can be delayed until after delivery for many patients, especially if the diagnosis is made during the third trimester of pregnancy.[91,92] If warranted, thyroid resection can be done under local anesthesia.[93] Moosa and Mazzaferi reported on 61 pregnant patients with thyroid cancer and 528 age-matched nonpregnant controls.[94] They reviewed diagnosis, treatment, and outcome for the two cohorts. Seventy-four percent of the pregnant patients had been discovered to possess an asymptomatic thyroid nodule during routine examinations. Twenty percent of the pregnant patients underwent thyroid surgery during the second trimester, while 77% of patients underwent surgery following delivery. Thirty percent of the patients received postoperative iodine-131 therapy; all of these treatments were administered postpartum. The presence of pregnancy or delayed surgery did not result in differences in cancer recurrence, distant recurrence, or death. Based upon these findings, Moosa and Mazzaferi concluded that treatment for thyroid cancer during pregnancy may be delayed until after delivery in most patients.[94] Additionally, Yasmeen et al. reviewed data from the California Cancer Registry of 595 women diagnosed with thyroid cancer within 9 months antepartum to 12 months postpartum, compared to matched nonpregnant counterparts, and no significant differences were found in overall survival, maternal or fetal outcomes.[95] Alves et al. performed a systematic review of four studies in total, including the two mentioned above, and there was no change in long term survival outcomes between pregnant and nonpregnant DTC patients.[96] Recommendations for papillary thyroid cancer when diagnosed early in the pregnancy, should be monitored by ultrasound and if it grows significantly (>50% growth) before 24–26 weeks, then surgery should be considered during the pregnancy. However, the more aggressive subtypes of medullary and anaplastic thyroid cancer should proceed to surgery.[90]

Cervical cancer

Evaluation of extent of disease for diagnosed cervical cancer includes physical examination and assessment of pelvic anatomic structures by MRI. Laparoscopic lymph node surgery has been reported.[97] Treatment options vary with disease stage, gestational age at diagnosis, and the desires of the patient. For stage I disease, Sorosky and colleagues have reported a favorable outcome with only planned follow-up observation until the third trimester.[98] They followed eight women with stage I disease, <2.5 cm in dimension, for a mean interval of 109 days. All patients underwent delivery via cesarean delivery, followed by radical hysterectomy. Serial MRIs were used to follow the disease for two patients, and no clinical disease progression was noted. After treatment, all patients were alive and free of disease at a mean follow-up of 37 months.

In a review of 22 patients with cervical cancer diagnosed during pregnancy or within 12 months postpartum, Allen and colleagues noted 20 live deliveries and only one disease recurrence.[99] Nine of 11 patients with microinvasive disease were treated with core biopsy only. Ten patients with stage IB or IIA disease were treated with radical hysterectomy, and one patient with stage IIIB disease received chemotherapy, radiation therapy, and simple hysterectomy as treatment. Allen recommended all pregnant women undergo cervical cytologic evaluation. Cone biopsy is safe in pregnancy and may be adequate treatment for microinvasive disease.[99]

Outcome and recurrence risk have been assessed in relation to method of delivery for women diagnosed with cervix cancer during pregnancy or within 6 months postpartum. Sood and colleagues followed 83 pregnant women with cervical cancer; 56 of these patients were diagnosed with during pregnancy, and 27 patients were diagnosed postpartum.[100] Since the risk of recurrence was increased in those diagnosed postpartum who delivered vaginally, Sood et al. concluded that women with cervical cancer should be delivered by cesarean. However, van der Vange and colleagues, in a case-control study, reported that mode of delivery had no effect on survival.[101] Overall, they noted no difference in survival of pregnant patients with cervical cancer compared to the nonpregnant group.

Systemic chemotherapy for cervical cancer can be effective when given during pregnancy. Most of the reported therapies have been platinum based and administered with several other agents such as vincristine and bleomycin.[102] However, neoadjuvant chemotherapy regimens have been described and include paclitaxel plus either cisplatin or carboplatin.[3,102,103] There are several case reports describing the use of neoadjuvant cisplatin-based regimens with either taxane or vinorelbine used in order to preserve the pregnancy until the fetus is viable with good maternal and fetal outcomes.[104–106]

Treatment of the pregnant patient with cervical cancer requires careful consideration of disease stage and gestational age. Early in pregnancy with early-stage disease, pregnancy termination followed by cancer treatment may be appropriate. Alternatively, planned delay in cancer treatment with careful monitoring of disease may allow for successful completion of the pregnancy.[98] Radiation therapy will likely cause fetal death and usually results in spontaneous abortion.[23]

Since a significant population of patients is diagnosed with cervical cancer while in childbearing age, the concern for preservation of fertility has led to the utilization of radical vaginal trachelectomy with pelvic lymphadenectomy, instead of radical hysterectomy, in select patients with stage I cervical cancer. Burnett and colleagues made this procedure available to 21 patients over a period of 6 years with 18 of 21 patients receiving radical trachelectomy in order to preserve fertility.[107] Within this group, one patient gave birth to healthy twins, delivered at 24 weeks, following superovulation treatment. One patient delivered a singleton term infant via cesarean hysterectomy; no residual disease was found in the cervix. The last patient most likely became pregnant in the week prior to the radical vaginal trachelectomy. She had spontaneous rupture of membranes at 20 weeks gestation, requiring hysterotomy for evacuation of the uterus with subsequent neonatal demise. Multiple other groups have described success in this procedure for fertility preservation.[108,109] There are still limited reports of this procedure done during pregnancy.[3,110]

Survival in cervical cancer patients diagnosed during pregnancy has had increasing data showing no significant difference in outcomes. Nguyen and colleagues concluded that tumor characteristics and maternal survival were not adversely affected by pregnancy, nor was pregnancy adversely affected by cervical cancer.[111] Similar conclusions were reached by van der Vange and colleagues in a case-control study. They reported on 23 patients diagnosed during pregnancy and 24 patients diagnosed within 6 months postpartum. Thirty-nine patients had early-stage disease. No difference in survival was noted for cases compared to controls. They noted that the delivery method had no effect on survival, thus concluding that prognosis for early-stage cervical cancer is similar in pregnant and nonpregnant women.[101,112] Zemlickis and colleagues reported on a long-term follow-up of cervical cancer outcome in a case-control study of pregnant women. No survival differences were observed. When compared to matched controls, patients with invasive cervical cancer were more likely to give birth to children who had lower birth weights. No adverse impact of pregnancy on cervix cancer outcome could be demonstrated.[113] More recently, Halaska et al. reported on a matched cohort study from 6 European centers with 132 pregnant patients with cervical cancer. With a median follow-up of 84 months, there was no difference in survival for patients diagnosed during a pregnancy versus those who were not pregnant.[114]

Hodgkin disease and non-Hodgkin lymphoma

The presentation of Hodgkin disease during pregnancy does not differ from that of the nonpregnant patient, with lymphadenopathy being the most common method of presentation.[115] The diagnosis is established by lymph node biopsy, with sufficient material to confirm specific type of disease.[116] Staging assessment, in addition to medical history and physical examination, can include an abdominal shielded chest radiograph, abdominal US, and MRI to document disease location and extent in order to assist treatment planning. For supradiaphragmatic disease, radiation therapy can be completed successfully while maintaining the pregnancy with uterine/fetal shielding.[24,26,116–118] Radiation therapy during pregnancy for stage IA and IIA Hodgkin disease has been reported by Woo and colleagues.[24] Sixteen patients received radiation to the neck (2), neck and mediastinum (3), or mantle.[119] Fetal radiation dose estimates were determined for nine patients. Reported doses ranged from 1.4 to 5.5 cGy for photon therapy and 10–13.6 cGy for cobalt therapy. There were 16 normal full-term infants, and the 10-year patient survival rate was 71%.[24] This outcome is similar to an earlier report by Jacobs and colleagues, who reported on the use of radiation therapy involving the neck and mediastinum during the second and third trimesters of pregnancy.[118] Supradiaphragmatic radiation therapy can be accomplished while maintaining a viable pregnancy. There are limited data regarding the impact of Hodgkin disease on pregnancy, and the effects of pregnancy upon disease prognosis. Anselmo and colleagues concluded that the prognosis of Hodgkin disease was not affected by pregnancy.[120] Tawil and colleagues, reporting on their experience with 12 patients with Hodgkin disease and pregnancy, concluded that pregnancy did not significantly affect the course of the malignancy, and the presence of this malignancy did not affect pregnancy outcome.[117] Examining pregnancy outcome, Zuazu and colleagues found no increase in the complication rate of pregnancy in 56 patients with leukemia or lymphoma. In those patients treated with systemic chemotherapy, there was no increase in incidence of fetal malformations.[121] In the Gelb series, patients were treated with a variety of systemic chemotherapy agent combinations, including MOPP (mechlorethamine, vincristine, procarbazine, prednisone), ABV (doxorubicin, bleomycin, vinblastine), COP (cyclophosphamide, vincristine, prednisone), and CHOP (cyclophosphamide, doxorubicin, vincristine, prednisone).[115] No fetal malformations were reported. Fifteen patients were alive and disease free. Gelb and colleagues concluded that otherwise indicated systemic therapy should not be delayed because of pregnancy.

Non-Hodgkin lymphoma during pregnancy presents at more advanced stage and has more aggressive biologic behavior than Hodgkin disease during pregnancy.[115,122,123] The clinical behavior of non-Hodgkin lymphoma appears to be the same with or without pregnancy.[115] Because the majority of patients present with advanced-stage disease, systemic chemotherapy is warranted. Combination chemotherapy has been reported to be used with some success. Agents used have included epirubicin, vincristine, prednisone, etoposide, cyclophosphamide, doxorubicin, and bleomycin in various combinations (VACOP-B, MACOP-B).[124–126] There have been several reports of the use of rituximab during pregnancy. Herold and colleagues utilized a combination of rituximab, doxorubicin, vincristine, and prednisolone to treat a female with bulky stage IIA NHL.[127] At the time of initiation of therapy, the patient was in her 21st week of pregnancy. She responded well to therapy and delivered a healthy infant at 35 weeks via cesarean section; the child demonstrated a normal B cell population. Kimby and colleagues treated a patient with Stage IIB NHL with weekly rituximab for four cycles.[128] The patient-reported conception occurrence between the first and second infusions of rituximab. She delivered a healthy baby girl at 40 weeks. The infant demonstrated a low granulocyte count at birth, but her hematologic parameters had recovered by 18 months of age. Since that time, there have been multiple reports of rituximab, cyclophosphamide, doxorubicin, vincristine, and prednisone (R-CHOP) during pregnancy for diffuse large B cell lymphoma with reports of fetal leukopenia but with only preterm birth complicating the pregnancy.[129,130]

In one reported multicenter, retrospective analyses, Evens et al. identified 90 patients diagnosed with either Hodgkin or non-Hodgkin lymphoma during pregnancy.[130] Six of the women terminated their pregnancy. Fifty-six women received chemotherapy during pregnancy that included R-CHOP as well as other modified regimens that included etoposide, bleomycin, dacarbazine, cytarabine, and cisplatin. Pretreatment also included steroids and growth factor support. One child was born with a malformation with microcephaly. There was an increase in induction of labor and therefore also c-sections and neonatal intensive care unti (NICU) admissions. The authors reported that the survival was in line with expected outcomes of similar lymphoma patients. In the largest series to date, Maggen et al. report on 134 patients with Hodgkin lymphoma. doxorubicin (Adriamycin) B—bleomycin. V—vinblastine. D—dacarbazine (DTIC) (ABVD) was the most common regimen given (92%). There were 2 still births. There was no statistically significant difference in survival when compared with nonpregnant lymphoma patients.[131] Aviles and colleagues reported the outcome of 16 patients treated for non-Hodgkin's lymphoma during pregnancy, including eight during the first trimester.[132] No congenital malformations were noted, and normal deliveries were reported. They concluded that pregnancy was not a contraindication to treating non-Hodgkin's lymphoma and that long-term remission was possible. Burkitt's lymphoma, anaplastic large-cell lymphoma, and T-cell lymphoma have also all been reported in association with pregnancy.[133–137]

Ovarian cancer

In a review of adnexal masses during pregnancy, one ovarian cancer was found in 125 patients.(98) There were 40 dermoids, 15 endometriomas, 14 cysts, 13 cystoadenomas, 9 tubal cysts, and 4 fibroids, indicating a 0.8% malignancy rate.[138] In a retrospective review, Sayedur and colleagues identified 9 cases of ovarian cancer and pregnancy over 24 years, an incidence of 0.08/1000 pregnant women. For pregnant women, adnexal masses are more frequent, likely to be benign and management decisions are becoming more complex.[139] US, percutaneous aspiration, and surgical intervention may be considered to provide diagnosis as well as prevention of torsion, rupture, and bleeding of large ovarian cysts.[140]

In a study by Platek and colleagues, 31 patients of 43,372 deliveries were found to have adnexal masses >6 cm persistent beyond 16 weeks of gestation.[141] No ovarian cancers were diagnosed. When malignancies have been found, germ cell tumors and epithelial cancers of low malignant potential were most common.[142] The pathology of ovarian cancer during pregnancy was reviewed by Dgani and colleagues.[143] They recorded data on 23 patients over a 24-year period. Borderline carcinomas were most frequent (35%), followed by invasive epithelial tumors (30%), dysgerminomas (17%), and granulosa cell tumors (13%). Early-stage disease was common; 74% of patients were stage I.

In the series of Sayedur and colleagues, seven of the nine patients had stage I epithelial tumors.[139] Five patients were treated with salpingo-oophorectomy, three with total abdominal hysterectomy, and bilateral salpingo-oophorectomy with omentectomy. They reported 100% survival for stage I disease and 78% 5-year survival overall. Conservative surgery for early-stage disease and low malignant potential tumors may preserve fertility. In the Dgani series, 14 of the 23 patients delivered live neonates.[143] Dgani concluded that the overall prognosis for ovarian cancer during pregnancy is better than ovarian tumors in general because of early stage at diagnosis and tumors of low malignant potential.

Chemotherapy for more advanced-stage disease has been reported primarily as case reports. Cisplatin, carboplatin, doxorubicin, bleomycin, cyclophosphamide, and, most recently, paclitaxel have all been given for treatment of ovarian cancer during pregnancy.[103,144–146]

Acute and chronic leukemia

Acute leukemia

Acute leukemia occurring during pregnancy presents unique circumstances because of bone marrow failure and the attendant cytopenias that may occur. Myeloid leukemias are more common than lymphoid. The presenting signs and symptoms are not different from those of the nonpregnant patient. The diagnosis is made by bone marrow aspiration, and standard classification is used for sub-typing and the initiation of therapy often cannot be delayed. In a series from the Mayo Clinic, 23 pregnant patients with acute leukemia, the majority of which were acute myeloid leukemia (AML), were treated between 1962 and 2016. Eighteen patients achieved a complete remission. Eleven of the pregnancies ended with a spontaneous or therapeutic abortion. Of the four patients diagnosed in the first trimester and delayed therapy >1 week, 2 died during induction therapy. No fetal malformations were noted in those treated with chemotherapy during pregnancy.[147]

Cardonick and Iacobucci performed an analysis of 152 patients who were treated for acute lymphoblastic leukemia (63 cases) or acute myelogenous leukemia (89 cases).[148] They found that six neonates developed congenital abnormalities and 12 neonates demonstrated IUGR. There were 11 cases of intrauterine fetal death and 2 neonatal deaths. All cases of abnormalities occurred in association with first-trimester usage of cytarabine or thioguanine, as monotherapy or in combination with an anthracycline. However, combinations of vincristine, mercaptopurine, doxorubicin or daunorubicin, cyclophosphamide, prednisone, and methotrexate were used in all trimesters.

Acute promyelocytic leukemia (APL) is of special interest because of the use of all-transretinoic acid (ATRA) in the treatment program. Retinoids have known teratogenic effects.[149] However, a number of case reports have documented fetal safety and favorable patient outcome with the use of ATRA for APL.[150,151]

Chronic leukemia

Pregnancy and chronic lymphocytic leukemia (CLL) is extraordinarily rare.[152,153] Welsh and colleagues reported a case of CLL with pregnancy and noted a substantial decrease in white blood cells after delivery.[153] They noted this apparent hematologic remission was not accompanied by clonal remission. Gurman described a case of a patient who became pregnant shortly after her diagnosis of CLL. She received no cytotoxic therapy, and she delivered a healthy infant at 39 weeks gestation.[34] Her third trimester was complicated by gestational diabetes and preeclampsia. Unlike the Welsh report, which demonstrated elevated numbers of lymphocytes in the intervillous space, the latter case demonstrated no lymphocytic infiltration of the placenta. Ali and colleagues treated a patient who was diagnosed with CLL during her 17th week of gestation.[154] She received three courses of leukapheresis at the 25th, 30th, and 38th week of gestation in order to maintain her WBC count below 100×10^9/l. She delivered a normal infant at 39 weeks of gestation.

Chronic myeloid leukemia has been treated during pregnancy with interferon α, hydroxyurea and leukapheresis, and leukapheresis alone.[155–158] No untoward effects of treatment on fetal growth, nor development or complications of labor and delivery have been reported.

Sustaining the pregnancy until delivery is feasible. Limited data suggest that pregnancy has no effect on CML long-term outcome; however, there are no case-control studies. Although limited data from animal studies suggest imatinib may have teratogenic properties, there is increasing, but conflicting data on imatinib use during pregnancy. Yilmaz et al. described three patients exposed to imatinib during pregnancy, all with healthy neonates at delivery.[159] Prabash et al. described two cases of normal births after imatinib exposure and continuation of imatinib therapy throughout the pregnancy.[160] Ault et al. described 19 pregnancies involving 18 patients who conceived while receiving imatinib. All female patients discontinued therapy at the time the pregnancy was discovered. Three pregnancies ended in spontaneous abortion and one with an elective abortion. Two of the 16 babies had abnormalities; one with hypospadias and another with rotation of the small intestine. The authors concluded that patients should use contraception as the discontinuation of imatinib may lead to loss of disease response. Another case report describes the development of a meningocele and death of the fetus exposed to imatinib.[161] Yadav et al. describe another woman who received hydroxyurea and imatinib during the third trimester with fetal complications of IUGR and oligohydramnios.[162] However, the child developed normally after delivery. Alizadeh et al. described 22 pregnancies in 14 patients or in the partner of a male patient exposed to tyrosine kinases for CML with only 1 with an atrial septal defect.[163] Therefore, patients should be encouraged to continue with contraception while on imatinib given these scant and conflicting reports, however, some patients have maintained imatinib therapy during pregnancy. This may be an option for some women, only after detailed and deliberative discussion with the treating team regarding risks and the limits of available information.

Melanoma

Surgical management remains the mainstay of treatment for newly diagnosed melanoma during pregnancy. There have been multiple reports of melanoma diagnosed during pregnancy. Johansson et al. describe the Swedish registry of 1019 women with pregnancy-associated melanoma.[164] Of these there was no difference in cause-specific mortality in pregnant versus nonpregnant patients. However, Bannister-Tyrrell et al. have described an Australian experience of 577 pregnancy-associated melanomas, of which 195 were diagnosed during pregnancy.[165] However, in this group there was an association with detection of the melanoma at more advanced stages.

Immunotherapy with checkpoint inhibition has dramatically changed treatment of melanoma and other immunogenic cancers. There remains limited data regarding exposure to checkpoint inhibitors during pregnancy. Bucheit et al. describe a patient who conceived a twin pregnancy on dual therapy with an anti-CTLA-4 and PD-1 therapy for metastatic melanoma and had a successful pregnancy.[166]

Transplacental malignancy and placental metastasis

A number of case reports have noted transplacental passage of malignancy from mother to neonate.[167–175] Catlin and colleagues reported a neonatal death related to the transplacental passage of maternal natural killer cell lymphoma.[167] Successful treatment of

Table 2 Placental metastases.

Tumor type (reference)
Small-cell lung cancer[174]
Melanoma[174]
Pancreas[176]
Breast[177]
Medulloblastoma[178]
Large-cell lung cancer[179]
B-cell lymphoma[180]
T-cell lymphoma[181]
Non-Hodgkin's lymphoma[182]
Large-cell lymphoma[135]

Table 3 Multidisciplinary approach to the pregnant patient with cancer.

Diagnosis and treatment planning	Considerations
Confirm diagnosis	Cytology, histology
Assess extent of disease	Staging, physical exam, organ function, metastatic disease
Disease-related prognosis independent of pregnancy	
Assess pregnancy	Comorbidities—age, diabetes, cardiac function
	Gestational age
	Expected delivery date
Review treatment options	*For patient*:
	Anticipated benefits for the patient
	"Cure," prolongation of life, improve or delay symptoms
	For fetus:
	Anticipated outcome
	Maintaining pregnancy
	Anticipated risks for fetus
Plan and implement treatment plan	
Reevaluate patient and fetus at frequent intervals	
Multidisciplinary treatment team members	Patient
	Obstetrician
	Oncologists-surgical, radiation, medical, gynecologist, radiation physicist
	Nurses
	Ethicists
	Social service
	Pastoral care

maternal transplacental small-cell lung cancer has been noted.[174] Teksam presented a striking case of a 33-week neonate who was emergently delivered after her mother was diagnosed with lung cancer. Due to the presence of placental metastases, the infant underwent initial screening with brain MRI and chest/abdomen CT, both of which were apparently normal. Unfortunately, serial examinations demonstrated development of a cerebellar tumor that significantly improved after chemotherapy, but the mass progressed a few months afterward. Biopsy and resection confirmed that the neoplasm was metastatic lung cancer. Additional metastatic lesions were identified in the frontal and temporal lobes on follow-up MRI.[175]

Leukemia cell identification in circulation in a neonate born to a mother with ALL has also been reported. However, leukemic cell engraftment and neonatal disease were not observed.[172] Acute monocytic leukemia transmission from mother to fetus has been documented.[170]

Alexander and colleagues reviewed 87 cases of fetal or placental metastases; they found that malignant melanoma affected 31% of these patients, making melanoma the most common malignancy to involve both the fetus and placenta.[171]

Dildy and colleagues reviewed placental metastases and reported 52 cases in 1989. Solid tumors and hematologic malignancies have been noted to involve the placenta (Table 2).[135,176–184] Systematic evaluation of the placenta at the time of delivery of the pregnant woman with cancer has not been routine. However, new technologies are being evaluated for easier identification of possible transplacental transfer of malignancies.

Conclusion

Cancer during pregnancy presents a unique opportunity for multispecialty oncologic and prenatal care. The gathering and discussion of data to be utilized in treatment planning requires careful coordination with obstetrical, surgical, and anesthesiology colleagues. Given the concern for the well-being of both the mother and fetus, support for and reassurance of the patient during the decision process becomes a paramount duty for physicians. It is possible to have a favorable outcome for mother and child. An outline of a sequential approach to multispecialty management for cancer and pregnancy is presented in Table 3.

Key references

The complete reference list can be found on Vital Source version of this title, see inside front cover.

1. Peccatori FA, Azim HA, Orecchia R, et al. Cancer, pregnancy and fertility: ESMO Clinical Practice Guidelines for diagnosis, treatment and follow-up. *Ann Oncol*. 2013;**24**:vi160–vi170.
2. Amant F, Berveiller P, Boere IA, et al. Gynecologic cancers in pregnancy: guidelines based on a third international consensus meeting. *Ann Oncol*. 2019;**30**: 1601–1612.
6. Andersson TML, Johansson ALV, Hsieh C-C, et al. Increasing incidence of pregnancy-associated breast cancer in Sweden. *Obstet Gynecol*. 2009; **114**:568–572. doi: 10.1097/AOG.0b013e3181b19154.
7. Dominici LS, Kuerer HM, Babiera G, et al. Wound complications from surgery in pregnancy-associated breast cancer (PABC). *Breast Disease*. 2010;**31**:1–5.
11. Hahn K, Johnson P, Gordon N, et al. Treatment of pregnant breast cancer patients and outcomes of children exposed to chemotherapy in utero. *Cancer*. 2006;**107**:1219–1226.
13. De Santis M, Straface G, Cavaliere AF, et al. Gadolinium periconceptional exposure: pregnancy and neonatal outcome. *Acta Obstet Gynecol Scand*. 2007;**86**:99–101.
16. Benveniste H, Fowler JS, Rooney WD, et al. Maternal-fetal in vivo imaging: a combined PET and MRI study. *J Nucl Med*. 2003;**44**:1522–1530.
23. Sood AK, Sorosky JI, Mayr N, et al. Radiotherapeutic management of cervical carcinoma that complicates pregnancy. *Cancer*. 1997;**80**:1073–1078.
24. Woo S, Fuller L, Cundiff J, et al. Radiotherapy during pregnancy for clinical stages IA–IIA Hodgkin's disease. *Int J Radiat Oncol Biol Phys*. 1992;**23**:407.
27. Islam MK, Saeedi F, Al-Rajhi N. A simplified shielding approach for limiting fetal dose during radiation therapy of pregnant patients. *Int J Radiat Oncol Biol Phys*. 2001;**49**:1469–1473.
33. Cardonick E, Gilmandyar D, Somer RA. Maternal and neonatal outcomes of dose-dense chemotherapy for breast cancer in pregnancy. *Obstet Gynecol*. 2012;**120**:1267–1272.
34. Germann N, Goffinet F, Goldwasser F. Anthracyclines during pregnancy: embryo-fetal outcome in 160 patients. *Ann Oncol*. 2004;**15**:146–150.
35. Cardonick E, Bhat A, Gilmandyar D, et al. Maternal and fetal outcomes of taxane chemotherapy in breast and ovarian cancer during pregnancy: case series and review of the literature. *Ann Oncol*. 2012;**23**:3016–3023.
36. Azim HA Jr, Santoro L, Russell-Edu W, et al. Prognosis of pregnancy-associated breast cancer: a meta-analysis of 30 studies. *Cancer Treat Rev*. 2012;**38**:834–842.
37. Litton J, Warneke C, Hahn K, et al. Case control study of women treated with chemotherapy for breast cancer during pregnancy as compared with non-pregnant breast cancer patients. *Oncologist*. 2013;**18**:369–376.

38. Aviles A, Neri N. Hematologic malignancies and pregnancy: a final report of 84 children who received chemotherapy in utero. *Clin Lymphoma*. 2001;**2**:173–177.
39. Van Calsteren K, Berteloot P, Hanssens M, et al. In utero exposure to chemotherapy: effect on cardiac and neurologic outcome. *J Clin Oncol*. 2006;**24**:e16–e17.
40. Abdel-Hady el S, Hemida RA, Gamal A, et al. Cancer during pregnancy: perinatal outcome after in utero exposure to chemotherapy. *Arch Gynecol Obstet*. 2012;**286**:283–286.
41. Murthy R, Theriault R, Barnett C, et al. Outcomes of children exposed in utero to chemotherapy for breast cancer. *Breast Cancer Res*. 2014;**16**:3414.
42. Cardonick EMD, Dougherty RMD, Grana GMD, et al. Breast cancer during pregnancy: maternal and fetal outcomes. *Cancer J*. 2010;**16**(1):76–82.
43. Loibl S, Han SN, von Minckwitz G, et al. Treatment of breast cancer during pregnancy: an observational study. *Lancet Oncol*. 2012;**13**:887–896.
44. Amant F, Vandenbroucke T, Verheecke M, et al. Pediatric outcome after maternal cancer diagnosed during pregnancy. *N Engl J Med*. 2015;**373**:1824–1834.
47. Murphy CG, Mallam D, Stein S, et al. Current or recent pregnancy is associated with adverse pathologic features but not impaired survival in early breast cancer. *Cancer*. 2012;**118**:3254–3259.
49. Liberman L, Giess C, Dershaw D, et al. Imaging of pregnancy associated breast cancer. *Radiology*. 1994;**191**:245–248.
51. Yang WT, Dryden MJ, Gwyn K, et al. Imaging of breast cancer diagnosed and treated with chemotherapy during pregnancy. *Radiology*. 2006;**239**:52–60.
54. Bottles K, Taylor R. Diagnosis of breast masses in pregnant and lactating women by aspiration cytology. *Obstet Gynecol*. 1985;**66**:76S–78S.
55. Keleher A, Wendt R, Delpassand E, et al. The safety of lymphatic mapping in pregnant breast cancer patients using Tc-99m sulfur colloid. *Breast J*. 2004;**10**:492–495.
56. Gentilini O, Cremonesi M, Toesca A, et al. Sentinel lymph node biopsy in pregnant patients with breast cancer. *Eur J Nucl Med Mol Imaging*. 2010;**37**:78–83.
58. Gropper A, Calvillo K, Dominici L, et al. Sentinel lymph node biopsy in pregnant women with breast cancer. *Ann Surg Oncol*. 2014;**21**:2506–2511.
59. Han SN, Amant F, Cardonick EH, et al. Axillary staging for breast cancer during pregnancy: feasibility and safety of sentinel lymph node biopsy. *Breast Cancer Res Treat*. 2018;**168**:551–557.
62. Mir O, Berveiller P, Goffinet F, et al. Taxanes for breast cancer during pregnancy: a systematic review. *Ann Oncol*. 2010;**21**(2):425–426. doi: 10.1093/annonc/mdp517.
70. Fanale M, Uyei A, Theriault R, et al. Treatment of metastatic breast cancer with trastuzumab and vinorelbine during pregnancy. *Clin Breast Cancer*. 2005;**6**:354–356.
74. Pant S, Landon MB, Blumenfeld M, et al. Treatment of breast cancer with trastuzumab during pregnancy. *J Clin Oncol*. 2008;**26**:1567–1569.
76. Shrim A, Garcia-Bournissen F, Maxwell C, et al. Trastuzumab treatment for breast cancer during pregnancy. *Can Fam Phys*. 2008;**54**:31–32.
77. Witzel ID, Muller V, Harps E, et al. Trastuzumab in pregnancy associated with poor fetal outcome. *Ann Oncol*. 2008;**19**:191–a–192.
86. Rouzier R, Werkoff G, Uzan C, et al. Pregnancy-associated breast cancer is as chemosensitive as non-pregnancy-associated breast cancer in the neoadjuvant setting. *Ann Oncol*. 2011;**22**:1582–1587.
102. Zagouri F, Sergentanis TN, Chrysikos D, et al. Platinum derivatives during pregnancy in cervical cancer: a systematic review and meta-analysis. *Obstet Gynecol*. 2013;**121**:337–343.
128. Kimby E, Sverrisdottir A, Elinder G. Safety of rituximab therapy during the first trimester of pregnancy: a case history. *Eur J Haematol*. 2004;**72**:292–295.
166. Bucheit AD, Hardy JT, Szender JB, et al. Conception and viable twin pregnancy in a patient with metastatic melanoma while treated with CTLA-4 and PD-1 checkpoint inhibition. *Melanoma Res*. 2020;**30**(4):423–425. doi: 10.1097/CMR.0000000000000657.
183. Baergen RN, Johnson D, Moore T, et al. Maternal melanoma metastatic to the placenta: a case report and review of the literature. *Arch Pathol Lab Med*. 1997;**121**:508–511.
184. Dunn JS Jr, Anderson CD, Brost BC. Breast carcinoma metastatic to the placenta. *Obstet Gynecol*. 1999;**94**:846.

69 Cancer and aging

Ashley E. Rosko, MD ■ Carolyn J. Presley, MD, MHS ■ Grant R. Williams, MD, MSPH ■ Rebecca L. Olin, MD, MSCE

> **Overview**
>
> Cancer is a disease of older adults; with over half of cancers diagnosed in adults 65 years and older. Older adults are also comprising a larger portion of cancer survivors, accounting for 62%. The therapeutic landscape and treatment approaches are highly variable as is the health of older adults. The unique factors that older adults face must be considered when developing treatment strategies for maximum care and quality of life.

Cancer is a disease predominately of older adults. Over half of cancers are diagnosed in those age 65 years and older, of which deaths are highest in this same population.[1] Cancer of any site is most frequently diagnosed among people aged 65–74.[1] The number of older adult cancer survivors is also increasing, accounting for 62% of cancer survivors; this demographic will grow in size as the US population age, life expectancies rise, and cancer survivorship rates increase.[2] Improving survival rates are a result of better cancer screening, advances in drug discovery, improved supportive care, and more tolerable therapeutic strategies for individuals with cancer. The dynamic therapeutic landscape is changing with highly variable treatment strategies beyond traditional chemotherapy; including targeted agents, immunotherapy, cellular therapy, and increasing access to allogeneic or autologous stem cell transplant. Similar to the heterogeneity in therapeutic strategies, oncologists recognize heterogeneity in health with aging. In order to reconcile differences in health with aging, national societies and guidelines have recommended that all older adults 65 years and older undergo a comprehensive geriatric assessment (CGA).[3] A geriatric assessment (GA) is a global evaluation of the health of older adults, comprising a multi-dimensional evaluation of functional status, fall history, social support, cognitive and psychologic status, sensory loss, nutritional status, and co-morbidities. The use of a GA aids in the clinical decision-making for patients with cancer and have been shown to predict mortality and toxicity, independent of performance status and age in solid tumors.[4,5] A GA aims to identify occult factors, unique to aging, that contribute to adverse events in cancer treatment.

Physiologic aging and cancer

Central to the approach of treatment decisions for older adults is understanding "right-fit" treatment decisions, neither over-treating nor undertreating an older adult with cancer. Treatment decisions for individuals with cancer are based on weighing the risks and benefits of therapy, personalized for the individual. With aging, individual health patterns are dynamic and may change with a cancer diagnosis. A personalized approach for an aging adult recognizes that chronologic age is not a good surrogate for health status. Physiologic changes, within organ systems, occur with aging for all individuals, and this process is called homeostenosis. Homestenosis was defined as the increased vulnerability to disease with aging and defined in the 1940s but is still relevant when approaching older adults with cancer today.[6] The rate of change in physiologic aging is unique to each person and each organ system and is influenced by genetics, behavior, and the environment. The trajectory of these changes is highly variable and can be challenging to characterize. Aging with pathology or "accelerated aging" is increasingly recognized as clinically distinct from "normal aging." Physiologic aging is associated with known changes across organ systems, here we characterize changes in cardiopulmonary status, renal function, hematologic/immune system, and the gastrointestinal tract.

Cardiopulmonary

The aging cardiovascular system is associated with decreased compliance of large vessels, fibrosis and calcification of cardiac valves, and changes in the conduction system. This can be associated with the development of cardiac morbidity including hypertension, heart failure, electrical conduction abnormalities, or valvular disease. Peak pulmonary aerobic activity has been reported to decline with age, as has diffusion capacity, but this may not yield clinically significant results.[7] For older adults with cancer, traditional therapeutic agents such as anthracyclines are known to result in cardiac impairment. Emerging data in targeted therapy also demonstrate changes within the cardiopulmonary system such as the development of arrhythmias with ibrutinib[8] or pulmonary toxicity associated with checkpoint inhibition.[9]

Renal

Serum creatinine is an unreliable metric to measure renal function with aging. Glomerular filtration rate (GFR)-estimating equations [modification of diet in renal disease (MDRD) or Cockcroft-Gault equation] have replaced serum creatinine as a better surrogate of renal function. Both structural and functional changes occur within the aging renal system. GFR declines with healthy aging at a rate of 0.75 mL/min/year per decade of life.[10] Given normal renal aging, many older adults are mislabeled as having chronic kidney disease with decreases in estimated GFR.[11] Many investigation agents and approved therapeutic regimens may not have specifically been studied in aging adults, and/or those with impaired renal function. Chemotherapeutic dosages that are excreted by glomerular filtration (water-soluble medications) require dosage adjustment.

Holland-Frei Cancer Medicine, Tenth Edition. Edited by Robert C. Bast, John C. Byrd, Carlo M. Croce, Ernest Hawk, Fadlo R. Khuri, Raphael E. Pollock, Apostolia M. Tsimberidou, Christopher G. Willett, and Cheryl L. Willman.
© 2023 John Wiley & Sons, Inc. Published 2023 by John Wiley & Sons, Inc.

Hematopoietic/immune system

Despite a decrease in bone marrow mass, most aging adults retain normal hematopoietic function throughout their lifespan with a normal hemoglobin, normal white blood cell count, and platelet parameters. However, changes in immunologic function with aging are well characterized and include alterations in both the innate and adaptive immune system. Distinct changes in the immune system are reported with aging and include the development of immunosenescence, changes in T-cells composition, alterations in proliferative capacity, and increased cytotoxicity. Immunosenescence has been defined as the age-related progressive decline in the ability to trigger or develop antibody and/or cellular responses against an infectious pathogen.[12] The aging immune system lends to increased susceptibility to infections and cancer development.

Gastrointestinal tract

Changes in gastric or intestinal motility and hepatobiliary perfusion change with normal aging. Gastric mucosa changes occur in half of adults with aging[13] most commonly due to *Helicobacter pylori*. Aging influences gastrointestinal tract motility and sensory function influencing transit, with a modest impact on absorption.[14] Innumerable cancer therapeutic agents are metabolized by the liver and confounded by poly-pharmacy common among aging adults. LiverTox[15] provides an online clinical registry of chemotherapeutic induced liver injury, in addition to evidence on dietary supplements and herbal products.

Biologic age

Biological age is a metric of functional reserve, physiologic decline, and estimates life expectancy. The cellular biological process that drives biologic aging processes are the known as the hallmarks of aging and include; genomic instability, telomere attrition, epigenetic alterations, loss of proteostasis, deregulated nutrient sensing, mitochondrial dysfunction, cellular senescence, stem cell exhaustion, and altered intercellular communication.[16] Defects in these pathways parallel that of cancer development. There is no simple way to assess biological age, and biomarkers of aging have been proposed to reflect the biology of aging and reproduce susceptibility to disease and loss of function. Criteria have also been developed by The American Federation for Aging Research (AFAR) recommending that the criteria for a biomarker of aging: (1) predict the rate of aging and mortality better than chronologic age; (2) reflect a biologic process that underlies the aging and not a marker of the disease itself; (3) safely tested; and (4) reproducible in humans and laboratory animal models.

Importantly for older adults with cancer, an accurate assessment of the physiologic age is warranted to drive treatment decisions that are personalized based on health. Understanding changes that occur normally across organ systems is important to characterize normal aging from accelerating aging. Biomarkers of aging afford one method to characterize physiologic aging and ongoing investigations, incorporating biomarkers in cancer clinical research, are under development. Importantly, functional age or frailty can also be readily assessed in routine oncology evaluation with the use of a GA to identify geriatric syndromes.

Geriatric syndromes in older adults with cancer

Geriatric syndromes are complex medical conditions highly prevalent in older adults that crosscut traditional organ-based medical conditions and are multifactorial, costly, and debilitating in nature. Common syndromes addressed include frailty, falls, dizziness, delirium, urinary incontinence, syncope, sleep disorders, pressure ulcers, and elder mistreatment.[17] Older adults with cancer are unique in that more health issues present per person compared to older adults without cancer.[18] Due to a new cancer diagnosis, geriatric syndromes may be overlooked, which could affect treatment tolerability and health outcomes. Among 12,480 Medicare beneficiaries studied, older adults with a history of cancer were more likely to experience one or more geriatric syndromes (60.3%) compared with older adults without cancer (53%). This not only puts older adults with cancer at a higher risk of further morbidity and mortality but increases their likelihood of hospitalizations and healthcare costs.[18] Along with a new cancer diagnosis, comes a barrage of diagnostic tests, multi-consultant appointments, new medications, and complicated treatment schedules. This significant treatment burden associated with a new cancer diagnosis compounds what older adults are already facing and can greatly challenge a medical system unprepared to address the multifactorial reality of geriatric care, particularly for frail older adults.

Frailty in older adults with cancer

The term "frail" is used to describe a subset of older patients with a critically reduced functional reserve that places them at risk for dependency, institutionalization, illness, hospitalization, and mortality.[19] A proposed definition of frailty is "a state of age-related physiologic vulnerability resulting from impaired homeostatic reserve and reduced capacity of the organism to withstand stress." Therefore, the clinical syndrome of frailty is proposed to be a dynamic consequence of a negative energy balance; for example, starting with undernutrition that leads to loss of muscle and bone mass and contributes to further decline in activity level and strength.[19] This, in combination with decreased reserve, contributes to the increased vulnerability of the frail patient. The result is failure to thrive, which is a syndrome of unexplained weight loss, decreased muscle mass, and metabolic abnormalities including a decrease in albumin, creatinine, cholesterol, and hemoglobin. Immune dysfunction and chronic inflammation may play a role in frailty. Markers of inflammation are associated with aging and frailty including the cytokine interleukin 6 (IL-6) and the acute phase reactant, C-reactive protein (CRP).[20] In addition, elevations in plasma D dimer have been associated with age. Both IL-6 and D dimer have been predictive of mortality and functional decline.[21,22]

A phenotype for frailty was developed in a prospective observational study of 5317 community-dwelling men and women age ≥65 years.[19] The "frailty phenotype" was defined as a clinical syndrome in which three or more of the following criteria are present: (1) unintentional weight loss ≥10 pounds in past year, (2) self-reported exhaustion, (3) weakness defined as the lowest twentieth percentile in grip strength adjusted for gender and body mass index, (4) slow walking speed defined as the lowest twentieth percentile on a timed walk of 15 feet, and (5) low physical activity defined as the lowest quintile of kilocalories per week.[19] Individuals with one or two of the criteria were categorized as an "intermediate or prefrail phenotype." Patients defined as frail or prefrail, compared with nonfrail, had a higher incidence of 3- and 7-year mortality, hospitalization, incident falls, progressive decline in ability to complete activities of daily living (ADL), and decreased mobility. On the basis of these criteria, 7% of community-dwelling individuals age 65 and older were frail and 47% were prefrail. The prevalence of frailty and prefrailty was greater in women than men and increased with age.[19] Frailty is also associated with an increased risk of recurrent falls, hip fracture, and any nonspine fractures.[23] As the "frailty phenotype" requires specific objective measurements that are not commonly employed in oncology, there is less data on its use in cancer care.

Another method of measuring frailty was developed by Rockwood and colleagues in which frailty is viewed as an accumulation of deficits.[24] This frailty index is based on the premise that while individual deficit may not have a discernible threat to mortality (or other outcomes), the accumulation of these individual deficits will add up to poorer outcomes in the older adult population. For example, in general populations of older people, the accumulation of deficits has been demonstrated to predict hospitalization, institutionalization, and death.[25] In comparison to the phenotype model developed by Fried and colleagues, which requires the knowledge of specific parameters, the deficits accumulation method can be used for virtually any data set which captures GA variables if enough variables are collected (recommended more than 30 health deficits be included).[26] Given the versatility of this method and its ability to be applied to the commonly utilized GAs, this is the primary definition used to date in older adults with cancer. A frailty index has been associated with increased chemotherapy toxicities, increased all-cause mortality, reduced health-related quality of life, and increased hospitalizations/long-term skilled nursing placement.[27,28] Compared to the frailty phenotype, use of the frailty index often identifies a higher proportion of frailty with estimates that are typically twofold higher.[29]

Frail older patients with cancer represent a unique subset of patients that pose challenging therapeutic decisions. The aforementioned geriatric measures of frailty have not been widely implemented in the care of older adults with cancer. An important initial step in evaluation of the frail patient is to determine whether the cancer is likely to decrease the patient's life expectancy. In a model proposed by Balducci and Stanta,[30] one would consider treatment of the cancer if it was impacting the patient's life expectancy or if it was causing a compromise in quality of life. The goal of treatment must be determined: cure, life prolonging, or palliation. Treatment decisions involve weighing the risks and benefits with the patient and caregiver. As the nation is aging, there will be a rise in the number of frail older patients with cancer. More clinical trials focusing on efficacy and tolerability of treatment within this patient population are needed.

In addition, there is a growing number of cancer survivors in the United States, many of whom are older adults.[31] How cancer and its many treatments impact the aging process is an area of growing interest. Several studies have suggested a pro-aging effect of cancer and its treatments with increases in frailty and other geriatric syndromes such as sarcopenia (loss of muscle mass).[32,33] In a seminal study of young adult childhood cancer survivors (average age of 34 years), the prevalence of frailty was similar to that of adults 65 years of age or older.[34] There is a growing need to understand the aging-related implications of cancer and cancer treatments in order to develop targeted interventions to improve long-term outcomes and integrate this into treatment decision-making particularly in the adjuvant setting.

Comorbidities in older adults with cancer

Comorbidity is defined as a concurrent medical problem that is a competing source of morbidity or mortality. In a study by Yancik and colleagues, summary data on comorbidity were collected on 7600 patients aged ≥55 years. The most common concurrent medical problems included hypertension (42.9%), heart-related conditions (39.1%), and arthritis (34.9%).[35] The number of comorbid conditions increased with age. Patients aged 55–64 had an average of 2.9 comorbid conditions, patients aged 65–74 had 3.6 comorbid conditions, and those 75 and older had 4.2 medical conditions.[35] The presence and profile of common comorbid conditions often vary by cancer type as well (see Figure 1).[36] A variety of tools are available to assess comorbid conditions, each with their own limitations and strengths, and no single measure is uniformly recommended; however, a systematic approach to assess comorbidity is critical.[37,38]

The presence of comorbid conditions has been strongly linked to reduced survival in older adults with cancer. While the absolute impact of comorbidity on survival varies by cancer type and severity of comorbid condition, patients with comorbidity have a 1.1- to 5.8-fold higher mortality risk.[39] The association between comorbidity and survival in patients with cancer is independent of a patient's functional status.[40] Therefore, each is an important domain to assess. The potential impact of a new disease as a competing cause of mortality decreases with increasing age secondary to the decrease in absolute projected life expectancy.[41] For example, consider the impact of a disease with a projected 50% mortality over 5 years in a 65-year-old person in comparison to an 85-year-old person. This disease will decrease the 65-year-old person's average life expectancy by approximately 10 years, whereas because the absolute projected life expectancy of an 85-year-old person is less than that of a 65-year-old person, it will decrease an 85-year-old person's average life expectancy by only about 2 years.[41] The number and severity of comorbid conditions increase with age and comorbid conditions also influence the likelihood of receipt and tolerance of chemotherapy. Data from the Surveillance, Epidemiology, and End Results-Medicare database demonstrates that older patients with colon cancer who have a history of heart failure, diabetes, or chronic obstructive pulmonary disease are less likely to receive adjuvant chemotherapy.[42]

The concept of multimorbidity, defined as the presence of several comorbid illnesses in which one single condition is not the dedicated focus, is of growing interest in the older adult population more broadly. The American Geriatrics Society (AGS) guiding principles for the care of older adults with multimorbidity created a conceptual framework for guiding clinical management of multimorbid patients.[43] These five guiding principles include (1) assessing patient preferences, (2) interpreting and applying the available evidence, (3) estimating prognosis, (4) considering treatment feasibility, and (5) optimizing therapies and care plans. These principles have been adapted to assist in guiding oncology decision-making in older adults with cancer.

A multidisciplinary approach: using a comprehensive geriatric assessment among older adults with cancer

The ideal care model for delivery of specialized care to the older adult with cancer requires multidimensional assessment and multidisciplinary management.[44] All older adults should undergo a CGA or GA screening to evaluate the possible need for a full evaluation.[45,46] These assessments can either be performed by a geriatric specialist trained in the nuances of the management of older adults or by use of systematic patient-reported and objective measures that can be obtained by the oncology team. In select high resource areas, it is ideal to involve a geriatrician as part of the multidisciplinary cancer team. This offers the advantage of incorporating a provider trained in the complex medical management of older adults within the clinic that can aid in treatment decisions

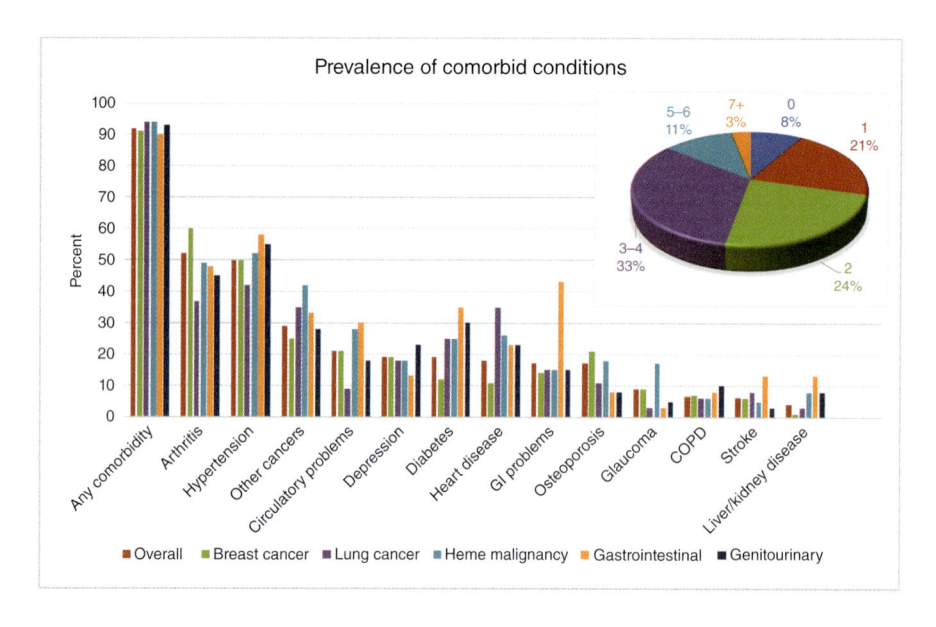

Figure 1 The prevalence of specific comorbid conditions overall and by cancer type and the overall distribution of comorbid conditions in a sample of 539 older adults from within the Carolina senior registry. Source: Williams et al.[36]

as well as provide referrals for GA-based interventions that may improve outcomes in vulnerable older adults. In contrast, in other clinical settings without access to a geriatric specialist, a GA can only be performed by the oncology team.[47] In these settings without access to a geriatric specialist, a patient-reported or nurse-led GA can be utilized; however, it is then up to the oncology team to incorporate these findings in treatment decision-making, identify appropriate GA-based interventions, and then provide appropriate referrals.[48,49]

A CGA is specifically designed to identify geriatric syndromes and other conditions that affect poor outcomes among older adults both with and without cancer. A CGA determines physiological rather than chronological age. It provides substantial information on functional status and deficits even among older adults deemed to have an excellent Eastern Cooperative Oncology Group Performance Status (ECOG PS).[50] Major components outlining a CGA include eight domains: functional status, physical performance, comorbidity, polypharmacy (PP), cognition, nutrition, psychological health, and social support. Though the cornerstone of geriatric medicine, these domains are often not addressed during busy oncology clinic appointments. While labor intensive, integrating a CGA into oncology care can not only improve health outcomes but can also improve patient and caregiver satisfaction and communication.[51]

Treatment decisions in older adults with cancer should be personalized and informed by individual estimates of the potential risks as well as the benefits of treatment. Employing a GA and other risk assessments can help obtain more objective estimates of survival and chemotherapy toxicity risk.[45,52,53] Similar in concept to staging a cancer, the oncology team should "stage the aging" to understand treatment tolerability and risks.[54,55] In addition, it is critically important to assess the patient's preferences and goals for treatment. Many older adults value functional independence over incremental increases in survival, and these preferences should be specifically elicited during treatment decision-making.[56,57] Lastly, the GA also can uncover many impairments that are overlooked by traditional oncologic evaluations, many of which have potential interventions.[58] For example, the presence of falls is often overlooked by the oncology team but is a well-known risk factor for chemotherapy toxicities and with many potential interventions such as physical or occupational therapy.[59,60]

Evidence-based use of cancer-specific geriatric screening tools

Cancer-specific geriatric screening tools have been developed to shorten the length of time required to evaluate a patient in lieu of a full CGA (see Table 1). These tools assess vulnerability and frailty and can inform risk of treatment toxicity. Similar to a CGA, they can enhance the prognostic value of routinely evaluating standard of care evaluation, such as the ECOG PS. Several studies demonstrate associations between the use of cancer-specific geriatric screening tools and global health outcomes. Though the preferred screening tool may vary depending on setting and situation, the G8 screening tool, made specifically for older adults with cancer, is one of the most studied tools internationally for multiple cancer types.[61] Based on the results of these geriatric screening tools, referral for a full GA within a dedicated geriatric oncology clinic or geriatrics clinic is recommended.

In one cancer-specific study, a CGA detected unknown geriatric problems in upwards of 51% of patients 70 years and older with a cancer diagnosis.[62] Within this cohort, 13.2% of patients had at least mild cognitive impairment and, since this particular population is at risk of delirium, it justified the need for specific attention and treatment plans. Once physicians were made aware of these results, geriatric interventions and adapted treatments took place in 25.7% and 25.3% of these patients, respectively. However, the prevalence of chemotherapy-related cognitive impairment is highly variable and warrants further research.[63] Regardless, cognitive impairments, such as memory loss, as well as mood disorders, such as depression, may affect patient understanding relating to disease, prognosis, and treatment plan. Due to the increase in oral chemotherapy agents and targeted therapy, a physician's awareness of a patient's CGA score relating to their psychological state could provide better insight into their ability to adhere to certain treatment plans.[64,65]

Table 1 Sampling of geriatric screening tools for older adults with cancer.

Tool	Population	Evaluates	Website
CARG	United States; all cancer types	Chemotherapy toxicity	https://www.mycarg.org/?page_id=2405
ESOGIA	France and Spain; advanced non-small-cell lung cancer	Integration of CGA in cancer treatment decision-making	https://ascopubs.org/doi/10.1200/JCO.2015.63.5839
CRASH	United States; all cancer types	Chemotherapy toxicity	https://moffitt.org/for-healthcare-providers/clinical-programs-and-services/senior-adult-oncology-program/senior-adult-oncology-program-tools
G8	All cancer types	Vulnerability	http://www.siog.org/files/public/g8_english_0.pdf
SIOG1	Prostate cancer	Frailty	http://www.siog.org/content/comprehensive-geriatric-assessment-cga-older-patient-cancer
VES-13	All cancer types	Vulnerability	https://www.rand.org/health-care/projects/acove/survey.html
EORTC QLQ-ELD-14	Europe; all cancer types	Health-related quality of life	https://www.eortc.org/app/uploads/sites/2/2018/08/Specimen-ELD14-English.pdf

Once cognitive function and medication-related vulnerabilities are brought to the attention of healthcare providers, there are more physician-initiated conversations pertaining to PP and potentially inappropriate medications (PIMs). Since PP and PIMs can increase the chance of adverse effects, such as hospitalizations and falls, these conversations are crucial in preventing adverse outcomes.[66] In addition, the results of an assessment can lead to referrals to appropriate geriatric programs, such as a fall clinic or geriatric daycare center, which can further prevent adverse effects during treatment.[67]

A CGA is instrumental in determining a personalized and appropriate course of treatment and has proven helpful in managing a number of geriatric syndromes that would otherwise result in increased hospital admission. For patients with cancer, a CGA assesses a number of possibilities that may give insight into potential outcomes following certain treatment courses and, ultimately, can assist in treatment decisions that may prevent unnecessary or excessive hospitalizations.[65]

Geriatric oncology screening tools and cancer-specific treatment outcomes

In addition to the presence of unidentified or under-identified geriatric syndromes, choosing appropriate treatment, whether surgery, radiation, and/or systemic therapy, is complicated for older adults with cancer due to the fact that they are chronically underrepresented in clinical trials. Geriatricians and geriatric oncologists use the CGA and cancer-specific geriatric screening tools to personalize cancer treatments to address the underlying heterogeneity of an aging oncology population. Several studies have demonstrated the usefulness of screening tools to assist with treatment decision-making and their association with treatment outcomes.

Surgery
Surgery is considered the gold-standard curative option for several cancer types including breast, prostate, lung, and colon cancers. Chronological age should not be the primary barrier for receipt of curative surgical treatment options. Physiologic age and risk can be determined using a CGA or abbreviated GA. A survey administered to oncologic surgeons evaluating the preferred course of treatment for older adults with cancer, more than 90% favored surgery. However, only 6.4% of surgeons from the same study used CGAs.[68] Despite the minimal use of CGAs in daily practice, they can provide valuable insight into a patient's experience postsurgery. For example, a study by Korc-Grodzicki et al. found that GAs are predictive of postoperative delirium in older adults undergoing major cancer surgery.[69] In addition, a study of patients with cancer 75 years and older, a higher Memorial Sloan Kettering-Frailty Index (MSK-FI) score was associated with short-term surgical outcomes, such as longer hospitalization and increased intensive care unit admissions. In addition, overall mortality was also associated with MSK-FI score, with a 20% 12-month risk of death for scores of 4 and higher.[70]

Systemic treatment
In cases where chemotherapy is preferred, a CGA can be helpful in predicting toxicity. The late Dr. Hurria et al. developed and implemented a cancer-specific chemotherapy toxicity tool that predicted high-grade treatment toxicities better than physician-graded performance status.[53] In the ESOGIA-GFPC-GECP 08-02 study, patients who were in the CGA-directed arm had fewer toxicities and improved quality of life; however, there was no difference in survival as compared to the standard of care arm. Though oncology research studies focus on survival as primary outcomes, the quality of life is sometimes more important to older adults than merely survival alone.[71] The INTEGRATED study demonstrated that the integration of a GA into routine cancer care whether chemotherapy, targeted therapy, or immunotherapy, resulted in fewer visits to the emergency room, fewer days in the hospital, a better ability to complete treatment, and improved quality of life.[72] These are just a few examples of how the incorporation of geriatric principles and risk stratification can improve outcomes that matter most to older adults with cancer.

Radiation
Radiation is used for older adults in both curative and palliative settings. Though current research on the role of a CGA in radiation treatment is limited, a pilot study conducted in older adults with head and neck cancer showed that patients were less likely to complete radiotherapy if the results of their G8 questionnaire deemed them vulnerable.[73] They are at higher risk for weight loss as compared to younger adults and may require treatment interruption due to common radiation-associated toxicities.[74] For older adults with lung cancer, the addition of chemotherapy to radiation therapy improves overall survival[75]; however, sequential versus concurrent chemoradiation may be associated with lower toxicity and equivalent survival.[76] A CALGB study determined there was no difference in breast cancer-specific mortality or 5-year overall survival when radiation was omitted for older women with low-risk stage I, estrogen receptor-positive breast cancer after lumpectomy, and received tamoxifen.[77] In summary, cancer treatment choice and delivery can be modified or informed

based on the results of dedicated geriatric oncology screening tools or a CGA when used in older adults regardless of treatment strategy or modality.

Survivorship in the older adult with cancer

Broadly, a cancer survivor is defined as any patient with a diagnosis of cancer, from the time of diagnosis onward.[78] However, practically, there is a need to distinguish between patients who receive curative-intent treatment and then may need to undergo surveillance and management of any residual toxicities (and may receive most of their care with their primary care physician), versus those who have ongoing active cancer, including metastatic disease, and receive ongoing therapy from their oncologist. Both groups of survivors have significant need for care coordination, but expectations and approaches may need to be different for these groups.

Older adult survivors are more likely to have comorbidities at the time of, and after, cancer diagnosis. One study found that on average, survivors reported having five comorbid conditions ever, and two comorbid conditions diagnosed after their cancer diagnosis.[79] Comorbidity burden is highest in the oldest survivors (≥ 85 years) and among lung cancer survivors.[31] Older adults may be more likely than younger adults to experience certain long-term effects of cancer and its treatment, such as fatigue, cognitive impairment, peripheral neuropathy, osteoporosis, and physical or functional limitations.[78] Evidence also suggests that older cancer survivors have more comorbidities than their counterparts of the same age without cancer.[80] Poly-pharmacy is another important and related consideration for the older cancer survivor. PP can decrease adherence and increase drug–drug interactions; medications such as benzodiazepines and opiates may remain on the patient's medication list after treatment has been completed. The American Society of Clinical Oncology (ASCO) has published a number of guidelines related to cancer survivorship, notably including guidelines for management of osteoporosis, cardiac dysfunction, chronic pain, neuropathy, and depression, as well as some disease-specific guidelines; however, these guidelines do not systematically address how the care of older adults survivors may be different than younger survivors.[81]

Beyond the management of comorbidities, long-term treatment toxicities, and PP, older adults require a focus on maintenance of physical function and fitness. Older adults generally decrease their level of physical activity during cancer diagnosis and treatment, and may not return to previous levels after treatment.[82] Increasing evidence suggests that maintaining physical activity is an effective method for treating physical decline associated with cancer and its treatment; however, overall there remain significant unknowns about how best to prescribe exercise, as well as the best way to study the utility of exercise in the older adult cancer survivor.[83]

One approach to the management of cancer survivors has been the survivorship care plan (SCP). The SCP is a document that lays out (1) a treatment summary; (2) surveillance plans if relevant, and which provider will be responsible for these; and (3) lifestyle information tailored to the needs of the survivor, including a focus on obesity, physical activity, and smoking. Although SCPs are strongly supported by the advocacy community and professional organizations, there is limited data proving their effectiveness at altering outcomes.[84] More research is needed to understand the advantages and disadvantages of SCPs, and in particular, this may be different for patients in the curative intent versus palliative treatment modes. As well, there is little data on the value of SCPs specifically for the older patient population. In 2015, a U13 meeting focusing on survivorship in the older adult was organized by the Cancer and Aging Research Group. The recommendations of this conference included further study of SCPs in older adults in order to better understand how best to tailor SCPs for older adults, how to involve caregivers in SCPs, use of GA to inform details of the SCP, and exploration of care delivery models that determine how best to share responsibility for chronic conditions and long-term toxicities between care providers.[85] GAs, in particular, should be routinely implemented in the care of the older adult cancer survivor, whether as part of a formal SCP or simply as an inherent part of clinical care.

Palliative care for the older adult with cancer

Similar to a discussion about survivorship, understanding the unique aspects of palliative care for older adults with cancer must begin with defining what we mean by palliative care. A helpful framework recognizes that palliative care includes (1) hospice care, which applies at the end of life, and (2) the remainder of palliative care services, which can be applied throughout the cancer care continuum, though still with an emphasis on care for patients with incurable cancers. The scope of palliative care includes goal setting, symptom management, and care of the caregiver.[86] Increasing evidence supports the value of early palliative care involvement,[87] with older adults being no exception.

With respect to goal setting, it is clear that the setting of realistic but meaningful goals relies significantly on effective communication about prognosis and treatment options. For older adults, effective communication can be challenging due to concurrent cognitive impairment, as well as cultural preferences regarding degree of involvement of family members, communication style, and religious and spiritual beliefs. The role of the caregiver in the care of an older adult with cancer is particularly crucial; the primary caregiver is often a spouse with health problems of his or her own, or an adult child, with professional and family responsibilities of his or her own. Caregivers themselves may suffer physical and emotional stress, and their assistance is part of the service that palliative care can provide.

Symptom management is an important area where management of the older adult with cancer may differ from younger patients. For example, pain is one of the most common symptoms experienced by cancer patients; differences in management for older adults include the need for vigilance surrounding use of opiates and nonsteroidal anti-inflammatories, as side effects of these approaches may be more pronounced in older patients.

Evidence suggests that older adults with cancer utilize palliative care to a lesser extent than their younger counterparts. The literature on barriers to palliative care and hospice care utilization in older adults has been systematically reviewed.[88] Based on 19 studies of older adults with cancer, demographic risk factors for decreased use of palliative care services included male sex, racial minority, being unmarried, and having low socioeconomic status or residing in rural areas. Interestingly, older age itself was not consistently associated with either increased or decreased use of palliative care services; of 12 studies evaluating this question, 6 found that advanced age increased the probability of palliative care usage, whereas 6 found that advanced age decreased this probability. Provider-related barriers included patients not feeling connected to providers, and not feeling adequately informed about treatment options. Further work is needed to determine the most practical and effective ways to overcome these barriers.

Conclusions

Improving outcomes for older adults with cancer requires a unique approach to aging in concert with cancer care. Attention to geriatric syndromes, multi-morbidity, shared decision-making, survivorship, and implementing a comprehensive GA can improve outcomes for older adults with cancer. As a field, important strides have been made in treatment decisions, symptom management, and identifying age-related deficits. However, in order to advance the science of cancer and aging and improve outcomes for older adults, a synchronized and systematic approach is needed. Importantly, gaps in knowledge are attributable to the under-enrollment of older adults in clinical trials and limited research in the field of aging biology as it applies to malignancy. Creating a shift in our culture towards dedicated research of aging adults with cancer is required to transform our own practice paradigms and advance the field of cancer and aging.

References

1. Howlader N, Noone AM, Krapcho M, et al. (eds). *SEER Cancer Statistics Review, 1975–2017*. Bethesda, MD, based on November 2019 SEER data submission, posted to the SEER web site, https://seer.cancer.gov/csr/1975_2017: *National Cancer Institute*; 2020.
2. Smith BD, Smith GL, Hurria A, et al. Future of cancer incidence in the United States: burdens upon an aging, changing nation. *J Clin Oncol*. 2009;**27**:2758–2765.
3. Mohile SG, Dale W, Somerfield MR, et al. Practical assessment and management of vulnerabilities in older patients receiving chemotherapy: ASCO guideline for geriatric oncology summary. *J Oncol Pract*. 2018;**14**:442–446.
4. Hamaker ME, Prins MC, Stauder R. The relevance of a geriatric assessment for elderly patients with a haematological malignancy–a systematic review. *Leuk Res*. 2014;**38**:275–283.
5. Hurria A, Gupta S, Zauderer M, et al. Development of a comprehensive geriatric assessment (CGA) measure for older patients (Pts) with cancer: a feasibility study. *J Clin Oncol*. 2004;**22**:769s.
6. Cowdry EV. *Problems of Ageing: Biological and Medical Aspects*, 2nd ed. Baltimore, MD: Williams & Wilkins; 1942.
7. Fleg JL, Morrell CH, Bos AG, et al. Accelerated longitudinal decline of aerobic capacity in healthy older adults. *Circulation*. 2005;**112**:674–682.
8. Stuhlinger MC, Weltermann A, Staber P, et al. Recommendations for ibrutinib treatment in patients with atrial fibrillation and/or elevated cardiovascular risk. *Wien Klin Wochenschr*. 2020;**132**:97–109.
9. Rashdan S, Minna JD, Gerber DE. Diagnosis and management of pulmonary toxicity associated with cancer immunotherapy. *Lancet Respir Med*. 2018;**6**:472–478.
10. Lindeman RD, Tobin J, Shock NW. Longitudinal studies on the rate of decline in renal function with age. *J Am Geriatr Soc*. 1985;**33**:278–285.
11. Gharbi MB, Elseviers M, Zamd M, et al. Chronic kidney disease, hypertension, diabetes, and obesity in the adult population of Morocco: how to avoid "over"- and "under"-diagnosis of CKD. *Kidney Int*. 2016;**89**:1363–1371.
12. Aiello A, Farzaneh F, Candore G, et al. Immunosenescence and its hallmarks: how to oppose aging strategically? a review of potential options for therapeutic intervention. *Front Immunol*. 2019;**10**:2247.
13. Sonnenberg A, Genta RM. Changes in the gastric mucosa with aging. *Clin Gastroenterol Hepatol*. 2015;**13**:2276–2281.
14. Soenen S, Rayner CK, Jones KL, et al. The ageing gastrointestinal tract. *Curr Opin Clin Nutr Metab Care*. 2016;**19**:12–18.
15. Hoofnagle JH, Serrano J, Knoben JE, et al. LiverTox: a website on drug-induced liver injury. *Hepatology*. 2013;**57**:873–874.
16. Lopez-Otin C, Blasco MA, Partridge L, et al. The hallmarks of aging. *Cell*. 2013;**153**:1194–1217.
17. Kuchel GA. Aging and homeostatic regulation. In: Halter JB, Ouslander JG, Studenski S, et al., eds. *Hazzard's Geriatric Medicine and Gerontology*, 7th ed. New York: McGraw-Hill Education; 2017.
18. Mohile SG, Fan L, Reeve E, et al. Association of cancer with geriatric syndromes in older medicare beneficiaries. *J Clin Oncol*. 2011;**29**:1458–1464.
19. Fried LP, Tangen CM, Walston J, et al. Frailty in older adults: evidence for a phenotype. *J Gerontol A Biol Sci Med Sci*. 2001;**56**:M146–M156.
20. Hubbard JM, Cohen HJ, Muss HB. Incorporating biomarkers into cancer and aging research. *J Clin Oncol*. 2014;**32**:2611–2616.
21. Cohen HJ, Harris T, Pieper CF. Coagulation and activation of inflammatory pathways in the development of functional decline and mortality in the elderly. *Am J Med*. 2003;**114**:180–187.
22. Cohen HJ, Pieper CF, Harris T, et al. The association of plasma IL-6 levels with functional disability in community-dwelling elderly. *J Gerontol A Biol Sci Med Sci*. 1997;**52**:M201–M208.
23. Ensrud KE, Ewing SK, Taylor BC, et al. Frailty and risk of falls, fracture, and mortality in older women: the study of osteoporotic fractures. *J Gerontol A Biol Sci Med Sci*. 2007;**62**:744–751.
24. Rockwood K, Mitnitski A. Frailty in relation to the accumulation of deficits. *J Gerontol A Biol Sci Med Sci*. 2007;**62**:722–727.
25. Rockwood K, Mitnitski A, Song X, et al. Long-term risks of death and institutionalization of elderly people in relation to deficit accumulation at age 70. *J Am Geriatr Soc*. 2006;**54**:975–979.
26. Searle SD, Mitnitski A, Gahbauer EA, et al. A standard procedure for creating a frailty index. *BMC Geriatr*. 2008;**8**:24.
27. Cohen HJ, Smith D, Sun CL, et al. Frailty as determined by a comprehensive geriatric assessment-derived deficit-accumulation index in older patients with cancer who receive chemotherapy. *Cancer*. 2016;**122**:3865–3872.
28. Guerard EJ, Deal AM, Chang Y, et al. Frailty index developed from a cancer-specific geriatric assessment and the association with mortality among older adults with cancer. *J Natl Compr Cancer Netw*. 2017;**15**:894–902.
29. van Deudekom FJ, van de Ruitenbeek M, Te Water W, et al. Frailty index and frailty phenotype in elderly patients with cancer. *Acta Oncol*. 2016;**55**:644–646.
30. Balducci L, Stanta G. Cancer in the frail patient. A coming epidemic. *Hematol Oncol Clin North Am*. 2000;**14**:235–250.
31. Bluethmann SM, Mariotto AB, Rowland JH. Anticipating the "silver tsunami": prevalence trajectories and comorbidity burden among older cancer survivors in the United States. *Cancer Epidemiol Biomark Prev*. 2016;**25**:1029–1036.
32. Williams GR, Chen Y, Kenzik KM, et al. Assessment of sarcopenia measures, survival, and disability in older adults before and after diagnosis with cancer. *JAMA Netw Open*. 2020;**3**:e204783.
33. Henderson TO, Ness KK, Cohen HJ. Accelerated aging among cancer survivors: from pediatrics to geriatrics. *Am Soc Clin Oncol Educ Book*. 2014:e423–e430.
34. Ness KK, Krull KR, Jones KE, et al. Physiologic frailty as a sign of accelerated aging among adult survivors of childhood cancer: a report from the St Jude Lifetime cohort study. *J Clin Oncol*. 2013;**31**:4496–4503.
35. Yancik R. Cancer burden in the aged: an epidemiologic and demographic overview. *Cancer*. 1997;**80**:1273–1283.
36. Williams GR, Deal AM, Lund JL, et al. Patient-reported comorbidity and survival in older adults with cancer. *Oncologist*. 2018;**23**:433–439.
37. Williams GR, Mackenzie A, Magnuson A, et al. Comorbidity in older adults with cancer. *J Geriatr Oncol*. 2016;**7**:249–257.
38. Extermann M. Measuring comorbidity in older cancer patients. *Eur J Cancer*. 2000;**36**:453–471.
39. Sogaard M, Thomsen RW, Bossen KS, et al. The impact of comorbidity on cancer survival: a review. *Clin Epidemiol*. 2013;**5**:3–29.
40. Extermann M, Overcash J, Lyman GH, et al. Comorbidity and functional status are independent in older cancer patients. *J Clin Oncol*. 1998;**16**:1582–1587.

70 Disparities in cancer care

Otis W. Brawley, MD, MACP

> **Overview**
>
> With the tremendous progress in cancer over the past half-century, increased emphasis has been placed on the study of outcomes. One glaring finding is that some populations have done better than others. This has led to the academic discipline of the study of disparities in health. The causes of cancer are both genetic and environmental; a few of the differences are due to differences in population biology. Most of the disparities are due to population differences in the practice and receipt of prevention and risk-reduction activities. Population differences also occur in receipt of quality treatment. It is estimated that at least one in five cancer deaths in the US is avoidable. The study of health disparities focuses on how to get adequate care to those who often do not receive it.

Over the past 50 years, tremendous progress has occurred in healthcare and especially in the prevention and treatment of cancer. This progress is best demonstrated by the nearly 30% decline in the age-adjusted cancer death rate since the early 1990s.[1] These improvements have led to an increasing appreciation of the differences in outcomes among subsets of the population; some populations have not benefited to the same extent as others.

The first studies to demonstrate that some populations have higher cancer death rates were published in the early 1970s.[2,3] These studies noted that Black or African-American populations have higher death rates compared to White or Caucasian populations.[4] The academic discipline is known as "health disparities" has grown to encompass differences among other racial/ethnic groups as well as considerations of geographic residence (northern United States vs southern United States, or rural vs urban) and socioeconomic status. As the field of health disparities has matured, its presence has also become a political issue. As such, the discipline has inspired legislation regarding healthcare reform and minority accrual to clinical trials.

The causes of cancer are both genetic and environmental. When populations and the differences between them are more fully appreciated, reasonable hypotheses can be generated about the factors that cause or prevent cancer, as well as the factors that make cancers more or less aggressive. With rigorous, careful study of well-defined populations, one can also increase knowledge about the efficacy and effectiveness of cancer prevention and treatment interventions.

Birth of the discipline

The US National Cancer Institute (NCI) established the Surveillance, Epidemiology, and End Results (SEER) program in the early 1970s as part of the implementation of the National Cancer Act of 1971. The program collects cancer incidence, mortality, and survival data by race and gender from well-defined population-based registries around the United States.[4] These data are publicly available at www.cancer.gov/statistics. The number of SEER registries has grown over the past half-century, but even today SEER does not provide a fully representative sample of the country for the calculation of US cancer rates.

SEER allows for special studies such as the NCI Black White Study, which began in the mid-1970s, lasted into the 1990s, and clearly documented racial disparities in cancer incidence, mortality, and survival when comparing these two populations.[4] The study also demonstrated differences in treatment patterns including that a higher proportion in the Black population received inappropriate or suboptimal cancer care. Before 2000, SEER did not collect socioeconomic information; however, it has recently expanded its collection of data to capture these data over patients' disease course.

The academic study of these differences among populations was first called *minority health research*, later called *special populations research*, and with the leadership of Surgeon General David Satcher in the late 1990s, became known as *health disparities research*.[5] More recently, the term *health equity* has gained favor. Today, the field no longer simply encourages healthcare workers to develop cultural competence and develop specific interventions to overcome health disparities or achieve health equity. It is now a transdisciplinary science that comprises clinicians, nurses, psychologists, social workers, geographers, epidemiologists, and others.

Defining health disparities

The NCI defines *cancer health disparities* as adverse differences in cancer incidence, cancer prevalence, cancer mortality, cancer survivorship, and burden of cancer or related health conditions that exist among specific populations in the US Translated, *disparities in health* is a concept of difference: some groups of people because they belong to a certain racial, ethnic or cultural group-do worse than others.[6]

Factors measured

A number of outcomes can be measured and compared. The most common outcomes include:

- *Incidence* – usually expressed as the number diagnosed with the disease in a given year per 100,000 people in the population. Incidence rates are the equivalent of the population's risk of developing a disease. Individuals from groups with a higher incidence of the disease have a higher risk of getting the disease.

Holland-Frei Cancer Medicine, Tenth Edition. Edited by Robert C. Bast, John C. Byrd, Carlo M. Croce, Ernest Hawk, Fadlo R. Khuri, Raphael E. Pollock, Apostolia M. Tsimberidou, Christopher G. Willett, and Cheryl L. Willman.
© 2023 John Wiley & Sons, Inc. Published 2023 by John Wiley & Sons, Inc.

- *Mortality* – usually expressed as the number of deaths caused by the disease in a given year per 100,000 people in the population. Mortality rates are the equivalent of the population's risk of death from the disease. Individuals from groups with the higher mortality rate of the disease have a higher risk of dying from that disease.
- Incidence and mortality are often age-adjusted to a standard population to remove the effects of two populations having different age distributions. Age is a risk factor for many cancers. When a population has a higher age-adjusted incidence rate in 1990 compared to 1960, the rise in age-adjusted rate represents the increasing importance of a risk factor other than an increased number of older people in the population driving up the rate. Non-age-adjusted rates are referred to as "crude rates."
- *Survival* – the time from diagnosis to death. Survival of a cohort is sometimes expressed as median survival, the time from diagnosis to the time when half of the patients in the cohort are still alive. Survival is often expressed as the proportion alive after a specified time period, usually 5 years after diagnosis.
- *Prevalence* – the proportion of a population that has a disease or disease risk factor at a given time point.

Differences in patterns of care (screening, diagnosis, or treatment) are also measured. For example, one can compare the proportions of patients from two different population subsets receiving high-quality treatment; and in many instances, there are substantive differences in access to high-quality care depending on race/ethnicity, geographic residence, or insurance status. Increasingly, disparities in comorbid disease, or *morbidity* due to disease and treatment (quality of life), are measured outcomes. Patient-reported outcomes (PROs) are also becoming more common.

Population categorization

The field began by looking at inequities in patterns of care among Black and White populations; however, it has evolved such that populations are now defined not only by race but also by ethnicity and culture, geographic origin, socioeconomic status (SES), area of residence, and other factors. It is extremely important to clearly define population characteristics when doing health disparities research.[7,8]

While *race* is perhaps the most common category used to define populations in health disparities work, it is also the most controversial. The concept of race was put forth more than 300 years ago. Initial categories were Caucasian, Negroid or African, and Mongoloid or Asian – all of which had to do with skin color, facial traits, and presumed geographic area of origin. Distinct racial groups do not exist; rather, they overlap. The anthropology community has never accepted race as a biological categorization.[9]

The US Office of Management and Budget (OMB) defines race and ethnicity to collect government data – a definition that is used in every decennial census.[10] The OMB defines five racial groups and two ethnicities, Hispanic or non-Hispanic; since the 1980 census, it requires that each of these are self-determined by the individual being counted, rather than assigned by someone else (Table 1). Per the OMB directive, these racial categories reflect the social definition of race and are not biological categorizations. Of note, these OMB racial definitions have changed over time. For example, during the 70 years before the 1950 census, the race-group assignment for a person from the Indian subcontinent of Asia who migrated to the United States was changed three times.

Table 1 US Office of Management and Budget definition of race and ethnicity, 2010.[a]

The OMB instructions for ascertainment of race and ethnicity are:
First, individuals are asked to designate ethnicity as:
- *Hispanic* or *latino* or
- *Not hispanic* or *latino*

  Hispanic or Latino is defined as a person of Cuban, Mexican, Puerto Rican, South or Central American, or other Spanish culture or origin, regardless of race

Second, individuals are asked to indicate one or more races that apply among the following:
- *American Indian or Alaska Native* – A person having origins in any of the original peoples of North and South America (including Central America) and who maintains tribal affiliation or community attachment
- *Asian* – A person having origins in any of the original peoples of the Far East, Southeast Asia, or the Indian subcontinent including, for example, Cambodia, China, India, Japan, Korea, Malaysia, Pakistan, the Philippine Islands, Thailand, and Vietnam
- *Black or African American* – A person having origins in any of the Black racial groups of Africa
- *Native Hawaiian or other Pacific Islander* – A person having origins in any of the original peoples of Hawaii, Guam, Samoa, or other Pacific Islands
- *White* – A person having origins in any of the original peoples of Europe, the Middle East, or North Africa

The 1997 OMB standards permit the reporting of more than one race. An individual's response to the race question is based upon self-identification

[a]Source: Modified from Karen et al.[11]

The NCI SEER program and the National Center for Health Statistics of the Centers for Disease Control and Prevention (CDC) publish health data using the OMB definitions at https://www.seer.cancer.gov. They are dependent on the US Census for the population size, which is the denominator when calculating incidence and mortality rates. Mortality trends using the OMB race and ethnicity criteria and as published by the NCI SEER program are plotted in Figure 1. The plots use the race/ethnicity definition from the 2010 census.

The terms *ethnicity* and *culture* as used in academic study are very broad and encompass human identity that is not static nor mutually exclusive, but rather is fluid and without definite boundaries. In social research, ethnic groups are distinguished by the nature and source of human variation, for example, the behavioral, diet, lifestyle, and other environmental influences on health. When used appropriately, populations of one nationality can have multiple ethnicities. Indeed, Hispanic Americans comprise numerous cultures.[13]

Ethnicity and *culture* can be better scientific descriptors than race as each relates to environmental influences that may increase or decrease the likelihood of an illness. Even such habits as how one smokes cigarettes or engages in sexual activity are influenced by ethnicity and culture. While *ethnicity* and *culture* are related to factors that cause cancer, ethnic, and cultural influences also affect one's acceptance of disease and how one seeks and accepts therapy for disease.[7]

Area of geographic origin is also a better scientific descriptor than race. Many confuse race with area of geographic origin and the two terms overlap. Race is a very broad category. For example, the category White or Caucasian encompasses at least 840 areas of geographic origin,[14] while the category Black or African includes at least 109 areas of geographic origin. Most people have several areas of geographic origin because of population co-mingling (genetic

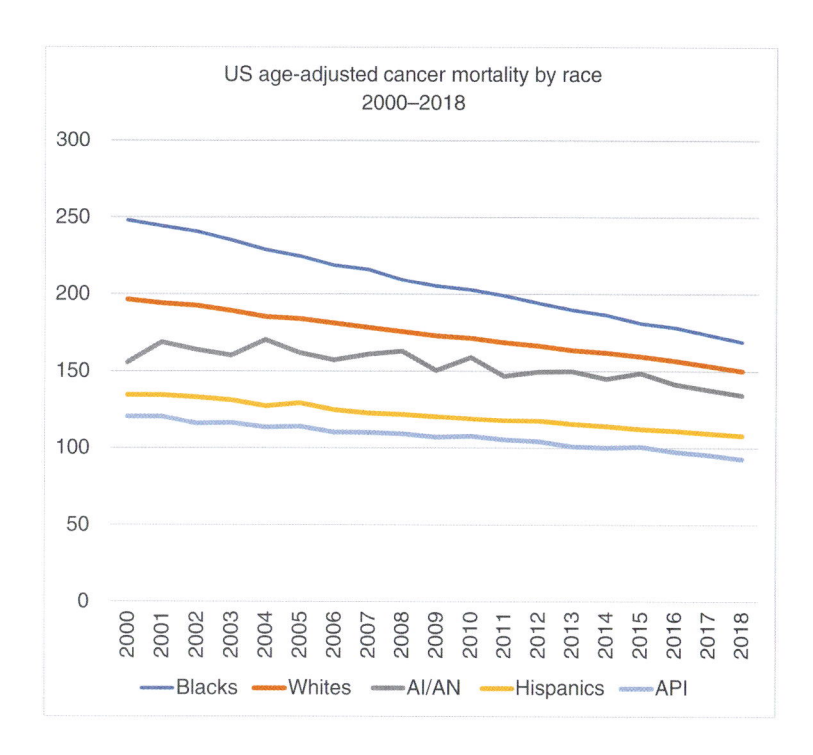

Figure 1 Mortality by race 2000 to 2018. Age-Adjusted US cancer mortality rates by year 2000 to 2018 by race and ethnicity. API, Asian Pacific Islander; AI/AN, American Indian, or Alaskan Native. Rates are age-adjusted to the 2000 standard. Source: Modified from Howlader et al.[12]

admixture) over the centuries. It has been appropriately said that trying to categorize people by racial category or area of geographic origin "is like trying to slice soup."[15]

A number of genetic traits correlate with *area of geographic origin*. For example, sickle cell disease is a genetic disease of people from the Mediterranean and sub-Saharan Africa. People from Spain, Italy, Greece, Turkey, Syria, and Lebanon have sickle cell disease; however, natives of southern Africa do not. Some who self-identify as White get sickle cell disease and others who consider themselves to be Black do not.[16]

While a genetic trait can have a higher prevalence among people from a specific geographic origin, rarely will the people of a specific area monopolize that trait. For example, cystic fibrosis is more common among, but not exclusive to, those originating in northern Europe. Alcohol dehydrogenase deficiency is common among, but not exclusive to, people from Japan. Glucose-6-phosphate dehydrogenase (G6PD) deficiency is common among, but not exclusive to, people of Mediterranean ancestry.[17]

Area of geographic origin can also correlate with environmental and infectious agents common to the area. For example, Hepatitis B is common among residents of Southeast Asia, which results in high liver cancer rates in that region.[18]

Ancestry – linked to race and area of geographic origin – is yet another way of categorizing populations. The influence of family allows for admixture within ancestry. While genetic influences often parallel ancestry, differences can occur as some genes are passed down more commonly than others. Some of the widely discussed Black/White differences in breast and prostate cancer incidence and mortality might better parallel ancestry or area of geographic origin rather than race.

Socioeconomic status (SES) – most commonly defined by education, income, insurance status, and occupation – is extremely important; however, controversy exists over how well SES can be used to determine the human condition. When comparing populations, researchers commonly use one or two SES measures in a model without fully considering the social-deprivation aspect of SES. Calculated during the decennial census in parts of the European Union, the social deprivation index takes into account more than a dozen markers of wealth, education, and social status to calculate a deprivation score. Nothing approximating that specificity exists in the US literature.

Both SES and social deprivation influence where we live, our birthing habits, our dietary choices, and even how or if we consume healthcare. Education is also influenced: Americans with less than a high school education are more than twice as likely to die of cancer as compared to those with a college education.[19] In the United States, educational status is more important than race in terms of risk of cancer death and death from a number of causes.[19-21] SES differences affect cancer stage at diagnosis, the distribution of pathologies, and the uptake of cancer care, especially cancer screening. At the population level, having SES advantages can lead to a higher proportion of wealthy people being diagnosed with early-stage, less aggressive disease compared to those who are poorer. Because wealthier individuals are more likely to participate in beneficial screening and to get high-quality care, they are more likely to have better health outcomes.

Birthing habits, which are related to SES, can influence the genetics of breast cancer. Data suggest that women who develop breast cancer and do not have children or had children after the age of age 30 are more likely to have estrogen-receptor-positive breast cancer. This group is generally college-educated and of middle- and upper-middle class. On the other hand, women who have children at an early age, do not breastfeed, and develop breast cancer are at a higher risk of having triple-negative (basal-like) breast cancer, which is harder to treat. This group is generally poorer and less educated.[22]

Low SES is often correlated with a higher risk of certain cancers because those who are poor often have a higher prevalence of

Table 2 Smoking prevalence by educational attainment, 2017.[a]

Educational attainment	Prevalence (%)
High school dropout	21.3
GED	35.3
High school graduate	19.6
Associates degree	15.5
	14.0
Undergraduate degree	7.1
	17.7
Graduate degree	4.1
	4.0

[a]Source: Data from Cornelius et al.[23]

habits associated with an increased cancer risk. For example, high caloric intake, lack of physical activity, and obesity – the triad of *energy balance* traits associated with more than a dozen cancers – are more common in the poor or less educated and are responsible for nearly one-third of all cancers in the United States. Those who are less educated and are poor tend to consume more calories each day from processed carbohydrates and other calorie-dense/nutrient-poor foods, which can be less expensive than some nutrient-rich foods. In another habit-related example, adults living below the poverty line are more likely to smoke compared to those from America's middle-class. There are also dramatic differences in smoking rates by education in the United States[23] (Table 2). As a result, smoking-related cancers are more common in poor- versus middle-class populations.

Relationships among population categories

Race may be better viewed as a characteristic and not a category. While much emphasis is placed on racial groups and outcome differences among those groups, this emphasis is partly due to the American obsession with race and the fact that most US population-based data are collected using the US OMB definition of race. Outcomes data based on ethnicity, SES, or ancestry are not easily obtained in the United States. While racial categories are not based in biology, they do have some relevance as a sociopolitical construct related to ethnicity, area of geographic origin, and SES. Put simply, race does matter, but not as an inherent immutable factor.

Unfortunately, the medical literature is filled with the medicalization of race.[24] A number of papers suggest that genetics defines racial differences, which cause differences in disease incidence, management, and outcomes for cancer and otherwise. Many of these papers should use the term *ancestry* (different from race), while others often ignore the clear correlations between race and SES, and that SES is likely the more influential disease-based variable.

More epidemiologic research that examines underlying factors and improves cancer risk-prediction models is called for to better understand the link between race and cancer risk. These models will be important as we move into the era of precision medicine and cancer interception.[25] Benevolent medical-racial profiling exists, as there is variation in cancer incidence and mortality by race for a number of cancers, even though race is a sociopolitical description. Substantial social issues are linked to risk of cancer. Self-identified race is, broadly, a marker of exposure across the life course.

Disparities in treatment patterns

Many early health-disparities studies described significant disparities in the quality of treatment received by different groups based on their race or socioeconomic status, suggesting that a number of factors lead to treatment differences. These include poverty, lack of insurance, social disenfranchisement, and discrimination.[26]

Some patients:

- Decline therapy due to culture-based discouragement around acceptance or cultural differences compared to the healthcare provider that result in mistrust;
- Decline therapy due to mistrust of those in medicine;
- Do not adhere to prescribed regimens due to illiteracy or lack of sufficient health literacy;
- Do not adhere to prescribed therapy due to the inconvenience of acquiring care, such as a lack of transportation;
- Cannot receive preferred or more aggressive therapies due to comorbid diseases associated with poverty; and/or
- Are not offered needed care due to discrimination based on race or SES.

The healthcare provider can often overcome these issues and provide the patient with the best service by being conscious of and concerned about the patient's needs. Many physicians/healthcare providers are now receiving training in culturally competent care. For example, the American Society of Clinical Oncology offers courses on communicating with patients from backgrounds different from the provider (https://elearning.asco.org/product-details/role-of-cultural-competency-in-reducing-cancer-disparities).[27]

Studies have identified disparities in quality of care received by minority and poor populations in the United States for breast-, colorectal-, lung-, prostate-, and bladder cancers, as well as other diseases.[26,28–32] Most research has occurred in breast cancer. For example, Lund et al. studied treatment patterns in metropolitan Atlanta over a 2-year period in 2000 and 2001.[33] While assessing women diagnosed with localized breast cancer, they found that 7% of Black and 2% of White women received no therapy within the first year after diagnosis. These women had sufficient access to care to receive both a screening mammogram and a suspicious-lesion biopsy, but none received therapy within 1 year of diagnosis.

The variables of minority race, lack of education, lack of insurance, and lower SES predict which patients are more likely to get inadequate care.[34,35] When these data are analyzed with logistic regression, less educated breast-cancer patients are more likely to receive nonstandard breast-cancer regimens and less likely to receive adequate chemotherapy dosing regardless of race. As well, obese breast-cancer patients are less likely to receive adequate dosing of chemotherapy and obesity is more common in minority and poor women.[36]

Disparities in quality of care can lead to disparities in prognosis and treatment

Unequal access to quality care due to race can cause differences in outcomes in unsuspecting ways and lead to erroneous assumptions. For example, Black compared to White American populations have disparate colorectal-cancer death rates. At each disease stage, Black people have higher mortality and inferior 5-year survival rates when compared to Whites. While this may suggest that colorectal cancer is more aggressive in Black people, the colorectal-cancer mortality rates of Black and White populations were very similar in the 1970s. This death-rate disparity has increased every year since 1981, and the mortality disparity is greater now than at any

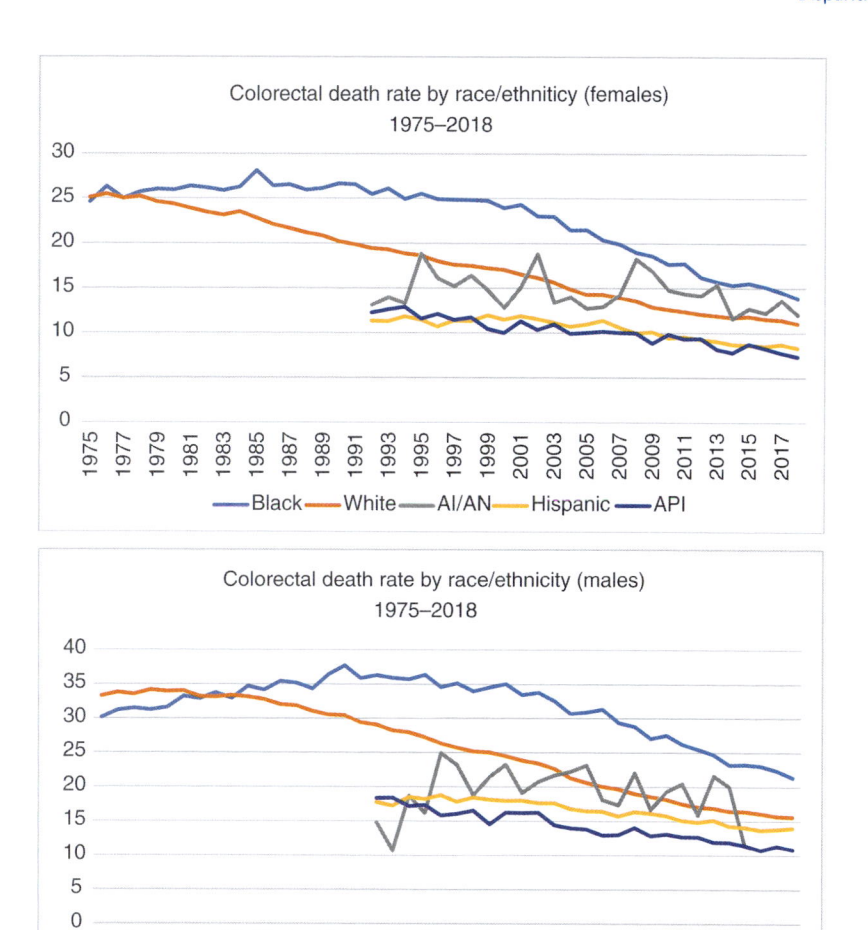

Figure 2 Colorectal cancer mortality by race and gender. Age-Adjusted US colorectal cancer mortality rates by sex, race, and ethnicity from 1975 to 2018 for Blacks and Whites. Data for other races and ethnicities were collected beginning in 1990. API, Asian Pacific Islander; AI/AN, American Indian, or Alaskan Native. Rates are age-adjusted to the 2000 standard. Source: Modified from Howlader et al.[12]

previous time, despite the decline in mortality rates for both races (Figure 2).

Patterns-of-care studies suggest that Black patients with stage 3 disease are less likely to receive adjuvant chemotherapy.[37] Other studies that show that these patients tend to be treated in hospitals that are overcrowded and resource-limited,[38] in which pathologists are often overworked and typically examine fewer nodes from each surgical specimen compared to hospitals where White patients receive treatment.[38,39] This primarily socioeconomic issue results in Black patients being less likely to have a thorough pathologic examination. As such, some Black patients diagnosed with stage 1 or 2 disease have true stage-3 colorectal cancer but receive less than optimal pathologic evaluation, which guides treatment decisions. These patients with true stage-3 disease should be treated with adjuvant chemotherapy. Instead, a higher proportion of Black, compared to White, patients are labeled as having a relapse of stage-2 colorectal-cancer – a major reason that many believe colorectal cancer is more aggressive in Black patients.[38]

In a classic "Will Rogers effect," Black, compared to White, patients at each cancer stage have inferior 5-year survival rates because of disparities in staging and treatment. Conversely, race-based outcome differences decrease dramatically when they are assessed within an equal-access healthcare system.[40] Regarding end-of-life services, palliative care is effective in moderating disease-, SES-, and treatment-related effects and is a key component in improving quality of life; however, those of White race and at higher education- and income status are more likely to receive palliative care.[41]

Genetic expression – race, ancestry, ethnicity, and culture

Within adequately staged patients receiving state-of-the-art care, small disparities in outcome by race often exist, with the survival rates of Black, compared to White, populations being slightly inferior. Elevated Microsatellite Alterations at Selected Tetranucleotide repeats (EMAST) – a marker of microsatellite instability that confers a poor prognosis – is more common among Blacks or African Americans.[42] Because EMAST appears to be an acquired defect associated with inflammation, the role of diet, the microbiome, and accumulation of EMAST are important issues when studying Black and White populations and colon-cancer disparities. In this example, diet, an environmental factor partially determined by ethnicity and culture, parallels race and affects the genetic expression and biologic behavior of the tumor.

Several extrinsic influences associated with race, ethnicity, culture, and even SES can affect genetic expression within a malignancy. A higher proportion of White American, compared to Black American, women are middle-class and college educated, who often delay childbirth to establish a career. Having a first-term pregnancy after the age of 30, or never having a child at all, is a risk factor, not just for breast cancer, but for estrogen-receptor-positive breast cancer – likely the reason that White American women have a higher incidence of breast cancer compared to Black American women.[43] In addition, growing evidence suggests that women who undergo childbirth at an early age, do not breastfeed, and then develop breast cancer, are more likely to develop triple-negative (basal-like) breast cancer. Social forces often discourage young black women from breastfeeding their infants. These forces include having to work or being provided – often to poor women – formula and free-formula coupons by formula vendors as they leave the hospital postchildbirth. Conversely, white middle-class culture encourages breastfeeding.[44]

Studies of White patients with breast cancer in the United States and Scotland suggest that middle-class social status in childhood is associated with a higher risk of estrogen-receptor-positive breast cancer among those who develop breast cancer decades later. On the other hand, poverty in childhood is associated with the acquisition of estrogen-receptor-negative or triple-negative (basal-like) disease, if one develops breast cancer in later life. Differences in diet and childhood patterns of weight gain are also thought to be causal. Duration of breastfeeding and number of children breastfed are correlated with a lower risk of basal-like breast cancer but not a reduced risk of luminal cancer, which has a better prognosis.[44–46]

In the United States, the Black and Hispanic female populations are disproportionately overweight or obese,[47] possibly due to ethnicity, culture, and SES. Obesity, or more specifically weight gain in adulthood, is a risk factor for postmenopausal breast cancer.[48] Differing pathologic trends seen in Black and White women may be due to these influences. Understanding the environmental influences associated with SES, ethnicity, and culture in the groups being compared can be especially useful in understanding epigenetics.

Populations and genetic differences

While evidence suggests that differences among broad, ill-defined population categories have been overemphasized, intrinsic genetic differences exist between well-defined populations. Race is not the appropriate way to define these populations; rather, intrinsic genetic markers better correlate with ancestry, area of geographic origin, and (sometimes) with ethnicity or culture. Genetic differences correlated or associated with race instead should be considered a familial or ancestral gene or a group of genes that is conserved among families. Even then, the prevalence of a polymorphism or gene may be higher in a specific population, but that population will rarely monopolize that gene.[49]

A closed society will conserve genetic traits within that society. Segregation on the basis of race, ethnicity or culture, area of geographic origin, or other factors can lead to preservation of a specific gene or group of genes in the segregated population,[50] as is demonstrated in several genetic diseases such as Tay–Sachs disease, cystic fibrosis, and sickle cell disease. While each of these diseases has a higher prevalence in specific groups, the disease is not exclusive to that group.

Perhaps the best example of segregation leading to a specific mutation being conserved in a population is seen in the study of BRCA mutations. Women with certain specific mutations of *BRCA1* and *BRCA2* – found in women of all races – are at a higher risk of developing breast- and ovarian cancer. Three specific mutations are common but not exclusive to people who identify themselves as being of Ashkenazi Jewish ancestry.[49,51] Population modeling suggests that these specific mutations – linked to a small number of individuals who were alive about 1200 years ago – are ancestral and common among Jewish families because of ethnic segregation.

Pharmacogenetics

Clinically relevant, drug-response variability exists due to differences in enzymes that metabolize drugs – differences that can vary by population. These populations can be categorized by race, ethnicity, ancestry, and area of geographic origin or sometimes by SES.[52] Extrinsic factors such as diet and the use of some medicines can lead to the up- or down-regulation of hepatic-enzyme expression through the same metabolic pathways as some drugs are metabolized. These enzymes are often involved in the detoxification of environmental toxins and carcinogens and thus, variations in detoxification enzymes may lead to variations in cancer risk.

The physician, interested in how his or her individual patient metabolizes prescribed drugs, sometimes uses a form of "population profiling" to assess for common drug-treatment issues. For example, approximately 10% of persons from certain areas of Southeast Asia develop severe cutaneous adverse reactions, such as Stevens–Johnson syndrome, when administered the antiseizure drug carbamazepine,[53] which might be a reasonable justification for avoiding use of carbamazepine in people whose ancestry includes an area of geographic origin in Malaysia, Burma, Singapore, or Thailand. Because the problem is especially prevalent among the population that lives within 150 km of the Thai-Burmese border, if carbamazepine must be used, careful monitoring or testing for certain allele frequencies of HLA-B*1502 might be in order.[54]

Tacrolimus – well-studied in renal transplant patients – is structurally related to several anticancer drugs and is metabolized by CYP3a.[55] Due to differences in polymorphisms of CYP3a, some Black or African-American patients receiving kidney transplants require higher tacrolimus doses, compared to those used in White patients, to reach trough concentrations. Even within a specific population, substantial variability exists in pharmacology. In Black patients, the 12-h serum tacrolimus concentration from one dose can vary by a factor of 3–5. Special attention to pharmacokinetics is needed in all patients treated with this drug.

Population differences of polymorphisms in *UGT1A1* affect the dosing and efficacy of certain cancer drugs, including irinotecan.[56] Indeed, some recommend pharmacogenetics testing before the use of this drug. Differences in *ABCG2* also affect the dosing and efficacy of topotecan, irinotecan, mitoxantrone, doxorubicin, and methotrexate.[57,58]

This is not a new concept, but rather is an old one reapplied in the genomics age. For decades we have appreciated that G6PD deficiency – the most common human-enzyme defect – is more common among people of Mediterranean or African origin. Those having the deficiency are at risk of hemolysis when taking sulfa antibiotics, certain antimalarials, and certain other drugs.

US government rules on minority inclusion in clinical trials

Numerous rules related to minority inclusion in clinical trials have been established because of concerns that racial minorities and women do not benefit equally, compared to White men, from trial participation in federally sponsored research. By legislation, OMB definitions of race and ethnicity are used to collect data that describe the populations enrolled in these trials. The clinical trialist with funding from the US National Institutes of Health (NIH) must annually report the race and gender of patients accrued to his/her clinical trials. While the NIH is the only federal entity required to collect these data, other agencies often collect it as well.

The NIH Revitalization Act of 1993, Public Law 103–43, mandates the inclusion of women and minorities in clinical research.[59] The law mandates that trials are "… designed and carried out in a manner sufficient to provide for valid analysis of whether the variables being studied in the trial affect women or members of minority groups, as the case may be, differently than other subjects in the trial". The stated goal of the legislation is to increase the opportunity for obtaining critically important information with which to enhance health and treat disease among all Americans, to detect and account for significant differences between genders or racial and ethnic groups where they exist, and to identify more subtle differences that might exist.

The NIH has interpreted this federal law as demanding diverse representation on federally sponsored trials, especially Phase III trials. The funded researcher must make a good-faith effort to accrue minorities and women at levels proportionate to the US population.

The legislation is controversial. Scientifically flawed, it calls for subset analysis to assess racial and ethnic differences and uses the terms *race* and *ethnicity* as if they define biologic categories. Furthermore, a cardinal rule of the clinical trial is that subset analysis is often wrong and should only be used to establish a hypothesis to be tested in a more rigorous study. A subset analysis is *post hoc*, retrospective, and underpowered. Power can be increased by oversampling, but this creates ethical concerns: a disproportionately greater number of minorities would be subject to the risk compared to the majority population.

Interestingly, the law was written just after publication of a subset analysis that suggested zidovudine was less effective in treating HIV in Black compared to White patients.[60] That publication caused a number of Black patients with HIV to either stop or refuse to start taking antiviral medicines. Indeed, because of this finding, rumors in the Black community – that anti-HIV therapies do not work for Black people – persist to this day. The original study did note that a higher proportion of Black participants had more advanced HIV disease and did not adhere to the prescribed regimen for social reasons. Factors associated with SES again caused the difference in outcome, which some interpreted as being due to inherent racial or biologic differences.[61]

The lawmakers who wrote the NIH Revitalization Act assumed that disparities existed because drugs and therapies used to treat major diseases were not tested in minorities and women. Some believed that diseases such as cancer behave differently in people of different races. Others believed that therapeutic drugs have different effects in Black versus White patients. Unfortunately, an important fact was ignored: many of the racial differences identified were because minority and poor patients did not receive beneficial treatments.[26] And treatments not administered certainly do not work.

If health disparities are to be overcome and if we are to have equity, we should embed thoughtful disparities-based research questions into cancer treatment, prevention, screening, and clinical trials to provide more robust statistical power to answer our questions.

Enrollment of diverse populations in clinical trials is important.[62] In the study of interventions and outcomes, consider how *efficacy* differs from *effectiveness*. Efficacy refers to how well an intervention works in an ideal clinical environment.[63] *Effectiveness* refers to how well that intervention works in a real-world situation. When research is implemented in the community, where most cancer care is provided, the results are more about effectiveness versus efficacy. Performing community-based research makes results more broadly pertinent to that population. Research about accrual to NCI-funded treatment-based studies has continued to show relative racial/ethnic balance in clinical-trial enrollment and refusal rates.[64] Indeed, increasingly research has shown that the population most often excluded from clinical study is the elderly of all races.[65] Appropriately, clinical-trial inclusion of elderly patients having comorbid age-associated diseases has become of interest to secure more realistic findings.

Summary

Health disparities- or health equity research and programs in the United States are paramount to carefully define the cancer-related risks and outcomes of various populations. Regardless of the specific definitions applied, differences in disease incidence and outcomes by population persist.

Importantly, a number of well-designed studies and meta-analyses show that equal treatment yields equal outcomes among equal patients.[66,67] When people with the same genetic markers are compared, race is not a factor in outcome, unless it is allowed to be. Rarely discussed are the numerous patterns-of-care studies that demonstrate unequal treatment in the United States by race and socioeconomic status.[68,69] This discussion often focuses on whether a particular breast-cancer drug is as effective in Blacks versus White women, not that a substantial proportion of Black or poor women do not get adequate treatment, as demonstrated in studies of surgical treatment as well as chemotherapy or radiation therapy.

With scientific progress, our understanding of cancer improves, so we may better appreciate its causes, biologic behaviors, and treatments. We are quickly moving into an era of personalized medicine in which genetics and genomics become very relevant. The advent of precision- and tailored medicine will make categorization using genes and polymorphisms even more important. The crude categories of race and ethnicity, and even SES, will still be important in terms of social issues such as access to care, exposures that cause cancer, and access to high-quality treatment.

Social interventions to overcome disparities and bring about equity include efforts to:

- Increase cultural competence and understanding of the patient by the healthcare provider
- Increase access to care through
  ○ Provision of insurance
  ○ Adequate staffing in community health centers
  ○ Attention to the patient's social situation
- Improve communications and educate those needing service using
  ○ Targeted messaging
  ○ Patient navigation

Key references

The complete reference list can be found on Vital Source version of this title, see inside front cover.

1. Siegel RL, Miller KD, Fuchs HE, Jemal A. Cancer statistics, 2021. *CA Cancer J Clin.* 2021;**71**:7–33.
2. Fontaine SA, Henschke UK, Leffall LD Jr, et al. Comparison of the cancer deaths in the black and white U.S.A. population from 1949 to 1967. *Med Ann Dist Columbia.* 1972;**41**:293–298.
4. Howard J, Hankey BF, Greenberg RS, et al. A collaborative study of differences in the survival rates of black patients and white patients with cancer. *Cancer.* 1992;**69**:2349–2360.
5. Satcher D. Our commitment to eliminate racial and ethnic health disparities. *Yale J Health Policy Law Ethics.* 2001;**1**:1–14.
6. DeSantis CE, Siegel RL, Sauer AG, et al. Cancer statistics for African Americans, 2016: progress and opportunities in reducing racial disparities. *CA Cancer J Clin.* 2016;**66**:290–308.
7. Foster MW, Sharp RR. Race, ethnicity, and genomics: social classifications as proxies of biological heterogeneity. *Genome Res.* 2002;**12**:844–850.
8. Ntzani EE, Liberopoulos G, Manolio TA, Ioannidis JP. Consistency of genome-wide associations across major ancestral groups. *Hum Genet.* 2012;**131**:1057–1071.
9. Baker JL, Rotimi CN, Shriner D. Human ancestry correlates with language and reveals that race is not an objective genomic classifier. *Sci Rep.* 2017;**7**:1572.
10. Friedman DJ, Cohen BB, Averbach AR, Norton JM. Race/ethnicity and OMB Directive 15: implications for state public health practice. *Am J Public Health.* 2000;**90**:1714–1719.
13. Teh BT. The importance of including diverse populations in cancer genomic and epigenomic studies. *Nat Rev Cancer.* 2019;**19**:361–362.
15. Nature Biotechnology. Slicing soup. *Nat Biotechnol.* 2002;**20**:637.
16. Mangla A, Ehsan M, Maruvada S. *Sickle Cell Anemia.* Treasure Island (FL): StatPearls; 2020.
17. Howes RE, Dewi M, Piel FB, et al. Spatial distribution of G6PD deficiency variants across malaria-endemic regions. *Malar J.* 2013;**12**:418.
18. Chen MS Jr,. Cancer health disparities among Asian Americans: what we do and what we need to do. *Cancer.* 2005;**104**:2895–2902.
19. Siegel RL, Jemal A, Wender RC, et al. An assessment of progress in cancer control. *CA Cancer J Clin.* 2018;**68**:329–339.
20. Siegel R, Ward E, Brawley O, Jemal A. Cancer statistics, 2011: the impact of eliminating socioeconomic and racial disparities on premature cancer deaths. *CA Cancer J Clin.* 2011;**61**:212–236.
21. Goding Sauer A, Siegel RL, Jemal A, Fedewa SA. Current prevalence of major cancer risk factors and screening test use in the United States: disparities by education and race/ethnicity. *Cancer Epidemiol Biomarkers Prev.* 2019;**28**:629–642.
22. Ambrosone CB, Zirpoli G, Ruszczyk M, et al. Parity and breastfeeding among African-American women: differential effects on breast cancer risk by estrogen receptor status in the Women's Circle of Health Study. *Cancer Causes Control.* 2014;**25**:259–265.
23. Cornelius ME, Wang TW, Jamal A, et al. Tobacco product use among adults – United States, 2019. *MMWR Morb Mortal Wkly Rep.* 2020;**69**:1736–1742.
24. Witzig R. The medicalization of race: scientific legitimization of a flawed social construct. *Ann Intern Med.* 1996;**125**:675–679.
26. Shavers VL, Brown ML. Racial and ethnic disparities in the receipt of cancer treatment. *J Natl Cancer Inst.* 2002;**94**:334–357.
27. Polite BN, Adams-Campbell LL, Brawley OW, et al. Charting the future of cancer health disparities research: a position statement from the American association for cancer research, the American cancer society, the American society of clinical oncology, and the National Cancer Institute. *Cancer Res.* 2017;**77**:4548–4555.
28. Green AK, Aviki EM, Matsoukas K, et al. Racial disparities in chemotherapy administration for early-stage breast cancer: a systematic review and meta-analysis. *Breast Cancer Res Treat.* 2018;**172**:247–263.
29. Liss DT, Baker DW. Understanding current racial/ethnic disparities in colorectal cancer screening in the United States: the contribution of socioeconomic status and access to care. *Am J Prev Med.* 2014;**46**:228–236.
31. Pollack CE, Armstrong KA, Mitra N, et al. A multidimensional view of racial differences in access to prostate cancer care. *Cancer.* 2017;**123**:4449–4457.
32. Wang EH, Yu JB, Abouassally R, et al. Disparities in treatment of patients with high-risk prostate cancer: results from a population-based cohort. *Urology.* 2016;**95**:88–94.
33. Lund MJ, Brawley OP, Ward KC, et al. Parity and disparity in first course treatment of invasive breast cancer. *Breast Cancer Res Treat.* 2008;**109**:545–557.
34. Griggs JJ, Culakova E, Sorbero ME, et al. Effect of patient socioeconomic status and body mass index on the quality of breast cancer adjuvant chemotherapy. *J Clin Oncol.* 2007;**25**:277–284.
35. Griggs JJ, Hawley ST, Graff JJ, et al. Factors associated with receipt of breast cancer adjuvant chemotherapy in a diverse population-based sample. *J Clin Oncol.* 2012;**30**:3058–3064.
36. Nyrop KA, Damone EM, Deal AM, et al. Obesity, comorbidities, and treatment selection in Black and White women with early breast cancer. *Cancer.* 2021;**127**:922–930.
37. Sineshaw HM, Ng K, Flanders WD, et al. Factors that contribute to differences in survival of black vs white patients with colorectal cancer. *Gastroenterology.* 2018;**154**:906–15.e7.
38. Rhoads KF, Ackerson LK, Ngo JV, et al. Adequacy of lymph node examination in colorectal surgery: contribution of the hospital versus the surgeon. *Med Care.* 2013;**51**:1055–1062.
39. Sineshaw HM, Sahar L, Osarogiagbon RU, et al. County-level variations in receipt of surgery for early-stage non-small cell lung cancer in the United States. *Chest.* 2020;**157**:212–222.
40. Feinstein AR, Sosin DM, Wells CK. The Will Rogers phenomenon. Stage migration and new diagnostic techniques as a source of misleading statistics for survival in cancer. *N Engl J Med.* 1985;**312**:1604–1608.
42. Grady WM, Carethers JM. Genomic and epigenetic instability in colorectal cancer pathogenesis. *Gastroenterology.* 2008;**135**:1079–1099.
43. Gordon NH. Association of education and income with estrogen receptor status in primary breast cancer. *Am J Epidemiol.* 1995;**142**:796–803.
44. John EM, Hines LM, Phipps AI, et al. Reproductive history, breast-feeding and risk of triple negative breast cancer: the Breast Cancer Etiology in Minorities (BEM) study. *Int J Cancer.* 2018;**142**:2273–2285.
46. Palmer JR, Viscidi E, Troester MA, et al. Parity, lactation, and breast cancer subtypes in African American women: results from the AMBER Consortium. *J Natl Cancer Inst.* 2014;**106**:dju237.
47. Ogden CL, Fryar CD, Martin CB, et al. Trends in obesity prevalence by race and hispanic origin-1999–2000 to 2017–2018. *JAMA.* 2020;**324**:1208–1210.
48. Islami F, Goding Sauer A, Miller KD, et al. Proportion and number of cancer cases and deaths attributable to potentially modifiable risk factors in the United States. *CA Cancer J Clin.* 2018;**68**:31–54.
49. Berman DB, Wagner-Costalas J, Schultz DC, et al. Two distinct origins of a common BRCA1 mutation in breast-ovarian cancer families: a genetic study of 15 185delAG-mutation kindreds. *Am J Hum Genet.* 1996;**58**:1166–1176.
50. Zhao F, Copley B, Niu Q, et al. Racial disparities in survival outcomes among breast cancer patients by molecular subtypes. *Breast Cancer Res Treat.* 2021;**185**:841–849.
51. Offit K, Gilewski T, McGuire P, et al. Germline BRCA1 185delAG mutations in Jewish women with breast cancer. *Lancet.* 1996;**347**:1643–1645.
52. Yasuda SU, Zhang L, Huang SM. The role of ethnicity in variability in response to drugs: focus on clinical pharmacology studies. *Clin Pharmacol Ther.* 2008;**84**:417–423.
53. Jaruthamsophon K, Tipmanee V, Sangiemchoey A, et al. HLA-B*15:21 and carbamazepine-induced Stevens-Johnson syndrome: pooled-data and in silico analysis. *Sci Rep.* 2017;**7**:45553.
54. Locharernkul C, Shotelersuk V, Hirankarn N. Pharmacogenetic screening of carbamazepine-induced severe cutaneous allergic reactions. *J Clin Neurosci.* 2011;**18**:1289–1294.
55. Vadivel N, Garg A, Holt DW, et al. Tacrolimus dose in black renal transplant recipients. *Transplantation.* 2007;**83**:997–999.
56. McLeod HL, Sargent DJ, Marsh S, et al. Pharmacogenetic predictors of adverse events and response to chemotherapy in metastatic colorectal cancer: results from North American Gastrointestinal Intergroup Trial N9741. *J Clin Oncol.* 2010;**28**:3227–3233.
58. Paulík A, Nekvindová J, Filip S. Irinotecan toxicity during treatment of metastatic colorectal cancer: focus on pharmacogenomics and personalized medicine. *Tumori.* 2020;**106**:87–94.
59. Freedman LS, Simon R, Foulkes MA, et al. Inclusion of women and minorities in clinical trials and the NIH Revitalization Act of 1993--the perspective of NIH clinical trialists. *Control Clin Trials.* 1995;**16**:277–285; discussion 86–89, 93–309.
60. Easterbrook PJ, Keruly JC, Creagh-Kirk T, et al. Racial and ethnic differences in outcome in zidovudine-treated patients with advanced HIV disease. Zidovudine Epidemiology Study Group. *JAMA.* 1991;**266**:2713–2718.
61. Hamilton JD, Hartigan PM, Simberkoff MS. The effect of zidovudine on patient subgroups. *JAMA.* 1992;**267**:2472–2473.
62. Regnante JM, Richie NA, Fashoyin-Aje L, et al. US cancer centers of excellence strategies for increased inclusion of racial and ethnic minorities in clinical trials. *J Oncol Pract.* 2019;**15**:e289–e299.
64. Langford AT, Resnicow K, Dimond EP, et al. Racial/ethnic differences in clinical trial enrollment, refusal rates, ineligibility, and reasons for decline among patients at sites in the National Cancer Institute's Community Cancer Centers Program. *Cancer.* 2014;**120**:877–884.

66 Tramontano AC, Chen Y, Watson TR, et al. Racial/ethnic disparities in colorectal cancer treatment utilization and phase-specific costs, 2000–2014. *PLoS One*. 2020;**15**:e0231599.

67 Fang P, He W, Gomez D, et al. Racial disparities in guideline-concordant cancer care and mortality in the United States. *Adv Radiat Oncol*. 2018;**3**:221–229.

68 Esnaola NF, Ford ME. Racial differences and disparities in cancer care and outcomes: where's the rub? *Surg Oncol Clin N Am*. 2012;**21**:417–437, viii.

71 Neoplasms in people living with human immunodeficiency virus

Chia-Ching J. Wang MD ■ Elizabeth Y. Chiao MD, MPH

Overview

People living with human immunodeficiency viruses (PLWH) are at increased risk for developing malignancies, particularly virally mediated cancers such as Kaposi sarcoma (KS), some types of lymphoma, and HPV-related cancers, such as cervical cancer and anal cancer. PLWH also have higher rates of alcohol and tobacco use, which increases their risk of non-virally mediated cancers, such as lung cancer and both oropharyngeal and non-oropharyngeal head and neck cancers. KS and lymphomas tend to occur at lower CD4 counts, and the incidences of these cancers have decreased since the advent of effective combination antiretroviral therapy (ART). However, the incidence for virally mediated cancers (such as anal cancer) other non-virally-mediated non-acquired immunodeficiency syndrome-defining cancers (such as lung cancer) have risen in the past decade in part because PLWH are living longer with wide-spread access to ART. In the past, PLWH with cancers often had lower survival and poorer outcomes due to severe immunodeficiency and poor performance status. In the modern ART era, survival and outcomes for individuals with human immunodeficiency virus (HIV)-associated lymphomas are generally similar to the HIV-negative population using standard rituximab-based multi-agent chemotherapy. For PLWH with other solid tumors, standard of care treatment is also currently recommended. Active areas of research for cancers in PLWH includes cancer prevention, immunotherapy, and continued development of new therapeutics to improve outcomes.

Introduction

Since the earliest clinical descriptions of the acquired immunodeficiency syndrome (AIDS) in 1991, the syndrome has been etiologically associated with malignancies, starting with Kaposi Sarcoma (KS).[1] After the discovery of the human immunodeficiency virus-1 (HIV), originally called human T-lymphotrophic virus III (HTLV-3), as the cause of AIDS, multiple other cancers, including intermediate-grade and high-grade non-Hodgkin's lymphoma (NHL), primary central nervous system lymphoma (PCNSL), and cervical cancers, were associated with AIDS and subsequently included in the US Centers for Disease Control and Prevention (CDC) definition of "AIDS-defining conditions."[2,3] Prior to wide-spread availability of combination antiretroviral therapy (ART), the International Agency on the Research of Cancer defined HIV itself as a biologic carcinogen.[4] The evidence suggests that HIV-specific proteins, including *Tat* and *Nef*, are cofactors in the carcinogenic process. In addition, HIV infection may also cause cancer indirectly through immune deficiency, particularly by accelerating the effect of oncogenic infections. Thus, people living with human immunodeficiency virus (PLWH) continue to have an increased risk of certain cancers similar to other immunodeficient populations, such as solid organ transplant recipients. The authors also hypothesize that immune surveillance may be impaired, in spite of ART, which may increase the risk for cancers that are particularly dependent on immune system surveillance (including cancers such as melanoma and lung). Furthermore, people living with HIV are also at higher risk for poor social determinants of health as well as exposure to other environmental carcinogens including smoking and alcohol.[5-7] Thus, HIV-related carcinogenesis is multifactorial and leads to both an increased risk of cancer and potential disparities in cancer outcomes (Figure 1).

The cancers for which PLWH are at the highest risk, as described by the highest standardized incidence ratios (the ratio of incident cancers among PLWH compared to the general population) are primarily virally mediated AIDS and non-AIDS Defining Cancers. However, PLWH remain at higher risk for lung cancer, as demonstrated in a review by Yarchoan and Uldrick[8] and shown in Table 1, as well as several other non-virally mediated cancers, including: non-oropharyngeal head and neck cancers and esophageal squamous cancer.[10,11]

Several other cancers that are not AIDS-defining and not virally mediated have also been found to have an increased incidence in PLWH. These include, but are not limited to, lung, melanoma, colorectal, and renal cancers. The increasing longevity of PLWH, as well as the prevalence of concurrent modifiable risk factors such as tobacco use in this population, may also influence the epidemiology of these malignancies. A meta-analysis of multiple HIV- and transplant-associated malignancies examining the relationship between virally mediated, non-virally mediated, and age-related cancers demonstrated the potentially similar epidemiologic and clinical characteristics between HIV- and transplant-associated immunosuppression.[5] As shown in Figures 2–5, the majority of virally mediated cancers, including cancers possibly associated with human papillomavirus (HPV), are elevated in both people living with HIV and post-transplant patients. In addition, the risk for cancers of the lung and kidney, melanoma, and leukemia are increased for both populations. While the most common age-related solid tumors (breast, colorectal, prostate) do not demonstrate an increased risk in immunosuppressed patients, certain other rarer tumors are only elevated in PLWH (brain and testis) or only in transplant patients (bladder and thyroid).

Epidemiology

After the introduction of combination ART in the mid-1990s, survival and the clinical outcomes of PLWH dramatically improved. In spite of global increased access to life-saving ART, which, when started before advanced immunosuppression (CD4 lymphocyte count >500 c/µL), has been shown to be associated with subsequent normal life expectancy, HIV-related morbidity

---

Holland-Frei Cancer Medicine, Tenth Edition. Edited by Robert C. Bast, John C. Byrd, Carlo M. Croce, Ernest Hawk, Fadlo R. Khuri, Raphael E. Pollock, Apostolia M. Tsimberidou, Christopher G. Willett, and Cheryl L. Willman.
© 2023 John Wiley & Sons, Inc. Published 2023 by John Wiley & Sons, Inc.

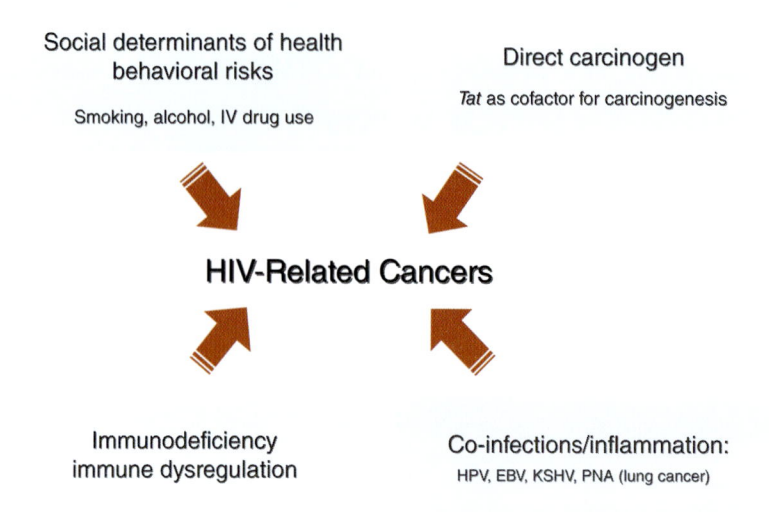

Figure 1 HIV-related carcinogenesis.

Table 1 HIV-associated cancers: the AIDS and non-AIDS defining cancers[a].

Cancer[b]	SIR after combination ART in the United States[c]	Role of immunosuppression from HIV infection	Etiologic viruses	Other causative factors
Non-Hodgkin's lymphoma	11.5	++ to ++++ for different types	EBV[d]	
Kaposi's sarcoma	498.1	+++	KSHV	
Cervical cancer	3.2	+	HPV	Tobacco
Lung cancer	2.0	+	?	Smoking, pulmonary infections
Anal cancer	19.1	+	HPV	
Hodgkin's lymphoma	7.7	++	EBV	
Oral cavity and pharyngeal cancer	1.6	0 to + for different types	HPV	Tobacco, alcohol
Hepatocellular carcinoma	3.2	0 or +	HBV, HCV	Alcohol, other hepatic insults
Vulvar cancer	9.4	+	HPV	
Penile cancer	5.3	+	HPV	

[a]Source: Yarchoan and Uldrick.[8]
[b]Shown are the principal tumors that are associated with an increase in the standardized incidence ratio (SIR) among persons with human immunodeficiency virus (HIV) infection in the United States. Plus signs (from 0 to ++++) indicate the relative association of the cancer with immunosuppression and low CD4+ counts, with 0 indicating no association and ++++ indicating a substantial association. ART denotes anti-retroviral therapy; EBV, Epstein–Barr virus; HBV, hepatitis B virus; HCV, hepatitis C virus; HPV, human papillomavirus; and KSHV, Kaposi's sarcoma–associated herpesvirus.
[c]The information in this column is from Hernández-Ramírez et al.[9]
[d]EBV is the cause of approximately 30–100% of the various forms of AIDS-defining non-Hodgkin's lymphoma; two exceptions are primary effusion lymphoma and large-B-cell lymphoma that develops in KSHV-related multicentric Castleman's disease, which are caused by KSHV. Approximately 80% of persons with primary effusion lymphoma are coinfected with EBV.

and mortality remains a public health issue. Some studies have estimated that the mortality rate for PLWH has decreased by 70% as result of the widespread availability of ART.[12] In addition, ART can decrease HIV transmission when ART is taken consistently and the HIV viral load is undetectable. However, in certain marginalized and vulnerable populations, the incidence of HIV has continued to increase in the past decade. Thus, although the incidence of HIV is decreasing, in 2019, the number of PLWH in the world has increased to 37 million.[13] Furthermore, in the United States, the prevalence of HIV has quadrupled in the last 15 years to an estimated 1.2 million,[14] with 45% of the PLWH over 50 years of age,[15] and as the population of PLWH increases, the cancer burden will continue to increase as well.

In addition to the aging population of PLWH, ART has also dramatically reduced the incidence of viral-mediated HIV-associated malignancies, such as KS and PCNSL.[7] However, as the incidence of AIDS-defining cancers has continued to decrease for PLWH, the incidence of non-AIDS defining cancers has continued to increase. A recent modeling study used the HIV/Cancer Registry Match, which is a record linkage study of HIV and cancer registries in nine US regions (www.hivmatch.cancer.gov). This analysis considered the 11 most common cancer types among PLWH and modeled the cancer burden by age from 2006 to 2030 (Figure 6).[16] Based on this projection, the epidemiology of cancer in PLWH will continue to evolve as the population ages and there is continued improvement in ART access.

Furthermore, although other cause-specific mortality rates have universally declined for PLWH, deaths associated with non-acquired immunodeficiency syndrome-defining cancers (NADC) remains the exception to that trend.[17,18] With the mortality burden of cancer among PLWH increasing over the past several years, cancer has become the leading cause of death among PLWH.[19,20] PLWH and cancer have been shown to have higher overall and cancer-specific mortality than the general population, with up to 30% of deaths attributable to cancer.[18,19,21–23] For example, Coghill et al.[24] demonstrated excess cancer mortality for PLWH and cancer compared with uninfected controls for lung cancer, NHL, breast cancer, and colorectal cancer. Other studies

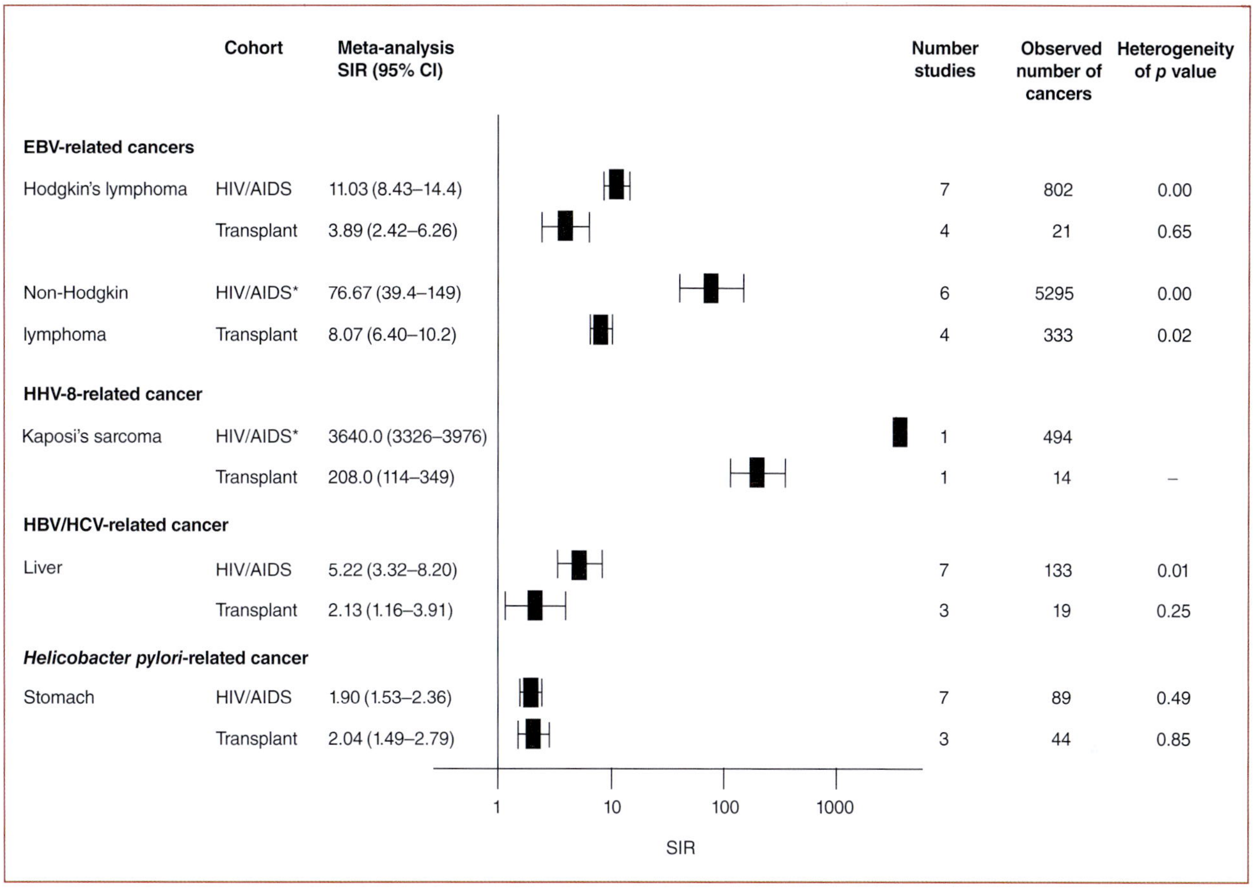

	Cohort	Meta-analysis SIR (95% CI)		Number studies	Observed number of cancers	Heterogeneity of p value
EBV-related cancers						
Hodgkin's lymphoma	HIV/AIDS	11.03 (8.43–14.4)		7	802	0.00
	Transplant	3.89 (2.42–6.26)		4	21	0.65
Non-Hodgkin lymphoma	HIV/AIDS*	76.67 (39.4–149)		6	5295	0.00
	Transplant	8.07 (6.40–10.2)		4	333	0.02
HHV-8-related cancer						
Kaposi's sarcoma	HIV/AIDS*	3640.0 (3326–3976)		1	494	
	Transplant	208.0 (114–349)		1	14	–
HBV/HCV-related cancer						
Liver	HIV/AIDS	5.22 (3.32–8.20)		7	133	0.01
	Transplant	2.13 (1.16–3.91)		3	19	0.25
***Helicobacter pylori*-related cancer**						
Stomach	HIV/AIDS	1.90 (1.53–2.36)		7	89	0.49
	Transplant	2.04 (1.49–2.79)		3	44	0.85

Figure 2 Standardized incidence ratios for cancers related to infection with Epstein–Barr virus, human herpesvirus 8, hepatitis B and C virus, and *Helicobacter pylori* in people with HIV/AIDS and in transplant recipients. EBV, Epstein–Barr virus; HBV, hepatitis B virus; HCV, hepatitis C virus; HHV8, human herpesvirus 8. *For AIDS-defining cancers, data from cohorts defined by an AIDS diagnosis included only those individuals who did not have that type of cancer at the time of AIDS. Source: Grulich et al.[5]

comparing cancer prognosis by HIV status have noted increased all-cause mortality among PLWH compared with the general population for Hodgkin's lymphoma (HL),[25–27] lung,[21,22,25,26,28,29] colorectal,[25,26] anal,[26,30] and prostate[21,26] cancers. Silverberg et al. demonstrated an increase in *cancer-specific* mortality for multiple cancers in PLWH in spite of adjustment for several common prognostic factors.[6,21]

The etiology of these outcome disparities is not completely understood. Several population-based studies have demonstrated differences in cancer treatment initiation by HIV status. In a Texas-based HIV/Cancer registry linkage study, Suneja et al.[22] compared 337 PLWH and 156,593 uninfected individuals with non-small cell lung cancer and found that PLWH were 60% less likely to receive lung cancer treatment. Another study of 174 PLWH and 3480 uninfected Medicare beneficiaries with lung cancer noted that, despite similar cancer treatment initiation rates, there was still a difference in survival by HIV status, suggesting other contributing factors to cancer outcome disparities.[23] Three studies utilized cancer registry data to measure treatment disparities for several common cancer types (Table 2), including two multi-state population-based studies[31,32] and a study conducted in the Kaiser Permanente Health System.[21] In general, PLWH had higher percentages without treatment for most cancers compared with uninfected controls, although there was variation across studies, suggesting the influence of access to cancer care, patient-specific or other risk factors. Furthermore, a survey of medical and radiation oncologists demonstrated that 20% of oncologists would not offer guideline-concordant cancer care to HIV-infected individuals, primarily because of concerns about safety and efficacy.[33] However, lack of treatment initiation may not be the only factor in poor cancer survival outcomes by PLWH. A recent study by Coghill et al.[34] have demonstrated that differences in cancer outcomes persist by HIV status even after accounting for differences by treatment initiation.

In order to address the observation that PLWH were less likely to initiate cancer treatment from population-based studies, in 2019, the National Comprehensive Cancer Network (NCCN) published treatment guidelines for PLWH and common cancers associated with HIV.[35] In most cases, individuals with HIV and cancer who are on ART should be treated according to standard guidelines for the general population. Coordinated care between medical oncologists, radiation oncologists, infectious disease physicians, and pharmacists should be provided for all patients undergoing therapy for cancer with HIV. However, there is some evidence that even with standard therapies, PLWH have poorer cancer outcomes. For example, a retrospective study of cervical cancer recurrence and mortality in Brazil demonstrated that while tumor responses at the end of chemotherapy and radiation were equivalent by HIV status, women with HIV who achieved complete responses (CRs) had twice the recurrence rate compared with women without HIV.[36] Another study in PLWH with cancer reported that chemoradiotherapy (CRT)/radiotherapy resulted in significantly reduced CD4

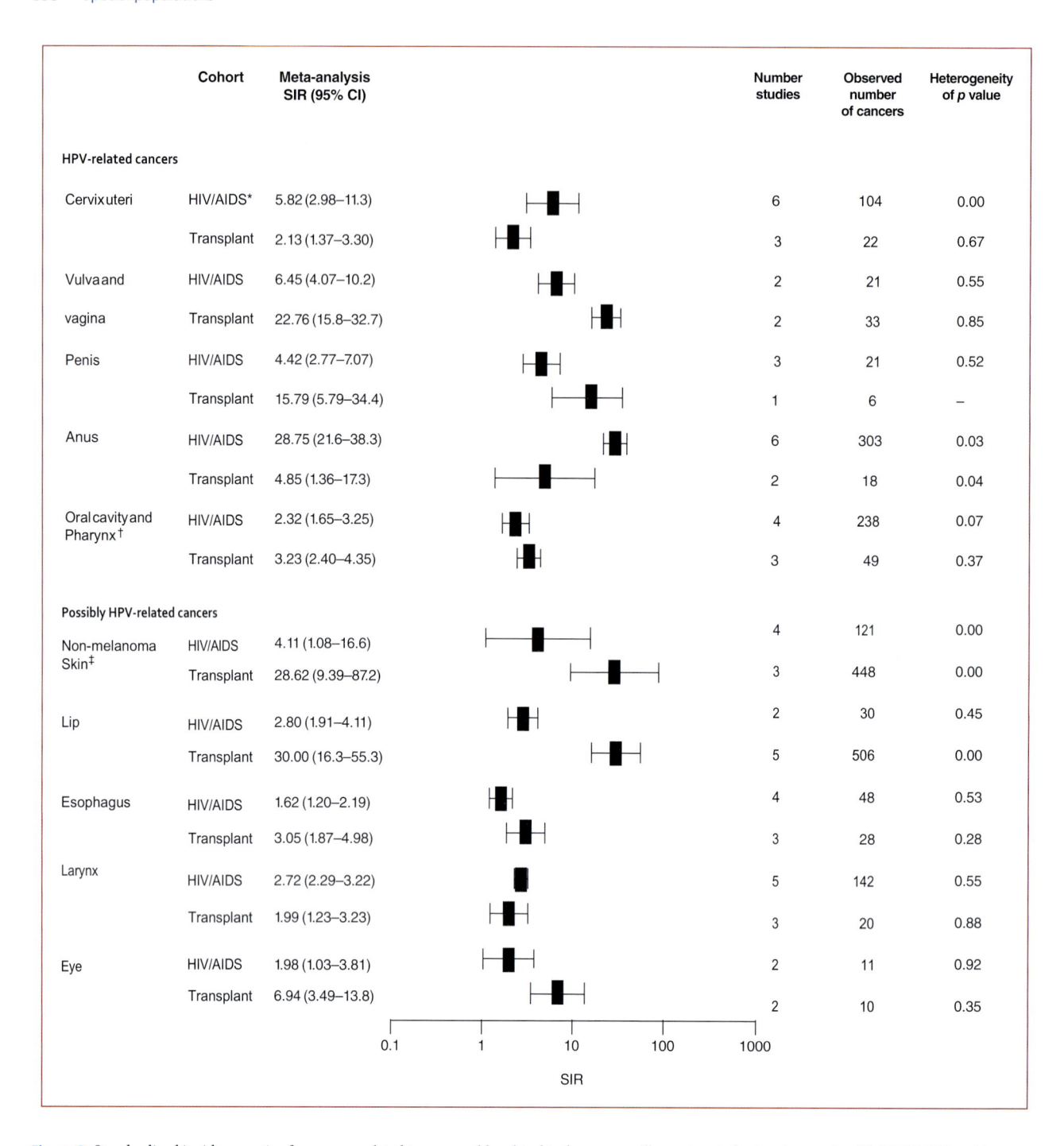

	Cohort	Meta-analysis SIR (95% CI)		Number studies	Observed number of cancers	Heterogeneity of p value
HPV-related cancers						
Cervix uteri	HIV/AIDS*	5.82 (2.98–11.3)		6	104	0.00
	Transplant	2.13 (1.37–3.30)		3	22	0.67
Vulva and vagina	HIV/AIDS	6.45 (4.07–10.2)		2	21	0.55
	Transplant	22.76 (15.8–32.7)		2	33	0.85
Penis	HIV/AIDS	4.42 (2.77–7.07)		3	21	0.52
	Transplant	15.79 (5.79–34.4)		1	6	–
Anus	HIV/AIDS	28.75 (21.6–38.3)		6	303	0.03
	Transplant	4.85 (1.36–17.3)		2	18	0.04
Oral cavity and Pharynx[†]	HIV/AIDS	2.32 (1.65–3.25)		4	238	0.07
	Transplant	3.23 (2.40–4.35)		3	49	0.37
Possibly HPV-related cancers						
Non-melanoma Skin[‡]	HIV/AIDS	4.11 (1.08–16.6)		4	121	0.00
	Transplant	28.62 (9.39–87.2)		3	448	0.00
Lip	HIV/AIDS	2.80 (1.91–4.11)		2	30	0.45
	Transplant	30.00 (16.3–55.3)		5	506	0.00
Esophagus	HIV/AIDS	1.62 (1.20–2.19)		4	48	0.53
	Transplant	3.05 (1.87–4.98)		3	28	0.28
Larynx	HIV/AIDS	2.72 (2.29–3.22)		5	142	0.55
	Transplant	1.99 (1.23–3.23)		3	20	0.88
Eye	HIV/AIDS	1.98 (1.03–3.81)		2	11	0.92
	Transplant	6.94 (3.49–13.8)		2	10	0.35

Figure 3 Standardized incidence ratios for cancers related to, or possibly related to, human papillomavirus infection, in people with HIV/AIDS and in transplant recipients. HPV, human papillomavirus. *For the AIDS-defining cancer (cervical cancer), data from cohorts defined by an AIDS diagnosis included only those individuals who did not have cervical cancer at the time of AIDS. [†]Excluding lip and nasopharynx. [‡]Any measure of non-melanoma skin. Source: Grulich et al.[5]

count compared with surgery, and subsequent increased risk of mortality.[37] Identifying optimized cancer care for PLWH and cancer has been challenging in the past because PLWH have traditionally been excluded from cancer clinical trials.[38] However, in the era of immunotherapy and improved outcomes from HIV due to ART, there has been a greater awareness and implementation of more modern clinical trial criteria, allowing enrollment of PLWH into clinical trials. Furthermore, the AIDS Malignancy Consortium, a National Cancer Institute (NCI)-funded clinical trials consortium, is focused on conducting clinical trials to improve cancer care outcomes for PLWH and cancer.

Kaposi sarcoma

KS is a rare, multi-centric, angio-proliferative tumor that was first described in 1872 by Moritz Kaposi, a Hungarian dermatologist. Although it was originally described as a relatively indolent skin tumor in elderly men,[39] subsequent epidemiologic investigations described multiple sub-types of KS, affecting different geographic and demographic populations. These subtypes included: Classic KS, occurring primarily in Mediterranean and Eastern European regions[40]; Endemic KS, which occurs primarily in Africa and is more aggressive[41]; Transplantation-associated KS; and HIV-related or "epidemic" KS.[42]

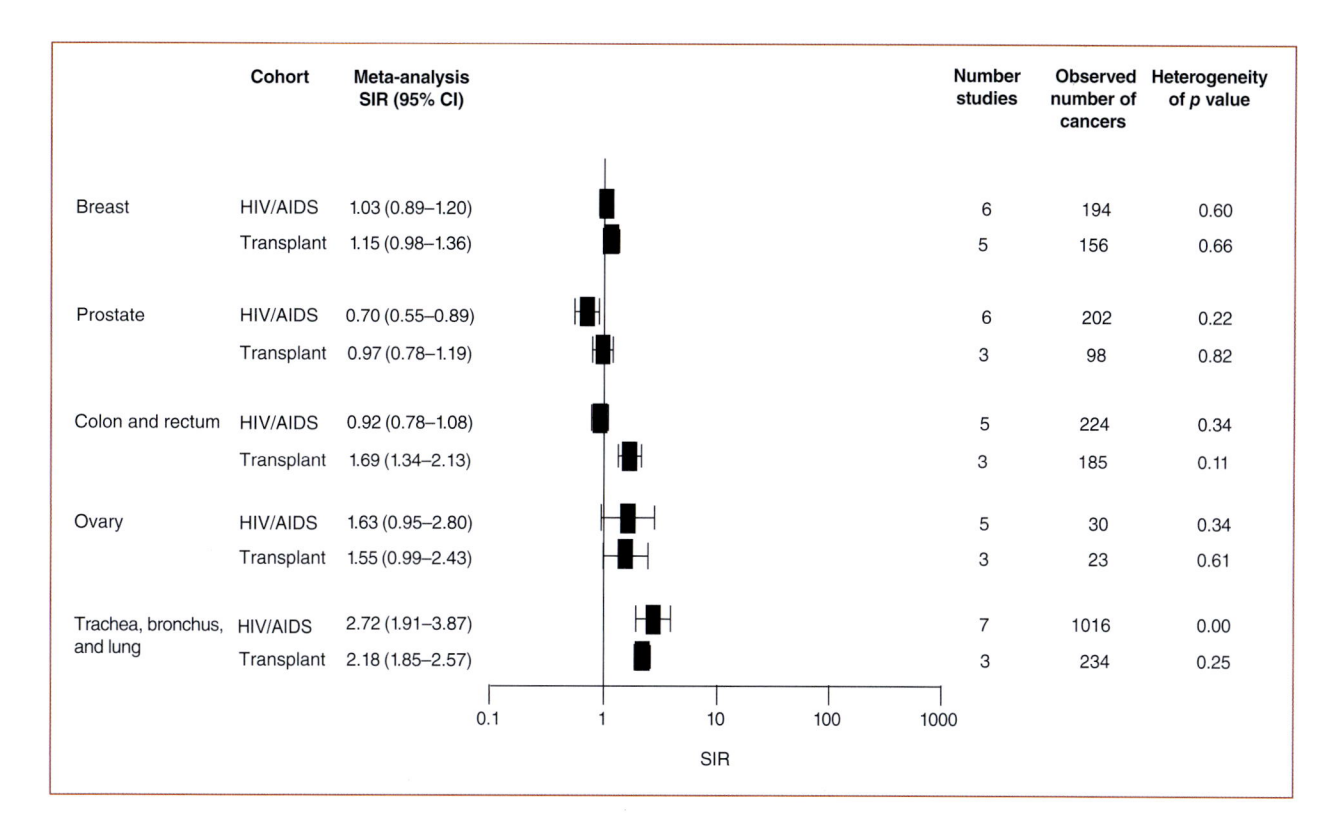

Cohort		Meta-analysis SIR (95% CI)	Number studies	Observed number of cancers	Heterogeneity of p value
Breast	HIV/AIDS	1.03 (0.89–1.20)	6	194	0.60
	Transplant	1.15 (0.98–1.36)	5	156	0.66
Prostate	HIV/AIDS	0.70 (0.55–0.89)	6	202	0.22
	Transplant	0.97 (0.78–1.19)	3	98	0.82
Colon and rectum	HIV/AIDS	0.92 (0.78–1.08)	5	224	0.34
	Transplant	1.69 (1.34–2.13)	3	185	0.11
Ovary	HIV/AIDS	1.63 (0.95–2.80)	5	30	0.34
	Transplant	1.55 (0.99–2.43)	3	23	0.61
Trachea, bronchus, and lung	HIV/AIDS	2.72 (1.91–3.87)	7	1016	0.00
	Transplant	2.18 (1.85–2.57)	3	234	0.25

Figure 4 Standardized incidence ratios for common epithelial cancers in people with HIV/AIDS and in transplant recipients. Source: Grulich et al.[5]

The increasing rate of KS was one of the earliest described manifestations of AIDS in 1981,[1] and it's epidemiologic trajectory continued to parallel the HIV epidemic prior to the advent of ART, with 30% of all AIDS patients developing KS.[43] Thus, the "epidemic KS" is synonymous or syndemic with HIV-related KS. Because it became apparent that certain sub-groups of PLWH, particularly men who have sex with men (MSM), had significantly higher risk for developing KS,[44] compared with a low risk of disease in intravenous drug users or other HIV groups,[45] an additional infectious agent as a cause for KS was hypothesized. Subsequently, using representational difference analysis, a novel gamma-herpesvirus was discovered and named "Kaposi sarcoma herpesvirus" (KSHV) or human herpes virus 8 (HHV-8), which was then identified as the etiologic agent of KS.[46,47] Over the last two decades, the epidemiology of KSHV demonstrates that its prevalence differs widely among geographic populations with low prevalence in the general population of northern Europe, North America, and most of Asia; while the prevalence is intermediate in the Mediterranean and parts of Latin and South America.[48] In contrast, KSHV seroprevalence is high in Sub-Saharan Africa (SSA), and transmission has been shown to occur early in life.[49] This likely contributes to the high endemic rates of KS is SSA. Of note, in Europe and North America, there are several sub-populations with much higher rates of KSHV seroprevalence, including among HIV-negative MSM, where the seroprevalence has been estimated at 14–26%, and up to 58% in MSM living with HIV.[50]

The syndemics of KS and HIV were also concomitantly affected by the widespread availability with ART, and the incidence of KS has substantially decreased in the past few decades. Shiels et al.[51] estimated that between 1990 and 2007, there were 85,922 cases of KS in the United States, but they noted that the proportion of AIDS-related KS decreased from 89% in 1990–1995 to 67% in 2001–2007 ($p < 0.001$). Furthermore, Silverberg et al.[7] estimated that the incidence of KS in North America decreased by 4% per year from 2005–2009 compared to 1996–1999. However, while the rates of KS in the United States continue to decline, a recent study of the US Cancer Statistics Registry found that the incidence of KS was significantly increasing in young men age 20–29, but incidence rates remained largely constant in men age 45–54, suggesting age-dependent changes in KS incidence rates.[52]

KSHV infection is a necessary component for KS pathogenesis. Similar to other herpesviruses, the HHV-8 genome encodes both lytic and latent genes. During latency, viral replication is dormant, and genes are infrequently expressed. Latent genes are encoded by *ORFK12* (kaposin), *ORF71* (vFLIP), *ORF72* (v-cyclin), ORF73 (latency-associated nuclear antigen[LANA]), *ORFK10.5* (vIRF3), and several viral micro ribonucleic acids (miRNAs).[53] KSHV is also unique because the virus carries homologs of human cellular gene products that are involved in inflammation, cell cycle regulation, and angiogenesis, such as viral cyclin-D1 (*CCND1*), vascular endothelial growth factor (*VEGF*), basic fibroblast growth factor (*FGF2*), and interleukin-6 (*IL6*).[54]

In addition, KS pathogenesis has been shown to be dependent on several other pathways involved in cellular proliferation, apoptosis and transformation pathways. For example, the TLR4 pathway, and its adaptor MyD88, and coreceptors CD14 and MD2[55] are constitutively activated in KSHV-transformed cells, resulting in chronic induction of IL-6, IL-1β, and IL-18. Subsequent activation of this pathway then leads to IL-6 mediated constitutive activation of the STAT3 pathway, which is itself an essential event for uncontrolled cellular proliferation and transformation. Furthermore, other HIV-specific proteins including regulatory transactivating (tat) protein has been shown to be released by HIV-infected cells. Furthermore, the interaction between HIV tat proteins causes uncontrolled proliferation of the KSHV-infected vascular or lymphatic endothelial cell, and prevents apoptosis of KS cells.[56,57]

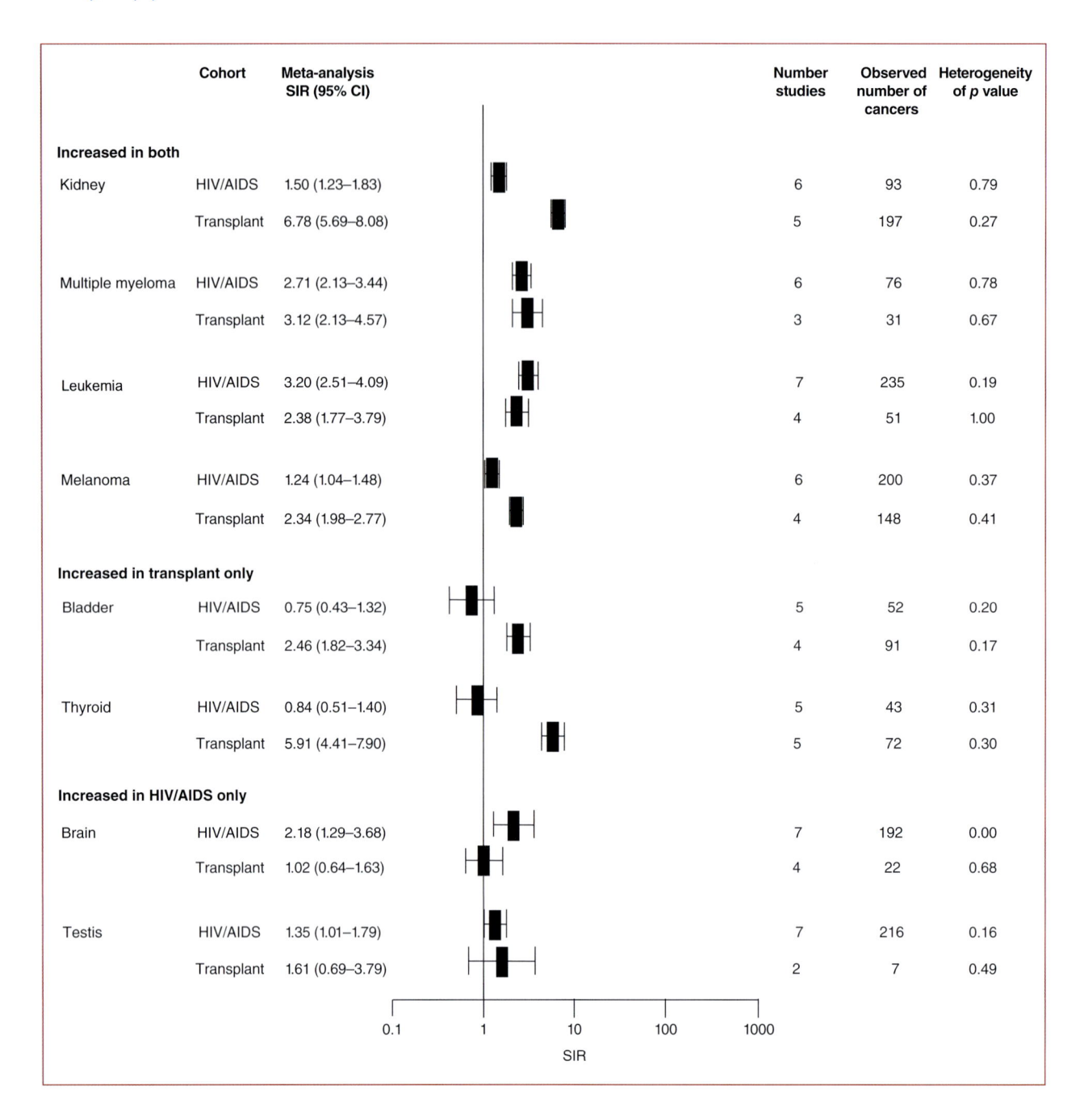

Cohort		Meta-analysis SIR (95% CI)	Number studies	Observed number of cancers	Heterogeneity of p value
Increased in both					
Kidney	HIV/AIDS	1.50 (1.23–1.83)	6	93	0.79
	Transplant	6.78 (5.69–8.08)	5	197	0.27
Multiple myeloma	HIV/AIDS	2.71 (2.13–3.44)	6	76	0.78
	Transplant	3.12 (2.13–4.57)	3	31	0.67
Leukemia	HIV/AIDS	3.20 (2.51–4.09)	7	235	0.19
	Transplant	2.38 (1.77–3.79)	4	51	1.00
Melanoma	HIV/AIDS	1.24 (1.04–1.48)	6	200	0.37
	Transplant	2.34 (1.98–2.77)	4	148	0.41
Increased in transplant only					
Bladder	HIV/AIDS	0.75 (0.43–1.32)	5	52	0.20
	Transplant	2.46 (1.82–3.34)	4	91	0.17
Thyroid	HIV/AIDS	0.84 (0.51–1.40)	5	43	0.31
	Transplant	5.91 (4.41–7.90)	5	72	0.30
Increased in HIV/AIDS only					
Brain	HIV/AIDS	2.18 (1.29–3.68)	7	192	0.00
	Transplant	1.02 (0.64–1.63)	4	22	0.68
Testis	HIV/AIDS	1.35 (1.01–1.79)	7	216	0.16
	Transplant	1.61 (0.69–3.79)	2	7	0.49

Figure 5 Standardized incidence ratios for other cancers occurring at increased rates in one or both populations. Source: Grulich et al.[5]

Tat protein also increases the production and release of matrix metalloproteinases (MMPs) from endothelial and inflammatory cells. MMPs contribute to the angiogenesis found in KS lesions.[58]

The histopathologic appearance of KS lesions consists of spindle-shaped tumor cells. In addition, there are often descriptions of fibrosis, inflammatory infiltrates, vascular slits, and hemosiderin seen on pathologic descriptions of lesion biopsies (see Figure 7).

Specific immunohistochemical staining of spindle cells for KSHV LANA is sensitive and specific, as is PCR detection of HHV-8 in the lesions.[60] Although 95% of KS presents as skin lesions (alone or in addition to visceral disease), visceral disease alone can occur. In addition, lymphadenopathy often accompanies skin disease, or can occur alone, as can visceral disease.

Although visceral disease occurs most commonly in the lung and gastrointestinal (GI) tract, at autopsy, almost every organ system can show involvement. In particular, silent bone lesions are commonly seen on imaging follow-up. Pulmonary disease is rarely silent and often presents with bronchospasm, dyspnea and hemoptysis. Endoscopically, KS most often presents as small submucosal vascular nodules. For this reason, it may be difficult to establish a diagnosis of GI KS by biopsy because it can be difficult to access the submucosa.[61] In patients with suspected pulmonary KS, violaceous endobronchial lesions can provide an empiric diagnosis of pulmonary KS because endobronchial biopsy is discouraged due to the risk of hemorrhage.[62]

Visceral KS is often rapidly progressive when it involves the lungs, with a median survival time of only 2–6 months in the

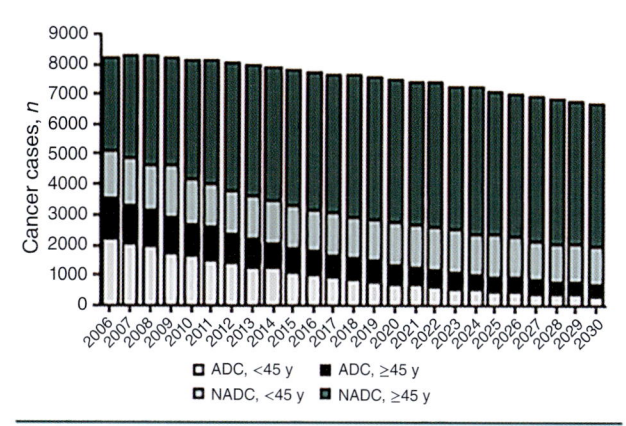

Black segments represent ADC, green segments represent NADC, dark bars represent cancer cases among persons aged ≥45 y, and light bars represent cancer cases among those aged <45 y. ADC, AIDS-defining cancer; NADC, non-AIDS-defining cancer.

Figure 6 Cancer burden projected through 2030 for PLWH. Source: Reprinted with permission from Shiels et al.[16]

Table 2 Selected NADCs w/o cancer treatment (%) by HIV status.

	Study	PLWH	Uninfected
Anal	Marcus et al.[21]	5	7
	Suneja et al.[31]	**7**	**10**
	Suneja et al.[32]	5	3
Prostate	Marcus et al.[21]	43	41
	Suneja et al.[31]	**28**	**24**
	Suneja et al.[32]	**24**	**7**
Colorectal	Marcus et al.[21]	8	7
	Suneja et al.[31]	**16**	**9**
	Suneja et al.[32]	**10**	**4**
Lung	Marcus et al.[21]	**36**	**24**
	Suneja et al.[31]	**40**	**28**
	Suneja et al.[32]	**33**	**14**
HL	Marcus et al.[21]	19	14
	Suneja et al.[31]	**29**	**21**
	Suneja et al.[32]	**17**	**8**

Bold indicates <0.05 by HIV status.

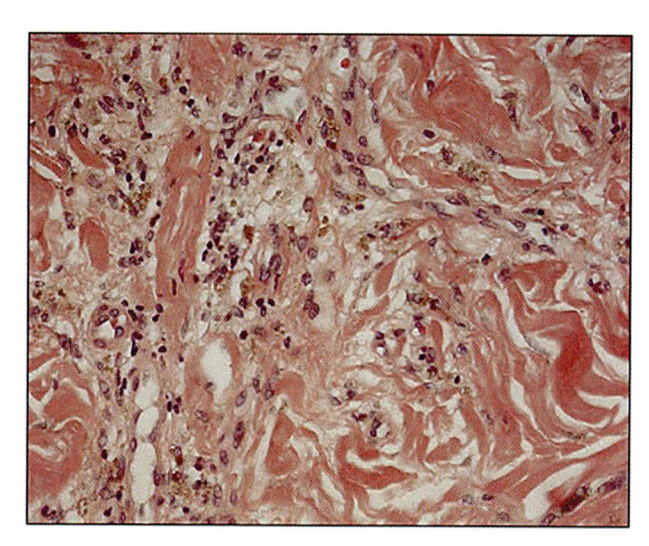

Figure 7 Histopathology of Kaposi's sarcoma showing vascular slits surrounded by spindle cells and hemosiderin deposits in macrophages. Source: Used with permission from Sanders et al.[59]

Table 3 KS ACTG staging criteria[a].

Tumor (T)	T_0: Tumor limited to skin and/or nodes and/or minimal oral disease
	T_1: Tumor associated edema or ulceration, Extensive oral KS, Gastrointestinal KS, or Visceral KS (other than non-nodal viscera)
Immune system (I)	I_0: CD4+ T-cell count ≥150 µL
	I_1: CD4+ T-cell count <150 µL
Systemic illness (S)	S_0: No prior OI, thrush or B symptoms[b]
	S_1: Prior OI, thrush, B symptoms, Karnofsky performance status <70%, or other HIV-related illnesses

For each risk factor the subscripts "0" and "1" represent good risk and poor risk respectively. In the era of effective antiretroviral therapy, T_1S_1 represents the poor risk patients and T_0S_0, T_0S_1, or T_1S_0 represent good risk patients.
[a]Source: Gonçalves et al.[65]
[b]B symptoms are characterized by fever, night sweats and ≥10% of body weight loss. ACTG, AIDS Clinical Trials Group; KS, Kaposi sarcoma; OI, opportunistic infection.

pre-ART era.[62] However, even in the post-ART era, respiratory failure is the most often cause of death in patients with pulmonary KS. Gastrointestinal KS has been reported in 40% of cases at initial diagnosis with any segment of the GI tract involved, and lesions in the oral cavity often correlates with GI tract involvement elsewhere. GI tract involvement can present with abdominal pain, nausea, vomiting, or GI bleeding,[63] but often presents without symptoms. Although screening endoscopy to detect occult disease may be warranted for patients at high risk for GI disease, this may only be needed for patients with advanced AIDS and evidence of occult GI bleeding.[64]

Because KS is a multi-centric disease, staging is based on the acquired immunodeficiency syndrome clinical trials group (ACTG)—rather than the standard tumor, nodal, metastatic (TNM)—staging system. The ACTG staging system (Table 3) is based on tumor burden (T), severity of immunosuppression (I), and the presence of systemic illness (S).[66] For tumor burden, patients with tumor-associated edema or ulceration, extensive oral KS, gastrointestinal KS, or KS in other non-nodal viscera are considered poor risk (T_1). Good risk (T_0) patients have disease confined to the skin, lymph nodes and non-nodular oral disease confined to the palate. The original staging criteria developed before availability of ART defined I_1 as a CD4+ T-cell count <200 cells/µL. However, in the ART era, low initial CD4 count often is associated with improved outcome because ART often rapidly reverses the low CD4 count, and in some patients, starting ART and CD4 count improvement alone treats their KS disease.[67] In addition, the staging system was updated to define I_1 as CD4<150 cells/µL.[65]

One of the most important components of KS treatment is ART, with the goal of CD4 count increases and HIV viral load suppression. ART has multiple mechanisms of action to treat KS including the inhibition of HIV replication, decreased production of the tat protein, and restored immunity to HHV-8. Furthermore, there are some *in vitro* data demonstrating anti-angiogenic activity of some protease inhibitors (PIs).[68] However, non-PI-containing ART regimens also lead to KS regression, and while there are no data demonstrating improved outcomes with PI-containing regimens, Kowalkowski et al.[69] demonstrated that after controlling for time on ART, the incidence of KS was significantly lower after taking a boosted PI-based regimen compared to other regimens, including non-nucleoside reverse transcriptase (NNRTI) and integrase inhibitor (II) regimens. While HIV viral load suppression is necessary for KS control, the use of ART alone is often inadequate for poor risk KS (any T_1 disease or T_1,S_1 disease), and the median time to response to ART alone is 3–9 months.[70] Furthermore, patients with low CD4 counts and KS may develop the paradoxical worsening of their KS which is related to the immune-related inflammatory syndrome (IRIS). It has been reported that approximately 12% of PLWH and KS develop IRIS after ART initiation.[71] The standard therapy for IRIS associated with other opportunistic infections (tuberculosis, Pneumocystis pneumoniae pneumonia, *Mycobacterium avium* complex infection) often require corticosteroids to treat IRIS, however, instead of corticosteroids to treat KS-IRIS, it should be treated with rapid initiation of systemic chemotherapy. Finally, another manifestation of poor-risk KS can be caused by an inflammatory cytokine syndrome characterized by high KSHV viral loads and IL-6 levels.[72] These patients often have significant edema and third-spacing of fluids, including ascites and pleural effusions, fever, low albumin, occasionally a syndrome consistent with sepsis. The main differential diagnoses for these KS-related inflammatory cytokine syndromes include Multicentric Castleman disease, Primary Effusion Lymphoma, and if no lymphoproliferative disease is identified, the Kaposi sarcoma Inflammatory Cytokine Syndrome (KICS).[73,74]

Currently, given the multi-centric nature of the disease, systemic chemotherapy remains the mainstay of KS therapy for poor risk (visceral involvement) and symptomatic KS disease. While long-term remissions are possible with both ART and systemic chemotherapy, the term "cure" is not a treatment goal because there are no curative therapies for either HIV or KSHV infections. The two approved single-agent IV chemotherapeutic agents for treatment of KS in the United States are liposomal doxorubicin and paclitaxel. Earlier in the pre-ART era, combination chemotherapy regimens were first used for KS treatment, including a regimen of doxorubicin, bleomycin, and vincristine. However, liposomal doxorubicin alone has an equivalent response rate with less toxicity.[75] Subsequently, a small randomized trial comparing the efficacy and outcomes of liposomal doxorubicin compared to paclitaxel demonstrated that both therapies improved symptoms such as pain and swelling in PLWH with advanced KS, and demonstrated comparable response rates, progression free survival rates and median survival. However, the paclitaxel arm had slightly higher rates of grade 3–5 toxicity, thus Paclitaxel is often used for first line therapy. Of note, although both Paclitaxel and Paclitaxel have high treatment response rates, approximately 30% of patients will only achieve stable disease and will need long-term therapy.

In low- and middle-income countries (LMICs), paclitaxel therapy is rarely available, but a recent study conducted by the acquired immunodeficiency syndrome clinical trials group/acquired immunodeficiency syndrome malignancy consortium (AMC) in 11 sites in Brazil, Kenya, Malawi, South Africa, Uganda, and Zimbabwe compared oral etoposide plus ART versus bleomycin and vincristine plus ART versus paclitaxel plus ART. The study was stopped early because the paclitaxel arm demonstrated superior progression-free survival (PFS) at week 48 compared to the other two arms. Although paclitaxel was associated with higher rates of hypersensitivity, myelosuppression, peripheral neuropathy, alopecia, and drug interactions with ART, the study established it as the standard treatment in LMICs.[76]

While radiotherapy had been a common treatment for KS in the past, complications such as severe mucositis, radiotherapy fibrosis, loss of skin compliance, and chronic lymphedema may occur with these treatments. Thus, because these types of complications can lead to recurrent cellulitis and, ultimately, deeper soft tissue infections and osteomyelitis, radiotherapy should be used with extreme caution. Radiotherapy is best suited for patients with a single or a few locally symptomatic areas or for symptomatic disease that requires rapid tumor reduction, particularly for facial edema or life-threatening upper airway or eye lesions. Other topical and intra-lesional therapies include aliretinoin gel, which demonstrated a 49% response in a phase 3 study[77]; intra-lesional vinblastine, which has been shown to have a 70% response rate, but is associated with pain and hyperpigmentation after treatment[78]; cryotherapy with liquid nitrogen or imiquimod topical therapy have been tried, but with poor response rates.

Novel therapies are needed, particularly for treatment of KS in LMICs. Inhibition of the (mTOR) signaling pathway with rapamycin, which is commonly utilized for transplant-related KS, has been examined in an AMC study.[79] Other agents that have shown variable responses include imatinib,[80] the MMP COL-3,[81] bevacizumab,[82] IL-12, and thalidomide.[83] Of note, a recent study showed that the immune modulating thalidomide-derivative, pomalidomide, was tolerable and lead to a 73% response rate, with activity in both AIDS-KS and HIV-unassociated KS.[84] Finally, there are several trials evaluating checkpoint inhibitors (CPIs), including a phase I trial of infusional nivolumab from AMC 095, and a phase I intra-lesional nivolumab trial at the University of California San Francisco (NCT03316274), both of which are currently enrolling patients.[85]

Lymphoma

Lymphomas are the principal hematologic malignancies occurring with increased frequency in association with HIV/AIDS. Multicentric Castleman disease, a polyclonal group of lymphoproliferative disorders, also occurs more frequently in PLWH.

Non-Hodgkin lymphoma

NHL has been considered an AIDS-defining condition since 1985[86] and remains the most common cancer that occurs in excess among HIV-infected individuals.[87] Most HIV-associated NHLs are aggressive B-cell neoplasms, with diffuse large B-cell lymphomas (DLBCL) and Burkitt/Burkitt-like lymphomas (BL) occurring most commonly. Following the introduction of effective combination antiretroviral therapy (cART), the incidence of HIV-associated NHL significantly decreased, with the most dramatic decline observed in primary central nervous system lymphoma (PCNSL).[88] The heterogeneity in the pathogenesis of lymphoma in people living with HIV is reflected in the multiple morphological subtypes. For instance, HIV-associated PCNSL are almost universally associated with Epstein–Barr virus (EBV) infection and tend to occur when the CD4 counts are lower than 50 cells/mcL.[89] In contrast, HIV-associated DLBCL is associated with EBV in 30–50% of cases and the CD4 counts are variable with germinal center-type typically occurring at higher CD4 counts than activated B-cell type.[90] HIV-associated Burkitt's lymphoma (BL) is associated with EBV in 25–40% of cases and tends to occur when CD4 counts are somewhat better preserved.[91]

Diffuse large B-cell lymphoma (DLBCL)

DLBCL is the most common lymphoid neoplasm in adults, accounting for approximately 30% of NHLs diagnosed annually.[92] DLBCL is also the most common form of HIV-associated NHL. Clinical trials have consistently demonstrated improved CR, PFS, and overall survival (OS) with R-CHOP (rituximab plus cyclophosphamide, doxorubicin, vincristine, and prednisone) or CHOP-like chemotherapy in immunocompetent individuals with DLBCL, and R-CHOP is now the standard of care for DLBCL in the general population.[93–96] In a randomized phase III trial conducted by the AMC (AMC 010 study) in patients with HIV-associated NHL ($N = 150$; 80% DLBCL; 9% BL), the addition of rituximab to CHOP (R-CHOP) was associated with improved CR rates (CR + unconfirmed CR [CRu]) compared with CHOP alone (58% vs 47%). Although median time to progression improved from 85 to 125 weeks ($p = NS$) there were no statistically significant differences in PFS (10 months vs 9 months) or OS (32 months vs 25 months). The infusional DA-EPOCH regimen (dose-adjusted etoposide, prednisone, vincristine, cyclophosphamide, and doxorubicin) was evaluated in a phase II study in previously untreated patients with HIV-associated NHL ($N = 39$; 79% DLBCL; 18% BL). Treatment with DA-EPOCH resulted in an overall response rate (ORR) of 87% with a CR in 74% of patients.[97] At a median follow-up of 53 months, PFS and OS rates were 73% and 60%, respectively. Only two of the patients with a CR experienced disease recurrence at last follow-up (for a disease-free survival [DFS] rate of 92%). OS was decreased among the patients with low baseline CD4 counts (≤100/mcL) compared with those having higher CD4 counts (16% vs 87%); this association was confirmed by multivariate analysis using a Cox proportional hazard model.[97]

In immunocompetent individuals, the more intensive, DA-EPOCH-R (DA-EPOCH + rituximab) was more toxic and did not improve PFS or OS compared with R-CHOP as front-line therapy for *de novo* DLBCL.[98] There is no randomized controlled trial comparing R-CHOP versus DA-EPOCH-R for HIV-associated DLBCL. However, retrospective pooled analyses of patients with HIV-associated NHL treated in the R-CHOP or DA-EPOCH-R protocols showed among the patients who were treated with concurrent DA-EPOCH-R, both PFS and OS were significantly improved compared with R-CHOP (after adjusting for International Prognostic Index and CD4 counts).[99,100] The incidence of treatment-related deaths was higher in patients with low baseline CD4 counts (<50/mcL) compared with those with higher CD4 counts (37% vs 6%; $p < 0.01$).[99] If the analysis was limited to DLBCL, treatment with DA-EPOCH-R resulted in improved OS compared with R-CHOP (HR 0.34, 95% CI 0.11–0.97; $p = 0.05$).[100] Despite the limits of the retrospective data that are currently available, at this time, many experts will likely recommend DA-EPOCH-R as the preferred regimen for HIV-associated DLBCL.

The treatment of relapsed or refractory lymphomas remains challenging. The standard of care in HIV-negative population is salvage therapy followed by high-dose chemotherapy and autologous hematopoietic stem-cell transplantation (AHSCT). In the cART era, several clinical trials have demonstrated that HIV-infected patients can safely and successfully undergo this treatment modality.[101–104] Treatment-related mortality is 3–5% across several conditioning regimens, and long-term outcomes in reported series appear comparable to HIV-negative patients.[101–104] BMT CTN0803 is a phase II study designed to prospectively assess OS after AHSCT in HIV-infected patients with chemotherapy-sensitive relapsed/refractory lymphomas treated with carmustine, etoposide, Ara-C, and melphalan (BEAM) conditioning. Preliminary data in 43 patients showed CR rate of 92%, with 1-year OS of 87% and cumulative incidence of treatment-related mortality of 5.2%.[105] Their OS was also similar to that of a control population from the Center for International Blood and Marrow Transplant Research (CIBMTR) database matched for age, performance status, disease, and disease status at AHSCT. For patients with relapsed/refractory HIV-associated NHL who can tolerate curative treatment regimens, AHSCT may offer the best chance for disease control. HIV infection alone should not preclude an attempt to obtain stem cells in candidates for AHSCT as the results are comparable to the HIV-negative population.

Burkitt lymphoma
Burkitt lymphoma (BL) is an aggressive NHL characterized by obligate *MYC* gene rearrangement or translocation, and it comprises at least 10% of HIV-associated NHL in the United States in a recent study.[106] PLWH with BL typically present with advanced disease but they have similar stage, marrow involvement, CNS involvement, and histology compared to the general population.[107,108] Recent studies suggest that HIV-infected patients with BL and preserved immune function may benefit from more intensive chemotherapeutic approaches with acceptable toxicities. The use of CODOX-M/IVAC (cyclophosphamide, vincristine, doxorubicin, high-dose methotrexate (HD-MTX)/ifosfamide, etoposide, high-dose cytarabine) in 14 PLWH showed that intensive chemotherapy regimens can be feasible and well-tolerated, with outcomes comparable to HIV-uninfected patients treated at a single institution during the same time period.[109] More recently, a larger prospective multi-center study investigated the safety and tolerability of rituximab with modified CODOX-M/IVAC in 34 PLWH. Twenty-seven patients experienced grade 3–5 toxicities (mainly hematologic and infectious); five patients did not complete treatment and there was one treatment-related death. There was only one CNS relapse, which occurred in someone with baseline CNS disease. The 1-year PFS was 69% (95% CI: 51–82%) and 2-year OS was 69% (95% CI, 51–82%),[110] comparable to that observed in the HIV-uninfected population.

For PLWH with significant co-morbidities and who do not have CNS involvement, less intensive chemotherapy for BL might be appropriate. In an uncontrolled prospective study of DA-EPOCH-R in patients with BL ($N = 30$; including HIV-associated BL, $n = 11$), the CR rate was 100% and both the PFS and OS rates at a median of 73 months of follow-up was 92%.[111] However, this study included mainly PLWH with low-risk BL and without leptomeningeal disease. Given the high risk of CNS disease in this patient population, the use of a combination regimen without CNS-penetrating agents should be approached with some caution until more clinical trial data become available from an ongoing multicenter study.

Primary central nervous system lymphoma (PCNSL)
PCNSL is a rare variant of NHL that is typically EBV-driven and nearly always restricted to patients with CD4 < 50 cells/mcL. It is rarely seen in PLWH benefiting from cART.[112] The current diagnostic algorithm calls for brain biopsy in all suspected cases whenever feasible. The first-line test in diagnostic evaluation of suspected PCNSL is magnetic resonance-based examination of the brain with gadolinium contrast. In addition, the presence of EBV in cerebrospinal fluid (CSF) and fluorodeoxyglucose (18F) positron emission tomography (FDG-PET) also offer important diagnostic information.[113]

In the cART era, HIV-infected patients are now being treated with HD-MTX or other similar regimens with improving outcomes. Among a small number of HIV-infected PCNSL patients, their median OS was 75 months if they received HD-MTX.[114] More recently, there have been case reports of HIV-infected PCNSL being successfully treated with durable remissions using high-dose chemotherapy and AHSCT.[115,116] However, infectious complications, as well as flare of opportunistic conditions, could be significant as patients have died from Toxoplasmosis and Klebsiella sepsis.[115]

Hodgkin lymphoma

The incidence of classical Hodgkin lymphoma (cHL) is approximately 50 per 100,000 person-years among PLWH, which is five- to 20-fold higher than in the background population.[117–119] Although the risk for developing cHL is substantially elevated by HIV infection, cHL is not an AIDS-defining condition. The risk of cHL has remained stable and the burden of disease has actually increased since the introduction of cART.[120–122] Nodular sclerosis subtype is less strongly associated with EBV than other subtypes, while mixed cellularity (often EBV positive) is the most common subtype among older adults.[123] Prior to cART, mixed cellularity was the commonest subtype.[124–126] In the cART era, likely due to improved immunity among HIV-infected populations, the nodular sclerosis subtype now accounts for nearly 50% of cases.[119] HIV may accelerate the development of the EBV-positive cHLs that occur at older ages, for example by leading to loss of immune control of EBV infection. cHL in PLWH also occurs with relatively high frequency during the first few months after initiation of cART as the CD4 cell counts are increasing and the HIV viral loads are decreasing, suggesting that HL may be driven by immune recovery rather than by CD4 cell count depletion.[127]

Historically, long-term outcomes for HIV-associated cHL without cART were poor.[128,129] In the cART era, high cure rates in HIV-associated cHL have recently been demonstrated. A recent retrospective comparison of 93 PLWH and 131 HIV-unrelated patients treated with ABVD (adriamycin, bleomycin, vinblastine, and dacarbazine) from 1997 to 2010 found similar outcomes in the two populations. HIV-infected patients received protease-inhibitor sparing cART and appropriate opportunistic infection prophylaxis. Only one toxic death was noted among PLWH. Five-year DFS and OS rates in HIV-infected versus uninfected patients, respectively, were 85% versus 87% and 81% versus 88%, with no statistically significant differences between groups.[130] ABVD remains the general standard-of-care first-line therapy for both early and advanced HIV-negative cHL, and limited existing evidence generally supports ABVD as a standard in HIV-associated cHL. Brentuximab vedotin, a CD30-directed immuno-conjugate of the antimitotic agent monomethyl auristatin E, was approved by the US Food and Drug Administration for refractory cHL.[131] The AMC in collaboration with the NCI Cancer Therapy Evaluation Program is testing the combination of brentuximab vedotin, doxorubicin, vinblastine, and dacarbazine.[132]

Multicentric Castleman disease (MCD)

MCD, a disease manifested by fever, diffuse lymphadenopathy and hepatosplenomegaly, is more common in HIV-infected individuals than the general population, and is associated with increased incidence of lymphoma in HIV-infected patients.[133] MCD is also present in 11–30% of patients with POEMS syndrome (polyneuropathy, organomegaly, endocrinopathy, M protein, skin changes) who have a documented clonal plasma cell disorder.[134]

Since the beginning of the HIV/AIDS epidemic, clinicians recognized that KS and MCD often coexist. Indeed, KS is present in up to 70% of individuals with MCD at diagnosis.[133] Several studies have shown that HHV-8 could be isolated from the lymph nodes of almost all PLWH with MCD, whereas HIV-negative MCD seldom expressed HHV-8.[135,136] Once MCD is confirmed, plasma HHV-8 DNA levels have also been demonstrated to correlate with symptomatic disease flare and may serve as a helpful biomarker to monitor disease activity and response to therapy.[137] Additionally, there appears to be a high degree of HHV-8 replication, with mostly lytic genes (such as viral IL-6) being active in infected cells in patients with MCD.[138,139] It is uncertain whether cART usage contributes to control of HIV-associated MCD. The incidence of HIV-associated MCD appears to be increasing in the cART era.[140] Among 48 patients diagnosed with MCD in the cART era, 44% were on cART at the time of MCD diagnosis, and of those, 20 had HIV viral loads less than 400 copies/mcL,[133] implying that well-controlled HIV infection does not eliminate the risk of MCD.

Currently, the most data for MCD treatment relate to the use of rituximab. As a single agent, rituximab at the standard dose of 375 mg/m[16] for 4 weeks for HIV-associated MCD results in response rates of 60–70%, with OS of 95% at 2 years, and DFS of 79% at 2 years.[141–143] More recently, chemotherapy combined with rituximab has also shown efficacy.[144–146] The rituximab-liposomal doxorubicin combination may be particularly useful for HIV-infected patients with MCD and concurrent KS, which tends to progress when patients are treated with rituximab alone.[146] Interestingly, in a retrospective series of 113 patients with HIV-associated MCD who had received chemotherapy, rituximab or a combination of the two as first-line therapy, fewer patients who received rituximab progressed to NHL.[147] Given the role of IL-6 in the pathogenesis of MCD, novel monoclonal antibodies targeting IL-6 and the IL-6 receptor are also being studied for the management of this disease. In Japan, tocilizumab was administered to 28 HIV-negative patients with MCD who were noted to have improved symptomatology, lymphadenopathy and inflammatory markers.[148] Siltuximab is a novel anti-IL-6 monoclonal antibody, which was used for treatment of MCD and unresectable unicentric CD in a phase I study. Interim results reported that 18 of 23 patients achieved clinical benefit, and 12 patients demonstrated objective tumor response. All 11 patients treated with the highest dose of 12 mg/kg achieved clinical benefit and eight achieved objective response.[149]

Cervical cancer

Cervical cancer continues to be included as an AIDS-defining cancer and remains the fourth most common cancer for women in the world. Due to differences in access to screening and prevention activities, cervical cancer remains the highest incidence cancer for women in many LMICs, and is the leading cause of death in many countries in SSA.[150] It has been hypothesized that the twin epidemics of HIV and high-risk (HR—which includes subtypes 16, 18 as well as up to 14 others and places those infected at substantially increased risk for cervical cancer) HPV infections along with limited access to cervical cancer screening have led to the large burden of the disease in SSA.

Although ART has not been shown to hasten the regression of cervical neoplasia or the clearance of HR HPV infection, improved immune function as a result of ART does decrease the risk of all HR HPV-related diseases. For example, in the pre-ART era, the observed increase in risk of cervical cancer among women living with human immunodeficiency viruses (WLWH) was approximately 4–8 times compared to the post-ART era where the risk is somewhat lower, as described above.[151,152] In addition, in areas of high cervical cancer incidence, such as SSA, women living with HIV have significantly higher rates of cervical cancer, with a standardized incidence ratio of 2.4, compared to HIV-negative women.

Studies conducted in both the pre-ART era and the ART era have found that WLWH have been shown to have more difficulty clearing HR HPV infections[153] and they are more likely than HIV-negative women to develop dysplasia and eventually cancer.[154,155] Furthermore, studies have shown that WLWH are more likely to have persistent HPV infection,[156,157] and larger, multifocal cervical intraepithelial lesions.[158] Of note, a study conducted by the women's interagency human immunodeficiency viruses cohort study (WIHS) highlighted the importance of cervical cytology cancer screening in WLWH in which cytologic exams were conducted every 6 months for a median follow-up of 10 years. They found that WLWH had a slightly increased risk for invasive cervical cancer (21.4 of 100,000 person-years), but not significantly increased compared to HIV-negative women (0 of 100,000 person-years, $p=0.59$).[153] Although the current specific CDC guidelines for screening WLWH is beyond the scope of this chapter, in general, the screening methodology is similar to HIV-negative women. In WLWH under age 30, cervical cytology is the primary form of screening and should occur within 1 year of sexual debut, but not after age 21. Women diagnosed with HIV between ages 21–29, should have cervical cytology within 1 year of their presentation to care with subsequent cervical cytology follow-up between 6 and 12 months. After three consecutive negative results on cervical cytology, cervical cytology can occur every 3 years. Women over the age of 30 can undergo testing with 6 month to yearly cytology alone or "co-testing" (screening with both HR HPV and cytology). If both HR HPV and cytology are negative, women can be re-screened in 3 years. If the HR HPV testing is positive, the subsequent follow-up is dependent on the types of HR HPV detected. Because the vast majority of advanced cervical intraepithelial neoplasia (CIN 2+) and invasive cancers are associated with HPV-16 or -18; if either are detected, those women are referred immediately for colposcopy.[159] For LMICs with no established national cervical cancer screening program, the World Health Organization has supported a "see-and-treat" approach with visual inspection of the cervix with acetic acid (VIA) to triage women to immediate treatment with cryotherapy without additional procedures such as colposcopy and biopsy.[160] In addition, HPV testing has been shown to have high sensitivity with lower specificity for the detection of cervical CIN2+ for WLWH. Studies among WLWH conducted in Zambia, South Africa, and Tanzania demonstrated that HR HPV testing had sensitivity ranging from 88% to 94% and with specificity ranging from 51% to 82%.[161,162]

The recommendations for treatment of CIN 2+ lesions do not differ for WLWH, although recurrence rates are high in this population, particularly among those with low CD4 counts and larger CIN lesions.[163] In high-income countries, the standard of care for treatment of CIN 2+ is a loop electrosurgical excision procedure (LEEP), which is an excisional procedure that needs to be administered by trained practitioners. Although cryotherapy, another ablative treatment option, is frequently used in LMICs because it is low cost and can be performed in primary care centers, a recent single institution randomized trial of 400 WLWH (200 in LEEP and 200 in cryotherapy arms) in Kenya, found a lower recurrence rate (relative risk 1.71, $p < 0.01$) for the LEEP arm compared to the cryotherapy arm.[164] In addition, the LEEP arm had slightly lower numbers of adverse events compared to the cryotherapy arm (30 vs 40, respectively). Furthermore, management of WLWH requires special precautions when using a VIA-based screen and treat model because these women are at higher risk for large lesions that are not eligible for treatment and invasive cancer.

Although cancer staging and treatment guidelines are similar for WLWH compared to HIV-negative women, there are certain nuances that clinicians need to consider. For similar reasons that PET/CT scans among HIV-positive lymphoma patients have reported high false positive rates and decreased accuracy for patients with higher HIV RNA detected in the plasma, PET/CT scans used for radiotherapy planning for WLWH and cervical cancer may be less predictive than for HIV-negative women.[165] A recent systematic review found that treatment response rates and survival with standard chemotherapy and radiation comparing WLWH and HIV-negative women are similar in the majority of studies. In addition, overall toxicity was found to be similar in three studies that specifically evaluated treatment toxicities.[166] However, one retrospective case-control study conducted in Brazil found that although WLWH and HIV-negative women demonstrated similar response rates after chemotherapy and radiation therapy, WLWH were more likely to have relapses at 2 years of follow-up as well as late cancer-specific and overall mortality compared to HIV-negative women.[36] The recent breakthrough of immunotherapy for the treatment of multiple cancer types suggests that the immune system is increasingly important in tumor control,[167] and radiotherapy may have both positive and negative effects (especially when combined with protease inhibitors).[168] Chronic HIV infection may complicate the immune response to chemotherapy and radiation, which could explain differences in long-term outcomes in WLWH compared to HIV-negative women. Of note, radiation therapy is only available in 28 of 54 African countries. Thus, in geographic locations without access to radiation therapy, both WLWH and HIV-negative women with locally advanced cervical cancer (LACC) are most frequently treated with neoadjuvant chemotherapy followed by radical hysterectomy. This approach has been associated with decreased 5-year DFS (69.3% vs 76.7%), but similar overall 5-year survival (75.4% vs 74.7%) compared to chemotherapy and radiotherapy for LACC in HIV-negative women.[114]

Non-AIDS-defining cancers

Anal cancer

Approximately 1% of women and 28% of men with anal cancer are HIV-infected.[169] Tumor size (T stage) and nodal status (N stage) are the most significant prognostic factors for patients with anal cancer. In a large series of 270 patients, the 5-year survival by stage was 86% for those with T1-2 disease versus less than 60% for T3-4 disease, and 76% for those with N0 disease versus 54% for those with node-positive disease.[170] In RTOG 98-11, tumor diameter >5 cm was associated with poorer 5-year DFS (72% vs 50%, $p=0.0003$; adjusted HR = 1.51, $p=0.0012$) and poorer 5-year OS (82% vs 57%, $p=0.0031$; adjusted HR = 1.39, $p=0.022$) when compared to tumor diameter 2–5 cm. Positive nodal involvement was associated with poorer 5-year DFS (61% vs 31%, $p = <0.0001$; adjusted HR = 1.82, $p = <0.001$) and poorer 5-year OS (74% vs 42%, $p = <0.0001$; adjusted HR = 1.88, $p = <0.001$) in the multivariate analysis.[171] In stratified analyses, positive nodal status had more adverse influence on DFS and OS than did tumor diameter. Patients with >5 cm tumor and positive nodal status had the worst DFS (only 30% at 3 years compared to 74% for the best group; <5 cm primary and N0) and OS (only 48% at 4 years compared to 81% for the best group; <5 cm primary and N0). Men had worse DFS (adjusted HR = 1.27, $p=0.0012$) and OS (adjusted HR = 1.38, $p=0.031$).

HIV-infected patients were excluded from these major trials on anal cancer. When CRT in standard doses of mitomycin or cisplatin with fluorouracil was first applied to HIV-infected patients in the pre-ART era, increased toxicity, requiring treatment breaks or dose reductions, and poorer clinical outcome were reported.[172,173] In five studies that included 53 HIV-infected patients, the incidence of grade 3–4 skin toxicity was 50–78%.[172–176] Pre-treatment CD4 count <200 was identified as a factor associated with poorer anal cancer control and increased treatment morbidity in a small retrospective cohort.[175] In the modern ART era, immune restoration with effective suppression of HIV viral load and elevation in CD4 count could be achieved in most HIV-infected patients, with improvement in therapy compliance and reduction in treatment-related side effects. Some studies show that HIV-infected patients had comparable disease control and survival to HIV-negative patients,[177–183] whereas others suggested that HIV-positive patients may do worse in terms of enhanced treatment-related toxicity and/or an increased risk for local relapse.[184–188] Wexler et al. reported the local failure rate was only 16% in their cohort, but 44% of patients had T1N0 disease,[181] which could reflect the fact that many of the referring providers are experienced in caring for HIV-infected individuals and more likely to examine patients for high-grade squamous intraepithelial lesions (HSIL) and anal cancer. Martin et al. reported their single-center experience with standard 5-FU/mitomycin CRT with long-term follow-up. Despite HIV-infected patients having higher nodal stages, the CR rates after CRT were higher than 80% in both HIV-infected and HIV-uninfected patients.[182] In contrast, one of the largest series of anal cancer patients (total = 107, HIV-infected and HIV-uninfected) showed that HIV-infected patients had significantly worse OS and colostomy free-survival compared with a similar cohort of HIV-negative patients, despite having a similar treatment approach, patient adherence and cancer stage.[188] There were also no differences in radiation-related acute toxicity based on HIV status. There are no clear explanations for the differences, or lack of differences, in the outcomes of anal cancer in HIV-infected versus HIV-negative populations. Almost all of these reports are limited by small patient numbers and the retrospective nature of the data.

Despite the effectiveness of CRT in primary treatment of anal cancer, the locoregional failure rate has been reported as 10–30%.[189,190] There are 10–20% of anal cancers that present with extra-pelvic disease at initial diagnosis,[191] and 25% of cases develop distant metastases.[192] For recurrent or metastatic anal cancer, treatment options are quite limited. Patients with biopsy-proven local recurrence of anal cancer can be treated with abdominoperineal resection and colostomy.[189] A small single-arm study of 19 patients showed cisplatin and 5-FU had a response rate of 66% for metastatic anal cancer.[193]

Lung cancer

Lung cancer is the leading cause of cancer mortality in the United States, and it has emerged as the leading non-acquired immunodeficiency syndrome-defining cancer (NADC) and is the most frequent cause of cancer deaths in HIV-infected persons.[122] The increased incidence of lung cancer in this population is believed to be mainly due to the higher rates of smoking, but other mechanisms may exist and are an area of active investigation. Prognosis of HIV-infected persons who develop lung cancer has been shown to be worse than uninfected persons in several studies, but it is not known if this is related to treatment disparities, lung cancer therapy intolerance, greater risk of treatment toxicity, or competing risks from AIDS and non-AIDS-related morbidity. Lung cancer prevention and early detection is also an emerging area of study for HIV-infected persons.

Early studies noted that a low CD4 count was associated with increased lung cancer incidence.[194] Inflammation, both locally in the lung and systemically, has also been investigated as a contributor to the increased lung cancer risk in PLWH. Preceding pneumonia (even when it occurred 5 years earlier) was an independent predictor of lung cancer.[195] HIV and smoking may have synergistic effects promoting lung inflammation, but this has not been linked to lung cancer risk.[196] Proinflammatory cytokines have also been found to be elevated prior to lung cancer diagnosis in HIV-infected persons.[197]

The effects of HIV infection on the tolerability, toxicity and effectiveness of lung cancer treatment are not well-known. A large ART-era analysis from the Veterans Affairs Health System found that HIV-infected patients had a postoperative mortality rate approximately twice that of uninfected individuals, and among patients with HIV infection, a CD4 cell count of $< 50/\mu L$ was associated with a substantially higher rate of mortality. However, this study did not include many patients who underwent lung cancer surgery.[198] An Italian study described lung cancer treatments in HIV-infected patients ($n = 68$) and found an expected frequency of major complications, but commented that HIV-infected patients received fewer cycles of chemotherapy than indicated.[199] In a cohort of patients at Kaiser Permanente California diagnosed with cancer from 1996 to 2011, those with HIV infection were less likely to receive treatment for lung cancer than HIV-uninfected patients (64% vs 76%, respectively).[21] The causes of these disparities remain unclear. Future research should further address lung cancer risk in this population, as well as identify and optimize effective prevention and treatment methods.

Hepatocellular carcinoma (HCC)

Over the last decade, HCC prevalence has increased among PLWH. In a US Veteran's Administration cohort of 24,000 individuals with HIV infection, the prevalence of HCC increased dramatically from 0.07% to 1.62% between 1996 and 2009 while the prevalence of HCC was much lower and remained stable in patients without hepatitis C virus (HCV) coinfection.[200] The epidemiology of cirrhosis and HCC in PLWH is dominated by the epidemiology of chronic HCV infection. The majority of persons with HCV in the United States were infected between 1965 and 1990, before availability of serological testing for HCV.[201] Because HCV infection takes an average of 30–40 years to cause cirrhosis or HCC, the patients infected between 1965 and 1990 would be expected to develop cirrhosis and HCC between 1995 and 2030. These epidemiologic features of HCV in the United States, together with the decline in competing AIDS-related mortality, largely explain the rise of HCC among HIV/HCV-coinfected patients. Interestingly, control of HIV replication does not appear to substantially reduce risk of HCC development.[202]

Prostate cancer

The relationship between HIV and prostate cancer is unclear. Studies have shown either no association,[203] increased[204] or decreased[205,206] incidence of prostate cancer in HIV-infected men. Since hypogonadism is relatively common among PLWH,[207] it would seem to support a lower incidence of prostate cancer. Hessol et al. found no statistically significant difference in prostate cancer mortality between people with AIDS and the general population, with a standardized mortality rate of 1.14 (95% CI: 0.52–1.75).[208] However, in a separate analysis from the SEER-Medicare database, HIV-infected men with prostate cancer were significantly more likely to experience relapse or death (HR, 1.32; 95% CI, 1.03–1.71; $p = 0.03$), and more likely to experience relapse or cancer-specific death (HR, 1.28; 95% CI, 0.92–1.78; $p = 0.15$) when compared

Table 4 Antiretroviral drug interaction resources.[a]

Resource	Website	Source
AIDSinfo	www.aidsinfo.nih.gov	U.S. Department of Health and Human Services (DHHS)
AIDSMeds	aidsmeds.com/	HIV+ patients and physicians
Clinical care options	clinicalcareoptions.com/	Clinical care options
FDA MedWatch	https://www.fda.gov/safety/medwatch-fda-safety-information-and-adverse-event-reporting-program	U.S. Food and Drug Administration (FDA)
HIV InSite	www.hivinsite.com	University of California San Francisco
HIVMA	www.hivma.org	HIV Medical Association
HIV medication guide	www.hivmedicationguide.com	J. Antony Gagnon, Pharm.D., B.Pharm., D.P.H., CDE, CAE and Rachel Therrien, Pharm., D.P.H.,MSC
Johns Hopkins POC IT Center: HIV Guide	www.hopkins-hivguide.org	Johns Hopkins University
The Internet's H1V/AIDS Oral Healthcare Resource	www.HIVdent.org	US nonprofit dentists, nurses, pharmacists
Medscape	www.medscape.com	WebMD Health Professional Network
Toronto General Hospital Immunodeficiency Clinic	www.tthhivclinic.com/	Toronto General Hospital
University of Liverpool HIV Drug Interactions Website	www.hiv-druginteractions.org	University of Liverpool HIV Pharmacology Group

[a]Source: Based on Rudek et al.[215]

with HIV-uninfected patients.[34] As the HIV population continues to age, the association of HIV infection with poor prostate cancer outcomes will become increasingly relevant, especially because prostate cancer is projected to become the most common malignant neoplasm in the HIV population in the United States by 2030.[16] Research on clinical strategies to improve outcomes in HIV-infected patients with cancer is warranted.

Breast cancer

There is a growing population of older women living with HIV. Among 16 million HIV-infected women aged 15+ years, an estimated 6325 were diagnosed with breast cancer in 2012, 74% of whom were in SSA. Among all breast cancers, HIV-infected women constituted less than 1% of the clinical burden, except in Eastern, Western and Middle Africa, where they comprised 4–6% of breast cancer patients under age 50, and in Southern Africa where this patient subgroup constituted 26% and 8% of breast cancers diagnosed under and over age 50, respectively.[209] Since these numbers are expected to increase in the next decade, early detection and treatment research targeted to this population is needed.

While there are no reliable data about the role of HIV infection on the risk or stage of breast cancer at presentation, more side effects seem to occur during the treatment of breast cancer in HIV-infected women. Hurley et al. found that chemotherapy was poorly tolerated in patients with HIV, suggesting that HIV/AIDS and ART may negatively affect chemotherapy tolerability with a greater degree of lymphocytopenia and neutropenia.[210] Parameswaran et al.[211] similarly reported that 56% of patients with HIV and breast cancer in New York required a dose reduction in chemotherapy, compared with 30% of uninfected patients.

General management issues

HIV-infected cancer patients require careful coordination of care between their HIV care provider and their oncologist. Typically, patients' ART is continued through their cancer therapy, although modifications may be needed. In general, patients with CD4 counts >200/μL are at low risk of AIDS-related complications, and their malignancy should be managed similarly to HIV-uninfected patients. In patients with CD4 ≤ 200/μL, there is a higher risk of treatment-related and opportunistic complications, as well as treatment-related mortality.[99] However, this high-risk group is not a homogenous population, and their risk assessment should include HIV viral load, sensitivity of the virus to available antiretroviral drugs and prior history of AIDS-related complications.

Drug–drug interactions

An effective antiretroviral regimen for treatment-naive patients generally consists of two nucleoside reverse transcriptase inhibitors (NRTI) combined with a third active antiretroviral drug from one of three drug classes: an integrase strand transfer inhibitor (ISTI), a non-nucleoside reverse transcriptase inhibitor (NNRTI), or a protease inhibitor (PI) with a pharmacokinetic enhancer (cobicistat or ritonavir).[212] The guideline-recommended NRTI combinations of emtricitabine and tenofovir (Truvada) or abacavir and lamivudine (Epzicom) are equally effective and likely to have minimal clinically relevant adverse effects on cancer therapy.[213] NNRTI is no longer favored due to the increased risk of transmitted resistance.[214] Ritonavir is a potent inhibitor of CYP3A4 and may have different effects on other CYP or UGT metabolizing enzymes and drug transporters. For more details on drug–drug interactions between common ART and chemotherapy, refer to Table 4 for updated resources. By comparison, ISTI has minimal drug–drug interactions, as it has little ability to alter drug-metabolizing enzymes.[216,217] At this time, ISTI-based regimens are the favored ART for HIV-infected patients with cancer that require chemotherapy.

Immunotherapy

Immunotherapy has changed the management of multiple types of malignancies with proven efficacy and a good safety profile in the majority of patients. However, people living with HIV have been excluded from almost all clinical trials of immune CPIs. This is due to many concerns, including unknown effects of immunotherapy on the T-cell repertoire, interactions with antiretroviral agents and the possibility of unmasking opportunistic infections. Additionally, it has been hypothesized that HIV-infected patients may not have sufficient T-cell immunity to benefit from PD-1 or PD-L1 blockade.[218]

Despite immune dysfunction due to HIV, cancer in HIV-infected individuals is often responsive to immunotherapy. Case reports and retrospective cohort studies from the United States and Europe have described an acceptable safety profile with the use of nivolumab, pembrolizumab and ipilimumab in HIV-infected patients, with reported tumor responses in cHL, melanoma and lung cancer.[219-221] A systematic review of CPIs in PLWH noted overall response and adverse event rates that were similar to the general population. In the subset of patients in whom viral load was measured, HIV remained suppressed in 93% of participants, and CD4 counts increased modestly. Notably, CPI use in KS was associated with an ORR of 63%.[222] A prospective phase I study of pembrolizumab in PLWH with a CD4 count ≥100/μL and advanced cancer demonstrated evidence of safety and activity in KS, NHL, lung cancer, and liver cancer.[218]

As people living with HIV are living longer, cancer has become a major cause of morbidity and mortality. Given the persistent immune abnormalities despite ART and the implications for cancer risk, immunotherapy may have a dual benefit by acting both on cancer cells and on HIV reservoir. In order to advance our understanding, PLWH must be included in immuno-oncology studies.

Key references

The complete reference list can be found on Vital Source version of this title, see inside front cover.

4. Krewski D, Bird M, Al-Zoughool M, et al. Key characteristics of 86 agents known to cause cancer in humans. *J Toxicol Environ Health B*. 2019;**22**(7–8):244–263.
5. Grulich AE, van Leeuwen MT, Falster MO, Vajdic CM. Incidence of cancers in people with HIV/AIDS compared with immunosuppressed transplant recipients: a meta-analysis. *Lancet*. 2007;**370**(9581):59–67.
7. Silverberg MJ, Lau B, Achenbach CJ, et al. Cumulative incidence of cancer among persons with HIV in North America: a cohort study. *Ann Intern Med*. 2015;**163**(7):507–518.
8. Yarchoan R, Uldrick TS. HIV-associated cancers and related diseases. *N Engl J Med*. 2018;**378**(22):2145.
9. Hernández-Ramírez RU, Shiels MS, Dubrow R, Engels EA. Cancer risk in HIV-infected people in the USA from 1996 to 2012: a population-based, registry-linkage study. *The lancet HIV*. 2017;**4**(11):e495–e504.
10. Hernandez-Ramirez RU, Shiels MS, Dubrow R, Engels EA. Cancer risk in HIV-infected people in the USA from 1996 to 2012: a population-based, registry-linkage study. *Lancet HIV*. 2017;**4**(11):e495–e504.
11. Thrift AP, Kramer JR, Hartman CM, et al. Risk and predictors of esophageal and stomach cancers in HIV-infected veterans: a matched cohort study. *J Acquir Immune Defic Syndr*. 2019;**81**(3):e65–e72.
13. World Health Organization. *Global Health Observatory (GHO) Data*, 2019; https://www.who.int/gho/hiv/en (accessed 21 July 2019).
14. HIV Surveillance Supplemental Report. Estimated HIV incidence and prevalence in the United States 2014–2018. Volume 25(1), 2020; https://www.cdc.gov/hiv/pdf/library/reports/surveillance/cdc-hiv-surveillance-supplemental-report-vol-25-1.pdf (accessed 1 August 2020).
15. Hall HI, An Q, Tang T, et al. Prevalence of diagnosed and undiagnosed HIV infection—United States, 2008–2012. *MMWR Morb Mortal Wkly Rep*. 2015;**64**(24):657–662.
16. Shiels MS, Islam JY, Rosenberg PS, et al. Projected cancer incidence rates and burden of incident cancer cases in HIV-infected adults in the united states through 2030. *Ann Intern Med*. 2018;**168**(12):866–873.
18. Smith CJ, Ryom L, Weber R, et al. Trends in underlying causes of death in people with HIV from 1999 to 2011 (D:A:D): a multicohort collaboration. *Lancet*. 2014;**384**(9939):241–248.
20. Kong CY, Sigel K, Criss SD, et al. Benefits and harms of lung cancer screening in HIV-infected individuals with CD4+ cell count at least 500 cells/mul. *AIDS*. 2018;**32**(10):1333–1342.
21. Marcus JL, Chao C, Leyden WA, et al. Survival among HIV-infected and HIV-uninfected individuals with common non-AIDS-defining cancers. *Cancer Epidemiol Biomark Prev*. 2015;**24**(8):1167–1173.
24. Coghill AE, Pfeiffer RM, Shiels MS, Engels EA. Excess mortality among HIV-infected individuals with cancer in the United States. *Cancer Epidemiol Biomark Prev*. 2017;**26**(7):1027–1033.
31. Suneja G, Shiels MS, Angulo R, et al. Cancer treatment disparities in HIV-infected individuals in the United States. *J Clin Oncol*. 2014;**32**(22):2344–2350.
33. Suneja G, Boyer M, Yehia BR, et al. Cancer treatment in patients with HIV infection and non-AIDS-defining cancers: a survey of US oncologists. *J Oncol Pract*. 2015;**11**(3):e380–e387.
34. Coghill AE, Suneja G, Rositch AF, et al. HIV infection, cancer treatment regimens, and cancer outcomes among elderly adults in the United States. *JAMA Oncol*. 2019;**5**(9):e191742.
35. Reid E, Suneja G, Ambinder RF, et al. Cancer in people living with HIV, version 1.2018, NCCN clinical practice guidelines in oncology. *J Natl Compr Cancer Netw*. 2018;**16**(8):986–1017.
36. Ferreira MP, Coghill AE, Chaves CB, et al. Outcomes of cervical cancer among HIV-infected and HIV-uninfected women treated at the Brazilian National Institute of Cancer. *AIDS*. 2017;**31**(4):523–531.
37. Calkins KL, Chander G, Joshu CE, et al. Immune status and associated mortality after cancer treatment among individuals with HIV in the antiretroviral therapy era. *JAMA Oncol*. 2019;**6**(2):227–235.
38. Uldrick TS, Ison G, Rudek MA, et al. Modernizing clinical trial eligibility criteria: recommendations of the american society of clinical oncology-friends of cancer research HIV working group. *J Clin Oncol*. 2017;**35**(33):3774–3780.
46. Chang Y, Cesarman E, Pessin MS, et al. Identification of herpesvirus-like DNA sequences in AIDS-associated Kaposi's sarcoma. *Science*. 1994;**266**(5192):1865–1869.
49. Newton R, Labo N, Wakeham K, et al. Determinants of gammaherpesvirus shedding in saliva among Ugandan children and their mothers. *J Infect Dis*. 2018;**218**(6):892–900.
52. White DL, Oluyomi A, Royse K, et al. Incidence of AIDS-related Kaposi sarcoma in all 50 United States From 2000 to 2014. *J Acquir Immune Defic Syndr*. 2019;**81**(4):387–394.
53. Dittmer DP, Damania B. Kaposi sarcoma-associated herpesvirus: immunobiology, oncogenesis, and therapy. *J Clin Invest*. 2016;**126**(9):3165–3175.
55. Gruffaz M, Vasan K, Tan B, et al. TLR4-mediated inflammation promotes KSHV-induced cellular transformation and tumorigenesis by activating the STAT3 pathway. *Cancer Res*. 2017;**77**(24):7094–7108.
59. Sanders CJ, Canninga-van Dijk MR, Borleffs JC. Kaposi's sarcoma. *Lancet*. 2004;**364**(9444):1549–1552.
60. Schneider JW, Dittmer DP. Diagnosis and treatment of Kaposi sarcoma. *Am J Clin Dermatol*. 2017;**18**(4):529–539.
61. Hengge UR, Ruzicka T, Tyring SK, et al. Update on Kaposi's sarcoma and other HHV8 associated diseases. Part 1: epidemiology, environmental predispositions, clinical manifestations, and therapy. *Lancet Infect Dis*. 2002;**2**(5):281–292.
65. Gonçalves PH, Uldrick TS, Yarchoan R. HIV-associated Kaposi sarcoma and related diseases. *AIDS*. 2017;**31**(14):1903–1916.
68. Sgadari C, Monini P, Barillari G, Ensoli B. Use of HIV protease inhibitors to block Kaposi's sarcoma and tumour growth. *Lancet Oncol*. 2003;**4**(9):537–547.
74. Polizzotto MN, Uldrick TS, Wyvill KM, et al. Clinical features and outcomes of patients with symptomatic kaposi sarcoma herpesvirus (KSHV)-associated Inflammation: prospective characterization of KSHV inflammatory cytokine syndrome (KICS). *Clin Infect Dis*. 2016;**62**(6):730–738.
76. Krown SE, Moser CB, MacPhail P, et al. Treatment of advanced AIDS-associated Kaposi sarcoma in resource-limited settings: a three-arm, open-label, randomised non-inferiority trial. *Lancet*. 2020;**395**(10231):1195–1207.
84. Polizzotto MN, Uldrick TS, Wyvill KM, et al. Pomalidomide for symptomatic Kaposi's sarcoma in people with and without HIV infection: a phase I/II study. *J Clin Oncol*. 2016;**34**(34):4125–4131.
85. Bender Ignacio RA, Lin LL, Rajdev L, Chiao E. Evolving paradigms in HIV malignancies: review of ongoing clinical trials. *J Natl Compr Cancer Netw*. 2018;**16**(8):1018–1026.
95. Pfreundschuh M, Trumper L, Osterborg A, et al. CHOP-like chemotherapy plus rituximab versus CHOP-like chemotherapy alone in young patients with good-prognosis diffuse large-B-cell lymphoma: a randomised controlled trial by the MabThera International Trial (MInT) Group. *Lancet Oncol*. 2006;**7**(5):379–391.
98. Bartlett NL, Wilson WH, Jung SH, et al. Dose-adjusted EPOCH-R compared with R-CHOP as frontline therapy for diffuse large B-cell lymphoma: clinical outcomes of the phase III intergroup trial alliance/CALGB 50303. *J Clin Oncol*. 2019;**37**(21):1790–1799.
150. Bray F, Ferlay J, Soerjomataram I, et al. Global cancer statistics 2018: GLOBOCAN estimates of incidence and mortality worldwide for 36 cancers in 185 countries. *CA Cancer J Clin*. 2018;**68**(6):394–424.
155. Clark E, Chen L, Dong Y, et al. Veteran women living with HIV have increased risk of HPV-associated genital tract cancers. *Clin Infect Dis*. 2020;**72**(9):e359–e366.
158. Ghebre RG, Grover S, Xu MJ, et al. Cervical cancer control in HIV-infected women: past, present and future. *Gynecol Oncol Rep*. 2017;**21**:101–108.
159. Panel on Antiretroviral Guidelines for Adults and Adolescents. Guidelines for the Use of Antiretroviral Agents in Adults and Adolescents with HIV. Department of Health and Human Services. Available at https://clinicalinfo.hiv.gov/sites/default/files/guidelines/documents/AdultandAdolescentGL.pdf. (accessed 10 October 2020).

161. Chibwesha CJ, Frett B, Katundu K, et al. Clinical performance validation of 4 point-of-care cervical cancer screening tests in HIV-infected women in Zambia. *Journal of Lower Genital Tract Disease*. 2016;**20**(3):218–223.
164. Greene SA, De Vuyst H, John-Stewart GC, et al. Effect of cryotherapy vs loop electrosurgical excision procedure on cervical disease recurrence among women with HIV and high-grade cervical lesions in Kenya: a randomized clinical trial. *JAMA*. 2019;**322**(16):1570–1579.
166. Shah S, Xu M, Mehta P, et al. Differences in outcomes of chemoradiation in women with invasive cervical cancer by human immunodeficiency virus status: a systematic review. *Pract Radiat Oncol*. 2020;**11**(1):53–65.
168. Rengan R, Mick R, Pryma DA, et al. Clinical outcomes of the HIV protease inhibitor nelfinavir with concurrent chemoradiotherapy for unresectable stage IIIA/IIIB non-small cell lung cancer: a phase 1/2 trial. *JAMA Oncol*. 2019;**5**(10):1464–1472.
182. Martin D, Balermpas P, Fokas E, et al. Are there HIV-specific differences for anal cancer patients treated with standard chemoradiotherapy in the era of combined antiretroviral therapy? *Clin Oncol (R Coll Radiol)*. 2017;**29**(4):248–255.
183. Sparano JA, Lee JY, Palefsky J, et al. Cetuximab plus chemoradiotherapy for HIV-associated anal carcinoma: a phase II AIDS malignancy consortium trial. *J Clin Oncol*. 2017;**35**(7):727–733.
196. Sigel K, Makinson A, Thaler J. Lung cancer in persons with HIV. *Curr Opin HIV AIDS*. 2017;**12**(1):31–38.
202. Park LS, Tate JP, Sigel K, et al. Association of viral suppression with lower AIDS-defining and non-AIDS-defining cancer incidence in HIV-infected veterans: a prospective cohort study. *Ann Intern Med*. 2018;**169**(2):87–96.
203. Godbole SV, Nandy K, Gauniyal M, et al. HIV and cancer registry linkage identifies a substantial burden of cancers in persons with HIV in India. *Medicine (Baltimore)*. 2016;**95**(37):e4850.
206. Sun D, Cao M, Li H, et al. Risk of prostate cancer in men with HIV/AIDS: a systematic review and meta-analysis. *Prostate Cancer Prostatic Dis*. 2020;**24**:24–34.
208. Hessol NA, Ma D, Scheer S, et al. Changing temporal trends in non-AIDS cancer mortality among people diagnosed with AIDS: San Francisco, California, 1996–2013. *Cancer Epidemiol*. 2018;**52**:20–27.
209. McCormack VA, Febvey-Combes O, Ginsburg O, Dos-Santos-Silva I. Breast cancer in women living with HIV: a first global estimate. *Int J Cancer*. 2018;**143**(11):2732–2740.
215. Rudek MA, Flexner C, Ambinder RF. Use of antineoplastic agents in patients with cancer who have HIV/AIDS. *Lancet Oncol*. 2011;**12**(9):905–912.
218. Uldrick TS, Goncalves PH, Abdul-Hay M, et al. Assessment of the safety of pembrolizumab in patients with HIV and advanced cancer-A phase 1 study. *JAMA Oncol*. 2019;**5**(9):1332–1339.
219. Chang E, Sabichi AL, Kramer JR, et al. Nivolumab treatment for cancers in the HIV-infected population. *J Immunother*. 2018;**41**(8):379–383.
220. Spano JP, Veyri M, Gobert A, et al. Immunotherapy for cancer in people living with HIV: safety with an efficacy signal from the series in real life experience. *AIDS*. 2019;**33**(11):F13–F19.
221. Tio M, Rai R, Ezeoke OM, et al. Anti-PD-1/PD-L1 immunotherapy in patients with solid organ transplant, HIV or hepatitis B/C infection. *Eur J Cancer*. 2018;**104**:137–144.
222. Cook MR, Kim C. Safety and efficacy of immune checkpoint inhibitor therapy in patients with HIV infection and advanced-stage cancer: a systematic review. *JAMA Oncol*. 2019;**5**(7):1049–1054.

72 Cancer survivorship
Lewis Foxhall, MD

> **Overview**
>
> Continued advances in early detection and treatment as well as an increased proportion of older individuals in the United States have supported an ever-expanding population of cancer survivors. Many live decades after completing treatment but with relatively frequent occurrence of persistent or late-occurring side effects of treatment that may impinge on quality of life. The occurrence of second cancers and an increasing prevalence of comorbid conditions with aging, psychosocial problems, and opportunities for general health improvement warrant careful attention by clinicians. This article examines the growing awareness of the common challenges faced by survivors and highlights recommended strategies for management of these conditions. Consideration of health-system-related barriers to optimum care will focus on potential improvements in practice, potentially offering improvements in quality of care for cancer survivors.

adult-onset cancer. A wide range of approaches to addressing the various components of survivorship care are used in settings ranging from comprehensive cancer centers to individual community oncology practices and primary care. Research has provided insights into pathways to improve care of survivors but evidence remains limited as to the best approach. While progress has been made in improving management of cancer survivors, many needs remain unmet. Fragmentation of the US health care system and lack of a clear delineation of roles and coordination among those caring for survivors continues to create missed opportunities, duplication of effort, and less than optimal outcomes. Information technology infrastructure supporting survivorship care is limited and quality measures need further assessment and refinement. There is, however, agreement on the potential benefits of improving care for this population and multiple innovative models are being used to enhance delivery of high quality, patient-centered, comprehensive survivorship care.

Introduction

The population of US cancer survivors is approaching 17 million and is projected to exceed 22 million over the next decade, driven by improvements in cancer treatment, screening, and early detection as well as demographic changes.[1] However, documentation of outcomes and generalized application of best practices in the management of this potentially vulnerable population remains a promising though challenging goal.

The term "cancer survivor" is intended to apply to individuals initially diagnosed with cancer and through the balance of life. This broadly encompasses those involved in the cancer journey, extending to family and caregivers, and has been used to provide encouragement by drawing a distinction with the term cancer victim. It further highlights survivorship as a phase of the cancer care continuum. While not universally embraced, this definition (developed by the National Coalition of Cancer Survivors) is broadly accepted by many cancer patients, families, and caregivers as well as by major organizations. The potential benefits of focusing on the care of these individuals include the opportunity to maximize the positive outcomes of the commonly challenging treatment they received and provide the best opportunity to optimize duration, function, and quality of life.

Much of the work related to improving care for those diagnosed as adults was predated by the research and implementation of strategies related to childhood cancer survivors, captured in *The Children's Oncology Group Long-Term Follow-Up Guidelines for Survivors of Childhood, Adolescent and Young Adult Cancers*.[2] These guidelines were critical in guiding work with the pediatric population and have served a formative role in developing recommendations for care of adult-onset cancer survivors. Discussion in this article primarily concerns management of individuals with

Raising awareness of cancer survivorship

The expansion of cancer survivorship programs in cancer centers and community settings has helped bring attention to the distinct needs of cancer survivors. The dissemination of professional and public education efforts improves engagement of clinicians and survivors themselves, though knowledge and implementation of recommended approaches in survivorship management remain at a much lower level than that related to treatment phases of care. Population-based surveys have identified an array of issues that may affect survivor's health and quality of life, including information needs in areas such as persistent side effects and symptoms related to treatment or the cancer itself, follow-up testing, wellness and health promotion, interpersonal and emotional challenges, financial and insurance problems, as well as sexual functioning and fertility. Common physical problems including fatigue, lymphedema, neuropathy, cardiac dysfunction, and others discussed below, also occur. These vary significantly by the treatment received and the type of cancer being treated and the comorbid conditions present.[3-5]

Background

In a 1985 essay, Dr. Fitzhugh Mullan shared his perspective as a young physician on the experience of being treated for and surviving cancer.[6] This essay has been cited as a cornerstone for the development of current thinking related to what is now considered a distinct phase of the cancer continuum. Dr. Mullan went on to collaborate with a small group of like-minded individuals to refine the concept of extended care for individuals with cancer including a focus on the time after completion of treatment now termed "survivorship." This collaborative became the National Coalition of Cancer Survivors and offered the following definition of cancer survivorship: an individual is considered a cancer survivor from the time of cancer diagnosis, through the balance of his or her life. The definition was intended to replace the term "cancer victim" and be empowering to individuals diagnosed with cancer whether they are still living with cancer or are considered to have no evidence of disease. This is said to be a definition and not a label that is intended to help clarify the distinct challenges and opportunities related to care beyond treatment for the various types of cancer.[7,8] Other definitions of cancer survivorship have been offered by various authors and the American Cancer Society (ACS) that focus on the content of survivorship management as well as the period of time after completion of treatment.[9]

Dr. Mullan described three phases of the cancer journey starting with "acute survival," which dealt with the diagnosis and treatment period along with care directed to the immediate complications of treatment. The next phase, "extended survival," involved the period after completion of treatment and the onset of "remission" with no apparent evidence of disease but including the protracted recovery from the effects of treatment and the cancer itself. This included significant psychological and social impacts to the patient and caregivers. The third phase, "permanent survival," dealt with the persistent impacts of the cancer experience. This phase included significant psychological and social impacts to both the patient and caregivers. The framing of his firsthand experience serves as an insightful, self-reported case study that significantly influenced the development of the formative period of the field of cancer survivorship over the ensuing three decades. Dr. Mullan died in November of 2019 at 77, having served a distinguished career that helped launch the cancer survivorship movement, and focused on improving health equity and social challenges in medical care and medical education.

The evolution of the current concepts of cancer survivorship care included significant research contributions led by the National Cancer Institute (NCI) Office of Cancer Survivorship, established in 1995, and its founding director Dr. Julia Roland. The cancer survivor population is heterogeneous and there has been a growing awareness by the public, health professionals, and policy leaders of the distinct needs and challenges they face. These challenges include potential for progression of persistent disease or recurrence of the original cancer, development of additional cancers, ongoing or late-occurring complications of treatment or the cancer itself, as well as issues related to comorbid conditions especially in older survivors. Further challenges include, at times, serious psychological conditions and social or financial issues related to treatment or difficulty returning to precancer employment or activities. Delivery of potentially beneficial behavioral interventions to reduce risk related to tobacco, diet, and physical activity and genetic counseling frequently are underused and may be limited by functional status, financial barriers, insufficient prioritization and assistance from health care providers, and lack of access to medical care.[10,11]

The unmet needs of survivors and the multiple health system barriers to optimum care were outlined in a series of reports from the then Institute of Medicine (IOM), Centers for Disease Control and Prevention, and the Presidents Cancer Panel. Key among these was the 2006 IOM report From *Cancer Patient to Cancer Survivor: Lost in Transition*.[12] The publication provided a delineation of physical and mental health concerns of survivors, described the role of survivorship care in the cancer control continuum and recommended practice and policy changes aimed at improving management of the survivor population. The recommendations of this report have directed much of the clinical and research effort over the last 15 years which have led to a better understanding of this phase of the continuum and the implementation of various approaches aimed at providing improved longevity and quality of life for cancer survivors. While significant progress has been accomplished in addressing the complex and highly interactive structure of the survivorship ecosystem, gaps in knowledge and opportunities for improved care and research remain as described by Nekhlyudov.[8]

Significance

The population of cancer survivors in the United States continues to increase driven by a growing and aging population, declining cancer mortality, and improved early detection and treatment. Recently, the ACS reported a 2.2% drop in cancer mortality from 2016 to 2017, the largest single-year drop ever recorded, with the mortality rate declining by 29% from 1991 to 2017.[13] This decline was accompanied by minimal change in incidence.[13] Improvements in early detection and treatment, including immunotherapy leading to better outcomes for previously untreatable types of cancer, further increase the prevalence of cancer survivors, now estimated at 16.9 million. The number is projected to grow to 22.1 million by 2030 (Table 1).[1] Globally, the reported number of survivors as of 2018 is 43.8 million though this is based on the number surviving 5 years. Most identified survivors reside in higher and upper middle income countries.[14]

The traditional gauge for having survived cancer has been the 5-year mark and this continues to be used as the basis of determining survival rates (Figure 1). Today, 69% of cancer survivors were diagnosed over 5 years ago.[1] This represents a change from the 49% overall survival at 5 years in 1975. Now, approximately 45% live 10 years or more and 18% live 20 years or more after

Table 1 Estimated numbers of US Cancer Survivors by gender and site for 2019 and 2030.[a]

Males		
Cancer site	2019	2030
Prostate	3,650,030	5,017,810
Colon and rectum	776,120	994,210
Melanoma of the skin	684,470	936,980
Urinary bladder	624,490	832,910
Non-Hodgkin lymphoma	400,070	535,870
Kidney and renal pelvis	342,060	476,910
Testis	287,780	361,690
Lung and bronchus	258,200	325,680
Leukemia	256,790	352,900
Oral cavity and pharynx	249,330	315,750
All sites	**8,138,790**	**10,995,610**
Females		
Cancer site	2019	2030
Breast	3,861,520	4,957,960
Uterine corpus	807,860	1,023,290
Colon and rectum	768,650	965,590
Thyroid	705,050	989,340
Melanoma of the skin	672,140	888,740
Non-Hodgkin lymphoma	357,650	480,690
Lung and bronchus	313,140	398,930
Cervix	283,120	288,710
Ovary	249,230	297,580
Kidney and renal pelvis	227,510	316,620
All sites	**8,781,580**	**11,174,200**

Estimates do not include *in situ* carcinoma of any site except urinary bladder and do not include basal cell or squamous cell skin cancers.
[a]Source: Data taken from Miller et al.[1]

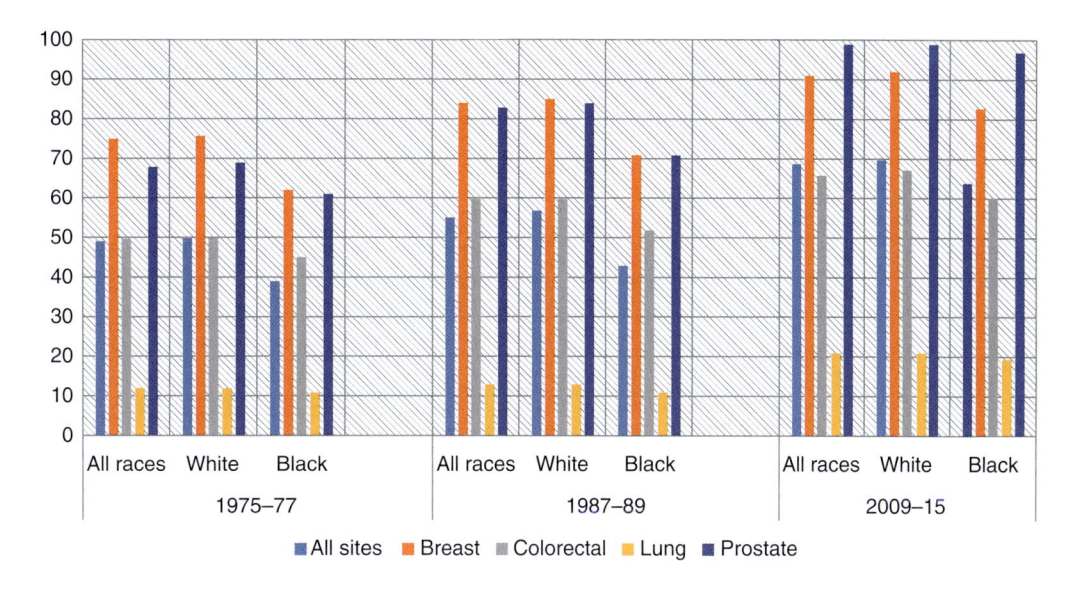

Figure 1 Trends in 5-year relative survival rates (%) for top 4 most common cancers, by Race, US, 1975–2015. Source: Data from American Cancer Society.[15]

diagnosis. Survival varies significantly by site, with much lower rates for pancreas (10%), lung and bronchus (21%), and ovary (48%). These statistics do not yet reflect the anticipated significant impact from newer, more effective treatment approaches, such as immunotherapy.

Racial and ethnic disparities in survival are noted across several sites, with reduced rates of survival in populations of African vs. European heritage. Across all cancer types, the differential averages 6% less, though larger differences of 21% and 19% are reported with regard to cancer of the uterine corpus and oral cavity and pharynx, respectively. Reflecting the higher incidence of cancer associated with aging, almost two-thirds of cancer survivors are 65 years or greater; and those over 80 years old now represent 20% of the survivor population.[1]

Components of survivorship care

The type and severity of problems encountered by cancer survivors are heterogeneous and vary by the type of cancer, treatments used, and comorbid conditions of the patient, but these can be organized into a group of categories or domains that can be strategically addressed. The following describes the categorization of the components of survivorship care aimed at addressing these problems based on the 2006 IOM report.[12] These components are included in the ASCO Core Curriculum for Cancer Survivorship Education.[16] A detailed listing of domains of care and published guidelines are included in Nekhlyudov et al.[8]

Surveillance for recurrence

A large observational study stratified various cancer types to define a high-risk period and mortality risk compared to a population baseline. Results indicated that the risk period was highly variable, and for many, exceeded the traditional 5-year surveillance period.[17] Recommendations for surveillance examinations, imaging, and laboratory testing are listed in cancer-specific guidelines for follow-up care, such as those from the National Comprehensive Cancer Network (NCCN) and ACS. These recommendations are based largely on expert consensus. Limited randomized studies examining the effectiveness of these recommendations have been published. Among these studies, the frequency and intensity of surveillance varied by the type of cancer and risk of recurrence, as well as time since completion of treatment. Evidence for long-term benefit of regular surveillance beyond the traditional 5-year period is limited. As with any intervention, the benefits of early detection of recurrence must be weighed against the potential harms of radiation used in imaging as well as the costs of testing. Regarding breast and colon cancer post-therapeutic surveillance, studies have shown varied outcomes, with no benefit in survival, quality of life, or morbidity from intensive screening in female breast cancer survivors without symptoms.[18] Improved 10-year survival outcomes in colorectal cancer survivors have been documented when hepatic metastatic disease is identified and resected, leading to an improved survival of 17–25%.[19] However, intensity of colorectal cancer follow-up testing with CEA and imaging was not associated with earlier time to detection of recurrence or overall survival in another large observational study.[20]

Screening for second primary cancers

Survivors may be at increased risk of a second or multiple additional cancers due to inherited genetic predisposition, chemotherapy, or radiation used for treatment of the primary cancer that may contribute to cellular proliferation and or immune suppression. Also, behavioral factors such as tobacco, diet, and physical inactivity, may increase risk, particularly if they were not sufficiently addressed as a component of the patient's primary cancer treatment.[21] Clinician advice for survivors to follow cancer screening recommendations for average-risk individuals or, when indicated, those for increased risk individuals, plays an important role in patient adherence to screening protocols.[22] For example, survivors who have received mantle radiation for childhood Hodgkin's disease should initiate screening at 25 years of age and follow more frequent screening for breast cancer, including MRI.[23] A thorough cancer family history is important and formal genetic consultation and testing may be recommended.

Identification and management of persistent long-term and late occurring effects of treatment and the cancer itself

Current cancer therapeutic modalities are more effective than in the past but have numerous potentially toxic side effects that must be managed during treatment. Some of these effects of treatment or the cancer may persist after completion of primary treatment, while other adverse effects may develop months or years later. These vary in relation to the specific cancer type, treatment type, and individual factors. Survivors should be queried as to the presence of these adverse consequences and appropriate support or referral can be used to mitigate the associated symptoms or physical dysfunction. Effects that occur in a significant proportion of survivors include but are not limited to the following: fatigue, chronic pain, peripheral neuropathy, vasomotor/menopausal symptoms, cognitive problems, osteoporosis, infertility, sexual dysfunction, insomnia, depression, and anxiety, as well as cardiac dysfunction. Persistent effects related to growing use of immune therapies will become more common as these treatment modalities are applied to a growing number of cancer types.[8,24-26] While numerous instruments are available to assist in identification and diagnosis of these conditions, there is no single comprehensive questionnaire that identifies these issues across the spectrum of survivorship care.[27] Various cancer survivorship management guidelines, such as those by the ACS (https://www.cancer.org/health-care-professionals/national-cancer-survivorship-resource-center/tools-for-health-care-professionals.html) and the American Society of Clinical Oncology (ASCO; https://www.asco.org/practice-policy/cancer-care-initiatives/prevention-survivorship/survivorship-compendium-0) related to management of these issues are useful in addressing these conditions.

Identification and management of psychosocial conditions

Fear of recurrence is a commonly noted concern along with anxiety and depression and may be associated with significant adverse impact on quality of life in some survivors. Screening for depression and other psychological problems and referral as needed to local resources is recommended. A systematic review of studies in Europe demonstrated highly variable rates of psychological symptoms in survivors, although they did not differ greatly from the general population.[28] Systematic distress screening with instruments such as the NCCN distress thermometer scale is included as a standard in American College of Surgeon (ACOS) accreditation. Caregivers and family members may also be impacted by psychological problems and these should be assessed and managed as needed.[28]

Reduce exposure to cancer risk factors, improve nutrition, and physical activity

Behavioral changes to modify exposure to tobacco and alcohol, improve nutrition, address obesity if present, and increase physical activity as tolerated, can reduce risk of second cancers and may have a positive impact on recurrence risk. Additionally, these measures can improve quality of life and help to mitigate some persistent symptoms, such as fatigue.[29-32]

Implementation of survivorship care—overcoming delivery system challenges

Acting on the recommendations of the 2006 IOM report,[12] a wide array of clinical programs and policy initiatives have been developed in an effort to achieve high-quality cancer survivorship care.

Models of survivorship care delivery

Several approaches to the organization of survivorship care delivery have been implemented in the United States and internationally. These include nurse-led models that may be multidisciplinary clinics in large cancer centers, individual or small programs, some of which focus on specific cancer sites, among others. Another approach aims to integrate primary care clinicians into survivorship care using a process of risk stratification to help determine if a particular patient may be better served in the oncology setting, primary care setting, or in a shared/combined environment.[33-35] A program combining support by oncology specialists and primary care has shown improved receipt of recommended interventions.[36,37] Approaches such as risk stratified shared care utilized in Australia and the United Kingdom have been effective and may be adaptable for the United States. These use guidelines to help direct care by oncology and generalist teams with a focus on care coordination and ongoing data collection for assessment.[33,38,39] The inclusion of rehabilitation, geriatric care, and other specialty services such as cardiology are other clinical areas that may be utilized to better address survivors' needs.

Evidence informing the relative benefits and harms of these and other approaches is quite limited and varies considerably.[40] Further evaluative research on clinical outcomes such as longevity and impact on quality of life are needed to identify best practices that could lead to defined standards of care.[41-43]

Self-management is an approach that is being utilized internationally in the United Kingdom, Canada, and Australia and to a limited degree in the United States.[44,45] International cancer survivorship care models have combined the risk-stratified model with the integration of self-management. In England, Northern Ireland, and Australia, demonstrations of this model have shown improved delivery of clinical services, psychosocial support, and improved patient satisfaction. Survivors are assessed for risk of recurrence, late effects, comorbidities, and the availability of local resources. Primary care clinicians are providing clinical services and supporting self-management through a care pathway that has been informed by individual patient data obtained from population-based registries. Adaptation of these models for use in the United States is under consideration, though concerns regarding the fragmentation of the US health care system resulting in limitations on communication and coordination of care across various specialty groups and primary care teams may limit effectiveness. Advances in technology related to self-monitoring, telemedicine, and distance education may facilitate such a transition.[46] Expansion of optimized survivorship care into middle and lower resource areas internationally following the effective implementation of early diagnostic and treatment regimens, will require the development of resource-stratified guidelines similar to those developed for other parts of the cancer care continuum for these settings.[47]

Summary of treatment and survivorship care plan

Challenges to implementing a high-quality system of care for cancer survivors persist. Experience with the various models of survivorship management, while supported by expert consensus, has not demonstrated the improvements in outcomes that were hoped for following publication of the IOM report.[12] The use of a synoptic summary of the patient's treatment coupled with an evidence-based care plan recommended in that report has proved challenging to implement. The primary use of these tools to inform improved communication and coordination among various health professional teams and the patient, while thought to be beneficial, have not been utilized widely or shown the expected benefits that were anticipated.[48,49] New models of survivorship care continue to be deployed and should be thoroughly evaluated for the potential benefits and possible harms that they may demonstrate in various settings and with various types of survivors.

The construct and use of the survivor treatment summary and care plan as one of the core recommendations in the original IOM report have evolved significantly. While evidence of its utility has been difficult to document, it is still considered an important tool in providing optimum survivorship care, but it should be aimed at improving communication and collaboration among professionals of the health care team and patients.[50] Implementation has been problematic and success has been limited even after its inclusion in the ACOS cancer center accreditation standards.[50-55] Barriers to implementation have included time constraints, lack of payment, and limited evidence of effectiveness.[56]

A phased approach to full implementation was added to the ACOS standards in 2016, but even this has been revised in the 2020 standards to include the treatment summary and care plan as an optional component of an overall survivorship program.[57] This change has been driven by a realization that the document itself may be best used as an aid to facilitate discussion among care providers and the survivor, especially at times of transition, such as at completion of active treatment or upon transfer of care to another provider.[58] Major organizations have developed summary and care plan templates and toolkits to facilitate adoption (Table 2).

Coordination of care

Survivorship care has traditionally been delivered by the treating oncology teams. With the recognition that many survivors continue to receive general care from existing primary care teams or establish relationships with primary teams at some point after treatment is completed, the need for coordination of care supported by shared communication among the clinical teams and patients has risen in importance. Efforts to improve the coordination of care for cancer survivors among the various professional groups providing support have been limited in their success. Fragmentation of the US health care system, poorly defined clinical roles, lack of standardized communication processes, and underdeveloped interoperability among information technology platforms have been persistent barriers to needed improvements in care coordination. All these factors lead to missed opportunities for improved care, misuse, and overuse of recommended services and support.

Improvement in survivorship care coordination and communication between oncology treatment teams and primary care team have been the focus of numerous studies. Lack of clarity as to the respective roles of each clinical team is a persistent theme across multiple settings. Discordance of views by each group highlights areas in need of better understanding and trust among these critical patient care teams, as well as the survivors.[37,59,60] Primary care clinicians have expressed willingness to participate in the care of survivors yet express needs in terms of knowledge of areas of survivorship care, including late and long-term effects. Oncology specialists prefer a specialist-based approach but may not be able to provide full primary care services, manage multiple comorbidities, or psychosocial support that are frequently needed by survivors. Additional headwinds created by inadequate integration of information technology support into EHRs and limited interoperability further impede implementation. Lack of a systematic mutually agreeable approach to address these concerns limits the degree to which the goal of high-quality coordinated care can be achieved.[61-63]

Achieving an effective future state of coordination and collaboration in service of improved outcomes for cancer survivors should address the identified barriers through a multilevel approach. Knowledge gaps may be addressed through programs for health professionals at undergraduate, postgraduate, and continuing education frameworks designed to build knowledge as well as enhance confidence in managing survivors. Professional education opportunities on survivorship topics have become more readily available including published textbooks and online offerings (Table 3). Mobile applications are also available and more are being developed to provide point of care access to guidelines and survivorship care information.

Deployment and evaluation of novel systems of care such as the proposed onco-generalist model, or combined risk-stratified shared care approach or adapting international models such as those used in the United Kingdom and Australia that include

Table 2 Summary and care plan templates.

Organization	Tool(s)	Link
American Society of Clinical Oncology	Survivorship care plan templates by cancer site, Treatment plan template, OncoLife Survivorship Care Plan, Journey Forward: Guiding Survivors as They Move Ahead, American Head and Neck Society care plan and treatment summary[a]	https://www.asco.org/practice-policy/cancer-care-initiatives/prevention-survivorship/survivorship-compendium
American Cancer Society	Life After Treatment Guide, Life After Treatment Guide—A Guide for American Indians & Alaska Natives	https://www.cancer.org/health-care-professionals/national-cancer-survivorship-resource-center/tools-for-cancer-survivors-and-caregivers.html
National Cancer Survivorship Resource Center	The National Cancer Survivorship Resource Center Toolkit: Implementing Clinical Practice Guidelines for Cancer Survivorship Care	https://smhs.gwu.edu/gwci/survivorship/ncsrc/national-cancer-survivorship-center-toolkit

[a] The ASCO portal provides links to a number of different tools created by different organizations.

Table 3 Resources for professional education on survivorship.

Organization	Tool(s)	Link
Australian Cancer Survivorship Centre	Cancer Survivorship e-learning course	https://education.eviq.org.au/courses/supportive-care/cancer-survivorship
Dana-Farber Cancer Institute	Cancer Survivorship in Primary Care	http://www.cancerpcp.org/
George Washington School of Medicine and Health Sciences	Cancer Survivorship E-Learning Series for Primary Care Providers	https://smhs.gwu.edu/gwci/survivorship/ncsrc/elearning
Princess Margaret Cancer Center	Princess Margaret Cancer Classes	https://pmcancerclasses.ca/ Currently have a "Introduction to Rehab and Cancer Survivorship" class in production
Stanford University	Health After Cancer: Cancer Survivorship for Primary Care	https://mededucation.stanford.edu/courses/health-after-cancer/
UT MD Anderson Cancer Center	Cancer Survivorship Algorithms	https://www.mdanderson.org/for-physicians/clinical-tools-resources/clinical-practice-algorithms/survivorship-algorithms.html
American Cancer Society	Cancer Survivorship Guidelines App	https://www.cancer.org/health-care-professionals/national-cancer-survivorship-resource-center/tools-for-health-care-professionals.html
University of Melbourne	Cancer Survivorship for Primary Care Practitioners	https://www.futurelearn.com/courses/cancer-survivorship
National Academies of Sciences, Engineering, and Medicine	Long-Term Survivorship Care After Cancer Treatment: Proceedings of a Workshop.	https://www.ncbi.nlm.nih.gov/books/NBK499470/
American Society of Clinical Oncology	Survivorship Compendium	https://www.asco.org/practice-policy/cancer-care-initiatives/prevention-survivorship/survivorship/survivorship-compendium
Oncology Nursing Society (Publisher)	Book	Cancer Survivorship: Interprofessional, Patient-Centered Approaches to the Seasons of Survival Edited By: Pamela Haylock	Carol Curtiss ISBN: 9781635930306. Copyright Year: 2019
Springer (Publisher)	Book	Rodriguez, M.A., & Foxhall, L.E. (Eds.). (2019). Handbook of Cancer Survivorship Care

self-management, should be tested for acceptance by clinicians and patients as well as effectiveness and benefit or harm. Attention to needed infrastructure enhancements related to integration into EHRs to establish patient registries and build point of service education, reminders, and best practice alerts is necessary to achieve better outcomes for patients and improved efficiency and effectiveness for clinicians. Further research to inform clinical guidelines and a learning system approach to their use will build confidence and aid adherence by clinicians and patients.[64–67]

Clinical practice guidelines for survivorship care

While evidence-based approaches are preferred, many of the existing survivorship guidelines do not follow strict evidence-based rules and most are based on expert consensus opinion. Major organizations have developed follow-up care guidelines for cancer survivors (Table 4).

Evaluating health care quality for cancer survivors

Evaluation of the impact of survivor care guidelines is dependent upon the development and use of standard metrics to measure effectiveness.[68] Development and use of clinical quality indicators for survivorship care have begun to be implemented. Assessment of the quality of survivorship care strategies are included in the IOM Report, *Delivering High-Quality Cancer Care: Charting a New Course for a System in Crisis 2013*.[69] The ASCO Quality Oncology Practice Initiative (QOPI®) focuses primarily on treatment but is beginning to develop measures that may include cancer survivor related care. The recently introduced mCODE format includes standardized measures that may be further developed for use in the survivor population. The development of patient-held electronic medical records facilitated by blockchain technology may provide a future opportunity to improve longitudinal evaluation as well as coordination and communication. Patient-reported outcome measures may also bring objective reporting methodology for

Table 4 Follow-up care guidelines for cancer survivors.

Organization	Tool(s)	Link
The Children's Oncology Group	Consensus and evidence-based guidelines for long-term care for those with childhood, adolescent, and young adult-onset cancers	https://childrensoncologygroup.org/index.php/survivorshipguidelines
National Comprehensive Cancer Network	NCCN Guidelines Version 1.2020:Survivorship	Members only: https://www.nccn.org/professionals/physician_gls/pdf/survivorship.pdf
American Cancer Society	Guidelines intended for primary care clinicians targeting selected commonly occurring cancer types; guidelines for nutrition and physical activity for survivors	https://www.cancer.org/health-care-professionals/american-cancer-society-survivorship-guidelines.html https://www.cancer.org/health-care-professionals/american-\ignorespacescancer-society-prevention-early-detection-guidelines/nupa-guidelines-for-cancer-survivors.html
MD Anderson Cancer Center	Consensus-based practice algorithms by cancer site	https://www.mdanderson.org/for-physicians/clinical-tools-resources/clinical-practice-algorithms/survivorship-algorithms.html
American College of Sports Medicine	Exercise guidelines for cancer survivors	https://www.acsm.org/docs/default-source/files-for-resource-library/exercise-guidelines-cancer-infographic.pdf?sfvrsn=c48d8d86_4

this phase of cancer care. A number of standardized instruments intended to regularly collect information and status directly from patients are playing a growing role in evaluation and improvement of survivorship care internationally and in the United States.[70–73]

A comprehensive, evidence-based framework for evaluating and improving quality in survivorship care by Nekhlyudov et al.[8] provides a guide to the systematic improvement of quality and effectiveness of care for cancer survivors.

Special populations

Adolescent and young adult (AYA) as well as older survivors face unique challenges in clinical care. Approximately 70,000 younger individuals between ages 15 and 30 years are diagnosed with cancer annually in the United States. Cancer is the leading cause of premature mortality in this age group. Many of the survivors in this population do not receive regular follow-up care and, more often than their peers without a cancer diagnosis, have a higher frequency of tobacco use, obesity, and chronic conditions resulting in worse states of physical and mental health. ASCO's Cancer Survivorship Committee has developed a list of resources for AYA cancer survivors.[74,75]

As the baby boomer population ages, the number of older cancer survivors has climbed, and now those 65 and older represent over 60% of total survivors and are expected to be over 70% by 2040. The older population experiences an average of five comorbidities that may impact longevity and quality of life after cancer. These conditions include a broad range of, at times, complex diseases that will require close attention as cancer survivors age.[76]

Financial impact

Much of the success of modern cancer treatment is due to improved chemotherapy agents and newer immunotherapies. While these are often highly effective, they are also very expensive and the financial impact of current treatment modalities can create financial hardship for survivors and their families. The Patient Protection and Affordable Care Act coverage provision and optional expansion of Medicaid have provided financial support to many survivors though these provisions may continue to be reduced.[77] Limits in insurance coverage and higher out-of-pocket costs place survivors in difficult financial situations prompting stress, and, at times, causing delay or avoidance of needed treatment due to cost. Patients under treatment and in the survivorship phase of care may benefit from counseling regarding these situations.[78–80] Caregivers and family members of cancer survivors while included in the definition of cancer survivorship may be called upon more frequently in situations related to financial burden. Their needs should be considered in all situations but may be particularly important when this added stress is present.[81] Socioeconomic issues were addressed through articles of the Affordable Care Act including improved access to insurance coverage for treatment and primary care, access for those with preexisting conditions such as cancer and chronic complications of treatment, exclusion of lifetime limits on coverage, especially important for childhood cancer survivors. Many of these advances though are threatened as health care policy in the United States is being reassessed. While newer treatment options are bringing successful outcomes to many, the cost of newer treatments has added a new complication of financial burden referred to as financial toxicity.

Summary

The steadily growing number of US cancer survivors is approaching 17 million. Many of these individuals can benefit from strategic medical management and supportive care. Survivorship care focuses on the period after completion of treatment and is guided by recommendations that target management of persistent and late-occurring effects of treatment and the cancer itself, screening for recurrence and second cancers, promotion of wellness, and primary prevention of cancer as well as psychosocial challenges faced by many patients.

Numerous clinical practice models have been established to address survivor needs including multidisciplinary clinics in major centers, individual oncology-based approaches, shared care including primary care clinicians, and programs with significant self-care components among others.

Completion and distribution of Summary of Treatment and Survivorship Care Plan documents were promoted but proved difficult to implement at scale. Current strategies include a balanced approach using a survivorship care team and multiple tools to organize and improve care.

Coordination and collaboration among oncology treatment specialists and primary care teams are encouraged. Utilization of electronic health record (EHR) infrastructure, education programs to address knowledge gaps, and improve self-efficacy are utilized to improve care delivery. Clinical practice guidelines are available and provide guidance to address survivor needs in a systematic fashion.

Significant numbers of survivors in advanced age groups who often have multiple comorbid conditions require close attention as do survivors in adolescent and young adult (AYA) age groups. Racial and ethnic disparities in survivor populations call for a higher level of intervention. Attention to the needs of caregivers and family members is warranted.

Key references

The complete reference list can be found on Vital Source version of this title, see inside front cover.

1 Miller KD, Nogueira L, Mariotto AB, et al. Cancer treatment and survivorship statistics, 2019. *CA Cancer J Clin.* 2019;**69**(5):363–385 https://doi.org/10.3322/caac.21565.
2 The Children's Oncology Group. *Long-Term Follow-Up Guidelines for Survivors of Childhood, Adolescent and Young Adult Cancers, Version 5.* Monrovia, CA, Children's Oncology Group; 2018 www.survivorshipguidelines.org.
4 Kent EE, Arora NK, Rowland JH, et al. Health information needs and health-related quality of life in a diverse population of long-term cancer survivors. *Patient Educ Couns.* 2012;**89**(2):345–352.
5 de Moor JS, Mariotto AB, Parry C, et al. Cancer survivors in the United States: prevalence across the survivorship trajectory and implications for care. *Cancer Epidemiol Biomarkers Prev.* 2013;**22**(4):561–570.
6 Mullan F. Seasons of survival: reflections of a physician with cancer. *N Engl J Med.* 1985;**313**:270–273.
8 Nekhlyudov L, Mollica MA, Jacobsen PB, et al. Developing a quality of cancer survivorship care framework: implications for clinical care, research and policy. *J Nat Cancer Inst.* 2019;**111**(11):djz089, first published online May 16, 2019.
9 Marzorati C, Riva S, Pravettoni G. Who is a cancer survivor? A systematic review of published definitions. *J Cancer Edu.* 2017;**32**:228–237. First published online Feb 8, 2016.
10 Nekhlyudov L, Ganz PA, Arora NK, Rowland JH. Going beyond being lost in transition: a decade of progress in cancer survivorship. *J Clin Oncol.* 2017;**35**(18):1978–1981. Published online 2017 Apr 24. doi: 10.1200/JCO.2016.72.1373.
11 National Academies of Sciences, Engineering, and Medicine. *Long-Term Survivorship Care After Cancer Treatment: Proceedings of a Workshop.* Washington, DC: The National Academies Press; 2018. https://doi.org/10.17226/25043.
12 National Research Council. *From Cancer Patient to Cancer Survivor: Lost in Transition.* Washington, DC: The National Academies Press; 2006. doi: https://doi.org/10.17226/11468.
13 Siegel RL, Miller KD, Jemal A. Cancer Statistics, 2020. *CA Cancer J Clin.* 2020;**70**:7–30. https://doi.org/10.3322/caac.21590.
15 American Cancer Society. *Cancer Facts & Figures 2020.* Atlanta, GA: American Cancer Society; 2020.

16. Shapiro CL, Jacobsen PB, Henderson T, et al. ReCAP: ASCO core curriculum for cancer survivorship education. *J Oncol Pract.* 2016;**12**(2):145, e108-17. Epub 2016 Jan 26. doi: 10.1200/JOP.2015.009449.

17. Dood RL, Zhao Y, Armbruster SD, et al. Defining survivorship trajectories across patients with solid tumors: an evidence based approach. *JAMA Oncol.* 2018;**4**(11):1519–1526. Published online 2018 Jun 2. doi: 10.1001/jamaoncol.2018.2761.

20. Snyder RA, Hu C-Y, Cuddy A, et al. Association between intensity of post-treatment surveillance testing and detection of recurrence in patients with colorectal cancer. *JAMA.* 2018;**319**(20):2104–2115. doi: 10.1001/jama.2018.5816.

21. Wood ME, Vogel V, Ng A, et al. Second malignant neoplasms: assessment and strategies for risk reduction. *J Clin Oncol.* 2012;**30**(30):3734–3745.

24. Shapiro CL. Cancer survivorship. *N Engl J Med.* 2018;**379**:2438–2450. doi: 10.1056/NEJMra1712502.

26. Gegechkori N, Haines L, Lin JJ. Long term and latent side effects of specific cancer types. *Med Clin North Am.* 2017;**101**(6):1053–1073. doi: 10.1016/j.mcna.2017.06.003.

29. Ligibel J, Alfano CM, Courneya KS, et al. American Society of Clinical Oncology position statement on obesity and cancer. *J Clin Oncol.* 2014;**32**(31):3568–3574. doi: 10.1200/JCO.2014.58.4680.

31. LoConte NK, Brewster AM, Kaur JS, et al. Alcohol and cancer: a statement of the American Society of Clinical Oncology. *J Clin Oncol.* 2018;**36**(1):83–93. doi: 10.1200/JCO.2017.76.1155.

32. Karam-Hage M, Cinciripini PM, Gritz ER. Tobacco use and cessation for cancer survivors: an overview for clinicians. *CA Cancer J Clin.* 2014;**64**(4):272–290. doi: 10.3322/caac.21231.

33. Oeffinger KC, McCabe MS. Models for delivering survivorship care. *J Clin Oncol.* 2006;**24**(32):5117–5124. doi: 10.1200/JCO.2006.07.0474.

34. McCabe MS, Partridge A, Grunfeld E, Hudson MM. Risk based health care, the cancer survivor, the oncologist, and the primary care physician. *Semin Oncol.* 2013;**40**(6):804–812. doi: 10.1053/j.seminoncol.2013.09.004.

35. Mayer DK, Alfano CM. Personalized risk-stratified cancer follow-up care: its potential for healthier survivors, happier clinicians and lower costs. *J Natl Cancer Inst.* 2019;**111**(5):442–448. doi: 10.1093/jnci/djy232.

37. Smith TG, Strollo S, Hu X, et al. Understanding long-term cancer survivors' preferences for ongoing medical care. *J Gen Int Med.* 2019;**34**(10):2091–2097. doi: 10.1007/s11606-019-05189-y Epub 2019 Jul 31.

38. Alfano CM, Mayer DK, Bhatia S, et al. Implementing personalized pathways for cancer follow-up care in the United States: proceedings from an American Cancer Society-American Society of Clinical Oncology summit. *CA Cancer J Clin.* 2019;**69**(3):234-247. doi: 10.3322/caac.21558. Epub 2019 Mar 8.

42. Halpern MT, Viswanathan M, Evans TS, et al. Models of cancer survivorship care: overview and summary of current evidence. *J Oncol Pract.* 2015;**11**(1):e19–e27. doi: 10.1200/JOP.2014.001403 Epub 2014 Sep 9.

50. Jacobsen P, DeRosa AP, Henderson TO, et al. Systematic review of the impact of cancer survivorship care plans on health outcomes and health care delivery. *J Clin Oncol.* 2018;**36**(20):2088–2100.

51. Mayer DK, Nekhlyudov L, Snyder CF, et al. ASCO clinical oncology clinical expert statement on cancer survivorship care planning. *J Oncol Prac.* 2014;**10**(6):345–351. doi: 10.1200/JOP.2014.001321.

55. Corsini N, Neylon K, Tian EJ, et al. Impact of treatment summaries for cancer survivors: a systematic review. *J Cancer Surviv.* 2020;**14**:405–416. doi: 10.1007/s11764-020-00859-x.

59. Klabunde CN, Han PKJ, Earle CC, et al. Physician roles in the cancer related follow-up care of cancer survivors. *Fam Med.* 2013;**45**(7):463–474.

60. Potosky AL, Han PKJ, Rowland JH, et al. Differences between primary care physicians and oncologists knowledge attitudes and practices regarding the care of cancer survivors. *J Gen Intern Med.* 2011;**26**(12):1403–1410. doi: 10.1007/s11606-011-1808-4 Epub 2011 Jul 22.

62. Lawrence RA, McLoone JK, Wakefield CE, Cohn RJ. Primary care physicians perspectives on their role in cancer care. *J Gen Intern Med.* 2016;**31**(10):1222–1236. doi: 10.1007/s11606-016-3746-7 Epub 2016 May 24.

66. Alfano CM, Mayer DK, Bhatia S, et al. Implementing personalized pathways for cancer follow up care in the US: proceedings from an American Cancer Society-ASCO summit. *CA Cancer J Clin.* 2019;**69**(3):234–247. doi: 10.3322/caac.21558 Epub 2019 Mar 8.

68. McCabe MS, Bhatia S, Oeffinger KC, et al. ASCO statement: achieving high-quality cancer survivorship care. *J Clin Oncol.* 2013;**31**(5):631–640. Published online 2013 Jan 7. doi: 10.1200/JCO.2012.46.6854.

69. Institute of Medicine. *Delivering High-Quality Cancer Care: Charting a New Course for a System in Crisis.* Washington, DC: The National Academies Press; 2013. doi: https://doi.org/10.17226/18359.

73. Bottomley A, Reijneveld JC, Koller M, et al. Current state of quality of life and patient reported outcomes research. *Eur J Cancer.* 2019;**121**:55–63. doi: https://doi.org/10.1016/j.ejca.2019.08.016.

76. Bluethmann SM, Mariotto AB, Rowland KH. Anticipating the "Silver Tsunami": prevalence trajectories and comorbidity burden among older cancer survivors in the US. *Cancer Epidemiol Biomarkers Prev.* 2016;**25**(7). doi: 10.1158/1055-9965.EPI-16-0133 Published July 2016.

82. Jefford M, Roland J, Grunfeld E, et al. Implementing improved post-treatment care for cancer survivors in England, with reflections from Australia, Canada and the USA. *Br J Cancer.* 2013;**108**:14–20.